The Complete Directory for People with Chronic Illness

2013/14

Eleventh Edition

The Complete Directory for People with Chronic Illness

Condition Descriptions
Associations
Publications
Research Centers
Support Groups
Web sites

A SEDGWICK PRESS Book

Grey House Publishing

R
616.044
COMPLETE
2013-14

PUBLISHER: Leslie Mackenzie
EDITOR: Richard Gottlieb
EDITORIAL DIRECTOR: Laura Mars

PRODUCTION MANAGER: Kristen Thatcher
PRODUCTION ASSISTANT: Brittany O'Brien

MARKETING DIRECTOR: Jessica Moody

A Sedgwick Press Book
Grey House Publishing, Inc.
4919 Route 22
Amenia, NY 12501
518.789.8700
FAX 518.789.0545
www.greyhouse.com
E-MAIL: books@greyhouse.com

While every effort has been made to ensure the reliability of the information presented in this publication, Grey House Publishing neither guarantees the accuracy of the data contained herein nor assumes any responsibility for errors, omissions or discrepancies. Grey House accepts no payment for listing; inclusions in the publication of any organization, agency, institution, publication, service or individual does not imply endorsement of the editors or publisher.

Errors brought to the attention of the publisher and verified to the satisfaction of the publisher will be corrected in future editions.

First edition published 1994
Eleventh edition published 2013
Printed in Canada
All rights reserved
The complete directory for people with chronic illness – 1994-2013

       1053 p.; 27.5 cm
       Other title: DCI
       ISSN: 1080-7659

1.   Chronic diseases – United States – Directories. 2. Chronic Diseases – Bibliography. 3. Chronic Disease – United States – Directories. 4. Social Support – United States – Directories. 5. Information Services – United States – Directories. 6. Rehabilitation – United States – Directories. I. Title: DCI.

RC108 .C645
616' .0025'73   96-640803
ISBN: 978-1-61925-114-4

Table of Contents

Introduction

Health care professionals estimate that 133 million Americans suffer from a chronic illness and, due to the aging of our population, this number will reach 171 million by 2030. This eleventh edition of *The Complete Directory for People with Chronic Illness* offers a comprehensive overview of 89 specific chronic illnesses from Addison's to Wilson's Disease. Each chapter includes an easy-to-understand medical description, plus a wide range of condition-specific support services and information resources that deal with the variety of issues concerning those with a chronic illness, as well as those who support the chronic illness community.

> *". . .The strength of this source is . . . in the information referral portion of each entry: the wide range of resources and organizations presented that can assist with additional information and support . . ."*
> **American Reference Books Annual**

"Chronic" comes from the Greek word *chronos* meaning time (Greek god Chronos is often depicted as Father Time). Chronic Illness Alliance defines chronic illness as . . . *an illness that is permanent or lasts a long time. It may get slowly worse over time [or] go away. It may cause permanent changes to the body [and] will certainly affect the person's quality of life.* National Center for Health Statistics defines chronic illness as *lasting 3 months or more.*

However you define chronic illness, this new edition provides thousands of ways to deal with the many aspects of chronic disease. It includes associations, state agencies, libraries & resource centers, research centers, magazines, newsletters, audio & video tapes, hot lines, support groups and web sites. In addition to chapters dealing with specific chronic conditions, this edition includes several chapters relevant to the chronic illness community in general, such as wish foundations and death and bereavement groups.

The Complete Directory for People with Chronic Illness provides critical information to those dealing for the first time with the stress and crucial need-to-know issues, as well as to those already coping with chronic disease. *How can I connect with others with diabetes? What cancer treatment is best for me? When do I need to protect my 2-year old with a heart condition from normal play? Why is my healthy child angrier than his chronically ill sibling?* You'll find ways to answer these questions and more in the pages of this edition.

In addition to patients and their families, this directory offers sought-after support for hospital and medical center personnel, especially discharge planners, social service workers, and disability coordinators. *The Complete Directory for People with Chronic Illness* is full of resources crucial for people with chronic illness as they transition from diagnosis to home, home to work, and work to community life.

The Complete Directory for People with Chronic Illness provides, in one source, **comprehensive, critical, immediate information** – from national associations to children's books. It is the perfect choice for those who find navigating the Internet overwhelming (we've done it for you), as well as for those who feel comfortable surfing the Net (we provide valuable, specific web sites).

Educational Material
- To access information by specific chronic illness, body system, or disorder category, the cross-referenced *Chronic Illness – Body System* chart in the front of the book makes it easy.
- *Next Steps After Your Diagnosis* is a detailed, 21-page article, with information and support resources in five important categories, listed below, plus critical phone numbers and web sites.
  1. Take the Time you Need
  2. Get the Support you Need
  3. Talk with Your Doctor
  4. Seek out Information
  5. Decide on a Treatment Plan

Arrangement
The 89 chronic condition chapters are arranged alphabetically by name of the disorder. Each chapter begins with a brief description of the illness, written in layman's terms, with probable causes, symptoms and treatment options.

Following each description are disease-specific resources. Chapters contain the following: **National Associations; State Agencies; Libraries & Resource Centers; Magazines, Newsletters, Pamphlets; Research Centers; Books for Adults; Books for Children; Support Groups & Hotlines; Audio & Video Resources; Web Sites.**

This reference work profiles 10,599 listings. This edition includes 8,222 fax numbers, 5,601 e-mails, 8,538 web sites, and 9,368 key executives. Brief descriptions and other details are included depending on the type of listing; Associations, for example, may include year founded and yearly dues, while Magazines may include frequency and number of pages.

In addition to the 89 chapters of chronic illnesses, *The Complete Directory for People with Chronic Illness* includes several supplemental chapters in the back of the book designed to provide value to individuals with chronic illness and their families: **General Resources** – information relevant to the general chronic illness community; **Wish Foundations** – organizations devoted to granting wishes of chronically and terminally ill individuals; and **Death & Bereavement** – support services for those who find themselves or a loved one close to death or grieving a loss.

Rounding out this directory are two indexes that allow users additional access to the information: **Entry Name Index** and **Geographic Index**.

The Complete Directory for People with Chronic Illness is also available for subscription on G.O.L.D. – Grey House OnLine Database. Subscribers to G.O.L.D. can access their subscription via the Internet and do customized searches that make finding information quicker and easier. Visit http://gold.greyhouse.com for more information.

CHRONIC ILLNESS — BODY SYSTEM

The following chart lists the chronic illness and its body system(s) or disorder category. Chronic conditions not listed do not fall into a specific system(s). A cross-reference chart follows that lists the information in reverse — body system or disorder categories followed by chronic illnesses.

CHRONIC ILLNESS	BODY SYSTEM/DISORDER CATEGORY
Addison's Disease	Endocrine
Aging	Cells & Tissues
AIDS/HIV	Immune, Infectious Disease
Allergies	Immune
Alzheimer's Disease	Nervous
Amyotrophic Lateral Sclerosis	Nervous
Arthritis	Muscular, Skeletal
Asthma	Respiratory
Ataxia	Nervous
Attention Deficit Hyperactivity Disorder	Behavioral, Developmental
Autistic Spectrum Disorders	Behavioral, Developmental
Brain Tumors	Nervous
Carpal Tunnel Syndrome	Muscular, Skeletal, Nervous
Celiac Disease	Gastrointestinal
Cerebral Palsy	Nervous, Muscular
Chronic Fatigue Syndrome	Immune
Chronic Pain	Nervous
Cooley's Anemia (Thalassemia)	Blood
Congential Heart Disease	Cardiovascular
Crohn's Disease	Gastrointestinal
Cystic Fibrosis	Respiratory, Gastrointestinal
Diabetes Mellitus	Endocrine
Down Syndrome	Developmental
Eating Disorders (Anorexia Nervosa, Bulimia)	Behavioral
Endometriosis	Reproductive
Fabry Disease	Gastrointestinal
Fibromyalgia Syndrome	Muscular, Skeletal
Gastrointestinal Disorders	Gastrointestinal
Gaucher's Disease	Gastrointestinal
Growth Disorders	Developmental
Head Injuries	Nervous
Hearing Impairment	Sensory
Heart Disease	Cardiovascular
Hemophilia	Blood
Hepatitis	Infectious Disease
Hydrocephalus	Nervous
Hypertension	Cardiovascular
Impotence	Reproductive
Incontinence	Urinary
Infertility	Reproductive
Kidney Disease	Gastrointestinal

CHRONIC ILLNESS	BODY SYSTEM/DISORDER CATEGORY
Liver Disease	Gastrointestinal
Lung Disease	Respiratory
Lupus Erythematosus	Cells & Tissues
Mental Illness: General	Behavioral
Mental Illness: Depression	Behavioral
Mental Illness: Schizophrenia	Behavioral
Migraine	Cardiovascular, Nervous
Multiple Sclerosis	Nervous
Muscular Dystrophy	Nervous
Myasthenia Gravis	Nervous
Neurofibromatosis	Nervous, Dermatologic
Osteogenesis Imperfecta	Skeletal
Osteoporosis	Skeletal
Paget's Disease	Skeletal
Parkinson Disease	Nervous
Post-Polio Syndrome	Muscular, Skeletal
Prader Willi Syndrome	Endocrine
Raynaud's Disease	Cardiovascular
Sarcoidosis	Cells & Tissues, Respiratory
Scleroderma	Cells & Tissues, Dermatologic
Scoliosis	Skeletal
Seizure Disorders	Nervous
Sexually Transmitted Diseases	Reproductive, Infectious Disease
Sickle Cell Disease	Blood
Sjogren's Syndrome	Cells & Tissues
Skin Disorders	Dermatologic
Sleep Disorders	Dermatologic
Spina Bifida	Nervous, Skeletal
Spinal Cord Injuries	Nervous
Stroke	Nervous
Substance Abuse	Behavioral
Tay Sachs Disease	Nervous
Thyroid Disease	Endorcrine
Tick-Borne Disease	Infectious Disease
Tourette Syndrome	Nervous
Tuberculosis	Respiratory, Infectious Disease
Tuberous Sclerosis	Nervous, Dermatologic
Turner Syndrome	Endocrine
Ulcerative Colitis	Gastrointestinal
Visual Impairment	Sensory
War Syndromes	Nervous
Wilson's Disease	Gastrointestinal

BY BODY SYSTEM/DISORDER CATEGORY

Behavioral
Attention Deficit Disorder; Autism; Eating Disorders; Mental Illness; Substance Abuse

Blood
Cooley's Anemia; Hemophilia; Sickle Cell Disease

Cardiovascular
Heart Disease; Hypertension; Migraine; Raynaud's Disease

Cells & Tissues
Aging; Lupus Erythematosus; Scleroderma; Sjogren's Syndrome

Dermatologic
Neurofibromatosis; Scleroderma; Skin Disorders; Tuberous Sclerosis

Developmental
Attention Deficit Disorder; Autism; Down Syndrome; Growth Disorders

Endocrine
Addison's Disease; Diabetes; Turner Syndrome

Gastrointestinal
Celiac Disease; Crohn's Disease; Cystic Fibrosis; Fabry Disease; Gastrointestinal Disorders; Gaucher's Disease; Kidney Disease; Liver Disease; Ulcerative Colitis

Immune
AIDS; Allergies; Chronic Fatigue Syndrome

Infectious Disease
AIDS; Hepatitis; Sexually Transmitted Diseases; Tick-Borne Disease; Tuberculosis

Muscular
Arthritis; Carpal Tunnel Syndrome; Cerebral Palsy; Fibromyalgia Syndrome; Post-Polio Syndrome

Nervous
Agent Orange Related Injuries; Alzheimer's Disease; Amyotrophic Lateral Sclerosis; Ataxia; Brain Tumors; Carpal Tunnel Syndrome; Cerebral Palsy; Charcot-Marie-Tooth Disorder; Chronic Pain; Gulf War Syndrome; Head Injuries; Hydrocephalus; Multiple Sclerosis; Muscular Dystrophy; Myasthenia Gravis; Neurofibromatosis; Parkinson Disease; Seizure Disorders; Spina Bifida; Spinal Cord Injuries; Stroke; Tourette Syndrome; Tuberous Sclerosis

Reproductive
Endometriosis; Impotence; Infertility; Sexually Transmitted Diseases

Respiratory
Asthma; Cystic Fibrosis; Lung Disease; Tuberculosis

Skeletal
Arthritis; Carpal Tunnel Syndrome; Fibromyalgia Syndrome; Osteognesis Imperfecta; Osteoporosis; Paget's Disease; Post-Polio Syndrome; Scoliosis; Spina Bifida

Sensory
Hearing Impairment; Visual Impairment

Urinary
Incontinence

Next Steps After Your Diagnosis: Finding Information and Support

Introduction

Your doctor* gave you a diagnosis that could change your life. This article can help you take the next steps.

Every person is different, of course, and every person's disease or condition will affect them differently. But research shows that after getting a diagnosis, many people have some of the same reactions and needs.

About this Article

Next Steps After Your Diagnosis offers general advice for people with almost any disease or condition. And it has tips to help you learn more about your specific problem and how it can be treated.

The information in this article is presented in a simple way to help you scan the material and read only what you need right now. Organizations, publications, and other resources are included if you would like to know more. The on-line version www.ahrq.gov/consumer/diaginfo.htm has many additional resources and their Internet links.

Five Basic Steps

This article describes five basic steps to help you cope with your diagnosis, make decisions, and get on with your life.

Step 1: Take the time you need.
Do not rush important decisions about your health. In most cases, you will have time to carefully examine your options and decide what is best for you.

Step 2: Get the support you need.
Look for support from family and friends, people who are going through the same thing you are, and those who have "been there." They can help you cope with your situation and make informed decisions.

---

* Your medical care might come from a doctor, nurse, physician assistant, or another kind of clinician or health care practitioner. To keep it simple, in this article we use the term "doctor" to refer to any of these professionals with whom you might interact.

Step 3: Talk with your doctor.

Good communication with your doctor can help you feel more satisfied with the care you receive. Research shows it can even have a positive effect on things such as symptoms and pain. Getting a "second opinion" may help you feel more confident about your care.

Step 4: Seek out information.

When learning about your health problem and its treatment, look for information that is based on a careful review of the latest scientific findings published in medical journals.

Step 5: Decide on a treatment plan.

Work with your doctor to decide on a treatment plan that best meets your needs.

As you take each step, remember this: Research shows that patients who are more involved in their health care tend to get better results and be more satisfied.

Step 1:
Take the time you need.

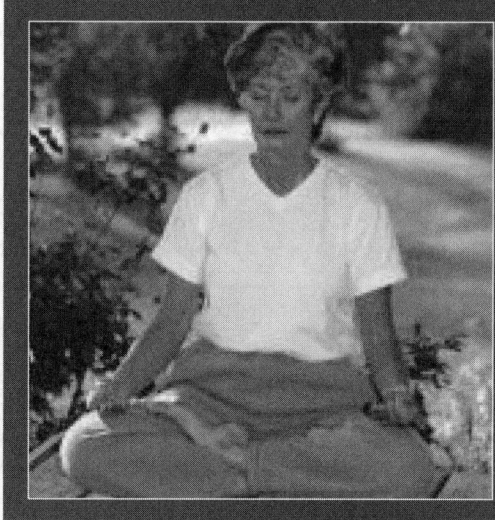

*Take time to breathe.
Don't panic, and don't
feel pressured into making
a rush decision.*

Alexis, cancer survivor

A diagnosis can change your life in an instant.

Like so many other people in your situation, you might be feeling one or more of the following emotions after getting your diagnosis:

- Afraid
- Alone
- Angry
- Anxious
- Ashamed
- Confused
- Depressed
- Helpless
- In denial

- Numb
- Overwhelmed
- Panicky
- Powerless
- Relieved (that you finally know what's wrong)
- Sad
- Shocked
- Stressed

It is perfectly normal to have these feelings. It is also normal, and very common, to have trouble taking in and understanding information after you receive the news – especially if the diagnosis was a surprise. And it can be even harder to make decisions about treating or managing your disease or condition.

Take time to make your decisions.

No matter how the news of your diagnosis has affected you, do not rush into a decision. In most cases, you do not need to take action right away. Ask your doctor how much time you can safely take.

Taking the time you need to make decisions can help you:

• Feel less anxious and stressed.

• Avoid depression.

• Cope with your condition.

• Feel more in control of your situation.

• Play a key role in decisions about your treatment.

Step 2:
Get the support you need.

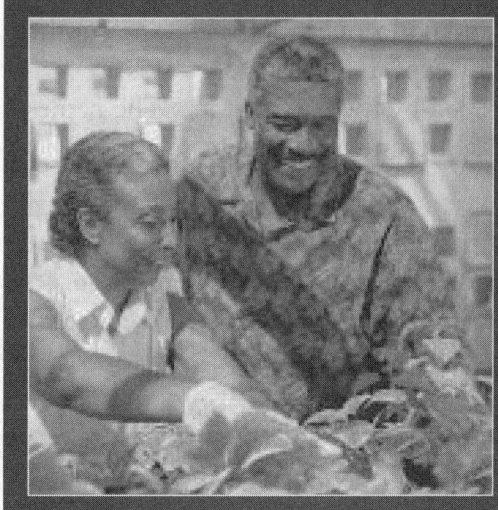

I was shocked when I was diagnosed with diabetes. The extra support I got from my friends and support group really helped me adjust to the new lifestyle I had to adopt.

Richard, person with diabetes

You do not have to go through it alone.

Sometimes the emotional side of illness can be just as hard to deal with as the physical side. You may have fears or concerns. You may feel overwhelmed. No matter what your situation, having other people to turn to will help you know you are not alone.

Here are the kinds of support you might want to seek:

Family and friends.

Talking to family and friends you feel close to can help you cope with your illness or condition. Just knowing that someone is there can be a comfort.

Sometimes it is hard to ask for help. And sometimes your family and friends want to help, but they do not want to intrude, or they do not know how to ask or what to offer. Think about specific ways people can help you. One idea is to ask someone to come with you to a doctor's appointment to help ask questions, take notes, and talk with you afterward.

If you do not have family or friends who can provide support, other people or groups can.

Support or self-help groups.

Support groups are made up of people with the same disease or condition who get together to share information and concerns and to help one another. Support groups may or may not be led by experts. Self-help groups are similar to support groups but usually are led by the participants. The names "support group" and "self-help group" sometimes are used to refer to either kind.

Research on support groups shows that participants feel less anxious, experience less depression, have a better quality of life, and have more success coping with their disease or condition. Similar findings have been reported for self-help groups.

On-line support or self-help groups.

The Internet has support or self-help groups for people whose concerns and situations may be similar to yours. You can also find "message boards," where you can post questions and get answers. These on-line communities can help you connect with people who can give you support and provide information.

But be careful. Not every idea or treatment you come across in these groups will be scientifically proven to be safe and effective. If you read about something interesting and new, check it out with your doctor.

Counselor or therapist.

A good counselor or therapist can help you cope with sadness, depression, and feelings of being overwhelmed. If you think this kind of help might be right for you, ask your doctor or other health care professional to recommend someone in your area.

People like you.

You might want to meet and talk with someone in your own situation. Someone who has "been there" can talk about the real-life outcomes of their treatment choices as well as how they have learned to live with their disease or condition. Some advocacy or support groups can help you make this kind of contact.

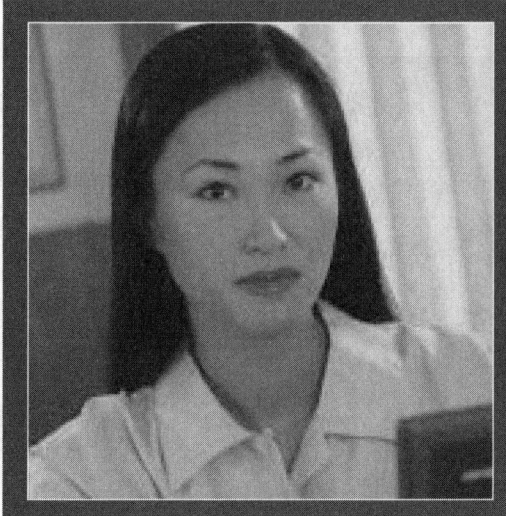

If only I had known what it would be like to live with the after-effects of this type of surgery, I might have chosen a different kind.

Susan, who underwent surgery for a digestive disease

Help is available.

Take advantage of the support that is available to you. See "Where to Find More Information" on page xxx for specific places to find support. An expanded list appears in the on-line version of this article at www.ahrq.gov/consumer/diaginfo.htm.

Step 3:
Talk with your doctor.

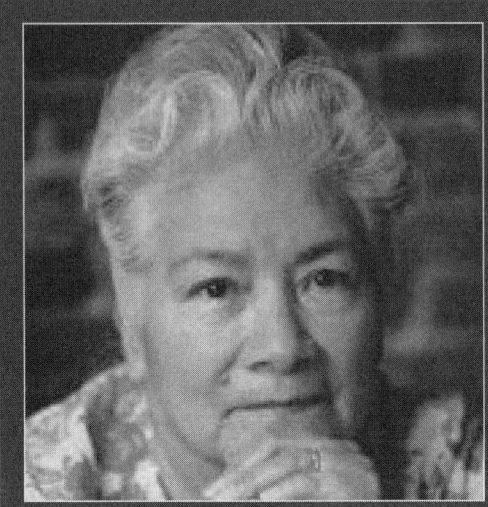

*I had trouble under-
standing what my doctor
was telling me. The words
were too technical, and there
was too much to absorb. I
finally asked her to slow
down and keep it simple.
That helped a lot.*

Dana, person with
heart disease

Your doctor is your partner in health care.

You probably have many questions about your disease or condition. The first
person to ask is your doctor.

It is fine to seek more information from other sources; in fact, it is important
to do so. But consider your doctor your partner in health care—someone
who can discuss your situation with you, explain your options, and help you
make decisions that are right for you.

It is not always easy to feel comfortable around doctors. But research has
shown that good communication with your doctor can actually be good for
your health. It can help you to:

- Feel more satisfied with the care you receive.

- Have better outcomes (end results), such as reduced pain and better
  recovery from symptoms.

Being an active member of your health care team also helps to reduce your
chances of medical mistakes, and it helps you get high-quality care.

Of course, good communication is a two-way street. Here are some ways to
help make the most of the time you spend with your doctor.

Prepare for your visit.

- Think about what you want to get out of your appointment. Write down all your questions and concerns. Some suggested questions are listed on page xxiii.

- Prepare and bring to your doctor visit a list of all the medicines you take.

- Consider bringing along a trusted relative or friend. This person can help ask questions, take notes, and help you remember and understand everything once you leave the doctor's office.

Give information to your doctor.

- Do not wait to be asked.

- Tell your doctor everything he or she needs to know about your health— even the things that might make you feel embarrassed or uncomfortable.

- Tell your doctor how you are feeling—both physically and emotionally.

- Tell your doctor if you are feeling depressed or overwhelmed.

Get information from your doctor.

- Ask questions about anything that concerns you. Keep asking until you understand the answers. If you do not, your doctor may think you understand everything that is said.

- Ask your doctor to draw pictures if that will help you understand something.

- Take notes.

- Tape record your doctor visit, if that will be helpful to you. But first ask your doctor if this is okay.

- Ask your doctor to recommend resources such as Web sites, booklets, or tapes with more information about your disease or condition.

Also see "Ten Important Questions to Ask Your Doctor After a Diagnosis," on page xxiii.

Do not hesitate to seek a second opinion.

A second opinion is when another doctor examines your medical records and gives his or her views about your condition and how it should be treated. You might want a second opinion to:

• Be clear about what you have.

• Know all of your treatment choices.

• Have another doctor look at your choices with you.

It is not pushy or rude to want a second opinion. Most doctors will understand that you need more information before making important decisions about your health.

Check to see whether your health plan covers a second opinion. In some cases, health plans require second opinions.

Here are some ways to find a doctor for a second opinion:

• Ask your doctor. Request someone who does not work in the same office, because doctors who work together tend to share similar views.

• Contact your health plan or your local hospital, medical society, or medical school.

• Use the Doctor Finder on-line service of the American Medical Association at www.ama-assn.org.

Get information about next steps.

• Get the results of any tests or procedures. Discuss the meaning of these results with your doctor.

• Make sure you understand what will happen if you need surgery.

• Talk with your doctor about which hospital is best for your health care needs.

Finally, if you are not satisfied with your doctor, you can do two things: (1) talk with your doctor and try to work things out, and/or (2) switch doctors, if you are able to. It is very important to feel confident about your care.

To learn more, see "Where to Find More Information" on page xxx. The online version of this article includes additional resources.

Ten Important Questions to Ask Your Doctor After a Diagnosis

These 10 basic questions can help you understand your disease or condition, how it might be treated, and what you need to know and do before making treatment decisions.

1. What is the technical name of my disease or condition, and what does it mean in plain English?

   _____

2. What is my prognosis (outlook for the future)?

   _____

3. How soon do I need to make a decision about treatment?

   _____

4. Will I need any additional tests, and if so what kind and when?

   _____

5. What are my treatment options?

   _____

6. What are the pros and cons of my treatment options?

   _____

7. Is there a clinical trial (research study) that is right for me? (See page xxiv.)

   _____

8. Now that I have this diagnosis, what changes will I need to make in my daily life?

   _____

9. What organizations do you recommend for support and information?

   _____

10. What resources (booklets, Web sites, audiotapes, videos, DVDs, etc.) do you recommend for further information?

    _____

Step 4:
Seek out information.

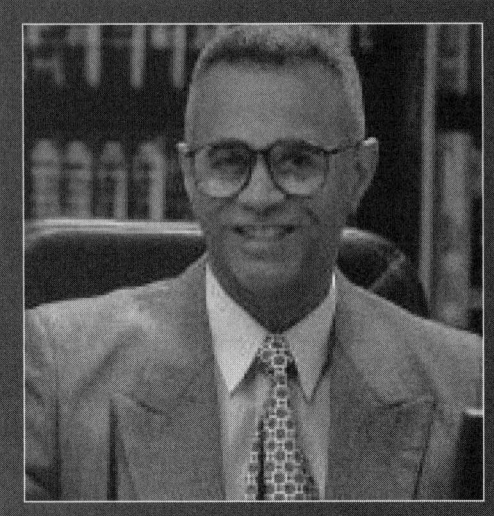

I'm really glad I took the time to research my options. It stopped me from jumping into a treatment that would have been completely wrong for me.

Seth, prostate cancer survivor

Now that you know your treatment options, you can learn which ones are backed up by the best scientific evidence. "Evidence-based" information—that is, information that is based on a careful review of the latest scientific findings in medical journals—can help you make decisions about the best possible treatments for you.

Evidence-based information comes from research on people like you.

Evidence-based information about treatments generally comes from two major types of scientific studies:

- **Clinical trials** are research studies on human volunteers to test new drugs or other treatments. Participants are randomly assigned to different treatment groups. Some get the research treatment, and others get a standard treatment or may be given a placebo (a medicine that has no effect), or no treatment. The results are compared to learn whether the new treatment is safe and effective.

- **Outcomes research** looks at the impact of treatments and other health care on health outcomes (end results) for patients and populations. End results include effects that people care about, such as changes in their quality of life.

Take advantage of the evidence-based information that is available.

Health information is everywhere—in books, newspapers, and magazines, and on the Internet, television, and radio. However, not all information is good information. Your best bets for sources of evidence-based information include the Federal Government, national nonprofit organizations, medical specialty groups, medical schools, and university medical centers.

Some resources are listed below, grouped by type of information. See "Where to Find More Information" on page xxx for additional ideas. The online version of Next Steps After Your Diagnosis lists many more, and includes links to Internet sites.

▆ Information.

Information about your disease or condition and its treatment is available from many sources. Here are some of the most reliable:

- **healthfinder®:** www.healthfinder.gov/organizations/OrgListing.asp
  The healthfinder® site—sponsored by the U.S. Department of Health and Human Services—offers carefully selected health information Web sites from government agencies, clearinghouses, nonprofit groups, and universities.

- **Health Information Resource Database:**
  www.health.gov/nhic/#Referrals
  Sponsored by the National Health Information Center, this database includes 1,400 organizations and government offices that provide health information upon request. Information is also available over the telephone at 800-336-4797.

- **MEDLINEplus®:** www.nlm.nih.gov/medlineplus
  MedlinePlus® has extensive information from the National Institutes of Health and other trusted sources on over 650 diseases and conditions. The site includes many additional features.

- **National nonprofit groups** such as the American Heart Association, American Cancer Society, and American Diabetes Association can be valuable sources of reliable information. Many have chapters nationwide. Check your phone book for a local chapter in your community. The Health Information Resource Database (www.health.gov/nhic/#Referrals) can help you find national offices of nonprofit groups.

- **Health or medical libraries** run by government, hospitals, professional groups, and other reliable organizations often welcome consumers. For a list of libraries in your area, go to the MedlinePlus® "Find a Library" page at http://www.nlm.nih.gov/medlineplus/libraries.html.

Current medical research.

You can find the latest medical research in medical journals at your local health or medical library, and in some cases, on the Internet. Here are two major online sources of medical articles:

- **MEDLINE/PubMed®:** http://www.ncbi.nlm.nih.gov/entrez/query.fcgi
  PubMed® is the National Library of Medicine's database of references to more than 14 million articles published in 4,800 medical and scientific journals. All of the listings have information to help you find the articles at a health or medical library. Many listings also have short summaries of the article (abstracts), and some have links to the full article. The article might be free, or it might require a fee charged by the publisher.

- **PubMed Central:** http://www.pubmedcentral.nih.gov/
  PubMed Central is the National Library of Medicine's database of journal articles that are available free of charge to users.

Clinical trials.

Perhaps you wonder whether there is a clinical trial that is right for you. Or you may want to learn about results from previous clinical trials that might be relevant to your situation. Here are two reliable resources:

- **ClinicalTrials.gov:** http://clinicaltrials.gov/ct/g
  ClinicalTrials.gov provides regularly updated information about federally and privately supported clinical research on people who volunteer to participate. The site has information about a trial's purpose, who may participate, locations, and phone numbers for more details. The site also describes the clinical trial process and includes news about recent clinical trial results.

- **Cochrane Collaboration:** www.cochrane.org
  The Cochrane Collaboration writes summaries ("reviews") about evidence from clinical trials to help people make informed decisions. You can search and read the review abstracts free of charge at http://www.cochrane.org/

reviews/index.htm. Or you can read plain-English consumer summaries of the reviews at www.informedhealthonline.org.

The full Cochrane reviews are available only by subscription. Check with your local medical or health library (see page xxxii) [link back to library section in on-line version] to see whether you can access the full reviews there.

Outcomes research.

Outcomes research provides research about benefits, risks, and outcomes (end results) of treatments so that patients and their doctors can make better informed decisions. The U.S. Agency for Healthcare Research and Quality (AHRQ) supports improvements in health outcomes through research, and sponsors products that result from research such as:

- **National Guideline Clearinghouse™:** www.guideline.gov
  The National Guideline Clearinghouse™ is a database of evidence-based clinical practice guidelines and related documents. Clinical practice guidelines are documents designed to help doctors and patients make decisions about appropriate health care for specific diseases or conditions. The clearinghouse was originally created by AHRQ in partnership with the American Medical Association and America's Health Insurance Plans.

Steer clear of deceptive ads and information.

While searching for information either on or off the Internet, beware of "miracle" treatments and cures. They can cost you money and your health, especially if you delay or refuse proper treatment. Here are some tip-offs that a product truly is too good to be true:

- Phrases such as "scientific breakthrough," "miraculous cure," "exclusive product," "secret formula," or "ancient ingredient."

- Claims that the product treats a wide range of ailments.

- Use of impressive-sounding medical terms. These often cover up a lack of good science behind the product.

- Case histories from consumers claiming "amazing" results.

- Claims that the product is available from only one source, and for a limited time only.

- Claims of a "money-back guarantee."

- Claims that others are trying to keep the product off the market.

- Ads that fail to list the company's name, address, or other contact information.

To learn more about finding evidence-based information, see "Where to Find More Information," page xxx. The on-line edition of this article has many additional resources.

Step 5:
Decide on a treatment plan.

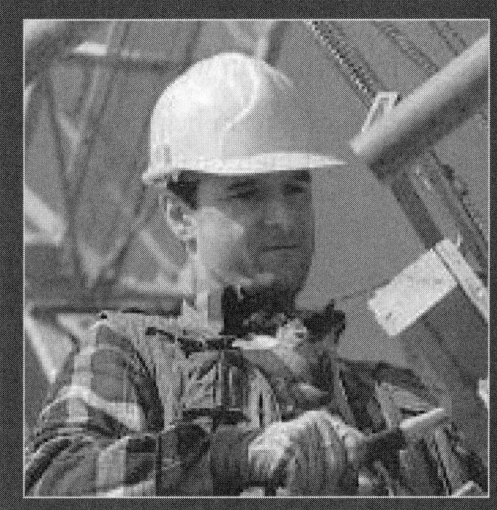

My doctor told me I had done one of the hardest but most important things a patient has to do: Face up to the diagnosis and make decisions. It feels good to be where I am now.

Bob, person with a
neurological disorder

At this point, you have learned about your disease or condition and how it can be treated or managed. Your information may have come from the following sources:

- Your doctor.

- Second opinions from one or more other doctors.

- Other people who are or were in the same situation as you.

- Information sources such as Web sites, health or medical libraries, and nonprofit groups.

Work with your doctor to make decisions.

When you are ready to make treatment decisions, you and your doctor can discuss:

- Which treatments have been found to work well, or not work well, for your particular condition.

- The pros and cons of each treatment option.

Make sure that your doctor knows your preferences and feelings about the different treatments – for example, whether you prefer medicine over surgery.

Once you and your doctor decide on one or more treatments that are right for you, you can work together to develop a treatment plan. This plan will include everything that will be done to treat or manage your disease or condition—including what you need to do to make the plan work.

Remember, being an active member of your health care team helps to reduce your chances of medical mistakes, and it helps you get high-quality care.

Take another deep breath.

You have taken important steps to cope with your diagnosis, make decisions, and get on with your life. Remember two things:

- Call on others for support as you need it.

- Make use of evidence-based information for any future health decisions.

Where to Find More Information

Get the support you need.

American Self-Help Group Clearinghouse
http://mentalhelp.net/selfhelp/

National Board for Certified Counselors (NBCC)
3 Terrace Way, Suite D
Greensboro, NC 27403-3660
336-547-0607.
www.nbcc.org

National Institute of Mental Health
Public Information and Communications Branch
6001 Executive Boulevard, Room 8184, MSC 9663
Bethesda, MD 20892-9663
Phone: 866-615-6464 (toll-free)
TTY: 301-443-8431
http://www.nimh.nih.gov/HealthInformation/GettingHelp.cfm

Talk to your doctor.

Be an Active Member of Your Health Care Team. Food and Drug Administration. 2004. http://www.fda.gov/cder/consumerinfo/active_member.htm. Phone: 888-INFO-FDA (888-463-6332).

Be Informed: Questions to Ask Your Doctor Before You Have Surgery. Agency for Healthcare Quality and Research. 1995. http://www.ahrq.gov/consumer/surgery.htm. Phone: 800-358-9295.

Five Steps to Safer Health Care. Agency for Healthcare Research and Quality. 2003. http://www.ahrq.gov/consumer/5steps.htm. Phone: 800-358-9295.

Getting a Second Opinion Before Surgery. Centers for Medicare & Medicaid Services. 2004. www.medicare.gov/Publications/Pubs/pdf/02173.pdf. Phone: 800-MEDICARE (800-633-4227).

How to Get a Second Opinion. National Women's Health Information Center. 2003. http://www.4woman.gov/pub/secondopinion.htm. Phone: 1-800-994-WOMAN.

Quick Tips – When Planning for Surgery. Agency for Healthcare Research and Quality. 2002. http://www.ahrq.gov/consumer/quicktips/tipsurgery.htm. Phone: 800-358-9295.

Quick Tips – When Talking with Your Doctor. Agency for Healthcare Research and Quality. 2002. http://www.ahrq.gov/consumer/quicktips/doctalk.htm. Phone: 800-358-9295.

Talking with Your Doctor: A Guide for Older People. National Institute on Aging. 2002. www.niapublications.org/pubs/talking/index.asp. Phone: 800-222-2225. |

Seek out information.

2005 Toll-Free Numbers for Health Information. National Health Information Center. www.health.gov/nhic/pubs/tollfree.htm. Phone: 800-336-4797.

AARP Health Guide. AARP. 2004. www.aarp.org/health/healthguide. Phone: 888-OUR-AARP (888-687-2277).

HON Code of Conduct (HONcode) for Medical and Health Web Sites Health on the Net Foundation. http://www.hon.ch/HONcode/

How to Evaluate Health Information on the Internet: Questions and Answers. National Cancer Institute. 2003. http://cis.nci.nih.gov/fact/ 2_10.htm. Phone: 800-4-CANCER (800-422-6237).

How to Find Medical Information. National Institute of Arthritis and Musculoskeletal and Skin Diseases. 2001. http://www.niams.nih.gov/hi/ topics/howto/howto.htm. Phone: 877-22-NIAMS (877-226-4267) (toll-free).

JAMA Patient Page: Health Information on the Internet. The Medem Network. http://www.medem.com/medlb/ article_detaillb.cfm?article_ID=ZZZLJLLLTMC&sub_cat=603

National Guideline Clearinghouse™. Agency for Healthcare Research and Quality. http://www.guideline.gov/

NOAH: New York Online Access to Health. http://www.noah-health.org/

A User's Guide to Finding and Evaluating Health Information on the Web. Medical Library Association. 2003. http://www.mlanet.org/resources/ userguide.html#1

Virtual Treatments Can Be Real-World Deceptions. Federal Trade Commission. 2001. http://www.ftc.gov/bcp/conline/pubs/alerts/ mrclalrt.htm

Your Guide to Choosing Quality Health Care. Agency for Healthcare Research and Quality. 2002. http://www.ahrq.gov/consumer/qntool.htm. Phone: 800-358-9295.

AHRQ consumer publications:

20 Tips to Help Prevent Medical Errors—Practical tips and questions to ask. (AHRQ 00-P038)

20 Tips to Help Prevent Medical Errors in Children (AHRQ 02-P034)

Five Steps to Safer Health Care—Shorter version of 20 Tips. (AHRQ 03-M007)

Ways You Can Help Your Family Prevent Medical Errors!—Easy-to-read version, with drawings. (AHRQ 01-0017)

Your Guide to Choosing Quality Health Care—Based on research about the information people want and need when choosing health plans, doctors, treatments, hospitals, and long-term care. (AHRQ 99-012)

Improving Health Care Quality: A Guide for Patients and Their Families—Short version of *Your Guide to Choosing Quality Health Care*. (AHRQ 01-0004)

Quick Checks for Quality—Checklist to use when choosing health plans, doctors, treatments, hospitals, and long-term care. (AHRQ 99-R027)

Quick Tips:
> *When Getting Medical Tests* (AHRQ 01-0040b)
> *When Getting a Prescription* (AHRQ 01-0040c)
> *When Planning for Surgery* (AHRQ 01-0040d)
> *When Talking with Your Doctor* (AHRQ 01-0040a)

To order AHRQ publications:

For electronic copies of these publications, go to the AHRQ Web site at www.ahrq.gov/consumer

For print copies, contact the AHRQ Publications Clearinghouse at 800-358-9295.

Description

1 Addison's Disease

Addison's disease is a rare disorder that stems from the malfunction of the adrenal glands located on top of the kidneys. In this disease, there is a deficiency of hormones produced by the adrenal cortex, the gland's firm outer layer. Most often, Addison's disease results from destruction of the adrenal gland. This glandular destruction may result from unusual infections, malignant tumors, an autoimmune process or other rare disorders. At least half of all cases of Addison's disease result from patient's developing antibodies against their own adrenal tissue (autoimmune process).

There can be increased water excretion in the urine and lowered blood pressure, which can lead to severe dehydration and other major complications. The symptoms of Addison's disease increase with the progression of the disease. Early signs may include fatigue, loss of appetite, low blood pressure (hypotension), weakness and significant loss from the kidneys of water and minerals. Other symptoms may include darkened scars and skin folds, as well as dark freckles on the head and shoulders. In the later stages, nausea may develop, as well as dizziness, further dehydration, low blood sugar (hypoglycemia) and mental changes including confusion.

Patients who are treated early have an excellent prognosis, but it is imperative that treatment be instituted immediately and vigorously. In order to counteract the hormonal loss, physicians prescribe steroid hormone replacement therapy. Certain doses of hormones need to be increased during times of illness and surgery. Treatment should never be stopped, even for a day, without the advice of a physician. Persons on treatment should wear an alert bracelet to let emergency medical providers know of their diagnosis.

National Agencies & Associations

2 Endocrine Society
8401 Connecticut Avenue   301-941-0200
Chevy Chase, MD 20815   888-363-6274
                                    Fax: 301-941-0259
          e-mail: societyservices@endo-society.org
                                    www.endo-society.org
Source of state-of-the-art research and clinical advancements in endocrinology and metabolism. Dedicated to promoting excellence in research education and clinical practice in the field of endocrinology. Prime advocate and integrative force for clinicians.
Teresa K. Woodruff, Ph.D., President
Richard J. Santen, M.D., President-Elect

3 National Adrenal Diseases Foundation
505 Northern Boulevard   516-487-4992
Great Neck, NY 11021   Fax: 516-829-5710
                e-mail: nadfsupport@nadf.us
                                    www.nadf.us
Nonprofit organization dedicated to offer support information and research for individuals having diseases of the adrenal glands. Goals of the organization include assisting patients through informational and educational activities as well as support programs.
Paul Margulies, M.D., FACP, F, Medical Director
Melanie G Wong, Executive Director

4 National Institute of Diabetes & Digestive & Kidney Diseases
National Institutes of Health
31 Center Drive   301-496-3583
Bethesda, MD 20892-2560   800-860-8747
                                    Fax: 703-738-4929
                e-mail: ndic@info.niddk.nih.gov
                                    www.diabetes.niddk.nih.gov
Conducts and supports research on many of the most serious diseases affecting public health. The Institute supports much of the clinical research on the diseases of internal medicine and related subspecialty fields as well as many basic science disciplines.
Griffin P. Rodgers, M.D., M.A.C.P., Director

Support Groups & Hotlines

5 National Health Information Center
PO Box 1133   310-565-4167
Washington, DC 20013   800-336-4797
                                    Fax: 301-984-4256
                e-mail: info@nhic.org
                                    www.health.gov/nhic
Offers a nationwide information referral service, produces directories and resource guides.

Magazines

6 Endocrine News
Endocrine Society
8401 Connecticut Avenue   301-941-0200
Chevy Chase, MD 20815   888-363-6274
                                    Fax: 301-941-0259
          e-mail: societyservices@endo-society.org
                                    www.endo-society.org
Endocrine News is the source of trends and insights for members of the endocrine community.
Monthly
Kelly E Mayo PhD, President
Scott Hunt, Executive Director

Newsletters

7 Addison News
6142 Territorial   www2.dmci.net/users/hoffmanrj
Pleasant Lake, MI 49272

8 NADF News
National Adrenal Diseases Foundation
505 Northern Boulevard   516-487-4992
Great Neck, NY 11021   Fax: 516-829-5710
                e-mail: nadfmail@aol.com
                                    www.nadf.us
Contains information on the latest research, question and answer column by an endocrinologist and helpful hints for those with Addison's Disease.
Quarterly Monthly
Melanie G Wong, Executive Director
Debbie Benish, Editor

Web Sites

9 Healing Well
                                    www.healingwell.com
An online health resource guide to medical news, chat, information and articles, newsgroups and message boards, books, disease-related web sites, medical directories, and more for patients, friends, and family coping with disabling diseases, disorders, or chronic illnesses.

10 Health Finder
                                    www.healthfinder.gov
A government Web site where you will find information and tools to help you and those you care about stay healthy.

11 Health Link USA
                                    www.healthlinkusa.com

Discussion forum for treatments, symptoms and causes of 700 health conditions, diseases and topics.

12   Helios Health

www.helioshealth.com

Online resource for your health information. Detailed information about specific health topics, access to expert advice from our Medical Advisory Board, and up-to-date health news.

13   Hormone Foundation

www.hormone.org

Educational resource for you, your loved ones, and your health professionals on the prevention, treatment, and cure of hormone-related conditions.

14   MedicineNet

www.medicinenet.com

An online resource for consumers providing easy-to-read, authoritative medical and health information.

15   Medscape

www.medscape.com

Search engine providing links to websites with information on illnesses, diseases and disorders.

16   National Adrenal Disease Foundation

www.medhelp.org

Non-profit organization dedicated to providing support, information and education to individuals having Addison's disease as well as other diseases of the adrenal glands.

17   WebMD

www.webmd.com

Information on Addison's disease, including an overview of the disease, symptoms and home treatment.

Description

18 # Aging

The elderly population in the United States is growing faster than any other segment of the population, and has done so since 1900. It is estimated that this trend will continue at least through the year 2050. In 2004, there were 36.3 million people in the U.S. One in eight persons is over 85 years, classified as 'old old.' By 2040, it is anticipated that one person in five will exceed 65 years of age, and the number of people over 85 will increase to four times their number today, representing the aging of the baby boomers.

Aging is not a disease, but part of the normal life cycle, and many seniors retain good health and live independently for long past the traditional age of retirement. In time, however, most will develop one or more chronic conditions; for those over 75 years of age, the most common conditions are hypertension, heart disease, hearing loss, arthritis, and cataracts. By the year 2030, 150 million Americans are expected to have a chronic condition, and 42 million will be limited in their ability to work or live independently. Treating this population will require many medical and nonmedical services, integrated to provide a comprehensive continuum of care. See also *Alzheimer's Disease.*

National Agencies & Associations

19 **American Association of Retired Persons**
601 E Street NW
Washington, DC 20049   888-687-2277
TTY: 877-434-7598
e-mail: member@aarp.org
www.aarp.org
AARP is the nation's leading organization for people age 50 and older. It serves their needs and interests through information and education, advocacy and community services provided by a network of local chapters and experienced volunteers.
Barry Rand, CEO
Robert G Romasco, President

20 **Commission on Accreditation of Rehabilitation Services**
6951 E Southpoint Road   520-325-1044
Tucson, AZ 85756   888-281-6531
Fax: 520-318-1129
carf.org
CARF reviews and grants accreditation services nationally and internationally at the request of a facility or program. Their standards are rigorous, so those services that meet them are among the best available.
Brian J. Boon, President/CEO
Amanda E. Birch, Adminsterator of Operations

21 **Gerontological Society of America**
1220 L Street NW   202-842-1275
Washington, DC 20005   Fax: 202-842-1150
e-mail: geron@geron.org
www.geron.org
Nonprofit professional organization with more than 5000 members in the field of aging. Provides researchers, educators, practitioners and policy makers with opportunities to understand, advance, integrate and use basic and applied research on aging populations.
Rita B. Effros, President
Suzanne R. Kunkel, Treasurer

22 **Institute for Life Course and Aging**
263 McCaul St.   416-978-0377
Toronto, Ontario, M5T1W-3J1   Fax: 416-978-4771
e-mail: aging@utoronto.ca
www.aging.utoronto.ca
The Institute is a research center under the auspices of the School of Graduate Studies at the University of Toronto.
Dr. Lynn McDonald, PhD., Director
Susan Murphy, Administration

23 **International Federation on Aging**
351 Christie Street   416-342-1655
Toronto, Ontario, M6GC6-3C3   Fax: 416-392-4157
e-mail: jbarratt@ifa-fiv.org
www.ifa-fiv.org
To inform, educate and promote policies and practice to improve the quality of life of older persons around the world.
Greg Shaw, Director, International & Corporate Rela
Dr. Jane Barratt, Secretory General

24 **Leading Age**
2519 Connecticut Avenue NW   202-783-2242
Washington, DC 20008-1520   Fax: 202-783-2255
e-mail: info@LeadingAge.org
www.leadingage.org/?
National association of more than 4 000 nonprofit nursing homes continuing care retirement communities independent living centers and community service providers serving more than 60,000 older Americans each year.
William L Minnix Jr, President and CEO
Katrinka Smith Sloan, COO and SVP Member Services

25 **National Council on Aging**
1901 L Street NW   202-479-1200
Washington, DC 20036   Fax: 202-479-0735
TTY: 202-479-6674
TDD: 202-479-6674
e-mail: info@ncoa.org
www.ncoa.org
The nation's first charitable organization dedicated to promoting the dignity, independence, well-being and contributions of older Americans. NCOA serves as a national voice and powerful advocate on behalf of older Americans.
James P Firman EdD, President/CEO
Jay Greenberg, Vice President

26 **Problems of the Elderly Committee**
1050 Connecticut Avenue   202-662-1000
Washington, DC 20003-1019   Fax: 202-662-1501
e-mail: crimjustice@abanet.org
www.abanet.org/crimjust
This Committee examines the issues that affect the elderly as victims of street crime, identity theft, financial exploitation and other crimes of which they are targets. The committee looks at issues arising from the aging prisons populations and the elders as perpetrators of crime, also.
Laurel G. Bellows, President
Robert M. Carlson, Chair Person

27 **Senior Resource**
4521 Campus Drive   858-793-7901
Irvine, CA 92612   877-793-7901
Fax: 858-792-9080
e-mail: questions@seniorresource.com
www.seniorresource.com
An agency that helps seniors to understand aging and gives different resources consisting of sociologic changes; metabolic changes; positive aging; and physical changes.
Bryan D Hatchell, Chair

28 **US Administration on Aging**
1 Massachusetts Avenue   202-619-0724
Washington, DC 20001   Fax: 202-357-3555
e-mail: aclinfo@acl.hhs.gov
www.aoa.gov
The Administration on Aging an agency in the US Department of Health and Human Services is one of the nation's largest providers

of home and community-based care for older persons and their caregivers.
Kathy Greenlee, Administrator
Sharon Lewis, Acting Principal Deputy

State Agencies & Associations

Alaska

29   **AARP Alaska State Office**
3601 C Street
Anchorage, AK 99503   866-227-7447
Fax: 907-341-2270
e-mail: ak@aarp.org
www.aarp.org/states/ak
AARP is a nonprofit nonpartisan membership organization for people age 50 and over. AARP is dedicated to enhancing the quality of life as one ages, in addition to facilitating social change and delivering value to members through information and advocacy.
Fred Jenkins, Development Director
George Hieronymus, AARP Alaska State President

Arizona

30   **AARP Arizona: Phoenix Collier Center**
Collier Center
201 E Washington Street
Phoenix, AZ 85004-2428   866-389-5649
Fax: 602-256-2928
e-mail: azaarp@aarp.org
www.aarp.org/states/az
AARP is a nonprofit nonpartisan membership organization for people age 50 and over. AARP is dedicated to enhancing the quality of life as one ages, in addition to facilitating social change and delivering value to members through information and advocacy.
Leonard J Kirschner PhD, Arizona AARP State President
David Mitchell, Arizona AARP State Director

Arkansas

31   **AARP Arkansas State Office: Little Rock**
1701 Centerview Drive
Little Rock, AR 72211   866-544-5379
Fax: 501-227-7710
e-mail: araarp@aarp.org
www.aarp.org/states/ar
AARP is a nonprofit nonpartisan membership organization for people age 50 and over. AARP is dedicated to enhancing the quality of life as one ages, in addition to facilitating social change and delivering value to members through information and advocacy.
Mary Dillard, Arkansas AARP State President
Pat Jones, Arkansas AARP State Media Relations

California

32   **AARP California State Office: Pasadena**
200 S Los Robles Avenue
Pasadena, CA 91101-2422   866-448-3615
Fax: 626-583-8500
e-mail: calosangeles@aarp.org
www.aarp.org/states/ca
AARP is a nonprofit nonpartisan membership organization for people age 50 and over. AARP is dedicated to enhancing the quality of life as one ages, in addition to facilitating social change and delivering value to members through information and advocacy.
Helen Russ, California AARP State President
Thomas A Porter, California AARP State Director

33   **AARP California State Office: Sacramento**
1415 L Street
Sacramento, CA 95814   866-448-3614
Fax: 916-446-2223
e-mail: casacramento@aarp.org
www.aarp.org/states/ca
AARP is a nonprofit nonpartisan membership organization for people age 50 and over. AARP is dedicated to enhancing the qual-

ity of life as one ages, in addition to facilitating social change and delivering value to members through information and advocacy.
Helen Russ, California State AARP President
Thomas A Porter, California State AARP Director

Colorado

34   **AARP Colorado State Office: Denver**
303 E 17th Avenue
Denver, CO 80203-5012   866-554-5376
Fax: 303-764-5999
e-mail: coaarp@aarp.org
www.aarp.org/states/co
AARP is a nonprofit nonpartisan membership organization for people age 50 and over. AARP is dedicated to enhancing the quality of life as one ages, in addition to facilitating social change and delivering value to members through information and advocacy.
Robert Martinez, Colorado AARP State President
Jon Looney, Colorado AARP State Director

Florida

35   **AARP Florida State Office: St. Petersburg**
400 Carillon Parkway
Saint Petersburg, FL 33716   866-595-7678
Fax: 727-369-5191
TTY: 727-561-9544
e-mail: flaarp@aarp.org
www.aarp.org/states/fl
AARP is a nonprofit nonpartisan membership organization for people age 50 and over. AARP is dedicated to enhancing the quality of life as one ages, in addition to facilitating social change and delivering value to members through information and advocacy.
Kathy Marma, Florida AARP State Media Relations
Thomas Thame MD, Florida AARP State Board of Directors

36   **Goodwill Industries-Suncoast**
Goodwill Industries-Suncoast
10596 Gandy Boulevard
St. Petersburg, FL 33702   727-523-1512
888-279-1988
Fax: 727-563-9300
TTY: 727-579-1068
e-mail: gw.marketing@goodwill-suncoast.org
www.goodwill-suncoast.org
A nonprofit, community-based organization whose mission is to help people achieve self-sufficiency through the dignity and power of work, serving people who are disadvantaged, disabled or elderly. The mission is accomplished through providing independent living skills, affordable housing, and training and placement in community employment.
Jay Mc Cloe, Director Resource Development

Georgia

37   **AARP Georgia: Atlanta**
999 Peachtree Street NE
Atlanta, GA 30309-4421   866-295-7281
Fax: 404-881-6997
e-mail: gaaarp@aarp.org
www.aarp.org/states/ga
AARP is a nonprofit nonpartisan membership organization for people age 50 and over. AARP is dedicated to enhancing the quality of life as one ages, in addition to facilitating social change and delivering value to members through information and advocacy.
Matthew McWilliams, Georgia AARP State Media Relations
Will Phillips, AARP Georgia Associate State Director

Hawaii

38   **AARP Hawaii State Office: Honolulu**
1132 Bishop Street
Honolulu, HI 96813   808-843-1906
866-295-7282
Fax: 808-843-1908
e-mail: oahuaarp@hawaii.rr.com
www.aarp.org/states/hi
AARP is a nonprofit nonpartisan membership organization for people age 50 and over. AARP is dedicated to enhancing the qual-

ity of life as one ages, in addition to facilitating social change and delivering value to members through information and advocacy.
Stuart TK Ho, AARP Hawaii Interim State President
Barbara Kim Stanton, Hawaii AARP State Director

Idaho

39   **AARP Idaho State Office: Meridian**
3830 E Gentry Way
Meridian, ID 83642   866-295-7284
Fax: 208-288-4424
e-mail: aarpid@aarp.org
www.aarp.org/states/id
AARP is a nonprofit nonpartisan membership organization for people age 50 and over. AARP is dedicated to enhancing the quality of life as one ages, in addition to facilitating social change and delivering value to members through information and advocacy.
Cheryl Tussey, Idaho AARP State Media Relations
Jim Wordelman, AARP Idaho State Director

Illinois

40   **AARP Illinois State Office: Chicago**
222 N LaSalle Street
Chicago, IL 60601-1033   866-448-3613
Fax: 312-372-2204
e-mail: aarpil@aarp.org
www.aarp.org/states/il
AARP is a nonprofit nonpartisan membership organization for people age 50 and over. AARP is dedicated to enhancing the quality of life as one ages, in addition to facilitating social change and delivering value to members through information and advocacy.
Evelyn Gooden, Illinois AARP State President
Gerardo Cardenas, Illinois AARP State Media Relations

Indiana

41   **AARP Indiana State Office: Indianapolis**
One N Capitol Avenue
Indianapolis, IN 46204-2025   866-448-3618
Fax: 317-423-2211
e-mail: inaarp@aarp.org
www.aarp.org/states/in
AARP is a nonprofit nonpartisan membership organization for people age 50 and over. AARP is dedicated to enhancing the quality of life as one ages, in addition to facilitating social change and delivering value to members through information and advocacy.
Martin DeAgostino, Indiana AARP State Media Relations
June Lyle, AARP Indiana State Director

Iowa

42   **AARP Iowa State Office: Des Moines**
600 E Court Avenue
Des Moines, IA 50309   866-554-5378
Fax: 515-244-7767
e-mail: iaaarp@aarp.org
www.aarp.org/states/ia
AARP is a nonprofit nonpartisan membership organization for people age 50 and over. AARP is dedicated to enhancing the quality of life as one ages, in addition to facilitating social change and delivering value to members through information and advocacy.
Ann Black, Iowa AARP State Media Relations
Bruce Koeppl, Iowa AARP State Director

Kansas

43   **AARP Kansas State Office: Topeka**
555 S Kansas
Topeka, KS 66603   866-448-3619
Fax: 785-232-8259
e-mail: ksaarp@aarp.org
www.aarp.org/states/ks
AARP is a nonprofit nonpartisan membership organization for people age 50 and over. AARP is dedicated to enhancing the quality of life as one ages, in addition to facilitating social change and delivering value to members through information and advocacy.
Mary Tritsch, Kansas AARP State Media Relations
Maren Turner, Kansas AARP State Director

Kentucky

44   **AARP Kentucky State Office: Louisville**
10401 Linn Station Road
Louisville, KY 40223   866-295-7275
Fax: 502-394-9918
e-mail: kyaarp@aarp.org
www.aarp.org/states/ky
AARP is a nonprofit nonpartisan membership organization for people age 50 and over. AARP is dedicated to enhancing the quality of life as one ages, in addition to facilitating social change and delivering value to members through information and advocacy.
Bill Harned, AARP Kentucky State President
Fred Smith, Executive Council Community Service

Louisiana

45   **AARP Louisiana State Office: Baton Rouge**
301 Main Street
Baton Rouge, LA 70825   866-448-3620
Fax: 225-387-3400
e-mail: la@aarp.org
www.aarp.org/states/la
AARP is a nonprofit nonpartisan membership organization for people age 50 and over. AARP is dedicated to enhancing the quality of life as one ages, in addition to facilitating social change and delivering value to members through information and advocacy.
Earl A White, AARP Louisiana State President
Julia Kenny, AARP Louisiana State Director

Maine

46   **AARP Maine State Office: Portland**
1685 Congress Street
Portland, ME 04102   866-554-5380
Fax: 207-775-5727
e-mail: me@aarp.org
www.aarp.org/states/me
AARP is a nonprofit nonpartisan membership organization for people age 50 and over. AARP is dedicated to enhancing the quality of life as one ages, in addition to facilitating social change and delivering value to members through information and advocacy.
Bruce Kinney, Maine AARP State Advocacy Coordinator
Phyllis Cohn, Maine AARP State Media Relations

Massachusetts

47   **AARP Massachusetts State Office: Boston**
1 Beacon Street
Boston, MA 02108   866-448-3621
Fax: 617-723-4224
e-mail: ma@aarp.org
www.aarp.org/states/ma
AARP is a nonprofit nonpartisan membership organization for people age 50 and over. AARP is dedicated to enhancing the quality of life as one ages, in addition to facilitating social change and delivering value to members through information and advocacy.
Charlie Desmond, AARP Massachusetts State President
Claire Redmond, Executive Council Member

Michigan

48   **AARP Michigan State Office: Lansing**
309 N Washington Square
Lansing, MI 48933   866-227-7448
Fax: 517-482-2794
TTY: 877-434-7598
e-mail: miaarp@aarp.org
www.aarp.org/states/mi
AARP is a nonprofit nonpartisan membership organization for people age 50 and over. AARP is dedicated to enhancing the quality of life as one ages, in addition to facilitating social change and delivering value to members through information and advocacy.
Steve Gools, AARP Michigan State Director
Stepheni Schlinker, Michigan AARP State Media Relations

Minnesota

49 **AARP Minnesota State Office: Saint Paul**
30 E Seventh Street
Saint Paul, MN 55101   866-554-5381
                                   Fax: 651-221-2636
                              e-mail: aarpmn@aarp.org
                              www.aarp.org/states/mn
AARP is a nonprofit nonpartisan membership organization for people age 50 and over. AARP is dedicated to enhancing the quality of life as one ages, in addition to facilitating social change and delivering value to members through information and advocacy.
Michele Kimball, AARP Minnesota State Director
Amy Gromer McDonough, AARP Minnesota State Media Relations

Missouri

50 **AARP Missouri State Office: Kansas City**
700 W 47th Street
Kansas City, MO 64112-1805   866-389-5627
                                   Fax: 816-561-3107
                              e-mail: moaarp@aarp.org
                              www.aarp.org/states/mo
AARP is a nonprofit nonpartisan membership organization for people age 50 and over. AARP is dedicated to enhancing the quality of life as one ages, in addition to facilitating social change and delivering value to members through information and advocacy.
John McDonald, AARP Missouri State Director
Anita K Parran, AARP Missouri State Media Relations

Montana

51 **AARP Montana State Office: Helena**
30 W 14th Street
Helena, MT 59601   866-295-7278
                                   Fax: 406-441-2230
                              e-mail: mtaarp@aarp.org
                              www.aarp.org/states/mt
AARP is a nonprofit nonpartisan membership organization for people age 50 and over. AARP is dedicated to enhancing the quality of life as one ages, in addition to facilitating social change and delivering value to members through information and advocacy.
Max Logan, AARP Montana Volunteer State President
Bob Bartholomew, AARP Montana State Director

Nebraska

52 **AARP Nebraska State Office: Lincoln**
301 S 13th Street
Lincoln, NE 68508   866-389-5651
                                   Fax: 402-323-6908
                              e-mail: neaarp@aarp.org
                              www.aarp.org/states/ne
AARP is a nonprofit nonpartisan membership organization for people age 50 and over. AARP is dedicated to enhancing the quality of life as one ages, in addition to facilitating social change and delivering value to members through information and advocacy.
Sunny Andrews, AARP Nebraska State President
Devorah Lanner, AARP Nebraska State Media Relations

Nevada

53 **AARP Nevada State Office: Las Vegas**
5820 S Eastern Avenue
Las Vegas, NV 89119   866-389-5652
                                   Fax: 702-938-3225
                              e-mail: nvaarp@aarp.org
                              www.aarp.org/states/nv
AARP is a nonprofit nonpartisan membership organization for people age 50 and over. AARP is dedicated to enhancing the quality of life as one ages, in addition to facilitating social change and delivering value to members through information and advocacy.
Deborah Moore, AARP Nevada Spokeswoman
Nancy Andersen, AARP Nevada State Volunteer Coordinator

New Hampshire

54 **AARP New Hampshire State Office-Manchester**
900 Elm Street
Manchester, NH 03101   866-542-8168
                                   Fax: 603-629-0066
                              e-mail: nh@aarp.org
                              www.aarp.org/states/nh
AARP is a nonprofit nonpartisan membership organization for people age 50 and over. AARP is dedicated to enhancing the quality of life as one ages, in addition to facilitating social change and delivering value to members through information and advocacy.
Kelly Clark, AARP New Hampshire State Director
Jamie Bulen, AARP New Hampshire State Media Relations

New Jersey

55 **AARP New Jersey State Office: Princeton**
101 Rockingham Row
Princeton, NJ 08540   866-542-8165
                                   Fax: 609-987-4634
                              e-mail: njaarp@aarp.org
                              www.aarp.org/states/nj
AARP is a nonprofit nonpartisan membership organization for people age 50 and over. AARP is dedicated to enhancing the quality of life as one ages, in addition to facilitating social change and delivering value to members through information and advocacy.
Sy Larson, AARP New Jersey State President
Jane Margesson, AARP New Jersey State Media Relations

New Mexico

56 **AARP New Mexico State Office: Sante Fe**
535 Cerrillos Road
Santa Fe, NM 87501   866-389-5636
                                   Fax: 505-820-2889
                              e-mail: nmaarp@aarp.org
                              www.aarp.org/states/nm
AARP is a nonprofit nonpartisan membership organization for people age 50 and over. AARP is dedicated to enhancing the quality of life as one ages, in addition to facilitating social change and delivering value to members through information and advocacy.
Louis Sarabia, AARP New Mexico State President
Stan Cooper, AARP New Mexico State Director

New York

57 **AARP New York State Office: Albany**
1 Commerce Plaza
Albany, NY 12260   866-227-7442
                                   Fax: 518-434-6949
                              e-mail: nyaarp@aarp.org
                              www.aarp.org
AARP is a nonprofit nonpartisan membership organization for people age 50 and over. AARP is dedicated to enhancing the quality of life as one ages, in addition to facilitating social change and delivering value to members through information and advocacy.
Marilyn Pinksy, State President

58 **AARP New York State Office: New York City**
780 3rd Avenue
New York, NY 10017   866-227-7442
                                   Fax: 212-644-6390
                              e-mail: nyaarp@aarp.org
                              www.aarp.org/states/ny
AARP is a nonprofit nonpartisan membership organization for people age 50 and over. AARP is dedicated to enhancing the quality of life as one ages, in addition to facilitating social change and delivering value to members through information and advocacy.
Lois Aronstein, AARP New York State Director
Madeleine Moore, AARP New York State President

North Carolina

59   **AARP North Carolina State Office: Raleigh**
1511 Sunday Drive
Raleigh, NC 27607   866-389-5650
                                          Fax: 919-755-9684
                                          TTY: 919-508-0290
                                          e-mail: ncaarp@aarp.org
                                          www.aarp.org/states/nc
AARP is a nonprofit nonpartisan membership organization for
people age 50 and over. AARP is dedicated to enhancing the quality of life as one ages, in addition to facilitating social change and
delivering value to members through information and advocacy.
Diana D Hatch, AARP North Carolina State President
Bob Garner, Communications Director

North Dakota

60   **AARP North Dakota State Office: Bismarck**
107 W Main Avenue
Bismarck, ND 58501   866-554-5383
                                          Fax: 701-255-2242
                                          e-mail: ndaarp@aarp.org
                                          www.aarp.org/states/nd
AARP is a nonprofit nonpartisan membership organization for
people age 50 and over. AARP is dedicated to enhancing the quality of life as one ages, in addition to facilitating social change and
delivering value to members through information and advocacy.
Betty Keegan, AARP North Dakota State President
Lyle Halvorson, AARP North Dakota State Media Relations

Ohio

61   **AARP Ohio State Office: Columbus**
17 S High Street
Columbus, OH 43215-3467   866-389-5653
                                          Fax: 614-224-9801
                                          e-mail: ohaarp@aarp.org
                                          www.aarp.org/states/oh
AARP is a nonprofit nonpartisan membership organization for
people age 50 and over. AARP is dedicated to enhancing the quality of life as one ages, in addition to facilitating social change and
delivering value to members through information and advocacy.
Kathy Keller, AARP Ohio State Media Relations
Joanne Limbach, AARP Ohio State President

Oklahoma

62   **AARP Oklahoma State Office: Edmond**
126 N Bryant Avenue
Edmond, OK 73034   866-295-7277
                                          Fax: 405-844-7772
                                          e-mail: ok@aarp.org
                                          www.aarp.org/states/ok
AARP is a nonprofit nonpartisan membership organization for
people age 50 and over. AARP is dedicated to enhancing the quality of life as one ages, in addition to facilitating social change and
delivering value to members through information and advocacy.
Robert Bristow, AARP Oklahoma State President
Marjorie Lyons, Executive Council Member

Oregon

63   **AARP Oregon State Office: Clackamas**
9200 SE Sunnybrook Boulevard
Clackamas, OR 97015-5762   866-554-5360
                                          Fax: 503-652-9933
                                          e-mail: oraarp@aarp.org
                                          www.aarp.org/states/or
AARP is a nonprofit nonpartisan membership organization for
people age 50 and over. AARP is dedicated to enhancing the quality of life as one ages, in addition to facilitating social change and
delivering value to members through information and advocacy.
Ray Miao, AARP Oregon State President
Don Bruland, Director

Pennsylvania

64   **AARP Pennsylvania State Office: Harrisburg**
30 N 3rd Street
Harrisburg, PA 17101   866-389-5654
                                          Fax: 717-236-4078
                                          e-mail: sgardner@aarp.org
                                          www.aarp.org/states/pa
AARP is a nonprofit nonpartisan membership organization for
people age 50 and over. AARP is dedicated to enhancing the quality of life as one ages, in addition to facilitating social change and
delivering value to members through information and advocacy.
J Shane Creamer, AARP Pennsylvania State President
Steve Gardner, AARP Pennsylvania State Media Relations

South Carolina

65   **AARP South Carolina Office: Columbia**
1201 Main Street
Columbia, SC 29201   866-389-5655
                                          Fax: 803-251-4374
                                          e-mail: scaarp@aarp.org
                                          www.aarp.org/states/sc
AARP is a nonprofit nonpartisan membership organization for
people age 50 and over. AARP is dedicated to enhancing the quality of life as one ages, in addition to facilitating social change and
delivering value to members through information and advocacy.
Charles A Johnson, AARP SC State President
Patrick Cobb, AARP SC State Media Relations

Tennessee

66   **AARP Tennessee State Office: Nashville**
150 4th Avenue N
Nashville, TN 37219   866-295-7274
                                          Fax: 615-313-8414
                                          e-mail: tnaarp@aarp.org
                                          www.aarp.org/states/tn
AARP is a nonprofit nonpartisan membership organization for
people age 50 and over. AARP is dedicated to enhancing the quality of life as one ages, in addition to facilitating social change and
delivering value to members through information and advocacy.
Margot Seay, AARP Tennessee State President
Rebecca Kelly, AARP Tennessee State Director

Texas

67   **AARP Texas State Office: Austin**
98 San Jacinto Boulevard
Austin, TX 78701   866-227-7443
                                          Fax: 512-480-9799
                                          e-mail: rayuso@aarp.org
                                          www.aarp.org/states/tx
AARP is a nonprofit nonpartisan membership organization for
people age 50 and over. AARP is dedicated to enhancing the quality of life as one ages, in addition to facilitating social change and
delivering value to members through information and advocacy.
Rafael Ayuso, AARP Texas State Media Relations
Bob Jackson, AARP Texas State Director

Utah

68   **AARP Utah State Office: Midvale**
6975 Union Park Center
Midvale, UT 84047   866-448-3616
                                          Fax: 801-561-2209
                                          e-mail: utaarp@aarp.org
                                          www.aarp.org/states/ut
AARP is a nonprofit nonpartisan membership organization for
people age 50 and over. AARP is dedicated to enhancing the quality of life as one ages, in addition to facilitating social change and
delivering value to members through information and advocacy.
Pat Gamble Hovey, Volunteer State President of AARP Utah
Ruby Hammel, Executive Council Advocacy Coordinator

Vermont

69   AARP Vermont State Office: Montpelier
199 Main Street
Burlington, VT 05401   866-227-7451
                                              Fax: 802-651-9805
                                        e-mail: vtaarp@aarp.org
                                        www.aarp.org/states/vt
AARP is a nonprofit nonpartisan membership organization for people age 50 and over. AARP is dedicated to enhancing the quality of life as one ages, in addition to facilitating social change and delivering value to members through information and advocacy.
Nancy C Lang, AARP Vermont State President
Dave Reville, AARP Vermont State Media Relations

Virginia

70   AARP Virginia State Office: Richmond
707 E Main Street
Richmond, VA 23219   866-542-8164
                                              Fax: 804-819-1923
                                        e-mail: vaaarp@aarp.org
                                        www.aarp.org/states/va
AARP is a nonprofit nonpartisan membership organization for people age 50 and over. AARP is dedicated to enhancing the quality of life as one ages, in addition to facilitating social change and delivering value to members through information and advocacy.
Bill Kallio, AARP Virginia State Director
Tony Hylton, AARP Virginia State Media Relations

Washington

71   AARP Washington State Office: Seattle
9750 3rd Avenue NE
Seattle, WA 98115   866-227-7457
                                              Fax: 206-517-9350
                                        e-mail: waaarp@aarp.org
                                        www.aarp.org/states/wa
AARP is a nonprofit nonpartisan membership organization for people age 50 and over. AARP is dedicated to enhancing the quality of life as one ages, in addition to facilitating social change and delivering value to members through information and advocacy.
John Barnett, AARP Washington State President
Doug Shadel, AARP Washington State Director

West Virginia

72   AARP West Virginia Office: Charleston
300 Summers Street
Charleston, WV 25301   866-227-7458
                                              Fax: 304-344-4633
                                        e-mail: wvaarp@aarp.org
                                        www.aarp.org/states/wv
AARP is a nonprofit nonpartisan membership organization for people age 50 and over. AARP is dedicated to enhancing the quality of life as one ages, in addition to facilitating social change and delivering value to members through information and advocacy.
Ruth Wagner, AARP West Virginia State President
Ginger Thomp McDaniel, AARP West Virginia State Media Relations

Wisconsin

73   AARP Wisconsin State Office: Madison
222 W Washington Avenue
Madison, WI 53703   866-448-3611
                                              Fax: 608-251-7612
                                        e-mail: wistate@aarp.org
                                        www.aarp.org/states/wi
AARP is a nonprofit nonpartisan membership organization for people age 50 and over. AARP is dedicated to enhancing the quality of life as one ages, in addition to facilitating social change and delivering value to members through information and advocacy.
Ethel Percy Andrus, Founder
Albert W Majkrzak, AARP Wisconsin State President

Wyoming

74   AARP Wyoming State Office: Cheyenne
2020 Carey Avenue
Cheyenne, WY 82009   866-663-3290
                                        e-mail: wy@aarp.org
                                        www.aarp.org/states/wy
AARP is a nonprofit nonpartisan membership organization for people age 50 and over. AARP is dedicated to enhancing the quality of life as one ages, in addition to facilitating social change and delivering value to members through information and advocacy.
Les Engelter, AARP Wyoming State President
Joanne Bowlby, AARP Wyoming State Media Relations

International

75   AARP Virgin Islands State Office: St Croix
4093 Diamond Ruby
Christiansted, VI 00820   866-389-5633
                                              Fax: 340-692-2544
                                        e-mail: viaarp@aarp.org
                                        www.aarp.org/states/vi/
AARP is a nonprofit, nonpartisan membership organization for people age 50 and over. AARP is dedicated to enhancing the quality of life as one ages in addition to facilitating social change and delivering value to members through information, advocacy and service.
Hugo Dennis, Jr., AARP Virgin Islands State President

Libraries & Resource Centers

76   Aging In America/Morningside House Nursing
1000 Pelham Pkwy South
Bronx, NY 10461   877-244-6469
                                        e-mail: admissiondept@aiamsh.org
                                        www.aginginamerica.org
Aging in America is a community-based, social service agency. Morningside House is a provider of specialized medical, nursing and rehabilitative services.
Dr William T Smith, President/CEO

Research Centers

77   Case Western Reserve University: Center on Aging and Health
10900 Euclid Avenue   216-368-4413
Cleveland, OH 44106   800-515-2774
                                              Fax: 216-368-3842
                                        e-mail: contact-cas@cwru.edu
                                        fpb.case.edu/Centers/UCAH
Research organization conducting supporting and facilitating research into the chronically ill aged person.
Diana L Morris, PhD, RN, FAAN, F, Executive Director
Evelyn Duffy, DNP, ANP/GNP-BC,, Associate Director

78   Center for the Study of Aging
706 Madison Avenue   518-465-6927
Albany, NY 12208-3604   Fax: 518-462-1339
                                        e-mail: iapaas@aol.com
                                        www.centerforthestudyofaging.org
Not-for-profit educational and research center for social and medical research on aging health exercise lifelong health and fitness and programs to improve the health and quality of life for older men and women.
Sara Harris, Executive Director
Debra Treadgold, President

79   Columbia University Center for Geriatrics Gerontology
College of Physicians and Surgeons
630 West 168th Street   212-305-3595
New York, NY 10032   Fax: 212-305-1343
                                        e-mail: psadmissions@columbia.edu
                                        www.cumc.columbia.edu/dept/ps
Clinical research in geriatric/gerontology and long-term care.
Lee Goldman MD, Dean

80 **Creighton University Center for Healthy Aging**
2500 California Plaza
Omaha, NE 68178
402-280-2700
Fax: 402-280-4623
e-mail: medadmissions@creighton.edu
medicine.creighton.edu/CAAD
Focuses on human development, aging and health care for the elderly.
Robert W. Dunlay, M.D., Dean
Michael D. White, M.D., Associate Dean for Medical Education

81 **Landon Center on Aging University of Kansas Medical Center**
University of Kansas Medical Center
3901 Rainbow Boulevard
Kansas City, KS 66160
913-588-5000
800-766-3777
Fax: 913-588-1201
e-mail: rnudo@kumc.edu
www2.kumc.edu/coa
Provides support for interdisciplinary research on the issue of age and aging.
Randolph J Nudo, Director
Linda Redford, Associate Director

82 **Purdue University: Center for Research on Aging**
1202 W. State Street
W Lafayette, IN 47907-2055
765-494-9692
Fax: 765-494-2180
e-mail: calc@purdue.edu
www.purdue.edu/aging
Social science research on aging health and health care delivery.
Kenneth F Ferraro, Director
David J Waters,, Assistant Director

83 **Roy M and Phyllis Gough Huffington Center on Aging**
Huffington Center on Aging
Baylor College of Medicine
Houston, TX 77030
713-798-5804
Fax: 713-798-6688
e-mail: Gretchen@bcm.tmc.edu
www.hcoa.org
Internal unit of Baylor College representing research into the biology of aging.
Robert E. Roush, Director
Nancy L Wilson, Assistant Director

84 **University of Pennsylvania Institute on Aging**
3615 Chestnut Street
Philadelphia, PA 19104-2676
215-898-3163
Fax: 215-573-5566
e-mail: aging@mail.med.upenn.edu
www.med.upenn.edu/aging
The mission of the IOA is to improve the health of the elderly by increasing the quality and quantity of clinical and basic research as well as educational programs focusing on normal aging and age-related diseases at the UPSM and across the entire Penn campus.
John Q Trojanowski, Acting Director
Steven E Arnold, Associate Director

Support Groups & Hotlines

85 **Aging Support Group**
Consultants for Aging Families
649 Remington Street
Fort Collins, CO 80524
970-498-0730
e-mail: nanceemc@aol.com
www.fortnet.org/CAF
A source of support, guidance, and accurate, thorough information to help manage the needs and preferences of your older family members.
Nancy McCambridge, Director

86 **Children of Aging Parents**
PO Box 167
Richboro, PA 18954
215-355-6611
800-227-7294
Fax: 215-355-6824
e-mail: info@caps4caregivers.org
www.caps4caregivers.org
A nonprofit, charitable organization that assists the nation's nearly 54 million caregivers of the elderly or chronically ill with reliable information, referrals and support, and to heighten public awareness.

87 **National Health Information Center**
PO Box 1133
Washington, DC 20013-1133
310-565-4167
800-336-4797
Fax: 301-984-4256
e-mail: info@nhic.org
www.health.gov/nhic
A health information referral service sponsored by the Office of Disease Prevention and Health Promotion. NHIC puts health professionals and consumers who have health questions in touch with those organizations that are best able to provide answers.

Books

88 **Activities for the Disabled, Elderly and Adults**
Haworth Press
10 Alice Street
Binghamton, NY 13904-1580
607-722-5857
800-429-6784
Fax: 607-722-0012
www.haworthpress.com
Learn how to effectively plan and deliver activities for a growing number of older people with developmental disabilities. It aims to stimulate interest and continued support for recreation program development and implementation among developmental disability and aging service systems.
136 pages Hardcover
ISBN: 1-560240-92-X

89 **Adult Children and Aging Parents**
American Counseling Association
5999 Stevenson Avenue
Alexandria, VA 22304-3302
703-823-9800
800-347-6647
Fax: 703-823-0252
www.counseling.org
Provides effective intervention strategies and suggestions for counselors who work with older persons, individually and with the family. Offers information on many vital topics such as Alzheimer's Disease, retirement, elder abuse and suicide.
216 pages
ISBN: 0-840354-48-7

90 **Aging and Family Therapy**
Haworth Press
10 Alice Street
Binghamton, NY 13904-1580
607-722-5857
800-429-6784
Fax: 607-722-0012
www.haworthpress.com
Here are creative strategies for use in therapy with older adults and their families. This book provides practitioners with information, insight, reference tools, and other sources that will contribute to more effective intervention with the elderly and their families.
244 pages Hardcover
ISBN: 0-866567-78-3

91 **Aging and Our Families**
Human Sciences Press
233 Spring Street
New York, NY 10013-1522
212-620-8000
800-221-9369
Handbook for family caregivers.
132 pages Paperback
ISBN: 0-898854-41-5

92 **Caregivers' Roller Coaster**
Loyola University Press
3441 N Ashland Avenue
Chicago, IL 60657-1355
773-281-1818
800-621-1008
www.loyolapress.com
A simply written self-help guide for caregivers of the frail elderly. Offers support for men and women, not trained professionals, who find themselves caring for aging family members in their own homes. Offers practical advice and information on Alzheimer's, Medicare, insurance and community services for the elderly.
150 pages
ISBN: 0-829407-45-6

93 **Caring for Those You Love: A Guide to Compassionate Care for the Aged**
Bethany Chaffin, author
Horizon Publishers & Distributors, Inc.

191 N 650 East
Bountiful, UT 84010-3628
801-295-9451
Fax: 801-298-1305
e-mail: hpservice09@hotmail.com
horizonpublishersbookstore.com
Includes helpful information on identifying the problems of the aged. It explains the best and most frequently used treatments prescribed for these problems, and tells how family members can help to meet the physical, emotional, and spiritual needs of aging parents and other loved ones.
108 pages
ISBN: 0-882902-70-9
Duane S Crowther, Owner/CEO
Jean D Crowther, Owner/CEO

94   Continuing Care Retirement Community Directory
American Assoc. of Homes & Services for the Aging
901 E Street NW
Washington, DC 20004-2037
800-508-9442
Fax: 301-206-9789
A national consumer's directory of continuing care retirement communities. This directory is a vital tool for individuals searching and evaluating a community for themselves or a loved one.

95   Court-Related Needs of the Elderly and Persons with Disabilities
Commission on the Mentally Disabled
1800 M Street NW
Washington, DC 20036-5802
202-331-2240
www.statejustice.org/
Report of the National Conference, examines the barriers of the judicial system impeding access for the elderly and persons with disabilities.

96   Creative Movements for Older Adults
Human Sciences Press
233 Spring Street
New York, NY 10013-1522
212-620-8000
800-221-9369
Exercises for the elderly.
172 pages Cloth
ISBN: 0-898854-14-8

97   Diagnosis and Treatment of Old Age
S Karger Publishers
26 W Avon Road
Farmington, CT 06085-1162
860-675-7834
800-828-5479
Fax: 860-675-7302
www.karger.ch/company/karger.htm#10
These papers furnish a concise update on the diagnosis and treatment of Alzheimer's disease.
112 pages Hardcover
ISBN: 3-805548-44-3

98   Elder Care
Center For Public Representation
PO Box 260049
Madison, WI 53726-0049
608-251-4008
800-369-0388
Fax: 608-251-1263
www.law.wisc.edu/pal
A compendium of alternatives for providing and financing long-term care. This practical guide provides the most comprehensive and comforting information to help navigate a number of consumer minefields.
224 pages
ISBN: 0-873371-13-5

99   Elderly in Modern Society
Vance Bibliographier
PO Box 229
Monticello, IL 61856-0229
217-762-3831
A bibliography of laws and human rights for the elderly.
15 pages
ISBN: 0-792001-10-9

100   Falling in Old Age
Reing Tideiksaar PhD, author
Springer Publishing Company
11 W 42nd Street
New York, NY 10036
212-431-4370
877-687-7476
Fax: 212-941-7842
e-mail: cs@springerpub.com
www.springerpub.com

This book provides an enormous body of fall-related research that has been organized by the author into easy, digestible information for geriatric health professionals. Extensively updated and revised for its second edition, the book has direct clinical applications and strategies for preventing and managing falls. It also contains new information on the physical, psychological, and social complications of falling.
412 pages Hardcover
ISBN: 0-826152-91-6

101   Family Carebook
CAREsource Program Development
505 Seattle Tower
Seattle, WA 98101-3021
206-625-9080
Guide to aging, the special needs of older adults, and the demands of providing care and support. Experts explain potential conflicts, planning opportunities and strategies for success.
475 pages Paperback
ISBN: 1-878866-12-5

102   From Theory to Therapy: The Development of Drugs for Alzheimer's Disease
Alzheimer's Association
225 N Michigan Avenue
Chicago, IL 60611-1696
800-272-3900
Fax: 866-699-1246
TDD: 312-335-8700
e-mail: media@alz.org
www.alz.org
Provides a layman's explanation of how experimental drugs are being developed and tested for Alzheimer's disease, and information about patient participation in clinical drug trials.

103   Geriatric Rehabilitation Preview
RTC on Aging
7601 E Imperial Highway
Downey, CA 90242-4155
310-940-7402
www.usc.edu/dept/gero/RRTConAging
Covers research, training activities, and other issues pertaining to the rehabilitation of elderly persons with disabilities.

104   Health Care of the Aged
Abraham Monk, PhD, author
Haworth Press
10 Alice Street
Binghamton, NY 13904-1580
607-722-5857
800-429-6784
Fax: 607-722-0012
www.haworthpress.com
Focusing on the need for developing new service delivery models for the aged, this book examines fiscal, political, and social criteria influencing this challenge of the 1990s. The aged are caught in the sweeping changes currently occurring in the financing, organizing and delivery of human health care services.
183 pages Hardcover
ISBN: 1-560240-65-5

105   Healthy Aging: Good Investment & Together We Care: Helping Caregivers Find Supp.
National Council on Aging
1901 L Street NW
Washington, DC 20036
202-479-1200
Fax: 202-479-0735
TDD: 202-479-6674
e-mail: info@ncoa.org
www.ncoa.org
Describes seven model programs that could be used in community-based organizations serving older adults.
2 Book Set
James P Firman, EdD, President/CEO

106   International Health Guide for Senior Citizen Travelers
Pilot Books
103 Cooper Street
Babylon, NY 11702-2368
516-422-2225
Fax: 516-669-4173
Covers essential pre-departure health planning such as advice on specific health concerns, disease prevention, specific travel problems, medical preparedness and assistance.
70 pages Paperback
ISBN: 0-875761-39-9
Anne Small, President

107 Living Well in a Nursing Home
Lynn Dickinson, Xenia Vosen, author
Hunter House Publishing
1515 1/2 Park Street   510-865-5282
Alameda, CA 94501   800-266-5592
                                              Fax: 510-865-4295
                              e-mail: ordering@hunterhouse.com
                                          www.hunterhouse.com
This book concentrates on the positive aspects of nursing homes,
providing tips, support and reassurance.
256 pages Paperback
ISBN: 0-897934-60-2

108 Mentally Impaired Elderly
Ellen D Taira, author
Haworth Press
10 Alice Street   607-722-5857
Binghamton, NY 13904-1580   800-429-6784
                                              Fax: 607-722-0012
                                          www.haworthpress.com
Provides effective support and sensitive care for the most vulnera-
ble segment of the elderly population, those with mental
impairment.
191 171 pages
ISBN: 1-560241-68-1

109 Mirrored Lives
Greenwood Publishing Group, Inc/Praeger Publishers
PO Box 6926
Portsmouth, NH 03802-6926   800-225-5800
                                              Fax: 877-231-6980
                               e-mail: service@greenwood.com
                                          www.greenwood.com
Discusses geriatric decline connected to nonterminal illness in old
age. Koch takes a sensitive but thorough look at the declining years
of his father.
240 pages
ISBN: 0-275936-71-6

110 Nursing Home Information Services
925 15th Street NW   202-347-8800
Washington, DC 20005-2301
Lists acceptable nursing homes across the nation and provides information about their costs, admission requirements, standards
and programs.

111 Nursing Home and You: Partners in Caring
American Assn. of Homes & Services for the Aging
901 E Street NW
Washington, DC 20004-2037   800-508-9442
                                              Fax: 301-206-9789
Offers information to nursing home staff and family members
about caring for persons with Alzheimer's Disease.

112 Older Americans Information Directory
Grey House Publishing
4919 Route 22   518-789-8700
Amenia, NY 12501   800-562-2139
                                              Fax: 518-789-0545
                                 e-mail: books@greyhouse.com
                                          www.greyhouse.com
An invaluable resource that offers up-to-date information on the
prevalent social, health and financial issues facing older Americans in the 21st century, as well as recreational and educational opportunities to enrich their lives.
1200 pages
ISBN: 1-592375-43-X
Leslie Mackenzie, Publisher

113 On Your Behalf
CAREsource Program Development
505 Seattle Tower   206-625-9080
Seattle, WA 98101
This book takes the mystery out of very important sets of legal options. It gives lay people as well as advisors, service providers, and
caregivers the information they need to understand their options
and the importance of individual choice.
16 pages Books & Video
ISBN: 1-878866-14-1

114 Physical Activity and the Aging
Human Kinetic Publishers
PO Box 5076
Champaign, IL 61825-5076   800-747-4457
                                              Fax: 217-351-1549
                                          www.humankinetics.com
North America's leading scholars examine the effects of aging on
motor function, cardiovascular function, balance, the nervous sys-
tem, changes in activity level, and possible reasons for activity
level changes.
208 pages
ISBN: 0-873222-20-2

115 Planning for Long-Term Care
National Council on Aging
1901 L Street NW   202-479-1200
Washington, DC 20036   Fax: 202-479-0735
                                             TDD: 202-479-6674
                                        e-mail: info@ncoa.org
                                                  www.ncoa.org
Identify the various long-term care resources within your family
and in your community using this thorough and readable guide.
160 pages
James P Firman, EdD, President/CEO

116 Read Easy
CAREsource Program Development
505 Seattle Tower   206-625-9080
Seattle, WA 98101
If books, audio tapes and computers can spark the imagination of
the young adult and the middle aged, why not seniors as well? All it
takes is commitment to make quality library resources and programs accessible and user-friendly to older readers. Read Easy is
an invaluable planning and operations guide, explaining senior
needs to library professionals and librarianship principles to
senior care professionals.
95 pages
ISBN: 1-878866-13-3

117 Resources for Elders with Disabilities
Resources for Rehabilitation
22 Bonad Road   781-368-9080
Winchester, MA 01890   Fax: 781-368-9096
                                        e-mail: orders@rfr.org
                                                   www.rfr.org
Provides information that enables elders, family members and
other caregivers, and service providers to locate appropriate services. Includes information about rehabilitation, laws that affect
elders with disabilities, and self-help groups. Published in large
print.

ISBN: 0-929718-31-3

118 Senior Center Self: Assessment & National Accreditation Manual
National Council on Aging
1901 L Street NW   202-479-1200
Washington, DC 20036   Fax: 202-479-0735
                                              TDD: 2024796674
                                        e-mail: info@ncoa.org
                                                  www.ncoa.org
Based upon compliance with standards (best practices) developed
by the National Institutes of Senior Centers. This program was de-
veloped under the auspices of NCOA's National Institute of Senior
Centers (NISC).
Book & CD Set
James P Firman, EdD, President/CEO

119 Senior Citizens and the Law
Center for Public Representation
PO Box 260049   608-251-4008
Madison, WI 53726-0049   800-369-0388
                                              Fax: 608-251-1263
An introduction to legal problems facing the elderly in Wisconsin.
This edition discusses legal problems associated with Social Secu-
rity, Medicare, SSI, guardianship and its alternatives, commu-
nity-based services, probate, taxes, private health insurance and
consumer protection.
176 pages
ISBN: 0-932622-29-1

120 Successful Models of Community Long Term Care Services for the Elderly
Haworth Press
10 Alice Street   607-722-5857
Binghamton, NY 13904-1580   800-429-6784
Fax: 607-722-0012
www.haworthpress.com
Experienced practitioners provide examples of successful community-based long term care service programs for the elderly.
174 pages
ISBN: 0-866569-87-9

121 Unloving Care
Harper Collins Publishers/Basic Books
10 E 53rd Street   212-207-7000
New York, NY 10022-5299   800-242-7737
Fax: 212-207-7203
www.harpercollins.com
A leading public health expert gives his account of the negative aspects of nursing homes.
305 pages
ISBN: 0-465088-81-3

Magazines

122 AARP Magazine
American Association of Retired Persons
601 East Street NW   202-434-3525
Washington, DC 20049   888-687-2277
e-mail: member@aarp.org
www.aarp.org
Celebrity interviews. Features on health and finance. Movie reviews and more. All with an eye toward the topics and issues you care about most.
A Barry Rand, CEO

123 Abstracts in Social Gerontology
National Council on Aging
1901 L Street NW   202-479-1200
Washington, DC 20036   Fax: 202-479-0735
TDD: 202-479-6674
e-mail: info@ncoa.org
www.ncoa.org
Detailed abstracts are provided for recent major journal articles, books, reports and other materials on many facets of aging, including adult education, demography, family relations, institutional care and work attitudes.
Quarterly
James P Firman, EdD, President/CEO

124 Innovations
National Council on Aging
1901 L Street NW   202-479-1200
Washington, DC 20036   Fax: 202-479-0735
TDD: 2024796674
e-mail: info@ncoa.org
www.ncoa.org
Explores significant developments in the field of aging through opinion articles, profiles and research summaries. Features articles on social trends, articles on specific aging programs and information on NCOA's activities. Members are free.
Quarterly
James P Firman, EdD, President/CEO

125 International Journal of Technology and Aging
Human Sciences Press
233 Spring Street   212-620-8000
New York, NY 10013-1522   800-221-9369
Fax: 212-463-0742
Designed to serve health-care professionals, researchers, academicians and industries concerned with the convergence of two recent trends, the dramatic advances in technology and the rapidly growing elderly population.

126 Modern Maturity
AARP

601 E Street NW
Washington, DC 20049-0003   800-424-3410
e-mail: member@aarp.org
www.aarp.org
Offers news and information of concern to those 50 and older. Features articles on current events, health, recreation, housing, family life, legislation and other issues.
6x Year

Newsletters

127 AARP Bulletin
American Association of Retired Persons
601 East Street NW
Washington, DC 20049   888-687-2277
www.aarp.org
Get daily news about the issues that matter to you.
Bill Novelli, AARP CEO

128 Best Practices
American Assoc. of Homes & Services for the Aging
2519 Connecticut Avenue NW   202-783-2242
Washington, DC 20008-1520   Fax: 202-783-2255
e-mail: info@aahsa.org
www.aahsa.org
Keeps nonprofit aging service providers informed of new trends and developments in quality of care for older persons.

129 Bulletin
AARP
601 E Street NW
Washington, DC 20049   800-424-3410
e-mail: member@aarp.org
www.aarp.org
11x Year

130 CAPSule
Children of Aging Parents
PO Box 167   215-355-6611
Richboro, PA 18954-0167   800-227-7294
Fax: 215-355-6824
e-mail: info@caps4caregivers.org
www.caps4caregivers.org
Newsletter devoted to assisting caregivers of the elderly.
12 pages Quarterly
Lenore Sherman, Executive Director
Karen Rosenberg, Director Senior Services

131 Capital Advantage
Capital Advantage Publishing
2731-A Prosperity Avenue   703-289-4670
Fairfax, VA 22031   Fax: 703-289-4678
e-mail: sales@capitaladvantage.com
www.capitaladvantage.com
Publishes articles on all aspects of aging including legislation, innovative programs and services.
Monthly

132 Center for the Study of Aging Newsletter
University of Pennsylvania Center for Aging Study
3615 Chestnut Street   215-898-3163
Philadelphia, PA 19104-4205   Fax: 215-573-8684
e-mail: www.med.upenn.edu/aging
ageweb@mail.med.upenn.edu
News and information concerning the University and Center aging activities, programs and seminars.

133 Elderly Health Services Letter
American Business Publishing
3100 Highway 138   732-681-1133
Wall Township, NJ 0771
Information on trends and developments in the expanding field of health services for the elderly.
Monthly
Robert Jenkins, Publisher

134 Geriatric Care News
DRS Geriatric Publishing Company

7435 SE 71st Street   206-232-9689
Mercer Island, WA 98040-5314
Newsletter for the elderly and their families.
Monthly
Denise Schramke, Publisher

135 Geriatrics
7500 Old Oak Boulevard   440-243-8100
Cleveland, OH 44130-3343
Articles for physicians and laypersons relating to care of middle-aged and elderly persons.
Monthly

136 Gerontology News
Gerontological Society of America
1030 15th Street NW   202-842-1275
Washington, DC 20005   Fax: 202-842-1150
                                          e-mail: geron@geron.org
                                                  www.geron.org
It reports on policy issues, legislative actions, Society events, research results, and recently released major reports on aging. Regular features include Washington Updates; Research Highlights; Grants Available; New Resources and Reports; Data Updates; and Calls for Papers, Nominations, and Manuscripts.
Carol Ann Schutz, Executive Director

137 Health After 50: Johns Hopkins Medical Letter
Johns Hopkins Medical Institutions
550 Broadway   410-955-3182
Baltimore, MD 21205-2011   800-829-9170
                                          e-mail: www.medjhu.edu
Health newsletter for people over 50.
10 pages Monthly
ISBN: 1-042188-2 -
Rodney Friedman, Publisher

138 Lifelong Health and Fitness
Center for the Study of Aging
706 Madison Avenue   518-465-4927
Albany, NY 12208-3604   Fax: 518-462-1339
                                          e-mail: iapaas@aol.com
                              www.centerforthestudyofaging-albany.org
A quarterly newsletter published by the Center for the Study of Aging.
8 pages Quarterly
Sara Harris, Executive Director

139 NCOA Week
National Council on Aging
1901 L Street NW   202-479-1200
Washington, DC 20036   Fax: 202-479-0735
                                              TDD: 202-479-6674
                                            e-mail: info@ncoa.org
                                                   www.ncoa.org
Breaking news of NCOA initiatives, crucial legislative and policy issues, research studies, developments in work and volunteering for older adults, benefits for seniors, trends in aging, grant opportunities, and more. Members only.
Weekly
James P Firman, EdD, President/CEO

140 Senior Focus
National Council on Aging
1901 L Street NW   202-479-1200
Washington, DC 20036   Fax: 202-479-0735
                                              TDD: 202-479-6674
                                            e-mail: info@ncoa.org
                                                   www.ncoa.org
Timely, objective, and practical information on health and wellness, lifestyle, and financial issues for seniors and people who work with them.
Bi-Monthly
James P Firman, EdD, President/CEO

141 Vital Aging Report
National Council on Aging

1901 L Street NW   202-479-1200
Baltimore, MD   Fax: 202-479-0735
                                              TDD: 202-479-6674
                                            e-mail: info@ncoa.org
                                                   www.ncoa.org
Packed with news about health and financial matters as well as United Senior's Health Council's innovative programs and research. The USHC is a program of the National Council on the Aging. Member price $17.50.
Quarterly
James P Firman, EdD, President/CEO

Pamphlets

142 American Perceptions of Aging in the 21st Century
National Council on Aging
1901 L Street NW   202-479-1200
Washington, DC 20036   Fax: 202-479-0735
                                              TDD: 2024796674
                                            e-mail: info@ncoa.org
                                                   www.ncoa.org
There are many interesting and important findings related to aging in America as reported by over 3000 respondents. This chartbook is intended as a handy reference for scholars, the press and advocates.
James P Firman, EdD, President/CEO

143 Care of the Elderly in America
Vance Bibliographies
PO Box 229   217-762-3831
Monticello, IL 61856-0229
A bibliography of aged care in America.
11 pages
ISBN: 1-555905-59-5

144 Exploring Care Options for a Relative with Alzheimer's Disease
American Assoc. of Homes & Services for the Aging
2519 Connecticut Avenue NW   202-783-2242
Washington, DC 20008-1520   800-508-9442
                                              Fax: 202-783-2255
                                          e-mail: www.aahsa.org
                                                 pub@aahsa.org

145 Medicare Health Plan Choices: Consumer Update
National Council on Aging
1901 L Street NW   202-479-1200
Washington, DC 20036   Fax: 202-479-0735
                                              TDD: 202-479-6744
                                            e-mail: info@ncoa.org
                                                   www.ncoa.org
Annually updated report contains important information about options that are available to Medicare beneficiaries. Medicare is changing, Medigap premiums are going up, and many Medicare HMOs are dropping service to seniors. Pamphlets available in single copies or packs of 50.
James P Firman, EdD, President/CEO

146 Nonprofit Housing and Care Options for Older People
American Assoc. of Homes & Services for the Aging
901 E Street NW
Washington, DC 20004-2037   800-508-9442
                                              Fax: 301-206-9789
Offers information on continuing care facilities, retirement communities and more for the elderly and relatives caring for Alzheimer's patients.

147 Time Out!
Alzheimer's Association
225 N Michigan Avenue
Chicago, IL 60611-1696   800-272-3900
                                              Fax: 866-669-1246
                                              TDD: 312-335-8700
                                            e-mail: media@alz.org
                                                    www.alz.org
Details the Association's position supporting a national respite care policy and recommends actions for federal and state policy makers.
1991 14 pages

Audio & Video

148 Aphasia: Struggling for Understanding
Filmakers Library
124 E 40th Street   212-808-4980
New York, NY 10016-1798   Fax: 212-808-4983
e-mail: info@filmakers.com
www.filmakers.com

What if your ability to speak or understand speech was taken away without warning, and you struggled to find words that just won't come? This film is about two people faced with the daunting task of learning to speak again, of regaining their humanity. DVD or VHS, Classroom Rental VHS also available for $65. 14 minutes in length.
DVD or VHS
Sue Oscar, Co-President

Web Sites

149 Alliance for Aging Research
www.agingresearch.org
Improving the health and independence of Americans as they age. Promotes medical and behavioral research into the aging process.

150 American Association of Retired Persons
www.aarp.org
AARP is the nation's leading organization for people age 50 and older. Information and education, advocacy, and community services provided by a network of local chapters and experienced volunteers throughout the country.

151 American Society on Aging
www.asaging.org
An association of diverse individuals bound together by a common goal: to support the commitment and enhance the knowledge and skills of those who seek to improve the quality of life of older adults and their families.

152 Gerontological Society of America
www.geron.org
Nonprofit professional organization with more than 5000 members in the field of aging. Provides researchers, educators, practitioners and policy makers with opportunities to understand, advance, integrate and use basic and applied research on aging to improve the quality of life as one ages.

153 Healing Well
www.healingwell.com
An online health resource guide to medical news, chat, information and articles, newsgroups and message boards, books, disease-related web sites, medical directories, and more for patients, friends, and family coping with disabling diseases, disorders, or chronic illnesses.

154 Health Finder
www.healthfinder.gov
Searchable, carefully developed web site offering information on over 1000 topics. Developed by the US Department of Health and Human Services, the site can be used in both English and Spanish.

155 Healthlink USA
www.healthlinkusa.com
Health information concerning treatment, cures, prevention, diagnosis, risk factors, research, support groups, email lists, personal stories and much more. Updated regularly.

156 Helios Health
www.helioshealth.com
Online resource for your health information. Detailed information about specific health topics, access to expert advice from our Medical Advisory Board, and up-to-date health news.

157 MedicineNet
www.medicinenet.com
An online resource for consumers providing easy-to-read, authoritative medical and health information.

158 Medscape
www.medscape.com

Medscape offers specialists, primary care physicians, and other health professionals the Web's most robust and integrated medical information and educational tools.

159 National Council on Aging
www.ncoa.org
Seniors Corner includes many resources and health related information on older Americans and their caregivers.

160 National Institute of Aging
www.nia.nih.gov
Conducts research on aging, behavioral and social research, neuroscience and neuropsychology, geriatrics, and clinical gerontology.

161 Research Center
www.resarch.aarp.org
Online center offering information on consumer issues, demographics, independent living and other items of interest to senior citizens.

162 US Administration on Aging
www.aoa.gov
An agency in the US Department of Health and Human Services, is one of the nation's largest providers of home and community-based care for older persons and their caregivers.

163 WebMD
www.webmd.com
WebMD provides valuable health information, tools for managing your health, and support to those who seek information.

Description

164 AIDS/HIV

AIDS, Acquired Immune Deficiency Syndrome, is an infectious disorder that suppresses the normal function of the human body's immune system. AIDS is a result of HIV (Human Immunodeficiency Virus) infection, which destroys the body's ability to fight infections. Specifically, the virus infects and later destroys T-cells, which are a part of the body's immune system that responds to invading organisms. This destructive process is slow and silent, which means that HIV can be contracted years before any symptoms appear. When enough T-cells have been destroyed, the body is invaded by organisms that wouldn't ordinarily be able to cause serious disease. An early symptom of HIV infection is usually an increasing number of infections. Weight loss, fever and night sweats are common. Certain cancers, especially lymphoma and Kaposi's sarcoma, also take advantage of the body's lowered resistance.

HIV transmission requires contact with body fluids and is usually spread from an infected person to a noninfected person by unprotected sexual intercourse, or by sharing needles. Mothers can give HIV infection to their children before and during childbirth and while breastfeeding.

Prevention of HIV infection is the best way to stop the AIDS epidemic. Unfortunately, progress on a vaccine has been disappointing, so avoiding contact with the virus is the primary method of prevention. Avoiding the riskier types of sexual intercourse will reduce one's risk, as will the use of a condom duringvaginal and anal sex. Injecting drug users should not share needles. The use of needle exchange programs has decreased the spread of HIV infection. Women with HIV are encouraged to avoid pregnancy. If pregnant, HIV positive women should stay on medicine directed against HIV and should not breastfeed. Today, infants born to HIV women are treated with medication immediately after birth and this has greatly reduced the incidence of vertical transmission of the infection from mother to child. Until anti-HIV drugs became available, infected persons usually had a rapid downhill course. Today, combination drug treatment can offer most infected persons a long period of relatively good health. However, the treatment regimen is often complex and expensive, involving three or four drugs which must be taken several times a day. Since skipping doses encourages growth of virus that is resistant to the drugs, it is very important to take the drugs exactly as directed.

National Agencies & Associations

165 AIDS Coalition of Cape Breton
150 Bentinck Street
Sydney, Nova Scotia, B1P-6H1
902-567-1766
Fax: 902-567-1766
e-mail: christineporter@accb.ns.ca
www.aidscoalitionofcapebreton.ca/index.h

Provides support and advocacy services for PLW HIV/AIDS (people living with HIV/AIDS). Services provided deal with social, legal, ethical and spiritual issues.
Christine Porter, Executive Director
Jo-Anne Rolls, PHA Program Coordinator

166 AIDS Committee of Durham
22 King Street West
Oshawa, Ontario, L1H-1A3
905-576-1445
877-361-8750
Fax: 905-576-4610
e-mail: info@aidsdurham.com
www.aidsdurham.com
To provide HIV/AIDS related services to the infected or affected and the general community in the region of Durham.
Doug Willoughby, President
Todd Shearing, Vice President

167 AIDS Committee of London
#30-186 King Street
London, Ontario, N6A-3C1
519-434-1601
866-920-1601
Fax: 519-434-1843
e-mail: info@hivaidsconnection.ca
www.aidslondon.com
Is a community-based, charitable organization providing HIV-related services to people living with and concerned about HIV/AIDS in London and area.
Brian Lester, Executive Director
Elizabeth Lam, Office Manager

168 AIDS Committee of Ottawa
251 Bank Street
Ottawa, Ontario, K2P-1X3
613-238-5014
Fax: 613-238-3425
e-mail: info@aco-cso.ca
www.aco-cso.ca
Works to empower people living with HIV/AIDS and the PLWHA (persons living with HIV/AID) community in Ottawa through promoting the well being and quality of life of those living with, or close affected by HIV/AIDS.
Kathleen Cummings, Executive Director
Elysia Sugden, Office Administrator

169 AIDS Committee of Toronto
399 Church Street
Toronto, Ontario, M5B-2J6
416-340-2437
Fax: 416-340-8224
www.actoronto.org
Delivers responsive, effective, and valued community-based HIV support services and education, prevention, outreach and fundraising programs that promote health, well-being, worth and rights of individuals and communities living with, affected by and at risk for HIV/AIDS, and increase awareness of HIV/AIDS.
Richard Willett, Co Chair
Hazelle Palmer, Executive Director

170 AIDS Committee of York Region
194 Eagle Street E
Newmarket, Ontario, L3Y-1J6
905-953-0248
800-243-7717
Fax: 905-953-1372
e-mail: edacyr@bellnet.ca
www.acyr.org
The AIDS Committee of York Region envisions an informed and compassionate society, which is supportive of people living with HIV/AIDS who are striving to overcome social and service challenges, working with them towards a healthy and empowered lifestyle.
Radha Bhardwaj, Acting Executive Director
Vibhuti Mehra, Executive Assistant/ Office Manager

171 AIDS Network
600 Williamson Street
Madison, WI 53703
608-252-6540
800-486-6276
Fax: 608-252-6559
TTY: 608-441-3542
e-mail: info@aidsnetwork.org
www.aidsnetwork.org
Provides critical AIDS care and prevention services. Sustained in these efforts by the resources expertise and passion of hundreds of volunteers and donors.
Mary Vasquez, President
Lana Chute, Vice President

172 AIDS New Brunswick
65 Brunswick Street
Fredericton, NB, E3B-1G5

506-459-7518
800-561-4009
Fax: 888-501-6301
e-mail: info@aidsnb.com
www.aidsnb.com

A provincial organization committed to facilitating community-based responses to the issues of HIV/AIDS. The aim is to promote and support the health and well-being of persons living with and affected by HIV/AIDS and to reduce the spread of HIV/AIDS in New Brunswick.
Stephen Alexander, Executive Director
Keri Ann Scott, Operation Coordinator

173 AIDS Niagara
Normandy Resource Center
St. Catharines, Ontario, L2R-3C9

905-984-8684
800-773-9843
Fax: 905-988-1921
e-mail: info@aidsniagara.com
www.aidsniagara.com

AIDS Niagara is dedicated to improving the quality of life for those infected and/or affected by HIV/AIDS.
Ash Shihora, Director
Francis Gregotski, Vice Chair

174 AIDS PEI
375 University Avenue
Charlottetown, PE, C1A-4N4

902-566-2437
Fax: 902-626-3400
e-mail: info@aidspei.com
www.aidspei.com

To create a supportive environment for Persons Living with AIDS/HIV, to increase public understanding of the impact of HIV/AIDS, and to reduce the incidence of HIV/AIDS in Prince Edward Island.
Leslie Labobe, Director
Mike Chipman, Chairperson

175 AIDS Thunder Bay
574 Memorial Avenue
Thunder Bay, Ontario, P7B 3-3Z2

807-345-1516
800-488-5840
Fax: 807-345-2505
e-mail: info@aidsthunderbay.org
www.aidsthunderbay.org

Provide quality, compassionate support, education and advocacy around HIV and AIDS, and related issues.
Dennis Eeles, President
Brent Trudel, Vice President

176 AIDS Treatment Data Network
57 Willoughby St.
Brooklyn, New York, NY 11201

347- 47- 740
TTY: 212-925-9560
e-mail: info@housingworks.org
www.housingworks.org

The Network is a national independent community-based not-for-profit organization that provides treatment access and advocacy, case management, supportive counseling and English and Spanish language information services to men women and children with HIV.
Natacha Baron, Associate Medical Director
Dr. Priya Parasher, Dental Director

177 AIDS United
1424 K Street, NW
Washington, DC 20005

202-408-4848
Fax: 202-408-1818
www.aidsunited.org

National organization dedicated to the development analysis cultivation and encouragement of sound policies and programs in response to the HIV epidemic. We do this through the dissemination of information and the building and use of advocacy.
Vignetta Charles, Ph.D., Senior Vice President
Michael Kaplan, President, CEO

178 AIDS.ORG
P.O. Box 69491
Los Angeles, CA 90069

323-656-6036
www.aids.org

The mission of AIDS.ORG is to help prevent HIV infections and to improve the lives of those affected by HIV and AIDS by providing education and facilitating the free and open exchange of knowledge at any easy-to-find centralized Web site.
Peter Dobson, Director
Alain Berrebi, Executive Director

179 AIDSinfo
PO Box 4780
Rockville, MD 20849-6303

1 3-1 3-5 28
800-448-0440
Fax: 301-315-2818
TTY: 888-480-3739
e-mail: contactus@aidsinfo.nih.gov
www.aidsinfo.nih.gov

AIDSinfo is a U.S. Department of Health and Human Services (DHHS) project that offers the latest federally approved information on HIV/AIDS clinical research, treatment and prevention, and medical practice guidelines for people living with HIV/AIDS, their families and friends, health care providers, scientists, and researchers.

180 ANKORS: Kootenay & Boundary HIV/AIDS and Hepatitis C Support Services
101 Baker Street
Nelson, BC, V1L-4H1

250-505-5506
800-421-2437
Fax: 250-505-5507
e-mail: information@ankors.bc.ca
www.ankors.bc.ca

ANKORS' mission is to respond to the evolving needs of those living with and affected by HIV/AIDS and Hepatitis C.
Cheryl Dowden, Executive Director
Gary Dalton, Community Care Team

181 Access AIDS Network
111 Elm Street
Sudbury, Ontario, P3C-1T3

705-688-0500
800-465-2437
Fax: 705-688-0423
e-mail: aaninfo@reseauaccessnetwork.com
www.accessaidsnetwork.com

A non-profit, community-based charitable organization, committed to promoting wellness, education, harm and risk reduction.
Richard Rainville, Executive Director
Christine Coutu, Clerical Intake Worker

182 Alberta Reappraising AIDS Society
Box 61037
Calgary, Alberta, T2N-4S6

403-289-6609
Fax: 403-206-7717
e-mail: aras@aras.ab.ca
www.aras.ab.ca

Promote critical discussion of the HIV/AIDS dogma.
David Crowe, President
Roger Swan, Treasurer

183 American Autoimmune Related Diseases Association
22100 Gratiot Avenue
Eastpointe, MI 48021

586-776-3900
800-598-4668
Fax: 586-776-3903
e-mail: aarda@aarda.org
www.aarda.org

Awareness, education, referrals for patients with any type of autoimmune disease.
Virginia T. Ladd, President/Executive Director
Stanley M. Finger, Chairman

184 American Civil Liberties Union AIDS Project
125 Broad Street
New York, NY 10004

212-549-2500
e-mail: media@aclu.org
www.aclu.org/HIVAIDS/HIVAIDSMain.cfm

Offers legislative and employment information public awareness materials and support for persons with HIV/AIDS and their families.
Susan Herman, President
Anthony D. Romero, Executive Director

185 American Federation of Teachers HIV/AIDS Education Project
555 New Jersey Avenue NW
Washington, DC 20001-2029

202-879-4400
www.aft.org

A group of education professionals with the main purpose of their work being the education and public awareness of HIV and AIDS.
Randi Weingarten, President
Lorretta Johnson, Secretary-treasurer

186 American Foundation for AIDS Research
120 Wall Street
New York, NY 10005-3908

212-806-1600
800-342-2437
Fax: 212-806-1601
TTY: 800-243-7889
e-mail: kevin.frost@amfar.org
www.amfar.org

Supports research in basic clinical prevention and public policy and publishes the HIV/AIDS Treatment Directory.
Kenneth Cole, Chairman
Patricia J. Matson, Vice Chairman

187 Asian & Pacific Islander Wellness Center Community HIV/AIDS Services
730 Polk Street
San Francisco, CA 94109

415-292-3400
Fax: 415-292-3404
TTY: 415-292-3410
e-mail: info@apiwellness.org
www.apiwellness.org

HIV Care Services is the only integrated HIV services program targeting A&PIs in Northern California. Integrates primary care with psychiatric mental health HIV treatment psychosocial support and, in response to evolving needs, targeted HIV prevention.
Lin Lin, President
Bart Akoki, Vice President

188 Asian and Pacific Island Wellness Center
730 Polk Street
San Francisco, CA 94109

415-292-3400
Fax: 415-292-3404
TTY: 415-292-3410
e-mail: info@apiwellness.org
www.apiwellness.org

Our mission is to educate support empower and advocate for Asian and Pacific Islander communities - particularly A&PIs living with or at-risk for HIV/AIDS.
Lin Lin, President
Bart Akoki, Vice President

189 Better Existence with HIV
1244 W. Thorndale
Chicago, IL 60660

773-293-4740
Fax: 773-293-4750
www.behiv.org

Private not-for-profit AIDS service organization. Only comprehensive AIDS service provider in all northern Cook County. Effectively combines direct service and prevention programs.
Eric Nelson, Executive Director
Julie Supple, Director of Programs

190 Black Coalition for AIDS Prevention
20 Victoria Street
Toronto, ON M5C-2N8

416-977-9955
Fax: 416-977-7664
e-mail: blackcap@black-cap.com
www.black-cap.com

A volunteer-driven, charitable, not-for-profit, community-based organization. Works in partnership with organizations and individuals who support in principle and practice our mission, philosophy and activities.
Angela Robertson, Chair
Trevor Grey, Co-Chair

191 British Columbia Persons with AIDS Society
1107 Seymour Street
Vancouver, BC, V6B-5S8

604-893-2200
800-994-2437
Fax: 604-893-2251
e-mail: info@positivelivingbc.org
www.positivelivingbc.org

Exists to enable persons living with AIDS and HIV disease to empower themselves through mutual support and collective action.
John Bishop, Chair
Claudette Cardinal, Vice chair

192 CDC National Prevention Information Network (NPIN)
PO Box 6003
Rockville, MD 20849-6003

301-519-0459
1 8-0 4-8 04
Fax: 888-282-7681
TTY: 888-480-3739
e-mail: info@cdcnpin.org
www.cdcnpin.org

The CDC National Prevention Information Network (NPIN) is the U.S. reference, referral, and distribution service for information on HIV/AIDS, sexually transmitted diseases (STD's), and tuberculosis (TB). NPIN produces, collects, catalogs, processes, stocks, and disseminates materials and information on HIV/AIDS, STD's, and TB to organizations and people working in those disease fields in international, national, state, and local settings.

193 Canadian Foundation for AIDS Research
200 Wellington Street West
Toronto, Ontario, ON M5V-3B8

416-361-6281
800-563-2873
Fax: 416-361-5736
www.canfar.ca

A national charitable foundation whose goal is to raise awareness in order to generate funds for research into all aspects of HIV infection and AIDS.
Andrew M Pringle, Chair
Salah J. Bachir, Deputy Chair

194 Central Alberta AIDS Network Society
4611-50th Avenue
Red Deer, AB T4N-3Z9

403-346-8858
877-346-8858
Fax: 403-346-2352
e-mail: Info@caans,org
www.caans.org

Central Alberta AIDS Network Society is a local charity and a Turning Point agency that offers support to individuals who are infected or affected by HIV/AIDS and provides prevention and education throughout Central Alberta.
Jennifer Vanderschae, Executive Director
Alma , Health Promotion Coordinator

195 Children Affected by AIDS Foundation
6033 W Century Boulevard
Los Angeles, CA 90045

310-258-0850
Fax: 310-258-0851
e-mail: caaf@caaf4kids.org
www.caaf4kids.org

The mission of the Children Affected by AIDS Foundation (CAAF) is to make a positive difference in the lives of children infected with HIV and affected by AIDS. CAAF accomplishes this by helping meet their diverse, special needs, advocating and educating.
Jayne Harkness, President
Joe Christina, Founder, Vice President

196 Children's AIDS Fund
PO Box 16433
Washington, DC 20041

703-433-1560
866-829-1560
Fax: 703-433-1561
e-mail: info@childrensaidsfund.org
www.childrensaidsfund.org

The Children's AIDS Fund works to limit suffering of children and their families caused by HIV disease by providing care services resourced referrals and education.
Anita Smith, President

197 Clinical Focus on Primary Immune Deficiency Diseases
Immune Deficiency Foundation
40 W Chesapeake Avenue
Towson, MD 21204

410-321-6647
800-296-4433
Fax: 410-321-9165
e-mail: info@primaryimmune.org
www.primaryimmune.org

Educational monograph is designed specifically for health care professionals and focuses on topics relevant to primary immune deficiency diseases.
Marcia Boyle, President & Founder
John Seymour, Vice Chair

198 Committee of Ten Thousand
236 Massachusetts Avenue NE
Washington, DC 20002

202-543-0988
800-488-2688
Fax: 202-543-6720
e-mail: cott-dc@earthlink.net
www.cott1.org

Represents people with hemophilia who contracted HIV/AIDS and Hepatitis C from tainted factory concentrates in the 1970s and 1980s. The only national advocacy and support agency for this seriously disabled community.
Corey S Dubin, President
Mary Lou Murphy, Co-Vice President

199   Continuum
255 Golden Gate Avenue
San Francisco, CA 94102
415-437-2900
Fax: 415-437-2550
TTY: 415-861-1399
e-mail: anne@continuumhiv.org
web.mac.com/tenderloinhealth
Empower and dignify the lives of underserved people with HIV and AIDS providing innovative health and human services that establish community, and reduce the rate of HIV infection.
Colm Hegarty, Director Development & Public Relations
Chiquita T Tuttle, Interim Executive Director

200   Deaf AIDS Project Family Service Foundation
Family Service Foundation
5301 76th Avenue
Landover Hills, MD 20784
301-459-2121
866-935-4658
Fax: 301-459-0675
TTY: 301-731-2116
e-mail: ssoulier@fsfinc.org
www.deafnonprofit.net/dap
The AIDS Administration established in 1987 as a division of the Maryland Department of Health and Mental Hygiene leads public health initiatives regarding HIV (Human Immunodeficiency Virus), the virus that causes AIDS.

201   Elizabeth Glaser Pediatric AIDS Foundation
1140 Connecticut Avenue NW
Washington, DC 20036
202-296-9165
888-499-4673
Fax: 202-296-9185
e-mail: info@pedaids.org
www.pedaids.org
Creates a future of hope for children and families worldwide by eradicating pediatric AIDS providing care and treatment to people with HIV/AIDS and accelerating the discovery of new treatments for other serious and life-threatening pediatric illnesses.
Charles Lyons, President/CEO
Susie Zeegan, Co-Founder

202   Farha Foundation
576, Sainte-Catherine Street E
Montreal, QC, H2L-2E1
514-270-4900
Fax: 514-270-5363
e-mail: farha@farha.qc.ca
www.farha.qc.ca
A fundraising organization, committed to help men, women and children living with HIV/AIDS.
Nancy Farha, Executive Director
Lucille Valade, Event Manager

203   Foundation for Children with AIDS
6221 Blue Grass Avenue
Harrisburg, PA 17112-2331
717-489-0206
888-683-8323
Fax: 717-489-0214
e-mail: info@AFCAids.org
www.helpchildrenwithaids.org
A national nonprofit organization founded to improve the quality of life for drug-effected and HIV-infected children and their families. The foundation raises funds for family and community-based services for children and their families affected by HIV.
Nick Cassino, President
Robert Maynard, Vice President

204   HIV West Yellowhead Services
Box 2427
Jasper, Alberta, T0E-1E0
780-852-5274
877-291-8811
Fax: 780-852-5273
e-mail: hivdirector@incentre.net
www.hivwestyellowhead.com
Encourage a positive, healthy lifestyle and provide accurate information to the people living and working in the region.
Allan Bearns, Chair
Nancy Taylor, Vice Chair

205   HIV/Hepatitis C in Prison (HIP) Committee
California Prison Focus
San Francisco, CA 94103
510-665-1935
e-mail: contact@prisons.org
www.prisons.org/hivin.htm
The HIV/HCV in Prison Committee of California Prison Focus works on behalf of prisoners to fight for consistent access to quality medical care including access to all new HIV and hepatitis C medications, diagnostic testing and combination therapies.
Michelle Foy, Contact
Judy Greenspan, Contact

206   Health Information Network
PO Box 30762
Seattle, WA 98113
206-784-5655
Fax: 206-784-3240
www.healthinfonetwork.org
Offers information public awareness and support for women with HIV/AIDS and the public in general.
Kathi Knowles, Executive Director

207   Health Information Network for Women and AIDS
Positive Women's Network
2817 Rockefeller Avenue
Everett, WA 98201
425-259-9899
888-651-8931
Fax: 425-259-9880
www.pwnetwork.org
A partnership of women living with and affected by HIV/AIDS supports women in making informed choices about HIV/AIDS and health.
Rhea Reynolds, President
Tayah E. H. Renfro, Vice President

208   Heart Touch™ Project
3400 Airport Avenue
Santa Monica, CA 90405
310-391-2558
Fax: 310-391-2168
e-mail: executive@hearttouch.org
www.hearttouch.org
Non-profit educational and service organization devoted to the delivery of compassionate and healing touch to home or hospital-bound men women and children.
Patrick Callahan, Executive Director
Jennifer Noguera, Director of Programs

209   Immune Deficiency Foundation
40 W Chesapeake Avenue
Towson, MD 21204-4841
410-321-6647
800-296-4433
Fax: 410-321-9165
e-mail: info@primaryimmune.org
www.primaryimmune.org
The only national charitable organization aimed at fighting the primary immune deficiency diseases. The founders included parents of children with primary immune deficiency immunologists who treat immune deficient patients and other individuals with an immune deficiency.
Marcia Boyle, President & Founder
John Seymour, Vice Chair

210   International Council of AIDS Service Organization
65 Wellesley Street E
Toronto Ontario, M4Y 1-1G7
416-921-0018
Fax: 416-921-9979
e-mail: icaso@icaso.org
www.icaso.org
A global network of non-governmental and community-based organizations.
Mary Ann Torres, Executive Director
Margaret Quish, Financial Manager

211   Life Force: Women Fighting AIDS
57 Willoughby Street
Brooklyn, NY 11201-4300
718-797-0937
Fax: 718-797-4011
e-mail: info@lifeforceinc.org
www.lifeforceinc.org
A support network offering prevention education awareness risk reduction workshops and support for woman with HIV/AIDS.
Sayida Self, Program Director
Linney Smith, Executive Director

212   Living Positive
9912-106 Street
Edmonton, Alberta, T5K-1C5
780-488-5768
800-210-9561
Fax: 780-702-8211
www.edmlivingpositive.ca
Dedicated to providing emotional, spiritual and psychological support to all those living with HIV.
Lance Hansen, Director
Deborah Norris, Chairperson

213 Medical Library Association
65 E Wacker Place
Chicago, IL 60601-7246

312-419-9094
Fax: 312-419-8950
e-mail: info@mlahq.org
www.mlahq.org

Non-profit educational organization of more than 1,100 institutions and 3,600 individual members in the health sciences information field, committed to educating health information professionals, supporting health information research and promoting access to information.
Ruth Holst, President
Carla J Funk, Executive Director

214 Multifaith Works
1401 East Jefferson Street
Seattle, WA 98122

206-324-1520
Fax: 206-324-2041
e-mail: info@rosehedge.org
www.multifaith.org

Non-profit non-denominational organization that provides housing and supportive services to people living with AIDS or other life-threatening illness and community education on issues of human diversity.
Paul Binder, President
Anthony Radovich, Secretary

215 NAMES Project Foundation AIDS Memorial Quilt
AIDS Memorial Quilt
204 14th Street NW
Atlanta, GA 30318-5304

404-688-5500
Fax: 404-688-5552
e-mail: info@aidsquilt.org
www.aidsquilt.org

International non-governmental non-profit organization that is the custodian of the AIDS Memorial Quilt a poignant memorial and powerful tool for use in preventing new HIV infections.
Robert Bush, Chair
Tom Gertz, Vice Chair

216 National AIDS Fund
1424 K Street, N.W
Washington, DC 20005-1511

202-408-4848
888-234-AIDS
Fax: 202-408-1818
www.aidsfund.org

The National AIDS Fund is one of America's largest philanthropic organizations dedicated to eliminating HIV/AIDS as a major health and social problem. The Fund's primary purpose is channeling critical resources to community-based organizations to fight HIV.
Mark Ishaug, President & CEO
Douglas Brooks, Senior Vice President

217 National AIDS Treatment Advocacy Project
580 Broadway
New York, NY 10012

212-219-0106
888-26N-ATAP
Fax: 212-219-8473
e-mail: info@natap.org
www.natap.org

Educate by sending out literature e-mail lists and give forums on how to prevent HIV or how to live with it.
Jules Levin, Executive Director
Jose Ernesto Nunez, Executive Assistant

218 National Coalition on Immune System Disorders
1090 Vermont Avenue NW
Washington, DC 20005-4953

202-371-8090
800-438-2996
Fax: 202-371-1945

Professional and lay organizations with a primary interest in the immune system and its diseases.
Robert R Humphreys, Executive Director

219 National Hospice & Palliative Care Organization (NHPCO)
1731 King Street
Alexandria, VA 22314

703-837-1500
800-646-6460
Fax: 703-837-1233
e-mail: nhpco_info@nhpco.org
www.nhpco.org

The nation's only advocate for terminally ill patients and their families. Founded in 1978, the NHPCO is the only organization devoted to hospice in the United States. Support is included from state hospice organizations, patients, families, communities, provider program members and professional/volunteer members.

Represents hospice care interests to Congress, regulatory agencies, courts, voluntary organizations and the public.
Donald Schumacher, President/CEO
Samira Beckwith, Treasurer

220 National Minority AIDS Education Training Center
Howard University
1840 7th Street NW
Washington, DC 20001-3029

202-865-8146
Fax: 202-667-1382
e-mail: gdowner@howard.edu
www.aetcnmc.org/index

Located at Howard University as a HIV/AIDS training and technical resource for providers of minority HIV-infected patients throughout the country. The NMAETC receives 100% of its funding through the MAI Initiative.
Goulda Downe PhD RD, Principal Investigator
David Luckett, Deputy Director

221 National Native American AIDS Prevention Center
720 S Colorado Boulevard
Denver, CO 80246

720-382-2244
Fax: 720-382-2248
e-mail: information@nnaapc.org
www.nnaapc.org

To address the impact of HIV/AIDS on American Indians Alaska Natives and Native Hawaiians through culturally appropriate advocacy research education and policy development in support of healthy Indigenous people.
D Shane Barnett, Chairperson
Mary Helen Deer, Vice Chairperson

222 National Prevention Information Network CDC NPIN
PO Box 6003
Rockville, MD 20849-6003

301-519-0459
1 8-0 4-8 04
Fax: 888-282-7681
TTY: 888-480-3739
e-mail: info@cdcnpin.org
www.cdcnpin.org

The CDC National Prevention Information Network (NPIN) is the U.S. reference referral and distribution service for information on HIV/AIDS, sexually transmitted diseases (STDs) and tuberculosis (TB).
Jay Laudato, Executive Director

223 National Prison Project/ACLU AIDS in Prison Project
125 Broad Street
New York, NY 10004

212-549-2500
e-mail: media@aclu.org
www.aclu.org

National Prison Project seeks to create constitutional conditions of confinement and strengthen prisoners' rights through class action litigation and public education. Our policy priorities include reducing prison overcrowding and improving prisoner medical care.
Susan N Herman, President
Anthony Romero, Executive Director

224 New England AIDS Education and Training Center
38 Chauncy Street
Boston, MA 02111-3318

617-262-5657
Fax: 617-262-5667
e-mail: aidsed@neaetc.org
www.neaetc.org

Our goal is to increase the number of health care providers effectively trained to counsel diagnose treat and manage the care of individuals with HIV infection and to assist in the prevention of high risk behavior which may lead to infection.
James Meenaghan, Project Manager
Helene Bednarsh, Director

225 North Bay Aids Committee
269 Main Street W
North Bay, Ontario, ON P1B2T-2T8

705-497-3560
800-387-3701
Fax: 705-497-7850
e-mail: acnba@efni.com
www.aidsnorthbay.com

To assist and support all persons infected or affected by HIV/AIDS and to limit the spread of the virus through education and outreach strategies.
Stacey L Mayhall, Executive Director
Kirk Titmus, Board Chair

226 Ontario HIV Treatment Network
1300 Yonge Street
Toronto, ON M41X3

416-642-6486
877-743-6486
Fax: 416-640-4245
e-mail: info@ohtn.on.ca
www.ohtn.on.ca

To optimize the quality of life of people living with HIV in Ontario and to promote excellence and innovation in treatment, research, education and prevention through a collaborative network of excellence representing consumers, providers, researchers and other stakeholders.
David Hoe, President
Claire Kendell, Vice President

227 Pediatric AIDS Foundation
11150 Santa Monica Boulevard
Los Angeles, CA 90025-3092

310-314-1459
Fax: 310-314-1469
e-mail: info@pedaids.org
www.pedaids.org

A national nonprofit organization confronting medical problems unique to children infected with HIV/AIDS. The foundation funds critically needed pediatric AIDS research and provides help to hospitals that serve the needs of children with HIV/AIDS.
Charles Lyons, President/CEO
Susie Zeegan, Co-Founder

228 Peel HIV/AIDS Network
160 Traders Boulevard E
Mississauga, Ontario, L4Z 3-4K1

905-361-0523
866-896-8700
Fax: 905-361-1004
e-mail: info@phan.ca
www.phan.ca

Committed to serving people living with and affected by HIV/AIDS and to limit the spread of the virus through support education advocacy and volunteerism.
Tania Fernandes, Board Co Chair
Sanya Khan, Board Secretary

229 Project Inform
1375 Mission Street
San Francisco, CA 94103

415-558-8669
800-822-7422
Fax: 415-558-0684
e-mail: support@projectforum.org
www.projectforum.org/HIVhealth/infoline

HIV Health Infoline has provided HIV treatment and access to care information, free of charge, to people living with HIV, their providers and support networks. Staffed by highly trained volunteers, the Infoline has the personal experiences and outside connections to answer questions about living healthfully with HIV.
Dana Van Gorder, Executive Director
Michael Allerton, President

230 Resources and Services Database Centers for Disease Control
Centers for Disease Control
1600 Clifton Road
Atlanta, GA 30333

800-232-4636
877-242-9760
Fax: 301-562-1050
TTY: (888) 232-63
e-mail: info@hivatwork.org
www.brta-lrta.org

Describes more than 16 000 organizations that provide HIV and AIDS prevention education and social services. These include public health departments community and social service organizations hospitals and clinics.

231 The AIDS Network
140 King Street East
Hamilton, ON, L8N-1B2

905-528-0854
866-563-0563
Fax: 905-528-6311
e-mail: info@aidsnetwork.ca
www.aidsnetwork.ca

Ruthann Tucker, Executive Director
Roxanne Ali, Director Program Services

232 Toronto People with AIDS Foundation
200 Gerard Street E
Toronto, Ontario, M5A-2E6

416-506-1400
Fax: 416-506-1404
e-mail: info@pwatoronto.org
www.pwatoronto.org

The Toronto People with AIDS Foundation exists to promote the health and well-being of all people living with HIV/AIDS by providing accessible, direct, and practical support services.
Cory Garlough, President
Brian Fior, Vice president

233 UNICEF USA
125 Maiden Lane
New York, NY 10038

212-686-5522
800-486-4233
Fax: 212-779-1679
e-mail: information@unicefusa.org
www.unicefusa.org

Supports child survival protection and development worldwide through education advocacy and fundraising for AIDS and other conditions.
Caryl M Stern, President and CEO
Edward G Lloyd, Executive Vice President and CFO

234 Well Project
112 Krog Street NE
Atlanta, GA 30307

404-474-3152
888-616-9355
e-mail: info@thewellproject.org
www.thewellproject.org

The Well Project is a not for profit corporation and an initiative conceived developed and administered by HIV+ women and those who are affected by this disease. Our Founder Dawn Averitt Bridge was diagnosed with HIV in 1988.
Dawn Averitt Bridge, Founder & Board President
Richard Averitt, CO Founder

235 Women Alive
1301 N. Willowbrook Avenue
Compton, CA 90222

310-605-1365
800-554-4876
Fax: 310-605-1366
e-mail: info@women-alive.org
www.women-alive.org

Coalition of, by and for women living with HIV/AIDS. Created ways to help women connect with each other, bring others out of isolation, exchange information about HIV treatments and take charge of their lives.
Alfredia Thomas, President
Carrie Broadus, Executive Director

236 Women's AIDS Network Women and Children's Service Program
Women and Children's Service Program
4 North Broad street
Trenton, NJ 08608

415-864-4376
www.njwan.org

Marylou Freund, President
Deborah Walker McCall, Associate Dean

State Agencies & Associations

Alabama

237 Alabama Department of Public Health
201 Monroe Street
Montgomery, AL 36104-3000

334-206-5364
800-228-0469
Fax: 334-206-2092
www.adph.org/aids

Offers health education and risk education activities including compiling a state community resource directory.
Danna Cargill, Office Manager
Jane B Cheeks, Division Director

Alaska

238 Alaska Department of Health and Social Services: AIDS/STD Program
3601 C Street
Anchorage, AK 99503-0249

907-269-8000
800-478-0084
Fax: 907-562-7802
e-mail: mollie_cross@health.state.ak.us
www.epi.hss.state.ak.us/hivstd

The HIV/STD Program addresses public health issues and activities with the goal of preventing sexually transmitted diseases (STDs) and HIV infection in Alaska as well as their impact on

health. AIDS program offers education to providers and organizations.
John Middaug PhD, Chief Dept of Public Health/Epidemiology
Mollie Cross, Prevention Community Planning Group

Arizona

239 Arizona Department of Health Services
150 N 18th Avenue   602-542-1025
Phoenix, AZ 85007   800-334-1540
                                           Fax: 602-542-0883
                                           www.azdhs.gov
Provides HIV and AIDS seropositive surveillance case investigation and analysis and AIDS health education and training for the public.
Margery Sheridan, Division Chief
Will Humble, Interim Director

240 Body Positive HIV and AIDS Research and Re Southwest Center for HIV/AIDS
1144 E McDowell Road   602-307-5330
Phoenix, AZ 85006   Fax: 602-307-5021
                    e-mail: cweiner@phoenixbodypositive.org
                                           http://swhiv.org/
Body Positive is a non-profit organization created by and for people infected and affected by HIV, that provides the community with the knowledge, resources and collective strength necessary for individuals to live long and well with HIV and to prevent the spread of the disease.
Ken Gabel, Chair
jessica Fotinoes, Vice Chair

241 Tucson Interfaith HIV/AIDS Network (TIHAN)
2660 North 1st avenue   520-299-6647
Tucson, AZ 85719   Fax: 520-784-0620
                                           e-mail: friends@tihan.org
                                           www.tihan.org
Serving interfaith communities of Tucson through compassionate care education training and spiritual support so that we can make more people aware of the health crisis which affects all of us. Also provide non-medical in-home help.
david Cormier, Treasurer
Catherine Davis, President

Arkansas

242 Arkansas Department of Health AIDS Prevention Program
AIDS Prevention Program
4815 West Markham Street   501-661-2000
Little Rock, AR 72205   800-462-0599
                                           www.healthyarkansas.com
Provides educational materials such as pamphlets and films conducts HIV and AIDS research and operates a speakers bureau.
Dr. Clark fincher, President
Paul Halverson, Director

California

243 Aids, Medicine and Miracles
3288 21st Street   415-252-7111
San Francisco, CA 94110-2423   Fax: 415-252-7117
                    e-mail: amminfo@aidsmedicineandmiracles.org
                            www.aidsmedicineandmiracles.org
Provides culturally sensitive counseling and education to stop the spread of HIV infection, and to help people face the emotional, psychological and social changes of living with HIV disease.
Gregg Cassin, Chair
Daniel Ramos, Secretary

244 California Collaborative Treatment Group CCTG Data Center
CCTG Data Center
3900 Fifth Avenue   619-543-5006
San Diego, CA 92103-1910   Fax: 619-298-1359
                                           e-mail: rhaubrich@ucsd.edu
                                           www.cctg.ucsd.edu
The CCTG is a multi-center clinical trials organization founded by Dr. Allen McCutchan in 1986. The primary mission of the CCTG is

to improve the scientific basis for HIV patient care and HIV prevention. CCTG develops treatment protocols and drug therapies.
Richard Haub MD, Investigator/Professor of Medicine
Allen McCutc MD, Investigator/Professor of Medicine

245 California Department of Health Services Office of Aids
Office of Aids
PO Box 997377,   916-445-4171
Sacramento, CA 95899   800-458-5231
                                           Fax: 916-440-7404
                                           www.dhs.ca.gov/aids
Works to develop strategies and implement programs for education and prevention testing and counseling supportive care and treatment and research to control the spread of HIV infection.
David Maxwell-Jolly, Director

246 Los Angeles County Department of Health Services
AIDS Programs
600 S Commonwealth Avenue   213-351-8000
Los Angeles, CA 90005   800-243-7889
                                           Fax: 213-738-0825
                                           e-mail: aids@ph.lacounty.org
                                           www.lapublichealth.org
Responsible for planning coordinating and implementing county wide HIV/AIDS efforts.
Charles L Henry, Director
Raymond H Johnson, Chief of Staff

247 San Francisco AIDS Foundation (SFAF)
1035 Market Street   415-487-3000
San Francisco, CA 94103   800-367-AIDS
                                           Fax: 415-487-8079
                                           TTY: 415-487-3012
                                           TDD: 415-487-8099
                                           e-mail: info@aidslifecycle.org
                                           www.sfaf.org
SFAF provides confidential array of services-including financial benefits counseling client advocacy housing assistance HIV prevention efforts and needle exchange.
Neil Giuliano, CEO
Nancy Durlester, VP Development

248 San Francisco Area AIDS Education and Training Center
UCSF Box 1365
50 Beale Street   415-597-9168
San Francisco, CA 94105-1365   Fax: 415-597-9386
                                           e-mail: sfaetc@ucsf.edu
                                           http://www.sfaetc.ucsf.edu/
Helps to improve the care of people living with HIV and AIDS by supporting state-of-the-art clinical consultation education and training for health care professionals and organizations in Sa Francisco San Mateo and Marin counties.
Jacqueline Tulsky, Medical Director
Ronald H Goldschmidt, Director

Colorado

249 CO Center for AIDS Research: University Colorado Health Sciences Center/CFAR
Division of Infectious Diseases
4200 E 9th Avenue   303-315-7233
Denver, CO 80262   Fax: 303-315-8681
                                           e-mail: colorado.cfar@uchsc.edu
                                           www.uchsc.edu/ccfar
Describes forms and patterns of use of complimentary and alternative medicine (CAM) for the treatment of HIV/AIDS.
Edward N Janoff MD, CFAR Director
Kristin Jones, CFAR Administrator

250 Mountain-Plains AIDS Education and Training Center (MPAETC)
12631 E 17th Avenue   303-724-0867
Aurora, CO 80045   Fax: 303-724-0875
                                           e-mail: info@mpaetc.org
                                           www.mpaetc.org
One of 12 regional AETCs funded nationwide by a grant from the U.S. Health Resources and Services Administration through the Ryan White Comprehensive AIDS Resources Emergency (CARE)

Act. Provides educational programs about HIV infection for healthcare providers.
Beth Mullin Rotach, Director
Lucy Bradley-Springe, Principal Investigator

Connecticut

251 Connecticut Department of Health Services AIDS Programs
AIDS Programs
410 Capitol Avenue   860-509-8000
Hartford, CT 06134   800-842-0038
                                              Fax: 860-509-7853
                                 e-mail: webmaster.dph@ct.gov
                                              www.dph.state.ct.us
Operates a speakers bureau provides training workshops seminars and counseling services conducts meetings and offers information and referral services.
Rosa M Biaggi, Director
William Gerrish, Communications

252 Northwestern Connecticut AIDS Project
100 Migeon Avenue   860-482-1596
Torrington, CT 06790-0985   800-381-2437
                                              Fax: 860-482-3606
                                   e-mail: general@nwctaids.org
                                www.freewebs.com/nwctaidsproject
A nonprofit organization offering support and a variety of services to people with AIDS and their loved ones. Provides education to all segments of the public about AIDS prevention and treatment.
Patricia Lafayette, Executive Director
Demetria McMilliAn, Program Director Client Services

Delaware

253 Delaware Department of Health and Social Services
Division of Public Health, HIV/STD Program
417 Federal Street   302-744-4700
Dover, DE 19901   888-459-2943
                                              Fax: 302-739-6659
                                   e-mail: dhssinfo@state.de.us
                          www.dhss.delaware.gov/dhss/dph/index.htm
Provides HIV counseling and testing prevention education and AIDS surveillance and studies.
Jamie Rivera, Director

District of Columbia

254 Washington DC Department of Health HIV/AIDS Administration
HIV/AIDS Administration
899 North Capitol Street NE
Washington, DC 20002   202-442-5955
                                              www.doh.dc.gov
Mission is to reduce the incidence of HIV/AIDS and number of deaths related to HIV/AIDS in the District of Columbia by the application of sound public health practices and initiatives through HIV disease surveillance tracking, monitoring, and intervention.
Mohammed Akhter, Director

Florida

255 Florida Department of Health Bureau of HIV/AIDS
Bureau of HIV/AIDS
4052 Bald Cypress Way   850- 24- 414
Tallahassee, FL 32399-1715   Fax: 850- 24- 444
                              e-mail: DiseaseControl@doh.state.fl.us
                                              www.doh.state.fl.us
Making voluntary HIV testing a routine part of medical care implementing new models for diagnosing HIV infections outside medical settings preventing new infections by working with persons diagnosed with HIV and their partners.
Tom Liberti, Bureau Chief
Janell Clemons, Administrative Assistant

256 Positive Voices
9526 NE 2nd Ave   786-873-8576
Miami, FL 33138   888-POS-CONN
                                              Fax: 786-623-0701
                           e-mail: email@positiveconnections.org
                                       www.positiveconnections.org

The Center for Positive Connections is a non-profit community based organization that is run for those infected our community. Our mission is to provide educational emotional holistic and social support at all individuals living with HIV/AIDS.
Dr. David Newman, President
Rec Ken Furguson, Vice President

Georgia

257 Georgia Department of Human Resources: Division of Public Health
AIDS Section
2 Peachtree Street NW   404-657-2700
Atlanta, GA 30303   800-551-2728
                                              Fax: 404-657-3100
                                   e-mail: gdphinfo@dhr.ga.us
                                       http://health.state.ga.us
Provides technical support and assistance to the Public Health Districts to prevent STD and HIV infection ensuring the availability of quality STD/HIV prevention and treatment by improving quality assurance guidelines and methods by providing appropriate training.
Katheryn K. Cheek, Board Chair
James W Curran, Dean

Hawaii

258 Hawaii Department of Health: Communicable Disease Division
AIDS/Sexually Transmitted Diseases Control Branch
1250 Punchbowl St   80 - 5 - 44
Honolulu, HI 96813-2317   Fax: 80 - 5 - 44
                              e-mail: janice.okubo@doh.hawaii.gov
                              www.hawaii.gov/health/about/admin
Offers research education surveillance and testing components. AIDS information and guidelines about the placement of infants children and adolescents who test positive for HIV in nursery or school settings are also available.
Chiyome Fuki MD, Director
Loretta Fuddy, Deputy Director

Idaho

259 Idaho Department of Health and Welfare The STD/AIDS Program
The STD/AIDS Program
450 W State Street 1st Floor   208-334-6527
Boise, ID 83720-0036   Fax: 208-332-7346
                                   e-mail: apsportal@dhw.idaho.gov
                                       www.healthandwelfare.idaho.gov
Program receives federal funding to support testing treatment and prevention services for Idaho's reportable sexually transmitted infections.
Richard Roberge, Chairman
Janet Penfold, Vice Chair

Illinois

260 AIDS Legal Council of Chicago
180 N Michigan Avenue   312-427-8990
Chicago, IL 60601   866-506-3038
                                              Fax: 312-427-8419
                                   e-mail: info@aidslegal.com
                                              www.aidslegal.com
Legal advice and services for persons who are HIV positive or have AIDS and their companions families etc.
Todd A Solomon, President
Dr. Matthew Feldhaus, Vice President

261 Chicago Department of Health
333 S State Street   312-747-9884
Chicago, IL 60604   Fax: 312-747-9765
                                              TTY: 312-747-2374
                                   e-mail: publichealth@cdph.org
                                              www.cityofchicago.org
Offers educational services audiovisual materials surveillance of HIV and AIDS counseling and referrals.
Carolyn Lopez, President
Bechara Choucair, Commissioner

262 **Illinois Department of Public Health: Division of Infectious Diseases**
535 W Jefferson Street   217-782-4977
Springfield, IL 62761   Fax: 217-782-3987
                              TTY: 800-547-0466
                              www.idph.state.il.us
Administers the AIDS Drug Assistance Program (ADAP). Currently nearly 3 300 clients use ADAP services each month accessing 10 000 prescriptions. Client approved for ADAP must re-apply on an annual basis in order to continue to receive services.
Damon Arnold, Director
Randy J Dunn, State Superintendent of Education

263 **Test Positive Aware Network (TPAN)**
5537 N Broadway Street   773-989-9400
Chicago, IL 60640-1405   Fax: 773-989-9494
                              e-mail: tpan@tpan.com
                              www.tpan.com
Empowers people living with HIV through peer-led programming support services information dissemination and advocacy. Provides services to the broader community to increase HIV knowledge and sensitivity and to reduce the risk of infection.
Bill Farrand, CEO/Dierctor of Client Services
Thomas Hart, President

Kansas

264 **Kansas Department of Health & Environment Epidemiology & Disease Prevention: HIV**
1000 SW Jackson   785-296-1500
Topeka, KS 66612-1274   Fax: 785-368-6368
                              e-mail: info@kdheks.gov
                              www.kdheks.gov
Conducts surveillance of HIV/AIDS in Kansas. Conducts Prevention Program with training for counselors and educators partial funding of counseling test sites and distribution of educational materials. Provides medications and primary care.
Sam Brownback, Governer
Robert Moser, Secretary

Louisiana

265 **Louisiana Department of Health & Hospitals : Office of Public Health**
Louisiana AIDS Prevention/Surveillance Program
628 N 4th Street   22 - 3 - 80
Baton Rouge, LA 70821-0629   Fax: 22 - 3 - 80
                              e-mail: avis.richard-griffin@la.gov
                              http://www.dhh.louisiana.gov/offices/?id
The HIV/AIDS Program was established in 1985 to provide leadership policy development and technical assistance including HIV/AIDS education prevention and services to parish health units and community based organizations throughout the state.
William Clark, Medical Director
William Hineman, Director/Program Manager II

Maine

266 **Maine Bureau of Health: Division of Disease Control**
HIV/STD Program
286 Water Street   207-287-8016
Augusta, ME 04333   800-821-5821
                              Fax: 207-287-3498
                              TTY: 800-606-0215
                              e-mail: chris.zukas-lessard@maine.gov
                              www.maine.gov/dhhs/boh/index.htm
Provides technical assistance to state agencies and private organizations regarding AIDS education and policy development.
Chris Zukas-Lessard, Deputy Director
Dora Anne Mills, Director

Massachusetts

267 **Massachusetts Department of Health HIV/AIDS Bureau**
HIV/AIDS Bureau

250 Washington Street   617-624-6000
Boston, MA 02108   800-235-2331
                              Fax: 617-624-5399
                              TTY: 617-437-1672
                              www.mass.gov/dph
Assisting in preventing the spread of the HIV epidemic and the development of appropriate cost-effective health and support services which will maintain patients in the least restrictive setting.
Kevin Cranston, Director
John Auerbach, Commissioner Department of Public Health

268 **New England AIDS Education & Training Center (NEHEC)**
38 Chauncy Street   617-262-5657
Boston, MA 02215-3318   Fax: 617-262-5667
                              e-mail: aidsed@neaetc.org
                              www.neaetc.org
The New England HIV Education Consortium (NEHEC), a HRSA minority AIDS initiative program, is a training and education program serving all six states in the New England region. The principal goal of NEHEC is to address the HIV-related training, educational, and support needs of the full, spectrum of providers as they provide state-of-the-art, quality and compassionate care to individuals living with HIV/AIDS.
Donna M Gallagher RNC/MS/ANP, Principal Investigator/Project Director
Barry Sandberg MS/MPA, Assistant Director/Administrator

Michigan

269 **Michigan Department of Community Health HIV/AIDS Prevention & Intervention Secti**
HIV/AIDS Prevention & Intervention Section
201 Townsend avenue   17 -73 -740
Lansing, MI 48913   888-826-6565
                              Fax: 517-241-5911
                              www.michigan.gov/mdch
Gives general public and high-risk education grants supporting educational materials programs and a hotline.
James K haven, Director Division HIV/AIDS-STD
Nick Lyon, Deputy Director

Minnesota

270 **Minnesota Department of Health: AIDS/STD Prevention Service**
Office of Infectious Diseases
P.O. Box 64975   651-201-5000
Minneapolis, MN 55164-9272   877-925-4189
                              Fax: 612-623-5743
                              e-mail: indepcweb@health.state.mn.us
                              www.health.state.mn.us
This division is to prevent death and disability from HIV and other sexually transmitted diseases by providing statewide leadership regarding the prevention of transmission and the availability of health and supportive services for infected persons.
Harry Hull, Director

Mississippi

271 **Mississippi Department of Public Health: STD/HIV Prevention Program**
570 E Woodrow Wilson Drive   601-576-7400
Jackson, MS 39216   866-458-4948
                              Fax: 601-576-7909
                              www.msdh.state.ms.us
Funds two statewide hotlines one for the general public and one for the gay community. Both offer health education and risk reduction activities of the Program include baseline evaluation of public knowledge about AIDS through surveys.
Joy Sennett, Director Communicable Disease Office

Missouri

272 **Missouri Department of Health: Bureau of AIDS Prevention**
912 Wildwood   573-751-6400
Jefferson City, MO 65102-0570   866-628-9891
                              Fax: 573-751-6010
                              e-mail: info@dhss.mo.gov
                              www.dhss.mo.gov

Human Immunodeficiency Virus (HIV) disease and infection and Acquired Immunodeficiency Syndrome (AIDS) surveillance monitors and analyzes data on the number of people infected with HIV and/or AIDS and identifies and tracks trends in disease incidence.
Margaret T Donnelly, Director
Bret Fischer, Director

Montana

273   Montana Deptartment of Health And Human Services
STD & HIV Prevention Program
1400 Broadway   406-444-4540
Helena, MT 59620   800-233-6668
                                       Fax: 406-444-1861
                                       www.dphhs.state.mt.us
This program receives a Federal grant through the Centers for Disease Control to carry out a health education/risk reduction program to detect and prevent the spread of HIV infection through a number of services.
Jane Smilie, Acting Administrator
Anna Whiting Sorrell, Director

Nevada

274   Nevada Department of Human Resources: Health Program Section
4126 Technology Way   775-684-4000
Carson City, NV 89706-2009   Fax: 775-684-4010
                                       e-mail: nvdhr@dhhs.nv.gov
                                       www.dhhs.nv.gov
Provides HIV counseling and testing a speakers bureau information and referrals resource materials including AIDS video recordings and education.
Harold Cook, Administrator
Mike Wilden, Director

275   TBAN
6955 N. Durango Dr. Ste   702-608- 247
Las Vegas, NV 89149-8333   Fax: 702-870-2474
                                       www.tban.com/
TBAN formerly The Tampa AIDS Network (TAN) is a community organization which provides prevention education emotional and physical support services and advocacy on behalf of all persons affected by HIV disease.
Mike Gardinear, President
Joe Russo, Treasurer

New Hampshire

276   New Hampshire Department of Health and Human Services
Division of Public Health Services
129 Pleasant Street   603-271-4502
Concord, NH 03301-4604   800-852-3345
                                       Fax: 603-271-4934
                                       TTY: 800-735-2964
                                       TDD: 8007352964
                                       www.dhhs.state.nh.us
HIV/AIDS Program receives both state and Federal funding pertaining to AIDS education risk reduction testing and surveillance.
Joyce J Welch, Program Coordinator
James Fredyma, Director

New Jersey

277   New Jersey Department of Health: Division of AIDS Prevention & Control
Division of HIV/AIDS Service (DHAS)
Po Box 360   609-292-7837
Trenton, NJ 08625-0360   800-367-6543
                                       www.state.nj.us/health
Serves to coordinate and direct primary HIV activities within the Department networking with other divisions and agencies to provide information and care programs to populations in need.
Laurence E Ganges, Assistant Commissioner
John Fasanella, Director

278   New Jersey Woman AIDS Network
4 North Broad Street   609-695-1200
Trenton, NJ 08608   800-747-1108
                                       Fax: 609-695-1201
                                       e-mail: office@njwan.org
                                       www.njwan.org
A leader in identifying issues facing women with HIV/AIDS educating service providers advocating for appropriate policies and building a multicultural women and HIV/AIDS movement.
Patryce Burgess, Interim Executive Director
Adrienne Smith, Program Coordinator

New Mexico

279   New Mexico Health Department: Public Health Division
HIV/AIDS/STD Prevention & Services Bureau
1190 S Saint Francis Drive   505-827-2613
Santa Fe, NM 87502-4182   800-545-2437
                                       Fax: 505-827-2530
                                       www.health.state.nm.us
Provides training programs and HIV education to the general public and professionals risk reduction information AIDS school curriculums classroom presentation information and an AIDS hotline.
Don Maestas, Director

New York

280   New York Department of Health, Office of Public Health: AIDS Institute
AIDS Institute
Empire State Plaza   518-474-9866
Albany, NY 12237-0001   866-881-2809
                                       Fax: 518-473-8814
                                       e-mail: hivpubs@health.state.ny.us
                                       www.health.state.ny.us
Awards grants and maintains relationships with regional AIDS service groups, crisis intervention, psychosocial counseling and legal, financial and housing assistance. The Institute also offers preventive education, risk reduction education, HIV counseling and testing and patient care.
Wendy V. Gould, Coordinator Educational Materials

North Carolina

281   North Carolina Department of Health & Natural Resources
HIV/STD Prevention & Care
2001 Mail Service Center   919-855-4800
Raleigh, NC 27699-1902   Fax: 919-870-4829
                                       e-mail: hivstdprevention@ncmail.net
                                       www.ncpublichealth.com
Oversee the AIDS surveillance program HIV counseling testing partner notification health education risk reduction and public information efforts in North Carolina.
Rebecca King, Chief
Jeffrey Engel, Director

Ohio

282   Ohio Department of Health: Division of Preventive Medicine
HIV/AIDS Surveillance Division
246 N High Street   614-466-3543
Columbus, OH 43215-0118   800-777-4775
                                       Fax: 614-644-1909
                                       TTY: 800-332-AIDS
                                       e-mail: Surveillance@odh.ohio.gov
                                       www.odh.ohio.gov
Consists of AIDS surveillance seroprevalence programs, health care worker education, health education and risk reduction projects.
John R. Kasich, Governor
Theodore E. Wymyslo, M.D., Director

Oklahoma

283   Oklahoma Department of Health: AIDS Division
1000 NE 10th   405-271-5600
Oklahoma City, OK 73117-1207   800-522-0203
                                       Fax: 405-271-5149
                                       www.health.state.ok.us

Provides prevention-related services and funding to the network of AIDS service delivery organizations, both public and private in Oklahoma. The Division provides services and training and certification of AIDS educators, surveillance, and seroprevalence staff.
Rocky D McElvany, Interim Commissioner of Health
Ken Feagins, Director

Oregon

284 Oregon Department of Human Resources Health Division HIV Program
Health Division, HIV Program
800 NE Oregon Street   971-673-1222
Portland, OR 97232   800-777-2437
                             Fax: 971-673-1299
                             TTY: 971-673-0372
                    e-mail: health.webmaster@state.or.us
                             www.oregon.gov/DHS/ph
HIV Program includes training workshops for AIDS trainers curriculum development or revision and an AIDS hotline through Cascade AIDS Project.
Veda Latin, HST Program Manager
Mitch Zahn, HIV Prevention Manager

Pennsylvania

285 Pennsylvania Department of Health: Bureau of HIV/AIDS
Division of HIV/AIDS
8th Floor West   717-783-4677
Harrisburg, PA 17120   877-PA -EALT
                             Fax: 717-772-6975
                       e-mail: c-hivepi@state.pa.us
                             www.portal.state.pa.us
The purpose of the Division of HIV/AIDS is to develop and implement a multi-dimensional coordinated strategy to prevent disease and change high-risk behaviors as well as provide resources and direction for sustaining preventive behavior and avoiding infection.
Janice P Kopelman MSW LSW, Director

286 Philadelphia Department of Public Health: AIDS Program
AIDS Activities Coordinating Office (AACO)
1101 Market Street   215-685-5600
Philadelphia, PA 19107   800-985-AIDS
                             Fax: 215-685-5293
                             www.phila.gov/health
Administers federal state and city funded HIV/AIDS programs in Philadelphia through collaborative service contracts with community-based organizations.
Marla Gold MD, Program Coordinator
Nan Feyler, Chief of Staff

Rhode Island

287 Rhode Island Department of Health: Division of Disease Prevention & Control
Office of AIDS/HIV
3 Capitol Hill   401-222-5960
Providence, RI 02908   800-381-AIDS
                             Fax: 401-222-2488
                             www.health.state.ri.us
Provides health education and risk reduction activities through its AIDS program. Services include professional conferences, providing assistance for in-service programs, presentation of two courses and organization of an AIDS minority program. Also, provides public health services in HIV/AIDS and Viral Hepatitis. The office develops policies, funds community programs and conducts surveillances.
Paul G. Loberti, Chief Administrator
Lucille Minuto, Assistant Administrator

South Carolina

288 South Carolina Department of Health & Environmental Control
Bureau of Preventive Health Services
2600 Bull Street
Columbia, SC 29201   803-898-3432
                             www.scdhec.net

Provides services to prevent the spread of sexually transmitted diseases (STD's) and HIV infection to reduce associated illness and death and to provide care and support resources for persons with HIV disease.
Jeff Jones MD, Director

Tennessee

289 Tennessee Department of Health: AIDS Program
Cordell Hull Building, 4th Floor
425 Fifth Avenue N   615-741-3111
Nashville, TN 37243   Fax: 615-741-2491
                       e-mail: tn.health@tn.gov
                             health.state.tn.us
Provides HIV/STD education and information, as well as collecting monitoring and distributing data. Provides assistance to individuals, and intervention and treatment services.
Bill Haslam, Governor
John J. Dreyzehner, MD, MPH, Commissioner

Texas

290 AIDS Outreach Center (AOC)
400 North Beach Street   817-335-1994
Fort Worth, TX 76111   Fax: 817-335-3617
                       e-mail: info@aoc.org
                             www.aoc.org
The staff and volunteers of the AIDS Outreach Center (AOC) provide a wide range of social services, outreach activities, testing and counseling, prevention education programs and public policy advocacy for men, women and children living with HIV, and their loved ones.
Shannon Hilgart, Executive Director
Michelle Barefield, Director of Prevention, Education and Ou

291 Houston Department of Health and Human Services: Bureau of HIV Prevention
8000 N Stadium Drive   713-794-9020
Houston, TX 77054-1823   Fax: 713-798-0830
                             TTY: 713-794-9092
                             www.houstontx.gov/health
Coordinates sexually transmitted disease surveillance, seroprevalence, contract tracing partner notification, public information, minority initiatives and health evaluation/risk reduction.
Stephen L Williams, Director

292 Texas Department of Health: Bureau of HIV and STD Prevention
HIV/STD Division
PO Box 149347   512-458-7111
Austin, TX 78756-3199   888-963-7111
                             TTY: 800-735-2989
                             TDD: 512-458-7708
                             www.dshs.state.tx.us
Mission is to prevent, treat, and/or control the spread of HIV, STD, and other communicable diseases to protect the health of the citizens of Texas.
David Lakey, Commissioner

Utah

293 Utah Department of Health: Bureau of Communicable Disease Control
Division of Epidemiology & Laboratory Services
288 N 1460 W   801-538-6129
Salt Lake City, UT 84114-2105 800-537-1046
                             Fax: 801-538-9923
                       e-mail: rrolfs@utah.gov
                             www.health.utah.gov/cdc
Secures and distributes funds for AIDS prevention services, provides educational programs and counseling to the general public, AIDS service organizations, health workers and groups at risk.
Teresa Garrett , MS, RN, Division Director, Chief Public Health N
Tamara Hampton, Administrative Assistant

Vermont

294 Vermont Department of Health: Health Surveillance HIV/AIDS/STD/TB Program
108 Cherry Street   802-863-7200
Burlington, VT 05402-0070   800-464-4343
                                        Fax: 802-865-7754
                                        TTY: 802-863-7235
                                        www.healthvermont.gov
Provides health education and risk reduction activities nurses and other professional training, AIDS presentations, educational and media campaigns and counseling and referrals.
Rod Copeland PhD, Director HIV/AIDS Program

Virginia

295 Virginia Department of Health: Division of HIV, STD, and Pharmacy Services
109 Governor Street   804-786-6267
Richmond, VA 23219   800-533-4148
                                        Fax: 804-786-7528
                                        e-mail: hiv-stdhotline@vdh.virginia.gov.
                                        www.vdh.virginia.gov
Supports local health departments and community-based organizations in the prevention, surveillance and treatment of HIV and other STD's, including their complications, through provision of education, information, and health care services.
Casey Riley, Director
Ashley Carter, HIV/STD Data and Statistics

Washington

296 Northwest AIDS Education and Training Center (AETC)
901 Boren Avenue   206-685-0198
Seattle, WA 98104   Fax: 206-221-4945
                                        e-mail: mfa4@u.washington.edu
                                        http://depts.washington.edu/nwaetc/
Located at the University of Washington, offering HIV treatment education, clinical consultation, capacity building and technical assistance to health care professionals and agencies in Washington, Alaska, Montana, Idaho, and Oregon.
Mary Annese, MPA, Evaluator
Laurie Conratt MBA, Director

297 Washington Department of Health: Division of HIV/AIDS Prevention Services
HIV Client Services
PO Box 47840   360-236-3434
Olympia, WA 98504-7840   877-376-9316
                                        Fax: 360-236-3400
                                        e-mail: brown.mcdonald@doh.wa.gov
                                        www.doh.wa.gov/cfh/HIV_AIDS/Prev_Edu
Provides information and referrals to local, state and national resources relating to HIV/AIDS provides informational and educational materials to individuals, agencies and organizations and actively works with print and broadcast media to promote HIV/AIDS awareness.
Paul Brown, HIV Data Manager
Brown McDonald, HIV Prevention Services Manager

West Virginia

298 West Virginia Department of Health & Human Resources
HIV/AIDS & STD Program
One Davis Square   304-558-0684
Charleston, WV 25301-3715   800-352-6513
                                        Fax: 304-558-1130
                                        e-mail: wvdhhrsecretary@wvdhhr.org
                                        www.wvdhhr.org
Provides the AIDS-related services in 15 public health HIV-counseling and testing centers which offer by appointment confidential or anonymous testing.
Martha Yeage Walker, Secretary

Wisconsin

299 Wisconsin Department of Health and Social Services: Division of Health
HIV/AIDS/Hepatitis Program

1 West Wilson Street   608-266-1865
Madison, WI 53703   877-865-3432
                                        Fax: 608-267-2832
                                        TTY: 888-701-1251
                                        e-mail: DHSwebmaster@wisconsin.gov
                                        www.dhs.wisconsin.gov
Coordinates counseling and testing sites activities and services to HIV-infected persons, produces a report that contains information and recommendations for health care workers, emergency medical technicians and food service workers.
Seth Foldy, Administrator and State Health Officer
Thomas Sieger, Deputy Administrator

Wyoming

300 Wyoming Department of Health HIV/AIDS/Hepatitis Program
HIV/AIDS/Hepatitis Program
401 Hathaway Building   307-777-7656
Cheyenne, WY 82002-0001   866-571-0944
                                        Fax: 307-777-7439
                                        www.health.wyo.gov
100 percent federally funded and responsible for the solicitation development and implementation of community AIDS prevention initiatives.
Thomas O. Forslund, Director and State Health Officer
Lee Clabbots, Deputy Director

Foundations

301 National Hemophilia Foundation
116 West 32nd Street   212-328-3700
New York, NY 10001   800-42H-ANDI
                                        Fax: 212-328-3777
                                        e-mail: handi@hemophilia.org
                                        www.hemophilia.org
The National Hemophilia Foundation is dedicated to finding better treatments and cures for bleeding and clotting disorders and to preventing the complications of these disorders through education, advocacy and research.
Jorge De la Riva, Chair
Ken Trader, Vice Chair

Libraries & Resource Centers

302 AIDS Library of Philadelphia
1233 Locust Street   215-985-4851
Philadelphia, PA 19107   Fax: 215-985-4492
                                        e-mail: library@aidslibrary.org
                                        www.aidslibrary.org
Improving access to health and support services, preventing HIV transmission, and raising the public awareness of HIV/AIDS related issues.
Allie Frase, Collection Management Librarian
Ben Remsen, Public Services

303 National Library of Medicine
8600 Rockville Pike   301-594-5983
Bethesda, MD 20894   888-346-3656
                                        Fax: 301-402-1384
                                        TDD: 800-735-2258
                                        e-mail: custserv@nlm.nih.gov
                                        www.nlm.nih.gov/
The National Library of Medicine (NLM), on the campus of the National Institutes of Health in Bethesda, Maryland, is the world's largest medical library. The Library collects materials in all areas of biomedicine and health care, as well as works on biomedical aspects of technology, the humanities, and the physical, life, and social sciences.
Dr Donald Lindberg, Director
Betsy L Humphreys, Deputy Director

Research Centers

304 CDC National Prevention Information Network (NPIN)
PO Box 6003   404-679-3860
Rockville, MD 20849-6003   800-458-5231
                                     Fax: 888-282-7681
                                     TTY: 800-243-7012
                                     e-mail: info@cdcnpin.org
                                     www.cdcnpin.org
The CDC National Prevention Information Network (NPIN) is the
U.S. reference, referral, and distribution service for information
on HIV/AIDS, sexually transmitted diseases (STDs), and tuberculosis (TB). NPIN produces, collects, catalogs, processes, stocks,
and disseminates materials and information on HIV/AIDS, STDs,
and TB to organizations and people working in those disease fields
in international, national, state, and local settings.
Kevin Fetnton, director
hazel D. Dean, Deputy Director

Alabama

**305 Centers for AIDS Research: University of Alabama at
Birmingham**
BBRB 256
Birmingham, AL 35294-1150   205-934-4011
                                    http://www.uab.edu
Provides expertise, resources, and services not otherwise readily
obtained through traditional funding mechanisms.
Robert P. Kimberly, Director
Cheryl A. Perry, Deputy Director

306 General Clinical Research Center: UAB
Room 907 Medical Education Building   205-934-4852
Birmingham, AL 35294   e-mail: ccts@uab.edu
                                        www.ccts.uab.org
AIDS and genetics research.
Burt Nabors, MD, Director
Stuart Frank, Co-Principal Investigator

**307 University of Alabama at Birmingham: National Cooperative
Drug/AIDS**
UAB Center for AIDS Research
BBRB 256
Birmingham, AL 35294-1150   205-934-4011
                                    http://www.uab.edu

Robert P. Kimberly, Director
Cheryl A. Perry, Deputy Director

California

308 AIDS Clinical Trials Unit CARES Clinic
CARES Clinic
2315 Stocktown blvd.   916-734-2011
Sacramento, CA 95817   800-2 U- DAV
                                    Fax: 916-325-1955
                                    e-mail: actu@ucdavis.edu
                                    www.ucdmc.ucdavis.edu/actu
The ACTU at Davis Medical Center is dedicated to offering the lat-
est in research clinical trials to HIV/AIDS patients throughout
Northern Central California.
Thomas S. Nesbitt, Vice Chancellor
david A Acosta, Associate Vice Chancellor

309 Adult Research Opportunities
220 Dickinson Street   619-543-8080
San Diego, CA 92103-8208   Fax: 619-543-5066
                                    www.avrctrials.org
A university-based nonprofit clinical trials unit. Conduct's pa-
tient-oriented research and educational programs on HIV and
other chronic infections. Studies have pioneered the development
of treatments that continue to change the course of the HIV
epidemic.
Constance Benson, Director
Richard S Garfein, Professor and Chairman

**310 Center for AIDS Prevention Studies AIDS Research Institute
University of C**
AIDS Research Institute, University of California

50 Beale Street   415-597-9100
San Francisco, CA 94105   Fax: 415-597-9213
                                    e-mail: CAPS.Web@ucsf.edu
                                    www.caps.ucsf.edu
The mission of the Center for AIDS Prevention Studies is to con-
duct domestic and international research to prevent the acquisition
of HIV and to optimize health outcomes among HIV-infected
individuals.
Stephen F Morin, Director
Susan Kegeles, Co-Director

**311 Center for Interdisciplinary Research in Immunology and
Diseases at UCLA**
UCLA School of Medicine
924 Westwood Blvd. #545
Los Angeles, CA 90095   310-825-6373
                                    dgsom.healthsciences.ucla.edu
Research into immunology and blood disorders with special focus
on AIDS and HIV infections.
Albert Glover, Director, Academic Affairs

312 Centers for AIDS Research: North-Central California
UC Davis, Division of Infectious Diseases
4150 V Street   916-734-8033
Sacramento, CA 95817   Fax: 916-734-7766
                                    e-mail: nccfar@ucdavis.edu
                                    www.ucdmc.ucdavis.edu/nccfar
Provides expertise resources and services not otherwise readily
obtained through more traditional funding mechanisms.
Richard B Pollard, Division Chief
Krystin E Cheung, Director

313 Centers for AIDS Research: USCD Center for AIDS Research
Center for AIDS Research
9500 Gilman Drive   858-534-5545
La Jolla, CA 92093-0716   Fax: 858-822-5840
                                    e-mail: cfar@ucsd.edu
                                    cfar.ucsd.edu
Provides expertise resources and services and services not other-
wise readily obtained through traditional funding mechanisms.
Douglas Richman, Director
Kim Schafer, Administrative Director

314 Centers for AIDS Research: University of California, Los Angeles
UCLA AIDS Institute
10940 Wilshire Blvd.   310-794-4419
Los Angeles, CA 90024-1678   Fax: 310-794-3955
                                    e-mail: ebayrd@mednet.ucla.edu
                                    www.uclaaidsinstitute.org
Provides expertise, resources, and services not otherwise readily
obtained through traditional funding mechanisms.
Irvin S.Y. Chen, Director
Dr. Thomas Coates, Associate Director

**315 City of Hope National Medical Center Drug Discover/AIDS
Group**
City of Hope
1500 E Duarte Road
Duarte, CA 91010   626-256-4673
                                    www.cityofhope.org
Developmental research into the treatment of AIDS.
Michael A Friedman MD, CEO
Robert Stone, President

316 Kaiser Foundation Research Institute
2000 Broadway
Oakland, CA 94612   510-891-3400
                                    www.dor.kaiser.org
Tracy A Lieu, Director
Alyce Adams, Health Care Delivery and policy

317 Stanford University General Clinical Research Center
GCRC Administration
300 Pasteur Drive   650-723-4000
Stanford, CA 94305-5251   Fax: 650-725-6698
                                    e-mail: gcrcstanford@stanford.edu
                                    www.med.stanford.edu/gcrc
The Stanford General Clinical Research Center (GCRC) is the ma-
jor clinical research facility for Stanford University School of
Medicine. With patient care units in Stanford University Hospital

and Lucile Packard Children's Hospital the center plays a crucial role in the school's bench-to-bedside research mission.
Ellen Jo Baron, Director
Branimir I Sikic, Program Director

318   Stanford University National Cooperative Drug Discovery/AIDS Group
School of Medicine
300 Pasteur Drive   650-723-4000
Stanford, CA 94305   Fax: 650-725-6698
                              e-mail: gcrcstanford@stanford.edu
                                          www.med.stanford.edu

Ellen Jo Baron, Director
Branimir I Sikic, Program Director

319   UCLA AIDS Clinical Research Center
1399 S Roxbury Drive   310-557-2273
Los Angeles, CA 90035   Fax: 310-557-3450
                                          www.uclacarecenter.org
Dr.A Eugene, Chancellor
David T Feinberg, President

320   UCSD Antiviral Research Center
220 Dickinson Street   619-543-8080
San Diego, CA 92103-8208   Fax: 619-543-5066
                                          www.avrctrials.org
Develops treatment protocols and drug therapies and recruits research volunteers for AIDS studies and HIV related disorders.
Jill Kunkel, Director
Michael Giancola, Screening Co-ordinator

321   USC Internal Medicine
1520 San Pablo Street
Los Angeles, CA 90033-1034   800-872-2273
                                       Fax: 213-224-6687
                                          www.usc.edu/health/internal
Research into internal medicine with specialties in cardiovascular endocrinology and diabetes gastrointestinal and liver disease geriatric medicine hematology infectious diseases nephrology oncology pulmonary and critical care and rheumatology and immunology.
Alexandra Levine, Head

322   University of California San Francisco Center for AIDS Prevention
Center for AIDS Prevention Studies (CAPS)
50 Beale Street   415-597-9100
San Francisco, CA 94105-3411   Fax: 415-597-9213
                                       e-mail: CAPS.web@ucsf.edu
                                          www.caps.ucsf.edu
The mission of the Center for AIDS Prevention Studies is to conduct domestic and international research to prevent the acquisition of HIV and to optimize health outcomes among HIV- infected individuals.
Stephen F Morin, Director
Susan Kegeles, Co-Director

323   University of California: Institute of Health Policy Studies
513 Parnassus Avenue   415-476-9000
San Francisco, CA 94143-410   Fax: 415-476-0705
                                       e-mail: claire.brindis@ucsf.edu
                                          www.ihps.medschool.ucsf.edu
Health policy and AIDS research.
Susan Desmond-Hellman, Chancellor
Phillip R. Lee, director

Colorado

324   Centers for AIDS Research: University of Colorado Health Sciences Center
Colorado Center for AIDS Research
4200 East 9th Avenue   303-315-7233
Denver, CO 80262   Fax: 303-315-8681
                                       e-mail: colorado.cfar@uchsc.edu
                                          www.uchsc.edu/ccfar
Describes forms and patterns of use of complimentary and alternative medicine (CAM) for the treatment of HIV/AIDS.
Robert T. Schooley, Director

District of Columbia

325   George Washington National Cooperative: Drug Discovery/AIDS Treatment
Department of Pharmacology & Physiology
2300 Eye Street NW   202-994-3541
Washington, DC 20037-2336   Fax: 202-994-2870
                                       e-mail: phmsmc@gwumc.edu
                                          www.gwumc.edu/pharm
Studies and researches natural products and synthetic anti-AIDS agents.
Susan Ceryak, Associate Research Professor
Jian-Zhong Guo, Associate Research Professor

326   Whitman Walker Clinic AIDS/Medical Services Programs
1701 14th Street NW   202-745-7000
Washington, DC 20009-3840   Fax: 202-745-0238
                                       e-mail: info@wwc.org
                                          www.wwc.org
A non-profit community-based health organization serving the Washington D.C. metropolitan region. Established by and for the gay and lesbian community our clinic is comprised of diverse volunteers and staff who provide or facilitate the delivery of high quality comprehensive accessible health care and community services. Especially committed to ending the suffering of all those infected and affected by HIV/AIDS.
Adam Falcone, Chair
June Crenshaw, Vice Chair

Florida

327   Department of Epidemiology and Health Policy Research: University of Florida
1329 SW 16th Street   352-265-8035
Gainesville, FL 32608   Fax: 352-265-8047
                                       e-mail: rdarbelles.ichp.ufl.edu
                                          www.ehpr.ufl.edu
Studies into child and adolescent health financing and organization of health care delivery systems community health chronic conditions transition from pediatric to adult health care access to health care for vulnerable populations quality of life and outcomes research.
Clifford J Crook, Chair
John C Bierly, Program Assistant

328   Tampa Bay Research Institute
10900 Roosevelt Boulevard N   727-576-6675
Saint Petersburg, FL 33716-2308   Fax: 727-577-9862
                              e-mail: development@tampabayresearch.org
                                          www.tampabayresearch.org
TBRI is the first independent biomedical research organization of its kind in Florida. Our scientists dedicate their lives work to conquering chronic and infectious diseases while gaining a better understanding of the immune system.
Clifford J Crook, Chair
John C Bierly, Program Assistant

329   University of South Florida Center for HIV Education and Research
13301 Bruce B Downs Boulevard   813-974-4430
Tampa, FL 33612-3807   866-352-2382
                                       Fax: 813-974-8451
                                       e-mail: Contact@FCAETC.org
                                          www.usfcenter.org
Serves health care professionals throughout Florida by providing education and information on the transmission control treatment and prevention of HIV and AIDS and by conducting related research and community outreach.
jeffery beal, Director
Debbie Cestaro, Project Co-ordinator

Georgia

330   AIDS School Health Education Database Centers for Disease Control
Centers for Disease Control

1600 Clifton Road
Atlanta, GA 30333
404-639-3534
800-232-4636
TTY: 888-232-6348
e-mail: cdcinfo@cdc.gov
www.cdc.gov

An information awareness resource produced by the Division of Adolescent and School Health. The database offers descriptions of various educational resources for professionals relevant to the education of children and youth about HIV infection and AIDS.
Thomas R. Frieden, Director
Ileana Arias, Principal Deputy Director

331 Center for AIDS Research: Emory University Rollins School of Public Health
1518 Clifton Road NE
Atlanta, GA 30322-4201
404-727-2924
Fax: 404-727-9853
e-mail: cfar@emory.edu
www.cfar.emory.edu

Provides expertise resources and services not otherwise readily obtained through more traditional funding mechanisms.
James W Curran, Director
Carlos del Rio, Co-Director for Clinical Science

332 Educational Materials Database Centers for Disease Control
Centers for Disease Control
1600 Clifton Road
Atlanta, GA 30333-4201
404-639-3534
800-232-4636
TTY: 888-232-6348
e-mail: cdcinfo@cdc.gov
www.cdc.gov

An information awareness resource produced by the Division of Adolescent and School Health. The database offers descriptions of various educational resources for professionals relevant to the education of children and youth about HIV infection and AIDS.
Thomas R. Frieden, Director
Ileana Arias, Principal Deputy Director

333 Emory University: National Cooperative Drug Discovery for AIDS Treatment
Emory Healthcare Pediatrics Department
201 Dowman Drive
Atlanta, GA 30322
404-727-6123
Fax: 404-727-5737
www.pediatrics.emory.edu

Barbara J Stoll MD, Professor, Chair
James W Wagner, President

334 Funding Database Centers for Disease Control
Centers for Disease Control
1600 Clifton Road
Atlanta, GA 30333
404-639-3534
800-232-4636
TTY: 888-232-6348
e-mail: cdcinfo@cdc.gov
www.cdc.gov

A listing of HIV and AIDS related funding opportunities for community-based and HIV and AIDS service organizations.
Thomas Friedman MD, Director
Harold Jaffe, MD, MA, Associate Director of Science

Illinois

335 Clinical Research Center Northwestern Center for Clinical Researc
Northwestern Center for Clinical Research
633 Clark Street,
Chicago, IL 60611
312-503-8649
e-mail: nucats@northwestern.edu
www.nucats.northwestern.edu

Colleen De Luca, Associate Director, Administration
Philip Greenland, Director

Indiana

336 Purdue University Center for AIDS Research
School of Pharmacy and Pharmaceutical Sciences
575 Stadium Mall Drive
W Lafayette, IN 47907-2091
765-494-1361
Fax: 765-494-7880
e-mail: oss@pharmacy.purdue.edu
www.pharmacy.purdue.edu

Steve Byrn, Department Head
Stanley L Hem, Associate Department Head

Maryland

337 Center for AIDS Research: Johns Hopkins University School of Medicine
733 N. Broadway
Baltimore, MD 21205-2196
410-955-3182
www.hopkinsmedicine.org/aidsresearch

Provides expertise resources and services not otherwise readily obtained through more traditional funding mechanisms.
Ronald R Peterson, ,President, JHH/HS
Edward D Miller, MD, Dean, CEO

338 Johns Hopkins University: Center for Communication Programs
Johns Hopkins Bloomberg School of Public Health
111 Market Place
Baltimore, MD 21202
410-659-6300
Fax: 410-659-6266
e-mail: info@jhuccp.org
www.jhuccp.org

Health communications family planning and AIDS prevention research.
Susan Krenn, Director
James bon tempo, Associate Director of Communican Science

339 University of Maryland Center for Research, Grants & Contracts
Family Studies Depatrment
1142 School of Public Health
College Park, MD 20742
301-405-3672
Fax: 301-314-9161
e-mail: fmst@umd.edu
www.hhp.umd.edu/FMST

Erin McClure, Co-ordinator
Doris Richardson, business Manager

340 University of Maryland Center for Studies Family Studies Depatrment
1142 School of Public Health
College Park, MD 20742
301-405-3672
Fax: 301-314-9161
e-mail: fmsc@umd.edu
www.sph.umd.edu/fmsc

Erin McClure, Co-ordinator
Doris Richardson, business Manager

341 University of Maryland: Medical Biotechnology Center
701 E. PRATT ST,
Baltimore, MD 21202-1513
410-706-8802
Fax: 410-706-8184
e-mail: hill@UMCES.edu
www.umbi.umd.edu

Offers research into AIDS and HIV infection including vaccine development.
W Jonathan Lederer, Director
Kadir Aslan, Assistant Professor

Massachusetts

342 Center for AIDS Research: Harvard Medical School, Division of AIDS
The Landmark Buiding
104 Mt. Auburn Street
Cambridge, MA 02138
617-384-9039
Fax: 617-495-8231
e-mail: aids@hms.harvard.edu
aids.med.harvard.edu/cfar.htm

Provides expertise resources and services not otherwise readily obtained through traditional funding mechanisms.
Bruce Walker, Director
Myron Essex, Associate Director

343 Center for Blood Research Harvard Medical School/CBR
Harvard Medical School/CBR
200 Longwood Avenue
Boston, MA 02115
617-278-3140
Fax: 617-278-3131
e-mail: kirchhausen@crystal.harvard.edu
www.idi.harvard.edu

Offers research into blood disorders including multidisciplinary studies on AIDS and hemophilia cancer and diabetes research as well.
Fredrick Alt, President/ Director
Stephen Carriuolo, Financial Manager

344 Centers for AIDS Research: University of Massachusetts Medical School
364 Plantation Street
Worcester, MA 01605
508-856-3159
e-mail: publicaffairs@umassmed.edu
www.umassmed.edu/cfar
Provides expertise, resources, and services not otherwise readily obtained through traditional funding mechanisms.
celia Schiffer, Director
Shan Lu, Co-Director

345 Dana Farber Cancer Institute National Drug Discovery Group for AIDS Treatment
Dana-Farber Cancer Institute
450 Brookline Avenue
Boston, MA 02215-5450
617-632-3000
800-408-3324
TTY: 617-632-5330
TDD: 617-632-5330
e-mail: dana-farbercontactus@dfci.harvard.edu
www.dana-farber.org
Edward Benz, President and CEO
Dorthy E Puhy, Executive Vice President and COO

346 Developmental Medicine Center Children's Hospital Boston
Children's Hospital Boston
300 Longwood Avenue
Boston, MA 02115
617-355-6000
Fax: 617-730-0633
TTY: 617-730-0152
www.childrenshospital.org
Studies developmental effects of infants at risk and development effects of congenital HIV infection.
James Mandell, CEO
Sandra Fenwick, President, COO

Michigan

347 University of Michigan: National Cooperative Drug/AIDS Group
School of Dentistry
1011 N University Avenue
Ann Arbor, MI 48109-1078
734-763-6933
Fax: 734-763-3453
e-mail: paulk@umich.edu
www.dent.umich.edu
Focuses on the design of new drugs to fight AIDS.
John C Drach PhD, Director
Paul H Krebsbach, Department Chair

348 Wayne State University Center for Health Research
College of Nursing
Center for Health Research
Detroit, MI 48202
313-577-4082
888-837- 08
Fax: 313-577-6949
e-mail: nursinginfo@wayne.edu
www.nursing.wayne.edu/CHR
Facilitates interdisciplinary health research across diverse settings where nursing is practiced and healthcare is provided.
Nancy T Artinian, Director
Barbara K Redman, Dean

New York

349 Aaron Diamond AIDS Research Center
455 First Avenue
New York, NY 10016
212-448-5000
Fax: 212-725-1126
e-mail: webinfo@adarc.org
www.adarc.org
Committed to finding solutions to end the AIDS epidemic. In the decade and a half since HIV was identified researchers have learned more about this virus than about any other in history.
David Ho, Director & CEO
Gerald Friedland MD, Chairman

350 Centers for AIDS Research: Albert Einstein College of Medicine
Albert Einstein College of Medicine
Jack and Pearl Resnick Campus
Bronx, NY 10461
718-430-2000
Fax: 718-430-2374
e-mail: information@einstein.yu.edu
www.aecom.yu.edu/cfar
Provides consultation and support to the medical and research community in the scientific evaluation of CAM therapies.
Allen M Spiegel MD, Dean
Matthew Scharff MD, CFAR Investigator

351 Centers for AIDS Research: Columbia University College of Physicians
Center for AIDS Research
630 W 168th Street
New York, NY 10032
212-305-1296
e-mail: jka8@columbia.edu
www.cumc.columbia.edu
Provides a comprehensive framework for training educational programs and research which addresses health promotion disease prevention symptom management and quality of life for individuals with HIV. The goal of the Center is to create innovative research and service approaches for the prevention and management of HIV. This objective is fulfilled through research program development and program evaluations.
Lee Goldman MD, Executive Vice President
Lee Bollinger, JD, President of the University

352 Centers for AIDS Research: NYU School of Medicine
522 First Avenue
New York, NY 10016
212-263-8527
e-mail: zinszh01@med.nyu.edu
www.hivinfosource.org/hivis/cfar
Provides expertise resources and services not otherwise readily obtained through traditional funding mechanisms.
Derya Unutmanz MD, Director
David levy, Associate Dean

353 General Clinical Research Center Mount Sinai School of Medicine
Mount Sinai School of Medicine
One Gustave L Levy Place
New York, NY 10029-6574
212-241-6500
Fax: 212-348-5811
e-mail: hugh.sampson@mssm.edu
www.mssm.edu/gcrc
Focuses on AIDS education and prevention.
Dennis S Charney, Executive Vice President
Kennith Davis, President

354 HIV Center for Clinical and Behavioral Studies
1051 Riverside Drive
New York, NY 10032
212-543-5969
Fax: 212-543-6003
e-mail: whiteme@pi.cpmc.comlumbia.edu
www.hivcenternyc.org
Interdisciplinary research center that investigates the behavioral causes and consequences of HIV/AIDS. Focusing on the intersections of HIV infection gender and sexuality; treatment strategies for infected populations; and innovative dissemination of scientific findings.
Anke A Ehrhardt, Director
Heino F L Meyer-Bahlbur, Associate Director

355 Institute for Clinical Research Weill Cornell Medical College
Weill Cornell Medical College
1300 York Avenue
New York, NY 10065
212-746-5454
Fax: 212-746-8970
e-mail: cto@med.cornell.edu
www.med.cornell.edu
The mission of the ICR is to support, advance and promote clinical and translational research enterprises at WCMC. As part of Research and Sponsored Programs (RASP) the ICR streamlines the clinical research process and offers a wide range of services, resources and training.
David J Skorton MD, President of the University
Michelle A Lewis, MS, Director (Research and Sponsored Program

356 SUNY at Buffalo National Cooperative Drug Discovery Group for AIDS Treatment
Department of Biochemistry
140 Farber Hall
Buffalo, NY 14214-3000
716-829-2727
Fax: 716-829-2725
e-mail: jluck@buffalo.edu
www.buffalo.edu
Kenneth M Blumenthal, Professor and Chairman
Elizabeth O'Brocta, Assistant to the Chairman

357 Spellman Center for HIV Related Disease The Spellman Center
The Spellman Center
415 W Fifty-First Street
New York, NY 10019
212-459-8130
www.stclaresny.org
David Kaufman, Director

358 State University of New York: SUNY Stony HIV Treatment Development Center
Center for Infectious Diseases
101 Nicolls Road   631-444-4000
Stony Brook, NY 11794-5120   Fax: 631-444-2493
                    e-mail: rsteigbigel@notes.cc.sunysb.edu
                            www.stonybrookmedicalcenter.org
Human immunodeficiency virus research.
Joyce Klien, Director
Laura Coppola, Assistant Director

North Carolina

359 Centers for AIDS Research: Univeristy of North Carolina at Chapel Hill
UNC Center For AIDS Research
Lineberger Cancer Center   919-966-8645
Chapel Hill, NC 27599   e-mail: cfar@med.unc.edu
                                                    cfar.med.unc.edu
Administrative and shared research support to synergistically enhance and coordinate high quality AIDS research projects.
Ronald Swanstrom, Director
Myron S Cohen, Associate Director

Ohio

360 Centers for AIDS Research: Case Western University
Department of Medicine
Division of Infectious Diseases   216-368-0271
Cleveland, OH 44106-5029   Fax: 216-368-3055
                                      e-mail: mxl6@case.edu
                                      www.clevelandactu.org
Provides administrative and shared research support to enhance and coordinate high quality AIDS research projects.
Michael M Lederman, Co-Director
Jonathan Karn, Associate Director

Pennsylvania

361 Centers for AIDS Research: University of Pennsylvania
Penn Center for AIDS Research
295 John Morgan Building   215-573-7354
Philadelphia, PA 19104-6140   Fax: 215-573-7356
                    e-mail: oliviere@mail.med.upenn.edu
                                            www.med.upenn.edu
Also the Children's Hospital and the Wistar Institute provides important services and research for high quality projects.
James A Hoxie, Director
Ronald G Collman, Co-Director

362 Temple University Clinical Research Center Office of Clinical Research
Office of Clinical Research
Medical Education and Research Buil   215-707-7000
Philadelphia, PA 19140   Fax: 215-201-2684
                                          e-mail: tusm@temple.edu
                                          www.temple.edu/medicine
CRC Unit provides space to perform clinical research on 4 West of Temple University Hospital. The CRC Unit has the potential for three rooms for inpatient/outpatient studies and an additional room for outpatient studies.
Antonio Giorgio MD, President

363 Thomas Jefferson University: Center for Research in Medical Education
Jefferson Medical College
1020 Walnut Street   215-955-6000
Philadelphia, PA 19107   Fax: 215-923-7583
                    e-mail: Joseph.Gonnella@jefferson.edu
                                            www.jefferson.edu/jmc
Joseph Gonne MD, Director
Robert L Barchi MD, President

Rhode Island

364 Centers for AIDS Research: Brown University
The Miriam Hospital

CFAR/RISE Building   401-793-4068
Providence, RI 02906   Fax: 401-793-4704
                          e-mail: vgodleski@lifespan.org
                                            www.lifespan.org/cfar
Provides expertise resources and services not otherwise readily obtained through traditional funding mechanisms.
Charles C J Carpenter, Director
Susan Cu-Uvin, HIV and Women Core Co-Director

South Carolina

365 Medical University of South Carolina Health Services Administration
Medical University of South Carolina
171 Ashley Avenue   843-792-1414
Charleston, SC 29425   800-424-6872
                                              Fax: 843-792-2601
                                                    www.musc.edu
Devoted to public health policy and health care management including AIDS research.
Raymond S Greenburg, President
Dr. Mark Sothman, Vice President

Tennessee

366 Centers for AIDS Research: Vanderbilt University Medical Center
Division of Infectious Disease
1161 21st Avenue S   615-322-8972
Nashville, TN 37232-2582 e-mail: richard.daquila@vanderbilt.edu
                                      www.mc.vanderbilt.edu/cfar
Provides expertise resources and services not otherwise readily obtained through more traditional funding mechanisms.
Richard D' Aquila, Director
G Fatima Lima Ph.D., Associate Director

Texas

367 Centers for AIDS Research: Baylor College of Medicine
Department of Molecular Virology & Microbiology
One Baylor Plaza   713-798-3006
Houston, TX 77030   Fax: 713-798-5019
                                          e-mail: jbutel@bcm.edu
                                                www.bcm.edu/cfar
A research center that is a branch of the Centers for AIDS Research.
Janet S Butel, Director
William T Shearer, Co-Director

Vermont

368 University of Vermont: Office of Health Promotion Research
1 S Prospect Street   802-656-4187
Burlington, VT 05401   Fax: 802-656-8826
                                              e-mail: ohpr@uvm.edu
                                              www.uvm.edu/~ohpr
Research done into public policy and human health including AIDS information and evaluation.
Anne L Dorwaldt, Assistant Director
Rachael Chicoine, AAS, Research Project Assistant

Washington

369 Centers for AIDS Research: University of Washington, Harborview Medical Center
Center For AIDS & STDs
325 Ninth Avenue   206-744-4239
Seattle, WA 98104-2499   Fax: 206-744-3693
                    e-mail: worthy@u.washington.edu
                                    www.depts.washington.edu/cfas
Provides administrative and shared research support to synergistically enhance and coordinate high quality AIDS research projects. CFARs accomplish this through core facilities that provide expertise resource and services not otherwise readily obtained through more traditional funding mechanisms.
King K Holmes, Director
Mary Fielder, Assistant to the Director

370 **HIV Prevention Trials Unit University of Washington/Seattle HPTU Si**
University of Washington/Seattle HPTU Site
Cabrini Medical Tower 901 Boren Av   206-520-3800
Seattle, WA 98104   Fax: 206-520-3801
e-mail: hptu@u.washington.edu
www.depts.washington.edu
A worldwide collaborative clinical trials network established by
the National Institutes of Health (NIH) to evaluate the safety and
efficacy of non-vaccine prevention interventions alone or in combination using HIV incidence as the primary endpoint.
Connie Celum, Principal Investigator

Support Groups & Hotlines

371 **AEGIS AIDS Education Global Information System**
PO Box 184   949-495-1952
San Juan Capistrano, CA 92693   Fax: 949-443-1755
e-mail: comments@aegis.org
www.aegis.org
A not-for-profit, tax-exempt, educational corpoation that adds
more than 3000 documents each month. Reach more than 10 mil-
lion users annually, including: the US Federal Government, US
Educational Institutions, and Nonprofit organizations both here
and abroad.
Vanessa Robison, President
Sister Mary Elizabeth, Assistant Operations Director

372 **AIDS Alabama**
3521 7th Avenue S   205-324-9822
Birmingham, AL 35222   800-592-2437
Fax: 205-324-9311
e-mail: maryanne@aidsalabama.org
www.aidsalabama.org
Devotes its energy and resources statewide to helping people with
HIV/AIDS live healthy, independent lives and works to prevent
the spread of HIV. It is our goal to provide housing for those with
HIV in the Birmingham area, secure and administer grants for care
of persons with HIV statewide, and specialize in targeted preven-
tion education programs.
Elaine Cottle, Executive Director

373 **AIDS Hotline of Central New York**
AIDS Community Resources
627 W Genesee Street   315-475-2430
Syracuse, NY 13204   800-475-2430
Fax: 315-472-6515
e-mail: information@aidscommunityresources.com
www.aidscommunityresources.com
A not-for-profit, community-based organization providing prevention, education and support services to those infected with and
affected by HIV/AIDS Serves Cayuga, Herkimer, Jefferson,
Lewis, Madison, Oneida, Onondaga, Oswego and St. Lawrences
counties in New York State.
Michael Crinnin, Executive Director

374 **AIDS Support Group of Cape Cod**
428 S Street   508-778-1957
Hyannis, MA 02610   866-990-2437
Fax: 508-778-4501
e-mail: info@asgcc.org
www.asgcc.org
Our mission is to provide services that maintain and enhance the
quality of life for persons living with HIV and AIDS on Cape Cod
and Martha's Vineyard and to provide health education, prevention and harm reduction outreach via timely and accurate information about HIV/AIDS, STIs and viral hepatitis.
Krystin St. Onge, Interim Director

375 **AIDSinfo**
US Department of Health and Human Services
PO Box 6303   301-315-2816
Rockville, MD 20849-6303   800-448-0440
Fax: 301-315-2818
TTY: 888-480-3739
e-mail: contactus@aidsinfo.nih.gov
www.aidsinfo.nih.gov
Offers the latest federally approved information on HIV/AIDS
clinical research, treatment and prevention, and medical practice
guidelines for people living with HIV/AIDS, their families and
friends, health care providers, scientists, and researchers.

376 **Alaskan Statewide AIDS Helpline**
1057 W Fireweed   907-263-2050
Anchorage, AK 99503   800-478-AIDS
Fax: 907-263-2051
www.alaskanaids.org
A key collaborator within the state of Alaska in the provision of
supportive services to persons living with HIV/AIDS and their
families and in the elimination of the transmission of HIV infection and its stigma.
Heather Davis, Executive Director
Maureen Suttman, Client Resource Services

377 **BABES Network-YWCA**
1118 Fifth Ave   206-720-5566
Seattle, WA 98101   888-292-1912
Fax: 206-720-5901
e-mail: the_staff@babesnetwork.org
www.babesnetwork.org
A peer-based program, a sisterhood of women facing HIV together.
Reduces isolation, promotes self-empowerment, enhances quality
of life and serves the needs of women facing HIV and their families
through peer support, advocacy, education and outreach
Rhonda Kimm, Advocacy Coordinator
Amelia Vader, Program Manager

378 **COMPASS Program**
c/o Institute for Urban Family Health
16 East 16th Street   212-924-7744
New York, NY 10003   Fax: 212-691-4610
e-mail: info@institute2000.org
www.institute2000.org/health/rwp.htm
Medical services include HIV testing and specialized HIV medical
care for adults in addition to women's health services including gynecology, PAP tests, family planning and birth control methods.
Mental health services includes individual, couples, and family
counseling and psychiatric evaluations and monitoring.
Neil Calman MD/ABFP/FAAFP, President/Chief Executive Officer
Weston Willett, Chief Information Officer

379 **Cascade AIDS Project Hotline**
200 SW Fifth Avenue   503-223-5907
Portland, OR 97204   Fax: 503-223-6437
e-mail: info@cascadeaids.org
www.cascadeaids.org
Provides HIV prevention and services information by phone and
internet to youth and adults across Orgeon and the Northwest.
Charles Washington, President
warren Jimanez, Vice President

380 **Dunshee House**
303-17th Avenue East   206-322-2437
Seattle, WA 98112   Fax: 206-322-1779
e-mail: josh@dunsheehouse.org
www.dunsheehouse.org
A non-profit organization, builds community and cultivates powerful, healthy lives by providing emotional support and personal
development services to those affected by HIV/AIDS, the Queer
communities, and those who love them.
Michael Kann, President
Adrienne Miller, Vice President

381 **HEAL**
Sidney Hillman Family Pracitce
16 E 16th Street   212-924-7744
New York, NY 10003-3105   e-mail: healweb@thorup.com
www.thorup.com/HEAL
The Health Education AIDS Liaison provides alternative and holistic support groups and resources for people with HIV.

382 **HIV/AIDS Prevention Program**
Centers for Disease Control and Prevention
1600 Clifton Road   404-639-3534
Atlanta, GA 30333   800-232-4636
TTY: 888-232-6348
e-mail: cdcinfo@cdc.gov
www.cdc.gov

An information awareness resource produced by the Division of Adolescent and School Health. The database offers descriptions of various educational resources for professionals relevant to the education of children and youth about HIV infection and AIDS.
Thomas R. Frieden, Director
Ileana Arias, Principal Deputy Director

383   Immunization Division Centers for Disease Control
1600 Clifton Road   404-639-3534
Atlanta, GA 30333-2303   800-232-4636
                                          TTY: 888-232-6348
                                    e-mail: cdcinfo@cdc.gov
                                               www.cdc.gov
An information awareness resource produced by the Division of Adolescent and School Health. The database offers descriptions of various educational resources for professionals relevant to the education of children and youth about HIV infection and AIDS.
Thomas R. Frieden, Director
Ileana Arias, Principal Deputy Director

384   King County Crisis Clinic
9725 3rdAvenue NE   206-461-3210
Seattle, WA 98115   866-427-4747
                                        Fax: 206-461-8368
                                        TDD: 206-461-3219
                                   e-mail: info@crisisclinic.org
                                           www.crisisclinic.org
A non-profit organization, we offer an array of support services available to everyone in King County, Washington.
Kathleen Southwick, Executive Director
Susan Gemmel, Director

385   Minnesota AIDS Project AIDSLine
1400 Park Avenue   612-341-2060
Minneapolis, MN 55404   800-248-7321
                                        Fax: 612-341-4057
                                        TTY: 888-820-2437
                             e-mail: mapaidsline@mnaidsproject.org
                                        www.mnaidsproject.org
A statewide, toll-free information and referral service that can answer your questions about HIV and connect you to resources that can help
Bill Tiedmann, Executive Director

386   National Health Information Center
PO Box 1133   310-565-4167
Washington, DC 20013-1133   800-336-4797
                                        Fax: 301-984-4256
                                     e-mail: info@nhic.org
                                       www.health.gov/nhic
A health information referral service sponsored by the Office of Disease Prevention and Health Promotion. NHIC puts health professionals and consumers who have health questions in touch with those organizations that are best able to provide answers.

387   Project Inform Hotline
273 Ninth Street   415-558-8669
San Francisco, CA 94103-2621   800-822-7422
                                        Fax: 415-558-0684
                               e-mail: web@projectinform.org
                                        www.projectinform.org
Represents HIV-positive people in the development of treatments and a cure, supports individuals to make informed choices about their HIV health, advocates for quality health care to respond to HIV and related conditions, and promotes medical strategies that prevent new infections.
Christopher Esposito, President
Ferdinand Garcia, Vice President

Books

388   ABC of AIDS
Michael W. Adler, author
BMJ Publishing Group

PO Box 281   800-2FO-NBMJ
Annapolis, MD 20701-0281   Fax: 800-2FA-XBMJ
                                      e-mail: bmjpg@pmds.com
                                              ww.bmjpg.com
118 pages Paperback
ISBN: 0-727915-03-7

389   AIDS & HIV Related Diseases
Harper Collins Publishers
10 East 53rd Street
New York, NY 10022   212-207-7000
                                       www.harpercollins.com
An education guide for professionals and the public which covers such topics as: Understanding HIV and its effect on the immune system; HIV transmission; The history of AIDS and HIV; HIV testing; The natural course of an HIV infection; Medical treatment and those who administer them; The people who have AIDS; AIDS education.
1996 246 pages
ISBN: 0-306450-85-2

390   AIDS & Other Manifestations of HIV Infection
Academic Press (Elsevier)
1183 Westline Industrial Drive
St Louis, MO 63146   800-545-2522
                                        Fax: 800-535-9935
                                 e-mail: usbkinfo@elsevier.com
                                           www.elsevier.com
An essential reference resource providing a comprehensive overview of the biological properties of this etiologic viral agent, its clinicopathological manifestations, the epidemiology of its infection, and present and future therapeutic options.
2004-4th Edi 1000 pages
ISBN: 0-127640-51-7
Gary Wormser, Editor

391   AIDS Alert
American Health Consultants
3525 Piedmont Road   404-262-5476
Atlanta, GA 30305   800-688-2421
                                        Fax: 800-284-3291
                                             www.ahcpub.com
The definitive source of AIDS news and advice for health care professionals. Covers up-to-the-minute developments and guidance on the entire spectrum of AIDS challenges, including treatment, education, precaustion, screening, diagnosis and policy.

392   AIDS and HIV Related Diseases
Josh Powell, author
Plenum Publishing Corporation
233 Spring Street   212-620-8000
New York, NY 10013   800-221-9369
                                        Fax: 212-463-0742
                                   e-mail: books@plenum.com
An education guide for professionals and the public which covers such topics as: Understanding HIV and its effect on the immune system; HIV transmission; The history of AIDS and HIV; HIV testing; The natural course of an HIV infection; Medical treatment and those who administer them; The people who have AIDS; AIDS education.
1996 243 pages
ISBN: 0-306450-85-2

393   AIDS and Persons with Developmental Disabilities
Commission on the Mentally Disabled
1800 M Street NW   202-331-2240
Washington, DC 20036
A discussion of federal and state laws that defines the rights and responsibilities of individuals with disabilities and service providers with respect to HIV infection.

394   AIDS in the Twenty-First Century: Disease and Globalization
Tony Barnett, Alan Whiteside, author
Palgrave Macmillan
175 Fifth Avenue   212-982-3900
New York, NY 10010   800-221-7945
                                        Fax: 212-777-6359
                                             www.palgrave.com

Presents compelling data and research which reveals the shocking social and economic impact of HIV/AIDS on a global scale
432 pages
ISBN: 1-403900-05-0

395 AIDS, Revised Edition
Alan E. Nourse, M.D., author

Franklin Watts c/o Grolier
90 Old Sherman Tpke   203-797-3500
Danbury, CT 06816   800-621-1115
                                                 Fax: 203-797-3197
                                                 www.grolier.com
This bestselling book has been updated with the latest findings and research into the AIDS epidemic. Includes new statistical information and findings on HIV and AIDS.
144 pages
ISBN: 0-531106-62-4

396 AIDS: A Communication Perspective
Lawrence Erlbaum Associates Publishers
10 Industrial Avenue   201-236-9500
Mahwah, NJ 07430-2262   Fax: 201-236-6396
                                                 www.erlbaum.com

ISBN: 0-805809-98-8

397 AIDS: Distinguishing Between Fact and Opinion
Teresa Opheim, author

Greenhaven Press
PO Box 9187
Farmington Hills, MI 48333-9187   800-877-GALE
                                                 Fax: 800-414-5043
                                                 www.galegroup.com/greenhaven
For beginning debaters, reports and classroom use this book offers three debates: Can AIDS be spread by casual contact? Should the Food and Drug Administration make AIDS drugs more available? Is AIDS a moral issue?.
36 pages
ISBN: 0-899086-33-0

398 AIDS: How it Works in the Body
Lorna Greenberg, author

Franklin Watts
96 Leonard Street   www.wattspub.co.uk
London EC2A 4XD,
For readers ages 9-12
64 pages School Binding

399 AIDS: Trading Fears for Facts: A Guide for Young People
Karen Hein, Theresa Foy Digernimo, author

Consumer Reports Books
101 Truman Avenue   www.consumerreports.org
Yonkers, NY 10703-1057
Listed for young adult readers.
232 pages Paperback
ISBN: 0-890437-21-1

400 Amfar AIDS Handbook: The Complete Guide to Understanding HIV and AIDS
Darrell Ward, author

W.W. Norton & Company, Inc.
500 Fifth Avenue   212-354-5500
New York, NY 10110   Fax: 212-869-0856
                                                 www.norton.com
Gives a greater understanding of HIV/Aids. The causes and effects, what new treatment options are being developed.
360 pages
ISBN: 0-393316-36-X

401 Black Death: AIDS in Africa
Susan Hunter, author

Macmillan
175 Fifth Avenue
New York, NY 10010   646-307-5151
                                                 us.macmillian.com
The untold story of AIDS in Africa, home to 80 percent of the 40 million people in the world currently infected with HIV. Brings the staggering statistics to life and paints for the first time a stunning picture of the most important political issue today.
256 pages
ISBN: 1-403967-17-2

402 Children and the AIDS Virus: A Book for Children, Parents, and Teachers
Rosmarie Hausherr, author

Clarion Books
For readers ages 4-8.
48 pages Library Binding
ISBN: 0-899198-34-1

403 Community Service Delivery for Children with HIV Infection and Families
Geneva, Woodruff & Christopher Hanson, author

South Shore Mental Health Center
6 Fort Street   617-847-1950
Quincy, MA 02169   e-mail: contactus@ssmh.org
                                                 www.ssmh.org
A manual providing guidelines for developing community-based, family-centered services for children with HIV infection and their families. Describes how services can be planned and delivered using guiding principles and practices of transagency case management.

404 Coping When You or a Friend is HIV-Positive
Pat Kelly, author

Hazelden Publishing & Educational Services
15251 Pleasant Valley Road   651-257-4010
Center City, MN 55012-0176   800-328-9000
                                                 Fax: 651-213-4577
                                                 e-mail: customersupport@hazeldon.org
                                                 www.hazelden.org
Provides compassionate counsel for teens who have been diagnosed with the virus.
136 pages Paperback
ISBN: 1-568381-77-8

405 Dancing Against the Darkness: A Journey Through America in the Age of AIDS
Steven Petrow, author

Rowman & Littlefield Publishing Group
4501 Forbes Blvd.   717-794-3800
Lanham, MD 20706   800-462-6420
                                                 Fax: 717-794-3803
                                                 e-mail: custserv@rowman.com
                                                 www.lexingtonbooks.com

218 pages Hardcover
ISBN: 0-669243-09-4

406 Everything You Need to Know About AIDS
Katherine White, author

Rosen Publishing Group
29 E 21st Street   212-777-3017
New York, NY 10010   800-237-9932
                                                 Fax: 888-436-4643
                                                 e-mail: customerservice@rosenpub.com
                                                 www.rosenpublishing.com
Without proper information, our teens remain at risk for AIDS. This volume presents balanced information on the disease and on safer sex precautions, in a language that readers can understand.
64 pages Library Binding
ISBN: 0-823933-14-8
Barbara Taylor, Author

407 Everything You Need to Know About Being HIV Positive
Amy Shire, author

Rosen Publishing Group
29 E 21st Street   212-777-3017
New York, NY 10010   800-237-9932
                                                 Fax: 888-436-4643
                                                 e-mail: customerservice@rosenpub.com
                                                 www.rosenpublishing.com

To teens who need to understand what thier options are when living with HIV on a day-to-day basis. This book explains the facts about HIV.
Hardcover
ISBN: 0-823926-14-1
Amy Shire, Author

408   Everything You Need to Know When a Parent has AIDS
Barbara Hermie Draimin, author

Rosen Publishing Group
29 E 21st Street   212-777-3017
New York, NY 10010   800-237-9932
                                                   Fax: 888-436-4643
                               e-mail: customerservice@rosenpub.com
                                           www.rosenpublishing.com
More and more teens have a parent who has AIDS. Teens must learn where they can turn for help in dealing with this difficult situation. By presenting stories of teens in the same situation, this book helps readers deal with their anger and grief.
64 pages Library Binding
ISBN: 0-823916-90-1
Barbara Hermie Draimin DSW, Author

409   Global AIDS: Myths and Facts, Tools for Fighting the AIDS Pandemic
Alexander Irwin, Joyce Millen, author

South End Press
7 Brookline Street   718-874-0089
Cambridge, MA 02139-4146   e-mail: info@southendpress.org
                                           www.southendpress.org
10 myths about HIV/AIDS treatment and prevention while calling for an international movement to fight the disease.
296 pages
ISBN: 0-896086-73-9

410   Guide to Living With HIV Infection
John G. Bartlett, Ann K. Finkbeiner, author

John's Hopkins University Press
2715 N Charles Street   410-516-6900
Baltimore, MD 21218-4363   800-537-5487
                                                   Fax: 410-516-6968
                                                   www.press.jhu.edu
The most complete source of medical, emotional, social, and practical advice available for those infected with HIV and their loved ones. Provides essential information for making decisions about treatment and testing in a world transformed by new research and pharmacotherapy.
1996 408 pages Paperback
ISBN: 0-801884-85-6

411   Invisible People: How the U.S. Has Slept Through the Global AIDS Pandemic
Greg Behrman, author

Free Press Publishing Co.
1010 W Cass St   813-254-5888
Tampa, FL 33606-1307
368 pages
ISBN: 0-743257-55-3

412   Living Well With HIV and AIDS
Allen L Gifford MD, Kate Loring RN, author

Bull Publishing Company
PO Box 1377
Boulder, CO 80306   800-676-2855
                                                   Fax: 303-545-6354
                                                   www.bullpub.com
Offers the latest information based on the HIV care guidelines from the Department of Health & Human Services and the Center for Disease Control. Disscuses a shift in treatments emphasis to the ways of managing side effects such as lypodystrophy, redistribution of body fat, cardiac risks, and concerns with vulnerability to other ailments called comorbidities
2005 328 pages Papberback
ISBN: 0-923521-86-8

413   Living on the Edge
Michael Kelly, author

HarperCollins Canada Limited/Order Department
1995 Markham Road
Ontario, Canada M1 B 5M8,   800-387-0117
                                                   Fax: 800-668-5788
A gritty, honest, biographical account of one young man's experience from the original diagnosis via the development of the illness, how Michael has learned to live with his illness and how it has affected him and all his friends who support him.
160 pages
ISBN: 0-551027-49-5

414   Local AIDS Sercices: The National Directory
US Conference of Mayors
1620 I Street NW   202-293-7330
Washington, DC 20006   Fax: 202-293-2352
                                                   e-mail: info@usmayors.org
                                                   www.usmayors.org
2,500 organizations that provide various information and services for AIDS coordinates and other health-related professionals.

415   Lynda Madaras Talks to Teens About AIDS
Lynda Madaras, author

Waterfront Books
98 Brookes Avenue   802-658-7477
Burlington, VT 05401   800-639-6063
                                           e-mail: helpkids@waterfrontbooks.com
                                                   www.waterfrontbooks.com
An informative book about the HIV virus and AIDS.
128 pages

416   Night Kites
M.E. Kerr, author

HarperCollins Children's Books
1350 Avenue of the Americas
New York, NY 10019   212-261-6500
                                                   www.harperchildrens.com
For young adults.
224 pages Paperback
ISBN: 0-064470-35-0

417   No Longer Immune: A Counselor's Guide to AIDS
American Counseling Association
5999 Stevenson Avenue   703-823-9800
Alexandria, VA 22304   800-347-6647
                                                   Fax: 703-823-0252
                                                   www.counseling.org
Covers a broad range of issues such as working with specific populations, handling pre- and posttesting situations, coping with fear, grief and survivor guilt, preventing caregiver burnout and dealing with countertransference.
295 pages Paperback
ISBN: 1-556200-64-1

418   Parent Education Program-HIV/AIDS: A Challenge to Us All
Pediatric AIDS Foundation
2950 31st Street   310-314-1459
Santa Monica, CA 90405-3092   800-499-4673
                                                   Fax: 310-314-1469
                                                   e-mail: info@pedcids.org
                                                   www.pedaids.org
This parent meeting kit with a guide book and two videos will help any adult set up a parent meeting on the subject of AIDS. This kit provides accurate information to parents about HIV/AIDS, allows parents to voice concerns and fears, gives examples of appropriate answers to your child's questions about HIV/AIDS and replaces fear with knowledge and compassion.

419   Predicting AIDS and Other Epidemics
Christopher Lampton, author

Franklin Watts
96 Leonard Street   www.wattspub.co.uk
London EC2A 4XD,
144 pages S & L Binding

420   Scarlet Letters
AIDS Project Los Angeles

The David Geffen Center
Los Angeles, CA 90005   213-201-1600
www.apla.org
A bilingual (Spanidh/English) journal targeted at HIV prevention providers in the U.S. The Scarlet Letters features opinion pieces and research-based essays by invited HIV/STD prevention experts.

421   **Teen Guide to AIDS Prevention**
Alan E. Nourse, author

Franklin Watts
96 Leonard Street   www.wattspub.co.uk
London EC2A 4XD,
For young adult readers.
61 pages S & L Binding

422   **We Have AIDS**
Elaine Landau, author

Franklin Watts
96 Leonard Street   www.wattspub.co.uk
London EC2A 4XD,
For young adult readers.
S & L Binding

423   **What Is AIDS?**
Anna Forbes, author

The Rosen Publishing Group
PowerKids Press   212-777-3017
New York, NY 10010   800-237-9932
Fax: 888-436-4643
www.powerkidspress.com

For reader levels ages 4-8.
1st Edition 24 pages Hardcover

424   **Women & AIDS**
Diane Richardson, author

Methuen
11-12 Buckingham Gate   www.methuen.co.uk
London SW1E 6LB,
The first sourcebook to provide the information women need by identifying the most accurate sources and providing valuable statistical data.
183 pages Paperback
ISBN: 0-416017-51-7

425   **Women and AIDS: A Practical Guide for Those Who Help Others**
Continuum Publishing Corporation
370 Lexington Avenue   212-532-3650
New York, NY 10017-6503
Tailored to women, this book grapples with attitudes and realities of AIDS.

426   **Women and Aids: Coping and Caring**
Plenum Publishing Corportation
233 Spring Street   212-620-8000
New York, NY 10013-1522   800-221-9369
Fax: 212-463-0742
e-mail: info@plenum.com

1996 263 pages
ISBN: 0-306452-58-8
Ann O'Leary, Editor

427   **You Have HIV: A Day at a Time**
Lynn S. Baker, author

W.B. Saunders Company
www.elsevierhealth.com

258 pages paperback
ISBN: 0-721636-06-3

Children's Books

428   **AIDS Overview Series**
Lucent Books

Thomson Gale
Farmington Hills, MI 48333-9187   800-877-4253
Fax: 800-414-5043
e-mail: gale.customerservice@thomson.com
www.gale.com/lucent
A straightforward account that teaches young adults all about the growing problem of AIDS.
1998 112 pages
ISBN: 1-560061-93-6

429   **AIDS Awareness Library**
Rosen Publishing Group
29 E 21st Street
New York, NY 10010   800-237-9932
Fax: 888-436-4643
e-mail: customerservice@rosepub.com
www.rosenpublishing.com

1996 24 pages
ISBN: 0-823974-06-1

430   **AIDS To the Point: Confronting Youth Issues**
Diana L. Hynson, author

Abingdon Press
201 8th Avenue S   615-749-6347
Nashville, TN 37202-0801   800-251-3320
Fax: 615-749-6577
www.abingdonpress.com
A resource that offers a practical means of talking with teens, individually or in a group, about AIDS. This volume offers teaching articles, ready-to-go programs for teens, leader's guides, worship resources, facts and figures, where to go for help and a section exclusively in Spanish. This is a volume in the To The Point: Confronting Youth Issues series of books.
96 pages Paperback
ISBN: 0-687782-20-1

431   **AIDS: How it Works in the Body**
Franklin Watts Grolier
90 Old Sherman Turnpike   203-797-3500
Danbury, CT 06816-0001   Fax: 203-797-3197
www.grolier.com
Focuses on the physiological effects AIDS has on the body, explains the causes of the disease, how the immune system works to defend the body and how the HIV virus affects the immune system.
64 pages Grades 5-7
ISBN: 0-531200-74-4

432   **AIDS: Trading Fears for Facts a Guide for Teens**
Consumer Reports Books
9180 La Saint Drive   914-378-2567
Fairfield, OH 45014   Fax: 914-378-2907
Written specifically for teenage readers and filled with illustrations, this book includes the current facts about AIDS, discusses how the virus is transmitted and precautions that should be taken.

433   **AIDS: Trading Fears for Facts: A Guide for Young People**
Consumer Reports Books
9180 La Saint Drive   914-378-2567
Fairfield, OH 45014   Fax: 914-378-2907
www.consumerreports.com
1993
ISBN: 0-890432-62-4

434   **Dancing Against the Darkness: A Journey Through America in the Age of AIDS**
Heath Publishing
125 Spring Street   617-822-6650
Lexington, MA 02421-7801
A professional in the field, this author has chosen people across the nation to interview and use as examples for how the AIDS epidemic has struck America and what kind of lives it has affected.
Grades 7-12

435   **Everything You Need to Know When a Parent Has AIDS**
Barbara Hermie Draimin, DSW, author

Rosen Publishing Group

29 E. 21st Street
New York, NY 10010

212-777-3017
800-237-9932
Fax: 888-436-4643
e-mail: rosenpub@tribeca.ios.com

More and more teens have a parent who has AIDS. Teens must learn where they can turn up for health in dealing with this difficult situation. By presenting stories of teens in the same situation, this book helps readers deal with their anger and grief.

ISBN: 0-823916-90-1

436 Impact of AIDS
Franklin Watts Grolier
90 Old Sherman Turnpike
Danbury, CT 06816-0001

203-797-3500
800-621-1115
Fax: 203-797-3197
www.grolier.com

Examines the effects of the HIV infection and discusses the efforts in finding a cure for AIDS.
64 pages Grades 5-7
ISBN: 0-531172-25-2

437 Night Kites
Harper Collins
55 Avenue Road
Hazelton, Toronto, M5R3L2,

416-975-9334
www.harpercollins.com

This book focuses on two brothers, one of whom is homosexual and how they interact in the face of AIDS and the intolerance of homosexuality among the many people they know.
Grades 8-12

438 Our Immune System
Sara LeBien, author
Immune Deficiency Foundation
40 W Chesapeake Avenue
Towson, MD 21204-4841

410-321-6647
800-296-4433
Fax: 410-321-9165
e-mail: idf@primaryimmune.org
www.primaryimmune.org

This storybook educates children about primary immunodeficiency diseases through delightful, eye-catching illustrations. The characters explain how the immune system works and describe the treatments for pediatric patients. Children will understand their own bodies and be better prepared to deal with their own primary immunodeficiency.
G. Richard Barr, Chairman
Marcia Boyle, Founder, Chairperson

439 Predicting AIDS and Other Epidemics
Franklin Watts Grolier
90 Old Sherman Turnpike
Danbury, CT 06816-0001

203-797-3500
800-621-1115
Fax: 203-797-3197
www.grolier.com

Surveys the efforts of scientists and researchers to predict the spread of epidemic diseases, including AIDS.
128 pages Grades 7-12
ISBN: 0-531107-85-0

440 Problem of AIDS
Franklin Watts Grolier
90 Old Sherman Turnpike
Danbury, CT 06816-0001

203-797-3500
800-621-1115
Fax: 203-797-3197
www.grolier.com

Part of the Let's Talk About series, this book addresses the questions and answers children and young adults have about AIDS.
32 pages Grades 3-5
ISBN: 0-531171-91-4

441 Teen Guide to AIDS Prevention
Franklin Watts Grolier
90 Old Sherman Turnpike
Danbury, CT 06816-0001

203-797-3500
800-621-1115
Fax: 203-797-3197
www.grolier.com

Directly addresses the questions and fears of teenagers by explaining clearly and simply what AIDS is, how it is spread, and the preventive measures young persons should take.
64 pages Grades 9-12
ISBN: 0-531109-66-6

442 We Have AIDS
Franklin Watts Grolier
90 Old Sherman Turnpike
Danbury, CT 06816-0001

203-797-3500
800-621-1115
Fax: 203-797-3197
www.grolier.com

This book goes beyond statistics and facts and focuses on the personal side of the disease. Offers source notes, a bibliography and an index.
128 pages
ISBN: 0-531108-98-8

443 What's a Virus, Anyway? The Kid's Book About AIDS
Waterfront Books
98 Brookes Avenue
Burlington, VT 05401-3326

802-658-7477

A simple introduction to help adults talk with children about the subject of AIDS.
67 pages

Magazines

444 AIDS Alert
American Health Consultants
3525 Piedmont Road
Atlanta, GA 30305

404-262-5476
800-688-2421
Fax: 404-262-5560
www.ahcpub.com

Covers up-to-the-minute developments and guidance on the entire spectrum of AIDS challenges, including treatment, education, precautions, screening, diagnosis and policy.

445 AIDS Clinical Care
New England Journal of Medicine
860 Winter Street
Waltham, MA 02451-1413

781-893-3800
800-843-6356
Fax: 781-893-0413
e-mail: nejcust@mms.org
www.massmed.org

Up to date information specifically targeted at physicians with AIDS patients.
Monthly

446 AIDS: A Year In Review
Lippincott Williams & Wilkins
Po Box 1620
Hagerstown, MD 21741

301-223-2300
800-638-3030
www.lww.com

447 AIDS: International Monthly Journal
Lippincott Williams & Wilkins
Po Box 1620
Hagerstown, MD 21741

301-223-2300
800-638-3030
www.lww.com

448 AIDS: The Disease State Management Resource
American Health Consultants
Po Box 740056
Atlanta, GA 30374

800-688-2421
Fax: 800-284-3291
www.ahcpub.com

449 Critical Path AIDS Project
2062 Lombard Street
Philadelphia, PA 19146-1315

215-545-2212
www.critpath.org

Articles and reprints on experimental treatments and alternative therapies, and a listing of Philadelphia-area resources.
Monthly

450 Institute on Health Care for the Poor and Underserved at Meharry Medical College
Sage Publications

1005 DB Todd Boulevard
Nashville, TN 37208

615-327-6819
800-669-1269
Fax: 615-327-6362
e-mail: vbrennan@mmc.edu

Offers health care and public health policy research focusing on poor and underserved populations.
100pages 4x a year
Dr. Amy Cato, Director
Dr. Virginia Brennan, Editor

451 Journal of Acquired Immune Deficiency Syndrome
Lippincott Williams & Wilkins
Po Box 1620
Hagerstown, MD 21741-2601

301-223-2300
800-638-3030
www.lww.com

An interdisciplinary journal providing a synthesis of AIDS-related information from all relevant clinical and basic sciences.
Monthly
ISBN: 0-894925-5 -
William A Hazeltine, Editor

452 Journal of the Medical Library Association
Medical Library Association
65 E Wacker Place
Chicago, IL 60601-7246

312-419-9094
Fax: 312-419-8950
e-mail: info@mlahq.org
www.mlahq.org

An international, peer-reviewed journal that aims to advance the practice and research knowledgebase of health science librarianship.
Quarterly
Carla J Funk, Executive Director
Elizabeth Lund, Publications Director

453 POZ Magazine
POZ Publishing
462 Seventh Avenue
New York, NY 10018-7424

212-242-2163
Fax: 212-675-8505
e-mail: poz-editor@poz.com
www.poz.com

A magazine for people living with, and affected by, HIV/AIDS.
60 pages BiMonthly
Regan Hofmann, Editor in Chief
Jennifer Morton, Managing Editor

454 Risky Business
San Francisco AIDS Foundation Materials Dept.
333 Valencia Street
San Francisco, CA 94103-3547

415-861-3397

A comic book style magazine providing accurate information about AIDS using humor and real-life situations. Contains stories that stress the importance of knowing how AIDS is transmitted and prevented.

455 Straight Talk: A Magazine for Teens About AIDS
Custom Publishing Division of Rodale Press
33 E Minor Street
Emmaus, PA 18098-0001

610-967-5171

A lively magazine that includes articles about teens with AIDS, teens involved in peer education and teens at risk for getting infected. Good information is presented in an interesting format for young adults.

456 Washington Update
Committee of Ten Thousand
500 Belmont Street
Brockton, MA 02301

508-587-2512
e-mail: cott-dc@earthlink.net
www.cott1.org

Is a primer on government related issues of importance to COTT's constituency. From health care legislation, to regulatory affairs to Administration policy for chronic diseases. A hands-on journal for grass roots health care advocacy in our Nation's capital.
Bi-Monthly
John Rider, Contact

Newsletters

457 AIDS Alert
American Health Consualnts

3525 Piedmont Road
Atlanta, GA 30305

404-262-5476
800-688-2421
Fax: 404-262-5560
e-mail: customerservice@ahcpub.com
www.ahcpub.com

Covers up-to-the-minute developments and guidance on the entire spectrum of AIDS challenges, including treatment, education, precautions, screening, diagnosis and policy.

458 AIDS Link
University of Cincinnati-Medical Center Info.
231 Bethesda Avenue
Cincinnati, OH 45267-0001

513-558-5661
Fax: 513-558-3136
medcenter.uc.edu/

Aimed at healthcare professionals working with HIV/AIDS inflicted patients.
Rebecca Atterrin, Editor

459 AIDS News
Northern California Chapter of the NHF
7700 Edgewater Drive
Oakland, CA 94621-3023

510-568-6243

Provides current information for people who need to cope mentally and physically with the issues of virus infection and transmission. Provides answers to questions about AIDS, ARC, HIV infection and transmission prevention.
BiMonthly

460 AIDS Policy and Law
LRP Publications
747 Dresher Road
Horsham, PA 19044-0980

www.lrp.com

A report on AIDS policy and law developments from the courts, NIH, federal and state AIDS agencies and advocacy organizations.
24 year

461 AIDS Treatment Data Network
611 Broadway
New York, NY 10012

212-260-8868
800-734-7104
Fax: 212-260-8869
www.atdn.org

Information bulletins covering new treatments, clinical trials, and more.

462 AIDS Treatment News
ATN Publications
PO Box 411256
San Francisco, CA 94141-1256

800-873-2812
www.atnonline.org

Reports on the developments in treatments for HIV disease and related infections. Also covers issues relating to research.
BiMonthly

463 AIDS Update
Dallas Gay Alliance
PO Box 190812
Dallas, TX 75219-0812

214-528-4233
Fax: 214-521-6424
e-mail: info@dgla.org
www.divanet.com/dgla/

Includes general information on AIDS issues and treatments.

464 AIDS Weekly Plus
Charles Henderson
Po Box 5528
Atlanta, GA 31107-0528   e-mail: info@hendersonnet.atl.ga.us

All aspects of AIDS epidemic coverage, including research, treatments, vaccine development, political and public policy.
46 year

465 AIDS/STD News Report
CD Publications
8204 Fenton Street
Silver Spring, MD 0910

301-588-6380
800-666-6380
Fax: 301-588-6385
e-mail: info@cdpublications.com
www.cdpublications.com

Formerly AIDS News Alert, provides grant listings from federal, private, and corporate sources; proposal writing tips; updates on successful programs, and the latest news on AIDS/STD federal/state legislation, research, and successful programs.

466 APICHA News
Asian & Pacific Islander Coalition on HIV/AIDS
400 Broadway
New York, NY 10013
212-334-7940
866-274-2429
Fax: 212-334-7956
e-mail: apicha@apicha.org
www.apicha.org
Provides information on prevention education, client services and advocacy for Asians and Pacific Islanders.
Quarterly
Therese R Rodriguez, CEO

467 APLA Update
AIDS Project Los Angeles
3550 Wilshire Boulevard
Los Angeles, CA 90010
213-201-1600
www.apla.org
Presents news about AIDS and programs of AIDS Project Angeles to people affected by the disease.
20 pages

468 BETA
San Francisco AIDS Foundation
995 Market Street 200
San Francisco, CA 94103
415-487-3000
e-mail: feedback@sfaf.org
www.sfaf.org
Medical information.
Quarterly

469 Being Alive
Being Alive People with HIV/AIDS Action Coalition
621 N San Vincente Boulevard
West Hollywood, CA 90069
310-289-2551
Fax: 310-289-9866
e-mail: info@beingalivela.org
www.beingalivela.org
Medical updates, plus information on AIDS advocacy, a calendar of local events and listings of AIDS support groups.

470 Being Alive Newsletter
Being Alive-People with HIV/AIDS Action Coalition
7531 Santa Monica Boulevard
West Hollywood, CA 90040
323-874-4322
Fax: 323-969-8753
e-mail: kevin@beingalivela.org
www.beingalivela.org
A regularly-published source of information and education for our peers living with HIV/AIDS and for the greater community. Standing articles cover timely issues such as HIV/AIDS treatment options, mental health, substance abuse, nutrition, advocacy, community referrals, and a variety of other topics. Additionally, we feature information on Being Alive events alongside other relevant community events.
Quarterly
Kevin Kurth, Executive Director/Editor

471 CORPUS
AIDS Project Los Angeles
The David Geffen Center
Los Angeles, CA 90005
213-201-1600
e-mail: info@apla.org
www.apla.org
A journal that uses art, cultural criticism, poetry, short stories and humor to reveal the challenges of HIV prevention in gay and bisexual communities.
Annually
Craig E Thompson, Executive Director

472 COTT News
Committee on Ten Thousand
500 Belmont Street
Brockton, MA 02301
508-587-2512
www.cott1.org
A range of information, reportage and viewpoints regarding issues and events of importance to grass roots health care advocacy and support.
John Rider, Contact

473 Center for AIDS Prevention Studies
AIDS Research Institute

74 New Montgomery
San Francisco, CA 94105
415-597-9100
Fax: 415-597-9213
e-mail: capsweb@psg.ucsf.edu
www.caps.ucsf.edu
Local, national, and international interdisciplinary research.

474 Community Health Funding Report
CD Publications
8204 Fenton Street
Silver Spring, MD 20910-4571
301-588-6380
800-666-6380
Fax: 301-588-6385
e-mail: chf@cdpublications.com
www.cdpublications.com
Covers grants for AIDS and sexually transmitted disease related programs from federal and private sources. Includes news on national and local issues affecting AIDS and STD's and case studies of successful fundraising programs. This biweekly newsletter describes changes in funding streams for community based health programs, including AIDS programs. It lists available federal and private grant opportunities, along with Washington News Medicare/Medicaid.
18 pages BiMonthly
Mike Gerecht, Publisher
Amy Bernstein, Editor

475 Cott Washington Update
Committee of Ten Thousand
236 Massachusetts Avenue NE
Washington, DC 20002-4971
202-543-0988
800-488-2688
Fax: 202-543-6720
www.cott1.org
Offers legislative updates, information on clinical trials, therapies, book reviews, business and politics, a readers forum and resources pertaining to HIV/AIDS.
10 pages Monthly
Corey Dubin, President
Dave Cavenaugh, Government Relations

476 FOCUS
UCSF AIDS Health Project
1930 Market Street
San Francisco, CA 94102
415-476-3902
www.ucsf-ahp.org
Reviews the counseling aspects of AIDS: how HIV-related counseling is affected by the medical, epidemiological, and social realities of AIDS, as well as the emotional response to the disease. It is written for mental health and health care providers working on the front lines and is of interest to researchers, policy makers, and program administrators.
10x/year
James W Dilley MD, Executive Director

477 Gay Men's Health Crisis
119 West 24th Street
New York, NY 10011
212-367-1000
www.gmhc.org
Not-for-profit, volueteer-supported and community-based organization committed to national leadership in the fight against AIDS.

478 HIV Counselor PERSPECTIVES
UCSF AIDS Health Project
1930 Market Street
San Francisco, CA 94102
415-476-3902
www.ucsf-ahp.org
An educational resource for HIV antibody test counselors, prevention case managers, and other health and mental health professionals, particularly those working in brief counseling venues.
4 year
James W Dilley MD, Executive Director

479 HIV Frontline
Center for AIDS Prevention Studies
University of California
San Francisco, CA 94114
415-552-6356
Fax: 415-597-9213
e-mail: CAPSweb@psg.ucsf.edu
www.caps.ucsf.edu
Monthly newsletter aimed at mental health and healthcare professionals who counsel people living with HIV/AIDS.
Monthly
Dr. Leon McKusick

480   IDF Advocate
Immune Deficiency Foundation
40 W Chesapeake Avenue
Towson, MD 21204   800-296-4433
e-mail: idf@primaryimmune.org
www.primaryimmune.org
Mailed to patients, family members, physicians, nurses, industry,
government and interested individuals.
3x/year
Marcia Boyle, President/Founder

481   Immune Deficiency Foundation Newsletter
Immune Deficiency Foundation
40 W Chesapeake Avenue   410-321-6647
Towson, MD 21204-4841   800-296-4433
Fax: 410-321-9165
e-mail: idf@primaryimmune.org
www.primaryimmune.org
Offers medical updates and technology news on the latest services,
products and treatments for persons with immune diseases.
Tamara Brown, Medical Programs Manager

482   In Focus
Project Inform
205 13th Street   415-558-8669
San Francisco, CA 94103-2461   800-822-7422
Fax: 415-558-0684
e-mail: web@projectinform.org
www.projectinform.org
The organizational newsletter of Project Inform.
20+ pages 3x/year
Skip Emerson, Executive Assistant

483   Just Kids
3 Corners
5th Avenue   212-634-4879
New York, NY 10014
Covers medical and social issues faced by HIV-positive children,
teens and their parents.
Annual

484   MLA News
Medical Library Association
65 East Wacker Place   312-419-9094
Chicago, IL 60601-7246   Fax: 312-419-8950
e-mail: info@mlahq.org
www.mlahq.org
Keeps you at the forefront of association matters and the profession as a whole. Regular departments include calendar, continuing
education, employment opportunities, international news, Internet
resources, personals, professional development, and technology.
Columns include consumer health, expert searching, hospital librarianship, leadership and management, and new members.
Members only.
Jean P Shipman, President

485   NMAC Update
National Minority AIDS Council
300 I Street NE
Washington, DC 20002-4389   202-544-1076
www.nmac.org
A newsletter reporting on public policy issues and information on
subjects in organizational management.
BiMonthly

486   OUTReach
The San Francisco AID Foundation
995 Market Street   415-487-8000
San Francisco, CA 94103   Fax: 415-487-8009
TDD: 415-487-8099
www.sfaf.org
Features concise articles on a wide range of HIV/AIDS topics.

487   PAACNOTES
101 W Grand Avenue   312-222-1326
Chicago, IL 60610-4272   800-243-3059
A news journal of the Physicians Coalition for AIDS Care featuring articles on clinical management, scientific research and a diverse range of legal, ethical and economic issues directly affecting
the care of persons with HIV disease.

488   PWA Rag
Prisoners With AIDS Rights Advocacy Group
1626 Wilcox Avenue   770-946-9346
Loa Angeles, CA 90028   e-mail: RAGNEWS@aol.com
www.hometown.aol.com
Contains articles, treatment updates, and resources for prisoners.

489   Positive Living
APLA
3550 Wilshire Boulevard   213-201-1600
Los Angeles, CA 90010   800-922-2438
Monthly

490   Positive Outlook
2655 Swann Avenue   813-877-5696
Tampa, FL 33609
Focuses on local people and issues in West Central Florida.
Quarterly

491   Positive Social Support Newsletter
Lambda Center
4228 Wisconsin Avenue NW   202-965-8434
Washington, DC 20016   877-252-6232
e-mail: contact@lambcenter.com
www.thelambdacenter.com
Sponsored by and for people with HIV.

492   Positive Voice Newsletter
National Association of People with AIDS (NAPWA)
8401 Colesville Road   240-247-0880
Silverspring, MD 20910   866-846-9366
Fax: 240-247-0574
e-mail: info@napwa.org
www.napwa.org

Frank J Oldham Jr, President/CEO
Peter Kronenberg, VP Communications/Editor

493   Positive Woman
PO Box 34372   202-898-0372
Washington, DC 20043-4372
Provides medical information, including alternative and holistic
therapies for HIV-positive women.
BiMonthly

494   Positively Aware
Test Positive Aware Network
5537 N Broadway Street   773-989-9400
Chicago, IL 60640   Fax: 773-989-9494
e-mail: tpan@tpan.com
www.tpan.com
An internationally known and respected magazine devoted to HIV
treatment, wellness, and optimum quality of life for those living
with HIV, as well as those who care for them.
Bi-monthly
Jeff Berry, Publications Director

495   RAP* Time
Rural Center for AIDS/STD Prevention
Indiana University   812-855-7974
Bloomington, IN 47405-3085   800-566-8644
Fax: 812-855-3936
e-mail: aids@indiana.edu
www.indiana.edu/~aids/
Summarizes current research concerning HIV/STD prevention,
particularly in rural settings.
William L Yarber HSD, Senior Director

496   STEP Perspective
Seattle Treatment Exchange Project
1123 E John Street   206-329-4857
Seattle, WA 98102-5711   800-869-7837
e-mail: info@stepproject.org
www.thebody.com
Updates on treatments for HIV and related diseases condensed
from journals, conferences and databases by the scientific review
committee.

497   Seasons
National Native American AIDS Prevention Center

436 14th Street
Oakland, CA 94612-2011   510-444-2051
                                    Fax: 510-444-1593
                        e-mail: information@nnaape.org
                                       www.nnaapc.org
Features articles and artwork by Native Americans impacted by
HIV/AIDS.
Quarterly

498   Treatment Issues
Department of Medical Information   212-337-1950
New York, NY 10011-3601
The gay men's health crisis newsletter of experimental AIDS ther-
apies.
10x Year

499   Up Front Drug Information
5701 Biscayne Boulevard   305-757-2566
Miami, FL 33137-2601
Provides information on drugs and drug referrals.

500   Walk Talk
AIDS Coalition Silicon Valley
Walk For AIDS Silicon Valley
San Jose, CA 95154   408-451-WALK
                                     Fax: 408-248-7423
                          e-mail: info@walkforaids.org
The AIDS Coalition Silicon Valley Newsletter highlighting Walk
for AIDS Silicon Valley fundraising events, issues and articles
about HIV/AIDS service providers in the County.

501   Wisconsin AIDS Update
Wisconsin AIDS/HIV Program, Department of Health
PO Box 309   608-267-5287
Madison, WI 53701-0309   e-mail: webmaildph@dhfs.state.wi.us
                                     www.dhfs.state.wi.us
Includes epidemiological and clinical care articles, selections
from the most important current abstracts in ATIN and a statewide
list of events and resources.
Quarterly

502   World/Mundo
PO Box 11535   415-658-6930
Oakland, CA 94611-0535
Contains letters, advice, events calendar, and information on sup-
port groups in Northern California.

Pamphlets

503   AIDS Medicines in Development
Pharmaceutical Research & Manufacturers of America
950 F Street NW   202-835-3400
Washington, DC 20004   Fax: 202-835-3414
                                        www.phrma.org
An annual chart of antivirals, as well as information on diagnostics
and vaccines.

504   AIDS and Hemophilia: Protecting Yourself and Others
Hemophilia Council of California: Bay Area Office
7700 Edgewater Drive   510-568-7074
Oakland, CA 94621   Fax: 510-568-2048
                             e-mail: hccoak@aol.com
Lori Drake, Mental Health Counselor/Health Educator

505   AIDS, the Law & You
AIDS Action Committee
131 Clarendon Street   617-536-7733
Boston, MA 02116-5145   800-424-2634
                                     Fax: 617-437-6445
                          e-mail: webmaster@aac.org
                                         www.aac.org
Discusses legal protection against AIDS-related discrimination,
HIV testing and the law.

**506   Americans with Disabilities Act: What it Means for People with
         AIDS**
American Civil Liberties Union AIDS Project
132 W 43rd Street
New York, NY 10036-6503   212-944-9800
                                        www.aclu.org

507   Basics of HIV Disease: Questions and Answers
National Hemophilia Foundation
116 W 32nd Street   888-463-6643
New York, NY 10001-3212   800-424-2634
                                     Fax: 212-328-3777
                                      www.hemophilia.org
This publication contains basic information about hemophilia and
HIV disease.
1992 28 pages
Alan Kinniburgh, PhD, CEO

508   Be Smart About HIV
American Red Cross
1616 Fort Myer Drive   703-312-8724
Arlington, VA 22209-3100   Fax: 703-312-8738
                                       www.redcross.org
This brochure offers very simple and informative information on
the HIV virus, in both English and Spanish.
1996
Sandra L Mertz, Product Manager

509   Children with AIDS: Guidelines for Parents and Caregivers
AIDS Task Force of Central New York
627 W Genesee Street   315-415-2430
Syracuse, NY 13204-2347
Offers general information on AIDS, diet and feeding, household
chores, and coping with the illness.

510   Clinical Focus
Immune Deficiency Foundation
40 W Chesapeake Avenue   410-321-6647
Towson, MD 21204-4841   800-296-4433
                                     Fax: 410-321-9165
                          e-mail: idf@primaryimmune.org
                                     www.primaryimmune.org
Biannual publication for medical professionals covering current
issues and information regarding clinical approaches to primary
immune deficiencies.
BiAnnual
Marcia Boyle, Founder/Chair

511   Clinical Focus on Primary Immune Deficiency Diseases
Immune Deficiency Foundation
40 W Chesapeake Avenue   410-321-6647
Towson, MD 21204-4841   800-296-4433
                                     Fax: 410-321-9165
                          e-mail: idf@primaryimmune.org
                                     www.primaryimmune.org
educational mongraph is designed specifically for health care professionals and focuses on topics relevant to primary immune deficiency diseases.
Marcia Boyle, Founder/Chair

512   Clinical Presentation of the Primary Immunodeficiency Diseases
Immune Deficiency Foundation
40 W Chesapeake Avenue   410-321-6647
Towson, MD 21204-4841   800-296-4433
                                     Fax: 410-321-9165
                          e-mail: idf@primaryimmune.org
                                     www.primaryimmune.org
A primer for physicians.
Tamara Brown, Medical Programs Manager

513   Clinical Trials: Talking it Over
NIAID, Office of Communications
Building 31   301-496-5717
Bethesda, MD 20892-0001
Educational pamphlet pertaining to clinical trials.

514   Condoms and Sexually Transmitted Diseases, Especially AIDS
Department of Health and Human Services
National Institutes of Health   202-673-7700
Bethesda, MD 20892-0001
Offers information on condoms and how various forms of protec-
tion can be used to prevent sexually transmitted diseases, espe-
cially HIV/AIDS.

515   Eating Defensively: Food Safety Advice for Persons with AIDS
AIDSinfo

PO Box 6303
Rockville, MD 20849-6303

301-519-0459
800-448-0440
Fax: 301-519-6616
TTY: 888-480-3739
e-mail: ContactUs@aidsinfo.nih.gov
www.aidsinfo.nih.gov

The food safety advice in this brochure is intended to help persons with HIV infection to reduce the risk of food poisoning, thereby avoiding an illness that could worsen their condition or even cause death.
1992

516   HIV Infection and AIDS
NAID Office of Communications
31 Center Drive
Bethesda, MD 20892-0001

301-496-5717

Offers information on transmission, treatment, early symptoms, diagnosis, prevention and research.

517   HIV and AIDS During Pregnancy
March of Dimes
233 Park Avenue South
New York, NY 10003

212-353-8353
Fax: 212-254-3518
e-mail: NY639@marchofdimes.com
www.marchdofdimes.com

518   HIV/AIDS in the Workplace
New York Business Group on Health
386 Park Avenue S
New York, NY 10016-8804

212-252-7440
e-mail: nybgh@nybgh.org
www.nybgh.org

Offers information on federal law and state law regarding HIV/AIDS in the workplace, universal risks, health insurance and other business costs.

519   Hope for Children with AIDS
Pediatric AIDS Foundation
2950 31st Street
Santa Monica, CA 90405-3092

310-394-1459
888-499-4673
Fax: 310-394-1469
e-mail: info@pedaids.org
www.pedaids.org

A brochure offering information on the latest research and advances in the area of pediatric AIDS.

520   How to Keep an Infusion Log
Immune Deficiency Foundation
40 W Chesapeake Avenue
Towson, MD 21204

800-296-4433
e-mail: idf@primaryimmune.org
www.primaryimmune.org

This brochure explains the value of keeping an immune globulin infusion log, as well as practical information on how to set up your personal records.
Marci Boyle, President/Founder

521   IDF Guide for Nurses on Immune Globulin Therapy for Primary Immunodeficiency
Immune Deficiency Foundation
40 W Chesapeake Avenue
Towson, MD 21204

800-296-4433
e-mail: idf@primaryimmune.org
www.primaryimmune.org

This guide provides direction for nurses to administer immune globulin replacement therapy in the safest and most effective way. Information includes: clinical uses for immune globulin replacement therapy; product selection and characteristics; infusions, complications and adverse events of IVIG and SCIG; concomitant medications; nursing interventions and responsibilities and helpful references and resources.
Marcia Boyle, President/Founder

522   IDF Patient and Family Handbook
Immune Deficiency Foundation
40 W Chesapeake Avenue
Towson, MD 21204

800-296-4433
e-mail: idf@primaryimmune.org
www.primaryimmune.org

For patients and family pmembers, contains information about the diagnosis and treatment of primary immunodeficiency diseases, the immune system, specific diseases, therapies, general care, health insurance and issues specific to adult, adolescent and pediatric patients.
R Michael Blaese MD, Editor
Jerry A Winkelstein MD, Editor

523   Immune Deficiency Foundation
40 W. Chesapeake Avenue
Towson, MD 21204

800-296-4433
e-mail: idf@primaryimmune.org
www.primaryimmune.org

Your partner for living with primary immune deficiency diseases. This brochure describes the IDF and its activities and services.

524   Infections Linked to AIDS
NAID Office of Communications
31 Center Drive
Bethesda, MD 20892-0001

301-496-5717

Offers information on infections related to HIV/AIDS and referral numbers of where to receive help.

525   Our Immune System
Sara LeBien, author

Immune Deficiency Foundation
40 W Chesapeake Avenue
Towson, MD 21204-4841

410-321-6647
800-296-4433
Fax: 410-321-9165
e-mail: idf@primaryimmune.org
www.primaryimmune.org

This storybook educates children about primary immunodeficiency diseases through delightful, eye-catching illustrations. The characters explain how the immune system works and describe the treatments for pediatric patients. Children will understand their own bodies and be better prepared to deal with their own primary immunodeficiency.

526   Taking the HIV (AIDS) Test: How to Help Yourself
NAID Office of Communications
31 Center Drive
Bethesda, MD 20892-0001

301-496-5717

Offers information on the AIDS test, how it works, how it can help and should it be taken.

527   Teeens, Sexually Transmitted Diseases & HIV/AIDS
4 Brighton Road
West Sussex, RH13 5BA UK,

e-mail: info@avert.org
www.avert.org

Designed for teens, and contains information on what STD's are, how to avoid becoming infected, safer sex, how to spot symptoms of STD's, STD treatment, information about HIV/AIDS, information about testing and treatment, and advice helplines.

528   Testing Positive for HIV
NAID Office of Communications
31 Center Drive
Bethesda, MD 20892-0001

301-496-5717

Information on what a positive HIV test means, how not to spread the disease to others, and various health and dieting tips.

529   Testing for HIV Infection
American Red Cross
1616 Fort Myer Drive
Arlington, VA 22209-3100
1996

703-312-8724
Fax: 703-312-8738

Sandra L Mertz, Product Manager

530   Women, Sex, and HIV
American Red Cross
1616 Fort Myer Drive
Arlington, VA 22209-3100
1992

703-312-8724
Fax: 703-312-8738

Sandra L Mertz, Product Manager

531   Your Job and HIV: Are There Risks?
American Red Cross
1616 Fort Myer Drive
Arlington, VA 22209-3100
1992

703-312-8724
Fax: 703-312-8738

Sandra L Mertz, Product Manager

Audio & Video

532 AIDS Work: Six Healthcare Workers Face the AIDS Crisis
Fanlight Productions
Icarus Films   718-488-8900
Brooklyn, NY 11201   800-876-1710
                                                     Fax: 718-488-8642
                                           e-mail: info@fanlight.com
                                                     www.fanlight.com
Two physicians and four nurses reflect on several decades of combined experiences in caring for patients with HIV/AIDS. They discuss facing fear, frustration, burnout and grief as they struggle to deliver compassionate care, as well as the rewards of caring for this population. This inspirational program is invaluable for stress management programs, and in preparing students and new workers for the realities they will face.
VHS
ISBN: 1-572952-20-2
Steve Guy, Producer

533 Does Anyone Die of AIDS Anymore?
Louise Hogarth, author
Fanlight Productions
Icarus Films   718-488-8900
Brooklyn, NY 11201   800-876-1710
                                                     Fax: 718-488-8642
                                           e-mail: info@fanlight.com
                                                     www.fanlight.com
The answer to this disturbing film's title question is a resounding yes! Despite the much-hyped advances in treatment which, for some patients, have transformed HIV from a death sentence to a chronic illness, tens of thousands of people are still dying of AIDS in the United States. And tens of thousands more will die, even in this rich and medically advanced nation, because of ignorance and denial which have resulted in a 'third wave' of HIV infection.
26 Minutes
ISBN: 1-572958-48-0
Nicole Johnson, Publicity Coordinator

534 Roger's Story: For Cori
Howard Shepps, author
Fanlight Productions
Icarus Films   718-488-8900
Brooklyn, NY 11201   800-876-1710
                                                     Fax: 718-488-8642
                                           e-mail: info@fanlight.com
                                                     www.fanlight.com
Forty-four year-old Roger shares the harrowing story of his 20-year struggle against heroin, and his recent diagnosis with AIDS.
1989 28 Minutes
ISBN: 1-572950-47-1

535 Too Little, Too Late
Micki Dickoff, author
Fanlight Productions
Icarus Films   718-488-8900
Brooklyn, NY 11201   800-876-1710
                                                     Fax: 718-488-8642
                                           e-mail: info@fanlight.com
                                                     www.fanlight.com
In this moving video, family members of people with AIDS share their pain and frustration, as well as the solace they have derived from having been able to help their loved one to a peaceful death.
1987 49 Minutes
ISBN: 1-572950-27-7

536 Undetectable: The New Face of AIDS
Jay Corcoran, author
Fanlight Productions
Icarus Films   718-488-8900
Brooklyn, NY 11201   800-876-1710
                                                     Fax: 718-488-8642
                                           e-mail: info@fanlight.com
                                                     www.fanlight.com
This gripping documentary follows six women and men, straight and gay, of different ethnic and cultural backgrounds, over a three-year period as they deal for the first time with hope. Though the new multi-drug therapies for HIV disease offer a possible reprieve from what was once a death sentence, those who are lucky enough to respond to the drugs nonetheless face both a grueling treatment regimen, and the complex physical and psychological challenges of rebuilding their lives.
2001 56 Minutes
ISBN: 1-572958-45-6

Web Sites

537 AIDS United
                                                     www.aidsunited.org
To end the AIDS epidemic in the United States. We will achieve this goal through national, regional and local policy/advocacy, strategic grantmaking, and organizational capacity building. With partners throughout the country, we will work to ensure that people living with and affected by HIV/AIDS have access to the prevention and care services they need and deserve.

538 AIDS.ORG
                                                          www.aids.org
The mission of AIDS.ORG is to help prevent HIV infections and to improve the lives of those affected by HIV and AIDS by providing education and facilitating the free and open exchange of knowledge at any easy-to-find centralized website.

539 Children Affected by AIDS Foundation
                                                          www.caaf.org
The only organization solely devoted to providing social, educational, recreation and other critical support programs to vulnerable children impacted by HIV/AIDS in the U.S. and other countries.

540 Committee of Ten Thousand
                                                         www.cott1.org
A grass-roots, peer-led, education, advocacy and support organization for persons with HIV disease. Dedicated to the belief that persons with HIV/AIDS and all chronic diseases can lead productive and healthy lives

541 HIV/Hepatitis C in Prison (HIP) Committee
                                                 www.prisons.org/hivin.htm
Fighting for consistent access to quality medical care including access to all new HIV and Hepatitis C medications, diagnostic testing and combination therapies.

542 Healing Well
                                                     www.healingwell.com
A social network and support community for patients, caregivers, and families coping with the daily struggles of diseases, disorders and chronic illness.

543 Health Finder
                                                     www.healthfinder.gov
Searchable, carefully developed web site offering information on over 1000 topics. Developed by the US Department of Health and Human Services, the site can be used in both English and Spanish.

544 Healthlink USA
                                                    www.healthlinkusa.com
Health information concerning treatment, cures, prevention, diagnosis, risk factors, research, support groups, email lists, personal stories and much more. Updated regularly.

545 Helios Health
                                                     www.helioshealth.com
Online resource for your health information. Detailed information about specific health topics, access to expert advice from our Medical Advisory Board, and up-to-date health news.

546 Immune Deficiency Foundation
                                                  www.primaryimmune.org
The national patient organization dedicated to improving the diagnosis, treatment and quality of life of persons with primary immunodeficiency diseases through advocacy, education and research.

547 MedicineNet
                                                     www.medicinenet.com
An online resource for consumers providing easy-to-read, authoritative medical and health information.

548   Medscape

www.medscape.com

Medscape offers specialists, primary care physicians, and other health professionals the Web's most robust and integrated medical information and educational tools.

549   National AIDS Information Clearinghouse

www.cdcnac.org

Provides information and materials for employers on national, state and local resources related to HIV/AIDS in the workplace.

550   National Minority AIDS Education Training

www.nmaetc.org

Located at Howard University, as a HIV/AIDS training and technical resource for providers of minority HIV-infected patients throughout the country. The NMAETC receives 100% of its funding through the MAI Initiative. The NMAETC in collaboration with other HRSA funded programs seeks to influence health care professionals who treat minority HIV-infected patients.

551   New England AIDS Education & Training Ctr.

www.neaetc.org

One of eleven regional education centers funded by the Ryan White CARE Act and sponsored regionally by the Office of Community Programs at the University of Massachusetts Medical Center. The AETC Program is administered by Health Resources and Services Administration (HRSA) HIV/AIDS bureau.

552   People with AIDS Health Group

www.Aidsinfonyc.org

PWA is a non-profit buyers club organized to assist people with AIDS in obtaining medications — as well as provide support groups committed to the self-empowerment of people living with AIDS. They offer three programs: Treatment Education and Support, Advocacy and Public Policy, and Early Treatment Access.

553   San Francisco Area AIDS Education Center

www.ucsf.edu/sfaetc

Helps to improve the care of people living with HIV and AIDS by supporting state-of-the-art clinical consultation, education, and training for health care professionals and organizations in San Francisco, San Mateo, and Marin counties.

554   Smart & Strong

www.smartstrong.com

A healthcare education company that supports providers and empowers HIV positive patients through publications, seminars and innovative educational programs.

555   WebMD

www.webmd.com

Information on AIDS related diseases, including articles and resources.

Description

556 # Allergies

Allergy means altered reactivity. Allergies are usually characterized by a hypersensitivity to substances, such as pollens, pet dander, certain foods, some medications and molds. Such substances (allergens) can trigger an allergic response in susceptible individuals. Symptoms of allergies may present in a wide spectrum ranging from the mild sneezing, runny nose and congestion of hayfever to life-threatening reactions, known as anaphylaxis. Additional allergic reactions include itchy, watery eyes, skin rashes and asthma. More severe symptoms may include a tingling sensation in the mouth, swelling of the tongue and throat, difficulty breathing, hives, vomiting abdominal cramps, diarrhea, drop in blood pressure, loss of consciousness, and cardiovascular collapse leading to death. Allergic symptoms typically appear within minutes to two hours after the person has been exposed to the allergen.

Approximately 35 million people suffer from allergies in the United States. The cause of allergies is unclear, although there may be a genetic link in some people.

Treatment for allergies depends upon the specific substance, beginning with avoidance. Strict avoidance of the allergy-causing food is the only way to avoid a food allergy reaction. There are no medications that cure food allergies. Most people outgrow their food allergies, although peanuts, nuts, fish and shellfish are often considered life-long allergies.

For non-food allergies, medications such as antihistamines and inhaled bronchodilators, as well as allergy shots to reduce the allergic response, may be prescribed by doctors. Epinephrine, also called adrenaline, is the medication of choice for controlling a severe reaction. Individuals at risk of an anaphylactic reaction should have a bracelet or necklace with that information. Those who are allergic to insect stings should carry and use a pre-filled syringe of epinephrine (epipen) for prompt self-treatment.

National Agencies & Associations

557 **Allergy & Asthma Network Mothers of Asthmatics**
8201 Greensboro Drive
Fairfax, VA 22102
703-641-9595
800-878-4403
Fax: 703-288-5271
e-mail: info@aanma.org
www.breatherville.org
Leading nonprofit membership organization dedicated to eliminating suffering and death due to asthma, allergies and related conditions through education, advocacy, community outreach and research.
Michael Amato, Founder/President
Maria Marchiano, Board

558 **Allergy Asthma Information Association**
295 The West Mall
Toronto, Ontario, M9C4z-4Z4
416-621-4571
800-611-7011
Fax: 416-621-5034
e-mail: admin@aaia.ca
www.aaia.ca

To develop societal awareness of the seriousness of allergic disease, including asthma, and to enable allergic individuals, their families and caregivers, to increase control over allergy symptoms by providing leadership in information, education, advocacy, in partnership with health care professionals, business, industry and government.
Sharon Van Gyzan, Chair
Louis Isabella, Treasurer

559 **American Academy of Allergy, Asthma & Immunology**
555 East Wells Street
Milwaukee, WI 53202-3823
414-272-6071
800-822-2762
Fax: 414-272-6070
e-mail: info@aaaai.org
www.aaaai.org
Strives to serve the public through information on asthma and allergies, as well as referrals to allergists. Also offers pollen and mold statistics from the Committee on Pollen & Molds.
Kay Whalen, Executive Director
Marianne Canter, Director of Communications

560 **American Academy of Environmental Medicine**
6505 E Central Avenue
Wichita, KS 67206
316-684-5500
Fax: 316-684-5709
e-mail: administrator@aaemonline.org
www.aaem.com
Offers names of Clinical Ecologists and Allergy Specialists in the United States.
Amy L Dean, President
Jennifer Armstrong, Secretary

561 **American College of Allergy, Asthma & Immunology**
85 West Algonquin Road
Arlington Heights, IL 60005
847-427-1200
Fax: 847-427-1294
e-mail: mail@acaai.org
www.acaai.org
This association focuses its attention on research and public awareness of allergies. Distributes informational brochures and pamphlets, offers referrals and counseling services, as well as patient care.
Richard W Webber, President
James L Sublet, Vice President

562 **American Dietetic Association**
120 South Riverside Plaza
Chicago, IL 60606-6995
312-899-0040
800-877-1600
Fax: 312-899-1979
e-mail: media@eatright.org
www.eatright.org
Offers information and support to allergy sufferers. Serves the public through the promotion of optimal nutrition, health, and well-being.
Patricia M Babjak, CEO
Judith Rodriguez, President

563 **Association of Birth Defect Children Birth Defect Research for Children**
976 Lake Baldwin Lane
Celebration, FL 32814
407-566-8304
e-mail: staff@birthdefects.org
www.birthdefects.org
Offers informational packets on childhood asthma and prevention.
Betty Mekdeci, Contact

564 **Asthma and Allergy Foundation of America**
8201 Corporate Drive
Landover, MD 20785
202-466-7643
800-727-8462
Fax: 202-466-8940
e-mail: info@aafa.org
www.aafa.org
Nonprofit patient organization dedicated to improving the quality of life for people with asthma and allergies and their caregivers, through education, advocacy and research.
Lynn Hanessian, Chair
Michael Abu Carrick, Vice Chair

565 **Canadian Society of Allergy and Clinical Immunology**
PO BOX 51045
Orleans, ON K1S-5N8
613-986-5869
Fax: 613-730-1116
e-mail: csaci@royalcollege.ca
www.csaci.ca

Is the advancement of the knowledge and practice of allergy, clinical immunology, and asthma for optimal patient care.
Dr Paul Keith, President
Dr.Sandy Kapur, Vice President

566   Eczema Association for Science and Education
4460 Redwwod Highway   415-499-3474
San Rafael, CA 94903-1953   800-818-7546
e-mail: info@nationaleczema.org
www.nationaleczema.org
Offers resources and information for allergy patients.
Jamie Hubber, Chair
Susan Tofte, Secretary

567   Food Allergy and Anaphylaxis Network
7925 Jones Branch Dr.
McLean, VA 22102-3309   800-929-4040
Fax: 703-691-2713
e-mail: faan@foodallergy.org
www.foodallergy.org
Increases public awareness about food allergies and anaphylaxis advances research and provides education, emotional support and coping strategies to patients; serves as the communication link between the food industry, the government and the airline industry.
John L Lehr, CEO
George Dahlman, Vice President of Advocacy & Government

568   Immune Deficiency Foundation
40 W Chesapeake Avenue   410-321-6647
Towson, MD 21204-4841   800-296-4433
Fax: 410-321-9165
e-mail: idf@primaryimmune.org
www.primaryimmune.org
The national patient organization dedicated to improving the diagnosis treatment and quality of life of persons with primary immunodeficiency diseases through advocacy education and research.
Marcia Boyle, President & Founder
John Seymour PhD LMFT, Vice Chair

569   National Institute of Allergy and Infectious Diseases
NIAID Office of Communications and Public Liason
6610 Rockledge Drive   301-496-5717
Bethesda, MD 20892-6612   866-284-4107
Fax: 301-402-3573
TDD: 800-877-8339
e-mail: clane@niaid.nih.gov
www.niaid.nih.gov
Conducts and supports research on allergies; focused on understanding what happens to the body during the allergic process. Educates patients and health care workers in controlling allergic disease; offers various research centers that conduct and evaluate educational programs focused on methods to control allergic diseases.
Anthony S Fauci, MD, Director

State Agencies & Associations

California

570   Asthma and Allergy Foundation of America: Southern California Chapter
5900 Wilshire Boulevard   323-937-7859
Los Angeles, CA 90036   800-624-0044
Fax: 323-937-7815
e-mail: Breathingmatters@aafa-ca.org
http://www.aafa.org/display.cfm?id=10&su
Dedicated to controlling and curing asthma and allergic diseases through education, a network of support groups, the support of research and specialized training, increasing public awareness and providing medication and treatment to the under served. Program highlights include the Breathmobile, asthma camps and air power games for children.
Michael Ingram, Executive Director

Florida

571   Asthma and Allergy Foundation of America: Florida Chapter
200 Orangewood Drive   727-738-1146
Dunedin, FL 34698   Fax: 727-736-4484
e-mail: cherylsmall@aafaflorida.org
www.aafa.org
Works to serve its community through programs, advocacy, education, research and national involvement.
John Little, Executive Director

Maryland

572   Asthma and Allergy Foundation of America: Maryland/Greater Washington, DC
1498 Reisterstown Rd   410-484-2054
Baltimore, MD 21208   800-727-9333
Fax: 410-484-2043
e-mail: aafamd@rcn.com
www.aafa-md.org
Serves the state of Maryland, District of Columbia and Northern Virginia areas. Dedicated to helping asthma and allergy sufferers successfully manage and control their disease through the education, referrals and research. Major activities include accredited child care provider course, school liaison, asthma camp, patient assistance, college scholarships for high school seniors and professional education courses. Breathmobile, Mobile Asthma Clinic, visiting schools in the city of Baltimore.
Susan Sweitzer, Executive Director

Massachusetts

573   Asthma and Allergy Foundation of America: New England Chapter
109 Highland Ave.   781-444-7778
Needham, MA 02494   877-227-8462
Fax: 781-444-7718
TTY: 877-227-8462
e-mail: aafane@aafane.org
www.asthmaandallergies.org
Serves Massachusetts, Rhode Island, Connecticut, Maine, New Hampshire and Vermont. Program highlights include speakers and exhibits, telephone information and referrals, tobacco control program, scholarship essay contest for high school juniors, advocacy for safer environments and training programs for school, daycare and health professionals.
Debbie Saryan, Executive Director
Sharon Schumack, Health Education Coordinator

Michigan

574   Asthma and Allergy Foundation of America: Michigan Chapter
2075 Walnut Lake Rd   248-406-4254
West Bloomfield, MI 48323-8768   888-444-0333
Fax: 248-757-2102
e-mail: aafamich@sbcglobal.net
www.aafamich.org
Serves the state of Michigan through public forums, work place educational programs, patient advocacy, Asthma Camp and telephone referrals and information.
Kathleen Felice Slonager, Executive Director
Dr. Rola Bokhari-Panza, President

Missouri

575   Asthma and Allergy Foundation of America: St. Louis Chapter
1500 S Big Bend   314-645-2422
St. Louis, MO 63117   Fax: 314-692-2022
e-mail: aafa@aafastl.org
www.aafastl.org
This chapter has provided children who suffer from asthma and allergies with life saving medications, equipment and educational and emotional support. The founders of the St. Louis chapter identified the apparent need in their community to help children effectively manage their asthma through the provision of medical resources, equipment and education.
Joy Kreiger, Executive Director

Oregon

576 Asthma and Allergy Foundation of America: Oregon Chapter
14530 SW 144th Avenue   503-524-2232
Tigard, OR 97224-1445   Fax: 208-474-6839
e-mail: hensches@teleport.com
Serving the state of Oregon.
Sandra L Henschel, Executive Director

Pennsylvania

**577 Asthma and Allergy Foundation of America: Southern
Pennsylvania Chapter**
470 Sentry Parkway East   610-397-1540
Blue Bell, NJ 19422   Fax: 856-224-5893
e-mail: aafasepa@verizon.net
http://www.aafa.org/
In the process of establishing a vital, new program that will aid
children with chronic asthma. Many parents, some who are without
medical insurance, are unaware of the availability of a medical
support system that can help their children. The Children at Risk
program will enable parents to have their children evaluated and
also receive a free one month supply of medication. Parents will
also receive information regarding available options for follow up
care and prescription coverage.
Marijo Washburn, Executive Director

Texas

**578 Asthma and Allergy Foundation of America: North Texas
Chapter**
3904 Justin Drive   817-297-3132
Ft. Worth, TX 76244   888-932-2232
Fax: 817-297-6564
e-mail: info@aafatexas.org
www.aafatexas.org
Offers many educational programs and services that touch patients, caregivers, physicians and allied health professionals, including: child care provider education programs, school nurse and
respiratory therapist education programs, work site allergy education programs, spacer and peak flow meter distribution to those in
need, a toll free hotline, prescription assistance information, free
educational materials in English and Spanish, an electronic
newsletter, professional education, etc.
Laura Steves, Executive Director

Washington

**579 Asthma and Allergy Foundation of America: Washington State
Chapter**
108 S Jackson Street   206-368-2866
Seattle, WA 98104   800-778-2232
Fax: 206-368-2941
e-mail: aafawa@aafawa.org
www.aafawa.org
Program highlights include trainings for health care professionals
on asthma and allergy management, working collaboratively with
other local and regional agencies to improve the quality of life for
those affected by asthma and allergies, organizing health fairs and
other public events and providing educational materials and
products.
Penny Nelson, Executive Director

Research Centers

580 Columbus Children's Research Institute
700 Children's Drive   614-722-2000
Columbus, OH 43205   Fax: 614-35-079
e-mail: John.Barnard@NationwideChildrens.org
www.nationwidechildrens.org
Research institute dedicated to enhancing the health of children by
engaging in the high quality cutting-edge research according to the
highest scientific and ethical standards.
John A Barnard, Research Institute President
Steve Allen MD, CEO

581 Creighton University Allergic Disease Center
601 N 30th Street   402-280-4403
Omaha, NE 68131-0001   Fax: 402-280-4803
e-mail: casalej@creighton.edu
medicine.creighton.edu/allergy/homepage.
Robert G Townley, Investigator
Thomas B Casale, Chief

582 Institute for Rehabilitation and Research
21720 Kingsland Blvd.
Katy, TX 77450   800-447-3422
Fax: 713-874-1798
e-mail: tirr.referrals@memorialhermann.org
www.tirr.memorialhermann.org
Carl Josehart, Chief Executive Officer
Gerard E. Francisco, Chief Medical Officer

583 Mayo Clinic and Foundation: Division of Allergic Diseases
Department of Immunology
200 First Street SW   507-284-2511
Rochester, MN 55905   Fax: 507-284-0161
TTY: 507-284-9786
e-mail: lee.theresa@mayo.edu
www.mayoclinic.org
Provides a focus for research into the causes prevention and man-
agement of allergic diseases.
John H Noseworthy MD, President
William C Rupp MD, Vice President, CEO

**584 National Jewish Center for Immunology and Respiratory
Medicine**
Goodman Building Room 611   303-398-1287
Denver, CO 80206   800-423-8891
Fax: 303-398-1806
www.nationaljewish.org
Basic and clinical research into the causes and treatments of asth-
matic disorders.
Tom Gart, Chairman
Michael Salem, President & CEO

585 Research Institute of Palo Alto Medical Foundation
795 El Camino Real
Palo Alto, CA 94301-2302   650-326-8120
www.pamf.org/research
Clinical and general medical sciences research including allergy
and immunology disorders.
Jane Risser, Director
Andrea Norcia, Assistant Director

586 Scripps Research Institute
10550 N Torrey Pines Road
La Jolla, CA 92037   858-784-1000
www.scripps.edu
William Burfitt, President
Alex Bruner, Executive Vice President and Chief Opera

587 Texas Children's Allergy and Immunology Clinic
Clinical Care Center
6701 Fannin Street   832-824-1000
Houston, TX 77030   800-364-5437
Fax: 832-825-3072
e-mail: pediai@texaschildrenshospital.org
www.texaschildrenshospital.org
Mark A Wallace, President & CEO
Mark W Kline MD, Physician In Chief

588 University of Florida: General Clinical Research Center
University of Florida
1600 SW Archer Road   352-273-5500
Gainesville, FL 32610-0322   888-635-0763
Fax: 352-273-5541
e-mail: thomprd@ufl.edu
www.med.ufl.edu
Studies on allergies and immunology.
Robert Thompson, Program Director

589 University of Kansas Allergy and Immunology Clinic
University of Kansas Medical Center

3901 Rainbow Boulevard 913-588-5000
Kansas City, KS 66160 TTY: 913-588-7963
TDD: 913-588-7963
e-mail: dstechsc@kumc.edu
www.kumc.edu

This service provides complete evaluation of patients with allergic diseases such as rhinitis and asthma immunological deficiencies food and drug intolerances and autoimmune dysfunctions.

Barbara F Atkinson MD, Executive Vice Chancellor
Shelley Gebar, RN, MHA, Chief of Staff

590 University of Michigan Montgomery: John M. Sheldon Allergy Society
Alllergy & Clinical Immunology
24 Frank Lloyd Wright Drive 734-232-2154
Ann Arbor, MI 48106-0380 Fax: 734-647-6263
e-mail: echoreed@med.umich.edu
www.med.umich.edu/sheldonsociety

Travis A Miller, President

591 University of Texas Southwestern Medical Center at Dallas
University of Texas Southwestern Medical Center
5323 Harry Hines Boulevard 214-648-3111
Dallas, TX 75390 Fax: 214-648-9119
e-mail: news@utsouthwestern.edu
www.utsouthwestern.edu

Immunodermatology department researching allergies and immune disorders.

Daniel K Podolsky MD, President

592 Warren Grant Magnuson Clinical Center
National Institute of Health
9000 Rockville Pike 301-496-2563
Bethesda, MD 20892 800-411-1222
Fax: 301-402-2984
TTY: 866-411-1010
e-mail: prpl@mail.cc.nih.gov
www.cc.nih.gov

Established in 1953 as the research hospital of the National Institutes of Health. Designed so that patient care facilities are close to research laboratories so new findings of basic and clinical scientists can be quickly applied to the treatment of patients. Upon referral by physicians, patients are admitted to NIH clinical studies.

Michael J Klag MD, Chair
David K Henderson MD, Clinical Director

Support Groups & Hotlines

593 ASTHMA Hotline
American Academy of Allergy, Asthma and Immunology
2275 East Bayshore Road 650-328-3123
Palo Alto, CA 53202 800-822-2762
Fax: 650-321-4457
www.aaai.org

Referral line offering information on allergy and asthma treatments, referrals to an allergy/immunology specialist, lay organization or support groups across the country.

594 National Health Information Center
PO Box 1133 310-565-4167
Washington, DC 20013-1133 800-336-4797
Fax: 301-984-4256
e-mail: info@nhic.org
www.health.gov/nhic

A health information referral service sponsored by the Office of Disease Prevention and Health Promotion. NHIC puts health professionals and consumers who have health questions in touch with those organizations that are best able to provide answers.

Books

595 Allergies A to Z
Facts on File
132 W 31st Street 212-967-8800
New York, NY 10001 800-322-8755
Fax: 800-678-3633
e-mail: custserv@factsonfile.com
www.factsonfile.com

This vital resource for the one in five Americans who suffer from alleries provides reliable, up-to-date information on every aspect of this condition.
Paperback

596 Allergy Alerts from Living with Allergies
American Allergy Association
PO Box 7273 650-322-1663
Menlo Park, CA 94026-7273

These alerts cover a wide range of areas from dyes in medications to medication interactions, food additives like sulfites, spelt, situations that could trigger asthma, problems with collagen and even fabric softeners.

597 Allergy Plants that Cause Sneezing and Wheezing
Asthma and Allergy Foundation of America
1233 20th Street NW 202-466-7643
Washington, DC 20036-2330 800-727-8462
Fax: 202-466-8940
www.aafa.org

Destined to be displayed on coffee tables, the spectacular photographs in this book actually show allergy sufferers what causes their sneezing and wheezing.
64 pages Paperback

598 Complete Book of Children's Allergies
Allergy Central Products
96 Danbury Road 203-438-9580
Ridgefield, CT 06877-4053 800-422-3878
Fax: 203-431-8963
www.allergycontrol.com

Major childhood allergies, recommendations for treatment.
Softcover

599 Cooking for the Allergic Child
Allergy Central Products
96 Danbury Road 203-438-9580
Ridgefield, CT 06877-4053 800-442-3878
Fax: 203-431-8963
www.allergycontrol.com

More than 300 recipes with nutrients analysis.
Softcover

600 Diets to Help Gluten and Wheat Allergy
HarperCollins Canada Limited/Order Department
1995 Markham Road
Scarborough, M1B 5M8, 800-387-0117
Fax: 800-668-5788

This book offers sound and practical advice on gluten allergy wheat sensitivity and Celiac disease.
96 pages
ISBN: 0-722529-10-4

601 Food Allergy: A Primer for People
Asthma and Allergy Foundation of America
1233 20th Street NW 202-466-7643
Washington, DC 20036-2330 800-727-8462
Fax: 202-466-8940
www.aafa.org

Food allergies demystified.
66 pages Hardcover

602 Human Exposure Assessment for Airborne Pollutants: Advances & Opportunity
National Academies Press
500 5th Street NW 202-334-3313
Washington, DC 20001 888-624-8373
Fax: 202-334-2451
e-mail: customer_service@nap.edu
www.nap.edu

Explores the need for strategies to address indoor and outdoor exposures and examines the methods and tools available for finding out where and when significant exposures occur.
344 pages
ISBN: 0-309042-84-0
Sandy Adams, Publishing Operations Director
Dottie Lewis, Publishing Services Director

603 Indoor Allergens: Assessing & Controlling Adverse Health Effects
National Academies Press

500 5th Street NW
Washington, DC 20055

202-334-3313
888-624-8373
Fax: 202-334-2793
e-mail: customer_service@nap.edu
www.nap.edu

This comprehensive and practical volume will be important to allergists and other health care providers; public health professionals; specialists in building design, construction, and maintenance; faculty and students in public health; and interested allergy patients.
350 pages
ISBN: 0-309048-31-6
Sandy Adams, Publishing Operations Director
Dottie Lewis, Publishing Services Director

604 Infant Formulas for Allergic Infants and Dietetic Concerns for Toddlers
American Allergy Association
PO Box 7273
Menlo Park, CA 94026-7273

650-322-1663

Offers information on reliable food labels, evaluations of infant formulas, FDA labeling requirements under the new law and more.

605 New Food Labels
American Allergy Association
PO Box 7273
Menlo Park, CA 94026-7273

650-322-1663

Offers clear-cut and precise information on new label word definitions.

606 Pollen Times: By State, By Month
American Allergy Association
PO Box 7273
Menlo Park, CA 94026-7273

650-322-1663

A comprehensive guide offering information on how to plan vacations while avoiding pollen problems.

607 Traveling with Allergies: Prepare and Avoid Problems
American Allergy Association
PO Box 7273
Menlo Park, CA 94026-7273

650-322-1663

Prepare for travel, recognize and minimize the risk, sidestep smoke, food allergies, pollen, mold, dander, weather and emergencies.

Children's Books

608 All About Allergies
Dutton Children's Books
375 Hudson Street
New York, NY 10014-3658

212-366-2000
Fax: 212-366-2262
www.pengiunputnam.com

1993 64 pages
ISBN: 0-525674-10-1

609 Allergies
Franklin Watts Grolier
90 Old Sherman Turnpike
Danbury, CT 06816-0001

203-797-3500
800-621-1115
Fax: 203-797-3197
www.grolier.com

Covers the major types of allergies, including those of the respiratory and gastrointestinal tracts.
112 pages Grades 7-12
ISBN: 0-531125-16-5

610 Living with Allergies
Franklin Watts Grolier
90 Old Sherman Turnpike
Danbury, CT 06816-0001

203-797-3500
800-621-1115
Fax: 203-797-3197
www.grolier.com

Shows how people with allergies are able to overcome their handicap to lead full and productive lives.
32 pages Grades 5-7
ISBN: 0-531108-57-0

Magazines

611 Allergy & Asthma Today
Allergy and Asthma Network Mothers of Asthmatics
8201 Greensboro Drive
McLean, VA 22102

800-878-4403
e-mail: info@aanma.org
www.aanma.org

The practical, family-friendly magazine for people living with asthma, allergies and other respiratory conditions. Award-winning and medically reviewed, packed with news and real-life inspiration and success stories, the ultimate resource for patients, families and healthcare providers.
40 pages Quarterly
Laurie Ross, Managing Editor

Newsletters

612 Advice From Your Allergist
American College of Allergy & Immunology
85 W Algonquin Road
Alrlington Heights, IL 60005

847-359-2800
www.allergy.mcg.edu

Offers information on the effects, triggers and causes of allergies including house dust, pets, hay fever, hives and exercise.

613 Food Allergy News
Food Allergy and Anaphylaxis Network
10400 Eaton Place
Fairfax, VA 22030-2208

703-691-3179
800-929-4040
Fax: 703-691-2713
e-mail: faan@foodallergy.org
www.foodallergy.org

Contains allergy free recipes, practical tips such as birthday party, trick-or-treating and travel tips, a dietitian's column, medical information and product information.
12 pages BiMonthly
Anne Munoz-Furlong, Founder

614 MA Report
Allergy and Asthma Network/Mothers of Asthmatics
2751 Prosperity Avenue
Fairfax, VA 22031

703-641-9595
800-878-4403
Fax: 703-573-7794
e-mail: editor@aanma.org
www.breatherville.org

Provides up-to-date medical news, emotional support and practical strategies for overcoming asthma and allergies.
8 pages 8x Year
Mary McGowan, Executive Director
Nancy Sander, Editor-in-Chief

Pamphlets

615 Allergic Diseases
National Institute of Allergy & Infectious Disease
31 Center Drive
Bethesda, MD 20892-2520

301-496-5717
www.niaid.nih.gov/default.htm

Offers information on allergies, who gets them, diagnosis and treatments for various types of allergic diseases.

616 Allergies and You
American Lung Association
1740 Broadway
New York, NY 10019-4315

212-315-8700

Answers basic questions about allergy, particularly as it relates to asthma.

617 Eating Without Packet
American Allergy Association
PO Box 7273
Menlo Park, CA 94026-7273

650-322-1663

Twelve information sheets describing the most common food allergens, specific problems with common foods and supplements, and the facts on milk ingredient labeling, milk allergies, and milk sensitivity. Included in the packet is a 16-page handbook, Understanding Calcium and Osteoporosis.

618 FAAN Flashbacks
Food Allergy and Anaphylaxis Network
10400 Eaton Place   703-691-3179
Fairfax, VA 22030-2208   800-929-4040
                                                        Fax: 703-691-2713
                                         e-mail: faan@foodallergy.org
                                                      www.foodallergy.org
Series of reprints on specific topics of Food Allergy News. Specific pamphlets offer information on wheat, milk, soy, egg, fish, peanuts, managing food allergy in schools and anaphylaxis.
Anne Munoz-Furlong, Founder

619 Food Allergy and Atopic Dermatitis
Food Allergy and Anaphylaxis Network
10400 Eaton Place   703-691-3179
Fairfax, VA 22030-2208   800-929-4040
                                                        Fax: 703-691-2713
                                         e-mail: faan@foodallergy.org
                                                      www.foodallergy.org
The purpose of this booklet is to provide tips and other sources of information to help parents raise a child who is afflicted with atopic dermatitis.
12 pages
Anne Munoz-Furlong, Founder

620 Guide to Gluten-Free Diets
American Allergy Association
PO Box 7273   650-322-1663
Menlo Park, CA 94026-7273
Offers information on safe substitutes for baking and cooking. Differentiates celiac disease from wheat allergy. Sources of gluten in diet with warnings on when to check with the manufacturer.

621 Helpful Hints for the Allergic Patient
American Academy of Allergy, Asthma and Immunology
611 E Wells Street   414-272-6071
Milwaukee, WI 53202-3889   800-822-2762
                                                        Fax: 414-272-6070
                                                             www.aaaai.org
An informational brochure good for someone who has just been diagnosed with allergies.
8 pages

622 Just One Little Bite Can Hurt! Important Facts About Anaphylaxis
Food Allergy and Anaphylaxis Network
10400 Eaton Place   703-691-3179
Fairfax, VA 22030-2208   800-929-4040
                                                        Fax: 703-691-2713
                                         e-mail: faan@foodallergy.org
                                                      www.foodallergy.org
Offers information on what anaphylaxis is, what the patient should do if they have a reaction and important medical safety tips regarding the illness.
8 pages Booklet
Anne Munoz-Furlong, Founder

623 Nutrition Guide to Food Allergies
Food Allergy and Anaphylaxis Network
10400 Eaton Place   703-691-3179
Fairfax, VA 22030-2208   800-929-4040
                                                        Fax: 703-691-2713
                                         e-mail: faan@foodallergy.org
                                                      www.foodallergy.org
Offers answers to the most commonly asked questions about food allergies, common allergy causing foods and resources for the patient.
24 pages
Anne Munoz-Furlong, Founder

624 Something in the Air: Airborne Allergens
National Institute of Allergy & Infectious Disease
9000 Rockville Pike   301-496-5717
Bethesda, MD 20892-0001
Offers information on the symptoms to airborne substances, pollen, mold, dust, animal, chemical allergies and treatments for them.

Audio & Video

625 Alexander, the Elephant Who Couldn't Eat Peanuts
Food Allergy and Anaphylaxis Network
11781 Lee Jackson Highway
                                                             800-929-4040
                                                        Fax: 703-691-2713
                                                      www.foodallergy.org
Helps children cope with their own allergies and teach other children about tolerance. Both videos combine colorful animation with interviews of real-life children with food allergies who talk about their experiences.
Jennifer Roeder, Marketing/Media Communications Director

626 Allergic Rhinitis
American Academy of Allergy, Asthma and Immunology
611 E Wells Street   414-272-6071
Milwaukee, WI 53202-3889   800-822-2762
                                                        Fax: 414-272-6070
                                                             www.aaaai.org
Allergic rhinitis, often called hay fever, affects the quality of life of millions of Americans. This video covers the causes and symptoms of seasonal and chronic allergic rhinitis, as well as environmental controls and treatments.
10-13 minutes

627 Allergic Rhinitis: Nothing to Sneeze At!
Asthma and Allergy Foundation of America
1233 20th Street NW   202-466-7643
Washington, DC 20036-2330   800-727-8462
                                                        Fax: 202-466-8940
                                                             www.aafa.org
The basics of allergic rhinitis, with a touch of humor. Common allergens, environmental control, skin testing and immunotherapy medications.
Videotape

628 Allergic Skin Reactions
American Academy of Allergy, Asthma and Immunology
611 E Wells Street   414-272-6071
Milwaukee, WI 53202-3889   800-822-2762
                                                        Fax: 414-272-6070
                                                             www.aaaai.org
In some people, allergy symptoms include itching redness, rashes, or hives. This video describes the symptoms, triggers, and treatment for common skin reactions such as dermatitis, hives and angioedema.
10-13 minutes

629 An Overview of Allergy
American College of Allergy & Immunology
800 E NW Highway   847-359-2800
Palatine, IL 60067-6580
Strengthen relationships with patients by providing them with the essential information they need.

630 Sinusitis and Sinus Surgery
Milner-Fenwick
2125 Greenspring Drive   410-252-1700
Timonium, MD 21093-3100   800-432-8433
                                                        Fax: 410-252-6316
                                       e-mail: sales@milnerfenwick.com
                                                    www.milner-fenwick.com
Discusses sinusitis symptoms, causes, evaluation and treatments. Animation depicts how sinuses function and how irritants, allergies, colds or structural abnormalities cause sinus blockages. Also explains the role of medical therapy and irrigation in managing acute sinusitis.
14 minutes
Dolores McKee, Advertising Director

Web Sites

631 American College of Allergy, Asthma & Immunology
                                                             www.acaai.org
A professional association of more than 5,000 allergists/immunologists and allied health professionals. Promotes excellence in the practice of the subspecialty of allergy and immunology.

632   American Lung Association

www.lungusa.org

The leading organization working to save lives by improving lung health and preventing lung disease through Education, Advocacy and Research.

633   Asthma and Allergy Foundation of America

www.aafa.org

The leading patient organization for people with asthma and allergies, and the oldest asthma and allergy patient group in the world. Dedicated to improving the quality of life for people with asthma and allergic disease through education, advocacy and research.

634   Birth Defect Research for Children

www.birthdefects.org

Provides parents and expectant parents with information about birth defects and support services for their children

635   Food Allergy and Anaphylaxis Network

www.foodallergy.org

To raise public awareness, to provide advocacy and education, and to advance research on behalf of all those affected by food allergies and anaphylaxis.

636   Healing Well

www.healingwell.com

A social network and support community for patients, caregivers, and families coping with the daily struggles of diseases, disorders and chronic illness.

637   Health Finder

www.healthfinder.gov

Government website where individuals can find information and tools to hel you and those you care about stay healthy.

638   Healthlink USA

www.healthlinkusa.com

Health information concerning treatment, cures, prevention, diagnosis, risk factors, research, support groups, email lists, personal stories and much more. Updated regularly.

639   Helios Health

www.helioshealth.com

Online resource for your health information. Detailed information about specific health topics, access to expert advice from our Medical Advisory Board, and up-to-date health news.

640   Immune Deficiency Foundation

www.primaryimmune.org

National patient organization dedicated to improving the diagnosis, treatment and quality of life of persons with primary immunodeficiency diseases through advocacy, education and research.

641   MedicineNet

www.medicinenet.com

An online resource for consumers providing easy-to-read, authoritative medical and health information.

642   Medscape

www.medscape.com

Medscape offers specialists, primary care physicians, and other health professionals the Web's most robust and integrated medical information and educational tools.

643   WebMD

www.webmd.com

Information on allergies, including articles and resources.

Description

644   Alzheimer's Disease

Alzheimer's disease is a degenerative neurologic disease that attacks the brain and impairs memory, thinking faculties and behavior. As the most common form of dementing illness, it afflicts 4 million adults and is twice as common in women as in men. It primarily affects older people.

In spite of diligent research, the cause of Alzheimer's disease is unknown. The disease runs in families in about 15 to 20 percent of cases, although the remainder may have some genetic component. There are multiple symptoms of Alzheimer's disease, the most pronounced being gradual memory loss. Other symptoms include the inability to perform routine tasks, loss of language skills, disorientation and personality changes. The diagnosis is largely based on an interview with the patient and family members and an examination of the patient, although brain imaging tests and blood tests may add helpful information.

The brain's cells communicate with each other through various chemicals called neurotransmitters. In Alzheimer's disease, levels of the neurotransmitter acetylcholine are decreased. Recently-released drugs which enhance the transmission of acetylcholine can cause at least limited improvement in memory during the early stages of Alzheimer's disease. A new drug, memantine, has been developed to slow the progression of advanced disease.

An extract of Ginkgo biloba may also slow memory loss and other symptoms. Some research suggests that certain activities that involve using the brain, such as reading and doing crossword puzzles, seem to reduce the risk. Because Alzheimer's disease severely affects both the patient and the family, proper planning, as well as medical and social programs tailored to the individual and to family members are essential. A well-structured and safe living environment is the best way to preserve the welfare and dignity of the person with Alzheimer's disease. See also *Aging*.

National Agencies & Associations

645   Alzheimer Society of Canada
20 Eglinton Avenue W   416-488-8772
Toronto, Ontario, M4R-1K8   800-618-8816
                                                                Fax: 416-322-6656
                                                        e-mail: info@alzheimer.ca
                                                                www.alzheimer.ca
Identified, develops and facilitates national priorities that enable its members to effectively alleviate the personal and social consequences of Alzheimer's disease and related disorders, promotes research and leads the search for a cure.
Richard Nakoneczny, President

646   Alzheimer's Disease Education and Referral Center
PO Box 8250   301-495-3311
Silver Spring, MD 20907-8250   800-222-2225
                                                                Fax: 301-495-3334
                                                        e-mail: niaic@nia.nih.gov
                                                        www.nia.nih.gov/alzheimers

A service of the National Institute on Aging the center distributes information on Alzheimer's disease on current research activities and on services available to patients and family members. Offers a free list of publications available upon request.

647   Alzheimer's Disease and Related Disorders Association
International Conference on Alzheimer's Disease
Montrose Avenue and Simonds Drive   847-324-0356
Chicago, IL 60613-7633   800-272-3900
                                                                Fax: 866-699-1246
                                                                TTY: 312-335-5886
                                                        e-mail: chicagowalk@alz.org
                                                                www.alz.org
Dedicated to research for the prevention cure and treatment of Alzheimer's disease and related disorders and to providing support and assistance to the afflicted patients and their families.
Harry Johns, President and CEO
Rachel Cleaveland, Local Contact

648   Benjamin B Greenfield National Alzheimer's Center
Montrose Avenue and Simonds Drive   847-324-0356
Chicago, IL 60613-7633   800-272-3900
                                                                Fax: 866-699-1238
                                                                TTY: 312-335-5886
                                                                TDD: 312-335-8700
                                                        e-mail: chicagowalk@alz.org
                                                                www.alz.org
Located at the national Alzheimer's Association in Chicago this library offers a sizable collection of videos on a variety of subjects that may interest the Alzheimer's patient family members and caregivers.
Edward Berube, Chair
Rachel Cleaveland, Local Contact

649   Interior Alzheimer Society
#217, 1889 Springfield Road   250-762-3312
Kelowna, BC, V1Y-5V5   Fax: 250-762-3312
                                                                e-mail: ias@silk.net
                                                        www.alzheimer-society.ca
A registered, independent, charitable non-profit society that was founded in 1981. Mission is to support, educate, and advocate for all those affected by Alzheimer disease in the Central Okanagan area of British Columbia: the patients, caregivers, patients' families and the community.

650   John Douglas French Alzheimer's Foundation
11620 Wilshire Boulevard   323-930-6228
Los Angeles, CA 90025-1781   800-477-2243
                                                                Fax: 310-479-0516
                                                        e-mail: bwelch@alz.org
                                                                www.jdfaf.org
Provides seed money for promising research including the cause cure and prevention of Alzheimer's disease. Also gives funding to scientists who might not otherwise be funded.
Michael M Minchin Jr, President
Brian Welch, Local Contact

State Agencies & Associations

Alabama

651   Alzheimer's Association: North Alabama Chapter
4747 Bob Wallace Avenue SW   256-880-1575
Huntsville, AL 35805-4872   800-272-3900
                                                                Fax: 256-880-8596
                                                        e-mail: cwhite2@alz.org
                                                                www.alz.org

Al Wiggins, Chair
Courtney White, Local Contact

652   Alzheimer's Association: Southeast Alabama Chapter
PO Box 609   334-677-6799
Dothan, AL 36302   800-272-3900
                                                                Fax: 334-671-3715
                                                                www.alz.org

Kay Jones, Executive Director

653 **Alzheimer's Association: Southwest Alabama Chapter**
PO Box 9272   334-660-5661
Mobile, AL 36691   800-272-3900
                                            Fax: 334-660-5667
                                                   www.alz.org

Bunnie Sutton, Executive Director

Alaska

654 **Alzheimer's Disease Resource Agency of Alaska**
1750 Abbott Road   907-561-3313
Anchorage, AK 99507   800-272-3900
                                            Fax: 907-561-3315
                                   e-mail: dnobre@alzalaska.org
                                                   www.alz.org

Jackie Brunton, President
Debbie Newsham, Vice President

Arizona

655 **Alzheimer's Association: Desert Southwest Chapter**
1028 E McDowell Road   602-528-0545
Phoenix, AZ 85006-2622   800-272-3900
                                            Fax: 602-528-0546
                                e-mail: deborah.schaus@alz.org
                                                   www.alz.org
Serving the state of Arizona and Southern Nevada offices in Phoenix, Tucson, Sun City, Prescott and Las Vegas.
Deborah Schaus, Executive Director
Dawn Boeck, Development Assistant

656 **Alzheimer's Association: Northern Arizona**
225 Grove Avenue   928-771-9257
Prescott, AZ 86301-2911   800-272-3900
                                            Fax: 520-771-9297
                                      e-mail: pwinkels@alz.org
                                                   www.alz.org

Don Connell, Regional Director
Patty Winkels, Local Contact

657 **Alzheimer's Association: Northern Nevada**
225 Grove Avenue   928-771-9257
Prescott, AZ 86301   800-272-3900
                                            Fax: 520-771-9297
                                      e-mail: pwinkels@alz.org
                                                   www.alz.org

Meg Fenzi, Regional Director
Patty Winkels, Local Contact

658 **Alzheimer's Association: Southern Arizona**
5132 East Pima Street   520-322-6601
Tucson, AZ 85712   800-272-3900
                                            Fax: 520-322-6739
                                        e-mail: kraach@alz.org
                                                   www.alz.org

Tormay Newman, Director
Kelly Raach, Local Contact

659 **Alzheimer's Association: Southern Arizona Region**
3003 S Country Club Road   520-322-6601
Tucson, AZ 85713   800-272-3900
                                            Fax: 520-322-6739
                                        e-mail: kraach@alz.org
                                                   www.alz.org

Heriberto Contreras, Regional Director
Kelly Raach, Local Contact

Arkansas

660 **Alzheimer's Arkansas Programs and Services**
400 President Clinton Ave   501-265-0027
Little Rock, AR 72205   800-272-3900
                                            Fax: 501-227-6303
                                       e-mail: sdavis@alz.org
                                                   www.alz.org

Phyllis Watkins, Executive Director
Susie Davis, Local Contact

661 **Alzheimer's Association: Western Arkansas Chapter**
121 Riverfront Drive   479-426-5541
Fort Smith, AR 72901-3454   800-272-3900
                                            Fax: 479-782-3185
                                       e-mail: sdavis@alz.org
                                                   www.alz.org

Rebecca Freeman, Executive Director
Susie Davis, Local Contact

California

662 **Alzheimer's Association San Diego/Imperial Chapter**
6632 Convoy Court   858-966-3319
San Diego, CA 92111   800-272-3900
                                            Fax: 858-492-4406
                                 e-mail: walksandiego@alz.org
                                                   www.alz.org
The leading voluntary health organization in Alzheimer care, support and research. The mission is to eliminate Alzheimer's disease through the advancement of research; to provide and enhance care and support for all affected; to advocate for policy change; and to reduce the risk of dementia through the promotion of brain health.
Lisa Bruner, Executive Director
Shelita Weinfield, Local Contact

663 **Alzheimer's Association: California Central Chapter: Ventura County Office**
80 North Wood Road   80 - 4 - 60
Camarillo, CA 93010   800-272-3900
                                            Fax: 805-485-4767
                            e-mail: nfeatherston@centralcoastalz.org
                                                   www.alz.org
The local chapter of the National Alzheimer's Association. The chapter stands by people with Alzheimer's disease, their families and professional caregivers through the following programs and services: a telephone help line, support groups, respite grants.
Norma Featherston, Area Director
Carol Swinney, Office Manager

664 **Alzheimer's Association: Greater Sacramento**
11th St. & N St.   916-930-9080
Sacramento, CA 95814   800-272-3900
                                            Fax: 916-930-9085
                                        e-mail: estone@alz.org
                                                   www.alz.org

Mary Gillon MPA, Regional Director
Erin Stone, Local Contact

665 **Alzheimer's Association: Greater North Valley Chapter**
1000 Woodland Ave   530-895-9661
Chico, CA 95928-3148   800-272-3900
                                            Fax: 530-872-7470
                                      e-mail: swatroba@alz.org
                                                   www.alz.org

Herb Williams, President
Suzanne Watroba, Local Contact

666 **Alzheimer's Association: Los Angeles Chapter**
133 N Sunol Drive   323-930-6228
Los Angeles, CA 90063-5017   800-272-3900
                                            Fax: 323-938-1036
                                        e-mail: bwelch@alz.org
                                                   www.alz.org

Earl Greinetz, President
Brian Welch, Local Contact

667 **Alzheimer's Association: Monterey County Chapter**
5 Custom House Plaza   831-647-9890
Monterey, CA 93940-5337   800-272-3900
                                            Fax: 831-655-9241
                                     e-mail: janderson@alz.org
                                                   www.alz.org

Herb Williams, President
Joy Anderson, Local Contact

668   Alzheimer's Association: North Bay Chapter
4340 Redwood Highway   415-472-4340
San Rafael, CA 94903   800-272-3900
Fax: 415-472-4350
e-mail: info@alznorcal.org
www.alz.org

Provides a continuum of services for Alzheimer's families, education and referral in Marin, Sonoma and Napa counties. To provide leadership and to eliminate Alzheimer's disease through the advancement of research while enhancing care and support services.
Herb Williams, President
Eduardo Salaz, Vice President

669   Alzheimer's Association: Orange County Chapter
17771 Cowan   949-955-9000
Irvine, CA 92614   800-272-3900
Fax: 949-757-3700
e-mail: helpoc@alz.org
www.alz.org

Dedicated to providing services, education and advocacy for individuals, families and the community affected by Alzheimer's disease and related memory disorders. Services include: 24/7 help line, support groups, family orientation program and care managers.
Norma Castellano, Program Specialist
Bobbie Babbage, Family Services Coordinator

670   Alzheimer's Association: Riverside/San Bernardino Counties Chapter
5900 Wilshire Boulevard   323-930-6228
Los Angeles, CA 90036   800-272-3900
Fax: 323-938-1036
e-mail: bwelch@alz.org
www.alz.org

Help line, support groups, information and education for caregivers and community.
400 Members
Earl Greinetz, President
Brian Welch, Local Contact

671   Alzheimer's Association: San Francisco Bay Area Chapter
1060 La Avenida   650-962-8111
Mountain View, CA 94043   800-272-3900
Fax: 650-962-9644
e-mail: info@alznorcal.org
www.alz.org

Herb Williams, President
Eduardo Salaz, Vice President

672   Alzheimer's Association: Santa Barbara Central Coast Chapter
3400 Calle Real   805-892-4259
Santa Barbara, CA 93105-8820   800-272-3900
Fax: 805-892-4250
e-mail: gbolton@alz.org
www.alz.org

The Alzheimer's Association California Central Coast Chapter serves families caring for people with Alzheimer's disease and related dementia throughout San Luis Obispo, Santa Barbara and Ventura Counties, offering a variety of educational and supportive programs.
Rhonda Spiegel, Executive Director
Genny Bolton, Local Contact

673   Alzheimer's Association: Santa Cruz County Chapter
1777-A Capitola Road   831-464-9982
Santa Cruz, CA 95062   800-272-3900
Fax: 831-464-8930
e-mail: info@alznorcal.org
www.alz.org

Herb Williams, President
Eduardo Salaz, Vice President

Colorado

674   Alzheimer's Association: Greater Grand Junction Area Chapter
2232 N 7th Street   970-256-1274
Grand Junction, CO 81501   800-272-3900
Fax: 970-256-0569
e-mail: walktoendalzWS@alzco.org
www.alz.org

Linda Mitchell, President/CEO
Lisa Miller, Local Contact

675   Alzheimer's Association: Rocky Mountain Chapter
455 Sherman Street   303-813-1669
Denver, CO 80203   800-272-3900
Fax: 303-813-1670
e-mail: jlorentz@alz.org
www.alz.org

Linda Mitchell, President/CEO
Jill Lorentz, Local Contact

676   American Homes for the Aging: Western
5010 Aspen Drive   303-795-5465
Littleton, CO 80123   Fax: 303-794-0487
Part of the national association representing retirement communities, nursing homes and community services for the elderly.

Connecticut

677   Alzheimer's Association: Connecticut Chapter
99 Trinity Street   860-956-9560
Hartford, CT 06106   800-272-3900
Fax: 860-956-9590
e-mail: walkhelpct@alz.org
www.alz.org

Works with all individuals and family members affected by Alzheimer's disease and related disorders; ensures humane systems of care and support and promotes research efforts to treat and cure Alzheimer's disease.
Christopher Rupp, Chairman
Daniel P Finke, Treasurer

678   Alzheimer's Association: South Central Connecticut Chapter
2911 Dixwell Avenue   203-230-1777
Hamden, CT 06518   800-272-3900
Fax: 203-230-1712
www.alz.org

Patricia Clark, Executive Director

Delaware

679   Alzheimer's Association: Delaware Chapter
240 N James Street   302-633-4420
Newport, DE 19804   800-272-3900
Fax: 302-633-4494
e-mail: Wendy.Campbell@alz.org
www.alz.org

Wendy L Campbell, President
Theresa Haenn, Vice President Development

District of Columbia

680   Alzheimer's Association: Greater Washington DC Chapter
2524 Pensylvania Avenue Southeast   703-359-4440
Washington, DC 20020   800-272-3900
Fax: 202-483-4164
e-mail: alzwalknca@alz.org
www.alz.org

Help line-telephone referral support groups, caregiver education, respite services. We have three offices serving DC and surrounding Maryland counties.

Abigail Reinecker, Local Contact

Florida

681 Alzheimer's Association: Broward County Chapter
201 E Sample Road 800-861-7826
Deerfield Beach, FL 33407 800-272-3900
Fax: 954-786-1538
e-mail: barbara.grasch@alz.org
www.alz.org

Barbara Grasch, Director of Program Services
Ellen Brown, CEO

682 Alzheimer's Association: East Central Florida Chapter
Wickham Road 407-951-7992
Melbourne, FL 32935 800-272-3900
Fax: 407-729-8044
e-mail: jgiovanni@alz.org
www.alz.org

Joan Giovanni, Local Contact

683 Alzheimer's Association: Florida Gulf Coast Chapter
9365 US Highway 19 N 727-578-2558
Pinellas Park, FL 33782 800-272-3900
Fax: 727-578-2286
e-mail: milnel@alzflgulf.org
www.alz.org

Provides information and services to families and professionals dealing with memory related disorders.
Gloria JT Smith, President/CEO
Paul Anderson, Vice President Finance

684 Alzheimer's Association: Greater Miami Chapter
501 Marlins Way 305-891-6228
Miami, FL 33125 800-272-3900
Fax: 305-751-5551
e-mail: snewman@alz.org
www.alz.org

Reni Rizzo, Community Education Coordinator
Sharon Newman, Local Contact

685 Alzheimer's Association: Greater Orlando Area Chapter
Ampitheatre at 300 Robinson St., Do 407-951-7992
Orlando, FL 32801 800-272-3900
Fax: 407-228-4201
e-mail: jgiovanni@alz.org
www.alz.org

Stu Gaines, Chair
Joan Giovanni, Local Contact

686 Alzheimer's Association: Greater Palm Beach Area Chapter
600 N Congress Avenue 561-478-3120
Delray Beach, FL 33445 800-272-3900
Fax: 561-278-4910
www.alz.org

687 Alzheimer's Association: Northeast Florida
4237 Salisbury Rd 904-281-9077
Jacksonville, FL 32216 800-272-3900
Fax: 866-281-9078
e-mail: mdrinks@alz.org
www.alz.org

Michelle Drinks, Local Contact

688 Alzheimer's Association: Northern Central Florida Chapter
1001 NW 34th St 904-281-9077
Gainesville, FL 32605 800-272-3900
Fax: 352-372-2038
e-mail: mdrinks@alz.org
www.alz.org

Michelle Drinks, Local Contact
Tish Sheesley, CEO

689 Alzheimer's Association: Northwest Florida Chapter
119 Hollywood Boulevard 850-302-0581
Ft. Walton Beach, FL 32548 800-272-3900
Fax: 850-302-0583
www.alz.org

690 Alzheimer's Association: Southwest Florida Chapter
4075 Tamiami 941-235-7470
Port Charlotte, FL 33952 800-272-3900
Fax: 941-235-7473
www.alz.org

691 Alzheimer's Association: Tampa Bay Chapter
601 N Old Coachman Rd 727-259-2317
Clearwater, FL 33765 800-272-3900
Fax: 941-380-5701
e-mail: farinasr@alzflgulf.org
www.alz.org

Gloria JT Smith, President/CEO
Rachel Farinas, Local Contact

692 Alzheimer's Association: Volusia/Flagler Branch
111 N Frederick Avenue 407-951-7992
Daytona Beach, FL 32114-5126 800-272-3900
Fax: 386-238-8293
e-mail: jgiovanni@alz.org
www.alz.org

Joan Giovanni, Local Contact

693 Alzheimer's Association: West Central Florida Chapter
PO Box 2070 813-848-8888
New Port Richey, FL 34656-2070 800-272-3900
Fax: 813-849-6124
www.alz.org

Georgia

694 Alzheimer's Association: Atlanta Chapter
1925 Century Boulevard 404-728-6066
Atlanta, GA 30345-4021 800-272-3900
Fax: 404-636-9768
e-mail: rrotunda@alz.org
www.alz.org

Bennett Watts, Chair
Robyn Rotunda, Local Contact

695 Alzheimer's Association: Augusta Chapter
1899 Central Avenue 706-731-9060
Augusta, GA 30904-5755 800-272-3900
Fax: 706-731-9099
e-mail: kim.franklin@alz.org
www.alz.org

Bennett Watts, Chair
Bruce Flechter, Treasurer

696 Alzheimer's Association: Central Georgia Chapter
277 Martin Luther King Jr Boulevard 478-746-7050
Macon, GA 31201-3498 800-272-3900
Fax: 478-746-6679
e-mail: kim.franklin@alz.org
www.alz.org

Bennett Watts, Chair
Bruce Flechter, Treasurer

697 Alzheimer's Association: Greater Columbus Chapter
5900 River Road 706-327-6838
Columbus, GA 31904-0185 800-272-3900
Fax: 706-494-0533
e-mail: cvogler@alz.org
www.alz.org

Bennett Watts, Chair
Christina Vogler, Local Contact

698 Alzheimer's Association: Greater Georgia Chapter
1925 Century Boulevard 404-728-6066
Atlanta, GA 30345-4021 800-272-3900
Fax: 404-636-9768
e-mail: rrotunda@alz.org
www.alz.org

Bennett Watts, Chair
Robyn Rotunda, Local Contact

699 Alzheimer's Association: Southeast Georgia Chapter
201 Television Circle
Savannah, GA 31406
912-920-2231
800-272-3900
Fax: 912-921-7960
e-mail: dheddendorf@alz.org
www.alz.org

Deborah Heddendorf, Local Contact

700 Alzheimer's Association: Southwest Georgia Chapter
1512-1 Gillionville Road
Albany, GA 31707
229-388-8219
800-272-3900
Fax: 229-888-2620
e-mail: dphillips@alz.org
www.alz.org

Maggie Keenan, Office Volunteer
Dan Phillips, Local Contact

Hawaii

701 Alzheimer's Association: Honolulu Chapter
1050 Ala Moana Boulevard
Honolulu, HI 96814
808-591-2771
800-272-3900
Fax: 808-591-9071
e-mail: ebatalon@alz.org
www.alz.org

Eric Batalon, Local Contact
Chris Shirai, Chairman

702 Alzheimer's Association: West Hawaii Chapter
PO Box 390247
Kailua Kona, HI 96739-0247
808-591-2771
800-272-3900
Fax: 808-322-0008
e-mail: ebatalon@alz.org
www.alz.org

Eric Batalon, Local Contact

Idaho

703 Alzheimer's Association: Greater Idaho Chapter
1111 S Orchard
Boise, ID 83705-2878
208-384-1788
800-272-3900
Fax: 208-385-7191
e-mail: suzette.albers-tunnell@alz.org
www.alz.org

Suzette Albers-Tunne, Executive Director

704 Alzheimer's Association: Northern Idaho Chapter
2003 Kootenai Health Way
Coeur D Alene, ID 83814
208-666-2996
800-272-3900
Fax: 509-473-3389
e-mail: pchristo@alz.org
www.alz.org

PJ Christo, Outreach Coordinator
Joel Loiacono, Executive Director

Illinois

705 Alzheimer's Association: Central Illinois Chapter
606 W Glen Avenue
Peoria, IL 61614-4831
309-681-1100
800-272-3900
Fax: 309-681-1101
e-mail: kgabbert@alz.org
www.alz.org

Nikki Vulgaris, Executive Director
Kari Gabbert, Local Contact

706 Alzheimer's Association: East Central Illinois Chapter
303 N. Hershey
Bloomington, IL 61704-7337
217-351-1726
800-272-3900
Fax: 217-351-2161
www.alz.org

Provides information, support, and referral services to families
and individuals facing Alzheimer's disease. Includes newsletter,
support groups, and education.

707 Alzheimer's Association: Four Rivers Chapter
401 N Wall Street
Kankakee, IL 60901
815-936-0464
800-272-3900
Fax: 815-936-9363
www.alz.org

708 Alzheimer's Association: Greater Illinois Chapter
4709 Golf Road
Skokie, IL 60076-1260
847-933-2413
800-272-3900
Fax: 847-933-2417
e-mail: info@alz.org
www.alz.org

**709 Alzheimer's Association: Greater Illinois Chapter: Carbondale
Office**
402 E Plaza Drive
Carterville, IL 62918-1429
618-985-1095
800-272-3900
Fax: 618-457-7830
e-mail: GI.Chapter@alz.org
www.alz.org

Jill Schoenborn, Coordinator Outreach & Development

710 Alzheimer's Association: Land of Lincoln Chapter
South Second Street & Southwind Roa
Springfield, IL 62703-4833
217-801-9352
800-272-3900
Fax: 217-726-5185
e-mail: tarnold@alz.org
www.alz.org

Jane Field, Office Manager
Tina Arnold, Local Contact

711 American Homes for the Aging: Midwest Regional Office
911 N Elm Street
Hinsdale, IL 60521-3641
630-323-6755
800-272-3900
Fax: 630-325-0749
www.alz.org

Regional office of the AHA, a national professional association of
nonprofit nursing homes, retirement communities and homes for
the aging.

Indiana

712 Alzheimer's Association: Central Indiana Chapter
601 W. New York Street
Indianapolis, IN 46202-1816
317-575-9620
800-272-3900
Fax: 317-582-0669
e-mail: IndianaWalk@alz.org
www.alz.org

Heather Allen Hershberger, Executive Director
Leslie Bush, Local Contact

713 Alzheimer's Association: Northern Indiana Chapter
922 E Colfax Avenue
S Bend, IN 46617-3112
57 - 2 - 41
800-272-3900
Fax: 57 - 2 - 42
e-mail: AlzServicesNI@sbcglobal.net
www.alz.org

Iowa

714 Alzheimer's Association: Big Sioux Chapter
401 Gordon Drive
Sioux City, IA 51101-3716
712-279-5802
800-272-3900
Fax: 712-277-8076
e-mail: tschroeder@alz.org
www.alz.org

Kim McCormick, Executive Director
Terri Schroeder, Local Contact

715 Alzheimer's Association: East Central Iowa Chapter
1570 42nd Street NE
Cedar Rapids, IA 52402
319-294-9699
800-272-3900
Fax: 319-294-0068
e-mail: amiller2@alz.org
www.alz.org

Kelly Hauer, Executive Director
Abbey Miller, Local Contact

716 Alzheimer's Association: Greater Iowa Chapter
1730 28th Street
W Des Moines, IA 50266

515-440-2722
800-272-3900
Fax: 515-440-6385
e-mail: Carol.Sipfle@alz.org
www.alz.org

Carol Sipfle, Executive Director
Holly Bradford, Finance Director

717 Alzheimer's Association: Heart of Iowa Chapter
3915 Mortensen Road
Ames, IA 50014-7259

515-440-6383
800-272-3900
Fax: 515-292-0125
e-mail: cmathany@alz.org
www.alz.org

Chantelle Mathany, Local Contact

718 Greater Iowa Chapter Alzheimer's Association Quadcity Office
736 Federal Street
Davenport, IA 52803-5750

563-324-1022
800-272-3900
Fax: 563-324-6267
e-mail: Jerry.Schroeder@alz.org
www.alz.org

Jerry Schroeder, Program Specialist
Julie Seier, Community Relations Coordinator

Kansas

719 Alzheimer's Association: Heart of America Chapter
3846 W 75th Street
Prairie Village, KS 66208-4126

913-831-3888
800-272-3900
Fax: 913-831-1916
e-mail: jan.horn@alz.org
www.alz.org

Debra R Brook, Executive Director
Michelle Niedens, Education Director

720 Alzheimer's Association: Sunflower Chapter
347 S Laura
Wichita, KS 67211-4109

316-267-7333
800-272-3900
Fax: 316-267-6369
e-mail: lbelton@alz.org
www.alz.org

Marsha Hills, Executive Director
Lanette Belton, Local Contact

Kentucky

721 Alzheimer's Association: Lexington/ Bluegrass Chapter
465 E High Street
Lexington, KY 40507

859-266-5283
800-272-3900
Fax: 859-268-4764
e-mail: amber.lakin@alz.org
www.alz.org

Debbie Lacy Goodman, VP Awareness & Community Relations
Amber Lakin, Local Contact

722 Alzheimer's Association: Louisville Chapter
6100 Dutchmans Lane
Louisville, KY 40205

502-451-4266
800-272-3900
Fax: 502-456-2701
e-mail: wvogel@alz.org
www.alz.org

Teri Shirk, Chapter President & CEO
Whitney Vogel, Local Contact

Louisiana

723 Alzheimer's Association: Northeast/Central Louisiana Chapter
2300 Sycamore
Monroe, LA 71201

318-861-8680
800-272-3900
Fax: 318-998-7360
e-mail: dhayes@alz.org
www.alz.org

Debbie Hayes, Local Contact

724 Alzheimer's Association: Greater New Orleans Chapter
DePaul Hospital
1040 Calhoun Street
New Orleans, LA 70118-5999

504-648-4084
800-272-3900
Fax: 504-895-0493
e-mail: charrell@alz.org
www.alz.org

Chet Harrell, Local Contact

725 Alzheimer's Services of the Capital Area
3772 N Boulevard
Baton Rouge, LA 70806

225-334-7494
800-548-1211
Fax: 225-387-3664
e-mail: info@alzbr.org
www.alzbr.org

The mission of Alzheimer's Services of the Capital Area is to provide education and support services to memory impaired individuals as well as caregivers and professionals; and to enhance community awareness of Alzheimer's disease and related disorders.
Barbara Auten, Executive Director

Maine

726 Alzheimer's Association: Maine Chapter
383 U.S. Route 1
Scarborough, ME 04074-2419

207-772-0115
800-272-3900
Fax: 207-289-3705
e-mail: laurie.trenholm@alz.org
www.alz.org

Joy Heptner, Executive Director
Liz Weaver, Program Director

727 Maine Alzheimer's Care Center
154 Dresden Avenue
Gardiner, ME 04345

207-626-1770

Maryland

728 Alzheimer's Association: Central Maryland Chapter
1850 York Road
Timonium, MD 21093-5122

410-561-9099
800-272-3900
Fax: 410-561-3433
e-mail: info.maryland@alz.org
www.alz.org

Cass Naugle, Executive Director
Teri Bennett, Helpline Coordinator

729 Alzheimer's Association: Eastern Shore Chapter
909 Progress Circle
Salisbury, MD 21804

410-543-1163
800-272-3900
Fax: 410-546-0184
e-mail: dmagarelli@alz.org
www.alz.org

Cass Naugle, Executive Director
Damian Magarelli, Local Contact

730 Alzheimer's Association: Western Maryland Chapter
101 Clarke Pl.
Frederick, MD 21701

301-696-0315
800-272-3900
Fax: 301-696-9061
e-mail: kweddle@alz.org
www.alz.org

To eliminate Alzheimer's disease through the advancement of research and to enhance care and support for individuals their families and caregivers.
Cathy Hanson, Program Coordinator
Kristen Weddle, Local Contact

Massachusetts

731 Alzheimer's Association: Massachusetts Chapter
311 Arsenal Street
Watertown, MA 02472

617-868-6718
800-272-3900
Fax: 617-868-6720
www.alz.org

Nonprofit, national, voluntary health organization dedicated to Alzheimer research and care. Provides 24 hour help line, support

groups, a wanderers prevention program early stage patient programs, family educators, professional training, and advocacy.
James Wessle MBA, President & CEO
Betsy Fitzgerald-Cam, Vice President Communications

732 Alzheimer's Association: Western Regional Office: Massachusetts Chapter
264 Cottage Street   413-787-1113
Springfield, MA 01104   800-272-3900
                                     Fax: 413-787-1109
                                     www.alz.org

Nonprofit organization serving family and professional caregivers in seven counties in southwest Michigan. Provides information on Alzheimer's and other diseases, educational programs, resource libraries. Train-the-trainer agency referral, autopsy liaison, and other services.
Marcia McKen Med, Manager
Annie Clattenburg, Coordinator Administrative Services

Michigan

733 Alzheimer's Association: East Central Michigan Chapter
G-3287 Beecher Road   810-720-2791
Flint, MI 48503   800-272-3900
                                     Fax: 810-720-3040
                                     www.alz.org

734 Alzheimer's Association: Greater Michigan Chapter
20300 Civic Center Drive   248-351-0280
Southfield, MI 48076   800-272-3900
                                     Fax: 248-351-0417
                                     www.alz.org
A national network of chapters, is the largest national voluntary health organization committed to finding a cure for Alzheimer's and helping those affected by the disease. Provides a wide range of services and programs for Alzheimer's and other dementia patients for their families and for the general public.

735 Alzheimer's Association: Greater Michigan Chapter: Upper Peninsula Region
1420 Pine Street   906-228-3910
Marquette, MI 49855-4521   800-272-3900
                                     Fax: 906-228-2455
                                     TTY: 877-204-6924
                                     e-mail: ralmen@alz.org
                                     www.alz.org
Pamela Parkkila, Director
Ruth Almen, Local Contact

736 Alzheimer's Association: Michigan Great Lakes Chapter: West Shore Region
1740 Village Drive   734-475-7043
Muskegon, MI 49442-5546   800-272-3900
                                     Fax: 231-780-1494
                                     e-mail: mglcwalk@alz.org
                                     www.alz.org
Providing caregiver support groups a help line informational materials community education and a quarterly newsletter.
Barb Betts, Program Coordinator
Stephanie Barnhill, Local Contact

737 Alzheimer's Association: Mid-Michigan Chapter
4604 N Saginaw Road   989-839-9910
Midland, MI 48640   800-272-3900
                                     Fax: 989-839-5910
                                     TTY: 877-204-6924
                                     e-mail: boneill@alz.org
                                     www.alz.org
Dawn Spicer, Director
Betty O'Neill, Local Contact

738 Alzheimer's Association: Northeast Michigan Chapter
526 W Chisholm St   989-356-4087
Alpena, MI 49707   800-272-3900
                                     Fax: 989-354-7879
                                     e-mail: sruetz@alz.org
                                     www.alz.org
Shawn Ruetz, Local Contact

739 Alzheimer's Association: Northwest Michigan Chapter
921 W. 11th. Street   616-459-4558
Traverse City, MI 49864   800-272-3900
                                     Fax: 231-922-1584
                                     e-mail: sruetz@alz.org
                                     www.alz.org
Shawn Ruetz, Local Contact

Minnesota

740 Alzheimer's Association: Minnesota/Dakotas
1 Twins Way   952-830-0512
Minneapolis, MN 55403   800-272-3900
                                     Fax: 952-830-0513
                                     e-mail: mnnd-walk@alz.org
                                     www.alz.org
Mary Birchard, Executive Director
Libby Wilhelmy, Local Contact

Mississippi

741 Alzheimer's Association: Mississippi Chapter
1900 Dunbarton Drive   601-987-0020
Jackson, MS 39216   800-272-3900
                                     Fax: 601-987-9020
                                     e-mail: rruello@alz.org
                                     www.alz.org
Barb Dobrosky, Program Director
Rachel Ruello, Local Contact

742 Alzheimer's Foundation of the South: Mississippi Division
PO Box 2394   228-867-6251
Gulfport, MS 39503   800-272-3900
                                     Fax: 228-864-8843
                                     e-mail: alzms@cs.com
                                     www.alz.org
Rosemary Hudgins, Executive Director

Missouri

743 Alzheimer's Association: Mid-Missouri Chapter
2400 Bluff Creek Drive   573-443-8665
Columbia, MO 65201   800-272-3900
                                     Fax: 573-499-9701
                                     e-mail: cbaker@alz.org
                                     www.alz.org
Linda Newkirk, Executive Director
Chris Baker, Local Contact

744 Alzheimer's Association: Northwest Missouri-Chapter
10th and Faraon   816-364-4467
St. Joseph, MO 64502-1241   800-272-3900
                                     Fax: 816-364-2553
                                     e-mail: brenda.gregg@alz.org
                                     www.alz.org

745 Alzheimer's Association: Southwest Missouri Chapter
1500 S Glenstone   417-886-2199
Springfield, MO 65804   800-272-3900
                                     Fax: 417-886-0337
                                     e-mail: nreed@alz.org
                                     www.alz.org
Rebecca Argilagos, President/CEO
Nate Reed, Local Contact

746 Alzheimer's Association: St. Louis Chapter
700 Clark Avenue   314-801-0465
Saint Louis, MO 63102-3214   800-272-3900
                                     Fax: 314-432-3824
                                     e-mail: stlwalksupport@alz.org
                                     www.alz.org
Joan D'Ambrose, President
Alyssa Vorhies, Local Contact

Montana

747 Alzheimer's Association: Greater Billings Area Chapter
2100 South Shiloh Road
Billings, MT 59101
406-252-3053
800-272-3900
Fax: 406-252-2933
e-mail: sshannon@alz.org
www.alz.org

Kelly Donovan, President
Sharon Shannon, Local Contact

Nebraska

748 Alzheimer's Association: Great Plains Chap ter
1500 S. 70th St
Lincoln, NE 68506
402-420-2540
800-272-3900
e-mail: mfeit@alz.org
www.alz.org

The Alzheimer's Association of the Great Plains is dedicated to supporting those with Alzheimer's disease and their families and friends through specialized programs and services, educating families, communities, and health professionals about Alzheimer's disease.
Karen Noel, President/CEO
Mark Feit, Local Contact

749 Alzheimer's Association: Lincoln/Greater Nebraska Chapter
1500 S. 70th St.
Lincoln, NE 68506
402-420-2540
800-272-3900
Fax: 402-420-2541
e-mail: mfeit@alz.org
www.alz.org

Karen Noel, President/CEO
Mark Feit, Local Contact

750 Alzheimer's Association: Omaha/Eastern Nebraska Chapter
3220 Farnam St
Omaha, NE 68131-2167
402-502-4301
800-272-3900
Fax: 402-502-7001
e-mail: cenoviso@alz.org
www.alz.org

Duane Gross, President and CEO
Cathy Enoviso, Local Contact

Nevada

751 Alzheimer's Association: Northern Nevada Chapter
1301 Cordone Avenue
Reno, NV 89502-6362
775-786-8061
800-272-3900
Fax: 775-786-1920
e-mail: info@alznorcal.org
www.alz.org

Herb Williams, President
Eduardo Salaz, Vice President

752 Alzheimer's Association: Southern Nevada Chapter
5190 S Valley View Boulevard
Las Vegas, NV 89118-6062
702-248-2770
800-272-3900
Fax: 702-248-2771
e-mail: achavez@alz.org
www.alz.org

Luis Carrillo, Regional Director
Albert Chavez, Local Contact

New Hampshire

753 Alzheimer's Association of Vermont and New Hampshire
10 Ferry Street
Concord, NH 03301-5004
603-226-5868
800-272-3900
Fax: 603-225-8126
www.alz.org

Robbie Nicol, Chair
Robert Dowd, First Vice Chair

New Jersey

754 Alzheimer's Association: Greater New Jersey Chapter
400 Morris Avenue
Denville, NJ 07834
973-586-4300
800-272-3900
Fax: 973-586-4342
www.alz.org

Provides programs and services to individuals with Alzheimer's disease, their families and caregivers, including education and training, support groups, a toll free telephone help line and respite assistance.

755 Alzheimer's Association: South Jersey Chapter
3 Eves Drive
Marlton, NJ 08053
856-797-1212
800-272-3900
Fax: 609-784-8486
e-mail: Wendy.Campbell@alz.org
www.alz.org

Wendy L Campbell, President & CEO
Theresa Haenn, Vice President Development

New Mexico

756 Alzheimer's Association: New Mexico Chapter
9500 Montgomery Boulevard NE
Albuquerque, NM 87111
505-266-4473
800-272-3900
Fax: 505-266-0108
e-mail: nlawrie@alz.org
www.alz.org

Agnes Vallejos, Executive Director
Nika Lawrie, Local Contact

New York

757 Alzheimer's Association: Sullivan/Delaware Chapter
PO Box 911
Monticello, NY 12701
941-794-3774
800-272-3900
www.alz.org

758 Alzheimer's Association: Central New York Chapter
441 W Kirkpatrick Street
Syracuse, NY 13204-1361
315-472-4201
800-272-3900
Fax: 315-472-4206
e-mail: gfletcher@alz.org
www.alz.org

Larry Malfitano, President
Grant Fletcher, Local Contact

759 Alzheimer's Association: Hudson Valley/ Rockland/Westchester NY Chapter
2 Jefferson Plaza
Poughkeepsie, NY 12601-4027
845-471-2655
800-272-3900
Fax: 845-471-8960
e-mail: info@alzhudsonvalley.org
www.alz.org

Elaine Sproat, President & CEO
Meg Boyce, Director of Programs & Services

760 Alzheimer's Association: Long Island Chapter
3281 Veterans Memorial Highway
Ronkonkoma, NY 11779-3521
631-580-5100
800-272-3900
Fax: 631-580-3100
e-mail: Info@alzheimersli.org
www.alz.org

Voluntary health agency that provides care and consultation, information and referral, education, national safe return program and support groups to individuals with Alzheimer's, their families and/or caregivers.
Mary Ann Malack-Ragona, Executive Director/CEO
Linda Cody, Director of Development

761 Alzheimer's Association: New York City Chapter
360 Lexington Avenue
New York, NY 10017
646-744-2900
800-272-3900
Fax: 212-490-6037
e-mail: helpline@alznyc.org
www.alz.org/nyc

Lou-Ellen Barkan, President/CEO
Jed A. Levine, Executive Vice President

762   Alzheimer's Association: Northeastern New York Chapter
4 Pine West Plaza   518-867-4999
Albany, NY 12205-2083   800-272-3900
                                                 Fax: 518-867-4997
                                          e-mail: infoneny@alz.org
                                                       www.alz.org
Regional affiliate of national association. Works to educate and
support families, while raising funds in support of research.
Paul A Wajda, Chair
Warren E Garling, Vice Chair

763   Alzheimer's Association: Putnam County Chapter
Robin Hill Corporate Park
15 Mount Ebo Road S   845-278-0343
Brewster, NY 10509-2164   800-272-3900
                                    e-mail: info@alzhudsonvalley.org
                                                       www.alz.org
Stuart Greif, Program Development Specialist

764   Alzheimer's Association: Rochester Chapter
85 Adams Street   585-760-5472
Rochester, NY 14608   800-272-3900
                                                 Fax: 585-760-5401
                                      e-mail: rochesterwalk@alz.org
                                                       www.alz.org
Chris Lacey, Local Contact
Judy Lemoncelli, Local Contact

765   Alzheimer's Association: Southern Tier Chapter
401 Hayes Avenue   607-785-7852
Endicott, NY 13760-5421   800-272-3900
                                                 Fax: 607-785-4004
                                          e-mail: alzcny@alzcny.org
                                                       www.alz.org
L Jane Hudreck, Regional Director

766   Alzheimer's Association: Western New York Chapter
2805 Wehrle Drive   716-626-0600
Williamsville, NY 14421   800-272-3900
                                                 Fax: 717-626-2255
                                  e-mail: Donna.McKenzie@alz.org
                                                       www.alz.org
David Cascio, President
Linda Sabo, Executive Director

767   Alzheimer's Foundation of Staten Island
789 Post Avenue   718-667-7110
Staten Island, NY 10310-6427   877-574-7068
                                                 Fax: 718-667-8431
                                     e-mail: info@sialzheimers.org
                                                www.sialzheimers.org
Not-for-profit health and human services organization, serving
people with Alzheimer's disease and related dementias.
Leilani Joven Pelletie, Executive Director
David Cascio, President

North Carolina

768   Alzheimer's Association: Eastern North Carolina Chapter
1305 Navaho Dr.   919-832-3732
Raleigh, NC 27609   800-272-3900
                                                 Fax: 919-832-7989
                                          e-mail: awatkins@alznc.org
                                                       www.alz.org
Dedicated to providing program services education for patients,
families and professional caregivers, advocacy and research.
Alice Watkins, Executive Director
Rita Bhan, Developmental Director

769   Alzheimer's Association: Western North Carolina Chapter
3800 Shamrock Drive   704-532-7390
Charlotte, NC 28215   800-272-3900
                                                 Fax: 704-532-5421
                                            e-mail: infonc@alz.org
                                                       www.alz.org
A nonprofit voluntary organization dedicated to improving the
quality of life for those with Alzheimer's and their families
through a broad range of programs, including patient and family

services, education, advocacy and support of research through
national programs.
Beth Croom MA, Director of Programs/Education
Teresa Hoover, Program Associate/Helpline Coordinator

North Dakota

770   Alzheimer's Association: Fargo/Moorhead Regional Center
5225 31st Ave South   701-277-9757
Fargo, ND 58104   800-272-3900
                                                 Fax: 701-277-9785
                                     e-mail: traie.dockter@alz.org
                                                       www.alz.org
Gretchen Dobervich, Regional Center Director
Traie Dockter, Local Contact

Ohio

771   Alzheimer's Association: Canton Chapter
408 Ninth St. SW
Canton, OH 44707   800-272-3900
                                                 Fax: 330-996-7757
                                           e-mail: geoachl@alz.org
                                                       www.alz.org
Pam Schuellerman, Executive Director
Andy Junn, Development Director

772   Alzheimer's Association: Central Ohio Chapter
330 Huntington Park Lane   614-442-2014
Columbus, OH 43215-2112   800-272-3900
                                                 Fax: 614-457-6634
                                             e-mail: jsega@alz.org
                                                       www.alz.org
Kenneth Strong, Executive Director
Jennifer Monroe-Sega, Local Contact

773   Alzheimer's Association: Clark/Champaign, Miami Valley Chapter
1700 S. Patterson Blvd.   937-291-3332
Dayton, OH 45409-2620   800-272-3900
                                                 Fax: 937-323-9259
                                  e-mail: walkmiamivalley@alz.org
                                                       www.alz.org
Judy Turner, Executive Director
Marie McLaughlin, Local Contact

774   Alzheimer's Association: Cleveland Area Chapter
23215 Commerce Park Drive   216-721-8457
Beachwood, OH 44122-1013   800-272-3900
                                                 Fax: 216-831-8585
                                         e-mail: helpline@alzclv.org
                                                       www.alz.org
Nancy B Udelson, Executive Director
Robert Bazzarelli, President

775   Alzheimer's Association: Greater Cincinnati Chapter
720 E. Pete Rose Way   513-721-4284
Cincinnati, OH 45202-1742   800-272-3900
                                                 Fax: 513-345-8446
                                     e-mail: diana.bosse@alz.org
                                                       www.alz.org
Committed to support education, advocacy and research on behalf
of those affected by Alzheimer's disease.
Clarissa Rentz, Executive Director
Diana Bosse, Local Contact

776   Alzheimer's Association: Greater East Ohio Chapter: Greater Youngstown Office
3695B Boardman-Canfield Rd   330-533-3300
Canfield, OH 44406-0321   800-272-3900
                                                 Fax: 330-533-3307
                                           e-mail: geoachl@alz.org
                                                       www.alz.org
Pam Schuellerman, Executive Director
Andy Junn, Development Director

777 Alzheimer's Association: Miami Valley Chapter
1700 S. Patterson Blvd.   937-291-3332
Dayton, OH 45409-3661   800-272-3900
Fax: 937-291-0463
e-mail: walkmiamivalley@alz.org
www.alz.org

Judy Turner, Executive Director
Marie McLaughlin, Local Contact

778 Alzheimer's Association: Northwest Ohio Chapter
75 N. Main St.   419-537-1999
Mansfield, OH 44902-7906   800-272-3900
Fax: 419-522-5318
e-mail: nvargas@alz.org
www.alz.org

Voluntary health organization committed to finding a cure for Alzheimer's and helping those affected by the disease.
Michael Malone, President
Nick Vargas, Local Contact

779 Alzheimer's Association: West Central Ohio Chapter
200 East High Street   419-537-1999
Lima, OH 45801-3468   800-272-3900
Fax: 419-222-6212
e-mail: tschindler@alz.org
www.alz.org

A voluntary health agency providing information Alzheimer's disease and related dementias, serving 7 counties: Allen, Auglaize, Hancock, Hardin, Mercer, Putnam and Van Wert. Offers support group meetings in each county and provides a toll-free help line.
Salli Bollin, Executive Director
Toni Schindler, Local Contact

Oklahoma

780 Alzheimer's Association: Oklahoma Chapter
2448 E. 81st Street   918-392-5012
Tulsa, OK 74137-7804   800-272-3900
Fax: 918-481-7745
TTY: 800-493-1411
e-mail: shauptman@alz.org

Dedicated to serving Alzheimer's patients, their families, and caregivers through education, outreach, programs, support services and public advocacy.
Judi A Ver Hoef, President/CEO
Sarah Hauptam, Local Contact

Oregon

781 Alzheimer's Association: Columbia-Willamet Chapter
1940 North Victory Boulevard   503-416-0209
Portland, OR 97217-1610   800-272-3900
Fax: 503-413-6909
e-mail: kara.busick@alz.org
www.alz.org

Judy McKellar, Executive Director
Kara Busick, Local Contact

782 Alzheimer's Association: Cascade/Coast Chapter
100 Day Island Road   503-416-0209
Eugene, OR 97401   800-272-3900
Fax: 541-345-5797
e-mail: kara.busick@alz.org
www.alz.org

Judy Clarke, Vice President
Kara Busick, Local Contact

783 Alzheimer's Association: Mary's Peak Chapter
1925 NW Circle Boulevard   541-752-1012
Corvallis, OR 97330-1312   800-272-3900
Fax: 541-757-1395
www.alz.org

784 Alzheimer's Association: Mid-Willamette Chapter
PO Box 12768   503-371-7728
Salem, OR 97309-0768   800-272-3900
Fax: 503-571-9842
e-mail: midwillamatte@alz.org
www.alz.org

Pennsylvania

785 Alzheimer's Association: Delaware Valley Chapter
1 Citizens Bank Way   215-561-2919
Philadelphia, PA 19148   800-272-3900
Fax: 215-561-4663
e-mail: keely.boyle@alz.org
www.alz.org

Wendy L Campbell, President
Keely Boyle, Local Contact

786 Alzheimer's Association: Greater Pennsylvania Chapter: SW Regional Office
Landmarks Building, 100 Station   412-261-5040
Pittsburgh, PA 15219   800-272-3900
Fax: 412-471-2722
e-mail: mlong@alz.org
www.alz.org

Education training, information, support groups, free newsletter, telephone support, services to caregivers and diagnosed individuals, as well as professionals.
Diane Balcom, President/CEO
Mellisa Long, Local Contact

787 Alzheimer's Association: Greater Mid-Ohio
1100 Liberty Avenue   412-261-5040
Pittsburgh, PA 15222   800-272-3900
Fax: 412-471-2722
e-mail: mlong@alz.org
www.alz.org

Education training information support groups free newsletter telephone support services to caregivers and diagnosed individuals as well as professionals.
Bob LeRoy, President/CEO
Mellisa Long, Local Contact

788 Alzheimer's Association: Laurel Mountains Chapter
194 Donohoe Road   412-261-5040
Greensburg, PA 15601-1095   800-272-3900
Fax: 724-837-4567
e-mail: aspreng@alz.org
www.alz.org

Abby Spreng, Local Contact

789 Alzheimer's Association: Northeast Pennsylvania Chapter
63 North Franklin Street   717-822-4278
Wilkes Barre, PA 18701   800-272-3900
Fax: 717-822-9915
www.alz.org

790 Alzheimer's Association: Northwest Pennsylvania Chapter
726 West Bayfront Parkway   814-456-9200
Erie, PA 16507   800-272-3900
Fax: 814-454-0414
e-mail: ahurd@alz.org
www.alz.org

Bob LeRoy, President/CEO
Amanda Hurd, Local Contact

791 Alzheimer's Association: South Central Pennsylvania Chapter
3544 North Progress Avenue   717-651-5020
Harrisburg, PA 17110   800-272-3900
Fax: 717-651-5066
e-mail: tchambers@alz.org
www.alz.org

Bob LeRoy, President/CEO
Tiffani Chambers, Local Contact

Rhode Island

792 Alzheimer's Association: Rhode Island Chapter
245 Waterman Avenue   401-421-0008
Providence, RI 02906   800-272-3900
Fax: 401-941-8988
e-mail: Donna.McGowan@alz.org
www.alz.org

Elizabeth Morancy, Executive Director
Marge Angilly, Program Director

South Carolina

793 Alzheimer's Association: Low Country Chapter
20 Patriots Point Road
Charleston, SC 29464
843-571-2641
800-272-3900
Fax: 843-571-6020
e-mail: kalmstedt@alz.org
www.alz.org

Ashton Houghton, VP of Development & Communications
Kim Almstedt, Local Contact

794 Alzheimer's Association: Mid-State South Carolina Chapter
3223 Sunset Blvd
W Columbia, SC 29169-7044
803-791-3430
800-272-3900
Fax: 803-791-8388
www.alz.org

Adelle Stanley, Program Director
Lynee Moore, Director of Development

795 Alzheimer's Association: Upstate South Carolina Chapter
3027 MLK Jr. Blvd
Anderson, SC 29625-5528
864-224-3045
800-272-3900
Fax: 864-225-1387
e-mail: kwilliams@alz.org
www.alz.org

Cindy Alewine, President/CEO
Kimberly Williams, Local Contact

Tennessee

796 Alzheimer's Association: Eastern Tennessee Chapter
1600 World's Fair Park Drive
Knoxville, TN 37916
865-200-6668
800-272-3900
Fax: 865-544-6249
e-mail: jim.ward@alz.org
www.alz.org

Janice Wade-Whitehea, Executive Director
Jim Ward, Local Contact

797 Alzheimer's Association: Highland Rim Chapter
201 W Lincoln Street
Tullahoma, TN 37388-1004
931-455-3345
800-272-3900
Fax: 931-455-5396
e-mail: swood@alz.org
www.alz.org

George Jensen, Chair
Sarah Wood, Local Contact

798 Alzheimer's Association: Memphis Area Office
500 North Pine Lake Drive
Memphis, TN 38134
901-565-0011
800-272-3900
Fax: 901-565-9550
e-mail: sgraham@alz.org
www.alz.org

George Jensen, Chair
Susan Graham, Local Contact

799 Alzheimer's Association: Middle Tennessee Chapter
4205 Hillsboro Pike
Nashville, TN 37215-2859
615-292-4938
800-272-3900
Fax: 615-386-9768
e-mail: ajackson1@alz.org
www.alz.org

George Jensen, Chair
Andrew Jackson, Local Contact

800 Alzheimer's Association: Northeast Tennessee Chapter
207 North Boone Street
Johnson City, TN 37604
423-928-4080
800-272-3900
Fax: 423-928-1152
e-mail: tracey.kendall@alz.org
www.alz.org
Provide support, education, advocacy and research to those affected by Alzheimer's disease and their families.
George Jensen, Chair
Bruce Duncan, Vice Chair

801 Alzheimer's Association: Southeast Tennessee Chapter
7625 Hamilton Park Drive
Chattanooga, TN 37421
423-265-3600
800-272-3900
Fax: 423-265-3611
e-mail: clowery@alz.org
www.alz.org

George Jensen, Chair
Cindy Lowery, Local Contact

Texas

802 Alzheimer's Alliance: Texarkana Area
104 Cypress
Texarkana, TX 75503-7812
903-223-8021
877-312-8536
Fax: 903-792-1792
e-mail: lindanickersonalz@cableone.net
www.alztexark.org

Linda Nickerson, Executive Director
Fran Long, Program Director

803 Alzheimer's Association: Capital of Texas Chapter
3520 Executive Center Drive
Austin, TX 78731
512-241-0420
800-272-3900
Fax: 512-241-0430
e-mail: Annie.lagow@alz.org
www.alz.org
The Alzheimer Association Greater Austin Chapter is dedicated to providing leadership to enhance care and support services for individuals and their families while promoting the advancement of research eliminate Alzheimer's disease.
Daniel Hamilton, Chair
Annie LaGow, Local Contact

804 Alzheimer's Association: El Paso Chapter
4687 N Mesa
El Paso, TX 79912-1147
915-544-1799
800-272-3900
Fax: 915-544-8746
e-mail: susie.gorman@alz.org
www.alz.org

Mitch Moss, Chair
Susie Gorman, Local Contact

805 Alzheimer's Association: Greater Beaumont Area Chapter
8750 Phelan Blvd.
Beaumont, TX 77706
409-833-1613
800-272-3900
Fax: 713-314-1315
e-mail: walk@alztex.org
www.alz.org

Richard Elbein, Chief Executive Officer
Clarissa Urban, Local Contact

806 Alzheimer's Association: Greater Dallas Chapter
4144 N Central Expressway
Dallas, TX 75204-4228
214-540-2413
800-272-3900
Fax: 214-827-2064
e-mail: dhill@alz.org
www.alz.org
Provides support and assistance to persons affected by Alzheimer's disease and related dementias and their families and caregivers. Serving Collin, Cooke, Dallas, Deaton, Ellis, Fanning, Grayson, Hunt, Kaufmau, Navarro and Rockwall counties.
John R Gilchrist Jr, Executive Director
Jack Broyles, Chairman

807 Alzheimer's Association: Greater East Texas Chapter
2900 Raguet
Nacogdoches, TX 75962
713-314-1343
800-272-3900
Fax: 936-569-0514
e-mail: walk@alztex.org
www.alz.org

Phil King, Chief Financial Officer
Jessica Abad-Serpas, Local Contact

808　**Alzheimer's Association: Greater Wichita Falls Chapter**
901 Indiana　　　　　　　　　　　940-767-8800
Wichita Falls, TX 76301-3206　　　　800-272-3900
　　　　　　　　　　　　　　　Fax: 940-322-6259
　　　　　　　　　　e-mail: patty.taylor@alz.org
　　　　　　　　　　　　　　　　　　www.alz.org

Theresa Hocker, Executive Director
Patty Taylor, Local Contact

809　**Alzheimer's Association: Houston and Southeast Texas Chapter**
400 Hamilton Street　　　　　　　　713-314-1340
Houston, TX 77002　　　　　　　　800-272-3900
　　　　　　　　　　　　　　　Fax: 713-314-1315
　　　　　　　　　　e-mail: walk@alztex.org
　　　　　　　　　　　　　　　　　　www.alz.org

Richard Elbein, CEO
Rasheeda Daugherty, Local Contact

810　**Alzheimer's Association: Northeast Texas Chapter**
211 Winchester　　　　　　　　　903-509-8323
Tyler, TX 75701-8732　　　　　　　800-272-3900
　　　　　　　　　　　　　　　Fax: 903-509-8373
　　　　　　　　　　e-mail: jana@alzalliance.org
　　　　　　　　　　　　　　　　　　www.alz.org

Jana Humphrey, Executive Director
Sherlon Spurling, Client Services Coordinator

811　**Alzheimer's Association: Rio Grande Valley Region**
222 E Van Buren　　　　　　　　956-440-0636
Harlingen, TX 78550　　　　　　　800-272-3900
　　　　　　　　　　　　　　　Fax: 956-440-9290
　　　　　　　　　　　　　　　　　　www.alz.org

A nonprofit organization designed to educate and support individuals with Alzheimer's, their families and caregivers.

812　**Alzheimer's Association: STAR Chapter, Midland Region**
4400 N Big Spring　　　　　　　　432-570-9191
Midland, TX 79705　　　　　　　　800-272-3900
　　　　　　　　　　　　　　　Fax: 432-683-2345
　　　　　　　　　　e-mail: derdwurm@alz.org
　　　　　　　　　　　　　　　　　　www.alz.org

Mitch Moss, Chair
Debbie Erdwurm, Local Contact

813　**Alzheimer's Association: South Central Texas**
7400 Louis Pasteur Drive　　　　　210-822-6449
San Antonio, TX 78229　　　　　　800-272-3900
　　　　　　　　　　　　　　　Fax: 210-824-8069
　　　　　　　　　　e-mail: bbenavidez@alz.org
　　　　　　　　　　　　　　　　　　www.alz.org

Mitch Moss, Chair
Belinda Benavides, Local Contact

814　**Alzheimer's Association: Tarrant County Chapter**
101 Summit Avenue　　　　　　　817-336-4949
Fort Worth, TX 76102　　　　　　　800-272-3900
　　　　　　　　　　　　　　　Fax: 817-336-4966
　　　　　　　　　　e-mail: lyn.downing@alz.org
　　　　　　　　　　　　　　　　　　www.alz.org

Offers support to those afflicted with Alzheimer's disease and their families through education, support groups, case management, telephone help line and referral to services (i.e. long term care, adult daycare, medical assistance, legal assistance etc.).
Theresa Hocker, Executive Director
Lyn Downing, Local Contact

Utah

815　**Alzheimer's Association: Utah Chapter**
296 E. Murray Park Ave　　　　　　801-265-1944
Salt Lake City, UT 84107　　　　　800-272-3900
　　　　　　　　　　　　　　　Fax: 801-269-1226
　　　　　　　　　　e-mail: Emartini@alz.org
　　　　　　　　　　　　　　　　　　www.alz.org

Nick Sussman, Program Director
Elaine Martini, Local Contact

Vermont

816　**Alzheimer's Association: Vermont Chapter**
300 Cornerstone Drive　　　　　　802-316-3839
Williston, VT 05495-1139　　　　　800-272-3900
　　　　　　　　　　　　　　　Fax: 802-229-5231
　　　　　　　　e-mail: ashley.witzenberger@alz.org
　　　　　　　　　　　　　　　　　　www.alz.org

Randy Brock, President and Chair
Ashley Witzenberg, Director of Development

Virginia

817　**Alzheimer's Association: Central Virginia Chapter**
1160 Pepsi Place　　　　　　　　434-973-6122
Charlottesville, VA 22901　　　　　800-272-3900
　　　　　　　　　　　　　　　Fax: 434-973-4224
　　　　　　　　　　e-mail: alzcwva@alz.org
　　　　　　　　　　　　　　　　　　www.alz.org

Sue Friedman, President and CEO
Brian Phelps, Chair

818　**Alzheimer's Association: Greater Richmond Chapter**
4600 Cox Road　　　　　　　　　804-967-2580
Glen Allen, VA 23060　　　　　　800-272-3900
　　　　　　　　　　　　　　　Fax: 804-967-2588
　　　　　　　　　e-mail: sherry.peterson@alz.org
　　　　　　　　　　　　　　　　　　www.alz.org

Alzheimer's Association provides support and services to those with Alzheimer's and their families services include: help line, support groups, educational programs for family and professional caregivers, monthly newsletter, lending library, and a speakers
Sherry Peterson, CEO
Marry Ann Johnson, Program Director

819　**Alzheimer's Association: National Capital Area Chapter**
3701 Pender Drive　　　　　　　703-359-4440
Fairfax, VA 22030　　　　　　　　800-272-3900
　　　　　　　　　　　　　　　Fax: 703-359-4441
　　　　　　　　　e-mail: Danielle.Otsuka@alz.org
　　　　　　　　　　　　　　　　　　www.alz.org

Provides support and services to those diagnosed with Alzheimer's disease and related disorders and their families. Services include information on the disease, care options, caregiving techniques and research, support groups, education and training, and advocacy.
Matthew B Aaron, Chair
Danielle Otsuka, Director of Development

820　**Alzheimer's Association: Piedmont-Valley Area Chapter**
1160 Pepsi Place　　　　　　　　434-973-6122
Charlottesville, VA 22901　　　　　800-272-3900
　　　　　　　　　　　　　　　Fax: 434-973-4224
　　　　　　　　　　e-mail: mhanson@alz.org
　　　　　　　　　　　　　　　　　　www.alz.org

Sue Friedman, President and CEO
Mary Pat Hanson, Local Contact

821　**Alzheimer's Association: Roanoke Salem Chapter**
3959 Electric Rd　　　　　　　　540-345-7600
Roanoke, VA 24018　　　　　　　800-272-3900
　　　　　　　　　　　　　　　Fax: 540-345-7900
　　　　　　　　　　e-mail: mhanson@alz.org
　　　　　　　　　　　　　　　　　　www.alz.org

Sue Friedman, President and CEO
Mary Pat Hanson, Local Contact

822　**Alzheimer's Association: Southeastern Virginia Chapter**
6350 Center Drive　　　　　　　757-459-2405
Norfolk, VA 23502　　　　　　　800-272-3900
　　　　　　　　　　　　　　　Fax: 757-461-7902
　　　　　　　　　　e-mail: InfoSEVA@alz.org
　　　　　　　　　　　　　　　　　　www.alz.org

Provides support to people with Alzheimer's disease or related dementia and their families; educates professionals and the public about Alzheimer's disease and related dementia; supports research into causes, improved diagnosis, therapies and cures.
Gino V Colombara, Executive Director
Patricia Far Lacey, Director of Education & Family Services

823 Alzheimer's Association: Southside Virginia Chapter
120 S Hill Avenue   434-447-3963
S Hill, VA 23970-0310   800-272-3900
                                Fax: 434-447-9024
                    e-mail: gino.colombara@alz.org
                                        www.alz.org

Gino V Colombara, Executive Director
June Rainey, Education & Family Services Coordinator

Washington

824 Alzheimer's Association: Inland Northwest Chapter
800 N. Howard St.   509-473-3390
Spokane, WA 99201   800-272-3900
                                Fax: 509-473-3389
                        e-mail: sdruffel@alz.org
                                        www.alz.org

Joel Loiacono, Executive Director
Sandi Druffel, Local Contact

825 Alzheimer's Association: Western & Central Washington Chapter
100 W. Harrison St   206-529-3898
Seattle, WA 98119   800-272-3900
                                Fax: 206-363-5700
                          e-mail: walk@alzwa.org
                                        www.alz.org

Nancy Dapper, Executive Director
Justine Stevens, Local Contact

West Virginia

826 Alzheimer's Association: Greater Mid-Ohio Valley Chapter
1920 Park Ave.   304-865-6775
Parkersburg, WV 26101   800-272-3900
                    e-mail: wendy.hamilton@alz.org
                                        www.alz.org

Jane Marks, Executive Director
Wendy Hamilton, Local Contact

827 Alzheimer's Association: N Central West Virginia Chapter
1299 Pineview Drive   304-599-1159
Morgantown, WV 26505-4543   800-272-3900
                                Fax: 304-291-2577
                        e-mail: wvinfo@alz.org
                                        www.alz.org

Jane Marks, Executive Director
Jane Siers, Development Director

828 Alzheimer's Association: South West Virginia Chapter
601 Morris St.   304-343-2717
Charleston, WV 25301   800-272-3900
                                Fax: 304-343-2723
                          e-mail: kford@alz.org
                                        www.alz.org

Jane Marks, Executive Director
Kaarmin Ford, Local Contact

Wisconsin

829 Alzheimer's Association: Greater Wisconsin Chapter
La Crosse & Second Streets   608-784-5011
La Crosse, WI 54601   800-272-3900
                                Fax: 608-784-4428
                      e-mail: bwilliams@alz.org
                                        www.alz.org

To eliminate Alzheimer's disease through the advancement of research; to provide and enhance care and support for all affected; and to reduce the risk of dementia through the promotion of brain health.
Brad Beckman, President
Brett Williams, Local Contact

830 Alzheimer's Association: Indianhead Chapter
Carson Park Dr   715-345-2969
Eau Claire, WI 54703-5996   800-272-3900
                                Fax: 715-345-2969
                        e-mail: kdavies@alz.org
                                        www.alz.org

Mary B Bouche, Executive Director
Kathy Davies, Local Contact

831 Alzheimer's Association: Lake Superior Chapter
US Highway 2 East   715-392-3255
Ashland, WI 54806-1652   800-272-3900
                                Fax: 715-682-6561
                        e-mail: fcarlson@alz.org
                                        www.alz.org

Kim Kinner, Executive Director
Freda Carlson, Local Contact

832 Alzheimer's Association: Midstate Wisconsin Chapter
1800 S Central Ave   715-845-7440
Marshfield, WI 54449   800-272-3900
                                Fax: 715-387-5727
                        e-mail: aswatek@alz.org
                                        www.alz.org

833 Alzheimer's Association: North Central Wisconsin Chapter
1205 Lincoln St   715-362-7779
Rhinelander, WI 54501   800-272-3900
                                Fax: 715-362-1879
                       e-mail: jstpierre@alz.org
                                        www.alz.org

Kim Kinner, Executive Director
Julie St. Pierre, Local Contact

834 Alzheimer's Association: Northeast Wisconsin Chapter
1265 Lombardi Ave   920-469-2110
Green Bay, WI 54304   800-272-3900
                                Fax: 920-498-2203
                       e-mail: bbartlett@alz.org
                                        www.alz.org

Kim Kinner, Executive Director
Beverly Bartlett, Local Contact

835 Alzheimer's Association: South Central Wisconsin Chapter
1 John Nolen Drive   608-203-8502
Madison, WI 53703   800-272-3900
                                Fax: 608-232-3407
                         e-mail: ehilker@alz.org
                                        www.alz.org

Provides support and assistance to the families of those impacted by Alzheimer's and related dementias, including educational programs, support groups, information and referral and advocacy.
150 Members
Paul Rusk, Executive Director
Emily Hilker, Local Contact

836 Alzheimer's Association: Southeast Wisconsin Chapter
2900 North Menomonee River Parkway   414-479-8800
Milwaukee, WI 53222   800-272-3900
                                Fax: 414-479-8819
                                TTY: 414-479-8466
                         e-mail: slatona@alz.org
                                        www.alz.org

To eliminate Alzheimer's disease through advancement of research and to enhance care and support for individuals, their families and caregivers. Individual consultation over the phone or in person. Extensive library of educational materials for loan or purchase.
Kendra Albers, Special Events Manager
Shelby LaTona, Development Coordinato

Wyoming

837 Alzheimer's Wyoming
900 Werner Court   307-265-7960
Casper, WY 82602   Fax: 307-265-7960
                      e-mail: alzawy@tribcsp.com
                         www.alzheimerswyoming.org

Alzheimer's Affiliation of Wyoming is an independent organization that makes presentations about Alzheimer's Disease; assists

Alzheimer support groups; provides funds for respite care; maintains a lending library; refers patients and their families to services.
Mary Hein, Executive Director

Foundations

838 Long Island Alzheimers Foundation
5 Channel Drive   516-767-6856
Port Washington, NY 11050   Fax: 516-767-6864
e-mail: info@liaf.org
www.liaf.org
To help lighten the burden and improve the quality of life for those suffering with Alzheimer's disease and related dementias, their caregivers and their families.
Fred Jenny, Executive Director
Sean Phillips, Director of Development

Research Centers

839 Aging and Alzheimer's Disease Center Oregon Health Sciences University
Oregon Health Sciences University
3181 SW Sam Jackson Park Road   503-494-8311
Portland, OR 97239-3098   Fax: 503-494-6695
e-mail: kaye@ohsu.edu
www.ohsu.edu/research/alzheimers
Researches causes and consequences of Alzheimer's disease and ways of clinical services. Publishes a newsletter twice a year.
Jeffrey Kaye, Director
Joan Benedict, Administrative Coordinator

840 Alzheimer's Disease Center Emory University/VA Medical Center
201 Dowman Drive   404-727-6069
Atlanta, GA 30322   Fax: 404-286-55
e-mail: emoryadrc@emory.edu
www.med.emory.edu/ADRC
Researchers work to translate advances into improved care and diagnosis for Alzheimer's patients.
Allan Levey, Director
Stuart Zola, Co-Director

841 Alzheimer's Disease Center Kentucky University
Sanders-Brown Center on Aging
1030 South Broadway   859-257-1412
Lexington, KY 40504-0230   Fax: 859-323-2866
e-mail: rdavi3@email.uky.edu
/www.mc.uky.edu/coa
Researchers work to translate advances into improved care and diagnosis for Alzheimer's patients.
Linda J. Van Eldik, Ph.D., Director
Vince J Kellen, Chief Information Officer

842 Alzheimer's Disease Center Mayo Clinic Mayo Medical School
Mayo Medical School
200 First Street SW   507-284-2511
Rochester, MN 55905   Fax: 507-538-0161
TDD: 507-2849786
e-mail: mayoADC@mayo.edu
www.mayoclinic.com
Researchers work to translate advances into improved care and diagnosis for Alzheimer's patients.
John H Noseworhty MD, President
William C Rupp MD, Vice President, CEO

843 Alzheimer's Disease Center Pennsylvania University School of Medicine
Ralston House
3615 Chestnut Street   215-662-7810
Philadelphia, PA 19104   Fax: 215-662-7812
e-mail: jason.karlawish@uphs.upenn.edu
www.pennadc.org
Researchers work to translate advances into improved care and diagnosis for Alzheimer's patients.
John Q Trojanowski, Director

844 Alzheimer's Disease Center: Boston University
Boston University School of Medicine

72 E Concord Street   617-638-5426
Boston, MA 02118   888-458-2823
Fax: 617-414-1197
e-mail: buad@bu.edu
www.bu.edu/alzresearch
Researchers work to translate advances into improved care and diagnosis for Alzheimer's patients.
Neil W Kowall, Director
Richard Fine, Associate Director

845 Alzheimer's Disease Center: Johns Hopkins University School of Medicine
Johns Hopkins University Department of Pathology
720 Rutland Avenue   410-502-5164
Baltimore, MD 21205   Fax: 410-955-9777
e-mail: edelman1@jhmi.edu
www.alzresearch.org
Researchers work to translate advances into improved care and diagnosis for Alzheimer's patients.
Marilyn Albert, Director
Philip Wong, Associate Director

846 Alzheimer's Disease Center: University of California, Davis
4860 Y Street   916-734-5496
Sacramento, CA 95817   e-mail: wjjagust@lbl.gov
alzheimer.ucdavis.edu/
Researchers work to translate advances into improved care and diagnosis for Alzheimer's patients.
Charles DeCarli MD, Clinical Core Director

847 Alzheimer's Disease Center: University of Alabama at Birmingham
1720 7th Avenue S   205-934-3847
Birmingham, AL 35294-0017   Fax: 205-975-7365
e-mail: adbrain@uab.edu
www.main.uab.edu/adc
Researchers work to translate advances into improved care and diagnosis for Alzheimer's patients.
Daniel C Marson, Director
J Michael Wyss, Associate Director

848 Alzheimer's Disease Center: Washington University
1660 S Columbian Way   206-764-2069
Seattle, WA 98108-1597   800-317-5382
Fax: 206-768-5456
e-mail: wamble@u.washington.edu
www.depts.washington.edu/adrcweb
Researchers work to translate advances into improved care and diagnosis for Alzheimer's patients.
Sydney Lewis, Education and Outreach Coordinator
Nancy Brown, Lead Psychometrist and Autopsy Coordinat

849 Alzheimer's Disease Research Center Washington University School of Medicine
Washington University School of Medicine
4488 Forest Park Avenue   314-286-2683
St Louis, MO 63108   Fax: 314-286-2763
e-mail: morrisj@abraxas.wustl.edu
www.adrc.wustl.edu
Researchers work to translate advances into improved care diagnosis and treatment for Alzheimer's patients.
John Morris, Director
Virginia D Buckles, Executive Director

850 Alzheimer's Disease Research Center Duke University
Bryan ADRC
2200 W Main Street Suite A200   919-668-0820
Durham, NC 27705   866-444-2372
e-mail: kwe@duke.edu
adrc.mc.duke.edu
Researchers work to translate advances into improved care and diagnosis for Alzheimer's patients.
Kathleen A Welsh-Bohmer, Director
James Robert Burke, Associate Director

851 Cognitive Neurology and Alzheimer's Disease Center
CNADC

320 E Superior Street
Chicago, IL 60611　312-908-9339
Fax: 312-908-8789
e-mail: CNADC-Admin@northwestern.edu
www.brain.northwestern.edu
Researchers work to translate advances into improved care and diagnosis for Alzheimer's patients.
Megan Atchu, MA, Research Administrator
Kevin Connolly, Business Administrator

852 Cornell University: Winifred Masterson Burke Medical Research-Dementia
1300 York Avenue
New York, NY 10065　212-746-5454
Fax: 212-821-0576
e-mail: publicaffairs@med.cornell.edu
www.med.cornell.edu
Clinical and basic studies in metabolic aspects of the nervous system especially Alzheimer's disease.
David J Skorton MD, President
Thomas H Blair lll, Senior Director Administrator

853 Duke University Center for the Study of Aging and Human Development
Duke University
Box 3003
Durham, NC 27710　919-660-7500
Fax: 919-668-0453
e-mail: webmaster@geri.duke.edu
www.geri.duke.edu
Basic and clinical research into geriatrics and gerontology focusing on a number of chronic diseases in the elderly including osteoporosis cancer heart disease infectious diseases Alzheimer's disease and other disorders leading to dysmobility.
Harvey Jay Cohen MD, Director
Linda K George, Associate Director

854 Duke University Clinical Research Institute
Headquarters
2400 Pratt Street
Durham, NC 27705　919-668-8700
www.dcri.duke.edu
Multidisciplinary clinical research into the cause and prevention of human diseases such as Alzheimer's.
Robert A Harrington, Director
Elizabeth Be Reed, Chief Operating Officer

855 Indiana University Center for Aging Research
The Center for Aging Research
1050 Wishard Blvd
Indianapolis, IN 46202-2872　317-630-6083
Fax: 317-423-5695
e-mail: nnienaber@regenstrief.org
www.medicine.iupui.edu/iucar/?
Researchers work to translate advances into improved care and diagnosis for Alzheimer's patients.
Christopher Callahan, Director
Douglas K Miller, Associate Director

856 Indiana University: Human Genetics Center of Medical & Molecular Genetics
School of Medicine
340 West 10th Street
Indianapolis, IN 46202-3082　317-274-8157
e-mail: kcornett@iupui.edu
www.medicine.iu.edu
Comprised of a core group of scientists with primary appointments in the Department and a group of molecular biologists from other departments who hold joint appointments in Medical and Molecular Genetics.
D Craig Brater MD, Dean
John F. Fitzgerald, MD, MBA, Executive Associate Dean

857 Institute for Basic Research in Developmental Disabilities
1050 Forest Hill Road
Staten Island, NY 10314-0001　718-494-0600
866- 94- 973
TTY: 866- 933-488
e-mail: ibr@opwdd.ny.gov
www.opwdd.ny.gov/institute-for-basic-res
James F Moran, Acting Commissioner

858 Long Island Alzheimers Foundation
5 Channel Drive
Port Washington, NY 11050　516-767-6856
Fax: 516-767-6856
e-mail: info@liaf.org
www.liaf.org
Researchers work to translate advances into improved care and diagnosis for Alzheimer's patients.
Fred Jenny, Executive Director
Anna Maria Warmuz, Executive Assistant

859 Massachusetts Alzheimers Disease Research Center
Massachusetts ADRC
16th Street
Charlestown, MA 02129　617-726-3987
Fax: 617-724-1480
www.madrc.org
Multi-institutional consortium of Harvard affiliated facilities encompasses five Core units: an Administrative Core a Clinical Core a Database Management and Statistics Core a Neuropathology Core and an Education and Information Transfer Core. The ADRC also supports four specific research projects funded for 3-5 years and annually designates three or four pilot research projects that are funded for 1 year.
John H Growdon, Clinic Director
Bradley T Hyman, Center Director

860 Medical College of Georgia Alzheimers Research Center
1120 15th Street
Augusta, GA 30912　706-721-0211
Fax: 706-721-7063
e-mail: jbuccafu@mcg.edu
www.mcg.edu/centers/alz
Clinical and basic research of Alzheimer's disease.
Jerry Buccaf MD, Director
J Warren Beach, Member

861 Michigan Alzheimer's Disease Research Center
University of Michigan
2101 Commonwealth Blvd.,
Ann Arbor, MI 48105-0316　734-936-4000
e-mail: sgilman@umich.edu
www.med.umich.edu/alzheimers
Researchers work to translate advances into improved care and diagnosis for Alzheimer's patients.
Sid Gilman MD, Director
Bruno Giordani Ph.D., Core Director

862 Mount Sinai School of Medicine: Alzheimers Disease Research Center
Alzheimer's Disease Research Center
One Gustave L Levy Place
New York, NY 10029-6574　212-241-6696
Fax: 212-369-2344
e-mail: mary.sano@mssm.edu
www.mssm.edu
Focuses on Alzheimer's disease research.
Mary Sano, Director
Samuel Gandy, Associate Director

863 Neurosciences Institute of the Neurosciences Research Program
The Neurosciences Institute
10640 John Jay Hopkins Drive
San Diego, CA 92121　858-626-2000
Fax: 858-626-2099
e-mail: info@nsi.edu
www.nsi.edu
Nonprofit organization focusing on Alzheimer's and related disorders.
Gerald M Edelman, President

864 Ohio State University Neuroscience Program
1835 Neil Avenue
Columbus, OH 43210　614-292-8185
Fax: 614-921-44
www.psy.ohio-state.edu
Specializes in brain disorders such as Alzheimer's disease.
Richard Petty, Chair
Scott Burch, Behavioral Neurosciences Area Assistant

865 Taub Institute for Research on Alzheimers Disease and the Aging Brain
630 West 168th Street
New York, NY 10032　212-305-1818
Fax: 212-342-2849
e-mail: taubinstitute@columbia.edu
www.alzheimercenter.org

Researchers work to translate advances into improved care and diagnosis for Alzheimer's patients.
Michael L Shelanski, Co-Director
Richard Mayeux MD, Co-Director

866   The Alzheimer's Disease & Memory Disorders Center
ADMDC
One Baylor Plaza   713-798-5971
Houston, TX 77030   Fax: 713-798-7434
e-mail: neurons@bcm.edu
www.bcm.edu/neurology/admdc
Researchers work to translate advances into improved care and diagnosis for Alzheimer's Disease and other memory disorders.
Eli M Mizrahi, Chair, Department of Neurology
Keith Davis, Department Administrator

867   The Sam and Rose Stein Institute for Research on the Aging
University of California San Diego
9500 Gilman Drive   858-534-6299
La Jolla, CA 92093-0664   Fax: 858-534-5475
e-mail: steininstitute@ucsd.edu
www.sira.ucsd.edu
Research on aging and Alzheimer's disease.
Debra Kaine, Director
Maureen Halp MS, Executive Director

868   University Alzheimer Center University of Alabama at Birmingham
University of Alabama at Birmingham
1530 3rd Avenue S   205-934-4011
Birmingham, AL 35294-1150   800-333-6543
Fax: 205-975-7365
TTY: 205-934-4642
e-mail: adbrain@uab.edu
main.uab.edu
Researchers work to translate advances into improved care and diagnosis for Alzheimer's patients.
Dr. Carol Garrison, President
Kristen N Burdick, Director of Executive Affairs

869   University Alzheimer Center UHC: Case Western Reserve University
12200 Fairhill Road   216-844-6400
Cleveland, OH 44120   Fax: 216-844-6446
e-mail: Kathy.Shaw@Case.Edu
www.ohioalzcenter.org
Researchers work to translate advances into improved care and diagnosis for Alzheimer's patients.
Alan Lerner, Co-Director
Kathleen A Smyth, Administrator

870   University of Chicago Dept of Neurology University of Chicago Hospital
University of Chicago Hospital
5841 S Maryland Avenue   773-702-6390
Chicago, IL 60637-1470   Fax: 773-702-9076
e-mail: cgomez@neurology.bsd.uchicago.edu
neurology.uchicago.edu
Covers Translational Neuroscience Research and research programs in neuroimmunology neuromuscular disease and neurovirology provided the initial foundation and brought national recognition.
Kenneth Goodell, Senior Executive Administrator
Judith Maratea, Administrative Assistant

871   University of Illinois Health Services Research
University of Illinois College of Medicine
1601 Parkview Avenue   815-395-0600
Rockford, IL 61107   Fax: 815-395-5887
e-mail: prrockford@uic.edu
www.uirockford.com
A unit of the University of Illinois College of Medicine at Rockford serves faculty students health care providers human services agencies and other community organizations throughout Illinois with demographic health social and economic data. The skills data and resources available to faculty and students at the college are also available to individuals and organizations needing assistance.
Joann Glacken, Research Support Services

872   University of Maryland: Division of Infectious Diseases
UM Baltimore Department of Medicine
655 West Baltimore Street   410-706-7410
Baltimore, ML 21201   Fax: 410-706-0235
e-mail: rredfield@ihv.umaryland.edu
www.medschool.umaryland.edu
Focuses research on elderly studies including drug use treatments and infectious diseases of the aged.
E. Albert Reece, Vice President
Richard Pierson III MD, Senior Associate Dean for Academic Affai

873   University of Miami: Center on Aging Center on Aging
Center on Aging
1695 NW 9th Avenue   305-355-9080
Miami, FL 33136   Fax: 305-355-9076
e-mail: ajaret@med.miami.edu
centeronaging.med.miami.edu
Focuses on aged disorders such as Alzheimer's research.
Sara J Czaja, Co-Director
Charles B. Nemeroff, M.D., Ph.D, Director

874   Yeshiva University: Resnick Gerontology Center
Albert Einstein College of Medicine
Jack and Pearl Resnick Campus   718-920-6722
Bronx, NY 10467   866-633-8255
Fax: 718-655-9672
e-mail: ljacobs@aecom.yu.edu
www.aecom.yu.edu
Alzheimer's disease and other dementia studies.
Allen M Spiegel MD, Dean
Amy R Ehrlich, Geriatrics Fellowship Program Director

Support Groups & Hotlines

875   Alzheimer's Association Autopsy Assistance Network
Alzheimer s Association
Western/Central Washington Chapter   206-363-5500
Seattle, WA 98125   800-848-7097
Fax: 206-363-5700
e-mail: rowena.rye@alz.org
http://alzwa.org/resources6.htm
The primary purposes of the Autopsy Assistance Network are: to provide families with information regarding autopsy; to assist in obtaining a confirmed diagnosis; provide tissue for Alzheimer's disease research; and establish diagnosis for purpose of clinical and epidemiological studies.
Nancy Dapper, Executive Director
Rowena Rye, Community Resources

876   Alzheimer's Support Group
Columbus Health Rehabilitation Center
2100 Midway Street   812-372-8447
Columbus, IN 47201   Fax: 812-375-5117
www.columbushrc.com/
The skilled Nursing Center includes a separate unit dedicated to the care of residents with Alzheimer's disease and other forms of dementia. The Alzheimer's program is designed to celebrate the spirit of their residents, striving to offer a comfortable and compassionate environment that emphasizes positive life experiences and active involvement in a daily routine.
Mike Spencer, Executive Director

877   National Health Information Center
PO Box 1133   310-565-4167
Washington, DC 20013   800-336-4797
Fax: 301-984-4256
e-mail: info@nhic.org
www.health.gov/nhic
Offers a nationwide information referral service, produces directories and resource guides.

Books

878   36-Hour Day
Hachette Book Group USA

3 Center Plaza
Boston, MA 02108

800-759-0190
Fax: 800-331-1664
e-mail: webmaster@hbgusa.com
www.hachettebookgroup.com

A family guide to caring for persons with Alzheimer's disease, related dementing illnesses, and memory loss later in life.
1999
ISBN: 0-446618-76-2

879   Alzheimer Early Stages

Daniel Kuhn MSW, author

Hunter House Publishers
1515 1/2 Park Street
Alameda, CA 94501

510-865-5282
800-266-5592
e-mail: ordering@hunterhouse.com
www.hunterhouse.com

First steps in caring and treatments. This book is for family members and friends of those recently diagnosed with Alzheimer's Disase.
288 pages Paperback
ISBN: 0-897933-97-4

880   Alzheimer's Disease

Springer Publishing Company
536 Broadway
New York, NY 10012-3955

212-431-4370
877-687-7476
Fax: 212-941-7842
e-mail: marketing@springerpub.com
www.springerpub.com

This volume presents the latest research and findings on Alzheimer's disease.
1996 224 pages Softcover
ISBN: 0-826196-22-5
Annette Imperati, Marketing Director

881   Alzheimer's Disease Orientation Kit

Alzheimer's Association
225 North Michigan Avenue
Chicago, IL 60611-1696

800-272-3900
Fax: 866-699-1246
TDD: 312-335-8700
e-mail: media@alz.org
www.alz.org

A collection of materials developed to familiarize the audience with Alzheimer's disease and its effects on the patient and family. Includes the Orientation to Alzheimer's Disease videotape, Learning Guide and Caregiver Packet.

882   Alzheimer's Disease: A Guide to Federal Programs

Alzheimer's Disease Education & Referral Center
PO Box 8250
Silver Spring, MD 20907-8250

800-438-4380
Fax: 301-495-3334
www.alzheimers.org

Directory of Alzheimer's disease programs sponsored by federal agencies. Lists agency by agency, it provides locations and telephone numbers for multisite activities and demonstration programs and lists information resources.

883   Alzheimer's Disease: Activity-Focused Care

Butterworth-Heinemann
225 Wildwood Avenue
Woburn, MA 01801

800-366-2665
Fax: 800-446-6520
www.bh.com

Information for professional and family caregivers on activity-focused care for Alzheimer's patients.
436 pages
ISBN: 0-750699-08-6

884   Alzheimer's Disease: Advances in Neurology

Raven Press
1185 Avenue of the Americas
New York, NY 10036-2601

212-930-9500
800-777-2295

304 pages
ISBN: 0-781700-81-7

885   Alzheimer's Disease: Questions and Answers

Merit Publishing International

5840 Corporate Way
West Palm Beach, FL 33407

561-697-1116
Fax: 561-477-4961
e-mail: meritpi@aol.com
www.meritpublishing.com

Answers questions about Alzheimer's, explains what it is, how it is diagnosed, causes, and how if affects functions of the brain.
1999
ISBN: 1-873413-52-1
Gene Evans, President
Martin Garrido, VP

886   Alzheimer's Disease: Thesaurus

Alzheimer's Disease Education & Referral Center
PO Box 8250
Silver Spring, MD 20907-8250

800-438-4380
Fax: 301-495-3334
www.alzheimers.org

To help librarians and others to save time and money when searing online for books, journal articles, videos and other materials related to Alzheimer's disease.
140 pages

887   Alzheimer's Disease: Treatment and Family Stress: Directions for Research

Superintendent of Documents
PO Box 371954
Pittsburgh, PA 15250-7954

202-512-2250

Presents a collection of papers giving current information on research investigations that increase the understanding of the nature and consequences of family caregiving.
486 pages

888   Alzheimer's, Stroke and 29 Other Neurological Disorders Sourcebook

Omnigraphics
615 Griswold Street
Detroit, MI 48226-3993

313-961-1340
800-234-1340
Fax: 800-875-1340
e-mail: customerservice@omnigraphics.com
www.omnigraphics.com

Provides vital information for the nontechnical reader focusing on Alzheimer's disease, stroke and various neurological disorders. Answers thousands of questions related to afflications of the central nervous system with each chapter reviving a particular disorder and offers in-depth discussions.

ISBN: 0-780806-66-2
Georgiann Lauginiger, Customer Service Manager

889   Care That Works: A Relationship Approach to Persons with Dementia

John's Hopkins University Press
2715 N Charles Street
Baltimore, MD 21218-4319

410-516-6900
800-537-5487
Fax: 410-516-6998
www.press.jhu.edu

Focuses on building and improving the relationship between the caregiver and the person with Alzheimer's.
272 pages
ISBN: 0-801860-26-1

890   Care of Alzheimer's Patients: A Manual for Nursing Home Staff

Lisa P Gwyther, author

Alzheimer's Association
225 North Michigan Avenue
Chicago, IL 60611-1696

800-272-3900
Fax: 866-699-1246
TDD: 312-335-8700
e-mail: media@alz.org
www.alz.org

A care guide for nursing home staff. A useful resource for any caregiver or professional.
122 pages

891   Caregiver Helpbook

Legacy Health System
1015 NW 22nd Avenue
Portland, OR 97210

503-413-6778
Fax: 503-413-6911
e-mail: kshannon@lhs.org
www.legacyhealth.org

A helpful guide with useful self care tools for family caregivers of frail or ill older adults.
300 pages Paperback
ISBN: 0-937915-54-6
Kathy Shannon, Manager/Caregiver

892 Caring for Alzheimer's Patients: A Guide for Family & Healthcare Providers
Plenum Publishing Corporation
233 Spring Street   212-620-8460
New York, NY 10013-1522   800-221-9369
                                                        Fax: 212-463-0742
                                  e-mail: books@plenum.com
Consists of five organizations that furnish information and resources concerning Alzheimer's Disease support groups and hospitals.
308 pages
ISBN: 0-306431-99-8

893 Complete Guide to Alzheimer's Proofing Your Home
Purdue University Press
509 Harrison Street   765-494-2038
West Lafayette, IN 47907-2025   800-247-6553
                                                        Fax: 765-496-2442
                                  e-mail: pupress@purdue.edu
                                       www.thepress.purdue.edu
Guide on how to modify homes of Alzheimer's patients to facilitate caregiving.
496 pages Paperback
ISBN: 1-557532-02-8

894 Confronting Alzheimer's Disease
American Assoc. of Homes and Services for Aging
2519 Connecticut Avenue NW   202-783-2242
Washington, DC 20008-2008   Fax: 202-783-2255
                                                        www.aahsa.org
A resource for administrators, professional caregivers and families dealing with Alzheimer's disease and related disorders.
225 pages

895 Court-Related Needs of the Elderly and Persons with Disabilities
Commission on the Mentally Disabled
1800 M Street NW   202-331-2240
Washington, DC 20036
Report of the National Conference, examines the barriers of the judicial system impeding access for the elderly and persons with disabilities.

896 Developing Support Groups for Individuals with Early-Stage Alzheimer's Disease
Robyn Yale, author
Health Professions Press
PO Box 10624   410-337-9585
Baltimore, MD 21285-0624   888-337-8808
                                                        Fax: 410-337-8539
                                       www.healthpropress.com
This one-of-a-kind, step-by-step guidebook has been used as a national and international model to meet the needs of people just diagnosed with Alzheimer's disease. Clinical and administrative issues include selecting group participants, training facilitators and managing unique group topics, interactions and dynamics.
256 pages Paperback
ISBN: 1-878812-62-2

897 Directory of Alzheimer's Disease Treatment Facilities & Home Health Care
Oryx Press
4041 N Central Avenue   602-265-2651
Phoenix, AZ 85012-3397   800-279-4663
                                                        www.oryxpress.com
A compilation of 1,500 specialized facilities with day care, residential care, diagnosis and treatment facilities.

898 Ginny: A Love Remembered
Iowa State Press
2121 State Street   515-292-0155
Ames, IA 50014   800-862-6657
                                                        Fax: 515-292-3348
                                  e-mail: orders@iowastatepress.com
                                       iowastatepress.com

This book tells the story of midwest cartoonist Bob Artley's life with his beloved wife and their 10 year battle together against Alzheimer's disease, which finally claimed her.
278 pages Hardcover
ISBN: 0-813821-04-5
Brad Nobiling, Credit Manager

899 Hospice Alternative
Harper Collins Publishers/Basic Books
10 E 53rd Street   212-207-7057
New York, NY 10022-5299   800-242-7737
                                                        Fax: 212-207-7203
An account of the hospice experience. An innovative and humane way of caring for the terminally ill.
256 pages
ISBN: 0-465030-61-0

900 Hospice Care for Patients with Advanced Progressive Dementia
Springer Publishing Company
536 Broadway   212-431-4370
New York, NY 10012   877-687-7476
                                                        Fax: 212-941-7842
                                  e-mail: marketing@springerpub.com
                                       www.springerpub.com
Discusses adpating hospice care for terminally ill patients with dementia. Topics include infections, eating difficulties, and providing palliative care.
320 pages Hardcover
ISBN: 0-826111-62-9
Annette Imperati, Marketing Director

901 I'm Just Not Myself Anymore: A Family Guide to Alzheimer's Disease
Northwestern University Press
625 Colfax Street   847-491-5313
Evanston, IL 60208-4210   Fax: 847-491-8150
                                  e-mail: nupress@nwu.edu
                                       www.northwestern.edu

1993 283 pages Paperback
ISBN: 1-880416-72-7

902 Interventions for Alzheimer's Disease: A Caregiver's Complete Reference
Ruth M Tappen, author
Health Professions Press
PO Box 10624   410-337-9585
Baltimore, MD 21285-0624   888-337-8808
                                                        Fax: 410-337-8539
                                       www.healthpropress.com
For professionals who plan, administer or provide services to Alzheimer's patients.
256 pages Paperback
ISBN: 1-878812-39-4

903 Key Elements of Dementia Care
Alzheimer's Association
225 North Michigan Avenue
Chicago, IL 60611-1696   800-272-3900
                                                        Fax: 866-699-1246
                                                        TDD: 312-355-8700
                                  e-mail: media@alz.org
                                       www.alz.org
Defines, describes, and illustrates dementia-capable care throughout the range of residential care settings.
1997 90 pages

904 Nursing Home and You: Partners in Caring for a Relative with Alzheimer's Disease
American Assn. of Homes & Services for the Aging
901 E Street NW   202-783-2242
Washington, DC 20004-2037   800-508-9442
                                                        Fax: 202-783-2255
Offers suggestions for families of nursing home residents on how to work with staff to foster smooth transitions.
32 pages

905 Occupational Therapy Practice Guidelines for Adults with Alzheimer's Disease
American Occupational Therapy Association

4720 Montgomery Lane
Bethesda, MD 20824-1220

301-652-2682
Fax: 301-652-7711
TDD: 800-377-8555
www.aota.org

21 pages
ISBN: 1-569001-46-4

906   Positive Interactions Program of Activities for People with Alzheimer's

Sylvia Nissenboim, author

Health Professions Press
PO Box 10624
Baltimore, MD 21285-0624

410-337-9585
888-337-8808
Fax: 410-337-8539
www.healthpropress.com

All interactions focus on preventing individual dignity and providing opportunities to experience meaningful involvement and satisfaction. Works in a variety of settings and promotes the OBRA quality of care guidelines.

176 pages 1997
ISBN: 1-878812-40-8
Christine Vroman, Editor

907   Rethinking Alzheimer's Care

Sam Fazio, Dorothy Seman, author

Health Professions Press
PO Box 10624
Baltimore, MD 21285-0624

410-337-9585
888-337-8808
Fax: 410-337-8539
www.healthpropress.com

Appropriate for all settings providing long-term care, adult day services, or assisted living, this fresh and humanistic approach to Alzheimer's care will encourage caregivers to rethink the disease experience and explore its possibilities, instead of its limitations.

200 pages Paperback
ISBN: 1-878812-62-9
Jane Stansell, Editor

908   Speaking Our Minds: Personal Reflections from Individuals with Alzheimer's

WH Freeman and Company
41 Madison Avenue
New York, NY 10010

212-576-9400
888-330-8477
Fax: 212-689-2383
www.whfreeman.com/generalreaders

Personal reflections of people with Alzheimer's disease.

161 pages Hardcover
ISBN: 0-716732-24-6

909   The Comfort of Home for Alheimer's Disease A Guide for Caregivers

M. Meyer, M. Mittelman, P. Derr, C. Epstein, author

CareTrust Publications LLC
PO Box 10283
Portland, OR 97296-0283

800-565-1533
Fax: 415-673-2005
e-mail: sales@comfortofhome.com
www.comfortofhome.com

Walks readers through all Alzheimer's stages and cover the basics from undertaning the difference between AD and normal aging, to coping with the behavioral symptoms that come with the diminishing reasoning skills. Additionally, Comfort talks about how to provide safe physical care around other medical conditions the Alzheimer's sufferer may have, due to normal aging. Not the least of all, Comfort provides self-care tips for the caregivers to remain emotionally and mentally healthy.

2008 288 pages
ISBN: 0-978790-30-8

910   Therapeutic Interventions in Alzheimer's

Aspen Publishers
7201 McKinney Circle
Frederick, MD 21705-0990

301-698-7100
800-638-8437
Fax: 301-695-7931
e-mail: customerservice@aspenpub.com
www.aspenpub.com

A program of functional skills for activities of daily living.

197 pages

911   Time for Alzheimer's: A True Story

Emerald Ink Publishing
7141 Office City Drive
Houston, TX 77087-3722

800-324-5663
www.emeraldink.com

Based on the author's personal experience in caring for her mother.

139 pages
ISBN: 1-885373-13-3

912   Understanding Alzheimer's Disease

University Press of Mississippi
3825 Ridgewood Road
Jackson, MS 39211-6492

601-432-6205
Fax: 601-432-6217
e-mail: press@ihl.state.ms.us
www.upress.state.ms.us

Aimed at people with Alzheimer's, family members, caregivers, health care and human service professionals. Describes Alzheimer's from early to advanced stages. Discusses the care of AD patients, ideas to help families care for the AD patient at home, reviews treatements for the psychiatric, behavioral and cognitive effects of AD and describes research efforts to better understand AD and develop effective therapies. Price $28 Hardcover, $12 Paperback.

1996 150 pages
ISBN: 0-878059-11-3
Kathy Burgess, Advertising/Marketing Services Manager

913   When We Become the Parent to Our Parents

MEA Productions
55 Binks Hill Road
Plymouth, NH 03264

603-536-2641
Fax: 603-536-4851
e-mail: me.allen@juno.com
www.maryemmallen.blogspot.com

Experiences of a woman who cared for her mother and aunt, both Alzheimer's patients.

62 pages
ISBN: 0-965167-51-8
Mary Emma Allen, Author

Children's Books

914   Grandpa Doesn't Know It's Me

Donna Guthrie, author

Alzheimer's Association
225 North Michigan Avenue
Chicago, IL 60611-1696

800-272-3900
Fax: 866-699-1246
TDD: 312-335-8700
e-mail: media@alz.org
www.alz.org

Geared to the concerns of a young child who has a relative with Alzheimer's disease.

26 pages

915   Grandpa's Music: A Story About Alzheimer's

Alison Acheson, author

Albert Whitman & Company
6340 Oakton Street
Morton Grove, IL 60053-2723

847-581-0033
800-255-7675
Fax: 847-581-0039
e-mail: mail@whitmanco.com
www.albertwhitman.com

Children's book using text and illustrations to show the effects of Alzheimer's disease.

ISBN: 0-807530-52-8
Pat McPartland, Sales
Joe Campbell, Customer Service

916   Just for Children: Helping You Understand Alzheimer's Disease

Alzheimer's Association
225 North Michigan Avenue
Chicago, IL 60611-1676

800-272-3900
Fax: 866-699-1246
TDD: 312-335-8700
e-mail: media@alz.org
www.alz.org

Information about Alzheimer's disease written especially for children.
1997 2 pages Pack of 100

917   Let's Talk About When Someone You Love Has Alzheimer's Disease
Rosen Publishing Group's PowerKids Press
29 E 21st Street   212-777-3017
New York, NY 10010   800-237-9932
                                        Fax: 888-436-4643
               e-mail: customerservice@rosenpub.com
                              www.rosenpublishing.com
This book sensitively helps children cope with this unsettling disease.

ISBN: 0-823923-06-1
Elizabeth Weitzman, Author

918   Through Tara's Eyes: Helping Children Cope with Alzheimer's Disease
American Health Assistance Foundation
15825 Shady Grove Road   301-948-3244
Rockville, MD 20850   800-437-2423
                                        Fax: 301-258-9454
                                            www.ahaf.org
Told from the perspective of Tara who has a grandmother with Alzheimer's disease but does not know anything is wrong with her grandmother.
36 pages

919   What's Wrong with Grandma? A Family Experience with Alzheimer's
Margaret Shawver, author
Prometheus Books
59 John Glenn Drive   716-691-0133
Amherst, NY 14228-2197   800-421-0351
                                        Fax: 716-691-0137
                  e-mail: marketing@prometheusbooks.com
                              www.prometheusbooks.com
The story of a family's struggle with Alzheimer's disease as told by the youngest child.
62 pages Paperback
ISBN: 1-159011-74-2
Lisa Risio, Marketing Production Manager

920   Window of Time
Associated Publishers Group
1501 Country Hospital Road   615-254-2450
Nashville, TN 37218   800-327-5113
                                        Fax: 615-254-2405
                        e-mail: vlill@apgbooks.com
                                         www.apgbooks.com
Illustrated book about the relationship between a grandfather with Alzheimer's and his grandson.
28 pages
ISBN: 0-963633-51-1

Magazines

921   Alzheimer Disease and Associated Disorders: An International Journal
Raven Press
1185 Avenue of the Americas   212-930-9500
New York, NY 10036-2601   800-777-2295
A leading international forum for reports of new research findings and new approaches to diagnosis and treatments. Contributions are offered from all scientific and medical fields.
Quarterly
ISBN: 0-89303H- -
Peter J Whitehouse

922   Mature Health
Haymarket Group, Ltd.
45 W 34th Street   212-239-0855
New York, NY 10001-3073
Magazine featuring articles on health aspects of aging, as well as articles on recreation and leisure.

923   Research & Practice
Alzheimer's Association
225 North Michigan Avenue
Chicago, IL 60611-1696   800-272-3900
                                        Fax: 866-699-1246
                                        TDD: 312-335-8700
                                  e-mail: media@alz.org
                                              www.alz.org
Provides practical information for healthcare professionals on the current status of prominent areas of Alzheimer research.
Quarterly
ISBN: 2-909342-84-0

Newsletters

924   Advances: Progress in Alzheimer Research and Care
Alzheimer's Association
225 North Michigan Avenue
Chicago, IL 60611-1696   800-272-3900
                                        Fax: 866-699-1246
                                        TDD: 312-335-8700
                                  e-mail: media@alz.org
                                              www.alz.org
Provides information related to research and caregiving.
Quarterly

925   Aging and Alzheimer's Disease Center Newsletter
Oregon Health Sciences University
3181 SW Sam Jackson Park Road   503-494-6976
Portland, OR 97201-3098   Fax: 503-494-7499
                                  e-mail: kaye@ohsu.edu
                         www.ohsu.edu/som-alzheimers
Researches causes and consequences of Alzheimer's disease and ways of clinical services.
2x Year
Jeffrey Kaye, Director

926   Alzheimer Disease and Associated Disorders
Charles Decarli, author
Lippincott Williams & Wilkins
16522 Hunters Green Parkway   301-223-2300
Hagerstown, MD 21740   800-638-3030
                                        Fax: 301-223-2398
                                  e-mail: orders@lww.com
                                              www.lww.com
A leading international forum for reports of new research findings and new approaches to diagnosis and treatment.
Quarterly Journal

927   Alzheimer's Association: Tarrant County Chapter
101 Summit Avenue   817-336-4949
Fort Worth, TX 76102   800-471-4422
                                        Fax: 817-336-4966
                         www.alz.org/northcentraltexas
Newsletter for those afflicted with Alzheimer's disease. Includes education, support groups, case management, telephone helpline and referral to services (i.e. long term care, adult daycare, medical assistance, legal assistance, etc.).
8 pages
Theresa Hocker, Executive Director
Susanna Luk-Jones, Director Services

928   LIAFLine Newsletter
Long Island Alzheimers Foundation
5 Channel Drive   516-767-6856
Port Washington, NY   Fax: 516-767-6864
                                   e-mail: info@liaf.org
                                             www.liaf.org
It is intended for caregivers, service providers and anyone interested in Alzheimer's Disease or the Foundation.
Fred Jenny, Executive Director

Pamphlets

929   10 Warning Signs of Alzheimer's Disease
Alzheimer's Association

225 N Michigan Avenue
Chicago, IL 60601-7633

312-335-8700
800-272-3900
Fax: 866-699-1246
TDD: 866-403-3073
e-mail: info@alz.org
www.alz.org

Contains a list of symptoms and answers to the most frequently asked questions.
Pack of 100
Harry Johns, President/CEO

930   Alzheimer's Disease
National Institutes of Health
5600 Fishers Lane
Rockville, MD 20857-0001

301-468-2600
www.nih.gov

Contains information on the diagnosis and treatment of Alzheimer's and on research that offers hope for the future. Included is a list of sources of help for both the patient and the family.

931   Alzheimer's Disease: The Basics
Alzheimer's Association
225 N Michigan Avenue
Chicago, IL 60601-7633

312-335-8700
800-272-3900
Fax: 866-699-1246
TDD: 312-335-5886
e-mail: info@alz.org
www.alz.org

Symptoms, diagnosis, treatments and more
32 pages
Harry Johns, President/CEO

932   Behaviors
Alzheimer's Association
225 N Michigan Avenue
Chicago, IL 60601-7633

312-335-8700
800-272-3900
Fax: 866-669-1246
TDD: 312-335-5886
e-mail: info@alz.org
www.alz.org

The most common behaviors and how to manage them.
12 pages
Harry Johns, President/CEO

933   Caregiver Stress
Alzheimer's Association
225 N Michigan Avenue
Chicago, IL 60601-7633

312-335-8700
800-272-3900
Fax: 866-699-1246
TDD: 312-335-5886
e-mail: info@alz.org
www.alz.org

Symptoms of caregiver stress and ways you can become a healthy caregiver.
6 pages
Harry Johns, President/CEO

934   Caring for Alzheimer's Patients
Human Sciences Press
233 Spring Street
New York, NY 10013-1522

212-620-8000
800-221-9369

This handbook is designed for families, friends, and health-care professionals coping with the myriad of problems encountered by those afflicted with Alzheimer's disease.
308 pages Cloth

935   Dementia Care Practice Recommendations Phases 1 and 2
Alzheimer's Association
225 N Michigan Avenue
Chicago, IL 60601-7633

312-335-8700
800-272-3900
Fax: 866-699-1246
TDD: 312-335-5886
e-mail: info@alz.org
www.alz.org

Covers fundamentals of dementia care and six key care practice areas: food and fluid consumption, pain management, social engagement, resident wandering, falls and physical restraint-free care.
32 pages
Harry Johns, President/CEO

936   Early-Onset Alzheimer's: I'M Too Young to Have Alzheimer's Disease
Alzheimer's Association
225 N Michigan Avenue
Chicago, IL 60601-7633

312-335-8700
800-272-3900
Fax: 866-699-1246
TDD: 312-335-5886
e-mail: info@alz.org
www.alz.org

Addresses unique challenges for diagnosed individuals who are younger than 65
12 pages
Harry Johns, President/CEO

937   Early-Stage Alzheimer's: If You Have Alzheimer's Disease What You Should Know
Alzheimer's Association
225 N Michigan Avenue
Chicago, IL 60601-7633

312-335-8700
800-272-3900
Fax: 866-669-1246
TDD: 312-335-5886
e-mail: info@alz.org
www.alz.org

Coping strategies and tips for living with Alzheimer's
16 pages
Harry Johns, President/CEO

938   Home Safety for People with Alzheimer's Disease
Alzheimer's Disease Education & Referral Center
PO Box 8250
Silver Spring, MD 20907

800-438-4380
Fax: 301-495-3334
e-mail: adear@nia.nih.gov
www.nia.nih.gov

For those who provide in-home care for people with Alzheimer's disease or related disorders. The goal is to improve home safety by identifying potential problems in the home and offering possible solutions to help prevent accidents.
32 pages

939   If You Have Alzheimer's Disease: What You Should Know, What You Should Do
Alzheimer's Association
225 North Michigan Avenue
Chicago, IL 60611-1696

800-272-3900
Fax: 866-699-1246
TDD: 312-335-8700
e-mail: media@alz.org
www.alz.org

Guide for the person with Alzheimer's disease. Includes suggestions of things to do that will help the person cope.
1994 Pack of 100

940   Just for Teens: Helping You Understand Alzheimer's Disease
Alzheimer's Association
225 North Michigan Avenue
Chicago, IL 60611-1696

800-272-3900
Fax: 866-699-1246
TDD: 312-335-8700
e-mail: media@alz.org
www.alz.org

Information about Alzheimer's disease aimed at teenagers.
Pack of 100

941   Late Stage Care
Alzheimer's Association
225 North Michigan Avenue
Chicago, IL 60611-1696

800-272-3900
Fax: 866-699-1246
TDD: 312-335-8700
e-mail: media@alz.org
www.alz.org

Suggestions for coping with caregiving problems that commonly occur late in the progression of Alzheimer's disease.
Pack of 100

942   Legal Plans
Alzheimer's Association

225 N Michigan Avenue
Chicago, IL 60601-7633

312-335-8700
800-272-3900
Fax: 866-699-1246
TDD: 312-335-5886
e-mail: info@alz.org
www.alz.org

Covers legal documents and how to find a lawyer.
16 pages
Harry Johns, President/CEO

943   MedicAlert & Alzheimer's Association Safe Return
Alzheimer's Association
225 N Michigan Avenue
Chicago, IL 60601-7633

312-335-8700
800-272-3900
Fax: 866-699-1246
TDD: 312-335-5886
e-mail: info@alz.org
www.alz.org

Enroll in the nationwide emergency response program that provides help when a person with dementia wanders or has a medical emergency.
1 pages
Harry Johns, President/CEO

944   Money Matters
Alzheimer's Association
225 N Michigan Avenue
Chicago, IL 60601-7633

312-335-8700
800-272-3900
Fax: 866-699-1246
TDD: 312-335-5886
e-mail: info@alz.org
www.alz.org

Identifies care costs and how to pay for them.
28 pages
Harry Johns, President/CEO

945   National Public Policy Program to Conquer Alzheimer's Disease
Alzheimer's Association
225 North Michigan Avenue
Chicago, IL 60611-1676

800-272-3900
Fax: 866-699-1246
TDD: 312-335-8700
e-mail: media@alz.org
www.alz.org

Summary of the Association's public policy goals, objectives and policies.
1997-Present 12 pages

946   Nutrition Screening Initiative
Nutrition Screening Initiative
2626 Pennsylvania Avenue NW
Washington, DC 20037-1618

202-625-1662
e-mail: nsi@gmmb.com
www.cafp.org

Offers information on nutrition pertaining to older Americans and illnesses such as Alzheimer's disease.

947   Partnering with Your Doctor: A Guide for Persons with Memory Problems
Alzheimer's Association
225 N Michigan Avenue
Chicago, IL 60601-7633

312-335-8700
800-272-3900
Fax: 866-699-1246
TDD: 312-335-5886
e-mail: info@alz.org
www.alz.org

Tips on working with your doctor to get the best care.
20 pages
Harry Johns, President/CEO

948   Phase 3: Dementia Care Practice Recommendations
Alzheimer's Association
225 N Michigan Avenue
Chicago, IL 60601-7633

312-335-8700
800-272-3900
Fax: 866-699-1246
TDD: 312-335-5886
e-mail: info@alz.org
www.alz.org

Covers minimizing physical, emotional and spiritual distress; maximizing well-being; snsuring communication with the resident, family and care team.
28 pages
Harry Johns, President/CEO

949   Practice Recommendations for Home Care Professionals
Alzheimer's Association
225 N Michigan Avenue
Chicago, IL 60601-7633

312-335-8700
800-272-3900
Fax: 866-699-1246
TDD: 312-335-5886
e-mail: info@alz.org
www.alz.org

Covers concrete, evidence-based practice suggestions for addressing issues unique to people with dementia living in the community.
68 pages
Harry Johns, President/CEO

950   Report of the Panel on Alzheimer's Disease
National Clearinghouse for Alcohol and Drug Abuse
PO Box 2345
Rockville, MD 20857

800-729-6686
www.health.org

52 pages

951   Respite Care Guide
Alzheimer's Association
225 N Michigan Avenue
Chicago, IL 60601-7633

312-335-8700
800-272-3900
Fax: 866-699-1246
TDD: 312-335-5886
e-mail: info@alz.org
www.alz.org

Find help when you need a break from caregiving.
19 pages
Harry Johns, President/CEO

952   Steps to Diagnosis
Alzheimer's Association
225 North Michigan Avenue
Chicago, IL 60611-1696

800-272-3900
Fax: 866-699-1246
TDD: 312-335-8700
e-mail: media@alz.org
www.alz.org

Educates individuals and their families on the importance of seeking a diagnosis, and the various test completed to obtain an accurate diagnosis.

953   Steps to Enhancing Communication
Alzheimer's Association
225 North Michigan Avenue
Chicago, IL 60611-1696

800-272-3900
Fax: 866-699-1246
TDD: 312-335-8700
e-mail: media@alz.org
www.alz.org

Offers caregivers techniques for improving their approach to listening to and communication with the individual with Alzheimer's disease.
1996 Pack of 100

954   Tax Credits and Deductions
Alzheimer's Association
225 N Michigan Avenue
Chicago, IL 60601-7633

312-335-8700
800-272-3900
Fax: 866-669-1246
TDD: 321-335-5886
e-mail: info@alz.org
www.alz.org

Outlines caregiving tax deductions and credits.
3 pages
Harry Johns, President/CEO

955   Terms & Tips: An Alzheimer Care Handbook
Marjorie Brandenburg, author

Alzheimer's Association

225 North Michigan Avenue
Chicago, IL 60611-1696

800-272-3900
Fax: 866-699-1246
TDD: 312-335-8700
e-mail: media@alz.org
www.alz.org

Offers an explanation for over 250 terms and offers practical caregiver ideas and tips. Primarily for people with dementia and their caregivers, family members, and all providers of hands-on assistance.
1995 84 pages

956 Treatments for Alzheimer's Disease
Alzheimer's Association
225 N Michigan Avenue
Chicago, IL 60601-7633

312-335-8700
800-272-3900
Fax: 866-699-1246
TDD: 312-335-5886
e-mail: info@alz.org
www.alz.org

Information about FDA-approved drugs.
3 pages
Harry Johns, President/CEO

957 Useful Information on Alzheimer's Disease
National Clearinghouse for Alcohol and Drug Abuse
PO Box 2345
Rockville, MD 20857-0001

800-729-6686
e-mail: www.webmaster@health.org
www.health.org

24 pages

958 You Are One of Us: Clergy/Church Connections to Alzheimer Families
Alzheimer's Disease Education & Referral Center
PO Box 8250
Silver Spring, MD 20907-8250

301-495-3311
800-438-4380
Fax: 301-495-3334
www.alzheimers.org

Describes how clergy and church members can help families by including patients and their relatives in church activities, visiting patients and developing church programs that support family caregivers.

Audio & Video

959 Alzheimer's Association Caregiver Resources
Alzheimer's Association
Western/Central Washington Chapter
Seattle, WA 98125

206-363-5500
800-848-7097
Fax: 206-363-5700
e-mail: rowena.rye@alz.org
http://alzwa.org/resources6.htm

A variety of numerous resources, materials and publications providing information for assisting those with Alzheimer's Disease including a documentation guide, informational fact sheets on topics such as bathing, dressing, eating and dealing with grief, in addition resources on long term care options and a newsletter.
Nancy Dapper, Executive Director
Rowena Rye, Community Resources

960 Alzheimer's Association Dementia Care Conference
Alzheimer's Association
225 North Michigan Avenue
Chicago, IL 60601-7633

312-335-5790
800-272-3900
Fax: 866-699-1246
TDD: 312-335-8700
e-mail: careconference@alz.org
www.alz.org/careconference/

Selected sessions from the conference discussing topics such as assisted living preconference, sexuality, intimacy and lifestyle changes, and activity intensive changing approaches to Alzheimer care.
Marisol Sukhu, Hotel/Events Information
Sheryl Trotz, Continuing Education & Presentations

961 Alzheimer's Association Safe Return Police Training Video
Alzheimer's Association Massachusetts Chapter

311 Arsenal Street
Watertown, MA 02472

617-868-6718
800-548-2111
Fax: 617-868-6720
e-mail: communications@alzmass.org
www.alzmass.org/

An educational package designed to help police officers recognize and respond appropriately to Alzheimer patients who may need assistance. Kit includes 1 videotape and 3 print pieces.
James Wessler, President/Chief Executive Officer
Betsy Fitzgerald, Director of Communications

962 Alzheimer's Association: Waves of Stone Video and Documentary
Alzheimer's Association Rhode Island Chapter
245 Waterman Street
Providence, RI 02906

401-421-3900
800-272-3900
Fax: 401-421-0115
e-mail: info@alz.org
http://www.alz-ri.org/Videoshtm.htm

PBS documentary on Alzheimer's disease that discusses both scientific research and caregiver issues.
1994 57 minutes
Elizabeth Morancy, Executive Director
Rita St Pierre, Program Director

963 Another Home for Mom
Lori Hope, author
Fanlight Productions
4196 Washington Street
Boston, MA 02131-1731

617-469-4999
800-937-4113
Fax: 617-469-3379
e-mail: fanlight@fanlight.com
www.fanlight.com

A gentle documentary following one couple as they confront the decision of whether to place the husbands mother, who has Alzheimer's disease, in a nursing home.
1989 27 Minutes
ISBN: 1-572950-77-3

964 Caring...Sharing: The Alzheimer's Caregiver
Fanflight Productions
47 Halifax Street
Boston, MA 02130

617-469-4949
800-937-4113
Fax: 617-469-3379
e-mail: fanlight@fanflight.com
www.fanlight.com

Examines what it means to be a caregiver. This program will be invaluable for any person or group involved in the care of the elderly.
38 minutes
ISBN: 1-572951-22-2

965 For Those Who Take Care: An Alzheimer's Disease Training Program for Nurses
Alzheimer's Disease Education & Referral Center
PO Box 8250
Silver Spring, MD 20907-8250

301-495-3311
800-438-4380
Fax: 301-495-3334
www.alzheimers.org

Guide for training nursing assistants and nurses' aides in long term care facilities, adult day care and private homes. Manual, text and student handouts. Produced by the University of Kentucky.

Web Sites

966 Alzheimer Research Forum

www.alzforum.org

The web's most dynamic scientific community dedicated to understanding alzheimer's disease and related disorders.

967 Alzheimer Support

www.alzheimersupport.com

Serves Alzheimer's sufferers and their loved ones by reporting the latest news in research and treatment, making hard-to-find, recommended nutritional supplements available at manufacturer-direct low prices, and, most importantly, donating profits from each purchase to fund Alzheimer's medical research.

968 Alzheimer's Association

www.alz.org

The leading, global voluntary health organization in Alzheimer care and support, and the largest private, nonprofit funder of Alzheimer research.

969 Alzheimer's Disease International

www.alz.co.uk/adi

The international federation of 73 Alzheimer associations around the world, in relations with the World Health Organization.

970 Healing Well

www.healingwell.com

A social network and support community for patients, caregivers, and families coping with the daily struggles of diseases, disorders and chronic illness.

971 Health Finder

www.healthfinder.gov

A government website where individuals can find information and tools to help you and those you care about stay healthy.

972 Healthlink USA

www.healthlinkusa.com

Health information concerning treatment, cures, prevention, diagnosis, risk factors, research, support groups, email lists, personal stories and much more. Updated regularly.

973 Helios Health

www.helioshealth.com

Online resource for your health information. Detailed information about specific health topics, access to expert advice from our Medical Advisory Board, and up-to-date health news.

974 MEDLINEplus Health Information

www.nlm.nih.gov/medlineplus

MedlinePlus has extensive information from the National Institutes of Health and other trusted sources on over 700 diseases and conditions.

975 MedicineNet

www.medicinenet.com

An online resource for consumers providing easy-to-read, authoritative medical and health information.

976 Medscape

www.medscape.com

Medscape offers specialists, primary care physicians, and other health professionals the Web's most robust and integrated medical information and educational tools.

977 Neurology Channel

www.neurologychannel.com

Find clearly explained, medically accurate information regarding conditions, including an overview, symptoms, causes, diagnostic procedures and treatment options. On this site it is possible to ask questions and get information from a neurologist and connect to people who have similar health interests.

978 WebMD

www.webmd.com

Information on Alzheimer's disease, including articles and resources.

Description

979 ## Amyotrophic Lateral Sclerosis

Amyotrophic Lateral Sclerosis, ALS, also called Lou Gehrig's disease, is a neurological disorder that affects the motor nerves in the brain and spinal cord. The cause of ALS is unknown. It is marked by progressive muscle weakness.

Initial symptoms may be subtle, but early signs of ALS can include twitching and cramping of muscles (particularly in the hands and feet), as well as difficulty in swallowing. As the disorder progresses, use of legs and arms, breathing, speaking, and swallowing become increasingly difficult.

Although the physical symptoms of ALS are most debilitating, the disease does not seem to impair intellectual functioning, although recent research indicates a significant number of people with ALS who have cognitive defects. Voluntary eye movement (blinking) and the senses also remain unaffected.

Currently, there is no cure for ALS. A regime of physical therapy and psychological support can help patients and their families.

National Agencies & Associations

980 **ALS Association National Office**
1275 K Street NW
Washington, DC 20005
818-880-9007
800-782-4747
Fax: 818-880-9006
e-mail: alsinfo@alsa-national.org
www.alsa.org
National nonprofit voluntary health organization dedicated solely to the fight against amytrophic lateral sclerosis. Its mission: to find a cure for and improve living with ALS. The four fronts of battle are: encouraging identifying funding and monitor
Jane H Gilbert, President/CEO
Lucie Bruijn PhD, Chief Scientist

State Agencies & Associations

Arizona

981 **Arizona Chapter of the ALS Association**
4643 E Thomas Road
Phoenix, AZ 85018
602-297-3800
866-350-2572
Fax: 602-297-3804
e-mail: ken@alsaz.org
webaz.alsa.org
This chapter provides newsletters and other information to help patients and their families find sources of supplies, referrals or counseling as needed. Provides monthly support meetings, public awareness information and fundraising.
Ken Brissa, President
Taryn Norley, Executive Director

California

982 **ALS Association: Bay Area Chapter**
565 Commercial Street
San Francisco, CA 94111
415-904-2572
800-209-0433
Fax: 415-904-2573
e-mail: fightALS@alsabayarea.org
www.webaz.alsa.org
ALS Association chapters are multifaceted grass roots organizations that carry out ALSA's mission and strategic goals at the community level. The chapter, with supporting services from the national office, actively pursues the association's goals.
Fred Fisher, Executive Director
Madelon M Thomson, Director Patient/Family Services

983 **ALS Association: Greater Los Angeles Chapter**
28720 Roadside Drive
Agoura Hills, CA 91301
818-865-8067
866-750-2572
Fax: 818-865-8066
e-mail: webmaster@alsala.org
www.alsala.org
ALS Association chapters are multifaceted grass-roots organizations that carry out ALSA's mission and strategic goals at the community level. The chapter — with supporting services from the National Office — actively pursues the Association's goals.
Cameron Ward, Chairman
Barbara Frova, Vice Chair

984 **ALS Association: Greater Sacramento Chapter**
2717 Cottage Way
Sacramento, CA 95825
916-979-9265
Fax: 916-979-9271
e-mail: lou@alssac.org
www.alssac.org
ALS Association chapters are multifaceted grass roots organizations that carry out ALSA's mission and strategic goals at the community level. The chapter, with supporting services from the national office, actively pursues the association's goals.
Scott Ehlen, President
Richard Kline, Vice President

985 **ALS Association: Greater San Diego CIO**
7920 Silverton
San Diego, CA 92126-6350
858-271-5547
Fax: 858-271-5687
e-mail: info@alsasd.com
www.alsasd.com
ALS Association chapters are multifaceted grass-roots organizations that carry out ALSA's mission and strategic goals at the community level. The chapter — with supporting services from the National Office — actively pursues the Association's goals.
Jane Mitchell, Chairman
John Fieberg, Vice Chairman

986 **Orange County Chapter of the ALS Association**
1232 Village Way
Santa Ana, CA 92705-2334
714-285-1088
Fax: 714-285-0305
e-mail: information@alsaoc.org
weboc.alsa.org
Provides information to ALS patients families and caregivers; offers support groups, information and referrals, a loan closet and public awareness information.
Mark Hershey, President
Chad Kessler, Vice President

Colorado

987 **ALS Association: Rocky Mountain Chapter**
7403 Church Ranch Blvd.
Westminster, CO 80021
303-832-2322
866-ALS-3211
Fax: 303-832-3365
e-mail: info@alsaco.org
www.alscolorado.org
The ALS Association chapters are multifaceted grass-roots organizations that carry out ALSA's mission and strategic goals at the community level. The chapter — with supporting services from the National Office — actively pursues the Association's goals.
Pam Rush-Negri, Executive Director
Leslie Ryan, Patient Services Director

Connecticut

988 **Connecticut Chapter of the ALS Association**
4 Oxford Road
Milford, CT 06460
203-874-5050
877-257-2281
Fax: 203-874-7070
e-mail: Lauren@alsact.org
www.alsact.org
The central source in Connecticut for services and education of ALS patients, families and caregivers. Provides ALS patients with

information concerning medical care and facilities, support groups, daily living aids and other services.
Lauren D'Alessandro, Executive Director
Chris Capobianco, President

District of Columbia

989 ALS Association: National Capital Area Chapter
7507 Standish Place   301-978-9855
Rockville, MD 20855   Fax: 301-978-9854
                                               e-mail: info@ALSinfo.org
                                                       www.alsinfo.org
Offers patient referrals, informational newsletters and brochures, patient support groups and meetings and fund raising for research into finding cures and treatments for ALS.
Ronnie Gunnerson, Executive Director
Wilson Krahnke, President

Florida

990 ALS Association: Florida Chapter
3242 Parkside Center Circle   813-637-9000
Tampa, FL 33619   888-257-1717
                                               Fax: 813-637-9010
                                       e-mail: cbright@als-florida.org
                                                       webfl.alsa.org
ALS Association chapters are multifaceted grass-roots organizations that carry out ALSA's mission and strategic goals at the community level. The chapter — with supporting services from the National Office — actively pursues the Association's goals.
Nancy Baily, President

991 ALS Association: Florida Chapter East Coast Regional Office
5005 W Laurel Street   813-637-9000
Tampa, FL 33607   888-257-1717
                                               Fax: 813-637-9010
                                       e-mail: office@als-florida.org
                                                       webfl.alsa.org
ALS Association chapters are multifaceted grass-roots organizations that carry out ALSA's mission and strategic goals at the community level. The chapter — with supporting services from the National Office — actively pursues the Association's goals.
Nancy Baily, President

Georgia

992 ALS Association of Georgia
1955 Cliff Valley Way   404-636-9909
Atlanta, GA 30329   888-636-9940
                                               Fax: 404-636-9949
                                               e-mail: info@alsaga.org
                                                       www.alsaga.org
Offers meetings, local support groups, patient support equipment loan and research for persons suffering from ALS.
Kent Murphy, Chair
Candace Wood, Executive Director

Illinois

993 Lois Insolia ALS Center at Northwestern Memorial Hospital
5550 West Touhyu   847-679-3311
Skokie, IL 60077   888-ALS-1107
                                               Fax: 847-679-9109
                                       e-mail: info@lesturnerals.org
                                                       www.lesturnerals.org
Utilizes a multidisciplinary approach in treating ALS. Trained specialists provide diagnostic, rehabilitative and supportive services that focus on assessment, care planning and education. Patients and loved ones are encouraged to attend the support groups offered. Provides in-home visits by ALS nurse consultants and social worker, support groups, a lending bank of equipment, and grant programs for financial aid.
Teepu Siddique MD, Director

Indiana

994 ALS Association: Indiana Chapter
6525 E 82nd Street   317-915-9888
Indianapolis, IN 46250   888-508-3232
                                               Fax: 317-573-9889
                                       e-mail: jlewellen@alsaindiana.org
                                                       webin.alsa.org
ALS Association chapters are multifaceted grass-roots organizations that carry out ALSA's mission and strategic goals at the community level. The chapter — with supporting services from the National Office — actively pursues the Association's goals.
Melissa Pershing, Executive Director
Abbie Vollmar, Director of Patient Services

Kansas

995 ALS Association: Keith Worthington Chapter
6950 Squibb Rd   913-648-2062
Mission, KS 66202   800-878-2062
                                               Fax: 913-642-2431
                                       e-mail: bcooper@alsa-midwest.org
                                                       www.alsa-midwest.org
ALS Association chapters are multifaceted grass-roots organizations that carry out ALSA's mission and strategic goals at the community level. The chapter — with supporting services from the National Office — actively pursues the Association's goals.
Beckie Cooper, Executive Director
Sally Dwyer, Program Director

996 ALS Association: Keith Worthington Chapter Central/Western Kansas Branch
526 South Market   316-612-0188
Wichita, KS 67202   800-878-2062
                                               Fax: 316-612-8768
                                       e-mail: kwille@alsa-midwest.org
                                                       www.alsa-midwest.org
ALS Association chapters are multifaceted grass-roots organizations that carry out ALSA's mission and strategic goals at the community level. The chapter — with supporting services from the National Office — actively pursues the Association's goals.
Kathleen Willie, Awareness and Development

Kentucky

997 ALS Association: Kentucky CIO
2807 Amsterdam Road   85 - 3 - 13
Villa Hills, KY 41017   800-406-7702
                                               Fax: 85 - 3 - 19
                                       e-mail: mbacon@alsaky.org
                                                       webky.alsa.org
ALS Association chapters are multifaceted grass-roots organizations that carry out ALSA's mission and strategic goals at the community level. The chapter — with supporting services from the National Office — actively pursues the Association's goals.
Mary Bacon, Executive Director
Jennifer Lepa, Administrative Coordinator

Massachusetts

998 ALS Association: Massachusetts Chapter, Wakefield Office
7 Lincoln Street   781-245-2133
Wakefield, MA 01880-3021   800-258-3323
                                               Fax: 781-245-5414
                                       e-mail: info@als-ma.org
                                       www.webma.alsa.org/site/PageServer?pagen
Offers informational brochures and newsletters to promote public awareness, support groups and meetings for patients and their families, and referral information for members in the Massachusetts area.
Rick J Arrowood

Michigan

999   ALS Association: Michigan Chapter
24359 Northwestern Highway   648-354-6100
Southfield, MI 48075   800-882-5764
     Fax: 248-354-6440
     e-mail: sueb@alsofmi.org
     www.alsofmichigan.org
ALS Association chapters are multi-faceted grass-roots organizations that carry out ALSA's mission. and strategic goals at the community level. The chapter — with supporting services from the National Office — actively pursues the Association's goals.
Sue Burstein-Kahn, Executive Director
Lisa Alteri, President

1000   ALS Association: West Michigan Chapter
678 Front Street   616-459-1900
Grand Rapids, MI 49504   800-387-7121
     Fax: 616-459-4522
     e-mail: stacey@alsa-michigan.org
     webmi.alsa.org
ALS Association chapters are multi-faceted grass-roots organizations that carry out ALSA's mission. and strategic goals at the community level. The chapter — with supporting services from the National Office — actively pursues the Association's goals.
Stacey Orsted, Executive Director
Katee Stahl, Administrative Assistant

Minnesota

1001   ALS Association: Minnesota Chapter
333 N Washington Avenue   612-672-0484
Minneapolis, MN 55401   888-672-0484
     Fax: 612-672-9110
     e-mail: info@alsmn.org
     webmi.alsa.org
ALS Association chapters are multifaceted grass-roots organizations that carry out ALSA's mission and strategic goals at the community level. The chapter — with supporting services from the National Office — actively pursues the Association's goals.
Sue Spaulding, Executive Director
Sandy Judge, Development Director

Missouri

1002   ALS Association: Keith Worthington Chapter Central Missouri Branch Office
2025 E. Chestnut Expressway   417-886-5003
Springfield, MO 65802   888-386-1200
     Fax: 417-886-5003
     e-mail: springfield@alsa-midwest.org
     www.alsa-midwest.org
ALS Association chapters are multifaceted grass-roots organizations that carry out ALSA's mission and strategic goals at the community level. The chapter — with supporting services from the National Office — actively pursues the Association's goals.
Paul Blackwell, Services Staff
Valerie Gustin, Awareness and Development

1003   ALS Association: St. Louis Regional Chapter
2258 Weldon Parkway   314-432-7257
Saint Louis, MO 63146   888-873-8539
     Fax: 314-432-2991
     e-mail: mhill@alsastl.org
     webstl.alsa.org
A chapter serving the Eastern Missouri and Southern Illinois regions dedicated solely to finding the cause and cure of ALS through research, patient support, information and referrals and public awareness.
Maureen Barber-Hill, President
Richard Palank, Board Chair

Nebraska

1004   ALS Association: Keith Worthington Chapter Nebraska Branch Office
10730 Pacific at Shaker Place   402-991-8788
Omaha, NE 68114   866-762-6361
     Fax: 402-991-3690
     e-mail: nebraska@alsa-midwest.org
     www.alsa-midwest.org
ALS Association chapters are multifaceted grass-roots organizations that carry out ALSA's mission and strategic goals at the community level. The chapter — with supporting services from the National Office — actively pursues the Association's goals.
Shannon Todd, Services Staff
Sherrie Hanneman, Awareness and Development

New Hampshire

1005   ALS Association: Northern New England Chapter
The Champlain Mill
10 Ferry Street   603-226-8855
Concord, NH 03301   866-257-6663
     Fax: 603-226-8890
     e-mail: executive.director@alsanne.org
     www.alsanne.org
ALS Association chapters are multifaceted grass-roots organizations that carry out ALSA's mission and strategic goals at the community level. The chapter — with supporting services from the National Office — actively pursues the Association's goals.
Kathleen L Phillips, Executive Director
Christine Richards, Patient Services Director

New Mexico

1006   ALS Association: New Mexico CIO
PO Box 16495   505-323-6348
Albuquerque, NM 87191-6495   e-mail: als@alsanm.org
     www.alsa-nm.org
ALS Association chapters are multifaceted grass-roots organizations that carry out ALSA's mission and strategic goals at the community level. The chapter — with supporting services from the National Office — actively pursues the Association's goals.
Chuck Borgman, President
Terie Baker, Executive Director

New York

1007   ALS Association: Greater New York Chapter
42 Broadway   212-619-1400
New York, NY 10004   800-672-8857
     Fax: 212-619-7409
     e-mail: als@als-ny.org
     www.als-ny.org
ALS Association chapters are multifaceted grass-roots organizations that carry out ALSA's mission and strategic goals at the community level. The chapter — with supporting services from the National Office — actively pursues the Association's goals.
Richard Rose, Chairman
Wendy Schriber, Vice Chairman

1008   ALS Association: Upstate New York CIO
890 7th N Street   315-413-0121
Liverpool, NY 13088   866-499-7257
     Fax: 315-413-0508
     e-mail: info@alsaupstateny.org
     webuny.alsa.org
ALS Association chapters are multifaceted grass-roots organizations that carry out ALSA's mission and strategic goals at the community level. The chapter — with supporting services from the National Office — actively pursues the Association's goals.
Katharine Loomis, Executive Director
Shiann Atuegbu, Patient Services Coordinator

Ohio

1009 ALS Association: Northeast Ohio Chapter
6155 Rockside Road   216-592-2572
Independence, OH 44131   888-592-2572
                                  Fax: 216-592-2575
                       e-mail: alsa@alsaohio.org
                                  webnoh.alsa.org
Offers telephone consultation services, support groups, caregivers support groups, equipment loan bank and a 24 hour telephone answering service for persons with ALS.
Mary Wilson Wheelock, Executive Director
Fred M DeGrandis, President

1010 ALS Association: Western Ohio Chapter
1170 Old Henderson Road   614-273-2572
Columbus, OH 43220   866-273-2572
                                  Fax: 614-273-2573
                       e-mail: alsohio@alsohio.org
                                  webcsoh.alsa.org
Offers telephone consultation services, support groups, caregivers support groups, equipment loan bank and a 24 hour telephone answering service for persons with ALS.
Marlin Seymour, Executive Director
Yvonne Dressman, Care Coordinator

Oregon

1011 ALS Association: Oregon & SW Washington CIO
700 NE Multnomah   503-238-5559
Portland, OR 97232   800-681-9851
                                  Fax: 503-296-5590
                          e-mail: info@alsa-or.org
                                  webor.alsa.org
The ALS Association chapters are multifaceted grass-roots organizations that carry out ALSA's mission and strategic goals at the community level. The chapter — with supporting services from the National Office — actively pursues the Association's goals.
Lance Christian, Executive Director
Aubrey McCauley, Development Director

Pennsylvania

1012 ALS Association: Greater Philadelphia Chapter
321 Norristown Road   215-643-5434
Ambler, PA 19002   877-434-7441
                                  Fax: 215-643-9307
                  e-mail: alsassoc@alsphiladelphia.org
                              www.alsphiladelphia.org
To lead the fight to treat and cure ALS through global research and nationwide advocacy while also empowering people with Lou Gehrig's Disease and their families to live fuller lives by providing them with compassionate care and support.
Joan Borowsky, Development Coordinator
Jeffrey Cline, Chief Development Officer

1013 ALS Association: Western Pennsylvania Chapter
416 Lincoln Avenue   412-821-3254
Pittsburgh, PA 15209   800-967-9296
                                  Fax: 412-821-3549
                    e-mail: mbernarding@alswp.org
                              webwpawv.alsa.org
The mission of this chapter is to provide services and education to ALS patients, families and caregivers through medical information, support groups, assisting health care providers and providing communication devices.
Michael Bernarding, Executive Director
Marie Folino, Patient Services Director

South Carolina

1014 ALS Association: Jim (Catfish) Hunter Chapter
120-101 Penmarc Drive   919-755-9001
Raleigh, NC 27603   877-568-4347
                                  Fax: 919-755-0910
                       e-mail: jerry@catfishchapter.org
                              www.catfishchapter.org
ALS association chapters are multifaceted grass roots organizations that carry out ALSA's mission and strategic goals at the community level. The chapter, with supporting services from the national office, actively pursues the association's goals.
Jerry Dawson RN BSN, President & CEO
Megan Gardner, Executive Director

Tennessee

1015 ALS Association: Middle Tennessee Chapter
522 E Iris Drive   61 - 3 - 55
Nashville, TN 37204   877-216-5551
                                  Fax: 615-331-5796
                  e-mail: cheri.sanders@alstn.org
                              webtn.alsa.org
ALS Association chapters are multifaceted grass-roots organizations that carry out ALSA's mission and strategic goals at the community level. The chapter — with supporting services from the National Office — actively pursues the Association's goals.
Cheri Sanders, Executive Director
Patty Lane, Patient Services Coordinator

Texas

1016 ALS Association: Greater Houston CIO
PO Box 271561   713-942-2572
Houston, TX 77277-1561   866-788-2572
                                  Fax: 218-497-2572
              e-mail: linda.richardson@alsa-houston.org
                              www.alsa-houston.org
ALS Association chapters are multi-faceted grass roots organizations that carry out ALSA's mission and strategic goals at the community level. he chapter — with supporting services from the National Office — actively pursues the Association's goals.
Linda Richardson, President
Georgia Mclain, Patient Services

1017 ALS Association: North Texas Chapter
1231 Greenway Drive   972-714-0088
Irving, TX 75038   877-714-0088
                                  Fax: 972-714-0066
                  e-mail: a.reid@alsanorthtexas.org
                              webntx.alsa.org
ALS Association chapters are multi-faceted grass roots organizations that carry out ALSA's mission and strategic goals at the community level. he chapter — with supporting services from the National Office — actively pursues the Association's goals.
David Chayer, Executive Director
Bonnie Walsh, Development Director

1018 ALS Association: South Texas Chapter
8600 Wurzbach   210-733-5204
San Antonio, TX 78240   877-257-4673
                                  Fax: 210-733-5206
                  e-mail: Information@alsasotx.org
                              www.alsasotx.org
ALS Association chapters are multi-faceted grass roots organizations that carry out ALSA's mission and strategic goals at the community level. he chapter — with supporting services from the National Office — actively pursues the Association's goals.
Bonnie Walsh, Executive Director
Julia Dyer, Development Associate

Washington

1019 ALS Association: Evergreen Chapter
19115 68th Avenue   425-656-1650
Kent, WA 98032   866-786-7257
                                  Fax: 425-656-1649
                  e-mail: BeckyMooreED@alsa-ec.org
                              webwa.alsa.org
The ALS Association chapters are multifaceted grass-roots organizations that carry out ALSA's mission and strategic goals at the community level. The chapter — with supporting services from the National Office — actively pursues the Association's goals.
Rebecca Moore, Executive Director
Sonja Zimmer, Patient Services Director

1020 ALS Association: Oregon & SW Washington CIO
700 NE Multnomah 503-238-5559
Portland, OR 97232 800-681-9851
Fax: 503-296-5590
e-mail: info@alsa-or.org
webor.alsa.org

The ALS Association chapters are multifaceted grass-roots organizations that carry out ALSA's mission and strategic goals at the community level. The chapter — with supporting services from the National Office — actively pursues the Association's goals.
Cindy Burdell, Director
Lance Christian, Executive Director

Wisconsin

1021 ALS Association: Southeast Wisconsin Chapter
2505 N 124th Street 262-784-5257
Brookfield, WI 53005 Fax: 262-784-5260
e-mail: info@alsawi.org
webwi.alsa.org

Begun in 1987 as a support group this chapter is managed by a Board of Directors from all walks of life and disciplines. All members share a dedication to carry out the mission of Hope Through Research and Support Through Caring. The goal is to help ALS
Melanie Roach-Bekos, Executive Director
Linda Lehmann, Office Manager

Research Centers

1022 ALS Center at UCSF
350 Parnassus Avenue 415-353-2108
San Francisco, CA 94117 Fax: 415-353-2524
e-mail: alscenter@ucsf.edu
www.neurology2.ucsf.edu
Research serves as a cornerstone for our patient programs allowing us to translate the most recent advancement in therapies drug development and clinical management into care for our patients.
Catherine Lomen-Hoer, Director
Carolyn Rodriguez, Clinical Coordinator

1023 ALS Clinic at Penn Neurological Institute ALS Association Greater Philadelphia Cha
ALS Association Greater Philadelphia Chapter
321 Norristown Road 215-643-5434
Ambler, PA 19002 Fax: 215-643-9307
e-mail: brenda@alsphiladelphia.org
www.pennhealth.com/als
A multidisciplinary center for the evaluation and treatment of amyotrophic lateral sclerosis (ALS) and related disorders.
Brenda Edelm LCSW BCD, Director of Patient Services
Lauren Elman, Associate Medical Director

1024 ALS Clinical Department of Neurology
College of Medicine of the University of Vermont
89 Beaumont Avenue 802-656-2154
Burlington, VT 05405-3456 Fax: 802-656-8577
e-mail: Rup.Tandan@uvm.edu
www.med.uvm.edu
Clinical care facility for ALS patients.
Daniel Mark Fogel, President
Robert Cioffi, Chair

1025 Center for ALS and Related Diorders The Cleveland Clinic DepartmentOf Neurol
The Cleveland Clinic DepartmentOf Neurology
9500 Euclid Avenue 216-444-5538
Cleveland, OH 44195-5227 800-223-2273
Fax: 216-445-4653
TTY: 216-444-0261
e-mail: andrewd@ccf.org
my.clevelandclinic.org
Clinical care and research facility for ALS patients.
Erik P Pioro, Director
Kathleen M Kelly, ALS Clinical Coordinator

1026 Les Turner Research Laboratory Northwestern University Medical School
Northwestern University Medical School

5550 W Touhy Avenue 847-679-3311
Skokie, IL 60077 888-ALS-1107
Fax: 847-679-9109
e-mail: info@lesturnerals.org
www.lesturnerals.org
Scientists and researchers dedicate their time to discover what causes ALS and find a cure for the disease. The international team of scientists at the Laboratory are internationally recognized for their accomplishments in the field of ALS research.
Harvey Gaffen, President
Wendy Abrams, Executive Director

1027 Mayo Clinic: Department of Neurology
200 First Street SW 507-284-2511
Rochester, MN 55905 Fax: 507-284-0161
TDD: 507-284-9786
www.mayo.edu

Ongoing research and treatment for ALS.
John H Noseworthy MD, President
William C Rupp, MD, Vice President, CEO

1028 Motor Neuron Disease Clinic University of Connecticut Health Center
University of Connecticut Health Center
263 Farmington Avenue 860-679-2000
Farmington, CT 06030 Fax: 860-679-1454
TTY: 860-679-2242
www.uchc.edu

Francisco L. Borges, Chairman
Sanford Cloud Jr., Chair

1029 Motor Neuron Disease Program University of Michigan Health System
University of Michigan Health System
1500 E Medical Center Drive 734-936-6641
Ann Arbor, MI 48109-316 Fax: 734-153-53
www.med.umich.edu
Regional clinic that is dedicated to the diagnosis of Amyotrophic Lateral Sclerosis and improving the well-being of patients who have this disease.
Ora Hirsh Pescovitz MD, Vice President
Douglas L Strong, CEO

1030 Neuromuscular and ALS Center The Clinical Academic Building
The Clinical Academic Building
125 Patterson Street 732-235-7331
New Brunswick, NJ 08901 Fax: 732-235-7344
e-mail: nmalsweb@umdnj.edu
www2.umdnj.edu/nmalsweb
A multidisciplinary program for the diagnosis evaluation and long-term management of a host of neuromuscular diseases found in adults.
Jerry Belsh MD, Director
Annmarie Coyne-West, Patient Care Coordinator

1031 New England Medical Center: ALS Laboratory
800 Washington Street 617-636-5000
Boston, MA 02111-1533 Fax: 617-636-8568
www.tuftsmedicalcenter.org
Specializes in Amyotrophic Lateral Sclerosis research.
Ellen Zane, President, CEO
Margret Vosburgh, Chief Operating Officer

1032 Solomon Park Research Institute
12815 NE 124th Street 425-650-2020
Kirkland, WA 98034 800-470-1817
Fax: 425-650-2028
e-mail: pclapshaw@soloman.org
www.solomon.org
Amyotrophic lateral sclerosis research.
Patric Clapshaw, Director
Sheila Dunagan, Office Manager

1033 Stem Cell Research Program University of Wisconsin-Madison
University of Wisconsin-Madison
1500 Highland Avenue 608-890-0173
Madison, WI 53705-2280 Fax: 608- 26- 526
e-mail: gilbert@waisman.wisc.edu
www.waisman.wisc.edu/scrp

The mission of this program is to understand the molecular mechanisms responsible for the proliferation and differentiation of stem cells and assess their safety and efficacy following transplantation into various disease models.
Jacalyn McHugh, Research Program Manager
Anita Bhattacharyya, Principal Ivestigator

1034 Virginia Mason Medical Center Neuroscience Institute
Virginia Mason Medical Center
1100 9th Avenue   206-341-1900
Seattle, WA 98101   888-862-2737
www.virginiamason.org

Clinical care and research.
Gary Kaplan, Chairman, CEO

Support Groups & Hotlines

1035 ALS Association Free Standing Support Groups
ALS Association National Office
27001 Agoura Road   818-880-9007
Calabasas Hills, CA 91301-5104   800-782-4747
                                    Fax: 818-880-9006
                                    e-mail: alsinfo@alsa-national.org
                                    www.alsa.org
We know of support groups in Alabama, California, Florida, Illinois, New York, Oklahoma, Oregon, Puerto Rico, Utah and Virginia.
Gary Leo, President
Sondi Scheck, VP Operations/Administration

1036 American Society of Human Genetics
9650 Rockville Pike   301-634-7000
Bethesda, MD 20814-3998   Fax: 301-634-7001
                                    e-mail: estrass@genetics.faseb.org
                                    www.faseb.org
This society will locate a genetic counselor in various areas across the United States for persons with ALS.

1037 Amyotrophic Lateral Sclerosis Toll Free Hotline
ALS Association
27001 Agoura Road   818-880-9007
Calabasas Hills, CA 91301-5104   800-782-4747
                                    Fax: 818-880-9006
                                    e-mail: alsinfo@alsanational.org
                                    www.alsa.org
Informs individuals with ALS and their families of services available through the ALS Association.
Gary Leo, President
Sondi Scheck, VP Operations/Administration

1038 Les Turner Amyotrophic Lateral Sclerosis Foundation
5550 West Touhy   847-679-3311
Skokie, IL 60077   888-257-1107
                                    Fax: 847-679-9109
                                    e-mail: info@lesturnerals.org
                                    www.lesturnerals.org
Support groups offer patients and family members a chance to not feel alone and frustrated in coping with ALS and offers them the support of professionals as well as others who are experiencing similar problems.
Claire Owen, Director Patient Services

1039 National Health Information Center
PO Box 1133   310-565-4167
Washington, DC 20013   800-336-4797
                                    Fax: 301-984-4256
                                    e-mail: info@nhic.org
                                    www.health.gov/nhic
Offers a nationwide information referral service, produces directories and resource guides.

Books

1040 Amyotrophic Lateral Sclerosis: Guide for Patients and Families
Hiroshi Mitsumoto MD, author
Demos Medical Publishing

11 W 42nd Street   212-683-0072
New York, NY 10036   800-532-8663
                                    e-mail: info@demosmedpub.com
                                    www.demosmedpub.com
Covers every aspect of the management of ALS, from clinical features of the disease, to diagnosis, to an overview of symptom management. Major sections deal with medical and rehabilitative management, living with ALS, managing advanced disease, end-of-life issues and resources that can provide support and assistance in this time of need.
450 pages
ISBN: 1-932603-72-7

1041 Complete Bedside Companion: No-Nonsense Advice to Caring for the Seriously Ill
Rodger McFarlane, Philip Bashe, author
Simon & Shuster
1230 Avenue of the Americas
New York, NY 10020   212-698-7000
                                    www.simonandschuster.com
Offers warmth, encouragement, and the medical, legal, financial, and emotional advice you need when caring for an ailing loved one.
1999 544 pages
ISBN: 0-684843-19-6

1042 Easy-to-Swallow, Easy-to-Chew Cookbook
Donna L Weihofen, JoAnne Robbins, Paula A Sullivan, author
Wiley Publishers
111 River Street   201-748-6000
Hoboken, NJ 07030-5774   Fax: 201-748-6088
                                    e-mail: info@wiley.com
                                    www.wiley.com
Presents a collection of more than 150 nutritious recipes that make eating enjoyable and satisfying for anyone who has difficulty chewing or swallowing. Also shares helpful tips and techniques to make eating easier for the elderly and those with such as Parkinson's, AIDS, or head and neck cancers.
256 pages
ISBN: 0-471200-74-1

1043 Journeys with ALS
DLRC Press
PO Box 61661   757-473-1130
Virginia Beach, VA 23466   800-776-0560
                                    e-mail: mary@davidlawrence.com
Compiled by an ALS patient, this book contains 33 first person journeys with ALS. Some are hopeful, some are sad, a few are angry. All are powerful, real-life examples of people doing their best to cope, often with humor and high spirits.
1998
ISBN: 1-880731-58-4

1044 Learning to Fall: the Blessings of an Imperfect Life
Philip Simmons, author
Random House
1745 Broadway   www.randomhouse.com
New York, NY 10019
Philip Simmons was just thirty-five years old in 1993 when he learned that he had ALS, or Lou Gehrig's disease, and was told he had less than five years to live. As a young husband and father, and at the start of a promising literary career, he suddenly had to learn the art of dying. Nine years later, he has succeeded, against the odds, in learning the art of living.
176 pages

1045 Life on Wheels: for the Active Wheelchair User
Gary Karp, author
O'Reilly Media
1005 Gravenstein Highway N   707-827-7000
Sebastopol, CA 95472   800-998-9938
                                    Fax: 707-829-0104
                                    e-mail: orders@oreilly.com
                                    www.oreilly.com
For people who want to take charge of their life experience. Describes medical issues (paralysis, circulation, rehab, cure research); day-to-day living (exercise, skin, bowel and bladder,

sexuality, home access, maintaining a wheelchair); and social issues (self-image, adjustement, friends, family, cultural attitudes, activism)
565 pages
ISBN: 1-565922-53-2

1046 Non Chew Cookbook
Wilson Publishing Company
5708 Nicollet Avenue S
Minneapolis, MN 55419
800-843-2409
e-mail: nonchew@excite.com
www.nonchewcookbook.com
Soft food recipes good for the whole family.

1047 Realities in Coping with Progressive Neuromuscular Diseases
Charles Press Publishers
PO Box 15715   215-561-2786
Philadelphia, PA 19103   Fax: 215-561-0191
e-mail: mailbox@charlespresspub.com
www.charlespresspub.com
Focuses on this fundamental question by bringing together the work of 51 eminent authorities on neurology, nursing, psychology, social work, psychiarty, respiratory therapy, pastoral care and other related disciplines.
248 pages Hardcover only
ISBN: 0-914783-20-3

Newsletters

1048 ALS Today
Les Turner ALS Foundation
5550 West Touhy   847-679-3311
Skokie, IL 60077   888-257-1107
Fax: 847-679-9109
e-mail: info@lesturnerals.org
www.lesturnerals.org
Offers information on clinical trials, medical updates, recipes, resources and support groups available from the foundation.
3 per year

1049 LINK
ALS Association
27001 Agoura Road   818-880-9007
Calabasas Hills, CA 91301-5104   800-782-4747
Fax: 818-880-9006
e-mail: alsinfo@alsa-national.org
www.alsa.org
Offers information on a national level to all patients and chapter members of the ALS Association. Medical updates, loan equipment, resources, hotlines, support groups and news of charity and fundraising events are included as well.

1050 Massachusetts Chapter of the ALS Association Newsletter
Massachusetts Chapter of the ALS Association
7 Lincoln Street   781-245-2133
Wakefield, MA 01880-3021   800-258-3323
Offers information on activities, events, charity and fundraising activities, resources and more for members.
BiMonthly
Ginny DelVecchio, President

1051 Peach Lines
ALS Association of Georgia
3795 Manor House Drive   770-642-7962
Marietta, GA 30062-5147
Chapter newsletter offering information on support groups, meetings, hotlines, resources and reviews the newest technology and daily living aids for persons with ALS in the Georgia area.
BiMonthly

1052 Reaching Out
Orange County Chapter of the ALS Association
16787 Beach Boulevard   949-587-9700
Huntington Beach, CA 92647-4848
Offers information on support groups, meetings, charity events, fundraising activities and more for ALS members in the Orange County area.
BiMonthly

1053 South Texas Chapter of the ALS Association Newsletter
2389 W Military Highway   210-493-1311
San Antonio, TX 78231
Offers chapter information on events, charities, memorials, tributes and resources for persons with ALS and their families.
BiMonthly

1054 ALS News & Views
Western Pennsylvania Chapter-ALS Association
1323 Forbes Avenue   412-261-5940
Pittsburgh, PA 15219-4725
Offers information on resources, medical articles, events, charities, fundraising activities and more for patients with ALS, families and caregivers in the western Pennsylvania region.
8 pages BiMonthly
Rita Patchan, Editor

Pamphlets

1055 Basic Home Care for ALS Patients
ALS Association
1275 K Street NW   818-880-9007
Washington, DC 20005   800-782-4747
Fax: 818-880-9006
e-mail: alsinfo@alsa-national.org
www.alsa.org
Provides basic information about home care for people affected by ALS. This booklet is intended as an introductory guide and should be used along with professional medical care from one's physician, nurse and social worker.
Jane H Gilbert, President/CEO

1056 Maintaining Good Nutrition with ALS
ALS Association
1275 K Street NW   www.alsa.org
Washington, DC 20005
Helps people with ALS overcome the obstacles to eating well. Discusses the importance of nutrition to people with ALS and makes suggestions for dealing with various eating problems.
Jane H Gilbert, President/CEO

Audio & Video

1057 Driving Force: A Story of Life
Production House
811 St. John's   847-433-3172
Highland Park, IL 60035   Fax: 847-433-9383
Inspiring video featuring Dr. Frank de Leon Jones, a pychiatrist and ALS patient. Despite his disease and the need for continuous medical ventilation, Dr. de Leon Jones continues his challenging medical practice and physical education responsibilities. This is a film of courage, persistence and love of life. It offers poignant messages for ALS patients, family and caregivers as well as healthcare providers. Available in VHS or DVD.
Howie Samuelson, Executive Director

1058 Living with ALS: Adapting to Breathing Changes/Use of Non Invasive Ventilation
ALS Association
1275 K Street NW   www.alsa.org
Washington, DC 20005
Describes how ALS impacts this vital body function and what can be done to help the person with ALS.
Jane H Gilbert, President/CEO

1059 Living with ALS: Adjusting to Swallowing Difficulties & Good Nutrition
ALS Association
1275 K Street NW   www.alsa.org
Washington, DC 20005
In this video we look at the impact of ALS on swallowing and one's ability to maintain good nutrition. Health care professionals provide guidelines and tips for diet changes and for decision-making regarding a feeding tube; patients and their families share their own experiences and demonstrate their ingenuity in adapting to the

changes that weakened swallowing muscles and structures can cause.
2003
Jane H Gilbert, President/CEO

1060 Living with ALS: Communication Solutions & Symptom Management
ALS Association
1275 K Street NW
Washington, DC 20005   www.alsa.org
Jane H Gilbert, President/CEO

1061 Living with ALS: Mobility, Activities of Daily Living, Home Adaptions
ALS Association
1275 K Street NW
Washington, DC 10005   www.alsa.org
This first video, Functioning When Your Mobility is Affected, covers a range of mobility issues that occur with ALS. Our goal is to help you maximize your mobility, independence, safety and comfort. Health care professionals, persons with ALS and their families not only provide information in this video, but also demonstrate equipment and techniques that can help you maximize your function.
Jane H Gilbert, President/CEO

1062 Ventilation: Decision Making Process
Les Turner ALS Foundation
5550 West Touhy   847-679-3311
Skokie, IL 60077   888-257-1107
                                            Fax: 847-679-9109
                              e-mail: info@lesturnerals.org
                                      www.lesturnerals.org
Designed for ALS patients, their family members and health professionals. Includes interviews with three ventilator dependent ALS patients, family members and the medical staff from Lois Insolia ALS Center at Northwestern University Medical School. Available for loan to ALS patients.
20 Minutes

Web Sites

1063 Healing Well
                                          www.healingwell.com
A social network and support community for patients, caregivers, and families coping with the daily struggles of diseases, disorders and chronic illness.

1064 Health Finder
                                          www.healthfinder.gov
A government web site where individuals can find information and tools to help you and those you care about stay healthy.

1065 Healthlink USA
                                          www.healthlinkusa.com
Health information concerning treatment, cures, prevention, diagnosis, risk factors, research, support groups, email lists, personal stories and much more. Updated regularly.

1066 Helios Health
                                          www.helioshealth.com
Online resource for your health information. Detailed information about specific health topics, access to expert advice from our Medical Advisory Board, and up-to-date health news.

1067 MedWebPlus
                                          www.medwebplus.com
An independently run site related to everything medical and a few things that aren't.

1068 MedicineNet
                                          www.medicinenet.com
An online resource for consumers providing easy-to-read, authoritative medical and health information.

1069 Medscape
                                          www.medscape.com
Medscape offers specialists, primary care physicians, and other health professionals the Web's most robust and integrated medical information and educational tools.

1070 Neurology Channel
                                          www.neurologychannel.com
Find clearly explained, medically accurate information regarding conditions, including an overview, symptoms, causes, diagnostic procedures and treatment options. On this site it is possible to ask questions and get information from a neurologist and connect to people who have similar health interests.

1071 WebMD
                                          www.webmd.com
Information on Amyotrophic Lateral Sclerosis, including articles and resources.

Description

1072 Arthritis

Arthritis is a nonspecific term meaning inflammation of one or more joints. There are over 100 kinds of arthritis, many of them associated with illnesses of other body systems, such as the skin, gut, or liver. Most cases of arthritis are chronic and involve multiple joints. The three most common are rheumatoid arthritis (RA), osteoarthritis (OA), sometimes called degenerative joint disease, and gouty arthritis, or gout. Juvenile Rheumatoid Arthritis (JRA) affects children.

Rheumatoid arthritis may strike either sex at any age, but typically affects women in the early adult years. It is marked by considerable inflammation, commonly of the hands and feet. RA may also involve the knee, elbow, shoulder, ankle and neck, as well as other body systems in addition to the joints. Osteoarthritis tends to occur later in life, related to repeated wear and tear most commonly on weight-bearing joints, such as the hip and knee. Osteoarthritis often occurs earlier in people who have injured their joints in sports. Gout, which typically affects men in midlife, reflects a disorder in the body's metabolism of uric acid. Its most common feature is excruciating pain in the big toe.

Joints affected by arthritis are typically painful, stiff, and swollen. Nonspecific treatment may be used for arthritis of any sort. This includes the nonsteroidal anti-inflammatory drugs (NSAIDs) and aspirin. Steroids can be injected into the knee in OA and be indicated in an oral form for RA. Severe casesof rheumatoid arthritis are generally treated with more specific drugs that attempt to alter the body's immune system. Gouty arthritis responds to drugs that alter the production and metabolism of uric acid. For any kind of arthritis, local application of heat and cold, as well as physical therapy, are often helpful. In certain cases, joint surgery is recommended.

National Agencies & Associations

1073 American Juvenile Arthritis Organization Arthritis Foundation
Arthritis Foundation
PO Box 7669
Atlanta, GA 30357-0669
404-872-7100
800-283-7800
Fax: 404-872-9559
e-mail: help@arthritis.org
www.arthritis.org
A council established by the Arthritis Foundation which serves the special needs of young people with arthritis and their families. Provides information, inspiration and advocacy by identifying the needs of children with arthritis and speaks out on their behalf.
David E Shuey, Chair
John H Klippel MD, President & CEO

1074 Arthritis & Autoimmunity Research Centre (AARC) Foundation
190 Elizabeth Street
Toronto, Ontario, M5G-2C4
416-340-3843
Fax: 416-340-3453
e-mail: aarc.foundation@aarcf-uhn.ca
uhn.info@uhn.on.ca
Increase awareness of this large family of diseases, which affects over four million Canadians.
Gerri Grant, Executive Director
Pippa Shaddick, Development Manager

1075 Arthritis Foundation
PO Box 7669
Atlanta, GA 30335-669
404-872-7100
800-283-7800
Fax: 404-872-0457
e-mail: help@arthritis.org
www.arthritis.org
A nonprofit organization that depends on volunteers to provide services to help people with arthritis. Supports research to find ways to cure and prevent arthritis and provides services to improve the quality of life for those affected by arthritis. Provides help through information, referrals, speakers bureaus, forums, self-help courses, and various support groups and programs nationwide.
David E Shuey, Chairman, CEO

1076 Arthritis Society
393 University Avenue
Toronto Ontario, M5G 1-1E6
416-979-7228
800-321-1433
Fax: 416-979-8366
e-mail: info@arthritis.ca
www.arthritis.ca
Promoting evaluating and funding research in the areas of causes prevention treatment and cures of arthritis.
Janet Yale, CEO/President
Derek Rodrigues, Chief Financial Officer (CFO)

1077 Myositis Association
1737 King Street
Alexandria, VA 22314
70 -29 -485
800-821-7356
Fax: 70 -53 -675
e-mail: tma@myositis.org
www.myositis.org
Involves swelling of the muscles. It is an inflammatory myopathies that is a disease of the muscle where there is swelling and loss of muscle.
Bob Goldberg, Executive Director
Theresa R Curry, Communications Manager

1078 National Arthritis and Musculoskeletal & Skin Diseases Information Clearinghouse
National Institutes of Health
31 Center Drive - MSC 2350
Bethesda, MD 20892-2350
301-496-8190
Fax: 301-480-2814
e-mail: niamsinfo@mail.nih.gov
www.niams.nih.gov
Our mission is to support research into the causes treatment and prevention of arthritis and musculoskeletal and skin diseases, the training of basic and clinical scientists to carry out this research and the dissemination of information on research programs.
Stephen I Katz MD PhD, Director
Robert H Carter, Deputy Director

1079 National Institute of Arthritis and Musculoskeletal and Skin Disease (NIAMS)
1 AMS Circle
Bethesda, MD 20892
301-495-4484
877-226-4267
Fax: 301-718-6366
TTY: 301-565-2966
e-mail: niamsinfo@mail.nih.gov
www.niams.nih.gov
The NIAMS Information Clearinghouse provides information about various forms of arthritis and rheumatic disease and bone, muscle, and skin diseases. It distributes patient and professional education materials and refers people to other sources of information.
Stephen I Katz MD, PhD, Director
Robert H Carter, Deputy Director

State Agencies & Associations

Alabama

1080 Alabama Chapter of the Arthritis Foundation
2700 Hwy 280 E
Birmingham, AL 35223-3775
205-979-5700
800-879-7896
Fax: 205-979-4172
e-mail: info.al@arthritis.org
www.arthritis.org

Founded in 1948 this chapter affects thousands of lives through programs services information and referrals public and professional education and more for residents of Alabama. Research is a great priority of the chapter which supports the advancement
Kristin Whitehurst, Regional VP
Lisa Hemphill, Regional Development Director

Arizona

1081   Arthritis Foundation: Central Arizona Chapter
1313 E. Osborn Road   602-264-7679
Phoenix, AZ 85014   800-477-7679
                                      Fax: 602-264-0563
                          e-mail: info.caz@arthritis.org
                                       www.arthritis.org
A nonprofit health agency serving the needs of Arizona residents with arthritis. This chapter provides arthritis self-help courses, aquatic programs, foundation clubs, a juvenile arthritis parent group, exercise programs and informational brochures.
Warren Rizzo, Chair
Robert Leslie, Vice Chair

Arkansas

1082   Arthritis Foundation: Arkansas Chapter
6213 Father Tribou Street   501-664-7242
Little Rock, AR 72205-3002   800-482-8858
                                      Fax: 501-664-6588
                           e-mail: info.ar@arthritis.org
                                       www.arthritis.org

Carla Davis, Secretary
Diane Denham, VP Finance/Administration

California

1083   Arthritis Foundation: Northern California Chapter
657 Mission Street   415-356-1230
San Francisco, CA 94105-4120   800-464-6240
                                      Fax: 415-356-1240
                          e-mail: info.nca@arthritis.org
                                       www.arthritis.org
Offers research into the causes of arthritis and more effective treatments; serves people in California with arthritis through information and referral services, exercise programs, self-help courses, education and other activities.
PJ Handelhand, President
Deborah Jackson, Senior VP

1084   Arthritis Foundation: San Diego Area Chapter
9089 Clairemont Mesa Boulevard   858-492-1090
San Diego, CA 92123-1288   800-422-8885
                                      Fax: 858-492-9248
                           e-mail: info.sd@arthritis.org
                                       www.arthritis.org
Offers various programs and services including professional seminars, a speakers bureau, public forums, exercise classes, patient and family support groups, arthritis self-help courses and medical research to the residents of the San Diego area living with arthritis.
Veronica Braun, President
Sandra Hayhurst, Director Health Promotion

1085   Arthritis Foundation: Southern California Chapter
800 W 6th Street   323-954-5750
Los Angeles, CA 90017-3775   800-954-2873
                                      Fax: 323-954-5790
                          e-mail: info.sac@arthritis.org
                                       www.arthritis.org

Cynthia Callihan, Administrative Assistant
Christeen Amloian, Assistant Controller

Colorado

1086   Arthritis Foundation: Rocky Mountain Chapter
2280 S Albion Street   303-756-8622
Denver, CO 80222-4906   800-475-6447
                                      Fax: 303-759-4349
                           e-mail: info.rm@arthritis.org
                                       www.arthritis.org

Serves Colorado, Montana, and Wyoming and is dedicated to finding solutions to over 100 forms of arthritis which affect 43 millions of people nationwide.
Kristie Archer, Programs Coordinator
Laura Rosseisen, President

Connecticut

1087   Arthritis Foundation: Southern New England Chapter
35 Cold Spring Road   860-563-1177
Rocky Hill, CT 06067   800-541-8350
                                      Fax: 860-563-6018
                          e-mail: info.sne@arthritis.org
                                       www.arthritis.org
A resource center for persons in Southern New England, Connecticut, Maine and Vermont with arthritis. Offers self-help courses, exercise programs, aquatic programs, Dial-A-Doctor help line, and physician referrals.
Stephen Evangelista, CEO
Gail Campbell, CFO

District of Columbia

1088   Arthritis Foundation: Metropolitan Washington Chapter
2011 Pennsylvania Avenue NW   202-537-6800
Washington, DC 20006   Fax: 202-537-6859
                          e-mail: info.mwa@arthritis.org
                                       www.arthritis.org
The mission of the Arthritis Foundation is to improve lives through leadership in the prevention control and cure of arthritis and related conditions.
Calaneet Balas, President/CEO
Jacquelyn Hair, Director of Operations

Florida

1089   Arthritis Foundation: Florida Chapter, Gulf Coast Branch
3816 W Linebaugh Avenue   813-968-7000
Tampa, FL 33618   800-850-9455
                                      Fax: 941-795-0348
                         e-mail: info.fl.b4@arthritis.org
                                       www.arthritis.org
Dedicated to improving the quality of life for those in the seven county area of Pinellas, Pasco, Citrus, Levy, Hillsborough, Hernando and Polk, who have one or more of over 100 conditions that comprise the disease known as arthritis. Provides patient education and referral services.
Alexa Simpkins, Events Coordinator
Alvi McConahay, Regional Executive Director

Georgia

1090   Arthritis Foundation: Georgia Chapter
2790 Peachtree Road   404-237-8771
Atlanta, GA 30305   800-933-7023
                                      Fax: 404-237-8153
                           e-mail: info.ga@arthritis.org
                                       www.arthritis.org
A statewide health organization dedicated to reducing the devastating effects of arthritis by offering programs for people with arthritis and their families, information and educational services for people with arthritis, medical professionals and the general public.
Andrea Collins, Vice President Mission Delivery
Christina Lennon, VP Resource Development

Illinois

1091   Arthritis Foundation: Greater Chicago Chapter
35 E Wacker Drive   312-372-2080
Chicago, IL 60601   800-795-0096
                                      Fax: 312-372-2081
                           e-mail: info.gc@arthritis.org
                                       www.arthritis.org
Offers self-help courses, wellness workshops, educational seminars, aquatic programs, brochures and publications for persons with arthritis in the state of Illinois.
Roxanne Bartol, Information Systems Coordinator
Tom Fite, President

1092 Arthritis Foundation: Greater Illinois Chapter
2621 N Knoxville Avenue   309-682-6600
Peoria, IL 61604-3623   Fax: 309-682-6732
e-mail: greaterillinois@arthritis.org
www.arthritis.org

Craig Rogers, Area Director

Indiana

1093 Arthritis Foundation: Indiana Chapter
615 N Alabama   317-879-0321
Indianapolis, IN 46204   800-783-2342
Fax: 317-876-5608
e-mail: info.in@arthritis.org
www.arthritis.org
Offers programs and services for the arthritis community of Indiana.

Jenny Conder, Area Vice President
BJ Farrell, Director of Development

Iowa

1094 Arthritis Foundation: Iowa Chapter
2600 72nd Street   515-278-0636
Des Moines, IA 50322-4724   866-378-0636
Fax: 515-278-2603
e-mail: info.ia@arthritis.org
www.arthritis.org

Julie Dalrymple, Program Coordinator
Doyle Monsma CFRE, President/CEO

Kansas

1095 Arthritis Foundation: Kansas Chapter
1999 N Amidon Avenue   316-263-0116
Wichita, KS 67203-2122   800-362-1108
Fax: 316-263-3260
e-mail: info.ks@arthritis.org
www.arthritis.org
Serves 103 counties and is governed by the Volunteer Board of Directors elected from throughout the state. Services offered include water exercise classes, arthritis support groups, children's summer camp, loan closet of hospital equipment and self-help programs.

Dennis Bender, Area VP
Valerie Fairchild, Program Director

Kentucky

1096 Arthritis Foundation: Kentucky Chapter
2908 Brownsboro Road   502-585-1866
Louisville, KY 40206   800-633-5335
Fax: 502-585-1657
e-mail: myoung@arthritis.org
www.arthritis.org
Serves residents of 117 counties in Kentucky and the counties of Floyd and Clark in Indiana. This chapter is a resource center for funding research education programs for health professionals, community education and support services for people with arthritis.

Barbara Perez, President/CEO
Annette Beach, Annual Giving Coordinator

Maryland

1097 Arthritis Foundation: Maryland Chapter
9505 Reisterstown Road   410-654-6570
Owings Mills, MD 21117   800-365-3811
Fax: 410-654-9270
e-mail: info.md@arthritis.org
www.arthritis.org
This chapter supports research both locally and nationally to help find causes better treatments and ways to prevent the many forms of arthritis. Offers various educational booklets and brochures, a referral service for physician referrals, and other support services.

Barbara Newhouse, CEO
Gail Norman, COO

Massachusetts

1098 Arthritis Foundation: Massachusetts Chapter
29 Crafts Street   617-244-1800
Newton, MA 02458-1287   800-766-9449
Fax: 617-558-7686
e-mail: info.ma@arthritis.org
www.arthritis.org
Offers essential information research programs and services for the close to one million Massachusetts residents with arthritis.

Suha Bekdash, Administrative Assistant
Carmen Quinonez, Finance Manager

Michigan

1099 Arthritis Foundation: Michigan Chapter Chapter and Metro Detroit
1050 Wilshire Drive   248-649-2891
Troy, MI 48084-1564   800-968-3030
Fax: 248-649-2895
e-mail: info.mi@arthritis.org
www.arthritis.org
Supports research to prevent, control, and cure arthritis and related diseases. The Foundation also helps improve the lives of people with arthritis and their families by offering self-help classes, exercise programs, support groups, information and referrals.

Mary Sue Langen, Development Manager
Michelle Glazier, President/CEO

Minnesota

1100 Arthritis Foundation: North Central Chapter
1876 Minnehaha Avenue West   651-644-4108
Saint Paul, MN 55104   800-333-1380
Fax: 651-644-4219
e-mail: info.mn@arthritis.org
www.arthritis.org
A nonprofit organization providing programs and services to anyone affected by arthritis in the Minnesota area. Offers aquatic programs support groups juvenile arthritis support groups, research, grants program and information and referrals.

Chris Davis, Community Development Coordinator
Deb Cassidy, Assistant to the President

Mississippi

1101 Arthritis Foundation: Mississippi Chapter
731 Avignon Drive   601-853-7556
Ridgeland, MS 39157   Fax: 601-853-7516
e-mail: cbaker@arthritis.org
www.arthritis.org
Many Mississippians volunteer their services to help the chapter with fund raising and program support. Programs include land and water based exercise classes, and support groups, direct assistance to needy individuals to purchase arthritis medications and services.

Cynthia Baker, Development Specialist
Pamela Snow, ProgramsDirector

Missouri

1102 Arthritis Foundation: Eastern Missouri Chapter
9433 Olive Boulevard   314-991-9333
Saint Louis, MO 63132   800-406-2491
Fax: 314-991-4020
e-mail: info.emo@arthritis.org
www.arthritis.org

Jan Bignall, Director of Development
Karen Shoulders, Director of Programs

1103 Arthritis Foundation: Western Missouri, Greater Kansas City
1900 W 75th Street   913-262-2233
Prairie Village, KS 66208   888-719-5670
Fax: 91 -26 -228
e-mail: info.wmo@arthritis.org
www.arthritis.org
The only organization in the area representing the National Office in support of its international research program and in providing

services throughout the bi-state area. Offers a wide range of services and programs to deal with the needs of persons with arthritis.
Sherri Hayes, Director of Operations
Alyson Watkins, Special Events Coordinator

Nebraska

1104 Arthritis Foundation: Nebraska Chapter
600 N 93rd Street   402-330-6130
Omaha, NE 68114   800-642-5292
Fax: 402-330-6167
e-mail: mpuccioni@arthritis.org
www.arthritis.org
For close to 40 years the Arthritis Foundation has been the source for help and hope to the 263 000 Nebraskans and residents of Pottawattamie County Iowa with arthritis. Provides a wide variety of services designed to help people better cope with arthritis.
Cindy Doerr, Program Director/Editor
Marzia Pucci Shields, Executive Director

New Jersey

1105 Arthritis Foundation: New Jersey Chapter
555 Route 1 South   732-283-4300
Iselin, NJ 08830   888-467-3112
Fax: 732-283-4633
e-mail: info.nj@arthritis.org
www.arthritis.org
Offers various programs for the residents of New Jersey including support groups, self-help courses, water exercise and arthritis fitness classes and informational public forums.
Linda Gruskiewicz, President & CEO
Tanya Barbarics, Director

New York

1106 Arthritis Foundation: Central New York Chapter
3300 Monroe Avenue   585-264-1480
Rochester, NY 14618   Fax: 585-264-1517
e-mail: info@uny@arthritis.org
www.arthritis.org
Melinda Merante, Executive Director
Nicole Mau, Director

1107 Arthritis Foundation: Long Island Chapter
501 Walt Whitman Road   631-427-8272
Melville, NY 11747-2189   Fax: 631-427-3546
e-mail: into.li@arthritis.org
www.arthritis.org
The mission of the Arthritis Foundation is to fund research to find the cause and cures for arthritis and to improve the quality of life for those affected. There is a wide range of programs available for patients.
Patrick T McAsey, President
Roshane Gillespie, Program Secretary

1108 Arthritis Foundation: New York Chapter
122 E 42nd Street   212-984-8700
New York, NY 10168-1898   Fax: 212-878-5960
e-mail: nfo.ny@arthritis.org
www.arthritis.org
Offers land exercise programs warm water resources and programs, self-help groups and courses, events and activities video clinics, peer support and a lending library to arthritis sufferers in the New York area.
Suzanne Bliss, President CEO

1109 Arthritis Foundation: Rockland/Orange Unit
Helen Hayes Hospital
Route 9W   845-947-3000
W Haverstraw, NY 10993   Fax: 845-429-9602
e-mail: ameyerowitz@arthritis.org
www.arthritis.org
Aviva Meyerowitz, Community Outreach Coordinator
Beatrice Jasanya, Community Outreach Coordinator

North Carolina

1110 Arthritis Foundation: Carolinas Chapter
4530 Park Road   704-529-5166
Charlotte, NC 28209   800-365-3811
Fax: 704-529-0626
e-mail: info.car@arthritis.org
www.arthritis.org
Barbara Newhouse, President CEO
Candy Fuller, Community Development Coordinator

Ohio

1111 Arthritis Foundation: Central Ohio Chapter
3740 Ridge Mill Drive   614-876-8200
Hilliard, OH 43026   Fax: 614-876-8363
e-mail: info.coh@arthritis.org
www.arthritis.org
Offers information and referral services, self-help courses, aquatics program equipment loans, clinics, home assessment and continuing education to help more than 350,000 people in Central Ohio, including over 5,000 children affected with the 100 types of arthritis
Stephanie Houck, Director of Special Events
David Painter, Director of Outreach

1112 Arthritis Foundation: Northeastern Ohio Chapter
4630 Richmond Road   216-831-7000
Cleveland, OH 44128-5525   800-245-2275
Fax: 216-831-1764
e-mail: info.neoh@arthritis.org
www.arthritis.org
Barb Cvelbar, Director of Health Promotion
Cheryl Carter, Director of Development

1113 Arthritis Foundation: Northwestern Ohio Chapter
35 E Wacker Drive   31 -37 -208
Chicago, IL 60601   800-735-0096
Fax: 31 -37 -208
e-mail: info.gc@arthritis.org
www.arthritis.org
Tom Fite, CEO

1114 Arthritis Foundation: Ohio River Valley Chapter
7124 Miami Avenue   513-271-4545
Cincinnati, OH 45243   800-383-6843
Fax: 513-271-4703
e-mail: info.orv@arthritis.org
www.arthritis.org
Barbara Perez, President/CEO
Edith Nixon, Chair

1115 Arthritis Foundation; Great Lakes Region, Northeastern Ohio
4630 Richmond Road   216-831-7000
Cleveland, OH 44128-5525   800-245-2275
Fax: 216-831-1764
e-mail: info.neoh@arthritis.org
www.arthritis.org
Mary L Kudasick, Regional VP

Oklahoma

1116 Arthritis Foundation: Oklahoma Chapter
710 W. Wilshire Blvd   405-936-3366
Oklahoma City, OK 73116   800-627-5486
Fax: 405-936-0617
e-mail: info.ok@arthritis.org
www.arthritis.org
Sherri O'Neil, Executive Director
Sherri Harris, Director Special Events

Pennsylvania

1117 Arthritis Foundation: Central Pennsylvania Chapter
3544 North Progress Avenue   717-763-0900
Harrisburg, PA 17110   800-776-0746
Fax: 717-763-0903
e-mail: info.cpa@arthritis.org
www.arthritis.org

Serves 28 counties in the central Pennsylvania area. More than 441,233 persons in the chapter area are affected with one of the forms of arthritis seriously enough to require medical care. The chapter offers research services, professional education and training, parent and community services and public health education.
Douglas Knepp, Interim Executive Director

Rhode Island

1118 Arthritis Foundation: Southern New England Chapter
35 Cold Spring Road   860-563-1177
Rocky Hill, CT 06067   800-541-8350
                                        Fax: 860-563-6018
                               e-mail: info.sne@arthritis.org
                                            www.arthritis.org
Offers programs and services for persons in the Rhode Island area who are living with arthritis.
Stephen Evangelista, CEO
Gail Campbell, CFO

Tennessee

1119 Arthritis Foundation: Southeast Region
421 Great Circle Road   615-254-6795
Nashville, TN 37228   800-454-4662
                                        Fax: 615-254-8316
                                e-mail: info.tn@arthritis.org
                                            www.arthritis.org
This chapter serves the residents of Tennessee by offering arthritis support through Life Improvement Series Classes, exercise programs, educational programs, free information, public forums and seminars.
David Popen Esq, CEO

Texas

1120 Arthritis Foundation: North Texas Chapter
4300 Macarthur   214-826-4361
Dallas, TX 75209-6524   800-442-6653
                                        Fax: 214-824-5842
                               e-mail: info.ntx@arthritis.org
                                            www.arthritis.org
With over 1.5 million people in the North Texas Chapter area with arthritis, the chapter's mission is to improve lives through leadership in the prevention, control and cure of arthritis and related diseases.
Carla Brandt, CFO/COO
Jane Hynes, Director Administration/Info Systems

Utah

1121 Arthritis Foundation: Utah/Idaho Chapter
448 E 400 S   801-536-0990
Salt Lake City, UT 84111   800-444-4993
                                        Fax: 801-536-0991
                              e-mail: info.utid@arthritis.org
                                            www.arthritis.org
A nonprofit organization serving individuals with arthritis and their families in Utah and Idaho by providing invaluable services, programs and activities.
Lisa B Fall, President
Leslie Nelson, Program Director

Vermont

1122 Arthritis Foundation: Northern New England Chapter
6 Chenell Drive   603-224-9322
Concord, NH 03301   800-639-2113
                                        Fax: 603-224-3778
                               e-mail: info.sne@arthritis.org
                                            www.arthritis.org

Stephen Evangelista, CEO
Margaret Duffy, Regional Program Director

Virginia

1123 Arthritis Foundation: Virginia Chapter
3805 Cutshaw Avenue   804-359-1700
Richmond, VA 23230   800-456-4687
                                        Fax: 804-359-4900
                                e-mail: info.va@arthritis.org
                                            www.arthritis.org
Founded in 1954 this chapter is a nonprofit voluntary health organization dedicated to finding the cause prevention and cure for the entire group of diseases called arthritis. Offered classes books and information to better manage arthritis.
Angela Courtney, Vice President Community Development
C Annie Magnant, President

Washington

1124 Arthritis Foundation: Washington/Alaska Chapter
3876 Bridge Way N   206-547-2707
Seattle, WA 98103   800-746-1821
                                        Fax: 206-547-2707
                               e-mail: tzuehl@arthritis.org
                                            www.arthritis.org
Offers arthritis help lines and information lines for residents of Washington state. Provides self-help courses arthritis aquatic programs and resources for persons living with various forms of arthritis.
Barbara Osen, North Puget Sound Branch Director
Kim Mellen, Campaign Coordinator

Wisconsin

1125 Arthritis Foundation: Wisconsin Chapter Foundation
1650 S 108th Street   414-321-3933
W Allis, WI 53214-4021   800-242-9945
                                        Fax: 414-321-0365
                                e-mail: info@wi@arthritis.org
                                            www.arthritis.org
Statewide programs offered. Including aquatics exercise programs, support groups, self-help courses, professional education, public education seminars, advocacy counsel, juvenile arthritis support programs and children's camp information and referral help.

Libraries & Resource Centers

1126 New York Chapter of the Arthritis Foundation
122 East 42nd Street   212-984-8700
New York, NY 10168-1898   Fax: 212-878-5960
                                e-mail: info.ny@arthritis.org
                                            www.arthritis.org
Offers people with arthritis, their families and all those with an interest in the rheumatic diseases, information on how to live every day to its fullest, even when affected by a chronic disease.

Research Centers

1127 Affiliated Children's Arthritis Centers of New England
New England Medical Center
750 Washington Street   617-636-7285
Boston, MA 02111-1533   Fax: 617-350-8388
Research organization comprised of a network of 15 territory pediatric centers throughout New England and based at the Floating Hospital of New England Medical Center.
Jane G Schaller MD, Coordinator

1128 Arthritis and Musculoskeletal Center: UAB Shelby Interdisciplinary Biomedical Rese
Shelby Interdisciplinary Biomedical Research Bldg
1825 University Boulevard   205-934-0245
Birmingham, AL 35294-2182   Fax: 205-934-1564
                                       e-mail: rpk@uab.edu
                                       www.main.uab.edu/amc
Arthritis and related rheumatic disorders are studied.
Robert Kimbe MD, Director
Jennifer A Croker, Executive Administrator

1129 Boston University Arthritis Center
580 Harrison Avenue 617-638-4590
Boston, MA 02118 Fax: 617-638-5226
e-mail: mikyork@bu.edu
www.bumc.bu.edu
The research efforts of the Rheumatology Section relate to basic biologic mechanisms in the pathogenesis of scleroderma vasculitis amyloidosis osteoarthritis and systemic lupus erythematosus. There are concordant research efforts in clinical investigation of these disorders including testing of novel therapies.
Karen H Antman, Dean
Paul Monach, Associate Fellowship Program Director

1130 Boston University Medical Campus General Clinical Research Center
72 E Concord Street 617-638-4542
Boston, MA 02118 Fax: 617-638-8890
e-mail: jkopp@bu.edu
www.ctsi.bu.edu
Integral unit of the University Hospital specializing in arthritis and connective tissue studies.
Courtney Alpert, Administrative Coordinator
Janice Kopp, Executive Director

1131 Brigham and Women's Orthopedica and Arthritis Center
Brigham and Women's Hospital
75 Francis Street 617-732-5500
Boston, MA 02115 800-BWH-9999
TTY: 617-732-6458
www.brighamandwomens.org
Research studies into arthritis and rheumatic diseases.
Matthew Lian MD, Director

1132 Central Missouri Regional Arthritis Center Stephen's College Campus
Stephen's College Campus
1205 University Ave 573-882-8097
Columbia, MO 65211 888-702-8818
Fax: 573-884-5509
TDD: 0
e-mail: phelpsam@missouri.edu
marrtc.missouri.edu
Research into arthritis and rheumatic diseases.
Liz Raine, MPH, CHES,, Health Educator
Beth Richards ,BS,TRS, Director

1133 Department of Pediatrics, Division of Rheumatology
Duke University School of Medicine
T909 Children's Health Center 919-684-6575
Durham, NC 27710-1 Fax: 919-684-6616
rheum.pediatrics.duke.edu
Clinical and laboratory pediatric rheumatoid studies.
Laura Schanberg MD, Cochairman
Egla Rabinovich MD, Co-Chairman

1134 Hahnemann University Hospital, Orthopedic Wellness Center
Hahnemann University Hospital
230 N Broad St 215-762-7000
Philadelphia, PA 19102-1511 Fax: 215-762-8109
www.hahnemannhospital.com
Research activity at Hahnemann University into the areas of arthritis.
Dr. Arnold Berman, Director

1135 Medical University of South Carolina
96 Jonathan Lucas Street 843-792-1991
Charleston, SC 29403 800-424-MUSC
Fax: 843-792-7121
www.muschealth.com
Offers basic and clinical research on various types of arthritis.
Richard M Silver, Division Director/Professor
Gary S Gilkeson, Vice Chairman Research

1136 Medical University of South Carolina: Division of Rheumatology & Immunology
96 Jonathan Lucas Street 843-792-1991
Charleston, SC 29403 Fax: 843-792-7121
www.musc.edu

Offers basic and clinical research on various types of arthritis.
Richard M Silver, Division Director/Professor
Gary S Gilkeson, Vice Chairman Research

1137 Multipurpose Arthritis and Musculoskeletal Disease Center
School of Medicine Rheumatology Division
545 Barnhill Drive 317- 27- 843
Indianapolis, IN 46202 Fax: 317-274-1437
medicine.iupui.edu
The mission of this center is to pursue major biomedical research interests relevant to the rheumatic diseases. Current areas of emphasis include articular cartilage biology pathogenesis and treatment of various forms of amyloidosis the pathogenesis of dermatomyositis and immunologic and biochemical markers of cartilage breakdown and repair.
Bernetta Hartman, Executive Assistant to the Chairman
Martin Friedman, VP Medicine Specialties Division, IUHP

1138 Oklahoma Medical Research Foundation
825 NE 13th Street 405-271-6673
Oklahoma City, OK 73104-5005 800-522-0211
Fax: 405-271-OMRF
e-mail: contact@omrf.org
www.omrf.ouhsc.edu
Focuses on arthritis and muscoloskeletal disease research.
Dr Paul Kincade, Head of OMRF's Immunobiology
Philip M Silverman PhD, Member

1139 Rehabilitation Institute of Chicago
345 E Superior Street 312-238-1000
Chicago, IL 60611 800-354-7342
TTY: 312-238-1059
www.ric.org
Expertise in treating a range of conditions from the most complex conditions including cerebral palsy spinal cord injury stroke and traumatic brain injury to the more common such as arthritis chronic pain and sports injuries.
Edward B Case, Executive Vice President and Chief Finan
Joanne C Smith, President and Chief Executive Officer

1140 Rosalind Russell Medical Research Center for Arthritis at UCSF
350 Parnassus Avenue 415-476-1141
San Francisco, CA 94117 Fax: 415-476-3526
e-mail: rrac@medicine.ucsf.edu
www.rosalindrussellcenter.ucsf.edu
Arthritis research and its probable causes.
Ephraim P Engelman MD, Director
David Wofsy, Associate Director

1141 University of Michigan: Orthopaedic Research Laboratories
University of Michigan Mott Hospital
109 Zina Pitcher Place 734-936-7417
Ann Arbor, MI 48109-2200 Fax: 734-647-0003
www.orl.med.umich.edu
Develops and studies the causes and treatments for arthritis including new devices and assistive aids.
Dr SA Goldstein, Director

1142 Warren Grant Magnuson Clinical Center
National Institute of Health
9000 Rockville Pike 301-496-2563
Bethesda, MD 20892 800-411-1222
Fax: 301-480-9793
TTY: 866-411-1010
e-mail: prpl@mail.cc.nih.gov
www.clinicalcenter.nih.gov
Established in 1953 as the research hospital of the National Institutes of Health. Designed so that patient care facilities are close to research laboratories so new findings of basic and clinical scientists can be quickly applied to the treatment of patients. Upon referral by physicians, patients are admitted to NIH clinical studies.
John Gallin, Director
David Henderson, Deputy Director for Clinical Care

Support Groups & Hotlines

1143   Arthritis Foundation Information Hotline
1330 W. Peachtree Street
Atlanta, GA 30309-0669
404-872-7100
e-mail: contactus@arthritis.org
www.arthritis.org
Offers information and referrals, counseling, physicians information and more to persons living with arthritis.
John H Klippel, President/CEO

1144   Kids on the Block Arthritis Programs
Arthritis Foundation
PO Box 19000
Atlanta, GA 31126-1000
404-872-7100
800-283-7800
Fax: 404-872-0457
State and local programs that use puppetry to help children understand what it is like for children and adults who have arthritis.

1145   National Health Information Center
PO Box 1133
Washington, DC 20013
310-565-4167
800-336-4797
Fax: 301-984-4256
e-mail: info@nhic.org
www.health.gov/nhic
Offers a nationwide information referral service, produces directories and resource guides.

Books

1146   250 Tips for Making Life with Arthritis Easier
Arthritis Foundation Distribution Center
PO Box 6996
Alpharetta, GA 30023-6996
800-207-8633
Fax: 770-442-9742
www.arthritis.com
Learn about helpful services you didn't know were available through you bank, post office, phone company, grocery store, and other businesses you frequent.
88 pages

1147   Arthritis 101: Questions You Have, Answers You Need
Arthritis Foundation Distribution Center
PO Box 6996
Alpharetta, GA 30009-6996
800-207-8633
Fax: 770-442-9742
www.arthritis.com
Expert reviewers answer questions about basic arthritis facts, treatments, research, surgery and more. Also, specific information about six common conditions: rheumatoid arthritis, osteoarthritis, osteoporosis, fibromyalgia, lupus and gout.
144 pages

1148   Arthritis Helpbook: A Tested Self-Management Program for Coping
Kate Lorig and James Fries, author
Da Capo Press
Order Department
Jackson, TN 38301
800-343-4499
Fax: 800-351-5073
www.perseusbooksgroup.com/dacapo
This book teaches people proven techniques to reduce pain and increase dexterity, build a calcium-rich diet and maintain a healthy weight, design an exercise program that matches their needs, find tips and gadgets that solve common problems, overcome fatigue, depression, and other troubling feelings associated with these health issues, and learn about all available arthritis medications and surgeries.
2006 288 pages 6th Edition
ISBN: 0-201409-63-1

1149   Arthritis Self-Help Products
Aids for Arthritis
35 Wakefield Drive
Medford, NJ 08055-3204
609-654-6918
www.aidsforarthritis.com
Offers lists of arthritis self-help devices.

1150   Arthritis Self-Management
RA Rapaport Publishing
150 W 22nd Street
New York, NY 10011-2421
212-989-0200
800-234-0923
Fax: 212-989-4786
e-mail: editor@arthritis-self-mgmt.com
Publishes practical, how to information, focusing on the day-to-day and long term aspects of arthritis in a positive and up-beat style. Gives subscribers up-to-date news, facts and advice to help them mai tain their wellness and make informed decisions regarding their health.
48+ pages Bi-Monthly
Christine Martin Grove, Editor
Ingrid Strauch, Executive

1151   Arthritis: What Exercises Work
Dava Sobel, Arthur C Klein, author
MacMillan
175 5th Avenue
New York, NY 10010
212-674-5151
800-221-7945
Fax: 212-420-9314
us.macmillan.com
The right exercises for your kind of arthritis, pain-level, age, occupation, and hobbies. The most effective exercises for arthritis available anywhere, supported by medical doctors and backed by the latest research.
200 pages
ISBN: 0-312130-25-1

1152   Arthritis: Your Complete Exercise Guide
Human Kinetics Press
PO Box 5076
Champaign, IL 61825-5076
217-351-5076
800-747-4457
Fax: 217-351-2674
www.humankinetics.com
1993 152 pages Paperback
ISBN: 0-873223-92-6
Steve Ruhlig, Marketing Director

1153   Bone Up on Arthritis
Arthritis Foundation
PO Box 6996
Alpharetta, GA 30009-6996
800-207-8633
Fax: 770-442-9742
www.arthritis.com
A self-help education packet designed for home-study use, this program can improve your pain and function levels by teaching proven self-help techniques.
w/Audio Tapes

1154   Clinical Care in the Rheumatic Disease
Arthritis Foundation Distribution Center
PO Box 6996
Alpharetta, GA 30023-6996
800-207-8633
Fax: 770-442-9742
www.arthritis.com
This book was written for all health professionals caring for people with rheumatic diseases and for students in these disciplines.
224 pages

1155   Educational Rights for Children with Arthritis: A Parents Manual
AJAO
1314 Spring Street NW
Atlanta, GA 30309-2810
404-872-7100
www.arthritis.org/
A self-instructional manual helping parents to identify and obtain school services needed by their child with arthritis. Covers laws and special services, explores strategies for working with school personnel and stresses good communication and advocacy techniques.

1156   Exercise Beats Arthritis
Bull Publishing Company
PO Box 1377
Boulder, CO 80306
800-676-2855
Fax: 303-545-6354
www.bullpub.com
Easy-to-follow program will help arthritis sufferers of all ages manage the problems of living with this condition. In depth look at

minimizing the pain and limitations of arthritis, keep their joints mobile, increase muscle strength, strengthen bones and ligaments, perform daily tasks more easily.
1998 144 pages
ISBN: 0-923521-45-3

1157 Help Yourself Cookbook
Arthritis Foundation
PO Box 6996
Alpharetta, GA 30023-6996　　　　　　800-207-8633
　　　　　　　　　　　　　　　　　Fax: 770-442-9742
　　　　　　　　　　　　　　　　　www.arthritis.com

158 pages

1158 Living With Rheumatoid Arthritis
John's Hopkins University Press
2715 N Charles Street　　　　　　　　410-516-6900
Baltimore, MD 21218-4319　　　　　　800-537-5487
　　　　　　　　　　　　　　　　　Fax: 410-516-6998
　　　　　　　　　　　　　　　　　www.press.jhu.edu
This book offers practical and usable answers to the questions of everyday life. The authors provide clear explanations of the causes, diagnosis and treatment of the disease and why medication, joint protection, physical activity and good nutrition are essential components of care.
1993 312 pages Paperback
ISBN: 0-801871-47-6

1159 Personal Guide to Living Well with Fibromyalgia
Arthritis Foundation Distribution Center
PO Box 6996
Alpharetta, GA 30023-6996　　　　　　800-207-8633
　　　　　　　　　　　　　　　　　Fax: 770-442-9742
　　　　　　　　　　　　　　　　　www.arthritis.com
With this guide you'll learn the latest information about fibromyalgia, what researchers have uncovered about its causes, and an overview of the best treatment options available. Helpful worksheets and tables allow you to manage your condition and document your progress.
224 pages

1160 Primer on the Rheumatic Diseases
John H Klippel, author

Springer Publishing
233 Spring Street　　　　　　　　　　212-460-1500
New York, NY 10013　　　　　　　Fax: 212-460-1575
　　　　　　　　　e-mail: service-ny@springer.com
　　　　　　　　　　　　　　　　　www.springer.com
Designed to provide up-to-date information about the major clinical syndromes. One of the most prestigious and comprehensive texts on arthritis and related diseases, including osteoarthritis, rheumatoid arthritis, osteoporosis, lupus, and more than one hundred others.
724 pages
ISBN: 0-387356-64-8

1161 Toward Healthy Living: A Wellness Journal
Arthritis Foundation Distribution Center
PO Box 6996
Alpharetta, GA 30023-6996　　　　　　800-207-8633
　　　　　　　　　　　　　　　　　Fax: 770-442-9742
　　　　　　　　　　　　　　　　　www.arthritis.com
This spiral-bound journal has ample pages where you can record your thoughts, plus scales to monitor your mood and pain. Throughout the book you will also find wisdom from a variety of famous and ordinary people - those who live with chronic ilness, and those whose life lessons can help you gain a more positive outlook on daily living.
144 pages

1162 Understanding Juvenile Rheumatoid Arthritis
American Juvenile Arthritis Organization
PO Box 19000
Atlanta, GA 31126-1000　　　　　　　800-283-7800
A manual for health professionals to use in teaching children with JRA and their families about disease management and self-care.
372 pages

1163 We Can: A Guide for Parents of Children with Arthritis
AJAO

1330 W Peachtree Street NW
Atlanta, GA 30309-2904　　　　　　　404-872-7100
　　　　　　　　　　　　　　　　　www.arthritis.org/
Offers parents tips for daily living and practical points for helping their child toward independent adulthood.

Children's Books

1164 Arthritis
Franklin Watts Grolier
90 Old Sherman Turnpike　　　　　　203-797-3500
Danbury, CT 06816-0001　　　　　　800-621-1115
　　　　　　　　　　　　　　Fax: 203-797-3197
　　　　　　　　　　　　　　　　www.grolier.com
This book offers a clear explanation of the various forms and effects of the disease of arthritis and what treatments are available.
96 pages Grades 7-12
ISBN: 0-531108-01-5

1165 JRA and Me
American Juvenile Arthritis Organization
PO Box 19000
Atlanta, GA 31126-1000　　　　　　　800-283-7800
A workbook for school-aged children who have juvenile arthritis. This book offers a variety of educational games, puzzles and worksheets to teach children about their illness and how to take care of themselves.
57 pages

1166 Living with Arthritis
Franklin Watts Grolier
90 Old Sherman Turnpike　　　　　　203-797-3500
Danbury, CT 06816-0001　　　　　　800-621-1115
　　　　　　　　　　　　　　Fax: 203-797-3197
　　　　　　　　　　　　　　　　www.grolier.com
Shows how people with arthritis can overcome their pain and lead productive, full lives.
32 pages Grades 5-7

1167 Yard Sale Coloring Book
American Juvenile Arthritis Organization
PO Box 19000
Atlanta, GA 31126-1000　　　　　　　800-283-7800
A coloring/activity book based on a Kids on the Block script, written for third and fourth grade students. It can be used with Kids on the Block performances, as a stand-alone piece or with a free lesson plan packet.

Magazines

1168 Arthritis Today
Arthritis Foundation
1330 W Peachtree Street NW　　　　　404-872-7100
Atlanta, GA 30309-2922　　　　　　　800-933-0032
　　　　　　　　　　　　　　Fax: 404-872-9559
The authoritative and respected source of information for persons with arthritis, their families and health professionals who manage their care. As the official magazine of the Arthritis Foundation, it is backed by the Foundation's experience of 44 years and leadership in the fight against arthritis. This magazine gives its readers the advice, information and inspiration they need to live better with arthritis.
Monthly

Newsletters

1169 AJAO Newsletter
American Juvenile Arthritis Organization
1330 W Peachtree Street NW
Atlanta, GA 31126-2904　　　　　　　404-872-7100
　　　　　　　　　　　　　　www.arthritis.org/answers
Offers information and updates about the organization's activities and events. Legislative information, medical updates, camp information and more for children living with arthritis.
Quarterly
Janet Austin MEd, Editor

1170 **Arthritis Accent**
Arthritis Foundation Southern N.E. Chapter
35 Cold Spring Road   860-563-1177
Rocky Hill, CT 06067-3166   800-541-8350
                                 Fax: 860-563-6018
Information on chapter events and activities.
Quarterly

1171 **Arthritis Foundation of Illinois**
Greater Chicago Chapter
29 East Madison   312-372-2080
Chicago, IL 60602   800-735-0096
                                 Fax: 312-372-2081
                         e-mail: info.gc@arthritis.org
                                    www.arthritis.org

Marilynn J Cason, Chairman

1172 **Arthritis Foundation: Newsletter of Nebraska Chapter**
10846 Old Mill Road   402-330-6130
Omaha, NE 68154   800-642-5292
                                 Fax: 402-330-6167
                    e-mail: mpuccioni@arthritis.org
                                    www.arthritis.org
Contains information on research, medication, different types of
arthritis and features on oustanding volunteers.
3x Year
Cindy Doerr, Program Director/Editor

1173 **Arthritis Foundation: Southern Arizona Chapter**
6464 E Grant Road   520-290-9090
Tucson, AZ 85715   800-444-5426
Offers updated information and news on chapter activities and
events for persons with arthritis.
Monthly
Richard M Brown EdD, CFRE, President

1174 **Arthritis News**
Arthritis Foundation - WI Chapter
1650 S 108th Street   414-321-3933
West Allis, WI 53214   800-242-9945
                                 Fax: 414-321-0365
                         e-mail: info.wi@arthritis.org
                                    www.arthritis.org
Offers information on activities, events, medical research, infor-
mation and referrals to persons living in the Wisconsin area that are
afflicted with arthritis.
Quarterly
Judy Haugsland, CEO

1175 **Arthritis Observer**
Rocky Mountain Chapter of the Arthritis Foundation
2280 S Albion Street   303-756-8622
Denver, CO 80222-4906   800-475-6647
                                 Fax: 303-759-4349
                         e-mail: info.m@arthritis.org
                                    www.arthritis.org
Offers chapter information and educational programs to the com-
munity as well as updates on fund-raising events, resources, publi-
cations and medical updates for the arthritis community.
Quarterly

1176 **Arthritis Reporter**
New York Chapter of the Arthritis Foundation
122 E 42nd Street   212-984-8700
New York, NY 10168-0002   Fax: 212-878-5960
                         e-mail: info.ny@arthritis.org
                                    www.arthritis.org
Chapter newsletter offering information on upcoming events, ac-
tivities and groups for the arthritis community.
Quarterly

1177 **Arthritis Update of Rhode Island**
Arthritis Foundation Rhode Island Office
Airport Office Park   401-739-3773
Warwick, RI 02886   Fax: 401-739-8990
                         e-mail: info.sne@arthritis.org
                                    www.arthritis.org
Offers information, activities, events and updates on the chapter.
Quarterly

1178 **Arthritis Volunteer**
Tennessee Chapter of the Arthritis Foundation
1719 W End Avenue   615-320-7626
Nashville, TN 37203-5123   Fax: 615-329-3982
Keeps members up-to-date on arthritis developments and on pro-
grams, services and special events in Tennessee.
Quarterly

1179 **Factor Fax**
Arthritis Foundation: Northeast California Chapter
3040 Explorer Drive   916-368-5599
Sacramento, CA 95827   800-571-3456
                                 Fax: 916-368-5596
                        e-mail: info.neca@arthritis.org
                                    www.arthritis.org
Offers information on all of the chapter's activites, events and re-
sources for the arthritis community of central California.
Patrick Dunlap, VP Events/Programs/Services
Edward Kelley, Motion Coordinator

1180 **Focus**
Arthritis Foundation: Central Ohio Chapter
3740 Ridge Mill Drive   614-876-8200
Hilliard, OH 43026-9231   Fax: 614-876-8363
                                    www.arthritis.org
Offers updated information on arthritis as well as news of the ser-
vices and activities of the chapter.
Quarterly
Irene Baird, President

1181 **Health Points**
TyH Publications
17007 E Colony Drive
Fountain Hills, AZ 85268   800-801-1406
                         e-mail: editor@e-tyh.com
National newsletter with articles on complementary therapy, latest
nutrition news, disability issues and much more. Focus is on
fibromyalgia, chronic fatigue, arthritis and chronic pain.
Quarterly

1182 **News Across Our Horizons**
Northern & Southern New England Chapter
35 Cold Spring Road   860-563-1177
Rocky Hill, CT 06060   800-541-8350
                                 Fax: 860-563-6018
                        e-mail: info.sne@arthritis.org
                                    www.arthritis.org
Chapter newsletter offering information on programs, activities
and events of the foundation, medical and research articles and resources for persons with arthritis.

1183 **Newsletter of the Central Pennsylvania Chapter**
Central Pennsylvania Chapter/Arthritis Foundation
17 S 19th Street   717-763-0900
Camp Hill, PA 17011-5459   800-776-0746
                                 Fax: 717-763-0903
                        e-mail: info.cpa@arthritis.org
                                    www.arthritis.org
Offers information on activities and events of the Chapter.
Quarterly

1184 **Spectrum**
Michigan Chapter of the Arthritis Foundation
1050 Wilshire Drive   248-649-2891
Troy, MI 48084-1564   800-968-3030
                                 Fax: 248-649-2895
                        e-mail: info.mi@arthritis.org
                                    www.arthritis.org
Promotes various activities and programs and provides current in-
formation about arthritis.

1185 **Volunteer Voice**
Kentucky Chapter of the Arthritis Foundation
410 W Chestnut Street   502-893-9771
Louisville, KY 40202-2368   800-633-5335
Newsletter offering information and updates on chapter activities,
events, camps, juvenile programs and government/legislative
information.

Pamphlets

1186 Americans with Disabilities Act Resource Manual
Arthritis Foundation
PO Box 7669 404-872-7100
Atlanta, GA 30357-0669 800-283-7800
Fax: 404-872-0457

1187 Ankylosing Spondylitis
Arthritis Foundation
PO Box 7669 404-872-7100
Atlanta, GA 30357-0669 800-283-7800
Fax: 404-872-0457

1188 Arthritis Answers: Basic Information About Arthritis
Arthritis Foundation
PO Box 7669 404-872-7100
Atlanta, GA 30357-0669 800-283-7800
Fax: 404-872-0457

1189 Arthritis Foundation Services
Arthritis Foundation
PO Box 7669 404-872-7100
Atlanta, GA 30357-0669 800-283-7800
Fax: 404-872-0457

1190 Arthritis Information: Advocacy and Government Affairs
Arthritis Foundation
PO Box 7669 404-872-7100
Atlanta, GA 30357-0669 800-283-7800
Fax: 404-872-0457

1191 Arthritis Information: Children
Arthritis Foundation
PO Box 7669 404-872-7100
Atlanta, GA 30357-0669 800-283-7800
Fax: 404-872-0457

List of materials for children with arthritis, their families and the health professionals who care for them.

1192 Arthritis and Diet Information Package
NAMSIC/National Institutes of Health
1 AMS Circle 301-495-4484
Bethesda, MD 20892-0001 877-226-4267
Fax: 301-718-6366
TTY: 301-565-2966
e-mail: niamsinfo@mail.nih.gov
www.nih.gov/niams/

Offers information on nutrition and diet pertaining to the arthritis community.
16 pages

1193 Arthritis and Employment: You Can Get the Job You Want
Arthritis Foundation
PO Box 7669 404-872-7100
Atlanta, GA 30357-0669 800-283-7800
Fax: 404-872-0457

1194 Arthritis and Inflammatory Bowel Disease
Arthritis Foundation
PO Box 7669 404-872-7100
Atlanta, GA 30357-0669 800-283-7800
Fax: 404-872-0457

1195 Arthritis and Pregnancy
Arthritis Foundation
PO Box 7669 404-872-7100
Atlanta, GA 30357-0669 800-283-7800
Fax: 404-872-0457

How arthritis affects pregnancy, managing pregnancy and a new baby.

1196 Arthritis and Vocational Rehabilitation
Arthritis Foundation
2970 Peachtree Road NW 404-237-8771
Atlanta, GA 30305 800-933-7023
Fax: 404-237-8153
e-mail: info.ga@arthritis.org
www.arthritis.org

1197 Arthritis in Children Information Package
NAMSIC/National Institutes of Health
1 AMS Circle 301-495-4484
Bethesda, MD 20892-0001 877-226-4267
Fax: 301-718-6366
TTY: 301-565-2966
e-mail: niamsinfo@mail.nih.gov
www.nih.gov/niams/

1198 Arthritis in Children and La Artritis Infantojuvenil
American Juvenile Arthritis Organization
PO Box 19000
Atlanta, GA 31126-1000 800-283-7800
A medical information booklet about juvenile rheumatoid arthritis. This booklet is written for parents or other adults and includes details about different forms of JRA, medications, therapies and coping issues.

1199 Arthritis on the Job: You Can Work With It
Arthritis Foundation
PO Box 7669 404-872-7100
Atlanta, GA 30357-0669 800-283-7800
Fax: 404-872-0457

1200 Arthritis: Do You Know?
Arthritis Foundation
PO Box 7669 404-872-7100
Atlanta, GA 30357-0669 800-283-7800
Fax: 404-872-0457

A brief overview of arthritis and the services of the Arthritis Foundation.

1201 Aspirin and Other Nonsteroidal Anti-Inflamatory Drugs
Arthritis Foundation
PO Box 7669 404-872-7100
Atlanta, GA 30357-0669 800-283-7800
Fax: 404-872-0457

1202 Back Pain
Arthritis Foundation
PO Box 7669 404-872-7100
Atlanta, GA 30357-0669 800-283-7800
Fax: 404-872-0457

1203 Behcet's Disease
Arthritis Foundation
PO Box 7669 404-872-7100
Atlanta, GA 30357-0669 800-283-7800
Fax: 404-872-0457

1204 Bursitis, Tendionitis and Other Soft Tissue Rheumatic Syndromes
Arthritis Foundation
PO Box 7669 404-872-7100
Atlanta, GA 30357-0669 800-283-7800
Fax: 404-872-0457

1205 CPPD Crystal Deposition Disease
Arthritis Foundation
PO Box 7669 404-872-7100
Atlanta, GA 30357-0669 800-283-7800
Fax: 404-872-0457

1206 Corticosteriod Medications
Arthritis Foundation
PO Box 7669 404-872-7100
Atlanta, GA 30357-0669 800-283-7800
Fax: 404-872-0457

1207 Diet and Arthritis
Arthritis Foundation
PO Box 7669 404-872-7100
Atlanta, GA 30357-0669 800-283-7800
Fax: 404-872-0457

1208 Ehlers-Danlos Syndrome
Arthritis Foundation
PO Box 7669 404-872-7100
Atlanta, GA 30357-0669 800-283-7800
Fax: 404-872-0457

1209 Exercise and Your Arthritis
Arthritis Foundation

PO Box 7669
Atlanta, GA 30357-0669
404-872-7100
800-283-7800
Fax: 404-872-0457
Types of exercise for people with arthritis and how to do them.

1210 Family
Arthritis Foundation
PO Box 7669
Atlanta, GA 30357-0669
404-872-7100
800-283-7800
Fax: 404-872-0457
Effects of arthritis on family life and ways to cope.

1211 Family: Making the Difference
Arthritis Foundation
PO Box 7669
Atlanta, GA 30357-0669
404-872-7100
800-283-7800
Fax: 404-872-0457

1212 Gold Treatment
Arthritis Foundation
PO Box 7669
Atlanta, GA 30357-0669
404-872-7100
800-283-7800
Fax: 404-872-0457

1213 Gout
Arthritis Foundation
PO Box 7669
Atlanta, GA 30357-0669
404-872-7100
800-283-7800
Fax: 404-872-0457

1214 Guide to Effective Volunteer Lobbying
Arthritis Foundation
PO Box 7669
Atlanta, GA 30357-0669
404-872-7100
800-283-7800
Fax: 404-872-0457

1215 Health, Life and Disability Insurance for People with Arthritis
Arthritis Foundation
PO Box 7669
Atlanta, GA 30357-0669
404-872-7100
800-283-7800
Fax: 404-872-0457
Information about these three types of insurance.

1216 Hydroxychloroquine
Arthritis Foundation
PO Box 7669
Atlanta, GA 30357-0669
404-872-7100
800-283-7800
Fax: 404-872-0457

1217 Individuals with Arthritis
Mainstream
1030 5th Street NW
Washington, DC 20001-2504
202-898-1400
Mainstreaming individuals with arthritis into the workplace.
12 pages

1218 Juvenile Dermatomyositis
Arthritis Foundation
PO Box 7669
Atlanta, GA 30357-0669
404-872-7100
800-283-7800
Fax: 404-872-0457
www.arthritis.org

1219 Living and Loving: Information About Sexuality and Intimacy
Arthritis Foundation
PO Box 7669
Atlanta, GA 30357-0669
404-872-7100
800-283-7800
Fax: 404-872-0457

1220 Managing Your Activities
Arthritis Foundation
PO Box 7669
Atlanta, GA 30357-0669
404-872-7100
800-283-7800
Fax: 404-872-0457

1221 Managing Your Fatigue
Arthritis Foundation
PO Box 7669
Atlanta, GA 30357-0669
404-872-7100
800-283-7800
Fax: 404-872-0457

1222 Managing Your Health Care
Arthritis Foundation
PO Box 7669
Atlanta, GA 30357-0669
404-872-7100
800-283-7800
Fax: 404-872-0457

1223 Managing Your Pain
Arthritis Foundation
PO Box 7669
Atlanta, GA 30357-0669
404-872-7100
800-283-7800
Fax: 404-872-0457

1224 Managing Your Stress
Arthritis Foundation
PO Box 7669
Atlanta, GA 30357-0669
404-872-7100
800-283-7800
Fax: 404-872-0457

1225 Methotrexate
Arthritis Foundation
PO Box 7669
Atlanta, GA 30357-0669
404-872-7100
800-283-7800
Fax: 404-872-0457

1226 Myositis
Arthritis Foundation
PO Box 7669
Atlanta, GA 30357-0669
404-872-7100
800-283-7800
Fax: 404-872-0457

1227 Osteoarthritis
Arthritis Foundation
PO Box 7669
Atlanta, GA 30357-0669
404-872-7100
800-283-7800
Fax: 404-872-0457
Offers introductions, examples, explanations and research pertaining to this type of arthritis.

1228 Osteonecrosis
Arthritis Foundation
PO Box 7669
Atlanta, GA 30357-0669
404-872-7100
800-283-7800
Fax: 404-872-0457

1229 Overcoming Rheumatoid Arthritis
Michigan Chapter of the Arthritis Foundation
1050 Wilshire Drive
Troy, MI 48084-1564
248-649-2891
800-968-3030
Fax: 248-649-2895
e-mail: info.mi@arthritis.org
www.arthritis.org
Provides extensive information about the disease and treatment, with an emphasis on what you can do for yourself.

1230 Penicillamine
Arthritis Foundation
PO Box 7669
Atlanta, GA 30357-0669
404-872-7100
800-283-7800
Fax: 404-872-0457

1231 Polyarteritis Nodosa and Wegener's Granulomatosis
Arthritis Foundation
PO Box 7669
Atlanta, GA 30357-0669
404-872-7100
800-283-7800
Fax: 404-872-0457

1232 Polymyalgia Rheumatica and Giant Cell Arthritis
Arthritis Foundation
PO Box 7669
Atlanta, GA 30357-0669
404-872-7100
800-283-7800
Fax: 404-872-0457

1233 Pseudoxanthoma Elasticum Fact Sheet
Arthritis Foundation
PO Box 7669
Atlanta, GA 30357-0669
404-872-7100
800-283-7800
Fax: 404-872-0457

1234 Psoriatic Arthritis Information Package
NAMSIC/National Institutes of Health

1 AMS Circle   301-495-4484
Bethesda, MD 20892-0001   877-226-4267
Fax: 301-718-6366
TTY: 301-565-2966
e-mail: niamsinfo@mail.nih.gov
www.nih.gov/niams/

1235 Q&A's About Arthritis and Rheumatic Disease
NIH/National Institutes of Health
1 AMS Circle   301-495-4484
Bethesda, MD 20892-0001   877-226-4267
Fax: 301-718-6366
TTY: 301-565-2969
e-mail: niamsinfo@mail.nih.gov
www.nih.gov/niams

This pamphlet offers information, technical articles and research on arthritis and related disorders. Also included are referral organizations to help patients uncover more information.

1236 Reflex Sympathetic Dystrophy Syndrome Fact Sheet
Arthritis Foundation
PO Box 7669   404-872-7100
Atlanta, GA 30357-0669   800-283-7800
Fax: 404-872-0457

1237 Reiter's Syndrome
Arthritis Foundation
PO Box 7669   404-872-7100
Atlanta, GA 30357-0669   800-283-7800
Fax: 404-872-0457

1238 Rheumatoid Arthritis Information Package
NAMSIC/National Institutes of Health
1 AMS Circle   301-495-4484
Bethesda, MD 20892-0001   877-226-4267
Fax: 301-718-6366
TTY: 301-565-2966
e-mail: niamsinfo@mail.nih.gov
www.nih.gov/niams

Offers an introduction and definition of rheumatoid arthritis, treatments, causes, objectives, daily living, resources and medical information.

1239 Surgery: Information to Consider
Arthritis Foundation
PO Box 7669   404-872-7100
Atlanta, GA 30357-0669   800-283-7800
Fax: 404-872-0457

1240 Thinking About Tomorrow: A Career Guide for Teens with Arthritis
Arthritis Foundation
PO Box 7669   404-872-7100
Atlanta, GA 30357-0669   800-283-7800
Fax: 404-872-0457

1241 When Your Student Has Arthritis: A Guide for Teachers
Arthritis Foundation
PO Box 7669   404-872-7100
Atlanta, GA 30357-0669   800-283-7800
Fax: 404-872-0457

A medical information booklet written for teachers or other adults who have arthritis. The booklet describes different forms of juvenile arthritis, how arthritis might affect the child at school, and how to help the child work around these problems.

Audio & Video

1242 FIT Video
Arthritis Foundation
550 Pharr Road   404-237-8771
Altlanta, GA 30023-6996   800-933-7023
Fax: 404-237-8153
e-mail: info.ga@arthritis.org
www.arthritis.org

1243 In Control
Arthritis Foundation

1330 W Peachtree Street NW   404-872-7100
Atlanta, GA 30309-2922   800-283-7800
Fax: 404-872-0457

An excellent at-home program which includes video, audio cassettes and the Arthritis Helpbook. Provides tools to help meet the challenges of arthritis.

1244 PACE I
Arthritis Foundation
PO Box 6996
Alpharetta, GA 30023-6996   800-207-8633

1245 PACE II
Arthritis Foundation
PO Box 6996
Alpharetta, GA 30023-6996   800-207-8633
Fax: 770-442-9742
www.arthritis.com

1246 Pathways to Better Living
Arthritis Foundation
PO Box 6996
Alpharetta, GA 30023-6996   800-207-8633
Fax: 770-442-9742
www.arthritis.com

1247 Pool Exercise Program
Arthritis Foundation Distribution Center
PO Box 6996
Alpharetta, GA 30023-6996   800-207-8633
Fax: 770-442-9742
www.arthritis.com

This video features water exercises that will help you increase and maintain joint flexibility, strengthen and tone muscles, and increase endurance. All exercises are performed in water at chest level. No swimming skills are necessary.

Web Sites

1248 American Juvenile Arthritis Organization
www.arthritis.com
Serves the special needs of young people with arthritis and their families. Provides information, inspiration and advocacy.

1249 Arthritis Foundation
www.arthritis.org
Provide services to help through information, referrals, speakers bureaus, forums, self-help courses, and various support groups and programs nationwide.

1250 Healing Well
www.healingwell.com
An online health resource guide to medical news, chat, information and articles, newsgroups and message boards, books, disease-related web sites, medical directories, and more for patients, friends, and family coping with disabling diseases, disorders, or chronic illnesses.

1251 Health Finder
www.healthfinder.gov
Searchable, carefully developed web site offering information on over 1000 topics. Developed by the US Department of Health and Human Services, the site can be used in both English and Spanish.

1252 Healthlink USA
www.healthlinkusa.com
Health information concerning treatment, cures, prevention, diagnosis, risk factors, research, support groups, email lists, personal stories and much more. Updated regularly.

1253 Helios Health
www.helioshealth.com
Online resource for your health information. Detailed information about specific health topics, access to expert advice from our Medical Advisory Board, and up-to-date health news.

1254 MedicineNet
www.medicinenet.com
An online resource for consumers providing easy-to-read, authoritative medical and health information.

1255 Medscape

www.medscape.com

Medscape offers specialists, primary care physicians, and other health professionals the Web's most robust and integrated medical information and educational tools.

1256 National Arthritis & Musculoskeletal & Skin Diseases Information Clearinghouse

www.nih.gov/niams

Provides clinical and public information and research to increase understanding of the many rheumatic diseases and related disorders. Also provides lists and order forms for their resources and materials.

1257 WebMD

www.webmd.com

Information on arthritis, including articles and resources.

Description

1258 # Asthma

Asthma is a respiratory disorder that causes shortness of breath, wheezing, coughing and chest tightness. About 12 million people in the U.S. have asthma, and its incidence is increasing. It is the leading cause of hospitalization for children; however, some children with asthma will outgrow the disorder by the time they are teenagers or adults. Asthma ranges from mild illness to life-threatening episodes.

Numerous environmental factors trigger an asthma attack including allergies, infections, exercise, cold weather and stress. Treatment consists of avoiding or minimizing factors that cause an asthma attack, for example pet dander and pollen.

In addition, several medications are used to relieve asthma symptoms by opening lung airways, known as bronchodilation. Many of these drugs can be inhaled so that they work directly on the lungs. Inhaled steroids may be used for long-term control. Research and new therapies are being directed at trying to find medications that will prevent asthma from occurring. See also *Lung Disease*.

National Agencies & Associations

1259 **Allergy & Asthma Network Mothers of Asthmatics**
2751 Prosperity Avenue   703-641-9595
Fairfax, VA 22031   800-878-4403
                             Fax: 30 -40 -298
                       e-mail: info@aanma.org
                          www.breatherville.org
A national nonprofit network of families with a desire to overcome allergies and asthma by producing the most accurate timely practical and livable alternatives to suffering.
Nancy Sander, Founder/President
Hiwote Aberra, Database/Member Services Coordinator

1260 **American Academy of Allergy, Asthma & Immunology**
555 East Wells Street   414-272-6071
Milwaukee, WI 53202-3823   800-822-2762
                             Fax: 414-272-6070
                       e-mail: info@aaaai.org
                              www.aaaai.org
Strives to serve the public through information on asthma and allergies, as well as referrals to allergists. Also offers pollen and mold statistics from the Committee on Pollen & Molds.
Thomas B Casale, Executive Vice President
Kay A Walen, Executive Director

1261 **American Lung Association**
1301 Pennsylvania Avenue NW   202-785-3355
Washington, DC 20004   800-LUN-GUSA
                             Fax: 202-452-1805
                       e-mail: info@lungusa.org
                              www.lungusa.org
The mission of the American Lung Association is to prevent lung disease and promote lung health. Founded in 1904 to fight tuberculosis, the American Lung Association today fights disease in all its forms, with special emphasis on asthma, tobacco control and environmental health.
Charles Dean O'Conner, President, CEO
Don Awerkamp, Director

1262 **Association of Birth Defect Children Birth Defect Research for Children**
800 Celebration Avenue   407-566-8304
Celebration, FL 34747   Fax: 407-566-8341
                       e-mail: staff@birthdefects.org
                            www.birthdefects.org
Non-profit organization that provides parents and expectant parents with information about birth defects and support services for their children. Sponsors the National Birth Defect Registry, a research project that studies associations between birth defects and genetics.
Betty Mekdeci, Executive Director
John Bragg, Administrative Assistant

1263 **Asthma Society of Canada**
124 Merton Street   416-787-4050
Toronto, Ontario, M4S 2-6K1   866-787-4050
                             Fax: 416-787-5807
                       e-mail: info@asthma.ca
                              www.asthma.ca
A national registered healthcare charity, operating within a civil society business structure.
Dr. Robert Oliphant, President, CEO
Zhen Liu, Office Manager

1264 **Asthma and Allergy Information Association**
8201 Coprorate Drive   202-466-7643
Lanover, MD 20785   800-727-8462
                             Fax: 202-466-8940
                       e-mail: info@aafa.org
                              www.aafa.org
A not-for-profit organization, is the leading patient organization for people with asthma and allergies, and the oldest asthma and allergy patient group in the world. AAFA provides practical information, community based services and support through a national network of chapters and support groups. AAFA develops health education, organizes state and national advocacy efforts and funds research to find better treatments and cures.
Christopher Cole, Chair

1265 **National Advisory Allergic and Infectious Disease Council**
6610 Rockledge Drive   301-496-2644
Bethesda, MD 20892-6612   866-284-4107
                             Fax: 301-402-7123
                             TDD: 800-877-8339
                    e-mail: ocpostoffice@niaid.nih.gov
                    www.niaid.nih.gov/Pages/default.aspx
The National Institute of Allergy and Infectious Diseases (NIAID) conducts and supports basic and applied research to better understand treat and ultimately prevent infectious immunologic and allergic diseases.
Anthony S Fauci MD, Director
H Clifford Lane MD, Acting Deputy Director

State Agencies & Associations

Alaska

1266 **Asthma and Allergy Foundation of America: Alaska Chapter**
PO Box 201927   907-696-4810
Anchorage, AK 99520-1927   Fax: 907-696-4810
                       e-mail: aafaalaska@gci.net
                            www.aafaalaska.com
Formed in April, 2001, the AAFA Alaska chapter is moving quickly to provide educational programs and information about asthma and allergies through classes, workshops and educational materials. Focused not only on reaching children and adults with asthma information, but also health care professionals, caregivers, childcare providers and school personnel.
Suzi Jackson, Executive Director
Kathleen Bell, RN, Secretary

California

1267 Asthma and Allergy Foundation of America: Southern California Chapter
3435 Wilshire Boulevard
Los Angeles, CA 90036
323-937-7859
800-624-0044
Fax: 323-937-7815
e-mail: aafasocal@aol.com
www.aafasocal.com

Dedicated to controlling and curing asthma and allergic diseases through education, a network of support groups, the support of research and specialized training, increasing public awareness and providing medication and treatment to the under served. Program highlights include the Breathmobile, asthma camps and air power games for children.
Francene Lifson, Executive Director

District of Columbia

1268 Asthma and Allergy Foundation of America: Washington Chapter
1233 20th Street
Washington, DC 20036
206-368-2866
800-727-8462
Fax: 206-368-2941
e-mail: Info@aafa.org
www.aafa.org

Program highlights include trainings for health care professionals on asthma and allergy management, working collaboratively with other local and regional agencies to improve the quality of life for those affected by asthma and allergies, organizing health seminars and education programs.
Mary Brasle, Director of Programs and Services
Amy Patterson, Director Administration/Governance

Massachusetts

1269 Asthma and Allergy Foundation of America: New England Chapter
220 Boylston Street
Chestnut Hill, MA 02467
617-965-7771
877-227-8462
Fax: 617-965-8886
TTY: 877-227-8462
e-mail: info@asthmaandallergies.org
www.asthmaandallergies.org

Serves Massachusetts, Rhode Island, Connecticut, Maine, New Hampshire and Vermont. Program highlights include speakers and exhibits, telephone information and referrals, tobacco control program, scholarship essay contest for high school juniors, advocacy for safer environments and training programs for school, daycare and health professionals.
Patricia Goldman, Executive Director
Sharon Schumack, Health Education Coordinator

Michigan

1270 Asthma and Allergy Foundation of America: Michigan Chapter
2075 Walnut Lake Road
West Bloomfield, MI 48323-8768
248-406-4254
888-444-0333
Fax: 248-757-2102
e-mail: aafamich@sbcglobal.net
www.aafamich.org

Serves the state of Michigan through public forums, work place educational programs, patient advocacy, Asthma Camp and telephone referrals and information.
Karen Katz, Executive Director
Dr. Rola Bokhari-Panza, President

Missouri

1271 Asthma and Allergy Foundation of America: Greater Kansas City Chapter
9140 Ward Parkway
Kansas City, MO 64114
816-333-6608
888-542-8252
Fax: 816-333-6684
e-mail: info@aafakc.org
www.aafakc.org

Provides college scholarships, Family Asthma Education Day, adult discussion groups, Superkids Asthma Day Camp for grades 1-5, professional education, ACT, health fair participation, breath-

ing machine, peak flow meter and spacer distribution programs. They also have a quarterly newsletter, an asthma action line, emergency medication assistance, assistance to local school districts, free educational materials, seminars for work site clinicians and daycare workers and the smoke-free dining group.
Noel Albert, Executive Director

1272 Asthma and Allergy Foundation of America: St. Louis Chapter
1500 South Big Bend
St. Louis, MO 63117
314-645-2422
Fax: 314-692-2022
e-mail: aafa@aafastl.org
www.aafastl.org/

The Asthma and Allergy Foundation of America (AAFA), St. Louis Chapter, was founded in 1981 by a group of volunteer board-certified allergists, including Dr. Phillip Korenblat of Washington University and Dr. Raymond Slavin of St. Louis University. AAFA St. Louis provides services to the community in helping children effectively manage their asthma through the provision of medical resources, equipment and education.
H. James Wedner, M.D, President
Bill Reichhardt, Vice President

New Jersey

1273 Asthma and Allergy Foundation of America: Southeast Pennsylvania Chapter
32 Caspertown Street
Gibbstown, NJ 08027
856-224-9547
Fax: 856-224-5893
e-mail: aafasepa@prodigy.net
www.aafa.org

In the process of establishing a vital, new program that will aid children with chronic asthma. Many parents, some who are without medical insurance coverage, are unaware of the availability of a medical support system that can help their children. The Children at Risk program will enable parents to have their children evaluated and also receive a free one month supply of medication. Parents will also receive information regarding available options for follow up care and prescription coverage.
Lynn Hanessian, Chair
Michele Abu Carrick ,LICSW, Co-Chair, Governance

Oregon

1274 Asthma and Allergy Foundation of America: Oregon Chapter
14530 Southwest 144th Avenue
Tigard, OR 97224-1445
503-579-8375
Fax: 208-474-6839
e-mail: hensches@teleport.com

Serving the state of Oregon.
Sandra L Henschel, President

Texas

1275 Asthma and Allergy Foundation of America
9101 Quarter Horse Lane
Fort Worth, TX 76123
817-297-3132
888-933-AAFA
Fax: 817-563-5696
e-mail: info@aafatexas.org
www.aafatexas.org

Offers many educational programs and services that touch patients, caregivers, physicians and allied health professionals, including: child care provider education programs, school nurse and respiratory therapist education programs, and work site allergy education.
Joan Hart, Executive Director
Jim Rosenthal, President

1276 Asthma and Allergy Foundation of America: North Texas Chapter
3904 Justin Drive
Ft. Worth, TX 76244
817-297-3132
888-933-AAFA
Fax: 817-563-5696
e-mail: aafantx@hotmail.com
www.aafatexas.org

Offers many educational programs and services that touch patients. caregivers, physicians and allied health professionals, including: child care provider education programs, school nurse and respiratory therapist education programs, work site allergy education programs, spacer and peak flow meter distribution to those in need, a toll free hotline, prescription assistance information, free

educational materials in English and Spanish, an electronic newsletter, professional education, etc.
Jim Roseenthal, President
Stephen J Apaliski MD, VP Publications

Foundations

1277 Asthma and Allergy Foundation of America
1233 20th Street NW
Washington, DC 20036
202-466-7643
800-727-8462
Fax: 202-668-40
e-mail: info@aafa.org
www.aafa.org
AAFA provides practical information, community based services and support through a national network of chapters and support groups. AAFA develops health education, organizes state and national advocacy efforts and funds research to find better treatments and cures
William McLin, Executive Director

Research Centers

1278 Brigham and Women's Hospital: Rheumatology Immunology, and Allergy Division
75 Francis Street
Boston, MA 02115
61 -73 -550
Fax: 617-525-1001
TTY: 617-732-6458
www.brighamandwomens.org
Internationally renowned for excellence in clinical care clinical investigation and basic research. A faculty of 36 board certified rheumatologists and allergists provide eldtive urgent and emergency consultations as necessary.
Michael B Brenner MD, Division Chief
Jonathan S Coblyn, Clinical Director Rheumatology

1279 Childrens Hospital Immunology Division Children's Hospital
Children's Hospital
300 Longwood Avenue
Boston, MA 02115
61 -35 -600
www.childrenshospital.org
Organizational research unit of the Children's Hospital that focuses on the causes prevention and treatments of asthma infections and allergies.
Dr. James Mandell, CEO
Sandra Fenwick, President & COO

1280 Clinical Immunology, Allergy, and Rheumatology
Tulane Medical School
1700 Perdido Street
New Orleans, LA 70112-1210
504-988-5187
Fax: 504-988-3686
e-mail: medsch@tulane.edu
www.som.tulane.edu/medciar
Mauel Lopez MD, Director

1281 Duke Asthma, Allergy and Airway Center
4309 Medical Park Drive
Durham, NC 27704
919-620-7300
www.aaac.duhs.duke.edu/
Raffeal Rau, President
Dr Monica Kraft, Director

1282 Johns Hopkins University: Asthma and Allergy Center
5501 Hopkins Bayview Circle
Baltimore, MD 21224-6801
410-550-2101
Fax: 410-550-3256
e-mail: jhuallergy@jhmi.edu
www.hopkinsmedicine.org/allergy
Studies of allergic diseases and individuals with allergic disease pulmonary diseases and diseases involving inflammation and immunological processes.
Bruce S Bochner, Director
Peter S Creticos, Clinical Director

1283 National Jewish Division of Immunology
National Jewish Medical and Research Center

1400 Jackson Street
Denver, CO 80206-2762
303-398-1337
80 -42 -889
Fax: 303-270-2125
e-mail: harbeckr@njc.org
www.njc.org
The only medical center in the country whose research and patient care resources are dedicated to respiratory and immunologic diseases.
John Cambier, Chairman
Ronald J Harbeck, Medical Director

1284 Northwestern University: Division of Allergy and Immunology
The Feinberg School of Medicine
251 East Huron Street
Chicago, IL 60611
312-926-6895
Fax: 312-926-6905
e-mail: rpschleimer@northwestern.edu
www.medicine.northwestern.edu
A referral center of local regional and national stature. Areas of clinical excellence include asthma allergic bronchopulmonary aspergillosis idiopathic anaphylaxis drug allergy occupational immunologic lung disease and allergen immunotherapy.
Douglas E Vaughan MD, Chair
James Foody MD, Vice Chair Clinical Affairs

1285 University of Virginia: General Clinical Research Center
University of Virginia Health System
2515 Lee Street
Charlottesville, VA 22908-0787
434-924-2394
Fax: 434-924-9960
e-mail: gcrc@virginia.edu
www.healthsystem.virginia.edu/
Focuses on asthmatic disorders.
Arthur Garso Jr MD MPH, Principal Investigator
Eugene J Barrett, Program Director

1286 University of Wisconsin: Asthma, Allergy and Pulmonary Research Center
600 Highland Avenue
Madison, WI 53792-2454
608-263-6400
Fax: 608-263-6401
www.medicine.wisc.edu
Sheri L Lawrence, MBA, Administrator
Sharon Gehl, MBA, Associate Administrator

Support Groups & Hotlines

1287 Allergy & Asthma Networks Hotline
Allergy and Asthma Network/Mothers of Asthmatics
2751 Prosperity Avenue
Fairfax, VA 22031
703-641-9595
800-878-4403
Fax: 703-573-7794
www.breatherville.org
Mary McGowan, Executive Director
Michael Amato, Chair

1288 Asthma and Allergy Foundation of America
1233 20th Street NW
Washington, DC 20036
202-466-7643
Fax: 202-466-8940
e-mail: info@aafa.org
www.aafa.org
The foundation was formed to alleviate suffering and loss from asthma and allergy disorders. The foundation offers a nationwide network of chapters and support groups and provides education and emotional support for persons with allergies and asthma. Also funds research for improved treatments and ultimately a cure.

1289 National Health Information Center
PO Box 1133
Washington, DC 20013
310-565-4167
800-336-4797
Fax: 301-984-4256
e-mail: info@nhic.org
www.health.gov/nhic
Offers a nationwide information referral service, produces directories and resource guides.

1290 Physician Referral and Information Line
American Academy of Allergy Asthma and Immunology
555 East Wells Street
Milwaukee, WI 53202-3889
414-272-6071
800-822-2762
Fax: 414-272-6070
www.aaaai.org

Referral line offering information on allergy and asthma, referral to an allergy/immunology specialist.

1291 Support for Asthmatic Youth
Asthma and Allergy Foundation of America
1080 Glen Cove Avenue   516-625-5735
Glen Head, NY 11545-1565   Fax: 516-625-2976
A network of educational/support groups for adolescents between the ages of 9 and 17. All meetings are free and feature guest speakers, informational programs, games and other fun activities.
Renee Theodorakis MA, Director Adolescent Services

Books

1292 Asthma Care Training for Kids
Asthma and Allergy Foundation of America
1233 20th Street NW   202-466-7643
Washington, DC 20036   Fax: 202-466-8940
                                 e-mail: info@aafa.org
                                        www.aafa.org
Designed to help children ages 7-12 and their parents take charge of their asthma. In a series of three action filled sessions, children and their parents meet separately with their peers to learn about asthma management.

1293 Asthma Organizer
Allergy and Asthma Network/Mothers of Asthmatics
2751 Prosperity Avenue   703-641-9595
Fairfax, VA 22031-4397   800-878-4403
                                 Fax: 703-573-7794
                         www.mothersofasthmatics.org
Includes daily symptom diary and forms to track medications, office visits and updates to your personal management plan. Information on peak flow monitoring, managing asthma at school, understanding asthma activators, and allergy-proofing also included. Available in Spanish.
Loose Leaf
Mary McGowan, Executive Director

1294 Asthma Resources Directory
Allergy and Asthma Network/Mothers of Asthmatics
2751 Prosperity Avenue   703-641-9595
Fairfax, VA 22031-4397   800-878-4403
                                 Fax: 703-573-7794
                         www.mothersofasthmatics.org
Comprehensive listings of thousands of products, services, and resources for allergy and asthma questions.
Mary McGowan, Executive Director

1295 Asthma Self-Help Book
Asthma and Allergy Foundation of America
1233 20th Street NW   202-466-7643
Washington, DC 20036   Fax: 202-466-8940
                                 e-mail: info@aafa.org
                                        www.aafa.org
A thorough, practical look at asthma that includes information from the National Heart, Lung and Blood Institute's 1991 Asthma Guidelines.

1296 Asthma in the School: Improving Control with Peak Flow Monitoring
Asthma and Allergy Foundation of America
1233 20th Street NW   202-466-7643
Washington, DC 20036   Fax: 202-466-8940
                                 e-mail: info@aafa.org
                                        www.aafa.org
Comprehensive and practical guide to help the school nurse monitor and assist students with asthma.

1297 Asthma in the Workplace
John H Dekker & Sons
2941 Clydon Street SW   616-538-5160
Grand Rapids, MI 49509   Fax: 616-538-0720
1993 664 pages
ISBN: 0-824787-99-4

1298 Asthma: The Complete Guide
Asthma and Allergy Foundation of America

1233 20th Street NW   202-466-7643
Washington, DC 20036-2330   800-727-8462
                                 Fax: 202-466-8940
                                        www.aafa.org
An excellent self-management guide for asthma and allergy patients and their families.
357 pages Paperback

1299 Breathing Disorders: Your Complete Exercise Guide
Human Kinetics
PO Box 5076   217-351-5076
Champaign, IL 61825-5076   800-747-4457
                                 Fax: 217-351-2674
                              www.humankinetics.com

1993 144 pages Paperback
ISBN: 0-873224-26-4
Steve Ruhlig, Marketing Director

1300 Bronchial Asthma: Principles of Diagnosis and Treatment
Humana Press
999 Riverview Drive   973-256-1699
Totowa, NJ 07512   Fax: 973-256-8341
                         e-mail: humana@humanapr.com
                                www.humanapress.com

2001 496 pages
ISBN: 0-896038-61-0

1301 Children with Asthma: A Manual for Parents
Allergy Control Products
PO Box 793   203-438-9580
Ridgefield, CT 06877-0793   800-422-3878
                                 Fax: 203-431-8963
                              www.allergycontrol.com
Known as the asthma bible, this second edition is sprinkled with anecdotes by patients and their parents.
296 pages Paperback

1302 Conquering Asthma
Michael Newhouse, MD, author
B.C Decker, Inc.
50 King Street E, Floor 2 PO Box620   905-522-7017
Ontario, Canada L8N 3K7,   800-568-7281
                                 Fax: 905-522-7839
                           e-mail: info@bcdecker.com
                                   www.bcdecker.com
This text shows asthmatics how to live a healthier and happier life hardly aware that they have asthma.
1998 107 pages Paperback
ISBN: 1-896998-01-1

1303 Coping with Asthma
Rosen Publishing Group
29 E 21st Street   212-777-3017
New York, NY 10010   800-237-9932
                                 Fax: 888-436-4643
                 e-mail: customerservice@rosenpub.com
                              www.rosenpublishing.com
This book prepares students by explaining to them the dangers of asthma, a condition which, when properly treated, is completely manageable.

ISBN: 0-823929-69-8
Carolyn Simpson, Author

1304 Understanding Asthma
Phil Lieberman, MD, author
University Press of Mississippi
3825 Ridgewood Road   601-432-6205
Jackson, MS 39211-6492   Fax: 601-432-6217
                     e-mail: kburgess@ihl.state.ms.us
                                www.upress.state.ms.us
A guide to how the disease behaves and how the latest therapies work.
1999 120 pages Paperback
ISBN: 1-578061-42-3
Kathy Burgess, Advertising/Marketing Services Manager

Children's Books

1305 All About Asthma
Asthma and Allergy Foundation of America
1233 20th Street NW   202-466-7643
Washington, DC 20036-2330   800-727-8462
                                   Fax: 202-466-8940
                                        www.aafa.org
Written by a 10-year-old with asthma, this cleverly illustrated book explains causes and symptoms, and ways to control asthma to lead a normal life.
39 pages Paperback

1306 Asthma
Franklin Watts Grolier
90 Old Sherman Turnpike   203-797-3500
Danbury, CT 06816-0001   800-621-1115
                                   Fax: 203-797-3197
                                        www.grolier.com
This book offers vital information on causes and treatments, plus advice on how to prevent flare-ups.
96 pages Grades 7-12
ISBN: 0-531106-97-7

1307 Asthma Challenge
Asthma and Allergy Foundation of America
1233 20th Street NW   202-466-7643
Washington, DC 20036   Fax: 202-466-8940
                                   e-mail: info@aafa.org
                                        www.aafa.org
An exciting new team game for large or small groups. Custom designed, full color, stand up board and two sets of pretested question cards. Teens and adults win AAFA Bucks as they test their knowledge in categories like Sneezes and Wheezes and Asthma Nuts and Bolts.

1308 Best of Superstuff Activity Booklet
American Lung Association
1740 Broadway
New York, NY 10019-4315   212-315-8700
For young children with asthma featuring a series of activities designed to help youngsters cope with asthma.
32 pages Ages 6-8

1309 Bronkie the Bronchiasaurus
Asthma and Allergy Foundation of America
1233 20th Street NW   202-466-7643
Washington, DC 20036-2330   800-727-8462
                                   Fax: 202-466-8940
                                        www.aafa.org
A Super Nintendo role-playing adventure in which players manage the asthma of two dinosaurs. They must avoid triggers, maintain their peak-flow and take daily medications. Only then can they use their strongest defense - the powerful breath blast. Designed for ages 7 to 15.

1310 Childhood Asthma: Learning to Manage
Asthma and Allergy Foundation of America
1233 20th Street NW   202-466-7643
Washington, DC 20036-2330   800-727-8462
                                   Fax: 202-466-8940
                                        www.aafa.org
Self-paced, entertaining activity books for home use featuring practical guidelines for managing childhood asthma with a focus on using peak flow meters.

1311 Clubhouse Kids Learn About Asthma
Asthma and Allergy Foundation of America
1233 20th Street NW   202-466-7643
Washington, DC 20036-2330   800-727-8462
                                   Fax: 202-466-8940
                                        www.aafa.org
Interactive CD-ROM helps children ages 4-12 learn about asthma at their own pace. Sound, animation and game-like features draw players into the life of Janie, who has just been diagnosed with asthma.

1312 I'm a Meter Reader
Allergy and Asthma Network/Mothers of Asthmatics

2751 Prosperity Avenue   703-641-9595
Fairfax, VA 22031-4397   800-878-4403
                                   Fax: 703-573-7794
                                   www.mothersofasthmatics.org
Provides expert advice on how a peak flow meter can help detect when an asthma attack can occur in an easy to understand format with colorful illustrations. Available in Spanish. Companion video, I'm a Meter Reader, available as part of a set for $12.00.
Ages 4-9
Mary McGowan, Executive Director
Nancy Sander, Editor-in-Chief

1313 Let's Talk About Having Asthma
Rosen Publishing Group's PowerKids Press
29 E 21st Street   212-777-3017
New York, NY 10010   800-237-9932
                                   Fax: 888-436-4643
               e-mail: customerservice@rosenpub.com
                                   www.rosenpublishing.com
This book talks about the cause and treatments for asthma as well as the precautions sufferers should take. Recommended for grades K-4.

ISBN: 0-823950-32-8

1314 Lion Who Had Asthma
Asthma and Allergy Foundation of America
1233 20th Street NW   202-466-7643
Washington, DC 20036-2330   800-727-8462
                                   Fax: 202-466-8940
                                        www.aafa.org
A beautifully illustrated book that encourages preschoolers to use their imaginations and take their asthma medications.
24 pages Hardcover

1315 Luke Has Asthma Too!
Allergy Control Products
PO Box 793
Ridgefield, CT 06877-0793   800-422-3878
                                   Fax: 203-431-8963
This gentle book will make for good reading with children, whether they have asthma or not.

1316 Scorpions
Harper & Row
10 E 53rd Street
New York, NY 10022-5299   212-207-7000
                                   www.harpercollins.com
This novel, while not wholly dedicated to examining the ramifications of asthma on a child's life, does incorporate the theme into a compelling narrative.
Grades 6-9

1317 So You Have Asthma Too!
Allergy and Asthma Network/Mothers of Asthmatics
2751 Prosperity Avenue   703-641-9595
Fairfax, VA 22031-4397   800-878-4403
                                   Fax: 703-573-7794
                                   www.mothersofasthmatics.org
A children's illustrated book, offering a clear description and understanding of childhood asthma. Available in Spanish. Also see companion video, SO YOU HAVE ASTHMA TOO!, available as part of a set for $12.00.
Mary McGowan, Executive Director
Nancy Sander, Editor-in-Chief

1318 Winning Over Asthma
Asthma and Allergy Foundation of America
1233 20th Street NW   202-466-7643
Washington, DC 20036-2330   800-727-8462
                                   Fax: 202-466-8940
                                        www.aafa.org
Simple coloring book explains asthma through a story about five-year-old Graham.
30 pages Paperback

Magazines

1319 Controlling Asthma
American Lung Association
1740 Broadway   212-315-8700
New York, NY 10019-4315
For parents of children with asthma, this newsmagazine tells how parents can help their child deal with the many problems presented by asthma.
16 pages

1320 Starting Strong-Staying Strong: A Resource Guide for Educational Support Groups
Asthma and Allergy Foundation of America
1233 20th Street NW   202-466-7643
Washington, DC 20036   800-727-8462
                                      Fax: 202-466-8940
                                  e-mail: info@aafa.org
                                          www.aafa.org
A resource guide to help educational support groups get organized, publicize and remain successful. Great for people who want to start an asthma or allergy support group and for existing group leaders who want to strengthen their programs. Filled with stories of success and struggle from other group leaders, medical advisors and group members across the country. A companion CD-ROM provides additional tips.
Guide + CD-ROM
William McLin, Executive Director
Mike Tringale, Director Marketing/Communications

Newsletters

1321 Advance
Asthma and Allergy Foundation of America
1233 20th Street NW   202-466-7643
Washington, DC 20036-2330   800-727-8462
                                      Fax: 202-466-8940
                                          www.aafa.org
A bi-monthly , 8 page newsletter for patients and their families filled with timely and useful information about managing asthma and allergies.
BiMonthly

1322 Allergy & Asthma ADVOCATE Newsletter
American Academy of Allergy, Asthma and Immunology
611 E Wells Street   414-272-6071
Milwaukee, WI 53202   800-822-2762
                                      Fax: 414-272-6070
                                          www.aaaai.org
Offers tips and medical information on allergies and asthma via articles written by allied health and physician AAAAI members.
6 pages Quarterly

1323 BReATHE
Asthma and Allergy Foundation of America
8201 Corporate Drive
Landover, MD 20785   800-727-8462
                                  e-mail: info@aafa.org
                                          www.aafa.org
E-newsletter filled with information on how to control asthma and allergies, with stories from patients who are living life without limits.
Bi-Monthly
William McLin, President/CEO
Angel Waldron, Sr Manager Marketing/Communications

1324 FreshAAIR
Asthma and Allergy Foundation of America
8201 Corporate Drive   202-466-7643
Landover, MD 20785   800-727-8462
                                      Fax: 202-466-8940
                                  e-mail: info@aafa.org
                                          www.aafa.org
Filled with information about asthma, seasonal allergies, food allergies, back-to-school tips for parents, educational materials and more.
Bi-Monthly
William McLin, President/CEO
Angel Waldron, Sr Manager Marketing/Communications

1325 Leaders Link
Asthma and Allergy Foundation of America
8201 Corporate Drive
Landover, MD 20785   800-727-8462
                                  e-mail: info@aafa.org
                                          www.aafa.org
Provides useful and timely insights on how to plan and lead asthma and allergy support group meetings, how to keep your support group active and strong, and useful ideas from other support groups.
Bi-Monthly
William McLin, President/CEO
Angel Waldron, Sr Manager Marketing/Communications

1326 MA Report
Allergy and Asthma Network/Mothers of Asthmatics
2751 Prosperity Avenue   703-641-9595
Fairfax, VA 22031-4397   800-878-4403
                                      Fax: 703-573-7794
                                www.mothersofasthmatics.com
Offers information on medical breakthroughs, patient care, public awareness, activities and events focusing on the allergy and asthma patient. This newsletter keeps a patient fully informed with medical articles written by experts in the field.
Monthly
Mary McGowan, Executive Director
Nancy Sander, Editor-in-Chief

Pamphlets

1327 About Asthma
American Lung Association
1740 Broadway   212-315-8700
New York, NY 10019-4315
A popular style pamphlet explaining symptoms, treatment and more for persons with asthma.
16 pages

1328 Adverse Reactions to Foods
American Academy of Allergy, Asthma and Immunology
611 E Wells Street   414-272-6071
Milwaukee, WI 53202-3889   800-822-2762
                                      Fax: 414-272-6070
                                          www.aaaai.org
A patient's guide to problem foods, food additives, diagnosis, and treatment.

1329 Allergies and You
American Lung Association
1740 Broadway   212-315-8700
New York, NY 10019-4315
Answers basic questions about allergy, particularly as it relates to asthma.

1330 Allergies to Animals
American Academy of Allergy, Asthma and Immunology
611 E Wells Street   414-272-6071
Milwaukee, WI 53202-3889   800-822-2762
                                      Fax: 414-272-6070
                                          www.aaaai.org

1331 Allergy & Asthma
American Academy of Allergy, Asthma and Immunology
611 E Wells Street   414-272-6071
Milwaukee, WI 53202-3889   800-822-2762
                                      Fax: 414-272-6070
                                          www.aaaai.org
An informational brochure discussing major topics of allerges and asthma.

1332 Allergy and Asthma: An Informational Brochure
American Academy of Allergy, Asthma and Immunology

611 E Wells Street
Milwaukee, WI 53202-3889

414-272-6071
800-822-2762
Fax: 414-272-6070
www.aaaai.org

Offers information on asthma, its symptoms, causes, diagnosis and treatments.

1333 Anaphylaxis
American Academy of Allergy, Asthma and Immunology
611 E Wells Street
Milwaukee, WI 53202-3889

414-272-6071
800-822-2762
Fax: 414-272-6070
www.aaaai.org

1334 Asthma Alert
American Lung Association
1740 Broadway
New York, NY 10019-4315

212-315-8700

Quick reference folders with information on asthma, the symptoms and what to do in an emergency.

1335 Asthma Handbook
American Lung Association
1740 Broadway
New York, NY 10019-4315

212-315-8700

Explains asthma, gives self-care methods for handling it and helps patients work more effectively with their doctor.
28 pages

1336 Asthma Lifelines
American Lung Association
1740 Broadway
New York, NY 10019-4315

212-315-8700

Promotional brochure providing descriptions of ALA asthma education materials.
12 pages

1337 Asthma and Allergies in Seniors
American Academy of Allergy, Asthma and Immunology
611 E Wells Street
Milwaukee, WI 53202

414-272-6071
800-822-2762
Fax: 414-272-6070
www.aaaai.org

1338 Asthma and Pregnancy
American Academy of Allergy, Asthma and Immunology
611 E Wells Street
Milwaukee, WI 53202-3889

414-272-6071
800-822-2762
Fax: 414-272-6070
www.aaaai.org

1339 Asthma and the School Child
American Academy of Allergy, Asthma and Immunology
611 E Wells Street
Milwaukee, WI 53202-3889

414-272-6071
800-822-2762
Fax: 414-272-6070
www.aaaai.org

1340 Atopic Dermatitis
American Academy of Allergy, Asthma and Immunology
611 E Wells Street
Milwaukee, WI 53202-3889

414-272-6071
800-822-2762
Fax: 414-272-6070
www.aaaai.org

This brochure offers information on symptoms, diagnosi, treatment, and prognosis.

1341 Being Close
National Jewish Center for Immunology
1400 Jackson Street
Denver, CO 80206-2762

303-388-4461

A booklet offering information to patients suffering from a respiratory disorder such as emphysema, asthma or tuberculosis, that discusses sexual problems and feelings.

1342 Childhood Asthma
American Academy of Allergy, Asthma and Immunology
611 E Wells Street
Milwaukee, WI 53202-3889

414-272-6071
800-822-2762
Fax: 414-272-6070
www.aaaai.org

1343 Childhood Asthma: A Guide for Parents
Asthma and Allergy Foundation of America
1233 20th Street NW
Washington, DC 20036-2330

202-466-7643
800-727-8462
Fax: 202-466-8940
www.aafa.org

This colorful booklet helps parents learn all about asthma in children.
32 pages

1344 Childhood Asthma: A Matter of Control
American Lung Association
1740 Broadway
New York, NY 10019-4315

212-315-8700

A guide for parents of children with asthma, this booklet covers topics such as identifying asthma signs and symptoms as well as controlling the condition.
28 pages

1345 Consumer Guide to Health Care Plans
American Academy of Allergy, Asthma and Immunology
611 E Wells Street
Milwaukee, WI 53202-3889

414-272-6071
800-822-2762
Fax: 414-272-6070
www.aaaai.org

Gives answers to some commonly asked questions on health care.

1346 Efficacy of Asthma Education, Selected Abstracts
American Lung Association
1740 Broadway
New York, NY 10019-4315

212-315-8700

Abstracts documenting the efficacy of asthma education programs for physicians and other health professionals.

1347 Exercise-Induced Asthma & Bronchospasm
American Academy of Allergy, Asthma and Immunology
611 E Wells Street
Milwaukee, WI 53202-3889

414-272-6071
800-822-2762
Fax: 414-272-6070
www.aaaai.org

This brochure covers testing, treatment, and other advice on how to deal with exercise-induced asthma.

1348 Facts About Asthma
American Lung Association
1740 Broadway
New York, NY 10019-4315

212-315-8700

Primary public information leaflet on asthma.
12 pages

1349 Facts About Peak Flow Meters
American Lung Association
1740 Broadway
New York, NY 10019-4315

212-315-8700

Discusses the use of a peak flow meter for adults and children with asthma.
8 pages

1350 Healthy Breathing
National Jewish Center for Immunology
1400 Jackson Street
Denver, CO 80206-2762

303-388-4461

Offers patients with lung or respiratory disorders information on exercise and healthy breathing.

1351 Helping Others Breathe Easier
Allergy and Asthma Network/Mothers of Asthmatics
2751 Prosperity Avenue
Fairfax, VA 22031-4397

703-641-9595
800-878-4403
Fax: 703-573-7794
www.mothersofasthmatics.org

Offers information on educational resources, support groups and the Network for persons afflicted with asthma or allergic disorders.
Mary McGowan, Executive Director
Nancy Sander, Editor-in-Chief

1352 Home Control of Allergies and Asthma
American Lung Association
1740 Broadway
New York, NY 10019-4315

212-315-8700

103

Discusses substances in the home that may trigger asthma and allergy problems and offers suggestions for controlling them.
12 pages

1353   Immunitherapy
American Academy of Allergy, Asthma and Immunology
611 E Wells Street   414-272-6071
Milwaukee, WI 53202-3889   800-822-2762
                                                           Fax: 414-272-6070
                                                           www.aaaai.org
This brochure offers information on administration, benefits, and potential side effects of immune therapy.

1354   Inhaled Medications for Asthma
American Academy of Allergy, Asthma and Immunology
611 E Wells Street   414-272-6071
Milwaukee, WI 53202-3889   800-822-2762
                                                           Fax: 414-272-6070
                                                           www.aaaai.org
This brochure gives helpful information on classes of inhaled medication, types of inhalation devices, spacers and holding chambers, how proper training is necessary.

1355   Latex Allergy
American Academy of Allergy, Asthma and Immunology
611 E Wells Street   414-272-6071
Milwaukee, WI 53202-3889   800-822-2762
                                                           Fax: 414-272-6070
                                                           www.aaaai.org

1356   Making the Most of Your Next Doctor Visit
American Academy of Allergy, Asthma and Immunology
611 E Wells Street   414-272-6071
Milwaukee, WI 53202-3889   800-822-2762
                                                           Fax: 414-272-6070
                                                           www.aaaai.org
A personal asthma management monitor. Includes personal tracking charts to help you along.
10 pages

1357   Many Faces of Asthma
American Lung Association
1740 Broadway   212-315-8700
New York, NY 10019-4315
Provides an overview of asthma as a major public health problem, describes what happens during asthma attacks and explains how asthma is treated and managed.
12 pages

1358   Nocturnal Asthma
National Jewish Center for Immunology
1400 Jackson Street   303-388-4461
Denver, CO 80206-2762
Offers information to patients about how to understand and manage asthma at night.

1359   Occupational Asthma
American Academy of Allergy, Asthma and Immunology
611 E Wells Street   414-272-6071
Milwaukee, WI 53202-3889   800-822-2762
                                                           Fax: 414-272-6070
                                                           www.aaaai.org
This brochure also contains a list of most common agents theat cause occupational asthma and who is at risk.

1360   Occupational Asthma: Lung Hazards on the Job
American Lung Association
1740 Broadway   212-315-8700
New York, NY 10019-4315
Discusses occupational asthma, a form of asthma in which airways overreact to various irritants in the workplace.

1361   Outpatient Treatment of Asthma
American Academy of Allergy, Asthma and Immunology
611 E Wells Street   414-272-6071
Milwaukee, WI 53202-3889   800-822-2762
                                                           Fax: 414-272-6070
                                                           www.aaaai.org

1362   Peak Flow Meter: A Thermometer for Asthma
American Academy of Allergy, Asthma and Immunology

611 E Wells Street   414-272-6071
Milwaukee, WI 53202-3889   800-822-2762
                                                           Fax: 414-272-6070
                                                           www.aaaai.org

1363   Pollen and Spores Around the World
American Academy of Allergy, Asthma and Immunology
611 E Wells Street   414-272-6071
Milwaukee, WI 53202-3889   800-822-2762
                                                           Fax: 414-272-6070
                                                           www.aaaai.org
Multi-paged brochure offering graphes and tables of pollen levels and different times of the year in different parts of the country.
10 pages

1364   Removing House Dust and Other Allergic Irritants From Your Home
American Academy of Allergy, Asthma and Immunology
611 E Wells Street   414-272-6071
Milwaukee, WI 53202-3889   800-822-2762
                                                           Fax: 414-272-6070
                                                           www.aaaai.org
This brochure covers some good ideas on how to reduce dust in the home.

1365   Role of the Allergist & Clinical Immunologist in Patient Care
American Academy of Allergy, Asthma and Immunology
611 E Wells Street   414-272-6071
Milwaukee, WI 53202-3889   800-822-2762
                                                           Fax: 414-272-6070
                                                           www.aaaai.org
An informational brochure containing definitions and addresses for further information.

1366   School Information Packet
Allergy and Asthma Network/Mothers of Asthmatics
2751 Prosperity Avenue   703-641-9595
Fairfax, VA 22031-4397   800-878-4403
                                                           Fax: 703-573-7794
                                                           www.mothersofasthmatics.org
Practical, medical, and legal information for school administrators and parents of students with asthma.
Mary McGowan, Executive Director
Nancy Sander, Editor-in-Chief

1367   Standards for the Diagnosis and Care of Patients with Asthma
American Lung Association
1740 Broadway   212-315-8700
New York, NY 10019-4315
Standards developed by the American Thoracic Society, the medical section of the ALA. For physicians.
24 pages

1368   Student Asthma Action Card
Asthma and Allergy Foundation of America
1233 20th Street NW   202-466-7643
Washington, DC 20036-2330   800-727-8462
                                                           Fax: 202-466-8940
                                                           www.aafa.org
Indispensable tool for familiarizing school personnel with asthma triggers, daily medications and emergency directions for each of their students with asthma.

1369   Superstuff
American Lung Association
1740 Broadway   212-315-8700
New York, NY 10019-4315
Kit specifically designed to help the elementary schoolchild with asthma to learn how to manage the condition. The kit contains teaching tools, puzzles, riddles, stories and games.

1370   Teens Talk to Teens About Asthma
Asthma and Allergy Foundation of America
1233 20th Street NW   202-466-7643
Washington, DC 20036-2330   800-727-8462
                                                           Fax: 202-466-8940
                                                           www.aafa.org
Quotes and thoughts from teens capture the essence of what it feels like to have asthma.

1371 There are Solutions for the Student with Asthma
American Lung Association
1740 Broadway   212-315-8700
New York, NY 10017
Leaflet telling how parents and school personnel can work together to make life easier for children with asthma.
4 pages

1372 Tips to Remember
American Academy of Allergy, Asthma and Immunology
611 E Wells Street   414-272-6071
Milwaukee, WI 53202-3889
A set of 23 tip sheets offering information on various topics including allergy and asthma treatments, pregnancy and asthma, animal allergies, sinusitis and more.

1373 Tips to Remember Brochures
American Academy of Allergy, Asthma and Immunology
611 E Wells Street   414-272-6071
Milwaukee, WI 53202-3889   800-822-2762
                            Fax: 414-272-6070
                                 www.aaaai.org
Thirty three colorful brochures offered on numerous topics in allergy, asthma, and immunology.

1374 Triggers of Asthma
American Academy of Allergy, Asthma and Immunology
611 E Wells Street   414-272-6071
Milwaukee, WI 53202-3889   800-822-2762
                            Fax: 414-272-6070
                                 www.aaaai.org
This brochure gives helpful information on what will cause an asthma attack.

1375 Understanding Asthma
National Jewish Center for Immunology
1400 Jackson Street   303-388-4461
Denver, CO 80206
Offers a brief introduction to asthma and then goes into the physiology of asthma, the triggers of asthma, and diagnosis and monitoring of asthma.
27 pages

1376 Understanding Immunology
National Jewish Center for Immunology
1400 Jackson Street   303-388-4461
Denver, CO 80206-2762
Offers information to patients and the public on the body's defenses. Explains how immunity develops, the basics of immunologic medicine and coping with respiratory disorders.

1377 Understanding Your Child with Asthma
National Jewish Center for Immunology
1400 Jackson Street   303-388-4461
Denver, CO 80206-2762   800-222-5264
Offers information on patient care, research, education and adult programs offered by the Association.

1378 Understanding the Pollen and Mold Season
American Academy of Allergy, Asthma and Immunology
611 E Wells Street   414-272-6071
Milwaukee, WI 53202-3889   800-822-2762
                            Fax: 414-272-6070
                                 www.aaaai.org

1379 Unproven Methods in Diagnosing and Treating Allergies
Asthma and Allergy Foundation of America
1233 20th Street NW   202-466-7643
Washington, DC 20036-2330   800-727-8462
                            Fax: 202-466-8940
                                 www.aafa.org

1380 Use of Steroids for Asthma and Allergies
American Academy of Allergy, Asthma and Immunology
611 E Wells Street   414-272-6071
Milwaukee, WI 53202-3889   800-822-2762
                            Fax: 414-272-6070
                                 www.aaaai.org

1381 What Every Patient Should Know About Asthma & Allergy Medications
American Academy of Allergy, Asthma and Immunology
611 E Wells Street   414-272-6071
Milwaukee, WI 53202-3889   800-822-2762
                            Fax: 414-272-6070
                                 www.aaaai.org

1382 What is an Allergic Reaction?
American Academy of Allergy, Asthma and Immunology
611 E Wells Street   414-272-6071
Milwaukee, WI 53202-3889   800-822-2762
                            Fax: 414-272-6070
                                 www.aaaai.org
This brochure gives helpful information on what will cause an allergic reaction.

1383 Your Child and Asthma
National Jewish Center for Immunology
1400 Jackson Street   303-388-4461
Denver, CO 80206-2762
A booklet offerring information to parents and family about their child with asthma. Offers information on diagnosis, treatments, triggers and family concerns.

Audio & Video

1384 Asthma Handbook Slides
American Lung Association
1740 Broadway   212-315-8700
New York, NY 10019-4315
Slides and script based on The Asthma Handbook for asthma patients and others.
Film

1385 Asthma Management
American Academy of Allergy, Asthma and Immunology
611 E Wells Street   414-272-6071
Milwaukee, WI 53202-3889   800-822-2762
                            Fax: 414-272-6070
                                 www.aaaai.org
Although there is currently no cure for asthma, attacks can be controlled by appropriate asthma management. This video describes what happens during an asthma attack, how your allergists diagnoses asthma, and ways your allergist can help you to manage your condition.
10-13 minutes

1386 Asthma and the Athlete
American Academy of Allergy, Asthma and Immunology
611 E Wells Street   414-272-6071
Milwaukee, WI 53202   800-822-2762
                            Fax: 414-272-6070
                                 www.aaaai.org
In the past, people with asthma were sometimes discouraged from exercising. Today we know that everyone, including asthmatics, can benefit from physical actilvity. This video details which exercises are best for those with asthma, and how an allergist can help asthmatic athletes to properly manage and treat their disease.
10-13 minutes

1387 Environmental Control Measures
American Academy of Allergy, Asthma and Immunology
611 E Wells Street   414-272-6071
Milwaukee, WI 53202-3889   800-822-2762
                            Fax: 414-272-6070
                                 www.aaaai.org
By conrtolling your environment, you can reduce your exposure to substances called allergens that trigger your allergic symptoms. This program depicts common outdoor and indoor allergens, methods an allergist uses to diagnose which substances you're allergic to, and how to reduce your exposure to allergic triggers.
10-13 minutes

1388 I'm a Meter Reader
Allergy and Asthma Network/Mothers of Asthmatics

2751 Prosperity Avenue   703-641-9595
Fairfax, VA 22031-4397   800-878-4403
      Fax: 703-573-7794
      www.mothersofasthmatics.org

Provides expert advice on how a peak flow meter can help detect when an asthma attack can occur in an easy to understand format. Companion book, I'm a Meter Reader, available as part of a set for $12.00.
Video
Mary McGowan, Executive Director
Nancy Sander, Editor-in-Chief

1389 Immunotherapy
American Academy of Allergy, Asthma and Immunology
611 E Wells Street   414-272-6071
Milwaukee, WI 53202-3889   800-822-2762
      Fax: 414-272-6070
      www.aaaai.org

Immunotherapy, of allergy shots, is a long-term allergy and asthma treatment program that helps control allergic symptoms and reduces the need for medications. Learn more about immunotherapy through this video, which includes information on allergy testing and how your allergist determines if immunotherapy is right for you.
10-13 minutes

1390 Managing Asthma in School: An Action Plan
Asthma and Allergy Foundation of America
1233 20th Street NW   202-466-7643
Washington, DC 20036-2330   800-727-8462
      Fax: 202-466-8940
      www.aafa.org

Gives the basics of asthma and a plan for school nurses, parents and physicians to work together.
14 minutes

1391 Managing Childhood Asthma
American Lung Association
Box 596-COL   212-245-8000
New York, NY 10001   800-586-4872
      Fax: 312-440-9374
      e-mail: webmaster@ala.org
      www.ala.org

What parents need to know to manage asthma. 22 minutes.
Video

1392 Pharmacologic Therapy of Pediatric Asthma
American Lung Association
1740 Broadway   212-315-8700
New York, NY 10019-4315

A Learning Resource Program developed by a joint committee of the American Thoracic Society and the ALA.
Film

1393 Regular Kid
American Lung Association
1740 Broadway   212-315-8700
New York, NY 10019-4315

This film shows how families and children cope with asthma problems. Proven asthma management strategies are presented through the experiences of four children with asthma, ranging in age from toddler to teenager.
Film

1394 So You Have Asthma Too!
Allergy and Asthma Network/Mothers of Asthmatics
2751 Prosperity Avenue   703-641-9595
Fairfax, VA 22031-4397   800-878-4403
      Fax: 703-573-7794
      www.mothersofasthmatics.org

Offers a clear description and understanding of childhood asthma.
Video
Mary McGowan, Executive Director
Nancy Sander, Editor-in-Chief

1395 Stinging Insect Allergy
American Academy of Allergy, Asthma and Immunology

611 E Wells Street   414-272-6071
Milwaukee, WI 53202-3889   800-822-2762
      Fax: 414-272-6070
      www.aaaai.org

Although many people are afraid of stinging insects such as bees, the stings of these insects actually cause some people to have serious allergic reactions. This video tells how to recognize and avoid stinging insects, what to do if you are stung and how to identify symptoms of an allergic reaction and get medical help.
10-13 minutes

1396 Understanding Allergic Reactions
American Academy of Allergy, Asthma and Immunology
611 E Wells Street   414-272-6071
Milwaukee, WI 53202-3889   800-822-2762
      Fax: 414-272-6070
      www.aaaai.org

During an allergic reaction, your body responds to a substance generally considered harmless to most people. This video portrays what happens in you body's immune system during an allergic reaction, how to avoid allergic substances, and methods your allergist uses to treat your allergies.
10-13 minutes

1397 What School Personnel Should Know About Asthma
American Lung Association
1740 Broadway   212-315-8700
New York, NY 10019-4315

Professionally produced videotape discussing the triggers, symptoms and management of childhood asthma.
Videotape

1398 You're in Charge: Teens with Asthma
Asthma and Allergy Foundation of America
1233 20th Street NW   202-466-7643
Washington, DC 20036-2330   800-727-8462
      Fax: 202-466-8940
      www.aafa.org

Designed for young adults dealing with the daily challenges of asthma management. Teens share their experiences and use of peak flow meters and prescribed medications.
10 minutes

Web Sites

1399 American Academy of Allergy, Asthma and Immunology
      www.aaaai.org
The largest professional medical organization devoted to the allergy/immunology specialty. Represents asthma specialists, clinical immunologists, allied health professionals and others with a special interest in the research and treatment of allergic disease.

1400 American College of Allergy, Asthma and Immunology
      www.acaai.org
A professional association of more than 5,000 allergists/immunologists and allied health professionals whose mission is to promote excellence in the practice of the subspecialty of allergy and immunology.

1401 American Lung Association
      www.lungusa.org
To save lives by improving lung health and preventing lung disease.

1402 Asthma and Allergy Foundation of America
      www.aafa.org
Dedicated to improving the quality of life for people with asthma and allergic diseases through education, advocacy and research.

1403 Gazoontite
      www.gazoontite.com
Provides links to websites involving asthma and also asthma-related products, such as books and guides.

1404 Healingwell
      www.healingwell.com
A social network and support community for patients, caregivers, and families coping with the daily struggles of diseases, disorders and chronic illness.

1405 Health Finder

www.healthfinder.gov

A government web site where individuals can find information and tools to help you and those you care about stay healthy.

1406 Healthlink USA

www.healthlinkusa.com

Health information concerning treatment, cures, prevention, diagnosis, risk factors, research, support groups, email lists, personal stories and much more. Updated regularly.

1407 Helios Health

www.helioshealth.com

Online resource for your health information. Detailed information about specific health topics, access to expert advice from our Medical Advisory Board, and up-to-date health news.

1408 MedicineNet

www.medicinenet.com

An online resource for consumers providing easy-to-read, authoritative medical and health information.

1409 Medscape

www.medscape.com

Medscape offers specialists, primary care physicians, and other health professionals the Web's most robust and integrated medical information and educational tools.

1410 WebMD

www.webmd.com

Provides links to over 100 articles involving asthma information.

Description

1411 Ataxia

Ataxia refers to a group of diseases that cause failure of muscular coordination, resulting in a staggered gait, the inability to stand or sit straight and the inability to make smooth, voluntary movements. All ataxias involve deterioration of the cerebellum and/or the brain and spinal structures that communicate with it. Conditions that are associated with ataxia may be hereditary or sporadic.

The most common hereditary ataxia is Friedreich's ataxia, which typically begins between 5 and 15 years of age. At first there is gait unsteadiness and slurred speech which progresses to weakness of the extremities. Some patients develop spinal deformity or cardiac problems. Other, less common hereditary ataxias generally begin during adult life. Sporadic cases also begin in adulthood and may be due to toxins, such as alcohol, or may be of unknown cause. Sporadic cases are often a symptom of some other disease, such as multiple sclerosis, stroke, or vitamin deficiencies. Although essentially all patients will become wheelchair-dependent at some point, the outlook for long-term survival is good.

Treatment for any of the ataxias is aimed at the underlying cause, but often supportive, with physical therapy, assistive devices, psychological support, career counseling and treatment of complications. Genetic counseling is appropriate for those with the hereditary forms and their families.

National Agencies & Associations

1412 National Ataxia Foundation
2600 Fernbrook Lane   763-553-0020
Minneapolis, MN 55447   Fax: 763-553-0167
e-mail: naf@ataxia.org
www.ataxia.org
The National Ataxia Foundation is dedicated to improving the lives of persons affected by ataxia through support education and research.
Michael Parent, Executive Director
Susan Hagen, Patient Services Director

1413 National Health Information Center
PO Box 1133   310-565-4167
Washington, DC 20013   800-336-4797
Fax: 301-984-4256
e-mail: info@nhic.org
www.health.gov/nhic
Offers a nationwide information referral service, produces directories and resource guides.

Support Groups & Hotlines

Alabama

1414 Alabama Ambassador: National Ataxia Foundation
123 Leigh Ann Road   256-828-4858
Hazel Green, AL 35750   e-mail: diannebw@aol.com
www.ataxia.org
Ambassadors are often in areas not served by a support group or chapter.
Dianne Blaine-Williamson, NAF Ambassador

1415 Alabama Support Group: National Ataxia Foundation
16 Oaks Circle   205-531-2514
Birmingham, AL 35244   e-mail: donnellyB6132@aol.com
www.ataxia.org
Becky Donnelly, Group Contact

Arizona

1416 Phoenix Area Support Group: National Ataxi a Foundation
2322 W Sagebrush Drive   480-726-3579
Chandler, AZ 85224-2155   e-mail: rtg22@cox.net
www.ataxia.org
Rita Garcia, Director

1417 Tucson Support Group: National Ataxia Foundation
7665 E Placita Luna Preciosa   520-885-8326
Tucson, AZ 85710   e-mail: bbeck15@cox.net
www.ataxia.org
Bart Beck, Director

California

1418 California Ambassador: National Ataxia Foundation
315 W Alamos   559-281-9188
Clovis, CA 93612   e-mail: mike betchel@yahoo.com
www.ataxia.org
Mike Betchel, NAF Ambassador

1419 Los Angeles Support Group: National Ataxia Foundation
339 W Palmer   818-246-5758
Glendale, CA 91204   e-mail: harryluther@sbcglobal.net
www.ataxia.org
Sid Luther, President

1420 Northern California Support Group: National Ataxia Foundation
26840 Eldridge Avenue   510-783-3190
Hayward, CA 94544   e-mail: rsisbig@aol.com
www.ataxia.com
Deborah Ominctin, Leader

1421 Orange County Support Group: National Ataxia Foundation
829 W Gary Ave   323-788-7751
Montebello, CA 90640   e-mail: dnavar@ucla.edu
www.ataxia.org
Daniel Navar, Group Leader

1422 San Diego Support Group: National Ataxia Foundation
2087 Granite Hills Drive   619-447-3753
El Cajon, CA 92019   e-mail: sdasg@cox.net
www.ataxia.org
Earl McLaughlin, Group Leader

Colorado

1423 Denver Support Group: National Ataxia Foundation
5902 W Maplewood Drive   303-973-8035
Littleton, CO 80123   e-mail: tom_sathre@acm.org
www.ataxia.org
Tom Sathre, Group Leader

Florida

1424 Florida Ambassador: National Ataxia Foundation
302 Beach Drive   850-654-2817
Destin, FL 30541   e-mail: csugars@cox.net
www.ataxia.org
Ambassadors are often in areas not served by a support group or chapter.
Christina Sugars, NAF Ambassador

1425 Northwest Florida Support Group: National Ataxia Foundation
54 Troon Terrace   904-273-4644
Ponte Vedra, FL 32082-3321   e-mail: jmcgranepvb@bellsouth.net
www.ataxia.org
June McGrane, Group Leader

1426 West Central FL Support Group: National Ataxia Foundation
9753 Elm Way
Tampa, FL 33635
813-453-1084
e-mail: flataxia@yahoo.com
www.ataxia.org

Crystal Frohna, Group Leader

Georgia

1427 Georgia Support Group: National Ataxia Foundation
320 Peters Street
Savannah, GA 30313
404-822-7451
e-mail: rookssgj@yahoo.com
www.ataxia.org

Greg Rooks, Group Leader

Illinois

1428 Chicago Area Support Group: National Ataxia Foundation
410 W Mahogany Ct
Palatine, IL 60067
847-496-7544
e-mail: caasg2@aol.com
www.ataxia.org

Craig Lisack, Group Leader

1429 Chicago Metro Support Group: National Ataxia Foundation
5633 N Kenmore
Chicago, IL 60660
773-334-1667
e-mail: cmarsh34@ameritech.net
www.ataxia.org

Chris Marsh, Group Leader

Indiana

1430 Southern Indiana Support Group: National Ataxia Foundation
1102 Ridgewood Drive
Huntingburg, IN 47542
812-630-4783
e-mail: monicasfaith@insightbb.com
www.ataxia.org

Monica Smith, Group Leader

Louisiana

1431 Louisiana Support Group: National Ataxia Foundation
2250 Gause Blvd
Slidell, LA 70431
985-643-0783
e-mail: ataxia1@earthlink.net
www.ataxia.org

Charlene Danielson, President
Camille Daglio, Vice-President

Maine

1432 Maine Support Group: National Ataxia Foundation
PO Box 113
Bowdoinham, ME 04008
e-mail: rollins@gwi.net
www.ataxia.org

Kelly Rollins, Group Leader

Maryland

1433 Chesapeake Area Support Group: National Ataxia Foundation
3200 Baker Circle
Adamstown, MD 21710-9666
301-644-1836
e-mail: carljlauter@erols.com
www.ataxia.org

Carl J Lauter, Group Leader

Massachusetts

1434 New England Area Support Group: National Ataxia Foundation
45 Juliette Street
Andover, MA 01810
978-475-8072
www.ataxia.org

Donna Gorzela, Group Leader

Michigan

1435 Detroit Support Group: National Ataxia Foundation
20217 Wyoming
Detroit, MI 48221
313-736-2827
e-mail: tinyt48221@yahoo.cpom
www.ataxia.org

Tanya Tunstul, Group Leader

Minnesota

1436 Minnesota Ambassador: National Ataxia Foundation
5179 Meadow Drive SE
Rochester, MN 55904
504-282-7127
e-mail: logoetz@gmail.com
www.ataxia.org

Lori Goetzman, NAF Ambassador

1437 Twin Cities Area Support Group: National Ataxia Foundation
2549 32nd Avenue S
Minneapolis, MN 55406
612-724-3487
e-mail: lschultz@bitstream.net
www.ataxia.org

Lenore Healy Schultz, Group Leader

Mississippi

1438 Mississippi Area Support Group: National Ataxia Foundation
PO Box 17005
Hattisburg, MS 39404
e-mail: daglio1@bellsouth.net
www.ataxia.org

Camille Daglio, Group Leader

Missouri

1439 Kansas City Support Group: National Ataxia Foundation
17700 E 17th Terrace Court S
Independence, MO 64057
816-257-2428
www.ataxia.org

Lois Goodman, Group Leader

1440 Mid Missouri Support Group: National Ataxia Foundation
1609 Cocoa Court
Columbia, MO 65202
573-474-7232
e-mail: rogercooley@localnet.com
www.ataxia.org

Roger Cooley, Contact

New York

1441 Central NY Area Support Group: National Ataxia Foundation
2849 Bingley Road
Cazenovia, NY 13035
e-mail: johnsons@summitsolutions.net
www.ataxia.org

Linda Johnson, President

1442 New York Ambassador National Ataxia Foundation
36 W Redoubt Rd
Fishkill, NY 12524
763-553-0020
e-mail: vrabsolutely@aol.com
www.ataxia.org

Valerie Ruggiero, NAF Ambassador

1443 Tri-State Area Support Group: National Ataxia Foundation
Northgate 6C
Bronxville, NY 10708
212-844-8711
e-mail: markmeghan@aol.com
www.ataxia.org

Mark Mitchell, Group Leader

Ohio

1444 Central Ohio Support Group: National Ataxia Foundation
7852 Country Court
Mentor, OH 44060
440-255-8284
e-mail: wurbanski@oh.rr.com
www.ataxia.org

Cecilia Urbanski, Group Leader

1445 North East Ohio Support Group National Ataxia Foundation
PO Box 148
Mesopotamia, OH 44439
440-693-4454
e-mail: kakah@windstream.net
www.ataxia.org

Joe Miller, President

1446 Ohio Ambassador: National Ataxia Foundation
1283 Westfield SW
North Canton, OH 44720
330-499-4060
e-mail: jkardos@juno.com
www.ataxia.org

James Kardos, NAF Ambassador

Oklahoma

1447 **Oklahoma Ambassador: National Ataxia Foundation**
5700 SE Hazel Road   918-331-9530
Bartlesville, OK 74006   e-mail: droopydog36@hotmail.com
                                                www.ataxia.org

Darrell Owens, NAF Ambassador

Oregon

1448 **Willamette Valley Support Group: National Ataxia Foundation**
Albany General Hospital   541-812-4162
Albany, OR 97321   Fax: 541-812-4614
                                      e-mail: malindam@samhealth.org
                                                www.ataxia.org

Malinda Moore, President

South Carolina

1449 **Carolinas Support Group: National Ataxia National Ataxia Foundation**
1305 Cely Road   864-220-3395
Easley, SC 29642   e-mail: cecerussell@hotmail.com
                                                www.ataxia.org

Cece Russell, Group Leader

Texas

1450 **Houston Support Group: National Ataxia Foundation**
9405 Highway 6 S   281-693-1826
Houston, TX 77083   e-mail: angelahcloud@aol.com
                                                www.ataxia.org

Angela Cloud, Group Leader

1451 **North Texas Support Group: National Ataxia Foundation**
7 Wentworth Court
Trophy Club, TX 76262   e-mail: cheve11e@sbcglobal.net
                                                www.ataxia.org

David Henry Jr, Group Leader

1452 **Texas Ambassador: National Ataxia Foundation**
356 Las Brisas Blvd   830-557-6050
Seguin, TX 78155-0193   e-mail: acemom@peoplepc.com
                                                www.ataxia.org

Charlene Danielson, President
Camilie Daglio, Vice-President

Utah

1453 **Utah Support Group: National Ataxia Foundation**
Moran Eye Clinic   801-585-2213
Salt Lake City, UT 84132   e-mail: julia.kleinschmidt@hsc.utah.edu
                                                www.ataxia.org

Dr Julia Kleinschmidt, Group Leader

Washington

1454 **Seattle Support Group: National Ataxia Foundation**
14104 107th Avenue   425-823-6239
Kirkland, WA 98034   e-mail: ataxiaseattle@comcast.net
                            www.ataxia.org/chapters/Seattle/default.
Milly Lewendon, Group Leader

1455 **Washington Ambassador National Ataxia Foundation**
PO Box 19045
Spokane, WA 99219   509-482-8501
                                                www.ataxia.org

Linda Jacoy, Ambassador

Books

1456 **Directory of National Genetic Voluntary Organizations**
Genetic Alliance
4301 Connecticut Avenue NW   202-966-5557
Washington, DC 20008-2369   800-336-4363
                                    Fax: 202-966-8553
                                e-mail: info@geneticalliance.org
                                            www.geneticalliance.org

Lists hundreds of organizations and associations dealing with genetic conditions.

1457 **Hereditary Ataxia: Guidebook for Managing Speech & Swallowing**
National Ataxia Foundation
2600 Fernbrook Lane N   763-553-0020
Minneapolis, MN 55447-4752   Fax: 763-553-0167
                                       e-mail: naf@mr.net
                                                www.ataxia.org

1458 **Living with Ataxia**
National Ataxia Foundation
2600 Fernbrook Lane N   763-553-0020
Minneapolis, MN 55447-4752   Fax: 763-553-0167
                                       e-mail: naf@mr.net
                                                www.ataxia.org

Compassionate resource for people who have or may be at risk of having ataxia, and for their families. This book explains the nature and causes of ataxia, the basic genetics that underlie many kinds of ataxia, discusses medical management of ataxia, provides practical advice for everyday living, points the way to many useful resources and assures that living a good life is an entirely reasonable aspiration, even with ataxia.
112 pages

1459 **Ten Years to Live**
National Ataxia Foundation
2600 Fernbrook Lane N   763-553-0020
Minneapolis, MN 55447-4752   Fax: 763-553-0167
                                       e-mail: naf@mr.net
                                                www.ataxia.org

Struggles of the Schut family with hereditary ataxia.

ISBN: 0-962716-63-1

Newsletters

1460 **Alert**
Alliance of Genetic Support Groups
4301 Connecticut Avenue NW   301-652-5553
Washington, DC 20008-2304   800-336-4363
                                e-mail: alliance@capaccess.org
                                www.medhelp.org/www/agsg2.htm
Functions as a vehicle of communication between the Alliance and its constituency. Provides timely and useful information on genetics research.
Monthly

1461 **GENES Information Services**
Genetic Network of the Empire State
Empire State Plaza   518-474-7148
Albany, NY 12201   Fax: 518-474-8590

1462 **Generations**
National Ataxia Foundation
2600 Fernbrook Lane N   763-553-0020
Minneapolis, MN 55447-4752   Fax: 763-553-0167
                                       e-mail: naf@mr.net
                                                www.ataxia.org

Provides the latest in ataxia research, information on coping, reference material, updates on chapters and support groups and personal stories on living with ataxia. With a readership of more than 25,000, this publication is distributed throughout the US and the world. This publication is for ataxia families, the medical community, ataxia researchers and interested individuals. This publication is free to NAF members.
Quarterly

1463 **Genexus**
Great Plains Genetic Service Network
The University of Iowa   319-356-2674
Iowa City, IA 52242   Fax: 319-356-3347

1464 **Great Lakes Genetic News**
Great Lakes Regional Genetics Group
1500 Highland Avenue   608-266-2907
Madison, WI 53705-2274   Fax: 608-263-3496

1465 MARGIN
Mid-Atlantic Regional Human Genetics Network
260 S Broad Street   215-456-7910
Philadelphia, PA 19102-5021   Fax: 215-456-7911

1466 MSRGSN Newsletter
Mountain States Regional Genetics Service Network
4300 Cherry Creek Drive S   303-692-2423
Denver, CO 80246   Fax: 303-782-5576
                e-mail: joyce.hooker@state.co.us
                                www.mostgene.org

8-12 pages
Joyce Hooker, Coordinator

1467 NERG News
New England Regional Genetics Group
PO Box 670   207-839-5324
Mount Desert, ME 04660-0670   Fax: 207-839-8637

1468 SERGG
Southeast Regional Genetics Group
PO Box 1642   404-778-8551
Decatur, GA 30031-1642   Fax: 404-778-8562
                        e-mail: mlane@sergginc.org
                                        sergginc.org

Pamphlets

1469 Alliance Brochure
Genetic Alliance
4301 Connecticut Avenue NW   202-966-5557
Washington, DC 20008-2304   Fax: 202-966-8553
                        e-mail: info@geneticalliance.org
                                www.geneticalliance.org
Explains the services and programs offered by the alliance.

1470 Ataxia Fact Sheet
National Ataxia Foundation
2600 Fernbrook Lane N   763-553-0020
Minneapolis, MN 55447-4752   Fax: 763-553-0167
                                e-mail: naf@mr.net
                                        www.ataxia.org
Describes ataxia as a symptom and its association with other medical problems as well as the hereditary types.

1471 Familial Spastic Paraplegia
National Ataxia Foundation
2600 Fernbrook Lane N   763-553-0020
Minneapolis, MN 55447-4752   Fax: 763-553-0167
                                e-mail: naf@mr.net
                                        www.ataxia.org
Defines this disorder and notes symptoms, causes and treatments.

1472 Frenkel's Exercises
National Ataxia Foundation
2600 Fernbrook Lane N   763-553-0020
Minneapolis, MN 55447-4752   Fax: 763-553-0167
                                e-mail: naf@mr.net
                                        www.ataxia.org
Describes an exercise program designed for those with ataxia.

1473 Friedrich's Ataxia
National Ataxia Foundation
2600 Fernbrook Lane N   763-553-0020
Minneapolis, MN 55447-4752   Fax: 763-553-0167
                                e-mail: naf@mr.net
                                        www.ataxia.org
Describes symptoms, diagnosis, genetics and hints on coping.

1474 Gene Testing for Ataxia
National Ataxia Foundation
2600 Fernbrook Lane N   763-553-0020
Minneapolis, MN 55447-4752   Fax: 763-553-0167
                                e-mail: naf@mr.net
                                        www.ataxia.org
Describes the latest information about who should consider it and where to have it done.

1475 Health Insurance
National Ataxia Foundation

2600 Fernbrook Lane N   763-553-0020
Minneapolis, MN 55447-4752   Fax: 763-553-0167
                                e-mail: naf@mr.net
                                        www.ataxia.org
Offers health insurance advice for persons with ataxia.

1476 Hereditary Ataxia: Brochure
National Ataxia Foundation
2600 Fernbrook Lane N   763-553-0020
Minneapolis, MN 55447-4752   Fax: 763-553-0167
                                e-mail: naf@mr.net
                                        www.ataxia.org
Describes recessive and dominant ataxias, information on how hereditary ataxia is transmitted and explanations of the NAF's role in education, service and prevention.

1477 Hereditary Ataxia: Fact Sheets
National Ataxia Foundation
2600 Fernbrook Lane N   763-553-0020
Minneapolis, MN 55447-4752   Fax: 763-553-0167
                                e-mail: naf@mr.net
                                        www.ataxia.org
Various ataxia fact sheets relating to specific forms of hereditary ataxia. Individual ataxia fact sheets include Friederich's ataxia and specific forms of spinocerebellar ataxias (SCAs).

1478 Incorporating Consumers into Regional Genetics Networks
Genetic Alliance
4301 Connecticut Avenue NW   202-966-5557
Washington, DC 20008-2304   Fax: 202-966-8553
                        e-mail: info@geneticalliance.org
                                www.geneticalliance.org

1479 Informed Consent: Participation In Genetic Research Studies
Genetic Alliance
4301 Connecticut Avenue NW   202-966-5557
Washington, DC 20008-2304   Fax: 202-966-8553
                        e-mail: info@genticalliance.org
                                www.geneticalliance.org
This booklet explains the nature of genetic research with its benefits and risks.

1480 Pen-Pal Directory
National Ataxia Foundation
2600 Fernbrook Lane N   763-553-0020
Minneapolis, MN 55447-4752   Fax: 763-553-0167
                                e-mail: naf@mr.net
                                        www.ataxia.org
National, state and international directory of others who are affected by ataxia. Available to NAF Pen-Pal members only. Application available.

1481 Students with Friedreich's Ataxia
National Ataxia Foundation
2600 Fernbrook Lane N   763-553-0020
Minneapolis, MN 55447-4752   Fax: 763-553-0167
                                e-mail: naf@mr.net
                                        www.ataxia.org
Worksheet for teachers, parents and others who need to understand the physical constraints of ataxia.

Audio & Video

1482 Together...There Is Hope
National Ataxia Foundation
2600 Fernbrook Lane N   763-553-0020
Minneapolis, MN 55447-4752   Fax: 763-553-0167
                                e-mail: naf@mr.net
                                        www.ataxia.org
Video discussing ataxias genetic patterns of inheritance and the National Ataxia Foundation and its research efforts.

Web Sites

1483 Healing Well
                                www.healingwell.com
An online health resource guide to medical news, chat, information and articles, newsgroups and message boards, books, dis-

ease-related web sites, medical directories, and more for patients, friends, and family coping with disabling diseases, disorders, or chronic illnesses.

1484 Health Finder

www.healthfinder.gov

Searchable, carefully developed web site offering information on over 1000 topics. Developed by the US Department of Health and Human Services, the site can be used in both English and Spanish.

1485 Healthlink USA

www.healthlinkusa.com

Health information concerning treatment, cures, prevention, diagnosis, risk factors, research, support groups, email lists, personal stories and much more. Updated regularly.

1486 Helios Health

www.helioshealth.com

Online resource for your health information. Detailed information about specific health topics, access to expert advice from our Medical Advisory Board, and up-to-date health news.

1487 MedicineNet

www.medicinenet.com

An online resource for consumers providing easy-to-read, authoritative medical and health information.

1488 Medscape

www.medscape.com

Medscape offers specialists, primary care physicians, and other health professionals the Web's most robust and integrated medical information and educational tools.

1489 National Ataxia Foundation

www.ataxia.org

Information on ataxia, ataxia research, listing of chapters and support groups and related links. Researchers may download NAF's ataxia reserch application guidelines and forms. Exerpts of articles in NAF's quarterly news publication, Generations. Online registration for NAF's annual membership meetings. Caladar of events on NAF activities. This site is for ataxia familes, the medical community, ataxia reserachers and interested individuals.

1490 WebMD

www.webmd.com

Information on Ataxia, including articles and resources.

Description

1491 Attention Deficit Hyperactivity Disorder

Attention Deficit-Hyperactivity Disorder, ADHD, and Attention Deficit Disorder, ADD, are neurologically based disorders. ADHD primarily affects children, with 2 to 4 percent of the school-age population in the United States having some symptoms. In about 25 percent of attention deficit cases, hyperactivity is not present, and it is thus labeled ADD. ADHD's three major symptoms are distractibility, impulsivity and hyperactivity. The dominant symptom of ADD is day dreaming or tuning out. ADHD is seen 10 times more frequently in boys than girls. Studies show that 90 percent have academic problems or are underachievers, although these difficulties may not begin until the middle school years.

While studies suggest that about 50 percent of children with these disorders will improve at puberty, both ADHD and ADD can exist throughout a lifetime and, in fact, may first be diagnosed in teen or adult years.

Often, an affected individual experiences difficulties that can impact learning, peer relations, family life, and self-esteem. These difficulties may manifest themselves through angry outbursts, self-imposed social isolation, blaming others, a quickness to fight, and a high sensitivity to criticism.

Treatment of ADHD and ADD include: education programs with resource or tutorial help; psychological programs to improve self-esteem and help families and individuals deal with associated stress; and medical therapy. Treatment must be individualized to address both intrinsic characteristics of the child and relevant environmental factors, and be coordinated with a variety of interventions within the school, home and community.

Many professionals agree that medication, when appropriate, combined with counseling, best controls symptoms. Stimulant medications, including the new longer active agents, are the drugs of choice. To identify children with this disorder and to develop the most appropriate treatment plan, parents will need to consult with a psychiatrist, pediatric neurologist, or pediatrician.

National Agencies & Associations

1492 Children & Adults with Attention Deficit Disorders
8181 Professional Place
Landover, MD 20785

301-306-7070
800-233-4050
Fax: 301-306-7090
www.chadd.org

CHADD's primary objectives are: to provide a support network for parents and caregivers; to provide a forum for continuing education; to be a community resource and disseminate accurate evidence-based information about AD/HD to parents, educators and adults.
E Clarke Ross, CEO
Ruth Hughes, Chief Program Officer Community Service

1493 Council for Exceptional Children
2900 Crystal Drive
Arlington, VA 22202-3557

703-620-3660
88 -23 -773
Fax: 703-264-9494
TTY: 866-915-5000
e-mail: service@cec.sped.org
www.cec.sped.org

Advocates appropriate policies standards and development for individuals with special needs. Provides professional development for special educators.
Bruce Ramirez, Executive Director
Joan Melner, Assistant Executive Director

1494 Feingold Association of the US
37 Shell Road
Rocky Point, NY 11778

631-369-9340
800-321-3287
Fax: 631-369-2988
e-mail: help@feingold.org
www.feingold.org

Helps families of children with learning and behavior problems including attention deficit disorder. Also helps chemically-sensitive and salicylate-sensitive adults. Program is based upon a diet which primarily eliminates certain synthetic food additives.

1495 Learning Disabilities Association of America
4156 Library Road
Pittsburgh, PA 15234-1349

412-341-1515
888-300-6710
Fax: 412-344-0224
e-mail: info@LDAAmerica.org
www.ldaamerica.org

An information and referral center for parents and professionals dealing with learning disabilities.
Barbara Lefler, Director of Affiliate Services
Patricia Lillie, President

1496 National Center for Learning Disabilities
381 Park Avenue S
New York, NY 10016-8806

212-545-7510
888-575-7373
Fax: 212-545-9665
www.ncld.org

One of the foremost nonprofit organizations committed to improving the lives of the estimated one in ten children with learning disabilities raising public awareness and understanding.
James H Wendorf, Executive Director
Sheldon H Horowitz EdD, Director/Professional Services

1497 National Dissemination Center for Children with Disabilities
1825 Connecticut Avenue NW
Washington, DC 20009

800-695-0285
Fax: 202-884-8441
TTY: 202-884-8200
e-mail: nichcy@aed.org
www.nichcy.org

Publishes free, fact filled newsletters. Arranges workshops. Advises parents on the laws entitling children with disabilities to special education and other services.
Dr Suzanne Ripley, Contact

Libraries & Resource Centers

1498 HEATH Resource Center
George Washington University
2134 G Street NW
Washington, DC 20052-0001

202-973-0904
800-544-3284
Fax: 202-994-3365
e-mail: askheath@gwu.edu
http://www.heath.gwu.edu/

The HEATH Resource Center of The George Washington University, Graduate School of Education and Human Development, is the national clearinghouse on postsecondary education for individuals with disabilities.
Dr Lynda West, Principal Investigator
Dr Joel Gomez, Co-Principal Investigator

Support Groups & Hotlines

1499 Attention Deficit Information Network
475 Hillside Ave   617-455-9895
Needham, MA 02194
Offers support and information to families of children with attention deficit disorder, adults with ADD and professionals through an international network of 60 parent and adult chapters.

1500 National Federation of Families for Children's Mental Health
9605 Medical Center Drive   240-403-1901
Rockville, MD 20850   Fax: 240-403-1909
e-mail: ffcmh@ffcmh.org
www.ffcmh.org
Provides advocacy at the national level for the rights of children and youth with emotional, behavioral and mental health challenges and their families; provides leadership and technical assistance to a nation-wide network of family run organizations; and collaborates with family run and other child serving organizations to transform mental health care in America.
Sandra Spencer, Executive Director
Andrea Barnes, Policy & Research Assistant

1501 National Health Information Center
PO Box 1133   310-565-4167
Washington, DC 20013-1133   800-336-4797
Fax: 301-984-4256
e-mail: info@nhic.org
www.health.gov/nhic
A health information referral service sponsored by the Office of Disease Prevention and Health Promotion. Puts health professionals and consumers who have health questions in touch with those organizations that are best able to provide answers.

Books

1502 ADHD Parenting Handbook: Practical Advice for Parents from Parents
Colleen Alexander-Roberts, author
Taylor Trade Publishing
4501 Forbes Boulevard   301-459-3366
Lanham, MD 20706   Fax: 301-429-5743
e-mail: custserv@nbnbooks.com
www.rlpgtrade.com
A compilation of practical advice and tips for handling day-to-day activities that routinely become problematic for ADHD children, such as getting dressed for school, going to bed, performing chores, completing homework, and playing with other children.
Paperback
ISBN: 0-878338-62-4

1503 ADHD in Schools: Assessment and Intervention Strategies
George J DuPaul, Gary Stoner, author
Guilford Publications
72 Spring Street
New York, NY 10012   800-365-7006
Fax: 212-966-6708
e-mail: info@guilford.com
www.guilford.com
Provides essential guidance for school-based professionals meeting the challenges of ADHD at any grade level. Comprehensive and practical, includes several reproducible assessment tools and handouts.
330 pages Paperback
ISBN: 1-593850-89-0

1504 ADHD: Handbook for Diagnosis & Treatment
Western Psychological Services
12031 Wilshire Boulevard   310-478-2061
Los Angeles, CA 90025-1201   800-648-8857
Fax: 310-478-7838
www.wpspublish.com
This second edition helps clinicians diagnose and treat Attention Deficit Hyperactivity Disorder. Written by an internationally recognized authority in the field, it covers the history of ADHD, its primary symptoms, associated conditions, developmental course

and outcome, and family context. A workbook companion manual is also available.
700 pages

1505 Attention Deficit Disorder: A Different Perception
Underwood-Miller
708 Westover Drive
Lancaster, PA 17601-1242   717-285-2255
www.vance.hw.nl/dbase/publisher
1993 180 pages Paperback
ISBN: 0-887331-56-4

1506 Attention Deficit Disorder: Learning Disabilities
Random House
25 Van Zant Street   410-848-1900
East Norwalk, CT 06855-1726   800-726-0600
Fax: 800-214-1438
www.randomhouse.com
Realities, myths, and controversial treatments. Section I tries to dispel the myths and discusses proven treatments for ADHD and LD. Section II explains how the scientific community evaluates new treatment methods, and Section III summarizes alternative treatments and discusses scientific evidence pertaining to its usefulness.
256 pages
ISBN: 0-385469-31-4

1507 Attention Deficit Hyperactivity Disorder: What Every Parent Wants to Know
Paul H Brookes Publishing Company
PO Box 10624   301-337-9580
Baltimore, MD 21285-0624   800-638-3775
Fax: 410-337-8539
e-mail: custserv@brookspublishing.com
www.brookespublishing.com
1993 320 pages Paperback
ISBN: 1-557661-41-3
Dante Washington, Customer Service Representative

1508 Coping with ADD/ADHD
Rosen Publishing Group
29 E 21st Street   212-777-3017
New York, NY 10010-6209   800-237-9932
Fax: 888-436-4643
e-mail: customerservice@rosenpub.com
www.rosenpublishing.com
At least 3.5 million American youngsters suffer from ADD. This book defines the syndrome and provides specific information about treatment and counseling.
150 pages Hardcover
ISBN: 0-823931-96-X

1509 Helping Your ADD Child With or Without Hyperactivity
John F Taylor PhD, author
Random House Inc.
Department of Library Marketing   800-733-3000
New York, NY 10017   800-726-0600
Fax: 212-940-7381
e-mail: crownpublicity@randomhouse.com
www.randomhouse.com
Inside this book you will find step-by-step tools for helping your ADD or ADHD child. From extensive screening for spotting the initial signs to the pros and cons of nutritional, psychological, and drug treatments.
2001
ISBN: 0-761527-56-7

1510 Hyperactive Children Grown Up
Gabrielle Weiss, Lily Trokenberg Hechtman, author
Guilford Publications
72 Spring Street
New York, NY 10012   800-365-7006
Fax: 212-966-6708
e-mail: info@guilford.com
www.guilford.com
Reports findings on the etiology, treatment, and outcome of attention deficits and hyperactivity at all stages of development.
473 pages Paperback
ISBN: 0-898625-96-7

1511 **LD Child and the ADHD Child**
Suzanne H Stevens, author

John F Blair Publishing
1406 Plaza Drive   336-768-1374
Winston-Salem, NC 27103   800-222-9796
                              Fax: 336-768-9194
                         e-mail: blairpub@aol.com
                              www.blairpub.com
Helps parents raise their LD and/or ADHD children so that they, too, can grow up to be okay-so that they will be happy, well-adjusted, and successful adults despite the learning and behavior patterns that make them different.
Paperback
ISBN: 0-895871-42-8

1512 **Managing Attention Deficit Hyperactivity Disorder in Children:**
Sam Goldstein, Michael Goldstein, author

Wiley Publishing
111 River Street   201-748-6000
Hoboken, NJ 07030-5774   Fax: 201-748-6088
                             e-mail: info@wiley.com
                                   www.wiley.com
A proven approach to the diagnosis and management of one of the most challenging childhood disorders. In this book the authors describe a proven multidisciplinary approach to the diagnosis and treatment of childhood ADHD, developed at the prestigous Neurology, Learning and Behavior Center in Salt Lake City.
1998 896 pages
ISBN: 0-471121-58-9

1513 **Maybe You Know My Kid: A Parent's Guide to Identifying ADHD**
Birch Lane Press
120 Enterprise Avenue S
Secaucus, NJ 07094-1902   800-447-2665
The author writes about her family experiences with their son, David, who has attention deficit disorder. Contains a comprehensive review of important issues plus descriptions of some helpful management techniques.
222 pages

1514 **Medications for Attention Disorders and Related Medical Problems**
Specialty Press
300 NW 70th Avenue   954-792-8100
Plantation, FL 33317   800-233-9273
                              Fax: 954-792-8545
                     e-mail: sales@addwarehouse.com
                             www.addwarehouse.com
A comprehensive handbook covering the history, characteristics, and causes of ADHD. The equal importance of appropriate academic programming, counseling, and medication are stressed throughout.
415 pages Hardcover

1515 **Parents Helping Parents: A Directory of Support Groups for ADD**
CibaGelgy, Pharmaceuticals Division
External Communications   908-277-5000
Summit, NJ 07901   Fax: 973-781-2601

1516 **Parents' Hyperactivity Handbook: Helping the Fidgety Child**
Plenum Press
233 Spring Street   212-620-8000
New York, NY 10013-1578   Fax: 212-463-0742
                            e-mail: info@plenum.com

1993 306 pages
ISBN: 0-306444-65-8

1517 **Rethinking Attention Deficit Disorders**
Miriam Cherkes-Julkowski, author

Brookline Books
PO Box 1209   617-734-6772
Brookline, MA 02445   800-666-2665
                              Fax: 617-734-3952
                             www.brooklinebooks.com

Gives the classroom teacher useful information that provides ideas and strategies for working with children suffering from ADD.
1997 Paperback
ISBN: 1-571290-37-0

1518 **The New ADD in Adults Workbook**
Lynn Weiss, PhD, author

Taylor Trade Publishing
4501 Forbes Boulevard   301-459-3366
Lanham, MD 20706   Fax: 301-429-5743
                       e-mail: custserv@nbnbooks.com
                                  www.rlpgtrade.com
Not only touches on and dispels the most recent clinical findings, but also emphasizes the bigger perspective, focusing on the empowerment and diversity issues facing all of us on the A.D.D. continuum today. Persuades readers to work through their challenges with practical, prescriptive exercises and insights.
Paperback
ISBN: 0-878338-50-0

1519 **You Mean I'm Not Lazy, Stupid or Crazy?**
Tyrell & Jerem Press
PO Box 20089
Cincinnati, OH 45220-0089   800-622-6611
A new self-help book is the first written by ADD adults for ADD adults. This comprehensive guide provides accurate information, practical how-tos and moral support.

1520 **Attention Deficit/Hyperactivity Disorder**
Guilford Publications
72 Spring Street   212-431-9800
New York, NY 10012-4068   800-365-7006
                              Fax: 212-966-6708
A second edition that is the handbook on the diagnosis and treatment of ADHD in the 1990s. A companion workbook is also available with forms that may be photocopied.
747 pages Hardcover
ISBN: 0-898624-43-6

Children's Books

1521 **Self-Control Games & Workbook**
Western Psychological Services
12031 Wilshire Boulevard   310-478-2061
Los Angeles, CA 90025-1201   800-648-8857
                              Fax: 310-478-7838
This game is designed to teach self-control in academic and social situations. Addresses a total of 24 impulsive, inattentive and hyperactive behaviors. The companion workbook reinforces the use of positive self-statements, and problem-solving techniques, instead of expressing anger.
Game

1522 **Shelley, the Hyperactive Turtle**
Deborah Moss, author

Woodbine House
6510 Bells Mill Road
Bethesda, MD 20817   800-843-7323
                              Fax: 301-897-5838
                     e-mail: info@woodbinehouse.com
                             www.woodbinehouse.com
Reassures young children who are going through the diagnostic process or who are having problems behaving at school or making friends because of AD/HD.
20 pages
ISBN: 1-890627-75-1

Magazines

1523 **Attention**
Children & Adults with Attention Deficit Disorder
8181 Professional Place   301-306-7070
Landover, MD 20785-7221   800-233-4050
                              Fax: 301-306-7090
                              TTY: 301-429-0641

Quarterly

Newsletters

1524 ADHD Report
Guilford Publications
72 Spring Street
New York, NY 10012   800-365-7006
                                 Fax: 212-966-6708
                           e-mail: info@guilford.com
                                    www.guilford.com
Examines the nature, diagnosis, and outcomes associated with the disorder, and provides a single reliable guide to the latest developments in the fields of clinical management and education. Includes research findings, as well as ongoing coverage of ADHD in the news.
16 pages BiMonthly

1525 Chadder
Children & Adults with Attention Deficit Disorder
8181 Professional Place   301-306-7070
Landover, MD 20785-7221   800-233-4050
                                 Fax: 301-306-7090
                                 TTY: 301-429-0641

Quarterly

1526 Challenge
Challenge
PO Box 488   978-462-0495
West Newbury, MA 01985-0688   800-233-2322
National newsletter on ADD/ADHD that carries interviews with nationally-known scientists, as well as physicians, psychologists, social workers, educators, and other practitioners in the field of ADHD.
12 pages BiMonthly
Jean C Harrison, Executive Director

1527 Pure Facts
Feingold Association of the US
PO Box 6550   703-768-3287
Alexandria, VA 22306-0550
Monthly newsletter with articles on nutrition and behavior and lists of approved brand-name foods.

Pamphlets

1528 ADHD
Learning Disabilities Association of America
4156 Library Road   412-341-1515
Pittsburgh, PA 15234-1349   888-300-6710
                                 Fax: 412-344-0224
                           e-mail: info@ldaamerica.org
                                    www.ldaamerica.org
A booklet for parents offering information on Attention Deficit Hyperactivity Disorders and learning disabilities.
Sheila Buckley, Executive Director

1529 Attention Deficit Disorders and Hyperactivity
Council for Exceptional Children
1110 N Glebe Road   703-620-3660
Arlington, VA 22201   888-232-7733
                                 Fax: 703-264-9494
                         e-mail: service@cec.sped.org
                                    www.cec.sped.org
Published by the Council for Exceptional Children.

1530 COGREHAB
Life Science Associates
1 Fennimore Road   631-472-2111
Bayport, NY 11705-2115   Fax: 631-472-8146
                     e-mail: lifesciassoc@pipeline.com
                         lifesciassoc.home.pipeline.com
Divided into six groups for diagnosis and treatment of attention, memory and perceptual disorders to be used by and under the guidance of a professional.
$95 - $1,950

1531 Fact Sheet: Attention Deficit Hyperactivity Disorder
Learning Disabilities Association of America

4156 Library Road   412-341-1515
Pittsburgh, PA 15234-1349   888-300-6710
                                 Fax: 412-344-0224
                           e-mail: info@ldaamerica.org
                                    www.ldaamerica.org
A pamphlet offering factual information on ADHD.
Sheila Buckley, Executive Director

1532 Helping Adolescents with ADHD and Learning Disabilities
Learning Disabilities Association of America
4156 Library Road   412-341-1515
Pittsburgh, PA 15234-1349   888-300-6710
                                 Fax: 412-344-0224
                           e-mail: info@ldaamerica.org
                                    www.ldaamerica.org

Sheila Buckley, Executive Director

Audio & Video

1533 ADD Stepping Out of the Dark
ADD Videos
PO Box 622   845-255-3612
New Paltz, NY 12561-0622   Fax: 845-883-6452
A powerful, effective video, ideal for health professionals, educators and parents providing a visual montage designed to promote an understanding and awareness of attention deficit disorder. Based on actual accounts of those who have ADD, including a neurologist, an office worker, and parents of children with ADD. The video allows the viewer to feel the frustration and lack of attention that ADD brings to many.
Video
Lenae Madonna, Producer

1534 ADHD in Adults
Guilford Publications
72 Spring Street   212-431-9800
New York, NY 10012-4068   800-365-7006
                                 Fax: 212-966-6708
This program integrates information on ADHD with the actual experiences of four adults who suffer from the disorder. Representing a range of professions, from a lawyer to a mother working at home, each candidly discusses the impact of ADHD on his or her daily life. These interviews are augmented by comments from family members and other clinicians who treat adults with ADHD.
Video

1535 ADHD in the Classroom: Strategies for Teachers
Rusell A Barkley, author

Guilford Publications
72 Spring Street
New York, NY 10012   800-365-7006
                                 Fax: 212-966-6708
                           e-mail: info@guilford.com
                                    www.guilford.com
Designed to help teachers create a learning environment that is responsive to the needs of all students, including those with ADHD.

1536 ADHD: What Do We Know?
Guilford Publications
72 Spring Street   212-431-9800
New York, NY 10012-4068   800-365-7006
                                 Fax: 212-966-6708
An introduction for teachers and special education practitioners, school psychologists and parents of ADHD children. Topics outlined in this video include the causes and prevalence of ADHD, ways children with ADHD behave, other conditions that may accompany ADHD and long-term prospects for children with ADHD.
Video

1537 Around the Clock
Guilford Publications
72 Spring Street   212-431-9800
New York, NY 10012-4068   800-365-7006
                                 Fax: 212-966-6708
This videotape provides both professionals and parents a helpful look at how the difficulties facing parents of ADHD children can be handled.

1538 Attention Deficit Disorder
Pro-Ed, Inc.
8700 Shoal Creek Boulevard   512-451-3246
Austin, TX 78757-6897   800-897-3202
                                                    Fax: 800-397-7633
                                         e-mail: info@proedinc.com
                                               www.proedinc.com/
A video and book providing helpful suggestions for both home and
classroom management of students with attention deficit disorder.
216 pages Paperback
ISBN: 0-890797-42-0
Krista Anderson, Technical Advisor
Matt Synatschk, Books & Materials Permissions Editor

1539 Educating Inattentive Children
Western Psychological Services
12031 Wilshire Boulevard
Los Angeles, CA 90025-1201   800-648-8857
                                                    Fax: 310-478-7838
An excellent resource for teachers who encounter inattention and
hyperactivity in the classroom. It helps teachers distinguish deliberate misbehavior from the incompetent, nonpurposeful behavior
of the inattentive child.
Video

1540 It's Just Attention Disorder
Western Psychological Services
12031 Wilshire Boulevard   310-478-2061
Los Angeles, CA 90025-1201   800-648-8857
                                                    Fax: 310-478-7838
This ground-breaking videotape takes the critical first steps in
treating attention-deficit disorder: it enlists the inattentive or hy-
peractive child as an active participant in his or her treatment.
Video

1541 Why Won't My Child Pay Attention?
Western Psychological Services
12031 Wilshire Boulevard   310-478-2061
Los Angeles, CA 90025-1201   800-648-8857
                                                    Fax: 310-478-7838
Practical and reassuring videotape, noted child psychologist tells
parents about two of the most common and complex problems of
childhood: inattention and hyperactivity.
Video

Web Sites

1542 Attention Deficit Information Network
                                        www.addinfonetwork.com
Offers support and information to families of children and adults
with ADD and to professionals.

1543 Healing Well
                                               www.healingwell.com
A social network and support community for patients, caregivers,
and families coping with the daily struggles of diseases, disorders
and chronic illness.

1544 Health Finder
                                               www.healthfinder.gov
A government web site, where individuals can find information
and tools to help you and those you care about stay healthy.

1545 Healthlink USA
                                               www.healthlinkusa.com
Health information concerning treatment, cures, prevention, diagnosis, risk factors, research, support groups, email lists, personal
stories and much more. Updated regularly.

1546 Helios Health
                                               www.helioshealth.com
Online resource for your health information. Detailed information
about specific health topics, access to expert advice from our Medical Advisory Board, and up-to-date health news.

1547 MedicineNet
                                               www.medicinenet.com
An online resource for consumers providing easy-to-read, authoritative medical and health information.

1548 Medscape
                                               www.medscape.com
Medscape offers specialists, primary care physicians, and other
health professionals the Web's most robust and integrated medical
information and educational tools.

1549 WebMD
                                               www.webmd.com
Information on Attention Deficit Disorder, including articles and
resources.

Description

1550 Autistic Spectrum Disorders

Autistic Spectrum Disorders, ASD, includes (from most to least severe) autism, high-functioning autism (HFA), Asperger's syndrome, and PDD-NOS (pervasive development disorder — not otherwise specified). ASD typically appear during the first three years of life. Autism involves severe impairment of social and communication development. HFA symptoms are less severe, but include delayed language development. Asperger's is similar to HFA, but with no speech delay. PPD-NOS describes autistic categories that do not fit into any of the above. ASD affects behavior, communication, social interaction and other neurological functions.

ASD has numerous symptoms, all of which reduce the child's ability to communicate and interact. Many autistic children have abnormal social relationships, impaired understanding, and uneven intellectual development with mental retardation in most cases. They may exhibit repetitive movement (i.e., rocking, spinning, and hand twisting), avoid making eye contact, and have impaired verbal skills. Occasionally, children with ASD will have decreased sensitivity to pain, and have abnormal responses to light, touch and sound. The disorder can include self-injury and bizarre behavior.

ASD is two to four times more common in boys than in girls. It is found in people of all ethnic backgrounds, and throughout the world. In 2009, nine in 1000 children were diagnosed with ASD, up from one in 500 just six years ago.

In some cases, ASD may be linked to damage to the brain or nervous system. Studies of twins with autism point to a possible genetic link. ASD has been associated with the following risk factors: pre- and perinatal birth complications; prenatal infections with certain viruses; abnormalities of the brain detected with a CT scan or MRI (although no specific defects in the brain structure have been consistently identified). More recently, usual childhood vaccines, environmental toxins, and pollutants are being questioned to explain the sharp rise in ASD cases in recent decades, but researchers have been unable to confirm these findings.

Although there are no known cures for ASD, experts advocate early and intense behavioral, developmental and speech therapy. Medications may alleviate some of the accompanying behavior problems, but provide minimal help for the disorder itself and are generally not used. There is strong emphasis on early diagnosis, early intervention, and individualized educational programs to provide the opportunity for maximum development for the child with Autistic Spectrum Disorder.

National Agencies & Associations

1551 ARRISE
9238 Parklane Avenue
Franklin Park, IL 60131-2836
847-451-2740

Provides information about autism.

1552 Autism Research Institute
4182 Adams Avenue
San Diego, CA 92116-2536
619-281-7165
866-366-3361
Fax: 619-563-6840
www.autism.com

A clearinghouse for research on autism and related disorders of learning and behavior. Conducts and compiles research findings to provide people with the latest research available.
Stephen M Edelson PhD, Director

1553 Autism Services Center
929 Fourth Avenue
Huntington, WV 25701-0507
304-525-8014
Fax: 304-525-8026
www.autismservicescenter.org

Provides educational information to the public and professional communities on autism provides case management activities and referrals for persons afflicted with autism and their families.
Ruth Christ Sullivan, Founder and Executive Director

1554 Autism Society of America
4740 East-West Hwy
Bethesda, MD 20814
301-657-0881
800-328-8476
Fax: 301-657-0869
e-mail: info@autism-society.org
www.autism-society.org

A national charitable organization with the mission of providing as much information as possible about autism and the various options, approaches, methods and systems available to parents of children with autism, family members and professionals.
Lee Grossman, President/CEO
Barbara Newhouse, Chief Operating Officer

1555 Autism Treatment Center of America
2080 S Undermountain Road
Sheffield, MA 01257
413-229-2100
877-766-7473
Fax: 413-229-3202
e-mail: correspondence@option.org
www.autismtreatmentcenter.org

Since 1983 the Autism Treatment Center of America has provided innovative training programs for parents and professionals caring for children challenged by Autism Autism Spectrum Disorders Pervasive Developmental Disorder (PDD) and other developmental disorders.
Barry Neil Kaufman, Co-Founder/Co-Creator Son-Rise Program
Bryn Hogan, Director Son-Rise Program

1556 Autism Treatment Center of America: Son-Rise Program
2080 South Undermountain Road
Sheffield, MA 01257
413-229-2100
877-766-7473
Fax: 413-229-3202
e-mail: correspondence@option.org
www.son-rise.org

Since 1983, the Autism Treatment Center of America has provided innovative training programs for parents and professionals caring for children challenged by Autism, Autism Spectrum Disorders, Pervasive Developmental Disorder (PDD) and other developmental difficulties. The Son-Rise Program teaches a specific yet comprehensive system of treatment and education designed to help families and caregivers enable their children to dramatically improve in all areas of learning.
Sean Fitzgerald, Assistant Director Son-Rise Program
Barry Neil Kaufman, Co-Founder

1557 Community Services for Autistic Adults & Children
8615 E Village Avenue
Montgomery Village, MD 20886
240-912-2220
Fax: 301-926-9384
e-mail: csaac@csaac.org
www.csaac.org

The Community Services for Autistic Adults & Children is a non-profit organization dedicated to helping those with autism. Since 1979 CSAAC has served over 150 individuals and helped people with autism find housing, employment and other community services.
Ian Paregol, Executive Director
Don Rodrick, Chief Financial Officer

1558 **National Institute of Neurological Disorders and Stroke**
NIH Neurological Institute   301-496-5751
Bethesda, MD 20824   800-352-9424
                                          Fax: 301-402-2186
                                          TTY: 301-468-5981
                                          www.ninds.nih.gov
The mission of NINDS is to reduce the burden of neurological disease - a burden borne by every age group, by every segment of society, by people all over the world.
Story C Landis, PhD, Director
Walter J Koroshetz, Deputy Director

State Agencies & Associations

Alabama

1559 **Autism Society of Alabama**
Birmingham, AL 35243   205-951-1364
                                          877-4AU-TISM
                                          Fax: 205-967-8244
                                          e-mail: info@autism-alabama.org
                                          www.autism-alabama.org
Ryan Thomas, President
Jennifer Muller, Executive Director

1560 **Autism Society of North Alabama**
PO Box 2902   256-776-0505
Huntsville, AL 35801   e-mail: sherron@northalabamaautism.org
                                          www.northalabamaautism.org
Teresa White, President
Carol Wright, Vice President

Arizona

1561 **Autism Society of Pima County**
PO Box 44156   520-770-1541
Tucson, AZ 85733-4156   Fax: 520-319-5979
         e-mail: az-pimacounty@autismsocietyofamerica.org
                                          www.tucsonautism.org
Peter Earhart, President
Stephanie Hill, Vice President

California

1562 **Autism Society of California**
PO Box 15247   562-943-3335
Long Beach, CA 90815-0600   800-700-0037
                                          e-mail: brubin698@earthlink.net
                                          www.autismsocietyca.org
Dean Wilson, President
Gregory Fletcher, First Vice President

Colorado

1563 **Autism Society of Colorado**
550 S Wadsworth Boulevard   720-214-0794
Lakewood, CO 80226-4169   Fax: 720-274-2744
         e-mail: co-colorado@autismsocietyofamerica.org
                                          www.autismcolorado.org
Betty Lehman, Executive Director
Lorri Park, ProgramsDirector

Connecticut

1564 **Autism Society of Connecticut**
PO Box 1404
Guilford, CT 06437   888-453-4975
                                          www.autismsocietyofct.org

Delaware

1565 **Autism Society of Delaware**
924 Old Harmony Road   302-224-6020
Newark, DE 19713   Fax: 302-224-6017
                                          e-mail: delautism@delautism.org
                                          www.delautism.org
Theda Ellis, Executive Director
Kim Siegel, Development Director

District of Columbia

1566 **Autism Society of District Columbia**
5167 7th Street NE   202-561-5300
Washington, DC 20011-2624   Fax: 202-561-8634
         e-mail: dc-washington@autismsocietyofamerica.org
                                          www.autism-society.org/chapter130
Scott Badesch, President/ChiefExecutive Officer
John Dabrowski, Chief Financial Officer

Florida

1567 **Autism Society of Greater Orlando**
4743 Hearthside Drive   407-855-0235
Orlando, FL 32837-5445   e-mail: contact@asgo.org
                                          www.asgo.org
Donna Lorman, President
Marzena Batignani, Vice President

Georgia

1568 **Autism Society of Greater Georgia**
PO Box 3707   770-904-4474
Suwanee, GA 30024   Fax: 770-904-4476
                                          www.asaga.com
Steve Doran, President
Cindy Pike, Executive Director

Hawaii

1569 **Autism Society of Hawaii**
PO Box 2995   808-282-3676
Honolulu, HI 96802-2995   e-mail: naomig122@hotmail.com
                                          www.autismhi.org
William Bolman, President
Jessica Wong-Sumida, M.A., J.D., Executive Director

Idaho

1570 **Autism Society of Treasure Valley**
PO Box 44831   208-336-5676
Boise, ID 83711-9404   Fax: 202-884-5582
                                          e-mail: Autism.asatvc@yahoo.com
                                          www.asatvc.org

Illinois

1571 **Autism Society of Illinois**
2200 S Main Street   630-691-1270
Lombard, IL 60148-5366   888-691-1270
                                          Fax: 630-932-5620
                                          e-mail: info@autismillinois.org
                                          www.autismillinois.org
Karen McDonough, Executive Director
Kym Bills, President

Indiana

1572 **Autism Society of Indiana**
4740 Kingsway Drive   317-695-0252
Indianapolis, IN 46205-0252   Fax: 317-815-0859
                                          e-mail: info@inautism.org
                                          www.autismsocietyofindiana.org
Joshua Carr, President
Kylee Hope, Vice-President

Iowa

1573 **Autism Society of Iowa**
4549 Waterford Drive   515-327-9075
W Des Moines, IA 50265-2059   888-722-4799
                                          Fax: 319-557-1169
                                          e-mail: autism50ia@aol.com
                                          www.autismia.org
James Ball, Ed.D., BCBA-D, Executive Chair
Ron E. Simmons, Vice Chair

Kansas

1574 Autism Society of Kansas Autism Society of America
Autism Society of America
PO Box 860984   913-706-0042
Shawnee, KS 66286-2325   Fax: 316-943-3292
e-mail: ks-johnsoncounty@autismsocietyofamerica.
www.autismsocietyoftheheartland.org

Bill Robinso, President
DeeDee Velasquez-Per, Board Member

Kentucky

1575 Autism Chapter of Bluegrass Chapter
243 Shady Lane
Lexington, KY 40503-2034   859-299-9000
www.asbg.org

Sara Spragens, President

1576 Autism Society of Western Kentucky
230 Second Street Suite 206   270-826-0510
Henderson, KY 42419-1647   e-mail: nboyett1956@yahoo.com
www.autism.org

Nancy Boyett, President

Louisiana

1577 Autism Society of Louisiana
5430 S Woodchase Court
Baton Rouge, LA 70808   800-955-3760
e-mail: pjmanco@cox.net
www.lastateautism.org

Pat Giamanco, President

Maine

1578 Autism Society of Maine
72B Main Street
Winthrop, ME 04364-1406   800-273-5200
Fax: 207-377-9434
e-mail: nancy@asmonline.org
www.asmonline.org

Kim Humphrey, President
Lynda Mazzola, Vice President

Maryland

1579 Autism Society of Baltimore-Chesapeake
PO Box 10822   410-655-7933
Parkville, MD 21234   e-mail: info@baltimoreautismsociety.org
www.baltimoreautismsociety.org

Debbie Page, Co-President:
Kay Holman, Vice-President:

Massachusetts

1580 Autism Society of Massachusetts
20 Alice Agnew Drive   877-622-2884
Attleboro Falls, MA 2763-2108   Fax: 774-643-6331
e-mail: asamasschapter@hotmail.com
www.nationalautismassociation.org

Jo Pike, Co-Founder President/Executive Director
Laura Bono, Founding Board Member

Michigan

1581 Autism Society of Michigan
1213 Center Street   517-882-2800
Lansing, MI 48906-5338   800-223-6722
Fax: 517-862-2816
e-mail: mi-michigan@autismsocietyofamerica.org
www.autism-mi.org

Kathy Johnson, President
Penny Bearden, Vice President

Minnesota

1582 Autism Society of Minnesota
2380 Wycliff Street   651-647-1083
St Paul, MN 55114-1257   Fax: 651-642-1230
e-mail: info@ausm.org
www.ausm.org

Pam Erickson, Executive Director
Laurie Dixon, Associate Director

Missouri

1583 Autism Society of Gateway Chapter
7777 Bonhomme Avenue   314-863-0077
St Louis, MO 63105   Fax: 314-863-7494
e-mail: PegiSues@aol.com
www.autism-society.org

Pegi Price, President
James Ball, Ed.D., BCBA-D, Executive Chair

Nebraska

1584 Autism Society of Nebraska
1672 Van Dorn Street   402-472-4346
Lincoln, NE 68502   877-375-0120
e-mail: autismsociety@autismnebraska.org
www.autismnebraska.org

Shawn Neff, President
Georgann Albin, Executive Director

Nevada

1585 Autism Society of Northern Nevada
3490 Southampton Drive   775-786-9315
Reno, NV 89509-8911   Fax: 775-786-0984
www.autism-society.org/chapter547

Paul Deane, Vice President
Dinah Deane, President

New Hampshire

1586 Autism Society of New Hampshire
PO Box 68   603-679-2424
Concord, NH 03302-0068   Fax: 301-657-0869
e-mail: info@nhautism.com
www.nhautism.com

Stacey Shannon, President

New Jersey

1587 Autism Society of Southwest New Jersey
10 Shadow Oak Court   856-722-8518
Mount Laurel, NJ 08054-2113   e-mail: CMedo@aol.com
www.autism-society.org

New Mexico

1588 Autism Society of New Mexico
PO Box 30955   505-332-0306
Albuquerque, NM 87190   e-mail: nmautism@nmautismsociety.org
www.nmautismsociety.org

Sarah Baca, Executive Director
Sharon Esch, President

New York

1589 Autism Society of Albany
PO Box 3487   518-355-2191
Schenectady, NY 12303   Fax: 518-355-2191
e-mail: info@albanyautism.org
www.albanyautism.org

Gordon Zuckerman, President
Jenny DeBellis, Treasurer

North Carolina

1590 Autism Society of North Carolina
505 Oberlin Road   919-743-0204
Raleigh, NC 27605-1345   800-442-2762
                                    Fax: 919-743-0208
                        e-mail: info@autismsociety-nc.org
                                www.autismsociety-nc.org

Scott Badesch, Chief Executive Officer
David Laxton, Director Communications

North Dakota

1591 Autism Society of North Dakota
628 6th Avenue   701-281-8254
Alice, ND 58031   e-mail: Jocelyn@AutismND.org
                                www.AutismND.org

Kris Wallman, President
Renie Chadwell, Vice President

Ohio

1592 Autism Society of Greater Cincinnati
PO Box 58385   513-561-2300
Cincinnati, OH 45258   Fax: 513-561-4748
                        e-mail: asgc@cinci.rr.com
                                www.autismcincy.org

Kay Brown, President
Sue Radabaugh, Vice President

1593 Autism Society of Ohio Tri-County Chapter
1749 S Raccoon Road
Austintown, OH 44515   330-720-2066
                                www.triautism.com

Terry Chapin, President
Jack Campbell, Vice President

Oklahoma

1594 Autism Society of Central Oklahoma
PO Box 720103   405-370-3220
Norman, OK 73070   e-mail: ASOCO-owner@yahoogroups.com
                                www.asofok.org

Jeremy Rand, Contact

Oregon

1595 Autism Society of Oregon
PO Box 396   503-636-1676
Marylhurst, OR 97036-0396   888-288-4761
                                    Fax: 503-636-1696
                        e-mail: info@oregonautism.com
                                www.oregonautism.com

Jenny Schoonbee, President
Genevieve Athens, Executive Director

Pennsylvania

1596 Autism Society of Greater Harrisburg
PO Box 101   717-732-8400
Enola, PA 17025-0856   800-277-2425
                        e-mail: georgia.rackley@verizon.net
                                www.autismharrisburg.com

Georgia Rackley, President
Sherry Christian, Vice President

Rhode Island

1597 Autism Society of Rhode Island
PO Box 16603   401-595-3241
Rumford, RI 02916   e-mail: LRego@asa-ri.org
                                www.asa-ri.org

Lisa Rego, President
Claudia Swiader, Vice President

South Carolina

1598 Autism Society of South Carolina
806 Twelfth Street   803-750-6988
W Columbia, SC 29169   800-438-4790
                                    Fax: 703-750-8121
                        e-mail: scas@scautism.org
                                www.scautism.org

Craig Stoxen, President & CEO
Tim Conroy, Chief Operating Officer & Vice President

South Dakota

1599 Autism Society of Black Hills
521 7th Street   605-737-0377
Rapid City, SD 57701-4347   e-mail: sheritony@rap.midco.net
                                www.autismsd.com

Sandy Burns, President
Sheri Perkins

Tennessee

1600 Autism Society of East Tennessee
PO Box 30015   865-824-2897
Knoxville, TN 37930   Fax: 865-824-2896
                        e-mail: asaetc@gmail.com
                                www.asaetc.org

Mike Manfredo, President
Roddey M. Coe, Vice President

Texas

1601 Autism Society of Dallas
10503 Metric Drive   214-208-0792
Dallas, TX 75243   e-mail: autismsociety_dallas@yahoo.com
                                www.autism-society.org

Carolyn Garver, Contact
Pamela Lane, President

Vermont

1602 Autism Society of Vermont Autism Society of America
Autism Society of America
PO Box 978
White River Junction, VT 05001-0978   800-559-7398
                e-mail: vt-vermont@autismsocietyofamerica.org
                                www.autism-info.org

Virginia

1603 Autism Society of Northern Virginia
PO Box 1334   703-495-8444
Vienna, VA 22183-1334   Fax: 703-571-8138
                        e-mail: info@asanv.org
                                www.asanv.org

Kymberly S DeLoatche, Executive Director
Christopher Waddell, President

Washington

1604 Autism Society of Washington
P. O. Box 503
Olympia, WA 98507   888-279-4968
                                    Fax: 253-503-1157
                        e-mail: info@autismsocietyofwa.org
                                www.autismsocietyofwa.org

Jeffrey Foster, President
Teresa McCann, Vice-President

West Virginia

1605 Autism Socity of West Virginia
PO Box 1024   304-272-9834
Wayne, WV 25570 e-mail: wv-westvirginia@autismsocietyofamerica.o
                                www.aswv.org

Kim Farley, President
Ginny Gattlieb, 1st VP

Wisconsin

1606 Autism Society of Wisconsin
1477 Kenwood Drive   920-558-4602
Menasha, WI 54952   888-428-8476
                                              Fax: 920-553-0034
                                    e-mail: asw@asw4autism.org
                                             www.asw4autism.org

Nancy Alar, President
Dale Prahl, Vice President

Libraries & Resource Centers

1607 Autism Services Center
Keith Albee Building
929 4th Avenue   304-525-8014
Huntington, WV 25710   Fax: 304-525-8026
                                       www.autismservicescenter.org
Serves people with autism, other developmental disabilities and
those who care for and about them.
John Fields, Director
Mike Grady, Chief Executive Officer

1608 Emory Autism Resource Center
Emory University School of Medicine
Justin Tyler Traux Building   404-727-8350
Atlanta, GA 30322-0001   Fax: 404-727-3969
                          e-mail: michael.j.morrier@emory.edu
                          www.psychiatry.emory.edu/PROGRAMS/autism
The Emory Autism Resource Center is a component of the Depart-
ment of Psychiatry and Behavioral Sciences of Emory University's
School of Medicine. It is the only Georgia resource that provides a
comprehensive continuum of services specially designed to meet
the needs of children and adults with autism and their families.
Gail G McGee, PhD, Director
Michael J Morrier, MA, Asst Director Research Manager

1609 Indiana Resource Center for Autism (IRCA)
Indiana Institute on Disability & Community
Indiana University-Bloomington   812-855-6508
Bloomington, IN 47408-2696   800-825-4733
                                              Fax: 812-855-9630
                                              TTY: 812-855-9396
                                  e-mail: prattc@indiana.edu
                                    www.iidc.indiana.edu/irca
The Indiana Resource Center for Autism staff conduct outreach
training and consultations, engage in research, and develop and
disseminate information focused on building the capacity of local
communities, organizations, agencies, and families to support
children and adults across the autism spectrum in typical work,
school, home, and community settings.
Dr Cathy Pratt PhD, Director

Research Centers

1610 Center for Neurodevelopmental Studies
5430 W Glenn Drive   623-915-0345
Glendale, AZ 85301   800-352-3792
                                              Fax: 623-937-5425
                                     e-mail: admin@ccnsaz.org
                                    www.thechildrenscenteraz.org
Effective treatment methods for autism and developmental disabil-
ities are subjects researched and studied at the Center.
Lorna Jean King, Founder
Kent Rideout, Executive Director

1611 Division TEACCH University of North Carolina at Chapel H
University of North Carolina at Chapel Hill
100 Renee Lynne Court   919-966-5156
Carrboro, NC 27510-6305   Fax: 919-966-4003
                                       e-mail: teacch@unc.edu
                                              www.teacch.com
This organization is the division for the treatment and education of
Autistic and related communication handicapped children.
Catherine Jones, Office Manager/Parent Intake Coordinator
Elaine Coonrod, Clinical Director

1612 Institute for Basic Research in Developmental Disabilities
1050 Forest Hill Road   718-494-0600
Staten Island, NY 10314-6356   Fax: 718-494-0833
                                          www.health.gov/NHIC/
Conducts research into neurodegenerative diseases, Alzheimer's
disease, developmental disabilities, fragile X syndrome, Down's
syndrome, autism, epilepsy and basic science issues underlying all
developmental disabilities.

1613 Institute on Communication and Inclusion at Syracuse University
University of Syracuse
370 Huntington Hall   315-443-9379
Syracuse, NY 13244-2340   Fax: 315-443-2274
                                        e-mail: icistaff@syr.edu
                                            http://ici.syr.edu
College offering facilitated learning research into communication
with persons who have autism or severe disabilities. Offers books
videos and public awareness information on the research projects.
Douglas Biklen, Dean

1614 National Alliance for Autism Research
1 East 33rd Street   212-252-8584
New York, NY 10016   Fax: 212-252-8676
                          e-mail: contactus@autismspeaks.org
                                          www.autismspeaks.org
The National Alliance for Autism Research has merged with Au-
tism Speaks to further reach for the goal of finding the causes the
best prevention and treatments and a cure for autism.
Peter H Bell, Executive Vice President
Mark Roithmayr, President

1615 State University of New York Health Sciences Center
SUNY Downstate Medical Center
450 Clarkson Avenue   718-270-1000
Brooklyn, NY 11203-2098   Fax: 718-270-1271
                                    e-mail: health@downstate.edu
                                          www.downstate.edu/
Child psychiatry research programs.
John C Larosa, President

1616 The West Virginia Autism Training Center Marshall University
Marshall University
1 John Marshall Drive   304-696-2332
Huntington, WV 25755   800-344-5115
                                    e-mail: wvatc@marshall.edu
                                          www.marshall.edu/coe/atc
The Autism Training Center was established through the efforts of
parents of children with autism throughout West Virginia to provide education training and treatment programs for West Virgin-
ians who have Autism Pervasive Developmental Disorder (NOS)
or Asperger's Disorder and have been formally registered with the
Center.

Support Groups & Hotlines

1617 Autism Society of America
4340 East-West Highway   301-657-0881
Bethesda, MD 20814   800-328-8476
                                          www.autism-society.org
Exists to improve the lives of all affected by autism by increasing
public awareness about the day-to-day issues faced by people in
the spectrum, advocating for apporporiate services for individuals
across the lifespan, and providing the latest information regarding
treatment, education, research and advocacy.
Lee Grossman, President/CEO
John Dabrowski, Chief Financial Officer

1618 Genetic Alliance
4301 Connecticut Avenue NW   202-966-5557
Washington, DC 20008-2369   800-336-4363
                                              Fax: 202-668-8533
                                    e-mail: info@geneticalliance.org
                                          www.geneticalliance.org
A nonprofit health advocacy organization committed to transforming through genetics and promoting an environment of openness
centered on the health of individuals, families and communities.
Sharon Terry, President/CEO

1619   National Autism Hotline Autism Services Center
Keith Albee Building
929 4th Avenue   304-525-8014
Huntington, WV 25710   Fax: 304-525-8026
                                        www.autismservicescenter.org
Serving people with autism, other developmental disabilities anf
those who care for and about them.
Mike Grady, CEO, Autism Services Center
Derek Hyman, President & Treasurer

1620   National Health Information Center
PO Box 1133   310-565-4167
Washington, DC 20013-1133   800-336-4797
                                                    Fax: 301-984-4256
                                              e-mail: info@nhic.org
                                              www.health.gov/nhic
A health information referral service sponsored by the Office of
Disease Prevention and Health Promotion. Puts health profession-
als and consumers who have health questions in touch with those
organizations that are best able to provide answers.

Books

1621   A Miracle to Believe In
Option Indigo Press
2080 S Undermountain Road   413-229-2100
Sheffield, MA 01257   800-714-2779
                                                    Fax: 413-229-8931
                                                    optionindigo.com
A group of people from all walks of life come together and are
transformed as they reach out, under the direction of the
Kaufmans, to help a little boy the medical world had given up as
hopeless.
379 pages
ISBN: 0-440201-08-2
Bears Kaufman, Founder
Samahria Kaufman, Founder

**1622   A Parent's Guide to Asperger's Syndrome & High-Functioning
Autism**
Guilford Press
72 Spring Street
New York, NY 10012   800-365-7006
                                                    Fax: 212-966-6708
                                              e-mail: info@guilford.com
                                                    www.guilford.com
For parents of children on the higher end of the autistic spectrum.
All educators, the authors provide the basic on diagnosis, causes,
and treatment.
2002 278 pages
ISBN: 1-572307-67-6

**1623   Activities for Developing Pre-Skill Concepts In Children with
Autism**
Toni Flowers, author
Autism Society of North Carolina Bookstore
505 Oberlin Road   919-743-0204
Raleigh, NC 27605-1345   800-442-2762
                                                    Fax: 919-743-0208
                                              e-mail: info@autismsociety-nc.org
                                                    www.autismsociety-nc.org
Chapters include auditory development, concept development, so-
cial development and visual-motor integration.

1624   Asperger Syndrome or High-Functioning Autism?
Eric Schopler, Gary B Mesibov, Linda J Kunce, author
Springer Publishing
233 Spring Street   212-460-1550
New York, NY 10013   800-777-4643
                                                    Fax: 212-460-1575
                                              e-mail: service-ny@springer.com
                                                    www.springer.com
The precise relationship between high-functioning autism and
Asperger Syndrome is still a subject of debate. Leaders in the field
provide a general overview of the disorder and present diverse

opinions on diagnosis and assessment-neuropsychological is-
sues-treatment, and related conditions.
428 pages Hardcover
ISBN: 0-306457-45-3

1625   Asperger's Syndrome: A Guide for Parents and Professionals
Taylor & Francis
325 Chestnut Street
Philadelphia, PA 19106   215-625-8900
                                                    www.tonyattwood.com
Offers insight into the identification and treatment of children on
the higher functioning end of ASD.
201 pages
ISBN: 1-853025-77-1

1626   Autism Society of North Carolina Bookstore
505 Oberlin Road   919-743-0204
Raleigh, NC 27605-1345   800-442-2762
                                                    Fax: 919-743-0208
                                              e-mail: info@autismaociety-nc.org
                                                    www.autismsociety-nc.org
Offers one of the largest selections of books about autism.

1627   Autism Through the Lifespan: The Eden Model
Woodbine House
6510 Bells Mill Road   301-897-3570
Bethesda, MD 20817-1636   800-843-7323
                                                    Fax: 301-897-5838
Presents Eden's comprehensive model for helping children and
adults with autism, offering services that extend over their entire
lifespan. An overview of what is known about autism today, discussions about Eden's approach to behavior modification, placement and treatment, curriculum from early childhood to adulthood,
staffing issues, integration, decision making, and parental roles.
Also contains dozens of examples and case histories that illustrate
the program's successes.
1998 383 pages Paperback
ISBN: 0-933149-28-x

1628   Autism Treatment Guide
Elizabeth King Gerlach, author
Autism Society of North Carolina Bookstore
505 Oberlin Road   919-743-0204
Raleigh, NC 27605-1345   800-442-2762
                                                    Fax: 919-743-0208
                                              e-mail: info@autismsociety-nc.org
                                                    www.autismsociety-nc.org
This 3rd edition offers many of the most current findings in treatments fo autism spectrum disorder. First published in 1993 and updated regularly, this concise handbook provides hundres of
resource listings and suggested readings pertaining to ASD. This
is a must-have reference book for parents and professionals
2003 157 pages Softcover

1629   Autism and Asperger Syndrome Preparing for Adulthood
Autism Society of North Carolina Bookstore
505 Oberlin Road   919-743-0204
Raleigh, NC 27605-1345   800-442-2762
                                                    Fax: 919-743-0208
                                              e-mail: info@autismsociety-nc.org
                                                    www.autismsociety-nc.org
Chapters include topics such as what becomes of adults with ASD,
interventions for ASD, problems af communication, social functioning in adulthood, sterotyped, ritualistic, and obsessional behaviors, secondary education, post-secondary education, finding
and coping with employment, psychiatric disturbances in adulthood, leagal issues, sexual relationships and marriage, and
enhancing independence.
2004 388 pages Softcover

1630   Autism in Adolescents and Adults
Eric Schopler, Gary B Mesibov, author
Springer Publishing

233 Spring Street
New York, NY 10013

121-460-1500
800-777-4643
Fax: 212-460-1575
e-mail: service-ny@springer.com
www.springer.com

456 pages Hardcover
ISBN: 0-306410-57-4

1631   Autism...Nature, Diagnosis and Treatment
Guilford Press
72 Spring Street
New York, NY 10012

800-365-7006
Fax: 212-966-6708
e-mail: info@guilford.com
www.guilford.com

Covers perspectives, issues, neurobiological issues and new directions in diagnosis and treatment.
417 pages
ISBN: 0-898627-24-9

1632   Autism: Explaining the Enigma
Uta Frith, author

Wiley Publishing
111 River Street
Hoboken, NJ 07030-5774

201-748-6000
Fax: 201-748-6088
e-mail: info@wiley.com
www.wiley.com

Includes a new chapter outlining recent developments in neuropsycgological research, and overviews one of the most important theoretical and practical consequences of Frith's original insights into this puzzling condition.
264 pages
ISBN: 0-631229-01-8

1633   Autism: Identification, Education and Treatment
Dianne Zager, author

Lawrence Earlbaum Associates
10 Industrial Avenue
Mahwah, NJ 07430

201-258-2200
800-926-6579
Fax: 201-236-0072
www.erlbaum.com

Chapters include medical treatments, early intervention and communication development in autism.
2005 608 pages
ISBN: 0-805845-79-8

1634   Autism: The Facts
Simon Baron-Cohen, Patrick Bolton, author

Oxford University Press
2001 Evans Road
Cary, NC 27513

800-445-9714
Fax: 919-677-1303
e-mail: custserv.us@oup.com
www.oup-usa.org

Explains in a clear, straightforward manner what is known about the condition. Written first and foremost as a guide for parents, but required reading for interested professionals, it covers the recognition and diagnosis of autism, its biological and physiological causes, and the various treatments and educational techniques available.
128 pages
ISBN: 0-192623-27-3

1635   Autistic Adults at Bittersweet Farms
Haworth Press
10 Alice Street
Binghamton, NY 13904-1580

607-722-5857
800-429-6784
Fax: 607-722-0012
www.haworthpress.com

A touching view of an inspirational residential care program for autistic adolescents and adults.
205 pages Paperback
ISBN: 1-560240-57-0

1636   Beyond Gentle Teaching
J.J McGee and F.J Menolascino, author

Springer

233 Spring Street
New York, NY 10013

212-460-1500
800-777-4643
Fax: 212-460-1575
e-mail: service-ny@springer.com
www.springer.com

252 pages Hardcover
ISBN: 0-306438-56-1

1637   Biology of the Autistic Syndromes
Christopher Gillberg and Mary Coleman, author

Blackwell Publishing, Inc.
Commerce Place
Malden, MA 02148

781-388-8200
800-862-6657
Fax: 781-388-8210
www.blackwellpublishing.com

Autism is not a disease but a syndrome of different diseases. In this completely reworked and updated 3rd edition, the authors adress the difficulties this presents for clinical diagnosis with diagnostic aids and clear guidlines for medical evaluation. This is an essential text text for clinicians and will also be of interest to parents of autistic children.
2000 340 pages
ISBN: 1-898683-22-0

1638   Children with Autism
Woodbine House
6510 Bells Mill Road
Bethesda, MD 20817

800-843-7323
e-mail: info@woodbinehouse.com
www.woodbinehouse.com

A must-have reference if for the both the new parent coping with a child's recent diagnosis and one who's an experienced advocate. Available online only.
368 pages Paperback

1639   Communication Unbound: How Facilitated Communication Is Challenging Views
Teachers College Press
1234 Amsterdam Avenue
New York, NY 10027

212-678-3929
Fax: 212-678-4149
e-mail: tcpress@tc.columbia.edu
www.teacherscollegepress.com

Addresses the ways in which we receive persons with autism in our society, our community and our lives.
1993 221 pages

1640   Diagnosis Autism: Now What? 10 Steps to Improve Treatment Outcomes
Lawrence P Kaplan, PhD, author

Autism Society of North Carolina Bookstore
505 Oberlin Road
Raleigh, NC 27605-1345

919-743-0204
800-442-2762
Fax: 919-743-0208
e-mail: info@autismsociety-nc.org
www.autismsociety-nc.org

This practical guide was written to help parents of children with autism spectrum disorder form successful pediatric partnerships with physicians and other healthcare practitioners involved in their child's diagnosis and treatment. Containing chrts and worksheets, sample questions, research resources, and numerous planning strategies, this guide will aid parents and caregivers as they strive to build collaborative relationships with their child's case management team.
2005

1641   Effective Teaching Methods for Autistic Children
Rosalind C Oppenheim, author

Charles C Thomas Publisher
2600 S 1st Street
Springfield, IL 62704-4730

217-789-8980
800-258-8980
Fax: 217-789-9130
e-mail: books@ccthomas.com
www.ccthomas.com

The Rimland School for Autistic Children in Evanston, Illinois, with a Foreward by Bernard Rimland. This enlightening monograph is seven chapters detailing the specific problems encountered in teaching autistic children. Anecdotal reports of seven such children bring to light the need for special training and provide an

insight into their handling. Related research is reviewed and discussed.
1974 116 pages Paperback
ISBN: 0-398028-58-3

1642 Encounters with Autistic States
Jason Aronson
PO Box 15100
York, PA 17405-7100   800-782-0015
                                      Fax: 201-840-7242
                                      www.aronson.com

Hardcover
ISBN: 0-765700-62-

1643 Handbook of Autism and Pervasive Developmental Disorders
Autism Society of North Carolina Bookstore
505 Oberlin Road   919-743-0204
Raleigh, NC 27605-1345   800-442-2762
                                      Fax: 919-743-0208
                          e-mail: info@autismsociety.org
                                      www.autismsociety.org
A list of contributors address such topics as characteristics of autistic syndromes and interventions.
2005 1317 pages 2 volumes

1644 Helping Children with Autism Learn: Treatment Approaches for Parents
Bryna Siegel, author
Oxford University Press
2001 Evans Road
Cary, NC 27513   800-445-9714
                                      Fax: 919-677-1303
                          e-mail: custserv.us@oup.com
                                      www.oup.com

512 pages
ISBN: 0-195325-06-0

1645 Hidden Child: The Linwood Method for Reaching the Autistic Child
Woodbine House
6510 Bells Mill Road   301-897-3570
Bethesda, MD 20817-1636   800-843-7323
                                      Fax: 301-897-5838
                        e-mail: info@woodbinehouse.com
                                      www.woodbinehouse.com
Chronicle of the Linwood Children's Center's successful treatment program for autistic children.
286 pages Paperback
ISBN: 0-933149-06-9

1646 I'm Not Autistic on the Typewriter
TASH
11201 Greenwood Avenue N
Seattle, WA 98133-8612   206-361-8870
An introduction to the facilitated communication training method.

1647 Keys to Parenting the Child with Autism
Marlene Targ Brill, M.Ed, author
Barrons Educational Series, Inc.
250 Wireless Boulevard
Hauppauge, NY 11788   800-645-3476
                                      Fax: 631-434-3723
                        e-mail: fbrown@barronseduc.com
                                      www.barronseduc.com
This book explains what autism is and how it is diagnosed.
2001 224 pages
ISBN: 0-764112-92-9

1648 Let Community Employment Be the Goal for Individuals with Autism
Autism Society of North Carolina Bookstore
505 Oberlin Road   919-743-0204
Raleigh, NC 27605-1345   800-442-2762
                                      Fax: 919-743-0208
                      e-mail: info@autismsociaty-nc.org
                                      www.autismsociety-nc.org
A guide designed for people who are responsible for preparing individuals with autism to enter the work force.
1993 66 pages Booklet

1649 Let Me Hear Your Voice A Family's Triumph Over Autism
Catherine Maurice, author
Autism Society of North Carolina Bookstore
505 Oberlin Road   919-743-0204
Raleigh, NC 27605-1345   800-442-2762
                                      Fax: 919-743-0208
                      e-mail: info@autismsociety-nc.org
                                      www.autismsociety-nc.org
The Maurice family's second and third children were diagnosed with autism. This book recounts their experience with a home program using behavior therapy.
1993 371 pages Softcover
ISBN: 0-679408-63-0

1650 Management of Autistic Behavior
Pro-Ed, Inc.
8700 Shoal Creek Boulevard   512-451-3246
Austin, TX 78757-6897   800-897-3202
                                      Fax: 800-397-7633
                          e-mail: info@proedinc.com
                                      www.proedinc.com
Comprehensive and practical book that tells what works best with specific problems.
450 pages Paperback
ISBN: 0-890791-96-1
Lindy Jordaan, Marketing Coordinator

1651 Navigating the Social World: A Curriculum for Individuals with Asperger's Syndrome
Jeanette McAfee, author
Future Horizons
721 W Abram Street
Arlington, TX 76013   800-489-0727
                                      Fax: 817-277-2270
                                      www.fhautism.com
Addresses the most urgent problems facing those with Asperger's Syndrome, high-functioning autism, and related disorders.
387 pages
ISBN: 1-885477-82-1

1652 Neurobiology of Autism
Johns Hopkins University Press
2715 N Charles Street   410-516-6936
Baltimore, MD 21218-4319   Fax: 410-516-6998
                                      www.jhupbooks.com
This book discusses recent advances in scientific research that point to a neurobiological basis for autism and examines the clinical implications of this research.
272 pages
ISBN: 0-801856-80-9

1653 News from the Border: A Mother's Memoir of Her Autistic Son
Houghton Mifflin Company/Order Processing
222 Berkeley Street   617-351-5000
Boston, MA 02116   800-225-3362
                                      www.hmco.com
A searingly honest account of the author's family experiences with autism. Raising an autistic child is the central, ongoing drama of her married life and this riveting account of acceptance and coping.
1993 384 pages Cloth

1654 Pervasive Developmental Disorders: Finding a Diagnosis and Getting Help
O'Reilly & Associates
1005 Gravenstein Highway N   707-829-0515
Sebastopol, CA 95472-3858   800-998-9938
                                      Fax: 707-829-0104
                                      www.oreilly.com
Published for parents and patients with PDD-NOS and atypical PDD.
Paperback
ISBN: 1-565925-30-0

1655 Please Don't Say Hello
Human Sciences Press
233 Spring Street   212-620-8000
New York, NY 10013-1522

Paul and his family moved into a new neighborhood. Paul's brother was autistic. The children thought that Eddie was retarded until they learned that there were skills that he could do better than they could.
1976 47 pages Paperback
ISBN: 0-898851-99-8

1656 Psychoeducational Profile (PEP-3): TEACCH Individualized Psychoeducational Assessm
Autism Society of North Carolina Bookstore
505 Oberlin Road   919-743-0204
Raleigh, NC 27605-1345   800-442-2762
                                                        Fax: 919-743-0208
                            e-mail: info@autismsociety-nc.org
                                        www.autismsociety-nc.org
This is the revised edition of Psychoeducational Profile, a widely recognized assessment tool used to identify the learning strengths and weaknesses of children with autism spectrum disorder (ASD). Developed by Division TEACCH clinicians, this instrument has been updated in several ways, including improved psychometric properties, revised function domains, new items and sub-tests, within-group comparison data, and the addition of key documentation.
2005

1657 Raising a Child with Autism: A Guide to Applied Behavior Analysis for Parents
Taylor & Francis
325 Chestnut Street   215-625-8900
Philadelphia, PA 19106   Fax: 215-625-2940
Applied behavior analysis activities that parents can use with ASD children. Inlcuded is helpful guidance for toilet training, daily living, and increasing communication and sibling interaction.
173 pages
ISBN: 1-853029-10-6

1658 Reaching the Autistic Child: A Parent Training Program
Martin Kozloff, author
Brookline Books/Lumen Editions
PO Box 1209   617-734-6772
Brookline, MA 02445   800-666-2665
                                                        Fax: 617-734-3952
                                        www.brooklinebooks.com
Detailed case studies of social and behavioral change in autistic children and their families show parents how to implement the principles for improved socialization and behavior.
1998 Softcover
ISBN: 1-571290-56-7

1659 Record Book for Individuals with Autism Spectrum Disorders
Marci Wheeler and Cathy Pratt, PhD, author
Autism Society of North Carolina Bookstore
505 Oberlin Road   919-743-0204
Raleigh, NC 27605-1345   800-442-2762
                                                        Fax: 919-743-0208
                            e-mail: info@autismsociety-nc.org
                                        www.autismsociety-nc.org
This valuable resource provides a method for organizing and documenting information that will help parents track their child's development. This record book is divided into several categories, including: developmental and family history, sleeping and eating patterns, medical history, education history, behavior problems, skill development, and vital information. The book contains reproducible pages that will help parents keep important information up to date.
2000 44 pages Spiral Bound

1660 Riddle of Autism: A Psychological Analysis
Jason Aronson
PO Box 15100
York, PA 17405-7100
                                                        800-782-0015
                                                        Fax: 201-840-7242
                                                        www.aronson.com
Dr. Victor examines the myths that cloud an understanding of this disorder and describes the meanings of its specific behavioral symptoms.
356 pages Softcover
ISBN: 1-568215-73-8

1661 Siblings of Children with Autism: A Guide for Families
Woodbine House
6510 Bells Mill Road   301-897-3570
Bethesda, MD 20817   800-843-7323
                                                        Fax: 301-897-5838
                                                www.woodbinehouse.com
Resource for families with autistic children and nonautistic siblings examines the perceptions, needs, compromises, and inevitable stresses that brothers and sisters face.
160 pages
ISBN: 1-890627-29-1

1662 TEACCH Transition Assessment Profile
Autism Society of North Carolina Bookstore
505 Oberlin Road   919-743-0204
Raleigh, NC 27605-1345   800-442-2762
                                                        Fax: 919-743-0208
                            e-mail: info@autismsociety-nc.org
                                        www.autismsociety-nc.org
This new assessment profile is a major revision of the AAPEP. This comprehensive test was developed for older children and adolescents with autism spectrum disorder, particularly those who have transition needs. This assessment tool is structured to satisfy those provisions in the 2004 Individuals with Disabilities Education Act, which requires that adolescents be evaluated and also provided with a transition plan.
2007 Kit

1663 Targeting Autism: What We Know, Don't Know and Can Do to Help Young Children
University of California Press
1445 Lower Ferry Road   205-978-5000
Ewing, NJ 08618   800-777-4726
                                                        Fax: 800-999-1958
                                                        www.ucpress.com
Provides strong overviews of current work being done with autism and addresses the diferent life cycles of children with the condition through preschool, elementary school, and adolescence.
240 pages
ISBN: 0-520234-80-4

1664 Tasks Galore for the Real World
Laurie Eckenrode, Pat Fennell, and Kathy Hearsey, author
Autism Society of North Carolina Bookstore
505 Oberlin Road   919-743-0204
Raleigh, NC 27605-1345   800-442-2762
                                                        Fax: 919-743-0208
                            e-mail: info@autismsociety-nc.org
                                        www.autismsociety-nc.org
These visually structured tasks are strategies that translate complex, everyday life skills into simpler, meaningful learning situations. The myriad of ideas in this guide will be valuable to anyone developing functional, daily living goals for a child or client.
2004

1665 Teach Me Language: A Language Manual for Children with Autism
Sabrina Freeman, PhD and Lorelei Dake, BA, author
Autism Society of North Carolina Bookstore
505 Oberlin Road   919-743-0204
Raleigh, NC 27605-1345   800-442-2762
                                                        Fax: 919-743-0208
                            e-mail: info@autismsociety-nc.org
                                        www.autismsociety-nc.org
This book contains behaviorally based exercises and drills that adress common language weaknesses in children and incorporate professional speech pathology methods. These exercises were designed for children who are attentive, able to follow simple directions, have learned the basics of low-level language, and are visual learners. The activities and exercises are appropriate for children and young adults ages 5-18.
1997 410 pages Spiral Bound

1666 Teaching Children with Autism: Strategies to Enhance Communication and Socializing
Kathleen Ann Quill, author
Thomson Delmar Learning

Attn: Order Fullfillment
Florence, KY 41022

800-347-7707
Fax: 800-487-8488
www.delmarlearning.com

This book describes teaching strategies and instructional adaptations which promote communication and socialization in children with autism. It offers specific strategies that capitalize on the individual strengths and learning styles of the autistic child.
1996
ISBN: 0-827362-69-2

1667   Teaching Community Skills and Behaviors to Students with Autism or Related Problems
Indiana Resource Center for Autism
2853 East 10th Street
Bloomington, IN 47408-2696

812-855-6508
Fax: 812-855-9630
TTY: 812-855-9396
e-mail: iidc@indiana.edu
www.iidc.indiana.edu/irca/fmain1.html

Emphasizing the needs of the person with autism and the philosophy of community integration, this book cover the process of successful community-based teaching.
1988 117 pages

1668   The Autism Sourcebook
Karen Siff Exkorn, author
Autism Society of North Carolina Bookstore
505 Oberlin Road
Raleigh, NC 27605-1345

919-743-0204
800-442-2762
Fax: 919-743-0208
e-mail: www.autismsociety-nc.org
www.autismsociety-nc.org

This comprehensive handbook is for parents of newly diagnosed children who are looking for information about ASD, its diagnosis, treatment options, and practical strategies in one in-depth text.
2005

1669   The Everything Parent's Guide to Children with Autism
Adelle Jameson Tilton, author
Autism Society of North Carolina Bookstore
505 Oberlin Road
Raleigh, NC 27605-1345

919-743-0204
800-442-2762
Fax: 919-743-0208
e-mail: info@autismsociety-nc.org
www.autismsociety-nc.org

This book offers a wealth of information and reassuring advice for parents of newly diagnosed children. It is filled with hundreds of helpful tips, unique insights, and real-life situations, this is an essential guide for parents and family members.
2004 285 pages Softcover

1670   Understanding the Nature of Autism A Guide to the Autism Spectrum Disorders
Janice E Janzen, author
Autism Society of North Carolina Bookstore
505 Oberlin Road
Raleigh, NC 27605-1345

919-743-0204
800-442-2762
Fax: 919-743-0208
e-mail: info@autismsociety-nc.org
www.autismsociety-nc.org

Straightforward and comprehensive information that can be used by parents and professionals to develop curricula and programs for children with autism spectrum disorder. This important resource is a standard text used by educators, parents, and caregivers.
2003 508 pages Softcover

1671   When Snow Turns to Rain
Woodbine House
6510 Bells Mill Road
Bethesda, MD 20817-1636

301-897-3570
800-843-7323
Fax: 301-897-5838
e-mail: info@woodbinehouse.com
www.woodbinehouse.com

A gripping personal account of one family's experiences with autism. Chronicles a family's journey from parental bliss to devasta-

tion, as they learn that their son has autism. This book delves into diagnosis, treatments and attitudes toward persons with autism.
1993 250 pages Paperback
ISBN: 0-933149-63-8

1672   Autism Spectrum Disorders: The Complete Guide
Chantal Sicile-Kira, author
Autism Society of North Carolina Bookstore
505 Oberlin Road
Raleigh, NC 27605-1345

919-743-0204
800-442-2762
Fax: 919-743-0208
e-mail: info@autismsociety-nc.org
www.autismsociety-nc.org

This reference guide was written to help parents, professionals, and other members of the community learn more about autism spectrum disorder, and it presents a thorough overview of the disorder, from diagnosis through adulthood.
2004 360 pages Softcover

Children's Books

1673   Joey and Sam
Illana Katz and Edward Ritvo, MD, author
Autism Society of North Carolina Bookstore
505 Oberlin Road
Raleigh, NC 27605-1345

919-743-0204
800-442-2762
Fax: 919-743-0208
e-mail: ASNC@aol.com

A unique and invaluable tool for teaching children about others who are different. This awrd-winning and heartwarming sibling storybook examines the similarities and differences in behavior and educational experiences of two brothers, one of whom has autism.
1993 Softcover
ISBN: 1-882388-00-3

1674   Russell is Extra Special
Charles A Amenta III. MD, author
Autism Society of North Carolina Bookstore
505 Oberlin Road
Raleigh, NC 27605-1345

919-743-0204
800-442-2762
Fax: 919-743-0208
e-mail: info@autismsociety-nc.org
www.autismsociety-nc.org

A sensitive portrayal of an autistic boy written by his father.
Hardcover

1675   Wild Boy of Aveyron
Harlan Lane, author
Harvard University Press
79 Garden Street
Cambridge, MA 02138

800-405-1619
Fax: 800-406-9145
e-mail: contact_HUP@harvard.edu
www.hup.harvard.edu

A dramatic account of a wild boy of nature and a young French doctor who shaped the modern education of retarded, deaf, and preschool children.
368 pages
ISBN: 0-674953-00-2

Newsletters

1676   Autism Research Review International
Autism Research Institute
4182 Adams Avenue
San Diego, CA 92116-2536

619-281-7165
Fax: 619-563-6840
www.autismresearchchinstitute.com

A quarterly newsletter published by the Autism Research Institute.
8 pages Quarterly
Dr. Bernard Rimland, Director

Pamphlets

1677 Avoiding Unfortunate Situations
Autism Society of North Carolina Bookstore
505 Oberlin Road   919-743-0204
Raleigh, NC 27605-1345   800-442-2762
                                Fax: 919-743-0208
                    e-mail: info@autismsociety-nc.org
                              www.autismsociety-nc.org
A collection of tips and information from and about people with autism and other developmental disabilities and their encounters with law enforcement agencies.

1678 Developing a Functional and Longitudinal Individual Plan
Nancy Dalrymple, author
Autism Society of North Carolina Bookstore
505 Oberlin Road   919-743-0204
Raleigh, NC 27605-1345   800-442-2762
                                Fax: 919-743-0208
                    e-mail: info@autismspectrum-nc.org
                              www.autismspectrum-nc.org
It is the author's view that a functional, longitudinal approach should be taken when educating persons with autism spectrum disorder, and that the developmentof an individualized plan should incorporate school, home, and community. This guide discusses the importance of defining strengths, striving for independent functioning, and determining which activitiesshould recieve priority in the areas of self-care, social and leisure activities, and employment.
1989 11 pages Booklet

1679 Enabling Communication in Children with Autism
Autism Society of North Carolina Bookstore
505 Oberlin Road   919-743-0204
Raleigh, NC 27605-1345   800-442-2762
                                Fax: 919-743-0208
                    e-mail: info@autismsociety-nc.org
                              www.autismsociety-nc.org
Based on a 2 year research project, the goal of this book is to help teachers develop more communication-enabling enviroments for children with atuism spectrum disorder who use little or no speech. The authors illustrate many communication-enabling strategies, including the minimal speech approach, proximal communication, prompting, and multipointing.
2001 207 pages Softcover

1680 Job Seeker Involvment in Securing Employment
Nancy Kalina, author
Indiana Resource Center for Autism
2853 East 10th Street   812-855-6508
Bloomington, IN 47408-2696   Fax: 812-855-9630
                                TTY: 812-855-9396
                         e-mail: iidc@indiana.edu
                www.iidc.indiana.edu/irca/fmain1.html
A walk through the job development process, from identifying job options and writing a resume to negotiating workplace supports with a potential employer. Each step provides opportunities for the peronal with autism, or another disability, to become actively involved in their job search process.
1997 22 pages

1681 Learning to be Independent and Responsible
Nancy Dalrymple, author
Indiana Resource Center for Autism
2853 East 10th Street   812-855-6508
Bloomington, IN 47408-2696   Fax: 812-855-9630
                                TTY: 812-855-9396
                         e-mail: iidc@indiana.edu
                www.iidc.indiana.edu/irca/fmain1.html
People with autism build trust in people and environments through successful interactions. Individualized, supportive programs, utilizing positive instructional and environmental supports that lead to increased opportunities, chouse, and motivation are described in this booklet.
1989 11 pages

1682 Parents as Trainers of Legislators, Other Parents and Researchers
Autism Services Center
101 Richmond Street   304-525-8014
Huntington, WV 25702-1513   Fax: 304-525-8026
Reprint offering information on parents of autistic children that learn early in their child's life how little professionals know about autism.

1683 Sex, Sexuality, and the Autism Specrtum
Wendy Lawson, author
Autism Society of North Carolina Bookstore
505 Oberlin Road   919-743-0204
Raleigh, NC 27605-1345   800-442-2762
                                Fax: 919-743-0208
                    e-mail: info@autismsociety-nc.org
                              www.autismsociety-nc.org
The author, a psychologist, who has Aspergers Syndrome, presents her unique perspective on sexuality and interpersonal relationships. Filled with honest insights and positive advice, this is a valuable guide for persons with ASD and the people who live and work with them.
2005 175 pages Softcover

1684 Son-Rise Method
Option Institute
2080 S Undermountain Road   413-229-2100
Sheffield, MA 01257-9643   Fax: 413-229-8931
                         e-mail: sonrise@option.org
                              www.son-rise.org
Describes a program Barry and Samahria Kaufman developed to help heal their once-autistic son.

1685 What Is Autism
Autism Society of America
7910 Woodmont Avenue   301-657-0881
Bethesda, MD 20814-3065   800-328-8476
                                Fax: 301-657-0869
                    e-mail: info@autism-society.org
                              www.autism-society.org
Offers a definition and introduction to autism, produces a wide range of autism information written for various audiences. Offers a quarterly magazine, national conference, nationwide chapter network and many other resources.

Audio & Video

1686 A Sense of Belonging: Including Students with Autism in their School Community
Indiana Resource Center for Autism
2853 East 10th Street   812-855-6508
Bloomington, IN 47408-2696   Fax: 812-855-9630
                                TTY: 812-855-9396
                         e-mail: iidc@indiana.edu
                www.iidc.indiana.edu/irca/fmain1.html
Highlights the efforts of two elementary and one middle school in Indiana in teaching students with autism in general education settings. Comments from parents, school administrators, classmates, and educators illustrate the role they each played in supporting students with autism in becoming active learners in their school community. Includes practical strategies for teaching the student with autism.
1997 20 minutes

1687 Autism: A Strange, Silent World
Filmakers Library
124 E 40th Street   212-808-4980
New York, NY 10016   Fax: 212-808-4983
                         e-mail: info@filmakers.com
                              www.filmakers.com
A comprehensive view of autism by focusing on three children of different ages, with very different behaviors. Also introduces us to a remarkable group of parents, teachers and therapists who strive to maximize
VHS/DVD
Sue Oscar, Co-President
Linda Gottesman, Co-President

1688 Autism: A World Apart
Karen Cunninghame, author
Fanlight Productions
4196 Washington Street   617-469-4999
Boston, MA 02131-1731   800-937-4113
                                   Fax: 617-469-3379
                        e-mail: fanlight@fanlight.com
                                      www.fanlight.com
In this documentary, three families show us what the textbooks and studies cannot, what it's like to live with autism day after day, raise and love children who may be withdrawn and violent and unable to make personal connections with their families.
DVD
ISBN: 1-572959-50-9

1689 Developing IEPs Under the New Idea Regulations
LRP Publications
747 Dresher Road
Horsham, PA 19044-2247   800-341-7874
                                   Fax: 215-784-9639
                         e-mail: custserve@lrp.com
                                        www.lrp.com
A practical, step-by-step approach makes it easy to understand the legal and educational issues surrounding IEPs.
26 minutes

1690 Discipline Under the New Idea: Practical Methods and Procedures
LRP Publications
747 Dresher Road
Horsham, PA 19044-2247   800-341-7874
                                   Fax: 215-784-9639
                         e-mail: custserve@lrp.com
                                        www.lrp.com
Provides practical explanation of the discipline methods and procedures school officials are permitted to use for students with disabilities.
26 minutes

1691 Embracing Play: Teaching Your Child with Autism
Woodbine House
6510 Bells Mill Road   301-897-3570
Bethesda, MD 20817   800-843-7323
                                   Fax: 301-897-5838
                            www.woodbinehouse.com
Guide for parents who incorporate applied behavior analysis with their child.
1993 47 minutes

1692 Functional Behavioral Assessments: How to Do Them Right!
LRP Publications
747 Dresher Road
Horsham, PA 19044-2247   800-341-7874
                                   Fax: 215-784-9639
                         e-mail: custserve@lrp.com
                                        www.lrp.com
Assist you in understanding why a behavior problem has occured, so you can maximize the effectiveness of a planned intervention.
18 minutes

1693 Getting Started with Facilitated Communication
Syracuse University, Facilitated Communication Ins
370 Huntington Hall   315-443-9379
Syracuse, NY 13244-2340   Fax: 315-443-9218
                             e-mail: fcstaff@syr.edu
                             soeweb.syr.edu/thefci/
Describes in detail how to help individuals with autism and/or severe communication difficulties to get started with facilitated communication.
Videotape

1694 Going to School with Facilitated Communication
Syracuse University, School of Education
805 S Krouse   315-443-2693
Syracuse, NY 13244-0001
A video in which students with autism and/or severe disabilities illustrate the use of facilitated communication focusing on basic principles fostering facilitated communication.
Videotape

1695 I Want My Little Boy Back
Autism Treatment Center of America
2080 S Undermountain Road   413-229-2100
Sheffield, MA 01257   800-714-2779
                                   Fax: 413-229-8931
                          e-mail: www.son-rise.org
                          information@son-rise.org
This BBC documentary follows an English family with a child with autism before, during, and after their time at the Son-Rise Program. It uniquely captures the heart of the Son-Rise Program and is extremely useful in understanding the program's techniques.
Lauren Astor, Public Relations Manager

1696 I'm Not Autistic on the Typewriter
Syracuse University, School of Education
805 S Krouse   315-443-2693
Syracuse, NY 13244-0001
A video introducing facilitated communication, a method by which persons with autism express themselves.
Videotape

1697 Invisible Wall: Autism
PRIMEDIA/Films Media Group
Films for Humanities & Sciences
Princeton, NJ 08543   800-257-5126
                                   Fax: 609-671-0266
              e-mail: custserv@filmsmediagroup.com
                                       www.films.com/
It features interviews with Ivar Lovaas, the creator of applied behavior analysis therapy.
2001 52 minutes
Dean B Nelson, Chairman & President
Kevin Neary, Chief Financial Officer

1698 Public Schools and Students with Autism: Components of a Defensible Program
LRP Publications
747 Dresher Road
Horsham, PA 19044-2247   800-341-7874
                                   Fax: 215-784-9639
                         e-mail: custserve@lrp.com
                                        www.lrp.com
This video assists you in understanding transition planning, documentation of student progress and proven strategies you can implement in your program.
13 minutes

1699 Standards and Inclusion: Can We Have Both?
LRP Publications
747 Dresher Road
Horsham, PA 19044-2247   800-341-7874
                                   Fax: 215-784-9639
                         e-mail: custserve@lrp.com
                                        www.lrp.com
Addresses the critical issues educators face when supporting students with disabilities in inclusive settings. Through dynamic, powerful presentations by two inclusion experts.
40 minutes

1700 Understanding Autism
Suzanne Newman, author
Fanlight Productions
4196 Washington Street   617-469-4999
Boston, MA 02131-1731   800-937-4113
                                   Fax: 617-469-3379
                        e-mail: fanlight@fanlight.com
                                      www.fanlight.com
Parents of children with autism discuss the nature and symptoms of this lifelong disability and outlines a treatment program based on behavior modification principles.
1993 19 Minutes
ISBN: 1-572951-00-1

Web Sites

1701 Autism Research Institute
                                  www.autism.com/ari/

A clearinghouse for research on autism and related disorders of learning and behavior. Conducts and compiles research findings to provide people with the latest research available.

1702 Autism Resources

www.autism-resources.com

Provides information and links regarding the developmental disabilities autism and Asperger's Syndrome.

1703 Autism Society of America

www.autism-society.org

Exists to improve the lives of all affected by autism by increasing public awareness about the day-to-day issues faced by people on the spectrum, advocating for appropriate services for individuals across the lifespan, and providing the latest information regarding treatment, education, research and advocacy.

1704 Autism Treatment Center of America

www.autismtreatment.com

the worldwide teaching center for The Son-Rise Program , a powerful and effective treatment for children and adults challenged by Autism, Autism Spectrum Disorders, Pervasive Developmental Disorder (PDD) , Asperger's Syndrome, and other developmental difficulties.

1705 Community Services for Autistic Adults & Children

www.csaac.org

A private, non-profit agency which provides direct services to children and adults with autism across the lifespan. CSAAC's mission is to enable individuals with autism to reach their highest potential and contribute as confident individuals to their community.

1706 Healing Well

www.healingwell.com

A social network and support community for patients, caregivers, and families coping with the daily struggles of diseases, disorders and chronic illness.

1707 Health Finder

www.healthfinder.gov

A government web site there individuals can find information and tools to help you and those you care about stay healthy.

1708 Healthlink USA

www.healthlinkusa.com

Health information concerning treatment, cures, prevention, diagnosis, risk factors, research, support groups, email lists, personal stories and much more. Updated regularly.

1709 Helios Health

www.helioshealth.com

Online resource for your health information. Detailed information about specific health topics, access to expert advice from our Medical Advisory Board, and up-to-date health news.

1710 MedicineNet

www.medicinenet.com

An online resource for consumers providing easy-to-read, authoritative medical and health information.

1711 Medscape

www.medscape.com

Medscape offers specialists, primary care physicians, and other health professionals the Web's most robust and integrated medical information and educational tools.

1712 National Alliance for Autism Research

www.naar.org

The first organization in the United States dedicated to funding and accelerating biomedical research focusing on autism spectrum disorders.

1713 National Institute of Mental Health

www.nimh.nih.gov

Mission is to transform the understanding and treatment of mental illnesses through basic and clinical research, paving the way for prevention, recovery, and cure.

1714 Son Rise Program

www.autismtreatmentcenter.org

Describes an effective, loving and respectful method for treating children with autism. It teaches parents and healing professionals how to set up a home based program using the child's motivation to reach their special child.

1715 WebMD

www.webmd.com

Information on Autism, including articles and resources.

Description

1716 Birth Defects

Birth defects, or congenital abnormalities, occur in 3 to 4 percent of newborns and can include structural defects of the heart, major blood vessels, kidneys, urinary tract, gastrointestinal tract, skeleton and nervous system. The incidence of specific abnormalities varies with the type of defect. These defects may be single or several defects may occur together, often known as a syndrome.

Although in many instances the cause of the defect is unknown, genetic factors may cause many single malformations and syndromes. Some syndromes, such as Down syndrome, result from chromosomal abnormalities. Factors during the pregnancy can sometimes result in defects, such as taking certain drugs (Coumadin, Dilantin), maternal illness (diabetes), and various infections (German measles, Rubella).

Prior to birth, ultrasound evaluation of the fetus and testing of the amniotic fluid surrounding it can identify some defects. If a defect is identified and is serious, parents can decide how or if they wish the pregnancy to proceed. Other abnormalities may not be identified until birth. Treatment and outcome vary greatly, depending on the type and severity of the defect. Parents and other family members need honest information and emotional support when caring for a child born with congenital defects. If genetic factors are suspected, the parents should receive genetic counseling. See also *Spina Bifida and Congenital Heart Disease.*

National Agencies & Associations

1717 Birth Defect Research for Children
800 Celebration Avenue   407-566-8304
Celebration, FL 34747   Fax: 407-566-8341
e-mail: staff@birthdefects.org.
www.birthdefects.org
A nonprofit organization that provides information about birth defects of all kinds to parents and professionals. Offers a library of medical books and files of information on less common categories of birth defects and is involved in research to discover causes and prevention.
Betty Mekdeci, Executive Director
John Bragg, Administrative Assistant

1718 CAPP National Parent Resource Center
95 Berkeley Street   617-482-2915
Boston, MA 02116   800-331-0688
Fax: 617-695-2939
e-mail: cec@cec.sped.org
www.cec.sped.org
A parent-run resource system designed to further the needs and goals of family-centered community-based coordinated care for children with special health needs and their families. Offers written materials, training packages, workshops and presentations.
Marilyn Friend, President
Mark Innocenti, Associate Director

1719 Cleft Palate Foundation
1504 E Franklin Street   919-933-9044
Chapel Hill, NC 27514-2820   800-24C-LEFT
Fax: 919-933-9604
e-mail: info@cleftline.org
www.cleftline.org
Major services are provided through CLEFTLINE, a 24 hour toll free hotline for anyone affected by a facial birth defect. We provide free educational materials referrals to local treatment and support groups and hope.
Nancy C Smythe, Executive Director
Samantha Jennings MSW, Family Services Director

1720 Cornelia de Lange Syndrome Foundation
302 W Main Street   860-676-8166
Avon, CT 06001   800-223-8355
Fax: 860-676-8337
e-mail: info@cdlsusa.org
www.cdlsusa.org
Provides information about birth defects caused by Cornelia de Lange Syndrome.
Liana Garcia-Fresher, Executive Director
Barbara Koontz, Information Coordinator

1721 Easter Seals
233 South Wacker Drive   312-726-6200
Chicago, IL 60606   800-221-6827
Fax: 312-726-1494
TTY: 312-726-4258
e-mail: info@easter-seals.org
www.easter-seals.org
Provides services to children and adults with disabilities as well as support to their families.
Reenie Kavalor, VP Medical/Rehabilitation Services
Stephen F Rossman, Chair

1722 Federation for Children with Special Needs
1135 Tremont Street   617-236-7210
Boston, MA 02120   800-331-0688
Fax: 617-572-2094
e-mail: fcsninfo@fcsn.org
www.fcsn.org
A center for parents and parent organizations to work together on behalf of children with special needs.
Deborah Allen, Director
Peter Brenna CPA, Board of Director

1723 March of Dimes Birth Defects Foundation
1275 Mamaroneck Avenue
White Plains, NY 10605   914-997-4488
www.marchofdimes.com
Our mission is to improve the health of babies by preventing birth defects premature birth and infant mortality. The March of Dimes carries out this mission through programs of research community services education and advocacy to save babies' lives.

1724 National Early Childhood Technical Assistance Center
Campus Box 8040 UNC-CH   919-962-2001
Chapel Hill, NC 27599-8040   Fax: 919-966-7463
TDD: 919-843-3269
e-mail: nectac@unc.edu
www.nectac.org
Assists states and other designated governing jurisdictions as they develop multidisciplinary, coordinated and comprehensive services for children with special needs.
Lynn Kahn, Director
Beverly Payne-Betts, Administrative Assistant

1725 National Foundation for Facial Reconstruction
333 East 30th Street   212-263-6656
New York, NY 10016   Fax: 212-263-7534
e-mail: info@nffr.org
www.nffr.org
The National Foundation for Facial Reconstruction addresses the plight of children with a facial disfigurement by supporting state of the art treatment, innovative research, psychosocial support and medical training that inspires a new generation of pediatric doctors.
Whitney Burnett, Executive Director
Michele B Golombuski, MS, Associate Executive Director

1726 Parent Professional Advocacy League
45 Bromfield Street   617-542-7860
Boston, MA 02108   866-815-8122
Fax: 617-542-7832
e-mail: info@ppal.net
www.ppal.net

An organization of families of children with mental emotional or behavioral needs and concerned professionals. PALS support groups are run in many areas across the country.
Earl N. "Ski Stuck, Chair
Anne Metzger, Treasurer

Research Centers

1727 Boston University Center for Human Genetics
715 Albany Street
Boston, MA 02118-2394
617-638-4640
Fax: 617-638-7092
e-mail: amilunski@bu.edu
www.bumc.bu.edu
Offers research into genetic disorders and growth disorders.
Dr Karen H Antman, Dean
Jeff Milunsky, Co-Director

1728 California Teratogen Information Service UC San Diego School of Medicine Dept of
UC San Diego School of Medicine Dept of Pediatrics
9500 Gilman Drive
La Jolla, CA 92093-828
619-294-6291
800-532-3749
Fax: 619-220-0228
e-mail: ctispregnancy@ucsd.edu
www.ctispregnancy.org
Statewide service operated by the California Teratogen Information Service (CTIS) and Clinical Research Program. Our goal is to promote healthy pregnancies through education and research.
Kenneth Lyon Jones MD, Medical Director
Christina D Chambers, Program Director

1729 Department of Reproductive Genetics: Magee Women's Hospital
200 Lothrop Street
Pittsburgh, PA 15213-2582
412-647-8748
800-533-8762
Fax: 412-641-1032
e-mail: dbrucha@mail.magee.edu
www.upmc.com
Obstetrical and gynecological teaching unit of the University of Pittsburgh School of Medicine. A full-service women's hospital and now has expanded to include a range of services for women and men.
W Allen Hogge, Clinical Investigator
Jie Hu, Assistant Investigator

1730 Division Of Developmental and Behavioral Pediatrics
Children's Hospital Medical Center of Cincinnati
3333 Burnet Avenue
Cincinnati, OH 45229-3039
513-636-4200
800-344-2462
TTY: 513-636-4900
www.cincinnatichildrens.org
The Division of Developmental and Behavioral Pediatrics provides services for infants children and adolescents from birth to age 21 who are experiencing developmental or behavioral problems.
David J Schonfeld, Director
Matthew W Zurad, Business Director

1731 Georgetown University Child Development Center
Box 571485
Washington, DC 20057-1485
202-687-5000
Fax: 202-687-8899
e-mail: gucdc@georgetown.edu
www.gucchd.georgetown.edu
The mission of the GUCCHD is to bring together policy, research and clinical practice for the betterment of individuals and families, especially children youth and those with special needs including: development disabilities and special health care needs, mental health needs, young children and those in the child welfare system.
John De Gioia, President
Neal Horen, Co-Director Training and Technical Assis

1732 Louisiana State University Genetics Section of Pediatrics
200 Clay Avenue
New Orleans, LA 70118
504-896-9524
Fax: 504-894-3997
e-mail: ylacas@lsuhsc.edu
www.medschool.lsuhsc.edu

Yves Lacassie, Section Head
Mary Camille Fournet, Research Associate

1733 New England Regional Genetics Group
PO Box 920288
Needham, MA 02492
781-444-0126
Fax: 781-444-0127
e-mail: mfgnergg@verizon.net
www.nergg.org
Human genetic services and educational planning pertaining to birth defects.
Mary-Frances Garber, Executive Director
Cindy Ingham, Co-Director

1734 Teratology OTIS
1295 N Martin
Tucson, AZ 85721-202
520-626-3547
866-626-6847
e-mail: contactus@otispregnancy.org
www.otispregnancy.org
Teratology Information Services are comprehensive and multidisciplinary resources for medical consultation on prenatal exposures. TIS interpret information regarding known and potential reproductive risks into risk assessments that are communicated to individuals of reproductive age and health care providers.
Dee Quinn, Executive Director
Lori Wolfe, President

1735 Thomas Jefferson University: Daniel Baugh Institute
329 Jefferson Alumni Hall
1020 Locust Street
Philadelphia, PA 19107
215-503-7823
Fax: 215-503-2636
e-mail: James.Schwaber@mail.dbi.tju.edu
www.dbi.tju.edu
Cares for both out and in-patients with complex problems involving a wide variety of infectious diseases. The Division has an active clinical research program bringing state-of-the-art treatments to patients.
James Schwaber, Director
Boris N Kholodenko, Director Computational Cell Biology

1736 University of Illinois at Chicago Craniofacial Center
College of Medicine
180 DENT M/C 588
Chicago, IL 60612
312-996-7546
Fax: 312-413-1157
e-mail: dreisber@uic.edu
www.uic.edu

David J Reisberg, Director

1737 University of Iowa Birth Defects and Genetic Disorders Unit
Iowa Registry for Congenital/Inherited Disorders
100 Oakdale Campus
Iowa City, IA 52242-5000
319-335-3500
866-274-4237
Fax: 319-335-4030
e-mail: ircid@uiowa.edu
www.uiowa.edu
Established through the joint efforts of the University of Iowa the Iowa Department of Public Health and the Iowa Department of Human Services to monitor birth defects in the state.
Paul A Romitti, Director
Kim Keppler-Noreuil, Clinical Director for Birth Defects

1738 University of Miami: Mailman Center for Child Development
1601 NW 12th Avenue
Miami, FL 33136-6820
305-243-6801
Fax: 305-243-5978
TTY: 305-243-5937
TDD: 305-243-5937
www.pediatrics.med.miami.edu
Focuses on birth defects and children's illnesses.
Dr Robert Stempfel Jr, Director

1739 Wayne State University: CS Mott Center for Human Growth and Development
275 E Hancock Street
Detroit, MI 48201
313-577-1485
Fax: 313-577-8554
home.med.wayne.edu
Human growth and development disorders.
Dr Robert Sokol, Director
Valerie M Parisi, Dean

1740 Wichita Medical Research & Education Foundation
3306 E Central Avenue
Wichita, KS 67208-3104
316-686-7172
Fax: 316-687-0033
e-mail: info@wichitamedicalresearch.org
www.wichitamedicalresearch.org

The Wichita Medical Research Foundation promotes research for the development of new medical skills and knowledge which serve patients from Wichita and throughout Kansas.
Peggy L Johnson, Executive Director/COO
William Hendry PhD, President

Support Groups & Hotlines

1741 CUNY: Teratogen Information Service
People
1219 N Forest Road   716-634-8132
Williamsville, NY 14221-3292   888-773-0753
                                   Fax: 716-634-3889
                                   www.people-inc.org

Mary Ann Kedron, Ph.D., Chairperson
Joseph J. Abdallah, Vice Chairperson

1742 Connecticut Pregnancy Exposure Information Service
UConn Health Partners
Division of Human Genetics   860-523-6419
West Hartford, CT 06119   800-325-5391
                                   humangenetics.uchc.edu
Provides up-to-date information on all types of exposures during pregnancy or breastfeeding for Connecticut residents or women who have Connecticut physicians.
Philip E Austin, President
James F Abromaitis, Commissioner

1743 Illinois Teratogen Information Service (IT IS)
680 N Lake Shore Drive   312-981-4354
Chicago, IL 60611   800-252-4847
                                   e-mail: itis@fetal-exposure.org
                                   www.fetal-exposure.org
A free statewide service that is financially supported by the Illinois Department of Public Health. Provides information regarding all types of exposures during pregnancy, and is available to women who are pregnant or planning a pregnancy, fathers, physicians, and other health care providers in the State of Illinois
Kristen L Dieter MS/CGC, Genetic Counselor/Coordinator ITIS
Eugene Pergament MD/Ph.D, Medical Geneticist

1744 Indiana Teratogen Information Service
Indiana University Medical Center
975 W Walnut Street
Indianapolis, IN 46202   317-274-2241
                                   www.genetics.medicine.iu.edu
A telephone inquiry service that provides central, up-to-date, information from computersized sources, professional articles and expert consultants
David D Weaver MD, Director

1745 Missouri Teratogen Information Service
University of Missouri Health Care
1 Hospital Drive   573-882-7299
Columbia, MO 65212-1   Fax: 573-882-1593
                                   e-mail: umhs-muhealth@missouri.edu
                                   www.muhealth.org/
The Missouri Teratogen Information Services (MOTIS) helps promote healthy pregnancies by providing, counseling, education and information.
James Ross, Chief Executive Officer
James C Poehling, Chief Operating Officer

1746 National Health Information Center
PO Box 1133   310-565-4167
Washington, DC 20013-1133   800-336-4797
                                   Fax: 301-984-4256
                                   e-mail: info@nhic.org
                                   www.health.gov/nhic
A health information referral service sponsored by the Office of Disease Prevention and Health Promotion. Puts health professionals and consumers who have health questions in touch with those organizations that are best able to provide answers.

1747 Nebraska Information Service
University of Nebraska Medical Center
985440 Nebraska Medical Center   402-559-5071
Omaha, NE 68198-5440   Fax: 402-559-7248

Teratogen Information Project
Beth Conover APRN, MS, Genetic Counselor
Kathleen Caldwell, Project Assistant

1748 New Jersey Pregnancy Risk Information Service
254 Easton Avenue   732-745-6659
New Brunswick, NJ 8901-1766
DebraLynn Day Salvatore, Medical Director

1749 PALS Support Groups
Parent/Professional Advocacy League
45 Bromfield Street   617-542-7860
Boston, MA 02108   866-815-8122
                                   Fax: 617-542-7832
                                   e-mail: info@ppal.net
                                   ppal.net
Promotes a strong voice for families of children and adolescents with mental health needs. Advocates for supports, treatment and policies that enale families to live in their communities in an environment of stability and respect.
Lisa Lambert, Executive Director
Christopher Anselmo, Project Coordinator

1750 Pregnancy Healthline: Pennsylvania Hospital
8th & Spruce Streets   215-829-3601
Philadelphia, PA 19107
Betsy Schick-Boschetto MSN

1751 Pregnancy Risk Line
Utah Department of Health
PO Box 141010   801-328-2229
Salt Lake City, UT 84114-1010   800-822-2229
                                   www.health.utah.gov/prl
Provides vauluable information to women who are pregnant, considering becoming pregnant, or breastfeeding, and to their healthcare providers.

1752 Pregnancy Safety Hotline
Western Pennsylvania Hospital
4800 Friendship Avenue
Pittsburgh, PA 15224-1722   412-687-7233
                                   www.wphs.org

Michael Kerr MS

1753 Teratogen Information Services
University of Florida Health Science Center
PO Box 100296
Gainesville, FL 32610-0296   352-392-3050
                                   www.health.ufl.edu

Donna H Poynor MA

1754 Teratogen and Birth Defects Information Project
University of South Dakota
414 E Clark Street   605-677-5011
Vermillion, SD 57069-2307   877-269-6837
                                   Fax: 605-677-6534
                                   e-mail: urelations@usd.edu
                                   www.usd.edu

James Abbott, University President
Rod Parry, Dean of the Medical School

1755 University of Iowa Teratogen Information Service
University of Iowa Teratogen
200 Hakins Drive   319-353-7877
Iowa City, IA 52242   800-777-8442
                                   www.uihealthcare.com

Donna Katen Bahensky, Chief Executive Officer
Anne Madenrice, Chief Operations Officer

1756 University of Nebraska Medical Center Tera Togen Project
Genetic Medicine-Munroe-Meyer Institute
985430 Nebraska Medical Center   402-559-6800
Omaha, NE 68198-5430   800-656-3937
                                   Fax: 402-559-6688
                                   e-mail: gbschaef@unmc.edu
                                   www.unmc.edu/dept/mmi/
The section of Genetic Medicine provides comprehensive services for a variety of patients and their families. Direct services include diagnosis, interpretation of risks, supportive counseling, and suggestions/referrals for further management. The department partic-

ipates in clinics, inpatient consultation, and the Teratogen Information Project.

G Bradley Schaefer MD/FAAP/FACMG, Director Genetics Department

1757 Vermont Pregnancy Risk Information Service
Vermont Regional Genetics Center
1 Mill Street
Burlington, VT 05401-1530   800-932-4609
Alan E Guttmacher MD

Books

1758 Bendectin Report
930 Woodcock Road   407-245-7035
Orlando, FL 32812   800-313-2232
                                www.birthdefects.org
Report on research connecting the anti-nausea medication, Bendectin, with birth defects. Includes latest judicial opinion confirming $24 million judgment in a Bendectin case.
90 pages

1759 Dursban Report
930 Woodcock Road   407-245-7035
Orlando, FL 32812   800-313-2232
                                www.birthdefects.org
Report on research and latest EPA findings on Dursban and health problems, including MCS and birth defects.
90 pages

1760 Environmental Birth Defect Digest
930 Woodcock Road   407-245-7035
Orlando, FL 32812   800-313-2232
                                www.birthdefects.org
Compendium of research briefs from the world medical literature, plus original articles covering birth defects associated with medications, radiation, chemicals, toxic sites, dioxin, pesticides, lead, mercury, Bendectin, aspartame and more.
42 pages

1761 Understanding Birth Defects
Franklin Watts Grolier
90 Old Sherman Turnpike   203-797-3500
Danbury, CT 06816-0001   800-621-1115
                                Fax: 203-797-3197
                                www.grolier.com
What birth defects are, their genetic and environmental origins and what can be done to help, plus the problems of low birth weight are discussed.
128 pages
ISBN: 0-531109-55-0

Children's Books

1762 Don't Feel Sorry for Paul
JB Lippincott
530 Walnut Street   215-521-8300
Philadelphia, PA 19105   Fax: 215-521-8902
                                www.ilkins.com
Paul is seven and was born with deformities of both hands and feet. Paul must wear a prosthesis on both feet so that he can walk. He has a third prosthesis for his right hand. The third prosthesis has a pair of hooks Paul uses as fingers.
94 pages Hardcover
ISBN: 0-397315-88-0

1763 God, the Universe and Hot Fudge Sundaes
Houghton, Mifflin & Company
222 Berkeley Street
Boston, MA 02108-3107   617-351-5000
                                www.hmco.com

Newsletters

1764 Birth Defect News
Birth Defect Research for Children

800 Celebration Ave   407-566-8304
Celebration, FL 34747   e-mail: staff@birthdefects.org
                                www.birthdefects.org

8 pages Quarterly
Betty Mekdeci, Executive Director

1765 NewsLine
Federation for Children with Special Needs
95 Berkeley Street   617-482-2915
Boston, MA 02116-6230   800-331-0688
Offers information for parents and families on resources, medical updates, activities, fund-raising events and association news for their disabled children.
Quarterly

1766 PAL News
Parent Professional Advocacy League
95 Berkeley Street   617-482-2915
Boston, MA 02116-6264   800-331-0688
Offers information on medical and technological updates in the area of research on birth defects, support groups and family resources for persons with disabled children.
Quarterly

Pamphlets

1767 After School...Then What? The Transition to Adulthood
Federation for Children with Special Needs
95 Berkeley Street   617-482-2915
Boston, MA 02116-6230   800-331-0688
Preparing for the transition after high school for children with special needs.

1768 Agent Orange and Birth Defects
930 Woodcock Road   407-245-7035
Orlando, FL 32812   800-313-2232
                                www.birthdefects.org
Research booklet, including the latest findings from the National Birth Defect Registry and government research connecting Agent Orange to birth defects.
42 pages

1769 Birth Defects & Genetics: The Genetics Revolution
March of Dimes Birth
233 Park Avenue South   212-353-8353
New York, NY 10003   Fax: 212-254-3518
                                e-mail: NY639@marchofdimes.com
                                www.marchofdimes.com
Offers information on genetic testing and what it means to the patient and family members.

1770 Childhood Illnesses in Pregnancy: Chicken Pox & Fifth Disease
March of Dimes
233 Park Avenue South   212-353-8353
New York, NY 10003   Fax: 212-254-3518
                                e-mail: NY639@marchofdimes.com
                                www.marchofdimes.com
Located on the March of Dimes website.

1771 Cleft Lip & Palate
March of Dimes
233 Park Avenue South   212-353-8353
New York, NY 10003   Fax: 212-254-3518
                                e-mail: NY639@marchofdimes.com
                                www.marchofdimes.com
Located on March of Dimes website.

1772 Club Foot and Other Foot Deformities
March of Dimes
233 Park Avenue South   212-353-8353
New York, NY 10003   Fax: 212-254-3518
                                e-mail: NY639@marchofdimes.com
                                www.marchofdimes.com

1773 Genetic Counseling
March of Dimes
233 Park Avenue South   212-353-8353
New York, NY 10003   Fax: 212-254-3518
                                e-mail: NY639@marchofdimes.com
                                www.marchofdimes.com

1774 Gulf War and Birth Defects
930 Woodcock Road   407-225-7035
Orlando, FL 32812   800-313-2232
                                    www.birthdefects.org
Information booklet on recent data from the National Birth Defect
Registry and other research related to Gulf War exposures and
birth defects.
30 pages

1775 How to Find More About Your Child's Birth Defect or Disability
Association for Birth Defect Children
5400 Diplomat Circle
Orlando, FL 32810-5603   800-922-9234
                                    www.birthdefects.org
An informational fact sheet that encourages parents who have a
child with a birth defect or disability to become the expert on the
child's disability with some suggestions on how to educate
themselves.

1776 Low Birthweight
March of Dimes
233 Park Avenue South   212-353-8353
New York, NY 10003   Fax: 212-254-3518
                          e-mail: NY639@marchofdimes.com
                                    www.marchofdimes.com
Fact Sheets: one or two page review written for the general public.

1777 PKU Quick Reference and Fact Sheet
March of Dimes
233 Park Avenue South   212-353-8353
New York, NY 10003   Fax: 212-254-3518
                          e-mail: NY639@marchofdimes.com
                                    www.marchofdimes.com
Phenylketonuria (PKU) is an inherited disorder that affects the
way the body is able to process food. If left untreated, it causes
mental retardation. How PKU is passed on and how it is treated are
outlined.

1778 Teaching Social Skills to Youngsters with Disabilities
Federation for Children with Special Needs
95 Berkeley Street   617-482-2915
Boston, MA 02116-6230   800-331-0688
Explains the importance of instruction and training to learn appro-
priate social behavior.

1779 Toxoplasmosis
March of Dimes
233 Park Avenue South   212-353-8353
New York, NY 10003   Fax: 212-254-3518
                          e-mail: NY639@marchofdimes.com
                                    www.marchofdimes.com
Fact Sheets: one or two page review written for the general public.

Audio & Video

1780 Genetics and Inherited Traits
March of Dimes
233 Park Avenue South   212-353-8353
New York, NY 10003   Fax: 212-254-3518
                          e-mail: NY639@marchofdimes.com
                                    www.marchofdimes.com

1781 Why My Child
5400 Diplomat Circle   407-629-1466
Orlando, FL 32810-5603   800-313-2232
                                    www.birthdefects.org
A 9 1/2 minute video that explores the feelings every parent has
when their child is born with a birth defect. Emmy-award-winning
producer, Karen Dorsett, has created a compelling video that begins with the parents' question, Why my child? and follows
through to concerns about links between birth defects and environmental exposures to drugs, pesticides, dioxin, radiation,
hazardous wastes, etc.

Web Sites

1782 Association for Birth Defect Children
                                    www.birthdefects.org

Provides parents and expectant parents with information about
birth defects and support services for their children.

1783 Healing Well
                                    www.healingwell.com
A social network and support community for patients, caregivers,
and families coping with the daily struggles of diseases, disorders
and chronic illness.

1784 Health Finder
                                    www.healthfinder.gov
A government web site where individuals can find information and
tools to help you and those you care about stay healthy.

1785 Healthlink USA
                                    www.healthlinkusa.com
Health information concerning treatment, cures, prevention, diagnosis, risk factors, research, support groups, email lists, personal
stories and much more. Updated regularly.

1786 Helios Health
                                    www.helioshealth.com
Online resource for your health information. Detailed information
about specific health topics, access to expert advice from our Medical Advisory Board, and up-to-date health news.

1787 March of Dimes Birth Defects Foundation
                                    www.marchofdimes.com
Help moms have full-term pregnancies and research the problems
that threaten the health of babies.

1788 MedicineNet
                                    www.medicinenet.com
An online resource for consumers providing easy-to-read, authoritative medical and health information.

1789 Medscape
                                    www.medscape.com
Medscape offers specialists, primary care physicians, and other
health professionals the Web's most robust and integrated medical
information and educational tools.

1790 WebMD
                                    www.webmd.com
Information on birth defects, including articles and resources.

Description

1791 Brain Tumors

Brain tumors are either primary (originate in the brain) or metastatic (travel from other cancer sites). About 29,000 people in the United States are diagnosed with primary brain tumors each year; approximately 50 percent of those are benign (noncancerous). Cancerous brain tumors originating in the brain make up roughly 2 percent of all cancers. They may occur at any age but are most common in early adult and middle life. Metastatic brain tumors (those that spread from other cancers) occur in 20 to 40 percent of all cancers.

There are many different types of brain tumors, each with a distinctive appearance under the microscope and a characteristic pattern of onset, progression, location and response to treatment. Depending on the exact site and rate of growth of the tumor, symptoms may include change in personality, moodiness, impaired vision and hearing, headaches, nausea, vomiting, seizures, lethargy and a varying degree of weakness. Some cancers have a genetic basis. In most cases, the cause of an individual's brain tumor is not known.

The treatment of brain tumors, as in many other cancers, consists of a combination of surgical removal, chemotherapy and radiation therapy. Steroids reduce swelling, and antiseizure medication is commonly given. If the disease or its treatment has caused damage to the brain's functioning, the patient may also need physical therapy, speech therapy, or general supportive care. The prognosis depends on the patient's age and on the location, extent and precise type of the tumor. See also *Head Injuries.*

National Agencies & Associations

1792 American Brain Tumor Association
2720 River Road
Des Plaines, IL 60018-4117
847-827-9910
800-886-2282
Fax: 847-827-9918
e-mail: info@abta.org
www.abta.org

Services includes over 40 publications which address brain tumors their treatment and coping with the disease. Materials address brain tumors in all age groups. Provide free social service consultations and a mentorship program for new brain tumor support groups.
Elizabeth M Wilson, Executive Director
Geri Jo Duda RN, Patient Services

1793 Brain Tumor Society
55 Chapel Street
Newton, MA 02458
617-924-9997
800-770-8287
Fax: 617-924-9998
e-mail: info@braintumor.org
www.braintumor.org

Exists to find a cure for brain tumors and strives to improve the quality of life of brain tumor patients and their families. Disseminates educational information and provides access to psycho-social support and raises funds.
N Paul TonThat, Chief Executive Officer
Carrie Treadwell, Director of Research

1794 National Brain Tumor Foundation
22 Battery Street
San Francisco, CA 94111-5520
415-834-9970
800-934-2873
Fax: 415-834-9980
e-mail: info@braintumor.org
www.braintumor.org

Nonprofit health organization which raises funds for research and provides information and support to patients, their family members and friends and health professionals. Sponsors national and regional conferences, patient and caregiver programs.
Harriet Patt MPH, Director of Patient Services
N. Paul TonThat, Executive Director

1795 National Brain Tumor Society
22 Battery Street
San Francisco, CA 94111-5520
415-834-9970
800-934-2873
Fax: 415-834-9980
e-mail: info@braintumor.org
www.braintumor.org

Nonprofit health organization which raises funds for research and provides information and support to patients, their family members and friends and health professionals. Sponsors national and regional conferences, patient and caregiver programs.
Gerogre Gellert, Chief Medical Officer
N. Paul TonThat, Executive Director

1796 National Institute of Neurological Disorders and Stroke
NIH Neurological Institute
Bethesda, MD 20824
301-496-5751
800-352-9424
Fax: 301-402-2186
TTY: 301-468-5981
www.ninds.nih.gov

The mission of NINDS is to reduce the burden of neurological disease - a burden borne by every age group, by every segment of society, by people all over the world.
Story C Landis, PhD, Director
Walter J Koroshetz, Deputy Director

Foundations

1797 Brain Tumor Foundation for Children
6065 Roswell Road NE
Atlanta, GA 30328
404-252-4107
Fax: 404-252-4108
e-mail: bfc@bellsouth.net
www.braintumorkids.org

Provides information and emotional support for families of children with brain tumors. They also raise funds for brain tumor research and provide a telephone network system of parents who offer emotional support.
Rick Sauers, Chairman/Co-Founder
R Hal Meeks, Jr, President

1798 Children's Brain Tumor Foundation
274 Madison Avenue
New York, NY 10016
212-448-9494
866-228-HOPE
Fax: 212-448-1022
e-mail: info@cbtf.org
www.cbtf.org

Children's Brain Tumor Foundation (CBTF) is a national organization whose mission is to improve the treatment, quality of life and long-term outlook for children with brain and spinal cord tumors through research, support, education, and advocacy to families and survivors. CBTF provides research and quality of life grants, offers information and support via our toll free line, written educational material, meet the unique needs of childhood brain tumor survivors.
Robert Budlow, President
Joseph B Fay, Executive Director

1799 Pediatric Brain Tumor Foundation
302 Ridgefield Court
Asheville, NC 28806
828-665-6891
800-253-6530
Fax: 828-655-6894
e-mail: pbtfus@pbtfus.org
www.pbtfus.org

Dedicated to finding the cause and cure of childhood brain tumors through the support of medical research. Increases public awareness, aids in early detection and treatment, supports a national database on all primary brain tumors. Helps to provide hope and

emotional support for the thousands of children and families affected by this life threatening disease.
Michael Traynor, President
Glenn Wilcox, Vice President

Research Centers

1800 Brain Research Center Children s Hospital National Medical Cen
Children s Hospital National Medical Center
111 Michigan Avenue NW   202-476-3000
Washington, DC 20010   800-884-5433
Fax: 202-884-5226
e-mail: tbear@cnmc.org
www.dcchildrens.com

Edwin K Zechman Jr, President
Mark L Batshaw, Chief Medical Officer

1801 Brain Research Foundation
111 W Washington Street   312-759-5150
Chicago, IL 60602   Fax: 312-759-5151
e-mail: info@theBRF.org
www.thebrf.org
Supports cutting-edge neuroscience research that will lead to novel treatments and prevention of neurological disease and disorders in children and adults. Deliver this commitment through seed grants, which provide early stage fundinf for innovative research projects, as well as educational programs for researchers and the general public.
Nathan Hansom, President
Terre A Constantine PhD, Executive Director

1802 Brain Tissue Resource Center McLean Hospital
McLean Hospital
115 Mill Street   617-855-2000
Belmont, MA 02478   800-272-4622
Fax: 617-855-3199
e-mail: mcleaninfo@mclean.harvard.edu
www.brainbank.mclean.org
A centralized resource for the collection and distribution of human brain specimens for brain research.
Francine M Benes, Director
Edward D Bird, Director Emeritus

1803 Central Brain Tumor Registry of the US
244 E Ogden avenue   630-655-4786
Hinsdale, IL 60521   Fax: 630-655-1756
e-mail: cbtrus@aol.com
www.cbtrus.org
Nonprofit resource for gathering and distributing current statistics on all primary brain tumors for the entire US. Includes data on benign borderline and malignant primary brain tumors.
Carol Kruchko, President /Administrator
Jeri Dolan, Executive Administrator

1804 University of California, San Francisco Brain Tumor Research Center
Department of Neurological Surgery
505 Parnassus Avenue   415-353-7500
San Francisco, CA 94143-0112   Fax: 415-353-2889
e-mail: garritye@neurosurg.ucsf.edu
www.neurosurgery.ucsf.edu
Continuously funded by grants from the National Institutes of Health Since 1072, the Brain Tumor Research Center at UCSF is internationally recognized as a major research and treatment center for adults and children with tumors of the brain and spinal cord. This center emphasizes translational research into the biology and behavior of brain tumors - research in which scientists and health care clinicians work in partnership to translate laboratory findings of new or improved forms of therapy.
Charles B Wilson, Director
Michael Gillis, Administrative Director

Support Groups & Hotlines

Alabama

1805 Pediatric Brain Tumor Support Group
Children's Hospital

1600 7th Avenue S   205-939-9090
Birmingham, AL 35233-1785
Groups for parents and siblings of brain tumor patients. Related to Children's Hospital of Alabama. Babysitting available.
Paula Teague

Arizona

1806 Arizona Brain Tumor Support Group
Barrow Neurological Ins of St. Joe's Hospital
350 W Thomas Road
Phoenix, AZ 85013   623-205-6446
www.braintumorfoundation.org
Lanette Veres, Director

1807 Southern Arizona Brain Tumor Support Group
Arizona Cancer Cetner
1515 N Campbell Avenue   520-694-4605
Tucson, AZ   e-mail: mdrozdoff@umcaz.edu
www.braintumorfoundation.org
Marsha Drozdoff, Contact

California

1808 Bereavement Group for Children
The Center for Attitudinal Healing
33 Buchanan Drive
Sausalito, CA 94965   415-331-6161
www.braintumor.org
Jimmy Pete, Contact

1809 Brain Tumor Society
National Brain Tumor Society
22 Battery Street   415-834-9970
San Francisco, CA 94111-5520   800-770-8287
Fax: 415-834-9980
e-mail: info@braintumor.org
www.braintumor.org
N Paul TonThat, Executive Director

1810 Brain Tumor Support Group: Duarte
City of Hope National Medical Center
1500 E Duarte Road
Duarte, CA 91010   626-256-4673
www.braintumor.org
Heather Ducksworth, Contact

1811 Brain Tumor Support Group: Fresno
Cancer Center at St. Agnes
7130 N Millbrook Avenue   559-450-5528
Fresno, CA 93720   e-mail: karen.kennedy@samc.com
www.braintumor.org
Karen Kennedy, Contact

1812 Brain Tumor Support Group: Fullerton
St. Jude Medical Plaza
2151 N Harbor Blvd   714-446-7182
Fullerton, CA 92835   e-mail: kathy.pearson@stjoe.org
www.braintumor.org
Kathy Pearson RN, Contact

1813 Brain Tumor Support Group: Newport Beach
Hoag Hospital
Advanced Technology Pavilion   949-764-6036
Newport Beach, CA 92663   e-mail: lberberet@hoaghospital.org
www.braintumor.org
Lori Berberet RN, Contact

1814 Brain Tumor Support Group: Orange
UC Irvine-Chao Family Comprehensive Cancer Center
101 The City Drive   714-456-8609
Orange, CA 92868   e-mail: bakerd@uci.edu
www.braintumor.org
N. Paul TonThat, Chief Executive Officer
Michele Rhee, Director of Program Initiatives

1815 Brain Tumor Support Group: Redding
American Cancer Society
3290 Bechelli Lane
Redding, CA 96002   530-222-1058
www.braintumor.org

1816 Brain Tumor Support Group: Sacramento
UC Davis Ambulatory Care Center
4860 Y Street   916-734-5613
Sacramento, CA 95817   e-mail: kksmith@ucdavis.edu
                                        www.braintumor.org

Karen Smith RN, Contact
Carolyn Guadagnolo LCSW, Contact

1817 Brain Tumor Support Group: San Diego
Kaiser's Pt Loma Medical Facility
3250 Fordham
San Diego, CA 92117   619-515-9908
                                        www.braintumor.org

Connie Campbell, Contact

1818 Brain Tumor Support Group: San Francisco
UCSF
521 Parnassus Avenue   415-990-4461
San Francisco, CA 94143   e-mail: mlovely@braintumor.org
                                        www.braintumor.org

Sharon Lamb RN, Contact
Mary Lovely RN, Contact

1819 Brain Tumor Support Group: Santa Barbara
Cancer Center of Santa Barbara
300 W Pueblo Street
Santa Barbara, CA 93105   805-563-5852
                                        www.braintumor.org

Rosario Campuzano, Contact

1820 Brain Tumor Support Group: Stanford
Stanford Cancer Center
875 Blake Wilbur Drive
Stanford, CA 94305   415-990-4461
                                  e-mail: mlovely@braintumor.org
                                        www.braintumor.org

Joanie Taylor RN, Contact
Sharon Lamb RN, Contact

1821 Brain Tumor Support Group: Westlake Village
The Wellness Community
530 Hampshire Road
Westlake Village, CA 91361   805-379-4777
                                        www.braintumor.org

Rebecca Dekker MFT, Contact

1822 Brain Tumor/Pituitary Patient Support Group
John Wayne Cancer Institute
2200 Santa Monica Blvd   949-515-9595
Santa Monica, CA 90404   e-mail: pituitarybuddy@hotmail.com
                                        www.braintumor.org

Sharmyn McGraw, Contact

1823 Children Living with Illness
The Center for Attitudinal Healing
33 Buchanan Drive   415-331-6161
Sausalito, CA 94965   Fax: 415-331-4545
                                        www.healingcenter.org

Don Goewey, Executive Director

1824 Glendale Adventist Medical Center Brain Tumor Support Group
Cancer Services
381 Merrill Avenue
Glendale, CA 91026   818-409-3530
                                        www.braintumor.org

Connie Munoz LCSW, Contact

1825 Heads Up!
Northridge Hospital Medical Center
18300 Roscoe Blvd   818-885-8500
Northridge, CA 91325   e-mail: robert.salazar@chw.edu
                                        www.braintumor.org

Wanda Martin, Contact
Robert Salazar, Additional Contact

1826 Neuro-Oncology Information and Support Group
Sister Mary Pia Regional Cancer Center
1800 N California Street
Stockton, CA 95204-6019   209-467-6550
                                        www.stjosephscares.org

For patients and family members living with primary and meta-static brain tumors as well as spinal cord tumors. Free child care and refreshments are provided.
Jim Linderman

1827 Neuroscience Institute Brain Tumor Hotline
Hospital of the Good Samaritan
637 Lucas Avenue
Los Angeles, CA 90017-1912   800-762-1692
                                        e-mail: info@goodsam.org
                                        www.goodsam.org

Diana Selover, LCSW

1828 Patient Services
22 Battery Street   415-834-9970
San Francisco, CA 94111-5520   800-934-2873
                                        Fax: 415-834-9980
                                  e-mail: info@braintumor.org
                                        www.braintumor.org

Quickly access brain tumor information and resources.
12 pages
George Gellert, Chief Medical Officer
N. Paul TonThat, Executive Director

1829 Peninsula Support & Education Group for Parents of Children with Brain Tumors
Parents Helping Parents
1400 Parkmoor Avenue   408-727-5775
San Jose, CA 95126-3222   855-727-5775
                                        Fax: 408-28- 111
                                  e-mail: info@php.com
                                        www.php.com

A comprehensive family resource center providing information, training, guidance and support to families of children with special needs and the professionals who serve them.
Suzanne Cistulli, Chair
Robert Badagliacco, Treasurer

1830 Support Group for Caregivers of Brain Tumor Patients
UCLA Medical Center
200 UCLA Medical Plaza   310-206-6731
Los Angeles, CA 90095   e-mail: cabe@mednet.ucla.edu
Cheryl Abe LCSW, Clinical Social Worker
Pamela Hoff LCSW, Clinical Social Worker

1831 Vital Options International
4419 Coldwater Canyon Avenue   818-508-5657
Studio City, CA 91604-1479   Fax: 818-788-5260
                                  e-mail: info@vitaloptions.org
                                        www.vitaloptions.org
A not-for-profit cancer communications, support, and advocacy organization with a mission, to facilitate a global cancer dialogue.
Selma R Schimmel, CEO/Founder
Juliana Lee, Production Manager

1832 Wellness Community Cancer Support Groups
San Francisco/East Bay
3276 Mc Nutt Avenue   925-933-0107
Walnut Creek, CA 94597   e-mail: emaslan@yahoo.com
                                        www.braintumor.org

Erika Maslan MFCC, Contact

1833 Wellness Community: South Bay Cities
109 W Torrance Blvd   www.braintumor.org
Redondo Beach, CA 90277
Tom May, Contact

1834 Wellness Community: West Los Angeles
2716 Ocean Park Blvd   www.braintumor.org
Santa Monica, CA 90405

1835 Support Group for Parents of Children with Brain Tumors
Oakland Children's Hospital
747 52nd Street   510-428-3885
Oakland, CA   800-400-PEDS
                                        www.kidsfirst.org

Trish Murphy

Colorado

1836 Brain Tumor Resource and Vital Encouragement
Childrens Hospital
1056 19th Avenue 303-861-8888
Denver, CO e-mail: webmaster@tchden.org
www.tchden.org
Pediatric focus. Education and support. Retreats for parents of brain tumor patients.
Jim Shmerling, DHA, FACHE, President & CEO

1837 Colorado Brain Tumor Support Group
Swedish Medical Center 303-806-7420
Englewood, CO 80113 e-mail: lgibson@thecni.org
www.braintumorfoundation.org
Lorre Gibson, Contact

Connecticut

1838 Connecticut Brain Tumor Support Group
20 York Street 203-785-7528
New Haven, CT 06510 Fax: 203-688-2395
www.braintumorfoundation.org
Angela Thomas LCSW, Contact

Delaware

1839 Pediatric Brain Tumor Support Group
Ronald McDonald House
PO Box 269 302-661-4077
Wilmington, DE 19899-3629 e-mail: izienberg@kidshealth.org
www.kidshealth.org
Niel Izienberg MD, Chief Executive Officer and Founder

District of Columbia

1840 National Health Information Center
PO Box 1133 310-565-4167
Washington, DC 20013-1133 800-336-4797
Fax: 301-984-4256
e-mail: info@nhic.org
www.health.gov/nhic
A health information referral service sponsored by the Office of Disease Prevention and Health Promotion. Puts health professionals and consumers who have health questions in touch with those organizations that are best able to provide answers.

1841 Washington DC Metropolitan Area Support Group
George Washington University
2150 Pennsylvania Aveneu NW 202-994-4035
Washington, DC 20037-3201
Margaret Fiore, RN

Florida

1842 Angels in the Sun Brain Tumor Support Group
Wellness Community
3900 Clark Road
Sarasota, FL 34233 941-921-5539
www.braintumorfoundation.org
John Kleinbaum, Program Director

1843 Brain Tumor Support Group
Miami Children's Hospital Foundation
3000 SW 62nd Avenue 305-662-8386
Miami, FL 33155 e-mail: maria.penate@mch.com
Maria Penate RN, Facilitator
Raquel Pasaron, Facilitator

1844 Florida Brain Tumor Association
PO Box 770182 954-755-4307
Coral Springs, FL 33077-0182 e-mail: sshetsky@fbta.info
www.fbta.info
Provides hope, support and education to brain tumor survivors, their families and friends; conquers brain tumors by funding research into their causes and cures; and enriches the quality of life of those touched by brain tumors
Sheryl Shetsky, President
Gary L Kornfeld, VP

1845 Florida Brain Tumor Support Group
Healthpark Medical Ctr, Meeting Rm
Ft Meyers, FL 33919 239-433-4396
www.braintumorfoundation.org
Dona Ross, Contact

1846 Florida Brain Tumor Support Group: Deerfield Beach
North Broward Medical Center 954-755-4307
Deerfield Beach, FL 33441 e-mail: sshetsky@fbta.info
www.fbta.info
Sheryl Shetsky, President
Gary L Kornfeld, VP

1847 Hollywood Area Brain Tumor Support Group
Memorial Regional Hospital 954-265-4725
Hollywood, FL 33021 e-mail: csurloff@mhs.net
www.floridabraintumor.com
Sheryl Shetsky, Founder & President
Gary L. Kornfeld, Vice President

1848 Sarasota Area Brain Tumor Support Group
Institute of Advanced Medicine
5880 Rand Avenue
Sarasota, FL e-mail: sposin@fbta.info
www.fbta.info
Sheryl R Shetsky, President
Gary L Kornfeld, VP

1849 West Palm Beach Area Brain Tumor Support Group
Good Samaritan Medical Center
West Palm Beach, FL 33401 561-655-5511
www.fbta.info
Sheryl R Shetsky, President
Gary L Kornfeld, VP

Georgia

1850 All Ages Support Group
Brain Tumor Foundation for Children
6065 Roswell Road NE 404-252-4107
Atlanta, GA 30328-4015 Fax: 404-252-4108
e-mail: info@braintumorkids.org
www.braintumorkids.org/
Patient Support Group Activities includes bowling, fishing, craft parties, picnics, sporting events, holiday parties, etc. These activities, social events and more are provided for children of all ages and their families.
Mary Campbell, Executive Director
R Hal Meeks Jr, President

1851 Emory Brain Tumor Support Group
Emory Clinic
Department of Neurosurgery
Atlanta, GA 30322 404-778-3091
www.neurosurgery.emory.edu/btsg/index
Meets the first Thursday of each month with the purpose of providing an opportunity for information-sharing and suport for brain tumor patients, as well as their family, friends and caregivers.
Maxine Brown, Contact

1852 Hearts and Minds
Piedmont Hospital
1968 Peachtree Road NW 404-373-5202
Atlanta, GA Fax: 404-605-5000
www.piedmonthospital.org
H.M McFarling, M.D, Chairman
Leslie A. Donahue, President & CEO

1853 SBTF Brain Tumor Support Group
PO Box 422471 404-843-3700
Atlanta, GA 30342 e-mail: info@sbtf.org
www.sbtf.org
To improve the quality of life for brain tumor patients and their families.
Costas Hadjipanayis, President
Jennifer Kee Giliberto, Vice President

Illinois

1854 Brain Tumor Support Group
Northwestern Memorial Hospital
675 N St. Clair   312-695-8143
Chicago, IL 60611   312-695-0990
e-mail: mmaher@nmff.org
www.cancer.northwestern.edu

Steven Rosen, Director
Leonidas Platanias, MD, PhD, Deputy Director

1855 Parents of Children with Brain Tumors PCBT
Children's Memorial Hospital
2300 Children's Plaza   773-880-4316
Chicago, IL 60614
Meets quarterly and publishes a monthly newsletter. Library available at meetings (at CMH). Educational speakers and family functions.
Gina Baldacci LCSW, Contact

Indiana

1856 Brain Tumor Support Group
Community Hospital East
1500 North Ritter Avenue   317-355-1411
Indianapolis, IN 46219   e-mail: m.w.kemf@att.net
www.ecommunity.com/east

Michael Kemf, Facilitator
Marsha Cline, Facilitator

1857 Primary Brain Cancer Support Group
Women's Cancer Center at Lutheran Hospital
7950 W Jefferson Boulevard   260-435-7959
Fort Wayne, IN 46804
Linda Jordan RN, Contact

Iowa

1858 Iowa Brain Tumor Support Group
University of Iowa Hospitals
Iowa City, IA 52242
Lori Roetlin, Contact   319-356-2557
Sue May, Additional Contact

1859 Neurological Center of Iowa
Iowa Clinic
5950 University Avenue   515-875-9100
Des Moines, IA 50266-1418   Fax: 515-241-6090
www.iowaclinic.com/

Networks people in similar situations.
Mark A. Reece, Chairman of the Board
Steven A. Keller, Chair Patient Care Committee

1860 Quad Cities Brain Tumor Support Group
Genesis Medical Center
1401 W Central Park   563-421-1907
Davenport, IA 52804   e-mail: ided@genesishealth.com
Deb Ide, Contact

Kansas

1861 Gray Matters Support: Kansas City
24050 W 57th Street
Shawnee, KS 66226   e-mail: graymatters2007@yahoo.com
Debbie Stephenson, Contact

1862 Headstrong Brain Tumor Support Group
Victory in the Valley
3755 E Douglas   316-682-7400
Wichita, KS 67218   e-mail: info@victoryinthevalley.com
www.victoryinthevalley.org

Cary Cozby, Golf Pro & CEO
Tim Farrell, President, RST Ventures, Inc

Kentucky

1863 Meningioma/Benign Brain Tumor Support Group
Michael Quinlan Brain Tumor Foundation

4012 Dupont Circle   502-896-1701
Louisville, KY 40207
Kathy Quinlan-Thompson, Contact

1864 Wellness Community: Kentucky
1717 Dixie Highway
Fort Wright, KY 41011   859-331-5568
www.cancersupportcincinnati.org

Rick Bryan, Executive Director
Gail Laule, Office Manager

Louisiana

1865 Brain Tumor Support Group
3939 Houma Boulevard, Doctor's Row   504-835-5715
Metairie, LA 70005   e-mail: gmom224@cox.net
www.braintumor.org

Meets on the third Sunday of each month at 1:30 p.m., call to confirm.
Gayle Johnson, Contact Person

Maine

1866 Brain Tumor Support Group of Maine
Maine Medical Center
22 Bramhall Street   207-871-4527
Portland, ME 04102
Meets on the second Tuesday of each month from 7:00 to 9:00 p.m.
Nancy Fortier LCSW, Contact

Maryland

1867 Brain Tumor Networking Group
10628 Falls Road
Lutherville, MD 21022   410-832-2719
www.loyolamedicine.org

Ronald Petrocelli, Chair
Michael Cathey, Vice Chair

1868 Brain Tumor Support Group: Maryland
NIH Clinical Research Center
9000 Rockville Pike   301-496-6380
Bethesda, MD 20892   e-mail: garrenn@mail.nih.gov
www.braintumor.org

Nancy Garren, Contact

1869 Brainiacs
Perryville Library   410-459-8157
Perryville, MD 21903
Liz Carrino, Contact

1870 Johns Hopkins Brain Tumor Education Group
Weinberg Building   410-502-2789
Baltimore, MD 21231
Liz Carrino, Contact

1871 Washington DC Metropolitan Area Brain Tumor Support Group
George Washington Ambulatory Center
I & 22nd Street   301-371-8660
Middletown, MD 21769
Lionel Chaiken, Contact
Jeff Schanz, Contact

Massachusetts

1872 Brain Tumor Patient and Caregiver Support Group
Dana Farber Cancer Institute
Boston, MA 02115   617-632-3634
Nancy Tharler LICSW, Contact

1873 Brain Tumor Support Group: Lahey
Lahey Clinic Medical Center
41 Mall Road
Burlington, MA 01805   617-726-1061
www.lahey.org

Michele Lucas MSW LICSW, Contact

1874 Brain Tumor Support Group: Worcester
UMass Memorial Medical Center-University Campus

55 Lake Avenue N
Worcester, MA 01655

508-334-7595
Fax: 800-697-2593
e-mail: ellen.sharenow@umassmemorial.org
www.braintumor.org

Ellen Sharenow PhD, Contact

1875 Neurological Support Group of St. Luke's Hospital
101 Page Street
New Bedford, MA 02740-3464
Diane Robinson RN

508-997-1515

1876 Parent Education/Support Group
Dana Farber Cancer Institute
44 Binney Street
Boston, MA 2115

617-632-3301
800-525-5068
e-mail: dana.farbercontactus@dfci.harvard.edu
www.dfci.harvard.edu

For parents of children with brain tumors. Please call for schedule.
Beverly Lavalley Run, Facilitator
Edward Benz Jr, President

Michigan

1877 Brain Tumor Networking Club
Gilda's Club Metro Detroit
3517 Rochester Road
Royal Oak, MI 48073
Kristen Bernat, Contact

248-577-0800
Fax: 248-577-0898

1878 Brain Tumor Support Group for Patients & Families
University of Michigan Medical Center
1500 E Medical Center Drive
Ann Arbor, MI 48109-0316
Christina Crandall, Contact
Kathy Wilson, Contact

734-936-9071

1879 Brain Tumor Support Group: Ann Arbor
St Joseph Mercy Hospital, Cancer Care Center
5301 E Huron River Drive
Ann Arbor, MI 48106

734-712-3658
www.sjmh.com

Paula Nedela RN, Contact

1880 Brain Tumor Support Group: West Bloomfield
Henry Ford Hospital
6777 W Maple
West Bloomfield, MI 48322
Sandy Remer RN, Contact

313-916-1796

Missouri

1881 Brain Cancer Support Group
St John's Hospital
Main Hospital
Springfield, MO 65804
Laura Flowers, Contact

417-820-3157
e-mail: laura.flowers@mercy.net

1882 Brain Tumor Support Group: Kansas City
St Luke's Hospital of Kansas City
4321 Washington Suite 4000
Kansas City, MO 64111
Michelle Martin, Contact

816-932-6015

1883 Brain Tumor Support and Networking Group
Wellness Community of Greater St. Louis
1058 Old Des Peres Road
Saint Louis, MO 63131

314-238-2000
e-mail: info@wellnesscommunitystl.org
www.wellnesscommunitystl.org/

Mitchell L Baris, Chair of the Board
Mary Jane Pieroni, CPA, Treasurer

Montana

1884 Cancer Patient/Caregiver Support Group
Wellness Community
1820 W Lincoln Street
Bozeman, MT 59715

406-582-1600
e-mail: twcmontana@qwest.net

Becky Robideaux, Contact

New Hampshire

1885 Brain Injury/Brain Tumor Support Group
Frisbie Memorial Hospital
Carroll Wiskel LMSW, Contact
Rochester, NH 03867

New Jersey

1886 Brain Tumor Support Group: New Jersey
90 Bergen Street
Newark, NJ 07103
LaDawn McClamb, Contact

973-972-1164
e-mail: mcclamls@umdnj.edu

1887 Brain Tumor Support Group: Toms River
Community Medical Center
99 Highway 37 W
Toms River, NJ 08755

732-557-8270
e-mail: slaniado@sbhcs.com

Sherry Laniado LCSW, Contact

1888 Central New Jersey Brain Tumor Support Group
St. Luke's Roman Catholic Church
300 Clinton Avenue
North Plainfield, NJ 07063
Patty Anthony RN, Contact
Virginia Shrodo, Contact

732-321-7000

New Mexico

1889 People Living Through Cancer Support Groups
3411 Candelaria NE
Albuquerque, NM 87107

505-242-3263
888-441-4439
Fax: 505-242-6756
e-mail: info@pltc.org
www.pltc.org

A not for profit organization that connects and supports cancer survivors and caregivers by transforming shared individual experiences into enduring hope.
Beth Brown, Executive Director
Mary Ellen Kurucz, Program Director

New York

1890 Brain Tumor Support Group for Patients and Families
Albany Medical Center
Office of NY Oncology/Hematology
Albany, NY 12208-3412

845-338-4820
e-mail: eehauser@gmail.com
www.braintumor.org/patients-family-frien

Emilie Hauser, Contact

1891 Brain Tumor Support Group: Long Island
230 Main St. Emma Clark Library
Setauket, NY
Billie Wilczek

516-747-8749

1892 Long Island Brain Tumor Support Group
Old Bethpage Public Library
999 Old Country Road
Plainview, NY 11803
Bob Crescenzo, Contact

516-996-3705

1893 Mount Sinai Medical Center Brain Tumor Support Group
Ruttenberg Care Center-Guggenheim Pavilion
1190 Fifth Ave
New York, NY 10029
Kathleen Maloney-Lutz RN, Contact

212-717-3527

1894 New York Brain Tumor Support Group
525 E 68th Street
New York, NY 10021

212-746-3986
e-mail: wem9011@nyp.org
www.braintumor.org

Wendy Mitchell LMSW, Contact

North Carolina

1895 Brain Tumor Support Group: Raleigh Area
Raleigh Community Hospital
3400 Wake Forest Road
Raleigh, NC 27609-7373

919-846-0923
www.raleighcommunity.com

Lectures, educational materials, and newsletter. Home and hospital visitation.
Louise Clark, Director

1896 Duke Pediatric Brain Tumor Family Support Program
Preston Robert Tisch Brain Tumor Center
Duke University Medical Center 919-684-5301
Durham, NC 27710 Fax: 919-684-6674
e-mail: korpi001@mc.duke.edu
www.cancer.duke.edu/btc/

Darell D. Binger, MD, PhD, Director
Allan H Friedman MD, Deputy Director

1897 Preston Robert Tisch Brain Tumor Center at Duke
Cornucopia Cancer Support Center
5517 Durham Chapel Hill Blvd 919-668-6178
Durham, NC 27707 e-mail: stephanie.english@duke.edu
www.cancer.duke.edu

Stephanie English MSW LCSW, Contact

Ohio

1898 Brain Tumor Support Group: Cincinnati
Wellness Community
4918 Cooper Road 513-791-4060
Cincinnati, OH 45242 Fax: 513-791-8239

1899 Southwest Ohio Brain Tumor Support Group
Kettering Medical Center
3535 Southern Boulevard 937-298-3399
Kettering, OH 45429-1221 e-mail: jean.ruppert@kmcnetwork.org
Ronald Petrocelli, M.D., Chair
Michael Cathey, Vice Chair

1900 Support Group for Parents of Children with Brain Tumors
Cincinnati Childrens Hospital Medical Center
Childrens Hospital Medical Center 513-636-4200
Cincinnati, OH 45229-3039 800-344-2462
www.cincinnatichildrens.org/default.htm

Thomas Boat, Director
Stephen Daniels, Associate Chair

Oregon

1901 Brain Tumor Education & Support Group
Legacy Good Samaritan Hospital Cancer Center
1130 NW 22nd Ave 503-413-7921
Portland, OR 97210

Wendy Talbot MSW LCSW, Contact
Selma Annala RT CLC, Contact

1902 Central Oregon Brain Tumor Support Group
900 SW 23rd Place 541-350-7243
Redmond, OR 97756 e-mail: rgklug@crestviewcable.com
Rubyanne Klug, Contact

Pennsylvania

1903 Brain Tumor Community Group
Lancaster General Health Campus
Wellness Conference Room 800-860-9949
Lancaster, PA 17601
Christine Burfete RN, Contact

1904 Brain Tumor Support Group: Johnstown
John P Murtha Neuroscience and Pain Institute
1450 Scalp Avenue 814-534-3797
Johnstown, PA 15904 e-mail: dlehew@conemaugh.org
www.braintumor.org

N. Paul TonThat, Chief Executive Officer
Michele Rhee, Director of Program Initiatives

1905 Brain Tumor Support Group: Philadelphia
University of PA Hospital-Neurological Institute
3400 Spruce Street 215-615-5240
Philadelphia, PA 19104
Alisha Amendt MSN CRNP, Contact
Arbena Merolli MSW, Contact

1906 Brain Tumor Support Group: Pittsburgh
Cancer Caring Center

4117 Liberty Avenue 412-622-1212
Pittsburgh, PA 15224 e-mail: indo@cancercaring.org

1907 Delware Valley Brain Tumor Support Group at Jefferson
Jefferson Health System
Bluemle Life Sciences Building 215-955-4429
Philadelphia, PA 19107
Ann Marie DiBona RN, Contact
Janis Haaf RN, Contact

1908 Pediatric Cancer Foundation of the Lehigh Valley
Camelot for Children
2354 W Emmaus Avenue 610-393-9215
Allentown, PA 18103
Nicole Ronco, Contact

Rhode Island

1909 Brain Tumor Support Group: Providence
Brown University Campus
BioMedical Center 401-789-0126
Providence, RI 02912
Judy Allenson, Contact
Betty Bentley, Contact

1910 Rhode Island Brain & Spine Tumor Foundation
Bethany Home
229 Medway Street 401-272-4177
Providence, RI 02906 e-mail: ribstf@gmail.com
Colin Shaw, Contact

South Carolina

1911 Brain Tumor Support Group: Charleston
Hollings Cancer Center
86 Jonathon Lucas Street 843-792-8257
Charleston, SC 29445 e-mail: lizzic@musc.edu
www.braintumor.org

Christa Lizzi RN, Contact

1912 Brain Tumor Support Group: Florence
Florence Neurosurgery and Spine
1204 E Cheves Street 843-206-1910
Florence, SC 29506 e-mail: info@florenceneurosurgery.com
www.braintumor.org

South Dakota

1913 Cancer Support Group
Sanford Cancer Cetner Oncology Clinic
1020 W 18th Street
Sioux Falls, SD 57104 605-328-8000
www.lls.org/aboutlls/chapters/mn/patient
Sue Halbritter RN NP, Contact

Tennessee

1914 Cancer Support Group: Knoxville
Wellness Community of East Tennessee
2230 Sutherland Avenue 865-546-4661
Knoxville, TN 37919 Fax: 865-522-0938
e-mail: info@wellnesscommunitytn.org
www.cancersupportet.org

Christi Branscom, President
Beth Lee, Secretary

1915 Cancer Support Group: Nashville
Gilda's Club Nashville
1707 Division Street 615-329-1124
Nashville, TN 37203 e-mail: info@gildasclubnashville.org

1916 Memphis Regional Brain Tumor Survivors Group
Methodist University Hospital
1265 Union Ave 904-757-0806
Memphis, TN 38104 e-mail: cherrywel2@comcast.net
Cherry Welborn, Contact

Texas

1917 Brain Tumor Support Group: El Paso
Rio Grande Cancer Foundation
10460 Vista Del Sol Drive   915-562-7660
El Paso, TX 79925   e-mail: juttar@rgcf.org
Jutta Ramirez, Contact
Robert Lefferts, Contact

1918 Central Texas Brain Tumor Support Group
Brain and Spine Center at Brackenridge Hospital
3rd Floor Boardroom   512-636-1578
Austin, TX 78701
Thomas Lewman, Contact

1919 Houston Area Brain Tumor Network
MD Anderson Cancer Center Brain & Spine Center
1515 Holcombe Blvd   713-794-1777
Houston, TX 77030   e-mail: spanju@mdanderson.org
Mark Anderson, Contact
Suki Panju, Contact

1920 South Texas Brain Tumor Foundation Support Group
San Antonio Employees Federal Credit Union
6000 NW Loop 410   210-670-9323
San Antonio, TX 78201
Susie Soriano, Contact

Utah

1921 Cancer Wellness House
59 S 1100 E   801-236-2294
Salt Lake City, UT 84102
Karen Elliott

Virginia

1922 Brain Tumor Support Group: Richmond
St Mary's Hospital
Education Center   877-284-3905
Richmond, VA 23226   e-mail: curebt@hotmail.com
          www.abta.org
Ronald Petrocelli, M.D., Chair
Michael Cathey, Vice Chair

1923 Valley Brain Tumor Support Group
Rehab2Health
Shenandoah Memorial Hospital   540-984-4921
Woodstock, VA 22664   e-mail: vbtsg@shentel.net
Valorie Hockman, Contact

Washington

1924 Brain Cancer Support Group: Port Orchard
2186 Yukon Harbor Rd SE   360-536-5042
Port Orchard, WA 98366   e-mail: ideas56@msn.com
Victoria Tierney MA RC, Contact

1925 Brain Cancer Support Group: Seattle
Northwest Hospital
Professional Building   206-297-2500
Seattle, WA 98133

1926 Virginia Mason Brain Tumor Support Group
1201 Terry Avenue   206-223-7552
Seattle, WA 98111
Michelle Handler RN, Contact

1927 Wenatchee Valley Brain Tumor Support Group
Wellness Place
1610 Fifth Street   509-679-9574
Wenatchee, WA 98801   e-mail: hastings9@charter.net
Jeff Hastings, Contact
Mary Lowe, Contact

West Virginia

1928 Brain Tumor Support Group: Southern West Virginia
First Presbyterian Church

16 Broad Street   304-744-0393
Charleston, WV 25301-2487
Jeri McDonald

Wisconsin

1929 Brain Tumor Support Group: John Sierzant Lutheran Hospital, Gunderson Clinic
1836 S Avenue   608-791-9862
LaCrosse, WI
Esther Lindeman RN

1930 LODAT: Brain Tumor Support Group
Children's Hospital of Wisconsin
Room 888
Milwaukee, WI   414-962-8984
          www.braintumor.org
Living One Day At a Time is a parent support group for families of chidren with cancer. Monthly newsletter, informational meetings, social activities for families, and bereavement support.
Frances Swigart

Books

1931 Brain Tumor Resource Directory
National Brain Tumor Foundation
22 Battery Street   415-834-9970
San Francisco, CA 94111-5520   800-934-2873
          Fax: 415-834-9980
          e-mail: nbtf@braintumor.org
          www.braintumor.org
Comprehensive reference for healthcare providers, the directory contains the names and phone numbers of various organizations that offer services and products of particular interest to brain tumor patients and their families.
Rob Tufel, Director Patient Services

1932 Death Be Not Proud: A Memoir
Harper Collins
10 E 53rd Street
New York, NY 10022   212-207-7000
          www.harpercollins.com
The father of a young man diagnosed with glioblastoma multiforme wrote this 50-year-old classic.

ISBN: 0-060929-89-8

1933 Resource Guide for Parents of Children with Brain and Spinal Cord Tumors
Children's Brain Tumor Foundation
274 Madison Avenue   212-448-9494
New York, NY 10016   866-228-HOPE
          Fax: 212-448-1022
          e-mail: info@cbtf.org
          www.cbtf.org
Contains practical information to sort out the complexities of medical procedures, interruptions in school and social life, and uncertainty about the future.
Robert Budlow, President
Joseph B Fay, Executive Director

1934 Support Group Directory
National Brain Tumor Foundation
22 Battery Street   415-834-9970
San Francisco, CA 94111-5520   800-934-2873
          Fax: 415-834-9980
          e-mail: nbtf@braintumor.org
          www.braintumor.org
Directory listing support groups in the US and Canada, pediatric support groups, online support groups and additional resources on the North American Brain Tumor Coalition. Available online only.
Rob Tufel, Director Patient Services

1935 That's Unacceptable: Surviving a Brain Tumor: My Personal Story
Rebecca L Libutti, author
Krystal Publishing

PO Box 221
Martinsville, NJ 08836

908-889-6038
800-833-9327
Fax: 908-889-6038
e-mail: RLibutti@aol.com
www.krystalpublishing.com

Written by a ten-year survivor of glioblastoma multiforme, the book's title was the author's first response to the initial discouragement she received about pursuing aggressive treatment.
198 pages Paperback
RL Libutti

1936   The Essential Guide to Brain Tumors
National Brain Tumor Foundation
22 Battery Street
San Francisco, CA 94111-5520

415-834-9970
800-934-2873
Fax: 415-834-9980
e-mail: nbtf@braintumor.org
www.braintumor.org

Full of information concerning the brain, how it functions, what causes tumors, types of brain tumors, managing symptoms, and even surviving brain tumorrs.
80 pages
Rob Tufel, Director Patient Services

1937   Understanding and Coping with Your Child's Brain Tumor
National Brain Tumor Foundation
22 Battery Street
San Francisco, CA 94111-5520

415-834-9970
800-934-2873
Fax: 415-834-9980
e-mail: nbtf@braintumor.org
www.braintumor.org

Guide for families contains information for parents of children with brain tumors, including information about diagnosis, tumor types, treatment methods, social and emotional support and more. It also contains a glossary, along with listings of organizations and resources.
52 pages
Rob Tufel, Director Patient Services

Children's Books

1938   My Name is Buddy
Dave Bauer, author
National Brain Tumor Foundation
22 Battery Street
San Francisco, CA 94111-5520

415-834-9970
800-934-2873
Fax: 415-834-9980
e-mail: nbtf@braintumor.org
www.braintumor.org

Unique book for children with brain tumors. The reader follows Buddy, a Golden Retriever, on his journey through a brain tumor diagnosis and treatment. This true story uses photographs and narrative to describe Buddy's experiences before and after surgery and talks about his feelings and fears as a brain tumor patient.
Rob Tufel, Director Patient Services

Newsletters

1939   Butterfly Bulletin
Brain Tumor Foundation for Children
6065 Roswell Road NE
Atlanta, GA 30328-4015

404-252-4107
Fax: 404-252-4108
e-mail: info@braintumorkids.org
www.braintumorkids.org

Reporting on news and events of the Brain Tumor Foundation for Children.
Quarterly
Rick Sauers, Chairman/Co-Founder
R Hal Meeks, Jr, President

1940   Caring Hand
Pediatric Brain Tumor Foundation
302 Ridgefield Court
Asheville, NC 28806

828-665-6891
800-253-6530
Fax: 828-655-6894
e-mail: pbtfus@pbtfus.org
www.pbtfus.org

The Caring Hand is a regular newsletter, distributed free of charge to patient families, caregivers and medical/social work professionals.
Michael Traynor, President
Glenn Wilcox, Vice President

1941   Childhood Brain Tumor Foundation Newsletter
Childhood Brain Tumor Foundation
20312 Watkins Meadow Drive
Germantown, MD 20876-4259

310-515-2900
877-217-4166
e-mail: cbtf@childhoodbraintumor.org
www.childhoodbraintumor.org

Seeking second opinions, access to healthcare, and combating discrimination.

1942   Helping Hand
Pediatric Brain Tumor Foundation
302 Ridgefield Court
Asheville, NC 28806

828-665-6891
800-253-6530
Fax: 828-655-6894
e-mail: pbtfus@pbtfus.org
www.pbtfus.org

The Helping Hand is a regular newsletter, distributed free of charge to Ride for Kids and supporters.
Michael Traynor, President
Glenn Wilcox, Vice President

1943   Message Line Newsletter
American Brain Tumor Association
2720 S River Road
Des Plaines, IL 60018-4117

847-827-9910
800-886-2282
Fax: 847-827-9918
e-mail: info@abta.org
www.abta.org

Describes research advances and announces updates to publications.
TriAnnual
Elizabeth Wilson, Executive Director
Geri Jo Duda, RN, Patient Services

1944   SEARCH
National Brain Tumor Foundation
22 Battery Street
San Francisco, CA 94111-5520

415-834-9970
800-934-2873
Fax: 415-834-9980
e-mail: nbtf@braintumor.org
www.braintumor.org

Newsletter that covers topics of current interest to brain tumor survivors and their families.
Quarterly
Rob Tufel, Director Patient Services

1945   TLC (Tips for Living And Coping)
American Brain Tumor Association
2720 S River Road
Des Plaines, IL 60018-4117

847-827-9910
800-886-2282
Fax: 847-827-9918
e-mail: info@abta.org
www.abta.org

E-bulletin of news, research and development finds, support and treatment information.

ISBN: 0-944093-37-X
Elizabeth Wilson, Executive Director
Geri Jo Duda, RN, Patient Services

Pamphlets

1946   Clinical Trial Fact Sheet
National Brain Tumor Foundation
22 Battery Street
San Francisco, CA 94111-5520

415-834-9970
800-934-2873
Fax: 415-834-9980
e-mail: nbtf@braintumor.org
www.braintumor.org

Lists of clinical trial by state, tumor type and/or treatment type.

1947   Coping with Your Loved One's Brain Tumor
National Brain Tumor Foundation

22 Battery Street
San Francisco, CA 94111-5520
415-834-9970
800-934-2873
Fax: 415-834-9980
e-mail: nbtf@braintumor.org
www.braintumor.org

Describes important coping stategies for caregivers and family members of a loved one with a brain tumor.
12 pages Booklet

1948   Dictionary for Brain Tumor Patients
American Brain Tumor Association
2720 S River Road
Des Plaines, IL 60018-4117
847-827-9910
800-886-2282
Fax: 847-827-9918
e-mail: info@abta.org
www.abta.org

Offers a dictionary of terms used in the diagnosis and everday living with brain tumors.
Paperback
ISBN: 0-944093-27-2
Elizabeth Wilson, Executive Director
Geri Jo Duda, RN, Patient Services

1949   Ependymoma
American Brain Tumor Association
2720 S River Road
Des Plaines, IL 60018-4117
847-827-9910
800-886-2282
Fax: 847-827-9918
e-mail: info@abta.org
www.abta.org

ISBN: 0-944093-40-X
Elizabeth Wilson, Executive Director
Geri Jo Duda, RN, Patient Services

1950   Glioblastoma Multiforme and Anaplastic Astrocytoma
American Brain Tumor Association
2720 S River Road
Des Plaines, IL 60018-4117
847-827-9910
800-886-2282
Fax: 847-827-9918
e-mail: info@abta.org
www.abta.org

ISBN: 0-944093-36-1
Elizabeth Wilson, Executive Director
Geri Jo Duda, RN, Patient Services

1951   Living with A Brain Tumor
American Brain Tumor Association
2720 S River Road
Des Plaines, IL 60018-4117
847-827-9910
800-886-2282
Fax: 847-827-9918
e-mail: info@abta.org
www.abta.org

A guide for brain tumor patients.
2004
ISBN: 0-944093-54-X
Elizabeth Wilson, Executive Director
Geri Jo Duda, RN, Patient Services

1952   Medulloblastoma
American Brain Tumor Association
2720 S River Road
Des Plaines, IL 60018-4117
847-827-9910
800-886-2282
Fax: 847-827-9918
e-mail: info@abta.org
www.abta.org

Paperback
ISBN: 0-944093-33-7
Elizabeth Wilson, Executive Director
Geri Jo Duda, RN, Patient Services

1953   Meningioma
American Brain Tumor Association

2720 S River Road
Des Plaines, IL 60018-4117
847-827-9910
800-886-2282
Fax: 847-827-9918
e-mail: info@abta.org
www.abta.org

ISBN: 0-944093-23-X
Elizabeth Wilson, Executive Director
Geri Jo Duda, RN, Patient Services

1954   Metastatic Brain Tumors
American Brain Tumor Association
2720 S River Road
Des Plaines, IL 60018-4117
847-827-9910
800-886-2282
Fax: 847-827-9918
e-mail: info@abta.org
www.abta.org

ISBN: 0-944093-26-4
Elizabeth Wilson, Executive Director
Geri Jo Duda, RN, Patient Services

1955   Oligodendroglioma and Mixed Glioma
American Brain Tumor Association
2720 S River Road
Des Plaines, IL 60018-4117
847-827-9910
800-886-2282
Fax: 847-827-9918
e-mail: info@abta.org
www.abta.org

Pamphlet
ISBN: 0-944093-43-4
Elizabeth Wilson, Executive Director
Geri Jo Duda, RN, Patient Services

1956   Organizing a Support Group
American Brain Tumor Association
2720 S River Road
Des Plaines, IL 60018-4117
847-827-9910
800-886-2282
Fax: 847-827-9918
e-mail: info@abta.org
www.abta.org

Elizabeth Wilson, Executive Director
Geri Jo Duda, RN, Patient Services

1957   Pituitary Tumors
American Brain Tumor Association
2720 S River Road
Des Plaines, IL 60018-4117
847-827-9910
800-886-2282
Fax: 847-827-9918
e-mail: info@abta.org
www.abta.org

Pamphlet
ISBN: 0-944093-44-2
Elizabeth Wilson, Executive Director
Geri Jo Duda, RN, Patient Services

1958   Primer of Brain Tumors
American Brain Tumor Association
2720 S River Road
Des Plaines, IL 60018-4117
847-827-9910
800-886-2282
Fax: 847-827-9918
e-mail: info@abta.org
www.abta.org

A patient's reference manual offering information on brain tumors.

ISBN: 0-944093-35-3
Elizabeth Wilson, Executive Director
Geri Jo Duda, RN, Patient Services

1959   Radiation Therapy of Brain Tumors: A Basic Guide
American Brain Tumor Association
2720 S River Road
Des Plaines, IL 60018-4117
847-827-9910
800-886-2282
Fax: 847-827-9918
e-mail: info@abta.org
www.abta.org

ISBN: 0-944093-28-0
Elizabeth Wilson, Executive Director
Geri Jo Duda, RN, Patient Services

1960 Returning to Work: Strategies for Brain Tumor Patients
National Brain Tumor Foundation
22 Battery Street   415-834-9970
San Francisco, CA 94111-5520   800-934-2873
                                                 Fax: 415-834-9980
                                      e-mail: nbtf@braintumor.org
                                                www.braintumor.org
Reviews brain tumor survivors rights with respect to returning to
work and suggests several strategies to make it an easier transition
to go back into the workplace.
16 pages Brochure
Rob Tufel, Director Patient Services

1961 Stereotactic Radiosurgery
American Brain Tumor Association
2720 S River Road   847-827-9910
Des Plaines, IL 60018-4117   800-886-2282
                                                 Fax: 847-827-9918
                                          e-mail: info@abta.org
                                                     www.abta.org

ISBN: 0-944093-42-6
Elizabeth Wilson, Executive Director
Geri Jo Duda, RN, Patient Services

1962 Understanding Brain Tumors: Glioblastoma Multiforme
National Brain Tumor Foundation
22 Battery Street   415-834-9970
San Francisco, CA 94111-5520   800-934-2873
                                                 Fax: 415-834-9980
                                      e-mail: nbtf@braintumor.org
                                                www.braintumor.org
Helps patients and caregivers understand more about the diagnosis
and treatment of glioblastoma multiforme.
16 pages
Rob Tufel, Director Patient Services

1963 Using A Medical Library
American Brain Tumor Association
2720 S River Road   847-827-9910
Des Plaines, IL 60018-4117   800-886-2282
                                                 Fax: 847-827-9918
                                          e-mail: info@abta.org
                                                     www.abta.org

Elizabeth Wilson, Executive Director
Geri Jo Duda, RN, Patient Services

1964 What You Need to Know About Brain Tumors
National Cancer Institute
Building 31   301-435-3848
Bethesda, MD 20892-0001   800-422-6237
                                                     www.nci.nih.gov
Offers factual information about brain tumors, possible causes,
primary and secondary tumors, symptoms, diagnosis, treatment,
side effects, followup care, support and medical terms.

1965 When Your Child Returns to School
American Brain Tumor Association
2720 S River Road   847-827-9910
Des Plaines, IL 60018-4117   800-886-2282
                                                 Fax: 847-827-9918
                                          e-mail: info@abta.org
                                                     www.abta.org
Guides parents and teachers through a successful return to school
when a child has had a brain tumor.
Paperback
ISBN: 0-944093-21-3
Elizabeth Wilson, Executive Director
Geri Jo Duda, RN, Patient Services

Audio & Video

1966 Conference Audiotapes
National Brain Tumor Foundation
22 Battery Street   415-834-9970
San Francisco, CA 94111-5520   800-934-2873
                                                 Fax: 415-834-9980
                                      e-mail: nbtf@braintumor.org
                                                www.braintumor.org

Audiotapes of keynote addresses and conference workshops from
NBTF's biennial National Brain Tumor Conferences where leading researchers, physicians and health professionals address a
range of issues affecting brain tumor survivors, such as new approaches to radiation and surgery, research and coping skills for
families.
Rob Tufel, Director Patient Services

1967 Strategies for Healing
National Brain Tumor Foundation
414 13th Street   510-839-9777
Oakland, CA 94612   800-934-2873
                                                 Fax: 510-839-9779
                                      e-mail: nbtf@braintumor.org
                                                www.braintumor.org
CD-Rom contains vital information about treatment options and
self-care for newly diagnosed patients and their families.
Rob Tufel, Director Patient Services

Web Sites

1968 American Brain Tumor Association
                                                     www.abta.org
Provide free social service consultations; a mentorship program
for new brain tumor support group leaders; a nationwide database
of established support groups; the Connections pen-pal program;
networking with organizations that provide services to patients
and families; a resource listing of physicians offering investgative
treatments.

1969 Brain Tumor Society
124 Watertown Street   617-924-9997
Watertown, MA 02472   800-770-8287
                                                 Fax: 617-924-9998
                                          e-mail: info@tbts.org
                                                     www.tbts.org
Disseminates educational information and provides access to psycho-social support and raises funds to advance carefully selected
scientific research projects, improve clinical care and find a cure.

1970 Healing Well
                                                     www.healingwell.com
An online health resource guide to medical news, chat, information and articles, newsgroups and message boards, books, disease-related web sites, medical directories, and more for patients,
friends, and family coping with disabling diseases, disorders, or
chronic illnesses.

1971 Health Finder
                                                     www.healthfinder.gov
Searchable, carefully developed web site offering information on
over 1000 topics. Developed by the US Department of Health and
Human Services, the site can be used in both English and Spanish.

1972 Healthlink USA
                                                     www.healthlinkusa.com
Health information concerning treatment, cures, prevention, diagnosis, risk factors, research, support groups, email lists, personal
stories and much more. Updated regularly.

1973 Helios Health
                                                     www.helioshealth.com
Online resource for your health information. Detailed information
about specific health topics, access to expert advice from our Medical Advisory Board, and up-to-date health news.

1974 MedicineNet
                                                     www.medicinenet.com
An online resource for consumers providing easy-to-read, authoritative medical and health information.

1975 Medscape
                                                     www.medscape.com
Medscape offers specialists, primary care physicians, and other
health professionals the Web's most robust and integrated medical
information and educational tools.

1976 National Brain Tumor Foundation
                                                     www.braintumor.org

Nonprofit health organization which raises funds for research and provides information and support to patients, their family members and friends and health professionals. Sponsors national and regional conferences, patient and caregiver programs, support groups, special patient programs including a teleconference series, a newsletter, a medical advice nurse and a wide variety of patient information about treatments, tumor types and coping. Also has a web site listing patient resources.

1977   Pediatric Brain Tumor Foundation of the US

www.ride4kids.org

Goal is to create an awareness about this growing disease among children and adults so that fundraising programs may continue to expand in increased laboratory research.

1978   WebMD

www.webmd.com

Information on Brain Tumors, including articles and resources.

Description

Cancer

Cancer is a general term for more than 100 diseases characterized by abnormal or uncontrolled growth of cells. The resulting mass, or disease, can invade and destroy surrounding normal tissue. Cancer cells from the tumor can also spread (metastasize) through the blood or lymph (plasmatic fluid) to start new cancers in other parts of the body. In 2010, about 1,529,560 new cancer cases were diagnosed, and about 569,490 Americans died from their disease. Cancer is the second leading cause of death in the U.S., exceeded only by heart disease. Although these figures seem bleak, most cancers are potentially curable if detected at an early stage.

Cancer, also called a malignancy (from Latin, meaning bad), can be either a solid tumor (carcinoma), such as lung cancer, or a disorder of blood cell formation, such as leukemia.

Cancer is caused by an interplay of internal and external factors, individually or in combination. Abnormal genes can cause multiple changes that affect cell growth. Environmental factors, such as cigarette smoke, (also called a carcinogen – causing cancer) and exposure to radiation, play a role. Many cancers can be prevented by health awareness. For example, 90 percent of the over one million skin cancers that will be diagnosed this year could be drastically reduced by protection from solar rays. Lung cancer, one of the most prevalent and hazardous cancers could be drastically reduced by eliminating tobacco use. The American Cancer Society estimates that 30 percent of all cancer deaths are related to cigarette smoking.

Cancer treatment may be curative – removes the tumor in the hope that it will not reoccur, or palliative – prolongs life and minimize discomfort when a cure is not possible. A treatment program typically includes a combination of surgery, radiation therapy, and chemotherapy. Immunotherapy is the newest form of treatment and uses agents known as biologic-response modifiers (BRM), to alter the immune system in its response to malignant growth. Brief descriptions of the more common cancers follow.

Brain Cancer

Brain cancer occurs at varying rates but overall it comprises approximately 5.6 cases per 100,000 populations each year. They are most common in early or middle adult life and incidence in the elderly population is increasing. Overall incidence is about equal in males and females.

The seriousness of brain tumors is determined by their size, location, and rate of growth. While brain cancer does not normally spread to others areas, many other cancers have the propensity of spreading throughout the nervous system dend producing metastatic tumors in the brain. In adults, these tumors are most commonly from cancer of the lung, breast, or skin (melanoma). Symptoms include headaches, seizures, behavior problems, changes in eating or sleeping habits, lethargy and clumsiness. See also Brain Tumors.

Breast Cancer

Breast cancer is the most common malignant tumor in women in the western hemisphere. Approximately 207,090 new cases of breast cancer in women were diagnosed in 2010. As many as one in nine women will develop breast cancer during her lifetime. Incidence of breast cancer increases under the following conditions: age; (two-thirds of cases develop after age 55); a close relative (mother, sister) with breast cancer; a previous history of breast cancer; a previous history of breast cancer; exposure to radiation. Other risk factors include not having children, early onset of menstruation, and estrogen replacement therapy.

Early detection can be lifesaving. Many breast cancers are self-diagnosed. More than 80 percent of breast cancers occur as a painless mass. Monthly breast self-examination for women of all ages is crucial. The American Cancer Society recommends that women aged 20-39 have a clinical breast examination performed every three years. Depending on the presence of known risk factors, patients should undergo mammography either yearly or every other year between 40 and 50 years, and yearly after age 50.

Warning signs that can aid women in detecting breast cancer include lumps, swelling, skin irritation, tenderness of the nipple, and dimpling of the skin. Treatments vary, depending on when the cancer is discovered and whether it has spread. Research has shown that the traditional radical mastectomy (removal of the entire breast) canoften be replaced by lumpectomy (removal of just the tumor), coupled with radiation therapy. Chemotherapy or hormonal manipulation is also prescribed in some cases. The five year survival rate for localized (not spread) breast cancer has improved in recent years from 78 percent to 97 percent.

Colon and Rectal Cancer

In western countries, colon and rectal (colorectal) cancer account for more new cases of cancer per year than any other anatomic site except the lung. The incidence begins to rise at age 40 and peaks at age 60 to 75. Incidence of colorectal cancer increases in people who eat low-fiber diets that are high in animal protein, fat, and refined carbohydrates.

Symptoms vary, depending on the location and size of the tumor. Vague signs include weight loss, reduced appetite, and general malaise. More specific signs include rectal bleeding, blood in the stool, or a change in bowel habits.

A digital rectal examination and testing the stool for the presence of blood are important screening tests. Flexible sigmoidoscopy in which the doctor inserts a thin, flexible tube into the rectum shows tumors in 60 percent of cases. A colonoscopy is performed when a tumor is believed to be higher up the colon. These procedures are used to visualize abnormalities and take tissue samples (biopsy).

Treatment consists of surgical removal of the tumor, followed by radiotherapy and/or chemotherapy.

Leukemia

Leukemia is a disorder characterized by uncontrolled growth of abnormal and immature white or red blood cells, and is divided into acute and chronic forms. Although leukemia is often thought of as a childhood disease, it strikes 10 times as many adults as children. New treatment, especially for acute leukemia in children has resulted in dramatic improvements in the 5- year survival rates. Today, the likelihood of disease remission is greater than 95 percent, with 30 percent chance of the disease reappearing.

Warning signs of leukemia are related to the disruption of the different cells in the blood: weakness and fatigue are caused by anemia (decreased red blood cells); easy bruising and hemorrhages (e.g. nosebleeds) from reduced clotting cells (platelets); and repeated infections from abnormal white cells. Generalized symptoms include weight loss and malaise.

Treatment for leukemia includes chemotherapy with a wide variety of anticancer drugs. Transfusions restore red cells and platelets, and frequent infections are treated with antibiotics. Bone marrow transplants, in which new blood cells are provided, are one of the most recent and successful advances in the treatment of this disease.

Liver Cancer

Liver cancer comprises only about 0.6 percent of all cancers diagnosed in the United States. Risk include hepatitis B infection, hepatitis C infection, and exposure to any agent that causes liver damage, including alcohol. The remaining patients have no underlying liver disorder.

Symptoms include abdominal pain, weight loss, and a mass on the upper right side of the abdomen. The outlook for patients with liver cancer is usually grim. Surgery provides the best hope, but is suitable in only a few cases. Most experts remain wary of the benefit of liver transplantation. See also Liver Disease.

Lung Cancer

Lung cancer is one of the most prevalent cancers with an estimated 170,000 new cases each year. The frequency is increasing rapidly. Originally a disease that primarily affected men older than 60, lung cancer has become the second most common cause of cancer in women.

Cigarette smoking and exposure to industrial substances, such as asbestos, are strongly linked to lung cancer. Recent research has shown that exposure to secondhand smoke increases the risk for this disease.

Warning signs of lung cancer are persistent coughing, shortness of breath,sputum streaked with blood, chest pain, and reoccurring pneumonia or bronchitis. Early detection is difficult, as symptoms do not appear until the disease is in advanced stages. Treatment includes surgical removal of the lung if the cancer has not spread (metastasized) and/or chemotherapy and radiation therapy. Survival rates depend on tumor size, location, and whether or not the disease has spread. Because lung cancer is so difficult to treat, public health efforts are focused on prevention. See also Lung Disease.

Oral Cancer

Oral cancer represents approximately 2 percent of all newly diagnosed cancers, and 1.5 percent of cancer deaths. Incidence is more than twice as high in men as in women, and is most frequently found in men over age 40. Risk factors include cigarette, pipe, and cigar smoking, as well as the use of chewing tobacco and excessive intake of alcohol.

Oral cancer symptoms include a sore that bleeds easily, or a lump, thickening, or persistent red or white patch in the mouth. Difficulties in chewing and swallowing are symptoms of progressive disease.

Oral cancer can affect any part of the mouth, and primary care physicians and dentists often detect the disease during routine check-ups. Treatment consists of surgical removal (frequently disfiguring), radiation therapy, or a combination of both.

Ovarian Cancer

Ovarian cancer develops in 1 in 70 women and accounts for 4 percent of cancers in women. Despite its low incidence, it is the cause of more deaths in women than any other female reproductive cancer. Incidence rates are highest in the industrialized nations.

Risk factors include prior history of breast cancer and not having had children. Women who become pregnant at an early age, who have early menopause, and who use oral contraceptives are at less risk.

Ovarian cancer symptoms usually do not appear until the disease is well developed. The most common sign is an enlarging abdomen from of accumulated fluid; digestive disturbance such as discomfort, gas and distention, may also occur.

Often an abdominal mass is discovered during a routine pelvic examination in women who are symptom free. Therefore, women age 18 or older, or earlier if they are sexually active should have annual check-ups. (The Pap smear detects cervical cancer, not ovarian cancer.) Once diagnosed, 78 percent of ovarian cancer patients survive longer than one year and more than 52 percent survive longer than five years. If the disease is diagnosed before it has spread to the other parts of the body, the five-year survival rate is 95 percent.

Treatment includes surgical removal, followed by varying combinations of chemotherapy. As in all cancers, early detection is the key to effective therapy.

Pancreatic Cancer

Pancreatic cancer is one of the most dangerous cancers because it is difficult to detect and responds poorly to anticancer therapy. The incidence of this tumor has been increasing during the 21st century with 43,140 cases diagnosed in 2010. Men are affected more commonly than women, and the average age of diagnosis is from 55 to 65 years.

There is an increased incidence in those who smoke, consume a fatty diet and, to a lesser extent, who are diabetics. Chronic inflammation of the pancreas, especially among alcoholics, is also a predisposing cause.

Pancreatic cancer runs a particularly silent course, with no symptoms until it has significant advanced. The overall 5- year survival rate for patients with pancreatic cancer is less than 5 percent. Surgery is the mainstay of therapy, but only is appropriate for 15 percent of patients; radiation and/or chemotherapy are often part of treatment.

Prostate Cancer

Approximately 1 in 6 men will develop prostate cancer by 85. Incidencerates are higher among blacks and increases with age.

Early prostate cancer is symptom free. Pain and difficulty urinating, are late signs of prostate cancer. More than 50 percent of patients have a nodule that can be felt by a digital examination.

The American Cancer Society recommends that beginning at age 50, the digital rectal examination and PSA (prostatespecific antigen) blood test should be performed annually to men with a life expectancy of at least 10 years, due to the slow growth of prostate cancer. African- American males, who are at a greater risk of developing prostate cancer, should start screening at age 45, as should men with a close relative (father, brother) was diagnosed with prostate cancer at a young age.

Surgery, radiation and hormones are all used to treat prostate cancer, depending on age and health of the patient and how far the disease has progressed.

Skin Cancer

There are over one million cases of skin cancer that are diagnosed each year. The vast majority of these cases, called basal cell or squamous cell cancers, appear on areas that are most exposed to the sun and are highly curable. Melanoma is the most serious skin cancer and accounts for 4 percent of cases. Diagnosis of melanomas has more than doubled since the mid-70s and is estimated now to develop in 1 of 50 Americans. Similar to the more benign skin cancers, melanoma develops as the result of excessive exposure to the sun and has a higher incidence among those who work outdoors. Persons with fair complexions are at particular risk.

The warning signs of skin cancer include a persistent skin lesion, especially those that change in the size, color or shape. Other signs include scaliness, oozing, bleeding, pain or spread of pigmentation.

Prevention plays a key role in the development of melanoma, especially avoiding the sun's ultraviolet rays between 10 a.m. and 3 p.m. Sunscreens and protective clothing should be worn by those who spend the majority of their time outside, those who easily sunburn, and all children. In addition, early detection is critical because, despite advances in treatment, including the use of biologic response modifiers, melanoma is difficult to cure.

Stomach Cancer

Stomach (or gastric) cancer is most common among those living in northern areas of the U.S., and poor African-American populations. Its incidence increases with age; more than 75 percent of patients are over 50 years of age.

Diet and infection are believed to play a role in the development of stomach cancer. It is also more common in persons with vitamin B12 deficiency (pernicious anemia). Other causes are under investigation.

Symptoms of stomach cancer are usually vague, and include indigestion, abdominal discomfort, bloating, heartburn, and weight loss.

Removal of the tumor when possible offers the only hope of cure. The prognosis is good if the tumor is limited, but most patients are not diagnosed until their disease has spread.

Testicular Cancer

Cancer of the testes accounts for approximately 1 percent of all male cancers. However, unlike most cancers, testicular cancer usually occurs in the 15 to 40 age group; with the average age at diagnosis is 32 years.

The cause of testicular cancer is uncertain, but the incidence is increased in men with cogenital crytorochidism (a failure of one or both testes to descend). Some researchers believe that getting an infection with a virus, such as mumps, may play a role.

Fortunately, testicular cancer is one of the most curable of all cancers, In order to discover it early, men must perform self examination at regular intervals to feel for local abnormal growths such as lumps or nodules. Pain in the scrotal sac can also occur, although more than 90 percent of patients have a painless, solid testicular swelling.

Treatment of testicular cancer may include surgical removal, radiation, and chemotherapy.

Urinary Tract Cancer

Urinary tract cancers comprise about 9 percent of new cancer cases each year in men and 4 percent in women. The two most common urinary tract cancers are of the bladder and kidney.

Overall, the incidence rate is three times greater among men than women, and usually occurs in patients who are 40-70 years of age. Smoking is the greatest risk factor, with smokers having twice the incidence of nonsmokers. African-Americans, those living in urban areas, and workers exposed to dye, rubber, or leather are also at higher risk.

Common symptoms of bladder cancer include microscopic or observable blood in the urine and painful, increased, and urgent urination. Pain the lower back may also be present. Bladder cancer may be treated by surgical removal of the tumor combined with chemotherapy.

Risk factors for kidney (renal) cancer are cigarette smoking (most important) and obesity in women. Symptoms are similar to those in bladder cancer and may also include weight loss, nausea, and vomiting.

Total removal of the cancerous kidney is the treatment of choice and is used in nearly 90 percent of cases; radiation therapy and chemotherapy are relatively ineffective. Biologic response modifiers are promising but must responses are limited in duration.

Uterine and Cervical Cancer

The overall incidence of cervical cancer has decreased over the past 40 years, due mainly to regular checkups and the use of the Pap smear test for early detection. Risk factors include intercourse at an early age, cigarette smoking, multiple sex partners, and history of a sexually transmitted disease. Infection with the virus that causes genital warts (HPV), is responsible for half of all cases of cervical cancer.

Warning signs include bleeding outside the normal menstrual cycle or after menopause. Cervical cancer in most patients is treated with surgery, radiation, or a combination of both. Due to a recently developed vaccine that is 100 percent effective against HPV, the rates of cervical cancer have sharply decreased.

The American Cancer Society recommends that all women who are, or have been, sexually annual Pap test and pelvic examination. After three or more consecutive satisfactory examinations with normal findings, the Pap test may be performed less frequently, after being discussed with your health care provider.

Uterine cancer has been increasing since the 1970s. Risk factors include obesity, diabetes, high blood pressure, late onset of menopause, and estrogen-only hormone replacement therapy. Symptoms for most women include some form of abnormal bleeding from the uterus. Treatment for uterine and cervical cancers include surgery, radiation therapy, hormone therapy and, occasionally, chemotherapy.

National Agencies & Associations

1979 American Bone Marrow Donor Registry
PO Box 8841
Mandeville, LA 70470-8841
985-626-1749
800-745-2452
Fax: 985-626-7414
e-mail: jakabmdr@bellsouth.net
www.abmdr.org
A registry of bone marrow donors. Provides information on donor searches and recruitment.

1980 American Cancer Society
1599 Clifton Road NE
Atlanta, GA 30329-4250
404-320-3333
800-ACS-2345
TTY: 800-228-4327
www.cancer.org
A nationwide community based voluntary health organization dedicated to eliminating cancer as a major health problem by preventing saving lives and diminishing suffering through research education advocacy and services. Provides free printed materials.
Stephen F Sener, President
J. Lenard Lichtenfeld, MD, MACP, Deputy Chief Medical Officer

1981 American Prostate Society
10 East Lee St.
Baltimore, MD 21202-3117
410-837-3735
877-859-3735
Fax: 410-837-8510
e-mail: ameripros@mindspring.com
www.americanprostatesociety.com
The only organization dedicated exclusively to using existing medical capabilities to reduce death due to prostate cancer and to reduce unnecessary or ineffective prostate therapies for prostate growth.

1982 American Society of Colon and Rectal Surgeons
85 W Algonquin Road
Arlington Heights, IL 60005-4460
847-290-9184
Fax: 847-290-9203
e-mail: ascrs@fascrs.org
www.fascrs.org
ASCRS Represents more than 1000 board certified colon and rectal surgeons and other surgeons dedicated to advancing and promoting the science and practice of the treatment of patients with cancer and other diseases affecting the colon and related areas.
David Beck MD, President
Steven Wexner MD, President Elect

1983 Americas Association for the Care of the Children
P.O. Box 2154
Boulder, CO 80306-2154
303-527-2742
www.aaccchildren.net
Carries out a variety of programs to promote the health of children. Publishes educational materials on child health of interest to parents, educators and health professionals.
Judi Jackson, President
Doreen Trees, Vice President

1984 Association for Research of Childhood Cancer
PO Box 251
Buffalo, NY 14225-0251
716-681-4433
e-mail: president@arocc.org
www.arocc.org
A nonprofit organization staffed by volunteers and formed in 1971 by parents who had lost children to pediatric cancer. Charter members raise funds by various projects in order to provide seed money to various pediatric research centers.
Anne O'Donnell, President

1985 Association for the Cure of Cancer of the Prostate
1250 4th Street
Santa Monica, CA 90401
310-570-4700
800-757-4700
Fax: 310-570-4701
e-mail: info@pcf.org
www.pcf.org
Goal is to find better treatments and a cure for recurrent prostate cancer. Pursues the mission by reaching out to individuals corpora-

tions and others to harness society's resources - both financial and human - to fight this deadly disease.
Mike Milken, Founder/Chairman
Neil DeFeo, Chairman, President and CEO

1986   Bone Marrow Foundation
30 E End Avenue   212-838-3029
New York, NY 10128   800-365-1336
                                         Fax: 21 -22 -008
                       e-mail: theBMF@BoneMarrow.org
                                  cmgm.stanford.edu
Goal is to improve the quality of life for bone marrow and stem cell transplant patients and their families by providing financial aid education and emotional support.
Christina Merrill, Founder and Executive Director
Lee Kozer, Director

1987   Breast Cancer Action
55 New Montgomery Street   415-243-9301
San Francisco, CA 94105   877-2ST-OPBC
                                         Fax: 415-243-3996
                             e-mail: info@bcaction.org
                                       www.bcaction.org
Breast Cancer Action carries the voices of people affected by breast cancer to inspire and compel the changes necessary to end the breast cancer epidemic.
Joyce Bichier, Deputy Director
Lori Baralt, Secretary

1988   Breast Cancer Society of Canada
420 East Street North Sarnia   519-336-0746
Sarnia, ON N7T6Y-6Y5   800-567-8767
                                         Fax: 519-336-5725
                                 e-mail: bcsc@bcsc.ca
                                          www.bcsc.ca
Is a registered charitable organization established in 1991 in Point Edwards Ontario. Our mandate is to fund vital Canadian research into improving the detection, prevention and treatment of breast cancer as well as to ultimately find a cure and create awareness through education.
Marsha Davidson, Executive Director
Raelene Peseski, President

1989   Burger King Cancer Caring Center
4117 Liberty Avenue   412-622-1212
Pittsburgh, PA 15224   Fax: 412-622-1216
                          e-mail: info@cancercaring.org
                                    www.cancercaring.org
Provides a wide variety of support services to cancer patients their families and friends including support groups, education classes, personal counseling and telephone help line.
Rebecca Whitlinger, Executive Director
Stephanie Samolovitch, MSW, LSW, Director Support Services

1990   Canadian Breast Cancer Network (CBCN)
300-331 Cooper Street   613-230-3044
Ottawa, Ontario, K2P-0G5   800-685-8820
                                         Fax: 613-230-4424
                                 e-mail: cbcn@cbcn.ca
                                          www.cbcn.ca
Is a survivor-directed, national network of organizations and individuals. CBCN is a national link between all groups and individuals concerned about breast cancer, and represents the concerns of all Canadians affected by breast cancer and those at risk.
Jackie Manthorne, CEO
Chantale Lavoie, Program Coordinator

1991   Canadian Cancer Society
55 St Clair Avenue West   416-961-7223
Toronto, ON M4V 2-3B1   Fax: 416-961-4189
                                e-mail: info@cancer.ca
                                        www.cancer.ca
A national community-based organization of volunteers whose mission is the eradication of cancer and the enhancement of the quality of life of people living with cancer.
Peter Goodhand, President/CEO

1992   CancerCare
Public Information Associates

275 7th Avenue   212-302-2400
New York, NY 10001   800-813-4673
                                         Fax: 212-712-8495
                           e-mail: info@cancercare.org
                                       www.cancercare.org
National nonprofit organization that provides free, professional support services for anyone affected by a cancer diagnosis.
Helen H Miller LCSW, Executive Director
John Rutigliano, Chief Operating Officer

1993   Candlelighters Childhood Cancer Foundation
10400 Connecticut Avenue   301-962-3520
Kensington, MD 20895   800-366-2223
                                         Fax: 301-962-3521
                                e-mail: staff@acco.org
                                   www.candlelighters.org
Founded by parents of children with cancer. Candlelighters helps families of pediatric and adolescent cancer patients cope with the educational and emotional needs of the disease. The organization is the largest distributor of free childhood cancer books and other materials.
Ruth Hoffman MPH, Executive Director
Amber Masso, Program Director

1994   Colon Cancer Canada
5915 Leslie Street   416-785-0449
Toronto, On, M2H-1J8   888-571-8547
                                         Fax: 416-785-0450
                       e-mail: info@coloncancercanada.ca
                                   www.coloncancercanada.ca
Raise public awareness for this deadly disease and to raise money for vital research.
Bunnie Schwartz, Co-Founder & President
Leah Archambault, Executive Officer Coordinator

1995   Colorectal Cancer Association of Canada
5 Place Ville Marie   514-875-7745
Montreal, QC, H3B-2G2   Fax: 514-875-7746
                             e-mail: admin@ccac-accc.ca
                                        www.ccac-accc.ca
Non-profit organization dedicated to improving the quality of life of patients and increasing awareness of the disease.
Barry D Stein, President
Heidi Watts, Program Director

1996   ENCORE YWCA-National Board
YWCA-National Board
726 Broadway   212-614-2827
New York, NY 10003-9502   800-953-7587
The YWCA's discussion and exercise program for women who have had breast cancer surgery. Designed to restore physical strength and emotional well-being.

1997   Foundation for Dignity
37 S 20th Street   215-567-2828
Philadelphia, PA 19103
Offers counseling and seminars concerning the employment rights of cancer patients and for human services workers. The society offers an extensive list of publications dealing with all aspects of cancer prevention and care.
Barbara Hoffman, Staff Attorney

1998   International Association of Laryngectomees
American Cancer Society
PO Box 691060   757-888-0324
Stockton, CA 95269-1060   866-425-3678
                                         Fax: 209-472-0516
                            e-mail: ialhq@larynxlink.com
                                          www.theial.com
Consists of local clubs worldwide that provides services and information to patients who have undergone laryngectomies and their families. Members are given information on first aid, postoperative care, rehabilitation, esophageal speech and other speech alternatives. Directories of speech instructors and self-care supplies for the surgical site are distributed.
Jack Henslee, Executive Director

1999 Leukemia and Lymphoma Society
1311 Mamaroneck Avenue   914-949-5213
White Plains, NY 10605   800-955-4572
                                       Fax: 914-949-6691
                                            www.lls.org
The Leukemia and Lymphoma Society is the world's largest volun-
tary health organization dedicated to funding blood cancer re-
search education and patient services.
Timothy S. Durst, Chair of the Board
James H. Davis, PhD, JD, Vice Chair

2000 Make Today Count
1235 E Cherokee   417-885-3324
Springfield, MO 65804-2263   800-432-2273
                                       Fax: 417-888-7426
                                   smsu.edu/nursing/community
An organization that helps patients and their families cope with
cancer and other serious diseases and improve their quality of life.
Connie Gores, Director
Chris Anderson, Executive Administrative Assistant

2001 National Alliance of Breast Cancer Organizations
9 E 37th Street
New York, NY 10016   888-806-2226
                                       Fax: 212-689-1213
                                  e-mail: nabcoinfo@aol.com
                                            www.nabco.org
A network of breast cancer organizations that provides information assistance and referral to anyone with questions about breast
cancer and acts as a voice for the interests and concerns of breast
cancer survivors and women at risk.

2002 National Cancer Institute
9609 Medical Center Drive
Bethesda, MD 20892-8322   800-422-6237
                              e-mail: cancergovstaff@mail.nih.gov
                                            www.cancer.gov
One of the largest organizations dealing solely with cancer in its
many forms. Offers educational information public awareness research grants and more for patients their families and health care
professionals. Information specialists answer cancer-related questions by phone, LiveHelp instant messaging,and e-mail.
Deborah Pearson RN MPH, Chief Public Inquiries Office

2003 National Cancer Institute of Canada
10 Alcorn Avenue   416-961-7223
Toronto, Ontario, M4V-3B1   Fax: 416-961-4189
                                  e-mail: research@cancer.ca
                                            www.ncic.cancer.ca
Was formed through a joint initiative of the Department of Na-
tional Health and Welfare and the Canadian Cancer Society.
Dr Elizabeth Eisenhauer, President

2004 National Coalition for Cancer Survivorship
1010 Wayne Avenue   301-650-9127
Silver Spring, MD 20910   888-650-9127
                                       Fax: 301-565-9670
                               e-mail: info@canceradvocacy.org
                                        www.canceradvocacy.org
Survivor led advocacy organization working exclusively on behalf
of people with all types of cancer and their families. Dedicated to
assuring quality and care for all Americans.
Thomas P Sellers, President/CEO

2005 National Foundation for Cancer Research
4600 EW Highway   301-654-1250
Bethesda, MD 20814   800-321-2873
                                       Fax: 301-654-5824
                                   e-mail: info@nfcr.org
                                            www.nfcr.org
Contracts with major universities for basic science cancer research
in the fields of biophysics, theoretical physics and biochemistry.
William Potter, President
David M Sotsky, Director

2006 National Hospice & Palliative Care Organization (NHPCO)
1731 King Street   703-837-1500
Alexandria, VA 22314   800-658-8898
                                       Fax: 703-837-1233
                                  e-mail: nhpcoinfo@nhpco.org
                                            www.nhpco.org
The nation's only advocate for terminally ill patients and their families. Founded in 1978, the NHPCO is the only organization devoted to hospice in the United States. Support is included from
state hospice organizations, patients, families, communities, provider program members and professional/volunteer members.
Represents hospice care interests to Congress, regulatory agencies, courts, voluntary organizations and the public.
J. Donald Schumacher, PsyD, President & CEO
Galen Miller, PhD, Executive Vice President

2007 National Institute on Aging Information Center
31 Center Drive MSC 2292   301-496-1752
Bethesda, MD 20892   800-222-2225
                                       Fax: 301-496-1072
                                       TTY: 800-222-4225
                                            www.nih.gov/nia
Concerned with the health problems of older Americans. The Cen-
ter offers free printed materials including fact sheets about going
to the hospital and about prostate problems.
Richard J Hodes MD, Director
Linda Addiso Hardy, Lead Extraml Support Asst

2008 National Kidney and Urologic Diseases Information
Clearinghouse
31 Center Drive,MSC 2560   301-496-3583
Bethesda, MD 20892-2560   800-891-5390
                                       Fax: 301-907-8906
                              e-mail: nkudic@info.niddk.nih.gov
                                        www.www2.niddk.nih.gov
A service of the Federal Government's National Institute for Diabetes and Digestive and Kidney Diseases. Offers free information
about benign prostate enlargement and other non-cancerous urinary tract problems.
Griffin P Rodgers, Director

2009 National Marrow Donor Program
3001 Broadway Street NE   612-627-5800
Minneapolis, MN 55413-1763   800-627-7692
                                            www.marrow.org
Created to improve the effectiveness of the search for bone marrow
donors so that a greater number of bone marrow transplants can be
carried out.
Jeffrey W Chell MD, CEO
Patricia A Coppo MS, COO

2010 National Ovarian Cancer Coalition
2501 Oak Lawn Avenue   214-273-4200
Dallas, TX 75219   888-OVA-RIAN
                                       Fax: 561-393-7275
                                 e-mail: NOCC@ovarian.org
                                            www.ovarian.org
Our mission is to raise awareness about ovarian cancer and to promote education about this disease. By dispelling myths and misun-
derstandings the coalition is committed to improve the overall
survival rate and quality of life for women with ovarian cancer.
Elizabeth Isham Cory, President
David Barley, CEO

2011 New Brunswick Innovation Foundation
440 King Street, Suite 602   506-452-2884
Fredericton, NB, E3B-5H8   877-554-6668
                                       Fax: 506-452-2886
                                   e-mail: info@nbif.ca
                                            www.nbif.ca
An independent corporation, has the mission to contribute to
building the province's innovation capacity.
Alfred W Lacey, President/CEO

2012 Rethink Breast Cancer
215 Spadina Avenue   416-920-0980
Toronto, ON M5T 2-2C7   Fax: 416-920-5798
                            e-mail: hello@rethinkbreastcancer.com
                                        www.rethinkbreastcancer.com

Is a charity helping young people who are concerned about and affected by breast cancer through innovative breast cancer education, research and support programs.
MJ DeCoteau MA, Executive Director

2013 Skin Cancer Foundation
149 Madison Avenue   212-725-5176
New York, NY 10016-8728   800-754-6490
                                           Fax: 212-725-5751
                                    e-mail: info@skincancer.org
                                           www.skincancer.org
Conducts public and medical education programs to help reduce skin cancer. Major goals are to increase public awareness of the importance of taking protective measures against the damaging rays of the sun and to teach people how to recognize the early signs.
Perry Robins MD, President

2014 Support for People with Oral and Head and Neck Cancer
PO Box 53   516-759-5333
Locust Valley, NY 11560-0053   800-377-0928
                                           Fax: 516-671-8794
                                      e-mail: info@spohnc.org
                                              www.spohnc.org
Nonprofit organization founded in 1991 to address the broad emotional physical and humanistic needs of oral and head and neck cancer patients.
Nancy E Leupold, President/Founder
James J. Sciubba DMD, PhD, Vice President

2015 Y-ME National Breast Cancer Organization
135 S LaSalle Street   312-986-8338
Chicago, IL 60603   800-221-2141
                                           Fax: 312-294-8597
                                    e-mail: askyme@y-me.org
                                                 www.y-me.org
Provides support information and education to anyone touched by breast cancer. Support and information are available 24 hours through the National Breast Cancer Hotline which is staffed by breast cancer survivors who are trained peer counselors.
Cindy Geoghegan, CEO
Ginny Finn, Executive Director

State Agencies & Associations

Alabama

2016 American Cancer Society: Alabama
1100 Ireland Way   205-879-2242
Birmingham, AL 35205   Fax: 205-930-8895
                          e-mail: scarlet.thompson@cancer.org
                          www.cancer.org/docroot/com/com_0.asp
The American Cancer Society is the nationwide community-based voluntary health organization dedicated to eliminating cancer as a major health problem by preventing cancer, saving lives and diminishing suffering from cancer, through research and education.
Scarlet Thom (205-930-8889), Media/Public Relations Alabama

2017 Leukemia and Lymphoma Society: Alabama Chapter
Leukemia Society of America
100 Chase Park S   205-989-0098
Birmingham, AL 35244   888-560-9700
                                           Fax: 205-989-0099
                               www.lls.org/aboutlls/chapters/al/
Dedicated to finding cures for leukemia and related cancers and to improving the quality of life for patients and their families.
Melanie Mooney, Executive Director
Kate McLean, Campaign Coordinator, Special Events

Alaska

2018 American Cancer Society: Alaska
3851 Piper Street   907-277-8696
Anchorage, AK 99508   Fax: 907-263-2073
                              e-mail: leslie.jones@cancer.org
                                               www.cancer.org
The American Cancer Society is the nationwide community-based voluntary health organization dedicated to eliminating cancer as a

major health problem by preventing cancer saving lives and diminishing suffering from cancer through research and education.
Leslie Jones, Media/Public Relations Alaska

Arizona

2019 American Cancer Society: Arizona
4212 N 16th Street   602-224-0524
Phoenix, AZ 85016   800-227-2345
                                           Fax: 602-778-7699
                          e-mail: meg.kondrich@cancer.org
                                               www.cancer.org
The American Cancer Society is the nationwide community-based voluntary health organization dedicated to eliminating cancer as a major health problem by preventing cancer saving lives, and diminishing suffering from cancer through research and education.
Meg Kondrich, Media/Public Relations Arizona

2020 International Holistic Center
PO Box 15103   928-771-2826
Phoenix, AZ 85060-5103   e-mail: ihcinc@cox.net
                                         www.holisticresources.org
Provides information and referrals concerning holistic health care in Arizona and beyond.
Stan Kalson, President

2021 Leukemia and Lymphoma Society: Mountain States Chapter
Leukemia Society of America
3877 N 7th Street   602-567-7600
Phoenix, AZ 85014   800-568-1372
                                           Fax: 602-567-7601
                                    www.leukemia-lymphoma.org
Dedicated to finding cures for leukemia and related cancers and to improving the quality of life for patients and their families. Serves New Mexico and the Greater El Paso, TX area.
Tim Metzer, Executive Director

Arkansas

2022 American Cancer Society: Arkansas
901 N University   501-664-3480
Little Rock, AR 72207   Fax: 501-603-5223
                             e-mail: jodie.spears@cancer.org
                                               www.cancer.org
The American Cancer Society is the nationwide community-based voluntary health organization dedicated to eliminating cancer as a major health problem by preventing cancer, saving lives, and diminishing suffering from cancer, through research and education.
Jodie Spears, Media/Public Relations Arkansas

2023 Health Resource
933 Faulkner Street   501-329-5272
Conway, AR 72034   800-949-0090
                                           Fax: 501-329-9489
                       e-mail: research@thehealthresource.com
                                        www.thehealthresource.com
A medical information service which provides clients with an individualized, in depth research report on his or her specific health problem. Reports include latest treatment options, mainstream, experimental and alternative and top specialists.
Janice Guthrie, Director/Researcher
Shirley Effinger, Researcher

California

2024 American Cancer Society Santa Clara County / Silicon Valley / Central Coast Region
747 Camden Avenue   408-871-1062
Campbell, CA 95008   Fax: 408-871-2993
                             e-mail: angie.carrillo@cancer.org
                                               www.cancer.org
The American Cancer Society is the nationwide community-based voluntary health organization dedicated to eliminating cancer as a major health problem by preventing cancer, saving lives and diminishing suffering from cancer, through research and education.
Angie Carillo, Media/Public Relations Silicon Valley

2025 American Cancer Society: Central Los Angeles
3333 Wilshire Boulevard   213-386-6102
Los Angeles, CA 90010   Fax: 213-480-0806
e-mail: katherine.spangle@cancer.org
www.cancer.org
The American Cancer Society is the nationwide community-based voluntary health organization dedicated to eliminating cancer as a major health problem by preventing cancer, saving lives, and diminishing suffering from cancer, through research and education.
Katie Spangle, Media/Public Relations Los Angeles Area

2026 American Cancer Society: East Bay/Metro Region
1700 Webster Street   510-832-7012
Oakland, CA 94612   Fax: 510-763-8826
e-mail: patty.guinto@cancer.org
www.cancer.org
The American Cancer Society is the nationwide community-based voluntary health organization dedicated to eliminating cancer as a major health problem by preventing cancer, saving lives, and diminishing suffering from cancer, through research and education.
Patty Guinto, Media/Public Relations East Bay Area

2027 American Cancer Society: Fresno/Madera Counties
2222 W Shaw Avenue   559-451-0722
Fresno, CA 93711   Fax: 559-451-0744
e-mail: erica.jones@cancer.org
www.cancer.org
The American Cancer Society is the nationwide community-based voluntary health organization dedicated to eliminating cancer as a major health problem by preventing cancer, saving lives, and diminishing suffering from cancer, through research and education.
Erica Jones, Media/Public Relations Fresno CA

2028 American Cancer Society: Inland Empire
6355 Riverside Ave   951-683-6415
Riverside, CA 92506   Fax: 951-682-6804
e-mail: beckie.mooreflati@cancer.org
www.cancer.org
The American Cancer Society is the nationwide community-based voluntary health organization dedicated to eliminating cancer as a major health problem by preventing cancer, saving lives, and diminishing suffering from cancer, through research and education.
Beckie Moore, Media/Public Relations Riverside Region

2029 American Cancer Society: Orange County
1940 E Deere Avenue   949-261-9446
Santa Ana, CA 92705-5718   Fax: 949-261-9419
e-mail: jennifer.horspool@cancer.org
www.cancer.org
The American Cancer Society is the nationwide community-based voluntary health organization dedicated to eliminating cancer as a major health problem by preventing cancer, saving lives, and diminishing suffering from cancer, through research and education.
Jennifer Horton, Media/Public Relations Orange County

2030 American Cancer Society: Sacramento County
1765 Challenge Way   916-446-7933
Sacramento, CA 95815   Fax: 916-64 -977
e-mail: maria.robinson@cancer.org
www.cancer.org
The American Cancer Society is the nationwide community-based voluntary health organization dedicated to eliminating cancer as a major health problem by preventing cancer, saving lives, and diminishing suffering from cancer, through research and education.
Maria Robinson, Media/Public Relations Sacramento County

2031 American Cancer Society: San Diego County
2655 Camino Del Rio N   619-299-4200
San Diego, CA 92108   800-227-2345
Fax: 619-296-0928
e-mail: robin.brown@cancer.org
www.cancer.org
The American Cancer Society is the nationwide community-based voluntary health organization dedicated to eliminating cancer as a major health problem by preventing cancer, saving lives, and diminishing suffering from cancer, through research and education.
Robin Brown, Media/Public Relations San Diego CA

2032 American Cancer Society: San Francisco County
201 Mission Street   415-394-7100
San Francisco, CA 94105   Fax: 415-495-1877
e-mail: patty.guinto@cancer.org
www.cancer.org
The American Cancer Society is the nationwide community-based voluntary health organization dedicated to eliminating cancer as a major health problem by preventing cancer, saving lives and diminishing suffering from cancer, through research and education.
Patty Guinto, Media/Public Relations San Francisco

2033 American Cancer Society: Santa Maria Valley
426 E Barcellus   805-922-2354
Santa Maria, CA 93454   Fax: 805-925-1424
e-mail: jeb.baird@cancer.org
www.cancer.org
The American Cancer Society is the nationwide community-based voluntary health organization dedicated to eliminating cancer as a major health problem by preventing cancer, saving lives and diminishing suffering from cancer, through research and education.
Jeb Baird, Media/Public Relations Santa Maria

2034 American Cancer Society: Sonoma County
1451 Guerneville Road   707-545-6720
Santa Rosa, CA 95403   Fax: 707-545-3179
e-mail: angie.carrillo@cancer.org
www.cancer.org
The American Cancer Society is the nationwide community-based voluntary health organization dedicated to eliminating cancer as a major health problem by preventing cancer, saving lives and diminishing suffering from cancer, through research and education.
Angie Carillo, Media/Public Relations Central Coast

2035 Cancer Control Society and Cancer.Book House
2043 N Berendo Street   213-663-7801
Los Angeles, CA 90027   Fax: 323-663-7757
www.cancercontrolsociety.com
An informational organization offering books, films, videos, clinic tours and lists of patients with cancer.
Lorraine Rosenthal, Co-Founder
Frank Cousineau, President

2036 City of Hope National Medical Center Beckman Research Institute
Beckman Research Institute
1500 E Duarte Road   626-256-4673
Duarte, CA 91010   800-826-4673
e-mail: tpogue@coh.org
www.cityofhope.org
City of Hope is an innovative biomedical research, treatment and educational institution dedicated to the prevention and cure of cancer and other life-threatening illness.
Stephen J Foreman, Chair

2037 Leukemia & Lymphoma Society: Orange, Riverside, And San Bernadino Counties
2020 E 1st Street   714-881-0610
Santa Ana, CA 92705   888-535-9300
Fax: 714-881-0616
www.leukemia-lymphoma.org
Dedicated to finding cures for leukemia and related cancers and to improving the quality of life for patients and their families.

2038 Leukemia and Lymphoma Society: San Diego/Hawaii Chapter
Leukemia Society of America
9150 Chesapeake Dr   858-277-1800
San Diego, CA 92123   888-535-9300
Fax: 858-277-1748
www.leukemia.org
Dedicated to finding cures for leukemia and related cancers and to improving the quality of life for patients and their families.
Keith Turner, Executive Director

2039 Leukemia and Lymphoma Society: Greater Sacramento Area Chapter
Leukemia Society of America
4604 Roseville Road   916-348-1793
North Highlands, CA 95660   Fax: 916-348-7864
www.leukemia.org

155

Dedicated to finding cures for leukemia and related cancers and to improving the quality of life for patients and their families.
Tracy Latino, Executive Director

2040 Leukemia and Lymphoma Society: Greater Los Angeles Chapter
Leukemia Society of America
6033 W Century Boulevard
Los Angeles, CA 90045
310-342-5800
Fax: 310-342-5801
www.leukemia-lymphoma.org
Dedicated to finding cures for leukemia and related cancers and to improving the quality of life for patients and their families.
Donna Lynch, Executive Director

2041 Leukemia and Lymphoma Society: Northern California Chapter
Leukemia Society of America
1390 Market Street
San Francisco, CA 94102
415-625-1100
Fax: 415-625-1155
e-mail: supportservices@lls.org
www.lls.org
Dedicated to finding cures for leukemia and related cancers and to improving the quality of life for patients and their families.

2042 Leukemia and Lymphoma Society: Orange, Riverside, And San Bernadino Counties
2020 E 1st Street
Santa Ana, CA 92705
714-881-0610
888-535-9300
Fax: 714-881-0616
www.lls.org
Dedicated to finding cures for leukemia and related cancers and to improving the quality of life for patients and their families.

2043 Leukemia and Lymphoma Society: Tri-County Chapter
Leukemia Society of America
2020 E 1st Street
Santa Ana, CA 92705
714-881-0610
888-535-9300
Fax: 714-881-0616
www.leukemia-lymphoma.org
Dedicated to finding cures for leukemia and related cancers and to improving the quality of life for patients and their families.
John Walter, President & CEO
Louis J DeGennaro, Chief Mission Officer

2044 National Health Federation
PO Box 688
Monrovia, CA 91017
626-357-2181
Fax: 626-303-0642
e-mail: contact-us@thenhf.com
www.thenhf.com
A nonprofit consumer-oriented organization devoted to health matters. Dedicated to preserving freedom of choice in health care issues, prevention of diseases and the promotion of wellness.
Scott Tips, President
Sylvia Provenza, Vice-President

2045 Regional Cancer Foundation
1200 Gough Street
San Francisco, CA 94109
415-775-9956
Fax: 415-346-8652
e-mail: mail@regionalcancerfoundation.org
www.regionalcancerfoundation.org
This foundation offers, at no charge, a second opinion consultation to individuals diagnosed with cancer. The patient and a family member or friend meet with an interdisciplinary panel of local cancer specialists with expertise in radiation therapy, chemotherapy, and cancer treatment plans.
William Gillis, CEO
Arhur J Inerfield, Chairman

2046 Rose Kushner Breast Cancer Advisory Center
PO Box 757
Malaga Cove, CA 90274
301-897-3445
Fax: 301-897-3444
e-mail: lkkushner@yahoo.com
www.rkbcac.org
Provides a mail service offering referrals to health professionals as well as information about detection, diagnosis, treatment and physical and psychological rehabilitation for patients with breast cancer.

Colorado

2047 American Cancer Society: Colorado
2255 S Oneida Street
Denver, CO 80224
303-758-2030
Fax: 303-759-1615
e-mail: lynda.solomon@cancer.org
www.cancer.org
The American Cancer Society is the nationwide community-based voluntary health organization dedicated to eliminating cancer as a major health problem by preventing cancer, saving lives and diminishing suffering from cancer, through research and education.
Lynda Solomo, Media/Public Relations Colorado
Joel Quevill, Media/Public Relations Colorado

Connecticut

2048 American Cancer Society: Connecticut
Meriden Executive Park
Meriden, CT 06450
203-379-4700
Fax: 203-379-5060
e-mail: simone.upsey@cancer.org
www.cancer.org
The American Cancer Society is the nationwide community-based voluntary health organization dedicated to eliminating cancer as a major health problem by preventing cancer, saving lives and diminishing suffering from cancer, through research and education.
Simone Upsey, Media/Public Relations NH/MS/NL Counties
Christian Me, Media/Public Relations LF/FF Counties

2049 Leukemia and Lymphoma Society: Connecticut Chapter
Leukemia Society of America
321 Research Parkway
Meriden, CT 06450
203-379-0445
888-282-9465
Fax: 203-379-0451
www.lls.org/aboutlls/chapters/ct/
Founded in 1949 to help serve and educate the communities and residents who have been touched by leukemia, lymphoma, multiple myeloma and Hodgkin's disease.
Jean Montano, Executive Director
Dina Mariani, Deputy Executive Director

2050 Leukemia and Lymphoma Society: Fairfield County Chapter
Leukemia Society of America
25 Third Street
Stamford, CT 06905
203-967-8326
Fax: 203-325-8559
www.lls.org
Dedicated to finding cures for leukemia and related cancers and to improving the quality of life for patients and their families.

Delaware

2051 American Cancer Society: Delaware
92 Reads Way
New Castle, DE 19720
302-324-4427
Fax: 302-324-4233
e-mail: dawn.ward@cancer.org
www.cancer.org
The American Cancer Society is the nationwide community-based voluntary health organization dedicated to eliminating cancer as a major health problem by preventing cancer, saving lives, and diminishing suffering from cancer, through research and education.
Dawn Ward, Media/Public Relations Delaware

2052 Leukemia and Lymphoma Society: Delaware Chapter
Leukemia Society of America
100 W 10th Street
Wilmington, DE 19801
302-661-7300
800-220-1617
Fax: 302-661-0363
www.leukemia-lymphoma.org
Our mission is to cure leukemia, lymphoma, Hodgkin's disease and myeloma and to improve the quality of life of patients and their families.
Timothy S Durst, Chairman
James Davis, Vice-Chair

District of Columbia

2053 American Cancer Society: District of Columbia
1875 Connecticut Avenue NW
Washington, DC 20009
202-483-2600
Fax: 202-483-1174
e-mail: angela.collins@cancer.org
www.cancer.org

The American Cancer Society is the nationwide community-based voluntary health organization dedicated to eliminating cancer as a major health problem by preventing cancer, saving lives, and diminishing suffering from cancer, through research and education.
Angela Colli, Media/Public Relations Washington DC

2054 American Institute for Cancer Research
1759 R Street NW
Washington, DC 20009
202-328-7744
800-843-8114
Fax: 202-328-7226
e-mail: aicrweb@aicr.org
www.aicr.org

Not-for-profit research and educational organization. Provides grants for research into the causes, development, prevention and treatment of cancer through diet and nutrition. Offers publications, research results, conferences and various public services.

2055 Center for Science in the Public Interest
1220 L Street N.W.
Washington, DC 20005
202-332-9110
Fax: 202-265-4954
e-mail: cspi@cspinet.org
www.cspinet.org

The nation's leading consumer group concerned with food and nutrition issues. Focuses on diseases that result from consuming too many calories, too much fat, sodium and sugar such as cancer and heart disease.
Don Allen, Director of Finance
Tom Gegax, Board of Directors

Florida

2056 American Cancer Society: Florida
2006 W Kennedy Boulevard
Tampa, FL 33606
813-254-3630
Fax: 813-349-4431
e-mail: cynthia.dunlap@cancer.org
www.cancer.org

The American Cancer Society is the nationwide community-based voluntary health organization dedicated to eliminating cancer as a major health problem by preventing cancer, saving lives, and diminishing suffering from cancer, through research and education.
C. Dunlap, Media/Public Relations Tampa Region
Kristen Redd, Media/Public Relations Tampa Region

2057 Leukemia & Lymphoma Society: Suncoast Chapter
3507 E Frontage Road
Tampa, FL 33607
813-963-6461
800-436-6889
Fax: 813-963-1306
www.lls.org

Serves patients with leukemia, lymphoma, multiple myeloma and Hodgkin's disease in Charlotte, Citrus, Collier, DeSoto, Hardee, Hernando, Hillsborough, Lee, Manatee, Pasco, Pinellas and Sarasota counties.

2058 Leukemia and Lymphoma Society: Southern Florida Chapter
Leukemia Society of America
3325 Hollywood Boulevard
Hallandale, FL 33021
954-961-3234
Fax: 954-961-7376
www.lls.org

Dedicated to finding cures for leukemia and related cancers and to improving the quality of life for patients and their families.

2059 Leukemia and Lymphoma Society: Central Florida Chapter
Leukemia Society of America
3319 Maguire Boulevard
Orlando, FL 32803-3720
407-898-0733
Fax: 407-896-8645
www.lls.org

Dedicated to finding cures for leukemia and related cancers and to improving the quality of life for patients and their families.

2060 Leukemia and Lymphoma Society: Northern Florida Chapter
Leukemia Society of America
9143 Phillips Highway
Jacksonville, FL 32256
904-538-0721
800-868-0072
Fax: 904-538-9245
www.lls.org

Dedicated to finding cures for leukemia and related cancers and to improving the quality of life for patients and their families.

2061 Leukemia and Lymphoma Society: Palm Beach Area Chapter
Leukemia Society of America
4360 Northlake Boulevard
Palm Beach Gardens, FL 33410
561-775-9954
888-478-8550
Fax: 561-775-0930
www.lls.org

Dedicated to finding cures for leukemia and related cancers and to improving the quality of life for patients and their families.

Georgia

2062 American Cancer Society: Georgia
50 Williams Street
Atlanta, GA 30303
404-315-1123
Fax: 404-315-9348
e-mail: elissa.mccrary@cancer.org
www.cancer.org

The American Cancer Society is the nationwide community-based voluntary health organization dedicated to eliminating cancer as a major health problem by preventing cancer, saving lives, and diminishing suffering from cancer, through research and education.
E. McCrary, Media/Public Relations Georgia

2063 Kidscope
2045 Peachtree Road
Atlanta, GA 30309
404-892-1437
www.kidscope.org

A nonprofit organization formed to help families and children better understand the effects from cancer in a parent. The name can also be read as Kids Cope - one of the goals being to improve the chances that a child will successfully cope with the diagnosis.
H Elizabeth King PhD, Board Member
Carol Webb PhD, Board Member

2064 Leukemia and Lymphoma Society: Georgia Chapter
Leukemia Society of America
3715 Northside Parkway
Atlanta, GA 30327
404-720-7900
800-399-7312
Fax: 404-720-7878
e-mail: dick.brown@lls.org
www.leukemia-lymphoma.org

Dedicated to finding cures for leukemia and related cancers and to improving the quality of life for patients and their families.
Dick Brown, Executive Director
Maureen Quin Davidson, Director TNT

Hawaii

2065 American Cancer Society: Hawaii
2370 Nuuanu Avenue
Honolulu, HI 96817
808-595-7544
800-ACS-2345
Fax: 808-595-7545
TTY: 866-228-4327
e-mail: milton.hirata@cancer.org
www.cancer.org

The American Cancer Society is the nationwide community-based voluntary health organization dedicated to eliminating cancer as a major health problem by preventing cancer, saving lives, and diminishing suffering from cancer, through research and education.
Milton Hirata, Media Relations Contact - Hawaii

Idaho

2066 American Cancer Society: Idaho
2676 Vista Avenue
Boise, ID 83705
208-345-2184
800-ACS-2345
Fax: 208-343-9922
TTY: 866-228-4327
e-mail: jim.ryan@cancer.org
www.cancer.org

The American Cancer Society is the nationwide community-based voluntary health organization dedicated to eliminating cancer as a major health problem by preventing cancer, saving lives, and diminishing suffering from cancer, through research and education.
Jim Ryan, Media Relations Contact - Idaho

Illinois

2067 American Cancer Society: Illinois
225 N Michigan Avenue 312-372-0471
Chicago, IL 60601 800-ACS-2345
Fax: 312-372-0910
TTY: 866-228-4327
e-mail: melissa.leeb@cancer.org
www.cancer.org
The American Cancer Society is the nationwide community-based
voluntary health organization dedicated to eliminating cancer as a
major health problem by preventing cancer, saving lives, and diminishing suffering from cancer, through research and education.
Melissa Leeb, Media Relations Contact - Illinois

2068 Leukemia and Lymphoma Society: Illinois Chapter
Leukemia Society of America
651 W Washington Boulevard 312-651-7350
Chicago, IL 60661 800-742-6595
Fax: 312-463-0980
e-mail: pam.swenk@lls.org
www.lls.org
Dedicated to finding cures for leukemia and related cancers and to
improving the quality of life for patients and their families.
Pam Swenk, Executive Director
Jennifer Hufnagel, Director Donor Development

Indiana

2069 American Cancer Society: Indiana
5635 W 96th Street 317-344-7800
Indianapolis, IN 46278 800-ACS-2345
Fax: 317-344-7810
TTY: 866-228-4327
e-mail: leslie.smith@cancer.org
www.cancer.org
The American Cancer Society is the nationwide community-based
voluntary health organization dedicated to eliminating cancer as a
major health problem by preventing cancer, saving lives, and diminishing suffering from cancer, through research and education.
Leslie Smith Babione, Media Relations Contact - Indianapolis
Katie Burton, Media/Public Relations Indiana

2070 Leukemia and Lymphoma Society: Indiana Chapter
Leukemia Society of America
941 E 86th Street 317-726-2270
Indianapolis, IN 46240 800-846-7764
Fax: 317-726-2280
e-mail: amy.kwas@lls.org
www.lls.org
Dedicated to finding cures for leukemia and related cancers and to
improving the quality of life for patients and their families.
Amy Kwas, Executive Director
Sarah Moore, Deputy Executive Director

Iowa

2071 American Cancer Society: Iowa
8364 Hickman Road 515-253-0147
Des Moines, IA 50325 800-ACS-2345
Fax: 515-253-0806
TTY: 866-228-4327
e-mail: chaarles.reed@cancer.org
www.cancer.org
The American Cancer Society is the nationwide community-based
voluntary health organization dedicated to eliminating cancer as a
major health problem by preventing cancer, saving lives, and diminishing suffering from cancer, through research and education.
Chuck Reed, Media Relations Contact - Iowa

2072 People Against Cancer
604 E Street 515-972-4444
Otho, IA 50569-0010 800-662-2326
Fax: 515-972-4415
e-mail: info@PeopleAgainstCancer.net
www.peopleagainstcancer.com
A nonprofit grassroots organization whose mission is to find the
best cancer therapy for people with cancer worldwide.
Frank Wiewel, Executive Director

Kansas

2073 American Cancer Society: Kansas City
6700 Antioch 913-432-3277
Merriam, KS 66024 800-ACS-2345
Fax: 913-432-1732
TTY: 866-228-4327
e-mail: christine.winter@cancer.org
www.cancer.org
The American Cancer Society is the nationwide community-based
voluntary health organization dedicated to eliminating cancer as a
major health problem by preventing cancer, saving lives, and diminishing suffering from cancer, through research and education.
Christine Winter, Media Relations Contact

2074 Leukemia and Lymphoma Society: Mid-America Chapter
Leukemia Society of America
6811 W 63rd Street 913-262-1515
Shawnee Mission, KS 66202 800-256-1075
Fax: 913-262-2167
e-mail: janna.lacock@lls.org
www.lls.org
Dedicated to finding cures for leukemia and related cancers and to
improving the quality of life for patients and their families.
Janna LaCock, Executive Director
Jill Ring, Development Director

2075 Leukemia and Lymphona Society: Kansas Chapter
Leukemia Society of America
300 N Main 316-266-4050
Wichita, KS 67202 800-779-2417
Fax: 316-266-4960
e-mail: kelly.gerstenkorn@lls.org
www.lls.org/ks
Cure leukemia, lymphoma, Hodgkin's disease and myeloma and
improve the quality of life for patients and their families.
Timothy S Durst, Chairman
James Davis, Vice-Chair

Kentucky

2076 American Cancer Society: Kentucky
701 W Muhammad Ali Boulevard 502-584-6782
Louisville, KY 40203 800-ACS-2345
Fax: 502-584-6767
TTY: 866-228-4327
e-mail: doug.dressman@cancer.org
www.cancer.org
The American Cancer Society is the nationwide community-based
voluntary health organization dedicated to eliminating cancer as a
major health problem by preventing cancer, saving lives, and diminishing suffering from cancer, through research and education.
Doug Dressman, Executive Director-Louisville

2077 Leukemia and Lymphoma Society: Kentucky Chapter
Leukemia Society of America
600 E Main Street 502-584-8490
Louisville, KY 40202-2661 800-955-2566
Fax: 502-589-5316
e-mail: karyl.ferman@lls.org
www.lls.org
Founded in 1975 to serve Kentucky and Southern Indiana
residents touched by leukemia and its related cancers. Goal is to
find a cure for leukemia and its related cancers and to improve the
quality of life for patients and their families.
Karyl D Ferman, Executive Director
Katie Anderson, Director Team in Training

Louisiana

2078 American Cancer Society: Louisiana
2605 River Road 504-469-0021
New Orleans, LA 70121 800-ACS-2345
Fax: 504-219-2290
TTY: 866-228-4327
e-mail: jewel.m.bush@cancer.org
www.cancer.org
The American Cancer Society is the nationwide community-based
voluntary health organization dedicated to eliminating cancer as a

major health problem by preventing cancer, saving lives, and diminishing suffering from cancer, through research and education.
Jewel M Bush, Media Relations Contact

Maine

2079 American Cancer Society: Maine
1 Bowdoin Mill Island   207-373-3700
Topsham, ME 04086   800-ACS-2345
                                                          Fax: 207-725-6680
                                                          TTY: 866-228-4327
                                          e-mail: susan.clifford@cancer.org
                                                              www.cancer.org
The American Cancer Society is the nationwide community-based voluntary health organization dedicated to eliminating cancer as a major health problem by preventing cancer, saving lives, and diminishing suffering from cancer, through research and education.
Susan Clifford, Media Relations Contact - Maine

Maryland

2080 American Cancer Society: Maryland
8219 Town Center Drive   410-931-6850
Baltimore, MD 21236   800-ACS-2345
                                                          Fax: 410-931-6875
                                                          TTY: 866-228-4327
                                          e-mail: dawn.ward@cancer.org
                                                              www.cancer.org
The American Cancer Society is the nationwide community-based voluntary health organization dedicated to eliminating cancer as a major health problem by preventing cancer, saving lives, and diminishing suffering from cancer, through research and education.
Dawn Ward, Media Relations Contact - Baltimore Area

2081 Leukemia and Lymphoma Society: Maryland Chapter
Leukemia Society of America
11350 McCormick Road   410-527-0220
Hunt Valley, MD 21031-2001   800-242-4572
                                                          Fax: 410-527-0510
                                          e-mail: sharon.yateman@lls.org
                                                                  www.lls.org
Dedicated to finding cures for leukemia and related cancers and to improving the quality of life for patients and their families.
Sharon E Yateman, Executive Director
Allyson Yospe, Deputy Executive Director

Massachusetts

2082 American Cancer Society: Boston
18 Tremont Street   617-556-7400
Boston, MA 02108   800-ACS-2345
                                                          Fax: 617-263-6825
                                                          TTY: 866-228-4327
                                          e-mail: kate.langstone@cancer.org
                                                              www.cancer.org
The American Cancer Society is the nationwide community-based voluntary health organization dedicated to eliminating cancer as a major health problem by preventing cancer, saving lives, and diminishing suffering from cancer, through research and education.
Kate Langstone, Media Relations Contact - Boston Area

2083 American Cancer Society: Central New England Region-Weston MA
9 Riverside Road   781-894-6633
Weston, MA 02493   800-ACS-2345
                                                          Fax: 781-314-2699
                                                          TTY: 866-228-4327
                                          e-mail: jessica.saporetti@cancer.org
                                                              www.cancer.org
The American Cancer Society is the nationwide community-based voluntary health organization dedicated to eliminating cancer as a major health problem by preventing cancer, saving lives, and diminishing suffering from cancer, through research and education.
Jessica Saporetti, Media Relations Contact

Michigan

2084 Leukemia and Lymphoma Society: Michigan Chapter
1421 E 12 Mile Road   248-581-3900
Madison Heights, MI 48071   800-456-5413
                                                          Fax: 248-581-3901
                                          e-mail: peggy.shriver@lls.org
                                                                  www.lls.org

Peggy Shriver, Executive Director
Robin R Rhea, Director Operations

Minnesota

2085 American Cancer Society: Duluth
130 W Superior Street   218-727-7439
Duluth, MN 55802   800-ACS-2345
                                                          Fax: 218-727-8069
                                                          TTY: 866-228-4327
                                          e-mail: janis.rannow@cancer.org
                                                              www.cancer.org
The American Cancer Society is the nationwide community-based voluntary health organization dedicated to eliminating cancer as a major health problem by preventing cancer, saving lives, and diminishing suffering from cancer, through research and education.
Janis Rannow, Media Relations Contact

2086 American Cancer Society: Mendota Heights Mendota Heights
Mendota Heights
2520 Pilot Knob Road   651-255-8100
Mendota Heights, MN 55120   800-ACS-2345
                                                          Fax: 651-255-8133
                                                          TTY: 866-228-4327
                                          e-mail: lou.harvin@cancer.org
                                                              www.cancer.org
The American Cancer Society is the nationwide community-based voluntary health organization dedicated to eliminating cancer as a major health problem by preventing cancer, saving lives, and diminishing suffering from cancer, through research and education.
Lou Harvin, Media Relations Contact
Janis Rannow, Media Relations Contact

2087 American Cancer Society: Rochester
2900 43 Street NW   507-287-2044
Rochester, MN 55901   800-ACS-2345
                                                          Fax: 507-287-2178
                                                          TTY: 866-228-4327
                                          e-mail: janis.rannow@cancer.org
                                                              www.cancer.org
The American Cancer Society is the nationwide community-based voluntary health organization dedicated to eliminating cancer as a major health problem by preventing cancer, saving lives, and diminishing suffering from cancer, through research and education.
Janis Rannow, Media Relations Contact

2088 American Cancer Society: Saint Cloud
3721 23rd Street S   320-255-0220
Saint Cloud, MN 56301   800-239-7028
                                                          Fax: 320-255-5517
                                                          TTY: 866-228-4327
                                          e-mail: janis.rannow@cancer.org
                                                              www.cancer.org
The American Cancer Society is the nationwide community-based voluntary health organization dedicated to eliminating cancer as a major health problem by preventing cancer, saving lives, and diminishing suffering from cancer, through research and education.
Janis Rannow, Media Relations Contact

2089 Leukemia and Lymphoma Society: Minnesota Chapter
5217 Wayzata Boulevard   763-852-3000
Golden Valley, MN 55426   888-220-4440
                                                          Fax: 763-852-3001
                                          e-mail: Murray.Schmidt@lls.org
                                                                  www.lls.org

Murray Schmidt, Executive Director
Vickie Shaw, Deputy Executive Director

Mississippi

2090 American Cancer Society: Jackson
1380 Livingston Lane 601-362-8874
Jackson, MS 39213 800-ACS-2345
Fax: 601-362-8876
TTY: 866-228-4327
e-mail: kelly.lindsay@cancer.org
www.cancer.org

The American Cancer Society is the nationwide community-based voluntary health organization dedicated to eliminating cancer as a major health problem by preventing cancer, saving lives, and diminishing suffering from cancer, through research and education.
Kelly Lindsay, Media Relations Contact

2091 Leukemia and Lymphoma Society: Mississippi Chapter
408 Fontaine Place 601-956-7447
Ridgeland, MS 39157 877-538-5364
Fax: 601-956-6957
e-mail: Travis.Lee@lls.org
www.lls.org

Travis Lee, Campaign Director Team in Training
Natalie Michael, Campaign Director Team in Training

Missouri

2092 American Cancer Society: Saint Louis
4207 Lindell Boulevard 314-286-8100
Saint Louis, MO 63108 800-ACS-2345
Fax: 314-286-8160
TTY: 866-228-4327
e-mail: christine.winter@cancer.org
www.cancer.org

The American Cancer Society is the nationwide community-based voluntary health organization dedicated to eliminating cancer as a major health problem by preventing cancer, saving lives, and diminishing suffering from cancer, through research and education.
Christine Winter, Media Relations Contact

Montana

2093 American Cancer Society: Montana
3550 Mullan Road 406-542-2191
Missoula, MT 59808 800-ACS-2345
Fax: 406-327-0146
TTY: 866-228-4327
e-mail: jim.ryan@cancer.org
www.cancer.org

The American Cancer Society is the nationwide community-based voluntary health organization dedicated to eliminating cancer as a major health problem by preventing cancer, saving lives, and diminishing suffering from cancer, through research and education.
Jim Ryan, Media Relations Contact

Nebraska

2094 American Cancer Society: Nebraska
9850 Nicholas Street 402-393-5800
Omaha, NE 68114 800-ACS-2345
Fax: 402-393-7790
TTY: 866-228-4327
e-mail: mike.lefler@cancer.org
www.cancer.org

The American Cancer Society is the nationwide community-based voluntary health organization dedicated to eliminating cancer as a major health problem by preventing cancer, saving lives, and diminishing suffering from cancer, through research and education.
Mike Lefler, Media Relations Contact

2095 Leukemia and Lymphoma Society: Nebraska Chapter
10832 Old Mill Road 402-344-2242
Omaha, NE 68154 888-847-4974
Fax: 402-344-2422
e-mail: pattie.gorham@lls.org
www.lls.org

Pattie Gorham, Executive Director
Tonya Schroeder, Patient Services Manager - Portland Area

Nevada

2096 American Cancer Society: Nevada
6165 S Rainbow Boulevard 702-798-6877
Las Vegas, NV 89118 800-ACS-2345
Fax: 702-798-0530
TTY: 866-228-4327
e-mail: paulette.anderson@cancer.org
www.cancer.org

The American Cancer Society is the nationwide community-based voluntary health organization dedicated to eliminating cancer as a major health problem by preventing cancer, saving lives, and diminishing suffering from cancer, through research and education.
Paulette Anderson, Media Relations Contact

New Hampshire

2097 American Cancer Society: New Hampshire Gail Singer Memorial Building
Gail Singer Memorial Building
2 Commerce Drive 603-472-8899
Bedford, NH 03110 800-ACS-2345
Fax: 603-472-7093
TTY: 866-228-4327
e-mail: peter.davies@cancer.org
www.cancer.org

The American Cancer Society is the nationwide community-based voluntary health organization dedicated to eliminating cancer as a major health problem by preventing cancer, saving lives, and diminishing suffering from cancer, through research and education.
Peter Davies, Media Relations Contact

2098 New Hampshire Cancer Pain Initiative
125 Airport Road 603-225-0900
Concord, NH 03301 e-mail: info@nhpain.org.
www.nhpain.org

Made up of concerned people who have joined together to promote the alleviation of cancer pain through education, research and advisory activities.

New Jersey

2099 American Cancer Society: New Jersey
2600 US Highway 1 732-297-8000
N Brunswick, NJ 08902 800-ACS-2345
Fax: 732-297-9043
TTY: 866-228-4327
e-mail: marjorie.kaplan@cancer.org
www.cancer.org

The American Cancer Society is the nationwide community-based voluntary health organization dedicated to eliminating cancer as a major health problem by preventing cancer, saving lives, and diminishing suffering from cancer, through research and education.
Marjorie Kaplan, Media Relations Contact

2100 CanHelp
PO Box 1678
Livingston, NJ 07039 800-364-2341
Fax: 888-800-0201
e-mail: joan@canhelp.com
www.canhelp.com

Offers reports for cancer patients on orthodox and alternative therapies and coaching/counseling to help with treatment decision-making and coping.
Patrick M McGrady, Founder
Joan Runfola LCSW, Director

2101 Leukemia and Lymphoma Society: Northern New Jersey Chapter
Leukemia Society of America
116 South Euclid Avenue 908-654-9445
Westfield, NJ 07090 Fax: 908-654-9496
e-mail: gina.panas@lls.org
www.lls.org

Dedicated to finding cures for leukemia and related cancers and to improving the quality of life for patients and their families.

2102 Leukemia and Lymphoma Society: Southern New Jersey Chapter
Leukemia Society of America

216 Haddon Avenue
Westmont, NJ 08108-2811

856-869-0200
888-920-8557
Fax: 856-869-7383
e-mail: gina.panas@lls.org
www.lls.org

Dedicated to finding cures for leukemia and related cancers and to improving the quality of life for patients and their families.

New Mexico

2103 American Cancer Society: New Mexico
10501 Montgomery Boulevard NE
Albuquerque, NM 87111

505-260-2105
800-ACS-2345
Fax: 505-266-9513
TTY: 866-228-4327
e-mail: john.weisgerber@cancer.org
www.cancer.org

The American Cancer Society is the nationwide community-based voluntary health organization dedicated to eliminating cancer as a major health problem by preventing cancer, saving lives, and diminishing suffering from cancer, through research and education.
John Weisgerber, Media Relations Contact

2104 Leukemia and Lymphoma Society: Mountain States Chapter
Leukemia Society of America
3411 Candelaria NE
Albuquerque, NM 87107

505-872-0141
888-286-7846
Fax: 505-872-2480
e-mail: gina.panas@lls.org
www.lls.org

Dedicated to finding cures for leukemia and related cancers and to improving the quality of life for patients and their families. Serves New Mexico and the Greater El Paso, TX area.
Deborah Hoffman, Executive Director
Mikki Aronoff, Patient Services Manager - Portland Area

New York

2105 American Cancer Society: Central New York Region/East Syracuse
6725 Lyons Street
E Syracuse, NY 13057

315-437-7025
800-ACS-2345
Fax: 315-437-8233
TTY: 866-228-4327
e-mail: kim.mcmahon@cancer.org
www.cancer.org

The American Cancer Society is the nationwide community-based voluntary health organization dedicated to eliminating cancer as a major health problem by preventing cancer, saving lives, and diminishing suffering from cancer, through research and education.
Kim McMahon, Media Relations Contact

2106 American Cancer Society: Long Island
75 Davids Drive
Hauppauge, NY 11788

631-436-7070
800-ACS-2345
Fax: 631-436-5380
TTY: 866-228-4327
e-mail: jennifer.cucurullo@cancer.org
www.cancer.org

The American Cancer Society is the nationwide community-based voluntary health organization dedicated to eliminating cancer as a major health problem by preventing cancer, saving lives, and diminishing suffering from cancer, through research and education.
Jennifer Cucurullo, Media Relations Contact

2107 American Cancer Society: New York City
132 W 32nd Street
New York, NY 10001-3983

212-586-8700
800-ACS-2345
Fax: 212-237-3855
TTY: 866-228-4327
e-mail: jennifer.cucurullo@cancer.org
www.cancer.org

The American Cancer Society is the nationwide community-based voluntary health organization dedicated to eliminating cancer as a major health problem by preventing cancer, saving lives, and diminishing suffering from cancer, through research and education.
Jennifer Cucurullo, Media Relations Contact

2108 American Cancer Society: Queens Region / Rego Park
97-99 Queens Boulevard
Rego Park, NY 11374

718-263-2224
800-ACS-2345
Fax: 718-261-0758
TTY: 866-228-4327
e-mail: jennifer.cucurullo@cancer.org
www.cancer.org

The American Cancer Society is the nationwide community-based voluntary health organization dedicated to eliminating cancer as a major health problem by preventing cancer, saving lives, and diminishing suffering from cancer, through research and education.
Jennifer Cucurullo, Media Relations Contact

2109 American Cancer Society: Westchester Region/White Plains
2 Lyon Place
White Plains, NY 10601

914-949-4800
800-ACS-2345
Fax: 914-397-8851
TTY: 866-228-4327
e-mail: jennifer.cucurullo@cancer.org
www.cancer.org

The American Cancer Society is the nationwide community-based voluntary health organization dedicated to eliminating cancer as a major health problem by preventing cancer, saving lives, and diminishing suffering from cancer, through research and education.
Jennifer Cucurullo, Media Relations Contact

2110 Foundation for Advancement in Cancer Therapy
Old Chelsea Station
New York, NY 10113

212-741-2790
www.fact-ltd.org

Distributes information on cancer prevention and nontoxic therapies for cancer.
Ruth Sackman, President/Co-founder
James H Davis, Vice Chair

2111 Leukemia & Lymphoma Society Chapter: New York City
475 Park Avenue S
New York, NY 10016

212-376-7100
800-955-4572
Fax: 212-448-9214
e-mail: ossom@lls.org
www.leukemia-lymphoma.org

Dedicated to finding cures for leukemia and related cancers and to improving the quality of life for patients and their families. Educational materials, support services and financial aid available. Volunteer opportunities.
Michael Osso, Executive Director
Sara Lipsky, Deputy Executive Director

2112 Leukemia & Lymphoma Society: Westchester/ Hudson Valley Chapter
1311 Mamaroneck Avenue
White Plains, NY 10605

914-949-0084
Fax: 914-949-0391
www.lls.org/wch

Mission is to cure leukemia, lymphoma, Hodgkin's disease and myeloma, and to improve the quality of life of patients and their families.
Dennis P Chillemi, Executive Director
Diandra Kodl, Deputy Executive Director

2113 Leukemia and Lymphoma Society Chapter: New York City
475 Park Avenue S
New York, NY 10016

212-376-7100
800-955-4572
Fax: 212-448-9214
e-mail: ossom@lls.org
www.leukemia-lymphoma.org

Dedicated to finding cures for leukemia and related cancers and to improving the quality of life for patients and their families. Educational materials, support services and financial aid available. Volunteer opportunities.
Michael Osso, Executive Director
Sara Lipsky, Deputy Executive Director

2114 Leukemia and Lymphoma Society: Central New York Chapter
Leukemia Society of America
401 N Salina Street
Syracuse, NY 13203

315-471-1050
800-690-8944
Fax: 315-471-6434
e-mail: chip.lockwood@lls.org
www.lls.org

161

Dedicated to finding cures for leukemia and related cancers and to improving the quality of life for patients and their families.
Chip Lockwood, Executive Director
Kristen Duggleby, Campaign Director Donor Relations

2115 Leukemia and Lymphoma Society: Long Island Chapter
Leukemia Society of America
555 Broadhollow Road   631-752-8500
Melville, NY 11747   Fax: 631-752-9066
e-mail: tammy.philie@lls.org
www.lls.org
Established to serve Long Islanders with leukemia, lymphoma, Hodgkin's disease and myeloma, their families and friends.
Tammy Philie, Executive Director
Nicole Kowaleski, Deputy Executive Director

2116 Leukemia and Lymphoma Society: Upstate New York Chapter
Leukemia Society of America
5 Computer Drive W   518-438-3583
Albany, NY 12205   866-255-3583
Fax: 518-438-6431
e-mail: Maureen.Thornton@lls.org
www.lls.org
Dedicated to finding cures for leukemia and related cancers and to improving the quality of life for patients and their families.
Maureen O'Brien-Thor, Executive Director
Raechel Hunt, Patient Services Manager - Portland Area

2117 Leukemia and Lymphoma Society: Western New York & Finger Lakes Chapter
Leukemia Society of America
4053 Maple Road   716-834-2578
Amherst, NY 14226   800-784-2368
Fax: 716-837-0335
e-mail: nancy.hails@lls.org
www.lls.org
Dedicated to finding cures for leukemia and related cancers and to improving the quality of life for patients and their families.
Nancy Hails, Executive Director
Luann Burgio, Deputy Executive Director

North Carolina

2118 American Cancer Society: North Carolina
8300 Health Park   919-334-5218
Raleigh, NC 27615   800-ACS-2345
Fax: 919-841-1422
TTY: 866-228-4327
e-mail: jbright@cancer.org
www.cancer.org
The American Cancer Society is the nationwide community-based voluntary health organization dedicated to eliminating cancer as a major health problem by preventing cancer, saving lives, and diminishing suffering from cancer, through research and education.
Jeff Bright, Media Relations Contact

2119 Leukemia and Lymphoma Society: Eastern North Carolina Chapter
Flagship Building
401 Harrison Oaks Boulevard   919-677-3993
Cary, NC 27513   800-936-9337
Fax: 919-677-3992
e-mail: tiffany.armstrong@lls.org
www.lls.org

Tiffany Armstrong, Executive Director
Loreal Massiah, Patient Services Manager - Portland Area

2120 Leukemia and Lymphoma Society: North Carolina Chapter
Leukemia Society of America
5950 Fairview Road   704-998-5012
Charlotte, NC 28210   800-888-9934
Fax: 704-998-5010
www.lls.org
Dedicated to finding cures for leukemia and related cancers and to improving the quality of life for patients and their families.
Tiffany Armstrong, Executive Director
Loreal Massiah, Patient Services Manager - Portland Area

North Dakota

2121 American Cancer Society: North Dakota
4646 Amber Valley Parkway   701-232-1385
Fargo, ND 58104   800-ACS-2345
Fax: 701-232-1109
TTY: 866-228-4327
e-mail: jim.ryan@cancer.org
www.cancer.org
The American Cancer Society is the nationwide community-based voluntary health organization dedicated to eliminating cancer as a major health problem by preventing cancer, saving lives, and diminishing suffering from cancer, through research and education.
Jim Ryan, Media Relations Contact

Ohio

2122 American Cancer Society: Ohio
870 Michigan Avenue
Columbus, OH 43215   888-227-6446
Fax: 877-227-2838
TTY: 866-228-4327
e-mail: robert.paschen@cancer.org
www.cancer.org
The American Cancer Society is the nationwide community-based voluntary health organization dedicated to eliminating cancer as a major health problem by preventing cancer, saving lives, and diminishing suffering from cancer, through research and education.
Robert Paschen, Media Relations Contact

2123 Leukemia and Lymphoma Society: Central Ohio Chapter
Leukemia Society of America
2225 City Gate Drive   614-476-7194
Columbus, OH 43219   800-686-CURE
Fax: 614-476-7189
e-mail: phil.tanner@lls.org
www.lls.org
Dedicated to finding cures for leukemia and related cancers and to improving the quality of life for patients and their families.
Phil Tanner, Executive Director
Dan Swisher, Office Manager

2124 Leukemia and Lymphoma Society: Northern Ohio Chapter
Leukemia Society of America
23297 Commerce Park   216-910-1200
Cleveland, OH 44122   800-589-5721
Fax: 216-910-1201
e-mail: frank.canning@lls.org
www.lls.org
Dedicated to finding cures for leukemia and related cancers and to improving the quality of life for patients and their families.
Frank Canning, Field Director
Nancy Toghill, Office Manager

2125 Leukemia and Lymphoma Society: Southern Ohio Chapter
Leukemia Society of America
4370 Glendale Milford Rd   513-698-2828
Cincinnati, OH 45242   Fax: 513-361-2109
e-mail: michelle.steed@lls.org
www.lls.org
Dedicated to finding cures for leukemia and related cancers and to improving the quality of life for patients and their families. This chapter serves a 22-county geographic area.
Michelle Steed, Executive Director
Gene Fisher, Operations Director

Oklahoma

2126 American Cancer Society: Oklahoma
6525 N Meridian   405-843-9888
Oklahoma City, OK 73116   800-ACS-2345
Fax: 405-848-0795
TTY: 866-228-4327
e-mail: christina.lindholm@cancer.org
www.cancer.org
The American Cancer Society is the nationwide community-based voluntary health organization dedicated to eliminating cancer as a major health problem by preventing cancer, saving lives, and diminishing suffering from cancer, through research and education.
Christina Li, Media/Public Relations

2127 Leukemia and Lymphoma Society: Oklahoma Chapter
Leukemia Society of America
500 N Broadway   405-943-8888
Oklahoma City, OK 73102   888-828-4572
                                          Fax: 405-943-8355
                        e-mail: sherry.martin@lls.org
                                              www.lls.org
Dedicated to finding cures for leukemia and related cancers and to
improving the quality of life for patients and their families.
Sherry Marti MSW LCSW, Patient Services Manager - Portland Area
Jill Hull, Campaign Director Team in Training

Oregon

2128 American Cancer Society: Oregon
330 SW Curry Street   503-295-6422
Portland, OR 97239   800-ACS-2345
                                          Fax: 503-228-1062
                                          TTY: 866-228-4327
                 e-mail: gretchen.rosenberger@cancer.org
                                           www.cancer.org
The American Cancer Society is the nationwide community-based
voluntary health organization dedicated to eliminating cancer as a
major health problem by preventing cancer, saving lives, and diminishing suffering from cancer, through research and education.
Gretchen Rosenberger, Media Relations Contact

2129 Leukemia and Lymphoma Society: Oregon Chapter
Leukemia Society of America
9320 SWBarbur Boulevard   503-245-9866
Portland, OR 97219   800-466-6572
                                          Fax: 503-245-9865
                         e-mail: Sarah.Varner@lls.org
                                              www.lls.org
Dedicated to finding cures for leukemia and related cancers and to
improving the quality of life for patients and their families.
Sarah Varner, Executive Director
Sue Sumpter, Patient Services Manager - Portland Area

Pennsylvania

2130 American Cancer Society: Harrisburg Capital Area Unit
Capital Area Unit
3211 N Front Street   215-985-5336
Harrisburg, PA 17110   888-227-5445
                                          Fax: 717-231-5784
                                          TTY: 866-228-4327
                         e-mail: john.held@cancer.org
                                           www.cancer.org
The American Cancer Society is the nationwide community-based
voluntary health organization dedicated to eliminating cancer as a
major health problem by preventing cancer, saving lives, and di-
minishing suffering from cancer, through research and education.
Colleen Fitz, Media Relations Contact
John Held, Media Relations Contact

2131 American Cancer Society: Philadelphia
1626 Locust Street   215-985-5336
Philadelphia, PA 19103   888-227-5445
                                          Fax: 215-985-5406
                                          TTY: 866-228-4327
                         e-mail: john.held@cancer.org
                                           www.cancer.org
The American Cancer Society is the nationwide community-based
voluntary health organization dedicated to eliminating cancer as a
major health problem by preventing cancer, saving lives, and di-
minishing suffering from cancer, through research and education.
John Held, Media Relations Contact
Colleen Fitz, Media/Public Relations

2132 American Cancer Society: Pittsburgh
320 Bilmar Drive   215-985-5336
Pittsburgh, PA 15205   888-227-5445
                                          Fax: 412-919-1101
                                          TTY: 866-228-4327
                          e-mail: dcatena@cancer.org
                                           www.cancer.org
The American Cancer Society is the nationwide community-based
voluntary health organization dedicated to eliminating cancer as a

major health problem by preventing cancer, saving lives, and diminishing suffering from cancer, through research and education.
Dan Catena, Media Relations Contact

**2133 Leukemia and Lymphoma Society: Central Pennsylvania
Chapter**
800 Corporate Circle   717-652-6520
Harrisburg, PA 17110   800-822-2873
                                          Fax: 717-652-8614
                        e-mail: beth.mihmet@lls.org
                                              www.lls.org

Elizabeth Mihmet, Executive Director
Danielle Bubnis, Patient Services Manager

**2134 Leukemia and Lymphoma Society: Eastern Pennsylvania
Chapter**
555 N Lane   610-238-0360
Conshohocken, PA 19428   800-482-CURE
                                          Fax: 484-530-0833
                       e-mail: ursula.raczak@lls.org
                                              www.lls.org

Lydia Hernandez-Vele, Executive Director
Ursula Raczak, Deputy Executive Director

**2135 Leukemia and Lymphoma Society: Western Pennsylvania/West
Virginia Chapter**
Leukemia Society of America
333 E Carson Street   412-395-2873
Pittsburgh, PA 15219-1439   800-726-2873
                                          Fax: 412-395-2888
                           e-mail: massaric@lls.org
                                              www.lls.org

Tina Massari, Executive Director
Jeanne Caliguiri, Development Director

Rhode Island

2136 American Cancer Society: Rhode Island
931 Jefferson Boulevard   401-722-8480
Warwick, RI 02886   800-ACS-2345
                                          Fax: 401-421-0535
                                          TTY: 866-228-4327
                   e-mail: jim.beardsworth@cancer.org
                                           www.cancer.org
The American Cancer Society is the nationwide community-based
voluntary health organization dedicated to eliminating cancer as a
major health problem by preventing cancer, saving lives, and diminishing suffering from cancer, through research and education.
Jim Beardsworth, Media Relations Contact

2137 Leukemia and Lymphoma Society: Rhode Island Chapter
1210 Pontiac Avenue   401-943-8888
Cranston, RI 02920   Fax: 401-943-1377
                           e-mail: koconisb@lls.org
                                              www.lls.org

Bill Koconis, Executive Director
Gloria Hincapie, Patient Services Manager

South Carolina

2138 American Cancer Society: South Carolina
128 Stonemark Lane   803-750-1693
Columbia, SC 29210   800-ACS-2345
                                          Fax: 803-750-4000
                                          TTY: 866-228-4327
                          e-mail: mjwardle@cancer.org
                                           www.cancer.org
The American Cancer Society is the nationwide community-based
voluntary health organization dedicated to eliminating cancer as a
major health problem by preventing cancer, saving lives, and diminishing suffering from cancer, through research and education.
Mary Jane Wardle, Media Relations Contact

2139 Leukemia and Lymphoma Society: South Carolina Chapter
1247 Lake Murray Boulevard   803-749-4299
Irmo, SC 29063   Fax: 803-749-4088
                                              www.lls.org

2140 Leukemia and Lymphoma Society: South/West
107 Westpark Boulevard
Columbia, SC 29210

803-731-4060
Fax: 803-731-4066
e-mail: paul.jeter@lls.org
www.lls.org

Paul Jeter, Executive Director
Cassandra Wineglass, Patient Services Manager

South Dakota

2141 American Cancer Society: South Dakota
4904 S Technopolis Drive
Sioux Falls, SD 57106

605-361-8277
800-ACS-2345
Fax: 605-361-8537
TTY: 866-228-4327
e-mail: charlotte.hofer@cancer.org
www.cancer.org

The American Cancer Society is the nationwide community-based voluntary health organization dedicated to eliminating cancer as a major health problem by preventing cancer, saving lives, and diminishing suffering from cancer, through research and education.
Charlotte Ho, Media Relations Contact

Tennessee

2142 American Cancer Society: Tennessee
2000 Charlotte Avenue
Nashville, TN 37203

615-327-0991
800-ACS-2345
Fax: 615-341-7335
TTY: 866-228-4327
e-mail: brian.gillespie@cancer.org
www.cancer.org

The American Cancer Society is the nationwide community-based voluntary health organization dedicated to eliminating cancer as a major health problem by preventing cancer, saving lives, and diminishing suffering from cancer, through research and education.
Brian Gillespie, Media Relations Contact

2143 Leukemia & Lymphoma Society: Tennessee Chapter
404 BNA Drive
Nashville, TN 37217

615-331-2980
800-332-2980
Fax: 615-331-2941
e-mail: winslowm@tn.leukemia-lymphoma.org
www.leukemia-lymphoma.org

Founded in 1982 to better serve the needs of Tennesseans. Offers contribution funded community services, family support groups, free educational materials and financial assistance for those affected by leukemia, Hodgkin's disease, myeloma and lymphomas.
Colleen Grady, Executive Director
Mary Winslow, Patient Services Manager

Texas

2144 American Cancer Society: Texas
2433 Ridgepoint Drive
Austin, TX 78754

512-919-1800
800-ACS-2345
Fax: 512-919-1846
TTY: 866-228-4327
e-mail: justine.hall@cancer.org
www.cancer.org

The American Cancer Society is the nationwide community-based voluntary health organization dedicated to eliminating cancer as a major health problem by preventing cancer, saving lives, and diminishing suffering from cancer, through research and education.
Justin Hall, Media Relations Contact

2145 Leukemia and Lymphoma Society: North Texas Chapter
Leukemia Society of America
8111 LBJ Freeway
Dallas, TX 75251

972-239-0959
800-800-6702
Fax: 972-239-0892
e-mail: Tina.Garcia@lls.org
www.lls.org

Dedicated to finding cures for leukemia and related cancers and to improving the quality of life for patients and their families.
Tina Garcia, Executive Director
Sarah Bayley, Donor Development Director

2146 Leukemia and Lymphoma Society: South/West Texas Chapter
Leukemia Society of America

431 Isom Road
San Antonio, TX 78216-4170

210-377-1775
800-683-2458
Fax: 210-344-3717
www.lls.org

Dedicated to finding cures for leukemia and related cancers and to improving the quality of life for patients and their families.
Jon Walter, President/CEO
Jimmy Nangle, CFO

2147 Leukemia and Lymphoma Society: Texas Gulf Coast Chapter
Leukemia Society of America
5005 Mitchelldale
Houston, TX 77092

713-680-8088
Fax: 713-683-9504
e-mail: BillieSue.Parris@lls.org
www.lls.org

Dedicated to finding cures for leukemia and related cancers and to improving the quality of life for patients and their families.
Billie Sue Parris, Executive Director
Jane Thompson, Office Manager

Utah

2148 American Cancer Society: Utah
941 E 3300 S
Salt Lake City, UT 84106

801-483-1500
800-ACS-2345
Fax: 801-483-1558
TTY: 866-228-4327
e-mail: patricia.monsoor@cancer.org
www.cancer.org

The American Cancer Society is the nationwide community-based voluntary health organization dedicated to eliminating cancer as a major health problem by preventing cancer, saving lives, and diminishing suffering from cancer, through research and education.
Patricia Monsoor, Media Relations Contact

Vermont

2149 American Cancer Society: Vermont
121 Connor Way
Williston, VT 05495

802-872-6300
800-ACS-2345
Fax: 802-872-6399
TTY: 866-228-4327
e-mail: chris.falk@cancer.org
www.cancer.org

The American Cancer Society is the nationwide community-based voluntary health organization dedicated to eliminating cancer as a major health problem by preventing cancer, saving lives, and diminishing suffering from cancer, through research and education.
Chris Falk, Media Relations Contact

Virginia

2150 American Cancer Society: Virginia
4240 Park Place Court
Glen Allen, VA 23060

804-527-3700
800-ACS-2345
Fax: 804-527-3797
TTY: 866-228-4327
e-mail: domenick.casuccio@cancer.org
www.cancer.org

The American Cancer Society is the nationwide community-based voluntary health organization dedicated to eliminating cancer as a major health problem by preventing cancer, saving lives, and diminishing suffering from cancer, through research and education.
Domenick Casuccio, Media Relations Contact

2151 Arlin J Brown Information Center
PO Box 251
Fort Belvoir, VA 22060-0251

540-752-9511

An information clearinghouse on types of cancer health methods and nontoxic cancer therapies.

2152 Leukemia and Lymophoma Society: National Capital Area Chapter
Leukemia Society of America
5845 Richmond Highway
Alexandria, VA 22303

703-399-2900
Fax: 703-399-2901
e-mail: donna.mckelvey@lls.org
www.lls.org

Serves the greater Washington DC metropolitan area including Northern Virginia Prince George's and Montgomery counties.
Gabrielle Urquhart, Executive Director
Beth Gorman, Deputy Director

Washington

2153 American Cancer Society: Washington
728 134th Street SW 425-741-8949
Everett, WA 98204 Fax: 425-741-9638
e-mail: liz.lamb-ferro@cancer.org
www.cancer.org
The American Cancer Society is the nationwide community-based voluntary health organization dedicated to eliminating cancer as a major health problem by preventing cancer, saving lives, and diminishing suffering from cancer, through research and education.
Liz Lamb-Ferro, Media Relations Contact

2154 Washington Leukemia and Lymphoma Society: Alaska Chapter
Leukemia Society of America
530 Dexter Avenue N 206-628-0777
Seattle, WA 98109 888-345-4572
Fax: 206-292-9791
e-mail: wachapter@lls.org
www.leukemia-lymphoma.org
Dedicated to finding cures for leukemia and related cancers and to improving the quality of life for patients and their families.
Anne Gillingham, Executive Director
Kimberly Conn, Deputy Executive Director

West Virginia

2155 American Cancer Society: West Virginia
301 RHL Boulevard 304-746-9950
Charleston, WV 25309 800-ACS-2345
Fax: 304-746-9962
TTY: 866-228-4327
e-mail: amy.wentz@cancer.org
www.cancer.org
The American Cancer Society is the nationwide community-based voluntary health organization dedicated to eliminating cancer as a major health problem by preventing cancer, saving lives, and diminishing suffering from cancer, through research and education.
Amy Wentz Berner, Media Relations Contact

Wisconsin

2156 American Cancer Society: Wisconsin
N19 W24350 Riverwood Drive 262-523-5500
Waukesha, WI 53188 800-ACS-2345
Fax: 262-523-5533
TTY: 866-228-4327
e-mail: peter.balistrieri@cancer.org
www.acscan.org/action/wi
The American Cancer Society is the nationwide community-based voluntary health organization dedicated to eliminating cancer as a major health problem by preventing cancer, saving lives, and diminishing suffering from cancer, through research and education.
Peter Balistrieri, Media Relations Contact
Christopher Hansen, President, ACS CAN

2157 Leukemia and Lymphoma Society: Wisconsin Chapter
Leukemia Society of America
200 S Executive Drive 262-790-4701
Brookfield, WI 53005 800-261-7399
Fax: 262-790-4706
e-mail: bede.barthpotter@lls.org
www.lls.org
Founded in 1963 to serve Wisconsites touched by leukemia, lymphoma, Hodgkin's disease and myeloma.
Bede Barth Potter, Executive Director
Karen Ropel, Deputy Executive Director

Wyoming

2158 American Cancer Society: Wyoming
333 S Beech Street 307-577-4892
Casper, WY 82601 800-ACS-2345
Fax: 307-234-0926
TTY: 866-228-4327
e-mail: joel.quevillon@cancer.org
www.acscan.org
The American Cancer Society is the nationwide community-based voluntary health organization dedicated to eliminating cancer as a major health problem by preventing cancer, saving lives, and diminishing suffering from cancer, through research and education.
John R Seffrin, CEO,ACS
Christopher Hansen, President, ACS CAN

Foundations

2159 Chemotherapy Foundation
183 Madison Avenue 212-213-9292
New York, NY 10016 Fax: 212-133-31
www.chemotherapyfoundation.com
The Chemotherapy Foundation is dedicated to developing more effective methods of treatment for the control and cure of cancer. They provide educational materials and provide funds for innovative chemotherapy research, and sponsor professional and public educational symposia.
Shirley Cox, Executive Director
Franco Muggia, Chairman & Medical Director

2160 Dermatology Foundation
1560 Sherman Avenue 847-328-2256
Evanston, IL 60201-4808 Fax: 847-328-0509
e-mail: dfgen@dermatologyfoundation.org
www.dermfnd.org
The Foundation focuses on funding research that will advance patient care, and help develop and retain tomorrow's teachers and clinical leaders in the specialty.
Sandra Rahn Benz, Executive Director
James H Davis, Vice Chair

2161 National Children's Cancer Society
One South Memorial Drive 314-241-1600
Saint Louis, MO 63102 800-882-6227
Fax: 314-241-1996
e-mail: krudd@children-cancer.org
www.children-cancer.org
Our mission is to improve the quality of life for children with cancer and their families worldwide. We serve as a financial, emotional, educational, and medical resource for those in need, at every stage of their illness and recovery. The NCCS provides direct financial assistance to families for expenses not covered by insurance during their treatment; including transportation, lodging, gas money, medical assistance, health insurance premiums, and phone cards.
Mark Slocomb, Chairman
Mark Stolze, President/CEO

Libraries & Resource Centers

2162 Cancer Federation
PO Box 1298 951-849-4325
Banning, CA 92220 Fax: 951-849-0156
e-mail: info@cancerfed.org
www.cancerfed.com
The Federation is a not-for-profit organization that provides information, counseling, educational materials and meetings for the cancer patients, their families and friends. Also, they fund research and scholarships.
John Steinbacher, Executive Director

2163 Cancer Information Service
National Cancer Institute

6116 Executive Boulevard
Bethesda, MD 20892-8322

301-435-3848
800-422-6237
TTY: 800-332-8615
http://cis.nci.nih.gov/

Kramer Barnett, Director
Adamson Kristin, Administrative Resource Center

2164 **Patient Advocates for Advanced Cancer Treatments (PAACT)**
PO Box 141695
Grand Rapids, MI 49514-1695

616-453-1477
Fax: 616-453-1846
e-mail: paact@paactusa.org
www.paactusa.org

Provides support and advocacy for prostate cancer patients, their families, and the general public at risk. Information relative to the advancements in the detection, diagnosis, evaluation, and treatment of prostate cancer. Information, referrals, phone help, conferences, newsletter.
Richard H. Profit, President
Saleem Durvesh, Executive Marketing Director

Research Centers

2165 **Purdue Cancer Center Purdue University**
Purdue University
201 S University Street
W Lafayette, IN 47907-2064

765-494-9129
Fax: 765-494-9193
e-mail: cancerresearch@purdue.edu
www.cancer.purdue.edu

Provide a forum for 75 of Purdue's best and brightest scientists to collaborate across campus and nationwide to prevent cancer to ease its detection and to cure it.
Timothy Ratliff, Director
Andrea Gregory-Kreps, Operations Manager

Alabama

2166 **Birmingham VA Medical Center: Research and Development**
700 S 19th Street
Birmingham, AL 35233

205-933-8101
866-487-4243
Fax: 205-933-4484
www.birmingham.va.gov

An acute tertiary care facility with particularly strong programs in both medicine and surgery andserves as the primary referral center for the state. We provide health care services to eligible veterans in the VA Southeast Network .
Steven L Keller, Acting Chairman
Rica Lewis-Payton, Medical Center Director

2167 **Breast Cancer Resource Foundation of Alabama**
PO Box 531225
Birmingham, AL 35253

205-996-5463
Fax: 205-975-2432
e-mail: jgalbrea@uab.edu
www.bcrfa.org

Dedicated to finding a cure for breast cancer.
Dianne Mooney, President
Jennifer Galbreath, Program Director

2168 **University of Alabama At Birmingham Comprehensive Cancer Center**
UAB Comprehensive Cancer Center
1802 6th Avenue S
Birmingham, AL 35294-3300

205-934-5077
800-UAB-0933
e-mail: info@ccc.uab.edu
www3.ccc.uab.edu

The Center provides advanced cancer care research and education based on stringent peer-reviewed data.
Edward E Partridge, Director and Associate Director for Comm
Kirby I Bland, Deputy Director

Arizona

2169 **Southwest Association for Education in Biomedical Research**
PO Box 210101
Tucson, AZ 85721-0101

520-621-3931
Fax: 520-621-3355
e-mail: swaebr@ahsc.arizona.edu
www.swaebr.org

The mission of the Southwest Association for Education in Biomedical Research is to develop and implement a strong proactive campaign to educate school children as well as the general public in the vital role biomedical research plays in their everyday lives.
Charles Atkinson, President

2170 **University of Arizona Cancer Center**
1515 N Campbell Avenue
Tucson, AZ 85724-1454

520-626-5279
800-327-2873
www.azcc.arizona.edu

Comprehensive cancer center for diagnosis treatment and prevention.
David S Alberts, Director
Paola Villar Werstler, Director Of Development

California

2171 **Burnham Institute Cancer Center The Burnham Institute for Medical Resear**
The Burnham Institute for Medical Research
10901 N Torrey Pines Road
La Jolla, CA 92037

858-646-3100
Fax: 858-646-3199
e-mail: info@sanfordburnham.org
www.sanfordburnham.org

Known for world-class capabilities in stem cell research and drug discovery technologies. Dedicated to revealing the fundamental molecular causes of disease and devising the innovative therapies of tomorrow.
Kristiina Vuori, President & CEO
Gary Raisl, Executive VP,CFO,Treasurer

2172 **Cancer Prevention Institute of California**
2201 Walnut Avenue
Fremont, CA 94538-2334

510-608-5000
800-511-2300
Fax: 510-608-5095
www.cpic.org

The North California Cancer Center is dedicated to understanding the causes prevention and detection of cancer and to improving the quality of life for individuals living with cancer.
Reed Goertler, Chief Operations Officer
Sally Glaser PhD, CEO

2173 **City of Hope Comprehensive Cancer Research Center**
1500 E Duarte Road
Duarte, CA 91010

626-256-4673
800-256-4673
Fax: 626-930-5394
e-mail: tkronitis@coh.org
www.cityofhope.org

Excellence in biomedical research patient-centered medical care and community outreach.
Theodore G Krontiris MD, Director
Richard Jove, Deputy Director

2174 **Geraldine Brush Cancer Research Institute California Pacific Medical Center**
California Pacific Medical Center
2333 Clay Street #201
San Francisco, CA 94115

415-600-6000
e-mail: cpmcadmin@sutterhealth.org
www.cpmc.org

Martin Brotman, President
Robert Tomasello, Chairman

2175 **Ida and Joseph Friend Cancer Resource Center**
1600 Divisadero St.
San Francisco, CA 94143-981

415-885-3693
800-444-2559
Fax: 415-885-3701
e-mail: cancerresource@ucsfmedctr.org
www.cancer.ucsf.edu/crc/

The Cancer Resource Center supports wellness and the healing process by providing patients and their loved ones with information emotional support and community resources. The CRC maintains a multimedia library provides access to specialized health databases and offers research assistance. We host diverse support groups and classes and direct people to other community resources. All CRC programs are free.
Frank Mccorm PhD, Director

2176 **Jonsson Comprehensive Cancer Center University of California At Los Angeles**
University of California At Los Angeles

8-684 Factor Building
Los Angeles, CA 90095-1781
310-825-5268
888-662-8252
Fax: 310-206-5553
e-mail: jcccinfo@mednet.ucla.edu
www.cancer.ucla.edu

UCLA's Jonsson Comprehensive Cancer Center (JCCC) has established an international reputation for developing new cancer therapies providing the best in experimental treatments and expertly guiding and training the next generation of medical researchers.
Judith Gasson, Director
James Economou, Executive Director

2177 Pediatric Cancer Research Laboratory Children's Hospital of Orange County
Children's Hospital of Orange County
1201 W.LA Veta Ave
Orange, CA 92868-3874
714-997-3000
Fax: 714-532-8380
www.choc.org

CHOC is the first hospital devoted exclusively to caring for children in Orange County.
Dr Mitchell Cairo, Director

2178 Rebecca and John Moores UCSD Cancer Center
3855 Health Sciences Drive
La Jolla, CA 92093-0658
585-534-7600
Fax: 858-534-7628
e-mail: dedavis@ucsd.edu
www.cancer.ucsd.edu

One of the just 39 centers in the US to hold a National Cancer Institute designation as a Comprehensive Cancer Center. As such it ranks among the top centers in the nation conducting basic and clinical cancer research providing advanced patient care and serving the community through outreach and education programs.
John Alksne, Professor Surgery
Michael Andre, Adjunct Professor Radiology

2179 Salk Institute Cancer Center
Salk Institute for Biological Studies
PO Box 85800
San Diego, CA 92186-5800
858-453-4100
Fax: 858-453-8534
e-mail: communications@salk.edu
www.salk.edu

The Cancer Center was established in 1970. It is one of only eight basic research cancer centers in the country designated by the National Cancer Institute. The center includes 22 faculty members 150 postdoctoral researchers 45 graduate students and 80 research assistants. It comprises about half of the research at the Salk Institute.
Walter Eckhart, Professor and Laboratory Head
William R Brody, President

2180 Santa Barbara Breast Cancer Institute
5333 Hollister Avenue
Santa Barbara, CA 93111-2341
805-964-8883
Otto Sartorius, Director

2181 Stanford University: Beckman Center for Molecular and Genetic Medicine
School of Medicine, Department of Biochemistry
291 Campus Drive Rm LK3C02
Stanford, CA 94305-5101
650-723-3622
Fax: 650-724-9733
cmgm.stanford.edu

Dr Paul Berg, Emeritus Professor Biochemistry
Philip A Pizzo MD, Dean

2182 USC/Norris Comprehensive Cancer Center
1441 Eastlake Avenue
Los Angeles, CA 90033-1048
323-865-3000
uscnorriscancer.usc.edu

Major regional and national resource for cancer research treatment prevention and education.
Peter A Jones, Director
Nikias C.L Max, President

2183 University of California Berkeley Cancer Research Laboratory
449 Life Science Addition
Berkeley, CA 94720-2751
510-642-4711
Fax: 510-642-5741
e-mail: crl@berkeley.edu
www.crl.berkeley.edu/?q=crl

Basic research with a special emphasis on mammary cancer and tumor immunotherapy.
Astar Winoto, Director
Judith Yee, Manager

2184 University of California: Los Angeles Bone Marrow Transplantation Program
200 UCLA Medical Plaza
Los Angeles, CA 90024
310-206-6889
www.healthcare.ucla.edu/transplant

Treatment of leukemia and anemia.
David W Golde MD, Director
Gabriel Danovitch, M.D., Medical Director, Proffessor of Medicine

Colorado

2185 AMC Cancer Research Center
1600 Pierce Street
Denver, CO 80214
303-233-6501
800-321-1557
Fax: 303-239-3400
e-mail: contactus@amc.org
www.amc.org

Offers research activities publications meetings educational activities public services testing services community-based cancer control programs and knowledge of cancer mortality rates.
Alice Norton, Executive Director
Gail Eckhardt, Clinical Science

2186 Colorado Cancer Research Program
2253 S Oneida Street
Denver, CO 80224
303-777-2663
888-785-6789
Fax: 303-777-2642
e-mail: ccrp@co-cancerresearch.org
www.co-cancerresearch.org

A nonprofit community-based cancer program established to provide community hospitals and physicians access to a wide range of cancer research trials in order to provide their patients with greater options for the treatment control and prevention.
Jane Hajovsky, Executive Director
Eduardo Pajon, Principal Investigator

2187 University of Colorado Cancer Center
13001 E 17th Place
Aurora, CO 80045
303-724-3155
800-473-2288
Fax: 303-724-3162
e-mail: CancerCenter.Webmaster@uchsc.edu
www.uccc.info

UCCC consortium is the hub for cancer research in Colorado. With eight programs 17 shared core resources and nearly 400 members from three universities and six institutions UCCC is responsible for the majority of cancer research in the Rocky Mountain region.
Dan Theodorescu MD PhD, Director
Laurie Gasper MD, Associate Director for Clinical Research

Connecticut

2188 Yale University Comprehensive Cancer Center
333 Cedar Street
New Haven, CT 06520-8028
203-785-4095
866-925-3226
Fax: 203-785-4116
www.yalecancercenter.org

A National Cancer Institute designated comprehensive cancer center for over 30 years Yale Cancer Center is one of only 40 Centers in the nation and the only comprehensive center in Southern New England.
Thomas Lynch, Director
Kevin Vest, PT, MBA, FACHE, Deputy Director

District of Columbia

2189 Georgetown University: Vincent T Lombardi Cancer Research Center
3800 Reservoir Road NW
Washington, DC 20057
202-444-4000
www.lombardi.georgetown.edu

Established in 1970 the Lombardi Comprehensive Cancer Center is named for the legendary Green Bay Packers and Washington

Redskins coach Vince Lombardi who was treated for cancer at Georgetown University Hospital.
Louis M Weiner, Director
Peter G Shields, Deputy Director

2190 Howard University Cancer Center
2041 Georgia Avenue NW   202-806-7697
Washington, DC 20060-0001   Fax: 202-462-8928
                         e-mail: ladams-campbell@howard.edu
                                   www.cancer.howard.edu

Reduce the burden of cancer through research education and service with emphasis on the unique ethnic and cultural aspects of minority and underserved populations.
Lucile Adams-Campbel, Director
Wayne A I Frederick, Interim Director

2191 Melanoma Research Foundation
1411 K Street NW   202-347-9675
Washington, DC 20005   800-673-1290
                                     Fax: 202-347-9678
                              e-mail: info@melanoma.org
                                       www.melanoma.org

Founded in October 1996 by melanoma patients and their families to support research which will lead to cure for melanoma. Strictly a volunteer organization - not one person will receive compensation for his or her efforts.
Steve Silverstein, President & CEO
william G Reilly, President/Owner

2192 Rambaugh-Goodwin Institute for Cancer Research
1850 NW 69th Avenue   954-587-9020
Plantation, FL 33313   Fax: 954-587-6378
                                  e-mail: info@rgicr.org
                                          www.rgicr.org

RGI is committed to rapidly developing anti-cancer therapies in conjunction with industrial and academic partners using efficient models of cancer growth and metastasis with the aim of moving novel compounds to market in the shortest time possible.
Claire Thuning-Robin, Director

2193 UM/Sylvester Comprehensive Cancer Center
1475 NW 12th Avenue   305-243-1000
Miami, FL 33136   800-545-2292
                                        www.sylvester.org

UMHC offers an outpatient clinic a 40-bed inpatient unit a comprehensive treatment unit the Mohs surgery center/dermatology clinic the Rosenfield GI Center a cardiology lab and clinic a radiology/imaging suite an interventional radiology clinic the Spine Institute clinics on-site laboratory and pharmacy the Courtelis Center for Psychosocial Oncology the Jill Selevan Chapel a cafeteria as well as administrative offices.
Joan Scheiner, Chair
Jayne S. Malfitano, Vice Chair

2194 Emory University: Georgia Center for Cancer Statistics
Rollins School of Public Health
201 Dowman Drive   404-727-6123
Atlanta, GA 30322   Fax: 404-727-7261
                              e-mail: gccs@sph.emory.edu
                                    www.sph.emory.edu/gccs

Serves as a cancer registry for five counties of metropolitan Atlanta and ten rural counties of central Georgia.
James W Wagner, President

2195 Emory University: Winship Cancer Institute
1365-C Clifton Road NE   404-778-1900
Atlanta, GA 30322   888-946-7447
                               www.winshipcancer.emory.edu

A clinical cancer center coordinating basic and clinical cancer research.
Walter Currans, Executive Director
Fadlo Khuri MD, Deputy Directory for Basic Research

2196 Pacific Health Research Institute
3375 Koapaka Street   808-524-4411
Honolulu, HI 96819   Fax: 808-524-5559
                                    e-mail: info@phrei.org
                                        www.phrihawaii.org

Located in Honolulu Hawaii Pacific Health Research Institute (PHRI) is the largest independent biomedical research institute in the state. Since its founding on 1960 as an independent not for profit 501(c)(3) research institute PHRI today has become a leader in biomedical research in the Pacific. Indeed its researchers are performing complex investigations aimed at conquering some of the most debilitating and lethal diseases that afflict humankind.
Vicki L Shambaugh, MA, MPH, Director
Helen Petrovitch, Executive Director

2197 University of Hawaii: Cancer Research Center
1236 Lauhala Street   808-586-2985
Honolulu, HI 96813   Fax: 808-586-2982
                               e-mail: cvogel@crch.hawaii.edu
                                            www.crch.org

The mission of the Cancer Research Center of Hawaii is to reduce the burden of cancer through research education and service with an emphasis on the unique ethnic culture and environmental characteristics of Hawaii and the Pacific.
Carl-Wilhelm Vogel, Professor (Researcher)
Michele Carbone, Interim Cancer Center Director

2198 Cancer and Leukemia Group B
230 W Monroe   773-702-9171
Chicago, IL 60606   Fax: 312-345-0117
                              e-mail: marciak@uchicago.edu
                                           www.calgb.org

Integral unit of the Institute specializing in leukemia research and prevention.
Marcia Kelly, Administrative Coordinator
Michael Kelly, Director Protocol Operations

2199 Kellogg Cancer Care Center Evanston Hospital
Evanston Hospital
2650 Ridge Avenue   847-570-2000
Evanston, IL 60201   888-364-6400
                                             www.enh.org

Integral unit of the Evanston Hospital this center researches treatment and diagnosis of cancer including phase 1 and phase 2 studies.
Mark R Neaman, President, CEO
Jeffery H Hillebrand, COO

2200 Leukemia Research Foundation
3520 Lake Avenue   847-424-0600
Wilmette, IL 60091-1064   888-558-5385
                                     Fax: 847-424-0606
                                 e-mail: info@lrfmail.org
                                www.leukemia-research.org

To conquer leukemia lymphoma and myelodysplastic syndromes by funding research into their causes and cures and to enrich the quality of life of those touched by these diseases.
Kevin Radelet, Executive Director
Cindy Kane, Senior Director of Development

2201 Oncology Hematology Associates of Central Illinois
8940 N Wood Sage Road   309-243-3000
Peoria, IL 61615-7828   866-662-6564
                                  www.illinoiscancercare.com

Research into cancer treatments.
Robert Cooper, Director
Paul A S Fishkin, Hematology Internal Medicine Medical O

2202 Robert H Lurie Comprehensive Cancer Center of Northwestern University
Galter Pavilion 675 N Street Clair   312-695-0990
Chicago, IL 60611   866-587-4322
                                     Fax: 312-695-1352
                           e-mail: cancer@northwestern.edu
                                  www.lurie.northwestern.edu

Lurie Cancer Center is a founding member of the National Comprehensive Cancer Network an exclusive alliance of 21 of the nation's leading cancer centers.
Steven T Rosen, Director
Leonidas Platanias, Deputy Director

2203 University of Chicago Cancer Research Center
5841 S Maryland Avenue   773-702-6180
Chicago, IL 60637   877-824-0600
                        e-mail: cancerresources@uccrc.org
                                www.cancer.uchicago.edu
The University of Chicago Cancer Research Center (UCCRC) employs a wealth of intellectual technological and financial resources to pursue a comprehensive collaborative research program involving more than 200 renowned scientists and clinicians.
Mary Ellen Connellan, Executive Director
Justin Ullman, President

2204 University of Chicago: Clinical Nutrition Research Unit
5841 S Maryland Avenue   773-702-6180
Chicago, IL 60637-1463   877-824-0600
                        e-mail: feedback@bsd.uchicago.edu
                                    www.uchicago.edu
Provide superior healthcare in a compassionate manner ever mindful of each patient's dignity and individuality.
Michael M Le Beau PhD, Director
James L Madara, CEO

Indiana

2205 Mary Margaret Walther Program Walther Cancer Institute
Walther Cancer Institute
9292 N Meridian Street   317-708-6101
Indianapolis, IN 46260   Fax: 317-708-6102
                                  e-mail: info@walther.org
                                        www.walther.org
Focuses research on all types of cancer studies.
Leonard J Betley, Chairman
James E Ruckle, President/CEO

Iowa

2206 Iowa Oncology Research Association
300 E Locust   515-244-7586
Des Moines, IA 50309   888-244-6061
                                     Fax: 515-244-3037
                                  e-mail: sherrijr@iora.org
                                           www.iora.org
Clinical cancer studies and research.
Sherri Rickabaugh, Administrator
Becky Berrett, Research Assistants

2207 University of Iowa: Holden Comprehensive Cancer Center
UI Hospitals and Clinics
University of Iowa   319-353-8620
Iowa City, IA 52242-1002   800-777-8442
                                     Fax: 319-353-8988
                        e-mail: cancer-center@uiowa.edu
                    www.uihealthcare.com/depts/cancercenter
The Holden Cancer Center promotes interactive high-quality cancer research high-quality health care related to the prevention detection and treatment of cancer and educates cancer professionals and the citizens of Iowa about cancer.
Jean E Robillard, Vice President for Medical Affairs
Kenneth P Kates, CEO

Kansas

2208 Kansas State University: Terry C Johnson Center for Basic Cancer Research
Center for Basic Cancer Research
1 Chalmers Hall   785-532-6705
Manhattan, KS 66506   Fax: 785-532-6707
                                e-mail: marcia@k-state.edu
                                www.k-state.edu/cancer.center
The mission of the Terry C. Johnson Center for Basic Cancer Research is to further the understanding of cancers by funding basic

cancer research and supporting higher education training and public outreach.
Rob Denell, Director
S Keith Chapes, Associate Director

Kentucky

2209 Henry Vogt Cancer Research Institute James Graham Brown Cancer Center
James Graham Brown Cancer Center
2301 S 3rd Street   502-852-5555
Louisville, KY 40208   800-334-8635
                                    e-mail: info@ulh.org
                            www.louisville.edu/hsc/centers
The overall goal of the scientists in the Henry Vogt Cancer Research Institute is to study mechanisms relevant to tumor cell biology at the basic and translational level in order to provide insights that will contribute to the ultimate prevention and cure of malignant diseases.
Donald M Miller, Director
John W Eaton, Deputy Director

2210 Kentucky Cancer Program
2365 Harrodsburg Road   859-219-0772
Lexington, KY 40504-3381   Fax: 859-219-0548
                                e-mail: dka@kcp.uky.edu
                                        www.kcp.uky.edu
The KCP provides a variety of cancer programs and services to health professionals the public patients and survivors.
Debra Armstong, Director
Diane Frasure, Administrative Associate

2211 University of Kentucky: Children Cancer Study Group
Markey Cancer Center
800 Rose Street   859-257-4500
Lexington, KY 40536-93   800-333-8874
                                     Fax: 859-323-2074
                            www.ukhealthcare.uky.edu/markey/
Kentucky Children's Hospital is the only children's hospital in the region. Patients range in age from infants through adolescents and have a variety of illness and injuries.
Michael Karpf, Executive Vice President for Health Affa
Frank Butler, VP for Medical Center Operations

2212 University of Kentucky: Lucille Parker Markey Cancer Center
800 Rose Street   859-247-4500
Lexington, KY 40536   800-333-8874
                                     Fax: 859-323-2074
                            www.ukhealthcare.uky.edu/markey/
The Markey Cancer Center mission is to eliminate the morbidity and mortality of cancer through a comprehensive program of research education clinical care and community outreach.
Alfred M Cohen MD FACS, Director
Michael Karpf, Executive Vice President for Health Affa

Louisiana

2213 Baton Rouge Regional Tumor Registry Mary Bird Perkins Cancer Center
Mary Bird Perkins Cancer Center
4950 Essen Lane   225-767-0847
Baton Rouge, LA 70809   Fax: 225-215-1215
                                      www.marybird.org
The Louisiana Tumor Registry is composed of a central office and regional registries that collect and process cancer incidence data from the state's eight established geographic regions. These eight geographic areas are based on Louisiana's historic health districts.
Todd D Stevens, President, CEO
J Gerald Jolly, Chairman

2214 Tulane University Pulmonary Diseases Critical Care and Enviromental Medicine
School of Medicine
1430 Tulane Avenue   504-988-5187
New Orleans, LA 70112   800-588-5300
                                e-mail: medsch@tulane.edu
                        www.som.tulane.edu/pulmdis/facilities
Provides state-of-the-art care to patients and teaching to trainees through several areas of academic excellence that include: Interstitial Lung Diseases; Asthma; Cystic Fibrosis; Sleep Disorders;

Interventional Pulmonology; Lung Cancer; Smoking Cessation; Critical Care; and Environmental Medicine.
Lee Hamm, MD, Senior Vice President and Dean
Roy Weiner, Associate Dean for Clinical Research

Maryland

2215 Frederick Cancer Research Center
PO Box B
Frederick, MD 21702-1201
301-846-1000
Fax: 301-846-1108
web.ncifcrf.gov
Direct research into the causes treatment and prevention of cancer AIDS and related diseases.
Craig W Reynolds, Associate Director
Jo Anne Barb, Secretary

2216 Johns Hopkins University: Sydney Kimmel Comprehensive Cancer Center
The Harry and Jeanette Weinberg Buidling
401 N Broadway
Baltimore, MD 21231-0005
410-955-5222
www.hopkinskimmelcancercenter.org
Johns Hopkins Kimmel Cancer Center has active programs in clinical research laboratory research education community outreach and prevention and control.
Ronald J Danielles, President
Edward Miller MD, Dean of Medical Faculty, CEO

2217 National Foundation for Cancer Research National Foundation for Cancer Research
National Foundation for Cancer Research
4600 E W Highway
Bethesda, MD 20814-3206
301-654-1250
800-321-2873
Fax: 301-654-5824
e-mail: info@nfcr.org
www.nfcr.org
NFCR promotes and facilitates collaboration among scientists to accelerate the pace of discovery from bench to bedside. NFCR is committed to Research for a Cure - cures for all types of cancers.
Franklin C Salisbury Jr, President
Sujuan BA, Phd., COO

2218 Warren Grant Magnuson Clinical Center
National Institute of Health
9000 Rockville Pike
Bethesda, MD 20892
301-496-4000
800-411-1222
Fax: 301-480-9793
TTY: 866-411-1010
e-mail: prpl@mail.cc.nih.gov
www.clinicalcenter.nih.gov/index.html
Established in 1953 as the research hospital of the National Institutes of Health. Designed so that patient care facilities are close to research laboratories so new findings of basic and clinical scientists can be quickly applied to the treatment of patients. Upon referral by physicians, patients are admitted to NIH clinical studies.
John Gallin, Clinical Center Director
David Henderson, Deputy Director for Clinical Care

Massachusetts

2219 Boston University Cancer Research Center
820 Harrison Avenue
Boston, MA 02118
617-638-8265
Fax: 617-638-6518
e-mail: sfenness@bu.edu
www.bumc.bu.edu/clinicaltrials
The Office of Clinical Research (OCR) was established on July 1 1998 to serve as the central focus for clinical research support conduct and training at Boston University Medical Center.
Douglas V Faller, Director
Salli Fennessey, Manager

2220 Dana-Farber Institute: Department of Biostatistics and Computational Biology
450 Brookline Avenue
Boston, MA 02115-5450
617-632-3000
Fax: 617-632-2444
e-mail: biostatistics@jimmy.harvard.edu
www.dana-farber.org

Integral unit of the Institute organized into laboratories of biostatistics computing and epidemiology.
Marvin Zelen, Researcher
Edward J Benz, President, CEO

2221 David H. Koch Institute for Integrative Ca ncer Research
MIT Center for Cancer
Koch Institute at MIT 76-158
Cambridge, MA 02142
617-253-6403
Fax: 617-324-2238
e-mail: cancer@mit.edu
www.ki.mit.edu
The mission of MIT Cancer Center is to apply tools of basic science and technology to determine how cancer is caused progresses and responds to treatment. Through this effort they have developed an increasingly complete understanding of the nature of cancer cells which has led directly to improved treatments for the disease.
Dr Tyler Jacks, Director
Dr Jaqueline Lees, Associate Director

Michigan

2222 Gershenson Radiation Oncology Center Barbara Ann Karmanos Cancer Institute
Barbara Ann Karmanos Cancer Institute
4100 John Road
Detroit, MI 48201
313-745-9191
800-527-6266
Fax: 313-745-2314
e-mail: info@karmanos.org
www.karmanos.org
Radiation therapy and cancer treatment and research.
Gerold Bepler, President

2223 Meyer L Prentis Comprehensive Cancer Center of Metropolitan Detroit
Barbara Ann Karmanos Cancer Institute
4100 John Road
Detroit, MI 48201
313-745-9191
800-527-6266
Fax: 313-745-2314
e-mail: info@karmanos.org
www.karmanos.org
Gerald Bepler, President

2224 Meyer L Prentis Comprehensive Cancer Cente Barbara Ann Karmanos Cancer Institute
4100 John Road
Detroit, MI 48201
313-745-9191
800-527-6266
Fax: 313-745-2314
e-mail: info@karmanos.org
www.karmanos.org
Gerald Bepler, President

2225 University of Michigan: Cancer Center Cancer Research Committee
Cancer Research Committee
1500 E Medical Center Drive
Ann Arbor, MI 48109-094
734-764-0039
800-865-1125
Fax: 734-936-9582
www.cancer.med.umich.edu
The U-M Comprehensive Cancer Center provides its patients diagnostic treatment and support services in a collaborative environment focused on excellence in patient care.
Eric R Fearon, Associate Director for Science
Max S Wicha, Director

2226 Wayne State University Center for Molecular Medicine and Genetics
Wayne State University School of Medicine
3127 Scott Hall
Detroit, MI 48201
313-577-5323
Fax: 313-577-5218
e-mail: sshaw@wayne.edu
www.genetics.wayne.edu
Research focusing on human conditions such as cancer and neuromuscular disorders.
Lawrence I Grossman, Professor/Director
Jeffrey A Loeb, Associate Director

Minnesota

2227 Mayo Comprehensive Cancer Center
200 First Street SW
Rochester, MN 55905-0001
507-284-2511
Fax: 507-284-0161
TTY: 507-284-9786
www.mayo.edu
Scientists and physician investigators conduct wide-ranging research to improve patient care while training the next generation of medical scholars.
Denis Cortese, President/Chief Executive Officer
Robert A Rizza, Director

2228 University of Minnesota Masonic Cancer Center
Division of Oncology
420 Delaware Street SE
Minneapolis, MN 55455
612-624-8484
800-226-2376
Fax: 612-626-3069
e-mail: ccinfo@umn.edu
www.cancer.umn.edu
The Masonic Cancer Center fosters this mission by creating a collaborative research environment focused on the causes prevention detection and treatment of cancer; applying that knowledge to improve quality of life for patients and survivors; and sharing its discoveries with other scientists students professionals and the community.
Brian Steeves, Deputy Director
Ann D Cieslak, Executive Director

Missouri

2229 Cancer Research Center
3501 Berrywood Drive
Columbia, MO 65201
573-875-2255
Fax: 873-443-1202
www.cancerresearchcenter.org
Not only does the Cancer Research Center offer research they also offer community outreach programs to educate church groups civic clubs and other organizations about their research and cancer prevention.
Dr. Abe Eisenstark, Research Director
Jack Bozarth, Director

Nebraska

2230 Lincoln Cancer Center
4600 Valley Road
Lincoln, NE 68510-4844
402-483-2827
Fax: 402-483-4184
Barb Morton, Director

2231 University of Nebraska at Omaha Eppley Institute for Research in Cancer
University of Nebraska
985950 Nebraska Medical Center
Omaha, NE 68198-5950
402-559-4090
e-mail: hmmaurer@unmc.edu
www.unmc.edu/eppley
To improve the health of Nebraska through premier educational programs innovative research the highest quality patient care and outreach to underserved populations.
Harold M Maurer, Chancellor
Thomas H Rosenquist, Vice Chancellor

New Hampshire

2232 Norris Cotton Cancer Center Dartmouth-Hitchcock Medical Center
Dartmouth-Hitchcock Medical Center
One Medical Center Drive
Lebanon, NH 03756
603-653-9000
800-639-6918
Fax: 603-653-9003
e-mail: cancercenter@dartmouth.edu
www.cancer.dartmouth.edu
The Cancer Center provides a positive environment for treatment cure and recovery for patients with all forms of cancer.
Mark Israel MD, Director
Burton L Eisenberg, Deputy Director

New Mexico

2233 University of New Mexico: Cancer Research and Treatment Center
1201 Camino de Salud NE
Albuquerque, NM 87131-5001
505-272-4946
800-432-6806
Fax: 505-925-0100
www.cancer.unm.edu
One of the nation's 60 premier National Cancer Institute (NCI)-Designated Cancer Centers and we have been named one of America's Best Cancer Hospitals by U.S. News & World Report. UNM Cancer Center provides cancer diagnosis and treatment to over 40% of the adults and virtually all of the children diagnosed with cancer each year in New Mexico.
Cheryl Willman, Director/CEO
John A Trotter, Deputy EVP for Health Sciences

2234 University of New Mexico: Center for Non-Invasive Diagnosis
Mind Imaging Center/University of New Mexico
1101 Yale Boulevard NE
Albuquerque, NM 87131-0001
505-277-0111
Fax: 505-272-4056
www.hsc.unm.edu
Cardiology and cancer research.
David Lepre, Executive Director

New York

2235 Ackerman Institute for the Family
149 E 78th Street
New York, NY 10075
212-879-4900
Fax: 212-744-0206
e-mail: ackerman@ackerman.org
www.ackerman.org
Independent nonprofit research organization specializing in family therapy teaching and clinical services.
Lois Braverman, President/CEO
Evan Imber-B PhD, Director

2236 Albany Medical College Joint Center for Cancer and Blood Disorders
43 New Scotland Avenue
Albany, NY 12208
518-262-3125
877-AMC-8008
Fax: 518-262-3165
TTY: 518-262-1180
www.amc.edu
Offers research in the fields of cancer and blood disorders focusing on radiotherapy pathology and surgery.
Herbert Abbott, General Pediatric
Kevin Costello, Internal Medicine

2237 Albert Einstein Cancer Center Albert Einstein College of Medicine
Albert Einstein College of Medicine
1300 Morris Park Avenue
Bronx, NY 10461
718-430-2302
Fax: 718-430-2000
e-mail: aecc@aecom.yu.edu
www.einstein.yu.edu/centers/cancer/
The goal of AECC is to foster basic clinical population-based and translational research that addresses all aspects of the cancer problem.
Allen M Spiegel MD, Dean
David Goldman, Director

2238 Association for Research of Childhood Cancer
PO Box 251
Buffalo, NY 14225-0251
716-681-4433
e-mail: president@arocc.org
www.arocc.org
The Association was chartered by New York State in that year as a not-for-profit corporation whose primary purpose was to fund the major pediatric research centers in Western New York.
Larry Lorenz, Vice President
Anne O'Donnel, President

2239 Bassett Research Institute
One Atwell Road
Cooperstown, NY 13326
607-547-3456
800-227-7388
e-mail: research.institute@bassett.org
www.bassett.org
Research institute committed to seeking new information and new strategies for preventing detecting and treating disease.
Wiliiam F Streck MD, President/CEO

2240 Cancer Institute of Brooklyn
927 49th Street
Brooklyn, NY 11219-2923
718-972-5816
Fax: 718-972-8693
Jo-Ann Hertz, Executive Director

2241 Cancer Research Institute: New York
One Exchange Plaza 55 Broadway
New York, NY 10006
212-688-7515
800-992-2623
Fax: 212-832-9376
e-mail: info@cancerresearch.org
www.cancerresearch.org
The Cancer Research Institute is the world's only non-profit organization dedicated exclusively to the support and coordination of laboratory and clinical efforts that will lead to the immunological treatment control and prevention of cancer.
Jill O'Donnel-Tormey, Executive Director
Leslie Anson, Assistant to the Executive Director

2242 Columbia University Comprehensive Cancer Center
630 W 168th Street
New York, NY 10032
212-305-4186
Fax: 212-305-6889
/www.cumc.columbia.edu/
Lee Goldman, President
Anne L Taylor, Vice Dean

2243 Medical Foundation of Buffalo Hauptman-Woodward Medical Research Insti
Hauptman-Woodward Medical Research Institute
700 Ellicott Street
Buffalo, NY 14203-1102
716-898-8600
Fax: 716-898-8660
www.hwi.buffalo.edu
Nonprofit organization devoted to cancer research.
Herbert A Hauptman PhD, President/Nobel Laureate
Eaton E Lattman, Executive Director & CEO

2244 Memorial Sloan-Kettering Cancer Center
1275 York Avenue
New York, NY 10065
212-639-2000
888-675-7722
e-mail: publicaffairs@mskcc.org
www.mskcc.org
Sloan-Kettering Institute has endeavored to lead the way in basic science research oftentimes translating those advances into clinical treatments.
Harold Varmus, President, CEO
Paul A Marks, President Emeritus

2245 New York University Cancer Institute New York University Medical Center
New York University Medical Center
530 First Avenue
New York, NY 10016
212-263-7300
888-769-8633
Fax: 212-263-0715
www.nyucancerinstitute.org
The mission of the NYU Cancer Institute is to decrease and eliminate cancer as a significant health problem throughout New York the national and the world by developing and maintaining excellent programs in patient care research education and prevention.
William Carroll, Director
Lauren E Hackett, Executive Director of Administration

2246 Roswell Park Cancer Institute National Cancer Institute
Elm & Carlton Streets
Buffalo, NY 14263
716-845-2300
877-275-7724
e-mail: askrpci@roswellpark.org
www.roswellpark.org
Roswell Park Cancer Institute has made fundamental contributions to reducing the cancer burden and has successfully maintained an exemplary leadership role in setting the national standards for cancer care research and education.
Donald L Trump MD, Director
Ann Gioia, Director

2247 State University of New York Health Science Center At Brooklyn
450 Clarkson Avenue
Brooklyn, NY 11203
718-270-1000
www.downstate.edu
Downstate includes Colleges of Medicine Nursing and Health Related Professions and a School of Graduate Studies as well as its own teaching hospital an M.P.H. Program and extensive research facilities.
John C LaRosa, President
John B Clark, Interim Chancellor

2248 University of Rochester: James P Wilmot Cancer Center
601 Elmwood Avenue
Rochester, NY 14642
585-275-5823
866-494-5668
Fax: 585-276-0158
www.urmc.rochester.edu
To use education science and technology to improve health transforming the patient experience with fresh ideas and approaches steeped in disciplined science and delivered by health care professionals who innovate take intelligent risks and care about the lives they touch.
Jonathan W. Friedberg M.D., Director
Gregory Connolly, M.D., Hematology Oncology

North Carolina

2249 Cancer Center of Wake Forest University at Bowman Gray School of Medicine
Wake Forest University School Of Medicine
Medical Center Boulevard
Winston-Salem, NC 27157
336-716-2011
800-446-2255
Fax: 336-716-9593
e-mail: medadmit@wfubmc.edu
www1.wfubmc.edu/cancer
Provide a superb education as well as personal support. Beyond the academic experiences offered at our medical school we encourage the development of our students as caring physicians dedicated to providing the very best care professionally and personally to all patients.
William B Applegate M D M P, Dean
John D McConnell, CEO

2250 Duke Comprehensive Cancer Center
2424 Erwin Road
Durham, NC 27705
919-684-3377
888-ASK-DUKE
Fax: 919-684-5653
www.cancer.duke.edu
One of only 39 centers in the country designated by the National Cancer Institute (NCI) as a 'comprehensive cancer center ' Duke combines cutting-edge research with compassionate care. Our team of nationally recognized physicians and staff treat nearly 6 000 new patients per year giving them the extensive experience that yields better results. In fact U.S. News & World Report rates Duke #7 in the nation for cancer care and best in the Southeast.
H Kim Lyerly, Director
Anthony Means, Deputy Director

2251 University of North Carolina UNC Lineberger Comprehensive Cancer Center
School of Medicine
450 est Dr
Chapel Hill, NC 27514
919-966-3036
866-869-1856
Fax: 919-966-3015
e-mail: lccc@med.unc.edu
www.unclineberger.org
The Center provides multidisciplinary programs for most cancers giving patients the benefit of many medical specialists in one place often in one visit.
H Shelton Earp, Director
Michael O'Malley, Associate Director

Ohio

2252 Case Western Reserve University: Ireland Cancer Center
University Hospitals of Cleveland
11100 Euclid Avenue
Cleveland, OH 44106
216-844-1529
888-844-8447
www.uhhospitals.org/irelandcancer
Thomas F Senty, CEO

2253 Children's Hospital Research Foundation
700 Childrens Drive
Columbus, OH 43205-2696
614-722-2000
800-792-8401
Fax: 61 -35 -079
e-mail: CommunityLink@NationwideChildrens.org
www.nationwidechildrens.org

Offers research activities into Reye's Syndrome genetics and children's cancer chemotherapy.
Richard McClead, Medical Director
Richard J Brilli, Chief Medical Officer

2254 Medical College of Toledo: Cancer Research Division
Department of Pathology
3000 Arlington Avenue 419-383-4000
Toledo, OH 43614-2595 800-321-8383
Fax: 419-383-6130
e-mail: utmc.webmaster@utoledo.edu
www.utmc.utoledo.edu

Researches into all aspects of cancer.
Jill Zyrek-Betts, Assistant Professor

2255 Ohio State University Comprehensive Cancer Center
Arthur G James Cancer Hospital
300 W 10th Avenue 614-293-7521
Columbus, OH 43210-1240 e-mail: michael.caligiuri@osumc.edu
www.osucc.osu.edu
A national and international leader in research, which translates to high-quality patient care and educational programs for residents of Ohio and beyond.
Michael A Caligiuri M D, Director
John C Byrd, Associate Director

2256 Ohio State University General Clinical Research Center
The Ohio State University 614-293-8750
Columbus, OH 43210 Fax: 614-293-3796
e-mail: william.malarkey@osumc.edu
www.crc.osu.edu
Provides facilities and financial support for inpatient and outpatient cancer research.
William Malaykey, Program Director
David Phillips, Administrative Director

2257 The Cancer Prevention Institute
23 Jasper St 937-227-9400
Dayton, OH 45409 877-274-4543
Fax: 937-297-6970
e-mail: info@pch-dayton.org
www.premiercommunityhealth.org
Nonprofit organization focusing research activities primarily on cancer prevention anti-cancer drugs early diagnosis of cancer and bone marrow toxicity. previously known as the Hipple Cancer Research Center.
Stephen McHugh, Treasurer
Diane Ewing, Chair

Oklahoma

2258 Natalie Warren Bryant Cancer Center St. Francis Hospital
St. Francis Hospital
6600 S Yale Avenue 918-488-6688
Tulsa, OK 74136 e-mail: webadministrator@saintfrancis.com
www.saintfrancis.com/locations/nwbcc
Jake Henry Jr, President/Chief Executive Officer
Barry Steichen, Executive Vice President/Chief Administr

2259 Oklahoma Medical Research Foundation Immunobiolgy & Cancer Research
Oklahoma Medical Research Foundation
825 North East 13th Street 405-271-6673
Oklahoma City, OK 73104-5005 800-522-0211
Fax: 405-271-7016
e-mail: OMRF-President@omrf.org
www.omrf.org
Dr. Stephen Prescott, President

2260 Samuel Roberts Noble Foundation Biomedical Division
Samuel Roberts Noble Foundation
2510 Sam Noble Parkway 580-223-5810
Ardmore, OK 73401 Fax: 580-224-6217
www.noble.org
One of the largest international offshore drilling contractors in the world.
Michael A Cawley, CEO/President
Bill Goddard, Trustee

Pennsylvania

2261 Abramson Cancer Center of the University of Pennsylvania
3535 Market Street
Philadelphia, PA 19104-3309 800-789-PENN
Fax: 215-349-5445
e-mail: craig@mail.med.upenn.edu
www.penncancer.com
National leader in cancer research patient care and education.
Douglas L Fraker MD, Deputy Director
Caryn Lerman, Interim Director

2262 Allegheny Singer Research Institute West Penn Allegheny Health System
West Penn Allegheny Health System
4800 Friendship Avenue 412-362-8677
Pittsburgh, PA 15224 877-284-2000
Fax: 412-359-8610
e-mail: tchakurd@wpahs.org
www.wpahs.org

Christopher Olivia MD, President, CEO

2263 Eastern Cooperative Oncology Group
1818 Market Street 215-789-3645
Philadelphia, PA 19103 800-4CA-NCER
Fax: 267-256-5291
www.ecog.dfci.harvard.edu
Studies into cancer including biological response modifiers and cancer studies.

2264 Fox Chase Cancer Center
333 Cottman Avenue 215-728-6900
Philadelphia, PA 19111-2497 888-369-2427
www.fccc.edu
Linda Fliescher MPH PhD, Assistant Vice President for Communicati
Theresa Berger MBE, Project Manager

2265 Temple University FELS Institute for Cancer Research
School of Medicine
3500 N Broad Street 215-707-7000
Philadelphia, PA 19140 Fax: 215-707-7000
www.temple.edu/medicine
Policies and programs are oriented toward research and training in cancer-related basic biological and biochemical sciences with progressive extension into the areas of molecular developmental and chemical biology to advance knowledge of the etiology and pathogenesis of cancer. A major goal of the Institute is to utilize the advances made in basic science programs to develop novel targeted therapies for the treatment of cancer.
John M Daly MD, Dean
Diane Omdal, Director, Research Administration

2266 University of Pittsburgh Cancer Institute
5150 Centre Avenue 412-647-2811
Pittsburgh, PA 15232 e-mail: PCI-INFO@upmc.edu
www.upci.upmc.edu
Since 1985 the UPCI has been committed to improving the understanding of how cancer develops; to characterizing new lifesaving approaches for cancer prevention detection diagnosis and treatment; and to educating future generations of scientists and clinicians.
Nancy E Davidson MD, Committee Chair
Adam Brufsky MD PhD, Associate Director

Rhode Island

2267 Brown University Division of Biology and Medicine
BioMed Research Admin, Brown Medical School
The Warren Alpert Medical School of 401-863-3330
Providence, RI 02912-0001 Fax: 401-863-2660
www.biomed.brown.edu
Interdisciplinary studies in biological and medical sciences including studies in health care problems and fields of research such as cancer and diabetes.
John Perry, Senior Associate Dean
Edward J Wing, Medicine / Biological Sciences

2268 Roger Williams Clinical Cancer Research Center
Roger Williams General Hospital

825 Chalkstone Avenue
Providence, RI 02908 401-456-2000
www.rwmc.com

Kenneth Belcher, President
Sheri L. Smith, Ph.D., Chair

South Carolina

2269 Children's Center for Cancer and Blood Disorders
University of South Carolina School of Medicine
7 Richland Medical Park
Columbia, SC 29203 803-434-7000
www.palmettohealth.org
Joint clinical and basic research of juvenile cancer and blood disorders.
Charles D Beaman Jr, CEO

Tennessee

2270 St. Jude Children's Research Hospital
262 Danny Thomas Place 901-495-3300
Memphis, TN 38105 Fax: 901-495-4011
e-mail: donors@stjude.com
www.stjude.org
One of the world's premier pediatric cancer research centers.
Harvey J Cohen, Chair
William Evan PharmD, Director/CEO

2271 University of Tennessee Memphis: Cancer Center
66 N. Pauline St 901-448-5150
Memphis, TN 38163-0001 Fax: 901-528-5033
Alvin M Mauer MD, Director

Texas

2272 Baylor University Bone Marrow Transplantation Research Center
Baylor Research Institute
3500 Gaston Avenue 214-820-2687
Dallas, TX 75246 800-422-9567
www.baylorhealth.com
Offers bone marrow transplantation research in leukemia studies.
John B McWhorter, President
Irving D Prengler, VP Medical Staff Affairs

2273 Cancer Therapy and Research Center
7979 Wurzbach Road 210-450-1000
San Antonio, TX 78229 800-340-2872
www.ctrc.net
The mission of the Cancer Therapy & Research Center is to conquer cancer through research prevention and treatment.
Ian M Thompson MD, Director

2274 San Antonio Cancer Institute
7703 Floyd Curl Drive 210-567-7000
San Antonio, TX 78229-3900 Fax: 210-567-2709
www.uthscsa.edu/
Dr Tyler J Curiel, Director
William L Henrich MD MACP, President

2275 Southwest Foundation for Biomedical Research
PO Box 760549
San Antonio, TX 78245-0549 210-258-9400
www.sfbr.org
Advancing the health of our global community through innovative biomedical research.
John R Hurd, Chairman
Lewis J Moorman III, Vice-Chairman

2276 University of Texas: MD Anderson Cancer Center
1515 Holcombe Boulevard 713-792-2121
Houston, TX 77030-4009 800-392-1611
www.mdanderson.org
To eliminate cancer in Texas the nation and the world through outstanding programs that integrate patient care research and prevention and through education for undergraduate and graduate students trainees professionals employees and the public.
John Mendelsohn, President -Executive Committee
Raymond DuBois, Executive Vice President

2277 University of Texas: Medical Branch at Galveston Cancer Center
301 University Boulevard 409-772-1011
Galveston, TX 77555 Fax: 409-747-1938
TTY: 409-772-4200
e-mail: public.affairs@utmb.edu
www.utmb.edu
The mission of The University of Texas Medical Branch at Galveston is to provide scholarly teaching innovative scientific investigation and state-of-the-art patient care in a learning environment to better the health of society.
B Mark Evers, Director
David L Calender, President

Utah

2278 Brigham Young University Cancer Research Center
181 Benson Science Building 801-422-3913
Provo, UT 84602 e-mail: cancer_research@byu.edu
www.cancerresearch.byu.edu
Provide a rigorous research training program for students.
Daniel L Simmons, Director
Cecil O. Samuelson, President

2279 Huntsman Cancer Institute University of Utah School of Medicine
University of Utah School of Medicine
2000 Circle of Hope 801-585-0303
Salt Lake City, UT 84112 877-585-0303
Fax: 801-585-5886
e-mail: public.affairs@hci.utah.edu
www.huntsmancancer.org
Understand cancer from its beginnings to use that knowledge in the creation and improvement of cancer treatments to relieve the suffering of cancer patients and to provide education about cancer risk prevention and care.
Mary C Beckerle, Executive Director
Wallace Akerley, Senior Director of Clinical Research

Vermont

2280 University of Vermont Cancer Center University of Vermont
University of Vermont
E-213 Given Buildinge 802-656-4414
Burlington, VT 05405 877-540-4673
Fax: 802-656-8788
e-mail: info@vermontcancer.org
www.vermontcancer.org

Richard Branda, Interim Director
Marianne Baggs, Assistant to the Director

Virginia

2281 Cancer Research Foundation of America
1600 Duke Street 703-836-4412
Alexandria, VA 22314-3421 800-227-2732
Fax: 703-836-4413
e-mail: mmcleod@crfa.org
www.preventcancer.org
Prevention and early detection of cancer through research education and community outreach to all populations including children and the underserved.
Carolyn R Aldige, President and Founder
Marcia Myers Carlucci, Chairman

2282 Virginia Commonwealth University: Massey Cancer Center
401 College Street 804-828-0450
Richmond, VA 23298-5017 877-4MA-SSEY
Fax: 804-828-8453
e-mail: massey@vcu.edu
www.massey.vcu.edu
The mission of the University of Central Arkansas is to maintain the highest academic quality and to ensure that its programs remain current and responsive to the diverse needs of those it serves.
Gordon D Ginder MD, Director
Steven Grant MD, Associate Director

Washington

2283 Fred Hutchinson Cancer Research Center
1100 Fairview Avenue N   206-288-7222
Seattle, WA 98109-1024   800-804-8824
                                     Fax: 206-288-1025
                          e-mail: hutchdoc@fhcrc.org
                                          www.fhcrc.org
At Fred Hutchinson Cancer Research Center our interdisciplinary teams of world-renowned scientists and humanitarians work together to prevent diagnose and treat cancer HIV/AIDS and other diseases.
Lee Hartwell, Director/President
Mark Groudine, Executive Vice President and Deputy Dire

West Virginia

2284 West Virginia University: Mary Babb Randolph Cancer Center
Mary Babb Randolph Cancer Center Clinic
One Medical Center Drive   304-293-4500
Morgantown, WV 26506   877-427-2894
                                     Fax: 304-598-4553
                          www.wvucancer.org/pages/
Premier cancer facility with a national reputation of excellence in cancer treatment prevention and research.
Augusto Ochoa, Director
Lori K Acciavatti, Professional Technologists

Wisconsin

2285 University of Wisconsin Paul P Carbone Comprehensive Cancer Center
600 Highland Avenue   608-263-6400
Madison, WI 53792-6164   800-622-8942
                                     Fax: 608-263-8613
                          e-mail: gxw@medicine.wisc.edu
                                     www.cancer.wisc.edu
The University of Wisconsin Paul P. Carbone Comprehensive Cancer Center is the only comprehensive cancer center in Wisconsin as designated by the National Cancer Institute. An integral part of the UW School of Medicine and public Health this cancer center unites more than 250 physicians and scientists who work together in translating discoveries from research laboratories into new treatments that benefit cancer patients.
George Wildi MD, Director
Kelly Sitkin, Development Director

Support Groups & Hotlines

2286 American Cancer Society: San Jose Prostate Cancer Support Group
3369 Union Avenue
San Jose, CA 95124-2033   408-559-8553
                                          www.cancer.org

2287 American Foundation for Urologic Disease: Us Too Line
1128 N Charles Street   301-727-2908
Baltimore, MD 21201-5506   800-828-7866
                          e-mail: admin@afud.org
                                          www.afud.org
Provides information and referrals for family members, victims and other individuals concerned with prostate cancer.

2288 American Institute for Cancer Research
1759 R Street NW   202-328-7744
Washington, DC 20009   800-843-8114
                                     Fax: 202-328-7226
                          e-mail: aicrweb@aicr.org
                                          www.aicr.org

Melvin Huston, Chairman
Lawrence Pratt, Vice-Chairman

2289 Cancer Information Service
National Cancer Institute
1100 Fairview Avenue North   206-667-4675
Seattle, WA 98109-1024   800-422-6237
                                     Fax: 206-667-7792
                                     TTY: 800-332-8615
                                          www.cancer.gov

Provides the latest and most accurate cancer information to patients, their families, the public, and health professionals. Also provides personalized responses to specific questions about cancer and assistance to smokers who want to quit.
Nancy Zbaren, Program Director

2290 Cancer Support Community
3276 Mc Nutt Avenue   925-933-0107
San Francisco, CA 94597-1909   Fax: 925-933-0249
                          www.cancersupportcommunity.net
Offers understanding, support and guidance to people with cancer and those who care about them.
James Bouquin, President & Executive Director
Margaret Stauffer, Vice President & Program Director

2291 Cancervive
11636 Chayote Street   310-203-9232
Los Angeles, CA 90049   800-486-2873
                                     Fax: 310-471-4618
                          e-mail: cancervivr@aol.com
                                          www.cancervive.org
Dedicated to providing support, public education and advocacy to those who have experienced this disease. The mission of Cancervive is to assist survivors to reclaim their lives after cancer.
Susan Nessim Keeney, Founder/President

2292 Center for Cancer Survival
104 W Anapamu Street   805-962-6221
Santa Barbara, CA 93101-3126
Nonprofit, nonmedical outreach education program teaching specific emotional, mental and spiritual skills for survival on their journey of recovery from cancer.
Richard Sheldon, Founder

2293 Collaborative Medicine Center
10 Willow Street   415-383-3197
Mill Valley, CA 94941-2895
Not specifically a cancer treatment center but works with cancer patients by using a variety of supportive modalities. The emphasis at the center is on helping people learn to support and activate their own healing processes.
Martin L Rossman MD

2294 Commonwealth Cancer Help Program
451 Mesa Road   415-868-0970
Bolinas, CA 94924   Fax: 415-868-2230
                          e-mail: commonweal@commonweal.org
                          www.commonweal.org/programs/cancer-help/
An educational program designed to help participants reduce the stress of cancer, explore health habits, be with others experiencing the same difficulties and consider information on established and complementary therapeutic options.
Michael Lerner, President
Susan Braun, Executive Director

2295 Corporate Angel Network
Westchester County Airport
One Loop Road   914-328-1313
White Plains, NY 10604-1215   866-328-1313
                                     Fax: 914-328-3938
                          e-mail: info@corpangelnetwork.org
                                     www.corpangelnetwork.org
To ease the emotional stress, physical discomfort and financial burden of travel for cancer patients by arranging free flights to treatment cetners, using the empty seats on corporate aircraft flying on routine business.
Peter H. Fleiss, Executive Director
Randall Greene, President & CEO

2296 Exceptional Cancer Patients/ECaP
532 Jackson Park Drive   814-337-8192
Meadville, CT 16335   Fax: 814-337-0699
            e-mail: info@ecap-online.org, info@mind-body.org
                                     www.ecap-online.org/home.htm
The mission of EcaP/Exceptional Cancer Patients is to provide exceptional resources, comprehensive professional training programs and extraordinary interdisciplinary retreats that help people

facing the challenges of cancer and other chronic illnesses discover their inner healing resources.
Bernie Siegal MD, Founder
Barry Bittman MD, Chief Executive Officer

2297   Gilda's Club: Grand Rapids
1806 Bridge Street NW   616-453-8300
Grand Rapids, MI 49504   Fax: 616-453-8355
                                              e-mail: info@gildasclubgr.org
                                                    www.gildasclubgr.org
A free cancer support community of children, adults, families and friends.
Leann Arkema, President/CEO
Davis Sesbastian, Chair

2298   Gilda's Club: New York City
502 Eigth Avenue   718-788-1600
Brooklyn, NY 11215   Fax: 718-788-0322
                                              e-mail: info@gildasclubnyc.org
                                                    www.gildasclubnyc.org
Creates welcoming communities of free support for everyone living with cancer - men, women, teens and children - along with their families and friends. The innovative program is an essential complement to medical care, providing networking and support groups, workshops, lectures and social activities, all free of charge.
Robert Easton, Chairman of the Board
Lily Safani, CEO

2299   Gilda's Club: Quad Cities
1234 E River Drive   319-326-7504
Davenport, IA 52803   877-926-7504
                                              Fax: 563-323-1658
                                              e-mail: qc@gildasclubqc.org
                                                    www.gildasclubqc.org
A cancer support community providing people living with cancer, and all who touch their lives, access to other people going through the same experience.
Claudia Robinson, CEO
Melissa Wright, Program Director

2300   Gilda's Club: South Florida
119 Rose Drive   954-763-6776
Fort Lauderdale, FL 33316   Fax: 954-763-6761
                                              e-mail: info@gildasclubsouthflorida.org
                                                    www.gildasclubsouthflorida.org
A free cancer support community for women, men, children, and teens with all types of cancer and their families and friends. Offer networking groups, lectures, workshops, specialized children's and teen programs, and social events in a nonresidential, non-medical, home-like setting.
Shelley Goren, CEO
Sara Howley Callari, Chair

2301   I Can Cope
American Cancer Society
1599 Clifton Road NE   404-320-3333
Atlanta, GA 30329-4250   800-227-2345
                                                    www.cancer.org
An educational program for people facing cancer, either personally, or as a friend or family caregiver. Helps dispel cancer myths by presenting straightforward facts and answers to your cancer-related questions

2302   International Association of Cancer Victors and Friends
7740 W Manchester Avenue   310-822-5032
Playa del Rey, CA 90293-8449   Fax: 310-822-4193
                                              e-mail: IACUF@Inetworld.net
Offers reports and information on alternative therapies and recent cancer studies.
Ann Cinquina

2303   JamesCare For Life Support Groups & Services
James Cancer Hospital & Solove Research Institute
300 W 10th Avenue   614-293-5066
Columbus, OH 43210   800-293-5066
                                              Fax: 614-293-2565
                                              e-mail: jamesline@osumc.edu
                                                    www.cancer.osu.edu

JamesCare for Life Cancer Support Groups and Services provides a wide range of resources and services to assist patients and families on their journey. This group offers support for patients and families to share experiences, express concerns, and learn more about the impact of cancer and available treatments.
Michael A Caligiuri, CEO
Jeff Walker, Senior Executive Director

2304   Look Good... Feel Better
American Cancer Society
1599 Clifton Road NE   404-320-3333
Atlanta, GA 30329-4250   800-227-2345
                                                    www.lookgoodfeelbetter.org
A community-based, free, national service. Teaches female cancer patients beauty tips to look better and feel good about how they look during chemotherapy and radiation treatments

2305   Lung Cancer Alliance Support Group
888 16th Street NW   202-463-2080
Washington, DC 20006   800-298-2436
                                              e-mail: kay@lungcanceralliance.org
                                                    www.lungcanceralliance.org
Dedicated solely to support and advocacy for all those living with or at risk for lung cancer.
T.Joseph Lopez, Chairman
Cheryl Healton, President & CEO

2306   National Foundation for Cancer Research Hotline
4600 E W Highway   301-654-1250
Bethesda, MD 20814   800-321-2873
                                              Fax: 301-654-5824
                                              e-mail: info@nfcr.org
                                                    www.nfcr.org
To support cancer research and public education relating to prevention, earlier diagnosis, better treatments and ultimately, a cure for cancer. Promotes and facilitates collaboration among scientists to accelerate the pace of discovery from bench to bedside.
Silas Deane, VP Marketing/Communications

2307   National Health Information Center
PO Box 1133   310-565-4167
Washington, DC 20013-1133   800-336-4797
                                              Fax: 301-984-4256
                                              e-mail: info@nhic.org
                                                    www.health.gov/nhic
A health information referral service sponsored by the Office of Disease Prevention and Health Promotion. Puts health professionals and consumers who have health questions in touch with those organizations that are best able to provide answers.
Ellen Langhans, Chairwoman
Linda Harris, Lead, Health Communication and e-health

2308   National Hospice Helpline
1731 King Street   703-837-1500
Alexandria, VA 22314   800- 64- 646
                                              Fax: 703-837-1233
                                              e-mail: nhcpo_info@nhpco.org
                                                    www.nhpco.org
Offers more information on hospice in general and offers referrals to a hospice program in your area.
Ronald Fried, Chair
Linda Rock, Vice Chair

2309   PDQ
National Cancer Institute
6116 Executive Boulevard   301-402-5874
Bethesda, MD 20892-8322   800-422-6237
                                                    www.cancer.gov
An NCI database that contains the latest information about cancer treatment, screening, prevention, genetics, supportive care, and complementary and alternative medicine, plus clinical trials.
Mark Greene MD, Editor-in-Chief

2310   Reach to Recovery
American Cancer Society
1599 Clifton Road NE   404-320-3333
Atlanta, GA 30329-4250   800-227-2345
                                                    www.cancer.org
Provides support for people recentlry diagnosed with breast cancer; people facing a possible diagnosis of breast cancer; those in-

terested in or who have undergone a lumpectomy or mastectomy; those considering breast reconstruction; those who have lymphedema; those who are undergoing or who have completed treatment such as chemotherapy and radiation therapy; people facing breast cancer recurrence or metastasis

2311 United Ostomy Associations of America Advocacy Hotline
PO Box 512
Northfield, MN 55057-0512   800-826-0826
                                   e-mail: info@uoaa.org
                                       www.ostomy.org
A national network for bowel and urinary diversion support groups in the United States. The goal is to provide a nonprofit association that will serve to unify and strengthen its member support groups, which are organized for the benefit of people who have, or will have intestinal or urinary diversions and their caregivers.
Dave Rudzin, President

2312 Wainwright House Cancer Support Programs
260 Stuyvesant Avenue   914-967-6080
Rye, NY 10580-3115
Weeklong residential retreats offered four times a year to cancer patients. Retreats are devoted to cancer patient education, health promotion and stress management.
Richard Grossman, Program Director

2313 Women's Suffrage for Prostate Cancer Awareness
743 Caribou Court
Sunnyvale, CA 94087-4229   800-776-2262
                                   e-mail: info@pcawomen.org
                                       www.pcawomen.org
Women have banded together here to help people cope with the effects of prostate cancer on their lives and educate others about it. Members understand problems of patients and families and are here to support and educate.
Judith P. Barnhard, CPA, Chairman
May Barnhard, PC, Chairman

Books

2314 3rd Opinion: International Directory to Complementary Therapy Centers
Avery Publishing Group
120 Old Broadway   516-741-2155
New Hyde Park, NY 11040-5000
Discusses over 300 alternative treatment cancer centers, educational centers, support groups and other research services.

2315 A Breast Cancer Journey: Your Personal Guidebook
American Cancer Society
1599 Clifton Road NE   404-320-3333
Atlanta, GA 30329-4250   800-227-2345
Helps women steer through the maze of information, empowering them to take control of their disease, treatment choices, health care team and life. Guidebook format encourages the reader to organize her information in a logical, easily accessible manner, record personal feelings and concerns and understand the details of practical matters such as paperwork and insurance, legal and sexual issues, side effects of treatment, and helping the entire family with support.
440 pages paperback
ISBN: 0-944235-20-4

2316 American Cancer Society Cancer Book
Doubleday & Company
666 5th Avenue
New York, NY 10103-0001   212-765-6500
                                       www.randomhouse.com
Publishes 135 cancer organizations, centers, support services and various programs.

2317 American Cancer Society's Guide to Complementary/Alternative Cancer Methods
American Cancer Society
1599 Clifton Road NE   404-320-3333
Atlanta, GA 30329-4250   800-227-2345
Helps the public, the consumer and patients and their families understand what works, what's dangerous, and how best to evaluate the hundreds of claims that can be found on the internet and in the

popular press. Each entry is researched and based on scientific evidence. Possible problems or complications are identified and clearly highlighted for easy reference. Covers a broad range, including herbs, vitamins, minerals, diet, manual healing and biological methods. Clear, understandable language.
464 pages hardcover
ISBN: 0-944235-20-4

2318 American Cancer Society's Guide to Pain Control
American Cancer Society
1599 Clifton Road NE   404-320-3333
Atlanta, GA 30329-4250   800-227-2345
Provides a wealth of information, including talking to your health care team about pain, understanding what pain is and where it comes from, current drug and non-drug treatments and dealing with the financial burden of pain treatment. Includes information on how to record, chart and rate pain, guidelines for pain management, a comprehensive list of medications and other methods of pain relief and an informative resource guide.
400 pages paperback
ISBN: 0-944235-20-4

2319 American Cancer Society's Healthy Eating Cookbook: A Celebration of Food...
American Cancer Society
1599 Clifton Road NE   404-320-3333
Atlanta, GA 30329-4250   800-227-2345
More than 200 pages of irresistable recipes that turn healthy eating into a celebration of good food. Features photos and recipes from a host of the American Cancer Society's celebrity friends and fans. Includes hundreds of recipes, celebrity photos and essays, a handy Smart Substitution reference section and numerous tips for healthy cooking, including smart shopping, using leftovers and eating out.
216 pages hardcover
ISBN: 0-944235-20-4

2320 Bowel Cancer
Oxford University Press
2001 Evans Road   212-726-6000
Cary, NC 27513-2010   800-451-7556
                                       Fax: 919-677-1303
                                       www.oup-usa.org
Offers information and public awareness on the disease of bowel cancer.
152 pages

2321 Breast Cancer
Branden Publishing Company
17 Station Street   617-734-2045
Brookline Village, MA 02147   Fax: 617-734-2046
                                       www.branden.com
Paperback
ISBN: 0-828319-49-9

2322 Cancer Dictionary
Facts on File
11 Penn Plaza   212-967-8800
New York, NY 10001   800-322-8755
                                       Fax: 800-678-3633
352 pages Paperback

2323 Cancer Facts and Figures
American Cancer Society
1599 Clifton Road NE   404-320-3333
Atlanta, GA 30329-4250   800-227-2345
Publishes over 57 treatment centers.

2324 Cancer Rates and Risks
National Cancer Institute
Building 31
Bethesda, MD 20892-0001   800-422-6237
This book is a compact guide to statistics, risk factors, and risks for major cancer sites.
136 pages

2325 Cancer Sourcebook
Karen Bellenir, author
Omnigraphics

Penobscot Building
Detroit, MI 48226-4105
313-961-1340
800-234-1340
Fax: 800-875-1340
www.omnigraphics.com/

Offers basic information on cancer types, symptoms, diagnostic methods, and treatments. Includes statistics on cancer occurrences worldwide and the risks associated with known carcinogens and activities.

2003 1119 pages
ISBN: 0-780806-33-6

2326 Cancer Therapy: Ind. Consumer's Guide to Non-Toxic Treatment & Prevention

Ralph W. Moss, author

Equinox Press
Cancer Decisions
Lemont, PA 16851
814-238-3367
800-980-1234
Fax: 814-238-5865
www.cancerdecisions.com

A must for cancer patients and their families who want: Practical information on the most promising non-toxic treatments; Scientific evidence in readable language; Well-documented resource lists and medical references.

523 pages
ISBN: 1-881025-06-3

2327 Cancer in the Family: Helping Children Cope with a Parent's Illness

American Cancer Society
1599 Clifton Road NE
Atlanta, GA 30329-4250
404-320-3333
800-227-2345

A diagnosis of cancer changes a family forever. Ordinary responsibilities become more demanding, and parents sometimes need assistance in balancing all of their children's needs. This book outlines steps to take to help children understand what happens when a parent has been diagnosed with cancer. Offers suggestions for talking to children, helping them cope, answering difficult questions, managing role changes and disruptions in routines, recognizing signs that your child needs help.

272 pages paperback
ISBN: 0-944235-20-4

2328 Caregiving: A Step-By-Step Resource for Caring for the Person w/Cancer at Home

American Cancer Society
1599 Clifton Road NE
Atlanta, GA 30329-4250
404-320-3333
800-227-2345

This practical guide offers manageable solutions to the myriad conditions and situations the caregiver may face, from physical to emotional conditions and dealing with health care providers and insurance carriers, to taking care of his or her own needs as well as those of the patient. East to use, this handy reference offers thorough, concise check-lists, questions to ask, signs and symptoms to note, and where to turn for more help.

336 pages paperback
ISBN: 0-944235-20-4

2329 Celebrate! Healthy Entertaining for Any Occasion

American Cancer Society
1599 Clifton Road NE
Atlanta, GA 30329-4250
404-320-3333
800-227-2345

You can celebrate in style without taking a break from healthy eating or delicious food. This book combines 20 festive, fun theme menus with easy recipes that don't sacrifice taste. Each menu offers a combination of approximately 8 manageable recipes, including appetizers, main dishes, side dishes, desserts and even beverages. Activities and decorating ideas in each section help make entertaining a breeze.

272 pages paperback
ISBN: 0-944235-20-4

2330 Choices: Realistic Alternatives in Cancer Treatment

Harper Collins
Avenue of the Americas
New York, NY 10019
800-331-3761
Fax: 800-822-4090

Covers a wide gamut of information that includes treatment centers, associations, research groups, and other facilities that are equipped to assist cancer patients and their families.

2331 Colorectal Cancer: A Compassionate Resource for Patients and Their Families

American Cancer Society
1599 Clifton Road NE
Atlanta, GA 30329-4250
404-320-3333
800-227-2345

Addresses the full range of issues that colorectal cancer patients and their families may face- from what to do when confronted with a diagnosis to the latest medical data, treatment and procedures. Describes the process of the digestive system and the organs involved when the body is affected by colorectal cancer. Dietary factors for preventing colorectal cancer are explained and information about surgery, chemotherapy and radiation treatment follows. Includes easy recipes and a diet plan.

290 pages paperback
ISBN: 0-944235-20-4

2332 Consumer's Guide to Cancer Drugs

American Cancer Society
1599 Clifton Road NE
Atlanta, GA 30329-4250
404-320-3333
800-227-2345

Created for patients, cancer survivors and caregivers. Provides detailed information for the more than 200 medicines used to treat cancer or the symptoms of cancer. Drugs are listed alphabetically by generic name and described in depth. Detailed descriptions include common side effects, precautions and other important facts. All generic and trade names are listed in the index for easy cross-reference. Easy-to-understand language.

448 pages paperback
ISBN: 0-944235-20-4

2333 Coping: A Young Woman's Guide to Breast Cancer Prevention

Rosen Publishing Group
29 E 21st Street
New York, NY 10010
212-777-3017
800-237-9932
Fax: 888-436-4643
e-mail: customerservice@rosenpub.com
www.rosenpublishing.com

Breast cancer research has revealed the genetic predisposition of some cancers. This guide explains the nature of cancer, the risk of cancer and the ways to reduce that risk, especially for young women with a family history of breast cancer.

ISBN: 0-825929-67-1

2334 Everyone's Guide to Cancer Therapy

Andrews McMeel Publishing, LLC
c/o Simon & Schuster, Inc.
Riverside, NJ 08075
800-943-9839
Fax: 800-943-9831
e-mail: MPrzybylski@amuniversal.com
www.andrewsmcmeel.com

How cancer is diagnosed, treated, and managed day to day.

2002 960 pages Paperback
ISBN: 0-740718-56-8

2335 Health Consequences of Smoking: Cancer & Chronic Lung Disease in the Workplace

DIANE Publishing Company
330 Pusey Avenue, Unit #3 Rear
Darby, PA 19023
610-461-6200
800-782-3833
Fax: 610-461-6130
e-mail: dianepublishing@gmail.com
www.dianepublishing.net

Examines the relationship between cigarette smoking and occupational exposures. Establishes that in order to protect the workers fully, forces of labor, management, insurers and government must become as engaged in attempts to reduce the prevalence of cigarette smoking as they are in occupational exposure. Tables and figure. Extensive bibliography, index.

542 pages Paperback
ISBN: 0-788123-11-4
Herman Baron, Publisher

2336 Healthy and Hearty Diabetic Cooking

Diabetes Self-Management Books
PO Box 11477
Des Moines, IA 50381-0001
800-664-9269
James Hazlett, Editor
Melissa Glim, Associate Editor

178

2337 Home Care Guide for Cancer
John's Hopkins University Press
2715 N Charles Street 410-516-6900
Baltimore, MD 21218-4319 800-537-5487
Fax: 410-516-6998
www.press.jhu.edu
This easy to use workbook was designed for home caregivers, patients, support groups and education programs; it features easy to read type and index for quick reference and advice on twenty common cancer caregiving problems.
1996 260 pages Paperback
ISBN: 0-943126-30-4

2338 I Choose to Fight: Tom Harper's Courageous Victory Over Cancer
Prentice Hall
15 Columbus Circle
New York, NY 10023-7707 212-373-8000
www.prenhall.com
A semi, auto-biographical account of Tom Harper's ordeal with testicular cancer, an afflication in young men.

2339 Informed Decisions: The Complete Book of Cancer Diagnosis, Treatment and Recovery
American Cancer Society
1599 Clifton Road NE 404-320-3333
Atlanta, GA 30329-4250 800-227-2345
Offers the latest information on every aspect of cancer, from detection to recovery. Covers everything from cancer causes and risk, screening and diagnostic tests, and treatment strategies to coping tips and questions to ask your doctor. Includes tips on how to effectively deal with the system and get the most advanced care in the country. Helps cancer patients and families make the right kinds of decisions- decisions that suit your particular needs and desires, and help you feel in control.
690 pages hardcover
ISBN: 0-944235-20-4

2340 Love Knot
Jones & Bartlett Publishers
40 Tall Pine Drive
Sudbury, MA 01776 978-443-5000
800-832-0034
Fax: 978-443-8000
e-mail: aberry@jbpub.com
www.jbpub.com
232 pages Paperback
ISBN: 0-763714-12-7
Joy Stark, Associate Marketing Manager

2341 My Prostate and Me: Dealing with Prostate Cancer
Addison Books
2719 Houston Avenue
Houston, TX 77009-7607 800-829-9653

2342 National Cancer Institute Fact Book
National Cancer Institute
Building 31
Bethesda, MD 20892-0001 800-422-6237
This book presents general information about the National Cancer Institute including budget data, grants and contracts and historical information.

2343 No Less a Woman
Firestone Touchstone Paperbacks/Simon & Schuster
200 Old Tappan Road
Old Tappan, NJ 07675-7005 800-999-5479
Offers intimate interviews that explore the major issues of coping and surviving breast cancer, from diagnosis and treatment to physical and psychological recovery. In their own words, ten women describe how they successfully adjusted to the changes in their bodies and their feelings about themselves.
288 pages
ISBN: 0-671868-99-3

2344 Organizing and Maintaining Support Groups for Parents
Candlelighters' Childhood Cancer Foundation
7910 Woodmont Avenue 301-657-8401
Bethesda, MD 20814-3015 800-366-2223
Benefits of self-help support groups, activities, referral systems and parent/professional relations.

2345 Prostate Cancer: A Survivor's Guide
Don Kaltenbach and Tim Richards, author
Dattoli Cancer Foundation
2803 Fruitville Road 941-365-5599
Sarasota, FL 24237 800-915-1001
Fax: 941-366-3786
e-mail: info@dattolifoundation.org
www.dattolifoundation.org
Written with the aid of leading prostate cancer specialists, this book clearly explains tests, the latest statistics and how to interpret them.
updated 2003 256 pages
ISBN: 0-964008-89-0

2346 Prostate Cancer: What Every Man and His Family Needs to Know
American Cancer Society
1599 Clifton Road NE 404-320-3333
Atlanta, GA 30329-4250 800-227-2345
Written by a team of internationally known and respected medical experts, this newly revised edition explains everything a man needs to know about prostate cancer, the most common form of cancer (excluding skin cancer) among American men.
322 pages paperback
ISBN: 0-944235-20-4

2347 Prostate Health Workbook
Newton Malerman, author
Hunter House Publishing
PO Box 2194 510-865-5282
Alameda, CA 94501 800-266-5592
Fax: 510-865-4295
e-mail: ordering@hunterhouse.com
www.hunterhouse.com
A practical guide for the prostate cancer patients.
2002 160 pages Paperback
Cristina Sverdrup, Customer Service Manager

2348 Singing from the Soul
Bone Marrow Foundation
981 1st Avenue 212-838-3029
New York, NY 10022-5102 800-365-1336
e-mail: thebmf@aol.com
www.bonemarrow.org
Jose Carreras' autobiography describes in eloquent detail his bone marrow transplant experience.

2349 Teratologies: A Cultural Study of Cancer
Routledge
270 Madison Avenue 212-216-7800
New York, NY 10016 Fax: 212-563-2269
www.routledge.com
A distinctively feminist look at how cancer is perceived, experienced and theorized in contemporary society. Beginning with powerful personal accounts of her own illness, as well as self-help manuals and patients' personal stories, Jackie Stacey explores changing beliefs about the causes and treatments of cancer in both biomedecine and its increasingly popular alternative counterparts.
304 pages

2350 The Mountain You've Climbed: A Parent's Guide to Childhood Cancer Survivorship
1015 Locust Street 314-241-1600
Saint Louis, MO 63101 Fax: 314-241-1996
e-mail: krudd@children-cancer.org
www.nationalchildrenscancersociety.org
This guide is designed to answer parent's questions regarding childhood cancer, address issues related to diagnosis and offer suggestions on how to integrate the cancer experience into all areas of the family's life. It addresses issues beginning from the time of diagnosis through the completion of treatment and beyond.
Mark Slocomb, Chairman
Mark Stolze, President/CEO

2351 Understanding Breast Cancer Genetics
Barbara T Zimmerman, PhD, author
University Press of Mississippi

3825 Ridgewood Road
Jackson, MS 39211-6492

601-432-6205
Fax: 601-432-6217
e-mail: kburgess@ihl.state.ms.us
www.upress.state.ms.us

Clinical explanations for the genetic causes of the disease women most greatly fear.
2004 128 pages Paperback
ISBN: 1-578065-79-8
Kathy Burgess, Advertising/Marketing Services Manager

2352 Understanding Cancer Therapies
Helen S L Chan, MD, author
University Press of Mississippi
3825 Ridgewood Road
Jackson, MS 39211-6492

601-432-6205
Fax: 601-432-6217
e-mail: kburgess@ihl.state.ms.us
www.upress.state.ms.us

A practical and hopeful guide to the many treatments available.
2006 144 pages Paperback
ISBN: 1-578066-89-1
Kathy Burgess, Advertising/Marketing Services Manager

2353 Understanding Colon Cancer
A Richard Adrouny, MD; FACP, author
University Press of Mississippi
3825 Ridgewood Road
Jackson, MS 39211-6492

601-432-6205
Fax: 601-432-6217
e-mail: kburgess@ihl.state.ms.us
www.upress.state.ms.us

For the general reader a concise manual of facts, warnings, prevention, treatments, and forecasts.
2002 168 pages Paperback
ISBN: 1-578062-03-9
Kathy Burgess, Advertising/Marketing Services Manager

2354 When a Parent Has Cancer: A Guide to Caring for Your Children
Harper Collins
10 E 53rd Street
New York, NY 10022

212-207-7000
www.harpercollins.com

ISBN: 0-060187-09-3

2355 Women and Cancer: A Compassionate Reource for Patients and Their Families
American Cancer Society
1599 Clifton Road NE
Atlanta, GA 30329-4250

404-320-3333
800-227-2345

Concise, thorough and up-to-date, this book provides women who have been diagnosed with cancer information about the four most common cancers of the reproductive system- breast, cervical, endometrial and ovarian cancer. Each chapter describes how each organ is structured and how it functions, and the risks and benefits of new drug therapies, radiation and chemotherapy, and surgical procedures. Includes patient stories and addresses the full range of issues faced by patients and their families.
290 pages paperback
ISBN: 0-944235-20-4

2356 Young People with Cancer: A Handbook for Parents
Barry Leonard, author
DIANE Publishing Company
330 Pusey Avenue, Unit #3 Rear
Darby, PA 19023

610-461-6200
800-782-3833
Fax: 610-461-6130
e-mail: dianepublishing@gmail.com
www.dianepublishing.net

Gives you information on all stages of your child's cancer. It tells you what to expect and suggests ways to prepare for different situations.
109 pages Paperback
ISBN: 0-756736-59-5
Herman Baron, Publisher

Children's Books

2357 Cancer
Franklin Watts Grolier
90 Old Sherman Turnpike
Danbury, CT 06816-0001

203-797-3500
800-621-1115
Fax: 203-797-3197
www.grolier.com

Discusses causes such as chemicals, viruses, radiation and oncogenes, as well as diagnosis, types of cancers, immune defenses and common treatments.
96 pages Grades 7-12
ISBN: 0-531108-03-1

2358 Cancer: Overview Series
Lucent Books
Thomson Gale
Farmington Hills, MI 48333-9187

800-877-4253
Fax: 800-414-5043
e-mail: gale.customerservice@thomson.com
www.gale.com/lucent

Questions are answered for young adults on the issues of cancer prevention and treatment.
1999 112 pages
ISBN: 1-560063-63-7

2359 Help Yourself: Tips for Teenagers with Cancer
National Cancer Institute
Building 31
Bethesda, MD 20892-0001

800-422-6237

This magazine-style booklet is designed to provide information and support adolescents with cancer.
37 pages

2360 Hospital Days: Treatment Ways
National Cancer Institute
Building 31
Bethesda, MD 20892-0001

800-422-6237

Coloring book helping to orient children with cancer to hospital and treatment procedures.
26 pages

2361 Kathy's Hats: A Story of Hope
Trudy Krisher, author
Albert Whitman & Company
6340 Oakton Street
Morton Grove, IL 60053-2723

847-581-0033
800-255-7675
Fax: 847-581-0039
e-mail: mail@awhitmanco.com
www.albertwhitman.com

When Kathy turns nine she learns she has cancer. When she loses her hair due to the chemotherapy, she feels ugly and awkward. This is a matter-of-fact book about a tough time and subject, and its calm and respectable treatment well serves a story that is indeed one of hope.
32 pages Hardcover
ISBN: 0-807541-16-6
Pat McPartland, Sales
Joe Campbell, Customer Service

2362 Kemo Shark
Kidscope
3400 Peachtree Road NE
Atlanta, GA 30326-1107

404-233-0001
www.kidscope.org

Color comic book designed to help children with the psychological and physiological changes in a family where a parent has cancer and chemotherapy.

2363 Kid's 1st Cookbook: Delicious-Nutritious Treats to Make Yourself
American Cancer Society
1599 Clifton Road NE
Atlanta, GA 30329-4250

404-320-3333
800-227-2345

Do creepy spiders, sloppy dogs and tornado swirls sound edible to you? They will to kids. Inside this beautifully illustrated hardcover edition are activities, colorful recipes and cooking tips that will turn meal preparation into exciting family fun. Kids of all ages can

take charge, don a chef's hat and create delicious and nutricious snacks and dishes for every meal.
96 pages hardcover
ISBN: 0-944235-20-4

2364 Living with Cancer
Franklin Watts Grolier
90 Old Sherman Turnpike   203-797-3500
Danbury, CT 06816-0001   800-621-1115
                                 Fax: 203-797-3197
                                 www.grolier.com
Shows how persons with cancer can overcome their illness and lead productive lives.
32 pages Grades 5-7
ISBN: 0-531108-59-7

2365 My Book for Kids with Cancer
Waterfront Books
98 Brookes Avenue
Burlington, VT 05401-3326   800-639-6063
                                 www.waterfrontbooks.com/
Frustrated because he couldn't find any books about kids who survived cancer, Jason decided to write his own.
32 pages

2366 Our Mom Has Cancer
American Cancer Society
1599 Clifton Road NE   404-320-3333
Atlanta, GA 30329-4250   800-227-2345
When Abigail and Adrienne's mom told them she had cancer, they were afraid. But when the girls couldn't find any books that explained what might happen to their mother and what they might expect, they wrote one themselves. The girls, ages 9 and 11, tell readers that when their mother was tired during treatment, friends and family pitched in to help cook and to push her in her wheelchair. When chemotherapy made their mom's hair fall out, they threw a hat party for her.
32 pages hardcover
ISBN: 0-944235-20-4

2367 Sammie's New Mask: A Coloring Book for Friends of Children with Cancer
1015 Locust Street   314-241-1600
Saint Louis, MO 63101   Fax: 314-241-1996
                      e-mail: krudd@children-cancer.org
                      www.nationalchildrenscancersociety.org
Sammie's New Mask is about a young girl named Sammie and her friend, Jack, who has cancer. This story addresses Sammie's concerns and common misconceptions about cancer. This coloring book is designed for children in kindergarten through third grade.
K-3rd Grade
Mark Slocomb, Chairman
Mark Stolze, President/CEO

2368 Sammy's Mommy Has Cancer: For Children Who Have a Loved One with Cancer
Sherry Kohlenberg, author

Magination Press (American Psychological Assoc.)
750 First Street NE   202-336-5510
Washington, DC 20002-4242   800-374-2721
                                 Fax: 202-336-5502
                                 TDD: 202-336-6123
                      e-mail: magination@apa.org
                      www.apamaginationpress.apa.org
Sherry Kohlenberg wrote this book after she was diagnosed with breast cancer for her son. It is a warm, sensitive, straightforward story that will help young children understand and accept the changes in their lives when a parent is diagnosed with a life threatening illness. Parents will welcome this valuable aid in explaining the illness to their children. Both the story and the introduction offer useful suggestions for involving children in the jiys and sorrows of good and bad days.
1993 32 pages Softcover
ISBN: 0-945354-55-X

2369 Silver Kiss
Delacorte
1540 Broadway   212-354-6500
New York, NY 10036-4039

This moving tale describes the feelings of Zoe as her mother dies of cancer and her family attempts to shield her from seeing the slow decline in her mother.
Grades 8-12

2370 Silver Linings: Living with Cancer
Vantage Press
516 W 34th Street   212-736-1767
New York, NY 10001-1395   Fax: 212-736-2273
Highly personal journey of one woman's battle with breast cancer for over thirty-five years. From operations, radiation treatments, and hormone therapy and her faith and hope while induring them.

ISBN: 0-533113-52-0

2371 The Mountain You've Climbed: A Young Adult Guide to Childhood Cancer Survivorship
1015 Locust Street   314-241-1600
Saint Louis, MO 63101   Fax: 314-241-1996
                      e-mail: krudd@children-cancer.org
                      www.nationalchildrenscancersociety.org
This guide is designed to answer questions and address issues related to cancer survivorship for people ages 15 to 24. As survivorship rates continue to increase, the knowledge regarding late-effects also continues to increase. This survivorship guide will answer questions as well as address healthy living styles for your future.
Ages 15-24
Mark Slocomb, Chairman
Mark Stolze, President/CEO

2372 They Never Want to Tell You: Children Talk About Cancer
Harvard University Press
79 Garden Street   617-495-2480
Cambridge, MA 02138   800-448-2242
                                 Fax: 800-962-4983
                                 www.hup.harvard.edu
A comprehensive book that focuses on eight children who share their various experiences with cancer.
Grades 7-12
ISBN: 0-674883-70-5

2373 Waiting for Johnny Miracle
Harper & Row
10 E 53rd Street   212-207-7000
New York, NY 10022-5299
This powerful book focuses on Becky, a 17-year-old girl who must face the fear of cancer after being diagnosed with a malignant tumor. This book brings up the painful issues that come with the pain, treatment and death of cancer.
Grades 8-12

2374 Why God Gave Me Pain
Loyola University Press
3441 N Ashland Avenue   773-281-1818
Chicago, IL 60657-1355
Using a girl's diary entries, this book expounds on the side effects of cancer as well as the psychological ramifications of the debilitating disease.

Magazines

2375 American Journal of Clinical Oncology: Cancer Clinical Trials
Raven Press
1185 Avenue of the Americas   212-930-9500
New York, NY 10036-2601   800-777-2295
Offers outstanding coverage of ongoing research in cancer treatment. This journal is the primary source for timely updates covering all aspects of cancer management.
BiMonthly
ISBN: 0-277373-2 -
Luther W Brady, Editor

2376 Cancer Detection and Prevention Journal
Elsevier

Journals Customer Service Dept.
Orlando, FL 32887-4800

877-839-7126
Fax: 407-363-1354
e-mail: usjcs@elsevier.com
www.elsevier.com

A peer-refereed journal devoted to cancer prevention by predictive and preventitive oncology. It is uniquely focused on advances in genetics, molecular medicine and biotechnologies that have an impact on clinical oncology modalities.
2002-present

2377 Cancer Nursing: An International Journal for Cancer Care
Lippincott Williams & Wilkins
PO Box 1600
Hagerstown, MD 21741-1600

800-638-3030
Fax: 301-223-2400
e-mail: orders@lww.com
www.lww.com

Addresses the whole spectrum of problems arising in the care and support of cancer patients- prevention and early detection, geriatric and pediatric cancer nursing, medical and surgical oncology, ambulatory care, nutritional support, psychosocial aspects of cancer, patient responces to all treatment modalities, and specific nursing interventions.
BiMonthly
ISBN: 0-162220-X -

2378 Diseases of the Colon and Rectum
American Society of Colon and Rectal Surgeons
85 W Algonquin Road
Arlington Heights, IL 60005

847-290-9184
Fax: 847-290-9203
e-mail: ascrs@fascrs.org
www.fascrs.org

Diseases of the Colon and Rectum (DCR) is the official journal of the American Society of Colon and Rectal Surgeons and is mailed to all members on a mothly basis as a member benefit. Non-member subscribers have access to the online version of DCR.
journal

2379 Pancreas
Raven Press
1185 Avenue of the Americas
New York, NY 10036-2601

212-930-9500
800-777-2295

Provides a central forum for communication of original works involving both basic and clinical research on the exocrine and endocrine pancreas and their consequences in the disease state.
8x Year
ISBN: 0-885317-7 -
Vay Liang W Go, Editor

2380 Practice Parameters
American Society of Colon and Rectal Surgeons
85 W Algonquin Road
Arlington Heights, IL 60005

847-290-9184
Fax: 847-290-9203
e-mail: ascrs@fascrs.org
www.fascrs.org

Parameters that have been published in the scientific journal Diseases of the Colon and Rectum, along with other scientific journals. They can be found on the website under Professionals.

2381 Roswellness Magazine
Roswell Park Cancer Institute
Elm & Carlton Streets
Buffalo, NY 14263

716-845-2300
877-275-7724
e-mail: askrpci@roswellpark.org
www.roswellpark.org

A consumer magazine promoting good health habits, cancer prevention and early detection, and the services of Roswell Park Cancer Institute.
2x/year
Donald L Trump MD, FACP, President/CEO
Candace Johnson PhD, Deputy Director

2382 Skin Cancer Foundation Journal
Skin Cancer Foundation
245 5th Avenue
New York, NY 10016-8728

212-725-5176
800-754-6490
Fax: 212-725-5751
e-mail: info@skincancer.org
www.skincancer.org

A collection of articles by physicians, scientists and lay writers on the subject.

Newsletters

2383 Candlelighters' Quarterly
Childhood Cancer Foundation
7910 Woodmont Avenue
Bethesda, MD 20814

301-657-8401
800-366-2223

Artlices on living with and treating pediatric/adolescent cancer, written by and for parents and professionals in the field. Includes reviews, resources, pen pal column, and more.

2384 Candlelighters' Youth Newsletter
Childhood Cancer Foundation
7910 Woodmont Avenue
Bethesda, MD 20814-3015

301-657-8401
800-366-2223

Offers information to teenagers and young adults on cancer issues, medical information, camps and programs.
Quarterly

2385 Exceptional Cancer Patients/ECaP Newsletter
Exceptional Cancer Patients/ECaP
532 Jackson Park Drive
Meadville, CT 16335

814-337-8192
Fax: 814-337-0699
e-mail: info@ecap-online.org, info@mind-body.org
www.ecap-online.org/home.htm

E-newsletter with inspirational articles
2x/year
Bernie Siegal MD, Founder
Barry Bittman MD, Chief Executive Officer

2386 Melanoma Newsletter
Skin Cancer Foundation
245 5th Avenue
New York, NY 10016-8728

212-725-5176
800-754-6490
Fax: 212-725-5751
e-mail: info@skincancer.org
www.skincancer.org

For medical investigators and practitioners.

2387 Nutrition Action Healthletter
Center for Science in the Public Interest
1875 Connecticut Avenue NW
Washington, DC 20009-5736

202-332-9110
Fax: 202-265-4954
e-mail: cspi@cspinet.org
www.cspinet.org

The nation's leading consumer group concerned with food and nutrition issues. Focuses on diseases that result from consuming too many calories, too much fat, sodium and sugar such as cancer and heart disease.
16 pages 10 per year
Stephen Schmidt, Editor

2388 Oncology Times: The News Center for the Cancer Care Team
Lippincott Williams & Wilkins
PO Box 1600
Hagerstown, MD 21741-1600

800-638-3030
Fax: 301-223-2400
e-mail: orders@lww.com
www.lww.com

Reports on breaking clinical news in oncology, radiology, surgery, chemotherapy, and biological and gene therapy, as well as the professional, political, reimbursement, and practice management issues that affect those treating cancer patients.
2x Monthly

2389 Options: New Directions in the War on Cancer
People Against Cancer
614 E Street
Otho, IA 50569-0010

515-972-4444
Fax: 515-972-4415
e-mail: info@peopleagainstcancer.com
www.peopleagainstcancer.com

Published by People Against Cancer.
8 pages
Frank Wiewel, Executive Director

2390 Phoenix: Newsletter
Candlelighters' Childhood Cancer Foundation

7910 Woodmont Avenue
Bethesda, MD 20814-3015
For adult survivors of childhood cancer.

301-657-8401
800-366-2223

2391   Sun and Skin News
Skin Cancer Foundation
245 5th Avenue
New York, NY 10016-8728

212-725-5176
800-754-6490
Fax: 212-725-5751
e-mail: info@skincancer.org
www.skincancer.org

Deals with skin cancer and related subjects in nontechnical terms.

2392   Support for People with Oral and Head and Neck Cancer
PO Box 53
Locust Valley, NY 11560-0053

516-759-5333
800-377-0928
Fax: 516-671-8794
e-mail: info@spohnc.org
www.spohnc.org

This a patient run support program. Other services include patient networking oportunities, a national newsletter, a resource library and insurance information and assistance.
Nancy E Leupold, President/Founder

2393   The Phoenix
United Ostomy Associations of America, Inc.
The Phoenix Magazine
Mission Viejo, CA 92690

949-600-7296
800-826-0826
e-mail: publisher@uoaa.org
www.uoaa.org

The Phoenix magazine is the official publication of the United Ostomy Associations of America, Inc. and is published four times a year- December, March, June, and September.
Quarterly

2394   Voice of Hope
National Children's Cancer Society
1015 Locust Street
Saint Louis, MO 63101

314-241-1600
Fax: 314-241-1996
e-mail: krudd@children-cancer.org
www.nationalchildrenscancersociety.org

It educates donors on how their support is furthering the N.C.C.S. mission, and acknowledges supporters. Distributed to donors of the N.C.C.S.
3x/year
Mark Slocomb, Chairman
Mark Stolze, President/CEO

Pamphlets

2395   Advanced Cancer: Living Each Day
National Cancer Institute
Building 31
Bethesda, MD 20892-0001

800-422-6237

Booklet delving into all aspects of everyday living with cancer. Offers information on coping, how children react, facing the unknown, living wills, additional resources and making treatment decisions.
30 pages

2396   After Breast Cancer: A Guide to Followup Care
National Cancer Institute
Building 31
Bethesda, MD 20892-0001

800-422-6237

Explains the importance of checking for possible signs of recurring cancer by receiving regular mammograms, getting breast exams from a doctor, and continuing monthly breast self-exams.
15 pages

2397   Basic Family Library
Candlelighters' Childhood Cancer Foundation
7910 Woodmont Avenue
Bethesda, MD 20814-3015

301-657-8401
800-366-2223

A bibliography of materials on childhood cancers, medical support, death and bereavement and materials for children.

2398   Brachytherapy and IMRT
Michael Dattoli, Jennifer Cash, and Don Kaltenbach, author
Dattoli Cancer Foundation
2803 Fruitville Road
Sarasota, FL 34237

941-365-5599
800-915-1001
Fax: 941-366-3786
e-mail: info@dattolifoundation.org
www.dattolifoundation.org

A primer on seed implants and Intensity Modulated Radiation Therapy (IMRT). This booklet provides a comprehensive overview of prostate cancer treatment protocols that utilize brachytherapy and IMRT either with or without hormonal therapy.
50 pages Booklet

2399   Breast Biopsy: What You Should Know
National Cancer Institute
Building 31
Bethesda, MD 20892-0001

301-496-4000

Offers information on what happens before, during and after a breast biopsy.

2400   Breast Cancer: Understanding Treatment Options
National Cancer Institute
Building 31
Bethesda, MD 20892-0001

800-422-6237

Summarizes the biopsy procedure and examines the pros and cons of various types of breast surgery. It discusses lumpectomy and radiation therapy as primary treatment.
19 pages

2401   Breast Exams: What You Should Know
National Cancer Institute
Building 31
Bethesda, MD 20892-0001

800-422-6237

Provides answers to questions about breast cancer and breast screening methods.
10 pages

2402   Camps for Children with Cancer and their Siblings
Candlelighters' Childhood Cancer Foundation
7910 Woodmont Avenue
Bethesda, MD 20814-3015

301-657-8401
800-366-2223

A listing by state of day and overnight camp programs, children served and programs.

2403   Cancer Tests You Should Know About: A Guide for People 65 and Over
National Cancer Institute
Building 31
Bethesda, MD 20892-0001

800-422-6237

Describes the cancer tests important for people age 65 and older. Informs men and women of the exams they should be requesting when they schedule checkups with their doctors.
14 pages

2404   Cancer of the Bladder: Research Report
National Cancer Institute
Building 31
Bethesda, MD 20892-0001

800-422-6237

Offers information on the types of bladder cancer, mortality rates, diagnosis, symptoms, therapies, rehabilitation, clinical trials, and selected references.

2405   Cancer of the Colon and Rectum: Research Report
National Cancer Institute
Building 31
Bethesda, MD 20892-0001

800-422-6237

Informative pamphlet offering factual statistics on causes and prevention, detection, diagnosis, staging, treatment, followup, clinical trials and selected references.

2406   Cancer of the Ovary: Research Report
National Cancer Institute
Building 31
Bethesda, MD 20892-0001

800-422-6237

2407   Cancer of the Pancreas: Research Report
National Cancer Institute

183

Building 31
Bethesda, MD 20892-0001   800-422-6237
Offers information on the various types of pancreatic cancer, treatments, surgical procedures, chemotherapy, biological therapy, hormone therapy, clinical trials and selected references.

2408   Cancer of the Uterus: Endometrial Cancer
National Cancer Institute
Building 31
Bethesda, MD 20892-0001   800-422-6237
Offers information on the description and function of the uterus, incidence and mortality, possible causes and prevention, detection, diagnosis, staging, treatment, clinical trials and selected references.

2409   Cancer of the Uterus: Research Report
National Cancer Institute
Building 31
Bethesda, MD 20892-0001   800-422-6237

2410   Candlelighters Guide to Bone Marrow Transplants in Children
Candlelighters' Childhood Cancer Foundation
7910 Woodmont Avenue   301-657-8401
Bethesda, MD 20814-3015   800-366-2223
For parents who are contemplating a BMT or harvest for their child or whose child is undergoing the procedure.

2411   Chemotherapy and You: A Guide to Self-Help During Treatment
National Cancer Institute
Building 31
Bethesda, MD 20892-0001   800-422-6237
Explains chemotherapy and addresses problems and concerns of patients undergoing this treatment.

2412   Chew or Snuff is Real Bad Stuff
National Cancer Institute
Building 31   301-435-3848
Bethesda, MD 20892-2580   800-422-6237
                                           www.nci.nih.gov
Designed for young adults, this brochure describes the health and social effects of using smokeless tobacco products.

2413   Clearing the Air: A Guide to Quitting Smoking
National Cancer Institute
Building 31
Bethesda, MD 20892-0001   800-422-6237
Offers hints on quitting smoking and cancer prevention.
24 pages

2414   Cutaneous Melanoma of the Head and Neck
American Academy of Otolaryngology
1 Prince Street   703-836-4444
Alexandria, VA 22314-3357   Fax: 703-683-5100
                                           www.entnet.org
Self-instruction package.
Paperback
ISBN: 1-567720-22-6

2415   Diet, Nutrition and Cancer Prevention: The Good News
National Cancer Institute
Building 31
Bethesda, MD 20892-0001   800-422-6237
Provides an overview of dietary guidelines that may assist individuals in reducing their risks for some cancers.
16 pages

2416   Diet, Nutrition and Cancer Prevention: A Guide to Food Choices
National Cancer Institute
Building 31
Bethesda, MD 20892-0001   800-422-6237
Describes what is known about diet, nutrition and cancer prevention. Provides information about foods that contain components like fiber, fat and vitamins that may affect a person's risk of getting certain cancers.

2417   Dilemmas of Providing Help in a Crisis: The Role of Friends & Parents
Candlelighters' Childhood Cancer Foundation
7910 Woodmont Avenue   301-657-8401
Bethesda, MD 20814-3015   800-366-2223

2418   Do the Right Thing: Get a Mammogram
National Cancer Institute
Building 31
Bethesda, MD 20892-0001   800-422-6237
Targets black women age 40 and older. Describes the importance of regular mammograms in the early detection of breast cancer.

2419   Eating Hints: Recipes and Tips for Better Nutrition During Cancer Treatment
National Cancer Institute
Building 31
Bethesda, MD 20892-0001   800-422-6237
Provides recipes that help patients meet their needs for good nutrition during treatment.

2420   Facing Forward: A Guide for Cancer Survivors
National Cancer Institute
Building 31
Bethesda, MD 20892-0001   800-422-6237
Presents a concise overview of important survivor issues, including ongoing health needs, psychosocial concerns, insurance and employment.
43 pages

2421   Facts About Lung Cancer
American Lung Association
1740 Broadway   212-315-8700
New York, NY 10019-4315

2422   Facts About Radon
American Lung Association
1740 Broadway   212-315-8700
New York, NY 10019-4315

2423   Help, Hope, Believe
National Children's Cancer Society
1015 Locust Street   314-241-1600
Saint Louis, MO 63101   Fax: 314-241-1996
                          e-mail: krudd@children-cancer.org
                          www.nationalchildrenscancersociety.org
N.C.C.S. Informational Brochure
3x/year
Mark Slocomb, Chairman
Mark Stolze, President/CEO

2424   Helping Children Cope While a Sibling Undergoes Bone Marrow Transplant
Bone Marrow Foundation
981 1st Avenue   212-838-3029
New York, NY 10022-5102   e-mail: thebmf@aol.com
                                           www.bonemarrow.org
Discusses the wide array of emotions felt by the entire family as a child receives a bone marrow transplant.

2425   If You've Thought About Breast Cancer
Rose Kushner Breast Cancer Advisory Center
PO Box 224
Kensington, MD 20895-0224   Fax: 301-897-3444

2426   Immune System: How it Works
National Cancer Institute
Building 31
Bethesda, MD 20892-0001   800-422-6237
Written for the high school level, this booklet explains the human immune system for the general public. It describes the sophistication of the body's immune responses, the impact of immune disorders and the relation of the immune system to cancer therapies.
28 pages

2427   Informed Consent: Does the Current Process Reflect Current Treatments
Candlelighters' Childhood Cancer Foundation
7910 Woodmont Avenue   301-657-8401
Bethesda, MD 20814-3015   800-366-2223

2428   Insurance Articles
Candlelighters' Childhood Cancer Foundation
7910 Woodmont Avenue   301-657-8401
Bethesda, MD 20814-3015   800-366-2223

Includes: Tips on securing health insurance for childhood cancer survivors and patients, Stay a step ahead of you insuruer, and others.

2429 Interpreting Your PSA and Related Prostate Cancer Blood Tests
Michael Dattoli, Jennifer Cash, and Don Kaltenbach, author

Dattoli Cancer Foundation
2803 Fruitville Road   941-365-5599
Sarasota, FL 34237   800-915-1001
                                      Fax: 941-366-3786
                          e-mail: info@dattolifoundation.org
                              www.dattolifoundation.org
Provides a comprehensive overview of the PSA (prostate specific antigen) blood test and other related lab tests including the PSA velocity, free and bound PSA, and the PAP (prostatic Acid Phosphatase) blood test.
2006 50 pages Booklet

2430 Leading Self-Help Groups: Report on Workshop for Leaders of Groups
Candlelighters' Childhood Cancer Foundation
7910 Woodmont Avenue   301-657-8401
Bethesda, MD 20814-3015   800-366-2223

2431 Letter to a Friend Whose Child is Newly Diagnosed with Cancer
Candlelighters' Childhood Cancer Foundation
7910 Woodmont Avenue   301-657-8401
Bethesda, MD 20814-3015   800-366-2223

2432 Managing Your Child's Eating Problems During Cancer Treatment
National Cancer Institute
Building 31
Bethesda, MD 20892-0001   800-422-6237
Contains information about the importance of nutrition, side effects of cancer and its treatment.
32 pages

2433 Mastectomy: A Treatment for Breast Cancer
National Cancer Institute
Building 31
Bethesda, MD 20892-0001   800-422-6237
Presents information about the different types of breast surgery, explains what to expect at the hospital and during the recovery period.
25 pages

2434 Melanoma: Research Report
National Cancer Institute
Building 31
Bethesda, MD 20892-0001   800-422-6237
Offers information on types of skin cancer, detection, diagnosis, staging, treatment, clinical trials, selected references and additional information for patients with skin cancer.

2435 Nutrition for Patients Receiving Chemotherapy/Radiation Treatment
National Cancer Institute
Building 31
Bethesda, MD 20892-0001   800-422-6237
Describes the importance of maintaining nutritional intake while receiving chemotherapy and radiation.

2436 Once a Year for a Lifetime
National Cancer Institute
Building 31
Bethesda, MD 20892-0001   800-422-6237
Targets all women age 40 and older describing the importance of regular mammograms in the early detection of breast cancer.

2437 Oral Cancers: Research Report
National Cancer Institute
Building 31
Bethesda, MD 20892-0001   800-422-6237
Describes types of oral cancer, causes and risk factors, symptoms, prevention, detection, diagnosis, treatment, staging, methods of treatments, followup care, clinical trials and selected references for more information.

2438 Pap Test: It Can Save Your Life
National Cancer Institute
Building 31
Bethesda, MD 20892-0001   800-422-6237
Easy-to-read pamphlet tells women of the importance of getting a Pap test, how often to get it done and where to go to get it.

2439 Preparing your Child for a Bone Marrow Transplant
Bone Marrow Foundation
981 1st Avenue   212-838-3029
New York, NY 10022-5102   e-mail: thebmf@aol.com
                                      www.bonemarrow.org
Discusses the wide array of emotions felt by the entire family as a child receives a bone marrow transplant.

2440 Questions and Answers About Breast Lumps
National Cancer Institute
Building 31
Bethesda, MD 20892-0001   800-422-6237
Describes some of the most common noncancerous breast lumps and what can be done about them.
22 pages

2441 Questions and Answers About Choosing a Mammography Facility
National Cancer Institute
Building 31
Bethesda, MD 20892-0001   800-422-6237
Lists questions to ask in selecting a quality mammography facility.

2442 Questions and Answers About DES Exposure During Pregnancy and Before Birth
National Cancer Institute
Building 31
Bethesda, MD 20892-0001   800-422-6237

2443 Questions and Answers About Metastatic Cancer
National Cancer Institute
Building 31
Bethesda, MD 20892-0001   800-422-6237
Presents information on detection, treatment methods and common areas of reoccurrence.

2444 Questions and Answers About Pain Control
National Cancer Institute
Building 31
Bethesda, MD 20892-0001   800-422-6237
Discusses pain control using both medical and nonmedical methods.

2445 Radiation Therapy and You: A Guide To Self-Help During Treatment
National Cancer Institute
Building 31
Bethesda, MD 20892-0001   800-422-6237
Explains radiation therapy and addresses concerns of patients receiving radiation treatment.

2446 Recurrence: What Do I Do Now?
Dattoli Cancer Foundation
2803 Fruitville Road   941-365-5599
Sarasota, FL 34237   800-915-1001
                                      Fax: 941-366-3786
                          e-mail: info@dattolifoundation.org
                              www.dattolifoundation.org
This booklet offers comprehensive information on the issues surrounding ruccurence: detection, risk categories, treatment options including radiation, brachytherapy, and hormone therapy.
58 pages Booklet

2447 Research Report: Adult Kidney Cancer and Wilms' Tumor
National Cancer Institute
Building 31
Bethesda, MD 20892-0001   800-422-6237

2448 Skin Cancers, Basal Cell and Squamous Cell Carcinomas: Research Report
National Cancer Institute
Building 31
Bethesda, MD 20892-0001   800-422-6237

185

Offers information on types of skin cancer, incidence and mortality, risk factors, prevention, symptoms, detection, diagnosis, staging, treatment, followup care and clinical trials.

2449 Students with Cancer: A Resource for the Educator
National Cancer Institute
Building 31
Bethesda, MD 20892-0001   800-422-6237
Designed for teachers who have students with cancer in their classrooms or schools.
22 pages

2450 Sunlight, Ultraviolet Radiation and the Skin
National Cancer Institute
Building 31
Bethesda, MD 20892-0001   800-422-6237

2451 Support Systems for Parents of Children with Cancer
Candlelighters' Childhood Cancer Foundation
7910 Woodmont Avenue   301-657-8401
Bethesda, MD 20814-3015   800-366-2223

2452 Taking Time: Support for People with Cancer & People Who Care for Them
National Cancer Institute
Building 31
Bethesda, MD 20892-0001   800-422-6237
Discusses the emotional sides of cancer. how to deal with the disease and learn to talk with friends, family members and others about cancer.

2453 Talking with Your Child About Cancer
National Cancer Institute
Building 31
Bethesda, MD 20892-0001   800-422-6237
Designed for the parent whose child has been diagnosed with cancer.
16 pages

2454 Testicular Cancer: Research Report
National Cancer Institute
Building 31
Bethesda, MD 20892-0001   800-422-6237

2455 Testicular Self-Examination
National Cancer Institute
Building 31
Bethesda, MD 20892-0001   800-422-6237
Contains information about risks and symptoms of testicular cancer and provides instructions on how to perform testicular self-examination.

2456 What You Need to Know About Bladder Cancer
National Cancer Institute
Building 31   301-496-4000
Bethesda, MD 20892-0001
Offers information on the history, symptoms, diagnosis, treatment, followup care, support groups, medical terms and resources for more information.

2457 What You Need to Know About Cancer
National Cancer Institute
Building 31
Bethesda, MD 20892-0001   800-422-6237
Offers information on signs and symptoms, diagnosis, treatment, early detection and advances in medical technology.

2458 What You Need to Know About Cancer of The Colon and Rectum
National Cancer Institute
Building 31
Bethesda, MD 20892-0001   800-422-6237
Offers information on symptoms, diagnosis, treatments, and support for cancer patients.

2459 What You Need to Know About Cervical Cancer
National Cancer Institute
Building 31
Bethesda, MD 20892-0001   800-422-6237
Areas covered include early detection, symptoms, treatments, diagnosis, followup care, support, medical terms and resources.

2460 What You Need to Know About Esophagal Cancer
National Cancer Institute
Building 31
Bethesda, MD 20892-0001   800-422-6237
Offers information on symptoms, causes, preventions, diagnosis, support, medical terms and available resources.

2461 What You Need to Know About Kidney Cancer
National Cancer Institute
Building 31
Bethesda, MD 20892-0001   800-422-6237
Offers factual information on diagnosis, symptoms, prevention, treatment and referral sources.

2462 What You Need to Know About Larynx Cancer
National Cancer Institute
Building 31
Bethesda, MD 20892-0001   800-422-6237
Offers information on what cancer is, symptoms, diagnosis, treatment options, side effects of medication, rehabilitation, learning to speak again, living with cancer, causes and preventions, medical terms and resources.

2463 What You Need to Know About Lung Cancer
National Cancer Institute
Building 31
Bethesda, MD 20892-0001   800-422-6237
Offers information on types of lung cancer, symptoms, diagnosis, treatments, support, medical terms and resources.

2464 What You Need to Know About Oral Cancers
National Cancer Institute
Building 31
Bethesda, MD 20892-0001   800-422-6237
Offers information on symptoms, diagnosis, treatments, rehabilitation, followup care, support, medical terms and resources for cancer patients.

2465 What You Need to Know About Ovarian Cancer
National Cancer Institute
Building 31
Bethesda, MD 20892-0001   800-422-6237
Early detection, symptoms, diagnosis, treatments, medical terms and resources for further information.

2466 What You Need to Know About Pancreatic Cancer
National Cancer Institute
Building 31
Bethesda, MD 20892-0001   800-422-6237
Offers information on symptoms, diagnosis, treatment, support, medical terms and resources.

2467 What You Need to Know About Prostate Cancer
National Cancer Institute
Building 31
Bethesda, MD 20892-0001   800-422-6237
Offers information on symptoms, diagnosis, treatment options, side effects of medications, followup care, living with cancer and support resources for patients.

2468 What You Need to Know About Skin Cancer
National Cancer Institute
Building 31
Bethesda, MD 20892-0001   800-422-6237
Offers information on types of skin cancer, symptoms, causes, prevention, treatment planning, treating skin cancer, research and medical terms.

2469 What You Need to Know About Testicular Cancer
National Cancer Institute
Building 31
Bethesda, MD 20892-0001   800-422-6237
Offers information on the symptoms, diagnosing of testicular cancer, side effects of treatments, followup care, support for patients, cancer research, medical terms and resources.

2470 What You Need to Know About Uterine Cancer
National Cancer Institute
Building 31
Bethesda, MD 20892-0001   800-422-6237

Offers information on symptoms, diagnosing cancer of the uterus, treatments, followup care, support for patients, medical terms and resources.

2471 What You Need to Know About...
National Cancer Institute
Building 31
Bethesda, MD 20892-0001   800-422-6237
This is a series of booklets, broken down in this directory. Each provides information about a specific type of cancer. These booklets discuss emotional issues, treatment, diagnosis, symptoms and questions to ask the doctor about cancer.

2472 What are Clinical Trials All About?
National Cancer Institute
Building 31
Bethesda, MD 20892-0001   800-422-6237
Explains clinical trials (studies of new cancer treatments) to help patients decide if they want to take part in a trial.

2473 When Cancer Recurs: Meeting the Challenge Again
National Cancer Institute
Building 31
Bethesda, MD 20892-0001   800-422-6237
Offers information on why cancer can recur, where cancers can recur, diagnosing recurrent cancer, treatment methods and resources that offer more help.

2474 When Someone in Your Family Has Cancer
National Cancer Institute
Building 31
Bethesda, MD 20892-0001   800-422-6237
Written for young people whose parent or sibling has cancer.
28 pages

2475 Who is This Person Who Helped Save My Life
Bone Marrow Foundation
981 1st Avenue   212-838-3029
New York, NY 10022-5102   e-mail: thebmf@aol.com
www.bonemarrow.org
Discusses the wide range of emotions for a patient in the process of searching for and identifying a donor.

2476 Why Do You Smoke?
National Cancer Institute
Building 31
Bethesda, MD 20892-0001   800-422-6237
Contains a self-test to determine why people smoke and suggest alternatives that can help them stop and prevent cancer.

2477 Wish Fulfillment Organizations
Candlelighters' Childhood Cancer Foundation
7910 Woodmont Avenue   301-657-8401
Bethesda, MD 20814-3015   800-366-2223
A list of groups granting wishes of children with life-threatening, chronic or terminal illnesses, with criteria and contacts.

2478 Young People with Cancer: A Handbook for Parents
National Cancer Institute
Building 31
Bethesda, MD 20892-0001   800-422-6237
Discusses the most common types of childhood cancer, treatments, and side effects and issues that may arise when a child is diagnosed with cancer.
86 pages

Audio & Video

2479 Beyond the Loss of the Breast
Fanlight Productions
4196 Washington Street   617-469-4999
Boston, MA 02131-1731   800-937-4113
Fax: 617-469-3379
e-mail: fanlight@fanlight.com
www.fanlight.com
This video addresses breast cancer throught the personal narratives and poetry of two women living with recurrent breast cancer and the film maker, whose mother died from metastatic disease.
1994 25 Minutes
ISBN: 1-572951-68-0

2480 Living with Ovarian Cancer
National Ovarian Cancer Coalition
500 NE Spanish River Blvd   561-393-0005
Boca Raton, FL 33431   888-682-7426
Fax: 561-393-7275
e-mail: nocc@ovarian.org
www.ovarian.org
Videotape for women who have been recently diagnosed with ovarian cancer. Created to orient and inform patients and their families; describes the experiences of individuals intimately connected with the disease.
Suzy Lockwood-Rayermann RN, Chair
Julene Fabrizio, President

2481 Not Just a Cancer Patient
Fanlight Productions
4196 Washington Street   617-469-4999
Boston, MA 02131-1731   800-937-4113
Fax: 617-469-3379
e-mail: fanlight@fanlight.com
www.fanlight.com
Focuses on several articulate teenagers who are undergoing cancer treatment to help caregivers understand the needs and feelings of this population.
1991 23 Minutes
ISBN: 1-572950-86-2

2482 Skin Cancer: Preventable and Curable
Skin Cancer Foundation
245 5th Avenue   212-725-5176
New York, NY 10016-8728   800-754-6490
Fax: 212-725-5751
e-mail: info@skincancer.org
www.skincancer.org

Web Sites

2483 American Academy of Dermatology
www.aad.org
An organization of doctors who specialize in diagnosing and treating skin problems.

2484 American Cancer Society
www.cancer.org
Provides free printed materials, offers a range of services to patients and their families.

2485 American Lung Association
www.lungusa.org
A voluntary organization interested in the prevention and control of lung disease.

2486 American Prostate Society
www.ameripros.org
Organization dedicated exclusively to using existing medical capabilities to reduce death due to prostate cancer and to reduce unnecessary or ineffective prostate surgery.

2487 American Society of Colon and Rectal Surgeons
www.fascrs.org
Represents more than 1000 board certified colon and rectal surgeons and other surgeons dedicated to advancing and promoting the science and practice of the treatment of patients with diseases and disorders affecting the colon, rectum and anus.

2488 Association for the Cure of Cancer of the Prostate
www.capcure.org

2489 Bone Marrow Foundation
www.bonemarrow.org

2490 Healing Well
www.healingwell.com
An online health resource guide to medical news, chat, information and articles, newsgroups and message boards, books, disease-related web sites, medical directories, and more for patients, friends, and family coping with disabling diseases, disorders, or chronic illnesses.

2491 Health Finder

www.healthfinder.gov

Searchable, carefully developed web site offering information on over 1000 topics. Developed by the US Department of Health and Human Services, the site can be used in both English and Spanish.

2492 Healthlink USA

www.healthlinkusa.com

Health information concerning treatment, cures, prevention, diagnosis, risk factors, research, support groups, email lists, personal stories and much more. Updated regularly.

2493 Helios Health

www.helioshealth.com

Online resource for your health information. Detailed information about specific health topics, access to expert advice from our Medical Advisory Board, and up-to-date health news.

2494 International Association of Eating Disorders Professionals

www.iaedp.com

Supplies printed information and sponsors meetings and other activities. Publishes a directory of speech instructors and maintains a list of sources for supplies for laryngectomee.

2495 Leukemia and Lymphoma Society

www.leukemia.org

A national voluntary health agency dedicated to curing leukemia, lymphoma, Hodgkin's disease and myeloma and to improving the quality of life of patients and their families.

2496 MedicineNet

www.medicinenet.com

An online resource for consumers providing easy-to-read, authoritative medical and health information.

2497 Medscape

www.medscape.com

Medscape offers specialists, primary care physicians, and other health professionals the Web's most robust and integrated medical information and educational tools.

2498 National Alliance of Breast Cancer Organizations

www.nabco.org

A network of breast cancer organizations that provides information, assistance and referral to anyone with questions about breast cancer and acts as a voice for the interests and concerns of breast cancer survivors and women at risk.

2499 National Ovarian Cancer Coalition

www.ovarian.org

Our mission is to raise awareness about ovarian cancer and to promote education about the disease.

2500 Support for People with Oral and Head and Neck Cancer

www.spohnc.org

Nonprofit organization founded in 1991 to address the broad emotional, physical and humanistic needs of oral and head and neck cancer patients.

2501 United Ostomy Association

www.uoa.org

A national network for bowel and urinary diversion support groups in the United States. Its goal is to provide a nonprofit association that will serve to unify and strengthen its member support groups, which are organized for the benefit of people who have, or will have intestinal or urinary diversions and their caregivers.

2502 WebMD

www.webmd.com

Information on Cancer, including articles and resources.

2503 Webhelp

www.webhelp.com

Provides links to information, including research, treatment, prevention, support, and more.

Description

2504 # Carpal Tunnel Syndrome

Carpal Tunnel Syndrome, CTS, is a painful, often debilitating condition caused by compression of the median nerve as it passes through the wrist (carpal tunnel) to the hand. CTS most commonly occurs in women aged 30 to 50 years. The incidence is highest among keyboard users, secretaries, musicians, assembly-line workers, and others who engage in repetitive handwork.

An initial indication of CTS is a feeling that the hand is asleep. Typically, the patient wakes at night with numbness and tingling of the affected hand. The most serious functional problem occurs when it becomes difficult or impossible to move the thumb into a grasping position with the other fingers. In advanced cases, pain associated with CTS may radiate up the arm to the shoulder. While job-related movement is the most common cause of CTS, people with underlying conditions, such as diabetes, gout, rheumatoid arthritis, obesity and pregnancy, are more prone to experience symptoms. Although less common, the onset of CTS can stem from trauma, such as a blow to the hand or wrist.

Diagnosis involves the Phalen Test, in which the hands are placed together, back to back and the wrist is flexed. This maneuver generally produces tingling of the hand in a patient with CTS. Diagnosis is confirmed by testing how quickly an impulse is transmitted along the median nerve.

The condition can most often be successfully treated based on an understanding of workplace movement issues — ergonomics. keyboard users, and those engaged in similar activities, should adjust their seats and backrests to assure that their arms are positioned comfortably during work sessions. For mild cases of CTS, a lightweight brace, especially worn at night, can decrease symptoms by holding the wrist stable. Marked improvement may arise from wearing a brace for a week or two. However, in many cases, it is recommended that the sufferer cease working until symptoms have improved. Exercises and deep-tissue massage can strengthen the wrist and hand.

Over-the-counter anti-inflammatory medications, such as ibuprofen and aspirin, can also reduce symptoms of mild Carpal Tunnel Syndrome. In more acute conditions, cortisone injections may be administered. When symptoms are severe and persistent, surgery may be required to reduce pressure on the nerves. The most common surgery is an open incision technique called open carpal tunnel release, which usually improves the condition dramatically. A newer and less invasive procedure is endoscopic carpal tunnel release, which uses a smaller incision and visualizes the operative field using a fiber optic camera.

National Agencies & Associations

2505 **American Academy of Orthopaedic Surgeons**
6300 N River Road   847-823-7186
Rosemont, IL 60018-4262   800-346-2267
Fax: 847-823-8125
e-mail: custserv@aaos.org
www7.aaos.org

The American Academy of Orthopaedic Surgeons provides education and practice management services for orthopaedic surgeons and allied health professionals. The Academy also serves as an advocate for improved patient care and to inform the public.
Joshua J Jacobs, President
Andrew N Pollak, Treasurer

2506 **American Chronic Pain Association**
PO Box 850
Rocklin, CA 95677   800-533-3231
Fax: 916-632-3208
e-mail: ACPA@pacbell.net
www.theacpa.org

ACPA mission is to facilitate peer support and education for individuals with chronic pain and their families so that these individuals may live more fully in spite of their pain and to raise awareness among the health care community and policy makers.
Penny Cowan, Executive Director
Mary Jane Bent, Development and Distance Education at th

2507 **American Society for Surgery of the Hand**
822 W. Washington Boulevard   312-880-1900
Chicago, IL 60607   Fax: 847-384-1435
e-mail: info@assh.org
www.assh.org

The mission of the ASSH is to advance the science and practice of hand and upper extremity surgery through education research and advocacy on behalf of patients and practitioners.
Mark C Anderson CAE, Executive VP, CEO
W. P. Andre Lee, President

2508 **Arthritis Trust of America**
7376 Walker Road   615-799-1002
Fairview, TN 37602-8141   e-mail: admin@arthritistrust.org
www.arthritistrust.org

The Arthritis Trust of America provides information about auto-immune or collagen tissue diseases such as Rheumatoid Arthritis and related diseases. They provide publications and physician referrals and when funds are available they fund research.
Perry A Chapdelaine BA MA, Executive Director
Cheryl Jacobsen, President

2509 **National Institute of Arthritis and Musculoskeletal and Skin Disease (NIAMS)**
1 AMS Circle   301-495-4484
Bethesda, MD 20892-3675   888-226-4267
Fax: 301-718-6366
TTY: 301-565-2966
e-mail: niamsinfo@mail.nih.gov
www.niams.nih.gov

The NIAMS Information Clearinghouse provides information about various forms of arthritis and rheumatic disease and bone, muscle, and skin diseases. It distributes patient and professional education materials and refers people to other sources of information.
Stephen I Katz MD, PhD, Director/Chairman
Lynda F Bonewald Ph.D, Lefkowitz Professor

Research Centers

2510 **Center for Neurology & Stroke Baptist Hospital Office**
Baptist Hospital Office
333 West Thomas Road   602-335-0300
Phoenix, AZ 85015   Fax: 602-249-3118
e-mail: info@cnsaz.com
www.cnsaz.com

Providing comprehensive testing and consulting for neurological disorders.

2511 **Michigan Hand Center**
1111 Leffingwell Avenue NE
Grand Rapids, MI 49525   616-459-7101
      800-582-7244
      Fax: 616-957-0444
e-mail: info@michiganhandcenter.com
www.oamichigan.com

Janid Pike, Director
Samuel Agnew, MD,FACS

2512 **National Institute of Arthritis & Musculoskeletal Skin Diseases**
National Institutes of Health
I AMS Circle   301-495-4484
Bethesda, MD 20892-3675   Fax: 301-718-6366
TTY: 301-565-2966
e-mail: niamsinfo@mail.nih.gov
www.niams.nih.gov

Support Groups & Hotlines

2513 **National Health Information Center**
PO Box 1133   310-565-4167
Washington, DC 20013-1133   800-336-4797
Fax: 301-984-4256
e-mail: info@nhic.org
www.health.gov/nhic
A health information referral service sponsored by the Office of Disease Prevention and Health Promotion. Puts health professionals and consumers who have health questions in touch with those organizations that are best able to provide answers.
Ellen Langhans, Chairwoman
Linda Harris, Lead, Health Communication and e-health

Books

2514 **Occupational Therapy Practice Guidelines for Adults with Carpal Tunnel Syndrome**
American Occupational Therapy Association
4720 Montgomery Lane   301-652-2682
Bethesda, MD 20824-1220   Fax: 301-652-7711
TDD: 800-377-8555
www.aota.org

13 pages Paperback
ISBN: 1-569001-47-2

2515 **Pain Free Typing Techniques: Simple Solutions to Prevent Strain Injury**
Howard Richman, author

Sound Feelings Publishing
18375 Ventura Boulevard   818-757-0600
Tarzana, CA 91356   e-mail: information@soundfeelings.com
www.soundfeelings.com
This 12 page booklet provides drug-free treatments and suggestions for repetitive motion disorder and cumulative trauma disorders. Unconventional concepts for increasing human performance are revealed, which help prevent computer-related illnesses including hand pain, wrist pain, and other keyboard ergonomics. Most repetitive motion disorders and overuse injuries can be improved by correcting certain angles and positions.
1999 12 pages Booklet
ISBN: 1-882060-80-6

Pamphlets

2516 **Carpal Tunnel Syndrome**
Arthritis Foundation
PO Box 7669   404-872-7100
Atlanta, GA 30357-0669   800-283-7800
Fax: 404-872-0457
Offers an introduction to Carpal Tunnel, causes, symptoms, diagnosis and resources.

Web Sites

2517 **Avoiding Carpal Tunnel Syndrome**
www.indiana.edu/~ucsstaff/cts.html

A guide for computer keyboard users, by Mark Sheehan, reprinted from the University Computing Times.

2518 **CTD Resource Network**
www.ctdrn.org
This is an organization providing educational material and charitable assistance related to the prevention and treatment of cumulative trauma disorders, also known as repetitive strain injuries.

2519 **Carpal Tunnel Syndrome Home Page**
www.ctsplace.com
Information about carpal tunnel syndrome (CTS) and how to prevent it.

2520 **Computer-Related Repetitive Strain Injury**
www.unl.edu/ee/eeshop/rsi.html#PREVENT
Contains advice on proper posture and equipment from Paul Marxhausen, an engineering electronics technician.

2521 **Health Finder**
www.healthfinder.gov
Searchable, carefully developed web site offering information on over 1000 topics. Developed by the US Department of Health and Human Services, the site can be used in both English and Spanish.

2522 **MedicineNet**
www.medicinenet.com
An online resource for consumers providing easy-to-read, authoritative medical and health information.

2523 **Neurology Channel**
www.neurologychannel.com
Find clearly explained, medically accurate information regarding conditions, including an overview, symptoms, causes, diagnostic procedures and treatment options. On this site it is possible to ask questions and get information from a neurologist and connect to people who have similar health interests.

2524 **RSI Resources**
www.geocities.com/HotSprings/1702
Information on carpal tunnel and other repetitive strain injuries.

Description

2525 # Celiac Disease

Celiac disease, also called celiac sprue, is a chronic disease in which the small bowel cannot absorb most nutrients. This inability, called malabsorption, is caused by inflammation of the bowel triggered by a sensitivity to gluten, a cereal protein found in wheat and rye, and less so in barley and oats.

The disease may appear when a child is first given wheat products, generally in the second year of life. Some cases, however, do not appear until a person is in their twenties, or later, with women showing symptoms 10 to 15 years earlier than men. Affected children will fail to grow normally. Adults may lose weight despite a voracious appetite. There is no typical presentation of celiac disease. However, painful abdominal distention and passage of large, loose stools are common; iron deficiency anemia and vitamin deficiencies may appear.

Family incidence is a valuable clue. Celiac disease is more common in people with Type I diabetes and certain forms of thyroid and skin disease. Blood tests are helpful in making the diagnosis, but the most definitive test is examination of a small sample of the inflamed bowel.

Withdrawal of dietary gluten is the treatment for celiac disease; eating even small amounts of gluten-containing foods can prevent remission and cause relapse. Vitamins and minerals may also have to be supplemented. See also *Gastrointestinal Disorders* and *Crohn's Disease.*

National Agencies & Associations

2526 **American Celiac Society**
PO Box 23455   504-737-3293
New Orleans, LA 70183   Fax: 973-669-8808
e-mail: americanceliacsociety@yahoo.com
www.americanceliacsociety.org
Nonprofit tax exempt organization that supports efforts in education research and mutual support. Helps to set up support groups sponsors conferences seek funding for education and research identify ingredients in foods and educate the public.
Annette Bentley, President
James Bentley, Vice-President

2527 **Canadian Celiac Association**
5025 Orbitor Drive Building 1   905-507-6208
Mississauga, ON, L4W 4-Y5   800-363-7296
Fax: 905-507-4673
e-mail: info@celiac.ca
www.celiac.ca

A national organization dedicated to providing services and support to persons with celiac disease and dermatitis herpetiformis through programs of awareness, advocacy, education and research.
Anne Wraggett, President
Bill Shank, Executive Vice President

2528 **Celiac Sprue Association: USA**
PO Box 31700   402-558-0600
Omaha, NE 68131-700   877-CSA-4CSA
Fax: 402-643-4108
e-mail: celiacs@csaceliacs.org
www.csaceliacs.org
Member based nonprofit support organization dedicated to helping individuals with celiac disease and dermatitis herpetiformis

worldwide through education information and research. Includes over 150 support contacts nationwide and Cel-Kids Network.
Mary Schluckebier, Executive Director
Diane Craig, President

2529 **Gluten Intolerance Group: GIG**
31214 124th Avenue SE   253-833-6655
Auburn, WA 98092-3667   Fax: 253-833-6675
e-mail: info@gluten.net
www.gluten.net

Provides instructional and general information materials as well as counseling and access to gluten-free products and ingredients to persons with celiac sprue and their families, operates telephone information and referral service and conducts educational seminars.
Cynthia Kupp RDCD, Executive Director

Support Groups & Hotlines

2530 **American Celiac Society Hotline**
Dietary Support Coalition
PO BOX 23455   504-737-3293
New Orleans, LA 70183
Provides practical assistance to members and individuals with celiac disease and information about the disease to the public.
Annette Bentley, President
James Bentley, Vice President

2531 **Celiac Disease Foundation**
20350 Ventura Boulevard   818-716-1513
Woodlands Hills, CA 91364-1838   Fax: 818-267-5577
e-mail: cdf@celiac.org
www.celiac.org/

Provides services and support to persons with celiac disease and dermatitis herpetiformis, through programs of awareness, education, advocacy and research; telephone information and referral services; medical advisory board annual educational conference and quarterly newsletters.
Marcia Riches, President
Richard Tasoff, Vice-President

2532 **National Health Information Center**
PO Box 1133   310-565-4167
Washington, DC 20013   800-336-4797
Fax: 301-984-4256
e-mail: info@nhic.org
www.health.gov/nhic

Offers a nationwide information referral service, produces directories and resource guides.
Ellen Langhans, Chairwoman
Linda Harris, Lead, Health Communication and e-health

Books

2533 **CSA/USA Cookbook Series**
Celiac Sprue Association/USA
PO Box 31700   402-558-0600
Omaha, NE 68131   877-272-4272
Fax: 402-643-4108
e-mail: celiacs@csaceliacs.org
www.csaceliacs.org

Three cookbooks compiled from CSA members' contributions. Each contains a section of cooking hints, information on adapting recipes and a variety of special topics related to cooking gluten-free.
34 pages Annual
Mary Schluckebier, Executive Director

2534 **Cooperative Gluten-Free Commercial Products Listing**
Celiac Sprue Association/USA
PO Box 31700   402-558-0600
Omaha, NE 68131   877-272-4272
Fax: 402-643-4108
e-mail: celiacs@csaceliacs.org
www.csaceliacs.org

Listing of gluten-free products compiled from written documentation recieved by the Celiac Sprue Association from manufacturers and distributors. Also includes vendor information for companies

specializing in gluten-free products and phone numbers of companies.
2006 Annual
Mary Schluckebier, Executive Director

2535 Diets to Help Gluten and Wheat Allergy
HarperCollins Canada Limited/Order Department
1995 Markham Road
Scarborough, ON M1B-5M8   800-387-0117
                                           Fax: 800-668-5788
This book offers sound and practical advice on gluten allergy wheat sensitivity and Celiac disease.
96 pages
ISBN: 0-722529-10-4

2536 Gluten Intolerance
American Dietetic Association
1120 Connecticut Avenue NW   202-775-8277
Washington, DC 20036   800-877-1600
                                           www.eatright.org
Resource and recipe book.

2537 The Gluten-Free Gourmet
Bette Hagman, author
Gluten Intolerance Group: GIG
31214 124th Avenue SE
Auburn, WA 98092-3667   253-833-6655
                                           Fax: 253-833-6675
                                           e-mail: info@gluten.net
                                           www.gluten.net

225 recipes.
272 pages
ISBN: 0-805064-84-2
Cynthia Kupper RDCD, Executive Director

Newsletters

2538 GIG Quarterly Magazine
Gluten Intolerance Group: GIG
31214 124th Avenue SE
Auburn, WA 98092-3667   253-833-6655
                                           Fax: 253-833-6675
                                           e-mail: info@gluten.net
                                           www.gluten.net
Member magazine. Offers updated medical and technological information for patients with celiac disease, their families and healthcare professionals.
Quarterly
Cynthia Kupper RDCD, Executive Director

2539 Lifeline
Celiac Sprue Association/USA
PO Box 31700   402-558-0600
Omaha, NE 68131   877-272-4272
                                           Fax: 402-643-4108
                                           e-mail: celiacs@csaceliacs.org
                                           www.csaceliacs.org
Quarterly newsletter for members; contains up-to-date research information, personal stories from celiacs, cooking tips, recipes and contact information for support chapters and resource units.
Mary Schluckebier, Executive Director

2540 Whooo's Report
American Celiac Society
PO Box 23455   504-737-3293
New Orleans, LA 70183   e-mail: amerceliacsoc@netscape.net
Provides practical assistance to members and individuals with celiac disease and information about the disease to the public.

Pamphlets

2541 Celiac Disease
Gluten Intolerance Group: GIG
31214 124th Avenue SE
Auburn, WA 98092-3667   253-833-6655
                                           Fax: 253-833-6675
                                           e-mail: info@gluten.net
                                           www.gluten.net
Offers facts and statistics on celiac disease.
Cynthia Kupper RDCD, Executive Director

2542 Celiac Disease: A Hidden Epidemic
Peter Greene, MD, author
Harper Collins Publishers
10 East 53rd Street
New York, NY 10022   212-207-7000
                                           www.harpercollins.com
An inside-out examination and explanation of Celiac Disease.
2006 352 pages
ISBN: 0-060766-93-X
Cynthia Kupper RDCD, Executive Director

2543 Dermatitis Herpetiformis
Gluten Intolerance Group: GIG
31214 124th Avenue SE   253-833-6655
Auburn, WA 98092-3667   Fax: 253-833-6675
                                           e-mail: info@gluten.net
                                           www.gluten.net
Offers facts and statistics on dermatitis herpetformis.
Cynthia Kupper RDCD, Executive Director

2544 Grains and Flours
Celiac Sprue Association/USA
PO Box 31700   402-558-0600
Omaha, NE 68131   877-272-4272
                                           Fax: 402-643-4108
                                           e-mail: celiacs@csaceliacs.org
                                           www.csaceliacs.org
A variety of different gluten-free flour mixtures, to experiment with and discover your favorite!
Mary Schluckebier, Executive Director

2545 Guide to Gluten-Free Diets
American Allergy Association
PO Box 7273   650-322-1663
Menlo Park, CA 94026-7273
Offers information on safe substitutes for baking and cooking. Differentiates celiac disease from wheat allergy. Sources of gluten in diet with warnings on when to check with the manufacturer.

2546 Patient Packet
Celiac Sprue Association/USA
PO Box 31700   402-558-0600
Omaha, NE 68131   877-272-4272
                                           Fax: 402-643-4108
                                           e-mail: celiacs@csaceliacs.org
                                           www.csaceliacs.org
A basic information packet for the newly-diagnosed celiac. Provided free of charge to individuals, physicians, dietitians, and family members.
Mary Schluckebier, Executive Director

2547 Quick Start Diet Guide
Gluten Intolerance Group: GIG
31214 124th Avenue SE   253-833-6655
Auburn, WA 98092-3667   Fax: 253-833-6675
                                           e-mail: info@gluten.net
                                           www.gluten.net
Packet available to download on website.
Cynthia Kupper RDCD, Executive Director

Audio & Video

2548 CD-A NIH Consensus Conference
Celiac Sprue Association/USA
PO Box 31700   402-558-0600
Omaha, NE 68131   877-272-4272
                                           Fax: 402-643-4108
                                           e-mail: celiacs@csaceliacs.org
                                           www.csaceliacs.org
Celiac Disease - A NIH Consensus Conference - Reaching Out to Improve the Health of Millions.
Mary Schluckebier, Executive Director

Web Sites

2549 Celiac Disease & Gluten-Free Diet Online Resource Center
                                           www.celiac.com

Internet based support organization that provides important resources and information for people on gluten-free diets due to celiac disease, gluten intolerance or wheat allergy.

2550   Celiac Disease Foundation

www.celiac.org/

Provides services and support to persons with celiac disease and dermatitus herpetiformis, through programs of awareness, education, advocacy and research; telephone information and referral services; medical advisory board; and special educational seminars and quarterly meetings.

2551   Celiac Sprue Association: USA

www.csaceliacs.org

Member based, nonprofit support organization dedicated to helping individuals with celiac disease and dermatitis herpetiformis worldwide through education, information and research. Includes over 90 support chapters, 50 resource units, and Cel-Kids Network. Sponsors an annual conference, publishes educational materials, conducts a summer youth camp and provides phone and on-line counseling.

2552   Gluten Intolerance Group: GIG

www.gluten.net

Provides instructional and general information materials, as well as counseling and access to gluten-free products and ingredients to persons with celiac sprue and their families, operates telephone information and referral service, conducts educational seminars for health professionals, conducts and supports research, offers leadership and assistance to contacts and provides for a gluten-free kids camp.

2553   Healing Well

www.healingwell.com

An online health resource guide to medical news, chat, information and articles, newsgroups and message boards, books, disease-related web sites, medical directories, and more for patients, friends, and family coping with disabling diseases, disorders, or chronic illnesses.

2554   Health Finder

www.healthfinder.gov

Searchable, carefully developed web site offering information on over 1000 topics. Developed by the US Department of Health and Human Services, the site can be used in both English and Spanish.

2555   Healthlink USA

www.healthlinkusa.com

Health information concerning treatment, cures, prevention, diagnosis, risk factors, research, support groups, email lists, personal stories and much more. Updated regularly.

2556   Helios Health

www.helioshealth.com

Online resource for your health information. Detailed information about specific health topics, access to expert advice from our Medical Advisory Board, and up-to-date health news.

2557   MedicineNet

www.medicinenet.com

An online resource for consumers providing easy-to-read, authoritative medical and health information.

2558   Medscape

www.medscape.com

Medscape offers specialists, primary care physicians, and other health professionals the Web's most robust and integrated medical information and educational tools.

2559   WebMD

www.webmd.com

Provides links to over 20 articles involving Celiac disease.

Description

2560 Cerebral Palsy

Cerebral palsy, CP, applies to disorders of voluntary movement resulting from damage to areas in the brain. CP can be caused by birth trauma, insufficient oxygen supplied to the infant at or before birth, premature birth or a severe systemic disease, such as meningitis, during early infancy. However, the exact cause is often difficult to establish.

Children with cerebral palsy may not be identified until they reach 1-2 years of age and may show only lagging motor development. Therefore, children known to be at risk should be followed closely. Increased spastic movements are the most common symptoms, but children may also show weakness, poor sense of balance, involuntary movements and abnormal walking. In more severe cases, difficulty in speaking and mental retardation may also be present.

Since there is no known cure for cerebral palsy, the goal of treatment is to develop maximal independence. Therapy may include physical and occupational rehabilitation, the use of leg braces, speech training and special orthopedic surgery. Parents need assistance and guidance in understanding their child's status and potential.

National Agencies & Associations

2561 American Academy for Cerebral Palsy and Developmental Medicine
555 E Wells St.   414-918-3014
Milwaukee, WI 53202   Fax: 414-276-2146
e-mail: info@aacpdm.org
www.aacpdm.org
A multidisciplinary scientific society devoted to the study of cerebral palsy and other childhood onset disabilities, promoting professional education for the treatment and management of these conditions and to improving the quality of life for people with the condition.
1550 members
Maureen O'Donnel, President
Scott Hoffinger, Treasurer

2562 Canadian Cerebral Palsy Sports Association
720 Belfast Rd   613-748-1430
Ottawa, Ontario, K1G 0-5K9   866-247-9934
Fax: 613-748-1355
e-mail: info@ccpsa.ca
www.ccpsa.ca
Is an athlete focused national organization administering and governing sport opportunities targeted to athletes with CP and related disabilities.
Sandy Hermiston, President
Marie Dannhaeuser, Executive Director

2563 Easter Seals
233 S Wacker Drive   312-726-6200
Chicago, IL 60606   800-221-6827
Fax: 312-726-1494
TTY: 312-726-4258
e-mail: info@easter-seals.org
www.easter-seals.org
Provides services to children and adults with disabilities as well as support to their families.
Stephen F Rossman, Chairman

2564 Independent Living Research Utilization Project
2323 S Shepherd   713-520-0232
Houston, TX 77019   Fax: 713-520-5785
TTY: 713-520-0232
e-mail: ilru@ilru.org
www.ilru.org
A national center for information training research and technical assistance in independent living. Goal is to expand the body of knowledge in independent living and to improve utilization of results of research programs and demonstration projects.
Lex Frieden, Director
Linda CoVan, Grant Coordinator

2565 National Rehabilitation Information Center
8201 Corporate Drive   301-459-5900
Landover, MD 20785   800-346-2742
Fax: 301-459-4263
TTY: 301-459-5984
e-mail: narincinfo@heitechservices.com
www.naric.com/
One of the three components of the office of Special Education and Rehabilitative Services. Operates in concert with the Rehabilitation Services Administration and the Office of Special Education Programs.
Mark Odum, Director
Jessica H. Chaiken, Media and Information Services Manager

2566 United Cerebral Palsy Associations
1660 L Street NW   202-776-0406
Washington, DC 20036   800-872-5827
Fax: 202-776-0414
TTY: 202-973-7197
e-mail: info@ucp.org
www.ucp.org
A network of approximately 119 state and local voluntary agencies which provide services conduct public and professional education programs and support research in cerebral palsy.
Stephen Bennett, President, CEO
Michael E Hill, Senior Vice President

State Agencies & Associations

Alabama

2567 United Cerebral Palsy of Alabama
301 EA Darden Drive   256-237-8203
Anniston, AL 36202   Fax: 256-235-2388
e-mail: executivedirector@ecaucp.org
www.ecaucp.org
United Cerebral Palsy provides information, advocacy, referral services for persons with disabilities and/or their families. UCP also operates an equipment loan program, conducts parent workshops, disseminates written literature on topics of interest.
Linda Johns, Executive Director
Shannon Priddy, Development Director

2568 United Cerebral Palsy of East Central Alabama
301 EA Darden Drive   256-237-8203
Anniston, AL 36202   Fax: 256-235-2388
e-mail: executivedirector@ecaucp.org
www.ecaucp.org
United Cerebral Palsy provides information, advocacy, referral services for persons with disabilities and/or their families. UCP also operates an equipment loan program, conducts parent workshops, disseminates written literature on topics of interest to people with disabilities.
Donald Turner, Chairman of the Board
John Rogers, Treasurer

2569 United Cerebral Palsy of Greater Birmingha m
120 Oslo Circle   205-944-3900
Birmingham, AL 35211   800-654-4483
Fax: 205-944-3990
e-mail: gedwards@ucpbham.com
www.ucpbham.com
United Cerebral Palsy provides information, advocacy, referral services for persons with disabilities and/or their families. UCP also operates an equipment loan program, conducts parent work-

shops, disseminates written literature on topics of interest to people with disabilities.
Gary Edwards, Executive Director
Jennifer H Ellison, Chief Development Officer

2570   United Cerebral Palsy of Huntsville & Tennessee Valley
2075 Max Luther Drive   256-852-5600
Huntsville, AL 35810   Fax: 256-852-6722
e-mail: tracyc@ucphuntsville.org
www.ucp.org
United Cerebral Palsy provides information, advocacy, referral services for persons with disabilities and/or their families. UCP also operates an equipment loan program, conducts parent workshops, disseminates written literature on topics of interest.
Cheryl Smith, Executive Director
Tim Reeves, President

2571   United Cerebral Palsy of Mobile
3058 Dauphin Square Connector   251-479-4900
Mobile, AL 36607   Fax: 251-479-4998
e-mail: info@ucpmobile.org
www.ucp.org
United Cerebral Palsy provides information, advocacy, referral services for persons with disabilities and/or their families. UCP also operates an equipment loan program, conducts parent workshops, disseminates written literature on topics of interest.
Glenn Harger, President/CEO
Susan Watson, VP/COO

2572   United Cerebral Palsy of Northwest Alabama
4212 Jackson Highway   256-381-4310
Sheffield, AL 35660   Fax: 256-381-4378
e-mail: alison@ucpshoals.org
www.ucpshoals.org
United Cerebral Palsy provides information, advocacy, referral services for persons with disabilities and/or their families. UCP also operates an equipment loan program, conducts parent workshops, disseminates written literature on topics of interest.
Alison Isbell, Director
Linda Williamson, Development Director/WEE-CARE Director

2573   United Cerebral Palsy of West Alabama
1100 UCP Parkway   205-345-3031
Northport, AL 35476   Fax: 205-345-3035
e-mail: lisasucp@comcast.net
www.ucpa.org
United Cerebral Palsy provides information, advocacy, referral services for persons with disabilities and/or their families. UCP also operates an equipment loan program, conducts parent workshops, disseminates written literature on topics of interest.
Lisa D Skelton, Executive Director
Brenda Ewart, Development Director

Alaska

2574   United Cerebral Palsy of Alaska/PARENTS
4743 E Northern Lights Boulevard   907-337-7678
Anchorage, AK 99508   800-478-7678
Fax: 907-337-7671
TTY: 907-337-7629
e-mail: parents@parentsinc.org
www.ucpa.org
Provides information, advocacy, referral services for persons with disabilities and/or their families. UCP also operates an equipment loan program, conducts parent workshops, disseminates written literature on topics of interest to people with disabilities.

Arizona

2575   United Cerebral Palsy of Central Arizona
1802 Parkside Lane   602-943-5472
Phoenix, AZ 85027   Fax: 602-943-4936
e-mail: info@ucpofaz.org
www.ucpa.org
United Cerebral Palsy provides information, advocacy, referral services for persons with disabilities and/or their families. UCP also operates an equipment loan program, conducts parent workshops, disseminates written literature on topics of interest.
Dan Rossi, Executive Director
Perry Bramlett, Chief Human Resources Officer

2576   United Cerebral Palsy of Southern Arizona
635 N Craycroft Road   520-795-3108
Tucson, AZ 85711   Fax: 520-795-3196
e-mail: staff@ucpsa.org
www.ucpsa.org
United Cerebral Palsy provides information, advocacy, referral services for persons with disabilities and/or their families. UCP also operates an equipment loan program, conducts parent workshops, disseminates written literature on topics of interest.
Cindy Mars, Executive Director
Gary Bahman, Finance Director

Arkansas

2577   United Cerebral Palsy of Central Arkansas
9720 N Rodney Parham Road   501-224-6067
Little Rock, AR 72227   Fax: 501-227-5591
e-mail: general@ucpcark.org
www.ucpark.org
United Cerebral Palsy provides information, advocacy, referral services for persons with disabilities and/or their families. UCP also operates an equipment loan program, conducts parent workshops, disseminates written literature on topics of interest.
Woody Connette, Chair
Ian Ridlon, Vice-Chairman

California

2578   United Cerebral Palsy of Central California
4224 North Cedar Avenue   559-221-8272
Fresno, CA 93726-3700   Fax: 559-221-9347
e-mail: info@ccucp.org
www.ccucp.org/
United Cerebral Palsy provides information, advocacy, referral services for persons with disabilities and/or their families. UCP also operates an equipment loan program, conducts parent workshops, disseminates written literature on topics of interest to people with disabilities.
Mark Lanier, Presdient
Carol Klonnger, Vice-President

2579   United Cerebral Palsy of Greater Sacrament o
191 Lathrop Way   916-565-7700
Sacramento, CA 95815   Fax: 916-565-7773
e-mail: ucp@ucpsacto.org
www.ucpsacto.org
UCP provides programs and services for people with all types of developmental disabilities. These services include: day programs for adults, an in-home respite service, transportation, independent living services, information and referral services.
Doug Bergman, President/CEO
Tanya Hartle, COO

2580   United Cerebral Palsy of Los Angeles & Ventura Counties
6430 Independence Avenue   818-782-2211
Woodland Hills, CA 91367   Fax: 818-909-9106
e-mail: mail@ucpla.com
www.ucpla.org
United Cerebral Palsy provides information, advocacy, referral services for persons with disabilities and/or their families. UCP also operates an equipment loan program, conducts parent workshops, disseminates written literature on topics of interest to people with disabilities.
Ronald S Cohen, Chief Executive Officer
Clark Jensen, Chief Operating Officer

2581   United Cerebral Palsy of Orange County
980 Roosevelt   949-333-6400
Irvine, CA 92602   Fax: 949-333-6400
e-mail: info@ucp-oc.org
www.ucp-oc.org
United Cerebral Palsy provides information, advocacy, referral services for persons with disabilities and/or their families. UCP also operates an equipment loan program, conducts parent workshops, disseminates written literature on topics of interest.
Paul Pulver, Executive Director
Lauren Mille Beeler, Director of Therapy Services

2582 United Cerebral Palsy of San Diego County
8525 Gibbs Drive   858-571-7803
San Diego, CA 92123   Fax: 858-571-0919
                                            e-mail: ucp@ucpsd.org
                                                      www.ucpa.org
United Cerebral Palsy provides information, advocacy, referral
services for persons with disabilities and/or their families. UCP
also operates an equipment loan program, conducts parent workshops, disseminates written literature on topics of interest.
David Carucci, Executive Director
Mary Krieger, Associate Executive Director

**2583 United Cerebral Palsy of San Joaquin, Calaveras & Amador
         Counties**
333 W Benjamin Holt Drive   209-956-0290
Stockton, CA 95207   Fax: 209-956-0294
                                         e-mail: slarson@ucpsj.org
                                                    www.ucp.org
United Cerebral Palsy provides information, advocacy, referral
services for persons with disabilities and/or their families. UCP
also operates an equipment loan program, conducts parent workshops, disseminates written literature on topics of interest to
people with disabilities.
Leslie Heier, Interim Executive Director
Theresa Galano-Burke, Executive Assistant

2584 United Cerebral Palsy of San Luis Obispo
3620 Sacramento Drive   805-543-2039
San Luis Obispo, CA 93401   877-UCP-CAR1
                                             Fax: 805-543-2045
                                          e-mail: shaftmt@aol.com
                                                    www.ucp-slo.org
United Cerebral Palsy provides information, advocacy, referral
services for persons with disabilities and/or their families. UCP
also operates an equipment loan program, conducts parent workshops, disseminates written literature on topics of interest to
people with disabilities.
Mark Shaffer, UCP Executive Director
Karl Winkler, UCP Administrative Assistant

2585 United Cerebral Palsy of Santa Barbara County
6430 Independence Avenue   818-782-2211
Woodland Hills, CA 91367   888-733-4227
                                             Fax: 818-909-9106
                                           e-mail: mail@ucpla.org
                                                     www.ucpla.org
United Cerebral Palsy provides information, advocacy, referral
services for persons with disabilities and/or their families. UCP
also operates an equipment loan program, conducts parent work-
shops, disseminates written literature on topics of interest.
Ellen Kessler, Chairperson
Nick Roxborough, President

2586 United Cerebral Palsy of Santa Clara & San Mateo Counties
512 E Maude Avenue   650-917-6900
Sunnyvale, CA 94085-4431   Fax: 650-948-8503
                                         e-mail: info@ucpscsm.org
                                                  www.ucpscsm.org/
United Cerebral Palsy provides information, advocacy, referral
services for persons with disabilities and/or their families. UCP
also operates an equipment loan program, conducts parent
shops, disseminates written literature on topics of interest.
Stephen Bennett, President/CEO National Office (DC)
Armetta Parker, Marketing/Communications Director (DC)

2587 United Cerebral Palsy of Stanislaus County
1213 13th Street   209-577-2122
Modesto, CA 95353   Fax: 209-577-2392
                                         e-mail: rlonczak@ucpstan.org
                                                    www.ucpstan.org
United Cerebral Palsy provides information, advocacy, referral
services for persons with disabilities and/or their families. UCP
also operates an equipment loan program, conducts parent workshops, disseminates written literature on topics of interest to
people with disabilities.
Robert S Lonczak, Executive Director
Jeanette Jones, ProgramCoordinator

2588 United Cerebral Palsy of the Golden Gate
1970 Broadway   510-832-7430
Oakland, CA 94612   Fax: 510-839-1329
                                         e-mail: info@ucpgg.org
                                                    www.ucp.org
United Cerebral Palsy provides information, advocacy, referral
services for persons with disabilities and/or their families. UCP
also operates an equipment loan program, conducts parent workshops, disseminates written literature on topics of interest.
Karen Glatze, Administrator
Dori Maxon, SNAP Program Director

2589 United Cerebral Palsy of the Inland Empire
35-325 Date Palm Drive   760-321-8184
Cathedral City, CA 92234   877-512-2224
                                             Fax: 760-321-8284
                                          e-mail: info@ucpie.org
                                                    www.ucpie.org
United Cerebral Palsy provides information, advocacy, referral
services for persons with disabilities and/or their families. UCP
conducts parent workshops, disseminates written literature on top-
ics of interest to people with disabilities.
Roger M Alexander, Chair
Micki James, Vice Chair

2590 United Cerebral Palsy of the North Bay
3835 Cypress Drive   707-766-9990
Petaluma, CA 94954   800-872-5827
                                             Fax: 202-776-0414
                                          e-mail: info@ucpnb.org
                                                    www.ucp.org
United Cerebral Palsy's mission is to advance the independence,
productivity and full citizenship of people with disabilities
through an affiliate network.
Margaret Farman, Executive Director
Ron Hamilton, Chief of Operations

Colorado

2591 United Cerebral Palsy of Colorado
801 Yosemite Street   303-691-9339
Denver, CO 80230-5708   866-701-2277
                                             Fax: 303-691-0846
                                                    www.cpco.org
United Cerebral Palsy provides information, advocacy, referral
services for persons with disabilities and/or their families. UCP
also operates an equipment loan program, conducts parent workshops, disseminates written literature on topics of interest.
Jim Reuter, Chairman of the Board
Judith I Ham, President/CEO

Connecticut

2592 United Cerebral Palsy of Eastern Connecticut
42 Norwich Road   860-447-3800
Quaker Hill, CT 06375   Fax: 860-443-8272
                                         e-mail: email@ucpect.org
                                                    www.ucp.org
United Cerebral Palsy provides information, advocacy, referral
services for persons with disabilities and/or their families. UCP
also operates an equipment loan program, conducts parent workshops, disseminates written literature on topics of interest to
people with disabilities.
Margaret Morrison, Executive Director
Patricia Mansfield, Executive Director

2593 United Cerebral Palsy of Greater Hartford
80 Whitney Street   860-236-6201
Hartford, CT 06105   Fax: 860-218-2454
                                         e-mail: jmcmahon@sunrisegroup.org
                                                    www.ucphartford.org
United Cerebral Palsy provides information, advocacy, referral
services for persons with disabilities and/or their families. UCP
also operates an equipment loan program, conducts parent workshops, disseminates written literature on topics of interest to
people with disabilities.
Pam Reid, Regional Administrator
Sean Thompson, In-Home Support Coordinator

2594   United Cerebral Palsy of Southern Connecticut
94-96 South Turnpike Road   203-269-3511
Wallingford, CT 06492   Fax: 203-269-7411
                                    e-mail: ucpasouthernct@yahoo.com
                                                    www.ucpa.org
United Cerebral Palsy provides information, advocacy, referral services for persons with disabilities and/or their families. UCP also operates an equipment loan program, conducts parent workshops, disseminates written literature on topics of interest to people with disabilities.

Delaware

2595   United Cerebral Palsy of Delaware
700 A River Road   302-764-2400
Wilmington, DE 19809-2746   Fax: 302-764-8713
                                         e-mail: wmccool@ucpde.org
                                    www.ucp.org/ucp_local.cfm/52
United Cerebral Palsy provides information, advocacy, referral services for persons with disabilities and/or their families. UCP also operates an equipment loan program, conducts parent workshops, disseminates written literature on topics of interest.
Michelle Welch, President
D Bruce McClenathan, Vice President

District of Columbia

2596   United Cerebral Palsy of Washington DC
1818 New York Avenue   202-526-0146
Washington, DC 20002   Fax: 202-526-0519
                                          e-mail: dcarter@ucpdc.org
                                                    www.ucpdc.org
United Cerebral Palsy provides information, advocacy, referral services for persons with disabilities and/or their families. UCP also operates an equipment loan program, conducts parent workshops, disseminates written literature on topics of interest.
Mark A Simione, Board President
Roderick Johnson, Board Secretary

2597   United Cerebral Palsy of Washington DC & Northern Virginia
1818 New York Avenue NE   202-526-0146
Washington, DC 20002   Fax: 202-526-0519
                                      e-mail: webmaster@ucpdcnova.org
                                                    www.ucpdc.org
United Cerebral Palsy provides information, advocacy, referral services for persons with disabilities and/or their families. UCP also operates an equipment loan program, conducts parent workshops, disseminates written literature on topics of interest to people with disabilities.
Mark Simione, President
George Connors, 1st Vice President

Florida

2598   United Cerebral Palsy of Central Florida
3305 S Orange Avenue   407-852-3300
Orlando, FL 32806   Fax: 407-852-3301
                                          e-mail: mbetts@ucpcdc.org
                                                    www.ucpcfl.org
United Cerebral Palsy provides information, advocacy, referral services for persons with disabilities and/or their families. UCP also operates an equipment loan program, conducts parent workshops, disseminates written literature on topics of interest.
Ilene E Wilkins, President & Chief Executive Officer
Jill Wisth, Chief Financial Officer

2599   United Cerebral Palsy of East Central Florida
1100 Jimmy Ann Drive   386-274-6474
Daytona Beach, FL 32117   Fax: 386-274-6532
                                            e-mail: info@ucpecf.org
                                                    www.ucp.org

Barry Pollack, President/CEO
Kelly Johanessen, VP of Operations

2600   United Cerebral Palsy of Florida
1830 Buford Court   850-922-5630
Tallahassee, FL 32308   Fax: 850-922-1258
                                       e-mail: gloriawe@earthlink.net
                                                    www.ucp.org

United Cerebral Palsy provides information, advocacy, referral services for persons with disabilities and/or their families. UCP also operates an equipment loan program, conducts parent workshops, disseminates written literature on topics of interest.

2601   United Cerebral Palsy of North Florida: Tender Loving Care
1241 NE Avenue   850-769-7960
Panama City, FL 32401   Fax: 850-769-1060
                                  e-mail: kimberly.mcmanus@comcast.net
                                                    www.ucp.org
United Cerebral Palsy provides information, advocacy, referral services for persons with disabilities and/or their families. UCP also operates an equipment loan program, conducts parent workshops, disseminates written literature on topics of interest to people with disabilities.

2602   United Cerebral Palsy of Northeast Florida
3311 Beach Boulevard   904-396-1462
Jacksonville, FL 32207   Fax: 904-396-1199
                                     e-mail: cpnefagency@hotmail.com

2603   United Cerebral Palsy of Northwest Florida
2912 North East Street   850-432-1596
Pensacola, FL 32501-1324   Fax: 850-432-1930
                                     e-mail: information@ucpnwfl.org
                                                    www.ucpnwfl.org/
The number one service provider in Northwest Florida for individuals with cerebral palsy and other developmental disabilities, UCP provides information ,advocacy and referral services for persons with disabilities and/or their families. Additionally, UCP offers individuals assistance with daily living skills training, computer training, basic education, speech, physical and occupational therapy, residential, supported living and finding long-term employment.
Brain Bell, Chair
Michelle Fielder, Vice-Chairman

2604   United Cerebral Palsy of Sarasota-Manatee
1090 S Tamiami Trail   941-957-3599
Sarasota, FL 34236   Fax: 947-957-3499
                                         e-mail: ucpwendy@aol.com
                                                 www.ucpsarasota.org
United Cerebral Palsy provides information, advocacy, referral services for persons with disabilities and/or their families. UCP also operates an equipment loan program, conducts parent workshops, disseminates written literature on topics of interest.
Barnett A Greenberg, Chairperson
Mark Famiglio, President

2605   United Cerebral Palsy of South Florida
2700 W 81st Street   305-325-1080
Hialeah, FL 33016   Fax: 305-325-1313
                                   e-mail: info@ucpsouthflorida.org
                                                    www.ucp.org
United Cerebral Palsy provides information, advocacy, referral services for persons with disabilities and/or their families. UCP also operates an equipment loan program, conducts parent workshops, disseminates written literature on topics of interest.
Joseph Aniello, President & CEO
Linda Gluck, Vice President & CFO

2606   United Cerebral Palsy of Tallahassee
1830 Buford Court   850-878-2141
Tallahassee, FL 32308   Fax: 850-922-1258
                                       e-mail: gloriawe@earthlink.net
                                                    www.ucp.org
United Cerebral Palsy provides information, advocacy, referral services for persons with disabilities and/or their families. UCP also operates an equipment loan program, conducts parent workshops, disseminates written literature on topics of interest.

2607   United Cerebral Palsy of Tampa Bay
2215 E Henry Avenue   813-239-1179
Tampa, FL 33610   800-749-5155
                                               Fax: 813-237-3091
                                    e-mail: kryals@advanceability.org
                                                 www.ucptampa.org
United Cerebral Palsy provides information, advocacy, referral services for persons with disabilities and/or their families. UCP also operates an equipment loan program, conducts parent work-

shops, disseminates written literature on topics of interest to people with disabilities.
Jim King, Executive Director
Dawn Gosselin, Executive Development Assistant / Events

Georgia

2608   United Cerebral Palsy of Georgia
3300 NE Expressway   770-676-2000
Atlanta, GA 30341   Fax: 770-455-8040
                                             e-mail: info@ucpga.org
                                                    www.ucp.org
United Cerebral Palsy provides information, advocacy, referral services for persons with disabilities and/or their families. UCP also operates an equipment loan program, conducts parent workshops, disseminates written literature on topics of interest to people with disabilities.
Diane Wilush, Executive Director
Kevin Walton, Associate Executive Director

Hawaii

2609   United Cerebral Palsy of Hawaii
414 Kuwili Street   808-532-6744
Honolulu, HI 96817-5050   800-606-5654
                                             Fax: 808-532-6747
                                     e-mail: ucpa@diverseabilities.org
                                                    www.ucpahi.org
United Cerebral Palsy provides information, advocacy, referral services for persons with disabilities and/or their families. UCP also operates an equipment loan program, conducts parent workshops, disseminates written literature on topics of interest.
Jerry Pupillo, President
Stephen Hink, 1st Vice President

Idaho

2610   United Cerebral Palsy of Idaho
5420 W Franklin Road   208-377-8070
Boise, ID 83705   888-289-3281
                                             Fax: 208-322-7133
                                          e-mail: info@ucpidaho.org
                                                    www.ucp.org
United Cerebral Palsy provides information, advocacy and referral services for persons with disabilities and/or their families.
Kim Kane, Executive Director
Kathy Griffin, Program Director

Illinois

2611   United Cerebral Palsy Land of Lincoln
101 N 16th Street   217-525-6522
Springfield, IL 67203   Fax: 217-525-9017
                                             e-mail: info@ucpll.org
                                                    www.ucp.org
United Cerebral Palsy provides information, advocacy, referral services for persons with disabilities and/or their families. UCP also operates an equipment loan program, conducts parent workshops, disseminates written literature on topics of interest.
Brenda L Yarnell, President/CEO
Kathy Leuelling, Chief Operating Officer

2612   United Cerebral Palsy of East Central Illinois
1023 N Water   217-428-5033
Decatur, IL 62523   Fax: 217-428-5094
                                                    ww.ucpa.org
United Cerebral Palsy provides information, advocacy, referral services for persons with disabilities and/or their families. UCP also operates an equipment loan program, conducts parent workshops, disseminates written literature on topics of interest.
Woody Connette, Chair

2613   United Cerebral Palsy of Greater Chicago
547 W Jackson   312-765-0419
Chicago, IL 60661   Fax: 312-765-0503
                                             TTY: 312-368-0179
                                         e-mail: pdulle@ucpnet.org
                                                    www.ucpnet.org

United Cerebral Palsy provides information, advocacy, referral services for persons with disabilities and/or their families. UCP also operates an equipment loan program, conducts parent workshops, disseminates written literature on topics of interest to people with disabilities.
Paul J Dulle, President/CEO
Peggy Childs, Executive Vice President

2614   United Cerebral Palsy of Illinois
310 E Adams   877-550-8274
Springfield, IL 62701   877-550-8274
                                             Fax: 217-528-9739
                                             TTY: 877-550-8274
                                         e-mail: cpil@sbcglobal.net
                                                    www.ucpillinois.org
United Cerebral Palsy provides information, advocacy, referral services for persons with disabilities and/or their families. UCP also operates an equipment loan program, conducts parent workshops, disseminates written literature on topics of interest to people with disabilities.
Don Moss, Executive Director
Alice Foss, Associate Director

2615   United Cerebral Palsy of Southern Illinois
9 Cusumano Professional Plaza Drive   618-244-2505
Mount Vernon, IL 62864   Fax: 618-244-3568
                                         e-mail: ucpsi@onemain.com
                                                    www.ucpa.org
United Cerebral Palsy provides information, advocacy, referral services for persons with disabilities and/or their families. UCP also operates an equipment loan program, conducts parent workshops, disseminates written literature on topics of interest to people with disabilities.

2616   United Cerebral Palsy of Will County
311 S Reed Street   815-744-3500
Joliet, IL 60436   Fax: 815-744-3504
                                         e-mail: ucpwill@ucpwill.org
                                                    www.ucp.org
United Cerebral Palsy provides information, advocacy, referral services for persons with disabilities and/or their families. UCP also operates an equipment loan program, conducts parent workshops, disseminates written literature on topics of interest to people with disabilities.
Samuel Mancuso, President & Chief Executive Officer
Stephanie Bergner, Family Support/Respite Administrator

2617   United Cerebral Palsy of the Blackhawk Region
7399 Forest Hills Road   815-636-7132
Rockford, IL 61111   Fax: 815-282-8835
                                         e-mail: ucpbr@aol.com
                                                    www.ucpa.org
United Cerebral Palsy provides information, advocacy, referral services for persons with disabilities and/or their families. UCP also operates an equipment loan program, conducts parent workshops, disseminates written literature on topics of interest to people with disabilities.

2618   United Cerebral Palsy: Eastern Seals
230 W Monroe Street   312-726-6200
Chicago, IL 60606   800-221-6827
                                             Fax: 312-726-1494
                                                    www.stsweb.indstate.edu
United Cerebral Palsy provides information, advocacy, referral services for persons with disabilities and/or their families. UCP also operates an equipment loan program, conducts parent workshops, disseminates written literature on topics of interest.
John Rogers, IT consultant
Tyler Howe, Project Manager

Indiana

2619   United Cerebral Palsy Association of Indiana
1915 West 18th Street   317-632-3561
Indianapolis, IN 46202-1016   Fax: 317-632-3338
                                         e-mail: donnar@ucpaindy.org
                                                    www.ucpa.org
United Cerebral Palsy provides information, advocacy, referral services for persons with Cerebral Palsy and/or their families. UCP also provides funding for equipment and operates an equipment

loan program, disseminates written literature on topics of interest to people with disabilities.
Donna L Roberts, Executive Director

2620   United Cerebral Palsy Associations
6100 N Keystone Avenue   317-632-3561
Indianapolis, IN 46220   Fax: 317-632-3338
                                             e-mail: donnar@ucpaindy.org
                                                      www.ucpaindy.org
United Cerebral Palsy provides information, advocacy, referral services for persons with Cerebral Palsy and/or their families. UCP also provides funding for equipment and operates an equipment loan program, disseminates written literature on topics of interest.
Donna L Roberts, Executive Director
Beth Allison, Case Manager

2621   United Cerebral Palsy of the Wabash Valley
621 Poplar Street   812-232-6305
Terre Haute, IN 47807   Fax: 812-234-3683
                                            e-mail: ucp.wv@verizon.net
                                                       www.ucpwv.org
United Cerebral Palsy provides information, advocacy, referral services for persons with disabilities and/or their families. UCP also operates an equipment loan program, conducts parent workshops, disseminates written literature on topics of interest to people with disabilities.
Jacquie Denehie, Executive Director
Brain Garcia, President

Kansas

2622   United Cerebral Palsy of Kansas
5111 E 21st Street   316-688-1888
Wichita, KS 67208   Fax: 316-688-5687
                                              e-mail: davej@cprf.org
                                                          www.ucp.org
United Cerebral Palsy provides information, advocacy, referral services for persons with disabilities and/or their families. UCP also operates an equipment loan program, conducts parent workshops, disseminates written literature on topics of interest.
Dave Jones, Executive Director
Amelia Ornelas, Office Manager

Louisiana

2623   United Cerebral Palsy of Baton Rouge McMains Children's Developmental Center
1805 College Drive   225-923-3420
Baton Rouge, LA 70808   Fax: 225-922-9316
                                          e-mail: jketcham@mcmainscdc.org
                                                      www.mcmainscdc.org
United Cerebral Palsy provides information, advocacy, referral services for persons with disabilities and/or their families. UCP also operates an equipment loan program, conducts parent workshops, disseminates written literature on topics of interest.
Janet Ketcham, Director
Norman Landry, President

2624   United Cerebral Palsy of Greater New Orleans
1000 Leonidas St & Leake Avenue   504-865-0003
New Orleans, LA 70118   Fax: 504-865-0300
                                             e-mail: info@ucpgno.com
                                                        www.ucpgno.org
United Cerebral Palsy provides information, advocacy, referral services for persons with disabilities and/or their families. UCP also operates an equipment loan program, conducts parent workshops, disseminates written literature on topics of interest to people with disabilities.
Tommy Freel, Chair
Joanne Rinardo, Treasurer

Maine

2625   United Cerebral Palsy of Northeastern Maine
700 Mount Hope Avenue   207-941-2952
Bangor, ME 04401   877-603-0030
                                                  Fax: 207-941-2955
                                          e-mail: office@ucpofmaine.org
                                                          www.ucp.org

United Cerebral Palsy provides information, advocacy, referral services for persons with disabilities and/or their families. UCP also operates an equipment loan program, conducts parent workshops, disseminates written literature on topics of interest to people with disabilities.
Bobbi-Jo Yeager, Executive Director
Tricia Kail, Director of Services

Maryland

2626   United Cerebral Palsy of Central Maryland
1700 Reistertown Road   410-484-4540
Baltimore, MD 21208-2935   Fax: 410-484-1807
                                                   TTY: 800-451-2452
                                              e-mail: info@ucp-cm.org
                                                          www.ucp.org
United Cerebral Palsy provides information, advocacy, referral services for persons with disabilities and/or their families. UCP also operates an equipment loan program, conducts parent workshops, disseminates written literature on topics of interest.
Diane Coughlin, President and CEO
Judy Cox, Assistant to the President

2627   United Cerebral Palsy of Prince Georges & Montgomery Counties
4409 Forbes Boulevard   301-459-0566
Lanham, MD 20706   Fax: 301-459-7691
                                                   TTY: 301-459-7691
                                                   TDD: 301-262-4982
                                            e-mail: ucppgmc@aol.com
                                                       www.ucppgmc.com
Provides information, advocacy, referral services for persons with disabilities and/or their families. UCP also operates an equipment loan program, conducts parent workshops, disseminates written literature on topics of interest to people with disabilities.
Charles McNelly, Executive Director
Diane Dekoladenu, Program Director

2628   United Cerebral Palsy of Southern Maryland
221 Chinquapin Round Road   410-280-2003
Annapolis, MD 21401   Fax: 410-269-5757
                                             e-mail: ucpinfo@ucpsm.org
                                                          www.ucpsm.org
United Cerebral Palsy provides information, advocacy, referral services for persons with disabilities and/or their families. UCP also operates an equipment loan program, conducts parent workshops, disseminates written literature on topics of interest to people with disabilities.

Massachusetts

2629   United Cerebral Palsy of Berkshire County
208 W Street   413-442-1562
Pittsfield, MA 01201   Fax: 413-499-4077
                                            e-mail: info@ucpberkshire.org
                                                          www.ucp.org
United Cerebral Palsy provides information, advocacy, referral services for persons with disabilities and/or their families. UCP also operates an equipment loan program, conducts parent workshops, disseminates written literature on topics of interest to people with disabilities.
Christine Singer, Executive Director
Joni Thomas, Director of Development

2630   United Cerebral Palsy of MetroBoston
71 Arsenal Street   617-926-5480
Watertown, MA 02472   Fax: 617-926-3059
                                          e-mail: ucpboston@ucpboston.org
                                                          www.ucp.org
United Cerebral Palsy provides information, advocacy, referral services for persons with disabilities and/or their families. UCP also operates an equipment loan program, conducts parent workshops, disseminates written literature on topics of interest.
Todd Kates, Executive Director
Roberta Jaro, Associate Executive Director

Michigan

2631 **United Cerebral Palsy of Metropolitan Detroit**
23077 Greenfield   248-557-5070
Southfield, MI 48075   Fax: 248-557-0224
e-mail: main@ucpdetroit.org
www.ucp.org
United Cerebral Palsy provides information, advocacy, referral services for persons with disabilities and/or their families. UCP also operates an equipment loan program, conducts parent workshops, disseminates written literature on topics of interest.
Leslynn Angel, President & CEO
Latoya Jones, Chief Financial Officer

2632 **United Cerebral Palsy of Michigan**
4970 Northwind Drive   517-203-1200
E Lansing, MI 48823   800-828-2714
Fax: 517-203-1203
e-mail: ucp@ucpmichigan.org
www.ucp.org
United Cerebral Palsy provides information, advocacy, referral services for persons with disabilities and/or their families. UCP also operates an equipment loan program, conducts parent workshops, disseminates written literature on topics of interest.
Linda Potter, Executive Director
Linda Carey, Office Manager

Minnesota

2633 **United Cerebral Palsy of Central Minnesota**
510 25th Avenue North   320-253-0765
St. Cloud, MN 56303-3255   Fax: 320-253-6753
e-mail: info@ucpcentralmn.org
www.ucpcentralmn.org
Provides information, advocacy, referral services for persons with disabilities and/or their families. UCP conducts parent workshops, disseminates free newsletter. Computers go round recycles quality used computers to persons with disabilities. UCP awards scholarship for post secondary education.
Shelly Gaetz, President
Sue Schlosser, Vice-President

2634 **United Cerebral Palsy of Minnesota**
1821 University Avenue W   651-646-7588
St Paul, MN 55104-2892   877-528-5678
Fax: 651-646-3045
e-mail: ucpmnStacey@hotmail.com
www.ucp.org
United Cerebral Palsy provides information, advocacy, referral services for persons with disabilities and/or their families. UCP also operates an equipment loan program, conducts parent workshops, disseminates written literature on topics of interest.
Stacey Vogele, Executive Director
Ramsey Lee, Events Coordinator

Missouri

2635 **United Cerebral Palsy of Greater Kansas City**
1044 Main Street   816-531-4454
Kansas City, MO 64105   Fax: 816-531-3383
e-mail: bscott@ucpkc.org
www.ucp.org
Provides information, advocacy, referral services for persons with disabilities and/or their families. UCP also operates residential programs and care management for seniors.
Bruce A Scott, President & CEO
Sam T Switzer, Senior Vice President & CFO

2636 **United Cerebral Palsy of Greater St. Louis**
13975 Mancester Rd   636-227-6030
Manchester, MO 63011-3999   Fax: 636-779-2270
e-mail: forkoshr@ucpstl.org
www.ucpheartland.org/
United Cerebral Palsy provides information, advocacy, referral services for persons with disabilities and/or their families. UCP also operates an equipment loan program, conducts parent workshops, disseminates written literature on topics of interest to people with disabilities.
Woody Connette, Chair
Lan Ridlon, Vice Chair

2637 **United Cerebral Palsy of Northwest Missouri**
3303 Frederick Avenue   816-364-3836
St. Joseph, MO 64506   Fax: 816-390-8546
e-mail: ucp@ucpnwmo.org
www.ucpa.org
United Cerebral Palsy provides information, advocacy, referral services for persons with disabilities and/or their families. UCP also operates an equipment loan program, conducts parent workshops, disseminates written literature on topics of interest to people with disabilities.
Jared Bronner, President
Shawn Drew, Vice-President

Nebraska

2638 **United Cerebral Palsy of Nebraska**
920 S 107th Avenue   402-502-3572
Omaha, NE 68114   800-729-2556
Fax: 402-502-6791
e-mail: jennyh@ucpnebraska.org
www.ucp.org
United Cerebral Palsy provides information, advocacy, referral services for persons with disabilities and/or their families. UCP also operates an equipment loan program, conducts parent workshops, disseminates written literature on topics of interest.
Carol Hahn, Executive Director
Anne Brodin, Financial & Services Director

Nevada

2639 **United Cerebral Palsy of Northern Nevada**
4068 S McCarran Boulevard   775-331-3323
Reno, NV 89502-7532   Fax: 775-331-7913
e-mail: upcnn@ucpnn.org
www.ucpnv.org
United Cerebral Palsy provides information, advocacy, referral services for persons with disabilities and/or their families. UCP also provides employment and supported living services and disseminates written literature on topics of interest.
E. Sue Saunders, Chairperson
Julie Ann Utley, Vice Chairperson

New Jersey

2640 **United Cerebral Palsy of Hudson County**
721 Broadway   201-436-2200
Bayonne, NJ 07002   Fax: 201-436-6642
e-mail: kkearney@ucpofhudsoncounty.org
www.ucp.org
United Cerebral Palsy provides information, advocacy, referral services for persons with disabilities and/or their families. UCP also operates an equipment loan program, conducts parent workshops, disseminates written literature on topics of interest to people with disabilities.
Nick Starita, Executive Director
Keith J Kearney, Associate Executive Director

2641 **United Cerebral Palsy of Morris-Somerset**
245 Main Street   908-879-2243
Chester, NJ 07930   Fax: 908-879-8363
e-mail: info@ucpnj.org
www.ucpa.org
United Cerebral Palsy provides information, advocacy, referral services for persons with disabilities and/or their families. UCP also operates an equipment loan program, conducts parent workshops, disseminates written literature on topics of interest.

2642 **United Cerebral Palsy of New Jersey**
1005 Whitehead Road Extension   609-392-4004
Ewing, NJ 08638   888-322-1918
Fax: 609-882-4054
TTY: 609-882-0620
e-mail: info@cpofnj.org
www.cpofnj.org
United Cerebral Palsy provides information, advocacy, referral services for persons with disabilities and/or their families. UCP

also operates an equipment loan program, conducts parent workshops, disseminates written literature on topics of interest.
Mathew Jacobs, President
Warren Kelemen, Vice-President

New York

2643 Center for the Disabled
314 S Manning Boulevard   518-437-5700
Albany, NY 12208   e-mail: bulgaro@cftd.org
                                 www.cfdsny.org
United Cerebral Palsy provides information, advocacy, referral services for persons with disabilities and/or their families. UCP also operates an equipment loan program, conducts parent workshops, disseminates written literature on topics of interest to people with disabilities.
Alan Krafchin, CEO/President
Patrick J Rielly, Chief Operating Officer

2644 Cerebral Palsy Associations of New York State
90 State Street   518-436-0178
Albany, NY 12207   Fax: 518-436-8619
                                 e-mail: AffiliateServices@cpofnys.org
                                 www.cpofnys.org
Provides information, advocacy, referral services for persons with disabilities and/or their families. CP also operates an equipment loan program, conducts parent workshops and disseminates written literature on topics of interest to people with disabilities.
Michael Alvaro, Executive Vice President
Susan Constantino, President & CEO

2645 Niagara Cerebral Palsy
9812 Lockport Road   716-297-0798
Niagara Falls, NY 14304   Fax: 716-297-0998
                                 e-mail: info@niagaracp.org
                                 www.ucpaofniagara.com
Provides educational, residential, vocational and recreational programs.

2646 Prospect Child And Family Center
133 Aviation Road   518-798-0170
Queensbury, NY 12804   Fax: 518-798-0533
                                 e-mail: pcfccent@prospectcenter.com
                                 www.prospectcenter.com

Gary Edie, President
Eli Socolof, Vice-President

2647 United Cerebral Palsy of Chemung County
1118 Charles Street   607-734-7107
Elmira, NY 14901   Fax: 607-734-7334
                                 www.chemungcp.com
United Cerebral Palsy provides information, advocacy, referral services for persons with disabilities and/or their families. UCP also operates an equipment loan program, conducts parent workshops, disseminates written literature on topics of interest to people with disabilities.
Mark Peters, Executive Director
Leisa Alger, Associate Executive Director

2648 United Cerebral Palsy of Fulton & Montgomery Counties
67 Division Street   518-842-3511
Amsterdam, NY 12010   Fax: 518-843-6042
                                 www.ucpa.org
United Cerebral Palsy provides information, advocacy, referral services for persons with disabilities and/or their families. UCP also operates an equipment loan program, conducts parent workshops, disseminates written literature on topics of interest to people with disabilities.

2649 United Cerebral Palsy of Greater Suffolk
250 Marcus Boulevard   631-232-0011
Hauppauge, NY 11788   Fax: 631-232-4422
                                 e-mail: info@ucp-suffolk.org
                                 www.ucp-suffolk.org
United Cerebral Palsy provides information, advocacy, referral services for persons with disabilities and/or their families. UCP also operates an equipment loan program, conducts parent workshops, disseminates written literature on topics of interest.
Stephen H Friedman, President & CEO
James Monnier, Board of Directors

2650 United Cerebral Palsy of Nassau County
380 Washington Avenue   516-378-2000
Roosevelt, NY 11575   Fax: 516-868-4089
                                 e-mail: info@ucpn.org
                                 www.ucpn.org
United Cerebral Palsy provides information, advocacy, referral services for persons with disabilities and/or their families. UCP also operates an equipment loan program, conducts parent workshops, disseminates written literature on topics of interest to people with disabilities.
Robert Masterson, President
Thomas Connolly, Executive Vice President

2651 United Cerebral Palsy of New York City
80 Maiden Lane   212-683-6700
New York, NY 10038-4811   800-GIV-EUCP
                                 Fax: 212-685-8394
                                 e-mail: info@ucpnyc.org
                                 www.ucpnyc.org
United Cerebral Palsy provides information, advocacy, referral services for persons with disabilities and/or their families. UCP also operates an equipment loan program, conducts parent workshops, disseminates written literature on topics of interest.
Edward R. Matthews, Chief Executive Officer
Gary Geresi, President

2652 United Cerebral Palsy of Putnam & Southern Dutchess Counties
40 John Barrett Road   845-878-9078
Patterson, NY 12563   Fax: 845-878-3203
                                 e-mail: hvcs@aol.com
                                 www.ucpa.org
United Cerebral Palsy provides information, advocacy, referral services for persons with disabilities and/or their families. UCP also operates an equipment loan program, conducts parent workshops, disseminates written literature on topics of interest to people with disabilities.

2653 United Cerebral Palsy of Queens: Queens Centers for Progress
81-15 164th Street   718-380-3000
Jamaica, NY 11432   Fax: 718-380-0483
                                 TTY: 718-969-0270
                                 e-mail: info@queenscp.org
                                 www.queenscp.org
Provides information advocacy and referral services for persons with disabilities and/or their families. Offers an equipment loan program parent workshops and written literature on topics of interest to people with disabilities.
George Wildi Berger, President
Joseph A Cristiano, Vice-President

2654 United Cerebral Palsy of Westchester County
1186 King Street   914-937-3800
Rye Brook, NY 10573   Fax: 914-937-0967
                                 www.cpwestchester.org
United Cerebral Palsy provides information advocacy referral services for persons with disabilities and/or their families. UCP also operates an equipment loan program conducts parent workshops disseminates written literature on topics of interest to people with disabilities.
Richard Osterer, President
Richard Eising, Executive Vice President

2655 United Cerebral Palsy of Western New York
7 Community Drive   716-894-0130
Buffalo, NY 14225   Fax: 716-894-8257
                                 e-mail: ucpawny1@aol.com
                                 www.ucpa.org
United Cerebral Palsy provides information advocacy referral services for persons with disabilities and/or their families. UCP also operates an equipment loan program conducts parent workshops disseminates written literature on topics of interest to people with disabilities.

2656 United Cerebral Palsy of the North Country
4 Commerce Lane   315-379-9667
Canton, NY 13617   Fax: 315-379-9388
                                 e-mail: ucpa@imcnet.net
                                 www.cpnorthcountry.org/
United Cerebral Palsy provides information advocacy referral services for persons with disabilities and/or their families. UCP also

operates an equipment loan program conducts parent workshops disseminates written literature on topics of interest to people with disabilities.

North Carolina

2657 Easter Seals UCP North Carolina & Virginia
2315 Myron Drive   919-783-8898
Raleigh, NC 27607   800-662-7119
                                        Fax: 919-782-5486
                        e-mail: QM@nc.eastersealsucp.com
                                    www.nc.easterseals.com
A lifelong partner to families managing disabilities and mental health challenges. Serves more than 20,000 individuals and their families annually through an array of services. Enhances the quality of life for individuals and maximizes their potential for engaging in their communities.
Connie L Cochran, President/CEO

Ohio

2658 United Cerebral Palsy of Central Ohio
440 Industrial Mile Road   614-279-0109
Columbus, OH 43228-2411   Fax: 914-279-2527
                        e-mail: tfitch@ucpofcentralohio.org
                                    www.ucpofcentralohio.org
United Cerebral Palsy provides information advocacy referral services for persons with disabilities and/or their families. UCP also operates an equipment loan program conducts parent workshops disseminates written literature on topics of interest to people with disabilities.
Charles Dyas, President/Executive Committee Chair
Diane Dierna, Vice-President

2659 United Cerebral Palsy of Cincinnati
3601 Victory Parkway   513-221-4606
Cincinnati, OH 45229   Fax: 513-872-5262
                        e-mail: sschiller@ucp-cincinnati.org
                                       www.ucp-cincinnati.org
United Cerebral Palsy provides information advocacy referral services for persons with disabilities and/or their families. UCP also operates an equipment loan program conducts parent workshops disseminates written literature on topics of interest to people with disabilities.
Susan Schiller, Executive Director, Development Director

2660 United Cerebral Palsy of Greater Cleveland
10011 Euclid Avenue   216-791-8363
Cleveland, OH 44106   Fax: 216-721-3372
                        e-mail: sdean@ucpcleveland.org
                                       www.ucpcleveland.org/
United Cerebral Palsy provides information, advocacy, referral services for persons with disabilities and/or their families. UCP also operates an equipment loan program, conducts parent workshops, disseminates written literature on topics of interest to people with disabilities.
Mathew Cox, Chair
Sean Wenger, Vice-Chairman

2661 United Cerebral Palsy of Greater Dane
10011 Euclid Avenue   216-791-8363
Cleveland, OH 44106   Fax: 216-721-3372
                        e-mail: sdean@ucpcleveland.org
                                       www.ucpcleveland.org
United Cerebral Palsy provides information advocacy referral services for persons with disabilities and/or their families. UCP also operates an equipment loan program disseminates written literature on topics of interest to people with disabilities.
Robert J Darden, President
Douglas A Neary, Vice President

Oklahoma

2662 United Cerebral Palsy of Oklahoma
10400 Greenbriar Place   405-759-3562
Oklahoma City, OK 73159   Fax: 405-917-7082
                                      e-mail: info@ucpok.org
                                               www.ucpok.org

United Cerebral Palsy provides information advocacy referral services for persons with disabilities and/or their families. UCP also operates an equipment loan program conducts parent workshops disseminates written literature on topics of interest to people with disabilities.

Oregon

2663 United Cerebral Palsy of Oregon & SW Washington
11731 NE Glenn Widing Drive   503-777-4166
Portland, OR 97220   800-473-4581
                                        Fax: 503-771-8048
                             e-mail: ucpa@ucpaorwa.org
                                                www.ucp.org
United Cerebral Palsy provides information advocacy referral services for persons with disabilities and/or their families. UCP also operates an equipment loan program conducts parent workshops disseminates written literature on topics of interest to people with disabilities.
Bud Thoune, Executive Director
Doug Taylor, Development and Marketing Director

Pennsylvania

2664 United Cerebral Palsy Central PA
44 S 38th Street   717-975-0611
Camp Hill, PA 17011   Fax: 717-975-0839
                        e-mail: kidscenter@ucpcentralpa.org
                                                www.ucp.org
United Cerebral Palsy provides information advocacy referral services for persons with disabilities and/or their families. UCP also operates an equipment loan program conducts parent workshops disseminates written literature on topics of interest to people with disabilities.
Jeffrey W Cooper, President/CEO
Jennifer Brubaker, Director of Administrative Services

2665 United Cerebral Palsy of Beaver, Butler & Lawrence Counties
101 Hindman Lane   724-482-4765
Butler, PA 16001   Fax: 724-283-5945
                                                www.ucpa.org
United Cerebral Palsy provides information, advocacy, referral services for persons with disabilities and/or their families. UCP also operates an equipment loan program, conducts parent workshops, disseminates written literature on topics of interest to people with disabilities.

2666 United Cerebral Palsy of Northwestern Pennsylvania
3745 W 12th Street   814-836-9113
Erie, PA 16505   Fax: 814-833-3919
                              e-mail: leaton@mecaup.com
                                                www.ucpa.org
United Cerebral Palsy provides information advocacy referral services for persons with disabilities and/or their families. UCP also operates a wheelchair ramp building program, conducts parent workshops and offers adaptive recreation activities.
Laura Eaton, Executive Director

2667 United Cerebral Palsy of Pennsylvania
908 N Second Street   717-441-6044
Harrisburg, PA 17102   866-761-6129
                                        Fax: 717-236-2046
                    e-mail: kimberlycossar@wannarassoc.com
                                                www.ucp.org
United Cerebral Palsy provides information advocacy referral services for persons with disabilities and/or their families. UCP also operates an equipment loan program conducts parent workshops disseminates written literature on topics of interest to people with disabilities.
Joan Martin, Executive Director
Vini Portzline, Policy Information Exchange

2668 United Cerebral Palsy of Philadelphia Vicinity
102 E Mermaid Lane   215-242-4200
Philadelphia, PA 19118   Fax: 215-247-4229
                                        TTY: 215-248-7620
                              e-mail: ucpkravitz@aol.com
                                               www.ucpphila.org
United Cerebral Palsy provides information advocacy referral services for persons with disabilities and/or their families. UCP also

operates an equipment loan program conducts parent workshops disseminates written literature on topics of interest to people with disabilities.

Gary J Weyhmuller, President
David J Barnhart, Vice President

2669 United Cerebral Palsy of Pittsburgh
4638 Centre Avenue   412-683-7100
Pittsburgh, PA 15213   Fax: 412-683-4160
                         e-mail: info@ucppittsburgh.org
                                      www.ucp.org

United Cerebral Palsy provides information advocacy referral services for persons with disabilities and/or their families. UCP also operates an equipment loan program conducts parent workshops disseminates written literature on topics of interest to people with disabilities

Al Condeluci, CEO
Joyce Redmerski, Chief Financial Officer

2670 United Cerebral Palsy of South Central Pennsylvania
788 Cherry Tree Court   717-632-5552
Hanover, PA 17331   800-333-3873
                                      Fax: 717-632-2315
                  e-mail: phoughton@ucpsouthcentral.org
                                      www.ucp.org

Provides early intervention, in home personal care and community integration services for children and adults with disabilities in York, Adams and Franklin counties.

Paulette Houghton, Executive Director
William Long, Director of Operations

2671 United Cerebral Palsy of Southern Alleghenies Region
119 Jari Drive   814-262-9600
Johnstown, PA 15904   877-371-1110
                                      Fax: 814-262-9650
                            e-mail: info@ucpsar.org
                                      www.alucp.org

United Cerebral Palsy provides information, advocacy, referral services for persons with disabilities and/or their families. UCP also operates an equipment loan program, conducts parent workshops, disseminates written literature on topics of interest.

Marie Polinsky, CEO
Mark Malzi, CFO

2672 United Cerebral Palsy of Southwestern Pennsylvania
190 N Main Street   724-229-0851
Washington, PA 15301   Fax: 724-229-9252
                           e-mail: info@ucpswpa.org
                                      www.ucp.org

United Cerebral Palsy provides information, advocacy, referral services for persons with disabilities and/or their families. UCP also operates an equipment loan program, conducts parent workshops, disseminates written literature on topics of interest.

2673 United Cerebral Palsy of Western Pennsylvania
2904 Seminary Drive   724-832-8272
Greensburg, PA 15601   Fax: 724-837-8278
                       e-mail: ucp@ucpofwesternpa.org
                                      www.ucpa.org

United Cerebral Palsy provides information, advocacy, referral services for persons with disabilities and/or their families. UCP also operates an equipment loan program, conducts parent workshops, disseminates written literature on topics of interest.

Rhode Island

2674 United Cerebral Palsy of Rhode Island
200 Main Street   401-728-1800
Pawtucket, RI 02860   Fax: 401-728-0182
                             e-mail: info@ucpri.org
                                      www.ucpri.org

United Cerebral Palsy provides information, advocacy, referral services for persons with disabilities and/or their families. UCP also operates an equipment loan program, conducts parent workshops, disseminates written literature on topics of interest to people with disabilities.

Peter Quattromani, Executive Director & CEO
Karl Provost, CFO

Tennessee

2675 United Cerebral Palsy of Middle Tennessee
1200 9th Avenue N   615-242-4091
Nashville, TN 37208   Fax: 615-242-3582
                      e-mail: request@ucpnashville.org
                                      www.ucpmidtn.org/

United Cerebral Palsy provides information, advocacy, referral services for persons with disabilities and/or their families. UCP also operates an equipment loan program, conducts parent workshops, disseminates written literature on topics of interest to people with disabilities.

Deana Claiborne, Executive Director
Diane Dietrich, Director of Development

2676 United Cerebral Palsy of the Mid-South
3239 players club Parkway   901-761-4277
Memphis, TN 38125   Fax: 901-761-7876
                         e-mail: ucp@ucpmemphis.org
                                      www.ucpmemphis.org

United Cerebral Palsy provides information, advocacy, referral services for persons with disabilities and/or their families. UCP also operates an equipment loan program, conducts parent workshops, disseminates written literature on topics of interest to people with disabilities.

Michael Nolen, Chief Executive Officer
Kelly Burrow, Executive Vice-President of Development

Texas

2677 United Cerebral Palsy of Greater Houston
4500 Bissonet   713-838-9050
Bellaire, TX 77401   Fax: 713-838-9098
                         e-mail: ucp@ucphouston.org
                                      www.ucpa.org

United Cerebral Palsy provides information, advocacy, referral services for persons with disabilities and/or their families. UCP also operates an equipment loan program, conducts parent workshops, disseminates written literature on topics of interest to people with disabilities.

2678 United Cerebral Palsy of Metropolitan Dallas
8802 Harry Hines Boulevard   214-247-4505
Dallas, TX 75235   800-999-1898
                                      Fax: 214-351-2610
                      e-mail: billknudsen@ucpdallas
                                      www.ucpdallas.org

United Cerebral Palsy provides information, advocacy, referral services for persons with disabilities and/or their families. UCP also operates an equipment loan program, conducts parent workshops, disseminates written literature on topics of interest to people with disabilities.

Bill Knudsen, President / Chief Executive Officer
Becky Adams, Chief Operations Officer

2679 United Cerebral Palsy of Tarrant County
1555 Merrimac Circle   817-332-7171
Fort Worth, TX 76107   Fax: 817-332-7601
                             e-mail: info@ucptc.org
                                      www.ucpa.org

United Cerebral Palsy provides information, advocacy, referral services for persons with disabilities and/or their families. UCP also operates an equipment loan program, conducts parent workshops, disseminates written literature on topics of interest to people with disabilities.

2680 United Cerebral Palsy of Texas
1016 La Posada Drive   512-472-8696
Austin, TX 78752   800-798-1492
                                      Fax: 512-472-8026
                          e-mail: info@ucptexas.org
                                      www.ucpa.org

United Cerebral Palsy provides information, advocacy, referral services for persons with disabilities and/or their families. UCP also operates an equipment loan program, conducts parent workshops, disseminates written literature on topics of interest.

Utah

2681 **United Cerebral Palsy of Utah**
PO Box 65219
S Salt Lake, UT 84165 801-266-1805
Fax: 801-266-2404
e-mail: shellyp@ucputah.org
www.ucpa.org
United Cerebral Palsy provides information, advocacy, referral services for persons with disabilities and/or their families. UCP also operates an equipment loan program, conducts parent workshops, disseminates written literature on topics of interest.

Virginia

2682 **Cerebral Palsy of Virginia**
5825 Arrowhead Drive
Virginia Beach, VA 23462 757-497-7474
Fax: 757-497-0868
e-mail: kap@cerebralpalsyofvirginia.org
www.cerebralpalsyofvirginia.org
Cerebral Palsy provides information, advocacy, referral services for persons with disabilities and/or their families. Cerebral Palsy also operates an equipment loan program, summer computer camp, art works job training program and much more.
Kathy Prendergast, Executive Director
Michelle Majority, Associate Executive Director

Washington

2683 **United Cerebral Palsy of Pierce County**
6315 S 19th Street
Tacoma, WA 98466-6217 253-565-1463
Fax: 253-565-1463
e-mail: info@ucp-sps.org
www.ucpa.org
United Cerebral Palsy provides information, advocacy, referral services for persons with disabilities and/or their families. UCP also operates an equipment loan program, conducts parent workshops, disseminates written literature on topics of interest to people with disabilities.

Wisconsin

2684 **United Cerebral Palsy of Greater Dane County**
2801 Coho Street
Madison, WI 53713 608-273-4434
Fax: 608-273-3426
e-mail: ucpgdc@ucpdane.org
www.ucpdane.org
Provides information, advocacy, referral services for persons with disabilities and/or their families. UCP also conducts parent workshops and disseminates written literature on topics of interest to people with disabilities.
Wade Harrison, President
Rich Cooper, Vice-President

2685 **United Cerebral Palsy of North Central Wisconsin**
108 Scott Street
Wausau, WI 54401 715-842-8700
800-472-4408
www.ucpa.org
United Cerebral Palsy provides information, advocacy, referral services for persons with disabilities and/or their families. UCP also operates an equipment loan program, conducts parent workshops, disseminates written literature on topics of interest to people with disabilities.

2686 **United Cerebral Palsy of Southeastern Wisconsin**
7519 W Oklahoma Avenue
Milwaukee, WI 53219 414-329-4500
888-482-7739
Fax: 414-329-4510
TTY: 414-329-4511
e-mail: info@ucpsew.org
www.ucpsew.org/
United Cerebral Palsy provides information, advocacy, referral services for persons with disabilities and/or their families. UCP also operates an equipment loan program, conducts parent workshops, disseminates written literature on topics of interest to people with disabilities.
Scott Andreson, Presdient
Emmett Prosser, Secretary

2687 **United Cerebral Palsy of Wisconsin**
206 Water Street
Eau Claire, WI 54703 715-832-1782
Fax: 715-832-8203
e-mail: ucp1ruth@sbcglobal net
www.ucpwcw.org/
United Cerebral Palsy provides information, advocacy, referral services for persons with disabilities and/or their families. UCP also operates an equipment loan program, conducts parent workshops, disseminates written literature on topics of interest to people with disabilities.
Connie Werlein, President
Randi Johnson, Vice-President

Research Centers

2688 **Orthopaedic Biomechanics Laboratory Shriners Hospital for Crippled Children**
Shriners Hospital for Crippled Children
2181 Westlawn Building
Iowa City, IA 52242-1100 319-335-7529
Fax: 319-335-7530
Offers research and studies into cerebral palsy.
Stephen R Skinner, Clinical Director

Support Groups & Hotlines

2689 **Family Support Network**
215 Centennial Mall S
Lincoln, NE 68508-1813 402-477-2992
800-245-6081

2690 **National Health Information Center**
PO Box 1133
Washington, DC 20013-1133 310-565-4167
800-336-4797
Fax: 301-984-4256
e-mail: info@nhic.org
www.health.gov/nhic
A health information referral service sponsored by the Office of Disease Prevention and Health Promotion. Puts health professionals and consumers who have health questions in touch with those organizations that are best able to provide answers.
Ellen Langhans, Chairwoman
Linda Harris, Lead, Health Communication and e-health

Books

2691 **An Introduction to Your Child Who Has Cerebral Palsy**
Medic Publishing Company
PO Box 89
Redmond, WA 98073-0089 425-881-2883
Information and answers to questions for parents of children with cerebral palsy.

2692 **Children with Cerebral Palsy**
Woodbine House
6510 Bells Mill Road
Bethesda, MD 20817-1636 301-897-3570
800-843-7323
Fax: 301-897-5838
e-mail: info@woodbinehouse.com
www.woodbinehouse.com
Explains what Cerebral Palsy is, and discusses its diagnosis and treatment. Also offers information and advice concerning daily care, early intervention, therapy, educational options and family life.
432 pages Paperback
ISBN: 0-933149-15-8

2693 **Discovery Book**
United Cerebral Palsy Association
1660 L Street NW
Washington, DC 20036-5602 202-776-0406
800-872-5827
Fax: 202-776-0414
ucpnatl@ucpa.org

2694 **Individuals with Cerebral Palsy**
Mainstream
1030 5th Street NW
Washington, DC 20001-2504 202-898-1400
e-mail: info@mainstreaminc.org
www.mainstreaminc.org

Mainstreaming individuals with cerebral palsy into the workplace.
12 pages

**2695   Occupational Therapy Practice Guidelines for Adults with
         Cerebral Palsy**
American Occupational Therapy Association
4720 Montgomery Lane   301-652-2682
Bethesda, MD 20824-1220   Fax: 301-652-7711
                                         TDD: 800-377-8555
                                              www.aota.org

15 pages
ISBN: 1-569001-59-6

Children's Books

2696   Can't You Be Still?
Gemma B Publishing
776 Corydon Avenue   204-452-7566
Winnipeg, MB, R3M 0Y1,   Fax: 204-475-9903
                                   e-mail: gempub@mts.net
                                          www.gemmab.mb.ca
On Ann's first day at school, the other students are both fascinated
and horrified by her cerebral palsy. She wins them over by helping
them jump into the water and swim. Available in Braille.
24 pages Paperback
ISBN: 0-969647-70-0
Sarah Yates, President

2697   Cerebral Palsy
Franklin Watts Grolier
90 Old Sherman Tpke   203-797-3500
Danbury, CT 06816-0001   800-621-1115
                                         Fax: 203-797-3197
                                              www.grolier.com

A look at the causes, detection, prevention, effects and treatment of
Cerebral Palsy.
112 pages Grades 7-12
ISBN: 0-531125-29-7

2698   Here's What I Mean To Say
Gemma B Publishing
776 Corydon Avenue   204-452-7566
Winnipeg, MB, R3M 0Y1   Fax: 204-475-9903
                                   e-mail: gempub@mts.net
                                          www.gemmab.mb.ca
In this books Ann's battle to read is assisted by an angel, who helps
her read the directions in Jay's computer game. Is the angel read or
is this the magic of reading? Available in Braille.
32 pages Paperback
ISBN: 0-969647-72-7
Sarah Yates, President

2699   Mine for Keeps
Little, Brown & Company
34 Beacon Street   617-227-0730
Boston, MA 02108-1415   800-343-9204
Sarah Jean Copeland was born with cerebral palsy. At four years of
age she was placed in a school for handicapped children but made
such good progress that she could return home. Coming home for
Sarah meant a new school, and new adjustments to her parents, two
sisters, and her brother. At first Sarah was scared and didn't think
she could do all the things she needed to do, but she soon learned
her fears were not well-founded.
186 pages Hardcover

2700   My Brother Matthew
Woodbine House
6510 Bells Mill Road
Bethesda, MD 20817-1636   800-843-7323
A book written from the point of view of the brother of Matthew, a
boy with multiple disabilities, David describes the incidents characterizing how life in his family changes.
28 pages Grades K-5
Sarah Strickler

2701   Nobody Knows!
Gemma B Publishing

776 Corydon Avenue   204-452-7566
Winnipeg, MB, R3M 0Y1,   Fax: 204-475-9903
                                   e-mail: gempub@mts.net
                                          www.gemmab.mb.ca
An adventure during which a frustrated Ann goes out to find some-
one who understand what she wants. She meets a turtle and an alli-
gator, who like her don't use words to communicate. Available in
Braille.
24 pages Paperback
ISBN: 0-969647-71-9
Sarah Yates, President

Newsletters

2702   Family Support Bulletin
United Cerebral Palsy Associations
1660 L Street NW   202-842-1266
Washington, DC 20036-1202   800-872-5827

Pamphlets

2703   Cerebral Palsy: Facts & Figures
United Cerebral Palsy Associations
1660 L Street NW
Washington, DC 20036   800-872-5827
                                         Fax: 202-776-0414
                                              www.ucp.org
Offers information on what cerebral palsy is, the effects, causes,
types, and prevention.

Audio & Video

2704   A Day At A Time
Filmakers Library
124 E 40th Street   212-808-4980
New York, NY 10016-1798   Fax: 212-808-4983
                                  e-mail: info@filmakers.com
                                          www.filmakers.com
The story of twin girls with Cerebral Palsy, whose family is deter-
mined that they have every opportunity to participate in and lead
normal lives. Winner of a number of awards. DVD or VHS $195,
Classroom Rental $75
VHS or DVD
Sue Oscar, Co-President

Web Sites

**2705   American Academy for Cerebral Palsy and Developmental
         Medicine**
                                              AACPDM.org
A multidisciplinary scientific society devoted to the study of cerebral palsy and other childhood onset disabilities, to promoting professional education for the treatment and management of these
conditions, and to improving the quality of life for people with
these disabilities.

2706   Healing Well
                                         www.healingwell.com
An online health resource guide to medical news, chat, information and articles, newsgroups and message boards, books, disease-related web sites, medical directories, and more for patients,
friends, and family coping with disabling diseases, disorders, or
chronic illnesses.

2707   Health Finder
                                         www.healthfinder.gov
Searchable, carefully developed web site offering information on
over 1000 topics. Developed by the US Department of Health and
Human Services, the site can be used in both English and Spanish.

2708   Healthlink USA
                                         www.healthlinkusa.com
Health information concerning treatment, cures, prevention, diagnosis, risk factors, research, support groups, email lists, personal
stories and much more. Updated regularly.

2709   Helios Health

www.helioshealth.com

Online resource for your health information. Detailed information about specific health topics, access to expert advice from our Medical Advisory Board, and up-to-date health news.

2710   MedicineNet

www.medicinenet.com

An online resource for consumers providing easy-to-read, authoritative medical and health information.

2711   Medscape

www.medscape.com

Medscape offers specialists, primary care physicians, and other health professionals the Web's most robust and integrated medical information and educational tools.

2712   National Institute of Neurological Disorders and Stroke

www.ninds.nih.gov

The mission of NINDS is to reduce the burden of neurological disease - a burden borne by every age group, by every segment of society, by people all over the world.

2713   National Rehabilitation Information Center

www.naric.com/

One of the three components of the office of Special Education and Rehabilitative Services.

2714   Neurology Channel

www.neurologychannel.com

Find clearly explained, medically accurate information regarding conditions, including an overview, symptoms, causes, diagnostic procedures and treatment options. On this site it is possible to ask questions and get information from a neurologist and connect to people who have similar health interests.

2715   United Cerebral Palsy Associations

www.ucpa.org

A network of approximately 119 state and local voluntary agencies which provide services, conduct public and professional education programs and support research in cerebral palsy.

2716   WebMD

www.webmd.com

Provides links to over 20 articles involving cerebral palsy.

Description

2717 Chronic Fatigue Syndrome

Chronic Fatigue Syndrome, CFS, is an illness characterized by longstanding fatigue that impairs daily functioning. It may be accompanied by sore throat, swollen glands, muscle and joint pain, headaches, sleeplessness, and impaired memory or concentration. Profound or life-altering fatigue—the disease's hallmark—usually comes on suddenly and persists for at least six months, and often for years.

The cause of CFS is controversial. One theory is that a chronic viral infection is involved. Allergic reactions have also been proposed, and various immunologic abnormalities have been reported. Another theory involves proposed disturbances in the hormonal (endocrine) system. Psychological factors may be the cause, although CFS is distinct from typical depression or anxiety. Because the cause is unknown, there is no single test or group of tests that can diagnose CFS. Therefore, the goal in evaluating an individual with presumed CFS is to exclude other treatable illnesses.

Given the difficulty in proving a diagnosis or understanding the cause of CFS, it is not surprising that many treatments have been offered for it. Antidepressants appear to be the most successful treatment studied so far; as many as 80 percent of patients report benefit. Other therapies, including nutritional supplements, hormones, antiviral drugs and steroids have been mostly disappointing.

Patients with CFS need emotional support from physicians and family, due to the debilitating nature of the disease. Individual and group therapy may help some individuals. See also *Fibromyalgia*.

National Agencies & Associations

2718 American Academy of Sleep Medicine
2510 North Frontage Road
Darien, IL 60561   630-737-9700
                              Fax: 630-737-9790
                              www.aasmnet.org
A unique multi-disciplinary organization for both individual members and center members. The individual member branch includes clinicians involved in the diagnosis and treatment of patients with disorders of sleep and alertness.
Amy Aronsky, Director
M Safwan Badr, President

2719 International Association for Chronic Fatigue
27 N Wacker Drive
Chicago, IL 60606   847-258-7248
                              Fax: 847-579-0975
                              e-mail: Admin@iacfsme.org
                              www.IACFS.net
A nonprofit organization of research scientists, physicians, licensed medical healthcare professionals and other individuals and institutions interested in promoting the stimulation, coordination and exchange of ideas for CFS research and patient care.
Newsletter
Fred Friedberg, President
Staci R Stevens, Vice President

2720 National Chronic Fatigue Syndrome and Fibromyalgia Association
PO Box 18426   816-737-1343
Kansas City, MO 64133-8426   Fax: 816-524-6782
                              e-mail: information@ncfsfa.org
                              www.ncfsfa.org
Compiles and provides peer reviewed, scientifically accurate educational materials to inform the public, health professionals, patients and their families about the nature and impact of chronic fatigue syndrome, fibromyalgia and related disorders. Offers a support group.
Orvalene Prewitt, President

2721 National Institute of Allergy and Infectious Diseases
Office of Communications
6610 Rockledge Drive   301-402-1663
Bethesda, MD 20892-6612   866-284-4107
                              Fax: 301-402-1020
                              TDD: 800-877-8339
                              e-mail: af10r@nih.gov
                              www.niaid.nih.gov
Offers information and educational materials on Chronic Fatigue Syndrome and other disorders.
Anthony S Fauci, MD, Director

2722 Option Institute
2080 South Undermountain Road   413-229-2100
Sheffield, MA 01257   800-714-2779
                              Fax: 413-229-8931
                              e-mail: participantsupport@option.org
                              www.option.org
Self-defeating beliefs, along with attitudes and judgments, can lead to a host of physical and psychological challenges, including Chronic Fatigue Syndrome. The Option Institute offers programs designed to help you gain new perspectives on the attitudes and judgments that may be affecting your life, especially those regarding and surrounding Chronic Fatigue Syndrome.
Barry Kaufman, Co-Founder
Samahria Ltye Kaufman, Co-Founder

Foundations

2723 National CFIDS Foundation
103 Aletha Road   781-449-3535
Needham, MA 02492   Fax: 781-449-8606
                              e-mail: info@ncf-net.org
                              www.ncf-net.org
The goals of the Foundation are to help fund medical research to find a cause, expedite treatments and eventually a cure for this devastating disease. The NCF also strives to provide information, education, and support to those people who have CFIDS (also known as chronic fatigue syndrome (CFS), myalgic encephalomyelitis (ME) and many other names)— as well as related illnesses such as Gulf War Illness (GWI) and Multiple Chemical Sensitivities (MCS). Provides guides, articles, and newsletters.
Gail Kansky, President
Prof. Alan Cocchetto, Medical Advisor

Support Groups & Hotlines

2724 Centers for Disease Control and Prevention
1600 Clifton Road
Atlanta, GA 30333   800-232-4636
                              TTY: 888-232-6348
                              e-mail: cdcinfo@cdc.gov
                              www.cdc.gov
Collaborating to create the expertise, information, and tools that people and their communities need to protect their health - through health promotion, prevention of disease, injury and disability, and preparedness for new health threats.
Thomas R Frieden MD MPH, Director

2725 Chronic Fatigue Syndrome & Fibromyalgia Support
7250 Clearvista Dr   317-252-9223
Indianapolis, IN 46256
Offers emotional support, education and information about CFS and FMS through statewide monthly meetings and a quarterly

newsletter. Provides 24-hour hotline and physician/attorney referrals. Financial assistance for members. Support group meets twice a month at Community Hospital North Professional Building and at other locations throughout Indiana.

2726 National Chronic Fatigue Syndrome and Fibromyalgia Association
PO Box 18426   816-737-1343
Kansas City, MO 64133   Fax: 816-524-6782
e-mail: information@ncfsfa.org
www.ncfsfa.org
To educate and inform the public about the nature and impact of Chronic Fatigue Syndrome and Fibromyalgia and related disorders.
Orvalene Prewitt, President

2727 National Health Information Center
PO Box 1133   310-565-4167
Washington, DC 20013-1133   800-336-4797
Fax: 301-984-4256
e-mail: info@nhic.org
www.health.gov/nhic
A health information referral service sponsored by the Office of Disease Prevention and Health Promotion. Puts health professionals and consumers who have health questions in touch with those organizations that are best able to provide answers.
Ellen Langhans, Chairwoman
Linda Harris, Lead, Health Communication and e-health

Books

2728 CFIDS in Children Packet
CFIDS Association of America
PO Box 220398
Charlotte, NC 28222-0398   800-442-3437
This packet contains articles about CFIDS and children.
60 pages

2729 CFS Cookbook
CFIDS Association of America
PO Box 220398
Charlotte, NC 28222-0398   800-442-3437
Gourmet recipes designed to combat the monotony associated with CFIDS, allergy and immune-compromised diets.
218 pages

2730 Chronic Fatigue Syndrome Cookbook: Delicious & Wellness-Enhancing Recipes
DIANE Publishing Company
330 Pusey Avenue, Unit #3 Rear   610-461-6200
Darby, PA 19023   800-782-3833
Fax: 610-461-6130
e-mail: dianepublishing@gmail.com
www.dianepublishing.net
These recipes help combat the boredom of the CFS diet usually recommended and still satisfy all of your nutritional requirements as a CFS sufferer. In addition, the book includes a comprehensive look at the do's and don't's of a CFS diet, quick recipes for those days when you are too tired to cook and an insightful medical introduction.
218 pages Hardcover
ISBN: 0-756753-28-7
Herman Baron, Publisher

2731 Chronic Fatigue Syndrome and the Yeast Connection
CFIDS Association of America
PO Box 220398
Charlotte, NC 28222-0398   800-442-3437
Dr. Crook explains the possible role of multiple entities, including yeast overgrowth, allergies and chemical sensitivities, in CFS and how each contributes to immune dysregulation.
386 pages

2732 Chronic Fatigue Syndrome: Information for Physicians
Barry Leonard, author
DIANE Publishing Company

330 Pusey Avenue, Unit #3 Rear   610-461-6200
Darby, PA 19023   800-782-3833
Fax: 610-461-6130
e-mail: dianepublishing@gmail.com
www.dianepublishing.net
Includes a historical perspective on chronic fatigue syndrome; epidemiology; clinical picture; evaluation of patients; patient management; etiologic theories; public health service resources; fact sheet; resources for patients, overview of the CFS research program; NIAID and NIAID/Johns Hopkins hospital study, which seeks volunteers, management strategies for CFS; the relationship between nuerally mediatec hypotension and CFS and fibromyalgia and CFS; solving diagnostic and therapeutic dilemmas.
60 pages Paperback
ISBN: 0-788143-78-6
Herman Baron, Publisher

2733 Chronic Fatigue Syndrome: The Limbic Hypothesis
CFIDS Association of America
PO Box 220398
Charlotte, NC 28222-0398   800-442-3437
A detailed thesis proposing CFS as a limbic system encephalopathy in the context of a dysregulated neuroimmune system.
259 pages

2734 Chronic Fatigue: Your Complete Exercise Guide
Human Kinetics Press
PO Box 5076   217-351-5076
Champaign, IL 61825-5076   800-747-4457
Fax: 217-351-2674
www.humankinetics.com

1993 144 pages Paperback
ISBN: 0-873223-93-4
Steve Ruhlig, Marketing Director

2735 Coping With CFS
CFIDS Association of America
PO Box 220398   704-365-2343
Charlotte, NC 28222-0398   800-442-3437
Fax: 704-365-9755
e-mail: info@cfids.org
www.cfids.org
Offers practical, established coping strategies for living better with CFIDS. Based on Dr. Friedberg's experiences as a person with CFIDS and a counselor to PWCs.
176 pages
Jon Sterling, Chairman
Kim Kenny, President/CEO

2736 Disability and Chronic Fatigue Syndrome
The Haworth Press
10 Alice Street   607-722-5857
Binghamton, NY 13904-1580   800-429-6784
Fax: 800-895-0582
e-mail: getinfo@haworthpressinc.com
www.haworthpressinc.com
Discusses the difficult subject of how to diagnose disability in chronic fatigue syndrome patients, how to determine the severity of a patient's disability, and how new disability guidelines would make more chronic fatigue patients eligible to apply for disability benefits.
121 pages Paperback
ISBN: 0-789005-01-8
Bill Cohen, Publisher
Sandy Jones, VP Marketing

2737 Doctor's Guide to Chronic Fatigue Syndrome
CFIDS Association of America
PO Box 220398
Charlotte, NC 28222-0398   800-442-3437
Written by one of the world's leading experts on CFIDS.
275 pages

2738 Fifty Things You Should Know About the Chronic Fatigue Syndrome Epidemic
St. Martin's Press

175 5th Avenue
New York, NY 10010-7848

212-674-5151
800-221-7945
Fax: 212-420-9314

1993
ISBN: 0-312950-43-8

2739 Hope and Help for Chronic Fatigue Syndrome
CFIDS Association of America
PO Box 220398
Charlotte, NC 28222-0398

704-365-2343
800-442-3437
Fax: 704-365-9755
e-mail: info@cfids.org
www.cfids.org

Insight into the experience of having CFIDS, the physical and emotional impact, difficulty in obtaining a diagnosis, available methods of treatment and key strategies for regaining control over your life.
216 pages
Jon Sterling, Chairman
Kim Kenny, President/CEO

2740 International Classification of Sleep Disorders
American Academy of Sleep Medicine
One Westbrook Corporate Center
Westchester, IL 60154

708-492-0930
Fax: 708-492-0943
www.aasmnet.org

A comprehensive manual for physicians and other healthcare professionals containing information on 84 sleep disorders. The extensive text describes the diagnostic features of each disorder and includes specific diagnostic and severity criteria for each disorder.
396 pages Paperback

2741 Living with CFS: A Personal Story of the Struggle for Recovery
CFIDS Association of America
PO Box 220398
Charlotte, NC 28222-0398

800-442-3437

Describes the pain associated with the author's loss of livelihood, impaired physical and mental functioning and the strain on his marriage and friendships, while maintaining hope for recovery.
224 pages
ISBN: 1-560250-75-5

2742 Living with ME
CFIDS Association of America
PO Box 220398
Charlotte, NC 28222-0398

800-442-3437
Fax: 704-365-9755

The author describes M.E. (mylagic encephalomyelitis - the British term for chronic fatigue syndrome), and discusses practical methods for coping and comments on various treatments.

2743 Music Appreciation
CFIDS Association of America
PO Box 220398
Charlotte, NC 28222-0398

800-442-3437

A full-length collection of poems by Skloot who has been disabled by CFIDS since 1988.
105 pages

2744 Night-Side: CFS and the Illness Experience
CFIDS Association of America
PO Box 220398
Charlotte, NC 28222-0398

704-365-2343
800-442-3437
Fax: 704-365-9755
e-mail: info@cfids.org
www.cfids.org

An honest and ultimately hopeful exploration of what it means to have your life shattered by disease.
190 pages
Jon Sterling, Chairman
Kim Kenny, President/CEO

2745 Recovering From the Chronic Fatigue Syndrome: A Guide to Self-Empowerment
Berkley Books
200 Madison Avenue
New York, NY 10016-3903

212-951-8800
www.penguinputman.com

This book teaches persons with CFIDS to take control of their illness and to help themselves find the road to recovery.
1993 224 pages Paperback
ISBN: 0-399518-07-0

2746 Running on Empty
CFIDS Association of America
PO Box 220398
Charlotte, NC 28222-0398

704-365-2343
800-442-3437
Fax: 704-365-9755
e-mail: info@cfids.org
www.cfids.org

Landmark guide to CFIDS has just been revised and re-released. A must read for the newly disgnosed.
315 pages
Jon Sterling, Chairman
Kim Kenny, President/CEO

2747 Self-Caring Fatigue
Rodale Press
33 E Minor Street
Emmaus, PA 18098-0099

610-967-5171
800-441-7761
Fax: 610-967-8963
e-mail: info@rodale.com
www.rodale.com

A step-by-step plan to uncover and eliminate the causes of chronic fatigue.
1993 320 pages
ISBN: 0-875961-61-4

2748 Solving the Puzzle of CFS
2730 Wilshire Boulevard
Santa Monica, CA 90403-4724

310-453-4424
Fax: 310-966-9196

Magazines

2749 CFIDS Chronicle
CFIDS Association of America
PO Box 220398
Charlotte, NC 28222-0398

704-362-2343
800-442-3437
Fax: 704-365-9755

The largest and most comprehensive periodical specifically pertaining to chronic fatigue syndrome information in the world.

2750 Feel Good Catalog
2895 W Oxford Avenue
Englewood, CO 80110-4370

303-790-1045
800-997-6789

Variety of items to ease pain.

2751 Journal SLEEP
American Academy of Sleep Medicine
One Westbrook Corporate Center
Westchester, IL 60154

708-492-0930
Fax: 708-492-0943
www.journalslep.org

Publishes articles ranging from clinical investigations of sleep/wake disorders and medical problems during sleep, to investigations of the basic physiological and biochemical events and anatomical structures involved in normal and abnormal sleep. Includes psychological and psycho-physiological research, as well as research in relevant areas of circadian and biological rhythms.
10x Year
ISBN: 0-161810-5 -

2752 Journal of the Chronic Fatigue Syndrome
Haworth Medical Press
10 Alice Street
Binghamton, NY 13904-1503

607-722-5857
800-429-6784
Fax: 607-722-0012
www.haworth.org

Peer reviewed medical journal containing CFIDS scientific abstract information. Appropriate for patients as well as medical professionals.
Quarterly
Nancy Klimas MD, Founding Co-Editor

Newsletters

2753 Health Points
TyH Publications
17007 E Colony Drive
Fountain Hills, AZ 85268   800-801-1406
e-mail: editor@e-tyh.com
National newsletter with articles on complementary therapy, latest nutrition news, disability issues and much more. Focus is on fibromyalgia, chronic fatigue, arthritis and chronic pain.
Quarterly

2754 Heart of America News
National Chronic Fatigue Syndrome & Fibromyalgia
PO Box 18426   660-313-2000
Kansas City, MO 64133-8426
Offers scientifically accurate information, medical updates, informational references, articles on coping and living with Chronic Fatigue Syndrome and more, based on peer-reviewed materials.
Quarterly

2755 National Forum
103 Aletha Road   781-449-3535
Needham, MA 02492   Fax: 781-449-8606
e-mail: info@ncf-net.org
www.ncf-net.org
The Forum's focus: CFIDS/ME, FMS, GWI, MCS and related illnesses.
Gail Kansky, President

2756 Syndrome Sentinel
Massachusetts CFIDS Association
808 Main Street
Waltham, MA 02451-8533   781-893-4415
www2.shore.net
This quarterly newsletter contains articles written by health-care professionals working with these conditions. Contributors include traditional and alternative experts, as well as personal stories from people with these chronic syndromes and their significant others.

2757 The National Forum
The National CFIDS Foundation
103 Aletha Road   781-449-3535
Needham, MA 02492   Fax: 781-449-8606
e-mail: info@ncf-net.org
www.ncf-net.org
Offers the latest information on CFIDS treatments being tried throughout the United States.

Pamphlets

2758 Americans with Disabilities Act: CFS and Employment
National Chronic Fatigue Syndrome & Fibromyalgia
PO Box 18426   660-313-2000
Kansas City, MO 64133-8426

2759 CFIDS Membership Packet
CFIDS Association of America
PO Box 220398
Charlotte, NC 28222-0398   800-442-3437
Fax: 704-365-9755
Offers pamphlets, brochures, information on local support groups for members.

2760 CFIDS in Children
CFIDS Association of America
PO Box 220398
Charlotte, NC 28222-0398   800-442-3437
Describes the special difficulties faced by children with CFIDS.

2761 CFS in the Workplace
National Chronic Fatigue Syndrome & Fibromyalgia
PO Box 18426   660-313-2000
Kansas City, MO 64133

2762 Chronic Fatigue Syndrome & School Success
National Chronic Fatigue Syndrome & Fibromyalgia
PO Box 18426   660-313-2000
Kansas City, MO 64133-8426

2763 Chronic Fatigue Syndrome in Children
National Chronic Fatigue Syndrome & Fibromyalgia
PO Box 18426   660-313-2000
Kansas City, MO 64133

2764 Chronic Fatigue Syndrome in Men
National Chronic Fatigue Syndrome & Fibromyalgia
PO Box 18426   660-313-2000
Kansas City, MO 64133-8426

2765 Chronic Fatigue Syndrome: A Pamphlet for Physicians
National Institute of Allergy & Infectious Disease
Building 31, Room 7A50
Bethesda, MD 20892-2520   301-496-5717
www.niaid.nih.gov
Offers information on epidemiology, clinical procedures, evaluations, patient management, neuropsychologic features and etiologic theories.

2766 Chronic Fatigue Syndrome: The Thief of Vitality
National Chronic Fatigue Syndrome & Fibromyalgia
PO Box 18426   660-313-2000
Kansas City, MO 64133-8426

2767 Coping Skills
National Chronic Fatigue Syndrome & Fibromyalgia
PO Box 18426   660-313-2000
Kansas City, MO 64133-8426

2768 Disability Packet
CFIDS Association of America
PO Box 220398
Charlotte, NC 28222-0398   800-442-3437
Includes nine Chronicle articles about disability benefits and how persons with CFIDS can secure Social Security Disability Insurance benefits.
42 pages

2769 Facts About Chronic Fatigue Syndrome
Centers for Disease Control & Prevention
Division of Viral Diseases   404-639-3311
Atlanta, GA 30333

2770 Fibromyalgia
National Chronic Fatigue Syndrome & Fibromyalgia
PO Box 18426   660-313-2000
Kansas City, MO 64133-8426

2771 March is Chronic Fatigue Syndrome Awareness Month Tips
National Chronic Fatigue Syndrome & Fibromyalgia
PO Box 18426   660-313-2000
Kansas City, MO 64133

2772 Neuropsychological Rehabilitation Suggestions/Techniques
National Chronic Fatigue Syndrome & Fibromyalgia
PO Box 18426   660-313-2000
Kansas City, MO 64133-8426

2773 School's Guide for Students with CFS
National Chronic Fatigue Syndrome & Fibromyalgia
PO Box 18426   660-313-2000
Kansas City, MO 64133-8426

2774 Social Security Disability Benefits Information
National Chronic Fatigue Syndrome & Fibromyalgia
PO Box 18426   660-313-2000
Kansas City, MO 64133-8426

2775 Suicide is Not an Option
National Chronic Fatigue Syndrome
PO Box 18426   660-313-2000
Kansas City, MO 64133-8426

2776 Understanding CFIDS
CFIDS Association of America
PO Box 220398
Charlotte, NC 28222-0398   800-442-3437
Provides an extensive overview of CFIDS and answers the most commonly asked questions about the disease.

2777 Understanding the Emotions Surrounding CFS
National Chronic Fatigue Syndrome & Fibromyalgia

PO Box 18426   660-313-2000
Kansas City, MO 64133-8426

Audio & Video

2778 Behavioral and Circadian Sleep Problems of Infancy and Childhood
American Academy of Sleep Medicine
One Westbrook Corporate Center
Westchester, IL 60154   Fax: 708-492-0943
                                            708-492-0930
                                            www.aasmnet.org
Addresses the problems of sleep disorders in children and outlines the types of disturbances, both of a medical and behavioral nature, that are commonly identified.
66 slides

2779 CFS and Self-Esteem
CFIDS Association of America
PO Box 220398
Charlotte, NC 28222-0398   800-442-3437
Addresses the sources of low self-esteem in persons with CFIDS and offers reassurance and practical techniques for increasing self-confidence.
Audiotape

2780 CFS: Addressing the Realities of a Chronic Illness
National Chronic Fatigue Syndrome & Fibromyalgia
PO Box 18426   660-313-2000
Kansas City, MO 64133-8426
This video offers reliable information featuring patients and a medical professional.

2781 CFS: Unraveling the Mystery
CFIDS Association of America
PO Box 220398
Charlotte, NC 28222-0398   800-442-3437
An excellent videotape for convincing skeptics that CFIDS is a real disease.
Videotape

2782 Chronic Fatigue Syndrome: For Those Who Care
CFIDS Association of America
PO Box 220398
Charlotte, NC 28222-0398   800-442-3437
An audiotape designed for friends and family of persons with CFIDS.
Audiotape

2783 Chronic Fatigue Syndrome: Information, Relaxation/Healing Exercise
CFIDS Association of America
PO Box 220398
Charlotte, NC 28222-0398   800-442-3437
Includes a comprehensive overview of CFS and relaxation/healing and imagery/stress reduction exercises for persons with CFIDS.
Audiotape

2784 Fibromyalgia
National Chronic Fatigue Syndrome & Fibromyalgia
PO Box 18426   660-313-2000
Kansas City, MO 64133
Videotape

2785 HHS Satelite Video on Chronic Fatigue Syndrome and Fibromyalgia Association
National Chronic Fatigue Syndrome and Fibromyalgia
PO Box 18426   660-313-2000
Kansas City, MO 64133-8426

2786 Living Hell: The Real World of Chronic Fatigue Syndrome
CFIDS Association of America
PO Box 220398
Charlotte, NC 28222-0398   800-442-3437
An emotional exposure of the tragedy of CFIDS.
Videotape

2787 Neurocognitive Aspects of CFS
CFIDS Association of America
PO Box 220398
Charlotte, NC 28222-0398   800-442-3437

A description of CFIDS-associated neurocognitive deficits and strategies for coping with them and the embarrassment and frustration they cause.
Audiotape

Web Sites

2788 American Association for Chronic Fatigue Syndrome
                                            www.aacfs.org
A non profit organization of research scientists, physicians, licensed medical healthcare professionals, and other indviduals and institutions interested in promoting the stimulation, coordination, and exchange of ideas for CFS research and patient care.

2789 CFIDS Association of America
                                            www.cfids.org
The nation's leading charitable organization devoted to conquering chronic fatigue syndrome by supporting research, education and public policy programs.

2790 Centers for Disease Control and Prevention
                                            www.cdc.gov
Offers information and educational materials on CFS.

2791 Healing Well
                                            www.healingwell.com
An online health resource guide to medical news, chat, information and articles, newsgroups and message boards, books, disease-related web sites, medical directories, and more for patients, friends, and family coping with disabling diseases, disorders, or chronic illnesses.

2792 Health Finder
                                            www.healthfinder.gov
Searchable, carefully developed web site offering information on over 1000 topics. Developed by the US Department of Health and Human Services, the site can be used in both English and Spanish.

2793 Healthlink USA
                                            www.healthlinkusa.com
Health information concerning treatment, cures, prevention, diagnosis, risk factors, research, support groups, email lists, personal stories and much more. Updated regularly.

2794 Helios Health
                                            www.helioshealth.com
Online resource for your health information. Detailed information about specific health topics, access to expert advice from our Medical Advisory Board, and up-to-date health news.

2795 Journal of Chronic Fatigue Syndrome
                                            www.cfs-news.org/jcfs.htm
Offers multidisciplinary original research, practical clinical management, case reports, and literature reviews to keep the entire health care delivery team well informed.

2796 MedicineNet
                                            www.medicinenet.com
An online resource for consumers providing easy-to-read, authoritative medical and health information.

2797 Medscape
                                            www.medscape.com
Medscape offers specialists, primary care physicians, and other health professionals the Web's most robust and integrated medical information and educational tools.

2798 Option Institute
                                            www.option.org/cfs.shtml
Self-defeating beliefs, along with attitudes and judgments, can lead to a host of physical and psychological challenges, including Chronic Fatigue Syndrome. The Option Institute offers programs designed to help you gain new perspectives on the attitudes and judgments that may be affecting your life, especially those regarding and surrounding Chronic Fatigue Syndrome.

2799 Sleepnet
                                            www.sleepnet.com
Links all the sleep information located on the internet. Provides a place for everyone to read and post questions, or responses.

2800 WebMD

www.webmd.com

Information on Chronic Fatigue Syndrome, including articles and resources.

Description

2801 Chronic Pain

Chronic pain is defined as pain persisting for more than one month after resolution of an acute injury or pain that persists or recurs for more than three months. The pain may begin for unknown reasons, or may begin with some injury or illness but persist long after the triggering event is gone. Human pain has physiological causes but also has psychological components differing for each person. Many Americans suffer from chronic pain. The annual cost, including treatment and lost work days, now hovers around $100 billion in the US.

Doctors and patients have tried almost every conceivable type of therapy for chronic pain. Drug treatments include narcotics (codeine and morphine), non-narcotic painkillers such as acetaminophen, and nonsteroidal anti-inflammatory drugs such as ibuprofen. Use of anti-depressants, either alone or in conjunction with pain medications, can be beneficial. Doctors may inject drugs to block the nerves that carry the pain signal, or may even cut the nerve. Physical measures include heat or cold application, application of electrical stimuli (TENS), stretching, and general conditioning exercises. Psychological treatment includes psychotherapy, meditation, hypnosis and biofeedback-relaxation. Because of the complexity of chronic pain and its treatment, some doctors have begun to specialize in management of pain, and have organized multidisciplinary pain clinics which offer expertise from anesthesiology, rheumatology, neurosurgery, psychology and physical therapy.

A realistic goal of therapy is to improve one's daily functioning; for instance, being able to return to work or pleasurable activities. Those able to achieve this status will often state that the pain is still there but that it does not bother them like it once did. Whatever the stage of one's condition, peer support is important, and is available from local in-person support groups or from Internet chat rooms and bulletin boards.

National Agencies & Associations

2802 American Chronic Pain Association

PO Box 850
Rocklin, CA 95677   800-533-3231
                                          Fax: 916-632-3208
                                  e-mail: ACPA@pacbell.net
                                          www.theacpa.org

ACPA mission is to facilitate peer support and education for individuals with chronic pain and their families so that these individuals may live more fully in spite of their pain; and to raise awareness among the health care community and policy makers.
Penny Cowan, Executive Director

2803 American Pain Society

4700 W Lake Avenue   847-375-4715
Glenview, IL 60025   866-574-2654
                                          Fax: 847-375-6479
                              e-mail: info@americanpainsociety.org
                                      www.americanpainsociety.org

A multidisciplinary organization of basic and clinical scientists practicing clinicians policy analysts and others. Mission is to advance pain-related research education treatment and professional practice.
Catherine H Underwood, Executive Director
Seddon R Savage MD, MS, President

2804 International Association for the Study of Pain

111 Queen Anne Avenue N   206-283-0311
Seattle, WA 98109-4955   Fax: 206-283-9403
                                  e-mail: iaspdesk@iasp-pain.org
                                          www.iasp-pain.org

The International Association for the Study of Pain is the leading professional forum for science practice and education in the field of pain.
Eija Anneli Kalso MD, President
Judith A Paice PhD, RN, President Elect

2805 International Pelvic Pain Society Women's Medical Plaza

Women's Medical Plaza
1100 E Woodfield Road   847-517-8712
Schaumburg, IL 60173   800-624-9676
                                          Fax: 847-517-7229
                                  e-mail: info@pelvicpain.org
                                          www.pelvicpain.org

Short range goal is to recruit organize and educate health care professionals actively involved with the treatment of patients who have chronic pelvic pain.
Fred Marion Howard, Chairman of the Board
Richard P Marvel MD, President

2806 Reflex Sympathetic Dystrophy Syndrome Association (RSDSA)

PO Box 502   203-877-3790
Milford, CT 06460   877-662-7737
                                          Fax: 203-882-8362
                                      e-mail: info@rsds.org
                                              www.rsds.org

Nonprofit professional and consumer organization founded to support research into the cause, treatment and cure of reflex sympathetic dystrophy syndrome. RSDSA also organizes support groups, promote awareness among health professionals and develop educational programs.
Paul R Charlesworth, President
James E Tyrrell Jr, Chairman of the Board

Support Groups & Hotlines

2807 National Health Information Center

PO Box 1133   310-565-4167
Washington, DC 20013-1133   800-336-4797
                                          Fax: 301-984-4256
                                      e-mail: info@nhic.org
                                          www.health.gov/nhic

A health information referral service sponsored by the Office of Disease Prevention and Health Promotion. Puts health professionals and consumers who have health questions in touch with those organizations that are best able to provide answers.
Ellen Langhans, Chairwoman
Linda Harris, Lead, Health Communication and e-health

Books

2808 ACPA Facilitator Guide & Materials

American Chronic Pain Association
PO Box 850   916-632-0922
Rocklin, CA 95677   800-533-3231
                                          Fax: 916-632-3208
                                  e-mail: acpa@pacbell.net
                                          www.theacpa.org

This guide will help you and others in your community organize an ACPA chapter. The manual contains how-to information on organizing an ACPA chapter, sharing responsibility for the group with others, finding a meeting place, conducting the first meeting, and generating public interest in your area. You must be an ACPA member to purchase this manual.
Penny Cowan, Executive Director

2809 ACPA Family Manual
Penny Cowan, author
American Chronic Pain Association
PO Box 850
Rocklin, CA 95677
916-632-0922
800-533-3231
Fax: 916-632-3208
e-mail: acpa@pacbell.net
www.theacpa.org
A manual designed with the needs of those who live with a person who has chronic pain.
149 pages
ISBN: 0-967387-82-5
Penny Cowan, Executive Director

2810 ACPA Journal Reflections of You
American Chronic Pain Association
PO Box 850
Rocklin, CA 95677
916-632-0922
800-533-3231
Fax: 916-632-3208
e-mail: acpa@pacbell.net
www.theacpa.org
A daily meditation and personal journal book which provides positive and motivating thoughts to stimulate your thinking and challenge you to personal growth. Your daily entries in the journal will help track your progress and show when you have reached your personal goal.
Penny Cowan, Executive Director

2811 ACSM's Exercise Management for Persons with Chronic Disease & Disabilities
Human Kinetics Press
PO Box 5076
Champaign, IL 61825-5076
217-351-5076
800-747-4457
Fax: 217-351-2674
www.humankinetics.com
1993 384 pages Hardcover
ISBN: 0-736038-72-8
Steve Ruhlig, Marketing Director

2812 Essential Guide to Chronic Illness: The Active Patient's Handbook
James W Long, author
DIANE Publishing Company
330 Pusey Avenue, Unit #3 Rear
Darby, PA 19023
610-461-6200
800-782-3833
Fax: 610-461-6130
e-mail: dianepublishing@gmail.com
www.dianepublishing.net
A comprehensive guide to dealing with nearly 50 chronic illness and conditions from acne to Zollinger-Ellison syndrome, including diabetes, menopause, migraines, rheumatoid arthritis and psoriasis.
625 pages Paperback
ISBN: 0-788169-03-3
Herman Baron, Publisher

2813 From Patient to Person: First Steps
American Chronic Pain Association
PO Box 850
Rocklin, CA 95677
916-632-0922
800-533-3231
Fax: 916-632-3208
e-mail: acpa@pacbell.net
www.theacpa.org
A workbook designed to help anyone who has a chronic pain problem to gain a better understanding of how one can begin to cope with all the problems that their pain creates.

ISBN: 0-967387-80-9
Penny Cowan, Executive Director

2814 Occupational Therapy Practice Guidelines for Adults with Low Back Pain
American Occupational Therapy Association
4720 Montgomery Lane
Bethesda, MD 20824-1220
301-652-2682
Fax: 301-652-7711
TDD: 800-377-8555
www.aota.org
15 pages
ISBN: 1-569001-49-9

2815 Occupational Therapy Practice Guidelines for Adults with Hip Fracture/Replacement
American Occupational Therapy Association
4720 Montgomery Lane
Bethesda, MD 20824-1220
301-652-2682
Fax: 301-652-7711
TDD: 800-377-8555
www.aota.org
10 pages
ISBN: 1-569001-48-0

2816 Staying Well: Advanced Pain Management for ACPA Members
American Chronic Pain Association
PO Box 850
Rocklin, CA 95677
916-632-0922
800-533-3231
Fax: 916-632-3208
e-mail: acpa@pacbell.net
www.theacpa.org
This workbook is designed for those who have a working knowledge of the basics of pain management. This workbook provides additional skills necessary to continue to move forward in the journey to wellness.

ISBN: 0-969387-81-7
Penny Cowan, Executive Director

2817 Understanding Chronic Pain
Angela Koestler, PhD; Ann Myers, MD, author
University Press of Mississippi
3825 Ridgewood Road
Jackson, MS 39211-6492
601-432-6205
Fax: 601-432-6217
e-mail: kburgess@ihl.state.ms.us
www.upress.state.ms.us
A handbook for people coping with chronic pain and suffering and for those who seek to understand and support them.
2002 184 pages Paperback
ISBN: 1-578064-40-6
Kathy Burgess, Advertising/Marketing Services Manager

2818 Your Pain is Real: Free Yourself from Chronic Pain, Breakthrough Med. Trtmnt.
DIANE Publishing Company
330 Pusey Avenue, Unit #3 Rear
Darby, PA 19023
610-461-6200
800-782-3833
Fax: 610-461-6130
e-mail: dianepublishing@gmail.com
www.dianepublishing.net
A complete, authoritative and hopeful book on the subject of chronic pain relief. Offers revolutionary ways to relieve all types and degrees of painful conditions. Also offers breakthrough medical treatments, clear guidelines for seeking expert care and the latest scientific findings on pain management.
252 pages Hardcover
ISBN: 0-756753-70-8
Herman Baron, Publisher

Newsletters

2819 American Chronic Pain Association
PO Box 850
Rocklin, CA 95677-0850
916-632-0922
800-533-3231
Fax: 916-632-3208
e-mail: ACPA@pacbell.net
www.theacpa.org
A nonprofit organization with over 400 chapters in the US, Canada, Australia, New Zealand and Russia. The purpose of this organization is to provide a support system for those suffering chronic pain through group activities.
Quart w/ mbrshp
Penny Cowan, Executive Founder & Director

2820 Health Points
TyH Publications
17007 E Colony Drive
Fountain Hills, AZ 85268
800-801-1406
e-mail: editor@e-tyh.com

National newsletter with articles on complementary therapy, latest nutrition news, disability issues and much more. Focus is on fibromyalgia, chronic fatigue, arthritis and chronic pain.
Quarterly

Audio & Video

2821 ACPA Relaxation Tapes
American Chronic Pain Association
PO Box 850   916-632-0922
Rocklin, CA 95677   800-533-3231
                                       Fax: 916-632-3208
                              e-mail: acpa@pacbell.net
                                      www.theacpa.org
Audio tapes offering information on pain relief, breath relaxation and autogenic relaxation. These tapes are designed to help persons regain control of their bodies through exercises in relaxation techniques. $10.00-$25.00.
Audio Tapes
Penny Cowan, Executive Director

2822 ACPA Video: 10 Steps from Patient to Person
American Chronic Pain Association
PO Box 850   916-632-0922
Rocklin, CA 95677   800-533-3231
                                       Fax: 916-632-3208
                              e-mail: acpa@pacbell.net
                                      www.theacpa.org
The video, featuring Penny Cowan, founder of the ACPA, discussed the value of a multidisiplinary pain management program and what is necessary to maintain wellness long term.
Penny Cowan, Executive Director

2823 Affirmation Tape
American Chronic Pain Association
PO Box 850   916-632-0922
Rocklin, CA 95677   800-533-3231
                                       Fax: 916-632-3208
                             e-mail: ACPA@pacbell.net
                                      www.theacpa.org
Designed to help you focus on positive things about yourself and builds self-esteem.
Penny Cowan, Executive Director

2824 Relaxation Tape
American Chronic Pain Association
PO Box 850   916-632-0922
Rocklin, CA 95677   800-533-3231
                                       Fax: 916-632-3208
                             e-mail: ACPA@pacbell.net
                                      www.theacpa.org
Tape one includes pain relief and breath relaxation. Tape two includes general relaxation and autogenic relaxation.
Penny Cowan, Executive Director

Web Sites

2825 American Chronic Pain Association
                                      www.theacpa.org
Facilitating peer support and education for individuals with chronic pain and their families so that these individuals may live more fully in spite of their pain.

2826 American Pain Society
                                         ampainsoc.org
Multidisciplinary organization of basic and clinical scientists, practicing clinicians, policy analysts, and others.

2827 Discovery Health
                                 health.discovery.com
A source of information on various health topics, including chronic pain and its symptoms and treatments.

2828 Healing Well
                                    www.healingwell.com
An online health resource guide to medical news, chat, information and articles, newsgroups and message boards, books, disease-related web sites, medical directories, and more for patients, friends, and family coping with disabling diseases, disorders, or chronic illnesses.

2829 Health Finder
                                    www.healthfinder.gov
Searchable, carefully developed web site offering information on over 1000 topics. Developed by the US Department of Health and Human Services, the site can be used in both English and Spanish.

2830 Healthlink USA
                                    www.healthlinkusa.com
Health information concerning treatment, cures, prevention, diagnosis, risk factors, research, support groups, email lists, personal stories and much more. Updated regularly.

2831 Helios Health
                                    www.helioshealth.com
Online resource for your health information. Detailed information about specific health topics, access to expert advice from our Medical Advisory Board, and up-to-date health news.

2832 International Pelvic Pain Society
                                      www.pelvicpain.org/
Short range goal is to recruit, organizae, and educate health care professionals actively invlved with the treatment of patients who have chronic opelvic pain.

2833 MedicineNet
                                    www.medicinenet.com
An online resource for consumers providing easy-to-read, authoritative medical and health information.

2834 Medscape
                                      www.medscape.com
Medscape offers specialists, primary care physicians, and other health professionals the Web's most robust and integrated medical information and educational tools.

2835 WebMD
                                        www.webmd.com
Information on chronic pain, including articles and resources.

Description

2836 Congenital Heart Disease

Congenital Heart Disease (CHD) represents the most common group of congenital (present from birth) anomalies. CHD can be thought of as a group of disorders that result from the abnormal formation of the heart in utero. The heart develops between the 2nd and 6th week of gestation, and may be affected by genetic mutation, maternal systemic medications or toxins (e.g. alcohol abuse). The incidence of CHD in the population is about 8 cases in 1,000 live births, or just under 1%. About half of these cardiac defects are considered to be minor and can be followed clinically while the other half fall into the categories of major CHD. This latter group often requires surgery early in life to either completely repair the heart defect or in some cases, to redirect blood through the cardiovascular system to palliate the structural abnormality.

CHD can be divided into three major categories: left to right shunting lesions, left heart obstructive lesions and those that lead to marked cyanosis (decreased oxygen delivery to the organs and tissues), the so called cyanotic heart diseases.

The left to right shunting lesions are the most common of the three groups and include the ventricular septal defect (VSD), the atrial septal defect (ASD), the atrioventricular septal defect (also referred to as the AV canal), and the patent ductus arteriosus. In all of these left to right shunting lesions, there is a progressive increase in the amount of blood sent from the left side of the heartacross the given defect (hole) into the right side that delivers blood to the lungs. There is as a result, too much blood entering the pulmonary circuit and this can lead to problems with breathing and feeding for infants in the first few months of life.

The more common left heart obstructive diseases include aortic stenosis, coarctation of the aorta and the hypoplastic left heart syndrome. Each of these can lead to a marked reduction in the amount of blood flow that is able to leave the left side of the heart and can be delivered to the organs and tissues. This leads to marked abnormalities in the way the organs and tissues function and can cause serious and emergent problems for infants in the first week or two of life.

Cyanotic heart disease are those cardiac malformations that lead to a bluish discoloration of the baby as there is insufficient oxygenated blood that is delivered to the body with or without inadequate blood delivered to the lungs to pick up oxygen. The more common disorders in this group are tetralogy of Fallot, Transposition of the great arteries, tricuspid atresia and truncus arteriosus.

With the remarkable advances in neonatal cardiac surgery and interventional cardiac catheterization, almost all of the cardiac malformations can be aggressively addressed with excellent results, even in the youngest and smallest of patients. Overall, survival from all cardiac surgeries in children with CHD is greater than 95%, and even for the most complex of CHD it is approaching 90%. These children often require long-term follow-up from a pediatric cardiologist, but the vast majority lead healthy active lives. See also *Birth Defects*.

National Agencies & Associations

2837 Adult Congenital Heart Association

6757 Greene Street
Philadelphia, PA 19119-3508

215-849-1260
888-921-ACHA
Fax: 215-849-1261
e-mail: Info@achaheart.org, www.achaheart.org

The Adult Congenital Heart Association (ACHA) is a nonprofit organization which seeks to improve the quality of life and extend the lives of adults with congenital heart defects through education, outreach, advocacy and promotion of research.
Amy Verstappen, President
Tim Clair, Chief Operating Officer

2838 Congenital Heart Information Network

101 N Washington Avenue
Margate City, NJ 08402-1195

609-822-1572
Fax: 609-822-1574
e-mail: mb@tchin.org
www.tchin.org

C.H.I.N. is a national organization that provides reliable information support services, financial assistance and resources to families of children with congenital heart defects and acquired heart disease and adults with congenital heart defects.
Mona Barmash, President

2839 Kids with Heart National Association for Children's Heart Disorders

1578 Careful Drive
Green Bay, WI 54307-2504

920-498-0058
800-538-5390
e-mail: michelle@kidswithheart.org
www.kidswithheart.org

Kids with Heart is a nonprofit organization founded in 1985 dedicated to providing support for families affected by congenital heart defects through surgical care packages.
Michelle Rin BA, President
Dean Rintamaki, Vice President

2840 Schneeweiss Adult Congenital Heart Disease Center

New York Presbyterian Hospital
161 Fort Washington Avenue
New York, NY 10032

212-305-6936
Fax: 212-305-0490
www.congenitalheart.hs.columbia.edu

We provide such diagnostic services such as echocardiography cardiac MRI and cardiac catheterization. Highly specialized care is provided by a team of physicians specifically interested in the problems of adults with congenital heart disease.
Marlon S Rosenbaum MD, Director
Jonathan Ginns, Adult Congenital Heart Disease

Web Sites

2841 Heartpoint

www.heartpoint.com
Heartpoint provides information about specific heart defects.

2842 MedicineNet

www.medicinenet.com
An online resource for consumers providing easy-to-read, authoritative medical and health information.

2843 Medline Plus

www.nlm.nih.gov/medlineplus
This website includes information about congenital heart disease and includes links regarding support and treatment.

2844 Yale: Congenital Heart Disease

info.med.yale.edu/intmed/cardio/chd
This web site provides in-depth information regarding various types of heart conditions.

Description

2845 Cooley's Anemia (Thalassemia)

Cooley's anemia, or beta-Thalassemia major, is an inherited disorder characterized by abnormal production of hemoglobin in the red blood cells. There are two forms of beta-Thalassemia: beta-Thalassemia minor, in which the person has no symptoms, and beta-Thalassemia major, or Cooley's anemia, which is a severe, debilitating disease. Although a baby who has Cooley's anemia appears normal at birth, growth rates are impaired, and puberty may be significantly delayed or absent. Without therapy, there is a general decline. The skin becomes pale or jaundiced, facial bones become more prominent and pronounced, and the spleen becomes enlarged.

While there is no cure for Cooley's anemia, there are treatments such as blood transfusions, which can reduce some symptoms of the disease. However, children with Cooley's anemia should receive as few transfusions as possible because of the danger of iron overload from the "heme" portion of hemoglobin. Chelation, or binding, of the excess iron associated with multiple, repetitive transfusions is important, and is accomplished with deferoxamine. Removal of the spleen may reduce transfusion requirements.

Because there is no cure for beta-Thalassemia major, genetic screening of at-risk populations is very important, notably for persons of Mediterranean, African and Southeast Asian ancestry. Prenatal diagnosis can also be performed.

National Agencies & Associations

2846 American Hellenic Educational Progressive Association
1909 Q Street NW
Washington, DC 20009
202-232-6300
Fax: 202-232-2140
e-mail: ahepa@ahepa.org
www.ahepa.org
The mission of the AHEPA Family is to promote Hellenism Education Philanthropy Civic Responsibility and Family and Individual Excellence.
Basil N Mossaidis, Executive Director

2847 Fanconi Anemia Research Foundation
1801 Willamette Street
Eugene, OR 97401
541-687-4658
888-326-2664
Fax: 541-687-0548
e-mail: info@fanconi.org
www.fanconi.org
Funds research and provides education and support services worldwide to families affected with Fanconi anemia a rare genetic aplastic anemia that leads to bone marrow failure acute myelogenous leukemia and squamous cell carcinomas.

State Agencies & Associations

California

2848 Cooley's Anemia Foundation (CAF): California
2629 Foothill Boulevard
La Crescenta, CA 91214
800-601-2821
Fax: 212-279-5999
e-mail: info@cooleysanemia.org
www.cooleysanemia.org
The Cooley's Anemia Foundation (CAF) is dedicated to serving people afflicted with various forms of thalassemia, most notably the major form of this genetic blood disease, Cooley's anemia/thalassemia major. CAF's mission is advancing the treatment and curing the disease.
Christine Giannamore, Coordinator
Gina Cioffi Esq, National Office Executive Director

Illinois

2849 Cooley's Anemia Foundation (CAF): Illinois Oakbrook Towers
Oakbrook Towers
40 N Tower Road
Altbrook, IL 62503
847-602-2616
800-522-7222
Fax: 212-279-5999
e-mail: info@cooleysanemia.org
www.cooleysanemia.org
The Cooley's Anemia Foundation (CAF) is dedicated to serving people afflicted with various forms of thalassemia most notably the major form of this genetic blood disease Cooley's anemia/thalassemia major. CAF's mission is advancing the treatment and curing the disease.
Bruce Rod, President Illinois Office
Gina Cioffi, National Office Executive Director

Maryland

2850 Cooley's Anemia Foundation (CAF): Capital Area
15321 Peach Orchard Avenue
Silver Spring, MD 20905
301-989-8947
800-522-7222
Fax: 212-279-5999
e-mail: info@cooleysanemia.org
www.cooleysanemia.org
The Cooley's Anemia Foundation (CAF) is dedicated to serving people afflicted with various forms of thalassemia most notably the major form of this genetic blood disease Cooley's anemia/thalassemia major. CAF's mission is advancing the treatment and curing the disease.
Carl C Vitaliti, President Capital Area Office
Gina Cioffi Esq, National Office Executive Director

Massachusetts

2851 Cooley's Anemia Foundation (CAF): Massachusetts Chapter
44 Joseph Road
Newton, MA 02460-1122
617-332-5952
800-522-7222
Fax: 212-279-5999
e-mail: info@cooleysanemia.org
www.cooleysanemia.org
The Cooley's Anemia Foundation (CAF) is dedicated to serving people afflicted with various forms of thalassemia most notably the major form of this genetic blood disease Cooley's anemia/thalassemia major. CAF's mission is advancing the treatment and curing the disease.
Rudi Viscomi, President Massachusetts Office
Gina Cioffi, National Office Executive Director

New Jersey

2852 Cooley's Anemia Foundation (CAF): New Jersey Chapter
29 Alyson Place
Bloomfield, NJ 07003
732-688-2279
800-522-7222
Fax: 212-279-5999
e-mail: info@cooleysanemia.org
www.cooleysanemia.org
The Cooley's Anemia Foundation (CAF) is dedicated to serving people afflicted with various forms of thalassemia most notably the major form of this genetic blood disease Cooley's anemia/thalassemia major. CAF's mission is advancing the treatment and curing the disease.
Christine Somma, President New Jersey Office
Gina Cioffi, National Office Executive Director

New York

2853 Cooley's Anemia Foundation (CAF): Rochester
585-482-5587
800-522-7222
Fax: 212-279-5999
e-mail: info@cooleysanemia.org
www.cooleysanemia.org

The Cooley's Anemia Foundation (CAF) is dedicated to serving people afflicted with various forms of thalassemia most notably the major form of this genetic blood disease Cooley's anemia/thalassemia major. CAF's mission is advancing the treatment and curing the disease.
Shirley Cammilleri, President Rochester Office
Gina Cioffi Esq, National Office Executive Director

2854 Cooley's Anemia Foundation (CAF): Buffalo
135 Wellington Road   716-834-8903
Buffalo, NY 14216   800-522-7222
                              Fax: 212-279-5999
                    e-mail: info@cooleysanemia.org
                              www.cooleysanemia.org
The Cooley's Anemia Foundation (CAF) is dedicated to serving people afflicted with various forms of thalassemia most notably the major form of this genetic blood disease Cooley's anemia/thalassemia major. CAF's mission is advancing the treatment and curing the disease.
Dennis Locurto, President Buffalo Office
Gina Cioffi Esq, National Office Executive Director

2855 Cooley's Anemia Foundation (CAF): Long Island
111 Cherry Valley Avenue   516-358-9100
Garden City, NY 11530   800-522-7222
                              Fax: 516-358-9101
                    e-mail: info@cooleysanemia.org
                              www.cooleysanemia.org
The Cooley's Anemia Foundation (CAF) is dedicated to serving people afflicted with various forms of thalassemia most notably the major form of this genetic blood disease Cooley's anemia/thalassemia major. CAF's mission is advancing the treatment and curing the disease.
Thomas Rotolo, President Long Island Office
Janice Cenzoprano, Vice President Long Island Office

2856 Cooley's Anemia Foundation (CAF): Queens
157-26 9th Avenue   718-746-7677
Beachurst, NY 11357   800-522-7222
                              Fax: 718-746-7678
                    e-mail: info@cooleysanemia.org
                              www.cooleysanemia.org
The Cooley's Anemia Foundation (CAF) is dedicated to serving people afflicted with various forms of thalassemia most notably the major form of this genetic blood disease Cooley's anemia/thalassemia major. CAF's mission is advancing the treatment and curing the disease.
Paul Tucci, President Queen Office
Abbey Chakalis, Events Manager

2857 Cooley's Anemia Foundation (CAF): Staten Island
16B Dreyer Avenue   718-761-5380
Staten Island, NY 10314   800-522-7222
                              Fax: 718-761-5381
                    e-mail: info@cooleysanemia.org
                              www.cooleysanemia.org
The Cooley's Anemia Foundation (CAF) is dedicated to serving people afflicted with various forms of thalassemia most notably the major form of this genetic blood disease Cooley's anemia/thalassemia major. CAF's mission is advancing the treatment and curing the disease.
Gina Cioffi Esq, National Office Executive Director
Craig Butler, National Office Communications Director

2858 Cooley's Anemia Foundation (CAF): Suffolk Chapter Office
740 Smithtown Bypass   631-863-0532
Smithtown, NY 11787   800-522-7222
                              Fax: 631-863-0535
                    e-mail: info@cooleysanemia.org
                              www.cooleysanemia.org
The Cooley's Anemia Foundation (CAF) is dedicated to serving people afflicted with various forms of thalassemia most notably the major form of this genetic blood disease Cooley's anemia/thalassemia major. CAF's mission is advancing the treatment and curing the disease.
Gina Cioffi Esq, National Office Executive Director
Craig Butler, National Office Communications Director

2859 Cooley's Anemia Foundation (CAF): Westches ter/Rockland Chapter
3 Samuel Purdy Lane   914-232-1808
Katonah, NY 10536   800-522-7222
                              Fax: 212-279-5999
                    e-mail: info@cooleysanemia.org
                              www.cooleysanemia.org
The Cooley's Anemia Foundation (CAF) is dedicated to serving people afflicted with various forms of thalassemia most notably the major form of this genetic blood disease Cooley's anemia/thalassemia major. CAF's mission is advancing the treatment and curing the disease.
Peter Chieco, President Westchester/Rockland Office
Janet Manning, Executive Director

Texas

2860 Cooley's Anemia Foundation (CAF): Texas
4504 Astor Road   214-324-6147
Mesquite, TX 75150-2320   800-522-7222
                              Fax: 214-324-0612
                    e-mail: info@cooleysanemia.org
                              www.cooleysanemia.org
The Cooley's Anemia Foundation (CAF) is dedicated to serving people afflicted with various forms of thalassemia most notably the major form of this genetic blood disease Cooley's anemia/thalassemia major.
Mateen Shah, President
Gina Cioffi Esq, National Office Executive Director

Foundations

2861 Cooleys Anemia Foundation
330 Seventh Avenue
New York, NY 10001   800-522-7222
                              Fax: 212-279-5999
                    e-mail: info@cooleysanemia.org
                              www.cooleysanemia.org
Our mission is advancing the treatment and cure for this fatal blood disease, enhancing the quality of life of patients and educating the medical profession, trait carriers and the public about Cooley's anemia/thalassemia major.
Gina Cioffi, Esq, National Executive Director
Craig Butler, Communications Director

Support Groups & Hotlines

2862 National Health Information Center
PO Box 1133   310-565-4167
Washington, DC 20013   800-336-4797
                              Fax: 301-984-4256
                    e-mail: info@nhic.org
                              www.health.gov/nhic
A health information referral service sponsored by the Office of Disease Prevention and Health Promotion. Puts health professionals and consumers who have health questions in touch with those organizations that are best able to provide answers.
Ellen Langhans, Chairwoman
Linda Harris, Lead, Health Communication and e-health

Books

2863 Genes, Blood & Courage
129-09 26th Avenue   212-598-0911
Flushing, NY 11354   800-522-7222
                              www.cooleysanemia.org

2864 What is Cooley's Anemia
129-09 26th Avenue   718-321-2873
Flushing, NY 11354   800-522-7222
                              Fax: 718-321-3340
                    e-mail: info@cooleysanemia.org
                              www.cooleysanemia.org
Patient and family handbook.
Jayne Restivo, National Executive Director

2865   What is Thalassemia?
Cooley's Anemia Foundation
129-09 26th Avenue   718-321-2873
Flushing, NY 11354   800-522-7222
                                          Fax: 718-321-3340
                          e-mail: info@cooleysanemia.org
                                    www.cooleysanemia.org
A guide to help thalassemics and their parents understand thalassemia, the reasons for treatment and the hope for the future.
Jayne Restivo, National Executive Director

Children's Books

2866   Coloring Book on Thalassemia
129-09 26th Avenue   718-321-2873
Flushing, NY 11354   800-522-7222
                                          Fax: 718-321-3340
                          e-mail: info@cooleysanemia.org
                                    www.cooleysanemia.org
Available in English, Italian, Greek and Chinese.
Jayne Restivo, National Executive Director

Magazines

2867   AHEPAN Magazine
American Hellenic Educational Progressive Assn
1909 Q Street NW   202-232-6300
Washington, DC 20009   Fax: 202-232-2140
                                e-mail: ahepa@ahepa.org
                                          www.ahepa.org
This magazine includes all of the AHEPA organizations.
Quarterly
Basil N Mossaidis, Executive Director

Newsletters

2868   Lifeline
Cooley's Anemia Foundation
129-09 26th Avenue   718-321-2873
Flushing, NY 11354   800-522-7222
                                          Fax: 718-321-3340
                          e-mail: info@cooleysanemia.org
                                    www.cooleysanemia.org
A newsletter published by Cooley's Anemia Foundation.
Jayne Restivo, National Executive Director

Pamphlets

2869   Desferal Q&A
129-09 26th Avenue   718-321-2873
Flushing, NY 11354   800-522-7222
                                          Fax: 718-321-3340
                          e-mail: info@cooleysanemia.org
                                    www.cooleysanemia.org
Guideline for home infusion.
Jayne Restivo, National Executive Director

2870   What is Thalassemia Trait?
Cooley's Anemia Foundation
129-09 26th Avenue   718-321-2873
Flushing, NY 11354   800-522-7222
                                          Fax: 718-321-3340
                          e-mail: info@cooleysanemia.org
                                    www.cooleysanemia.org
This booklet offers information on the thalassemia trait.
1995
Jayne Restivo, National Executive Director

Audio & Video

2871   TAG Annual Patient/Family Conference Video
Cooley's Anemia Foundation

Thalassemia Action Group
New York, NY 10001   800-522-7222
                                          Fax: 212-279-5999
                              e-mail: TAG@cooleysanemia.org
                                   www.cooleysanemia.org/
Video from the Thalassemia Action Group/TAG Annual Patient/Family Conference held in March of each year.
Gina Cioffi Esq, National Executive Director
Craig Butler, Communications Director

2872   To Live
Cooley's Anemia Foundation
330 Seventh Avenue
New York, NY 10001   800-522-7222
                                          Fax: 212-279-5999
                           e-mail: info@cooleysanemia.org
                                   www.cooleysanemia.org/
An informative and educational video from Cooley's Anemia Foundation.
Gina Cioffi Esq, National Executive Director
Craig Butler, Communications Director

2873   You're Not Alone
Cooley's Anemia Foundation
330 Seventh Avenue
New York, NY 10004   800-522-7222
                                          Fax: 212-279-5999
                           e-mail: info@cooleysanemia.org
                                    www.cooleysanemia.org
An informative and educational video from Cooley's Anemia Foundation.
Gina Cioffi Esq, National Executive Director
Craig Butler, Communications Director

Web Sites

2874   Healing Well
                                    www.healingwell.com
An online health resource guide to medical news, chat, information and articles, newsgroups and message boards, books, disease-related web sites, medical directories, and more for patients, friends, and family coping with disabling diseases, disorders, or chronic illnesses.

2875   Health Finder
                                    www.healthfinder.gov
Searchable, carefully developed web site offering information on over 1000 topics. Developed by the US Department of Health and Human Services, the site can be used in both English and Spanish.

2876   Healthlink USA
                                    www.healthlinkusa.com
Health information concerning treatment, cures, prevention, diagnosis, risk factors, research, support groups, email lists, personal stories and much more. Updated regularly.

2877   Helios Health
                                    www.helioshealth.com
Online resource for your health information. Detailed information about specific health topics, access to expert advice from our Medical Advisory Board, and up-to-date health news.

2878   MedicineNet
                                    www.medicinenet.com
An online resource for consumers providing easy-to-read, authoritative medical and health information.

2879   Medscape
                                    www.medscape.com
Medscape offers specialists, primary care physicians, and other health professionals the Web's most robust and integrated medical information and educational tools.

2880   WebMD
                                    www.webmd.com
Information on Cooley's Anemia (Thalassemia), including articles and resources.

Description

2881 Crohn's Disease

Crohn's disease is a chronic inflammation in the lining of the digestive tract, generally in the small bowel or part of the colon. The cause is unknown, although the disease is more common in some families and racial groups. Although not a proven cause, periods of emotional stress have been linked with flare-ups of the disease. Onset is typically before age 30, with the peak incidence between 14 and 24 years.

Common symptoms include diarrhea, weight loss, fever, abdominal pain and loss of appetite. If the disease is extensive it may cause deficiencies of essential vitamins and other nutrients. Sometimes inflammation occurs outside the gut, attacking the eyes, joints or skin. Local complications include bowel perforation with formation of abscesses or fistulas which drain out to the skin. Established chronic Crohn's disease is characterized by lifelong exacerbations. These patients carry an increased risk of cancer of the small bowel and colon/rectum.

Therapy depends on the location of the disease and on its severity. Although no specific therapy is known, drug treatment can range from simple anti-diarrheal medications to anti-inflammatory drugs and immunosuppressives. Surgery may be necessary to treat complications. In all cases, careful attention should be paid to the patient's nutritional status and psychological well-being. See also *Gastrointestinal Disorders* and *Celiac Disease*.

National Agencies & Associations

2882 CCFA Camps Across America Crohn's & Colitis Foundation of America
Crohn's & Colitis Foundation of America
386 Park Avenue S   212-685-3440
New York, NY 10016   800-932-2423
                                      Fax: 212-779-4098
                                   e-mail: info@ccfa.org
                                          www.ccfa.org
A chance for children with Crhon's disease or ulcerative colitis to have a camping experience. Because CCFA camps are offered by chapters across the country every camp has its own flavor and style. Activities, as well as the length of stay may vary from child to child.
Richard Geswell, President

2883 Crohn's & Colitis Foundation of America
386 Park Avenue S   212-685-3440
New York, NY 10016   800-932-2423
                                      Fax: 212-779-4098
                                   e-mail: info@ccfa.org
                                          www.ccfa.org
CCFA's mission is to cure and prevent Crohn's disease and ulcerative colitis through research and to improve the quality of life of children and adults affected by this disease through education and support. The foundation offers patient and professional support.
Richard Geswell, President

2884 Ileitis and Colitis Educational Foundation
Central DuPage Hospital
25 N Winfield Road   630-933-1600
Winfield, IL 60190   Fax: 630-933-1300
                                      TTY: 630-933-4833
                        e-mail: cdh_information@cdh.org
                                           www.cdh.org

Offers support groups fund-raising activities educational materials and public awareness campaigns pertaining to these disorders.
Luke McGuinness, President, CEO
Richard A Mark, Vice Chair

2885 International Foundation for Functional Gastrointestinal Disorders (IFFGD)
PO Box 170864   414-964-1799
Milwaukee, WI 53217-8076   888-964-2001
                                      Fax: 414-964-7176
                                   e-mail: iffgd@iffgd.org
                                          www.iffgd.org
Nonprofit education, support and research organization devoted to increasing awareness and understanding of functional gastrointestinal disorders, including irritable bowel syndrome (IBS), constipation, diarrhea, pain, and incontinence. Mission is to inform, assist and support people affected by these disorders.
Nancy J Norton, President

2886 National Institute of Diabetes, Digestive & Kidney Diseases
National Institute of Health
1 Information Way   800-860-8747
Bethesda, MD 20892-3560   Fax: 703-738-4929
                                      TTY: 866-569-1162
                          e-mail: ndic@info.niddk.nih.gov
                                    www.diabetes.niddk.nih.gov
Conducts and supports research on many of the most serious diseases affecting public health. The Institute supports much of the clinical research on the diseases of internal medicine and related subspecialty fields as well as many basic science disciplines.
Dr. Griffin Rodgers, Acting Director

2887 Pediatric Crohn's and Colitis Association
PO Box 188   617-489-5854
Newton, MA 02468   e-mail: questions@pcca.hypermart.net
                                    www.pcca.hypermart.net
Focuses on all aspects of pediatric and adolescent Crohn's disease and ulcerative colitis, including medical, nutritional, psychological and social factors. Activities include information sharing, educational forums, newsletters and hospital outreach programs.

2888 Reach Out for Youth with Ileitis and Colitis
PO Box 857   631-293-3102
Melville, NY 11747   TTY: 631-293-3103
                          e-mail: info@reachoutforyouth.org
                                    www.reachoutforyouth.org
Provides educational seminars and individual and group support to patients and their families. Fundraising efforts support the center's programs, clinical and laboratory research, and purchase of state-of-the-art equipment.
Susan Spellman, Founder and Executive Director

2889 United Ostomy Association
PO Box 512
Northfield, MN 55057   800-826-0826
                                      Fax: 507-645-5168
                                    e-mail: info@uoa.org
                                           www.uoa.org
A national network for bowel and urinary diversion support groups in the United States. Its goal is to provide a nonprofit association that will serve to unify and strengthen its member support groups, which are organized for the benefit of people who have, or will have intestinal or urinary diversions and their caregivers.
David Rudzin, President
Daine Miterko, UOAA Advocacy Chair

2890 World Ostomy and Continence Nurses Society
15000 Commerce Parkway
Mt Laurel, NJ 08054   888-224-9626
                                      Fax: 856-439-0525
                                e-mail: wocn_info@wocn.org
                                          www.wocn.org
Membership comprises nurses that specialize in enterostomal therapy.
Phyllis Kupsick, MSN, FNP-BC, CW, President
Carolyn Watts, MSN, RN, CWON, President-Elect

State Agencies & Associations

Alabama

2891 CCFA Alabama Chapter
244 Goodwin Crest Drive
Birmingham, AL 35259
205-941-9900
800-249-1993
Fax: 205-941-1411
e-mail: ptalty@ccfa.org OR info@ccfa.org
www.ccfa.org/chapters/alabama/
Crohn's and Colitis Foundation of America is a non-profit, volunteer-driven organization dedicated to finding the cure for Crohn's disease and ulcerative colitis.
Pat Talty, Executive Director

Arizona

2892 CCFA Southwest Chapter: Arizona
8098 Via de Negocio
Scottsdale, AZ 85258
480-246-3676
877-259-2104
Fax: 480-246-3679
e-mail: southwest@ccfa.org
www.ccfa.org/chapters/southwest/
Crohn's and Colitis Foundation of America is a non-profit volunteer-driven organization dedicated to finding the cure for Crohn's disease and ulcerative colitis.
Kathie Gadberry, Executive Director
Bernadette Sewer, Development Coordinator

California

2893 CCFA California: Greater Los Angeles Chapter
1640 S Sepulveda Boulevard
Los Angeles, CA 90025
310-478-4500
866-831-9157
Fax: 310-478-4546
e-mail: losangeles@ccfa.org
www.ccfa.org/chapters/losangeles/
Crohn's and Colitis Foundation of America is a non-profit volunteer-driven organization dedicated to finding the cure for Crohn's disease and ulcerative colitis.
Iyad Zabaneh, Development Coordinator
Kerri Yoder, Education Manager

Colorado

2894 CCFA Rocky Mountain Chapter
1777 S Bellaire Street
Denver, CO 80222
303-639-9163
866-768-2232
Fax: 303-568-0424
e-mail: rockymountain@ccfa.org
www.ccfa.org/chapters/rockymountain/
Crohn's and Colitis Foundation of America is a non-profit volunteer-driven organization dedicated to finding the cure for Crohn's disease and ulcerative colitis.
Nancy Freimuth, Walk Manager
Mackenzie Lyle, Interim Executive Director

Connecticut

2895 CCFA Central Connecticut Chapter
P O Box 275
Branford, CT 06405
203-208-3130
e-mail: mgrande@ccfa.org
www.ccfa.org/chapters/centralct/
Crohn's and Colitis Foundation of America is a non-profit volunteer-driven organization dedicated to finding the cure for Crohn's disease and ulcerative colitis.
Sally Connolly, Board President

2896 CCFA Northern Connecticut Affiliate Chapter
PO Box 370614
W Hartford, CT 06137-0614
212-679-1570
800-932-2423
Fax: 212-679-3567
e-mail: info@ccfa.org
www.ccfa.org/chapters/northernct/
Crohn's and Colitis Foundation of America is a non-profit volunteer-driven organization dedicated to finding the cure for Crohn's disease and ulcerative colitis.
Marilyn Hagg Blohm, Executive Director National Headquarters
Jeff Neale, Public Relations National Headquarters

Florida

2897 CCFA Florida Chapter
2250 N Druid Hills Road
Boca Raton, FL 30329-2391
404-982-0616
877-664-2929
Fax: 404-982-0656
e-mail: kkeohane@ccfa.org
www.ccfa.org/chapters/florida/
Crohn's and Colitis Foundation of America is a non-profit volunteer-driven organization dedicated to finding the cure for Crohn's disease and ulcerative colitis.
Deborah Barnard, Development Manager
Lacy Woods, Administrator

Georgia

2898 CCFA Georgia Chapter
2250 N Druid Hills Road
Atlanta, GA 30329
404-982-0616
800-472-6795
Fax: 404-982-0656
e-mail: georgia@ccfa.org
www.ccfa.org/chapters/georgia/
Crohn's and Colitis Foundation of America is a non-profit volunteer-driven organization dedicated to finding the cure for Crohn's disease and ulcerative colitis.
Marcia Greenburg, Executive Director
Karen Rittenbaum, Development Director

Illinois

2899 CCFA Illinois: Carol Fisher Chapter
2250 E Devon Avenue
Des Plaines, IL 60018
847-827-0404
800-886-6664
Fax: 847-827-6563
e-mail: Illinois@ccfa.org
www.ccfa.org/chapters/illinois/
Crohn's and Colitis Foundation of America is a non-profit volunteer-driven organization dedicated to finding the cure for Crohn's disease and ulcerative colitis.
Marianne Floriano, Executive Director
Kristina Sickles, Development Coordinator

Indiana

2900 CCFA Indiana Chapter
931 E 86th Street
Indianapolis, IN 46240
317-259-8071
800-332-6029
Fax: 317-259-8091
e-mail: indiana@ccfa.org
www.ccfa.org/chapters/indiana/
Crohn's and Colitis Foundation of America is a non-profit volunteer-driven organization dedicated to finding the cure for Crohn's disease and ulcerative colitis.
Scott Baumruck, Development Director
Dawn Drinkut, Development Assistant

Iowa

2901 CCFA Iowa Chapter
PO Box 1184
Johnston, IA 50131-0016
515-664-8961
Fax: 319-277-6293
e-mail: iowa@ccfa.org
www.ccfa.org/chapters/iowa/
Crohn's and Colitis Foundation of America is a non-profit volunteer-driven organization dedicated to finding the cure for Crohn's disease and ulcerative colitis.
Tony Kline, Chapter President
Abbie Hansen, Vice President Communications

Kansas

2902 CCFA Mid-America Chapter: Kansas
1034 S Brentwood
St Louis, MO 63117
314-863-4747
800-783-8006
Fax: 314-863-4749
e-mail: sskodak@ccfa.org
www.ccfa.org/chapters/midamerica/

Crohn's and Colitis Foundation of America is a non-profit volunteer-driven organization dedicated to finding the cure for Crohn's disease and ulcerative colitis.
Steve Skodak, Executive Director
Andi Harrington, Development Manager

Louisiana

2903   CCFA Louisiana Chapter
7611 Maple Street   504-861-3433
New Orleans, LA 70118   866-382-2232
                                       Fax: 504-861-3466
                              e-mail: lams@ccfa.org
                              www.ccfa.org/chapters/louisiana
Crohn's and Colitis Foundation of America is a non-profit volunteer-driven organization dedicated to finding the cure for Crohn's disease and ulcerative colitis.
David Lee Thomas, Development Director
Gail C Smith, Development Assistant

Maryland

2904   CCFA Maryland Chapter
10400 Little Patuxent Parkway   443-276-0861
Columbia, MD 21044   800-618-5583
                                       Fax: 443-276-0865
                              e-mail: maryland@ccfa.org
                              www.ccfa.org/chapters/md-southde
Crohn's and Colitis Foundation of America is a non-profit volunteer-driven organization dedicated to finding the cure for Crohn's disease and ulcerative colitis.
Robert J Milanchus, Regional Executive Director
Mary Glagola, President

Massachusetts

2905   CCFA New England Chapter: Massachusetts
280 Hillside Avenue   781-449-0324
Needham, MA 02494   800-314-3459
                                       Fax: 781-449-0325
                              e-mail: ne@ccfa.org
                              www.ccfa.org/chapters/ne
Crohn's and Colitis Foundation of America is a non-profit volunteer-driven organization dedicated to finding the cure for Crohn's disease and ulcerative colitis.
Jess Adani, Development Manager
Kristin Patmos, Education Manager

Michigan

2906   CCFA Michigan Chapter: Farmington Hills
31313 N Western Highway   248-737-0900
Farmington Hills, MI 78334   Fax: 248-737-0904
                              e-mail: michigan@ccfa.org
                              www.ccfa.org/chapters/michigan
Crohn's and Colitis Foundation of America is a non-profit volunteer-driven organization dedicated to finding the cure for Crohn's disease and ulcerative colitis.
Bernard L Riker, Executive Director
Gilda Hauser, Development Manager

Minnesota

2907   CCFA Minnesota Chapter
1885 University Avenue W   651-917-2424
Saint Paul, MN 55104   888-422-3266
                                       Fax: 651-917-2425
                              e-mail: Minnesota@ccfa.org
                              www.ccfa.org/chapters/minnesota
Crohn's and Colitis Foundation of America is a non-profit volunteer-driven organization dedicated to finding the cure for Crohn's disease and ulcerative colitis.
Maggie Brown, Take Steps Manager
Ruby Lanoux, Development Manager

Missouri

2908   CCFA Mid-America Chapter: Missouri
1034 S Brentwood   314-863-4747
Saint Louis, MO 63117   800-783-8006
                                       Fax: 314-863-4749
                              e-mail: info@ccfa.org
                              www.ccfa.org/chapters/midamerica
Crohn's and Colitis Foundation of America is a non-profit volunteer-driven organization dedicated to finding the cure for Crohn's disease and ulcerative colitis.
Steve Skodak, Executive Director
Andi Harrington, Development Manager

New Jersey

2909   CCFA New Jersey Chapter
45 Wilson Avenue   732-786-9960
Manalapan, NJ 07726   Fax: 732-786-9964
                              e-mail: newjersey@ccfa.org
                              www.ccfa.org/chapters/newjersey
Crohn's and Colitis Foundation of America is a non-profit volunteer-driven organization dedicated to finding the cure for Crohn's disease and ulcerative colitis.
Rosemarie Golombos, Executive Director
Barbara Fedorchak, Chapter Development Manager

New York

2910   CCFA Greater New York Chapter: National Headquarters
386 Park Avenue S   800-932-2423
New York, NY 10016-8804   800-932-2423
                                       Fax: 212-679-3567
                              e-mail: info@ccfa.org
                              www.ccfa.org
Crohn's and Colitis Foundation of America is a non-profit volunteer-driven organization dedicated to finding the cure for Crohn's disease and ulcerative colitis.
Marilyn Hagg Blohm, Executive Director
Jeff Neale, Public Relations/Media Director

2911   CCFA Long Island Chapter
585 Stewart Avenue   516-222-5530
Garden City, NY 11530   Fax: 516-222-5535
                              e-mail: longisland@ccfa.org
                              www.ccfa.org/chapters/longisland
Crohn's and Colitis Foundation of America is a non-profit volunteer-driven organization dedicated to finding the cure for Crohn's disease and ulcerative colitis.
Marilyn Hagg Blohm, Executive Director National Office
Jeff Neale, Public Relations/Media National Office

2912   CCFA Rochester/Southern Tier Chapter
2117 Buffalo Road   585-617-4771
Rochester, NY 14624   800-932-2423
                              e-mail: rochester@ccfa.org
                              www.ccfa.org/chapters/rochester
Crohn's and Colitis Foundation of America is a non-profit volunteer-driven organization dedicated to finding the cure for Crohn's disease and ulcerative colitis.
Marilyn Hagg Blohm, Executive Director National Headquarters
Jeff Neale, Public Relations

2913   CCFA Upstate/Northeastern New York Chapter
4 Normanskill Boulevard   518-439-0252
Delmar, NY 12054   e-mail: upstateny@ccfa.org
                              www.ccfa.org/chapters/upstateny
Crohn's and Colitis Foundation of America is a non-profit volunteer-driven organization dedicated to finding the cure for Crohn's disease and ulcerative colitis.
Linda Winston, Chapter President
Peter Purcel MD, Medical Advisory Chair

2914   CCFA Western New York Chapter
2714 Sheridan Drive   716-833-2870
Tonawanda, NY 14150-0224   800-932-2423
                              e-mail: jpetri@ccfa.org
                              www.ccfa.org/chapters/westernny

Crohn's and Colitis Foundation of America is a non-profit volunteer-driven organization dedicated to finding the cure for Crohn's disease and ulcerative colitis.
Marilyn Hagg Blohm, Executive Director National Headquarters
Jeff Neale, Public Relations

North Carolina

2915 CCFA Carolinas Chapter
2901 N Davidson Street   704-332-1611
Charlotte, NC 28205   877-332-1611
Fax: 704-332-1612
e-mail: carolinas@ccfa.org
www.ccfa.org/chapters/carolinas
Crohn's and Colitis Foundation of America is a non-profit volunteer-driven organization dedicated to finding the cure for Crohn's disease and ulcerative colitis.
Angela Parks, Development Director
Julie Perkins, Special Events/Development Manager

2916 CCFA South Carolina Chapter
2901 N Davidson Street   704-332-1611
Charlotte, NC 28205   877-632-1611
Fax: 704-332-1612
e-mail: carolinas@ccfa.org
www.ccfa.org/chapters/carolinas
Crohn's and Colitis Foundation of America is a non-profit volunteer-driven organization dedicated to finding the cure for Crohn's disease and ulcerative colitis.
Angela Parks, Development Manager
Tewanna Sanders, Education & Support Manager

Ohio

2917 CCFA Central Ohio Chapter
5008 Pine Creek Drive   614-865-1933
Westerville, OH 43081   800-625-5977
Fax: 614-865-1934
e-mail: centralohio@ccfa.org
www.ccfa.org/chapters/centralohio
Crohn's and Colitis Foundation of America is a non-profit volunteer-driven organization dedicated to finding the cure for Crohn's disease and ulcerative colitis.
Janelle Gasaway, Take Steps Manager
Kelly Bush, Development Coordinator

2918 CCFA Northeast Ohio Chapter
23775 Commerce Park Road   216-831-2692
Beachwood, OH 44122   866-345-2232
Fax: 216-831-2792
e-mail: neohio@ccfa.org
www.ccfa.org/chapters/neohio
Crohn's and Colitis Foundation of America is a non-profit volunteer-driven organization dedicated to finding the cure for Crohn's disease and ulcerative colitis.
Kristin Knipp, Development Coordinator
Patty Kaplan, Development Manager NE Ohio Chapter

2919 CCFA Southwest Ohio Chapter
8 Triangle Park Drive   513-772-3550
Cincinnati, OH 45246   877-283-7513
Fax: 513-772-7599
e-mail: SWOhio@ccfa.org
www.ccfa.org/chapters/swohio
Crohn's and Colitis Foundation of America is a non-profit volunteer-driven organization dedicated to finding the cure for Crohn's disease and ulcerative colitis.
Rachel Spradlin, Take Steps Manager
Jenny Southers, Development Manager SE Ohio Chapter

Oklahoma

2920 CCFA Oklahoma Chapter
4504 E 67th Street   918-523-8540
Tulsa, OK 74136   800-658-1533
Fax: 918-523-8560
e-mail: jsummers@ccfa.org
www.ccfa.org/chapters/oklahoma

Crohn's and Colitis Foundation of America is a non-profit volunteer-driven organization dedicated to finding the cure for Crohn's disease and ulcerative colitis.
Judy Summers, Regional Executive Director
Christopher Woods, President

Pennsylvania

2921 CCFA Philadelphia/Delaware Valley Chapter
367 E Street Road   215-396-9100
Trevose, PA 19053   888-340-4744
Fax: 215-396-1170
e-mail: Philadelphia@ccfa.org
www.ccfa.org/chapters/philadelphia
Crohn's and Colitis Foundation of America is a non-profit volunteer-driven organization dedicated to finding the cure for Crohn's disease and ulcerative colitis.
Barbara Berman, Executive Director
Suzanne Rhodeside, Development Director

2922 CCFA Western Pennsylvania/West Virginia Chapter
300 Penn Center Boulevard   412-823-8272
Pittsburgh, PA 15235   877-823-8272
Fax: 412-823-8276
e-mail: wpawv@ccfa.org
www.ccfa.org/chapters/wpawv
Crohn's and Colitis Foundation of America is a non-profit volunteer-driven organization dedicated to finding the cure for Crohn's disease and ulcerative colitis.
10-12 pages
Jamie Rhoades, Development Manager
Susan Kukic, Executive Director

Tennessee

2923 CCFA Tennessee Chapter
95 White Bridge Road   615-356-0444
Nashville, TN 37205   866-814-2232
Fax: 615-356-0445
e-mail: tennessee@ccfa.org
www.ccfa.org/chapters/tennessee
Crohn's and Colitis Foundation of America is a non-profit volunteer-driven organization dedicated to finding the cure for Crohn's disease and ulcerative colitis.
Michelle J Chianese, Education & Support Manager
Nicole Boisvert, Walk Manager

Texas

2924 CCFA Houston Gulf Coast/South Texas Chapter
5120 Woodway   713-572-2232
Houston, TX 77056   800-785-2232
Fax: 713-572-2433
e-mail: infohouston@ccfa.org
www.ccfa.org/chapters/houston
Crohn's and Colitis Foundation of America is a non-profit volunteer-driven organization dedicated to finding the cure for Crohn's disease and ulcerative colitis.
Brandy Bendele, Walk Manager
Erin Fagan, Development Manager

2925 CCFA North Texas Chapter
12801 N Central Expressway   972-386-0607
Dallas, TX 75243   Fax: 972-386-0509
e-mail: ntexas@ccfa.org
www.ccfa.org/chapters/ntexas
Crohn's and Colitis Foundation of America is a non-profit volunteer-driven organization dedicated to finding the cure for Crohn's disease and ulcerative colitis.
Rachel Wallace, Development Manager
Sharon Seagraves, Executive Director

2926 CCFA Greater Washington DC/Virginia Chapter
4085 Chain Bridge Road   703-865-6130
Fairfax, VA 22314   877-807-5271
                                                   Fax: 703-865-8873
                          e-mail: washingtondc@ccfa.org
                          www.ccfa.org/chapters/washingtondc
Crohn's and Colitis Foundation of America is a non-profit volunteer-driven organization dedicated to finding the cure for Crohn's disease and ulcerative colitis.
Eileen Pugh, Executive Director
Stephanie Campbell, Development Coordinator

2927 CCFA Washington State Chapter
9 Lake Bellevue Drive   425-451-8455
Bellevue, WA 98005   877-703-6900
                                                   Fax: 425-451-1708
                          e-mail: northwest@ccfa.org
                          www.ccfa.org/chapters/northwest
Crohn's and Colitis Foundation of America is a non-profit volunteer-driven organization dedicated to finding the cure for Crohn's disease and ulcerative colitis.
Linda Huse, Executive Director
Jennifer Simmons, Development Manager

2928 CCFA Wisconsin Chapter
1126 S 70th Street   414-475-5520
W Allis, WI 53214   877-586-5588
                                                   Fax: 414-475-5502
                          e-mail: wisconsin@ccfa.org
                          www.ccfa.org/chapters/wisconsin
Crohn's and Colitis Foundation of America is a non-profit volunteer-driven organization dedicated to finding the cure for Crohn's disease and ulcerative colitis.
Jan Lenz, Executive Director
Nadine Davis, Development Coordinator

Libraries & Resource Centers

2929 National Digestive Diseases Information Clearinghouse
2 Information Way
Bethesda, MD 20892-3570   800-891-5389
                                                   Fax: 703-738-4929
                                                   TTY: 866-569-1162
                          e-mail: nddic@info.niddk.nih.gov
                          www.digestive.niddk.nih.gov
Established to increase knowledge and understanding about digestive diseases among people with these conditions and their families, health care professionals, and the general public. To carry out this mission, NDDIC works closely with a coordinating panel of representatives from Federal agencies, voluntary organizations on the national level, and professional groups to identify and respond to informational needs about digestive diseases.
Kathy Kranzfelder, Director

Research Centers

2930 Hahnemann University, Krancer Center for Inflammatory Bowel Disease Research
230 N Broad St   215-762-7000
Philadelphia, PA 19102   Fax: 215-762-8109
                          www.hahnemannhospital.com
Research into the causes and treatments of ulcerative colitis and Crohn's disease.
Dr. Harris Clearfield, Director

Support Groups & Hotlines

2931 Crohn's & Colitis Foundation of America Hotline
Crohn's & Colitis Foundation of America

386 Park Avenue S
New York, NY 10016   800-932-2423
                          e-mail: info@ccfa.org
                          www.ccfa.org
Our mission is to cure and prevent Crohn's disease and ulcerative colitis through research and to improve the quality of life of children and adults affected by these digestive disease through education and support. Known collectively as inflammatory bowel disease (IBD), these painful chronic illnesses affect up to one million Americans, including approximately 100,000 children under the age of 18.
Maura Breen, Chairman
Paul Salerno, Treasurer

2932 National Health Information Center
PO Box 1133   310-565-4167
Washington, DC 20013   800-336-4797
                                                   Fax: 301-984-4256
                          e-mail: info@nhic.org
                          www.health.gov/nhic
A health information referral service sponsored by the Office of Disease Prevention and Health Promotion. NHIC puts health professionals and consumers who have health questions in touch with those organizations that are best able to provide answers.

Books

2933 Crohn's Disease and Ulcerative Colitis Fact Book
Crohn's & Colitis Foundation of America
386 Park Avenue S   212-685-3440
New York, NY 10016-8804   800-932-2423
                                                   Fax: 212-779-4098
                          e-mail: info@ccfa.org
                          www.ccfa.org
Written in layman's language, this first complete guide is helpful in understanding and coping with inflammatory bowel diseases.

2934 Managing Your Child's Crohn's Disease or Ulcerative Colitis
Crohn's & Colitis Foundation of America
386 Park Avenue S   212-685-3440
New York, NY 10016-8804   800-932-2423
                                                   Fax: 212-779-4098
                          e-mail: info@ccfa.org
                          www.ccfa.org
Full-length book on Crohn's disease and ulcerative colitis, specifically targeted for parents of children and teenagers; includes topics on cause and diagnosis, treatment, surgery, hospitalization, diet and nutrition, school and social issues and resources for the patient.
$16.95 Members

2935 Ostomy Book: Living Comfortably with Colostomies, Ileostomies and Urostomies
Barbara Dorr Mullen and Kerry Anne McGinn, author

Bull Publishing Company
PO Box 1377thur Boulevard
Boulder, CO 80306   800-676-2855
                                                   Fax: 303-545-6354
                          www.bullpub.com
This book provides complete information on everything from details of surgery to the management of the appliances. Just as importantly, it is a beautifully told story of the entire expereince from diagnosis through rehabilitation to looking forward to a full and happy life.

ISBN: 0-923521-12-7

2936 People...Not Patients: Source Book for Living with Bowel Disease
Chron's & Colitis Foundation of America
386 Park Avenue S   212-685-3440
New York, NY 10016-8804   800-932-2423
                                                   Fax: 212-779-4098
                          e-mail: info@ccfa.org
                          www.ccfa.org
Contains the essential information you need to help you cope with Chron's disease and ulcerative colitis after you leave the doctor's office.

2937 Treating IBD
Crohn's & Colitis Foundation of America
386 Park Avenue S   212-685-3440
New York, NY 10016-8804   800-932-2423
                                          Fax: 212-779-4098
                                      e-mail: info@ccfa.org
                                               www.ccfa.org
Patient's guide to the medical and surgical management of Inflammatory Bowel Disease, this book gives information on treating
crohn's disease and ulcerative colitis, including drug therapies,
advances in nutritional care, and recently developed surgical
alternatives.

2938 Understanding Crohn Disease and Ulcerative Colitis
Jon Zonderman, Ronald S Vender, MD, author
University Press of Mississippi
3825 Ridgewood Road   601-432-6205
Jackson, MS 39211-6492   Fax: 601-432-6217
                              e-mail: kburgess@ihl.state.ms.us
                                        www.upress.state.ms.us
For patients and caregivers an overview of the nature and treat-
ments of inflammatory bowel disease.
2000 128 pages Paperback
ISBN: 1-578062-03-9
Kathy Burgess, Advertising/Marketing Services Manager

Magazines

2939 Colon and Rectal Surgery
International Academy of Proctology
PO Box 1716   765-342-3686
Martinsville, IN 46151   Fax: 765-342-4173
Information for professionals involved with colon and rectal sur-
gery.
George Donnally MD

2940 Digestive Health Matters
Intl. Foundation for Gastrointestinal Disorders
PO Box 170864   414-964-1799
Milwaukee, WI 53217-0864   888-964-2001
                                          Fax: 414-964-7176
                                      e-mail: iffgd@iffgd.org
                                               www.iffgd.org
Quarterly journal focuses on upper and lower gastrointestinal dis-
orders in adults and children. Educational pamphlets and
factsheets are available. Patient and professional membership.

2941 Foundation Focus
Crohn's & Colitis Foundation of America
386 Park Avenue S   212-685-3440
New York, NY 10016-8804   800-932-2423
                                          Fax: 212-779-4098
                                      e-mail: info@ccfa.org
                                               www.ccfa.org
Magazine for CCFA supporters.

2942 Phoenix Magazine
United Ostomy Association of America
PO Box 512
Northfield, MN 55057   800-826-0826
                                          Fax: 507-645-5168
                                       e-mail: info@uoa.org
                                                www.uoa.org
America's leading ostomy patient magazine providing colostomy,
ileostomy, urostomy and continent diversion information, man-
agement techniques, new products and much more.
Quarterly
David Rudzin, President

Newsletters

2943 Crohn's Disease, Ulcerative Colitis, and School
Pediatric Crohn's & Colitis Association
PO Box 188   617-489-5854
Newton, MA 02468   e-mail: questions@pcca.hypermart.net
                                          pcca.hypermart.net

Information on Crohn's Disease and Ulcerative Colitis, including
medical, nutritional, psychological and social factors.

2944 IBD File
Crohn's & Colitis Foundation of America
386 Park Avenue S   212-685-3440
New York, NY 10016-8804   800-932-2423
                                          Fax: 212-779-4098
                                      e-mail: info@ccfa.org
                                               www.ccfa.org
Offers updated information and the latest medical news about
Crohn's Disease and Colitis.

2945 Inflammatory Bowel Disease
Gastro-Intestinal Research Foundation
70 E Lake Street   312-332-1350
Chicago, IL 60601   Fax: 312-332-4757
                                      e-mail: girf@girf.org
                                                www.girf.org
Newsletter and patient pamphlet.

2946 Inner Circle
Reach Out for Youth with Ileitis and Colitis
84 Northgate Circle   516-293-3102
Melville, NY 11747   Fax: 516-293-3103
Provides information to patients with ileitis and colitis and their
families.

2947 Inside Story
Reach Out for Youth with Ileitis and Colitis
84 Northgate Circle   516-293-3102
Melville, NY 11747   Fax: 516-293-3103
Provides information to patients with ileitis and colitis and their
families.

Pamphlets

2948 ABC's of Pediatric Inflammatory Bowel Disease
Pediatric Crohn's & Colitis Association
PO Box 188   617-489-5854
Newton, MA 02468   e-mail: questions@pcca.hypermart.net
                                          pcca.hypermart.net
Information on Pediatric Inflammatory Disease, including medi-
cal, nutritional, psychological and social factors.

2949 CCFA: A Case for Support
Crohn's & Colitis Foundation of America
386 Park Avenue S   212-685-3440
New York, NY 10016-8804   800-932-2423
                                          Fax: 212-779-4098
                                      e-mail: info@ccfa.org
                                               www.ccfa.org
Reviews the work of the Crohn's and Colitis Foundation of America, sponsors a nationally recognized research program, which
seeks to improve treatment and ultimately find the cure for inflammatory bowel disease.

2950 Coping with Crohn's and Colitis is Tough
Crohn's & Colitis Foundation of America
386 Park Avenue S   212-685-3440
New York, NY 10016-8804   800-932-2423
                                          Fax: 212-779-4098
                                      e-mail: info@ccfa.org
                                               www.ccfa.org
Offers information on the Crohn's and Colitis Association. Also
offers factual information and statistics on the diseases.

2951 Crohn's Disease
NDDIC
2 Information Way   301-654-3810
Bethesda, MD 20892-0001   800-891-5389
                                          Fax: 301-907-8906
                              e-mail: nddic@info.niddlc.nin.gov
                                           www.niddk.nih.gov
October 1992

**2952 Guide for Children and Teenagers to Crohn's Disease/Ulcerative
Colitis**
Crohn's & Colitis Foundation of America

386 Park Avenue S
New York, NY 10016-8804

212-685-3440
800-932-2423
Fax: 212-779-4098
e-mail: info@ccfa.org
www.ccfa.org

Offers important information on these illnesses to children and teens.

2953 Ileostomy Guide
United Ostomy Associations of America, Inc.
PO Box 66
Fairview, TN 37062-0066

800-826-0826
e-mail: info@uoaa.org
www.uoaa.org

Written for persons who have recently had an ileostomy, this guidebook covers a spectrum of topics including basic facts about ileostomies, information for patients, helpful ideas and practical tips.
28 pages

2954 Questions & Answers About Diet and Nutrition
Crohn's & Colitis Foundation of America
386 Park Avenue S
New York, NY 10016-8804

212-685-3440
800-932-2423
Fax: 212-779-4098
e-mail: info@ccfa.org
www.ccfa.org

Raises important facts about how diet and nutrition affect persons with Crohn's Disease.

2955 Questions and Answers About Complications
Crohn's & Colitis Foundation of America
386 Park Avenue S
New York, NY 10016-8804

212-685-3440
800-932-2423
Fax: 212-779-4098
e-mail: info@ccfa.org
www.ccfa.org

Medical facts and complications from surgery.

2956 Questions and Answers About Crohn's Disease & Ulcerative Colitis
Crohn's & Colitis Foundation of America
386 Park Avenue S
New York, NY 10016-8804

212-685-3440
800-932-2423
Fax: 212-779-4098
e-mail: info@ccfa.org
www.ccfa.org

Offers information on the illness and answers the most frequently asked questions about Crohn's Disease. Also includes a glossary of IBD terms.

2957 Questions and Answers About Emotional Factors in Ileitis and Colitis
Crohn's & Colitis Foundation of America
386 Park Avenue S
New York, NY 10016-8804

212-685-3440
800-932-2423
Fax: 212-779-4098
e-mail: info@ccfa.org
www.ccfa.org

Answers some of the most commonly asked questions about ileitis and colitis and the role of emotional factors in their cause and course.

2958 Questions and Answers About Pregnancy in Ileitis and Colitis
Crohn's & Colitis Foundation of America
386 Park Avenue S
New York, NY 10016-8804

212-685-3440
800-932-2423
Fax: 212-779-4098
e-mail: info@ccfa.org
www.ccfa.org

Answers questions about inflammatory bowel disease concerning conception, pregnancy, delivery and nursing.

2959 Questions and Answers About Surgery
Crohn's & Colitis Foundation of America
386 Park Avenue S
New York, NY 10016-8804

212-685-3440
800-343-3637
Fax: 212-779-4098
e-mail: info@ccfa.org
www.ccfa.org

Answers questions and offers basic facts about surgery for persons suffering from Crohn's Disease and Ulcerative Colitis.

2960 Teacher's Guide to Crohn's Disease and Ulcerative Colitis
Crohn's & Colitis Foundation of America
386 Park Avenue S
New York, NY 10016-8804

212-685-3440
800-932-2423
Fax: 212-779-4098
e-mail: info@ccfa.org
www.ccfa.org

The purpose of this brochure is to increase the support and encouragement given to young people with Crohn's disease and ulcerative colitis by teachers who understand their illness.

2961 Crohn's Disease, Ulcerative Colitis and Your Child
Crohn's & Colitis Foundation of America
386 Park Avenue S
New York, NY 10016-8804

212-685-3440
800-932-2423
Fax: 212-779-4098
e-mail: info@ccfa.org
www.ccfa.org

Answers questions about IBD in children, providing information on early signs, growth and developments, treatments and special problems in school.

Web Sites

2962 Crohn's & Colitis Foundation of America

www.ccfa.org
CCFA provides educational and patient support services to both the lay and medical communities and plans to provide grants dedicated to pediatric research.

2963 Healing Well

www.healingwell.com
An online health resource guide to medical news, chat, information and articles, newsgroups and message boards, books, disease-related web sites, medical directories, and more for patients, friends, and family coping with disabling diseases, disorders, or chronic illnesses.

2964 Health Finder

www.healthfinder.gov
Searchable, carefully developed web site offering information on over 1000 topics. Developed by the US Department of Health and Human Services, the site can be used in both English and Spanish.

2965 Healthlink USA

www.healthlinkusa.com
Health information concerning treatment, cures, prevention, diagnosis, risk factors, research, support groups, email lists, personal stories and much more. Updated regularly.

2966 MedicineNet

www.medicinenet.com
An online resource for consumers providing easy-to-read, authoritative medical and health information.

2967 Medscape

www.medscape.com
Medscape offers specialists, primary care physicians, and other health professionals the Web's most robust and integrated medical information and educational tools.

2968 National Digestive Diseases Information Clearinghouse

www.niddk.nih.gov
Offers various educational information, resources and reprints focusing on Colitis, Ulcerative Colitis and Crohn's disease.

2969 Pediatric Crohn's and Colitis Association

pcca.hypermart.net/
Focuses on all aspects of pediatric and adolescent Crohn's disease and ulcerative colitis, including medical, nutritional, psychological and social factors. Activities include information sharing, educational forums, newsletters and hospital outreach programs, as well as support of research.

2970 **United Ostomy Association**

www.uoa.org

A national network for bowel and urinary diversion support groups in the United States. Its goal is to provide a nonprofit association that will serve to unify and strengthen its member support groups, which are organized for the benefit of people who have, or will have intestinal or urinary diversions and their caregivers.

2971 **WebMD**

www.webmd.com

Information on Crohn's disease, including articles and resources.

Description

2972 Cystic Fibrosis

Cystic fibrosis, CF, is an inherited disease of the exocrine (mucus-producing) glands, primarily affecting the gastrointestinal and respiratory tracts. The mucus that is secreted by persons with the disease is especially thick, thus blocking, rather than lubricating, passageways in the lungs and digestive tract. CF is the most common life-shortening genetic disease in the white population, occurring in 1 in 3,000 live births in the United States, but it occurs in people of all ethnic and racial backgrounds.

In the newborn with CF, thick fecal material may cause partial obstruction of the intestine, which then may contort and rupture. Later in life, blockage of secretions from the pancreas results in frequent, foul-smelling, fatty stools, distention of the abdomen and slowed growth. Damage to the lung occurs as thick mucus secretions plug airways. Fifty percent of all patients develop breathing problems marked by a chronic cough, wheezing and repeated lung infections.

The course of CF is usually determined by the degree to which the lungs are affected, and varies greatly from patient to patient. The prognosis is poor, but advances in therapy have helped many survive well into adulthood. Treatment usually includes aggressive use of antibiotics and other drugs to prevent lung complications, physical therapy, adequate nutrition and psychosocial support.

The first CF gene therapy research began in 1993, and scientists have identified mutations in a CF regulator genethat cause cells to produce abnormally thick mucus. Gene therapy to replace the defective gene with a functional copy is currently under study. Genetic screening is now available.

National Agencies & Associations

2973 Cystic Fibrosis Worldwide
50 Elm Street
Southbridge, MA 01550
508-764-2730
Fax: 508-765-8883
e-mail: information@cfww.org
www.cfww.org

IACFA is a non profit organization headquartered in Zurich Switzerland. The purpose and direction of the organization is to assist in improving the quality of life by identifying common problems and attempting to define possible solutions.
Christine Noke, Executive Director
Mitch Messer, President

Foundations

2974 Cystic Fibrosis Foundation
6931 Arlington Road
Bethesda, MD 20814
301-951-4422
800-344-4823
Fax: 301-951-6378
e-mail: info@cff.org
www.cff.org

The mission of the Cystic Fibrosis Foundation is to assure the development of the means to cure and control cystic fibrosis and to improve the quality of life for those with the disease.
Catherine C. McLoud, Chairman
Robert J Beall, Ph.D., President/CEO

Libraries & Resource Centers

2975 Children's Hospital of Orange County
455 S Main Street
Orange, CA 92868-3874
714-997-3000
e-mail: mail@choc.org
www.choc.org

Our mission is to nuture, advance and protect the health and well-being of children.
Kimberly C Cripe, President/CEO

Research Centers

Arizona

2976 Cystic Fibrosis Center: Phoenix Childrens Hospital
1919 E Thomas Road
Phoenix, AZ 85016
602-546-1000
888-908-5437
Fax: 602-460-23
www.phoenixchildrens.com

Robert Meyer, President and Chief Executive Officer
Bruce Morgenstern, Medical Staff President

Arkansas

2977 Arkansas Cystic Fibrosis Center Arkansas Children's Hospital
Arkansas Children's Hospital
1 Children's Way
Little Rock, AR 72202
501-364-1100
Fax: 501-364-3930
TTY: 501-364-1184
e-mail: pedspulmonary@uams.edu
www.arpediatrics.org

Provide high-quality specialized care to patients from comprehensive diagnosis to ongoing treatment.
John L Carroll, Division Chief
Dennis E Schellhase, Director

California

2978 Children's Hospital of Los Angeles
4650 Sunset Boulevard
Los Angeles, CA 90027
323-660-2450
e-mail: webmaster@chla.usc.edu
www.childrenshospitalla.org

Provides the highest quality healthcare for children who are the sickest and most seriously injured in our region and beyond.
Richard D Cordova, President/CEO
Rodney B Hanners, Senior Vice President & Chief Operating

2979 Childrens Hospital at Oakland
747 52nd Street
Oakland, CA 94609
510-428-3000
www.childrenshospitaloakland.org

The mission of Children's Hospital Oakland is to ensure the delivery of the highest quality pediatric care for all children through regional primary and subspecialty networks; a strong education and teaching program a diverse workforce state of the art research programs and facilities; and nationally recognized child advocacy efforts.
Bertram Lubin, President and Chief Executive Officer
Kathleen Hogue Gonzalez, Vice President, Research Administration

2980 Cystic Fibrosis Center: Cedars-Sinai Medical Center
Cedars-Sinai Medical Center
8700 Beverly Boulevard
Los Angeles, CA 90048
310-423-3277
800-233-2771
Fax: 310-423-4131
www.cedars-sinai.edu

2981 Cystic Fibrosis Center: University of California at San Francisco
400 Parnassus Avenue
San Francisco, CA 94122-0106
415-353-2961
Fax: 415-476-9278
e-mail: ucsf.org?
pulmonary.ucsf.edu

Provides comprehensive evaluation as well as inpatient and outpatient care for patients with cystic fibrosis.
Mary Ellen Kleinhenz, Adult CF Director
Dennis Niels MD, Pediatric CF Director

2982 Cystic Fibrosis Research
2672 Bayshore Parkway   650-404-9975
Mountain View, CA 94043   Fax: 650-404-9981
                                          e-mail: cfri@cfri.org
                                                  www.cfri.org
Cystic Fibrosis Research exists to fund research to provide educational and personal support and spread awareness of Cystic Fibrosis a life threatening genetic disease.
Carroll Jenkins, Executive Director
David Soohoo, Director of Programs

2983 Memorial Miller Children's Hospital Cystic Fibrosis Center
2801 Atlantic Avenue   562-933-2000
Long Beach, CA 90806   Fax: 562-933-8501
                          e-mail: enussbaum@memorialcare.org
                                    www.memorialcare.org/miller
provides a multidisciplinary approach to asthma cystic fibrosis sleep disorders and the entire spectrum of chronic and acute lung and airway disorders in children.
Eliezer Nuss, Medical Director
Barry Arbuckle, President

2984 Stanford CF Center Packard Children's Hospital At Stanford
Packard Children's Hospital At Stanford
725 Welch Road   650-497-8000
Palo Alto, CA 94304-1601   e-mail: jkirby@leland.stanford.edu
                                          cfcenter.stanford.edu

Colleen Dunn, Administrator
Cassie Everson, Research Coordinator

Colorado

2985 Denver Childrens Hospital
1830 Franklin Street   72 -77 -136
Denver, CO 80218   800-624-6553
                                          Fax: 303-832-9245
                                          TTY: 720-777-9390
                                  www.thechildrenshospital.org

Frank Accurs, Director
Jim Schmerling, President, CEO

Connecticut

2986 University of Connecticut Health Center
263 Farmington Avenue   860-679-2000
Farmington, CT 06030-0001   TTY: 860-679-2242
                                          TDD: 860-679-2242
                                  e-mail: president@uconn.edu
                                                  www.uchc.edu

Philip E Austin, President
Cato T Laurencin, Vice President for Health Affairs

2987 Yale University Cystic Fibrosis Research Center
Yale Pediatrics
333 Cedar Street   203-432-4771
New Haven, CT 06510   e-mail: sheila.rivera@yale.edu
                                          www.yalepediatrics.org
One of only two in the state of Connecticut the CF Center in the Children's Hospital at the Yale-New Haven Hospital offers a multidisciplinary team approach to provide the most comprehensive state of the art care of CF patients.
Marie Egan, Director
Richard C Levin, President

District of Columbia

2988 Metropolitan DC Cystic Fibrosis Center Children s Hospital National Medical Cen
Children s Hospital National Medical Center
111 Michigan Avenue NW   202-476-5000
Washington, DC 20010-2970   TTY: 800-855-1155
                                  e-mail: tbear@cnmc.org
                                  www.childrensnational.org
An active clinical and basic science research program that exists within the center.
Roberta Alessi, Senior Vice President
Mark Batshaw, Executive Vice President and Chief Acade

Florida

2989 Cystic Fibrosis Center: All Children's Hospital
Department of Pulmonology
501 6th Street S   727-898-7451
Saint Petersburg, FL 33701   800-456-4543
                                          Fax: 727-767-4218
                                                  www.allkids.org

Anthony D Kriseman, Pulmonology
Joseph (Jay) Fleece III, Chair

2990 Miami Childrens Hospital Division of Pulmonology
3100 SW 62nd Avenue   305-666-6511
Miami, FL 33155-3309   800-432-6837
                                          Fax: 305-663-8417
                                          e-mail: info@mch.com
                                                  www.mch.com
Division evaluates and treats many respiratory disorders including asthma chronic lung disease cystic fibrosis pneumonia and tuberculosis. The Division is strongly committed to a multidisciplinary medical approach to these complex disorders.
Moises Simps, Director
M Narendra Kini, President, CEO

2991 Nemours Childrens Clinic
807 Childrens Way   904-390-3600
Jacksonville, FL 32207   Fax: 904-390-3699
                                                  www.nemours.org
Nemours Children's Clinic is one integrated multispecialty group practice with locations in four states seeing patients from across the US and the world.
David J Bailey, President, CEO
Robert Bridges, Executive Vice-President

Georgia

2992 Department of Pediatrics Medical College of Georgia
1120 15th Street   706-721-3466
Augusta, GA 30912   Fax: 706-721-7311
                          e-mail: pwalling@ georgiahealth.edu
                                  www.mcg.edu/pediatrics

Dr William Kanto Jr, Chairperson Pediatrics

2993 Emory University: Cystic Fibrosis Center
201 Dowman Drive   404-727-6123
Atlanta, GA 30322-1028   Fax: 404-727-4828
                                  e-mail: lwolfen@emory.edu
                                                  www.emory.edu

Lindy Wolfen MD, Director
Jim Wagner, President

Illinois

2994 Comer Children's Hospital at the University of Chicago
5841 S Maryland Avenue   773-702-1000
Chicago, IL 60637   888-824-0200
                                                  www.uchospitals.edu

2995 Comer Children's Hospital at the Universit
5721 S Maryland Avenue   773-702-1000
Chicago, IL 60637   888-824-0200
                                  www.uchicagokidshospital.org
To provide superior healthcare in a compassionate manner ever mindful of each patient's dignity and individuality.

2996 Cystic Fibrosis Center: Childrens Memorial Hospital
2300 Childrens Plaza   773-880-4000
Chicago, IL 60614-3363   800-543-7362
                          e-mail: cf@childrensmemorial.org
                                  www.childrensmemorial.org
The Cystic Fibrosis Center at Children's Memorial Hospital has been a CFF-accredited CF care center since 1963. It is committed to providing exemplary care to each patient and family focused on individualized preventative care active management of lung health and nutrition and patient family education.
Susanna McCo, Director
Patrick M Magoon, President, CEO

2997 Cystic Fibrosis Center: Park Ridge Lutheran General Children's Hospital
Lutheran General Children's Hospital

1775 Dempster Street
Park Ridge, IL 60068

847-723-154
Fax: 847-696-3041
www.advocatehealth.com/lgch

James H Skogsbergh, President, CEO

2998 Loyola University Medical Center: Department of Pediatrics
2160 S 1st Avenue
Maywood, IL 60153

708-327-9120
888-584-7888
www.loyolamedicine.org

Vicki Keough, Dean and Professor

2999 Saint Francis Medical Center Peoria Pulmonary Association
530 NE Glen Oak Avenue
Peoria, IL 61637

309-655-2000
www.osfsaintfrancis.org

Dr. Denise Mammolito, President

Indiana

3000 The Riley Cystic Fibrosis Center
1701 North Senate Boulevard
Indianapolis, IN 46202

317-962-2000
800-248-1199
www.rileychildrenshospital.com

The Riley Cystic Fibrosis Center is the only Cystic Fibrosis Foundation accredited Cystic Fibrosis Center in the state. The Center provides state-of-the-art CF care at Riley and across the state.
Daniel Fink, President, CEO

Iowa

3001 Blank Childrens Hospital Pediatric Pulmonology Clinic
Children's Health Center
1212 Pleasant Street
Des Moines, IA 50309

515-241-6548
www.blankchildrens.org

David Starke, President, CEO
Ken Cheyne, Medical Director

3002 Pediatric Allergy & Pulmonary Division University of Iowa Healthcare
University of Iowa Healthcare
200 Hawkins Drive
Iowa City, IA 52242

319-356-2296
e-mail: allerpulm@uiowa.edu
www.uihealthcare.com/depts/med/pediatric

The Division of Allergy and Pulmonology offers evaluation and management of allergic disorders in children with too many infections and acute and chronic breathing disorders of childhood and adolescence.
Jody Kurtt RN, Director

Kansas

3003 Kansas University Medical Center: Cystic Fibrosis Center
3901 Rainbow Boulevard
Kansas City, KS 66160

913-588-5000
800-332-4199
TDD: 913-588-7963
e-mail: gperry@kumc.edu
www2.kumc.edu

Barbara F Atkinson, Executive Vice Chancellor

3004 St. Joseph Medical Center Cystic Fibrosis Care and Teaching Center
929 N. St. Francis
Wichita, KS 67214

316-268-5000
Fax: 316-583-90
e-mail: contact@viachristi.org
www.viachristi.org

Kay Glasner, Director
Maria Loving, Public Relations Specialist

Kentucky

3005 Kentucky University: Cystic Fibrosis Center
800 Rose Street
Lexington, KY 40536-0298

859-257-1000
800-333-8874
Fax: 859-257-7706
www.ukhealthcare.uky.edu

The cystic fibrosis team works with more than 175 patients and is dedicated to working with the most advanced therapies to improve the life of every patient.
Jamshed F Kanga, Director
Dr. Michael Karpf, Executive Vice President

3006 Kosair Childrens Cystic Fibrosis Center
Suite 201
Louisville, KY 40202-2021

502-629-6000
www.nortonhealthcare.com

The Cystic Fibrosis Center is one of 120 centers in the United States accredited by the National Cystic Fibrosis Foundation. Specialists provide diagnosis and multidisciplinary care for cystic fibrosis patients of all ages. Professional education and training is also provided.
Nemie Eid, Medical Director
Stephen A Williams, President, CEO

Louisiana

3007 Ernest N Morial Asthma, Allergy & Respiratory Disease Center
Louisiana State University School of Medicine
1901 Perdido Street
New Orleans, LA 70112-3932

504-568-4634
888-695-8647
Fax: 504-568-4295
e-mail: dthoma2@lsumc.edu
www.lsuhsc.edu

Warren R Summer, Director
Larry H. Hollier, President and Chief Operating Officer

Maine

3008 Central Maine Cystic Fibrosis Center
300 Main Street
Lewiston, ME 04240-7027

207-795-0111
Fax: 207-795-2303
www.cmhc.org

Ralph V Harder, Director
Peter Chkale, Chief Executive Officer

3009 Maine Medical Center: Cystic Fibrosis Clinical Center
22 Bramhall Street
Portland, ME 04102-3175

207-662-0111
877-339-3107
Fax: 207-775-6024
TTY: 207-662-4900
www.mmc.org

Richard W Peterson, President, CEO

3010 Maine Medical Center: Cystic Fibrosis Clin
22 Bramhall Street
Portland, ME 04102-3175

207-662-0111
877-339-3107
Fax: 207-775-6024
TTY: 207-662-4900
www.mmc.org

Richard W Peterson, President, CEO

Maryland

3011 Cystic Fibrosis Center: National Institute of Health NIDDK
Building 31 Room 9A06
Bethesda, MD 20892-2560

301-496-3583
www2.niddk.nih.gov

Dr Griffin Rodgers, Acting Director

3012 Cystic Fibrosis Foundation
6931 Arlington Road
Bethesda, MD 20814

301-951-4422
800-344-4823
Fax: 301-951-6378
e-mail: info@cff.org
www.cff.org

The mission of the Cystic Fibrosis Foundation a nonprofit donor-supported organization is to assure the development of the means to cure and control cystic fibrosis and to improve the quality of life for those with the disease.
Robert J Beall, President and CEO

Massachusetts

3013 Baystate Medical Center Wesson Memorial Unit
Wesson Memorial Unit

759 Chestnut Street
Springfield, MA 01199
413-794-0000
e-mail: Marian.Panto@bhs.org
www.baystatehealth.com
BMC serves as a regional resource for specialty medical care and research while providing comprehensive primary medical services to the community.
Mark R Tolosky, President & Chief Executive Officer
Paula S Dennison, Senior Vice President Human Resources

3014   Childrens Hospital Medical Center Cystic Fibrosis Center
300 Longwood Avenue
Boston, MA 02115
617-355-6000
Fax: 617-730-0373
TTY: 617-730-0152
www.childrenshospital.org
The Cystic Fibrosis Center at Children's Hospital Boston is one of the oldest and largest cystic fibrosis centers in the United States and was founded by Dr. Harry Schwachman one of the earliest physician investigators to help characterize the disorder.
Terry Spence, Director
Sandra Fenwick, President, CEO

3015   Cystic Firbrosis Center: Tufts New England Medical Center
Pediatric Pulmonology and Allergy Department
800 Washington Street
Boston, MA 02111
617-636-5000
www.nemc.org
We strive to heal to comfort to teach to learn and to seek the knowledge to promote health and prevent disease.
Ellen Zane, President and Chief Executive Officer
Margaret Vosburgh, Chief Operating Officer

3016   Massachusetts General Hospital
55 Fruit Street
Boston, MA 02114-2622
617-726-2000
Fax: 617-726-6989
TTY: 617-724-8800
TDD: 617-724-8800
www.massgeneral.org
Peter L Slavin, President
David Torchi, Chairman and Chief Executive Officer

3017   University of Massachusetts Memorial Medical Center
55 Lake Avenue N
Worcester, MA 01655
508-334-1000
www.umassmemorial.org
UMass Memorial Medical Center is the region's trusted academic medical center committed to improving the health of the people of Central New England through excellence in clinical care service teaching and research.
Walter Ettinger, President
George Brenckle, Senior Vice President and Chief Informat

Michigan

3018   East Lansing Cystic Fibrosis Center Michigan State University
Michigan State University
1200 E Michigan Avenue
Lansing, MI 48912
517-364-5440
Fax: 517-364-5413
phd.msu.edu
Eliane F Eakin, Director
H Dele Davies, Department Chair

3019   Kalamazoo Center for Medical Studies Michigan State University
Michigan State University
1000 Oakland Drive
Kalamazoo, MI 49008-1202
269-337-4400
800-275-5267
Fax: 269-337-4234
e-mail: programs@kcms.msu.edu
www.med.wmich.edu
John M. Dunn, Chairman of the Board
Paul A. Spaude, President & CEO

3020   University of Michigan: Cystic Fibrosis Center
A Alfred Taubman Health Care Center
1500 E Medical Center Drive
Ann Arbor, MI 48109-0318
734-936-4000
Fax: 734-936-7635
TTY: 800-649-3777
TDD: 800-649-3777
www.med.umich.edu
Samya Z Nasr, Director
Douglas L Strong, CEO

Minnesota

3021   University of Minnesota: Cystic Fibrosis Center
University of Minnesota Hospital
420 Delaware Street SE
Minneapolis, MN 55455
612-624-0962
800-688-5252
Fax: 612-624-0696
e-mail: cfcenter@umn.edu
www.med.umn.edu/peds/cfcenter/home.html
The mission was to develop approaches to understanding and treating the complications of CF.
Warren E Regelmann, Co-Director
Jordan M Dunitz, Co-Director

Mississippi

3022   University of Mississippi Medical Center
2500 N State Street
Jackson, MS 39216-4500
601-984-5046
Fax: 601-984-1973
www.umc.edu

Suzanne Mill, Director
Daniel W Jones, Chancellor

Missouri

3023   Children's Mercy Hospital Children's Mercy Hospitals & Clinics
Children's Mercy Hospitals & Clinics
2401 Gilham Road
Kansas City, MO 64108
816-234-3000
866-512-2168
Fax: 816-842-6107
TTY: 816-234-3816
e-mail: webmaster@cmh.edu
www.childrensmercy.org
Children's Mercy Hospital provides the highest level of medical care technology services equipment and facilities in promoting the health and well-being of children in the region from birth through adolescence.
Randall L O'Donnell PhD, President/CEO
V Fred Burry, Executive Medical Director/Executive Vic

3024   University of Missouri Columbia Cystic Fibrosis Center
University of Missouri/Dept of Child Health
One Hospital Drive N712
Columbia, MO 65212-1
573-882-6882
Fax: 573-821-54
e-mail: clarksonb@health.missouri.edu
www.ch.missouri.edu/cysticfibrosis.htm
Peter Konig, Director
Melissa Lawson, Division Director

3025   Washington University: Cystic Fibrosis Center
St. Louis Children's Hospital
660 S Euclid Avenue
Saint Louis, MO 63110
314-454-2694
888-678-4357
Fax: 314-454-2515
www.medschool.wustl.edu/
Dedicated to the treatment of patients with cystic fibrosis (CF) for more than 4 decades. The Cystic Fibrosis Clinical Center and affiliated programs has developed into a premier clinical and research program.
Thomas Ferko, Director

Nebraska

3026   University of Nebraska Medical Center Cystic Fibrosis Center
The Nebraska Medical Center
Omaha, NE 68198-5190
402-552-2000
800-922-0000
Fax: 402-559-7062
e-mail: necfcntr@unmc.edu
www.unmc.edu

Harold M Maurer, Chancellor
Hari Bandla, Associate Professor

Nevada

3027   Children's Lung Specialists
3838 Meadow Lane
Las Vegas, NV 89107
702-598-4411
Fax: 702-598-1988
e-mail: cls@childrens-lung-specialists.com
www.childrens-lung-specialists.com

231

The certified Cystic Fibrosis Center of Southern Nevada.
Ruben MD, Director/President/Owner
Craig Nakamu, Assistant Director

New Hampshire

3028   New Hampshire Cystic Fibrosis Care Teaching and Research Center
DarthmouthHitchcock Medical Center
One Medical Center Drive
Lebanon, NH 03756

603-650-5000
Fax: 603-500-07
TTY: 603-650-8034
www.dhmc.org

William Boyl, Director
Dennis Stoke, Director

New Jersey

3029   Monmouth Medical Center: Cystic Fibrosis & Pediatric Pulmonary Center
Monmouth Medical Center
95 Old Short Hills Road
West Orange, NJ 7052

732-222-5200
888-724-7123
Fax: 908-222-4472
e-mail: info@sbhcs.com
www.sbhcs.com

Peri Kamalakar, Director of Pediatric Hematology/Oncolog

3030   Monmouth Medical Center: Cystic Fibrosis & Monmouth Medical Center
368 Lakehurst Road
Toms River, NJ 08755

732-222-5200
888-724-7123
Fax: 908-222-4472
e-mail: info@sbhcs.com
www.sbhcs.com

Peri Kamalakar, Director of Pediatric Hematology/Oncolog

3031   New Jersey Medical School
185 S Orange Avenue
Newark, NJ 07101-1709

973-972-4595
Fax: 973-972-5965
e-mail: webnjms@umdnj.edu
njms.umdnj.edu

The mission of New Jersey Medical School is to educate students physicians and scientists to meet society's current and future healthcare needs through patient-centered education; pioneering research; innovative clinical rehabilitative and preventive care; and collaborative community outreach.
Maria L. Soto-Greene, MD, Vice Dean
Robert L Johnson MD, Dean

New York

3032   Albany Medical College Pediatric Pulmonary & Cystic Fibrosis Center
Department of Pediatrics
43 New Scotland Avenue
Albany, NY 12208

518-262-3125
877-262-8008
Fax: 518-262-6884
www.amc.edu

Scott Scroed, Division Chief

3033   Armond V Mascia Cystic Fibrosis Center NY Medical College
Division of Pediatrics Pulmonology
New York Medical College
Valhalla, NY 10595

914-594-4000
Fax: 914-594-4336
e-mail: pedpulm@nymc.edu
www.nycmc.edu

Provides comprehensive inpatient and outpatient consultation and management for children suffering from a broad variety of respiratory problems. They are the only accredited Cystic Fibrosis center in the Hudson Valley. The center is dedicated to teaching research and patient care.
Allen Dozer, Chief
Karl P Alder MD, President, CEO

3034   CF & Pediatric Pulmonary Care Center
Mount Sinai Hospital

One Gustave L Levy Place
New York, NY 10029-6574

212-241-6500
800-637-4624
Fax: 212-876-3255
www.mountsinai.org

Center staff perform outpatient and inpatient consultations with an integrated multidisciplinary team of professionals who are dedicated specifically to the practice of Pediatric Pulmonary Medicine.
Dennis S Charney, Dean, Executive Vice President

3035   Childrens Lung and Cystic Fibrosis Center
Women and Children's Hospital of Buffalo
140 Hodge Avenue
Buffalo, NY 14222-2099

716-878-7000
Fax: 716-888-3945
e-mail: AMTaylor@kaleidahealth.org
www.wchob.org

Services for infants children and teenagers with cystic fibrosis and other chronic respiratory conditions.
Annise Taylor, Manager
Cheryl Klass, President

3036   Cystic Fibrosis Center St. Vincent's Hospital & Medical Center
St. Vincent's Hospital & Medical Center of NY
36 7th Avenue
New York, NY 10011-6600

212-604-8895
Fax: 212-604-3899
www.svcmc.org

Maria Berdel, Co-Director
Patricia Wal MD, Co-Director

3037   Pulomonolgy Morgan Stanley Children's Hospital
Morgan Stanley Children's Hospital
3959 Broadway
New York, NY 10032-3702

212-305-5437
877-NYP-WELL
www.childrensnyp.org

Meyer Kattan, Director

3038   State University of NY Hospital: Upstate Medical Center
750 E Adams Street
Syracuse, NY 13210-1834

315-464-5540
877-464-5540
TDD: 315-464-5769
www.upstate.edu/uh

Stephen R Goodman, Vice President
David R. Smith, President

North Carolina

3039   UNC Cystic Fibrosis Center Department of Pediatrics
Department of Pediatrics
7011 Thurston-Bowles Building
Chapel Hill, NC 27599-7248

919-966-1077
Fax: 919-966-7524
www.med.unc.edu/cystfib/CFcent.htm

A large multidisciplinary group focused on the pathogenesis and other lung diseases.
Richard C Boucher, Director
Margaret Lei, Director

3040   Western Michigan University School of Medi cine
350 Hanes House
Durham, NC 27710

919-684-3364
888-275-3853
Fax: 919-684-2292
www.pulmonary.duke.edu

Provides primary and consultative care for patients with various lung diseases on an inpatient and outpatient basis.
Monica Kraft, Division Chief
Gina Brewer, Administrative Assistant

North Dakota

3041   St. Alexius Medical Heart and Lung Clinic
900 E Broadway Avenue
Bismarck, ND 58501

701-530-7000
877-530-5550
Fax: 701-530-8984
TTY: 701-530-5555
TDD: 701-530-5555
www.st.alexius.org

Specializes in services such as cardiac consultation cardiac surgery cardiac catheterization electrophysiology angioplasty intracoronary stents rotoblade asthma emphysema cystic fibrosis chronic lung disease. lung cancer allergy and anesthesia.
John Castleberry, Chair
Sr. Nancy Miller, OSB, President

Ohio

3042 Case Western Reserve University: Cystic Fibrosis Center
10900 Euclid Avenue 216-368-2000
Cleveland, OH 44106-2624 Fax: 216-844-5916
e-mail: Mds11@case.edu
www.case.edu

Barbara Snyder, President

3043 Columbus Children's Hospital: Cystic Fibrosis Center
700 Childrens Drive 614-722-2000
Columbus, OH 43205-0296 Fax: 614-722-4755
www.nationwidechildrens.org

Dr Steve Allen, CEO
Elizabeth D Allen, Physician

3044 Lewis H Walker MD: Cystic Fibrosis Center
Children's Hospital Medical Center of Akron
One Perkins Square 330-543-1000
Akron, OH 44308-1062 800-262-0333
TTY: 330-543-8080
www.akronchildrens.org/respiratory
One of six CF centers in the state of Ohio providing comprehensive care for patients who suffer from this disease. The center which is part of the Robert T. Stone Respiratory Center actively participates in clinical trials to research new drug therapies to manage cystic fibrosis.

Nathan Krayn, Director Cystic Fibrosis Center
William H Considine, President, CEO

3045 Pediatric Pulmonary Center The Children's Medical Center of Dayton
The Children's Medical Center of Dayton
1 Children's Plaza 937-641-3000
Dayton, OH 45404-1815 800-228-4055
Fax: 937-641-4500
www.childrensdayton.org

David Kinsaul, President, CEO
Robert Fink, Medical Director

3046 University of Cincinnati College of Medicine Division of Pediatrics
Children s Hospital Medical Center
3333 Burnet Avenue 513-636-4200
Cincinnati, OH 45229-3039 800-344-2462
Fax: 513-636-0345
TTY: 513-636-4900
e-mail: thomas.boat@cchmc.org
www.cincinnatichildrens.org
The University of Cincinnati Department of Pediatrics consists entirely of staff members from Cincinnati Children's Hospital Medical Center one of the nation's leading pediatric research and teaching institutions.

Michael Fisher, President, CEO
Thomas F Boat, Professor of Pediatrics

Oklahoma

3047 University of Oklahoma: Cystic Fibrosis Center
Department of Pediatrics
940 NE 13th Street 405-271-4401
Oklahoma City, OK 73104 Fax: 405-271-8710
e-mail: brenda-freese@ouhsc.edu
www.oumedicine.com

James A Royall, Professor/Chief Pediatric Pulmonology
Terrence L Stull MD, Chairman

Oregon

3048 Oregon Health & Science University
3181 SW Sam Jackson Park Road 503-494-8311
Portland, OR 97239-3098 e-mail: contactus@ohsuhealth.com
www.ohsuhealth.com
Oregon Health & Science University is a leading health and research university that strives for excellence in patient care education research and community service.

Joseph Rober, President
Steven D Stadum, Executive Vice President

Pennsylvania

3049 Cystic Fibrosis Center: Polyclinic Medical Center
Polyclinic Medical Center
PO Box 8700 717-231-8900
Harrisburg, PA 17105-8700 800-334-1007
Fax: 717-782-4679
www.pinnaclehealth.org

Muttiah Gane, Director
Michael A Young, FACHE, President/CEO

3050 Pediatric Pulmonary and Cystic Fibrosis Center
St. Christopher's Hospital for Children
3601 A Street 215-427-5000
Philadelphia, PA 19134 888-STC-RIS
Fax: 215-427-5555
www.stchristophershospital.com
A team of pediatric pulmonary medicine experts treats children with a wide range of acute and chronic lung diseases such as cystic fibrosis bronchopulmonary dysplasia apnea respiratory infections bronchiolitis congenital malformations including chest wall deformities and pneumonia.

Laurie Varlo, Director

3051 University of Pennsylvania: Penn Lung Center
Hospital of The University of Pennsylvania
3 Ravdin Suite F 215-662-4000
Philadelphia, PA 19104 800-789-7366
www.pennhealth.com
Penn Lung Center of the University of Pennsylvania Health System is a multidisciplinary resource for consultation second opinion diagnosis and ongoing treatment of patients with lung disease.

Leslie A Litzky, Associate Professor of Pathology and Lab
Maryl Kreide, Assistant Professor of Medicine

3052 University of Pittsburgh Cystic Fibrosis Center: Children's Hospital
Department of Cell Biology And Physiology
S362 BST 412-648-9362
Pittsburgh, PA 15261 Fax: 412-648-8330
e-mail: cdpweb@pitt.edu
www.cbp.pitt.edu/centers/cfrc.html
The primary goal of the Center is to focus the attention of new and established investigators on multidisciplinary approaches designed to improve the understanding and treatment of cystic fibrosis (CF).

Raymond A Frizzell, Director
Carol A Bertrand, Research Assistant Professor

Rhode Island

3053 Rhode Island Hospital: Cystic Fibrosis Center
Department of Pediatrics
593 Eddy Street 401-444-4000
Providence, RI 02903 Fax: 401-444-2168
e-mail: mschechter@lifespan.org
www.lifespan.org

Michael S Schechter, Director
George A Vecchione, President, CEO

South Carolina

3054 Medical University of South Carolina: Cystic Fibrosis Center
171 Ashley Avenue 803-792-1414
Charleston, SC 29403 800-424-6872
Fax: 843-876-1435
www.musc.edu/cfcenter
The objectives of the Cystic Fibrosis Center at MUSC are to offer unsurpassed care to patients with cystic fibrosis to teach medical students house staff medical care providers and general public about cystic fibrosis and to learn about cystic fibrosis through clinical and laboratory research.

Isabel Virella-Lowell, MD, Director
W Stuart Smith, Vice President, Executive Director

Tennessee

3055 Memphis Cystic Fibrosis Center LeBonheur Children's Medical Center
LeBonheur Children's Medical Center

848 Adams Ave
Memphis, TN 38103
901-287-5437
e-mail: info@lebonheur.org
www.lebonheur.org
Meri Armour, President, CEO

3056 Vanderbilt Children's Hospital
2200 Childrens Way
Nashville, TN 37232
615-936-1000
866-936-7811
www.vanderbiltchildrens.com
Children's Hospital provides top-level care while including the family as an essential element of a child's treatment plan.
Luke Gregory, Chief Executive Officer
Jonathan Gitlin, Vice Chancellor

Texas

3057 Cook Children's Medical Center: Cystic Fibrosis Clinic
4214 Andrews Highway
Midland, TX 79701
432-570-5693
www.cookchildrens.org
James C Cunningham MD, Director
Paula Webb, Vice President of Nursing Services

3058 Cystic Fibrosis Care and Teaching Center Children's Medical Center
Children's Medical Center
1935 Medical District Dr
Dallas, TX 75235
214-456-7000
Fax: 214-456-2563
www.childrens.com
The Dallas Cystic Fibrosis Care and Teaching Center manages the outpatient and inpatient care of approximately 400 infants children adolescents and adults.
Claude Prest MD, Director
Brenda Urbanczyk, Practice Administrator

3059 Cystic Fibrosis-Lung Disease Center: Santa Rosa Children's Hospital
CHRISTUS Center for Children and Families
333 N Santa Rosa
San Antonio, TX 78207
210-704-2011
Fax: 210-704-2651
www.santarosahealth.org
Serving more than 150 000 children each year CSRCH is a 200-plus bed facility and is the only academic Children's hospital in San Antonio partnering with The University of Texas Health Science Center at San Antonio while collaborating with private pediatricians to provide comprehensive pediatric services at one location since 1959.
Donna Beth Willey-Courand MD, Director
Patrick Carrier, President, CEO

3060 Texas Childrens Cystic Fibrosis Care Center
Texas Children's Clinical Care Center
6701 Fannin Street
Houston, TX 77030
832-824-1000
800-364-5437
Fax: 832-825-3072
e-mail: pulmonarymedicine@texaschildrenshospital
www.texaschildrenshospital.org
Provides comprehensive clinical services to help patients families and referring physicians deal with the many problems cystic fibrosis causes.
Mark A. Wallace, President and Chief Executive Officer
Dr. Mark Kline, Physician-in-Chief

3061 Tri-Services Military Cystic Fibrosis Center
Brooke Army Medical Center/Pediatrics Department
3851 Roger Brooke Drive
Fort Sam Houston, TX 78234-6320
210-916-3400
Fax: 210-916-3076
e-mail: ted.cieslak@cen.amedd.army.mil
www.bamc.amedd.army.mil
COL Ted Cieslak, Chief of Pediatrics
Joseph Caravalho, Commanding Officer

Utah

3062 University of Utah Intermountain Cystic Fibrosis Center
University Hospital & Clinics

50 N. Medical Drive
Salt Lake City, UT 84132
801-581-2121
800-824-2073
Fax: 801-585-5350
e-mail: judy.carle@hsc.utah.edu
www.med.utah.edu
Barbara A Chatfield MD, Director Pediatric Program
Loris Betz, Senior VP, Executive Dean

Vermont

3063 Medical Center Hospital of Vermont Cystic Fibrosis Center
Cystic Fibrosis Center
111 Colchester Avenue
Burlington, VT 05401-7152
802-847-0000
800-358-1144
Fax: 802-555-2323
www.fahc.org
Tom Lahiri MD, Director
Melinda L Estes, President, CEO

Virginia

3064 Eastern Virginia Medical School Children's Hospital of The King's Daught
Children's Hospital of The King's Daughters
601 Children's Lane
Norfolk, VA 23507
757-668-7000
e-mail: healthinfo@chkd.org
www.chkd.org
Provider of quality children's health services
James D. Dahling, President and Chief Executive Officer
Kathy Abshire, Vice President, Finance

3065 University of Virginia School of Medicine Cystic Fibrosis Center
Department of Pediatrics
PO Box 800793
Charlottesville, VA 22908
434-924-2250
800-251-3627
Fax: 434-243-6618
www.healthsystem.virginia.edu
Comprehensive care for children and adults with cystic fibrosis.
Steven T DeKosky MD, Vice President, Dean
Sharon L Hostler, Senior Associate Dean

Washington

3066 University of Washington: Cystic Fibrosis Center
University of Washington Medical Center/Adult Prog
1959 NE Pacific Street
Seattle, WA 98195
206-598-6116
Fax: 206-598-4610
www.washington.edu
UW Medicine works to improve the health of the public by advancing medical knowledge
Ronald Gibson, Center Director
Ronald Gibson, Professor and Center Director

West Virginia

3067 West Virginia University Cystic Fibrosis Center
Pediatrics Department
PO Box 9214
Morgantown, WV 26506-9214
304-293-1201
Fax: 304-293-1216
e-mail: kmoffett@hsc.wvu.edu
www.hsc.wvu.edu
The Hospital providing the full range of services including allergy/immunology cardiology child development critical care cystic fibrosis endocrinology adolescent medicine gastroenterology genetics and metabolic disease hematology/oncology neonatology nephrology neurology and apnea evaluation. Services provided by faculty with joint appointments include ophthalmology urology orthopedics psychiatry surgery and cardiothoracic surgery.
Kathryn S Moffett MD, Director
Giovanni Piedimonte, Chair

Wisconsin

3068 Medical College of Wisconsin: Cystic Fibrosis Clinic
Children's Hospital of Wisconsin
PO Box 1997
Milwaukee, WI 53201-1997
414-266-2000
877-266-8989
www.chw.org

Children's Hospital and Health System is an independent health care system dedicated solely to the health and well-being of children.
Robert Kliegman MD, Executive VP
Peter J Bartz, Cardiology Pediatric

3069 University of Wisconsin-Madison: Cystic Fibrosis/Pulmonary Center
Clinical Science Center
600 Highland Avenue
Madison, WI 53792
608-263-6400
800-323-8942
www.uwhealth.org
UW Health represents the academic medical care providers of the University of Wisconsin-Madison and its affiliated organizations.
Michael J Rock, Faculty
Prasad S Dalvie, Radiology

Support Groups & Hotlines

3070 National Health Information Center
PO Box 1133
Washington, DC 20013-1133
310-565-4167
800-336-4797
Fax: 301-984-4256
e-mail: info@nhic.org
www.health.gov/nhic
A health information referral service sponsored by the Office of Disease Prevention and Health Promotion. Puts health professionals and consumers who have health questions in touch with those organizations that are best able to provide answers.

Books

3071 Cystic Fibrosis: A Guide for Patient and Family
Raven Press
1185 Avenue of the Americas
New York, NY 10036-2601
212-930-9500
800-777-2295
253 pages Softcover
ISBN: 0-397516-53-3

3072 Understanding Cystic Fibrosis
Karen Hopkin, PhD, author
University Press of Mississippi
3825 Ridgewood Road
Jackson, MS 39211-6492
601-432-6205
Fax: 601-432-6217
e-mail: kburgess@ihl.state.ms.us
www.upress.state.ms.us
A useful guide for families and patients.
1998 128 pages Paperback
ISBN: 0-878059-67-9
Kathy Burgess, Advertising/Marketing Services Manager

Children's Books

3073 Give Me One Wish
Norton Publishers
500 5th Avenue
New York, NY 10110-0002
212-354-5500
800-233-4830
www.scholastic.com/
This book reads like a novel because it re-enacts the author's daughter's bout with cystic fibrosis.
Grades 10-12

3074 Robyn's Book: A True Diary
Scholastic
730 Broadway
New York, NY 10003-9511
212-505-3000
800-325-6149
This book chronicles the life of the author and her battle with cystic fibrosis.
Grades 7-12

3075 Toothpick
Holiday
40 E 49th Street
New York, NY 10017-1105
212-688-0085

This book uses relationships between two different teenagers to parallel the life of a person with cystic fibrosis.
Grades 6-9

Newsletters

3076 Better Breathing Bulletin
American Lung Association of Connecticut
45 Ash Street
East Hartford, CT 06108-3294
860-289-5401
800-586-4872
Fax: 860-289-5405
www.alact.org
This newsletter is aimed at persons with chronic lung problems.
John E Zinn, President/CEO

3077 Commitment
Cystic Fibrosis Foundation
6931 Arlington Road
Bethesda, MD 20814-5231
301-951-4422
800-344-4823
Fax: 301-951-6378
e-mail: info@cff.org
www.cff.org
Offers general information on cystic fibrosis, fund-raising features, public policy and news from across the nation on cystic fibrosis.

Pamphlets

3078 Consumer Fact Sheet
Cystic Fibrosis Foundation
6931 Arlington Road
Bethesda, MD 20814-5231
301-951-4422
800-344-4823
Fax: 301-951-6378
e-mail: info@cff.org
www.cff.org
Offers a brief introduction to cystic fibrosis, symptoms, causes, treatments and offers illustrations pertaining to drainage positions.

3079 Cystic Fibrosis: A Guide for Parents
American Lung Association
1740 Broadway
New York, NY 10019-4315
212-315-8700
Comprehensive booklet covering topics such as treatment, social aspects, inheritance, genetics and outlook for the future.
24 pages

3080 For Adults with Cystic Fibrosis: Facts on Reproduction
National Maternal and Child Health Clearinghouse
2070 Chain Bridge Road
Vienna, VA 22182-2588
703-442-9051
888-275-4772
Fax: 703-821-2098
e-mail: ask@hrsa.gov
www.ask.hrsa.gov
The purpose of this booklet is to review the reproductive issues that are unique to individuals with cystic fibrosis.

3081 Foundation Facts
Cystic Fibrosis Foundation
6931 Arlington Road
Bethesda, MD 20814-5231
301-951-4422
800-344-4823
Fax: 301-951-6378
e-mail: info@cff.org
www.cff.org
Offers information on the fund-raising and grants offered and supported by the foundation.

3082 Here's Everything You'll Need to Save Money with the CFF Health Services
CFF Home Health & Pharmacy Services
6931 Arlington Road
Bethesda, MD 20814-5223
800-342-6967
Fax: 800-233-3504
Offers information on the Cystic Fibrosis Foundation's home health services.

3083 Home Line
Cystic Fibrosis Foundation

6931 Arlington Road
Bethesda, MD 20814-5231

301-951-4422
800-344-4823
Fax: 301-951-6378
e-mail: info@cff.org
www.cff.org

Offers information on services and programs offered by the foundation.

Audio & Video

3084 Alex: The Life of a Child
Cystic Fibrosis Foundation
6931 Arlington Road
Bethesda, MD 20814

301-951-4422
800-344-4823
Fax: 301-951-6378
e-mail: info@cff.org
www.cff.org

The story of Alexandra Deford, a young girl who lost her battle with CF at the age of 8, has touched the hearts of millions and has helped to put a face to this disease. Alex's courage and strength is a true inspiration, and in the decades since her death, much progress has been made in the fight against CF. VHS only.
1986 1 Hr 35 Minutes
Robert J Beall, PhD, President/CEO

3085 Embers of the Fire
Mary Kondrat, author
Fanlight Productions
4196 Washington Street
Boston, MA 02131-1731

617-469-4999
800-937-4113
Fax: 617-469-3379
e-mail: fanlight@fanlight.com
www.fanlight.com

Offers a straight forward explanation of the disease with a primary focus on the stories of several courageous young people with cystic fibrosis during a week at summer camp. Addresses their fears of rejection, isolation and death while demonstrating the ways they have learned to lead fulfilling lives.
1992 28 Minutes
ISBN: 1-572950-98-6

3086 Expanding the Horizon of Hope: 50 Years of Progress
Cystic Fibrosis Foundation
6931 Arlington Road
Bethesda, MD 20814

301-951-4422
800-344-4823
Fax: 301-951-6378
e-mail: info@cff.org
www.cff.org

This film highlights the progress that has been made in CF research and care over the past 50 years, as well as the challenges that still lie ahead. It pays tribute to all who are involved in the CF effort—from researchers and clinicians, to patients and their families, to volunteers, donors and staff. DVD only.
2005 60 Minutes
Robert J Beall, PhD, President/CEO

3087 Faces of Cystic Fibrosis
Cystic Fibrosis Foundation
6931 Arlington Road
Bethesda, MD 20814

301-951-4422
800-344-4823
Fax: 301-951-6378
e-mail: info@cff.org
www.cff.org

Through the words of people with CF and their family members, hear the story of how the fight against CF has evolved into a story of hope and optimism that was never possible before...and how none of this would be possible without the dedication and efforts of volunteers. Available in VHS/DVD.
2001 11 Minutes
Robert J Beall, PhD, President/CEO

3088 Information About the Sweat Test
Cystic Fibrosis Foundation
6931 Arlington Road
Bethesda, MD 20814

301-951-4422
800-344-4823
Fax: 301-951-6378
e-mail: info@cff.org
www.cff.org

See and hear some basic information about the sweat test, the standard diagnostic test for CF. It is intended to help families better understand the sweat testing procedure and what to expect when the test is conducted. VHS only.
3.47 Minutes
Robert J Beall, PhD, President/CEO

Web Sites

3089 Healing Well
www.healingwell.com
An online health resource guide to medical news, chat, information and articles, newsgroups and message boards, books, disease-related web sites, medical directories, and more for patients, friends, and family coping with disabling diseases, disorders, or chronic illnesses.

3090 Health Finder
www.healthfinder.gov
Searchable, carefully developed web site offering information on over 1000 topics. Developed by the US Department of Health and Human Services, the site can be used in both English and Spanish.

3091 Healthlink USA
www.healthlinkusa.com
Health information concerning treatment, cures, prevention, diagnosis, risk factors, research, support groups, email lists, personal stories and much more. Updated regularly.

3092 Helios Health
www.helioshealth.com
Online resource for your health information. Detailed information about specific health topics, access to expert advice from our Medical Advisory Board, and up-to-date health news.

3093 MedicineNet
www.medicinenet.com
An online resource for consumers providing easy-to-read, authoritative medical and health information.

3094 Medscape
www.medscape.com
Medscape offers specialists, primary care physicians, and other health professionals the Web's most robust and integrated medical information and educational tools.

3095 WebMD
www.webmd.com
Provides links to over 45 articles involving cystic fibrosis.

Description

3096 Diabetes Mellitus

Diabetes mellitus is a condition in which the body lacks enough insulin to control its own blood glucose (sugar) level. Ordinarily, the pancreas releases enough of this hormone to let the body's cells absorb and metabolize glucose. In Type I diabetes (formerly called juvenile-onset diabetes and affecting 10 percent of diabetic patients), the pancreas simply stops producing insulin. In Type II, commonly affecting overweight individuals older than 40, the pancreas might release normal, reduced, or even elevated levels of insulin, but the body's cells are resistant to the insulin's action. In either case, blood glucose levels rise (hyperglycemia) until the kidney starts to dump sugar into the urine. The patient may experience excessive thirst and urination, hunger, weakness and weight loss. In extreme cases, when there is either insufficient insulin or the body undergoes stress, or strenuous exercise, some components of the blood become seriously altered and the patient may lapse into a coma. Long-term complications include an increased risk of coronary heart disease and other vascular diseases, such as stroke, vision loss and kidney failure.

Type I appears to be caused by a genetic predisposition that may express itself after an acute insult, often a viral infection. Genetic factors are important in Type II diabetes which runs strongly in families. It is much more common in obese people, as well as among African-Americans, Hispanics and Native Americans.

Prevention of acute and long-term complications requires careful management including maintaining the proper diet and exercise, blood glucose monitoring and medications. Thorough education of the patient and relevant family members is absolutely critical.

Some individuals with Type II diabetes can control their disease through diet, exercise and weight loss alone. Some will have to take oral medication that helps the pancreas make more insulin or makes the body more sensitive to insulin. Some Type II diabetics, and all Type I diabetics, need to take insulin. Research has shown that tight control of diabetes through frequent blood testing and proper adjustment of the dosage of insulin is most beneficial. Insulin is generally given in multiple injections throughout the day, with preparations varying by length of effectiveness. Closest control of glucose levels is achieved by giving insulin through a continuously-connected insulin pump. Pancreas transplantation is considered only for patients who also need some other organ, generally a kidney.

National Agencies & Associations

3097 American Association of Diabetes Educators
200 W Madison Street
Chicago, IL 60606
800-338-3633
e-mail: aade@aadenet.org
www.aadenet.org

An independent multidisciplinary organization of health professionals involved in teaching persons with diabetes. The mission is to enhance the competence of health professionals who teach persons with diabetes and advance the specialty practice of diabetes.
Donna Tomky, President
Tami Ross, VP

3098 American Diabetes Association
1701 N Beauregard Street
Alexandria, VA 22311
804-225-8038
888-342-2383
Fax: 804-225-8211
e-mail: askada@diabetes.org
www.diabetes.org

The nation's leading voluntary organization concerned with diabetes and its complications. The mission of the organization is to prevent and cure diabetes and to improve the lives of persons with diabetes. Offers a network of offices nationwide.
Julie Heverly, Area Director
Larry Hausner, CEO

3099 Diabetes Exercise and Sports Association
310 West Liberty
Louisville, KY 40202
502-581-0207
800-898-4322
Fax: 502-581-0206
e-mail: desa@diabetes-exercise.org
www.diabetes-exercise.org

Exists to enhance the quality of life for people with diabetes through exercise and physical fitness.
Paula Harper, Founder
Guy Hornsby, Chair

3100 Juvenile Diabetes Foundation: International
26 Broadway
New York, NY 10004
800-533-2873
Fax: 212-785-9595
e-mail: info@jdrf.org
www.jdf.org

Focuses energies on fund-raising, referrals, educational materials and information pertaining to juvenile diabetes.
Jeffery Brewer, President

3101 National Certification Board for Diabetes Educators
330 E Algonquin Road
Arlington Heights, IL 60005
847-228-9795
877-239-3233
Fax: 847-228-8469
e-mail: info@ncbde.org
www.ncbde.org

The Board for Diabetes Educators is dedicated to promoting excellence in the field of diabetes education through the development maintenance and protection of the certified Diabetes Educator credential and the certification process.
Samuel Abbate, Chair
Lance Hoxie, Chief Executive Officer

3102 National Diabetes Action Network for the Blind
National Federation of the Blind
200 East Wells Street
Baltimore, MD 21230
410-659-9314
Fax: 410-685-5653
e-mail: nfb@nfb.org
www.nfb.org

Leading support and information organization of persons losing vision due to diabetes. Provides personal contact and resource information with other blind diabetics about non-visual techniques of independently managing diabetes and monitoring glucose levels.
Marc Maurer, President
Fredric Schroeder, First Vice President

3103 National Institute of Diabetes, Digestive & Kidney Diseases
National Institutes of Health
1 Information Way
Bethesda, MD 20892-2560
800-860-8747
Fax: 703-738-4929
TTY: 866-569-1162
e-mail: ndic@info.niddk.nih.gov
www.diabetes.niddk.nih.gov

Conducts and supports research on many of the most serious diseases affecting public health. The Institute supports much of the clinical research on the diseases of internal medicine and related subspecialty fields as well as many basic science disciplines.
Dr. Griffin Rodgers, Acting Director

State Agencies & Associations

Alabama

3104 American Diabetes Association: Alabama
3918 Montclair Road   205-870-5172
Birmingham, AL 35213   888-DIA-BETE
                                   Fax: 205-879-2903
                                   e-mail: acasey@diabetes.org
                                   www.diabetes.org

Aimee Casey, Executive Director
Stephanie Willis, Director

3105 Juvenile Diabetes Research Foundation: Birmingham
14 Office Park Circle   205-871-0333
Birmingham, AL 35223   Fax: 205-871-0355
                                   e-mail: alabama@jdf.org
                                   www.jdrf.org/alabama

Karin Scott, Executive Director
Sarah Hendren, Special Events Manager

Alaska

3106 American Diabetes Association: Alaska
801 W Fireweed Lane   907-272-1424
Anchorage, AK 99503   888-DIA-BETE
                                   Fax: 907-272-1428
                                   e-mail: mcassano@diabetes.org
                                   www.diabetes.org

Michelle Cassano, Executive Director
Phoebe O'Connell, Manager

Arizona

3107 American Diabetes Association: Arizona
8125 N 23rd Avenue   602-861-4731
Phoenix, AZ 85021   Fax: 602-995-1344
                                   www.diabetes.org

Edyth Haro, Manager
Lynda Brown, Special Events Manager

3108 American Diabetes Association: Arizona, Border Area
333 W Ft Lowell Rd   520-795-3711
Tucson, AZ 85705   888-DIA-BETE
                                   Fax: 520-795-1179
                                   e-mail: fgomez@diabetes.org
                                   www.diabetes.org

Fred Gomez, Executive Director
Heidi Goldsmith, Manager

3109 American Diabetes Association: Atlanta Met
8125 N 23rd Avenue   602-861-4731
Phoenix, AZ 85021   Fax: 602-995-1344
                                   e-mail: kbisko@diabetes.org
                                   www.diabetes.org

Karen Bisko, Executive Director
Suzanne Miller, Director

3110 American Diabetes Association: Northern Arizona
5333 N 7th Street   602-861-4731
Phoenix, AZ 85014   Fax: 602-995-1344
                                   e-mail: llandon@diabetes.org
                                   www.diabetes.org

Laura Landon, Executive Director
Suzanne Miller, Programs Director

3111 Juvenile Diabetes Research Foundation: Phoenix Chapter
4343 E Camelback Road   602-224-1800
Phoenix, AZ 85018   Fax: 602-224-1801
                                   e-mail: desertsouthwest@jdrf.org
                                   www.jdrf.org/arizona

Marci Zimmerman, Executive Director
Valerie Jones, Associate Executive Director

Arkansas

3112 American Diabetes Association: Arkansas
320 Executive Court   501-221-7444
Little Rock, AR 72205   888-DIA-BETE
                                   Fax: 501-221-3138
                                   e-mail: rselig@diabetes.org
                                   www.diabetes.org

Rick Selig, Director
Charlotte Williams, Associate Manager

3113 Juvenile Diabetes Research Foundation: Northwest Arkansas Branch
4241 Gabel Dr   479-443-9190
Fayetteville, AR 72703   Fax: 479-443-2692
                                   e-mail: nwarkansas@jdrf.org
                                   www.nwark.jdrf.org

Deb Euculano, Special Events Manager

California

3114 American Diabetes Association: California
2720 Gateway Oaks Drive   916-924-3232
Sacramento, CA 95833   888-DIA-BETE
                                   Fax: 916-924-0529
                                   e-mail: AskADA@diabetes.org
                                   www.diabetes.org/

The American Diabetes Association is a nonprofit health organization providing diabetes research, information and advocacy. Founded in 1940, the American Diabetes Association conducts programs in all 50 states and the District of Columbia.
Michael D Farley CFRE, Chief Community Relations Officer
Richard Kahn PhD, Chief Scientific/Medical Officer

3115 Diabetes Society of Santa Clara Valley
4040 Moorpark Avenue   408-241-1922
San Jose, CA 95117   888-DIA-BETE
                                   Fax: 408-241-1972
                                   e-mail: Info@thediabetessociety.org
                                   www.diabetes.org

The Diabetes Society is dedicated to providing education and information to those who have diabetes educating the general public about the seriousness of this disease, and supporting research aimed at preventing complications and finding a cure.
Douglas Metz DPM/MPH, Executive Director
Thomas Smith, Program/Camp Director

3116 Juvenile Diabetes Research Foundation: Bakersfield Chapter
712 19th Street   661-636-1305
Bakersfield, CA 93301   Fax: 661-636-1307
                                   e-mail: Bakersfield@jdrf.org
                                   www.jdrf-bakersfield.org

The Juvenile Diabetes Research Foundation International (JDRF) is a charitable funder and advocate of type 1 (juvenile) diabetes research worldwide. The mission of JDRF is to find a cure for diabetes and its complications through the support of research.
Allison Perkins Thomas, Bakersfield Branch Manager
Arnold Donald, President/CEO Corporate Office (NY)

3117 Juvenile Diabetes Research Foundation: Inl and Empire Chapter
1001 East Cooley Drive   909-424-0100
Colton, CA 92324   Fax: 909-424-0044
                                   e-mail: inlandempire@jdrf.org
                                   www.inlandempire.jdrf.org

The Juvenile Diabetes Research Foundation International (JDRF) is a charitable funder and advocate of type 1 (juvenile) diabetes research worldwide. The mission of JDRF is to find a cure for diabetes and its complications through the support of research.
Jamie Brunelle, Board of Directors
Evelyn Edinin, Board of Directors

3118 Juvenile Diabetes Research Foundation: Los Angeles Chapter
800 West Sixth Street   213-233-9901
Los Angeles, CA 90017   Fax: 213-622-6276
                                   e-mail: losangeles@jdrf.org
                                   www.jdrf.org/losangeles

The Juvenile Diabetes Research Foundation International (JDRF) is a charitable funder and advocate of type 1 (juvenile) diabetes re-

search worldwide. The mission of JDRF is to find a cure for diabetes and its complications through the support of research.
Mark Rieck, Executive Director
Dennis Ellman Esq, Board of Directors President

3119 Juvenile Diabetes Research Foundation: Nor thern California Inland Chapter
1329 Howe Avenue   916-920-0790
Sacramento, CA 95825   Fax: 916-920-0367
e-mail: northernca@jdrf.org
www.jdrf.org/norcal
The Juvenile Diabetes Research Foundation International (JDRF) is a charitable funder and advocate of type 1 (juvenile) diabetes research worldwide. The mission of JDRF is to find a cure for diabetes and its complications through the support of research.
Victoria Webster, Executive Director
Molly Atkinson, Special Events Coordinator

3120 Juvenile Diabetes Research Foundation: Ora nge County Chapter
17992 Mitchell South   949-553-0363
Irvine, CA 92614   Fax: 949-553-8813
e-mail: orangecounty@jdrf.org
www.jdrfoc.org
The Juvenile Diabetes Research Foundation International (JDRF) is a charitable funder and advocate of type 1 (juvenile) diabetes research worldwide. The mission of JDRF is to find a cure for diabetes and its complications through the support of research.
Louise Cummings, Executive Director
John Giovannone, President

3121 Juvenile Diabetes Research Foundation: San Diego Chapter
5677 Oberlin Drive   858-597-0240
San Diego, CA 92121   Fax: 858-597-2072
e-mail: sandiego@jdrf.org
www.jdrf-sandiego-news.org
The Juvenile Diabetes Research Foundation International (JDRF) is a charitable funder and advocate of type 1 (juvenile) diabetes research worldwide. The mission of JDRF is to find a cure for diabetes and its complications through the support of research.
Linda Riley, Executive Director
Katherine Griswold, Special Events Manager

Colorado

3122 American Diabetes Association: Denver
2480 W 26th Avenue   720-855-1102
Denver, CO 80211   Fax: 720-855-1302
e-mail: AskADA@diabetes.org
www.diabetes.org/
The American Diabetes Association is a nonprofit health organization providing diabetes research, information and advocacy. Founded in 1940 the American Diabetes Association conducts programs in all 50 states and the District of Columbia.
Michael D Farley CFRE, Chief Community Relations Officer
Richard Kahn, Chief Scientific/Medical Officer

3123 Juvenile Diabetes Research Foundation: Colorado Springs Chapter
3710 Sinton Road   719-633-8110
Colorado Springs, CO 80907   Fax: 719-633-8155
e-mail: lpage@jdrf.org
www.jdrfcoloradosprings.org
The Juvenile Diabetes Research Foundation International (JDRF) is a charitable funder and advocate of type 1 (juvenile) diabetes research worldwide. The mission of JDRF is to find a cure for diabetes and its complications through the support of research.
Lynn Page, Branch Manager
Andi Chernushin, President

3124 Juvenile Diabetes Research Foundation: Roc ky Mountain Chapter
5613 DTC Parkway   303-779-0525
Greenwood Village, CO 80111   Fax: 303-720-1630
e-mail: RockyMountain@jdrf.org
www.jdrf.org/rockymountain
The Juvenile Diabetes Research Foundation International (JDRF) is a charitable funder and advocate of type 1 (juvenile) diabetes re-

search worldwide. The mission of JDRF is to find a cure for diabetes and its complications through the support of research.
James Buckles, Executive Director
Nancy L Walters, Special Events Director

Connecticut

3125 American Diabetes Association: Connecticut
306 Industrial Park Road   203-639-0385
Middletown, CT 06457   888-DIA-BETE
Fax: 860-632-5098
e-mail: AskADA@diabetes.org
www.diabetes.org
The American Diabetes Association is a nonprofit health organization providing diabetes research, information and advocacy. Founded in 1940 the American Diabetes Association conducts programs in all 50 states and the District of Columbia.
Michael D Farley CRFE, Chief Community Relations Officer
Richard Kahn, Chief Scientific/Medical Officer

3126 Juvenile Diabetes Research Foundation: Greater New Haven Chapter
2969 Whitney Avenue   203-248-1880
Hamden, CT 06518   Fax: 203-248-1820
e-mail: newhaven@jdf.org
www.jdrf.org/greaternewhaven
The Juvenile Diabetes Research Foundation International (JDRF) is a charitable funder and advocate of type 1 (juvenile) diabetes research worldwide. The mission of JDRF is to find a cure for diabetes and its complications through the support of research.
Mary K Kessler, Executive Director
Will Martinez, Board of Directors President

3127 Juvenile Diabetes Research Foundation: Fai rfield County Chapter
200 Connecticut Avenue   203-854-0658
Norwalk, CT 06854   Fax: 203-854-0798
e-mail: fairfield@jdrf.org
www.jdrf.org/fairfieldcounty
The Juvenile Diabetes Research Foundation International (JDRF) is a charitable funder and advocate of type 1 (juvenile) diabetes research worldwide. The mission of JDRF is to find a cure for diabetes and its complications through the support of research.
Barbara Rose, Executive Director
Michelle Tighe, Special Events Coordinator

3128 Juvenile Diabetes Research Foundation: Nor th Central CT and Western MA
18 North Main Street   860-561-1153
West Hartford, CT 06107   Fax: 860-561-3440
e-mail: northcentralct@jdrf.org
www.jdrf.org/index.cfm?page_id=100619
The Juvenile Diabetes Research Foundation International (JDRF) is a charitable funder and advocate of type 1 (juvenile) diabetes research worldwide. The mission of JDRF is to find a cure for diabetes and its complications through the support of research.
Mary Ann Slomski, Executive Director
Ellen Kellie, Special Events Coordinator

Delaware

3129 American Diabetes Association: Delaware
100 W 10th Street   302-656-0030
Wilmington, DE 19801   888-342-2383
Fax: 302-656-7331
e-mail: AskADA@diabetes.org
www.diabetes.org
The American Diabetes Association is a nonprofit health organization providing diabetes research, information and advocacy. Founded in 1940 the American Diabetes Association conducts programs in all 50 states and the District of Columbia.
Michael D Farley CFRE, Chief Community Relations Officer
Richard Kahn, Chief Scientific/Medical Officer

3130 Juvenile Diabetes Research Foundation: Del aware
100 West 10th Street   302-888-1117
Wilmington, DE 19801   Fax: 302-888-1878
e-mail: delaware@jdrf.org
www.jdrf.org/delaware

The Juvenile Diabetes Research Foundation International (JDRF) is a charitable funder and advocate of type 1 (juvenile) diabetes research worldwide. The mission of JDRF is to find a cure for diabetes and its complications through the support of research.
Ellen Rubesin, Executive Director
Stephanie Bucksner, Special Events Coordinator

District of Columbia

3131 American Diabetes Association: District of Columbia
1025 Connecticut Avenue NW 202-331-8303
Washington, DC 20036 888-342-2383
Fax: 202-331-1402
e-mail: AskADA@diabetes.org
www.diabetes.org
The American Diabetes Association is a nonprofit health organization providing diabetes research, information and advocacy. Founded in 1940 the American Diabetes Association conducts programs in all 50 states and the District of Columbia.
Michael D Farley CFRE, Chief Community Relations Officer
Richard Kahn, Chief Scientific/Medical Officer

3132 Juvenile Diabetes Research Foundation: Cap itol Chapter
1400 K Street NW 202-371-0044
Washington, DC 20005 Fax: 202-371-0046
e-mail: capitol@jdrf.org
www.jdrfcapitol.org
The Juvenile Diabetes Research Foundation International (JDRF) is a charitable funder and advocate of type 1 (juvenile) diabetes research worldwide. The mission of JDRF is to find a cure for diabetes and its complications through the support of research.
Pam Gatz, Executive Director
Carrie Hamilton, Special Events Director

Florida

3133 American Diabetes Association: Northeast F lorida/Southeast Georgia
8384 Baymeadows Road 904-730-7200
Jacksonville, FL 32256 888-342-2383
Fax: 940-730-7933
e-mail: AskADA@diabetes.org
www.diabetes.org
The American Diabetes Association is a nonprofit health organization providing diabetes research, information and advocacy. Founded in 1940 the American Diabetes Association conducts programs in all 50 states and the District of Columbia.
Sheri Criswell, Executive Director
Richard Kahn, Chief Scientific/Medical Officer

3134 American Diabetes Association: Seattle
1101 N Lake Destiny Road 407-660-1926
Maitland, FL 32751 Fax: 407-660-1080
e-mail: AskADA@diabetes.org
www.diabetes.org
The American Diabetes Association is a nonprofit health organization providing diabetes research, information and advocacy. Founded in 1940 the American Diabetes Association conducts programs in all 50 states and the District of Columbia.
Pauline Lowe, Executive Director
Richard Kahn, Chief Scientific/Medical Officer

3135 American Diabetes Association: South Coast Regional/Central Florida
1101 North Lake Destiny Road 407-660-1926
Maitland, FL 32751 888-342-2383
Fax: 407-660-1080
e-mail: AskADA@diabetes.org
www.diabetes.org
The American Diabetes Association is a nonprofit health organization providing diabetes research, information and advocacy. Founded in 1940, the American Diabetes Association conducts programs in all 50 states and the District of Columbia, reaching hundreds of communities.
Michael D Farley CFRE, Chief Community Relations Officer
Richard Kahn, Chief Scientific/Medical Officer

3136 Juvenile Diabetes Research Foundation: Cen tral Florida Chapter
279 Douglas Avenue 407-774-2166
Altamonte Springs, FL 32714 Fax: 407-774-2168
e-mail: centralflorida@jdrf.org
www.jdrf.org/centralflorida
The Juvenile Diabetes Research Foundation International (JDRF) is a charitable funder and advocate of type 1 (juvenile) diabetes research worldwide. The mission of JDRF is to find a cure for diabetes and its complications through the support of research.
Kendra Presley, Special Events Manager
Gwen Bell, Office Manager

3137 Juvenile Diabetes Research Foundation: Flo rida Sun Coast Chapter
3333 Clark Road 941-929-0621
Sarasota, FL 34231 Fax: 941-929-0602
e-mail: floridasuncoast@jdrf.org
www.jdrf.org/index.cfm
The Juvenile Diabetes Research Foundation International (JDRF) is a charitable funder and advocate of type 1 (juvenile) diabetes research worldwide. The mission of JDRF is to find a cure for diabetes and its complications through the support of research.
Sara Rankin, Executive Director
Jeannie Kawcak, Special Events Coordinator

3138 Juvenile Diabetes Research Foundation: Gre ater Palm Beach County Chapter
1450 Centrepark Boulevard 561-686-7701
West Palm Beach, FL 33401 Fax: 561-686-7702
e-mail: greaterpalmbeach@jdrf.org
www.jdrf.org/greaterpalmbeach
The Juvenile Diabetes Research Foundation International (JDRF) is a charitable funder and advocate of type 1 (juvenile) diabetes research worldwide. The mission of JDRF is to find a cure for diabetes and its complications through the support of research.
Lora Hazelwood, Executive Director
Esther Swann, Special Events Coordinator

3139 Juvenile Diabetes Research Foundation: Nor th Florida Chapter
8400 Baymeadows Way 904-739-2101
Jacksonville, FL 32256 Fax: 904-739-2693
e-mail: northflorida@jdrf.org
www.jdrf.org/northflorida
The Juvenile Diabetes Research Foundation International (JDRF) is a charitable funder and advocate of type 1 (juvenile) diabetes research worldwide. The mission of JDRF is to find a cure for diabetes and its complications through the support of research.
Brooks Biagini, Executive Director
Wendy Smit, Special Events Assistant

3140 Juvenile Diabetes Research Foundation: Sou th Florida Chapter
3411 NW 9th Avenue 954-565-4775
Fort Lauderdale, FL 33309 Fax: 954-565-4767
e-mail: southflorida@jdrf.org
www.jdrf.org/chapters/FL/South-Florida
The Juvenile Diabetes Research Foundation International (JDRF) is a charitable funder and advocate of type 1 (juvenile) diabetes research worldwide. The mission of JDRF is to find a cure for diabetes and its complications through the support of research.
Ingrid Velarde, Special Events Coordinator
Katelyn Tolzien, Special Events Coordinator

3141 Juvenile Diabetes Research Foundation: Tam pa Bay Chapter
5959 Central Avenue 727-344-2873
Saint Petersburg, FL 33710 Fax: 727-384-9009
e-mail: tampabay@jdrf.org
www.jdf.org
The Juvenile Diabetes Research Foundation International (JDRF) is a charitable funder and advocate of type 1 (juvenile) diabetes research worldwide. The mission of JDRF is to find a cure for diabetes and its complications through the support of research.
Arnold Donald, President/CEO Corporate Office
Robin Harding, EVP Development & COO

3142 American Diabetes Association: Atlanta Met ro
17 Executive Park   404-320-7100
Atlanta, GA 30329   888-342-2383
                                          Fax: 404-320-0025
                              e-mail: AskADA@diabetes.org
                                          www.diabetes.org
The American Diabetes Association is a nonprofit health organiza-
tion providing diabetes research, information and advocacy.
Founded in 1940 the American Diabetes Association conducts
programs in all 50 states and the District of Columbia, reaching
hundreds of communities
Michael Gault, Senior Executive Director
Richard Kahn, Chief Scientific/Medical Officer

3143 American Diabetes Association: Savannah
5105 Paulsen Street   912-353-8110
Savannah, GA 31405   888-343-2383
                                          Fax: 912-353-9114
                              e-mail: AskADA@diabetes.org
                                          www.diabetes.org
The American Diabetes Association is a nonprofit health organiza-
tion providing diabetes research, information and advocacy.
Founded in 1940 the American Diabetes Association conducts
programs in all 50 states and the District of Columbia.
Maria Center, Director
Richard Kahn, Chief Scientific/Medical Officer

3144 Juvenile Diabetes Research Foundation: Geo rgia Chapter
400 Perimeter Center Terrace   404-420-5990
Atlanta, GA 30346   Fax: 404-420-5995
                                 e-mail: georgia@jdrf.org
                                      www.jdrfgeorgia.org/
The Juvenile Diabetes Research Foundation International (JDRF)
is a charitable funder and advocate of type 1 (juvenile) diabetes research worldwide. The mission of JDRF is to find a cure for diabetes and its complications through the support of research.
Rob Shaw, Executive Director
Scott Whiteside, EVP/General Manager

3145 American Diabetes Association: Hawaii
1500 S Beretania Street   808-947-5979
Honolulu, HI 96826   888-342-2383
                                          Fax: 808-947-5978
                              e-mail: AskADA@diabetes.org
                                          www.diabetes.org
The American Diabetes Association is a nonprofit health organiza-
tion providing diabetes research, information and advocacy.
Founded in 1940 the American Diabetes Association conducts
programs in all 50 states and the District of Columbia.
Majken Mechling, Executive Director
Richard Kahn, Chief Scientific/Medical Officer

3146 Juvenile Diabetes Research Foundation: Haw aii Chapter
1019 Waimanu Street   808-988-1000
Honolulu, HI 96814   Fax: 808-597-8758
                                  e-mail: hawaii@jdrf.org
                                              www.jdf.org
The Juvenile Diabetes Research Foundation International (JDRF)
is a charitable funder and advocate of type 1 (juvenile) diabetes research worldwide. The mission of JDRF is to find a cure for diabetes and its complications through the support of research.
Arnold Donald, President/CEO Corporate
Robin Harding, EVP/Develpment & COO Corporate

3147 American Diabetes Association: Greater Ill inois
2580 Federal Drive   217-875-9011
Decatur, IL 62526   888-342-2383
                                          Fax: 217-875-6849
                              e-mail: AskADA@diabetes.org
                                          www.diabetes.org
The American Diabetes Association is a nonprofit health organiza-
tion providing diabetes research, information and advocacy.
Founded in 1940 the American Diabetes Association conducts

programs in all 50 states and the District of Columbia, reaching
hundreds of communities.
Donna Scott, Executive Director
Richard Kahn, Chief Scientific/Medical Officer

3148 American Diabetes Association: Northern Il linois
30 North Michigan Avenue   312-346-1805
Chicago, IL 60602   888-343-2383
                                          Fax: 312-346-5342
                              e-mail: AskADA@diabetes.org
                                          www.diabetes.org
The American Diabetes Association is a nonprofit health organiza-
tion providing diabetes research, information and advocacy.
Founded in 1940, the American Diabetes Association conducts
programs in all 50 states and the District of Columbia, reaching
hundreds of communities.
Michael D Farley CFRE (Corporate), Chief Community Relations
Officer
Richard Kahn, Chief Scientific/Medical Officer

3149 Juvenile Diabetes Research Foundation: Gre ater Chicago
Chapter
500 North Dearborn Street   312-670-0313
Chicago, IL 60610   Fax: 312-670-0250
                                 e-mail: illinois@jdrf.org
                                       www.jdrfillinois.org
The Juvenile Diabetes Research Foundation International (JDRF)
is a charitable funder and advocate of type 1 (juvenile) diabetes re-
search worldwide. The mission of JDRF is to find a cure for diabe-
tes and its complications through the support of research.
Amy Franze, Executive Director
Janine Tobola, Director Office Operations

3150 American Diabetes Association: Northern In diana/Northern
Ohio
6415 Castleway W Drive   317-352-9226
Indianapolis, IN 46250   888-342-2383
                                          Fax: 317-594-0748
                              e-mail: AskADA@diabetes.org
                                          www.diabetes.org
The American Diabetes Association is a nonprofit health organiza-
tion providing diabetes research, information and advocacy.
Founded in 1940 the American Diabetes Association conducts
programs in all 50 states and the District of Columbia.
Jennifer Pferrer, Executive Director
Richard Kahn, Chief Scientific/Medical Officer

3151 Diabetes Youth Foundation of Indiana
7311 Tousley Drive   317-750-9310
Indianapolis, IN 46256-9212   Fax: 317-243-4418
                             e-mail: dyfjulie@yahoo.com
                                      www.dyfofindiana.org
This nonprofit group whose mission is to improve the lives of chil-
dren with diabetes and their families.
Julie Shutt, Executive Director
Rick Crosslin, Camp Director

3152 Juvenile Diabetes Research Foundation: Ind iana State Chapter
8465 Keystone Crossing   317-202-0352
Indianapolis, IN 46240   Fax: 317-202-0357
                             e-mail: indianastate@jdrf.org
                                      www.jdrf.org/indiana
The Juvenile Diabetes Research Foundation International (JDRF)
is a charitable funder and advocate of type 1 (juvenile) diabetes research worldwide. The mission of JDRF is to find a cure for diabetes and its complications through the support of research.
Henry Rodriguez MD, Chapter President

3153 Juvenile Diabetes Research Foundation: Nor thern Indiana
Chapter
2004 Ironwood Circle   574-273-1810
South Bend, IN 46635   Fax: 574-273-1870
                           e-mail: northernindiana@jdrf.org
                                              www.jdrf.org
The Juvenile Diabetes Research Foundation International (JDRF)
is a charitable funder and advocate of type 1 (juvenile) diabetes re-

search worldwide. The mission of JDRF is to find a cure for diabetes and its complications through the support of research.
Arnold Donald, President/CEO Corporate
Robin Harding, EVP/Development & COO Corporate

The Juvenile Diabetes Research Foundation International (JDRF) is a charitable funder and advocate of type 1 (juvenile) diabetes research worldwide. The mission of JDRF is to find a cure for diabetes and its complications through the support of research.
Twynette S Davidson, Executive Director
Joe Salvagne, Chapter President

Iowa

3154 American Diabetes Association: Cedar Rapid s District
St Luke's Resource Center   319-247-5124
Cedar Rapids, IA 52406   888-342-2383
                                                Fax: 319-247-5125
                                          e-mail: AskADA@diabetes.org
                                                  www.diabetes.org
The American Diabetes Association is a nonprofit health organization providing diabetes research, information and advocacy. Founded in 1940 the American Diabetes Association conducts programs in all 50 states and the District of Columbia.
Jennifer Petsche, Manager
Richard Kahn, Chief Scientific/Medical Officer

3155 Juvenile Diabetes Research Foundation: Eas tern Iowa Chapter
701 10th Street SE   319-393-3850
Cedar Rapids, IA 52403   Fax: 319-393-3852
                                          e-mail: easterniowa@jdrf.org
                                              www.jdrf.org/easterniowa
The Juvenile Diabetes Research Foundation International (JDRF) is a charitable funder and advocate of type 1 (juvenile) diabetes research worldwide. The mission of JDRF is to find a cure for diabetes and its complications through the support of research.
Ann Elise Walsh, Special Events Manager
Mary Henry, Special Events Coordinator

3156 Juvenile Diabetes Research Foundation: Gre ater Iowa Chapter
5444 NW 96th Street   515-986-1512
Johnston, IA 50131   Fax: 515-986-1513
                                          e-mail: greateriowa@jdif.org
                                              www.jdrf.org/greateriowa
The Juvenile Diabetes Research Foundation International (JDRF) is a charitable funder and advocate of type 1 (juvenile) diabetes research worldwide. The mission of JDRF is to find a cure for diabetes and its complications through the support of research.
Jean Howieson, Special Events Director
Judy Greaves, Office Administrator

Kansas

3157 American Diabetes Association: Kansas
837 S Hillside   316-684-6091
Wichita, KS 67211   888-342-2383
                                                Fax: 316-684-5675
                                          e-mail: AskADA@diabetes.org
                                                  www.diabetes.org
The American Diabetes Association is a nonprofit health organization providing diabetes research, information and advocacy. Founded in 1940 the American Diabetes Association conducts programs in all 50 states and the District of Columbia.
Sarah Beth Webb, Director
Richard Kahn, Chief Scientific/Medical Officer

Kentucky

3158 American Diabetes Association: Kentucky
161 St Matthews Avenue   502-452-6072
Louisville, KY 40207   888-342-2383
                                                Fax: 502-893-2698
                                          e-mail: AskADA@diabetes.org
                                                  www.diabetes.org
The American Diabetes Association is a nonprofit health organization providing diabetes research, information and advocacy. Founded in 1940 the American Diabetes Association conducts programs in all 50 states and the District of Columbia.
Samantha Carroll, Associate Director
Richard Kahn, Chief Scientific/Medical Officer

3159 Juvenile Diabetes Research Foundation: Kentuckiana Chapter
133 Evergreen Road   502-485-9397
Louisville, KY 40243   866-485-9397
                                                Fax: 502-485-9591
                                          e-mail: kentuckiana@jdrf.org
                                         www.jdf.org/chapters/ky/kentuckiana

Louisiana

3160 American Diabetes Association: Louisana
2644 S Sherwood Forest Boulevard   225-216-3980
Baton Rouge, LA 70816   888-342-2383
                                                Fax: 225-295-7005
                                          e-mail: AskADA@diabetes.org
                                                  www.diabetes.org
Paige Grogan, Associate Manager
Lori Koonce, Associate Manager

3161 Juvenile Diabetes Research Foundation: Bat on Rouge Chapter
9457 Brookline Avenue   225-932-9511
Baton Rouge, LA 70809   Fax: 225-932-9514
                                          e-mail: batonrouge@jdrf.org
                                              www.jdrf.org/batonrouge
Kristy Andries, President/Development Chair
Danielle Graham, Special Events Assistant

3162 Juvenile Diabetes Research Foundation: Lou isiana Chapter
2201 Veterans Memorial Bouelvard   504-828-2873
Metairie, LA 70002   Fax: 504-828-4922
                                          e-mail: louisiana@jdrf.org
                                              www.jdrf.org/louisiana
Sam Robinson, President Board of Directors
Becky Spinnato, Vice President Fundraising

3163 Juvenile Diabetes Research Foundation: Shr eveport Chapter
2001 East 70th Street   318-798-1195
Shreveport, LA 71105   Fax: 318-798-1194
                                          e-mail: jburns@jdrf.org
                                              www.jdrf.org/shreveport
Jeff Knutson, President Board of Directors
Craig Floyd, Vice President Fundraising

Maine

3164 American Diabetes Association: Maine
80 Elm Street   207-774-7717
Portland, ME 04101   888-342-2383
                                                Fax: 207-774-7714
                                          e-mail: AskADA@diabetes.org
                                                  www.diabetes.org
Emily Silevinac, Associate Manager
Ryan Williams, Associate Manager

3165 Juvenile Diabetes Research Foundation: New England/Maine Chapter
33 Silver Street   207-761-0133
Portland, ME 04101   Fax: 207-761-1687
                                   e-mail: maine@jdrf.org OR eburgo@jdrf.org
                                                  www.jdrf.org/maine
Heidi Daniels, New England Chapter Executive Director
Emily Hampton Burgo, Branch Manager

Maryland

3166 American Diabetes Association: Maryland
800 Wyman Park Drive   410-265-0075
Baltimore, MD 21211   888-342-2383
                                                Fax: 410-235-4048
                                          e-mail: AskADA@diabetes.org
                                                  www.diabetes.org
Kathy Rogers, Executive Director
Dotty Raynor, Director

3167 Juvenile Diabetes Research Foundation: Mar yland Chapter
200 East Joppa Road   410-823-0073
Towson, MD 21286   Fax: 410-823-0416
                                          e-mail: maryland@jdrf.com
                                              www.jdrf.org/maryland/
Rebecca Maude, Executive Director
Dotty Raynor, Outreach Manager

Massachusetts

3168 American Diabetes Association: Boston
330 Congress Street   617-482-4580
Boston, MA 02210   888-342-2383
                                Fax: 617-482-1824
                    e-mail: AskADA@diabetes.org
                                www.diabetes.org

Christopher Boynton, Executive Director
Lori Glowacki, Director of Special Events

3169 Juvenile Diabetes Research Foundation: New England/Bay State Chapter
20 Walnut Street   781-431-0700
Wellesley, MA 02481   Fax: 781-431-8836
                      e-mail: baystate@jdrf.org
                              www.jdrf.org/baystate

Heidi Daniels, New England Chapter Executive Director
Virginia Irving, Associate Executive Director

Michigan

3170 American Diabetes Association: Michigan
3940 Broadmoor Avenue SE   616-458-9341
Grand Rapids, MI 49512   888-342-2383
                                Fax: 616-575-9930
                    e-mail: AskADA@diabetes.org
                                www.diabetes.org

Darla Hill, Coordinator
Sharice Purman, Director

3171 Juvenile Diabetes Research Foundation: Metropolitan Detroit/SE Michigan
24359 Northwestern Highway   248-355-1133
Southfield, MI 48075-2020   Fax: 248-355-1188
                    e-mail: metrodetroit@jdrf.org
                              www.jdrfdetroit.org

Rita L Combest, Development Director
Susan Kossik, Development Manager

3172 Juvenile Diabetes Research Foundation: Wes t Michigan Chapter
5075 Cascade Road SE   616-957-1838
Grand Rapids, MI 49546   Fax: 616-957-1169
                   e-mail: westmichigan@jrdf.org
                            www.jdrf.org/westmichigan

Annette Guilfoyle, Executive Director
Maxine Gray, Special Events Coordinator

Minnesota

3173 American Diabetes Association: Minnesota
Parkdale Center   763-593-5333
Saint Louis Park, MN 55416   888-342-2383
                                Fax: 952-582-9000
                    e-mail: AskADA@diabetes.org
                                www.diabetes.org

Jenni Hargraves, Executive Director
Becky Barnett, Associate Manager

3174 Juvenile Diabetes Research Foundation: Min nesota Chapter
2626 East 82nd Street   952-851-0770
Bloomington, MN 55425   800-663-1860
                                Fax: 952-851-0766
                      e-mail: minnesota@jdrf.org
                             www.jdrf.org/minnesota

Jackie Casey, Executive Director
Angie McCarthy, Special Events Manager

Mississippi

3175 American Diabetes Association: Mississippi
16 Northtown Drive   601-932-1118
Jackson, MS 39211   888-342-2383
                                Fax: 601-932-1988
                    e-mail: AskADA@diabetes.org
                                www.diabetes.org

The nation's leading voluntary health organization providing diabetes research, information and advocacy. Our mission is to pre-

vent and cure diabetes and to improve the lives of all people affected by diabetes.
Mary D Fortune, Executive Vice President
Stephanie J Coghlan MBA, Senior Regional Director

Missouri

3176 American Diabetes Association: Missouri
1944-A Sunshine   417-890-8400
Springfield, MO 65804   888-342-2383
                                Fax: 417-890-8484
                    e-mail: AskADA@diabetes.org
                                www.diabetes.org

Renee Paulsell, Executive Director
Jennifer Cotner-Jone, Associate Director

3177 Juvenile Diabetes Research Foundation: St. Louis Chapter
225 S Meramec Avenue   314-726-6778
Clayton, MO 63105   Fax: 314-726-6778
                    e-mail: metrostlouis@jdrf.org
                                www.jdrfstl.org

M Marie Davis, Executive Director
William Schmitt, Corporate Development

Montana

3178 American Diabetes Association: Montana
3203 3rd Avenue N   406-256-0616
Billings, MT 59101   888-342-2383
                                Fax: 406-896-0289
                    e-mail: AskADA@diabetes.org
                                www.diabetes.org

Karen Talmadge, Chair
Laurelean Gaines, President

Nebraska

3179 American Diabetes Association: Nebraska
14216 Dayton Circle   402-571-1101
Omaha, NE 68137   888-342-2383
                                Fax: 402-572-8141
                    e-mail: AskADA@diabetes.org
                                www.diabetes.org

Shawn Murphy, Executive Director
Kortney Krill, Associate Manager

3180 Juvenile Diabetes Research Foundation: Lin coln Chapter
1540 S 70th Street   402-484-8300
Lincoln, NE 68506   Fax: 402-484-8302
                       e-mail: lincoln@jdrf.org
                              www.jdrf.org/lincoln

Deb Gokie, Executive Director
Maggie Pavelka, Special Events Assistant

3181 Juvenile Diabetes Research Foundation: Oma ha Council Bluffs Chapter
9202 W Dodge Road   402-397-2873
Omaha, NE 68114   Fax: 402-572-3343
                        e-mail: omaha@jdrf.org
                              www.jdrf.org/omaha

Shawn Reynolds, Executive Director
Melissa Shapiro, Special Events Coordinator

Nevada

3182 American Diabetes Association: Nevada
2785 E Desert Inn Road   702-369-9995
Las Vegas, NV 89121   888-342-2383
                                Fax: 702-369-3717
                    e-mail: AskADA@diabetes.org
                                www.diabetes.org

Mary Stokes, Manager
Carly Rohrer, Associate Manager

3183 Juvenile Diabetes Research Foundation: Nevada Chapter
5542 S Fort Apache Road
Las Vegas, NV 89148
702-732-4795
Fax: 702-732-1635
e-mail: nevada@jdf.org
www.jdrf.org/nevada

Stuart Mason, Nevada Chapter Co-Founder
Flora Mason, Nevada Chapter Co-Founder

3184 Juvenile Diabetes Research Foundation: Nor thern Nevada Branch
5335 Kietzke Lane
Reno, NV 89511
775-786-1881
Fax: 775-827-0131
e-mail: northernnevada@jdrf.org
www.jdrf.org/northernnevada

Molly Dillon, Branch Manager
Arnie Pitts, Board of Directors President

New Hampshire

3185 American Diabetes Association: New Hampshire
249 Canal Street
Manchester, NH 03101
603-627-9579
888-342-2383
Fax: 603-669-1477
www.diabetes.org

3186 Juvenile Diabetes Research Foundation: New England/New Hampshire Chapter
2 Wellman Avenue
Nashua, NH 03064
603-595-2595
Fax: 603-595-2073
e-mail: newhampshire@jdrf.org
www.jdrf.org/newhampshire

Brooke Edwards, Special Events Coordinator
Heidi Daniels, New England Chapter Executive Director

New Jersey

3187 American Diabetes Association: New Jersey
CentrePoint II Suite 103
Bridgewater, NJ 08807
732-469-7979
888-342-2383
Fax: 732-469-4887
e-mail: AskADA@diabetes.org
www.diabetes.org

James Roberts, Executive Director
Pamela Hooper, Director

3188 Juvenile Diabetes Research Foundation: South Jersey Chapter
1415 Route 70 E
Cherry Hill, NJ 08034
856-429-1101
Fax: 856-429-1105
e-mail: southjersey@jdrf.org
www.jdrf.org/southjersey

Stephen Blocher, Executive Director
Robin Berger, Special Events Coordinator

3189 Juvenile Diabetes Research Foundation: Cen tral Jersey Chapter
740 Broad Street
Shrewsbury, NJ 07702
732-219-6654
Fax: 732-219-8722
e-mail: centraljersey@jdrf.org
www.jdrf.org/chapters/NJ/Central-Jersey

Lori McLane, Executive Director
Beckie Burlew, Special Events Coordinator

3190 Juvenile Diabetes Research Foundation: Mid -Jersey Chapter
28 Kennedy Boulevard
East Brunswick, NJ 08816
732-296-7171
Fax: 732-296-1433
e-mail: midjersey@jdrf.org
www.jdrf.org/NJ/Mid-Jersey

Elizabeth Giardina Preston, Chapter Executive Director
Sandra Hilsenrath, Special Events Coordinator

3191 Juvenile Diabetes Research Foundation: Roc kland County/Northern New Jersey
560 Sylvan Avenue
Englewood Cliffs, NJ 07632
201-568-4838
Fax: 201-568-5360
e-mail: rockland@jdrf.org
www.jdrf.org/northernnj

Douglas Rouse, Executive Director
Allison Hartstone, Special Events Coordinator

New Mexico

3192 American Diabetes Association: New Mexico
2625 Pennsylvania NE
Albuquerque, NM 87110
505-266-5716
888-342-2383
Fax: 505-268-4533
e-mail: AskADA@diabetes.org
www.diabetes.org

Betsey Robinson, Associate Director
Lisa Johnson, Manager

3193 Juvenile Diabetes Research Foundation: Albuquerque
2501 San Pedro NE
Albuquerque, NM 87110
505-255-4005
Fax: 505-260-1430
e-mail: newmexico@jdrf.org
www.jdrf.org/newmexico

Joann Perrine, Branch Manager
Elizabeth Romero, Fundraising Assistant

New York

3194 American Diabetes Association: New York
Pine W Plaza Building 2
Albany, NY 12205
518-218-1755
888-342-2383
Fax: 518-218-0114
e-mail: AskADA@diabetes.org
www.diabetes.org

Amy R Young, District Director
Karen Dooley, Associate Manager

3195 Juvenile Diabetes Research Foundation
Executive Office/Corporate Headquarters
120 Wall Street
New York, NY 10005-4001
212-725-4925
800-533-2873
Fax: 212-785-9595
e-mail: info@jdrf.org
www.jdrf.org/

Allan J Lewis, President/Chief Executive Officer
Amy C Franze, EVP Development

3196 Juvenile Diabetes Research Foundation: Long Island/South Shore Chapter
532 Broadhollow Road
Melville, NY 11747
631-414-1126
Fax: 631-414-1133
e-mail: longisland@jdrf.org
www.jdrf.org/longisland

Barbara Rogus, Executive Director
Christina Colandro, Special Events Manager

3197 Juvenile Diabetes Research Foundation: Buf falo/Western New York Chapter
331 Alberta Drive
Buffalo, NY 14226
716-833-2873
Fax: 716-833-0199
e-mail: westernny@jdrf.org
www.jdrf.org/westernny

Karen Swierski, Executive Director
Jennifer Hickok, Special Events Manager

3198 Juvenile Diabetes Research Foundation: Hud son Valley Chapter
Hollowbrook Office Park
Wappinger Falls, NY 12590
845-297-8600
Fax: 845-297-7887
e-mail: hudsonvalley@jdrf.org
www.letscurediabetes.com

Charlie Lawrence, Branch Manager
Linda Delia, Events Assistant

3199 Juvenile Diabetes Research Foundation: New York Chapter
432 Park Avenue S
New York, NY 10016
212-689-2860
Fax: 212-689-4038
e-mail: newyorkchapter@jdrf.org
www.nyc.jdrf.org

Mania Boyder, New York City Chapter Executive Director

3200 Juvenile Diabetes Research Foundation: Nor theastern New York
6 Greenwood Drive
East Greenbush, NY 12061
518-477-2873
Fax: 518-477-7004
e-mail: northeastny@jdrf.org
www.jdrf.org/NortheasternNY

Bev Kennedy, Executive Director
Darlene Robbiano, Special Events Manager

3201 Juvenile Diabetes Research Foundation: Roc hester Branch/Western New York Chapter
1200-A Scottsville Road
Rochester, NY 14624

585-546-1390
Fax: 585-546-1404
e-mail: rochester@jdrf.org
www.jdrf.org/rochester

Mary Anne Fox, Executive Director
Lisa Swindon, Senior Development Coordinator

3202 Juvenile Diabetes Research Foundation: Wes tchester County Chapter
30 Glenn Street
White Plains, NY 10603

914-686-7700
Fax: 914-686-7701
e-mail: westchester@jdrf.org
www.jdrf.org/westchester

Katherine Cintron, Executive Director
Dejan Popovich, Special Events Coordinator

North Carolina

3203 American Diabetes Association: North Carolina
222 South Church Street
Charlotte, NC 28202

704-373-9111
888-342-2383
Fax: 704-373-9113
www.diabetes.org

Dianne Roth, Executive Director

3204 Juvenile Diabetes Research Foundation: Triangle/Eastern North Carolina Chapter
2210 Millbrook Road
Raleigh, NC 27604

919-431-8330
Fax: 919-431-8373
e-mail: triangle@jdrf.org
www.jdrftriangle.org

Jim Burson, Chapter President
Courtney Davies, Executive Director

3205 Juvenile Diabetes Research Foundation: Cha rlotte Chapter
205 Regency Executive Park Drive
Charlotte, NC 28217

704-561-0828
Fax: 704-561-9920
e-mail: charlotte@jdrf.org
www.gwc.jdrf.org

Brenning Johnston, Volunteer Coordinator

3206 Juvenile Diabetes Research Foundation: Pie dmont Triad Chapter
1401-B Old Mill Circle
Winston-Salem, NC 27103

336-768-1027
Fax: 336-768-1029
e-mail: piedmont@jdrf.org
www.jdrf.org/triad

Brad Calloway, President Board of Directors
Tom Brinkley, VP Fundraising & Development

North Dakota

3207 American Diabetes Association: Nashville
1323 23rd Street S
Fargo, ND 58103

701-234-0123
Fax: 701-235-3080
e-mail: AskADA@diabetes.org
www.diabetes.org

Stephanie Chimeziri, Associate Director

3208 American Diabetes Association: North Dakota
1323 23rd Street South
Fargo, ND 58103

701-234-0123
888-342-2383
Fax: 701-235-3080
www.diabetes.org

Ohio

3209 American Diabetes Association: Ohio
4500 Rockside Road
Independence, OH 44131

216-328-9989
888-342-2383
Fax: 216-328-0007
e-mail: AskADA@diabetes.org
www.diabetes.org

Jill Pupa, Executive Director
Patti Clair, Associate Director

3210 Juvenile Diabetes Research Foundation/JDRF
1293-H Lyons Road
Dayton, OH 45458

937-439-2873
Fax: 937-439-4086
e-mail: dayton@jdrf.org
www.jdrf.org/dayton

Karen Myers, Executive Director
Vicky Williams, Office Manager

3211 Juvenile Diabetes Research Foundation: Mid-Ohio Chapter
1550 Old Henderson Rd
Columbus, OH 43220

614-464-2873
Fax: 614-464-2877
e-mail: midohio@jdrf.org
www.jdrf.org/midohio

Staci Perkins, Executive Director
Roberta Smedes, Office Manager

3212 Juvenile Diabetes Research Foundation: Akr on/Canton Chapter
5000 Rockside Road
Canton, OH 44131

888-718-3061
Fax: 216-328-8340
e-mail: jcallahan@jdrf.org
www.jdrf.org/chapters/OH/Northeast-Ohio

Laura E Maciag, Executive Director
Danielle Thompson, Special Events Manager

3213 Juvenile Diabetes Research Foundation: Gre ater Cincinnati Chapter
8041 Hosbrook Road
Cincinnati, OH 45236-3830

513-793-3223
Fax: 513-936-5333
e-mail: cincinnati@jdrf.org
www.jdrf.org/cincinnati

Bill Rice, Executive Director
Bethe Ferguson, Special Events Coordinator

3214 Juvenile Diabetes Research Foundation: Tol edo/Northwest Ohio Chapter
3450 W Central Avenue
Toledo, OH 43606

419-873-1377
800-533-2873
Fax: 419-720-6339
e-mail: northwestohio@jdrf.org
www.jdrf.org/northwestohio

Megan Meyer, Executive Director
Marna Cousino, Special Events Coordinator

Oklahoma

3215 American Diabetes Association: Oklahoma
3000 United Founders Boulevard
Oklahoma City, OK 73112

405-840-3881
888-342-2383
Fax: 405-840-3899
e-mail: AskADA@diabetes.org
www.diabetes.org

Diane Sarantakos, Executive Director
Andrea Barnett, Associate Manager

3216 Juvenile Diabetes Research Foundation: Cen tral Oklahoma Chapter
2601 NW Expressway
Oklahoma City, OK 73112

405-810-0070
888-533-9255
Fax: 405-810-0078
e-mail: oklahoma@jdrf.org
www.jdrf.org/centralok

Renee MacDonald, Executive Director
Shannon Scott, Special Events Coordinator

3217 Juvenile Diabetes Research Foundation: Tul sa Green County Chapter
4606 E 67th Street
Tulsa, OK 74136

918-481-5807
Fax: 918-481-5823
e-mail: tulsa@jdrf.org
www.jdrf.org/tulsa-green

Brandi Sullivan, Executive Director
Angela Peterson, Special Events Coordinator

Oregon

3218 American Diabetes Association: Oregon
2350 Oakmont Way   541-343-0735
Eugene, OR 97401   888-342-2383
                                    Fax: 541-342-1491
                              e-mail: AskADA@diabetes.org
                                    www.diabetes.org

Cynthia Benton, Associate Director

**3219 Juvenile Diabetes Research Foundation: Ore gon/SW
Washington Chapter**
7460 SW Hunziker Street   503-643-1995
Portland, OR 97223   866-598-9074
                                    Fax: 503-598-9087
                       e-mail: oregon-washington@jdrf.org
                                    www.jdrf.org/oregon

Ashleigh Farleigh, Special Events Manager
Debbie Secor, Special Events Assistant

Pennsylvania

3220 American Diabetes Association: Pennsylvania
3544 Progress Avenue   717-657-4310
Harrisburg, PA 17110   888-342-2383
                                    Fax: 717-657-4320
                                    www.diabetes.org

3221 American Diabetes Association: Western Pennsylvania
300 Penn Center Boulevard   412-824-1181
Pittsburgh, PA 15235   888-342-2383
                                    Fax: 412-824-2191
                              e-mail: AskADA@diabetes.org
                                    www.diabetes.org

Terri Seidman, Area Manager
Steven Shivak, Executive Director

**3222 Juvenile Diabetes Research Foundation: Central Pennsylvania
Chapter**
119 Aster Drive   717-901-6489
Harrisburg, PA 17112   Fax: 717-901-6573
                              e-mail: centralpa@jdrf.org
                                    www.jdrf.org/centralpa

Susan Harral, Executive Director
Kate Severs, Special Events Assistant

3223 Juvenile Diabetes Research Foundation: Ber ks County Chapter
619 Wellington Avenue   610-775-4169
West Lawn, PA 19609
Tammy A. Edwards, Contact

**3224 Juvenile Diabetes Research Foundation: Nor thwestern
Pennsylvania Chapter**
1700 Peach St   814-452-0635
Erie, PA 16501   Fax: 814-452-0645
                              e-mail: northwestpa@jdrf.org
                                    www.jdrf.org/northwestpa

Douglas K White, Executive Director
Amy Bement, Special Events Assistant

3225 Juvenile Diabetes Research Foundation: Phi ladelphia Chapter
225 City Line Avenue   610-664-9255
Bala Cynwyd, PA 19004   Fax: 610-664-9585
                              e-mail: philadelphia@jdrf.org
                                    www.jdrf.org/philadelphia

Ellen Rubesin, Executive Director
Kathy Farren, Special Events Director

3226 Juvenile Diabetes Research Foundation: Wes tern Pennsylvania
960 Penn Avenue   412-471-1414
Pittsburgh, PA 15222   888-528-8788
                                    Fax: 412-471-1417
                              e-mail: westernpa@jdrf.org
                                    www.jdrf.org/westernpa

David R Donahue, Executive Director
Kimberly A McElroy, Office Manager

Rhode Island

3227 American Diabetes Association: Rhode Island
146 Clifford St   401-351-0498
Providence, RI 02903   888-342-2383
                                    Fax: 401-351-1674
                                    www.jdf.org

South Carolina

3228 American Diabetes Association: South Carolina
2711 Middleburg Drive   803-799-4246
Columbia, SC 29204   888-342-2383
                                    Fax: 803-799-5792
                                    www.diabetes.org

3229 Juvenile Diabetes Research Foundation: Palmetto Chapter
810 Dutch Square Blvd   803-782-1477
Columbia, SC 29210   Fax: 803-782-8975
                              e-mail: palmetto@jdrf.org
                          www.jdrfpalmetto.org/about.aspx

Michael Slapnik, President
Dana Bruce, Executive Director

3230 Juvenile Diabetes Research Foundation: Low Country Chapter
520 Folly Road   843-345-0369
Charleston, SC 29412   Fax: 843-406-7957
                              e-mail: dmenefee@jdrf.org
                                    www.jdrf.org/lowcountry
Pam Nestor McAdams, Events/Walk Director South Coastal Chptr

South Dakota

3231 Juvenile Diabetes Research Foundation: Sio ux Falls Chapter
PO Box 88540   605-338-2295
Sioux Falls, SD 57109-8540

Tennessee

3232 American Diabetes Association: Nashville
4205 Hillsboro Road   615-298-3066
Nashville, TN 37215   888-342-2383
                                    Fax: 615-292-5357
                              e-mail: AskADA@diabetes.org
                                    www.diabetes.org

Glenda Berry, Executive Director
Harlyn Hardin, Director of Programs

3233 American Diabetes Association: Tennessee
5583 Murray Road   901-682-8232
Memphis, TN 38119   888-342-2383
                                    Fax: 901-682-8170
                              e-mail: AskADA@diabetes.org
                                    www.diabetes.org

John Carroll, Director
Daniele Cain, Coordinator

3234 Juvenile Diabetes Research Foundation: East Tennessee Chapter
355 Trane Lane   865-544-0768
Knoxville, TN 37919   Fax: 865-544-4312
                              e-mail: EastTennessee@jdrf.org
                                    www.easttennessee.jdrf.org

**3235 Juvenile Diabetes Research Foundation: Mid dle Tennessee
Chapter**
105 Westpark Drive   615-383-6781
Nashville, TN 37027   Fax: 615-383-4284
                              e-mail: MidTennessee@jrdf.org
                                    www.midtennessee.jdrf.org

Joe Bide, Vice President

Texas

3236 American Diabetes Association: Texas
4150 International Plaza
Fort Worth, TX 76109   817-332-7110
                                    888-342-2383
                                    Fax: 817-732-6244
                                    www.diabetes.org

3237 Juvenile Diabetes Research Foundation: South Central Texas Chapter
8700 Crownhill Boulevrad
San Antonio, TX 78209

210-822-5336
Fax: 210-822-1443
e-mail: scentraltexas@jdrf.org
www.sctx-jdrf.org

Doug Koskie, President
Brigitte West, Secretary

3238 Juvenile Diabetes Research Foundation: Dal las Chapter
9400 North Central Expressway
Dallas, TX 75231-5063

214-373-9808
Fax: 214-373-6337
e-mail: dallas@jrdf.org
www.jdrfdallas.org

Dave Johnson, President
Michael Keith, Treasurer

3239 Juvenile Diabetes Research Foundation: Gre ater Fort Worth/ Arlington Chapter
3840 Hulen Street
Fort Worth, TX 76107-2127

817-332-2601
Fax: 817-332-5641
e-mail: grfortworth@jdrf.org
www.jdf.org

3240 Juvenile Diabetes Research Foundation: Hou ston/Gulf Coast Chapter
2425 Fountain View
Houston, TX 77057

713-334-4400
Fax: 713-334-4040
e-mail: houston@jdrf.org
www.jdf.org

3241 Juvenile Diabetes Research Foundation: Wes t Texas Chapter
Clay Desta Towers, 10 Desta Drive
Midland, TX 79705

432-570-5643
Fax: 432-682-0765
e-mail: westtexas@jdrf.org
www.jdf.org

Utah

3242 American Diabetes Association: Utah
1245 E Brickyard Road
Salt Lake City, UT 84106

801-363-3024
888-342-2383
Fax: 801-363-3031
www.diabetes.org

Vermont

3243 American Diabetes Association: Vermont
1 Kennedy Drive
S Burlington, VT 05403

802-654-7716
888-342-2383
Fax: 802-658-9145
www.diabetes.org

Virginia

3244 American Diabetes Association: Richmond
4335 Cox Road
Glen Allen, VA 23060

804-225-8038
888-342-2383
Fax: 804-270-4742
www.diabetes.org

3245 American Diabetes Association: Virginia
870 Greenbrier Circle
Chesapeake, VA 23320

757-424-6662
888-342-2383
Fax: 757-420-0490
www.diabetes.org

3246 Juvenile Diabetes Research Foundation: Gre ater Blue Ridge Chapter
3959 Electric Road
Roanoke, VA 24018

540-772-1975
888-849-0510
Fax: 540-772-6672
e-mail: greaterblueridge@jdrf.org
www.jdrfgreaterblueridge.org

Mary Lou Bruce, Board President
Annette Kirby, Secretary

Washington

3247 American Diabetes Association: Seattle
Metropolitan Park E
Seattle, WA 98101

206-282-4616
888-342-2383
Fax: 206-903-8107
www.diabetes.org

Linda Henderson, Executive Director
Sarah Popelka, Director

3248 American Diabetes Association: Washington
1200 Sixth Avenue
Spokane, WA 99204

509-624-7478
888-342-2383
Fax: 509-624-7212
www.diabetes.org

3249 Juvenile Diabetes Research Foundation: Seattle Guild
1215 Fourth Avenue
Seattle, WA 98161-1101

206-343-0873
Fax: 206-343-7015
e-mail: terickson@jdrf.org
www.jdrfnorthwest.org

Nadie Heichel, Executive Director
Becky Baumgardner, Office Manager

3250 Juvenile Diabetes Research Foundation: Sea ttle Chapter
1333 N Northlake Way
Seattle, WA 98103-8900

206-545-1510
Fax: 206-545-1511
www.jdf.org

3251 Juvenile Diabetes Research Foundation: Spo kane County Area Chapter
9 South Washington
Spokane, WA 99201

509-459-6307
Fax: 509-459-6392
e-mail: inlandnw@jdrf.org
http://www.jdrf.org/index.cfm

Kay C Dightman, Contact

West Virginia

3252 American Diabetes Association: West Virginia
PO Box 238
Hurricane, WV 25526

304-768-2596
888-342-2383
Fax: 304-562-1887
e-mail: rahearn@diabetes.org
diabetes.org

Karen Talmadge, Chair
Lurelean Gaines, President

3253 Juvenile Diabetes Research Foundation: Hun tington Chapter
PO Box 2903
Huntington, WV 25728

304-525-4533

Wisconsin

3254 American Diabetes Association: Wisconsin
1701 North Beauregard Street Alexan
Monona, WI 53713

608-222-7785
888-342-2383
Fax: 608-222-7795
e-mail: bfolco@diabetes.org
www.diabetes.org

Barb Folco, Manager
Jay Kemp, Coordinator

3255 Juvenile Diabetes Research Foundation: Southeastern Chapter
3333 North Mayfair Road
Wauwatosa, WI 53222

414-453-4673
Fax: 414-453-4919
e-mail: southeastwi@jdrf.org
www.sewi.jdrf.org/

3256 Juvenile Diabetes Research Foundation: Gre ater Madison Chapter
434 S. Yellowstone Drive
Madison, WI 53719

608-833-2873
Fax: 608-833-9214
e-mail: westernwi@jdrf.org
www.jdrfwesternwisconsin.org/

Douglas Berry, President
Aaron Weinbe Swenson, Treasurer

3257 Juvenile Diabetes Research Foundation: Nor theast Wisconsin Chapter
1800 Appleton Road   920-997-0038
Menasha, WI 54952-0101   Fax: 920-997-0039
                                           e-mail: northeastwi@jdrf.org
                                                      www.jdrf.org
Julie Kersten, Executive Director
Dana Paschen, Special Events Coordinator

Libraries & Resource Centers

3258 Diabetes Control Program
California Department of Health Services
PO Box 997413   916-552-9888
Sacramento, CA 95899-7413   Fax: 916-552-9988
                                           http://www.caldiabetes.org/
Our mission is to prevent diabetes and its complications in California's diverse communities.
Susan Lopez-Payan, Interim Chief

3259 Division of Diabetes Translation
National Center for Chronic Disease Prevention
1600 Clifton Rd   800-232-4636
Atlantia, GA 30333-3717   Fax: 770-488-5966
                                           TTY: 888-232-6348
                                           e-mail: cdcinfo@cdc.gov
                                                      www.cdc.gov/diabetes
The Division of Diabetes Translation's (DDT) goal is to reduce the burden of diabetes in the United States. The division works to achieve this goal by combining support for public health-oriented diabetes prevention and control programs (DPCPs) and translating diabetes research findings into widespread clinical and public health practice.

3260 Health Science Library
Marshall University
1600 Medical Center Drive
Huntington, WV 25701   304-691-1700
                                           www.musom.marshall.edu/library
The Health Sciences Library's primary mission is serving the informational needs of the students, faculty, and staff at Marshall University and the Cabell-Huntington Hospital. The Library also plays an important role in providing information services to hospitals and healthcare professionals in the Huntington and the Tri-State area.
Edward Dzierzak, Director

3261 Joslin Center at University of Maryland Medicine
22 S Greene Street
Baltimore, MD 21201   800-492-5538
                                           TDD: 800735225800
                                           e-mail: joslin@umms001.ab.umd.edu
                                                      www.umm.edu/joslindiabetes
The Joslin Center at University of Maryland Medicine meets the highest standards of care for people with diabetes. Its programs reflect a philosophy which have been the hallmark of Joslin's care — a comprehensive team approach to diabetes treatment with programs designed to help children and adults with diabetes take charge of their own health and well-being.
Thomas W Donner, MD, Director

3262 Naomi Berrie Diabetes Center at Columbia University Medical Center
Russ Berrie Medical Science Pavillion
1150 St. Nicholas Avenue   212-851-5494
New York, NY 10032   Fax: 212-851-5459
                                           e-mail: diabetes@columbia.edu
                                                      nbdiabetes.org
The special focus of the Naomi Berrie Diabetes Center is on families — a concept that differentiates it from almost every other diabetes treatment facility in America. People with diabetes are strongly encouraged to involve their entire families in the treatment process.
Robin Goland, MD, Co-Director
Rudolph Liebel, Co-Director

3263 National Diabetes Information Clearinghous e
One Information Way
Bethesda, MD 20892-3560   800-860-8747
                                           Fax: 703-738-4929
                                           TTY: 866-8569-116
                                           e-mail: ndic@info.niddk.nih.gov
                                                      diabetes.niddk.nih.gov
To serve as a diabetes informational, educational, and referral resource for health professionals and the public. NDIC is a service of the NIDDK.

3264 Schulze Diabetes Institute
University of Minnesota
420 Delaware Street SE   612-626-3016
Minneapolis, MN 55455   e-mail: diitinfo@umn.edu
                                                      www.med.umn.edu
Formerly the Diabetes Institute for Immunology and Transplantation
David Sutherland MD, PhD, Director
Bernard Hering, Director

3265 Tallahassee Memorial Diabetes Center
Tallahassee Memorial Health Care
1300 Miccosukee Road   850-431-5404
Tallahassee, FL 32308   800-662-4278
                                           Fax: 850-431-6325
                                           www.tmh.org/diabetes
TMH provides comprehensive, patient-centered services to both children and adults. The Diabetes Center uses a team approach that involves the patient, physicians, nurse educators, registered dietitians with access to a diabetes counselor and registered pharmacists and social worker.
Richard M Bergenstal, MD, Medical Director

Research Centers

3266 Barbara Davis Center for Childhood Diabetes
13001 E 17th Place   303-724-2323
Aurora, CO 80045-6511   Fax: 303-724-6839
                                           e-mail: george.eisenbarth@uchsc.edu
                                                      www.uchsc.edu/misc/diabetes
Research and educational organization.
Marian Rewers, Clinical Director
George S Eisenbarth, Executive Director

3267 Baylor College of Medicine: Children's General Clinical Research Center
One Baylor Plaza   713-798-4780
Houston, TX 77030   Fax: 713-790-1345
                                           e-mail: pedi-webmaster@bcm.edu
                                                      www.bcm.edu/pediatrics
Offers research into juvenile aspects of immunology and infectious diseases including diabetes research activities.
Lisa Bomgaars, Medical Director
Mark A Ward, Director

3268 Benaroya Research Institute Virginia Mason Medical Center
Virginia Mason Medical Center
1201 9th Avenue   206-583-6525
Seattle, WA 98101-2795   Fax: 206-223-7543
                                           e-mail: info@benaroyaresearch.org
                                                      www.benaroyaresearch.org
Immunology and diabetes research.
Robert B Lemon, Chair
Gerald Nepom, Director

3269 Diabetes Education and Research Center The Franklin House
The Franklin House
PO Box 897   215-829-3426
Philadelphia, PA 19105   Fax: 215-829-5807
                                           e-mail: webmaster@dibeteseducationandresearchcen
                                                      www.diabeteseducationandresearchcenter.o
Is a non-profit organization serving the needs of people living in Philadelphia PA and surrounding communities. The goal of the Foundation is to improve the health of people with diabetes.

3270 Diabetes Research and Training Center: University of Alabama at Birmingham
Department of Medicine

1530 3rd Avenue S
Birmingham, AL 35294-1150

205-934-4011
Fax: 205-934-4389
TTY: 205-934-4642
www.main.uab.edu

The DRTC works to develop and evaluate new models of diabetes care and to facilitate translational diabetes research.
Dr Carol Garrison, President
William Ferniany, CEO

3271 Division on Endocrinology Northwestern University Feinberg School
Northwestern University Feinberg School of Medicin
251 East Huron Street
Chicago, IL 60611

312-926-6895
Fax: 312-503-7757
e-mail: help@medicine.northwestern.edu
www.medicine.northwestern.edu

Nonprofit organization focusing research activities on endocrinology metabolism nutrition and specializing in diabetes.
Joe Bass, MD, PhD, Chief of the Division of Endocrinology
Grazia Aleppo, MD, Director, Endocrinology Clinical Practic

3272 Endocrinology Research Laboratory Cabrini Medical Center
Cabrini Medical Center
227 E 19th Street
New York, NY 10003-7457

212-222-7464
e-mail: info@cabrininy.org
www.cabrininy.org

Focuses on the effects of insulin and insulin-like growth factors on human body functions.
Dr Leonid Poretsky, Director

3273 Indiana University: Area Health Education Center
714 N Senate Avenue
Indianapolis, IN 46202

317-278-8893
Fax: 317-278-0392
e-mail: ahec@iupui.edu
www.ahec.iupui.edu

A collaborative statewide system for community-based primary health care professions education that fosters the continuing improvement of health care services for all citizens in Indiana.
Richard D Kiovsky, MD, Director
Jonathan C Barclay, Associate Director

3274 Indiana University: Center for Diabetes Research
340 West 10th Street
Indianapolis, IN 46202-3082

317-274-8157
Fax: 317-274-1437
e-mail: rconsidi@iupui.edu
www.medicine.iu.edu

Our goal is to promote the training of scientists whose research will develop new understandings of the basis of the disease and its complications and to cultivate basic science research that can speed the discovery of more effective therapies.
Robert Considine, Associate Professor of Medicine
D Craig Brater MD, Dean

3275 Indiana University: Pharmacology Research Laboratory
Division of Clinical Pharmacology
1001 W 10th Street
Indianapolis, IN 46202

317-630-8795
Fax: 317-630-8185
e-mail: tamllewi@iupui.edu
www.medicine.iupui.edu/clinpharm

We will train highly skilled compassionate and altruistic professionals both generalists and specialists to be future leaders in medical practice academia and industry.
David A Flockhart, Division Director
John T Callaghan, Associate Professor of Medicine

3276 International Diabetes Center at Nicollet
3800 Park Nicollet Boulevard
Saint Louis Park, MN 55416-2533

952-993-3393
888-825-6315
Fax: 952-993-1302
e-mail: idcdiabetes@parknicollet.com
www.parknicollet.com/diabetes

Research center which improves the quality of life of individuals with diabetes and those at risk of developing diabetes by undertaking clinical care education research and outreach activities that stimulate and support health.
Richard Berg MD, Executive Director

3277 Joslin Diabetes Center
One Joslin Place
Boston, MA 02215-5306

617-732-2400
800-567-5461
Fax: 617-322-40
e-mail: diabetes@joslin.harvard.edu
www.joslin.org

An internationally recognized leader in diabetes and endocrine disease treatment research and patient and professional education affiliated with Harvard Medical School. In addition to its headquarters in Boston's Longwood Medical area Joslin has affiliated treatment centers across the nation. Established in 1898.
John L Brooks, Chairman of the Board
Martin J Abrahamson, Senior VP, Medical Director

3278 Metabolic Research Institute
1515 N Flagler Drive
West Palm Beach, FL 33401

561-802-3060
Fax: 561-802-3260
e-mail: moreinformation@metabolic-institute.com
www.metabolic-institute.com

The Metabolic Research Institute specializes in clinical studies involving endocrinology disorders complications of endocrinology disorders metabolic problems and selected renal disease.
William A Kaye, Co-Director
Barry Horowitz, Co-Director

3279 Sansum Diabetes Research Institute
2219 Bath Street
Santa Barbara, CA 93105-4321

805-682-7638
Fax: 805-682-3332
e-mail: info@sansum.org
www.sansum.org

A research institute devoted to the prevention treatment and cure of diabetes.
Lois Jovanovich, CEO & Chief Scientific Officer
Wendy Bevier, Associate Investigator

3280 University of Chicago: Comprehensive Diabetes Center
5841 S Maryland Avenue
Chicago, IL 60637

773-702-2371
800-989-6740
e-mail: diabetes@uchospitals.edu
www.kovlerdiabetescenter.org

The University of Chicago Kovler Diabetes Center offers a unique fully comprehensive approach to diagnosing and treating diabetes. Focuses on children adolescents and adults with diabetes as well as individuals at the highest risk for serious complications.
Louis H Philipson, Medical Director
Christopher Rhodes, Kovler Diabetes Center Pediatric Program

3281 University of Colorado: General Clinical Research Center, Pediatric
13001 E 17th Place
Aurora, CO 80045

720-777-2957
Fax: 72-77-727
e-mail: CTRCAdmin@tchden.org
www.uchsc.edu/pedsgcrc

Focuses on developmental studies and diabetes research.
Ronald J Sokol, Program Director
Philip S Zeitler, Associate Program Director

3282 University of Iowa: Diabetes Research Center
Department of Internal Medicine
200 Hawkins Drive
Iowa City, IA 52242

319-353-7842
www.int-med.uiowa.edu

The Diabetes Research Center combines the talents of experienced clinical investigators molecular biologists and vascular physiologists in an integrated multidisciplinary approach toward the study and treatment of abnormalities of vascular reactivity which characterize diabetes mellitus.
Ken Kates, Chief Executive Officer
John Swenning, Associate Director

3283 University of Kansas Cray Diabetes Center
3901 Rainbow Boulevard
Kansas City, KS 66160-7376

913-588-5000
Fax: 913-588-4023
TTY: 913-588-7963
e-mail: geaks@kumc.edu
www.kumc.edu

The KU Medical Center is a complex institution whose basic functions include research education patient care and community service involving multiple constituencies at state and national levels.
Barbara Atkinson, Executive Vice Chancellor

3284 University of Massachusetts: Diabetes and Endocrinology Research Center
55 Lake Avenue N
Worcester, MA 01655
508-856-8989
e-mail: evelyn.vignola@umassmed.edu
www.umassmed.edu
UMMS has exploded onto the national scene as a major center for research, and in the past four decades, UMMS researchers have made pivotal advances in HIV, cancer, diabetes, infectious disease and in understanding the molecular basis of disease.
Micheal F Collins MD, Senior VP
Michael P Czech, Professor and Chair

3285 University of Miami: Diabetes Research Institute
200 S Park Road
Hollywood, FL 33021
954-964-4040
800-321-3437
Fax: 954-964-7036
e-mail: info@drif.org
www.diabetesresearch.org
The Diabetes Research Institute (DRI) is an innovator in many fields of diabetes research but one of its primary strengths lies in islet cell transplantation, a cellular therapy that restores insulin production to normalize blood sugar control.
Thomas D Stern, Chairman
Camillo Ricordi, DRI Scientific Director

3286 University of New Mexico General Clinical Research Center
University of New Mexico Hospital
The University of New Mexico
Albuquerque, NM 87131-2240
505-277-0111
Fax: 505-272-0266
e-mail: mburge@salud.unm.edu
hsc.unm.edu/som/gcrc
Diabetes research.
Steve McKernan, CEO
Richard Larson, Vice President for Research

3287 University of Pennsylvania Diabetes and Endocrinology Research Center
700 Clinical Research Building (CRB
Philadelphia, PA 19104
215-898-4365
Fax: 215-898-5408
e-mail: gburgese@mail.med.upenn.edu
www.med.upenn.edu/idom/derc
The Penn Diabetes and Endocrinology Research Center (DERC) participates in the nationwide inter-disciplinary program established over two decades ago by the NIDDK to foster research and training in the areas of diabetes and related endocrine and metabolic disorders.
Mitchell A Lazar, Director
Morris J Birnbaum, Co Director

3288 University of Pittsburgh: Department of Molecular Genetics and Biochemistry
200 Lothrop Street
Pittsburgh, PA 15261
412-648-9570
Fax: 412-624-8997
e-mail: info@mmg.pitt.edu
www.mgb.pitt.edu
MMG students and fellows routinely publish their research in outstanding journals, present their science at international conferences and go on to achieve positions at prestigious laboratories and institutions.
J Richard Chaillet, Associate Professor
Bruce A McClane, Professor

3289 University of Tennessee: General Clinical Research Center
1265 Union Avenue
Memphis, TN 38104
901-516-2212
Fax: 901-516-7013
e-mail: bsalpert@utmem.edu
www.utmem.edu/crc
Congress directed the National Institutes of Health to establish clinical research centers throughout the United States to launch an all-out attack on human diseases.
Bruce S Alpert MD, Program Director
Teresa Carr, Research Nurses

3290 University of Texas General Clinical Research Center
7400 Merton Minter Boulevard
San Antonio, TX 78229
409-772-1950
Fax: 409-772-8097
e-mail: public.affairs@utmb.edu
www.utmb.edu/gcrc

Focuses on diabetes and infectious disease research.
Michael Lich MD, Program Director
Garland D Anderson, Principal Investigator

3291 University of Washington Diabetes: Endocrinology Research Center
DVA Puget Sound Health Care System
1660 S Columbian Way
Seattle, WA 98108
206-616-4860
Fax: 206-764-2693
e-mail: derc@u.washington.edu
www.depts.washington.edu/diabetes
The primary purpose of the DERC is to facilitate and enhance the diabetes-related research of approximately 100 Affiliate Investigators at the University of Washington
Jerry P Palmer MD, Director
David E Cummings, Deputy Director

3292 Vanderbilt University Diabetes Center
1211 Medical Center Drive
Nashville, TN 37232
615-322-5000
Fax: 615-936-1667
e-mail: dc.brown@vanderbilt.edu
www.mc.vanderbilt.edu/diabetes/vdc
The Vanderbilt Diabetes Center provides complete care for children and adults with diabetes under one roof
Joe C Davis, Chair in Biomedical Sciences
Alvin C Powers, Director Vanderbilt Diabetes Center

3293 Veterans Affairs Medical Center: Research Service
500 Foothill Drive
Salt Lake City, UT 84148
801-582-1565
Fax: 801-584-1289
www.va.gov
Diabetes and cancer research.
James Floyd, Director
Byron Bair, Director

3294 Warren Grant Magnuson Clinical Center
National Institute of Health
9000 Rockville Pike
Bethesda, MD 20892
301-496-4000
800-411-1222
Fax: 301-480-9793
TTY: 866-411-1010
e-mail: prpl@mail.cc.nih.gov
clinicalcenter.nih.gov
Established in 1953 as the research hospital of the National Institutes of Health. Designed so that patient care facilities are close to research laboratories so new findings of basic and clinical scientists can be quickly applied to the treatment of patients. Upon referral by physicians, patients are admitted to NIH clinical studies.
John Gallin, Director
David Henderson, Deputy Director for Clinical Care

3295 Washington University: Diabetes Research and Training Center
School of Medicine
660 S Euclid Avenue
Saint Louis, MO 63110
314-362-0558
Fax: 314-747-2692
e-mail: apermutt@wustl.edu
drtc.im.wustl.edu
DRTC investigators were involved in conducting 60 investigator-initiated diabetes-related clinical research protocols on the WU GCRC
Jean Schaffer MD, Professor of Medicine
Kristin E Mondy, Medicine/Infectious Diseases

Support Groups & Hotlines

3296 American Diabetes Association National Center
1701 N Beauregard Street
Alexandria, VA 22311
800-342-2383
Fax: 703-549-6995
e-mail: askada@diabetes.org
www.diabetes.org
To prevent and cure diabetes and to improve the lives of all people affected by diabetes.
John W Griffin Jr, Chair of the Board
Larry Hausner, CEO

3297 Diabetes Society
1165 Lincoln Avenue
San Jose, CA 95125
408-287-3785
Fax: 408-287-2701
e-mail: ckassouf@diabetessociety.org
www.diabetessociety.org
The Diabetes Society was organized in 1963 as the result of efforts by a group of mothers of children with diabetes. Today, the Diabetes Society offers its services to the estimated 140,000 people with diabetes in the Santa Clara Valley.
Greg Price, Board President
Carol Kassouf, CEO

3298 Juvenile Diabetes International Hotline
Juvenile Diabetes Research Foundation Int'l
26 Broadway
New York, NY 10004
800-533-2873
Fax: 212-785-9595
e-mail: info@jdrf.org
www.jdf.org
The leading charitable funder and advocate of type 1 (juvenile) diabetes research worldwide.
Robert Wood Johnson IV, Chairman
Jeffrey Brewer, President/CEO

3299 National Health Information Center
PO Box 1133
Washington, DC 20013
310-565-4167
800-336-4797
Fax: 301-984-4256
e-mail: info@nhic.org
www.health.gov/nhic
A health information referral service sponsored by the Office of Disease Prevention and Health Promotion. Puts health professionals and consumers who have health questions in touch with those organizations that are best able to provide answers.

Books

3300 101 Tips for Improving Your Blood Sugar
American Diabetes Association
1660 Duke Street
Alexandria, VA 22314-3447
800-232-3472
Fax: 703-549-6995
www.diabetes.org
Tips for 101 common situations and questions to reduce the risk of complications from blood sugar at the wrong level.
122 pages

3301 Balance Your Act: A Book for Adults with Diabetes
Pritchett & Hull
3440 Oakcliff Road
Atlanta, GA 30340-3079
800-774-1124
1993 96 pages Paperback
ISBN: 0-939838-14-1

3302 Buyer's Guide
American Diabetes Association
1660 Duke Street
Alexandria, VA 22314-3447
800-232-3472
Fax: 703-549-6995
www.diabetes.org
A catalog listing all manufacturers of insulin, syringes, pumps, test strips, monitors and more.

3303 Caring for the Diabetic Soul
American Diabetes Association
1660 Duke Street
Alexandria, VA 22314-3447
800-232-3472
Fax: 703-549-6995
www.diabetes.org
Restoring emotional balance for yourself and your family.
213 pages

3304 Clinical Practice Recommendations
American Diabetes Association
1660 Duke Street
Alexandria, VA 22314-3447
800-232-3472
Fax: 703-549-6995
www.diabetes.org

Features all current position and consensus statements of the American Diabetes Association.

3305 Complete Weight Loss Workbook
American Diabetes Association
1660 Duke Street
Alexandria, VA 22314-3447
800-232-3472
Fax: 703-549-6995
www.diabetes.org
A unique, brisk, practical workbook that offers a series of fresh, memorable tests, checklists, worksheets, mini-cases, calculation exercises, mental reminders, and other practical aids to losing weight and staying fit for good.
252 pages

3306 Computer Planned Menus for Health Professionals
American Diabetes Association
1660 Duke Street
Alexandria, VA 22314-3447
800-232-3472
Fax: 703-549-6995
www.diabetes.org
Input a patient's dietary prescription, food preferences, and budget, and the program produces individualized menus. Professional version includes license to distribute these customized menus.

3307 Control Diabetes the Easy Way
Random House Trade Books
400 Hahn Road
Westminster, MD 21157-4663
800-733-3000
Fax: 800-659-2436

ISBN: 0-679778-03-9

3308 Convenience Food Facts
American Diabetes Association
1660 Duke Street
Alexandria, VA 22314-3447
800-232-3472
Fax: 703-549-6995
www.diabetes.org
Helps to serve appetizing convenience foods low in sodium, cholesterol, and fat.
459 pages Softcover

3309 Cooking a la Heart
American Diabetes Association
1660 Duke Street
Alexandria, VA 22314-3447
800-232-3472
Fax: 703-549-6995
www.diabetes.org
Recipes that include a complete nutrient profile with diabetic exchanges.

3310 Diabetes & Pregnancy: What to Expect
American Diabetes Association
1660 Duke Street
Alexandria, VA 22314-3447
800-232-3472
Fax: 703-549-6995
www.diabetes.org
Information concerning an unborn baby's development, tests to expect, labor and delivery, birth control, and more.

3311 Diabetes A to Z
American Diabetes Association
1660 Duke Street
Alexandria, VA 22314-3447
800-232-3472
Fax: 703-549-6995
www.diabetes.org
Dictionary-style guidebook discussing basic terms and issues concerning diabetes. Third edition.
202 pages

3312 Diabetes Care Made Easy
Chronimed Publishing
PO Box 59032
Minneapolis, MN 55459-0032
612-513-6475
800-848-2793
Fax: 612-443-2806
Written and designed for both adults and for children with limited reading skills, this easy-to-read book explains how to exercise and

eat for better health, prevent foot problems, test blood sugar, cope with emotions, take insulin, and more. Also available in Spanish.
180 pages Paperback
ISBN: 1-885115-31-8

3313 Diabetes Education Goals
American Diabetes Association
1660 Duke Street
Alexandria, VA 22314-3447   800-232-3472
Fax: 703-549-6995
www.diabetes.org
Features advice on how to assess, plan, and evaluate patient education and counseling programs. Covers both short-term and in-depth goals. Focuses on the education process and assessing the unique needs of each patient.
64 pages Softcover

3314 Diabetes Low-Fat & No-Fat Meals in Minutes
John Wiley and Sons, Inc.
Customer Service-Consumer Accounts
Indianapolis, IN 46256   877-762-2974
Fax: 800-597-3299
e-mail: consumers@wiley.com
www.wiley.com
Includes more than 250 recipes, 60 days of diabetic menus, and 16 pages of full-color photographs. Each recipe features a complete nutrition analysis, including diabetic exchanges.
1998 352 pages
ISBN: 1-565610-84-9

3315 Diabetes Medical Nutrition Therapy
American Diabetes Association
1660 Duke Street
Alexandria, VA 22314-3447   800-232-3472
Fax: 703-549-6995
www.diabetes.org
A professional guide to management and nutrition education resources. Provides in-depth coverage of nutrition assessment, goal setting, intervention, and outcome evaluation. Information is provided on specific resources and case studies are cited for practical examples.
Softcover

3316 Diabetes Mellitus: A Practical Handbook
Bull Publishing Company
PO Box 1377
Boulder, CO 80306   800-676-2855
Fax: 303-545-6354
www.bullpub.com
This helpful and user friendly practical guide addresses the everyday concerns of all diabetics.
2002 Paperback
ISBN: 0-923521-72-0

3317 Diabetes Self-Management
RA Rapaport Publishing
150 W 22nd Street   212-989-0200
New York, NY 10011-2421   800-234-0923
Fax: 212-989-4786
e-mail: editor@diabetes-self-mgmt-com
Publishes practical, how to information, focusing on the day-to-day and long term aspects of diabetes in a positive and upbeat style. Gives subscribers up-to-date news, facts and advice to help them maintain their wellness and make informed decisions regarding their health.
Ingird Strauch, Executive
Richard A. Rapaport, Publisher

3318 Diabetes Sourcebook
Dawn D Matthews, author
Omnigraphics
615 Griswold   313-961-1340
Detroit, MI 48226-4105   800-234-1340
Fax: 800-875-1340
www.omnigraphics.com
This Sourcebook contains information for people seeking to understand the risk factors, complications, and management of the different types of diabetes. It includes information about testing.

diagnosis, medications, and other topics related to living with diabetes.
2003 622 pages
ISBN: 0-780806-29-8

3319 Diabetes Teaching Guide for People Who Use Insulin
Joslin Diabetes Center
1 Joslin Place   617-732-2400
Boston, MA 02215-5306   Fax: 617-732-2562
e-mail: diabetes@joslin.harvard.edu
www.joslin.org
Discusses the causes of diabetes, the role of diet and exercise, meal planning and complications. Also provide information on drawing blood, mixing and injecting insulin.

3320 Diabetes Youth Curriculum: A Toolbox for Educators
Chronimed Publishing
PO Box 59032   612-513-6475
Minneapolis, MN 55459-0032   800-848-2793
Fax: 612-443-2806
Program consisting of two volumes: the Curriculum and the Resource and Activities Guide (listed separately). Divided into sections dealing with general development concepts and specific guidelines for ages 6 to 8, 9 to 11, and 12 to 16.
136 pages Paperback
ISBN: 0-937721-49-2

3321 Diabetes: A Guide to Living Well
American Diabetes Association
7 Washington Square   518-218-1755
Albany, NY 12205   888-342-2383
Fax: 518-218-0114
e-mail: ADAorders@pbd.com
www.diabetes.org
Offers a guide to helping the person with diabetes design a program of individualized self-care and gain the willingness to follow it. Also tells how to deal with diet, exercise, stress, emotions, negative beliefs, and self-image.
242 pages Paperback
ISBN: 1-580402-09-7

3322 Diabetes: Your Complete Exercise Guide
Human Kinetics Publishers
PO Box 5076   217-351-1549
Champaign, IL 61825-5076   800-747-4457
Fax: 217-351-5076
Part of the Cooper Clinic and Research Institute Fitness Series providing exercise rehabilitation for persons with diabetes.
144 pages Paperback
ISBN: 0-873224-27-2

3323 Diabetes: Your Questions Answered
Paul Drury and Wendy Gatling, author
Elsevier
Book Customer Service Department
St. Louis, MO 63146   800-545-2522
Fax: 800-535-9935
e-mail: usbkinfo@elsevier.com
www.elsevier.com
This new volume in the popular Your Questions Answered series uses a question-and-answer format to provide easy access to hands-on guidance on the management of diabetes. Its succinct, practical coverage explores the latest evidence-based practice guilines and their interpretation. Case vignettes illustrate the clinical relevance of the material.
2004 380 pages Softcover
ISBN: 0-443073-89-9

3324 Diabetic Gourmet
Diabetes Self-Management Books
PO Box 10676
Des Moines, IA 50336-0676   800-664-9269

3325 Diabetic's Guide to Health and Fitness
Human Kinetics Publishers
PO Box 5076   217-351-1549
Champaign, IL 61825-5076   800-747-4457
Fax: 217-351-5076
272 pages Paperback
ISBN: 0-880113-47-2

3326   Direct and Indirect Costs of Diabetes in the US
American Diabetes Association
1660 Duke Street
Alexandria, VA 22314-3447   800-232-3472
                                      Fax: 703-549-6995
                                        www.diabetes.org
Examines the specific costs of diabetes, as well as all the costs of health care for people with diabetes and compares those costs with the total cost of health care for the US population without diabetes.
32 pages Softcover

3327   Dr. Bernstein's Diabetes Solution
Richard K Bernstein, MD, author
Little, Brown and Company
Publicity Department
New York, NY 10020   800-759-0190
                      e-mail: publicity@littlebrown.com
                        www.hachettebookgroupusa.com
A complete guide to achieving normal blood sugars with strong emphasis on diet and up-to-date information on products, insulins, and oral agents.
512 pages Hardcover
ISBN: 0-316099-06-6

3328   Easy & Elegant Entrees
American Diabetes Association
1660 Duke Street
Alexandria, VA 22314-3447   800-232-3472
                                      Fax: 703-549-6995
                                        www.diabetes.org
Recipes that are low in fat and calories.

3329   Exchanges for All Occasions
American Diabetes Association
1660 Duke Street
Alexandria, VA 22314-3447   800-232-3472
                                      Fax: 703-549-6995
                                        www.diabetes.org
Meal planning suggestions for traveling, entertaining, camping, dining out, and more.

3330   Family Cookbook: Volumes I-IV
American Diabetes Association
1660 Duke Street
Alexandria, VA 22314-3447   800-232-3472
                                      Fax: 703-549-6995
                                        www.diabetes.org
Unforgettable recipes for the whole family. Great for diabetics.

3331   Fitness Book: For People with Diabetes
American Diabetes Association
1660 Duke Street
Alexandria, VA 22314-3447   800-232-3472
                                      Fax: 703-549-6995
                                        www.diabetes.org
Advice on learning to exercise to lose weight, exercise safely, increase your competitive edge, get your mind and body ready to exercise, and more.
149 pages

3332   Great Starts & Fine Finishes
American Diabetes Association
1660 Duke Street
Alexandria, VA 22314-3447   800-232-3472
                                      Fax: 703-549-6995
                                        www.diabetes.org
Healthy select cookbook offering great meals in minutes.

3333   Healthy Eater's Guide to Family & Chain Restaurants
American Diabetes Association
1660 Duke Street
Alexandria, VA 22314-3447   800-232-3472
                                      Fax: 703-549-6995
                                        www.diabetes.org
Advice on safe choices from fast-food menus, complete with nutrition values and exchanges.

3334   Healthy Homestyle Cookbook
American Diabetes Association

1660 Duke Street
Alexandria, VA 22314-3447   800-232-3472
                                      Fax: 703-549-6995
                                        www.diabetes.org
Lay-flat binding for hands-free reference.
181 pages

3335   How to Cook for People with Diabetes
American Diabetes Association
1660 Duke Street
Alexandria, VA 22314-3447   800-232-3472
                                      Fax: 703-549-6995
                                        www.diabetes.org
One hundred and fifty recipes featuring unusual techniques.
205 pages

3336   If Your Child Has Diabetes: An Answer Book for Parents
Putnam Publishing Group
200 Madison Avenue   212-951-8400
New York, NY 10016-3903
Provides information and recommendations for parents of children with diabetes on subjects such as school, recreation, medical and life insurance and employment as well as general information about diabetes.

3337   Intensified Insulin Management for You
Chronimed Publishing
PO Box 59032   612-513-6475
Minneapolis, MN 55459-0032   800-848-2793
                                      Fax: 612-443-2806
Manual helping those with diabetes to understand and use an intensified insulin regimen under the guidance of their health care provider. A personalized program for advanced diabetes self-care that focuses on emotional and intellectual goals as well as on how diet and exercise fit into an intensified regimen.
85 pages Paperback
ISBN: 0-937721-84-0

3338   Intensive Diabetes Management
American Diabetes Association
1660 Duke Street
Alexandria, VA 22314-3447   800-232-3472
                                      Fax: 703-549-6995
                                        www.diabetes.org
Delivers practical advice on how to help your patients achieve better glucose control through intensified management.
128 pages Softcover

3339   Learning to Live Well with Diabetes
Chronimed Publishing
PO Box 59032   612-513-6475
Minneapolis, MN 55459-0032   800-848-2793
                                      Fax: 612-443-2806
Updated and revised edition reflects the latest medical advances, technologies, and research. In straight-forward language, it explains how to take charge of your diabetes and live an active, healthy life.
525 pages Paperback
ISBN: 0-937721-79-4

3340   Life with Diabetes: A Series of Teaching Outlines
American Diabetes Association
1660 Duke Street
Alexandria, VA 22314-3447   800-232-3472
                                      Fax: 703-549-6995
                                        www.diabetes.org
Presents a comprehensive curriculum for diabetes education. Each outline includes a statement of purpose, prerequisites for attending the session, materials needed for teaching the session, recommended teaching method, a content outline, instructor notes, an evaluation and documentation plan, and suggested readings related to each topic.

3341   Managing Type II Diabetes
Chronimed Publishing
PO Box 59032   612-513-6475
Minneapolis, MN 55459-0032   800-848-2793
                                      Fax: 612-443-2806
Revised and updated guide for people with Type II diabetes. Offers the latest medical advances and practical advice. Includes tips on

dealing with emotions, finding motivation to manage diabetes, preventing and treating complications, monitoring blood glucose, and more.
192 pages Paperback
ISBN: 1-885115-26-1

3342 Managing Your Gestational Diabetes
Chronimed Publishing
PO Box 59032   612-513-6475
Minneapolis, MN 55459-0032   800-848-2793
                                         Fax: 612-443-2806
Gives answers to questions on weight gain, injecting insulin, and preventing complications.
128 pages Paperback
ISBN: 1-565610-52-0

3343 Manual of Pediatric Nutrition
B.C Decker, Inc.
50 King Street E, Floor 2 PO Box620   905-522-7017
Ontario, Canada L8N 3K7,   800-568-7281
                                         Fax: 905-522-7839
                                         e-mail: info@bcdecker.com
                                         www.bcdecker.com
A comprehensive guide that provides an overview of nutritional care for both healthy and ill pediatric patients.
2005 500 pages
ISBN: 1-550093-08-8

3344 Maximizing the Role of Nutrition in Diabetes Management
American Diabetes Association
1660 Duke Street
Alexandria, VA 22314-3447   800-232-3472
                                         Fax: 703-549-6995
                                         www.diabetes.org
Integrates medical, nutritional, and behavioral sciences and recognizes the importance of each in total diabetes care.
64 pages Softcover

3345 Medical Management of Pregnancy Complicated by Diabetes
American Diabetes Association
1660 Duke Street
Alexandria, VA 22314-3447   800-232-3472
                                         Fax: 703-549-6995
                                         www.diabetes.org
Information on every aspect of pregnancy and diabetes, providing precise protocols for treatment. Techniques for managing blood glucose levels from the time of conception through every stage of pregnancy.
136 pages Softcover

3346 Medical Management of Type I Diabetes
American Diabetes Association
1660 Duke Street
Alexandria, VA 22314-3447   800-232-3472
                                         Fax: 703-549-6995
                                         www.diabetes.org
Instruction on all issues impacting patients with Type 1 diabetes, including: blood glucose regulation, nutrition, exercise, blood pressure, blood lipid levels, and other key elements.
176 pages Softcover

3347 Medical Management of Type II Diabetes
American Diabetes Association
1660 Duke Street
Alexandria, VA 22314-3447   800-232-3472
                                         Fax: 703-549-6995
                                         www.diabetes.org
Complete overview of Type II diabetes, including diagnosis and classification, pathogenesis, and prevention/treatment of complications.
112 pages Softcover

3348 Month of Meals Set of 5
American Diabetes Association
1660 Duke Street
Alexandria, VA 22314-3447   800-232-3472
                                         Fax: 703-549-6995
                                         www.diabetes.org

Each planner offers twenty-eight day's worth of tasty selections including a holiday planner, ethnic meals, fast foods, meat and potatoes, and vegetarian dishes. Available individually.
5 planners

3349 Outsmarting Diabetes
Richard S Beaser, author
John Wiley and Sons, Inc.
Customer Service-Consumer Accounts
Indianapolis, IN 46256   877-762-2974
                                         Fax: 800-597-3299
                                         e-mail: consumers@wiley.com
                                         www.wiley.com
Shows how intensive control can dramatically reduce the effects of insulin-dependent diabetes and the risk of long-term complications.
256 pages Paperback
ISBN: 0-471346-94-4

3350 Pumping Insulin
John Walsh PA, CDE and Ruth Roberts, MA, author
Torrey Pines Publishing
The Diabetes Mall   619-497-0900
San Diego, CA 92103   800-988-4772
                                         Fax: 619-497-0900
                                         www.diabetesnet.com
Features information for achieving excellent blood sugar control, correcting pump problems quickly, and lowering risks for complications.
322 pages Paperback

3351 Quick and Easy Meals and Menus
Diabetes Self-Management Books
PO Box 11066
Des Moines, IA 50380-0001   800-664-9269

3352 Quick and Healthy Recipes & Ideas
American Diabetes Association
1660 Duke Street
Alexandria, VA 22314-3447   800-232-3472
                                         Fax: 703-549-6995
                                         www.diabetes.org
More than 190 recipes with complete nutrition information for each.

3353 Quick and Hearty Main Dishes
American Diabetes Association
1660 Duke Street
Alexandria, VA 22314-3447   800-232-3472
                                         Fax: 703-549-6995
                                         www.diabetes.org
Offers recipes for main courses.

3354 Raising a Child with Diabetes: A Guide for Parents
American Diabetes Association
1660 Duke Street
Alexandria, VA 22314-3447   800-232-3472
                                         Fax: 703-549-6995
                                         www.diabetes.org
You'll learn how to help your child adjust to insulin to allow for favorite foods, have a busy schedule and still feel healthy and strong, negotiate the twists and turns of being different, and much more.

3355 Real Life Parenting of Kids with Diabetes
Virginia Nasmyth Loy, author
McGraw-Hill Companies
Returns Department
Dubuque, IA 52002   877-833-5524
                                         Fax: 609-308-4484
                                         e-mail: pbg.ecommerce_custserv@mcgraw-hill.com
                                         www.mcgraw-hill.com
Virginia Loy had engineered successful management of her two sons' diabetes for 12 years at the time of publication. She is offering her organized, experienced, and practical advice to parents, for helping children to cope with and manage their diabetes from elementary school through college.
2001 188 pages Paperback
ISBN: 1-580400-83-3

3356   Resource and Activities Guide
Chronimed Publishing
PO Box 59032   612-513-6475
Minneapolis, MN 55459-0032   800-848-2793
                                           Fax: 612-443-2806
For use with the Diabetes Youth Curriculum. Contains 300 educational activities that correspond with the text in the Curriculum and can easily be removed for photocopying.
260 pages Loose Leaf
ISBN: 0-937721-50-6

3357   Right from the Start
American Diabetes Association
1660 Duke Street
Alexandria, VA 22314-3447   800-232-3472
                                           Fax: 703-549-6995
                                           www.diabetes.org
Addresses issues such as: learning to take charge, coping, changing one's eating habits, getting fit, self-testing, family issues, preventive care, finances, as well as resources to turn to for further information and support. Available for both Type 1 and Type 2.
Pkg. of 25

3358   Savory Soups and Salads
American Diabetes Association
1660 Duke Street
Alexandria, VA 22314-3447   800-232-3472
                                           Fax: 703-549-6995
                                           www.diabetes.org
Offers exciting recipes for quick and healthy side dishes.

3359   Simple and Tasty Side Dishes
American Diabetes Association
1660 Duke Street
Alexandria, VA 22314-3447   800-232-3472
                                           Fax: 703-549-6995
                                           www.diabetes.org
Healthy recipes for the diabetic.

3360   Special Celebrations and Parties Cookbook
American Diabetes Association
1660 Duke Street
Alexandria, VA 22314-3447   800-232-3472
                                           Fax: 703-549-6995
                                           www.diabetes.org
Offers a list of more than 150 holiday recipes.

3361   Take-Charge Guide to Type I Diabetes
American Diabetes Association
1660 Duke Street
Alexandria, VA 22314-3447   800-232-3472
                                           Fax: 703-549-6995
                                           www.diabetes.org
Offers answers to the most important questions regarding Type 1 diabetes.

3362   Therapy for Diabetes Mellitus and Related Disorders
American Diabetes Association
1660 Duke Street
Alexandria, VA 22314-3447   800-232-3472
                                           Fax: 703-549-6995
                                           www.diabetes.org
Guides through the treatment of specific problems of persons with diabetes. Represents the views and experience of leading clinicians in a concise, practical approach to treatment.
384 pages

3363   Type 2 Diabetes: Your Healthy Living Guide
American Diabetes Association
1660 Duke Street
Alexandria, VA 22314-3447   800-232-3472
                                           Fax: 703-549-6995
                                           www.diabetes.org
A thorough guide to staying healthy with Type 2. Includes everything from choosing a health care team and eating and exercising properly to self-monitoring, insulin, dealing with complications, and keep mentally fit.
180 pages

3364   Using Insulin
Torrey Pines Press

The Diabetes Mall   619-497-0900
San Diego, CA 92103   800-988-4772
                                           Fax: 619-497-0900
                                           www.diabetesnet.com
How to take charge of your blood sugars in diabetes. Information on feeling better, improving your health, and achieving peace of mind.
316 pages Paperback

3365   Voice of the Diabetic
811 Chern Street   573-875-8911
Columbia, MO 65201   e-mail: epc@roudley.com
                                           www.nfb.org
Personal stories and practical guidelines by blind diabetics and medical professionals, medical news, resource column and a recipe corner.

3366   Weight Management for Type II Diabetes
John Wiley and Sons, Inc.
Customer Service-Consumer Accounts
Indianapolis, IN 46256   877-762-2974
                                           Fax: 800-597-3299
                                    e-mail: consumers@wiley.com
                                           www.wiley.com
An interactive, personalized guide that helps you manage your weight and your diabetes by making gradual lifestyle changes. Details how to set reasonable goals, keep pace with an exercise program, design your own meal plan, manage stress, and more.
1997 224 pages Paperback
ISBN: 0-471347-50-7

3367   When Diabetes Complicates Your Life
Chronimed Publishing
PO Box 59032   612-513-6475
Minneapolis, MN 55459-0032   800-848-2793
                                           Fax: 612-443-2806
Directly addresses the subject of diabetic complications. This revised edition includes chapters on nerves and circulation, kidneys, and eyes. Enhancements to the new edition include a chapter on vitamins, herbs, and supplements, and reference to the latest research.
Feb 1998 208 pages Paperback
ISBN: 1-565611-27-6

Children's Books

3368   Diabetes
Franklin Watts Grolier
90 Old Sherman Turnpike   203-797-3500
Danbury, CT 06816-0001   800-621-1115
                                           Fax: 203-797-3197
                                           www.grolier.com
Looks at the differences between juvenile and adult-onset diabetes, discusses the history of the disease, causes, complications and treatments.
128 pages Grades 7-12
ISBN: 0-531108-82-1

3369   Dinosaur Tamer
American Diabetes Association
1660 Duke Street
Alexandria, VA 22314-3447   800-232-3472
                                           Fax: 703-549-6995
                                           www.diabetes.org
Twenty-five fictional stories that will entertain, enlighten, and ease your child's frustrations about having diabetes. Each tale evaporates the fear of insulin shots, blood tests, going to diabetes camp, and more.
Ages 8-12

3370   Even Little Kids Get Diabetes
Connie Pirner, author
Albert Whitman & Company
6340 Oakton Street   847-581-0033
Morton Grove, IL 60053-2723   800-255-7675
                                           Fax: 847-581-0039
                                    e-mail: mail@awhitmanco.com
                                           www.albertwhitman.com

A preschooler tells how it was discovered when she was only two, that she has this common disease and describes her daily treatment and the precautions her family must observe.
24 pages Hardcover
ISBN: 0-807521-58-8
Pat McPartland, Sales
Joe Campbell, Customer Service

3371 Everyone Likes to Eat
John Wiley and Sons, Inc.
Customer Service-Consumer Accounts
Indianapolis, IN 46256   877-762-2974
                              Fax: 800-597-3299
                    e-mail: consumers@wiley.com
                              www.wiley.com
Revised and up-to-date second edition. How children can eat most of the foods they enjoy and still take care of their diabetes. Intended for elementary-school-age children, this guide is filled with activities, puzzles, and problem-solving exercises.
128 pages Paperback
ISBN: 0-471346-82-1

3372 Grilled Cheese
American Diabetes Association
1660 Duke Street
Alexandria, VA 22314-3447   800-232-3472
                              Fax: 703-549-6995
                              www.diabetes.org
Story designed to ease children's fears and frustrations of having diabetes.

3373 Kiss the Candy Days Good-bye
Delacorte Press
1540 Broadway   212-354-6500
New York, NY 10036-4039
This book focuses on Jimmy who is surprised to learn he has diabetes after seeming so healthy and fit. The story contains information on symptoms and the dangers of untreated diabetes.
Grades 6-8

3374 Living with Diabetes
Franklin Watts Grolier
90 Old Sherman Turnpike   203-797-3500
Danbury, CT 06816-0001   800-621-1115
                              Fax: 203-797-3197
                              www.grolier.com
Shows how persons with diabetes can control their illness and lead productive lives.
32 pages Grades 5-7
ISBN: 0-531108-44-9

3375 Shira: A Legacy of Courage
Doubleday
666 5th Avenue   212-354-6500
New York, NY 10103-0001
A biographical account of Shira Putter's fight with a rare form of diabetes. Using the victim's diary, this book is both powerful and poignant, as well as an educational resource for all people struggling with diabetes.
Grades 4-9

3376 Sun, the Rain and the Insulin
American Diabetes Association
1660 Duke Street
Alexandria, VA 22314-3447   800-232-3472
                              Fax: 703-549-6995
                              www.diabetes.org
Author chronicles a week at a summer diabetes camp, using her expertise and experience to capture the journey and the fight to cope that all people go through when diabetes hits the family.

Magazines

3377 Countdown
Juvenile Diabetes Foundation International
432 Park Avenue S   212-889-7575
New York, NY 10016-8013   Fax: 212-725-7259
Offers the latest news and information in diabetes research and treatment to everyone from an international arena of diabetes in-

vestigators to parents of small children with diabetes, from physicians to school teachers, from pharmacists to corporate executives.
Sandy Dylak, Editor

3378 Diabetes
American Diabetes Association
1660 Duke Street
Alexandria, VA 22314-3447   800-232-3472
                              Fax: 703-549-6995
                              www.diabetes.org
A peer-reviewed journal focusing on laboratory research.
Monthly

3379 Diabetes Care
American Diabetes Association
1660 Duke Street
Alexandria, VA 22314-3447   800-232-3472
                              Fax: 703-549-6995
                              www.diabetes.org
A peer-reviewed journal emphasizing reviews, commentaries and original research on topics of interest to clinicians.
Monthly

3380 Diabetes Forecast
American Diabetes Association
1660 Duke Street
Alexandria, VA 22314-3447   800-232-3472
                              Fax: 703-549-6995
                              www.diabetes.org
The monthly lifestyle magazine for people with diabetes, featuring complete, in-depth coverage of all aspects of living with diabetes.
Monthly

3381 Diabetes Spectrum: From Research to Practice
American Diabetes Association
1701 N Beauregard Street
Alexandria, VA 22311   800-232-3472
                              Fax: 703-549-6995
                              www.diabetes.org
A journal translating research into practice and focusing on diabetes education and counseling.
Quarterly

3382 Joslin Magazine
Joslin Diabetes Center
1 Joslin Place   617-732-2400
Boston, MA 02215-5306   Fax: 617-732-2562
                    e-mail: diabetes@joslin.harvard.edu
                              www.joslin.org

3383 Voice of the Diabetic
Ed Bryant, author
National Federation of the Blind
1800 Johnson Street   410-659-9314
Baltimore, MD 21230-4998   Fax: 410-685-5653
                    e-mail: subscribe@diabetes.nfb.org
                              www.nfb.org
The leading publication in the diabetes field. Each issue addresses the problems and concerns of diabetes, with a special emphasis for those who have lost vision due to diabetes. Available in print and on cassette.
28 pages Quarterly
Eileen Ley, Director of Publishing
Elizabeth Lunt, Editor

Newsletters

3384 Clinical Diabetes
American Diabetes Association
1660 Duke Street
Alexandria, VA 22314-3447   800-232-3472
                              Fax: 703-549-6995
                              www.diabetes.org
A bimonthly newsletter providing practical treatment information for primary care physicians.
BiMonthly

3385 Diabetes Advisor
American Diabetes Association
1701 N Beauregard Street   703-549-1500
Alexandria, VA 22311   800-232-3472
                                            Fax: 703-836-7439
                                  e-mail: askada@diabetes.org
                                            www.diabetes.org
Offers informative articles and research in the area of diabetes for
professionals and patients. Offers facts and research on diagnosis,
symptoms, technology and the newest devices for persons with di-
abetes, as well as referral and hotline numbers.
Bi-Monthly
John G Graham IV, CEO

3386 Diabetes Dateline
National Diabetes Information Clearinghouse
1 Information Way   301-654-3327
Bethesda, MD 20205   800-860-8747
                                            Fax: 301-907-8906
                              e-mail: ndic@info.niddck.nih.gov
                                            www.niddk.nih.gov
BiAnnually

3387 Diabetes Educator
American Association of Diabetes Educators
444 N Michigan Avenue   312-644-2233
Chicago, IL 60611-3959   Fax: 312-644-4411
Offers information to health professionals working with persons
with diabetes.
James J Balija, Executive Director

3388 Kid's Corner
American Diabetes Association
1660 Duke Street
Alexandria, VA 22314-3447   800-232-3472
                                            Fax: 703-549-6995
                                            www.diabetes.org
A mini-magazine for kids that offers word searches, puzzles and
jokes - plus an encouraging story in each issue about kids with diabetes.
8 pages Quarterly

Pamphlets

3389 Dental Tips for Diabetics
National Diabetes Information Clearinghouse
1 Information Way   301-654-3327
Bethesda, MD 20892-0001   800-860-8747
                                            Fax: 301-907-8906
                              e-mail: ndic@info.niddk.nih.gov
                                            www.niddk.nih.gov
Discusses the relationship between diabetes and periodontal disease. Describes the symptoms of periodontal problems and preventive measures.

3390 Diabetes Dateline
National Diabetes Information Clearinghouse
1 Information Way   301-654-3327
Bethesda, MD 20892-0001   Fax: 301-907-8906
                                       e-mail: ndic@aerie.com
This bulletin features news about current issues in diabetes research and control, special events, patient and professional meeting, and new publications available from NDIC and other
organizations.
Quarterly

3391 Diabetes and Brief Illness
Chronimed Publishing
PO Box 59032   612-513-6475
Minneapolis, MN 55459-0032   800-848-2793
                                            Fax: 612-443-2806
This booklet gives self-care instructions and eating suggestions to
prevent development of ketoacidosis during brief illness that dis-
rupts normal eating.
12 pages Pack of 10

3392 Diabetes and Exercise
Chronimed Publishing
PO Box 59032   612-513-6475
Minneapolis, MN 55459-0032   800-848-2793
                                            Fax: 612-443-2806
Exercise and weight loss tips and precautions for those with both
insulin and non-insulin-dependent diabetes.
36 pages Pack of 10

3393 Diabetes in Pregnancy
March of Dimes
233 Park Avenue South   212-353-8353
New York, NY 10003   Fax: 212-254-3518
                              e-mail: NY639@marchofdimes.com
                                         www.marchofdimes.com
Fact Sheets: one or two page review written for the general public.

3394 Diabetic Foot Care
American Diabetes Association
1660 Duke Street
Alexandria, VA 22314-3447   800-232-3472
                                            Fax: 703-549-6995
                                            www.diabetes.org
Booklet discussing early detection and prompt treatment of diabetic foot problems.
12 pages

3395 Gestational Diabetes: What To Expect
American Diabetes Association
7 Washington Square   518-218-1755
Albany, NY 12205   888-342-2383
                                            Fax: 518-218-0114
                                 e-mail: ADAorders@pbd.com
                                            www.diabetes.org
A complete comprehensive guide for women with gestational diabetes. Explains the stages in your baby's development, the types of
prenatal testing you may recieve, and what to expect during labor,
delivery, and beyond.
100 pages
ISBN: 1-580402-33-X

3396 Healthy Eating
Chronimed Publishing
PO Box 59032   612-513-6475
Minneapolis, MN 55459-0032   800-848-2793
                                            Fax: 612-443-2806
Offers simple guidelines for choosing healthful foods, lowering
fat intake, and timing meals and snacks. Available in Spanish.
Pack of 10

3397 Healthy Food Choices
American Diabetes Association
1660 Duke Street
Alexandria, VA 22314-3447   800-232-3472
                                            Fax: 703-549-6995
                                            www.diabetes.org
Pamphlet containing the basics of good nutrition.

3398 Hypoglycemia The Other Sugar Disease
Anita Flegg, author
Book Coach Press
3-390 MacKay Street   613-746-3334
Ontario, Canada K1M 2C4,   e-mail: info@bookcoachpress.com
                                         www.bookcoachpress.com
This book is filled with dozens of real-life practical tips and will
give you the tools to feel better and take control of your life.

3399 Insulin-Dependent Diabetes
National Diabetes Information Clearinghouse
1 Information Way   301-654-3327
Bethesda, MD 20892-0001   Fax: 301-654-3327
                                       e-mail: ndic@aerie.com
Explains diabetes and how it develops and describes the differences between the two major forms of diabetes, insulin-dependent
and noninsulin-dependent.

3400 Low Blood Sugar
Chronimed Publishing
PO Box 59032   612-513-6475
Minneapolis, MN 55459-0032   800-848-2793
                                            Fax: 612-443-2806
Pack of 10

3401 Noninsulin-Dependent Diabetes
National Diabetes Information Clearinghouse
1 Information Way   301-654-3327
Bethesda, MD 20892-0001   Fax: 301-907-8906
                                      e-mail: ndic@aerie.com
Describes the symptoms and diagnosis of noninsulin-dependent diabetes; diabetes management, including diet, oral drugs, and insulin; glucose monitoring; and complications.
1992 35 pages

3402 Recognizing and Treating Low Blood Sugar (Hypoglycemia)
Chronimed Publishing
PO Box 59032   612-513-6475
Minneapolis, MN 55459-0032   800-848-2793
                                      Fax: 612-443-2806
The causes, symptoms, and treatment of low blood sugar are clearly presented in this booklet, including guidelines for using glucagon.
12 pages Pack of 10

3403 Taking Care of Gestational Diabetes
International Diabetes Center at Park Nicollet
3800 Park Nicollet Boulevard   952-993-3874
Minneapolis, MN 55416-2699   888-637-2675
                                      Fax: 952-993-0501
                                      e-mail: idccustsvc@parknicollet.com
                                      www.idcpublishing.com
Available in Spanish. Empowering women to make healthy choices for a healthy pregnancy, a healthy baby, and a healthy lifestyle. This book covers food planning, testing, targets, medications and more.
242 pages

3404 Understanding Gestational Diabetes
National Diabetes Information Clearinghouse
1 Information Way   301-654-3327
Bethesda, MD 20892-0001   Fax: 301-907-8906
                                      e-mail: ndic@aerie.com
A guide for women who develop diabetes during pregnancy. It discusses symptoms and diagnosis of gestational diabetes, risk factors, tests during pregnancy and daily management including the use of insulin and blood gluclose monitoring.
44 pages

Audio & Video

3405 ADA Clinical Education Series on CD-Rom
American Diabetes Association
1660 Duke Street
Alexandria, VA 22314-3447   800-232-3472
                                      Fax: 703-549-6995
                                      www.diabetes.org
Features complete texts of Medical Management of Type 1 Diabetes, Medical Management of Type 2 Diabetes, Therapy for Diabetes Mellitus and Related Disorders, 2nd Ed., and Medical Management of Pregnancy Complicated by Diabetes, 2nd Ed.
CD-Rom

3406 Black Experience
American Diabetes Association
300 Research Parkway   203-639-0385
Meriden, CT 06450-7137   800-342-2383
                                      Fax: 203-639-0292
                                      www.diabetes.org/
Designed to increase awareness of diabetes in the black community.
L Butcher, District Director

3407 Diabetes & Exercise Video
American Diabetes Association
1660 Duke Street
Alexandria, VA 22314-3447   800-232-3472
                                      Fax: 703-549-6995
                                      www.diabetes.org
A video offering information on how to maintain good health and exercise in controlling diabetes.

3408 Label Reading and Shopping
American Diabetes Association/Conn. Affiliate

300 Research Parkway   203-639-0385
Meriden, CT 06450-7137   800-842-6323
                                      Fax: 203-639-0292
                                      www.diabetes.org/
Provides practical information on how to shop and what to look for on labels.
Videotape

3409 Living Well with Diabetes
American Diabetes Association/Conn. Affiliate
300 Research Parkway   203-639-0385
Meriden, CT 06450-7137   800-842-6323
                                      Fax: 203-639-0292
                                      www.diabetes.org/
Presents two patient role models who are successfully following a treatment plan for noninsulin dependent diabetes.
Videotape

3410 On Top of My Game: Living with Diabetes
American Diabetes Association/Conn. Affiliate
300 Research Parkway   203-639-0385
Meriden, CT 06450-7137   800-842-6323
                                      Fax: 203-639-0292
                                      www.diabetes.org/
Six patients and their families share their day-to-day frustrations and successes in managing diabetes.
Videotape

3411 Physicians Guide to Type I Diabetes
American Diabetes Association/Conn. Affiliate
300 Research Parkway   203-639-0385
Meriden, CT 06450-7137   800-842-6323
                                      Fax: 203-639-0292
                                      www.diabetes.org/
Principles of good care in the diagnosis and management of Type I.
Videotape

3412 Survival Skills for Diabetic Children
Ajn Company
555 W 57th Street   212-582-8820
New York, NY 10019-2961   800-226-6256
                                      Fax: 212-586-5462
How to provide insulin-dependent children with education, supervision, and support.
1988 28 minutes

3413 Understanding Diabetes: A User's Guide to Novolin
American Diabetes Association/Conn. Affiliate
300 Research Parkway   203-639-0385
Meriden, CT 06450   800-842-6323
                                      Fax: 203-639-0292
                                      www.diabetes.org/
Basic information about diabetes and the role insulin plays in blood glucose control.
Videotape

Web Sites

3414 American Association of Diabetes Educators
                                      www.aabenet.org
The mission is to enhance the competence of health professionals who teach persons with diabetes, advance the specialty practice of diabetes education, and to improve the quality of diabetes education and care for all those affected by diabetes.

3415 American Diabetes Association
                                      www.diabetes.org
Offers a network of 52 affiliates with over 55,000 volunteers, including a professional membership of more than 10,000 physicians, social workers, nutritionists, educators and nurses.

3416 Diabetes Dictionary
                                      www.niddk.nih.gov
Provides research funding and support for basic and clinical research in the areas of type 1 and type 2 diabetes and other metabolic disprders.

3417 Diabetes Exercise and Sports Association
                                      www.diabetes-exercise.org

Exists to enhance the quality of life for people with diabetes through exercise and physical fitness.

3418 Healing Well

www.healingwell.com

An online health resource guide to medical news, chat, information and articles, newsgroups and message boards, books, disease-related web sites, medical directories, and more for patients, friends, and family coping with disabling diseases, disorders, or chronic illnesses.

3419 Health Finder

www.healthfinder.gov

Searchable, carefully developed web site offering information on over 1000 topics. Developed by the US Department of Health and Human Services, the site can be used in both English and Spanish.

3420 Healthlink USA

www.healthlinkusa.com

Health information concerning treatment, cures, prevention, diagnosis, risk factors, research, support groups, email lists, personal stories and much more. Updated regularly.

3421 Helios Health

www.helioshealth.com

Online resource for your health information. Detailed information about specific health topics, access to expert advice from our Medical Advisory Board, and up-to-date health news.

3422 MedicineNet

www.medicinenet.com

An online resource for consumers providing easy-to-read, authoritative medical and health information.

3423 Medscape

www.medscape.com

Medscape offers specialists, primary care physicians, and other health professionals the Web's most robust and integrated medical information and educational tools.

3424 National Diabetes Information Clearinghous e

www.niddk.nih.gov/health/diabetes/ndic

Offers various materials, resources, books, pamphlets and more for persons and families in the area of diabetes.

3425 WebMD

www.webmd.com

Information on diabetes, including articles and resources.

Description

3426 Down Syndrome

Down syndrome is a collection of inherited abnormalities caused by an extra chromosome. Instead of having the normal number of chromosomes (46), children with Down syndrome have an extra chromosome 21. (Because there are three copies of chromosome 21 instead of the normal two, Down syndrome is often called trisomy 21). This chromosomal abnormality results in altered growth and development. Approximately 4,000 children are born with Down syndrome every year in the United States. The overall incidence is about 1 in every 700 live births, but there is a marked variability depending on maternal age. In the early childbearing years, the incidence is about 1/2000 live births; for mothers over 40, it rises to at least 1/100 if not more frequent with advancing age.

Down syndrome is associated with a wide variety of clinical signs, although most individuals do not possess all of them. Common findings include decreased muscle tone, slanting eyes with folds of skin in the inside corners, white spots appearing in the irises of the eyes, and single creases across the palms of one or both hands. Physically, children with Down syndrome have broad feet with short toes, short ears and necks, small heads and small oral cavities. Mental development in the child with Down syndrome is impaired; the mean IQ is approximately 50. Hearing and speech abilities may also be hampered. However, many children with Down syndrome can reach surprisingly high levels of achievement. Congenital heart disease is found in nearly half of patients, and there is an increased susceptibility to acute leukemia. Today, most patients survive well into adulthood, although problems such as Alzheimer's Disease and psychiatric illness may increase with age.

It is essential that parents enroll their children with Down syndrome in an infant development program. These programs advise parents on how to help a child with Down syndrome in language, cognitive, social and motor skills.

National Agencies & Associations

3427 ARC The ARC of the United States
The ARC of the United States
1660 L Street NW   301-565-3842
Washington, DC 20036   800-433-5255
Fax: 301-565-3843
e-mail: info@thearc.org
www.thearc.org
Works to include all children and adults with cognitive intellectual and developmental disabilities in every community.
Mohan Mehra, President
Nancy Webster, Vice President

3428 Aleh Foundation Aleh Institutions USA
Aleh Institutions USA
5317 13th Avenue   718-851-4596
Brooklyn, NY 11219   800-317-2534
Fax: 718-851-4597
e-mail: shlomo@alehfoundation.com
www.alehfoundation.org

Founded in 1983, the Aleh Rehabilitation Center has served as a residential facility to close to 200 children with multiple, physical and mental disabilities. These children and their families benefit from a wide range of services in a caring, supportive atmosphere.
Rabbi Shlomo Braun, Founder & Director

3429 Canadian Down Syndrome Society
5005 Dalhousie Drive NW   403-270-8500
Calgary Alberta, T3N-5R8   800-883-5608
Fax: 403-270-8291
e-mail: info@cdss.ca
www.cdss.ca
Resource linking parents and professionals through advocacy education and providing information.
Krista J Flint, Executive Director

3430 National Association for Down Syndrome
PO Box 206   630-325-9112
Wilmette, IL 60091   e-mail: info@nads.org
www.nads.org
A non-for-profit organization founded in Chicago in 1961 by parents of children with Down syndrome who felt a need to create a better environment and bring about understanding and acceptance of people with Down syndrome.
Jackie Rotondi, President
Diane Urhausen, Executive Director

3431 National Dissemination Center for Children with Disabilities
1825 Connecticut Avenue NW   202-884-8200
Washington, DC 20009   800-695-0285
Fax: 202-884-8441
TTY: 202-884-8200
e-mail: nichcy@aed.org
www.nichcy.org
Publishes free, fact filled newsletters. Arranges workshops. Advises parents on the laws entitling children with disabilities to special education and other services.
Dr Suzanne Ripley, Contact

3432 National Down Syndrome Congress
1370 Center Drive   770-604-9500
Atlanta, GA 30338   800-232-6372
Fax: 770-604-9898
e-mail: info@ndsccenter.org
www.NDSCcenter.org
The mission of the NDSC is to provide information, advocacy, and support concerning all aspects of life for individuals with Down Syndrome.
Brooks Robertson, President
Sue Joe, Resources Specialist

3433 National Down Syndrome Society
666 Broadway   212-460-9330
New York, NY 10012   800-221-4602
Fax: 212-979-2873
e-mail: info@ndss.org
www.ndss.org
NDSS supports researchers seeking the causes of and answers to many of the medical genetic behavioral and learning problems associated with Down syndrome. Also sponsors symposia and conferences for parents and professionals provides advocacy.
Jon Colman, President
Betsy Goodwin, Founder

3434 National Early Childhood Technical Assistance System
University of North Carolina, Chapel Hill
Campus Box 8040 UNC-CH   919-962-2001
Chapel Hill, NC 27599-0001   Fax: 919-966-7463
e-mail: nectac@unc.edu
www.nectac.org
Assists states and other entities in developing comprehensive services for children with special needs through the age of eight and their families.
Lynne Kahn, Director & Principal Investigator
Joan Danaher, Associate Director Information Resources

State Agencies & Associations

California

3435 Down Syndrome Association of Los Angeles
16461 Sherman Way
Van Nuys, CA 91406
818-786-0001
Fax: 818-786-0004
e-mail: info@dsala.org
www.dsala.org
Offers information on Down syndrome, counseling, resources, facts, laws and other forms of information.
Gail Williamson, Executive Director
Sandra Baker, Office Administrator/Spanish Coordinator

Colorado

3436 Mile High Down Syndrome Association
2121 S Oneida Street
Denver, CO 80224
303-797-1699
Fax: 303-756-6144
e-mail: info@mhdsa.org
www.mhdsa.org

Mac Macsovits, Executive Director
Melissa Davis, Volunteer Coordinator

Connecticut

3437 Connecticut Down Syndrome Congress
263 Farmington Avenue
Farmington, CT 06030-0485
205-351-1157
888-486-8537
e-mail: manager@ctdownsyndrome.org
www.ctdownsyndrome.org
Sheryl Knapp, Secretary
Walter Glomb, President

Florida

3438 Gold Coast Down Syndrome Organization
2255 Glades Road
Boca Raton, FL 33431
561-912-1231
Fax: 561-912-1232
e-mail: gcdso@bellsouth.net
www.goldcoastdownsyndrome.org
Gold Coast Down syndrome Organization is a private nonprofit corporation dedicated to making the future brighter for people with Down syndrome in Palm Beach County, Florida.
Sue Killan, President
Tina Trujillo, Secretary

3439 Goodwill Industries-Suncoast
Goodwill Industries-Suncoast
10596 Gandy Boulevard
St. Petersburg, FL 33702
727-523-1512
888-279-1988
Fax: 727-577-2749
e-mail: gw.marketing@goodwill-suncoast.rog
www.goodwill-suncoast.org
A nonprofit community based organization whose purpose is to improve the quality of life for people who are disabled, disadvantaged and/or aged. This mission is accomplished through a staff of over 1,200 employees providing independent living skills, affordable housing, career assessment and planning, job skills, training, placement, and job retention assistance with useful employment. Annually, Goodwill Industries-Suncoast serves over 30,000 people in Citrus, Hernando, Levy, Marion and more.
Martin W Gladysz, Chair
R Lee Waits, President/CEO

Georgia

3440 Down Syndrome Association of Atlanta
2221 Peachtree Rd
Atlanta, GA 30309
404-320-3233
Fax: 404-228-7475
e-mail: contactus@AtlantaDSAA.org
www.dsaatl.org

Hawaii

3441 Hawaii Down Syndrome Congress
419 Keoniana Street
Honolulu, HI 96815
808-949-1999
e-mail: Conkay@AOL.com
www.downscity.com

Constance K Smith, President

Indiana

3442 Indiana Down Syndrome Foundation
2625 N. Meridian Street #49
Indianapolis, IN 46208
317-925-7617
888-989-9255
Fax: 317-925-7619
e-mail: info@dsindiana.org
www.indianadsf.org

Lisa Tokarz-Guiterre, Executive Director
Jeff Huffman, President

Massachusetts

3443 Massachusetts Down Syndrome Congress
20 Burlington Mall Road
Melrose, MA 02176
781-221-0024
800-664-MDSC
Fax: 781-221-0011
e-mail: mdsc@mdsc.org
www.mdsc.org
Maureen Gallagher, Executive Director
Sarah Cullen, Outreach Coordinator

Minnesota

3444 Down Syndrome Association of Minnesota
656 Transfer Road
St Paul, MN 55114
651-603-0720
800-511-3696
Fax: 651-603-0726
e-mail: dsamn@dsamn.org
www.dsamn.org
A non-profit organization dedicated to ensuring that all individuals with Down syndrome and their families receive the support necessary to participate in, contribute to and achieve the fulfillment of life in their community.
Craig Parker, President
Kathleen Forney, Executive Director

New York

3445 Association for Children with Down Syndrome
4 Fern Place
Plainview, NY 11803
516-933-4700
Fax: 516-933-9524
e-mail: msmith@acds.org
www.acds.org
Nonprofit educational program that combines national information and research dissemination with direct services at the local level. Services include early intervention, pre-school, recreation programs and residential homes.
Michael M Smith, Executive Director
Cecilia Barry, Principal

Ohio

3446 Down Syndrome Association of Greater Cincinnati
644 Linn Street
Cincinnati, OH 45203-1734
513-761-5400
Fax: 513-761-5401
e-mail: dsagc@dsagc.com
www.dsagc.com
The mission of the Down Syndrome Association of Greater Cincinnati is to provide information resources and support to individuals with Down syndrome, their families, and their communities.
Janet Gora, Executive Director
Nora Lindsay Quinn, Event Coordinator

Tennessee

3447 Down Syndrome Association of Middle Tennessee
111 N Wilson Boulevard   615-386-9002
Nashville, TN 37205-2411   Fax: 615-386-9754
                                  e-mail: dsamt@bellsouth.net
                                               www.dsamt.org
A nonprofit organization of families whose mission is to enhance
the quality of life for all individuals with Down Syndrome by providing information and support to families professionals and the
community.
Sheila Moore, Executive Director
Erin Kice, Program Coordinator

Texas

3448 Down Syndrome Guild of Dallas
701 N Central Expressway   214-267-1374
Richardson, TX 75080-1174   Fax: 972-234-2510
                                www.downsyndromedallas.org

Kelly Drablos, President
Tamara White, Secretary

3449 Texas Association on Mental Retardation
TAMR Headquarters   512-349-7470
Austin, TX 78755   Fax: 512-349-2117
                              e-mail: pat.holder@tamr-web.com
                                            www.tamr-web.com
An organization made up of professionals, parents, consumers and
advocates. Our goal is to create an accessible system of services
and resources which support personal choice and promotes lives of
dignity and self-determination.
Pat Holder

Virginia

3450 Down Syndrome Association of Hampton Roads
The Endependence Center   757-466-3696
Norfolk, VA 23502   e-mail: DSAHR@verizon.net
                                               www.dsahr.org
The Down Syndrome Association of Hampton Roads is a
not-for-profit organization serving the needs of individuals with
Down Syndrome and their families. The association is supported
by a board of directors, an advisory board and dedicated
volunteers.
Andrea Anderson, President
Florence Thacker, Secretary

Wisconsin

3451 Down Syndrome Association of Wisconsin
3211 South Lake Drive   414-327-3729
Milwaukee, WI 53235   866-327-3729
                                           Fax: 414-327-1329
                                        e-mail: info@dsaw.org
                                                www.dsaw.org
An organization created by families for families of individuals and
for individuals with Down Syndrome. Our primary mission is to
provide each person with Down Syndrome the support needed to
achieve personal goals and develop self-esteem.
Tom Oday, President
Nicole Cook, Treasurer

Libraries & Resource Centers

3452 Adult Down Syndrome Center of Lutheran General Hospital
1999 Dempster Street
Park Ridge, IL 60068   847-318-2303
                                       www.advocatehealthc.com
The Adult Down Syndrome Center is a comprehensive medical resource providing multidisciplinary medical and psychosocial care
for adults with Down syndrome, with an emphasis on health
promotion.
Brian Chicoine MD, Medical Director

3453 Ann Whitehill Down Syndrome Program
Riley Hospital for Children

702 Barnhill Drive
Indianapolis, IN 46202   800-248-1199
                                               www.iuhealth.org
Brings together specialists from many areas to address the medical
and psychosocial needs of children with Down Syndrome. We also
refer the family to local resources for therapy and developmental
programs.
Evans Parker, President
William Cast, CEO

3454 Blick Clinic for Developmental Disabilities
640 W Market Street   330-762-5425
Akron, OH 44303-1465   Fax: 330-762-4019
                               e-mail: blickclinic@blickclinic.com
                                             www.blickclinic.com
Blick Clinic is a private, non-profit outpatient clinic which began
by a group of parents of children with developmental disabilities
and a few volunteer professionals. Together, they developed the
Clinic into a single, comprehensive source of diagnostic, evaluation, treatment, and support group services to persons with
developmental disabilities.

3455 Center for Disabilities and Development
University of Iowa Hospitals and Clinics
100 Hawkins Drive   319-353-6900
Iowa City, IA 52242-1011   877-686-0031
                                           Fax: 319-356-8284
                                           TTY: 877-686-0032
                              e-mail: CDD-Webmaster@uiowa.edu
                                     www.healthcare.uiowa.edu/cdd
Provides comprehensive health care and services to people with
disabilities of all ages and their families through a combination of
outpatient, impatient, and community based programs. UHS provides information, evaluation, treatment recommendations, and
training related to aging and disabilities. UHS provides both
preservice and inservice training programs for service providers
and others who provide services to individuals with disabilities.

3456 Children's Hospital of Philadelphia
34th St & Civic Center Boulevard
Philadelphia, PA 19104-4399   215-590-1000
                                                www.chop.edu
The oldest hospital dedicated exclusively to pediatrics, strives to
be the world leader in the advancement of healthcare for children
by integrating excellent patient care, innovative research and quality professional education into all of its programs.

3457 Children's Neurodevelopment Center
Hasbro Children's Hospital
167 Point Street
Providence, RI 02903   401-444-3500
                                               www.lifespan.org/
The Children's Neurodevelopment Center (CNDC) at Hasbro
Children's Hospital provides evaluation and treatment of children
with neurological, genetic, developmental, metabolic and behav-
ioral disorders.
Timothy J. Babineau, President and Chief Executive Officer
Kenneth E. Arnold, Senior Vice President and General Counse

3458 Dartmouth-Hitchcock Medical Center - Genetics and Development
One Medical Center Drive   603-653-1400
Lebanon, NH 03756-0001   Fax: 603-653-3585
                          www.employees.dartmouth-hitchcock.org
Dartmouth-Hitchcock Clinic is committed to a regional, integrated, comprehensive healthcare system, which can evolve under
physician leadership, lay administrative support and public trustee
guidance. DHC and its partnering DHMC organizations are recognized as leaders in using scientific methods to improve health care
delivery.
Carol B Andrew EdD, MS
Mary Beth Dinulos, MD

3459 Developmental Evaluation Clinic
Westchester Institute for Human Development
Cedarwood Hall   914-493-8150
Valhalla, NY 10595-1681   e-mail: wihd@wihd.org
                                                www.wihd.org
WIHD envisions a future where all people, including children and
adults living with disabilities, fully participate in society, live

healthy and productive lives, and have access to culturally appropriate services and supports, emerging technologies, competent professionals, caring families, caregivers, and communities.

3460   Developmental Medicine Center (DMC)
Children's Hospital Boston
300 Longwood Avenue   617-355-6000
Boston, MA 02115   Fax: 617-730-0373
                                    TTY: 617-730-0152
                                    www.childrenshospital.org
Provides developmental evaluation and treatment services for children aged birth to adolescence with a wide range of developmental, behavioral and learning difficulties
Leonard A Rappaport MD, MS, Program Director
Sandra Fenwick, President, CEO

3461   Down Syndrome Center of Western Pennsylvania
One Children's Hospital Drive   412-692-5325
Pittsburgh, PA 15224-2524   Fax: 412-692-5723
                                    www.chp.edu
The Down Syndrome Center of Western Pennsylvania has a lending library of books, videos, audio cassettes and periodicals; provides current information about Down syndrome to families and professionals; maintains a file of articles on issues relating to Down Syndrome and publishes a quarterly newsletter in conjunction with the Down Syndrome Group of Western Pennsylvania.
Dr William Cohen, MD, Director

3462   Down Syndrome Clinic of Houston
6701 Fannin Street, 16th Floor   832-822-3478
Dallas, TX 75235-7701   Fax: 832-825-3399
          e-mail: downsyndrome@texaschildrenshospital.org
                                    www.texaschildreshospital.org
The mission of the Down Syndrome Clinic of Houston is to help individuals with Down syndrome reach his or her fullest potential. We accomplish our goal by offering a clinic where children receive complete evaluations by a multidisciplinary team. Families will obtain needed strategies for management of common concerns.
Nirupama Madduri, MD, Chief of Service
Jennifer Chung, Clinic Coordinator

3463   Dr. Gertrude A Barber National Institute
136 E Avenue   814-453-7661
Erie, PA 16507-1899   Fax: 814-455-1132
          e-mail: BNIerie@barberinstitute.org
                                    www.barberinstitute.org
We believe that all persons have the capacity for growth and fulfillment, and to that end they must be afforded every opportunity to attain the greatest use of thier potential within themselves and their community.
John Barber, JD, President/CEO
Maureen Barber-Carey, EdD, Executive Vice President

3464   Jane and Richard Thomas Center for Down Syndrome
Cincinnati Center for Developmental Disorders
3333 Burnet Avenue   513-636-4200
Cincinnati, OH 45229-3039   800-344-2462
                                    Fax: 513-636-0527
                                    TTY: 513-636-4900
                                    www.cincinnatichildrens.org
The Jane and Richard Thomas Center for Down Syndrome conducts research and offers interdisciplinary evaluations and intervention for infants, children, adolescents and young adults with Down syndrome. By providing a range of comprehensive services within one center, families can now spend less time pursuing services through multiple agencies and professionals.
David J Schonfeld MD, Division Head
Michael Fisher, President and CEO

3465   Kennedy Krieger Institute
707 N Broadway   443-923-9200
Baltimore, MD 21205-1888   800-873-3377
                                    Fax: 410-550-9292
          e-mail: info@kennedykrieger.org
                                    www.kennedykrieger.org
Kennedy Krieger Institute is an internationally recognized facility located in Baltimore, Maryland dedicated to improving the lives of children and adolescents with pediatric developmental disabilities through patient care, special education, research, and professional

training. Our clinical programs offer an interdisciplinary approach in treatment tailored to the individual needs of each child.
Gary W Goldstein, President

3466   LaRabida Children's Hospital: Developmental Disabilities & Delays
6501 South Promontory Drive   773-363-6700
Chicago, IL 60649   e-mail: info@larabida.org
                                    www.larabida.org
La Rabida Children's Hospital is dedicated to excellence in caring for children with chronic illness, disabilities, or who have been abused, allowing them to achieve their fullest potential through expertise and innovation within the health care and academic communities.
Paula Kienberger Jaudes, MD, President/CEO

3467   Marcus Institute for Development and Learning
1920 Briarcliff Road   404-727-9450
Atlanta, GA 30329   Fax: 404-727-9598
          e-mail: Marcus_Info@MarcusInstitute.org
                                    www.marcus.org
Our mission is to provide information, services and programs to people with developmental disabilities and their families, as well as those who live and work with them. We offer integrated state-of-the-art clinical, behavioral, educational and family support services through a single organization to reduce the stress and aggravation for families who may have a child with mild to severe disabilities.
Charles M Shaffer, Jr, President/CEO
Dr Claire Coles, Director Fetal Alcohol Center

3468   MeritCare Children's Hospital Down Syndrome Outpatient Service
Coordinated Treatment Center
736 Broadway   701-234-6600
Fargo, ND 58122-4420   800-828-2901
                                    Fax: 701-234-6965
                                    www.meritcare.com
MeritCare Children's Hospital offers a multidisciplinary outpatient service to help accommodate the special medical developmental, behavioral, family and community needs of patients with Down Syndrome.

3469   Mt. Washington Pediatric Clinic
1708 W Rogers Avenue   410-578-8600
Baltimore, MD 21209-4596   Fax: 410-466-1715
                                    www.mwph.org
The primary purpose of the Mt. Washington Pediatric Hospital and its affiliates is to sponsor and promote the provision of the highest quality pediatric health care services in a nurturing environment.
Sheldon J Stein, President/CEO
Robert H Imhoff, III, VP Development

3470   Santa Rosa Medical Center
PO Box 7330
San Antonio, TX 78207-0330   210-228-2386
                                    www.srmcfl.com
Philip Wright, CEO

3471   UCSF Children's Hospital Health Library
505 Parnassus Avenue
San Francisco, CA 94143   415-476-1000
                                    www.ucsfhealth.org
This Health Library is an online resource to supplement information your doctors, nurses and pharmacists may provide. Our library includes a medical dictionary and an online calendar of our health events. We have news about our research advances and treatments, patient education materials and listings of other helpful Web sites.
Mark Laret, CEO

3472   University of Maryland: Department of Pediatrics
22 South Greene Street   410-328-8667
Baltimore, MD 21201   Fax: 410-328-3981
                                    http://www.umm.edu/pediatrics/
Recognized throughout Maryland and the mid-Atlantic region as a valuable resource for critically and chronically ill children, the University of Maryland Hospital for Children combines state-of-the-art medicine with family-centered care.

3473 University of Washington: Experimental Education Unit
Box 357925
Seattle, WA 98195-7925
206-543-4011
Fax: 206-543-8480
www.eeuweb.org
The Experimental Education Unit (EEU) is a state-certified special education school that serves children from birth to age 7 with diverse abilities. Faculty at the EEU conduct research projects, and provide training opportunities to undergraduate and graduate students, educators, and other professionals.
Rick Neel, Director

Research Centers

3474 Institute for Basic Research in Developmental Disabilities
44 Holland Avenue
Albany, NY 12229-0001
718-494-0600
866-946-9733
Fax: 718-494-0833
TTY: 866-933-4889
www.omr.state.ny.us
Conducts research into neurodegenerative diseases Alzheimer's disease developmental disabilities fragile X syndrome Down's Syndrome autism epilepsy and basic science issues underlying all developmental disabilities.
W Ted Brown, Director
Raju K Pullarkat, Chair Developmental Biochemistry

3475 Kennedy Krieger Institute - Down Syndrome
10 Center Drive
Bethesda, MD 20892
301-496-4000
888-554-2080
Fax: 443-923-9138
TTY: 443-923-2645
e-mail: webmaster@kennedykrieger.org
clinicalcenter.nih.gov
Dedicated to improving the lives of children and adolescents with pediatric developmental disabilities through patient care special education research and professional training.
John Gallin, Director
Char Koller, Research

3476 National Institute of Child Health and Human Development
PO Box 3006
Rockville, MD 20847
800-370-2943
Fax: 301-984-1473
TTY: 888-320-6942
e-mail: NICHDInformationResourceCenter@mail.nih.
www.nichd.nih.gov
Duane Alexander MD, Director

Support Groups & Hotlines

3477 Down Syndrome Association of Greater Cinci nnati
644 Linn Street
Cincinnati, OH 45203-1734
513-761-5400
Fax: 513-761-5401
e-mail: janet@dsagc.com
www.dsagc.com

Janet Gora, Executive Director
Collette Maddy, Office Coordinator

3478 National Down Syndrome Congress
1370 Center Drive
Atlanta, GA 30338
770-604-9500
800-232-6372
Fax: 770-604-9898
e-mail: info@ndsccenter.org
www.ndsccenter.org
Provides information, advocacy and support concerning all aspects of life for individuals with Down syndrome.
David Tolleson, Executive Director
Jim Faber, President

3479 National Down Syndrome Society Hotline
666 Broadway
New York, NY 10012
212-460-9330
800-221-4602
Fax: 212-979-2873
e-mail: info@ndss.org
www.ndss.org
NDSS supports researchers seeking the causes of and answers to many of the medical, genetic, behavioral and learning problems associated with Down syndrome; sponsors symposia and conferences for parents and professionals; performs advocacy; provides information and refferal through a toll-free number; and develops and disseminates educational materials.
Jon Colman, President
Patricia Baker, Program Manager

3480 Parents of Children with Down Syndrome
Arc of Montgomery County
11600 Nebel Street
Rockville, MD 20852-2538
301-984-5777
Fax: 301-816-2429
TTY: 301-881-1548
e-mail: asachs@arcmontmd.org
www.arcmontmd.org/
Activities include formal and informal meetings, parent-to-parent support, contacting new parents of down syndrome children to offer support and information on community resources, providing information on doctors, hospitals and professionals.
Petere Holden, Executive Director
John Slavcoff, President of the Board

Books

3481 ACDS Infant, Toddler & Pre-school Curriculum for Children
Association for Children with Down Syndrome
4 Fern Place
Plainview, NY 11803
516-933-4700
Fax: 516-933-9524
e-mail: msmith@acds.org
www.acds.org
This curriculum is user friendly for parents, educators, related service professionals and other caregivers. It provides checklists and teaching strategies to facilitate aquisition of skills in cognition, self-help, socialization, speech and language, gross and fine motor skills plus much more.
Michael M. Smith, Executive Director

3482 Babies with Down Syndrome
Woodbine House
6510 Bells Mill Road
Bethesda, MD 20817-1636
800-843-7323
Praised as the finest book ever written for new parents, this book covers everything they need to know about rearing these beautiful and special children in a loving environment.
237 pages Paperback
ISBN: 0-933149-02-6

3483 Bethy and the Mouse: God's Gifts in Special Packages
Faith and Life Press
718 Main Street
Newton, KS 67114-0344
316-283-5100
A father's account of his special children, Bethy with Down Syndrome and The Mouse who has been born with microcephaley. A tender story of a father's love.
164 pages Paperback
ISBN: 0-873031-11-3

3484 Breast Feeding the Baby with Down Syndrome
LaLeche League International
957 Plum Grove Road
Schaumburg, IL 60173-4048
847-519-7730
Fax: 847-963-0460
e-mail: llli@llli.org
www.llli.org
16 pages Pamphlet

3485 Cara: Growing with a Retarded Child
Temple University Press
USB Room 305, Broad & Oxford
Philadelphia, PA 19122
215-204-8787
www.temple.edu/tempress
The author offers information and experiences on raising her daughter, Cara, who has Down syndrome.

3486 Communication Skills in Children with Down Syndrome
Woodbine House
6510 Bells Mill Road
Bethesda, MD 20817
800-843-7323
Offers parents a chance to learn what to expect as communication skills progress from infancy through early teenage years. Discus-

sions are included on speech and language therapy, hearing problems, school performance and intelligibility issues.
150 pages Paperback
ISBN: 0-933149-53-0

3487 **Current Approaches to Down's Syndrome**
Greenwood Publishing Group, Inc/Praeger Publishers
PO Box 6926
Portsmouth, NH 03802-6926   800-225-5800
                              Fax: 877-231-6980
                    e-mail: service@greenwood.com
                              www.greenwood.com
An exploration of current initiatives relating to Down syndrome in the medical, educational and social fields.
447 pages
ISBN: 0-275902-12-9
David Lane, Editor
Brian Stratford, Editor

3488 **Differences in Common: Straight Talk on Mental Retardation/Down Syndrome**
Woodbine House
6510 Bells Mill Road
Bethesda, MD 20817   800-843-7323
A collection of essays by the mother of an adult son who has Down syndrome. Focuses on mainstreaming, terminology, parent groups and advocacy.
M Trainer, Editor

3489 **Down Syndrome: A Review of Current Knowledge**
Jean-Adolphe Rondal, Juan Perera, and Lynn Nadek, author
John Wiley and Sons, Inc.
Customer Service-Consumer Accouts
Indianapolis, IN 46256   877-762-2974
                              Fax: 800-597-3299
                    e-mail: consumers@wiley.com
                              www.wiley.com

1999 350 pages Hardcover
IT Lott, Editor
E McCoy, Editor

3490 **Down Syndrome: An Update and Review for Primary Care Physicians**
Dartmouth-Hitchcock Medical Center
1 Medical Center Drive   603-650-5000
Lebanon, NH 03756-0001
An excellent medical review of Down syndrome intended for physicians.
WC Cooley, Editor

3491 **Down Syndrome: The Facts**
Oxford University Press
2001 Evans Road   212-726-6000
Cary, NC 27513-2010   800-451-7556
                              Fax: 919-677-1303
                              www.oup-usa.org
A book for parents who have a child with Down syndrome written by a pediatrician who works with Down syndrome children.
M Selikowitz, Editor

3492 **From 17 Months to 17 Years...A Look at Down Syndrome**
Bonnie Lavender
RR-1, Box 102C   315-287-2973
Richville, NY 13681
Includes profiles of six families who have children with Down syndrome. Offers photographs and accompanying text that detail each family's experiences with Down syndrome.
B Lavender, Editor
GJ Lega, Editor

3493 **Medical and Surgical Care for Children with Down Syndrome**
Woodbine House
6510 Bells Mill Road
Bethesda, MD 20817-1636   800-843-7323
Provides detailed and easy-to-understand information for parents on a wide range of medical conditions and treatments including: heart disease, recurrent infections, thyroid problems, eye problems, skin conditions, ear, nose and throat problems, orthopedic

conditions, leukemia, facial and dental concerns and neurological problems.
320 pages Paperback
ISBN: 0-933149-54-9

3494 **Parent's Guide to Down Syndrome: Toward a Brighter Future**
Siegfried M Pueschel, MD, PhD, JD, MPH, author
Brookes Publishing Company
Customer Service Department
Baltimore, MD 21285-0624   800-638-3775
                              Fax: 410-337-8539
                    e-mail: custserv@brookespublishing.com
                              www.brookespublishing.com
A comprehensive reference book especially for new parents but useful and informative to seasoned parents as well. Range of topics include a history of Down syndrome, physical characterisitcs, developmental expectations, early intervention, feeding the young child and the school years.
2001 338 pages Paperback
ISBN: 1-557664-52-8

3495 **Parents of Children with Down Syndrome**
11600 Nebel Street   301-984-5792
Rockville, MD 20852-2538   Fax: 301-816-2429
Activities include formal and informal meetings, parent-to-parent support, contacting new parents of down syndrome children to offer support and information on community resources, providing information on doctors, hospitals and professionals.

3496 **Paul**
Miriam Perrone
440 Park Avenue   912-638-8551
Saint Simons Island, GA 31522-4357
How a determined mother carved a semi-independent life for her now-grown Down's syndrome child.

3497 **Show Me No Mercy**
PO Box 801
Nashville, TN 37202-0801
A father of a young adult man with Down syndrome relates the experience of his attempt to be reunited with his son after a family tragedy separates them.
R Perske, Editor

3498 **Since Owen**
Johns Hopkins University Press
2715 N Charles Street   410-516-6900
Baltimore, MD 21211-2105   Fax: 410-516-6968
                              www.press.jhu.edu
A well written book displaying understanding from a veteran parent communicating with other parents of children with disabilities.
466 pages
Charles R Callanan, Editor

3499 **Teaching the Infant with Down Syndrome: A Guide for Parents & Professionals**
Pro-Ed, Inc.
8700 Shoal Creek Boulevard   512-451-3246
Austin, TX 78757-6897   800-897-3202
                              Fax: 800-397-7633
                    e-mail: info@proedinc.com
                              www.proedinc.com
A manual providing teaching ideas and activities that can be used to assist an infant's development.
MJ Hanson, Editor

3500 **To Give an Edge: A Guide for New Parents of Children with Down's Syndrome**
Viking Press
7000 Washington Avenue S   612-941-8780
Eden Prairie, MN 55344-3580
A guide for new parents designed to provide information about the disorder and how other parents of children with Down syndrome have coped.
JE Rynders, Editor
JM Horrobin, Editor

3501 **Understanding Down's Syndrome An Introduction for Parents**
Brookline Books

PO Box 1209
Brookline, MA 02445

617-734-6772
800-666-2665
Fax: 617-734-3952
www.brooklinebooks.com

The author provides answers and explanations to the countless questions directed to him during his twenty years' involvement with Down syndrome individuals and their families.
Softcover
ISBN: 1-571290-09-5

Children's Books

3502 Our Brother Has Down's Syndrome: An Introduction for Children
Firefly Books
250 Sparks Avenue   416-499-8412
Willowdale, M2H 2S4,   e-mail: service@fireflybooks.com
                                                      www.fireflybooks.com
Two young sisters tell about their little brother with Down syndrome in this color picture book.
21 pages
S Cairo, Editor

3503 Secret Place of the Stairs
Harper & Row
10 E 53rd Street   212-207-7000
New York, NY 10022-5299
A story that weaves many themes, including the institutionalizing of the protagonist's sister, her parents' divorce and her own expectations.
Grades 7-10

3504 We Can Do It!
Macmillan
866 3rd Avenue
New York, NY 10022-6221   212-702-7865
                                                      www.macmillan.com
A colorful book of photographs that show the daily activities of young children with different developmental delays, including Down syndrome.
L Dwight, Editor

Magazines

3505 Down Syndrome, Papers and Abstracts for Professionals
200 Rabbit Road   301-963-1857
Gaithersburg, MD 20878
Quarterly review of research literature pertaining to Down syndrome.

3506 Exceptional Parent Magazine
209 Harvard Street   617-730-5800
Brookline, MA 02446-5071   Fax: 617-730-8742
A publication dealing with many issues affecting exceptional children and their families.
Monthly

Newsletters

3507 Down Syndrome News
National Down Syndrome Congress
7000 Peachtree Dunwoody Rd NE
Atlanta, GA 30328-1655   770-604-9500
                                                     800-232-6372
                              e-mail: NDSC.center@aol.com
                                      www.ndsccenter.org
Contains book reviews, articles and items of interest to those touched by Down syndrome.
10x Annually
Frank J Murphy, Executive Director

3508 Down Syndrome Today
Down Syndrome Today Publications
PO Box 212
Holtsville, NY 11742-0212   516-654-3242

Offers information, articles, resources and materials for the parent and professional working and nurturing patients and persons with Downs syndrome.
Debra Hoeft, Publisher

3509 National Down Syndrome Society Update
666 Broadway   212-460-9330
New York, NY 10012-2317   800-221-4602
                                               Fax: 212-979-2873
                                                      www.ndss.org
Offers information on the activities of the society, new breakthroughs in medical technology, articles offering state of the art information to families and individuals with Down syndrome, and answers to questions about the illness.
12 pages Quarterly
Fran Goldstein, Editor

3510 On the Up with Down Syndrome
Carole Shafer, author
Down Syndrome Association of Wisconsin
9401 West Beloit Road   414-327-3729
Milwaukee, WI 53227   866-327-3729
                                               Fax: 414-327-1329
                               e-mail: thomtalent@aol.com
                                                      www.dsaw.org
Offers the exchange of ideas and experiences. Free to our members. Membership is $20.00/year.
Quarterly
Ron Irwin, Board President
Robbin Lyons, Newsletter Contact

Pamphlets

3511 Alzheimer's Disease and Down Syndrome
National Down Syndrome Society
666 Broadway   212-460-9330
New York, NY 10012-2317   800-221-4602
                                                      www.ndss.org
1995

3512 Down Syndrome
March of Dimes
233 Park Avenue South   212-353-8353
New York, NY 10003   Fax: 212-254-3518
                            e-mail: NY639@marchofdimes.com
                                      www.marchofdimes.com

3513 Heart and Down Syndrome
National Down Syndrome Society
666 Broadway   212-460-9330
New York, NY 10012-2317   800-221-4602
                                                      www.ndss.org
1995

3514 Life Planning and Down Syndrome
National Down Syndrome Society
666 Broadway   212-460-9330
New York, NY 10012-2317   800-221-4602
                                                      www.ndss.org

3515 Neurology of Down Syndrome
National Down Syndrome Society
666 Broadway   212-460-9330
New York, NY 10012-2317   800-221-4602
                                                      www.ndss.org
1995

3516 New Parents
Association for Children with Down Syndrome
4 Fern Place   516-933-4700
Plainview, NY 11803   Fax: 516-933-9524
                                  e-mail: msmith@acds.org
                                                      www.acds.org
Bibliography compiled for parents who have just given birth to a child with Down syndrome. Free upon reciept of a stamped, self-addressed envelope.
Michael Smith, Executive Director

3517 **Sexuality in Down Syndrome**
National Down Syndrome Society
666 Broadway   212-460-9330
New York, NY 10012-2317   800-221-4602
                                      www.ndss.org

1995

3518 **Speech and Language in Children and Adolescents with Down Syndrome**
National Down Syndrome Society
666 Broadway   212-460-9330
New York, NY 10012-2317   800-221-4602
                                      www.ndss.org

1995

Audio & Video

3519 **Adaptation to the Initial Crisis**
Lawren Productions
930 Pitner Avenue   847-328-6700
Evanston, IL 60202-1556   800-421-2363
A family learns to adapt to the birth of a child with a handicap.

3520 **Bernardsville Beginnings**
National Down Syndrome Society
666 Broadway   212-460-9330
New York, NY 10012-2317   800-221-4602
                                      Fax: 212-979-2873
                                      www.ndss.org
Follows Alison through her first full year in a first grade inclusion program. Step-by-step account of teaching staff preparation, classroom experiences, a portrayal of one girl's successful adjustment, and a whole class matured by the experience.
23 minutes

3521 **Bittersweet Waltz**
National Down Syndrome Society
666 Broadway   212-460-9330
New York, NY 10012-2317   800-221-4602
                                      Fax: 212-979-2873
                                      e-mail: info@ndss.org
                                      www.ndss.org
Experience of Alec and his first year included in a regular fifth grade class. From a point of view of a parent, a child, and the school administration.
18 minutes

3522 **Colin and Ricky**
Lawren Productions
930 Pitner Avenue   847-328-6700
Evanston, IL 60202-1556   800-421-2363
A young boy comes to deal with his disappointment surrounding the birth of his baby brother with Down syndrome.

3523 **Congratulations: An Introduction to Down Syndrome for Parents/Family/Friends**
New Challenges
96 Ogden Avenue   914-287-0723
White Plains, NY 10605
Film for parents which addresses some of the most commonly asked questions about raising a child with Down syndrome.

3524 **Daddy's Girl**
Carle Media
110 W Main Street   217-384-4838
Urbana, IL 61801-2715
A film starring a twelve-year-old actress with Down syndrome, dealing with her divorced father's inability to accept the fact that his daughter has Down syndrome.
Carolyn Baxley

3525 **Down Syndrome: See the Potential**
Down Syndrome Association of Charlotte
PO Box 3136
Charlotte, NC 28210   800-232-6372
Video highlighting the capability of children with Down syndrome.

3526 **Gifts of Love**
National Down Syndrome Society
666 Broadway   212-460-9330
New York, NY 10012-2317   800-221-4602
                                      Fax: 212-979-2873
                                      www.ndss.org
Four families of children with Down syndrome talk about their feelings and experiences with their children, particularly during the first six years. All the children live at home and attend programs in their communities.
25 minutes

3527 **Infant Motor Development: A Look at the Phases**
Communication Skill Builders/Therapy Skill Builder
3830 E Bellevue   520-323-7500
Tucson, AZ 85733
A video depicting development in and activities for infants birth through 12 months.

3528 **New Expectations**
Lawren Productions
930 Pitner Avenue
Evanston, IL 60202-1556   800-421-2363
Focuses on the emotional and technical aspects of Down syndrome. Highlights four persons at various life stages from infancy to adulthood in the areas of education and employment.

3529 **New Set of Fears, a New Set of Hopes**
Meyer Children's Rehabilitation Institute
Resource Center, 444 S 44th Street   402-559-7467
Omaha, NE 68131   800-232-6372
Explores the way a family adjusts as they go through the life cycle with their child who has Down syndrome.

3530 **Opportunities to Grow**
National Down Syndrome Society
666 Broadway   212-460-9330
New York, NY 10012-2317   800-221-4602
                                      Fax: 212-979-2873
                                      e-mail: info@ndss.org
                                      www.ndss.org
Sequel to Gifts of Love video shows how people with Down syndrome, ages 6 to 26, participate equally in all phases of community life. Vignettes of 15 young men and women illustrate how inclusion, education, computer facilitation, socialization programs, and employment training help them to fulfill their potential.
25 minutes

3531 **Stepping Stones**
AIT
PO Box A
Bloomington, IN 47402-0120   800-457-4509
Series of video programs on teaching basic skills to at-risk, special needs and normally developed children.

3532 **Thanks Mom and Dad: Profiles of Patrick**
University of Washington
CDMRC Mail Stop WJ-10   206-543-4011
Seattle, WA 98195-0001   800-232-6372
Documentary on the life of Patrick, a young man with Down syndrome from birth through his graduation from high school.

3533 **You Don't Outgrow Down Syndrome**
National Association for Down Syndrome
PO Box 4542   630-325-9112
Oak Brook, IL 60522-4542   800-232-6372
                                      www.nads.org
Winner of the second annual International Rehabilitation Film Festival.

Web Sites

3534 **Aleh Foundation**
                                      www.aleh.org
Aleh Rehabilitation Center has served as a residential facility to close to 200 children with multiple, physical and mental disabilities.

3535 **Down Syndrome**
                                      www.downsyn.com

A resource for new paretns of children with Down syndrome. Provides a personnel perspective from parents who also have children with Down syndrome.

3536 Healing Well

www.healingwell.com

An online health resource guide to medical news, chat, information and articles, newsgroups and message boards, books, disease-related web sites, medical directories, and more for patients, friends, and family coping with disabling diseases, disorders, or chronic illnesses.

3537 Health Finder

www.healthfinder.gov

Searchable, carefully developed web site offering information on over 1000 topics. Developed by the US Department of Health and Human Services, the site can be used in both English and Spanish.

3538 Healthlink USA

www.healthlinkusa.com

Health information concerning treatment, cures, prevention, diagnosis, risk factors, research, support groups, email lists, personal stories and much more. Updated regularly.

3539 Helios Health

www.helioshealth.com

Online resource for your health information. Detailed information about specific health topics, access to expert advice from our Medical Advisory Board, and up-to-date health news.

3540 MedicineNet

www.medicinenet.com

An online resource for consumers providing easy-to-read, authoritative medical and health information.

3541 Medscape

www.medscape.com

Medscape offers specialists, primary care physicians, and other health professionals the Web's most robust and integrated medical information and educational tools.

3542 National Down Syndrome Society

www.ndss.org

NDSS works to obtain a better understanding of Down syndrome, the potential of people with Down syndrome, to support research about the condition, and to provide information and referral services for families and professionals.

3543 WebMD

www.webmd.com

Information on Down Syndrome, including articles and resources.

Description

3544 Eating Disorders (Anorexia Nervosa, Bulimia)

Anorexia nervosa and bulimia nervosa are eating disorders characterized by a disturbed sense of body image and an irrational fear of obesity. They are manifested by abnormal patterns relating to food and by self-induced, marked weight loss.

Anorexia is a psychiatric disorder in which dieting and a desire for thinness leads to excessive weight loss. About 95 percent of persons with this disorder are female, although males can be affected. The onset usually occurs during adolescence and some sufferers are in their 60s. Anorexia nervosa is characterized by self-starvation, food preoccupation and rituals, compulsive exercising, and often a resulting absence of menstrual cycles. The cause is unknown, although social factors appear to play an important role, including advertisements that equate thinness with desirability. Denial is a prominent feature, and sufferers usually resist treatment.

Bulimia is characterized by recurring episodes of binge eating followed by efforts to avoid weight gain, such as purging through self-induced vomiting or abuse of laxatives and/or diuretics (water pills). Unlike patients with anorexia, those with bulimia usually have normal weight. Binges are often triggered by psychological stress and carried out in secret. Warning signs of bulimia include eating uncontrollably, frequent use of the bathroom, erosion of dental enamel of the front teeth (from vomiting), and painless swollen salivary glands. Bulimia may coexist with anorexia.

Anorexia nervosa is associated with a 10 percent death rate, generally from a sudden disturbance of heart rhythm. Fortunately, most sufferers will eventually return to a normal or near-normal body weight, although many continue to struggle with body image and unhealthy eating patterns. Treatment for both illnesses is similar, beginning with the need to restore body weight. Initial treatment may require hospitalization for physical stabilization. Long-term psychological treatment and behavior modification is often necessary and focuses on behavioral and emotional growth for both the individual with the eating disorder and their family. See also *Obesity*.

National Agencies & Associations

3545 Academy for Eating Disorders
111 Deer Lake Road
Deerfield, IL 60015-1577

847-498-4274
Fax: 847-480-9282
e-mail: info@aedweb.org
www.aedweb.org

AED is an association of multidisciplinary professionals promoting effective treatment, developing prevention initiatives, advocating for the field, stimulating research and sponsoring an annual conference.
Pamela K. Keel, PhD, FAED, President
Carla Slawson, MBA, Executive Director

3546 American Dietetic Association
120 S Riverside Plaza
Chicago, IL 60606-6995

312-899-0040
800-877-1600
e-mail: media@eatright.org
www.eatright.org

ADA offers nutrition information consumer tips nutrition fact sheets consumer frequently asked questions and referrals to registered dieticians.
Patricia M Babjak, Chief Executive Officer
Judith C Rodriguez, President

3547 Anna Westin Foundation
PO Box 268
Chaska, MN 55318

952-361-3051
e-mail: kitty@annawestinfoundation.org
www.annawestinfoundation.org

The Anna Westin Foundation is dedicated to the prevention and treatment of eating disorders. They are committed to preventing the tragic loss of life to anorexia nervosa and bulimia and to raising public awareness of those dangerous illnesses.
Kitty Westin, President

3548 Anorexia Nervosa & Bulimia Association
1500 Ouellette Avenue
Windsor, ON N8X 1-1C0

519-969-0227
e-mail: info@bana.ca
www.bana.ca

Facilitate advocate and coordinate support for any individual directly or indirectly affected by eating disorders and to raise public awareness through improved communication and the provision of education within our community.
Steven Richards, President
Sarah Woodruff, Vice-President

3549 Dads and Daughters
34 E Superior Street
Duluth, MN 55802

218-772-3942
888-824-DADS
Fax: 218-728-0314
e-mail: info@dadsanddaughters.org
www.thedadman.com

Provides tools to strengthen father-daughter relationships and transform pervasive cultural messages that value daughters more for how they look than who they are.
Gregg Rutter, Development Director
David Sadker, Author of Teachers

3550 Eating Disorders Action Group
6156 Quinpool Road
Halifax Nova Scotia, B3L 1-3Z9

902-443-9944
e-mail: reception@edag.ca
www.edag.ca

A community based charitable organization dedicated to promoting healthy body image and self esteem and to supporting individuals who experience disordered eating.

3551 Eating Disorders Anonymous
PO Box 55876
Phoenix, AZ 85078-5876

www.4eda.org

EDA provides information about local support group meetings.

3552 Eating Disorders Coalition for Research, Policy and Action
720 7th Street NW
Washington, DC 20001-4303

202-543-9570
Fax: 202-543-9570
e-mail: manager@eatingdisorderscoalition.org
www.eatingdisorderscoalition.org

Advocates at the federal level on behalf of people with eating disorders their families and professionals working with these populations. Promotes federal support for improved access to care.
David Jaffe, Executive Director
Jeanine Cogan, Policy Director

3553 Healthy Weight Network
402 S 14th Street
Hettinger, ND 58639

701-567-2646
Fax: 701-567-2602
e-mail: hwj@healthyweight.net
www.healthyweight.net

Promotes information and resources pertaining to the Health at Any Size paradigm.
Frances M Berg MS, Founder/Editor

3554 **International Association of Eating Disorders Professionals**
PO Box 1295   309-346-3341
Pekin, IL 61555-1295   800-800-8126
Fax: 309-346-2874
e-mail: iaedpmembers@earthlink.net
www.iaedp.com

IAEDP Offers professional counseling and assistance to the medical community, courts, law enforcement officials and social welfare agencies.
Mary Bellofatto, President
Emmett R Bishop, Immediate Past President

3555 **Jessie's Hope Society**
11739 23rd Street   604-466-4877
Maple Ridge, BC V2X-5X8   877-288-0877
Fax: 604-466-4897
e-mail: info@jessieshope.org
www.jessieshope.org

Promote positive body image by fostering in youth within communities and across cultures throughout British Columbia.
Connie Coniglio, Chair
Mimi Hudson, Secretary

3556 **National Association of Anorexia Nervosa and Associated Disorders**
750 E Diehl Road   630-577-1330
Naperville, IL 60563   Fax: 847-433-4632
e-mail: anadhelp@anad.org
www.anad.org

Works to prevent eating disorders and provides numerous programs — all free — to help victims and families including hotlines, support groups, referrals, information packets and newsletters. Educational/prevention programs include presentations and early detection.
Vivian Hanse Meehan, Founder/President
Laura Discipio, Executive Director

3557 **National Eating Disorder Information Centr e**
ES 7-421, 200 Elizabeth Street   416-340-4156
Toronto, Ontario, M5G-2C4   866-633-4220
Fax: 416-340-4736
e-mail: nedic@uhn.on.ca
www.nedic.ca

Promotes healthy lifestyles, including both healty eating and appropriate, enjoyable exercise.
Merryl Bear MEd, Director
Jessica Rust, Administrative Coordinator

3558 **National Eating Disorders Association**
603 Stewart Street   206-382-3587
Seattle, WA 98101   800-931-2237
Fax: 206-829-8501
e-mail: info@NationalEatingDisorders.org
www.nationaleatingdisorders.org

Our mission is to eliminate eating disorders and body dissatisfaction through prevention efforts education referral and support services advocacy training and research.
Lynn S Grefe MA, Chief Executive Officer
Molly Bauthues, Communications Manager

3559 **National Eating Disorders Screening Program**
One Washington Street   781-239-0071
Wellesley Hills, MA 02481   Fax: 781-431-7447
e-mail: smhinfo@mentalhealthscreening.org
www.mentalhealthscreening.org

Offers eating disorders screening.
Douglas G Jacobs MD, President/Medical Director

3560 **National Women's Health Information Center**
8270 Willow Oaks Corporate Drive
Fairfax, VA 22031   800-994-9662
Fax: 703-560-6598
TTY: 888-220-5446
TDD: 888-220-5446
e-mail: Wanda.jones@hhs.gov
www.4woman.gov

Government agency with free health information for women.
Wanda K Jones PhD, Deputy Assistant Secretary for Health
Frances E Ashe-Goins, Deputy Director

3561 **Weight-Control Information Network National Institutes of Health**
National Institutes of Health
1 WIN Way   202-828-1025
Bethesda, MD 20892-3665   877-946-4627
Fax: 202-828-1028
e-mail: win@info.niddk.nih.gov
www.win.niddk.nih.gov/index.htm

Information on obesity weight-control and nutrition.
BiAnnual

State Agencies & Associations

Connecticut

3562 **Renfrew Center of Connecticut**
1445 E. Putnam Avenue
Wilton, CT 06897   800-736-3739
Fax: 203-563-9936
e-mail: foundation@renfrew.org
www.renfrewcenter.com

Florida

3563 **Renfrew Center of Miami**
151 Majorca Avenue
Coral Gables, FL 33134   800-REN-FREW
Fax: 305-445-2729
e-mail: info@renfrewcenter.com
www.renfrewcenter.com

3564 **Renfrew Center of South Florida**
7700 Renfrew Lane
Coconut Creek, FL 33073   800-736-3739
Fax: 954-698-9007
e-mail: info@renfrewcenter.com
www.renfrewcenter.com

Maryland

3565 **St. Joseph's Medical Center**
7601 Osler Drive
Towson, MD 21204   410-337-1000
www.stjosephtowson.com

John Tolmie, President/CEO

Massachusetts

3566 **Massachusetts Eating Disorder Association**
92 Pearl Street   617-558-1881
Newton, MA 02458   866-343-MEDA
Fax: 617-558-1771
e-mail: info@medainc.com
www.medainc.org

A nonprofit organization dedicated to the treatment and prevention of eating disorders. MEDA provides help line resource and referral, assessments, client consultations, individual therapy, support groups and an intensive evening treatment program.
100+ Members
Rebecca Manley, Founder
Beth Mayer, CEO

New Jersey

3567 **American Anorexia Bulimia Association: New Jersey Chapter**
10 Station Place   609-252-0202
Metuchen, NJ 08840   Fax: 609-688-1544
e-mail: njaaba@NJAABA.org
www.njaaba.org

3568 **Renfrew Center of Northern New Jersey**
174 Union Street
Ridgewood, NJ 07450   800-736-3739
Fax: 201-652-6253
e-mail: info@renfrewcenter.org
www.renfrewcenter.com

New York

3569 Renfrew Center of New York
11 E 36th Street
New York, NY 10016   800-736-3739
                                           Fax: 212-686-1865
                                e-mail: info@renfrewcenter.org
                                        www.renfrewcenter.com

3570 Westchester Task Force on Eating Disorders/American Anorexia Bulimia
3 Mount Joy Avenue   914-472-3701
Scarsdale, NY 10583-2632

Pennsylvania

3571 American Anorexia Bulimia Association of Philadelphia
PO Box 1287   215-221-1864
Langhorne, PA 19047   Fax: 215-702-8944
                                           www.aabaphila.org

3572 Pennsylvania Educational Network for Eating Disorders
4801 McKnight Road
Pittsburgh, PA 15237   412-215-7967
                                               www.pened.org
PENED is a nonprofit organization providing education, support, and referral information to the general and professional public.
Anita Sincro Maier, Therapist
Ralph F. Wilps, Therapist

3573 Renfrew Center of Bryn Mawr
735 Old Lancaster Road
Bryn Mawr, PA 19010   800-736-3739
                                           Fax: 610-527-9361
                                e-mail: info@renfrewcenter.org
                                        www.renfrewcenter.com

3574 Renfrew Center of Philadelphia
475 Spring Lane
Philadelphia, PA 19128   800-REN-FREW
                                           Fax: 215-482-7390
                                   e-mail: info@renfrew.org
                                        www.renfrewcenter.com

Research Centers

3575 Academy for Eating Disorders
111 Deer Lake Road   847-498-4274
Deerfield, IL 60015-1577   Fax: 847-480-9282
                                     e-mail: info@aedweb.org
                                              www.aedweb.org
Disseminate knowledge regarding eating disorders to members of the Academy other professionals and the general public
Debra Katzman, President
Susie Orbach, Board of Advisor

3576 Center for the Study of Anorexia and Bulimia
1841 Broadway at 60th Street   212-333-3444
New York, NY 10023   Fax: 212-333-5444
                                               www.icpnyc.org
The Institute is composed of a group of 150 professionally trained licensed psychotherapists who offer a full range of psychotherapeutic services including individual and group psychotherapy and psychoanalysis in addition to more specialized treatment services.
Jim M Pollack CSW, Executive Director/Director of Treatment
Ron Taffel, Chair

3577 Division of Digestive & Liver Diseases of Cloumbia University
630 W 168th Street   212-305-5960
New York, NY 10032-3784   Fax: 212-305-8466
                                e-mail: hjw14@columbia.edu
                                        www.cumc.columbia.edu
The Division's faculty members are devoted to research and the clinical care of patients with gastrointestinal, liver and nutritional disorders. The Division is also responsible for the Gastroenterology Training Program at the medical center and for teaching medical students, interns, residents, fellows and attending physicians aspects of gastrointestinal and liver diseases.
Howard J Worman MD, Division Director
Karen Wisdom, Director

3578 Harris Center for Education and Advocacy in Eating Disorders
2 Longfellow Place   617-726-8470
Boston, MA 02114   Fax: 617-726-1595
                                e-mail: dherzog@partners.org
                                        www.harriscentermgh.org
Conducts research provides a newsletter and information.
David B Herzog MD, Director
David B Herzog, Director

Support Groups & Hotlines

3579 AABA Support Group
Chippenham Medican Center
7101 Jahnke Rd.   804-320-3911
Richmond, VA 23225
Elliot Spanier, Contact

3580 About Kids GI Disorders
IFFGD
PO Box 170864   414-964-1799
Milwaukee, WI 53217-8076   888-964-2001
                                           Fax: 414-964-7176
                                     e-mail: iffgd@iffgd.org
                                        www.aboutkidsgi.org
About Kids is the pediatric branch of the International Foundation for Functional Gastrointestinal Disorders (IFFGD), a registered nonprofit education and research organization founded in 1991. Their mission is to inform, assist, and support those affected by gastrointestinal (GI) disorders, addressing issues of digestive health in children through support of education and research. IFFGD promotes awareness among the public, health care providers, researchers, and regulators.
Nancy J Norton, President/Founder

3581 Association of Gastrointestinal Motility D isorders
AGMD International Corporate Headquarters
12 Roberts Drive   781-275-1300
Bedford, MA 01730   Fax: 781-275-1304
                                e-mail: digestive.motility@gmail.com
                                        www.agmd-gimotility.org
A non-profit international organization which serves as an integral educational resource concerning digestive motility diseases and disorders. Also functions as an important information base for members of the medical and scientific communities. Also provides a forum for patients suffering from digestive motility diseases and disorders as well as their families and members of the medical, scientific, and nutritional communities.
Mary Angela DeGrazia-DiTucci, President/Patient/Founder

3582 Coconut Creek Eating Disorders Support Group
Renfrew Center
7700 NW 48th Avenue   954-698-9222
Coconut Creek, FL 33073-3508   877-367-3383
                                           Fax: 954-698-9007
                                               www.renfrew.org

Samuel Menagad, Director

3583 Eating Disorder Resource Center
330 W 58th Street   212-989-3987
New York, NY 10019   e-mail: info@edrcnyc.org
                                               www.edrcnyc.org
A specialized treatment program for women and men who were suffering from bulimia. Now EDRC treats eating disorders of all kinds, offering individual, group, family and couples treatment for those challenged by bulimia, binge eating disorder, anorexia and other kinds of body dysmorphia.
Judith Brisman, Director & Founder
Senna Lauer, Marketing Assistant

3584 **Eating Disorders Association of New Jersey**
10 Station Place
Metuchen, NJ 08840   800-522-2230
                                                   Fax: 732-906-9307
                                              e-mail: info@edanj.org
                                                    www.edanj.org
A non-profit state organization whose mission is to provide supportive services and resources to indivudals affected by eating disorders, including family members and friends.

3585 **First Presbyterian Church in the City of New York Support Groups**
First Presbyterian Church in the City of New York
12 West 12th Street   212-675-6150
New York, NY 10011   e-mail: fpcnyc@fpcnyc.org
                                                    www.fpcnyc.org
The First Presbyterian Church in the City of New York provides numerous programs and supports groups for both adults and children including an educational program for autistic children.
Jon M Walton, Senior Pastor
Sarah Segal Mccaslin, Associate Pastor

3586 **Holliswood Hospital Psychiatric Care, Serv ices and Self-Help/Support Groups**
87-37 Palermo Street   718-776-8181
Holliswood, NY 11423   800-486-3005
                                                   Fax: 718-776-8572
                                   e-mail: HolliswoodInfo@libertymgt.com
                                              www.holliswoodhospital.com/
The Holliswood Hospital, a 110-bed private psychiatric hospital located in a quiet residential Queens community, is a leader in providing quality, acute inpatient mental health care for adult, adolescent, geriatric and dually diagnosed patients. Holliswood Hospital treats patients with a broad range of psychiatric disorders. Additionally, specialized services are available for patients with psychiatric diagnoses compounded by chemical dependency, or a history of physical or sexual abuse.
Susan Clayton, Support Group Coordinator
Angela Hurtado, Support Group Coordinator

3587 **National Health Information Center**
PO Box 1133
Washington, DC 20013   310-565-4167
                                                     800-336-4797
                                                   Fax: 301-984-4256
                                               e-mail: info@nhic.org
                                                  www.health.gov/nhic
A health information referral service sponsored by the Office of Disease Prevention and Health Promotion. Puts health professionals and condumers who have health questions in touch with those organizations that are best able to provide answers.

3588 **Pediatric/Adolescent Gastroesophageal Reflux Association**
PO Box 7728
Silver Spring, MD 20901   301-601-9541
                                                     888-887-7729
                                             e-mail: gergroup@aol.com
                                                    www.reflux.org
Provides information and support to parents, patients and doctors about Gastroesophageal Reflux.
Beth Anderson, Director

3589 **Richmond Support Group**
Warwick Medical & Professional Ctr   804-320-7881
Richmond, VA

Books

3590 **Anorexia Nervosa & Recovery: A Hunger for Meaning**
The Haworth Press
10 Alice Street   607-722-5857
Binghamton, NY 13904   800-429-6784
                                             e-mail: getinfo@haworth.com
                                                    www.haworth.com

1993 146 pages Paperback
ISBN: 0-918393-95-7

3591 **Bearly Any Fat Cookbook**
Obesity Foundation

5600 S Quebec Street   303-850-0328
Englewood, CO 80111-2202   e-mail: editor@obesity.org
                                                    www.obesity.org
Perfect cookbook to assist anyone in a weight reduction program.

3592 **Body Betrayed**
American Psychiatric Press
1400 K Street NW   202-682-6268
Washington, DC 20005-2403   Fax: 202-789-2648
A book concentrating on women, eating disorders and treatments.
440 pages Hardcover
ISBN: 0-880485-22-1

3593 **Bulimia: A Guide to Recovery**
Gurze Books
PO Box 2238
Carlsbad, CA 92018-9883   800-756-7533
                                                   Fax: 760-434-5476
                                             e-mail: gzcatl@aol.com
                                                    www.bulimia.com
This intimate guidebook offers a complete understanding of bulimia and a plan for recovery. It includes a two-week program to stop bingeing, things-to-do instead of bingeing, a two-week guide for support groups, specific advice for loved ones and Eating Without Fear, Hall's story of self-cure which has inspired thousands of other bulimics.
280 pages Paperback
ISBN: 0-936077-31-X

3594 **Conversations with Anorexics**
Jason Aronson
PO Box 15100
York, PA 17405-7100   800-782-0015
                                                   Fax: 201-840-7242
                                                    www.aronson.com
A Compassionate and Hopeful Journey through the Therapeutic Process.
238 pages
ISBN: 1-568212-61-5

3595 **Coping with Eating Disorders**
Rosen Publishing Group
29 E 21st Street   212-777-3017
New York, NY 10010   800-237-9932
                                                   Fax: 888-436-4643
                                  e-mail: customerservice@rosenpub.com
                                               www.rosenpublishing.com
This book offers practical suggestions on coping with eating disorders.

ISBN: 0-823929-74-4
Barbara Moe, Author

3596 **Cult of Thinness**
Oxford University Press
2001 Evans Road   212-726-6000
Cary, NC 27513-2010   800-451-7556
                                                   Fax: 919-677-1303
                                                    www.oup-usa.org

1996 256 pages
ISBN: 0-195082-41-9

3597 **Deadly Diet: Recovering from Anorexia & Bulimia**
New Harbinger Publications
5674 Shattuck Avenue
Oakland, CA 94609-1662   800-748-6273
                                                   Fax: 510-652-5472
                                                www.newharbinger.com

1993 265 pages Paperback
ISBN: 1-879237-42-3

3598 **Eating Diorders Resource Catalogue**
Gurze Books
PO Box 2238
Carlsbad, CA 92018-9883   800-756-7533
                                                   Fax: 760-434-5476
                                                    www.bulimia.com
This catalogue of resources contains over 140 books, videos and audiotapes, lists of national organizations and treatment facilities and basic facts about eating disorders. It is widely distributed by

individuals who are suffering, their loved ones, the health care professionals who treat them and educators who are working towards prevention.
24 pages Annual

3599   Eating Disorder Sourcebook
Gurze Books
PO Box 2238
Carlsbad, CA 92018-2238   800-756-7533
                                    Fax: 760-434-5476
                                e-mail: gzcatl@aol.com
                                       www.bulimia.com
An ideal book for someone with a loved one who has an eating disorder but who knows little about this subject, this new release presents a clear overview of basic issues.
222 pages Paperback

3600   Eating Disorders Resource Catalogue
Gurze Books
PO Box 2238
Carlsbad, CA 92018-9883   800-756-7533
                                    Fax: 760-434-5476
                                       www.bulimia.com
This catalogue of resources contains over 140 books, videos and audiotapes, lists of national organizations and treatment facilities and basic facts about eating disorders. It is widely distributed by individuals who are suffering, their loved ones, the health care professionals who treat them and educators who are working towards prevention.
28 pages Annual

3601   Eating Disorders-Overview Series
Lucent Books
Thomson Gale
Farmington Hills, MI 48333-9187   800-877-4253
                                    Fax: 800-414-5043
                     e-mail: gale.customerservice@thomson.com
                                    www.gale.com/lucent
This book examines how eating disorders can be identified, who is affected by them, and how they can be treated.
2001
ISBN: 1-560066-59-8

3602   Eating Disorders: When Food Turns Against You
Franklin Watts Grolier
90 Old Sherman Tpke
Danbury, CT 06816-0001   203-797-3500
                                    Fax: 203-797-3197
                                       www.grolier.com
1993 96 pages
ISBN: 0-531111-75-0

3603   Emotional Eating: A Practical Guide to Taking Control
Free Press
866 3rd Avenue
New York, NY 10022   800-223-7445
                                    Fax: 800-943-9831
                                    www.simonsays.com
1003 200 pages
ISBN: 0-029002-15-0

3604   Encyclopedia of Obesity and Eating Disorders
Facts on File
11 Penn Plaza   212-967-8800
New York, NY 10001   800-322-8755
                                    Fax: 800-678-3633
From abdominoplasty to Zung Rating Scale, this volume defines and explains these disorders, along with medical and other problems associated with them.
272 pages Hardcover

3605   Endorphins: Eating Disorders & Other Addictive Behavior
WW Norton & Company
500 5th Avenue   212-354-5500
New York, NY 10110-0054   800-233-4830
                                    Fax: 800-458-6515
                                       www.wwnorton.com
1993 320 pages
ISBN: 0-393701-56-5

3606   Etiology and Treatment of Bulimia Nervosa
Jason Aronson

PO Box 15100
York, PA 17405-7100   800-782-0015
                                    Fax: 201-767-1576
                                       www.aronson.com
352 pages Softcover
ISBN: 1-568213-39-5

3607   Evaluation and Management of Eating Disorders
Human Kinetics Publishers
PO Box 5076   217-351-1549
Champaign, IL 61825-5076   800-747-4457
                                    Fax: 217-351-5076
368 pages Cloth
ISBN: 0-873229-11-8

3608   Fear of Being Fat
Jason Aronson
PO Box 15100
York, PA 17405-7100   800-782-0015
                                    Fax: 201-840-7242
                                       www.aronson.com
366 pages
ISBN: 0-876688-99-7

3609   Getting Better Bit(e) by Bit(e)
Gurze Books
PO Box 2238
Carlsbad, CA 92018-2238   800-756-7533
                                    Fax: 760-434-5476
                                e-mail: gzcatl@aol.com
                                       www.bulimia.com
This practical book on recovery from bulimia and binge eating is packed with lists, exercises, case studies, discussions, insights and specific things to do. This book also addresses the day-to-day problems faced by eating disorder sufferers and concentrates on key behavior changes necessary for progress.
143 pages Paperback

3610   Going Backwards
Scholastic
730 Broadway   212-505-3000
New York, NY 10003-9511   800-325-6149
A story that weaves the themes of acceptance, death, mortality and family loyalty to present a controversial plot.
Grades 7-10

3611   Golden Cage: The Enigma of Anorexia Nervosa
Gurze Books
PO Box 2283
Carlsbad, CA 92018-2283   800-756-7533
                                    Fax: 760-434-5476
                                e-mail: gzcatl@aol.com
                                       www.bulimia.com

3612   Group Psychotherapy for Eating Disorders
American Psychiatric Press
1400 K Street NW   202-682-6268
Washington, DC 20005-2403   Fax: 202-789-2648
The first book to fully explore the use of group therapy in the treatment of eating disorders.
353 pages Hardcover
ISBN: 0-880484-19-5

3613   Helping Athletes with Eating Disorders
Human Kinetics Publishers
PO Box 5076   217-351-1549
Champaign, IL 61825-5076   800-747-4457
                                    Fax: 217-351-5076
Gives readers the information they need to identify and address major eating disorders such as: anorexia, bulimia nervosa, and eating disorders not otherwise specified.
208 pages Cloth
ISBN: 0-873223-83-7

3614   Hope and Recovery: A Mother-Daughter Story About Anorexia Nervosa & Bulimia
Franklin Watts Grolier
90 Old Sherman Tpke
Danbury, CT 06816-0001   800-621-1115
                                    Fax: 800-374-4329

Mother and daughter tell a story of a young woman's recovery from the horror of an eating disorder. This compelling account shows how anorexia and bulimia can affect an entire family.
192 pages
ISBN: 0-531111-40-7

3615 Hungry Self: Women, Eating and Identity
Gurze Books
PO Box 2283
Carlsbad, CA 92018-2283　　　　　　　800-756-7533
　　　　　　　　　　　　　　　　　　Fax: 760-434-5476
　　　　　　　　　　　　　　　e-mail: gzcatl@aol.com
　　　　　　　　　　　　　　　　　　www.bulimia.com

3616 Insights in the Dynamic Psychotherapy of Anorexia and Bulimia
Jason Aronson
400 Keystone Industrial Park
Dunmore, PA 18512-1523　　　　　　　800-782-0015
　　　　　　　　　　　　　　　　　　Fax: 201-840-7242
　　　　　　　　　　　　　　　　　　www.aronson.com

320 pages Hardcover
ISBN: 0-876685-68-8

3617 It's Not Your Fault
Gurze Books
PO Box 2238
Carlsbad, CA 92018-2238　　　　　　　800-756-5476
　　　　　　　　　　　　　　　　　　Fax: 760-434-5476
　　　　　　　　　　　　　　　e-mail: gzcatl@aol.com
　　　　　　　　　　　　　　　　　　www.bulimia.com
In this comprehensive, medically sound guide to overcoming eating disorders, Dr. Marx defines the warnings signs of eating disorders, explores causes, at risk populations, the role of drug therapy and advises patients and families where and how they can find help.

3618 Making Peace with Food
Gurze Books
PO Box 2238
Carlsbad, CA 92018-2238　　　　　　　800-756-7533
　　　　　　　　　　　　　　　　　　Fax: 760-434-5476
　　　　　　　　　　　　　　　e-mail: gzcatl@aol.com
　　　　　　　　　　　　　　　　　　www.bulimia.com
This unique, full sized workbook is designed to help anyone who experienced compulsive eating, yo-yo dieting, food and body anxiety, or associated eating disorders. Filled with ideas, workbook pages, exercises and resources, Kano's book is an excellent aid to clarifying and overcoming your personal diet/weight struggle.
224 pages Paperback

3619 Meals Without Squeals Sense
Bull Publishing
PO Box 1377
Boulder, CO 80306　　　　　　　　　800-676-2855
　　　　　　　　　　　　　　　　　　Fax: 303-545-6354
　　　　　　　　　　　　　　　　　　www.bullpub.com
Straight forward information on childrens growth accompanies age specific, child tested recipes. Explained is how common feeding problems can be solved and show ways to offer children positive experiences with food.
2006 288 pages
ISBN: 1-933503-00-4

3620 My Name is Caroline
Doubleday
666 Fifth Avenue　　　　　　　　　212-354-6500
New York, NY 10103
A poignant tale of one woman's battle with bulimia throughout her life as a successful student, athlete, scholar and musician.
Grades 10-12

3621 Obesity: Theory and Therapy
Raven Press
1185 Avenue of the Americas　　　　212-930-9500
New York, NY 10036-2601　　　　　800-777-2295
A classic reference for clinicians dealing with obesity, this volume provides the most up-to-date research, preclinical and clinical information.
500 pages
ISBN: 0-881678-84-8

3622 Practice Guidelines for Eating Disorders
American Psychiatric Press
1400 K Street NW　　　　　　　　　202-682-6268
Washington, DC 20005-2403　　　　Fax: 202-789-2648
Designed for health care professionals, this guideline includes information on all aspects of anorexia nervosa and bulimia nervosa, including self-induced vomiting, use of laxatives and vigorous exercise to prevent weight gain.
38 pages Paperback
ISBN: 0-890423-00-8

3623 Psychodynamic Technique in the Treatment of the Eating Disorders
Jason Aronson
PO Box 15100
York, PA 17405-7100　　　　　　　800-782-0015
　　　　　　　　　　　　　　　　　Fax: 201-840-7242
　　　　　　　　　　　　　　　　　www.aronson.com

440 pages Hardcover
ISBN: 0-876686-22-6

3624 Self-Starvation
Jason Aronson
PO Box 15100
York, PA 17405-7100　　　　　　　800-782-0015
　　　　　　　　　　　　　　　　　Fax: 201-840-7242
　　　　　　　　　　　　　　　　　www.aronson.com

312 pages Softcover
ISBN: 1-568218-22-2

3625 Starving to Death in a Sea of Objects
Jason Aronson
PO Box 15100
York, PA 17405-7100　　　　　　　800-782-0015
　　　　　　　　　　　　　　　　　Fax: 201-840-7242
　　　　　　　　　　　　　　　　　www.aronson.com
How emancipation becomes security for anorexics.
464 pages Softcover
ISBN: 0-876684-35-5

3626 Surviving an Eating Disorder: Perspectives & Strategies
Gurze Books
PO Box 2238
Carlsbad, CA 92018-2238　　　　　　800-756-7533
　　　　　　　　　　　　　　　　　Fax: 760-434-5476
　　　　　　　　　　　　　　　e-mail: gzcatl@aol.com
　　　　　　　　　　　　　　　　　www.bulimia.com

Parents, spouses and friends of individuals with food problems will find practical guidelines in this book for helping themselves and their loved ones.
222 pages Paperback

3627 Treating Bulimia: A Psychoeducational Approach
American Anorexia/Bulimia Association
165 W 46th Street　　　　　　　　　212-575-6200
New York, NY 10036-2501　　　　e-mail: amanbu@aol.com
　　　　　　　　　　　　　www.members.aol.com/amanbu

3628 When Food is Love
Gurze Books
PO Box 2238
Carlsbad, CA 92018-2238　　　　　　800-756-7533
　　　　　　　　　　　　　　　　　Fax: 760-434-5467
　　　　　　　　　　　　　　　e-mail: gzcatl@aol.com
　　　　　　　　　　　　　　　　　www.gurze.com
Drawing on her own personal experience, Roth explores similarities between eating and loving such as fantasizing, wanting the forbidden, creating drama, control issues, and the experience of relationship.
205 pages Paperback

3629 Withering Child
University of Georgia Press
330 Research Drive　　　　　　　　404-542-2830
Athens, GA 30602　　　　　　　　　800-266-5842
　　　　　　　　　　　　　　　　　Fax: 709-369-6131
　　　　　　　　　　　　e-mail: books@ugapress.uga.edu
　　　　　　　　　　　　　　　www.uga.edu/ugapress

1993 288 pages
ISBN: 0-820315-60-5

Children's Books

3630 **Billy's Story**
Metro Intergroup of Overeaters Anonymous
117 W 26th Street   212-206-8621
New York, NY 10001

3631 **I Was a Fifteen-Year-Old Blimp**
Harper & Row
10 E 53rd Street   212-207-7000
New York, NY 10022-5299
This story focuses on Gabby, a teenage girl who overhears others discuss her weight and takes radical steps to become popular.
Grades 6-9

Magazines

3632 **BASH Magazine**
Bulimia Anorexia Self-Help/Behavior Adaptation
PO Box 39903
Saint Louis, MO 63139-8903   800-762-3334
A journal of eating and mood disorders.
Monthly

Newsletters

3633 **AABA Newsletter**
American Anorexic and Bulemic Association
165 W 46th Street   212-575-6200
New York, NY 10036-2501
This newsletter is published three times a year and is mailed to the members of the AABA. The AABA is a tax-exempt, nonprofit organization with a membership of professionals, sufferers of eating disorders, and their family and friends.

3634 **Eating Disorders Review**
Gurze Books
PO Box 2238
Carlsbad, CA 92018-9883   800-756-7533
                                     Fax: 760-434-5476
                                     e-mail: gzcatl@aol.com
                                     www.bulimia.com
Presents current clinical information for the professional treating eating disorders. Features summeries of relevant research from journals and unpublished studies, abstracts, nutritional notes, questions and answers, book reviews and reproducible client handouts.
8 pages BiMonthly
Joel Yager MD, Editor-in-Chief
Liegh Cohn, Publisher

3635 **National Association of Anorexia Nervosa and Associated Disorders Newsletter**
PO Box 7   847-831-3438
Highland Park, IL 60035   Fax: 847-433-4632
                                     e-mail: anad20@aol.com
                                     www.anad.org

2 pages Quarterly
Vivian Hansen Meehan, President
Dawn Ries, Administrator

3636 **WIN Notes**
Weight-control Information Network
1 WIN Way   202-828-1025
Bethesda, MD 20892-3665   877-946-4627
                                     Fax: 202-828-1028
            e-mail: win@mathewsgroup.com
          www.niddk.nih.gov/health/nutrit/win.htm
Addresses the health information needs of individuals with weight-control problems. Available on the WIN web site.
BiAnnual

3637 **Working Together**
Anorexia Nervosa and Associated Disorders
PO Box 7   847-831-3438
Highland Park, IL 60035-0007   Fax: 847-433-4632

Designed for individuals, families, group leaders and professionals concerned with eating disorders. Provides updates on treatments, resources, conferences, programs, articles by therapists, recovered victims, group members and leaders.
Quarterly
Dawn Ries, Administrator

Pamphlets

3638 **Applying New Attitudes & Directions**
Anorexia Nervosa and Associated Disorders
PO Box 7   847-831-3438
Highland Park, IL 60035-0007   Fax: 847-433-4632
                                     e-mail: anad20@aol.com
Self-help booklet offering an eight-step program to recovery with suggestions, information and recovery stories.
Dawn Ries, Administrator

Audio & Video

3639 **Bulimia: A Guide to Recovery**
Gurze Books
PO Box 2238
Carlsbad, CA 92018-2238   800-756-7533
                                     Fax: 760-434-5476
                                     e-mail: gzcatl@aol.com
                                     www.bulimia.com
This newly rediscovered tape is an inspirational talk by Lindsey Hall on the relationship between bulimia, self-esteem and love. This was one of Lindsey's last public appearances, where she addressed a 1991 eating disorers conference in Colorado Springs.
Audio tape

Web Sites

3640 **Anorexia Nervosa & Related Eating Disorders**
                                     www.anred.com
Comprehensive site on eating disorders and related issues.

3641 **GERD Information Resource Center**
                                     www.gerd.com
A resource center with educational resources on Gastroesophageal Reflux Disease (GERD).

3642 **Gastroenterology Therapy Online**
                                     www.gastrotherapy.com
An informational website with resources for many kinds of diseases.

3643 **Healing Well**
                                     www.healingwell.com
An online health resource guide to medical news, chat, information and articles, newsgroups and message boards, books, disease-related web sites, medical directories, and more for patients, friends, and family coping with disabling diseases, disorders, or chronic illnesses.

3644 **Health Finder**
                                     www.healthfinder.gov
Searchable, carefully developed web site offering information on over 1000 topics. Developed by the US Department of Health and Human Services, the site can be used in both English and Spanish.

3645 **Healthlink USA**
                                     www.healthlinkusa.com
Health information concerning treatment, cures, prevention, diagnosis, risk factors, research, support groups, email lists, personal stories and much more. Updated regularly.

3646 **Helios Health**
                                     www.helioshealth.com
Online resource for your health information. Detailed information about specific health topics, access to expert advice from our Medical Advisory Board, and up-to-date health news.

3647 **MedicineNet**
                                     www.medicinenet.com

An online resource for consumers providing easy-to-read, authoritative medical and health information.

3648 Medscape

www.medscape.com

Medscape offers specialists, primary care physicians, and other health professionals the Web's most robust and integrated medical information and educational tools.

3649 National Association for Anorexia Nervosa and Associated Disorders

www.anad.org

ANAD provides educational/prevention programs include presentations and early detection packets for schools and community groups, sponsoring local and national training conferences for health professionals, and working with electronic and print media. Undertakes and encourages research, fights insurance discrimination.

3650 National Eating Disorders Association

www.NationalEatingDisorders.org

National nonprofit organization dedicated to increasing the awareness and prevention of eating disorders.

3651 WebMD

www.webmd.com

Information on Eating Disorders, including articles and resources.

3652 Weight-control Information Network

www.niddk.nih.gov/health/nutrit/win.htm

WIN addresses the health information needs of individuals through the production and dissemination of educational materials. In addition, WIN is developing communication strategies for a pilot program to encourage at-risk individuals to achieve and maintain a healthy weight by making changes in their lifestyle.

Description

3653 # Endometriosis

Endometriosis is a hormonal condition in which the tissue that normally lines the inside of the uterus (endometrium) is also found outside the uterus, generally on the outer surface of pelvic organs. These cells respond to the woman's hormonal cycles, and swell and bleed at the time of menses. This causes pain, generally worse with each period, pelvic masses and alterations of the menstrual cycle. The pain may be aggravated by intercourse or defecation. Although the reported incidence varies, endometriosis is commonly found in 10 to 15 percent of women between the ages of 25 and 44 years. It is estimated that 25 to 50 percent of infertile women have this disorder.

Treatment depends on the severity of the symptoms and the age and reproductive wishes of the patient. The pain associated with mild cases may be treated with non-steroidal anti-inflammatory drugs. More severe cases may respond to suppression of ovarian function. Laparoscopic surgery may destroy some of the collection of tissue, and is often used in hopes of improving fertility. Hysterectomy (removal of the uterus) is used for intractable cases, especially in women who do not desire future pregnancy.

National Agencies & Associations

3654 **American Association of Gynecologic Laproscopists**
6757 Katella Avenue 714-503-6200
Cypress, CA 90630-4505 800-554-2245
Fax: 714-503-6201
e-mail: lmichels@aagl.org
www.aagl.com
Our global commitment to women's healthcare is embodied in our continuing medical education of physicians and professionals to further promote the well documented high standards of minimally invasive gynecologic surgery.
Linda Michels, Executive Director
Franklin D Loffer, EVP/Medical Director

3655 **American Society for Reproductive Medicine**
1209 Montgomery Highway 205-978-5000
Birmingham, AL 35216-2809 Fax: 205-978-5005
e-mail: asrm@asrm.com
www.asrm.com
A private, nonprofit medical organization devoted to advancing the knowledge, understanding and expertise in all phases of reproductive medicine and biology. Offers patient education brochures, recommended readings and support. Publishes professional journal and consumer publications.
Robert W Rebar, MD, Executive Director
Andrew LaBarbera, Scientific Director

3656 **Endometriosis Association**
630 Ibis Drive 561-274-7442
Delray Beach, FL 33444 800-239-7280
Fax: 561-274-0931
e-mail: exec-comm@endocenter.org
www.endocenter.org
Nonprofit international organization dedicated to helping women and girls suffering from endometriosis. Services include chapter and support groups, crisis/counseling assistance, education of the public and medical community materials including books and videos.
Ann Koerner, Operations Manager

3657 **Endometriosis Association International**
8585 N 76th Place 414-355-2200
Milwaukee, WI 53223 800-992-3636
Fax: 414-355-6065
www.endometriosisassn.org
Offers a 24 hour crisis call hotline, support groups, education in the form of literature including fact sheets, brochures, newsletters, articles educational videos, books and research.
Mary Lou Ballweg, President/Executive Director
Carolyn Keith, Co-Founder

3658 **Hysterectomy Educational Resources & Services (HERS) Foundation**
422 Bryn Mawr Avenue 610-667-7757
Bala Cynwyd, PA 19004 888-750-4377
Fax: 610-677-8096
e-mail: hersfdn@earthlink.net
www.hersfoundation.com
A nonprofit foundation which provides information about the alternatives to hysterectomy, the risks of the alternatives, and the consequences of the surgery. HERS provides telephone counseling by appointment for a fee of $5.00 per quarter hour. The fee can be waived if necessary. HERS also provides copies of a medical journals, a quarterly newsletter, and a free lending library of books, videos and audio tapes.

3659 **International Pelvic Pain Society Women's Medical Plaza**
Women's Medical Plaza
1100 E Woodfield Road 847-517-8712
Schaumburg, IL 60173 800-624-9676
Fax: 847-517-7229
e-mail: info@pelvicpain.org
www.pelvicpain.org
Short range goal is to recruit organize and educate health care professionals actively involved with the treatment of patients who have chronic pelvic pain.
Fred Marion Howard, Chairman of the Board
Howard Taylo Sharp, President

3660 **National Women's Health Network**
1413 K Street 202-682-2640
Washington, DC 20005 Fax: 202-682-2648
e-mail: nwhn@nwhn.org
www.womenshealthnetwork.org
Nonprofit organization that does not accept financial support from pharmaceutical or tobacco companies or medical device manufacturers. Advocates for national policies that protect and promote all women's health and provides evidence-based independent information.
Bindiya Patel, Chairperson
Malika Redmond, Action Vice Chair

Foundations

3661 **Fertility Research Foundation**
877 Park Avenue 212-744-5500
New York, NY 10021 888-439-2999
Fax: 212-744-6536
e-mail: info@frfbaby.com
www.frfbaby.com
Offers information on treatment and the latest research on male and female infertility.
Masood Khatamee MD, Executive Director

Libraries & Resource Centers

3662 **National Womens Health Resource Center**
157 Broad Street
Red Bank, NJ 07701 877-986-9472
Fax: 732-249-4671
e-mail: info@healthywomen.org
www.healthywomen.org
The not-for-profit National Women's Health Resource Center (NWHRC) is the leading independent health information source for women. NWHRC develops and distributes up-to-date and ob-

jective women's health information based on the latest advances in medical research and practice.
Elizabeth Battaglino Cahill, Executive Vice President
Amber McCracken, Director Communications

Research Centers

3663 Dartmouth Medical School: Microbiology Department
Department of Microbiology & Immunology
1 Rope Ferry Road   603-650-1200
Hanover, NH 03755-1404   877-DMS-1797
                                       Fax: 603-650-1202
e-mail: microbiology@dartmouth.edu
www.dms.dartmouth.edu
Dartmouth Medical School is a beacon of discovery and learning stimulating inquiry and harnessing ingenuity for new solutions and better health
Ann Hill, Administrative Assistant
Gregory J MacDonald, Assistant Professor of Medicine

3664 Endometriosis Association Research Program : Vanderbuilt University
1211 Medical Center Drive   615-322-5000
Nashville, TN 37232   Fax: 615-343-8881
www.mc.vanderbilt.edu

Heather Arnold, Senior Secretary

3665 Endometriosis Reseach Center and Women's Hospital
The Endometriosis Research Center
630 Ibis Drive   561-274-7442
Delray Beach, FL 33444   800-239-7280
                                       Fax: 561-274-0931
www.endocenter.org
A nonprofit organization dedicated to establishing a center to conduct research and provide women education and treatment.
Ann Koerner, Operations Manager

3666 University of Tennessee: Division of Reproductive Endocrinology
956 Court Avenue
Memphis, TN 38163   901-528-5859
www.utmem.edu/obgyn/reproductive.htm
Studies into endometriosis.
Dr. Jon Buster, Chief
Kennard Brown, Executive Vice Chancellor & Chief Operat

Support Groups & Hotlines

3667 National Health Information Center
PO Box 1133   310-565-4167
Washington, DC 20013   800-336-4797
                                       Fax: 301-984-4256
e-mail: info@nhic.org
www.health.gov/nhic
A helath information referral service sponsored by the Office of Disease Prevention and Health Promotion. Puts health professionals and consumers who have health questions in touch with those organizations that are best able to provide answers.

3668 RESOLVE Helpline
1760 Old Meadow Road   703-556-7172
McLean, VA 22102   Fax: 703-506-3266
www.resolve.org
A nationwide network mandated to promote reproductive health and to ensure equal access to all family building options for men and women experienceing infertility or other reproductive disorders.
Barbara Collura, President/ CEO
Margaret Cha Berardelli, Director

Books

3669 Alternatives for Women with Endometriosis Guide by Women for Women
Third Side Press

225 W Farragut   773-271-3029
Chicago, IL 60625-1863   Fax: 773-271-0459
                                       e-mail: thirdside@aol.com
174 pages
ISBN: 1-879427-12-5

3670 Coping with Endometriosis
Avery Putnam Penguin
375 Hudson Street   212-366-2000
New York, NY 10014   800-847-5515
                                       Fax: 800-775-4829
e-mail: online@penguinputnam.com
www.penguinputnam.com
Educates readers about the disease, focusing on the particular psychological and emotional concerns that those suffering from endometriosis may have.
322 pages
ISBN: 1-583330-74-7

3671 Endometriosis Sourcebook
Endometriosis Association
8585 N 76th Place   414-355-2200
Milwaukee, WI 53223   800-992-3636
                                       Fax: 414-355-6065
e-mail: endo@endometriosisassn.org
www.EndometriosisAssn.org
Comprehensive, authorative and up-to-date resource that includes information about treatment options, strategies for coping with the disease and its effects on you and those around you.
473 pages Paperback
ISBN: 0-809232-63-4
Mary Lou Ballweg, Founder/Executive Director

3672 Endometriosis and Infertility and Traditio nal Chinese Medicine
Blue Poppy Press
5441 Western Avenue   303-447-8372
Boulder, CO 80301   800-487-9296
                                       Fax: 303-245-8362
e-mail: honora@bluepoppy.com
www.bluepoppy.com/press
An easy to understand guide to Chinese medicine as it relates to endometriosis and infertility.
105 pages Paperback
ISBN: 0-936185-14-7
Honora Wolfe, Marketing Director

3673 Endometriosis: A Key to Healing through Nutrition
Endometriosis Association
8585 N 76th Place   414-355-2200
Milwaukee, WI 53223   800-992-3636
                                       Fax: 414-355-6065
e-mail: endo@endometriosisassn.org
www.endometriosisassn.org
An excellent resource tool to help patients begin making changes in their diets.
Mary Lou Ballweg, Founder/Executive Director

3674 Endometriosis: A Natural Approach
Ulysses Press
PO Box 3440   510-601-8301
Berkeley, CA 94703   800-377-2542
                                       Fax: 510-601-8307
e-mail: ulysses@ulyssespress.com
www.ulyssespress.com
This is a solid resource, written in a clear, basic tone, for anyone who needs information about the widespread disease known as endometriosis. Chapters cover all aspects of endometriosis, from what it is and what causes it, to diagnosis, natural therapies, and conventional treatments.
120 pages
ISBN: 1-569750-88-2

3675 Endometriosis: Advanced Management and Surgical Techniques
Springer Verlag
175 5th Avenue   212-460-1500
New York, NY 10010   800-777-4643
                                       Fax: 212-473-6272
e-mail: service@springer-ny.com
www.springer-ny.com

This book provides a practical, clinical, and thorough examination of both the medical and surgical treatment of this disease.

3676   Endometriosis: Complete Reference for Taking Charge of Your Health
Contemporary Books/McGraw-Hill Companies
130 E Randolf Street   312-233-7596
Chicago, IL 60601   Fax: 312-233-7570
An authoritative guide on endometriosis, including its prevention and relationship with other diseases. Special sections are dedicated to endo and menopause, endo and teenagers, endo and nutrition, endo and cancer as well as endo and environmental toxins.

Newsletters

3677   Endometriosis Association Newsletter
Endometriosis Association
8585 N 76th Place   414-355-2200
Milwaukee, WI 53223   800-992-3636
                                      Fax: 414-355-6065
                    e-mail: endo@endometriosisassn.org
                              www.EndometriosisAssn.org
Contains research updates and latest health news that affects women and girls with endometriosis. Regular features such as crisis call helpers, news and announcements, and request for contact provide networking and support assistance.
10 pages Bi-Monthly
Mary Lou Ballweg, Executive Director

Pamphlets

3678   Infertility: Causes and Treatment
American College/Obstetricians and Gynecologists
409 12th Street SW   304-725-8410
Washington, DC 20024   800-762-2264
                                      Fax: 304-728-2171
                                           www.acog.com
To obtain a free copy of this publication, please send a self-addressed stamped #10 envelope and request by title.

Audio & Video

3679   Monroe Institute Surgical Support Tapes
Endometriosis Association
8585 N 76th Place   414-355-2200
Milwaukee, WI 53223-2633   800-992-3636
                                      Fax: 414-355-6065
                    e-mail: endo@endometriosisassn.org
                              www.EndometriosisAssn.org
Anxiety is normal for women before surgery, so women with endometriosis will be happy to hear this wonderful series of audiotapes specifically developed for relaxation.
Audiotape
Mary Lou Ballweg, Founder/Executive Director

Web Sites

3680   American Society for Reproductive Medicine
                                           www.asrm.com
Devoted to advancing the knowledge, understanding and expertise in all phases of reproductive medicine and biology. Offers patient education brochures, recommended readings and support.

3681   Endometriosis Association
                              www.EndometriosisAssn.org
Nonprofit organization dedicated to helping women and girls suffering from endometriosis. Services include chapter and support groups, crisis/counseling assistance, education of the public and the medical community. Materials, including books, video/audiotapes, CDs, newsletters and articles mostly based on data from the Association's research registries and its extensive research program, including a flagship scientific team at Vanderbuilt University School of Medicine.

3682   Endometriosis Research Center
                                         www.endocenter.org
Maintain and offer a vast database of unbased and fact-based materials on every aspect of Endometriosis to practitioners, researchers, patients and all those interested in the disease.

3683   Endometriosis Support Group
                              www.geocities.com/HotSprings/5422
Online support group and question forum for endometriosis.

3684   Healing Well
                                       www.healingwell.com
An online health resource guide to medical news, chat, information and articles, newsgroups and message boards, books, disease-related web sites, medical directories, and more for patients, friends, and family coping with disabling diseases, disorders, or chronic illnesses.

3685   Health Finder
                                       www.healthfinder.gov
Searchable, carefully developed web site offering information on over 1000 topics. Developed by the US Department of Health and Human Services, the site can be used in both English and Spanish.

3686   Healthlink USA
                                       www.healthlinkusa.com
Health information concerning treatment, cures, prevention, diagnosis, risk factors, research, support groups, email lists, personal stories and much more. Updated regularly.

3687   Helios Health
                                       www.helioshealth.com
Online resource for your health information. Detailed information about specific health topics, access to expert advice from our Medical Advisory Board, and up-to-date health news.

3688   International Pelvic Pain Society
                                       www.pelvicpain.org/
Short range goal is to recruit, organize, and educate health care professionals actively involved with the treatment of patients who have chronic pelvic pain.

3689   MedicineNet
                                       www.medicinenet.com
An online resource for consumers providing easy-to-read, authoritative medical and health information.

3690   Medscape
                                       www.medscape.com
Medscape offers specialists, primary care physicians, and other health professionals the Web's most robust and integrated medical information and educational tools.

3691   Universe of Women's Health
                                           www.obgyn.net
A comprehensive website dedicated to women's health.

3692   WebMD
                                           www.webmd.com
Information on Endometriosis, including articles and resources.

Description

3693 **Fabry Disease**

Fabry disease is an inherited fat storage disorder caused by deficiency of an enzyme involved in the biodegradation of lipids (fats). As abnormal storage of the fatty compound increases with time, blood vessels become narrowed, leading to decreased blood flow. The problem occurs in all blood vessels in the body, but affects in particular the skin, kidneys, heart, brain and nerves.

In children, Fabry begins with pain and burning sensations in hands and feet that is worse with exercise and hot weather. Other symptoms include a dark red rash around the waist, decreased ability to perspire and cloudiness of the cornea, which usually does not affect vision.

As those with Fabry's grow older, they may have impaired circulation, leading to early heart attacks and strokes. As kidneys become more involved, many patients require kidney transplants or dialysis. Gastrointestinal symptoms include frequent bowel movements shortly after eating. Patients with Fabry disease usually survive into adulthood but have a reduced life expectancy.

Currently, there is no cure for Fabry disease and treatment typically deals with controlling its symptoms. Pain in hands and feet respond to several medications. Gastrointestinal hyperactivity may be controlled by taking a nutritional supplement. Enzyme replacement therapy was given a dramatic boost in 2003 when the FDA approved a new synthetic enzyme. It is given intravenously and reduces lipid (fat) accumulation in many types of cells.

National Agencies & Associations

3694 **Association for Neuro-Metabolic Disorders**
3901 Rainbow Boulevard   913-588-5000
Kansas City, KS 66160   800-334-7980
                                         TTY: 913-588-7963
                                  e-mail: VOLK4OLKS@aol.com
                                             www.kumc.edu
Serves as an advocate organization for families of patients with neuro-methabolic disorders such as phenylketonuria, maple syrup urine disease, galactosemia and biotinidase. Provides educational information for parents and children and provides networking.
Barbara F Atkinson MD, Executive Vice Chancellor

3695 **Genetic and Rare Diseases Information Center**
Genetic and Rare Diseases Informati   301-251-4925
Gaithesburg, MD 20898-8126   888-205-2311
                                         Fax: 301-251-4911
                                         TTY: 888-205-3223
                                  e-mail: GARDinfo@nih.gov
                             www.rarediseases.info.nih.gov/GARD
Provides free and immediate access to accurate, reliable information about genetic and rare diseases. Also provides assistance to patients and families, health professionals and other interested parties.
Stephen C. Groft, Director
P.J. Brooks, Health Scientist Administrator

3696 **International Center for Fabry Disease Mt. Sinai School of Medicine**
Mt. Sinai School of Medicine
One Gustave L Levy Place   212-241-6500
New York, NY 10029   866-322-7963
                                  e-mail: fabry.disease@mssm.edu
                                             www.mssm.edu
Clinical research center attended by a staff of physicians and nurses specially trained to understand and meet the needs of individuals with Fabry disease. Services offered to both men and women of all ages include diagnosis, evaluation and treatment consultation.
Robert J Desnick PhD MD, Professor and Chair
Dennis Charney, Executive VP

3697 **National Institute of Neurological Disorders and Stroke (NINDS)**
NIH Neurological Institute   301-496-5751
Bethesda, MD 20824   800-352-9424
                                         Fax: 301-496-0296
                                         TTY: 301-468-5981
                                             www.ninds.nih.gov
The mission of NINDS is to reduce the burden of neurological disease - a burden borne by every age group, by every segment of society, by people all over the world.
Story C Landis PhD, Director
Walter J Koroshetz, Deputy Director

3698 **National Organization for Rare Disorders (NORD)**
55 Kenosia Avenue   203-744-0100
Danbury, CT 06813-1968   800-999-6673
                                         Fax: 203-798-2291
                                         TDD: 203-797-9590
                                  e-mail: orphan@rarediseases.org
                                             www.rarediseases.org
The National Organization for Rare Disorders(NORD), a 501(c)3 organization, is a unique federation of voluntary health organizations dedicated to helping people with rare orphan diseases and assisting the organizations that serve them. NORD is committed to the identification, treatment, and cure of rare disorders through programs of education, advocacy, research, and service.
Frank Sasinowski, Chair
Carolyn Asbury, Vice Chair

3699 **National Tay-Sachs and Allied Disease Association**
2001 Beacon Street   800-906-8723
Brighton, MA 02135   800-906-8723
                                         Fax: 617-277-0134
                                  e-mail: info@ntsad.org
                                             www.ntsad.org
A mutual support group coordinated by staff and volunteers who are parents of affected children of affected adults. One of several programs supported and sponsored by the association.
Bradley L Campbell, President
Stewart Altman, Vice President

Research Centers

3700 **Lysosomal Disease Center at the University of Pittsburgh**
E1650 Biomedical Science Tower
Pittsburgh, PA 15261   800-334-7980
                                                  pitt.edu
Offers diagnosis management treatment and genetic counseling for people with or at risk for lysosomal storage disease and their families.
John A Barrenger MD PhD, Director
Erin O'Rourk, Manager

3701 **National Gaucher Disease Foundation**
2227 Idlewood Road   770-934-2910
Tucker, GA 30084   800-504-3189
                                         Fax: 770-934-2911
                                  e-mail: rhonda@gaucherdisease.org
                                             www.gaucherdisease.org
Provides information and assistance for those affected by Gaucher disease.
Rhonda P Buyers, CEO/Executive Director
Barbara Lichtenstein, Programs Director National Gaucher Care

Support Groups & Hotlines

3702 Fabry Support & Information Group
108 NE 2nd Street Suite C   660-463-1355
Concordia, MO 64020   Fax: 660-463-1356
                                     e-mail: info@fabry.org
                                              www.fabry.org
To raise awareness of Fabry disease and its symptoms. The website provides mutual self-help by linking patients and family members/caregivers. In this way they can support and encourage one another.
J Johnson, Founder

Web Sites

3703 A World of Genetic Societies
                                     www.faseb.org/genetics
Listing of genetic professional societies, many with searchable databases.

3704 Alliance of Genetic Support Groups
                                     www.geneticalliance.org
Coalition of individuals, professionals and genetic support organizations.

3705 Fabry Support & Information Group
                                              www.fabry.org
Discussion page, information about disease, newsletters, patient biographies, links.

3706 Gene Clinics
                                          www.geneclinics.org
Searchable, expert-authored, peer reviewed disease database.

3707 International Center for Fabry Disease
                                 www.mssm.edu/crc/Fabry/fabry.html
Associated with Mt. Sinai, with information about Fabry including a program to family tree.

3708 International Storage Disease Collaborative
                             www.pediatrics.med.umn/edu/isdcsg/
This study group focuses on stem cell and bone marrow transplantation. Has discussion page/general information.

3709 MedicineNet
                                           www.medicinenet.com
An online resource for consumers providing easy-to-read, authoritative medical and health information.

3710 Morbus Fabry
                                              home.t-online.de
Fabry information and links to other sites.

3711 NIH's National Institute of Neurological Disorders & Strokes
                                           www.ninds.nih.gov
Description of disease, therapies.

3712 National Organization for Rare Disorders (NORD)
                                          www.rarediseases.org
The NORD is a unique federation of voluntary health organizations dedicated to helping people with rare orphan diseases and assisting the organization that serve them.

3713 National Society of Genetic Counselors
                                                      nsgc.org
Society website with searchable membership database.

3714 OMIM: Fabry Disease
                                          www.ncbi.nlm.nih.gov
Description of disease and links to research papers written.

3715 Pediatric Database: Fabry Disease
                                              www.icondata.com
Description of disease.

3716 Support-Group.Com: Fabry Disease
                                           www.support-group.com
Fabry Disease discussion forum.

Description

3717 Fibromyalgia Syndrome

Fibromyalgia syndrome, FMS, also called fibrositis or fibromyositis, is a condition of widespread muscular pain and fatigue. It strikes mostly women between the ages of 20 and 50, and may affect as many as one in 20 adult females. The pain ranges from mild discomfort to complete disability and may vary from day to day. Physical over-exertion, changes in weather, drafty environments, stress, depression, and hormonal changes can all contribute to flare-ups in FMS symptoms.

In addition to widespread pain, FMS also causes a decreased sense of energy, disturbances of sleep, and varying degrees of anxiety and depression. Other medical conditions sometimes associated with fibromyalgia include tension headaches, migraine, irritable bowel syndrome, premenstrual tension syndrome, chronic fatigue syndrome, cold intolerance, and restless leg syndrome.

A physician's diagnosis of FMS is usually based on the following criteria: widespread musculoskeletal pain; tenderness at 11 or more of 18 specific tender points, which are exquisitely more tender than adjacent sites; and scans of the brain. Fibromyalgia may remit spontaneously with decreased stress but can recur at frequent intervals or become chronic.

There is currently no commonly accepted cure for this condition. Aspirin and other drugs used to treat musculoskeletal pain partially improve symptoms. Antidepressant drugs, taken in low doses, have been shown to provide restorative sleep. Patients may also benefit from regular aerobic exercises, local applications of heat, gentle massage and reduced stress in their lives. See also *Chronic Fatigue Syndrome*.

National Agencies & Associations

3718 American Fibromyalgia Syndrome Association
6380 East Tanque Verde   520-733-1570
Tucson, AZ 85715   Fax: 520-290-5550
e-mail: kthorson@afsafund.org
www.afsafund.org
Nonprofit organization whose primary mission is to seed research in FMS and CFS. We acknowledge that patient and physician education, public awareness and advocacy are all important ingredients in aiding the lives of people with FMS and CFS.
Kristen Thorson, President
Steve Thorson, VP

3719 FM-CFS Canada
99 Fifth Avenue   www.fm-cfs.ca
Ottawa, Ontario, K1S-5P5
Dedicated to advancing Fibromyalgia (FM) and Chronic Fatigue Syndrome (CFS) education, research and treatment.
Graham Mayes, President/Director
Ed Napke, VP/Director

3720 National Chronic Fatigue Syndrome and Fibromyalgia Association
PO Box 18426   816-737-1343
Kansas City, MO 64133   Fax: 816-524-6782
e-mail: information@ncfsfa.org
www.ncfsfa.org

Offering a support group, medical and patient information plus research.
Orvalene Prewitt, President

3721 National Chronic Fatigue Syndrome and Fibr
PO Box 18426   816-737-1343
Kansas City, MO 64133   Fax: 816-524-6782
e-mail: information@ncfsfa.org
www.ncfsfa.org
Offering a support group medical and patient information plus research.
Orvalene Prewitt, President

3722 National Fibromyalgia Association
2121 S Towne Centre Place   714-921-0150
Anaheim, CA 92806   Fax: 714-921-6920
e-mail: kfox@fmaware.org
www.fmaware.org
Develops and extends programs dedicated to improving the quality of life for people with Fibromyalgia by increasing the awareness of the public media government and medical communities. Supports an ongoing media presence and assist local support groups.
Lynne Matallana, Founder/President
Rae Marie Gleason, Executive Director

3723 National Fibromyalgia Partnership (NFP)
PO Box 160
Linden, VA 22642   866-725-4404
Fax: 866-666-2727
e-mail: mail@fmpartnership.org
www.fmpartnership.org
The NFP is a 501(c)(3) non-profit, membership organization which publishes medically accurate information on Fibromyalgia to patients, health care professionals and the public. Information and resources not listed in this volume are available in print and/or on the NFP Web site. It also provides support and start-up information to support groups.
Tamara K Liller, President & Director of Publications
Jacqueline M Yencha, Vice-President, Asst Dir of Publications

3724 National Hemophilia Foundation/Hemophilia and AIDS/HIV Network (HANDI)
116 W 32nd Street   212-328-3700
New York, NY 10001   Fax: 212-328-3777
www.hemophilia.org
Dedicated to the treatment and the cure of hemophilia AIDS and other blood related disorders. This foundation wished to improve the quality of life of all those affected through promotion and support of research education and other services.
Val Bias, CEO
Neil Frick, Vice President

3725 National ME/FM Action Network
National ME/FM Action Network   613-829-6667
Suite 512, K2H8V- 8V7   Fax: 613-829-8518
www.mefmaction.net
A non-profit organization dedicated to advancing the recognition and understanding of Myalgic Encephalomyelitis/Chronic Fatigue Syndrome (ME/CFS) and Fibromyalgia Syndrome (FMS) through education, advocacy, support, and research.
Lydia E. Neilson, Founder and Chief Executive Officer
Margaret Parlor, President

3726 Option Institute
2080 S Undermountain Road   413-229-2100
Sheffield, MA 01257   800-714-2779
Fax: 413-229-8931
e-mail: participantsupport@option.org
www.option.org
Self-defeating beliefs along with attitudes and judgments can lead to a host of physical and psychological challenges, including Fibromyalgia. The Option Institute offers programs designed to help you gain new perspectives on the attitudes and judgments that can hamper progress.
Barry Kaufman, Co-Founder
Samahria Lyt Kaufman, Co-Founder

Libraries & Resource Centers

3727 Fibromyalgia Resources Group
103 Sherwood Hill Road 845-278-5944
Brewster, NY 10509 Fax: 845-278-2641
e-mail: kindness@fibrobetsy.com
Personalized patient service searches and distributes information on patient recommended, fibromyalgia literate doctors world wide. Information packet is included with each doctor list emailed. Doctor recommendations are welcome.
Betsy Jacobson, President

Support Groups & Hotlines

3728 Fibromyalgia Network
PO Box 31750 520-290-5508
Tucson, AZ 85751-1750 800-853-2929
Fax: 520-290-5550
e-mail: inquiry@fmnetnews.com
www.fmnetnews.com
Provides individuals with ad-free, patient-focused information that can be use today.

3729 National Chronic Fatigue Syndrome and Fibromyalgia Association Support Group
PO Box 18426 816-737-1343
Kansas City, MO 64133 Fax: 816-524-6782
e-mail: information@ncfsfa.org
www.ncfsfa.org
To educate and inform the public about the nature and impact of Chronic Fatigue Syndrome and Fibromyalgia and related disorders.
Orvalene Prewitt, President

3730 National Health Information Center
PO Box 1133 310-565-4167
Washington, DC 20013 800-336-4797
Fax: 301-984-4256
e-mail: info@nhic.org
www.health.gov/nhic
A health information referral service sponsored by the Office of Disease Prevention and Health Promotion. Puts health professionals and consumers who have health questions in touch with those organizations that are best able to provide answers.

3731 Rocky Mountain CFIDS/FMS Association
7020 E Girard Avenue 303-423-7367
Denver, CO 80224 e-mail: link@rmcfa.org
www.rmcfa.org
An educational resource for patients, medical professionals and those affected by these diseases.
Tim Smith, President
Mike Munoz, Executive Director

Books

3732 All About Fibromyalgia
Oxford University Press
198 Madison Avenue 212-726-6033
New York, NY 10016-4314 800-451-7556
Fax: 212-726-6447
www.oup-usa.org

ISBN: 0-195147-53-7

3733 Delicate Balance: Living Successfully with Chronic Illness
Perseus Books Group
5500 Central Avenue
Boulder, CO 80301 800-386-5656
Fax: 303-449-3356
e-mail: info@perseuspublishing.com
www.perseuspublishing.com
Up to date and practical advice and inspiration for the millions of Americans who struggle daily against chronic illness. From locating a suitable healthcare provider and making sense of the powerful emotions that accompany chronic illness, to seeking accomodations from the Americans with Disabilities Act, this book is helpful and hopeful.
312 pages
ISBN: 0-738203-23-8

3734 Fibromyalgia
NAMSIC/National Institutes of Health
1 AMS Circle 301-495-4484
Bethesda, MD 20892-0001 877-226-4267
Fax: 301-718-6366
TTY: 301-565-2966
e-mail: niamsinfo@mail.nih.gov
www.nih.gov/niams

3735 Fibromyalgia & Other Central Pain Syndromes
Daniel Wallace, Daniel Clauw, author
Lippincott Williams & Wilkins
16522 Hunters Green Parkway
Hagerstown, MD 21740-2116 800-638-3030
Fax: 301-223-2400
www.lww.com
Devoted to fibromyalgia and other centrally mediated chronic pain syndromes. Leading experts examine the latest research findings on these syndromes and present evidence-based reviews of current controversies.
2005
ISBN: 0-781752-61-2

3736 Fibromyalgia Guidelines: The Concensus Diagnosis & Treatment Protocols
FM-CFS Canada
99 Fifth Avenue www.fm-cfs.ca/fm
Ottawa, ON K1S-5P5
This entire special issue of the Journal of Musculoskeletal Pain [JMP] is devoted to presentation of what will likely to be called the Canadian Consensus Document on Fibromyalgia Syndrome (FMS). The document encompasses a very broad scope, involving a clinical case definition, diagnosis, and management of FMS.
130 pages

3737 Fibromyalgia Relief Book: 213 Ideas for Improving Your Quality of Life
Walker & Company
435 Hudson Street 212-727-8300
New York, NY 10014 Fax: 212-727-0984
e-mail: orders@walkerbooks.com
www.walkerbooks.com

208 pages Paperback
ISBN: 0-802775-53-5
Josh Wood, Sales Director

3738 Fibromyalgia Supporter
Anadem Publishing Company
3620 N High Street
Columbus, OH 43214 800-633-0055
Fax: 614-262-6630
e-mail: anadem@anadem.com
www.anadem.com

3739 Fibromyalgia Survivor
Anadem Publishing Company
3620 N High Street
Columbus, OH 43214 800-633-0055
Fax: 614-262-6630
e-mail: anadem@anadem.com
www.anadem.com

ISBN: 0-964689-12-X

3740 Fibromyalgia Syndrome and Chronic Fatigue Syndrome in Young People
Fibromyalgia Network
PO Box 31750
Tucson, AZ 85751-1750 800-853-2929
Fax: 520-290-5550
www.fmnetnews.com

Guide for parents.

3741 Fibromyalgia and Chronic Myofascial Pain Syndrome: a Survivor Manual
New Harbinger Publishers
5674 Shattuck Avenue
Oakland, CA 94609
800-748-6273
Fax: 510-652-5472
www.newharbinger.com
Written from the perspective of myofacial pain syndrome.
432 pages

3742 Fibromyalgia, Managing the Pain
Anadem Publishing Company
3620 N High Street
Columbus, OH 43214-3611
800-633-0055
Fax: 614-262-6630
e-mail: anadem@anadem.com
www.anadem.com
Comprehensive guide to the syndrome, including chapters on diagnosis, medication, physical medicine treatments, occupational adjustments, advice on flare ups and some medical and legal aspects of FMS.

3743 Inside Fibromyalgia
Anadem Publishing Company
3620 N High Street
Columbus, OH 43214
614-262-2539
800-633-0055
Fax: 614-262-6630
e-mail: anadem@anadem.com
www.anadem.com
Written by a physician who has fibromyalgia. From the newest medications to alternative therapies and everything in between, Dr. Pellegrino helps you develop a plan for healing today and tomorrow.
Paperback
ISBN: 1-890018-36-8

3744 Laugh at Your Muscles
Anadem Publishing Company
3620 N High Street
Columbus, OH 43214-3611
800-633-0055
Fax: 614-262-6630
e-mail: anadem@anadem.com
www.anadem.com

3745 Taking Charge of Fibromyalgia
FMS Educational Systems
500 Bushway Road
Wayzata, MN 55391
419-841-3435
Fax: 419-841-3435
e-mail: info@fmsedsys.com
www.fmsedsys.com
Written by three professionals who have fibromyalgia and who often update the book.

3746 Taking Control of TMJ: Your Total Wellness Program
Robert O Uppgaard, DDS, author
New Harbinger Publications
5674 Shattuck Avenue
Oakland, CA 94609
800-748-6273
Fax: 510-652-5472
www.newharbinger.com
Six-step wellness program helps readers understand what TMJ is and provides exercises to improve jaw functioning, relieve pain and deal with trigger points, eliminate harmful habits, deal with contributing stress, and evaluate and improve your diet and exercise habits. Additional chapters cover the connection between TMJ, whiplash, and fibromyalgia.
2004 200 pages Paperback
ISBN: 1-572241-26-8

3747 Understanding Post-Traumatic Fibromyalgia
Anadem Publishing Company
3620 N High Street
Columbus, OH 43214-3611
800-633-0055
Fax: 614-262-6630
e-mail: anadem@anadem.com
www.anadem.com
Anyone with post-traumatic fibromyalgia will benefit from reading this book focusing exclusively on this condition.

Magazines

3748 FM Monograph
National Fibromyalgia Partnership
PO Box 160
Linden, VA 22642
866-725-4404
Fax: 866-666-2727
e-mail: mail@fmpartnership.org
www.fmpartnership.org
Publishes a print quarterly (available online and in booklet form in English, Spanish, and French) which provides information on fibromyalgia symptoms, diagnosis, treatment, and research. Comprehensive resource packets and reprints are also available on a variety of subjects. Technical support is provided to fibromyalgia support organizations worldwide.
Quarterly
Tamara Liller, President

3749 Fibromyalgia AWARE
National Fibromyalgia Association
2238 N Glassell Street
Orange, CA 92865
714-921-0150
Fax: 714-921-6920
e-mail: nfa@FMaware.org
www.FMaware.org
Official publication of the National Fibromyalgia Association. Available to members and contributors.

3750 Fibromyalgia Frontiers
National Fibromyalgia Partnership (NFP)
PO Box 160
Linden, VA 22642
866-725-4404
Fax: 866-666-2727
e-mail: mail@fmpartnership.org
www.fmpartnership.org
Publishes a print quarterly (available online and in booklet form in English, Spanish, and French) which provides information on fibromyalgia symptoms, diagnosis, treatment, and research. Comprehensive resource packets and reprints are also available on a variety of subjects. Technical support is provided to fibromyalgia support organizations worldwide. Included with membership into NFP.
Quarterly
Tamara Liller, President

3751 Journal of Musculoskeletal Pain
Haworth Medical Press
10 Alice Street
Binghamton, NY 13904-1503
607-722-5857
800-429-6784
Fax: 607-722-0012
e-mail: getinfo@haworthpress.com
www.haworthpress.com
Peer reviewed medical journal containing FMS scientific abstract information. Appropriate for medical professionals as well as amateur.
Quarterly

Newsletters

3752 Fibromyalgia Clinic Kentfield Rehabilitation Newsletter
Fibromyalgia Clinic
25 Sir Francis Drake Boulevard
Kentfield, CA 94904
415-485-3530

3753 Florida Fibromyalgia News
FMS Association of Florida
PO Box 14848
Gainesville, FL 32604-4848
352-371-2750
Quarterly newsletter.

3754 Health Points
TyH Publications
17007 E Colony Drive
Fountain Hills, AZ 85268
800-801-1406
e-mail: editor@e-tyh.com
National newsletter with articles on complementary therapy, latest nutrition news, disability issues and much more. Focus is on fibromyalgia, chronic fatigue, arthritis and chronic pain.
Quarterly

3755 Healthwatch
CFIDS and Fibromyalgia Health Resource
2040 Alameda Padre Serra
Santa Barbara, CA 93103   800-366-6056
                                      Fax: 805-965-0042
               e-mail: cutomerservice@prohealthinc.com
                                   www.immunesupport.com
Healthwatch serves fibromyalgia and chronic fatigue syndrome
sufferers by focusing on reporting the latest news in research and
treatment, making hard-to-find nutritional supplements available
at low prices, and raising needed funds for medical research.

3756 Journal of Musculoskeletal Medicine
Cliggott Publishing Company
55 Holly Hill Lane   203-661-0600
Greenwich, CT 06830-6074
This journal provides a unique and efficient monthly update on the
management of musculoskeletal disorders. Offers articles regarding orthopedics, rheumatology, sports medicine, etc.

3757 To Your Health and Healthpoints
To Your Health
17007 E Colony Drive
Fountain Hills, AZ 85268   800-801-1406
                                      Fax: 480-837-1875
                                          www.e-tyh.com
Resource catalogue and newspaper for FMS, CFIDS, arthritis, and
chronic pain. Features vitamins and health products developed
specifically for FMS and CFIDS making hard-to-find, recommended nutritional supplements available to fibromyalgia and
chronic fatigue syndrome sufferers at a manufacturer-direct low
price.

Audio & Video

3758 Audio Cassette Program on Fibromyalgia
Arthritis Foundation/Research Cassettes
111 E Wacker Drive   312-616-3470
Chicago, IL 60601-3713
Covers treatment and research taped during a patient education
forum.

3759 Fibromyalgia Interval Training
Arthritis Foundation Distribution Center
PO Box 6996
Alpharetta, GA 30023-6996   800-207-8633
                                      Fax: 770-442-9742
                                        www.arthritis.com
Designed for people with fibromyalgia, the video features warm
water exercises in shallow and deep water, including warmup,
stretching, upper and lower body exercises, aerobics, strengthing,
cool-down and relaxation. Designed to help you manage the pain,
stiffness and fatigue of fibromyalgia.

3760 Fibromyalgia Stretch Video & Strength and Toning Video
Oregon Fibromyalgia Foundation
1221 SW Yamhill
Portland, OR 97205   503-228-3217
                                          www.myalgia.com
These videos offer comprehensive stretching and strength and toning regimens developed by exercise physiologist Sharon Clark
PhD, FNP, specifically for people with FMS. Fibromyalgia patients are shown demonstrating these unique stretching and
strength and toning programs. Prices are per video and do not include shipping and handling.

3761 Fibromyalgia: Face to Face
Ontario Fibromyalgia Association
250 Cloor Street E   416-979-7228
Toronto, Ontario, M4W
A 14 minute insight into living with FMS from people, including
children, who are coping with this syndrome.

3762 Improving Muscle Tone and Strength
Oregon Fibromyalgia Foundation
1221 SW Yamhill   503-228-3217
Portland, OR 97205
A video developed by exercise physiologist Sharon Clark, PhD,
RN, specifically for people with fibromyalgia.

Web Sites

3763 American Fibromyalgia Research Association
                                         www.afsafund.org
Charitable organization whose primary mission is to seed research
in FMS and CFS. We acknowledge that patient and physician education, public awareness and advocacy are all important ingredients in aiding the lives of people with FMS and CFS.

3764 FM/CFS Canada
                                            www.fm-cfs.ca
Dedicated to advancing Fibromyalgia (FM) and Chronic Fatigue
Syndrome (CFS) education, research and treatment.

3765 Healing Well
                                        www.healingwell.com
An online health resource guide to medical news, chat, information and articles, newsgroups and message boards, books, disease-related web sites, medical directories, and more for patients,
friends, and family coping with disabling diseases, disorders, or
chronic illnesses.

3766 Health Finder
                                         www.healthfinder.gov
Searchable, carefully developed web site offering information on
over 1000 topics. Developed by the US Department of Health and
Human Services, the site can be used in both English and Spanish.

3767 Healthlink USA
                                       www.healthlinkusa.com
Health information concerning treatment, cures, prevention, diagnosis, risk factors, research, support groups, email lists, personal
stories and much more. Updated regularly.

3768 Helios Health
                                        www.helioshealth.com
Online resource for your health information. Detailed information
about specific health topics, access to expert advice from our Medical Advisory Board, and up-to-date health news.

3769 MedicineNet
                                        www.medicinenet.com
An online resource for consumers providing easy-to-read, authoritative medical and health information.

3770 Medscape
                                          www.medscape.com
Medscape offers specialists, primary care physicians, and other
health professionals the Web's most robust and integrated medical
information and educational tools.

3771 My Fibromyalgia & Chronic Fatigue Syndrome
                                           www.fms-help.com
A woman's personal story about her battle with fibromyalgia.

3772 National Fibromyalgia Association
                                           www.fmaware.org
Information for fibromyalgia patients and the general public.

3773 National Fibromyalgia Partnership (NFP)
PO Box 160
Linden, VA 22642   866-725-4404
                                      Fax: 866-666-2727
                          e-mail: mail@fmpartnership.org
                                   www.fmpartnership.org
The NFP is a 501(c)(3) non-profit, membership organization
which publishes medically accurate information on fibromyalgia
to patients, health care professionals and the public. Information
and resources not listed in this volume are available in print and/or
on the NFP website. It also provides support and start-up
informaiton to support groups. Additional website:
www.frontiersnews.org
Tamara K Liller, President & Director of Publications
Jacqueline M Yencha, Vice-President, Asst Dir of Publications

3774 Neurology Channel
                                       www.neurologychannel.com
Find clearly explained, medically accurate information regarding
conditions, including an overview, symptoms, causes, diagnostic
procedures and treatment options. On this site it is possible to ask

questions and get information from a neurologist and connect to people who have similar health interests.

3775 Option Institute
Option Institute

www.option.org/fibromyalgia.html

Self-defeating beliefs, along with attitudes and judgments, can lead to a host of physical and psychological challenges, including Fibromyalgia. The Option Institute offers programs designed to help you gain new perspectives on the attitudes and judgments that may be affecting your life, especially those regarding and surrounding Fibromyalgia.

3776 WebMD

www.webmd.com

Information on Fibromyalgia Syndrome, including articles and resources.

Description

3777 Gastrointestinal Disorders

The digestive tract is responsible for taking food into the body, processing it into simple chemicals that can be absorbed to nourish the body, and expelling the remainder.

Motility disorders of the gastrointestinal (GI) tract are conditions in which there is a failure of normal top-to-bottom movement of gastric contents. In reflux, the food content moves from the stomach back into the esophagus, irritating that organ and causing heartburn, the most common symptom. This is known as GERD, or gastro-esophageal reflux disease, and sometimes causes choking or coughing. Complications include inflammation and even ulceration of the esophagus. It is a problem in infants, but also occurs in adults especially with advancing age. Occasionally, an ulcer may develop in a segment of the GI tract, typically in the stomach or duodenum. An infectious agent, H. pylori, plays a central role in peptic ulcer disease. In achalasia, the normal movement of food down the GI tract by peristalsis is disrupted, and contents of the esophagus are unable to move into the stomach. As a result, the person chokes on food or liquid. Chest pain and coughing at night may also occur.

Other motility disorders reflect the bowel's inability to move its contents forward properly. Children may be born with Hirschprung's disease in which peristalsis is absent or abnormal in the large bowel, resulting in partial or complete obstruction. The most common motility disorder in adults is called irritable bowel syndrome; also known as functional bowel or spastic colitis, it causes variable degrees of abdominal pain and bloating, diarrhea and/or constipation.

Outpouchings in the walls of the lower GI tract, called diverticula, sometimes trap nutrient waste, and may become infected, bleed, and rupture. Finally, the digestive tract may fail in its primary task of absorbing nutrients, known as malabsorption syndromes. Rarely it will absorb too much of something. In hemochromatosis, for instance, the bowel takes in too much iron from the diet, and the excess is stored in and damages the liver, pancreas, heart, and gonads. More commonly, the body absorbs too little nutrient rather than too much. For instance, celiac disease, or sprue, is a disorder caused by intolerance to gluten, a cereal protein in wheat rye, barley, and oats. Lactose intolerance is an inability to digest a carbohydrate in dairy products. Treatment for malabsorption syndromes includes dietary modifications and, in more serious cases, supplementation with intravenous feedings known as parenteral nutrition.

National Agencies & Associations

3778 American College of Gastroenterology
PO Box 342260
Bethesda, MD 20827-2260   301-263-9000
www.acg.gi.org

ACG serves clinical and scientific information needs of member physicians and surgeons who specialize in digestive and related disorders. Emphasis is on scholarly practice, teaching and research.
Delbert H Chumley MD, President
Edgar Achkar, Director

3779 American Dietetic Association
120 S Riverside Plaza   312-899-0040
Chicago, IL 60606-6995   800-877-1600
e-mail: media@eatright.org
www.eatright.org

ADA serves the public through the promotion of optimal nutrition health and well-being.
Patricia M Babjak, Chief Executive Officer
Judith Rodriguez, President

3780 American Gastroenterological Association National Office
National Office
4930 Del Ray Avenue   301-654-2055
Bethesda, MD 20814   Fax: 301-654-5920
e-mail: member@gastro.org
www.gastro.org

AGA fosters the development and application of the science of gastroenterology by providing leadership and aid including patient care, research, teaching, continuing education, scientific communication and matters of national health policy.
Ian L Taylor MD, President
Loren Lane, Vice President

3781 American Hemochromatosis Society
4044 W Lake Mary Boulevard   407-829-4488
Lake Mary, FL 32746-2012   888-655-4766
Fax: 407-333-1284
e-mail: mail@americanhs.org
www.americanhs.org

Educates the public, the medical community and the media by distributing the most current information available on hereditary hemochromatosis (HH) including DNA screening for HH and pediatric HH; also facilitates patient empowerment through an online network.
Sandra Thomas, President/Founder

3782 American Motility Society
45685 Harmony Lane   734-699-1130
Belleville, MI 48111   Fax: 734-699-1136
e-mail: admin@motilitysociety.org
www.motilitysociety.org

Promotes research and sponsors professional education seminars about gastrointestinal motility topics including disorders of esophageal, gastric, small intestinal, and colonic function; and sponsors biennial meetings (even years), syposia and courses.
Michael Cami MD, President
Lori Ennis, Executive Director

3783 American Pancreatic Association
PO Box 14906   612-626-9797
Minneapolis, MN 55414   Fax: 612-625-7700
e-mail: apa@umn.edu
www.american-pancreatic-association.org

Provides forum for presentation of scientific research related to the pancreas.
Martin Freeman, President
Ashok Saluja, Secretary-Treasurer

3784 American Pseudo-Obstruction and Hirschsprung's Disease Society
1825 Connecticut Avenue NW   202-884-8200
Washington, DC 20009   800-695-0285
Fax: 202-884-8441
TTY: 202-884-8200
e-mail: nichcy@aed.org
www.nichcy.org

Promotes public awareness of gastrointestinal motility disorders in particular intestinal pseudo-obstruction and Hirschsprung's disease; provides education and support to individuals and families of children who have been diagnosed with these disorders.

3785 American Society for Gastrointestinal Endoscopy
1520 Kensington Road
Oak Brook, IL 60523
630-573-0600
800-353-2743
Fax: 630-573-0691
e-mail: info@asge.org
www.asge.org
ASGE provides information training and practice guidelines about gastrointestinal endoscopic techniques.
M Brian Fennerty, President
Gregory G Ginsberg, President-Elect

3786 American Society for Parenteral and Enteral Nutrition (ASPEN)
8630 Fenton Street
Silver Spring, MD 20910-3805
301-587-6315
Fax: 301-587-2365
e-mail: aspen@nutr.org
www.nutritioncare.org
Offers information and continuing medical education to professionals involved in the care of parenterally and enterally fed patients. Membership includes complimentary subscriptions to two peer reviewed journals.
Charles Ston Vanway, President
Tom Jaksic, Vice President

3787 American Society of Adults with Pseudo-Obstruction
International Corporate Headquarters
19 Carrol Road
Woburn, MA 01801-6161
781-935-9776
Fax: 781-933-4151
ASAP educates the general public and medical community about chronic intestinal pseudo-obstruction (CIP) and other related digestive motility disorders; serves as an integral source of information for patients of all ages with CIP and related disorders.

3788 Center for Digestive Disorders: Central
25 N Winfield Road
Winfield, IL 60190
630-933-1600
877-933-4234
Fax: 630-933-1300
TTY: 630-933-4833
e-mail: cdh_information@cdh.org
www.cdh.org
Multifaceted program to meet the needs of people who suffer from gastrointestinal problems; offers literature, videotapes and educational meetings and, if medical care is needed, appropriate referrals are made.
Luke McGuinness, President/CEO
Jim Spear, Executive Vice President/CFO

3789 Cyclic Vomiting Syndrome Association
10520 W Bluemound Road
Milwaukee, WI 53226
414-342-7880
Fax: 414-342-8980
e-mail: cvsa@cvsaonline.org
www.cvsaonline.org
CVSA provides opportunities for patients, families and professionals to offer and receive support and share knowledge about cyclic vomiting syndrome; actively promotes and facilitates medical research about nausea and vomiting.
Kathleen Adams, President, Co Founder
Jennifer Dhuse, Secretary

3790 Digestive Disease National Coalition
507 Capitol Court NE
Washington, DC 20002
202-544-7497
Fax: 202-546-7105
e-mail: ddnc@hmcw.org
www.ddnc.org
Informs the public and the health care community about digestive disorders; seeks Federal funding for research education and training; and represents members' interests regarding Federal and State legislation that affects digestive diseases research.
Linda Aukett, Chairperson
James DeGerome, President

3791 International Academy of Proctology
2209 John R Wooden Drive
Martinsville, IN 46151
765-342-3686
Fax: 765-342-4173
Encourages study of diseases of the colon and accessory organs of digestion and conducts seminars.

3792 International Foundation for Functional Gastrointestinal Disorders
700 W.Viginia St
Milwaukee, WI 53204-8076
414-964-1799
888-964-2001
Fax: 414-964-7176
e-mail: iffgd@iffgd.org
www.iffgd.org
IFFGD is a nonprofit education support and research organization devoted to increasing awareness and understanding of functional gastrointestinal disorders, including irritable bowel syndrome (IBS), constipation, diarrhea, pain, and incontinence.
Nancy J Norton, President

3793 Iron Overload Diseases Association
525 Mayflower Road
W Palm Beach, FL 33405
561-586-8246
866-768-8629
Fax: 561-842-9881
e-mail: iod@ironoverload.org
www.ironoverload.org
Conducts professional education symposiums and exhibits at medical meetings; serves and counsels hemochromatosis patients and families; offers doctor referrals; promotes patient advocacy concerning insurance, Medicare, blood banks, and the FDA.
Roberta Crawford, Founder/President

3794 National Digestive Diseases Information Clearinghouse
Two Information Way
Bethesda, MD 20892-3570
800-891-5389
Fax: 703-738-4929
TTY: 866-569-1162
e-mail: nddic@info.niddk.nih.gov
www.digestive.niddk.nih.gov
Offers various educational information, public resources and reprints, public awareness materials and more on digestive disorders.
Griffin P Rodgers MD MACP, Director

3795 North American Society for Pediatric Gastroenterology and Nutrition
PO Box 6
Flourtown, PA 19031
215-233-0808
Fax: 215-233-3918
e-mail: naspghan@naspghan.org
www.naspghan.org
Promotes research and provides a forum for professionals in the areas of pediatric GI liver disease, gastroenterology, and nutrition. Associated with fellow organizations in Europe and Australia (ESPGAN, AUSPGAN).
Margaret K Stallings, Executive Director
Philip M Sherman, President

3796 Pediatric Adolescent Gastroesophageal Reflux Association
PO Box 7728
Silver Spring, MD 20907
301-601-9541
888-887-7729
e-mail: gergroup@aol.com
www.reflux.org
PAGER's mission is to: (l) gather and disseminate information on pediatric gastroesophageal reflux (GER) and related disorders; (2) provide educational and emotional support to patients with GER, their families, and professionals; (3) promote awareness of GER within both the medical community and the general public; and (4) promote research into the causes, treatments and eventual cure for pediatric GER.
Beth Anderson, Director

3797 Society for Surgery of the Alimentary Tract
900 Cummings Center
Beverly, MA 01915
978-927-8330
Fax: 978-524-8890
www.ssat.com
SSAT provides a forum for exchange of information among physicians specializing in alimentary tract surgery.
David W Rattner, President
David M Mahvi, President-Elect

3798 Society of American Gastrointestinal Endoscopic Surgeons
11300 W Olympic Boulevard
Los Angeles, CA 90064
310-437-0544
Fax: 310-437-0585
www.sages.org

SAGES encourages study and practice of gastrointestinal endoscopy laparoscopy and minimal access surgery.

Jo Buyske, President
Steven D Schwaitzberg, President-Elect

3799 Society of Gastroenterology Nurses and Associates
401 N Michigan Avenue   312-321-5165
Chicago, IL 60611-4267   800-245-7462
                                  Fax: 312-673-6694
                       e-mail: sgna@smithbucklin.com
                                      www.sgna.org

SGNA provides members with continuing education opportunities practice and training guidelines and information about trends and development in the field of gastroenterology.

Peggy Gauthier, President
Leslie Stewart, President-Elect

3800 United Ostomy Association
PO Box 512
Northfield, MN 55057   800-826-0826
                                  Fax: 507-645-5168
                             e-mail: info@uoaa.org
                                      www.uoaa.org

A national network for bowel and urinary diversion support groups in the United States. Its goal is to provide a nonprofit association that will serve to unify and strengthen its member support groups, which are organized for the benefit of people who have, or will have intestinal or urinary diversions and their caregivers.

Dave Rudzin, President
Diane Miterko, Chair

Foundations

3801 American Porphyria Foundation
4900 Woodway   713-266-9617
Houston, TX 77056   866-APF-3635
                                  Fax: 713-840-9552
                       e-mail: porphyrus@aol.com
                         www.porphyriafoundation.com

The APF is dedicated to improving the health and well-being of individuals and families affected by porphyria. Our mission is to enhance public awareness about porphyria, develop educational programs and distributing educational material for patients and physicians and support research to improve treatment and ultimately lead to a cure.

Desiree H Lyon, Executive Director
James Young, Chairman

3802 Gastro-Intestinal Research Foundation
70 East Lake Street   312-332-1350
Chicago, IL 60601-5907   Fax: 312-332-4757
                             e-mail: girf@girf.org
                                      www.girf.org

Provides funds for equipment, laboratories and the support of investigators and young physicians in the University of Chicago Gastroenterology Section, a group of full-time dedicated doctors who seek solutions to all kinds of gastrointestinal illnesses, affecting the esophagus, the stomach, the small intestine, the large intestine, the liver, the gallbladder, and the pancreas.

Jennifer Hanauer, Director
Stephen Wright, GIRF Staff

3803 Oley Foundation
43 New Scotland Ave   518-262-5079
Albany, NY 12208-3478   800-776-6539
                                  Fax: 518-262-5528
                                      www.oley.org

Promotes and advocates education and research in home parenteral and enteral nutrition; provides support and networking to patients through information clearinghouse and regional volunteer networks; sponsors meetings and conferences, including annual patient/clinician conference; maintains speakers bureau.

Joan Bishop, Executive Director
Cathy Harrington, Administrative Assistant

Research Centers

3804 Baylor College of Medicine: General Clinical Research Center for Adults
One Baylor Plaza   713-798-4951
Houston, TX 77030   e-mail: dbier@bcm.edu
                               www.bcm.edu/pediatrics

Endocrinology, genetics and gastroenterology research.

Dennis M Bier MD, Program Director
Paul Klotman, President

3805 Digestive Disorders Associates Ridgely Oaks Professional Center
Ridgely Oaks Professional Center
621 Ridgely Avenue   41 -22 -488
Annapolis, MD 21401   800-273-0505
                                  Fax: 410-224-6971
                                 TTY: 800-735-2258
                                       www.dda.net

Specialize in the diagnosis and treatment of diseases of the entire digestive system including esophagus stomach small and large intestine colon liver pancreas and gall bladder.

Michael S Epstein, Founder
Charles E King, Doctor

3806 Gastrointestinal Research Foundation
70 E Lake Street   312-332-1350
Chicago, IL 60601-5915   Fax: 312-332-4757
                             e-mail: info@girf.org
                                      www.girf.org

Founded to help combat gastrointestinal diseases. Raises funds to support research at the Center for study of the Digestive Diseases at the University of Chicago Medical Center and to support advanced training for scientists. Sponsors educational activities for the public.

Martin N Sandler, Co-Founder
Steven R Davidson, Co-Chairman

3807 University of California: Davis Gastroenterology & Nutrition Center
Pediatric GI Medical Center
4900 Broadway
Sacramento, CA 95820-2214   91- 73- 904
                                www.ucdmc.ucdavis.edu

Research into gastrointestinal mobility and electro-physiology nutrition support and references for the public and patient evaluations.

Bonnie Hyatt, Assistant Director
Jenny Carrick, Senior Director of Communications and Ma

3808 University of California: Los Angeles Center for Ulcer Research
LA Medical Center
Building 115 Room 117   310-312-9284
Los Angeles, CA 90073   Fax: 310-268-4963
                       e-mail: cureadmn@mednet.ucla.edu
                                www.cure.med.ucla.edu

Offers basic and clinical research related to peptic ulcer disease including causes checks and balances and stress-ulcer relationships.

Enrique Rozengurt, Director
Emeran Mayer, Co-Director

3809 University of Michigan Michigan Gastrointestinal Peptide Research Ctr.
U-M Health System
1500 E Medical Center Drive   734-936-4000
Ann Arbor, MI 48109   Fax: 734-763-2535
                        e-mail: GutPeptide@umich.edu
                              www.med.umich.edu/mgpc

Research into gastroenterology including chemistry of gut hormones is studied.

Chung Owyang MD, Director
Juanita Merc MD PhD, Associate Director

3810 University of Pennsylvania: Harrison Department of Surgical Research
3400 Spruce Street   215-662-4000
Philadelphia, PA 19104   800-789-PENN
                                  Fax: 215-615-0471
                       e-mail: julie.koehler@uphs.upenn.edu
                      www.uphs.upenn.edu/surgery/res/harrisonr

Offers research and studies on surgical transplantations gastrointestinal physiology.

Julie Hagan Koehler MBA, Business Director
Georgina Suarez, Administrative Assistant

Support Groups & Hotlines

3811 National Health Information Center
PO Box 1133
Washington, DC 20013 310-565-4167
800-336-4797
Fax: 301-984-4256
e-mail: info@nhic.org
www.health.gov/nhic
A health information referral service sponsored by the Office of Disease Prevention and Health Promotion. Puts health professionals and consumers who have health questions in touch with those organizations that are best able to provide answers.

3812 Pull-thru Network
2312 Savoy Street
Hoover, AL 35226-1528 205-978-2930
e-mail: ptnmail@charter.net
www.pullthrough.org
Dedicated to the needs of those born wutith anorectal malformation or colon disease and any of the associated diagnoses.

Magazines

3813 ASAP Forum
ASAP International Corporate Headquarters
19 Carroll Road
Woburn, MA 01801 781-935-9776
Fax: 781-933-4151
e-mail: asapgi@sprynet.com
Educates the general public and medical community about chronic intestinal pseudo-obstruction (CIP) and other related digestive motility disorders; serves as an integral source of information for patients of all ages with CIP and related disorders, their families, and members of the medical community.

3814 American Journal of Gastroenterology
American College of Gastroenterology
4900B 31st St S
Arlington, VA 22206-1656 703-820-7400
Fax: 703-931-4520
www.acg.gi.org
Serves clinical and scientific information needs of member physicians and surgeons, who specialize in digestive and related disorders. Emphasis is on scholarly practice, teaching, and research.
Thomas F Fise, Executive Director

3815 American Journal of Gastrointestinal Surgery
Society for Surgery of the Alimentary Tract
13 Elm Street
Manchester, MA 01944 978-526-8330
Fax: 978-526-4018
e-mail: ssat@prri.com
www.ssat.com
Provides information for physicians specializing in gastrointestinal surgery.

3816 Clinical Perspectives in Gastroenterology
American Gastroenterological Association
7910 Woodmont Avenue
Bethesda, MD 20814 301-654-2055
Fax: 301-654-5920
e-mail: aga001@801.com
www.gastro.org
Focuses on research, medical and professional developments in the science of gastroenterology.
Robert Greenberg, Executive VP

3817 Digestive Health Matters
Intl. Foundation for Gastrointestinal Disorders
PO Box 170864
Milwaukee, WI 53217-0864 414-964-1799
888-964-2001
Fax: 414-964-7176
e-mail: iffgd@iffgd.org
www.iffgd.org
Quarterly journal focuses on upper and lower gastrointestinal disorders in adults and children. Educational pamphlets and factsheets are available. Patient and professional membership.

3818 Gastroenterology
American Gastroenterological Association
7910 Woodmont Avenue
Bethesda, MD 20814-3002 301-654-2055
Fax: 301-654-5920
e-mail: aga001@801.com
www.gastro.org
Focuses on research, medical and professional developments in the science of gastroenterology.
Robert Greenberg, Executive VP

3819 Gastroenterology Nursing
Society of Gastroenterology Nurses and Associates
401 N Michigan Avenue
Chicago, IL 60611 312-321-5165
800-245-7462
Fax: 312-321-5194
e-mail: sgna@sba.com
www.sgna.org
Provides members with information about trends and development in the field of gastroenterology nursing.

3820 Gastrointestinal Endoscopy
American Society for Gastrointestinal Endoscopy
1520 Kensington Road
Oak Brook, IL 60523 630-573-0600
Fax: 630-573-0691
www.asge.org
Provides information, training, and practice guidelines about gastrointestinal endoscopic techniques.

3821 Journal of Parenteral and Enteral Nutrition
ASPEN
8630 Fenton Street
Silver Spring, MD 20910-3805 301-587-6315
Fax: 301-587-2365
e-mail: aspen@nutr.org
www.nutritioncare.org
Offers information to professionals involved in the care of parenterally and enterally fed patients.
100 pages BiMonthly
Adrian Nickel, Director Communications/Marketing

3822 Journal of Pediatric Gastroenterology and Nutrition
N American Society for Pediatric Gastroenterology
6900 Grove Road
Thorofare, NJ 08086 609-848-1000
Fax: 609-848-5274
www.jpgn.org/
Provides information for professionals in the areas of pediatric GI liver disease, gastroenterology, and nutrition.

3823 Journal of the American Dietetic Association
American Dietetic Association
216 W Jackson Boulevard
Chicago, IL 60606-6995 312-899-0040
800-877-1600
Fax: 312-899-1979
www.eatright.org
Professional journal of the ADA.

3824 Nutrition in Clinical Practice
ASPEN
8630 Fenton Street
Silver Spring, MD 20910-3805 301-587-6315
Fax: 301-587-2365
e-mail: aspen@nutr.org
www.nutritioncare.org
Offers information to professionals involved in the care of parenterally and enterally fed patients.
100 pages BiMonthly
Adrian Nickel, Director Communications/Marketing

3825 Pancreas
American Pancreatic Association
10833 LeConte Avenue
Los Angeles, CA 90095-6904 310-825-4976
Fax: 310-206-2472
e-mail: hreber@surgery.medch.ucla.edu
Provides information on scientific research related to the pancreas.
Howard A Reber MD

3826 Phoenix Magazine
United Ostomy Association of America

PO Box 512
Northfield, MN 55057
800-826-0826
Fax: 507-645-5168
e-mail: info@uoaa.org
www.uoa.org

America's leading ostomy patient magazine providing colostomy, ileostomy, urostomy and continent diversion information, management techniques, new products and much more.
Quarterly
David Rudzin, President

Newsletters

3827 ADA Courier
American Dietetic Association
216 W Jackson Boulevard
Chicago, IL 60606-6995
312-899-0040
800-877-1600
Fax: 312-899-1979
www.eatright.org

Information for the public on the promotion of optimal nutrition, health, and well-being.

3828 APF Newsletter
PO Box 22712
Houston, TX 77227
713-266-9617
Fax: 713-840-9552
e-mail: porphyrus@aol.com
www.porphyriafoundation.com

Provides updates on treatment and research, as well as informative articles on patients and specialists who treat porphyria. It's mailed to all Sponsors of the APF.
Desiree H Lyon, Executive Director

3829 ASAP Capsule
ASAP International Corporate Headquarters
19 Carroll Road
Woburn, MA 01801
781-935-9776
Fax: 781-933-4151
e-mail: asapp@sprynet.com

Professional membership newsletter for ASAP, an organization which educates the general public and medical community about chronic intestinal pseudo-obstruction (CIP) and other related digestive motility disorders; serves as an integral source of information for patients of all ages with CIP and related disorders, their families, and members of the medical community.

3830 ASAP Digest
ASAP International Corporate Headquarters
19 Carroll Road
Woburn, MA 01801
781-935-9776
Fax: 781-933-4151
e-mail: asapgi@sprynet.com

General membership newsletter for ASAP. Educates the general public and medical community about chronic intestinal pseudo-obstruction (CIP) and other related digestive motility disorders; serves as an integral source of information for patients of all ages with CIP and related disorders, their families, and members of the medical community.

3831 Clinical Updates
American Society for Gastrointestinal Endoscopy
1520 Kensington Road
Oak Brook, IL 60523
630-573-0600
Fax: 630-573-0691
www.asge.org

Provides information, training, and practice guidelines about gastrointestinal endoscopic techniques.
Quarterly

3832 Code V
Cyclic Vomiting Syndrome Association (CVSA)
13180 Caroline Court
Elm Grove, WI 53122-1732
614-837-2586
Fax: 614-837-6543
e-mail: drwaites@infinet.com
www.beaker.iupui.edu/cvsa

Newsletter for members of the CVSA.

3833 Hemochromatosis Awareness
Hemochromatosis Foundation
PO Box 8569
Albany, NY 12208
518-489-0972
Fax: 518-489-0227
www.hemochromatosis.org

Provides information to the public, families, professionals and government agencies about hereditary hemochromatosis (HH); conducts and raises funds for research; encourages early screening for HH; holds symposiums and meetings; and offers genetic counseling along with support for patients, families, and professionals.
Margit Krikker MD, Medical Director

3834 Ironic Blood
Iron Overload Diseases Association
433 Westward Drive
North Palm Beach, FL 33408-5123
561-840-8512
Fax: 561-842-9881
e-mail: iod@ironoverload.org
www.ironoverload.org

Information for hemochromatosis patients and families.

3835 Lifeline Letter
Oley Foundation
Albany Medical Center
Albany, NY 12208-3478
518-262-5079
800-776-6539
Fax: 518-262-5528
e-mail: bishopj@mail.amc.edu
www.oley.org

Information on home parenteral and enteral nutrition for patients and the public.
16 pages Bi-Monthly
Joan Bishop, Executive Director

3836 Ostomy Quarterly
United Ostomy Association
PO Box 66
Fairview, TN 37062
800-826-0826
e-mail: info@uoa.org
www.uoa.org

First person stories, ostomy management advice from an ET and MD, organization news and ostomy product information.
72 pages Quarterly

3837 Pull-thru Network News
Pull-thru Network
4 Woody Lane
Westport, CT 06880
203-221-7530
e-mail: Pullthrunw@aol.com
members.aol.com/pullthrunw/Pullthru.html

Provides information to patients and families of children who have had or will have pull-through surgery to correct an imperforate anus or associated malformation, Hirschsprung's disease, or other fecal incontinence problems.

3838 SGNA News
Society of Gastroenterology Nurses and Associates
401 N Michigan Avenue
Chicago, IL 60611
312-321-5165
800-245-7462
Fax: 312-321-5194
e-mail: sgna@sba.com
www.sgna.org

Provides members with information about trends and development in the field of gastroenterology.

3839 WIN Notes
Weight-control Information Network
1 WIN Way
Bethesda, MD 20892-3665
202-828-1025
877-946-4627
Fax: 202-828-1028
e-mail: win@mathewsgroup.com
www.niddk.nih.gov/health/nutrit/win.htm

Addresses the health information needs of individuals with weight-control problems. Available on the WIN web site.
BiAnnual

Pamphlets

3840 Acute Intermittent Porphyria
American Prophyria Foundation
PO Box 22712
Houston, TX 77227
713-266-9617
www.enterprise.net

An informational brochure published by the American Porphyria Foundation.

3841 Common Questions About Porphyria
American Prophyria Foundation
PO Box 22712
Houston, TX 77227 713-266-9617
www.enterprise.net
An informational brochure published by the American Porphyria Foundation.

3842 Diet and Nutrition in Porphyria
American Prophyria Foundation
PO Box 22712
Houston, TX 77227 713-266-9617
www.enterprise.net
An informational brochure published by the American Porphyria Foundation.

3843 Drugs and Porphyria
American Prophyria Foundation
PO Box 22712
Houston, TX 77227 713-266-9617
www.enterprise.net
An informational brochure published by the American Porphyria Foundation.

3844 Erythropoietic Protoporphyria
American Prophyria Foundation
PO Box 22712
Houston, TX 77227 713-266-9617
www.enterprise.net
An informational brochure published by the American Porphyria Foundation.

3845 Hematin
American Prophyria Foundation
PO Box 22712
Houston, TX 77227 713-266-9617
www.enterprise.net
An informational brochure published by the American Porphyria Foundation.

3846 Iron Overload Alert
Iron Overload Diseases Association
433 Westward Drive 561-840-8512
North Palm Beach, FL 33408-5123 Fax: 561-842-9881
e-mail: iod@ironoverload.org
www.ironoverload.org
Information for hemochromatosis patients and families.

3847 Issues in Women's Gastrointestinal Health
Gastro-Intestinal Research Foundation
70 E Lake Street 312-332-1350
Chicago, IL 60601 Fax: 312-332-4757
e-mail: girf@girf.org
www.girf.org
Patient education pamphlet.

3848 Porphyria Cutanea Tarda
American Prophyria Foundation
PO Box 22712
Houston, TX 77227 713-266-9617
www.enterprise.net
An informational brochure published by the American Porphyria Foundation.

Audio & Video

3849 A Day in the Life of a Child
Albany Medical Center 518-262-5079
Albany, NY 12208-3478 800-776-6539
Fax: 518-262-5528
www.oley.org
In this video you are welcomed into the household of the Miller family. The Millers have three children, one of whom is tube fed. Jessica has been dependent on tube-feedings since birth, and her family is prepared to show you just what that means. They share tips for keeping a sterile environment in a house with three children, and tips for helping Jessica fit in with her peers.
Joan Bishop, Executive Director

3850 Cleveland Clinic Teaching Conference
Hemochromatosis Foundation
PO Box 8569 518-489-0972
Albany, NY 12208 Fax: 518-489-0227
www.hemochromatosis.org
Provides information to the public, families, and professionals about hereditary hemochromatosis.

3851 Family Teaching Conference
Hemochromatosis Foundation
PO Box 8569 518-489-0972
Albany, NY 12208 Fax: 518-489-0227
www.hemochromatosis.org
Provides information to the public, families, and professionals about hereditary hemochromatosis.

3852 Life with Mic-Key
Albany Medical Center 518-262-5079
Albany, NY 12208-3478 800-776-6539
Fax: 518-262-5528
www.oley.org
Serves as an informative and introductory guide for adapting to life with a Mic-key low profile feeding tube. Low profile means that the Mic-key tube lies very close to the patient's body and does not stick out. It's slim design allows more air to circulate around the stoma site and makes it easy to care for. The Mic-key tube uses a balloon to hold it in place and comes with several important accessories, including two types of extensions sets and an anti-reflux valve.
10 Minutes
Joan Bishop, Executive Director

3853 Mealtime Notions - The 'Get Permission' Approach to Mealtimes and Oral Motor
Marsha Dunn Klein, MED, OTR/L, author
Albany Medical Center 518-262-5079
Albany, NY 12208-3478 800-776-6539
Fax: 518-262-5528
www.oley.org
This video explores the development of trusting feeding relationships, understanding the child's pace, and strategies for increasing permissive behavior. Tools discussed in this video include an introduction to the sensory continuum, a description of the around the bowl technique, and tips for removing the stress from your child's mealtime.
10 Minutes
Joan Bishop, Executive Director

Web Sites

3854 American College of Gastroenterology (ACG)
www.acg.gi.org
Serves clinical and scientific information needs of member physicians and surgeons, who specialize in digestive and related disorders. Emphasis is on scholarly practice, teaching, and research.

3855 American Gastroenterological Association (AGA)
www.gastro.org
Fosters the development and application of the science of gastroenterology by providing leadership and aid, including patient care, research, teaching, continuing education, scientific communication, and matters of national health policy pertaining to gastroenterology.

3856 American Hemochromatosis Society
www.americanhs.org
Educates the public, the medical community, and the media by distributing the most current information available on hereditary hemochromatosis (HH), including DNA screening for HH and pediatric HH; also facilitates patient empowerment through an online network.

3857 American Porphyria Foundation
PO Box 22712 713-266-9617
Houston, TX 77227 Fax: 713-840-9552
e-mail: porphyrus@aol.com
www.porphyriafoundation.com

Advances awareness, research, and treatment of the porphyrias; provides self-help services for members; and provides referrals to porphyria treatment specialists.
Karl E Anderson, MD, Chairman

3858   American Pseudo-Obstruction and Hirschsprung's Disease Society

Promotes public awareness of gastrointestinal motility disorders, in particular intestinal pseudo-obstruction and Hirschsprung's Disease; provides education and support to individuals and families of children who have been diagnosed with these disorders through parent-to-parent contact, publications, and educational symposia; and encourages and supports medical research in the area of gastrointestinal motility disorders.

3859   American Society for Gastrointestinal Endoscopy

www.asge.org

ASGE provides information, training, and practice guidelines about gastrointestinal endoscopic techniques.

3860   American Society of Abdominal Surgeons

www.gis.net/~absurg/

ASAS sponsors extensive continuing education program for physicians in the field of abdominal surgery and maintains library.

3861   Background on Functional Gastrointestinal Disorders

www.med.unc.edu

Statistical background information on gastrointestinal disorders.

3862   Children's Motility Disorder Foundation

www.motility.org

CMDF works to increase awareness of pediatric motility disorders in the general public and among the physicians most likely to encounter children suffering from these conditions, such as pediatricians and family practice doctors. Supports medical research regarding the causes, treatment, and potentially life-threatening disorders.

3863   Cyclic Vomiting Syndrome Association

www.cvsaonline.org/

CVSA provides opportunities for patients, families, and professionals to offer and receive support and share knowledge about cyclic vomiting syndrome; actively promotes and facilitates medical research about nausea and vomiting; increases worldwide public and professional awareness; and serves as a resource center for information.

3864   Gastrointestinal Research Foundation

www.girf.org

Founded to help combat gastrointestinal diseases. Raises funds to support research at the Center for the study of the Digestive Diseases at the University of Chicago Medical Center and to support advanced training for scientists. Sponsors educational activities for the public.

3865   Healing Well

www.healingwell.com

An online health resource guide to medical news, chat, information and articles, newsgroups and message boards, books, disease-related web sites, medical directories, and more for patients, friends, and family coping with disabling diseases, disorders, or chronic illnesses.

3866   Health Finder

www.healthfinder.gov

Searchable, carefully developed web site offering information on over 1000 topics. Developed by the US Department of Health and Human Services, the site can be used in both English and Spanish.

3867   Healthlink USA

www.healthlinkusa.com

Health information concerning treatment, cures, prevention, diagnosis, risk factors, research, support groups, email lists, personal stories and much more. Updated regularly.

3868   Helios Health

www.helioshealth.com

Online resource for your health information. Detailed information about specific health topics, access to expert advice from our Medical Advisory Board, and up-to-date health news.

3869   Hemochromatosis Foundation

www.hemochromatosis.org

Provides information to the public, families, and professionals about hereditary hemochromatosis (HH); conducts and raises funds for research; encourages early screening for HH; holds symposiums and meetings; and offers genetic counseling along with support for patients, families, and professionals.

3870   International Foundation for Functional Gastrointestinal Disorders

www.iffgd.org

IFFGD is a nonprofit education, support and research organization devoted to increasing awareness and understanding of functional gastrointestinal disorders, including irritable bowel syndrome (IBS), constipation, diarrhea, pain, and incontinence. Mission is to inform, assist and support people affected by these disorders.

3871   MedicineNet

www.medicinenet.com

An online resource for consumers providing easy-to-read, authoritative medical and health information.

3872   Medscape

www.medscape.com

Medscape offers specialists, primary care physicians, and other health professionals the Web's most robust and integrated medical information and educational tools.

3873   National Digestive Diseases Information Clearinghouse

www.niddk.nih.gov

Offers various educational information, public resources and reprints, public awareness materials and more on digestive disorders.

3874   North American Society for Pediatric Gastroenterology and Nutrition

www.naspgn.org

Promotes research and provides a forum for professionals in the areas of pediatric GI liver disease, gastroenterology, and nutrition. Associated with fellow organizations in Europe and Australia (ESPGAN, AUSPGAN).

3875   Nutrition in Clinical Practice

www.clinnutr.org

Offers information to professionals involved in the care of parenterally and enterally fed patients.

3876   Oley Foundation

www.wizvax.net/oleyfdn

Promotes and advocates education and research in home parenteral and enteral nutrition; provides support and networking to patients through information clearinghouse and regional volunteer networks; sponsors meetings and conferences, including annual patient/clinician conference; maintains speakers bureau.

3877   Pediatric Adolescent Gastroesophageal Assn

www.reflux.org

Discussions led by local experts, family medical histories and check swabs, supervised nap room and separate activity room for kids, trained babysitters available.

3878   Pediatric/Adolescent Gastroesophageal Reflux Association

www.reflux.org

PAGER gathers and disseminates information on pediatric gastroesophageal reflux and related disorders; provides support and education to patients, their families, and the public; promotes the general welfare of patients, their families, and the public; promotes the general welfare of patients with gastroesophageal reflux and their families; and promotes public awareness of the condition.

3879   Pull-thru Network

members.aol.com/pullthrunw/Pullthru.html

Provides emotional support and information to patients and families of children who have had or will have pull-through surgery to correct an imperforate anus or associated malformation, Hirschsprung's disease, or other fecal incontinence problems; sponsors online discussion groups. A chapter of the United Ostomy Association.

3880   Society for Surgery of the Alimentary Tract

www.ssat.com

SSAT provides a forum for exchange of information among physicians specializing in alimentary tract surgery.

3881   Society of American Gastrointestinal Endoscopic Surgeons

www.sages.org

SAGES encourages study and practice of gastrointestinal endoscopy, laparoscopy, and minimal acces surgery.

3882   WebMD

www.webmd.com

Information on Gastrointestinal Disorders, including articles and resources.

Description

3883 ## Gaucher's Disease

Gaucher's disease is an inherited disorder of metabolism of fats. These metabolic products can not be broken down properly because of a deficiency of an enzyme called glucocerebroside. Symptoms can include fatigue, anemia, bleeding problems (such as nosebleeds and easy bruising), enlargement of the spleen and/or liver, bone pain, easily fractured bones and brown pigmentation of the skin. The degree of symptoms and complications vary by age of onset and the degree of involvement of the disorder's clinical forms. Diagnosis is based on finding Gaucher's typical cells in the bone marrow.

The treatment for Gaucher's disease is enzyme replacement, called Cerezyme, administered intravenously. Removal of the spleen and blood transfusions may be necessary. Current research is aimed at genetic therapy.

National Agencies & Associations

3884 **National Foundation for Jewish Genetic Diseases**
One Gustave L Levy Place   212-241-6500
New York, NY 10029-6574   Fax: 212-241-6947
                                 www.mssm.edu/jewish_genetics
This foundation was created to raise funds for and to inform the public about genetic diseases which afflict descendants of eastern and central European Jews. It sponsors medical symposia from time to time.
R J Desnick PhD MD, Center Director
Dennis S Charney, Executive VP

3885 **National Gaucher Foundation**
2227 Idlewood Road
Tucker, GA 33008   800-504-3189
                                      Fax: 770-934-2911
                           e-mail: ngf@gaucherdisease.org
                                  www.gaucherdisease.org
National foundation providing information and assistance for those affected by Gaucher disease as well as education and outreach to increase public awareness.
Robin A Ely MD, President/Medical Director
Rhonda P Buyers, CEO/Executive Director

3886 **National Organization for Rare Disorders (NORD)**
55 Kenosia Avenue   203-744-0100
Danbury, CT 06813-1968   800-999-6673
                                      Fax: 203-798-2291
                                      TDD: 203-797-9590
                           e-mail: orphan@rarediseases.org
                                    www.rarediseases.org
The NORD is a unique federation of voluntary health organizations dedicated to helping people with rare orphan diseases and assisting the organizations that serve them.
Frank Sasinowski, Chair
Carolyn Asbury, Vice Chair

Research Centers

3887 **Children's Gaucher Research Fund**
8110 Warren Court   916-797-3700
Granite Bay, CA 95746-2123   Fax: 916-797-3707
                        e-mail: research@childrensgaucher.org
                                  www.childrensgaucher.org
A nonprofit organization that raises funds to coordinate support research to find a cure for Type 2 and Type 3 Gaucher Disease.
Roscoe Brady, Scientific Advisory Board
Gregory Grabowski, Scientific Advisory Board

3888 **Comprehensive Gaucher Treatment Center at Tower Hermatology Oncology**
9090 Wilshire Boulevard   310-888-8680
Beverly Hills, CA 90211   888-248-4456
                                      Fax: 310-285-7298
                           e-mail: info@gaucherwest.com
                                      www.gaucherwest.com
The Comprehensive Gaucher Treatment Center at Tower Hermatology Oncology under the direction of Dr. Barry Rosenbloom provides clinical evaluations for the diagnosis and treatment of patient's with Gaucher disease. We provide a multi-disciplinary program that includes Hermatology Genetics Orthopedics and Radiology. To ensure continuity of care we provide assistance to other physicians regarding testing diagnosis evaluation and management of the Gaucher patient.
Barry Rosenbloom, Director
Cheryl Elzinga, Gaucher Coordinator

3889 **LAC/USC Imaging Science Center**
1975 Zonal Avenue   323-442-1900
Los Angeles, CA 90089-9034   Fax: 323-442-2722
                               e-mail: nestrada@usc.edu
                              www.usc.edu/schools/medicine
Provides a Gaucher Disease radiology consultant: Michael R Terk MD.and Muskuloskeletal Imaging.
Coreen Rodgers, COO
Sherri Sammon, Associate Director

Support Groups & Hotlines

3890 **Brave Kids**
151 Sawgrass Corners Drive   904-280-1895
Ponte Vedra Beach, FL 32082   800-568-1008
                                      Fax: 904-280-1897
                               e-mail: info@bravekids.org
                                       www.bravekids.org
An organization that offers support for parents and children suffering from serious health problems.
Kristen Fitzgerald, Founder

3891 **National Health Information Center**
PO Box 1133   310-565-4167
Washington, DC 20013   800-336-4797
                                      Fax: 301-984-4256
                                  e-mail: info@nhic.org
                                    www.health.gov/nhic
Offers a nationwide information referral service, produces directories and resource guides.

Newsletters

3892 **Gaucher Disease Newsletter**
National Gaucher Foundation
11140 Rockville Pike   301-816-1515
Rockville, MD 20852-3151   800-925-8885
Offers information on the latest research, treatments and technology for persons affected by Gaucher Disease. Also includes legislative and medical information.
Quarterly

Pamphlets

3893 **Gaucher Disease Fact Sheet**
National Gaucher Foundation
11140 Rockville Pike   301-816-1515
Rockville, MD 20852-3151   800-925-8885
Offers information on what Gaucher Disease is, the symptoms, risks, treatments and the workings of the National Gaucher Foundation.

3894 **Living with Gaucher Disease**
National Gaucher Foundation
11140 Rockville Pike   301-816-1515
Rockville, MD 20852-3151   800-925-8885

A guide for parents, families and relatives that teach them how to deal with and cope with a diagnosis of Gaucher Disease.
24 pages

Audio & Video

3895   Pain & Hope
National Gaucher Foundation
11140 Rockville Pike   301-816-1515
Rockville, MD 20852-3151   800-925-8885
A patient and family perspective on Gaucher Disease.

Web Sites

3896   Gaucher Disease Homepage
                                           www.gaucherdisease.org
Information on Gaucher disease, including symptoms, treatment, prevalence, resources, support, and news.

3897   Healing Well
                                                   www.healingwell.com
An online health resource guide to medical news, chat, information and articles, newsgroups and message boards, books, disease-related web sites, medical directories, and more for patients, friends, and family coping with disabling diseases, disorders, or chronic illnesses.

3898   Health Finder
                                                     www.healthfinder.gov
Searchable, carefully developed web site offering information on over 1000 topics. Developed by the US Department of Health and Human Services, the site can be used in both English and Spanish.

3899   Healthlink USA
                                                   www.healthlinkusa.com
Health information concerning treatment, cures, prevention, diagnosis, risk factors, research, support groups, email lists, personal stories and much more. Updated regularly.

3900   Helios Health
                                                     www.helioshealth.com
Online resource for your health information. Detailed information about specific health topics, access to expert advice from our Medical Advisory Board, and up-to-date health news.

3901   MedicineNet
                                                   www.medicinenet.com
An online resource for consumers providing easy-to-read, authoritative medical and health information.

3902   Medscape
                                                     www.medscape.com
Medscape offers specialists, primary care physicians, and other health professionals the Web's most robust and integrated medical information and educational tools.

3903   WebMD
                                                         www.webmd.com
Information on Gaucher's disease, including articles and resources.

Description

3904 ## Growth Disorders

There are many conditions that make a child grow more slowly than average. Any sort of severe chronic illness, especially one involving the digestive system, may cause this. Certain genetic conditions such as Turner syndrome, a sex chromosome abnormality or achondroplasia (skeletal maldevelopment) will predictably limit growth and eventual adult height. Endocrine, or hormonal, causes of short stature include underactivity of the thyroid gland (hypothyroidism) or pituitary gland, where growth hormone (GH) is normally formed. Finally, there are many cases where the child's height is significantly below that of peers, yet none of these conditions is present. This may reflect two parents who are themselves quite short, or may be completely unexplained.

If slow growth is related to low levels of GH, therapy with synthetic GH is extremely effective. Regular injections will be necessary for a prolonged period until an acceptable height is reached.

Regardless of the underlying cause, a child whose disorder is recognized at birth or who is not growing as quickly as the rest of his or her peers should receive a complete evaluation by a pediatric endocrinologist or other growth specialist.

National Agencies & Associations

3905 **Dwarf Athletic Association of America**
708 Gravenstein Highway N
Sebastopol, CA 95472
972-317-8299
888-598-3222
Fax: 972-966-0184
e-mail: daaa@flash.net
www.daaa.org
Develops, promotes and provides quality amateur level athletic opportunities for dwarf athletes in the US. Our mission is to encourage people with dwarfism to participate in sports regardless of their level of skill.
Amy B Andrews, Board President
Mike Cekanor, Board VP

3906 **Genetic Alliance**
4301 Connecticut Avenue NW
Washington, DC 20008
202-966-5557
Fax: 202-966-8553
e-mail: info@geneticalliance.org
www.geneticalliance.org
Improves health through the authentic engagement of communities and individuals. The goal is to build capacity within the genetics community. Transform health through genetics, and promote an environment of opennes cetnered on the health of individuals, families and communities.
Sharon F Terry MA, President/CEO
Greg Biggers, Entrepreneur-In-Residence

3907 **Little People of America**
250 El Camino Real
Tustin, CA 92780
714-368-3689
888-LPA-2001
Fax: 714-368-3367
e-mail: info@lpaonline.org
www.lpaonline.org
Focuses research, support and information on persons who are short in stature.
Lois Gerage-Lamb, President
Bill Bradford, Senior VP

3908 **Little People's Research Fund (LPRF)**
616 Old Edmondson Avenue
Catonsville, MD 21228
410-747-1100
800-232-LPRF
Fax: 410-747-1374
e-mail: lprf@lprf.org
www.lprf.org
LPRF supports research into the disabling conditions of skeletal dysplasia (dwarfism), promotes patient care and education of the medical community as well as the general public. It assists families by sponsoring clinics in various states.
Steven E Kopits MD, Medical Advisor

3909 **National Institute of Child Health and Human Development**
PO Box 3006
Rockville, MD 20847
800-370-2943
Fax: 866-760-5947
TTY: 888-320-6942
e-mail: NICHDInformationResourceCenter@mail.nih.
www.nichd.nih.gov
Duane Alexander MD, Director

Foundations

3910 **Human Growth Foundation**
997 Glen Cove Avenue
Glen Head, NY 11545
516-671-4041
800-451-6434
Fax: 516-671-4055
e-mail: hgf1@hgfound.org
www.hgfound.org
Our mission is to help children, and adults with disorders of growth and growth hormone through research, education, support, and advocacy. The Foundation is dedicated to helping medical science to better understand the process of growth. It is composed of concerned parents and friends of children, and adults, with growth problems; and, interested health professionals.
Patricia D Costa, Executive Director
Pisit Pitukcheewanont, President

3911 **MAGIC Foundation for Children's Growth**
6645 West North Avenue
Oak Park, IL 60302
708-383-0808
800-362-4423
Fax: 708-383-0899
e-mail: dianne@magicfoundation.org
www.magicfoundation.org
Provides support services for the families of children afflicted with a wide variety of chronic and/or critical disorders, syndromes and that affect a child's growth.
Dianne Tamburrino, Executive Director
Susan Smith, Director Medical Education

3912 **March of Dimes Birth Defects Foundation**
1275 Mamaroneck Avenue
White Plains, NY 10605
914-997-4488
www.marchofdimes.com
Our mission is to improve the health of babies by preventing birth defects, premature birth, and infant mortality.

Research Centers

3913 **Case Western Reserve University: Bolton Brush Growth Study Center**
2123 Abington Road
Cleveland, OH 44106-4905
216-368-4649
Fax: 216-368-3204
e-mail: mgh4@po.cwru.edu
dental.cwru.edu/bolton-brush
Investigations and research into the growth and development of the human body. Extensive collection of longitudinal human growth data.
Mark G Hans, Director
Aaron Weinbe, Associate Professor and Chairman

3914 **International Skeletal Dysplasia Registry Medical Genetics Institute**
Medical Genetics Institute
8700 Beverly Boulevard
Los Angeles, CA 90048
310-423-3277
800-233-2771
Fax: 310-423-0462
www.csmc.edu

Provides patient services for skeletal dysplasia patients particularly research in dwarfism.
David L Rimoin MD PhD, Director
Xiao-Ning Chen, Research Scientist

3915 **New Jersey Institute of Technology Center for Biomedical Engineering**
University Heights   973-596-8449
Newark, NJ 07102-1982   Fax: 973-596-6056
e-mail: william.c.hunter@njit.edu
www.njit.edu
Offers research into facial and bone disorders.
Robert A Altenkirch, President
Joel Bloom, Vice President

3916 **WM Krogman Center for Research in Child Growth and Development**
3101 Walnut Street   215-898-1470
Philadelphia, PA 19104-6003   e-mail: mannj@upenn.edu
www.upenn.edu
Focuses research and studies on growth disorders and birth defects.
Amy Gutmann, President

Support Groups & Hotlines

3917 **National Health Information Center**
PO Box 1133   310-565-4167
Washington, DC 20013   800-336-4797
Fax: 301-984-4256
e-mail: info@nhic.org
www.health.gov/nhic
Offers a nationwide information referral service, produces directories and resource guides.

Books

3918 **Growing Children: A Parent's Guide**
Human Growth Foundation
997 Glen Cove Avenue   516-671-4041
Glen Head, NY 11545   800-451-6434
Fax: 516-671-4055
e-mail: hgf1@hgfound.org
www.hgfound.org
Offers parents information on the normal pattern of their child's growth, growth charts, recognition of growth problems, evaluation of growth problems and resources for more information.
Patricia D Costa, Executive Director

3919 **Short and OK**
Human Growth Foundation
997 Glen Cove Avenue   516-671-4041
Glen Head, NY 11545   800-451-6434
Fax: 516-671-4055
e-mail: hgf1@hgfound.org
www.hgfound.org
Guide for parents of short children offering information on behavior issues, medical issues and psychological warning signs.
54 pages
Patricia D Costa, Executive Director

Pamphlets

3920 **Achondroplasia**
Human Growth Foundation
997 Glen Cove Avenue   516-671-4041
Glen Head, NY 11545   800-451-6434
Fax: 516-671-4055
e-mail: hgf1@hgfound.org
www.hgfound.org
Signs, causes and prevention of achondroplasia.
Patricia D Costa, Executive Director

3921 **Growth Hormone Testing**
Human Growth Foundation

997 Glen Cove Avenue   516-671-4041
Glen Head, NY 11545   800-451-6434
Fax: 516-671-4055
e-mail: hgf1@hgfound.org
www.hgfound.org
What to expect during the testing period.
Patricia D Costa, Executive Director

3922 **Intrauterine Growth Retardation**
Human Growth Foundation
997 Glen Cove Avenue   516-671-4041
Glen Head, NY 11545   800-451-6434
Fax: 516-671-4055
e-mail: hgf1@hgfound.org
www.hgfound.org
Explains some of the reasons for an infant's failure to grow normally in intrauterine life.
Patricia D Costa, Executive Director

3923 **Most Frequently Asked Questions with Growth Hormone Deficiency**
Human Growth Foundation
997 Glen Cove Avenue   516-671-4041
Glen Head, NY 11545   800-451-6434
Fax: 516-671-4055
e-mail: hgf1@hgfound.org
www.hgfound.org
Provides a brief overview for parents about Growth Hormone Deficiency.
Patricia D Costa, Executive Director

3924 **Septo-Optic Dysplasia**
Human Growth Foundation
997 Glen Cove Avenue   516-671-4041
Glen Head, NY 11545   800-451-6434
Fax: 516-671-4055
e-mail: hgf1@hgfound.org
www.hgfound.org
Also known as DeMorsier Syndrome. Describes the disease and the different treatments that can lead to the significant improvement in the quality of life.
Patricia D Costa, Executive Director

Web Sites

3925 **Alliance of Genetic Support Groups**
A coalition of voluntary genetic support groups, consumers and professionals addressing the needs of individuals and families affected by genetic disorders from a national perspective.

3926 **Atomz**
www.pediatricservices.com
A search engine providing over 60 links to sites involving various growth disorders.

3927 **Healing Well**
www.healingwell.com
An online health resource guide to medical news, chat, information and articles, newsgroups and message boards, books, disease-related web sites, medical directories, and more for patients, friends, and family coping with disabling diseases, disorders, or chronic illnesses.

3928 **Health Finder**
www.healthfinder.gov
Searchable, carefully developed web site offering information on over 1000 topics. Developed by the US Department of Health and Human Services, the site can be used in both English and Spanish.

3929 **Healthlink USA**
www.healthlinkusa.com
Health information concerning treatment, cures, prevention, diagnosis, risk factors, research, support groups, email lists, personal stories and much more. Updated regularly.

3930 **Helios Health**
www.helioshealth.com
Online resource for your health information. Detailed information about specific health topics, access to expert advice from our Medical Advisory Board, and up-to-date health news.

3931   Human Growth Foundation

www.HGFound.org

Organization committed to expanding and accelerating research into growth hormone deficiency. Provides education and support to those affected by growth disorders and their families and fosters the exchange of information with the medical community.

3932   MedicineNet

www.medicinenet.com

An online resource for consumers providing easy-to-read, authoritative medical and health information.

3933   Medscape

www.medscape.com

Medscape offers specialists, primary care physicians, and other health professionals the Web's most robust and integrated medical information and educational tools.

3934   OHSU Homepage Search

www.ohsu.edu

A search which provides several links for information on growth disorders.

3935   WebMD

www.webmd.com

Information on growth disorders, including articles and resources.

Description

3936 **Head Injuries**

Head Injuries, or Traumatic Brain Injuries, cover a range of severity. Currently, there are 5.3 million Americans living with a disability because of a head or brain injury. Concussion, the most common injury, is the momentary loss of consciousness. It usually resolves without any major complications. Damage can result from penetration of the skull or from acceleration/deceleration of the brain that occurs in severe automobile accidents. Injuries can include brain bruising and bleeding into the brain, resulting in swelling that can be life threatening because the skull, as a rigid structure, cannot expand.

Postconcussion syndrome commonly follows a mild injury and can include temporary headaches, dizziness, mild mental slowing and sleepiness. A moderate head or brain injury results in loss of consciousness usually lasting from minutes to a few hours, followed by a few days or weeks of confusion. Loss of consciousness for greater than two minutes implies a worse outcome. Cognitive and psychological impairments lasting many months or even permanently are usual consequences of moderate injury. A severe injury almost always results in prolonged unconsciousness or coma lasting days to weeks or longer. People who sustain a severe head or brain injury often have brain contusions, hematomas (a collection of blood) and/or damage to the nerve fibers or axons. Many people who sustain a severe brain injury make significant improvements in the first year or two. After that improvement tends to slow down, but may continue for years. Some physical and/or cognitive impairments are permanent. See also *Brain Tumors*.

National Agencies & Associations

3937 **American Brain Tumor Association**
2720 River Road   847-827-9910
Des Plaines, IL 60018-4117   800-886-2282
                                    Fax: 847-827-9918
                                 e-mail: info@abta.org
                                        www.abta.org

Services includes over 40 publications which address brain tumors their treatment and coping with the disease. Materials address brain tumors in all age groups. Provide free social service consultations and a mentorship program for new brain tumor support groups.
Elizabeth M Wilson, Executive Director
Geri Jo Duda, Patient Services

3938 **Brain Injury Association**
1608 Spring Hill Road   703-761-0750
Vienna, VA 22182   800-444-6443
                                    Fax: 703-761-0755
                                 e-mail: info@biausa.org
                                        www.biausa.org

The BIA's mission is to create a better future through brain injury prevention research education and advocacy. Offers information on state and national offices treatment and rehabilitation conferences prevention financial development and more.
Susan H Connors, President/CEO
Mary S Reitter, EVP/COO

3939 **Dynamic Rehab**
1800 W Big Beaver Road   281-485-4144
Troy, MI 48084   888-DYN-MIC
                                    Fax: 281-485-4196
                         e-mail: dynmaicrehab@sbcglobal.net
                                      www.dynamicrehab.net

Primary focus is the production and distribution of motivational videotapes and workshops.
Greta Ludwig PT, Owner/Physical Therapist
Teresa Turner, Owner/Physical Therapist

3940 **FASST, Friends & Survivors Standing Together**
21100 W. Capitol Drive
Pewaukee, WI 53072   Fax: 262-790-9670

Nonprofit organization supporting brain injured people and their caregivers. Information, support groups and more.

3941 **Family Caregiver Alliance/National Center on Caregiving**
180 Montgomery Street   415-434-3388
San Francisco, CA 94104   800-445-8106
                                    Fax: 415-434-3508
                              e-mail: info@caregiver.org
                                      www.caregiver.org

Caregiver information and assistance via phone or e-mail; fact sheets and publications describing and documenting caregiver needs and services.
Kathleen Kelly, Executive Director
Ping Hao, President

3942 **International Brain Injury Association**
5909 Ashby Manor Place   703-960-0027
Alexandria, VA 22313   Fax: 703-960-6603
                            e-mail: chaynes@hdipub.com
                                 www.internationalbrain.org

Provides scientific and medical leadership worldwide in the field of brain injury.
Nathan Zasler, Chairman
Margaret Roberts, Executive Director/Administration

3943 **Rainbow House**
4149 W 26th Street
Chicago, IL 60623   773-521-1815
                                   www.rainbow-house.org

Rainbow House is a Chicago-based nonprofit organization whose mission is to end domestic violence. Rainbow House has offered domestic violence prevention programs support and outreach services and resources to survivors across the City of Chicago.
Angel Beltran, Chair
Rosy Mares, Vice Chair

3944 **TPN: The Perspective Network**
PO Box 121012   770-844-6898
W Melbourne, FL 32912-1012   Fax: 770-844-6898
                                   e-mail: TPN@tbi.org
                                         www.tbi.org

The Perspective Network provides forums and resources for persons with families, caregivers, friends and the professionals who serve them. Their goals are to promote a sense of community and to increase public awareness of brain injury.

State Agencies & Associations

Alabama

3945 **Alabama Head Injury Foundation**
3100 Lorna Road   205-823-3818
Hoover, AL 35216   800-433-8002
                                    Fax: 205-823-4544
                            e-mail: ahif1@bellsouth.net
                                    http://www.ahif.org

Services provided to Alabamians with traumatic brain injury or spinal cord injury include information, housing, respite care, recreation programs, resource coordination.
Keith Belt, President
Charles D Priest, Executive Director

Arizona

3946   Brain Injury Association of Arizona
5025 E Washington Street   602-508-8024
Phoenix, AZ 85034   888-500-9165
Fax: 602-508-8285
e-mail: info@biaaz.org
www.biaaz.org

Information and resources for brain injury survivors and their families. Support group listings available. Educational training, conference for families and survivors, neuro-specific resources and helpline.
Lisa Counters, President
Rebecca Armendariz, VicePresident

Arkansas

3947   Brain Injury Association of Arkansas
PO Box 26236   501-374-3585
Little Rock, AR 72221-6236   800-444-6443
Fax: 501-918-6595
e-mail: info@brainassociation.org
www.brainassociation.org

Dana Austen, President
Kortney Coats, Vice President

Colorado

3948   Brain Injury Association of Colorado
4200 W Conejos Place   303-355-9969
Denver, CO 80204   800-955-2443
Fax: 303-355-9968
e-mail: informationreferral@biacolorado.org
www.biacolorado.org

William Levis, President
Gavin Attwood, Executive Director

Connecticut

3949   Brain Injury Association of Connecticut
200 Day Hill Road   86 - 2 - 02
Windsor, CT 06095   800-278-8242
Fax: 86 - 2 - 05
e-mail: general@biact.org
www.biact.org

500 Members
Paul A Slager, President
Julie Peters, Executive Director

Delaware

3950   Brain Injury Association of Delaware
840 Walker Road   302-346-2083
Dover, DE 19904   800-411-0505
Fax: 888-258-3694
e-mail: biadresourcecenter@cavtel.net
www.biausa.org/Delaware

Devon Dorman, President
Esther Curtis, Executive Director

Florida

3951   Brain Injury Association of Florida
1637 Metropolitan Boulevard   850-410-0103
Tallahassee, FL 32308   800-992-3442
Fax: 850-410-0105
e-mail: biaftalla@biaf.org
www.biaf.org

Valerie E Breen, President/CEO

3952   Choices for Work Program Goodwill Industries-Suncoast
Goodwill Industries-Suncoast
10596 Gandy Boulevard   727-523-1512
St Petersburg, FL 33702   888-279-1988
Fax: 727-563-9300
TTY: 727-579-1068
e-mail: gw.marketing@goodwill-suncoast.com
www.goodwill-suncoast.org

A nonprofit community based organization whose purpose is to improve the quality of life for people who are disabled, disadvantaged and/or aged. This mission is accomplished through a staff of over 1,200 employees providing independent living skills, affordable housing, career assessment and job skills training and opportunities.
Deborah A. Passerini, President
Oscar J. Horton, Chair

3953   Pensacola Brain Injury TBI/ABI Support Group
TBI/ABI Support Group
2001 N E Street   850-457-2870
Pensacola, FL 32507   e-mail: hens8250@bellsouth.net
pensacolabrainnetwork.com/sys-tmpl/door

Survivors and caregivers oriented association. Publishes monthly magazine.
Peggy Henshall, Support Group Coordinator

Hawaii

3954   Brain Injury Association of Hawaii
420 Kuwili Street   808-791-6942
Honolulu, HI 96817-1474   Fax: 808-454-1975
e-mail: biahi@hawaiiantel.net
www.biausa.org/Hawaii

Ian Mattoch, President
Mary Wilson, Executive Director

Idaho

3955   Brain Injury Association of Idaho
PO Box 414   208-342-0999
Boise, ID 83701-0414   888-374-3447
Fax: 208-333-0026
e-mail: info@biaid.org
www.biaid.org

Michelle Featherston, President

Illinois

3956   Brain Injury Association of Illinois
PO Box 64420   312-726-5699
Chicago, IL 60664-0420   800-699-6443
Fax: 312-630-4011
e-mail: info@biail.org
www.biail.org

Philicia L Deckard, Executive Director
Irene Pedersen, Founder

Indiana

3957   Brain Injury Association of Indiana
9531 Valparaiso Court   317-356-7722
Indianapolis, IN 46268   866-854-4246
Fax: 31 - 8 - 17
e-mail: info@biai.org
www.biausa.org/Indiana

Anna Garrett, Executive Director
Laura C Trexler, TBI Grant Program Director

Iowa

3958   Brain Injury Association of Iowa
7025 Hickman Road   319-466-7455
Urbandale, IA 50322   800-444-6443
Fax: 800-381-0812
e-mail: info@biaia.org
www.biaia.org

Geoffrey Lauer, Executive Director

Kansas

3959 Brain Injury Association of Kansas and Greater Kansas City
6405 Metcalf Avenue
Overland Park, KS 66202
913-754-8883
800-444-6443
Fax: 816-842-1531
e-mail: info@biaks.org
www.biaks.org

Rob Flores, President
Betsy Johnson, Executive Director

Kentucky

3960 Brain Injury Association of Kentucky
7410 New Lagrange Roadd
Louisville, KY 40222
502-493-0609
800-592-1117
Fax: 502-426-2993
www.biak.us

Chell Austin, Executive Director
Wes Wilkinson, Development Director

Maine

3961 Brain Injury Association of Maine
13 Washington Street
Waterville, ME 04901
207-861-9900
800-275-1233
Fax: 207-861-4617
e-mail: info@biame.org
www.biame.org

Mary Lombardo, President
Leslie DuVall, Director of Operations

Maryland

3962 Brain Injury Association of Maryland
2200 Kernan Drive
Baltimore, MD 21207
410-448-2924
800-221-6443
Fax: 410-448-3541
e-mail: info@biamd.org
www.biamd.org

Patricia Janus, President
Diane Tripplet, Executive Director

Massachusetts

3963 Brain Injury Association of Massachusetts
30 Lyman Street
Westborough, MA 01581
508-475-0032
800-242-0030
Fax: 508-475-0400
e-mail: biama@biama.org
www.biama.org

Shahriar Khaksari, President
Arlene Korab, Executive Director

Michigan

3964 Brain Injury Association of Michigan
7305 Grand River
Brighton, MI 48114-2334
810-229-5880
800-444-6443
Fax: 810-229-8947
e-mail: info@biami.org
www.biami.org

Our mission is to enhance the lives of those affected by brain injury through education, advocacy, research and local support groups and to reduce the incidence of brain injury through prevention.
Katie Knight, Program Coordinator
Michael F Dabbs, President

Minnesota

3965 Brain Injury Association of Minnesota
34 13th Avenue NE
Minneapolis, MN 55413
612-378-2742
800-669-6442
Fax: 612-378-2789
e-mail: info@braininjurymn.org
www.braininjurymn.org

20-24 pages
Andrew Kiragu, Board Chairman

Mississippi

3966 Brain Injury Association of Mississippi
2727 Old Canton
Jackson, MS 39296-5912
601-981-1021
800-444-6443
Fax: 601-981-1039
e-mail: info@msbia.org
www.msbia.org

Howard T Katz, Chairman
Lee Jenkins, Executive Director

Missouri

3967 Brain Injury Association of Missouri
10270 Page Avenue
Saint Louis, MO 63132-1322
314-426-4024
800-444-6443
Fax: 314-426-3290
e-mail: info@biamo.org
www.biamo.org

Information and referral services and support groups through the state of Missouri.
John Bennett, President of the Board
Terrie Price, VP

Montana

3968 Brain Injury Association of Montana
1280 S 3rd W
Missoula, MT 59801
406-541-6442
800-241-6442
Fax: 406-541-4360
e-mail: biam@biamt.org
www.biamt.org

Bobbi Perkins, President
Kristen Morgan, Program Director

New Hampshire

3969 Brain Injury Association of New Hampshire
109 N State Street
Concord, NH 03301
603-225-8400
800-773-8400
Fax: 603-228-6749
e-mail: mail@bianh.org
www.bianh.org

Brant Elkind, President
Steven Wade, Executive Director

New Jersey

3970 Brain Injury Association of New Jersey
825 Georges Road
N Brunswick, NJ 08902
732-745-0200
800-669-4323
Fax: 732-745-0211
e-mail: info@bianj.org
www.bianj.org

Barbara Parker, President

New Mexico

3971 Brain Injury Association of New Mexico
3234 Candelaria NE
Albuquerque, NM 87107
505-292-7414
88 - 2 - 74
Fax: 505-271-8983
e-mail: info@braininjurynm.org
www.braininjurynm.org

John Tiwald, Board President
Mark Pedrotty, VP

New York

3972 Brain Injury Association of New York State
10 Colvin Avenue
Albany, NY 12206-1242
518-459-7911
800-228-8201
Fax: 518-482-5285
e-mail: info@bianys.org
www.bianys.org

Marie Cavallo, President
Judith Avner, Executive Director

3973 RRTC on Community Integration of Persons with TBI
2323 S Shepherd
Houston, TX 77019
713-630-0526
800-732-8124
Fax: 713-630-0529
e-mail: terri.hudler-hull@memorialhermann.org
www.tbicommunity.org

Karen A Hart PhD, Director Of Training
Sunil Kothari, Medical Director

North Carolina

3974 Brain Injury Association of North Carolina
2113 Cameron Street
Raleigh, NC 27605
919-833-9634
800-377-1464
Fax: 919-833-5415
e-mail: bianc@bianc.net
www.tbicommunity.org

Cindy Boyd, Board Chairman
Sandra Farmer, President

Ohio

3975 Brain Injury Association of Ohio
855 Grand View Avenue
Columbus, OH 43215-1123
614-481-7100
866-644-6242
Fax: 614-481-7103
e-mail: help@biaoh.org
www.biaoh.org

Jon Fishpaw, President
Suzanne Minnich, Executive Director

Oklahoma

3976 Brain Injury Association of Oklahoma
PO Box 88
Hillsdale, OK 73743-0088
580-233-4363
800-444-6443
Fax: 580-233-4546
e-mail: brainhelp@braininjuryoklahoma.org
www.braininjuryoklahoma.org

Tracy Grammer, President
Gary Clarke, Chairman

Oregon

3977 Brain Injury Association of Oregon
PO Box 549
Molalla, OR 97038
503-740-3155
800-544-5243
Fax: 503-961-8730
e-mail: info@biaoregon.org
www.biaoregon.org

Tootie Smith, President
Sherry Stock, Executive Director

Pennsylvania

3978 Brain Injury Association of Pennsylvania
950 Walnut Bottom Road
Carlisle, PA 17015
717-657-3601
866-635-7097
Fax: 717-692-5567
e-mail: info@biapa.org
www.biapa.org

Drew Nagele, Chairman of Board Development Committee
Stewart L Cohen, Chairman

Rhode Island

3979 Brain Injury Association of Rhode Island
935 Park Avenue
Cranston, RI 02910-2743
401-461-6599
Fax: 401-461-6561
e-mail: braininjuryctr@biaofri.org
www.biaofri.org

Michael Baker, Co-President
Colleen McCarthy, Co-President

South Carolina

3980 Brain Injury Association of South Carolina
800 Dutch Square Boulevard
Columbia, SC 29210
803-731-9823
877-TBI-FACT
Fax: 803-731-4804
e-mail: scbraininjury@bellsouth.net
www.biausa.org/sc

Elaine Phillips, President
Joyce Davis, Executive Director

Tennessee

3981 Brain Injury Association of Tennessee
955 Woodland St
Nashville, TN 37206
615-248-5878
877-757-2428
Fax: 615-383-1176
e-mail: biaoftn@yahoo.com
www.biaoftn.org

Guynn Edwards, President
Pam Bryan, Executive Director

Texas

3982 Brain Injury Association of Texas
316 W 12th Street
Austin, TX 78701
512-326-1212
800-392-0040
Fax: 512-478-3370
e-mail: info@biatx.org
www.biatx.org

Jane Boutte, President

Utah

3983 Brain Injury Association of Utah
1800 S W Temple
Salt Lake City, UT 84115
801-484-2240
800-281-8442
Fax: 801-484-5932
e-mail: biau@sisna.com
www.biau.org

Teresa Such-Niebar, President
Ron S Roskos, Executive Director

Vermont

3984 Brain Injury Association of Vermont
92 S Main Street
Waterbury, VT 05676
802-244-6850
877-856-1772
Fax: 802-244-4005
e-mail: support1@biavt.org
www.biavt.org

Marsha Bancroft, President
Trevor Squirrell, Executive Director

Virginia

3985 Brain Injury Association of America's National Family Helpline
1608 Spring Hill Road
Vienna, VA 22182
703-761-0750
800-444-6443
Fax: 703-761-0755
e-mail: FamilyHelpline@biausa.org
www.biausa.org

Greg Oshanick, Chairman
Susan Conners, President and CEO

3986 Brain Injury Association of Virginia
1506 Willow Lawn Drive
Richmond, VA 23230
804-355-5748
800-444-6443
Fax: 804-355-6381
e-mail: info@biav.net
www.biav.net

Anne McDonnell, Executive Director
Lynette Scott, Program Director

Washington

3987 Brain Injury Association of Washington
800 Jefferson Street
Seattle, WA 98104
206-388-0900
800-523-5438
Fax: 206-388-0901
e-mail: info@biawa.org
www.biawa.org

Richard Adler, President
Gene van den Bosch, Executive Director

West Virginia

3988 Brain Injury Association of West Virginia
PO Box 574
Institute, WV 25112-0574
304-766-4892
800-356-6443
Fax: 304-766-4940
e-mail: mdavis@brainman.com
www.biausa.org/WVirginia

Michael W Davis, Board of Director
Linda Arthur, Board of Director

Wisconsin

3989 Brain Injury Association of Wisconsin
21100 W Capitol Drive
Pewaukee, WI 53072
262-790-9660
800-882-9282
Fax: 262-790-9670
e-mail: admin@execpc.com
www.biaw.org

Advocacy, education, prevention, information, resources, and support groups in regards to traumatic brain injury.
David Voss, President
Mark Warhus, Executive Director

Wyoming

3990 Brain Injury Association of Wyoming
111 W 2nd Street
Casper, WY 82601
307-473-1767
800-643-6457
Fax: 307-237-5222
e-mail: biaw@tribcsp.com
www.biausa.org/Wyoming

Larry Plemmons, President
Jack Nokes, Director

Foundations

3991 Brain Trauma Foundation
708 Third Avenue
New York, NY 10017-4201
212-772-0608
Fax: 212-772-2035
e-mail: info@braintrauma.org
www.braintrauma.org

Our goal at the Brain Trauma Foundation is to improve the outcome of TBI patients through Guideline development, clinical research, professional education, and quality improvement programs.
Quarterly
Jamshid Ghajar, MD, President
Pamela Drexel, Executive Director

Libraries & Resource Centers

Michigan

3992 Wayne State University: Gurdjian-Lissner Biomechanics Laboratory
Department of Neurological Surgery
4160 John R Street
Detroit, MI 48201
313-831-0777
877-486-7978
Fax: 313-966-0368
e-mail: neurosurgery@med.wayne.edu
www.neurosurgery.med.wayne.edu

Head and neck injury research.
Murali Guthikonda, MD, FACS, Professor (Clinician-Educator) and Chair
Patti Bekowies, MBA, Chief Administrative Officer

Research Centers

3993 Brady Institute Jamaica Hospital Medical Center
Jamaica Hospital Medical Center
8900 Van Wyck Expressway
Jamaica, NY 11418-2897
718-206-6000
Fax: 718-206-6559
www.jamaicahospital.org

The James and Sarah Brady Institute for Traumatic Brain Injury.
David P Rosen, President & CEO
Neil Foster Phillips, Chairman

3994 Dana Alliance for Brain Initiatives
745 Fifth Avenue
New York, NY 10151
212-223-4040
Fax: 212-317-8721
e-mail: danainfo@dana.org
www.dana.org

A non-profit organization of more than 250 neuroscientists which was formed to help provide information about the personal and public benefits of brain research.
Jane Nevins, Vice President
Edward F Rover, President

3995 Institute for Rehabilitation and Research
21720 Kingsland Blvd.
Katy, TX 77450
28- 57- 555
800-447-3422
Fax: 713-874-1798
e-mail: tirr.referrals@memorialhermann.org
www.tirr.org

John Kajander, President

3996 New York University Medical Center Head Trauma Program
Reet
New York, NY 10010-4020
212-998-9819
Fax: 212-340-7158
Research pertaining to young adults suffering from head injuries.
Dr Yehuda Ben-Yishay, Coordinator

3997 Ohio State University Laboratory of Psychobiology
1835 Neil Avenue
Columbus, OH 43210-1222
614-292-8185
Fax: 614-292-4537
www.psy.ohio-state.edu/labs

Studies done on recovery of function after brain damage.
Laura Peterson, Lab Coordinator
James Walton, Research Associate

3998 Rehabilitation Institute of Michigan
261 Mack Avenue
Detroit, MI 48201
313-745-1203
Fax: 313-745-2376
www.rimrehab.org

Physical medicine and rehabilitation medicine.
William H Restum PhD, President
Horacio Varg Jr, Interim Executive Director

3999 Thomas Jefferson University Ischemia-Shock Research Center
1020 Locust Street
Philadelphia, PA 19107-6731
215-503-4400
Fax: 215-503-9920
e-mail: jgsbs-info@jefferson.edu
www.jefferson.edu

Promotes research into head injuries and clinical studies.

4000 Thomas Jefferson University Ischemia-Shock
1020 Walnut Street
Philadelphia, PA 19107
215-955-6000
Fax: 215-923-7932
www.jefferson.edu

Promotes research into head injuries and clinical studies.

4001 Tulane University: US-Japan Biomedical Research Laboratories
1430 Tulane Avenue
New Orleans, LA 70112
504-988-5187
Fax: 504-394-7169
e-mail: medsch@tulane.edu
www.tulane.edu/som/

Focuses research efforts on neuroendocrinology and neurosciences.
Benjamin P Sachs, MB, BS, Senior Vice President, Dean
Mary Brown, MBA, Vice President

4002 **UCLA Neuropsychiatric Institute**
760 Westwood Plaza   310-825-2631
Los Angeles, CA 90095   800-825-9989
                                                   Fax: 310-825-9179
                                        e-mail: pwhybrow@mednet.ucla.edu
                                                   www.semel.ucla.edu
Devote to teach research and patient care in psychiatry neuroscience and related fields.
Peter Whybrow, Director

4003 **University of California: Irvine Brain Imaging Center**
101 The City Drive S   949-824-7872
Irvine, CA 92697-3960   Fax: 949-824-7873
                                            e-mail: BIC@msx.hsis.uci.edu
                                                   www.bic.uci.edu
Offers PET scan analysis of brain functions focusing on brain damage brain tumors and head injuries.
Steven L Small, PhD, MD, Director
David B Keator, MCS, Technical Director

4004 **University of California: San Francisco Laboratory for Neurotrauma**
1001 Potrero Avenue
San Francisco, CA 94110-3518   415-206-8313
                                                   www.ucsf.edu
Research done into traumatic brain and head injuries.
Lawrence H Pitts MD

4005 **University of Memphis: Department of Psych ology**
Memphis State University
202 Psychology Building   901-678-2000
Memphis, TN 38152   Fax: 901-678-2579
                                         e-mail: psycadvise@memphis.edu
                                              www.memphis.edu/psychology/
Evaluation and development of assessment and treatment procedures for neurologically impaired persons.
Guy Mittleman, Professor Director of CAPR
Frank Andrasik, Professor, Chair

4006 **Virginia Commonwealth University: Rehab Research and Training Center**
1314 W Main Street   804-828-1851
Richmond, VA 23284-2011   Fax: 804-828-2193
                                                   TTY: 804-828-2494
                                                   www.vcu.edu/rrtcweb/
Focuses research on traumatic brain and head injuries.
Paul Wehman, Director
Jeanne Dalton, Public Relations Assistant Specialist

Support Groups & Hotlines

4007 **National Health Information Center**
PO Box 1133   301-565-4167
Washington, DC 20013   800-336-4797
                                                   Fax: 301-984-4256
                                                   e-mail: info@nhic.org
                                                   www.health.gov/nhic
Offers a nationwide information referral service, produces directories and resource guides.

Alabama

4008 **Alabama Head Injury Foundation Helpline**
3100 Lorna Road   205-823-3818
Hoover, AL 35216-5451   800-433-8002
                                                   Fax: 205-823-4544
                                             e-mail: ahif1@bellsouth.net
                                                   www.ahif.org/
The Alabama Head Injury Foundation (AHIF) was founded by professionals and families in 1983 to increase public awareness of Traumatic Brain Injury (TBI) and to stimulate the development of supportive services. AHIF provides accessible resources, services and programs that meet the unique needs of individuals with traumatic brain injury (TBI) as well as spinal cord injury (SCI) in certain programs.
Charles D Priest, Executive Director
Janet Massey, Executive Assistant

Arizona

4009 **Brain Injury Association of Arizona**
5025 E Washington Street   602-508-8024
Phoenix, AZ 85034   888-500-9165
                                                   Fax: 602-508-8285
                                                   e-mail: info@biaaz.org
                                                   www.biaaz.org
Information and resources for brain injury survivors and their families. Support group listings available. Educational training, conference for families and survivors, neuro-specific resources and helpline.
Kim Halloran, Executive Director
Jeanne Andersen, Information & Referral Manager

Arkansas

4010 **Brain Injury Association of Arkansas Helpl ine**
PO Box 26236   501-374-3585
Little Rock, AR 72221-6236   866-610-4841
                                                   Fax: 501-918-6595
                                         e-mail: info@brainassociation.org
                                                   www.bia-ar.org
Founded in 1980, the Brain Injury Association of America (BIAA) is a national organization serving and representing individuals, families and professionals who are touched by a life-altering, often devastating, traumatic brain injury (TBI). BIAA provides information, education and support through its network of chartered state affiliates, local chapters and support groups across the country to assist the 5.3 million Americans currently living with traumatic brain injury and their families.
Dana Austen, President Arkansas State Office
Kortney E Gold, Vice President

California

4011 **Brain Injury Association of California Hel pline**
3501 Mall View Road   661-872-4903
Bakersfield, CA 93306   Fax: 661-873-2508
                                           e-mail: calbiainfo@yahoo.com
                                                   www.biacal.org/
Founded in 1980, the Brain Injury Association of America (BIAA) is a national organization serving and representing individuals, families and professionals who are touched by a life-altering, often devastating, traumatic brain injury (TBI). BIAA provides information, education and support through its network of chartered state affiliates, local chapters and support groups across the country to assist the 5.3 million Americans currently living with traumatic brain injury and their families.
Paula Daoutis, Administrative Director
Ursula Pesta, Project Coordinator

4012 **Jodi House**
625 Chapala St.   805-563-2882
Santa Barbara, CA 93101   Fax: 805-563-3982
                                             e-mail: info@jodihouse.org
                                                   www.jodihouse.org
Jodi House is a community-based, post-rehabilitation day program that provides opportunities for social interaction, life skill training, recreation, and support for adults living with acquired brain injury (i.e. from head trauma, tumor, and stroke) and their families.
Gayle Cummings, Co-President
Timothy Morton-Smith, Co-President/Vice President of Finance

Colorado

4013 **Brain Injury Association of Colorado Helpline**
1385 South Colorado Boulevard   303-355-9969
Denver, CO 80222   800-955-2443
                                                   Fax: 303-355-9968
                                             e-mail: biacolo@aol.com
                                                   www.BIAColorado.org

Dannis Schanel, LCSW, CBIST, President
Gavin Attwood, Exececutive Director

Connecticut

4014 Brain Injury Association of Connecticut Helpline
200 Day Hill Road   860-219-0291
Windsor, CT 06095-1304   800-278-8242
                                   Fax: 860-219-0568
                          e-mail: general@biact.org
                             www.biact.homestead.com/
Supports persons with brain injuries and their families by promoting services to facilitate full inclusion within their local community and to increase awareness and understanding of brain injury and its prevention through community education.
500 Members
Paul A. Slager, Esq., President
Dr. Johnny Magwood, BSME, MBA, DBA, Vice President

Delaware

4015 Brain Injury Association of Delaware Helpl ine
32 West Loockerman Street   302-346-2083
Dover, DE 19904   800-411-0505
                                   Fax: 302-678-3183
                    e-mail: biadresourcecenter@cavdel.net
                                 www.biaofde.org//
Founded in 1980, the Brain Injury Association of America (BIAA) is a national organization serving and representing individuals, families and professionals who are touched by a life-altering, often devastating, traumatic brain injury (TBI). BIAA provides information, education and support through its network of chartered state affiliates, local chapters and support groups across the country to assist the 5.3 million Americans currently living with traumatic brain injury and their families.
Elizabeth Furber, President Delaware State Office
Timothy J Walker, Vice President

Florida

4016 Brain Injury Association of Florida
1637 Metropolitan Blvd   850-410-0103
Tallahassee, FL 32308   800-992-3442
                                   Fax: 850-410-0105
                              e-mail: admin@biaf.org
                                     www.biaf.org

Gary Clarke, Chairman
Valerie Breen, President/CEO

Hawaii

4017 Brain Injury Association of Hawaii
420 Kuwili Street   808-436-8977
Honolulu, HI 96817   e-mail: biahi@hawaiiantel.net
                               www.biausa.org/Hawaii
Dedicated to serving those affected by brain injury throughgh advocacy, prevention, and support
Mary Wilson, Executive Director
Ian Mattoch, President

Illinois

4018 American Brain Tumor Association Patient Line
8550 W. Bryn Mawr Ave   773-577-8750
Chicago, IL 60631-4117   800-886-2282
                                   Fax: 773-577-8738
                              e-mail: info@abta.org
                                     www.abta.org
Offers emergency support, information and referrals for patients and their families.
Ronald Petrocelli, MD, Chair
Elizabeth M Wilson, President, CEO

4019 Brain Injury Association of Illinois Helpline
PO Box 64420   312-726-5699
Chicago, IL 60664-420   800-699-6443
                                   Fax: 312-630-4011
                              e-mail: info@biail.org
                                     www.biail.org
Works with all people with brain inquiries and their families with professionals who serve them. Provides camp oppurtunities, support groups, educational seminars, information and referrals and a quarterly newsletter.
Irene Pedersen, Founder
Philicia L Deckard, Executive Director

Indiana

4020 Brain Injury Association of Indiana Helpli ne
9531 Valparaiso Court   317-356-7722
Indianapolis, IN 46268   866-854-4246
                                   Fax: 317-802-1768
                               e-mail: info@biai.org
                                     www.biai.org
Founded in 1980, the Brain Injury Association of America (BIAA) is a national organization serving and representing individuals, families and professionals who are touched by a life-altering, often devastating, traumatic brain injury (TBI). BIAA provides information, education and support through its network of chartered state affiliates, local chapters and support groups across the country to assist the 5.3 million Americans currently living with traumatic brain injury and their families.
Nancy Ritter, Chairperson
Anna Garrett, Executive Director

Iowa

4021 Brain Injury Alliance of Iowa Helpline
Brain Injury Association of America
7025 Hickman Road   319-272-2312
Urbandale, IA 50322   855-444-6443
                                   Fax: 319-272-2109
                               e-mail: info@biaia.org
                                     www.biaia.org

Geoffrey Lauer, Executive Director
Natasha Retz, Director of Programs and Services

Kansas

4022 Brain Injury Association of Kansas and Greater Kansas City Helpline
6701 W. 64th Street   913-754-8883
Overland Park, KS 66202   800-783-1356
                                   Fax: 816-842-1531
                    e-mail: rabramowitz@biaks.org
                                     www.biaks.org

Whitney Sunderland, President
Robin Abramowitz, Executive Director

Kentucky

4023 Brain Injury Alliance of Kentucky
7321 New LaGrange Road   502-493-0609
Louisville, KY 40222   800-592-1117
                                   Fax: 502-426-2993
                       e-mail: chell.austin@biak.us
                                     www.biak.us
Founded in 1980, the Brain Injury Association of America (BIAA) is a national organization serving and representing individuals, families and professionals who are touched by a life-altering, often devastating, traumatic brain injury (TBI). BIAA provides information, education and support through its network of chartered state affiliates, local chapters and support groups across the country to assist the 5.3 million Americans currently living with traumatic brain injury and their families.
Andrew Horne, President Kentucky State Office
Chell Austin, Executive Director

Louisiana

4024 Brain Injury Association of Louisiana Help line
c/o National Headquarters Office
8325 Oak Street   504-982-0685
New Orleans, LA 70118   800-444-6443
                                   Fax: 703-761-0755
                              e-mail: info@biala.org
                                     www.biala.org/
Founded in 1980, the Brain Injury Association of America (BIAA) is a national organization serving and representing individuals, families and professionals who are touched by a life-altering, often

devastating, traumatic brain injury (TBI). BIAA provides information, education and support through its network of chartered state affiliates, local chapters and support groups across the country to assist the 5.3 million Americans currently living with traumatic brain injury and their families.
Janet Clark, Chairman
Tommy Lotz, Executive Director

Maryland

4025 Brain Injury Association of Maryland Helpl ine
Kernan Hospital
2200 Kernan Drive   410-448-2924
Baltimore, MD 21207   800-221-6443
                                  Fax: 410-448-3541
                           e-mail: info@biamd.org
                                    www.biamd.org
Founded in 1980, the Brain Injury Association of America (BIAA) is a national organization serving and representing individuals, families and professionals who are touched by a life-altering, often devastating, traumatic brain injury (TBI). BIAA provides information, education and support through its network of chartered state affiliates, local chapters and support groups across the country to assist the 5.3 million Americans currently living with traumatic brain injury and their families.
Mark Huslage, President Maryland State Office
Bryan Thomas Pugh, Executive Director

Massachusetts

4026 Brain Injury Association of Massachusetts Helpline
30 Lyman Street   508-475-0032
Westborough, MA 01581   800-242-0030
                                  Fax: 508-475-0400
                               TTY: 508-948-0593
                          e-mail: biama@biama.org
                                     www.biama.org
Founded in 1980, the Brain Injury Association of America (BIAA) is a national organization serving and representing individuals, families and professionals who are touched by a life-altering, often devastating, traumatic brain injury (TBI). BIAA provides information, education and support through its network of chartered state affiliates, local chapters and support groups across the country to assist the 5.3 million Americans currently living with traumatic brain injury and their families.
Teresa Hayes, President Massachusetts State Office
Mathew Martino, Executive Board

4027 VALT Support Group (Vital Active Life After Trauma)
53 Linden Street   617-277-6327
Brookline, MA 02149

Michigan

4028 Brain Injury Association of Michigan Helpline
7305 Grand River   810-229-5880
Brighton, MI 48114-2334   800-444-6443
                                  Fax: 810-229-8947
                            e-mail: info@biami.org
                                     www.biami.org
Deborah Newton, Chair
Michael F Dabbs, President

Minnesota

4029 Brain Injury Alliance of Minnesota
34 13th Avenue North East   612-378-2742
Minneapolis, MN 55413   800-669-6442
                                  Fax: 612-378-2789
                      e-mail: info@braininjurymn.org
                               www.braininjurymn.org
Tom Gode, Executive Director

Mississippi

4030 Brain Injury Association of Mississippi Helpline
2727 Old Canton Road   601-981-1021
Jackson, MS 39216-5912   800-444-6443
                                  Fax: 601-981-1039
                          e-mail: ljenkins@msbia.org
                                    www.msbia.org/
Howard T Katz, MD, Chair
Lee Jenkins, Executive Director

Missouri

4031 Brain Injury Association of Missouri Helpline
2265 Schuetz Road   314-426-4024
St Louis, MO 63146-1322   800-444-6443
                                  Fax: 314-426-3290
                            e-mail: info@biamo.org
                                     www.biamo.org
Information and referral services and support groups throughout the state of Missouri.
Eric Hart, Psy.D, Board President
Stephanie Cooper, Executive Director

Montana

4032 Brain Injury Alliance of Montana
1280 South 3rd Street West   406-541-6442
Missoula, MT 59801   800-241-6442
                                  Fax: 406-243-2349
                          e-mail: kristen@biamt.org
                                     www.biamt.org
Kristen Morgan, MSW, Program Director
Molly Walsh, Outreach Coordinator

New Hampshire

4033 Brain Injury Association of New Hampshire
Brain Injury Association of America
109 N State Street   603-225-8400
Concord, NH 03301-4447   800-773-8400
                                  Fax: 603-228-6749
                            e-mail: mail@bianh.org
                                     www.bianh.org
Laura Flashman, PhD, President
Steven D Wade, Executive Director

New Jersey

4034 Brain Injury Alliance of New Jersey
Brain Injury Association of America
825 Georges Road   732-745-0200
North Brunswick, NJ 08902   800-669-4323
                                  Fax: 732-745-0211
                            e-mail: info@bianj.org
                                     www.bianj.org
Edward Kim, MD, MBA, Chairperson
Barbara Geiger-Parker, President/CEO

New Mexico

4035 Brain Injury Alliance of New Mexico
3232 Candelaria NE   505-292-7414
Albuquerque, NM 87107   888-292-7415
                                  Fax: 505-271-8983
                    e-mail: braininjurynm@msn.com
                                www.braininjurynm.org
Founded in 1980, the Brain Injury Association of America (BIAA) is a national organization serving and representing individuals, families and professionals who are touched by a life-altering, often devastating, traumatic brain injury (TBI). BIAA provides information, education and support through its network of chartered state affiliates, local chapters and support groups across the country to assist the 5.3 million Americans currently living with traumatic brain injury and their families.
John Tiwald, Board President New Mexico State Office
Mark Pedrotty, PhD, Vice President

New York

4036 Brain Injury Association of New York State Helpline
10 Colvin Avenue
Albany, NY 12206-1242

518-459-7911
800-228-8201
Fax: 518-482-5285
e-mail: info@bianys.org
www.bianys.org

Marie Cavallo, Ph.D, President
Judith Avner, Executive Director

4037 Cafe Plus
216 W Manlius Street
East Syracuse, NY 13057

315-446-3124
e-mail: cafeplus@dreamscape.com
www.dreamscape.com/cafeplus

For people who have survived a head-injury or some type of head trauma.
David Listowski, Manager

4038 Hy Feinstein Clubhouse
Long Island Head Injury Association
300 Kennedy Drive
Hauppauge, NY 11788

631-543-2245
Fax: 631-543-2261
e-mail: lgiordano@headinjuryassoc.org
www.headinjuryassociation.org/feinstein

The LIHIA provides a place for people with head injury to participate in meaningful work, to have the opportunity to meet and build friendships and ultimately seek employment within the community.
Stuart Gleiber, President
Leonard Feinstein, Vice President

North Carolina

4039 Brain Injury Association of North Carolina Helpline
2113 Cameron Street
Raleigh, NC 27605

919-833-9634
800-377-1464
Fax: 919-833-5415
e-mail: bianc@bianc.net
www.bianc.net/

Susan Baker, Director of Finance
Cindy Boyd, Fundraising Chair

North Dakota

4040 Brain Injury Association of North Dakota
1225 South 12th Street
Bismarck, ND 58504

877-525-2724
Fax: 701-845-1175
e-mail: braininjurynd@gmail.co
www.braininjurynd.com/

Founded in 1980, the Brain Injury Association of America (BIAA) is a national organization serving and representing individuals, families and professionals who are touched by a life-altering, often devastating, traumatic brain injury (TBI). BIAA provides information, education and support through its network of chartered state affiliates, local chapters and support groups across the country to assist the 5.3 million Americans currently living with traumatic brain injury and their families.
April Fairfield, Executive Director
Rebecca Quinn, Eastern Region Contact

Ohio

4041 Brain Injury Association of Ohio
855 Grandview Avenue
Columbus, OH 43215-1000

614-481-7100
800-444-6443
Fax: 614-481-7103
e-mail: help@biaoh.org
www.biaoh.org

Stephanie Ramsey, President
Jon Fishpaw, First Vice President

Oklahoma

4042 Brain Injury Association of Oklahoma Helpl ine
3015 E. Skelly Dr.
Tulsa, OK 74105-0088

918-789-0406
800-765-6809
Fax: 918-712-9019
e-mail: braininjuryoklahoma@gmail.com
www.braininjuryoklahoma.org

Founded in 1980, the Brain Injury Association of America (BIAA) is a national organization serving and representing individuals, families and professionals who are touched by a life-altering, often devastating, traumatic brain injury (TBI). BIAA provides information, education and support through its network of chartered state affiliates, local chapters and support groups across the country to assist the 5.3 million Americans currently living with traumatic brain injury and their families.
Adam Sherman, PhD, President Oklahoma State Office
Mary Dobbs, Vice-President

Oregon

4043 Brain Injury Alliance of Oregon
Brain Injury Association of America
2145 NW Overton Street
Portland, OR 97210

503-413-7707
800-544-5243
Fax: 503-413-6849
e-mail: biaor@biaoregon.org
www.biaoregon.org

Non-profit providing information and referral, support groups, prevention, education, training, and advocacy for those with brain injury, families, and professionals.
Ralph Wiser, President
Chuck McGilvrary, Vice-President

Rhode Island

4044 Brain Injury Association of Rhode Island H elpline
935 Park Avenue
Cranston, RI 02910-2743

401-461-6599
Fax: 401-461-6561
e-mail: braininjuryctr@biaofri.org
www.biausa.org/RI/

Founded in 1980, the Brain Injury Association of America (BIAA) is a national organization serving and representing individuals, families and professionals who are touched by a life-altering, often devastating, traumatic brain injury (TBI). BIAA provides information, education and support through its network of chartered state affiliates, local chapters and support groups across the country to assist the 5.3 million Americans currently living with traumatic brain injury and their families.
Michael L. Baker, Co-President
Sharon Brinkworth, Executive Director

Tennessee

4045 Brain Injury Association of Tennessee Help line
955 Woodland Street
Nashville, TN 37206

615-248-2541
800-444-6443
Fax: 615-383-1176
e-mail: biaoftn@yahoo.com
www.braininjurytn.org/

Founded in 1980, the Brain Injury Association of America (BIAA) is a national organization serving and representing individuals, families and professionals who are touched by a life-altering, often devastating, traumatic brain injury (TBI). BIAA provides information, education and support through its network of chartered state affiliates, local chapters and support groups across the country to assist the 5.3 million Americans currently living with traumatic brain injury and their families.
Guynn Edwards, President Tennessee State Office
Pam Bryan, Executive Director

Utah

4046 Brain Injury Alliance of Utah
Brain Injury Association of America
5280 Commerce Dr.
Murray, UT 84107

801-716-4993
800-281-8442
Fax: 801-716-4995
e-mail: info@biau.org
www.biau.org/

Antonietta Anna Russo, Ph.D., President
Ron S Roskos, Executive Director

Vermont

4047   Brain Injury Association of Vermont Helpli ne
92 South Main Street   802-244-6850
Waterbury, VT 05676   877-856-1772
Fax: 802-244-4005
e-mail: support1@biavt.org
www.biavt.org
Founded in 1980, the Brain Injury Association of America (BIAA) is a national organization serving and representing individuals, families and professionals who are touched by a life-altering, often devastating, traumatic brain injury (TBI). BIAA provides information, education and support through its network of chartered state affiliates, local chapters and support groups across the country to assist the 5.3 million Americans currently living with traumatic brain injury and their families.
Marsha Bancroft, President Vermont State Office
Trevor Squirrell, Executive Director

Virginia

4048   Brain Injury Association of Virginia Helpline
1506 Willow Lawn Dr   804-355-5748
Richmond, VA 23230-5018   800-444-6443
Fax: 804-355-6381
e-mail: info@biav.net
www.biav.net
Nonprofit organization providing information and resources related to brain injury to individuals with brain injuries, their families and professionals who deal with brain injury.
Kimberly Moore, President
Anne McDonnell, Executive Director

Washington

4049   Brain Injury Association of Washington Hel pline
P.O. Box 3044   206-467-4800
Seattle, WA 98114   877-982-4292
Fax: 206-467-4808
e-mail: info@braininjurywa.org
www.braininjurywa.org/
Founded in 1980, the Brain Injury Association of America (BIAA) is a national organization serving and representing individuals, families and professionals who are touched by a life-altering, often devastating, traumatic brain injury (TBI). BIAA provides information, education and support through its network of chartered state affiliates, local chapters and support groups across the country to assist the 5.3 million Americans currently living with traumatic brain injury and their families.
Mark T Long, President Washington State Office
Deborah Crawley, Executive Director

4050   Brain Injury Resource Center
Brain Injury Resource Center
PO Box 84151   206-621-8558
Seattle, WA 98124-5451   Fax: 206-329-4355
e-mail: brain@headinjury.com
www.headinjury.com
Disseminates head injury information and provides referrals to facilitate adjustment to life following head injury. Organizes seminars for professionals, head injury survivors, and their families.
Constance Miller MA, Founder/President
B Parker Lindner MPA, Communications Specialist

West Virginia

4051   Brain Injury Association of West Virginia Helpline
Brain Injury Association of America
PO Box 574   304-400-4506
Institute, WV 25112-574   800-356-6443
Fax: 304-766-4940
e-mail: mdavis@brainman.com
Michael W Davis, President

Wisconsin

4052   Brain Injury Alliance of Wisconsin
21100 W. Capitol Dr.   262-790-9660
Brookfield, WI 53072   800-882-9282
Fax: 262-790-9670
e-mail: admin@execpc.com
www.biaw.org
Founded in 1980, the Brain Injury Association of America (BIAA) is a national organization serving and representing individuals, families and professionals who are touched by a life-altering, often devastating, traumatic brain injury (TBI). BIAA provides information, education and support through its network of chartered state affiliates, local chapters and support groups across the country to assist the 5.3 million Americans currently living with traumatic brain injury and their families.
Audrey Nelson, President Wisconsin State Office
Lori Schultz, Executive Director

Wyoming

4053   Brain Injury Alliance of Wyoming
111 West 2nd Street   307-473-1767
Casper, WY 82601   800-643-6457
Fax: 307-237-5222
e-mail: director@wybia.org
www.wybia.org/
Dorothy Cronin, Director

Books

4054   An Educational Challenge: Meeting the Needs of Students with Brain Injury
Brain Injury Association
105 N Alfred Street   703-236-6000
Alexandria, VA 22314   800-444-6443
Fax: 703-236-6001

4055   Brain Injury Glossary
HDI Publishers
10600 NW Freeway, Suite 202
Houston, TX 77219   800-321-7037
Fax: 713-956-2288
Contains glossary and descriptions of health care providers.

4056   Brainlash
Demos Medical Publishing
386 Park Avenue S   212-683-0072
New York, NY 10016   Fax: 212-683-0118
e-mail: orderdept@demospub.com
www.demosmedpub.com
Maximize your recovery from mild brain injury.
376 pages
ISBN: 1-888799-37-4
Dr. Diana M Schneider

4057   Coming Home: A Discharge Manual for Families of Persons with a Brain Injury
HDI Publishers
10600 NW Freeway, Suite 202
Houston, TX 77219   800-321-7037
Fax: 713-956-2288

4058   Communication Disorders Following Traumatic Brain Injury
Pro-Ed, Inc.
8700 Shoal Creek Boulevard   512-451-3246
Austin, TX 78757-6897   800-897-3202
Fax: 800-397-7633
e-mail: info@proedinc.com
www.proedinc.com
For graduates and professionals, this text takes a holistic approach toward treating the client with traumatic brain injury.
439 pages Paperback
ISBN: 0-890792-95-X
Lindy Jordaan, Marketing Coordinator

4059   Dano Cerebral: Guia Para Familias y Cuidadores
Brain Injury Association/HDI Publishers/Catalogue

PO Box 131401
Houston, TX 77219   800-321-7037
     Fax: 713-526-7787
This book, written in Spanish, is a thorough, well-researched guide for people with brain injury, their families and caregivers. Up-to-date information covers such topics as Intensive Care- admittance and discharge; Mechanics of brain injury; Coma; Consequences of brain injury; Mental and Emotional symptoms among many others.
158 pages 1994

4060 From the Ashes
Phoenix Project
PO Box 84151   206-329-1371
Seattle, WA 98124-5451
A self-help book that addresses the trauma that comes with a head injury and introduces methods of building a fulfilling and productive life.
108 pages

4061 Handbook of Head Truma: Acute Care to Recovery
Plenum Publishing Corporation
233 Spring Street   212-620-8000
New York, NY 10013-1522   800-221-9369
     Fax: 212-463-0742
     e-mail: books@plenum.com
466 pages
ISBN: 0-306439-47-6

4062 Head Injury and the Family: A Life and Living Perspective
St. Lucie Press
100 E Linton Boulevard   407-274-9906
Delary Beach, FL 33483   Fax: 407-274-9927
One of the best books written in this area. Easy to read, written with family, caregivers and patients in mind. Includes exercises and vignettes.

4063 Integrating Community Resources
HDI Publishers
10600 NW Freeway, Suite 202
Houston, TX 77219   800-321-7037
     Fax: 713-956-2288

4064 Living with Brain Injury: A Guide for Families
Brain Injury Association/HDI Publishers/Catalogue
PO Box 131401
Houston, TX 77219   800-321-7037
     Fax: 713-526-7787
This book will help readers- families, persons with brain injury and professionals alike- through this uncharted territory. topics include: How brain injury is caused and how it can be treated: Physical, cognitive and behavioral symptoms; Questions family members commonly ask.
145 pages 1998

4065 National Directory of Brain Injury Rehabilitatiom
Brain Injury Association
105 N Alfred Street   703-236-6000
Alexandria, VA 22314   800-444-6443
     Fax: 703-236-6001
Desk reference for professionals listing brain injury rehabilitation programs and individual service providers nationwide.

4066 National Directory of Head Injury Rehabilitation Services
Brain Injury Association
105 N Alfred Street   703-236-6000
Alexandria, VA 22314   800-444-6443
     Fax: 703-236-6001

4067 Planning for the Future
Brain Injury Association
105 N Alfred Street   703-236-6000
Alexandria, VA 22314   800-444-6443
     Fax: 703-236-6001
This book provides a meaningful life for a child with a disability after your death.

4068 Recovery from Brain Damage in the Elderly
Aspen Publishers
PO Box 990
Frederick, MD 21705-0990   800-638-8437

Recovery and rehabilitation techniques in the area of brain damage in the elderly.

4069 Sexuality and the Person with Traumatic Brain Injury
Brain Injury Association
105 N Alfred Street   703-236-6000
Alexandria, VA 22314   800-444-6443
     Fax: 703-236-6001

4070 Stress Management Following Head Injury: Strategies for Families and Caregivers
Brain Injury Association
105 N Alfred Street   703-236-6000
Alexandria, VA 22314   800-444-6443
     Fax: 703-236-6001

4071 TBI Tool Kit
HDI Publishers
10600 NW Freeway, Suite 202
Houston, TX 77219   800-321-7037
     Fax: 713-956-2288

4072 Traumatic Brain Injury Rehabilitation: Brain Injury Consortium Monograph Series
St. Lucie Press
100 E Linton Boulevard   407-274-9906
Delray Beach, FL 33483   Fax: 407-274-9927
Assistive technology, under the Americans with Disabilities Act, is that designed for and used by individuals with the intent of eliminating, ameliorating, or compensating for functional limitations. Coverage includes impaired functions that limit vocational outcome, behavior concerns in the workplace, maximizing a client's residual knowledge skills, use of computers and adapting work environments.

4073 Traumatic Head Injury: Cause, Consequence and Challenge
Brain Injury Association/HDI Publishers/Catalogue
PO Box 131401
Houston, TX 77219   800-321-7037
     Fax: 713-526-7787
A resource book on traumatic brain injury which translates technical medical information on brain injury into simple, easy-to-understand language for persons with brain injury and their families. Covered topics: a general overview of brain injury; similarities and differences among people with brain injury; types and consequences of brain injury; recovery and rehabilitation; accepting and coping with change.
60 pages 1993

4074 Why Did it Happen on a School Day: My Family's Experience with Brain Injury
Brain Injury Association
105 N Alfred Street   703-236-6000
Alexandria, VA 22314   800-444-6443
     Fax: 703-236-6001

4075 Working After Brain Injury
HDI Publishers
10600 NW Freeway, Suite 202
Houston, TX 77219   800-321-7037
     Fax: 713-956-2288

Magazines

4076 Journal of Head Trauma Rehabilitation
Aspen Publishers
1600 Research Boulevard   301-251-8500
Rockville, MD 20850-3129   800-638-8437
     www.aspenpub.com
Scholarly journal designed to provide information on clinical management and rehabilitation of the head-injured for the practicing professional.

4077 Mouth Magazine
PO Box 558   785-272-2578
Topeka, KS 66601-0558   Fax: 785-272-7348
     www.mouthmag.org
Bi-monthly magazine with subscription.

Newsletters

4078 BIAW News
Brain Injury Association of Wisconsin
21100 W Capitol Drive   262-790-9660
Pewaukee, WI 53072   800-882-9282
                                  Fax: 262-790-9670
                        e-mail: admin@execpc.com
                                       www.biaw.org

David Voss, President
Mark Warhus, Executive Director

4079 Brain Injury Source
Brain Injury Association
105 N Alfred Street   703-236-6000
Alexandria, VA 22314   Fax: 703-236-6001
                               e-mail: BIAV@visi.net
                                      www.biausa.org
Written for and by professionals in the field. Blends professionally written articles on information and research in brain injury with a user friendly format that incorporates graphics and charts to effectively deliver the messages. Full color.
50+ pages Quarterly

4080 Brain Waves
Brain Injury Association of Florida
1637 Metropolitan Boulevard   850-410-0103
Tallahassee, FL 32308   800-992-3442
                                  Fax: 850-410-0105
                          e-mail: biaftalla@biaf.org
                                        www.biaf.org
Each issue highlights a topic related to TBI and TBI resources.
Bi-Annually
Valerie E Breen, President/CEO

4081 Brainstorm
Brain Injury Association of Arizona
777 E Missouri   602-323-9165
Phoenix, AZ 85014   888-500-9165
                                  Fax: 602-508-8285
                           e-mail: info@biaaz.org
                                       www.biaaz.org
A newsletter serving persons with brain injury, their families and professionals.
8 pages Quarterly
Mary Bradley, Board President
Mattie Cummins, Executive Director

4082 TBI Challenge!
Brain Injury Association of America
105 N Alfred Street   703-236-6000
Alexandria, VA 22314-3010   Fax: 703-236-6001
                                      www.biausa.org
Exclusively for and about persons with brain injury. Provides information to individuals with brain injury and their families. Professionals will benefit from the perspectives provided in Kid's Corner, Relatively Speaking, Ask the Lawyer, Information and Resources and Ask the Doctor.
bimonthly

Pamphlets

4083 A Survey of Accredited and Other Rehabilitation Facilities
Brain Injury Association
105 N Alfred Street   703-236-6000
Alexandria, VA 22314   800-444-6443
                                  Fax: 703-236-6001
Education, training and cognitive rehabilitation in barin injury programs.

4084 About Head Injuries
Channing L Bete Company
200 State Road
South Deerfield, MA 01373   800-628-7733
Covers basic information including identifying the members of the treatment team and how to take care of yourself as a caregiver.

4085 Adolescents with Closed Head Injuries: A Report of Initial Cognitive Deficits
Brain Injury Association
105 N Alfred Street   703-236-6000
Alexandria, VA 22314   800-444-6443
                                  Fax: 703-236-6001

4086 Basic Questions About Head Injury & Disability
Brain Injury Association
105 N Alfred Street   703-236-6000
Alexandria, VA 22314   800-444-6443
                                  Fax: 703-236-6001

4087 Behavioral and Psychosocial Sequelae of Pediatric Head Injury
Brain Injury Association
105 N Alfred Street   703-236-6000
Alexandria, VA 22314   800-444-6443
                                  Fax: 703-236-6001

4088 Brain Damage is a Family Affair
Brain Injury Association
105 N Alfred Street   703-236-6000
Alexandria, VA 22314   800-444-6443
                                  Fax: 703-236-6001

4089 Brain Injuries: A Guide for Families & Caretakers
Brain Injury Association
105 N Alfred Street   703-236-6000
Alexandria, VA 22314   800-444-6443
                                  Fax: 703-236-6001

4090 Brain Injury: A Home Based Cognitive Rehabilitation Program
HDI Publishers
10600 NW Freeway, Suite 202
Houston, TX 77219   800-321-7037
                                  Fax: 713-956-2288

4091 Catastrophic Injury Cases: The Relationship of Traumatic Brain Injury
Brain Injury Association
105 N Alfred Street   703-236-6000
Alexandria, VA 22314   800-444-6443
                                  Fax: 703-236-6001

4092 Children with Disabilities: Understanding Sibling Issues
Brain Injury Association
105 N Alfred Street   703-236-6000
Alexandria, VA 22314   800-444-6443
                                  Fax: 703-236-6001

4093 Counseling Head Injured Patients: Guidelines for Community Health Workers
Brain Injury Association
105 N Alfred Street   703-236-6000
Alexandria, VA 22314   800-444-6443
                                  Fax: 703-236-6001

4094 Education Concerns for the Traumatically Head Injured Student
Brain Injury Association
105 N Alfred Street   703-236-6000
Alexandria, VA 22314   800-444-6443
                                  Fax: 703-236-6001

4095 From One Family Member to Another
Brain Injury Association
105 N Alfred Street   703-236-6000
Alexandria, VA 22314   800-444-6443
                                  Fax: 703-236-6001
A mother tells the story of her son's injury and recovery. Gives suggestions for structuring the home environment.

4096 Guide to Selecting and Monitoring Head Injury Rehabilitation Services
Brain Injury Association
105 N Alfred Street   703-236-6000
Alexandria, VA 22314   800-444-6443
                                  Fax: 703-236-6001

4097 Head Injury Survivor on Campus: Issues & Resources
Brain Injury Association

105 N Alfred Street   703-236-6000
Alexandria, VA 22314   800-444-6443
                  Fax: 703-236-6001

4098 Head Injury: A Booklet for Families
Brain Injury Association
105 N Alfred Street   703-236-6000
Alexandria, VA 22314   800-444-6443
                  Fax: 703-236-6001

4099 Head Injury: A Guide for Families
HDI Publishers
10600 NW Freeway, Suite 202
Houston, TX 77219   800-321-7037
                  Fax: 713-956-2288
Structured by problem with examples and practical coping strategies.

4100 Hearing Loss Following Head Injury
Brain Injury Association
105 N Alfred Street   703-236-6000
Alexandria, VA 22314   800-444-6443
                  Fax: 703-236-6001

4101 Hiring Persons with a Brain Injury: What to Expect
HDI Publishers
10600 NW Freeway, Suite 202
Houston, TX 77219   800-321-7037
                  Fax: 713-956-2288

4102 Individual Psychotherapy with the Brain Injured Adult
Brain Injury Association
105 N Alfred Street   703-236-6000
Alexandria, VA 22314   800-444-6443
                  Fax: 703-236-6001
Review of literature on substance abuse and head injury. Includes statistics, and treatment options, strategies and extensive bibliography.

4103 Information General Sobre: Lesion Cerebral
Brain Injury Association
105 N Alfred Street   703-236-6000
Alexandria, VA 22314   800-444-6443
                  Fax: 703-236-6001

4104 Introductory Information for Families
Brain Injury Association
105 N Alfred Street   703-236-6000
Alexandria, VA 22314   800-444-6443
                  Fax: 703-236-6001
A collection of readings on basic information about TBI and a guide for selecting rehabilitation facilities.

4105 Know Your Brain
Nat'l Institute of Neurological Disorders & Stroke
PO Box 5801
Bethesda, MD 20824   800-352-9424
                  Fax: 301-402-2186
                  www.ninds.nih.gov
Basic information about the brain, neuroscience research, and disorders of the brain.

4106 Legal and Financial Issues for Families
Brain Injury Association
105 N Alfred Street   703-236-6000
Alexandria, VA 22314   800-444-6443
                  Fax: 703-236-6001
Packet designed for families that explores some of the legal and financial issues faced after TBI.

4107 Life After Brain Injury: Who am I
HDI Publishers
10600 NW Freeway, Suite 202
Houston, TX 77219   800-321-7037
                  Fax: 713-956-2288
A well-structured book. Dicusses specific problems areas. Includes good examples and gives lists of practical coping strategies.

4108 Mild Brain Injury: Damage and Outcome
Brain Injury Association

105 N Alfred Street   703-236-6000
Alexandria, VA 22314   800-444-6443
                  Fax: 703-236-6001

4109 Neuropsychology of Attention and Memory
Brain Injury Association
105 N Alfred Street   703-236-6000
Alexandria, VA 22314   800-444-6443
                  Fax: 703-236-6001

4110 Persisting Problems After Mild Head Injury: A Review of the Syndrome
Brain Injury Association
105 N Alfred Street   703-236-6000
Alexandria, VA 22314   800-444-6443
                  Fax: 703-236-6001

4111 Post-Traumatic Headaches: Subtypes & Behavioral Treatments
Brain Injury Association
105 N Alfred Street   703-236-6000
Alexandria, VA 22314   800-444-6443
                  Fax: 703-236-6001

4112 Recovery and Cognitive Retraining After Craniocerebral Trauma
Brain Injury Association
105 N Alfred Street   703-236-6000
Alexandria, VA 22314   800-444-6443
                  Fax: 703-236-6001

4113 Relationships Between Personality Disorders
Brain Injury Association
105 N Alfred Street   703-236-6000
Alexandria, VA 22314   800-444-6443
                  Fax: 703-236-6001
Social Disturbances and physical disability following TBI.

4114 Resources List of Organizations
Brain Injury Association
105 N Alfred Street   703-236-6000
Alexandria, VA 22314   800-444-6443
                  Fax: 703-236-6001

4115 Severe Brain Injury
Brain Injury Association
105 N Alfred Street   703-236-6000
Alexandria, VA 22314   800-444-6443
                  Fax: 703-236-6001
This pamphlet is in hand out format and would be appropriate for use in clinic or hospital setting.

4116 Spouses of Persons Who Are Brain Injured: Overlooked Victims
Brain Injury Association
105 N Alfred Street   703-236-6000
Alexandria, VA 22314   800-444-6443
                  Fax: 703-236-6001

4117 Stress Management Following Head Injury: Strategies for Families & Caregivers
Brain Injury Association
105 N Alfred Street   703-236-6000
Alexandria, VA 22314   800-444-6443
                  Fax: 703-236-6001

4118 Subarachnoid Hemorrhage & Aneurysm
University Hospital & Clinics
One Hosptial Drive   314-882-4141
Columbia, MO 65212
This pamphlet includes easy to read, general information plus a glossary and schematic diagrams. This pamphlet would be most appropriate for use with recently head injured patients.

4119 Substance Abuse Task Force White Paper
Brain Injury Association
105 N Alfred Street   703-236-6000
Alexandria, VA 22314   800-444-6443
                  Fax: 703-236-6001
Review of literature on substance abuse and head injury. Includes statistics, and treatment options, strategies and extensive bibliography.

4120 Susan's Dad: A Child's Story of Head Injury
Brain Injury Association

105 N Alfred Street
Alexandria, VA 22314

703-236-6000
800-444-6443
Fax: 703-236-6001

4121 **Teaching Persons with A Brain Injury: What to Expect**
HDI Publishers
10600 NW Freeway, Suite 202
Houston, TX 77219

800-321-7037
Fax: 713-956-2288

4122 **Unseen Injury: Minor Head Injury**
Brain Injury Association
105 N Alfred Street
Alexandria, VA 22314

703-236-6000
800-444-6443
Fax: 703-236-6001

4123 **What is Anoxic Brain Injury**
Brain Injury Association
105 N Alfred Street
Alexandria, VA 22314

703-236-6000
800-444-6443
Fax: 703-236-6001

4124 **When Your Child Goes to School After an Injury**
Brain Injury Association
105 N Alfred Street
Alexandria, VA 22314

703-236-6000
800-444-6443
Fax: 703-236-6001

4125 **When Your Child is Seriously Injured: The Emotional Impact on Families**
Brain Injury Association
105 N Alfred Street
Alexandria, VA 22314

703-236-6000
800-444-6443
Fax: 703-236-6001

4126 **Working After A Head Injury**
HDI Publishers
10600 NW Freeway, Suite 202
Houston, TX 77219

800-321-7037
Fax: 713-956-2288

Audio & Video

4127 **A Fate Better than Death**
Brain Injury Association
105 N Alfred Street
Alexandria, VA 22314

703-236-6000
800-444-6443
Fax: 703-236-6001

Video features 4 young adults with traumatic brain injury. Focuses on support groups.

4128 **Neuropsychological Assessment: What it Does & Does Not Do**
Brain Injury Association
105 N Alfred Street
Alexandria, VA 22314

703-236-6000
800-444-6443
Fax: 703-236-6001

This pamphlet is in hand out format and would be appropriate for use in clinic or hospital setting.

4129 **Peter Wegner Is Alive and Well and Living in Providence**
Filmakers Library
124 E 40th Street
New York, NY 10016-1798

212-808-4980
Fax: 212-808-4983
e-mail: info@filmakers.com
www.filmakers.com

Peter Wegner was a professor at Brown University when he recveived an award in London and was hit by a bus there. The film follows the challenges and decisions faced by his family, in dealing with the serious brain injuries sustained. Comatose, brain surgery, how can a person decide the right path for their loved one? Winner of American Psychology Award. DVD or VHS $195, Classroom Rental $55
VHS or DVD
Sue Oscar, Co-President

4130 **Unseen Injury: Minor Head Injury**
Brain Injury Association
105 N Alfred Street
Alexandria, VA 22314

703-236-6000
800-444-6443
Fax: 703-236-6001

Designed specifically for viewing by family members.

4131 **Surviving Coma: The Journey Back**
Brain Injury Association
105 N Alfred Street
Alexandria, VA 22314

703-236-6000
800-444-6443
Fax: 703-236-6001

21 minutes

Web Sites

4132 **Agency for Healthcare: Research Facility**

www.ahcpr.gov

Mission is to improve quality, safety, efficiency, and effectiveness of healthcare for all Americans.

4133 **American Brain Tumor Association**

www.abta.org

Provides a mentorship program for new brain tumor support group leaders; a nationwide database of established support groups; the Connections pen-pal program; networking with organizations that provide services to patients and families; a resource listing of physicians offering investgative treatments.

4134 **Brain Injury Association**

www.biausa.org

Seeking to improve the quality of life for people with brain injuries and their families through information and resource referral, legislative advocacy, prevention awareness, and professional education. BIA's mission is to create a better future through brain injury prevention, research, education and advocacy.

4135 **Brain Research Institute: Medicine School University of California, Los Angeles**

medicine.ucsd.edu

BRI is an organized research unit.

4136 **Headinjury.Com**

www.headinjury.com

Maintained by the Head Injury Hotline, a non-profit clearinghouse founded and operated by head injury activist. The primary goal are to empower through education, resources and support. The basic premise is that the medical system is deeply flawed and that the brain injury rehab industry is no exception. The site integrates resources from diverse organizations including support groups, rehabilitation and research sites.

4137 **Healing Well**

www.healingwell.com

An online health resource guide to medical news, chat, information and articles, newsgroups and message boards, books, disease-related web sites, medical directories, and more for patients, friends, and family coping with disabling diseases, disorders, or chronic illnesses.

4138 **Health Finder**

www.healthfinder.gov

Searchable, carefully developed web site offering information on over 1000 topics. Developed by the US Department of Health and Human Services, the site can be used in both English and Spanish.

4139 **Healthlink USA**

www.healthlinkusa.com

Health information concerning treatment, cures, prevention, diagnosis, risk factors, research, support groups, email lists, personal stories and much more. Updated regularly.

4140 **Helios Health**

www.helioshealth.com

Online resource for your health information. Detailed information about specific health topics, access to expert advice from our Medical Advisory Board, and up-to-date health news.

4141 **MedicineNet**

www.medicinenet.com

An online resource for consumers providing easy-to-read, authoritative medical and health information.

4142 **Medscape**

www.medscape.com

Medscape offers specialists, primary care physicians, and other health professionals the Web's most robust and integrated medical information and educational tools.

4143 **Neurology Channel**

www.neurologychannel.com

Find clearly explained, medically accurate information regarding conditions, including an overview, symptoms, causes, diagnostic procedures and treatment options. On this site it is possible to ask questions and get information from a neurologist and connect to people who have similar health interests.

4144 **Road Less Traveled**

www.lesstravel.org

Dedicated to survivors and families of victims of Traumatic Brain Injury.

4145 **TBI Help**

www.tbihelp.com

Information concerning head injury.

4146 **Traumatic Brain Injury**

community-2.webtv.net

This site is dedicated to survivors and all who wish to learn more about traumatic brain injury.

Description

4147 Hearing Impairment

Approximately 21 million Americans have some degree of hearing impairment or Deafness. This common problem affects people of all ages, and the loss can range from mild to severe.

Hearing loss is divided into four categories: conductive, sensorineural, mixed and central. Conductive hearing loss is caused by a defect in the external ear canal or middle ear, and can be helped by hearing aids, medical treatment or surgery. Sensorineural hearing loss results from damage to the inner ear and to the primary nerve that transmits sound waves to the brain. Mixed hearing loss is a combination of conductive and sensorineural defects. Central hearing loss results from impairment of brain function.

Hearing loss may be present at birth or begin later in life. Causes include infections (such as meningitis), injury, prolonged noise exposure, hereditary diseases and side effects of certain drugs. Amplification of sound with hearing aids helps almost all persons with mild-to-severe conductive or sensorineural hearing loss. Profoundly deaf persons who cannot be helped by hearing aids may benefit from a cochlear implant, a specialized device inserted into the inner ear. Children with hearing impairments may have slow or inaccurate speech development, or problems with concentration. Early diagnosis usually helps children improve their auditory ability, through the use of hearing aids, educational programs and speech therapy. Hearing loss in adults, if moderate or severe, is usually obvious to the patient family members. In young children, however, the problem is easily overlooked and the opportunity for early intervention can be lost.

National Agencies & Associations

4148 ABLEDATA
8630 Fenton Street
Silver Spring, MD 20910
301-608-8998
800-227-0216
Fax: 301-608-8958
TTY: 301-608-8912
e-mail: abledata@macrointernational.com
www.abledata.com
An information and referral service that uses computer listings and a large file system to answer requests related to assistive devices. Houses a large file system library and contacts with other sources which enables them to answer just about any question.
Katherine Belknap, Project Director
Steve Lowe, Associate Project Manager/Webmaster

4149 ADARA
PO Box 480
Myersville, MD 21773
501-224-6678
Fax: 501-868-8812
TTY: 501-868-8850
e-mail: adaraorg@comcast.net
www.adara.org
Professional networking for excellence in service delivery with individuals who are deaf or hard of hearing. A partnership of national organizations, local affiliates, professional sections and individual members working together to support social services.
Barry Critchfield, President
Michelle Niehaus, President-Elect

4150 Academy of Doctors of Audiology
3493 Lansdowne Dr.
Lexington, KY 40517
866-493-5544
Fax: 859-271-0607
www.audiologist.org
Encourages audiology training programs to include pertinent aspects of hearing aid dispensing in their curriculum.
Nancy N Green, President
Brian Urban, President-Elect

4151 Academy of Rehabilitative Audiology
PO Box 952
DeSoto, TX 75123
e-mail: ara@audrehab.org
www.audrehab.org
Provides professional education research and interest in programs for hearing handicapped persons.
Kathleen Cienkowski, Ph.D., President
Linda Thibodeau, Ph.D., President-Elect

4152 American Academy of Audiology
11480 Commerce Park Drive
Reston, VA 20191
703-790-8466
800-222-2336
Fax: 703-790-8631
e-mail: infoaud@audiology.org
www.audiology.org
A professional organization of individuals dedicated to providing high quality hearing care to the public. Provides professional development education and research and provides increased public awareness of hearing disorders and audiologic services.
Bettie Borton, President
Erin Miller, President-Elect

4153 American Academy of Otolaryngology: Head
1650 Diagonal Road
Alexandria, VA 22314-3357
703-836-4444
Fax: 703-684-4288
TTY: 703-519-1585
e-mail: executiveservices@entnet.org
www.entnet.org
The missions of the AAO-HNS and its foundation are to advance the art and science of otolaryngology-head and neck surgery through state-of-the-art education, research and learning; and to unite, serve and represent the interests of its members and their families.
James L. Netterville, President
Richard W. Waguespack, President-Elect

4154 American Association of the Deaf-Blind
PO Box 2831
Kensington, MD 20891-3803
301-495-4403
Fax: 301-495-4404
TTY: 301-495-4402
e-mail: AADB-Info@aadb.org
www.aadb.org
Promotes better opportunities and services for deaf-blind people. The mission of this organization is to assure that a comprehensive, coordinated system of services is accessible to all deaf-blind people, enabling them to achieve their maximum potential.
600 Members
Jill Gaus, President
Lynn Jansen, Vice President

4155 American Auditory Society
PO Box 779
Pennsville, NJ 08070
877-746-8315
Fax: 650-763-9185
e-mail: amaudsoc@comcast.net
www.amauditorysoc.org
Publishes Ear & Hearing and The Bulletin of the American Auditory Society.
Linda Hood, PhD, President
Darla M. Eastlack, Executive Director

4156 American Hearing Research Foundation
310 W. Lake Street
Elmhurst, IL 60126-4539
630-617-5079
Fax: 630-563-9181
e-mail: sparmet@american-hearing.org
www.american-hearing.org
Supports medical research and education into the causes prevention and cures of deafness, hearing losses and balance disorders.

Also keeps physicians and the public informed of the latest developments in hearing research and education.
Richard G. Muench, Chairman
Alan G. Micco, President

4157 American Society for Deaf Children
800 Florida Avenue NE, #2047   202-644-9204
Washington, DC 20002-3695   800-942-2732
Fax: 410-795-0965
TTY: 717-334-8808
e-mail: asdc@deafchildren.org
www.deafchildren.org
A nonprofit parent-helping-parent organization promoting a positive attitude toward signing and deaf culture. Also provides support encouragement and current information about deafness to families with deaf and hard of hearing children.
Beth S Benedict PhD, President
Joseph Finnegan, VP

4158 American Speech-Language-Hearing Association
2200 Research Boulevard   301-296-5700
Rockville, MD 20850   800-638-8255
Fax: 301-296-8580
TTY: 301-296-5650
e-mail: actioncenter@asha.org
www.asha.org
A professional and scientific organization for speech-language pathologists and audiologists concerned with communication disorders. Provides informational materials and a toll-free HELPLINE number for consumers to inquire about speech, language or hearing disorders.
Patricia A. Prelock, PhD, President
Elizabeth S. McCrea, PhD, President -Elect

4159 American Tinnitus Association
522 SW Fifth Avenue   503-248-9985
Portland, OR 97204-0005   800-634-8978
Fax: 503-248-0024
e-mail: tinnitus@ata.org
www.ata.org
Provides information about tinnitus and referrals to local contacts/support groups nationwide. Also provides a bibliography service, funds scientific research related to tinnitus and offers workshops to professionals. Works to promote public education.
Thomas J. Lobl, PhD, Chair
Melanie F. West, Vice-Chair

4160 Association of Late-Deafened Adults
8038 Macintosh Lane   815-332-1515
Rockford, IL 61107   866-402-2532
Fax: 877-907-1738
TTY: 815-332-1515
e-mail: info@alda.org
www.alda.org
Serves as a resource and information center for late-deafened adults and works to increase public awareness of the special needs of late-deafened adults.
Mary Lou Mistretta, President
Dave Litman, President-Elect

4161 Auditory-Verbal International
1390 Chain Bridge Road   703-739-1049
McLean, VA 22101   Fax: 703-739-0395
TTY: 703-739-0874
e-mail: audiverb@aol.com
www.auditory-verbal.org
Dedicated to helping children who have hearing losses learn to listen and speak. Promotes the Auditory-Verbal Therapy approach which is based on the belief that the overwhelming majority of these children can hear and talk by using their residual hearing ability.
Chellie Lisenby, Executive Director
Steven R Rech, President

4162 Better Hearing Institute
1444 I Street NW   202-449-1100
Washington, DC 20005   800-327-9355
Fax: 202-216-9646
TTY: 703-642-0580
e-mail: mail@betterhearing.org
www.betterhearing.org
A nonprofit educational organization that implements national public information programs on hearing loss and available medical, surgical, hearing aid and rehabilitation assistance for millions with uncorrected hearing problems.
Sergei Kochk PhD, Executive Director
Renee La Mura, Administrative Director

4163 CAPCOM
6707 Old Dominion Drive   202-363-0535
McLean, VA 22101   800-241-2232
TTY: 703-749-1876
Conducts research on the special needs of the hearing impaired including senior citizens. Presents workshops on law and the deaf and on promoting productive working relationships for the hearing impaired employees of agencies and corporations.

4164 Canine Assistance for the Disabled CADI
CADI
3958 Union Road   314-892-2554
Saint Louis, MO 63125   e-mail: supportdogs@MSN.com
The mission of Support Dogs Inc. is to give people with disabilities greater independence and improve lives through the help of a support or touch dog and promote canines as partners through abilities education.

4165 Center on Employment: Rochester Institute of Technology
National Technical Institute for the Deaf
52 Lomb Memorial Drive   585-475-6400
Rochester, NY 14623-5604   Fax: 585-475-7570
TTY: 585-475-6400
e-mail: ntidcoe@rit.edu
www.ntid.rit.edu/nce
Operated by the National Technical Institute for the Deaf at Rochester Institute of Technology, the NTIC Center on employment was established to promote successful employment of RIT's deaf students and graduates.
John Macko, Director
Lorie Fidurko, Office Assistant

4166 Cochlear Implant Association
5335 Wisconsin Avenue NW   202-895-2781
Washington, DC 20015-2052   Fax: 202-895-2782
e-mail: pwms.cici@worldnet.att.net
Provides information and support to implant users and their families, professionals and the general public.
John McCelland, President
Lorie Singer, VP

4167 Convention of American Instructors of the Deaf
PO Box 377   817-354-8414
Bedford, TX 76095-0377   TTY: 817-354-8414
e-mail: caid@swbell.net
www.caid.org
An organization that promotes professional development communication and information among educators of deaf individuals and other interested people.
Keith Mousley, President
Larry Quinsland, Ph.D, Vice-President

4168 Council on Education of the Deaf College of Education
College of Education
343 A Erickson Hall   330-672-0735
East Lansing, MI 48824-0001   Fax: 330-672-2498
TTY: 330-672-2396
e-mail: catalyst@kent.edu
www.deafed.net/PageText.asp?hdnPageId=58
Offers information and referral services to the hearing impaired.
Dr Karen Dilka, Executive Director
Dr Carmel Collum Yarger, President

4169 **Deaf Artists of America**
302 Goodman Street N
Rochester, NY 14607-1148　　　　Fax: 716-244-3690
　　　　　　　　　　　　　　TTY: 315-224-3460
www.deafed.net/publisheddocs/sub/ivc39.h
Organized to bring support and recognition to deaf and hard of
hearing artists. The goals are to publish information about deaf artists, provide cultural and educational opportunities, exhibit and
market deaf artists' work and collect and disseminate information.
Tom Willard, Executive Director

4170 **Deaf REACH**
3521 12th Street NE　　　　　　　202-832-6681
Washington, DC 20017　　　　　Fax: 202-832-8454
　　　　　　　　　　　　　　TTY: 202-832-6681
e-mail: lweinstock@deaf-reach.org
www.deaf-reach.org
Offers group homes for mentally ill adults, day programs for the
developmentally disabled deaf, referrals case management and
housing placement. Serves adults with disabilities, specifically
deaf and/or low-income.
Annette Reichman, President
Jon Tomar, VP

4171 **Deafness Research Foundation**
641 Lexington Avenue　　　　　　212-328-9480
New York, NY 10022　　　　　　　866-454-3924
　　　　　　　　　　　　　　Fax: 212-328-9484
　　　　　　　　　　　　　　TTY: 888-435-6104
e-mail: info@drf.org
www.drf.org
The nation's largest voluntary health organization entirely committed to public awareness and support for basic and clinical research into deafness and hearing disabilities. Sponsors a broad
program of innovative research and education.
Elizabeth Thorp, President, CEO
Clifford Tallman, Principal

4172 **Deafness and Communicative Disorders Branch**
Department of Education
400 Maryland Ave., SW　　　　　202-205-8730
Washington, DC 20202-2736　　　800-872-5327
　　　　　　　　　　　　　　Fax: 800-437-0833
　　　　　　　　　　　　　　TTY: 202-205-8352
e-mail: annette.reichman@ed.gov
www.ed.gov/offices/OSERS/RSA.html
Promotes improved and expanded rehabilitation services for deaf
and hard of hearing people and individuals with speech or lan-
guage impairments.
Annette Reichman, Branch Chief

4173 **Dogs for the Deaf**
10175 Wheeler Road　　　　　　　541-826-9220
Central Point, OR 97502　　　　　800-990-3647
　　　　　　　　　　　　　　Fax: 541-826-6696
　　　　　　　　　　　　　　TTY: 541-826-9220
　　　　　　　　　　　　　　TDD: 541-826-9220
e-mail: info@dogsforthedeaf.org
www.dogsforthedeaf.org
Trains ear dogs to alert deaf persons to certain sounds. Dogs are
chosen from pet adoption shelters and assigned on the basis of a
prioritized waiting list. Four to five months of training teaches
them to alert their masters to a number of sounds.
Robin Dickson, President/CEO
Vaughn Maurice, General Manager

4174 **EAR Foundation**
1817 Patterson Street　　　　　　615-627-2724
Nashville, TN 37203　　　　　　　800-545-4327
　　　　　　　　　　　　　　Fax: 615-627-2728
　　　　　　　　　　　　　　TTY: 615-627-2724
　　　　　　　　　　　　　　TDD: 615-627-2724
e-mail: info@earfoundation.org
www.earfoundation.org
A national non-profit organization committed to the goal of better
hearing and balance through public and professional education
programs including The Meniere's Network and the Young Ears
program. The Meniere's Network is a national network of patient
outreach.
Amy Nielsen, Associate Director

4175 **Hands Organization: Advocacy Network for the Deaf and
Hearing Impaired**
Advocacy Network For The Deaf And Hearing Impaired
PO Box 17755　　　　　　　　　773-978-8552
Chicago, IL 60617-0755　　　　　TTY: 773-978-8552
Advocacy for the deaf and hearing impaired; information and re-
ferrals educational events sign language summer youth camps and
newsletters.

4176 **Hear Now: Starkey Hearin Foundation**
The Starkey Hearing Foundation
6700 Washington Avenue S
Eden Prairie, MN 55344　　　　　866-354-3254
　　　　　　　　　　　　　　Fax: 952-828-6900
e-mail: info@StarkeyFoundation.org
www.sotheworldmayhear.org
Committed to making technology accessible to deaf and hard of
hearing individuals throughout the United States. Also raises
funds to provide hearing aids, cochlear implants and related services to children and adults who have hearing losses.
Richard Brown, President
Brady Forseth, Executive Director

4177 **Hearing Education and Awareness for Rocker s**
1405 Lyon Street　　　　　　　　415-409-3277
San Francisco, CA 94115　　　　　Fax: 415-552-4296
　　　　　　　　　　　　　　TTY: 415-476-7600
e-mail: hear@hearnet.com
www.hearnet.com
Educates the public about the real dangers of hearing loss resulting
from repeated exposure to excessive noise levels.
Kathy Peck, Executive Director
John Doyle, Secretary

4178 **Hearing Loss Association of America**
7910 Woodmont Avenue　　　　　301-657-2248
Bethesda, MD 20814-3079　　　　Fax: 301-913-9413
　　　　　　　　　　　　　　TTY: 301-657-2248
e-mail: info@hearingloss.org
www.hearingloss.org
Promotes awareness and information about hearing loss communication assistive devices and alternative communication skills
through publications exhibits and presentations.
Diana D. Bender, Ph.D, President
Anna Gilmore Hall, Executive Director

4179 **Helen Keller National Center for Deaf/Blind Youth and Adults**
141 Middle Neck Road　　　　　　516-944-8900
Sands Point, NY 11050-1299　　　Fax: 516-944-7302
　　　　　　　　　　　　　　TTY: 516-944-8637
e-mail: hkncinfo@hknc.org
www.hknc.org
The national center and its 10 regional offices providing diagnostic evaluations comprehensive vocational and personal adjustment
training and job preparation and placement for people who are
deaf/blind from every state and territory.

4180 **House Ear Institute**
2100 W 3rd Street　　　　　　　　213-483-4431
Los Angeles, CA 90057　　　　　　800-388-8612
　　　　　　　　　　　　　　Fax: 213-483-8789
　　　　　　　　　　　　　　TTY: 213-484-2642
　　　　　　　　　　　　　　TDD: 213-484-2642
e-mail: info@hei.org
www.hei.org
A national non-profit otologic research and educational institute
that provides information on hearing and balance disorders.
John W House MD, President
James D Boswell, CEO

4181 **International Hearing Dog**
5901 E 89th Avenue　　　　　　　303-287-3277
Henderson, CO 80640　　　　　　Fax: 303-287-3425
　　　　　　　　　　　　　　TTY: 303-287-3277
　　　　　　　　　　　　　　TDD: 303-287-3277
e-mail: info@hearingdog.org
www.ihdi.org

Trains dogs to hear for deaf persons - telephones, doorbells, babies etc.
Samuel Cheris, Chairman
Valerie Foss-Brugger, President/ Executive Director

4182 International Hearing Society
16880 Middlebelt Road   734-522-7200
Livonia, MI 48154   800-521-5247
                                  Fax: 734-522-0200
                          e-mail: tom.higgins8@verizon.net
                                       www.ihsinfo.org
A nonprofit professional association which represents Hearing Instrument Specialists in the United States, Canada and several other countries. The society is recognized for promoting and maintaining the highest possible standards for its members.
Thomas Higgins, President
Kathleen Mennillo, Executive Director

4183 John Tracy Clinic
806 W Adams Boulevard   213-748-5481
Los Angeles, CA 90007-2505   800-522-4582
                                  Fax: 213-749-1651
                                  TTY: 213-747-2924
                                       www.jtc.org/
An educational facility for preschool age children who have hearing losses and their families. In addition to on-site services worldwide correspondence courses in English and Spanish are offered to parents whose children are of preschool age and are hard of hearing.
Michael D. Barker, Chair
J. Gaston Kent, President and Chief Executive Officer

4184 Listening and Spoken Language Knowledge Ce nter
3417 Volta Place NW   202-337-5220
Washington, DC 20007   Fax: 202-337-8314
                                  TTY: 202-337-5221
                          e-mail: info@agbell.org
                 www.listeningandspokenlanguage.org/
The world's oldest and largest membership organization promoting the use of spoken language by children and adults who are hearing impaired. Members include parents of children with hearing loss, adults who are deaf or hard of hearing and educators.
Lyn Robertson, Ph.D., President
Alexander T Graham, Executive Director/CEO

4185 National Association of the Deaf
8630 Fenton Street   301-587-1788
Silver Spring, MD 20910-4500   Fax: 301-587-1791
                          e-mail: nad.info@nad.org
                                       www.nad.org
The nation's largest constituency organization safeguarding the accessibility and civil rights of 28 million deaf and hard of hearing Americans in education, employment, health care and telecommunications. A private, nonprofit organization.
Christopher Wagner, President
Howard A Rosenblum, CEO

4186 National Captioning Institute
3725 Concorde Parkway   703-917-7600
Chantilly, VA 20151   Fax: 703-917-9853
                                  TTY: 703-917-7600
                          e-mail: jagudelo@ncicap.org
                                       www.ncicap.org
Advocates captioned television for people who want to see, as well as hear, the dialogue of a television program. It not only enables deaf and hard-of-hearing people to understand all of a program's content but it is also beneficial for new Americans learning English.
Gene Chao, President, CEO
Drake Smith, Chief Technology Officer

4187 National Center for Voice and Speech: Univ ersity of Iowa
The University Of Iowa
250 Hawkins Drive   319-335-6600
Iowa City, IA 52242   Fax: 319-335-6603
                          e-mail: ingo-titze@uiowa.edu
                                       www.ncvs.org
This is a consortium of institutions focusing on voice and speech disorders. The members of this consortium are the University of Iowa, the Denver Center for Performing Arts, the University of Wisconsin-Madison and the University of Utah.
Ingo Titze PhD, Executive Director
Eric Hunter, Deputy Executive Director

4188 National Consortium on Deaf-Blindness
Teaching Research
345 N Monmouth Avenue
Monmouth, OR 97361   800-438-9376
                                  Fax: 503-838-8150
                                  TTY: 800-854-7013
                          e-mail: info@nationaldb.org
                                       www.nationaldb.org
Collects organizes and disseminates information related to children and youth who are deaf-blind and connects consumers of deaf-blind information to sources of information about deaf-blindness assistive technology and deaf-blind people.
John Reiman
Kathy McNulty

4189 National Dissemination Center for Children
1825 Connecticut Avenue NW   202-884-8200
Washington, DC 20009   800-695-0285
                                  Fax: 202-884-8441
                                  TTY: 202-884-8200
                          e-mail: nichcy@fhi360.org
                                       www.nichcy.org
Publishes free fact filled newsletters. Arranges workshops. Advises parents on the laws entitling children with disabilities to special education and other services.
Bruce Ramirez, Executive Director
John Westbrook, Director

4190 National Family Association for Deaf-Blind
141 Middle Neck Road
Sands Point, NY 11050   800-225-0411
                                  Fax: 516-883-9060
                          e-mail: NFADB@aol.com
                                       www.nfadb.org
NFADB advocates for all persons who are deaf-blind of any chronological age and cognitive ability, supports national policy to benefit people who are deaf-blind, encourages the founding and strengthening of family organizations in each state and shares information.
Susan Green, President
Cynthia Jackson-Glenn, Treasurer

4191 National Institute on Deafness and other Communication Disorders
National Institutes Of Heath
31 Center Drive   301-496-7243
Bethesda, MD 20892-2320   800-241-1044
                                  Fax: 301-402-0018
                                  TTY: 800-241-1055
                          e-mail: nidcdinfo@nidcd.nih.gov
                                       www.nidcd.nih.gov
A national resources center for information about hearing, balance, smell, taste, voice, speech and language.
Dr. James F Battey, Jr., M.D., Ph.D, Director
Marin Allen PhD, Chief Office of Health Communication

4192 National Organization for Hearing Research
P.O. Box 421   610-649-6114
Narberth, PA 19072   Fax: 610-668-1428
                                  TTY: 610-664-3135
                          e-mail: info@nohrfoundation.org
                                       www.nohrfoundation.org
This organization is a nonprofit private foundation seeking to fund exceptional researchers with $5 000 seed money grants.

4193 Rainbow Alliance of the Deaf
309 Millside Drive
Columbus, OH 43230   e-mail: president@rad.org
                                       www.rad.org
A national organization serving the deaf gay and lesbian community. Represents approximately 24 chapters throughout the United States Canada and Europe.
Larry Pike, President
Steven Schumacher, Secretary

4194 Registry of Interpreters for the Deaf
333 Commerce Street
Alexandria, VA 22314

703-838-0030
Fax: 703-838-0454
TTY: 703-838-0459
e-mail: ridinfo@rid.org
www.RID.org

A membership organization with almost 4 000 members including professional interpreters and translators persons with deafness or hearing impairments and professionals in related fields.
Brenda Walker Prudhom, President/Board of Directors
Shane H. Feldman, Executive Director

4195 Society of Hearing Impaired Physicians
1999 Mowry Avenue
Fremont, CA 94538-1622

510-797-2939
Fax: 510-797-0168
e-mail: fphship@aol.com

This Society aids and assists physicians medical students and prospective medical students whose hearing impairment may necessitate different tools and/or approaches to medical practice and training.

4196 Telecommunications for the Deaf
8630 Fenton Street
Silver Spring, MD 20910

301-589-3786
Fax: 301-589-3797
TTY: 301-589-3006
e-mail: info@tdi-online.org
www.tdi-online.org

A nonprofit consumer advocacy organization promoting full visual and other access to information and telecommunications for people who are deaf, hard of hearing, deaf-blind and speech impaired.
Claude Stout, Executive Director
Scott Recht, Business Manager

4197 Tripod
1727 W Burbank Boulevard
Burbank, CA 91506

818-972-2080
Fax: 818-972-2090
TTY: 818-972-2080
e-mail: info@tripod.org
www.tripod.org

TRIPOD is a nonprofit organization dedicated to providing support and services for deaf and hard of hearing children and their families. TRIPOD offers model local educational programs, Montessori, bilingual parent, infant, toddler and preschool programs.

4198 USA Deaf Sports Federation
PO Box 910338
Lexington, KY 40591-0338

605-367-5760
Fax: 605-782-8441
TTY: 605-367-5761
e-mail: HomeOffice@usdeafsports.org
www.usdeafsports.org

A governing body for all deaf sports and recreation in the United States.
Jack C. Lamberton, President
Chris Kaftan, Secretary

State Agencies & Associations

Alabama

4199 Alabama Institute for Deaf and Blind
205 East South Street
Talladega, AL 35160

256-761-3200
Fax: 256-761-3344
TTY: 256-761-3200
e-mail: mascia.john@aidb.state.al.us
www.aidb.org

Dr. John Mascia, President
Dr. Frieda Meacham, Vice President, Instructional Programs

Arizona

4200 Arizona Association of the Deaf
5025 N Central Avenue
Phoenix, AZ 85012

e-mail: tposedly@aol.com
www.azadinc.org

This organization shall be organized and operated exclusively to promote the welfare of deaf and hard of hearing residents of the state of Arizona in education, economic, security, social equality, and just rights and privileges as citizens.
Tom Buell, President
Joy Saunders, Vice President

Arkansas

4201 Arkansas Association of the Deaf
26 Corporate Hill Drive
Little Rock, AR 72205

e-mail: hdketchum@aol.com
www.arkad.org

The mission of the Arkansas Association of the Deaf is to promote the educational, economic, and social welfare of Arkansans who are deaf or hard of hearing.
Holly Ketchum, President
Billie Jordan, 1st Vice President

District of Columbia

4202 Shiloh Senior Center for the Hearing Impaired
913 P Street NW
Washington, DC 20001

202-232-1425
TTY: 202-667-9779

Senior programs, sponsored by the DC Office on Aging in co-ordination with grantee: Shiloh Baptist Church serving the entire Metro Washington area's deaf and hard-of-hearing senior citizens.

Florida

4203 Florida Association of the Deaf
7852 Mansfield Hollow Rd.
Delray Beach, FL 33446

e-mail: june@fadcentral.org
www.fadcentral.org

The mission of the Florida Association of the Deaf is to promote, protect, and preserve the rights and quality of life of Deaf and hard of hearing individuals in the state of Florida.
June McMahon, President
Lissette Molina, Vice President

Georgia

4204 Georgia Association of the Deaf
PO Box 615
Hiram, GA 30141-1616

e-mail: turqcat9992000@yahoo.com
www.gadeaf.org

Julie Burton, President
Russell Fleming, Vice President

Illinois

4205 Illinois Association of the Deaf
PO Box 1275
Oak Park, IL 60304

773-237-1877
Fax: 847-740-2319
TTY: 847-740-2319
e-mail: botz@iadeaf.org
www.iadeaf.org

The Illinois Association of the Deaf is a non-profit, political, educational, social economic, welfare of the deaf, and cultural organization made up of deaf, hard of hearing, and hearing members.
Angela Botz, President
Crystal Kelley Schwartz, Vice-President

Kansas

4206 Kansas Association of the Deaf
PO Box 10085
Olathe, KS 66051

785-273-0612
Fax: 785-273-9063
e-mail: president@deafkansas.org
www.deafkansas.org

The mission of the Kansas Association of the Deaf a state-wide, non-profit organization is to assure that an extensive, organized system of services is accessible to all deaf or hard of hearing people in Kansas.
Ann Cooper, President
Pam Siebert, Vice-President

Kentucky

4207 Kentucky Association of the Deaf
1707 Richmond Drive
Louisville, KY 40205-1407
Fax: 606-272-7747
TTY: 606-223-3999
e-mail: president@kydeaf.org
www.kydeaf.org

The mission of the Kentucky Association of the Deaf is to advocate for the deaf and hard of hearing in Kentucky by promoting equality, accessibility, and quality of life through employment, services, education and welfare.
Sharon White, President
Arlen Finke, Vice-President

Louisiana

4208 Louisiana Association of the Deaf
3112 Valley Creek Drive
Baton Rouge, LA 70808
225-341-6406
Fax: 225-923-1235
TTY: 225 923-1266
e-mail: info@lad1908.org
www.lad1908.org

Lou Cannon, President
Cindy Robillard, VP

Massachusetts

4209 Massachusetts State Association of the Deaf
PO Box 276
Reading, MA 01867
781-388-9114
Fax: 781-388-9015
TTY: 781-388-9115
e-mail: MSADeaf@aol.com
www.msad.org

The Massachusetts State Association of the Deaf is a statewide nonprofit organization serving the estimated 350 000 deaf and hard of hearing Massachusetts citizens and their families.
Justine Barros, President
Michelle Donatello, Vice President

Michigan

4210 Michigan Deaf Association
6093 133rd Ave
Saugatuck, MI 49453
Fax: 586-775-0906
e-mail: info@mideaf.org
www.mideaf.org

MDA is a non-profit, tax exempt organization with a mission to help improve the lives of Deaf and Hard of Heating citizens of Michigan. MDA is affiliated with he National Association of the Deaf whose mission is to promote, protect, and preserve the rights of the deaf and hearing impaired communities.
Scot A Pott, President
Kat Vogtmann, 1st Vice-President

New York

4211 Center for Hearing and Communication
50 Broadway
New York, NY 10004
917-305-7700
Fax: 917-305-7888
TTY: 917-305-7999
e-mail: inf@lhh.org
www.chchearing.org

A private not-for-profit rehabilitation agency for infants, children and adults who are hard of hearing and deaf. The League's mission is to improve the quality of life for people with all degrees of hearing loss.
Laurie Hanin, Executive Director
Ellen Lafargue, Director Audiology

North Carolina

4212 North Carolina Association of the Deaf
1200 Revolution Mill Drive
Greensboro, NC 27405
919-773-2974
Fax: 919-834-0127
e-mail: NCAD2011@gmail.com
www.ncadeaf.org

Christina Bryant, Chairperson

North Dakota

4213 North Dakota Association of the Deaf
1115 11th Avenue North
Fargo, ND 58102
e-mail: rolewitz @ hotmail.com
www.nddeaf.org

The North Dakota Association of the Deaf is actively involved in issues affecting Deaf citizens in North Dakota.
Michele Rolewitz, President
Cody Duncan, Vice President

Oklahoma

4214 Oklahoma Association of the Deaf
2737 Sunnybrook Lane
Enid, OK 73703
e-mail: Mlznull@aol.com
www.ok-oad.org

The purpose of Oklahoma Association of the Deaf is to promote the interests of the deaf and to advance the social, educational, cultural and economic well-being of the deaf.
Lynn Null, President
Ka Ann Varner, Vice President

Oregon

4215 Oregon Association of the Deaf
999 Locust Street NE
Salem, OR 97301
e-mail: contact@deaforegon.com
www.deaforegon.com

The Oregon Association of the Deaf is a non-profit organization working toward a better life for the deaf. Their mission is to create an opportunity for the Deaf of Oregon to join together in planning, devising, conducting and participating in activities.
Daniel Sloan, Committee
Wendy Stanley, Committee

Rhode Island

4216 Rhode Island Association of the Deaf
PO Box 40853
Providence, RI 02940
e-mail: riadsec@gmail.com
www.riadeaf.blogspot.in/

Heather Niedbala, Vice-President
Neil Leahey, Treasurer

Texas

4217 Texas Association of the Deaf
PO Box 1982
Manchaca, TX 78652-3570
e-mail: steve@deaftexas.org
www.deaftexas.org

Texas Association of the Deaf is an organization for persons who are deaf or hard of hearing. It is a membership organization to provide information and education including surveys and studies to bring the viewpoint on various issues affecting the lives of the deaf and hearing impaired.
Steve C Baldwin, President
Chris Kearney, VP

Virginia

4218 Virginia Association of the Deaf
5251 College Drive
Dublin, VA 24084
757-587-9555
Fax: 757-461-5376
TTY: 757-461-7527
e-mail: vadpresident007@yahoo.com
www.vad.org

LaDonna Larsen, President
Chuck Kelley, VP

Wisconsin

4219 Wisconsin Association of the Deaf
PO Box 114
Delavan, WI 53115-4230
608-825-9791
TTY: 414-607-3297
e-mail: wisdeaf@gmail.com
www.wisdeaf.org/

The mission of the Wisconsin Association of the Deaf is to ensure that a comprehensive and coordinated system of resources is ac-

cessible to Wisconsin people who are deaf or hard of hearing, enabling them to achieve their maximum potential.
Jenny Buechner-Madison, President
Steph Buell, Vice President

Wyoming

4220 Deaf Association of Wyoming
PO Box 20107   307-635-1125
Cheyenne, WY 82003   e-mail: president@dawyoming.org
                                          www.dawyoming.org
The Deaf Association of Wyoming is a state non-profit organizations; which is associated with the Association of the Deaf. Membership is open to all deaf persons, parents of deaf children, interpreters, professionals who work with deaf and all interested parties.
Heather Parsons, President
Bill Bitner, VP

Libraries & Resource Centers

4221 Captioned Films/Videos
National Association of the Deaf
8630 Fenton Street   301-587-1788
Silver Spring, MD 20910-4500   Fax: 301-587-1791
                                              TTY: 301-587-1789
                                                     www.nad.org
The mission of the National Association of the Deaf is to promote,protect,and preserve the rights and quality of life of eaf and hard of hearing individuals in the United States of America.
Jason Stark, Director-Described and Captioned Media P

4222 Captioned Media Program
National Association of the Deaf
8630 Fenton Street   301-587-1788
Silver Spring, MD 20910-4500   Fax: 301-587-1791
                                              TTY: 301-587-1789
                                                     www.nad.org
Free loans of educational and entertainment captioned films and videos for deaf and hard of hearing people.
Jason Stark, Director

4223 Friends of Libraries for Deaf Action USA
2930 Craiglawn Road   202-727-2255
Silver Spring, MD 20904-1816   Fax: 301-572-5168
                                              TTY: 301-572-5168
                                        e-mail: folda86@aol.com
                                                     www.folda.net/
Library services for people with disabilities.
Alice L Hagemeyer, President
Merrie A Davidson, Associate

4224 Library Services to the Deaf Community
District of Columbia Public Library
901 G Street NW   202-727-2145
Washington, DC 20001   TTY: 202-727-2255
                                e-mail: library_deaf_dc@yahoo.com
                                                     www.dclibrary.org
Assures that the deaf community is aware of existing library and information services by the District of Columbia Public Library; promotes public awareness about the deaf community, deaf history and culture, American Sign Language, and assistive technology for people with hearing loss.
John W Hill Jr, President
Bonnie R Cohen, VP

4225 Listening and Spoken Knowledge Center
3417 Volta Place NW   202-337-5220
Washington, DC 20007-2737   Fax: 202-337-8314
                                              TTY: 202-337-5221
                                          e-mail: info@agbell.org
                            www.listeningandspokenlanguage.org/
Contains one of the world's largest historical collections of publications, documents and information on deafness. In addition to the main collection, which includes books, periodicals and indexed clipping files dating from the turn of the century, the library also

houses a significant archival collection dealing with the history of deafness since the 16th century.
Lyn Robertson, Ph.D., President
Alexander T Graham, Executive Director/CEO

4226 Wallace Memorial Library
Rochester Institute of Technology
90 Lomb Memorial Drive
Rochester, NY 14623   585-475-2562
                  www.rit.edu/alumni/benefits/library.php
Information on physical disabilities and deafness.
Chandra McKenzie, Assistant Provost/Director

Research Centers

4227 Boys Town National Research Hospital
555 N 30th Street   402-498-6511
Omaha, NE 68131   800-320-1171
                                          Fax: 402-498-6331
                                          TTY: 800 320-1171
                                    www.boystownhospital.org
An internationally recognized center for state-of-the-art research diagnosis treatment of patients with ear diseases hearing and balance disorders cleft lip and palate and speech/language problems. Also includes programs such as Parent/Child Workshops Center for Childhood Deafness Register for Heredity Hearing Loss Center for Hearing research Center for Abused Handicapped and summer programs for gifted deaf teens and college students.
John K Arch, Executive VP
Edward M. Kolb, Medical Director

4228 Center for Hearing Loss in Children Boystown National Research Hospital
Boystown National Research Hospital
555 N 30th Street   402-498-6511
Omaha, NE 68131-2136   800-282-6657
                                          Fax: 402-498-6331
                                          TTY: 800 320-1171
                                  e-mail: chilic@boystown.org
                                    www.boystownhospital.org
The Center for Hearing Loss in Children unites professionals from a variety of disciplines to focus on research training information dissemination and continuing education in the area of childhood deafness.
John K Arch, Executive VP
Edward M. Kolb, Medical Director

4229 Central Institute for the Deaf
825 S Taylor Avenue   314-977-0132
Saint Louis, MO 63110-1502   877-444-4574
                                          Fax: 314-977-0023
                                          TTY: 314-977-0037
                                      e-mail: rfeder@cid.edu
                                                     www.cid.edu
Central Institute for the Deaf is a private nonprofit auditory-oral school for children who have hearing impairments. We teach children with hearing loss birth-12 to listen talk and succeed in the mainstream.
Ned Lemkemeier, President
Robin M Feder, Executive Director

4230 City University of New York Center for Research in Speech and Hearing
365 Fifth Avenue   212-817-7000
New York, NY 10016-4309   877-428-6942
                                          Fax: 212-817-1537
                                  e-mail: strangepin@aol.com
                                                     www.gc.cuny.edu
Programmable research of digital and auditory hearing aids and sensory aids for the speech and hearing impaired person.
Dr. William Kelly, President
Marilyn Marzolf, Chief of Staff

4231 Civitan International Research Center
1530 3rd Avenue S   205-934-8900
Birmingham, AL 35294-0001   800-UAB-CIRC
                                          Fax: 205-975-6330
                                                     www.circ.uab.edu

Studies of deaf children.
Dr Harald Sontheimer, Director
Dr Alan Percy, Medical Director

4232 Cleveland Hearing and Speech Center
11635 Euclid Avenue   216-231-0787
Cleveland, OH 44106-4319   Fax: 216-231-2135
TTY: 216-231-5266
e-mail: jkeatley@chsc.org
www.chsc.org
Offers research and studies into speech language and hearing disorders.
David J Abood, President
Bernard P Henri PhD, Executive Director

4233 David T Siegel Institute for Communicative Disorders
Humana Hospital-Michael Reese
3033 S Cottage Grove Avenue   773-791-2900
Chicago, IL 60616-3346   Fax: 773-791-4014
Conducts behavioral research on language development and sign language for the deaf.
Edward Applebaum, Chief Service

4234 Eaton-Peabody Laboratory of Auditory Physiology
Massachusetts Eye & Ear Institute
243 Charles Street   617-573-3745
Boston, MA 02114-3002   Fax: 617-720-4408
e-mail: eplweb@mit.edu
research.meei.harvard.edu/EPL
Auditory system and auditory information processing including ear-brain interactions in normal and pathologic hearing.
John Fernandez, President, CEO
Thane Benson, Consultant

4235 Gallaudet University: Center for Auditory and Speech Sciences
800 Florida Avenue NE   202-651-5000
Washington, DC 20002-3660   866-637-0102
Fax: 202-651-5295
TTY: 202-651-5005
e-mail: publicrelations@gallaudet.edu
www.gallaudet.edu
Develops new hearing tests that use speech sounds to measure hearing loss.
Dr T Alan Hurwitz, President
Deborah DeStefano, Special Assistant to the President

4236 Hear Center
301 E Del Mar Boulevard   626-796-2016
Pasadena, CA 91101   Fax: 626-796-2320
e-mail: info@hearcenter.org
www.hearcenter.org
Auditory and verbal program designed to help hearing impaired children infants and adults lead normal and productive lives. Seeks to develop auditory techniques to aid people who have communication problems due to deafness.
Ellen Simon, Executive Director
Deborah Lorino, Office Manager

4237 Houston Ear Research Foundation
7737 SW Freeway   713-771-9966
Houston, TX 77074-1867   800-843-0807
Fax: 713-771-0546
TTY: 800-843-0807
e-mail: info@houstoncochlear.org
www.houstoncochlear.org
Aims to improve health care and education for deaf and hearing-impaired children.
Jan Gilden, Clinical Audiologist
Mary Lynn McDonald

4238 Loyola University of Children: Parmly Hearing Institute
1032 W Sheridan Road   773-274-3000
Chicago, IL 60660   Fax: 773-508-2719
e-mail: webmaster@luc.edu
www.luc.edu
Engage in the comparative study of sensory systems including hearing vision speech perception vestibular function and the special senses of the lateral-line organ and electroreception in fish.
Richard Fay, PhD, Director
Dr William Yost, Professor of Psychology

4239 Northern Illinois University Research and Training Center
1425 W Lincoln Highway   815-753-1000
DeKalb, IL 60115-2825   800-892-3050
Fax: 815-753-6520
e-mail: helpdesk@niu.edu
www.niu.edu
Conducts research resource development and training/technical assistance projects geared toward enhancing the employment independent living and quality of life outcomes for traditionally underserved people who are deaf.
Douglas D Baker, President

4240 Ohio State University Otological Research Laboratories
410 W 10th Avenue   614-293-8103
Columbus, OH 43210   800-293-5123
Fax: 614-293-5506
e-mail: OSUCareConnection@osumc.edu
www.medicalcenter.osu.edu
Clinical and basic research in otology.
Larry Anstine, CEO
Peter Geier, Chief Operating Officer

4241 Ohio University Therapy Associates: Hearing, Speech and Language Clinic
W218 Grover Center   740-593-1000
Athens, OH 45701   Fax: 740-593-0287
e-mail: webteam@ohio.edu
www.ohio.edu/hearingspeech
Focuses on hearing and speech impairments.
Brooke Hallowell, Director
Davida Parsons, Clinical Director

4242 Oregon Health Sciences University Oregon Hearing Research Center Tinnitus Clinic
3181 S W Sam Jackson Park Road   503-494-7954
Portland, OR 97239-3098   Fax: 503-945-5656
TTY: 503-494-0910
e-mail: ohrc@ohsu.edu
www.ohsu.edu/xd/health/services/ent/serv
The first medical clinic in the world established exclusively for the treatment of chronic tinnitus. During the last 25 years we have successfully treated more than 7 000 patients with severe tinnitus. The Clinic also treats patients with hyperacusis (hypersensitivity to sounds).
William Martin PhD, Director
Baker Yong-Bing Shi, MD, PhD, Assistant Professor

4243 Regional Resource Center on Deafness Western Oregon State College
Western Oregon State College
345 N Monmouth Avenue   503-838-8444
Monmouth, OR 97361   877-877-1593
TTY: 503-838-8000
e-mail: rrcd@wou.edu
www.wou.edu/education/sped/rrcd.php
Improve the employment and independent living status of deaf and hard-of-hearing people by increasing the number of rehabilitation professionals and their community partners nationwide who have the necessary knowledge and communication skills to serve this population.
Cheryl Davis, Director
Konnie Sayers, Administrative Assistant

4244 Rehabilitation Engineering on Hearing Enha ncement
Lexington Center
800 Florida Avenue NE   202-651-5335
Washington, DC 20002   Fax: 202-651-5324
TTY: 202-651-5335
e-mail: info@hearingresearch.org
www.hearingresearch.org
A federally funded center that conducts research into hearing aid technology and alternate technologies.
Matthew H Bakke Ph D, Director
James J Mahshie PhD, Director

4245 Research and Training Center for Persons Who are Deaf or Hard of Hearing
University of Arkansas

26 Corporate Hill Drive
Little Rock, AR 72205-3822
501-686-9691
Fax: 501-686-9698
TTY: 501-686-9691
e-mail: dwatson@uark.edu
www.uark.edu/depts/rehabres

Rehabilitation of deaf and hearing impaired individuals.
Douglas Watson, Director
Glenn B Anderson, Professor Director of Training

4246 Rochester Institute of Technology: Nationa l Technical Institute for the Deaf
Lyndon Baines Johnson Building
52 Lomb Memorial Drive
Rochester, NY 14623
585-475-6400
Fax: 585-475-5978
TTY: 585-475-6400
e-mail: gbuckley@ntid.rit.edu
www.ntid.rit.edu

Provides technical and professional education and training for deaf students.
Dr Gerard Buckley, President

4247 Scottish Rite Center for Childhood Language Disorders
2800 - 16th Street NW
Washington, DC 20009-3602
202-232-8155
Fax: 202-483-8169
dcsr.org

Association offering speech-language evaluations and treatment hearing screening and consultation and referrals to children ages birth to 18 years with hearing or speech disorders.
Dr Tommie L Robinson, Director

4248 Speech Simulation Research Foundation
PO Box 824
Nassawadox, VA 23413-0824
757-442-2755

Focuses on hearing and speech disorders.
Monte Penney, Director

4249 State University College at Fredonia Youngerman Clinic
W123 Thompson Hall
Fredonia, NY 14063
716-673-3203
Fax: 716-673-3332
e-mail: melissa.sidor@fredonia.edu
www.fredonia.edu

Studies communication disorders including hearing and speech.
Melissa Sidor, Director

4250 State University College at Plattsburgh Auditory Research Laboratory
101 Broad Street
Plattsburgh, NY 12901-2170
518-564-2000
www.plattsburgh.edu

Dr John Ettling, President
Anne Hansen, Vice-President

4251 Syracuse University Institute for Sensory Research
Syracuse University
621 Skytop Road
Syracuse, NY 13244-1
315-443-4164
Fax: 315-443-1184
e-mail: rlsmith@syr.edu
www.isr.syr.edu

Sensory processing and hearing disorders.
Robert L Smith, Director

4252 Temple University Speech and Hearing Science Laboratories
1801 N Broad Street
Philadelphia, PA 19122
215-204-7000
e-mail: president@temple.edu
www.temple.edu

Speech and hearing studies.
Neil D Theobald, President
Kevin G Clark, Senior Advisor to the President/Interim

4253 Temple University: Section of Auditory Research
1801 N Broad Street
Philadelphia, PA 19122
215-204-7000
Fax: 215-707-6417
e-mail: president@temple.edu
www.temple.edu

Neil D Theobald, President
Kevin G Clark, Senior Advisor to the President/Interim

4254 The University of Memphis: School of Commu nication Sciences and Disorders
Memphis State University

101 Wilder Tower
Memphis, TN 38152-3520
901-678-2111
800-669-2678
Fax: 901-251-82
e-mail: recruitment@memphis.edu
www.memphis.edu/ausp

Offers research into hearing loss and deafness as well as speech impairments.
Shirley C Raines, President
Walt Manning, Associate Director

4255 Trace Center University of Wisconsin: Madison
University of Wisconsin: Madison
1550 Engineering Drive
Madison, WI 53706-2274
608-262-6966
Fax: 608-262-8848
TTY: 608-263-5408
e-mail: info@trace.wisc.edu
trace.wisc.edu

Research and development center working with communication control and computer access technologies for people with disabilities.
Gregg C Vanderheiden, Center Director
Julie Gamradt, Communication Director

4256 University of Alabama Speech and Hearing Center
5721 USA Drive N
Mobile, AL 36688-2
251-445-9378
Fax: 251- 44- 937
e-mail: sh-cntr@jaguar1.usouthal.edu
www.southalabama.edu/alliedhealth/speech

Providing undergraduate master's and doctoral programs that challenge the student to achieve the highest standards of academic learning scientific inquiry and clinical excellence.
Robert E Moore, Chair
Elizabeth M Adams, Assistant Professor of Audiology

4257 University of Chicago: Temporal Bone Laboratory for Ear Research
5841 S Maryland Avenue
Chicago, IL 60637-1463
773-702-1000
888-824-0200
Fax: 773-702-6809
www.uchospitals.edu

Focuses on hearing impairments and deafness research.
Dr Raul Hinojasa, Director

4258 University of Maine: Communication Science s & Disorders
5724 Dunn Hall
Orono, ME 04469-5724
207-581-2006
Fax: 207-581-2060
e-mail: Luanne.Wasson@umit.maine.edu
www.umaine.edu/comscidis

Speech disorders of adults and children including hearing impairments and deafness.
Judy Stickles, Clinic Director
Amy Engler Booth, Audiologist

4259 University of Michigan Communicative Disorders Clinic
412 Maynard Street
Ann Arbor, MI 48109-2054
734-764-1817
Fax: 734-764-7084
e-mail: kkellogg@chartermi.net
www.umich.edu/comdis

Focuses on communicative disorders including hearing impairments and speech disorders.
Mary Sue Coleman, President
Joerg Lahann, Assistant Professor of Biomedical Engine

4260 University of Michigan: Kresge Hearing Research Institute
1150 W Medical Center Drive
Ann Arbor, MI 48109-0500
734-764-8111
Fax: 734-764-0014
TTY: 734-764-8110
e-mail: josef@umich.edu
www.khri.med.umich.edu

Focuses on hearing and auditory disorders.
Josef M Miller, Director
Sue Kelch, Research Administrator

4261 University of Nebraska: Lincoln
1400 R Street
Lincoln, NE 68588
402-472-7211
Fax: 402-472-7697
e-mail: jbernthal1@unl.edu
www.unl.edu

Focuses on hearing impairments and deaf research.
Harvey Perlman, Chancellor
Marjorie Kostelnik, Dean Education Human Science

4262   University of North Carolina at Chapel Hill Division of Speech & Hearing
321 S. Columbia Street   919-966-1007
Chapel Hill, NC 27599-1   Fax: 919-966-0100
e-mail: idiana@med.unc.edu
www.med.unc.edu/ahs/sphs
The Division of Speech and Hearing Sciences prepares clinical practitioners in speech-language pathology and audiology to be scholars teachers and researchers in both the theoretical and applied aspects of human communication sciences and disorders.
Jackson Roush, PhD, Director
Lee McLean, PhD, Professor and Associate Dean

4263   University of Oklahoma: Health Sciences Ce nter
University of Oklahoma
1100 N Lindsey   405-271-4000
Oklahoma City, OK 73104   Fax: 405-713-60
www.ouhsc.edu
Dr. Dewayne Andrews, Senior Vice President and Provost
Kenneth D Rowe, Vice President for Administration and Fi

4264   University of Texas at Dallas Callier Center for Communication Disorders
1966 Inwood Road   214-905-3000
Dallas, TX 75235-7205   Fax: 214-905-3022
TDD: 214-905-3012
e-mail: roeser@callier.utdallas.edu
www.callier.utdallas.edu
Focuses on communication and behavioral disorders including hearing impairments and deafness research.
Tom Campbell, Executive Director
Phillip L Wilson, Head of Audiology

4265   University of Washington Department of Speech & Hearing Sciences
1417 NE 42nd Street   206-685-7400
Seattle, WA 98105-6246   Fax: 206-543-1093
e-mail: sphscadv@u.washington.edu
www.depts.washington.edu/sphsc/
Communication sciences and disorders.
Joan Hanson, Clinic Manager
Mary Wood, Assistant to the Chair

4266   Yeshiva University: Institute of Communication Disorders
Montefiore Medical Center
500 West 185th Street   212-960-5400
New York, NY 10033   Fax: 718-515-8235
e-mail: mfried@montefiore.org
www.yu.edu
Studies on communicative disorders including speech and hearing.
Richard M Joel, President
Josh Joseph, VP, Chief of Staff

Support Groups & Hotlines

4267   Aurora of Central New York
518 James Street   315-422-7263
Syracuse, NY 13203-2282   Fax: 315-422-4792
TTY: 315-422-9746
TDD: 315-422-9746
e-mail: auroracny@auroraofcny.org
Professional counseling services helps to assist individuals and their families deal with the trauma of hearing or vision loss.
Debra Chaken, Executive Director

4268   Beginnings for Parents of Children Who are Deaf or Hard of Hearing
302 Jefferson Street   919-715-4092
Raleigh, NC 27605   800-541-4327
Fax: 919-715-4093
TTY: 919-715-4092
e-mail: raleigh@ncbegin.org
www.ncbegin.org/

Beginnings provides support to parents of deaf and hard-of-hearing children in an unbiased, family-centered atmosphere. In addition, Beginnings also offers impartial information on communication options, placement and educational programs, and workshops for professional personnel who work with deaf and hard-of-hearing children. Advocacy and support for young people from birth to age 21 is available.
Jim Johnson, President
Dr Joni Y Alberg, Executive Director

4269   Children of Deaf Adults
PO Box 30715
Santa Barbara, CA 93130-0715   805-682-0997
www.coda-international.org
Promotes family awareness and individual growth in hearing children of deaf parents.
Carmel Batson, President
Millie Brother, Founder

4270   Children's Rights Program
Alexander Graham Bell Association
3417 Volta Place NW   202-337-5220
Washington, DC 20007   866-337-5220
Fax: 202-337-8314
e-mail: info@agbell.org
www.agbell.org
Actively advocates for the legal rights of children with hearing impairments and for legislation to upgrade the delivery of services to children and adults who are hearing impaired.
Gerri A Hanna, Director Advocacy/Policy

4271   Dial-a-Hearing Screening Test
PO Box 1880   610-544-7700
Media, PA 19063   800-222-3277
Fax: 610-543-2802
e-mail: dahst@aol.com
Hearing help information center. Provides local phone number for Dial-a-Hearing Screening Test and hearing information.
George Biddle, Executive Director

4272   International Hearing Society
International Hearing Society (IHS)
16880 Middlebelt Road   734-522-7200
Livonia, MI 48154   800-521-5247
Fax: 734-522-0200
e-mail: chelms@ihsinfo.org
http://ihsinfo.org/IhsV2/Home/Index.cfm
Hearing Aid Helpline, a service of International Hearing Society (IHS), provides a referral service for locating qualified hearing healthcare professionals. IHS is a professional association representing Hearing Instrument Specialists worldwide engaged in the practice of testing human hearing, selecting, fitting and dispensing of hearing instruments. Founded in 1951, the Society conducts programs in competency accreditation, education, training promoting specialty-level certification.
Thomas Higgins, President
Todd Beyer, Secretary

4273   John Tracy Clinic on Deafness
806 W Adams Boulevard   213-748-5481
Los Angeles, CA 90007-2599   800-522-4582
Fax: 213-749-1651
www.jtc.org
Hotline.
Michael D Barker, Chair
J.Gaston Kent, President & CEO

4274   National Health Information Center
PO Box 1133   310-565-4167
Washington, DC 20013   800-336-4797
Fax: 301-984-4256
e-mail: info@nhic.org
www.health.gov/nhic
Offers a nationwide information referral service, produces directories and resource guides.

4275   Project Eyes and Ears
1844 T Street SE   202-889-7045
Washington, DC 20020-4635   Fax: 202-889-6312

Disseminates information about resources to families and service providers, provides transition services for pre-kindergarten children who are deaf-blind and integrates children into normalized settings.
Janice Wellborn

Books

4276 A Child with Hearing Loss in Your Classroom? Don't Panic!
Alexander Graham Bell Association
3417 Volta Place NW   202-337-5220
Washington, DC 20007-2737   Fax: 202-337-8270
                                                    TTY: 202-337-5220
Designed for mainstream teachers, this booklet discusses educational needs for students with hearing impairments. It especially focuses on students' language skills and their abilities to follow directions, learn new concepts, and comprehend reading. Candid advice about getting support from professionals, implementing and mantaining an IEP, improving classroom acoustic environments and using the PATERR approach.
1993 25 pages

4277 A New Civil Right: Telecommunications Equality for Deaf and Hard of Hearing
Karen Peltz Strauss, author
Hearing Loss Association of America
7910 Woodmont Avenue   301-657-2248
Bethesda, MD 20814-3079   Fax: 301-913-9413
                                                    TTY: 301-657-2249
                                    e-mail: info@hearingloss.org
                                                    www.hearingloss.org
This book provides a compelling picture of the challenges and the realization that FCC regulation is required for people with hearing loss to receive the functional equivalence of what everyone else takes for granted.
2006 Hardcover
Jerry Portis, Executive Director
Brenda Battat, Assistant Executive Director

4278 A Quiet World: Living with Hearing Loss
David G Myers, author
Hearing Loss Association of America
7910 Woodmont Avenue   301-657-2248
Bethesda, MD 20814-3079   Fax: 301-913-9413
                                                    TTY: 301-657-2249
                                    e-mail: info@hearingloss.org
                                                    www.hearigloss.org
A social psychologist, teacher, and author. The Author's gradual hearing loss caused serious trouble in his career and in his relationships with loved ones as he approached 50. He tells the story of his journey from denial to acceptance to an exploration of the technologies that offer help.
2000 Hardcover
Jerry Portis, Executive Director
Brenda Battat, Assistant Executive Director

4279 ASL PAH! Deaf Students' Essays About their Language
Sign Media
4020 Blackburn Lane   301-421-0268
Burtonsville, MD 20866-1167   800-475-4756
                                                    Fax: 301-421-0270
                                                    TTY: 301-421-4460
                                    e-mail: signmedia@aol.com
                                                    www.signmedia.com
Tape/text combination featuring student essays on the role of ASL in their lives. The tape offers additional insights from the student authors. The text is not a transcript of the tape.
1979 Paperback/Video
ISBN: 0-932130-14-3
Barabara Olmert, Director Marketing

4280 ASL in Schools: Policies and Curriculum
Gallaudet University
11030 S Langley Avenue
Chicago, IL 60628-3819   800-621-2736
                                                    Fax: 800-621-8476
                                                    TTY: 888-630-9347
                                                    www.gallaudet.edu

Conference participants questioned experts on bilingual education for deaf students and discussed policy issues faced by educators across the United States.
139 pages

4281 Academic Acceptance of ASL
Gallaudet University
11030 S Langley Avenue
Chicago, IL 60628-3819   800-621-2736
                                                    Fax: 800-621-8476
                                                    TTY: 888-630-9347
                                                    www.gallaudet.edu
This monograph presents a dozen articles that demonstrate clearly and convincingly that the study of ASL affords the same educational values and the same intellectual rewards as the study of any other foreign language.
196 pages

4282 Access for All: Integrating Deaf, Hard of Hearing and Hearing Preschoolers
Gallaudet University
11030 S Langley Avenue
Chicago, IL 60628-3819   800-621-2736
                                                    Fax: 800-621-8476
                                                    TTY: 888-630-9347
                                                    www.gallaudet.edu
Describes a model program for integrating the Deaf and hard of hearing children in early education.
150 pages Book & Video

4283 American Deaf Culture
Gallaudet University
11030 S Langley Avenue
Chicago, IL 60628-3819   800-621-2736
                                                    Fax: 800-621-8476
                                                    TTY: 888-630-9347
                                                    www.gallaudet.edu
This book presents a collection of classic articles which have been selected to provide a variety of perspectives on language and culture of deaf people in America.
132 pages

4284 American Deaf Culture: An Anthology
Sign Media
4020 Blackburn Lane   301-421-0268
Burtonsville, MD 20866-1167   800-475-4756
                                                    Fax: 301-421-0270
                                                    TTY: 301-421-4460
                                    e-mail: signmedia@aol.com
                                                    www.signmedia.com
Features deaf and hearing authors offering their experience and perspectives on cultural values, ASL, social interaction in the Deaf community, education, folklore and more.
Paperback
ISBN: 0-932130-09-7
Barbara Olmert, Director Marketing
Sherman Wilcox, Editor

4285 American Sign Language: A Beginning Course
National Association of the Deaf
8630 Fenton Street   301-587-1788
Silver Spring, MD 20910-4500   Fax: 301-587-1791
                                                    TTY: 301-587-1789
                                                    www.nad.org
An interactive approach to teaching and learning American Sign Language, with 700 sign illustrations, each accompanied by an object drawing.
199 pages Paperback
ISBN: 0-913072-64-8
Donna Morris, Publications Manager

4286 An Invisible Condition: The Human Side of Hearing Loss
SHHH Publications
7910 Woodmont Avenue   301-657-2248
Bethesda, MD 20814-3572   Fax: 301-913-9413
Offers editorials from the SHHH Journal that have shaped the past decade of self help with their focus on the plight and hopes and the aspirations of hard of hearing people everywhere.

4287 Angels and Outcasts: An Anthology of Deaf Characters in Literature
Gallaudet University
11030 S Langley Avenue
Chicago, IL 60628-3819

Fax: 800-621-2736
Fax: 800-621-8476
TTY: 888-630-9347
www.gallaudet.edu

Collection of writings by and about deaf people revealing attitudes and prejudices common to western cultures.
375 pages

4288 Approaching Equality
TJ Publishers
817 Silver Spring Avenue   301-585-4440
Silver Spring, MD 20910-4617   800-999-1168
Fax: 301-585-5930
TTY: 301-585-4441
e-mail: tjpubinc@aol.com

Written by the former chair of the Commission on the Education of the deaf, this book reviews the dramatic developments in the education of deaf children.
112 pages Softcover
ISBN: 0-932666-39-6
Angela K Thames, President
Jerald A Murphy, VP

4289 Assessment & Management of Mainstreamed Hearing-Impaired Children
Pro-Ed, Inc.
8700 Shoal Creek Boulevard   512-451-3246
Austin, TX 78757-6897   800-897-3202
Fax: 800-397-7633
e-mail: info@proedin.com
www.proedinc.com

The theoretical and practical considerations of developing appropriate programming for hearing-impaired children who are being educated in mainstream educational settings are presented in this book.
415 pages Hardcover
ISBN: 0-890794-58-8
Linda Jordan, Marketing Coordinator

4290 Assessment of Hearing Impaired People
Gallaudet University
11030 S Langley Avenue
Chicago, IL 60628-3819

800-621-2736
Fax: 800-621-8476
TTY: 888-630-9347
www.gallaudet.edu

This is a comprehensive review of 62 tests used by educational institutions, rehabilitation agencies, and mental health centers.
128 pages Softcover

4291 At Home Among Strangers
Gallaudet University
11030 S Langley Avenue
Chicago, IL 60628-3819

800-621-2736
Fax: 800-621-8476
TTY: 888-630-9347
www.gallaudet.edu

Details the history and culture of the deaf community.
336 pages

4292 Basic Course in Manual Communication
National Association of the Deaf
8630 Fenton Street   301-587-1788
Silver Spring, MD 20910-4500   Fax: 301-587-1791
TTY: 301-587-1789
www.nad.org

Over 700 signs are grouped according to shape, location, and movement. Also includes dialogues for practice.
158 pages Paperback
Donna Morris, Publications Manager

4293 Basic Sign Communication: Student Materials
National Association of the Deaf

8630 Fenton Street   301-587-1788
Silver Spring, MD 20910-4500   Fax: 301-587-1791
TTY: 301-587-1789
www.nad.org

Includes study and reference materials for all three levels of Basic Sign Communication.
232 pages Paperback
ISBN: 0-913072-56-7
Donna Morris, Publications Manager

4294 Basic Sign Communication: Vocabulary
National Association of the Deaf
8630 Fenton Street   301-587-1788
Silver Spring, MD 20910-4500   Fax: 301-587-1791
TTY: 301-587-1789
www.nad.org

Features sections on Sign Vocabulary, Numbers, and Classifiers. Contains 1000 illustrated signs, organized alphabetically by gloss for quick reference.
162 pages Paperback
ISBN: 0-913072-55-9
Donna Morris, Publications Manager

4295 Basic Vocabulary and Language Thesaurus for Hearing Impaired Children
Alexander Graham Bell Association
3417 Volta Place NW   202-337-5220
Washington, DC 20007-2737   Fax: 202-337-8270
TTY: 202-337-5220

This simple thesaurus lists spontaneous vocabulary used by normally hearing children and lets patients and teachers check so that children with hearing losses have mastered these words.
1977 76 pages

4296 Basic Vocabulary: American Sign Language for Parents and Children
TJ Publishers
817 Silver Spring Avenue   301-585-4440
Silver Spring, MD 20910-4617   800-999-1168
Fax: 301-585-5930
TTY: 301-585-4441
e-mail: tjpubinc@aol.com

Carefully selected words and signs include those families use every day. Alphabetically organized vocabulary incorporates developmental lists helpful to both deaf and hearing children and over 1,000 clear sign language illustrations.
240 pages Softcover
ISBN: 0-932666-00-0
Angela K Thames, President
Jerald A Murphy, VP

4297 Being in Touch
Gallaudet University
11030 S Langley Avenue
Chicago, IL 60628-3819   800-621-2736
Fax: 800-621-8476
TTY: 888-630-9347
www.gallaudet.edu

Provides information on hearing and vision loss.
80 pages

4298 Best Practices in Educational Interpreting
Sign Enhancers
2625 SE Hawthorne Boulevard   503-304-4501
Portland, OR 97214-2941   Fax: 503-304-1063
TTY: 503-304-4501
e-mail: sign@signenhancers.com
www.signenhancers.com

Specific recommendations of best practices for working in preschool through graduate school. Case studies focus on real-life situations with suggested solutions and questions for further thought.
269 pages
ISBN: 0-205263-11-9

4299 Between Friends
Beltone Electronics Corporation
4201 W Victoria Street
Chicago, IL 60646-6772   773-583-3600
www.beltone.com

For hearing aid wearers: quizzes, jokes, health, recipes and financial items.

6 pages
Renee Rockoff, Editor

4300 Black and Deaf in America
TJ Publishers
817 Silver Spring Avenue   301-585-4440
Silver Spring, MD 20910-4617   800-999-1168
                                         Fax: 301-585-5930
                                         TTY: 301-585-4441
                                  e-mail: tjpubinc@aol.com
An in depth look at some of the problems of the black deaf community, including undereducation and underemployment. This book includes an important chapter on signs used in the black community and presents interviews with prominent Black deaf individuals who share their joys, fears and hope for the future.

91 pages Softcover
ISBN: 0-932666-18-3
Angela K Thames, President
Jerald A Murphy, VP

4301 Blueprint for Conversational Competence
Alexander Graham Bell Association
3417 Volta Place NW   202-337-5220
Washington, DC 20007-2737   Fax: 202-337-8270
                                         TTY: 202-337-5220
A book that develops conversational skills in children with hearing impairments.

175 pages

4302 Book of Name Signs
Gallaudet University
11030 S Langley Avenue
Chicago, IL 60628-3819   800-621-2736
                                         Fax: 800-621-8476
                                         TTY: 888-630-9347
                                           www.gallaudet.edu
This text discusses the rules for ASL name sign formulation and their appropriate uses and presents a list of over 400 name signs.

112 pages

4303 Broken Ears: Wounded Hearts
Gallaudet University
11030 S Langley Avenue
Chicago, IL 60628-3819   800-621-2736
                                         Fax: 800-621-8476
                                         TTY: 888-630-9347
                                           www.gallaudet.edu
An intimate journey into the lives of a deaf, multihandicapped child and her young hearing parents.

186 pages Hardcover

4304 CUED Speech Resource Book for Parents of Deaf Children
Alexander Graham Bell Association
3417 Volta Place NW   202-337-5220
Washington, DC 20007-2737   Fax: 202-337-8270
                                         TTY: 202-337-5220
A comprehensive book describing cued speech, getting started, your child's rights in and out of school and families expectations with special attention on siblings and peer relationships.

832 pages Hardcover

4305 Can't Your Child Hear?
Gallaudet University
11030 S Langley Avenue
Chicago, IL 60628-3819   800-621-2736
                                         Fax: 800-621-8476
                                         TTY: 888-630-9347
                                           www.gallaudet.edu
Is deafness a difference to be accepted or a defect to be corrected? This comprehensive reference will help parents, as well as educators and other professionals, recognize their options in understanding and handling a child who is deaf.

340 pages Softcover

4306 Chelsea: The Story of a Signal Dog
Gallaudet University

11030 S Langley Avenue
Chicago, IL 60628-3819   800-621-2736
                                         Fax: 800-621-8476
                                         TTY: 888-630-9347
                                           www.gallaudet.edu
A story of a young deaf couple and their dog who acts as their ears.

169 pages

4307 Choices in Deafness
Woodbine House
6510 Bells Mill Road
Bethesda, MD 20817-1636   800-843-7323
Serving as an invaluable guide to the world of deaf education, this expanded edition covers a wide variety of communication options for children with hearing impairments. By providing medical, audiological, and educational information. It also contains numerous case studies. This indispensible book is an outstanding resource for parents.

1996 212 pages
ISBN: 0-933149-09-3

4308 Chuck Baird
Gallaudet University
11030 S Langley Avenue
Chicago, IL 60628-3819   800-621-2736
                                         Fax: 800-621-8476
                                         TTY: 888-630-9347
                                           www.gallaudet.edu
Contains 35 full-color plates of the artwork of the deaf artist.

55 pages

4309 Classroom Notetaker
Alexander Graham Bell Association
3417 Volta Place NW   202-337-5220
Washington, DC 20007-2737   Fax: 202-337-8270
                                         TTY: 202-337-5220
This detailed manual for instructors, administrators and staff note takers promotes classroom notetaking within long-term educational programs as vital for students who are deaf and hard of hearing from elementary school to college. This book will help readers to sell a notetaking program to schools and will give a good foundation for designing and implementing a notetaking program in a school or college.

1996 150 pages

4310 Closer Look: The English Program at the Model Secondary School for the Deaf
Gallaudet University
11030 S Langley Avenue
Chicago, IL 60628   800-621-2736
                                         Fax: 800-621-8476
                                         TTY: 888-630-9347
                                           www.gallaudet.edu
Program highlighting student-centered activities using carefully selected novels and literature texts to enhance students' reading comprehension and writing abilities through interaction with real literature.

67 pages

4311 Cochlear Implant Auditory Training Guidebook
Alexander Graham Bell Association
3417 Volta Place NW   202-337-5220
Washington, DC 20007-2737   Fax: 202-337-8270
                                         TTY: 202-337-5220
This guidebook full of reproducible masters was designed for parents and professionals working with children ages four and up who have cochlear implants. It includes an easy to follow hierarchy for listening goals and a quick placement test to help you find where to start.

236 pages

4312 Cochlear Implantation for Infants and Children
Alexander Graham Bell Association
3417 Volta Place NW   202-337-5220
Washington, DC 20007-2737   Fax: 202-337-8270
                                         TTY: 202-337-5220
This comprehensive text presents the surgical, medical, audiological speech and language and habilitation aspects of cochlear implants in infants and children.

1997 263 pages

4313 Cognition, Education and Deafness
Gallaudet University
11030 S Langley Avenue
Chicago, IL 60628-3819
800-621-2736
Fax: 800-621-8476
TTY: 888-630-9347
www.gallaudet.edu

The work of 54 authors is gathered in this definitive collection of current research on deafness and cognition. The articles are grouped into seven sections: cognition, problem solving, thinking processes, language development, reading methodologies, measurement of potential and intervention programs.
260 pages Hardcover

4314 Communicate with Me: Conversation Skills for Deaf Students
Gallaudet University
11030 S Langley Avenue
Chicago, IL 60628-3819
800-621-2736
Fax: 800-621-8476
TTY: 888-630-9347
www.gallaudet.edu

Students learn how to begin and end conversations, choose appropriate topics and maintain subjects.
160 pages

4315 Communication Access for Persons with Hearing Loss
Mark Ross, author
Hearing Loss Association of America
7910 Woodmont Avenue
Bethesda, MD 20814-3079
301-657-2248
Fax: 301-913-9413
TTY: 301-657-2249
e-mail: info@hearingloss.org
www.hearingloss.org

Communication access for persons with hearing loss covers both visual and hearing techniques devoted to persons with hearingloss, ranging from mild to profound.
Jerry Portis, Executive Director
Brenda Battat, Assistant Executive Director

4316 Communication Issues Among Deaf People
Gallaudet University
11030 S Langley Avenue
Chicago, IL 60628-3819
800-621-2736
Fax: 800-621-8476
TTY: 888-630-9347
www.gallaudet.edu

Monograph discussing important aspects of communication including total communication and the value of ASL.
138 pages

4317 Communication Issues Among Deaf People: Eyes, Hands and Voices
National Association of the Deaf
8630 Fenton Street
Silver Spring, MD 20910-4500
301-587-1788
Fax: 301-587-1791
TTY: 301-587-1789
www.nad.org

Includes over thirty relevant articles reflecting a wide range of perceptions and attitutes on communication among deaf people.
145 pages
Donna Morris, Publications Manager

4318 Communication Rules for Hard of Hearing People
Hearing Loss Association of America
7910 Woodmont Avenue
Bethesda, MD 20814-3079
301-657-2248
Fax: 301-913-9413
TTY: 301-657-2249
e-mail: info@hearingloss.org
www.hearingloss.org

To open the world of communication to people with hearing loss through education, information, support and advocacy.
Jerry Portis, Executive Director
Brenda Battat, Assistant Executive Director

4319 Communication and Adult Hearing Loss
Alexander Graham Bell Association
3417 Volta Place NW
Washington, DC 20007-2737
202-337-5220
Fax: 202-337-8270
TTY: 202-337-5220

This informative book was written for anyone who wants to communicate more effectively with a person with adult hearing loss.
1993 136 pages

4320 Comprehensive Signed English Dictionary
Harris Communications
6541 City W Parkway
Eden Prairie, MN 55344-3248
612-906-1180
Fax: 612-946-0924

Complete dictionary offers 3100 signs, including signs reflecting contemporary vocabulary.
457 pages

4321 Consumer Handbook on Dizziness and Vertigo
Dennis Poe, MD, author
Hearing Loss Association of Amercia
7910 Woodmont Avenue
Bethesda, MD 20814-3079
301-657-2248
Fax: 301-913-9413
TTY: 301-657-2249
e-mail: info@hearingloss.org
www.hearingloss.org

Learn the differences between dizziness and vertigo.
Hardcover
ISBN: 0-966182-64-2

4322 Conversational Sign Language II: An Intermdiate Advanced Manual
Harris Communications
6541 City W Parkway
Eden Prairie, MN 55344-3248
612-906-1180
Fax: 612-946-0924

This book presents English words and their American Sign Language equivalents.
218 pages

4323 Dancing Without Music
Gallaudet University
11030 S Langley Avenue
Chicago, IL 60628-3819
800-621-2736
Fax: 800-621-8476
TTY: 888-630-9347
www.gallaudet.edu

Investigates being deaf and its social ramifications.
320 pages

4324 Deaf Children in Public Schools Placement, Context, and Consequences
Gallaudet University
11030 S Langley Avenue
Chicago, IL 60628-3819
800-621-2736
Fax: 800-621-8476
TTY: 888-630-9347
www.gallaudet.edu

Assesses the progress of three second-grade deaf students to demonstrate the importance of placement, context, and language in their development.
August 1997 250 pages
ISBN: 1-563680-62-9

4325 Deaf Culture, Our Way
Gallaudet University
11030 S Langley Avenue
Chicago, IL 60628-3819
800-621-2736
Fax: 800-621-8476
TTY: 888-630-9347
www.gallaudet.edu

A revised edition of Silence is Golden, Sometimes, this new edition contains sections on Classic Humor, Bathroom Tales, Classic Hazards and New Technology.
115 pages

4326 Deaf Empowerment, Emergence, Struggle and Rhetoric
Gallaudet University
11030 S Langley Avenue
Chicago, IL 60628-3819
800-621-2736
Fax: 800-621-8476
TTY: 888-630-9347
www.gallaudet.edu

Examines the rhetorical foundation that motivated Deaf people to work for social change during the past two centuries. Assesses the

goal of a multicultural society and offers suggestions for community building through a new humanitarianism.
July 1997 192 pages Hardcover
ISBN: 1-563680-61-0

4327   Deaf Heritage: A Narrative History of Deaf America
National Association of the Deaf
8630 Fenton Street   301-587-1788
Silver Spring, MD 20910-4500   Fax: 301-587-1791
                                                      TTY: 301-587-1789
                                                             www.nad.org
In-depth history of Deaf America contains pictures, vignettes, and biographical profiles.
483 pages Paperback
Donna Morris, Publications Manager

4328   Deaf Heritage: Student Text and Workbook
National Association of the Deaf
8630 Fenton Street   301-587-1788
Silver Spring, MD 20910-4500   Fax: 301-587-1791
                                                      TTY: 301-587-1789
                                                             www.nad.org
Each chapter is followed by a vocabulary section and workbook activities including questions and follow-up activities for students.
115 pages Paperback
Donna Morris, Publications Manager

4329   Deaf History Unveiled: Interpretations from the New Scholarship
Gallaudet University
11030 S Langley Avenue
Chicago, IL 60628-3819   800-621-2736
                                                      Fax: 800-621-8476
                                                      TTY: 888-630-9347
                                                           www.gallaudet.edu
Essays written by internationally renowned deaf studies scholars.
316 pages

4330   Deaf Like Me
Gallaudet University
11030 S Langley Avenue
Chicago, IL 60628-3819   800-621-2736
                                                      Fax: 800-621-8476
                                                      TTY: 888-630-9347
                                                           www.gallaudet.edu
Written by the uncle and father of a deaf girl, this is an account of parents coming to terms with deafness.
292 pages

4331   Deaf President Now! The 1988 Revolution at Gallaudet University
Gallaudet University
11030 S Langley Avenue
Chicago, IL 60628-3819   800-621-2736
                                                      Fax: 800-621-8476
                                                      TTY: 888-630-9347
                                                           www.gallaudet.edu
This book chronicles the events leading up to the revolution in which deaf people won social change for themselves and all disabled people.
240 pages

4332   Deaf Sport: The Impact of Sports Within the Deaf Community
Gallaudet University
11030 S Langley Avenue
Chicago, IL 60628-3819   800-621-2736
                                                      Fax: 800-621-8476
                                                      TTY: 888-630-9347
                                                           www.gallaudet.edu
Describes the full ramifications of athletics for deaf people.
224 pages

4333   Deaf Students and the School-to-Work Transition
Gallaudet University
11030 S Langley Avenue
Chicago, IL 60628-3819   800-621-2736
                                                      Fax: 800-621-8476
                                                      TTY: 888-630-9347
                                                           www.gallaudet.edu

Studies severely and profoundly hearing impaired students as they leave high school and enter the work force.
278 pages

4334   Deaf Studies Curriculum Guide
Gallaudet University
11030 S Langley Avenue
Chicago, IL 60628-3819   800-621-2736
                                                      Fax: 800-621-8476
                                                      TTY: 888-630-9347
                                                           www.gallaudet.edu
Designed to help students explore the history, language and culture of deaf people.
250 pages

4335   Deaf Women: A Parade Through the Decades
Gallaudet University
11030 S Langley Avenue
Chicago, IL 60628-3819   800-621-2736
                                                      Fax: 800-621-8476
                                                      TTY: 888-630-9347
                                                           www.gallaudet.edu
A compilation of information, history, anecdotes and research that showcases many deaf women from all walks of American life.
192 pages

4336   Deaf and Hard of Hearing Individuals
Mainstream
1030 5th Street NW   202-898-1400
Washington, DC 20001-2504
Mainstreaming deaf individuals into the workplace.
12 pages

4337   Deaf in America: Voices from a Culture
Gallaudet University
11030 S Langley Avenue
Chicago, IL 60628-3819   800-621-2736
                                                      Fax: 800-621-8476
                                                      TTY: 888-630-9347
                                                           www.gallaudet.edu
Written by authors who are themselves deaf.
134 pages

4338   Deafness and Child Development
Gallaudet University
11030 S Langley Avenue
Chicago, IL 60628-3819   800-621-2736
                                                      Fax: 800-621-8476
                                                      TTY: 888-630-9347
                                                           www.gallaudet.edu
Provides rational, informed and balanced approaches to the effects of deafness in child development.
236 pages

4339   Deafness: 1993-2013
National Association of the Deaf
8630 Fenton Street   301-587-1788
Silver Spring, MD 20910   Fax: 301-587-1791
                                                      TTY: 301-587-1789
                                                             www.nad.org
Over 30 articles cover such topics as magnet schools, deaf identity, technology, multicultural education, communication, leadership, and sign language research.
Paperback
Donna Morris, Publications Manager

4340   Deafness: A Personal Account
Faber & Faber
19 Union Square W   781-721-1427
New York, NY 10003-3304   e-mail: contact@faber.co.uk
                                                           www.faber.co.uk
Poet, critic and translator David Wright's enduring memoir (now with a substantial new introduction by the author) describes with humor and insight his early life, his development as a poet, and little-known history of deaf education.
202 pages

4341   Deafness: An Autobiography
Gallaudet University

11030 S Langley Avenue
Chicago, IL 60628-3819

800-621-2736
Fax: 800-621-8476
TTY: 888-630-9347
www.gallaudet.edu/~gupress

This book is intended to explore the author's own experiences with deafness, and satisfy the curiosity about the condition of deaf people.
238 pages

4342 Deafness: Historical Perspectives
National Association of the Deaf
8630 Fenton Street
Silver Spring, MD 20910

301-587-1788
Fax: 301-587-1791
TTY: 301-587-1789
www.nad.org

Focuses on the history of deaf people. Topics cover a spectrum from a history of deaf theaters, to a genealogy of our first deaf families, to a conversation with a ghost.
Paperback
Donna Morris, Publications Manager

4343 Deafness: Life and Culture II
National Association of the Deaf
8630 Fenton Street
Silver Spring, MD 20910

301-587-1788
Fax: 301-587-1791
TTY: 301-587-1789
www.nad.org

Continues to explore the variety and diversity of the deaf experience.
133 pages Paperback
ISBN: 0-913072-79-6
Donna Morris, Publications Manager

4344 Directory of Auditory-Oral Programs
Alexander Graham Bell Association
3417 Volta Place NW
Washington, DC 20007-2737

202-337-5220
Fax: 202-337-8270
TTY: 202-337-5220

This directory lists auditory/oral programs in public and private schools, auditory-oral programs in speech and hearing centers and therapists who offer private tutoring and auditory-oral therapy.
67 pages

4345 Discovering Sign Language
Gallaudet University
11030 S Langley Avenue
Chicago, IL 60628-3819

800-621-2736
Fax: 800-621-8476
TTY: 888-630-9347
www.gallaudet.edu/~gupress

Here is a book of information about deaf people and sign communication.
104 pages Softcover

4346 Douglas Tilden, the Man and His Legacy
Gallaudet University
11030 S Langley Avenue
Chicago, IL 60628-3819

800-621-2736
Fax: 800-621-8476
TTY: 888-630-9347
www.gallaudet.edu/~gupress

A beautiful tribute to the Deaf sculptor, Douglas Tilden.
216 pages

4347 Ear Book
Gallaudet University
11030 S Langley Avenue
Chicago, IL 60628-3819

800-621-2736
Fax: 800-621-8476
TTY: 888-630-9347
www.gallaudet.edu/~gupress

A how-to book on obtaining and using an otoscope, recognizing and managing common ear disorders, when to call the doctor and when your child needs ear tubes.
136 pages Softcover

4348 Ear Gear: A Student Workbook on Hearing and Hearing Aids
Gallaudet University

11030 S Langley Avenue
Chicago, IL 60628-3819

800-621-2736
Fax: 800-621-8476
TTY: 888-630-9347
www.gallaudet.edu/~gupress

Attractive workbook designed to teach elementary-age children about hearing loss and the use of hearing aids.
75 pages

4349 Educating Deaf Children Bilingually
Gallaudet University
11030 S Langley Avenue
Chicago, IL 60628-3819

800-621-2736
Fax: 800-621-8476
TTY: 888-630-9347
www.gallaudet.edu/~gupress

Discusses perspectives and practices of educating deaf children with goals of age-level achievement.
120 pages

4350 Educating the Deaf: Psychology, Principles and Practices
Gallaudet University
11030 S Langley Avenue
Chicago, IL 60628-3819

800-621-2736
Fax: 800-621-8476
TTY: 888-630-9347
www.gallaudet.edu/~gupress

Offers extensive coverage of the background and history of the education of the deaf, as well as specific information on working with multihandicapped students.
383 pages

4351 Education and Deafness
Longman Publishing Group
95 Church Street
White Plains, NY 10601-1515

914-993-5000

This comprehensive introduction to educating students with hearing impairments provides extensive coverage of the interrelated issues that affect the teaching of these students. It concentrates on the severely to profoundly hearing impaired but includes an entire chapter devoted to students whose impairments are less severe (hard-of-hearing students).
320 pages Paperback
ISBN: 0-801300-26-6

4352 Educational and Development Aspects of Deafness
Gallaudet University
11030 S Langley Avenue
Chicago, IL 60628-3819

800-621-2736
Fax: 800-621-8476
TTY: 888-630-9347
www.gallaudet.edu/~gupress

Book detailing the ongoing revolution in the education of deaf children.
415 pages

4353 Empowerment and Black Deaf Persons
Gallaudet University
11030 S Langley Avenue
Chicago, IL 60628-3819

800-621-2736
Fax: 800-621-8476
TTY: 888-630-9347
www.gallaudet.edu/~gupress

Conference proceedings focusing on the guidance and training of African American deaf individuals.
175 pages

4354 Encyclopedia of Deafness and Hearing Disorders
Facts on File
11 Penn Plaza
New York, NY 10001

212-967-8800
800-322-8755
Fax: 800-678-3633

A comprehensive guide to all aspects of hearing impairments.

4355 Eye-Centered: A Study of Spirituality of Deaf People
NCOD
814 Thayer Avenue
Silver Spring, MD 20910-4500

301-587-7992

The findings of the five-year De Sales Project conducted by The National Catholic Office for the Deaf.

4356 FM Auditory Trainers: A Winning Choice for Students, Teachers and Parents
Alexander Graham Bell Association
3417 Volta Place NW   202-337-5220
Washington, DC 20007-2737   Fax: 202-337-8270
                                   TTY: 202-337-5220
A practical guide to the selection and use of FM trainers in class or at home.
67 pages

4357 For Teachers of the Hearing Impaired
Gallaudet University
11030 S Langley Avenue
Chicago, IL 60628-3819   800-621-2736
                                   Fax: 800-621-8476
                                   TTY: 888-630-9347
                                   www.gallaudet.edu/~gupress
Contains practical articles by and for teachers of hearing impaired children.

4358 Foundations of Spoken Language for Hearing Impaired Children
Alexander Graham Bell Association
3417 Volta Place NW   202-337-5220
Washington, DC 20007-2737   Fax: 202-337-8270
                                   TTY: 202-337-5220
This guide traces the individual progress of a child's speech development.
1978 87 pages

4359 Free Hand: Education of the Deaf
TJ Publishers
817 Silver Spring Avenue   301-585-4440
Silver Spring, MD 20910-4617   800-999-1168
                                   Fax: 301-585-5930
                                   TTY: 301-585-4441
                                   e-mail: tjpubinc@aol.com
Based on the proceedings of a 1990 symposium on the educational uses of ASL, A Free Hand presents papers by prominent educators, researchers and linguists in the changing role of American sign language in the classroom.
204 pages Softcover
ISBN: 0-932666-40-X
Angela K Thames, President
Jerald A Murphy, VP

4360 GA and SK Etiquette
Gallaudet University
11030 S Langley Avenue
Chicago, IL 60628-3819   800-621-2736
                                   Fax: 800-621-8476
                                   TTY: 888-630-9347
                                   www.gallaudet.edu/~gupress
This booklet presents guidelines for proper usage of the TDD.
53 pages

4361 Gallaudet Encyclopedia of Deaf People and Deafness
Gallaudet University
11030 S Langley Avenue
Chicago, IL 60628-3819   800-621-2736
                                   Fax: 800-621-8476
                                   TTY: 888-630-9347
                                   www.gallaudet.edu/~gupress
Three-volume set of research and information on deaf people and deafness.
1400 pages

4362 Growing Together: Information for Parents of Deaf & Hard of Hearing Children
Gallaudet University
11030 S Langley Avenue
Chicago, IL 60628-3819   800-621-2736
                                   Fax: 800-621-8476
                                   TTY: 888-630-9347
                                   www.gallaudet.edu/~gupress
This publication answers questions often asked by parents of children with a hearing loss.
92 pages

4363 Handtalk Zoo
Macmillan Publishing Company
866 3rd Avenue   212-702-2000
New York, NY 10022-6221   800-257-5755
                                   www.mcp.com
Wonderful photographs are used to show children at the zoo communicating with sign language.
28 pages Hardcover
ISBN: 0-027008-01-0

4364 Hearing Aid Handbook
Gallaudet University
11030 S Langley Avenue
Chicago, IL 60628-3819   800-621-2736
                                   Fax: 800-621-8476
                                   TTY: 888-630-9347
                                   www.gallaudet.edu/~gupress
A complete guide for wearers and clinicians for the use and maintenance of hearing aids.
172 pages Paperback

4365 Hearing Impaired Children and Youth and Developmental Disabilities
Gallaudet University
11030 S Langley Avenue
Chicago, IL 60628-3819   800-621-2736
                                   Fax: 800-621-8476
                                   TTY: 888-630-9347
                                   www.gallaudet.edu/~gupress
Offers insights from 24 experts to help clarify relationships between hearing impairments and developmental difficulties.
416 pages

4366 Hearing Loss Help
Impact Publications
9104 Manassas Drive   703-361-7300
Manassas Park, VA 20111-5211   Fax: 703-335-9469
                                   e-mail: info@impactpublications.com
                                   www.impactpublications.com
Self-help guide provides factual information on how we hear, and on the causes and symptoms of hearing loss. Gives practical information on ways to improve everyday communication and create better listening conditions, and covers assistive listening devices.

4367 Hearing Loss and Hearing Aids: A Bridge to Healing
Richard Carmen, author
Hearing Loss Association of America
7910 Woodmont Avenue   301-657-2248
Bethesda, MD 20814-3079   Fax: 301-913-9413
                                   TTY: 301-657-2249
                                   e-mail: info@hearingloss.org
                                   www.hearingloss.org
The Consumer Handbook on hearing loss and hearing aids.
Softcover
ISBN: 0-966182-61-8
Jerry Portis, Executive Director
Brenda Battat, Assistant Executive Director

4368 Hispanic Deaf
Gallaudet University
11030 S Langley Avenue
Chicago, IL 60628-3819   800-621-2736
                                   Fax: 800-621-8476
                                   TTY: 888-630-9347
                                   www.gallaudet.edu/~gupress
Hispanic students now make up the largest minority in education for deaf students. This timely collection includes articles by many of the professionals most closely involved with the education of this very special population.
213 pages Hardcover

4369 History of Special Education: From Isolation to Integration
Gallaudet University
11030 S Langley Avenue
Chicago, IL 60628-3819   800-621-2736
                                   Fax: 800-621-8476
                                   TTY: 888-630-9347
                                   www.gallaudet.edu/~gupress
Comprehensive volume examining the facts and events that shaped this field in Western Europe, United States and Canada.
464 pages

4370 Hollywood Speaks
Gallaudet University
11030 S Langley Avenue
Chicago, IL 60628-3819   800-621-2736
                                        Fax: 800-621-8476
                                        TTY: 888-630-9347
                                        www.gallaudet.edu/~gupress
How deafness has been treated in movies and how it provides yet
another window onto social history in addition to a fresh angle
from which to view Hollywood.
167 pages Hardcover

4371 Hometown Heroes: Successful Deaf Youth in America
Gallaudet University
11030 S Langley Avenue
Chicago, IL 60628-3819   800-621-2736
                                        Fax: 800-621-8476
                                        TTY: 888-630-9347
                                        www.gallaudet.edu/~gupress
A lively book showcasing more than 40 deaf and hard-of-hearing
teenagers in the United States.
108 pages

4372 How Hearing Impacts Relationships
Richard Carmen, author
Hearing Loss Association of America
7910 Woodmont Avenue   301-657-2248
Bethesda, MD 20814-3079   Fax: 301-913-9413
                                        TTY: 301-657-2249
                                        e-mail: info@hearingloss.org
                                        www.hearingloss.org
At last families of loved ones with untreated hearing loss can know
they are not alone and what options are available.
Softcover
ISBN: 0-966182-63-4
Jerry Portis, Executive Director
Brenda Battat, Assistant Executive Director

4373 How the Student with Hearing Loss Can Succeed in College
Alexander Graham Bell Association
3417 Volta Place NW   202-337-5220
Washington, DC 20007-2737   Fax: 202-337-8270
                                        TTY: 202-337-5220
This revised book details how students who are deaf or hard of
hearing and professionals must work together for students in college to be successful.
1996 304 pages

4374 How to Survive a Hearing Loss
Gallaudet University
11030 S Langley Avenue
Chicago, IL 60628-3819   800-621-2736
                                        Fax: 800-621-8476
                                        TTY: 888-630-9347
                                        www.gallaudet.edu/~gupress
This book presents the results of the author's intensive research
about hearing and the ear.
241 pages

4375 Hug Just Isn't Enough
Gallaudet University
11030 S Langley Avenue
Chicago, IL 60628-3819   800-621-2736
                                        Fax: 800-621-8476
                                        TTY: 888-630-9347
                                        www.gallaudet.edu/~gupress
Photos of deaf children and excerpts from interviews with parents
of deaf youngsters.

4376 I Didn't Hear the Dragon Roar
Gallaudet University
11030 S Langley Avenue
Chicago, IL 60628-3819   800-621-2736
                                        Fax: 800-621-8476
                                        TTY: 888-630-9347
                                        www.gallaudet.edu/~gupress
The remarkable true story of a deaf woman's journey from Hong
Kong to Katmandu.
251 pages

4377 IDEA Advocacy for Children Who are Deaf or Hard of Hearing
Alexander Graham Bell Association
3417 Volta Place NW   202-337-5220
Washington, DC 20007-2737   Fax: 202-337-8270
                                        TTY: 202-337-5220
This book offers up to date information about the 1997 Individuals
with Disabilities Education Act which affects children who are
deaf or hard of hearing.
1997 96 pages

**4378 Implications and Complications for Deaf Students of Full
Inclusion Movement**
Gallaudet University
11030 S Langley Avenue
Chicago, IL 60628-3819   800-621-2736
                                        Fax: 800-621-8476
                                        TTY: 888-630-9347
                                        www.gallaudet.edu/~gupress
A collection of papers discussing the full inclusion movement.
80 pages

4379 In Silence: Growing Up Hearing in a Deaf World
Gallaudet University
11030 S Langley Avenue
Chicago, IL 60628-3819   800-621-2736
                                        Fax: 800-621-8476
                                        TTY: 888-630-9347
                                        www.gallaudet.edu/~gupress
Author's story of growing up as a hearing child of deaf parents.
335 pages

4380 In This Sign
Gallaudet University
11030 S Langley Avenue
Chicago, IL 60628-3819   800-621-2736
                                        Fax: 800-621-8476
                                        TTY: 888-630-9347
                                        www.gallaudet.edu/~gupress
A modern classic following a family of deaf parents and their hearing impaired child through several decades of growth and pain,
tragedy and triumph.
275 pages

4381 Inclusion?
Gallaudet University
11030 S Langley Avenue
Chicago, IL 60628-3819   800-621-2736
                                        Fax: 800-621-8476
                                        TTY: 888-630-9347
                                        www.gallaudet.edu/~gupress
This book defines quality education for deaf and hard of hearing
students.
213 pages

4382 International Directory of Periodicals Related to Deafness
Gallaudet University
11030 S Langley Avenue
Chicago, IL 60628-3819   800-621-2736
                                        Fax: 800-621-8476
                                        TTY: 888-630-9347
                                        www.gallaudet.edu/~gupress
Offers information on more than 500 magazines and journals related to deafness.
150 pages

4383 International Telephone Directory for TDD Users
Gallaudet University
11030 S Langley Avenue
Chicago, IL 60628-3819   800-621-2736
                                        Fax: 800-621-8476
                                        TTY: 888-630-9347
                                        www.gallaudet.edu/~gupress
Offers 12,000 TDD members and organizations serving deaf people.
190 pages

4384 Introduction to Communication
Gallaudet University

11030 S Langley Avenue
Chicago, IL 60628-3819

800-621-2736
Fax: 800-621-8476
TTY: 888-630-9347
www.gallaudet.edu/~gupress

Curriculum materials exploring the areas of sound, hearing and interpersonal communication.
100 pages

4385 Invisible Condition: The Human Side of Hearing Loss

Howard E Stone, author

Hearing Loss Association of America
7910 Woodmont Avenue
Bethesda, MD 20814-3079

301-657-2248
Fax: 301-913-9413
TTY: 301-657-2249
e-mail: info@hearingloss.org
www.hearingloss.org

A collection of 14 years of editorials by the author from the SHHH Journal. An inspiration book that transcends hearing loss.
1993
Jerry Portis, Executive Director
Brenda Battat, Assistant Executive Director

4386 Its Your Turn Now: Using Dialogue Journals with Deaf Students
Gallaudet University
11030 S Langley Avenue
Chicago, IL 60628-3819

800-621-2736
Fax: 800-621-8476
TTY: 888-630-9347
www.gallaudet.edu/~gupress

Based on years of experience, this book reviews teachers' questions and answers.
130 pages

4387 Journey Into the Deaf World
DawnSignPress
6130 Nancy Ridge Drive
San Diego, CA 92121-3223

858-625-0600
800-549-5350
Fax: 858-625-2336
TTY: 858-625-0600
e-mail: comments@dawnsign.com
www.dawnsign.com

Provides explanation about the nature and meaning of the deaf world. Comprehensive work discusses latest findings and theories for deaf studies students and professionals working with deaf people.
528 pages Paperback
ISBN: 0-915035-63-4
Barry Howland, Marketing Director

4388 Journey Out of Silence

Dora Tinglestad Weber, author

Hearing Loss Association of America
7910 Woodmont Avenue
Bethesda, MD 20814-3079

301-657-2248
Fax: 301-913-9413
TTY: 301-657-2249
e-mail: info@hearingloss.org
www.hearingloss.org

Dora Weber, who made a long and arduous journey out of silence, shares her experiences in an effort to encourage those who are hearing impaired and to increase the sensitivity of those who are not.
Softcover
ISBN: 1-890676-30-6
Jerry Portis, Executive Director
Brenda Battat, Assistant Executive Director

4389 Joy of Signing
Gospel Publishing House
1445 N Boonville Avenue
Springfield, MO 65802-1894

417-862-2781
Fax: 417-862-7566
e-mail: jclore@ag.org
www.GospelPublishing.com

Illustrated sign language text with descriptions of the origin of selected signs and examples of how each is used. Second edition.
352 pages
Judy Clore, Promotions Coordinator

4390 Kaleidoscope of Deaf America
Harris Communications
6541 City W Parkway
Eden Prairie, MN 55344-3248

612-906-1180
Fax: 612-946-0924

Puts you in touch with the trends, the events and the thinking that is shaping your future.
79 pages

4391 Kendall Demonstration Elementary School Curriculum Guides
Gallaudet University
11030 S Langley Avenue
Chicago, IL 60628-3819

800-621-2736
Fax: 800-621-8476
TTY: 888-630-9347
www.gallaudet.edu/~gupress

These guides provide detailed information to help teachers organize curriculum, structure classes and develop individualized education programs.
18 months+

4392 Kid-Friendly Parenting with Deaf and Hard of Hearing Children
Gallaudet University
11030 S Langley Avenue
Chicago, IL 60628-3819

800-621-2736
Fax: 800-621-8476
TTY: 888-630-9347
www.gallaudet.edu/~gupress

A step-by-step guide offering parents hundreds of ideas and play activities for children ages 3 to 12.
336 pages

4393 Learning to Hear Again
Alexander Graham Bell Association
3417 Volta Place NW
Washington, DC 20007-2737

202-337-5220
Fax: 202-337-8270
TTY: 202-337-5220

This audiologic rehabilitation curriculum guide is designed to help audiologists and speech language pathologist provide rehabilitation and education for adults with hearing losses. The authors are practicing audiologists and have used these methods successfully in individual and group sessions. This comprehensive manual comprises lesson plans, activities and materials ready to be duplicated and distributed to clients.
1996 224 pages

4394 Learning to See: American Sign Language as a Second Language
Gallaudet University
11030 S Langley Avenue
Chicago, IL 60628-3819

800-621-2736
Fax: 800-621-8476
TTY: 888-630-9347
www.gallaudet.edu/~gupress

Provides a comprehensive introduction to the history and structure of ASL to the deaf community.
134 pages

4395 Least Restrictive Environment: The Paradox of Inclusion
LRP Publications
PO Box 980
Horsham, PA 19044-0980

800-341-7874
Fax: 215-784-9639
e-mail: custserv@lrp.com
www.lrp.com

Analyzes relevant federal law and the inclusion reform movement, and discusses the premise that an effort to force one generic placement on all children will create more problems than thought imaginable.
Paperback

4396 Legal Rights for the Deaf and Hard of Hearing
Hearing Loss Association of America
7910 Woodmont Avenue
Bethesda, MD 20814-3079

301-657-2248
Fax: 301-913-9413
TTY: 301-657-2249
e-mail: info@hearingloss.org
www.hearingloss.org

A comprehensive analysis of recent laws passed to protect the rights of and guarantee equal access for people with hearing loss.

The book explains in layman's terminology how legislation affects individuals with disabilities in everyday life.
2002 Softcover
Jerry Portis, Executive Director
Brenda Battat, Assistant Executive Director

4397 Legal Rights of Hearing-Impaired People
Gallaudet University
11030 S Langley Avenue
Chicago, IL 60628-3819
800-621-2736
Fax: 800-621-8476
TTY: 888-630-9347
www.gallaudet.edu/~gupress
Includes updated interpretations of legislation affecting hearing-impaired people, including chapters dealing with the ADA.
297 pages

4398 Lessons in Laughter: The Autobiography of a Deaf Actor
Gallaudet University
11030 S Langley Avenue
Chicago, IL 60628-3819
800-621-2736
Fax: 800-621-8476
TTY: 888-630-9347
www.gallaudet.edu/~gupress
Born deaf of deaf parents, Bernard Bragg dreamed of using sign language to act. This book recounts how he starred in his own television show.
237 pages

4399 Let's Learn About Deafness
Gallaudet University
11030 S Langley Avenue
Chicago, IL 60628-3819
800-621-2736
Fax: 800-621-8476
TTY: 888-630-9347
www.gallaudet.edu/~gupress
Hands-on school classroom activities for the deaf student.
82 pages

4400 Listen to Me: Auditory Exercises for Adults
Alexander Graham Bell Association
3417 Volta Place NW
Washington, DC 20007-2737
202-337-5220
Fax: 202-337-8270
TTY: 202-337-5220
Helps hard of hearing teenagers and adults to listen, lip read, pick up clues from conversations and remember what they have heard.
65 pages

4401 Listen with the Heart: Relationships and Hearing Loss
Hearing Loss Association of America
7910 Woodmont Avenue
Bethesda, MD 20814-3079
301-657-2248
Fax: 301-913-9413
TTY: 301-657-2249
e-mail: info@hearingloss.org
www.hearingloss.org
Written for family and friends as well as professionals. It is an excellent text for college and graduate level courses in psychology, mental health counseling, speech and hearing, special education, and deaf education.
Jerry Portis, Executive Director
Brenda Battat, Assistant Executive Director

4402 Listening
National Catholic Office for the Deaf
7201 Buchnan Street
Landover Hills, MD 20784-4500
301-577-1684
e-mail: nco@erols.com
www.ncod.org
Published as a pastoral service for the hearing impaired.

4403 Listening & Talking
Alexander Graham Bell Association
3417 Volta Place NW
Washington, DC 20007-2737
202-337-5220
Fax: 202-337-8270
TTY: 202-337-5220
This guide promotes spoken language in young hearing-impaired children.
191 pages

4404 Listening to Learn: A Handbook for Parents with Hearing-Impaired Children
Alexander Graham Bell Association

3417 Volta Place NW
Washington, DC 20007-2737
202-337-5220
Fax: 202-337-8270
TTY: 202-337-5220
Developed by teachers, this handbook provides parents with the essential steps necessary to develop effective spoken communication with their children.
98 pages

4405 Listening: Ways of Hearing in a Silent World
Hannah Merker, author
Hearing Loss Association of America
7910 Woodmont Avenue
Bethesda, MD 20814-3079
301-657-2248
Fax: 301-913-9413
TTY: 301-657-2249
e-mail: info@hearingloss.org
www.hearingloss.org
This book is about one woman's evocative account of her perceptions and remembrance of sound.
1999
Jerry Portis, Executive Director
Brenda Battat, Assistant Executive Director

4406 Literature Journal
Gallaudet University
11030 S Langley Avenue
Chicago, IL 60628-3819
800-621-2736
Fax: 800-621-8476
TTY: 888-630-9347
www.gallaudet.edu/~gupress
This book includes extensive examples of student and teacher entries taken from actual journals of deaf high school students.
44 pages

4407 Living with Hearing Loss
Marcia B Dugan, author
Hearing Loss Association of America
7910 Woodmont Avenue
Bethesda, MD 20814-3079
301-657-2248
Fax: 301-913-9413
TTY: 301-657-2249
e-mail: info@hearingloss.org
www.hearingloss.org
Living with Hearing Loss takes the reader from A to Z on the kinds and causes of hearing loss and its common early signs. Topics Include: Seeking Professional Evaluations, Hearing Aids, Assistive Technology, Speechreading, Communication Tips, Cochlear Implants, Dealing with Tinnitus, and resources.
2003
ISBN: 1-563681-34-0
Jerry Portis, Executive Director
Brenda Battat, Assistant Executive Director

4408 Looking Back: A Reader on the History of Deaf Communities & Sign Language
Gallaudet University
11030 S Langley Avenue
Chicago, IL 60628-3819
800-621-2736
Fax: 800-621-8476
TTY: 888-630-9347
www.gallaudet.edu/~gupress
Renowned researchers from around the world present provocative findings in six areas relating to the deaf culture.
558 pages

4409 Loss for Words
Gallaudet University
11030 S Langley Avenue
Chicago, IL 60628-3819
800-621-2736
Fax: 800-621-8476
TTY: 888-630-9347
www.gallaudet.edu/~gupress
The author's touching story of her life as an interpreter for her parents, head of her household by the age of eight and a teacher and helper to both of her deaf parents.
208 pages

4410 Mainstreaming Deaf and Hard of Hearing Students
Gallaudet University

800 Florida Avenue NE
Washington, DC 20002-3695

202-651-5000
800-621-2736
Fax: 800-621-8476
TTY: 888-630-9347
www.gallaudet.edu/~gupress

Gallaudet University is the world leader in liberal education and career development for deaf and hard-of-hearing undergraduate students.
40 pages

4411   Man Without Words
Gallaudet University
11030 S Langley Avenue
Chicago, IL 60628-3819

800-621-2736
Fax: 800-621-8476
TTY: 888-630-9347
www.gallaudet.edu/~gupress

Author relates her experiences teaching sign language to a 27 year old deaf Mexican man who had no education and no language.
203 pages

4412   Martimer
APSEA-RCHI
Box 308
Amherst, NS, B4H 3Z6,

902-667-3808
Fax: 902-667-0893

Periodical describing programs and services provided by the APSEA Resource Center for the Hearing Impaired.
Phyllis Cameron, Editor

4413   Mask of Benevolence: Disabling the Deaf Community
Gallaudet University
11030 S Langley Avenue
Chicago, IL 60628-3819

800-621-2736
Fax: 800-621-8476
TTY: 888-630-9347
www.gallaudet.edu/~gupress

Written by a doctor who does not view deafness as a handicap but rather a different state of hearing.
310 pages

4414   Meeting Halfway in ASL
MSM Productions
PO Box 23380
Rochester, NY 14692-3380

716-442-6370
Fax: 716-442-6371
TTY: 716-442-6370
e-mail: Books@deaflife.com
www.deaflife.com

Illustrated photographic sign-language book containing 1,300 photos.

ISBN: 0-963401-67-
Matthew Moore, Publisher

4415   Meeting the Challenge: Hearing-Impaired Professionals in the Workplace
Gallaudet University
11030 S Langley Avenue
Chicago, IL 60628-3819

800-621-2736
Fax: 800-621-8476
TTY: 888-630-9347
www.gallaudet.edu/~gupress

Provides information on communication methods, educational backgrounds and job search tactics used by more than 1500 participants and their current employment conditions.
236 pages

4416   Mental Health Services for Deaf People
Gallaudet University
11030 S Langley Avenue
Chicago, IL 60628-3819

800-621-2736
Fax: 800-621-8476
TTY: 888-630-9347
www.gallaudet.edu/~gupress

Contains information on over 350 mental health programs and services for deaf people across the United States.
210 pages

4417   Missing Words: The Family Handbook on Adult Hearing Loss
Gallaudet University

11030 S Langley Avenue
Chicago, IL 60628-3819

800-621-2736
Fax: 800-621-8476
TTY: 888-630-9347
www.gallaudet.edu/~gupress

Written by a mother who lost her hearing and her daughter, learning to cope.
304 pages

4418   Mother Father Deaf: Living Between Sound and Silence
Harvard University Press
79 Garden Street
Cambridge, MA 02138-1423

617-495-2480
800-448-2242
Fax: 800-962-4983
www.hup.harvard.edu

Based on interviews with 150 adult hearing children of deaf parents who chart the sometimes difficult middle ground between spoken and signed language.

4419   Moving Toward the Standards
Gallaudet University
11030 S Langley Avenue
Chicago, IL 60628-3819

800-621-2736
Fax: 800-621-8476
TTY: 888-630-9347
www.gallaudet.edu/~gupress

A national action plan for mathematics education reform for the deaf.
55 pages

4420   Music in Motion
Modern Signs Press
PO Box 1181
Los Alamitos, CA 90720-1181

562-596-8548
800-572-7332
Fax: 562-795-6614
TTY: 562-493-4168
e-mail: modsigns@aol.com
www.modsigns.com

Includes guitar notes and glossary of sign descriptions for 325-word vocabulary.
109 pages
ISBN: 0-916708-07-1

4421   NAD Deaf Awareness Kit
National Association of the Deaf
8630 Fenton Street
Silver Spring, MD 20910

301-587-1788
Fax: 301-587-1791
TTY: 301-587-1789
www.nad.org

Includes information that can be used both during Deaf Awareness Week and year-round to recognize the accomplishments and heritage of the deaf community.
Donna Morris, Publications Manager

4422   Never the Twain Shall Meet: The Communications Debate
Gallaudet University
11030 S Langley Avenue
Chicago, IL 60628-3819

800-621-2736
Fax: 800-621-8476
TTY: 888-630-9347
www.gallaudet.edu/~gupress

Should sign language be used in the education of Deaf children or should they be forced to deal with a hearing, speaking world on its own terms?
129 pages

4423   Next Step
Gallaudet University
11030 S Langley Avenue
Chicago, IL 60628-3819

800-621-2736
Fax: 800-621-8476
TTY: 888-630-9347
www.gallaudet.edu/~gupress

A national conference focusing on issues related to substance abuse in the deaf and hard of hearing population.
209 pages

4424   No Sound
Harris Communications

6541 City W Parkway
612-906-1180
Eden Prairie, MN 55344-3248
Fax: 612-946-0924

A moving, highly informative autobiography of Julius Wiggins, founder and president of the newspaper Silent News. Second edition.
211 pages

4425 No Walls of Stone: An Anthology of Literature by Deaf Writers
Gallaudet University
11030 S Langley Avenue
Chicago, IL 60628-3819
800-621-2736
Fax: 800-621-8476
TTY: 888-630-9347
www.gallaudet.edu/~gupress

Short fiction, essays, verse and drama written by the deaf and hard of hearing writer.
240 pages
Jill Jepson, Editor

4426 None So Deaf
Gallaudet University
11030 S Langley Avenue
Chicago, IL 60628-3819
800-621-2736
Fax: 800-621-8476
TTY: 888-630-9347
www.gallaudet.edu/~gupress

A student history of education of deaf people and the development of sign language.
51 pages Paperback

4427 Odyssey of Hearing Loss: Tales of Triumph
Michael A Harvey, PhD, author
Hearing Loss Association of America
7910 Woodmont Avenue
301-657-2248
Bethesda, MD 20814-3079
Fax: 301-913-9413
TTY: 301-657-2249
e-mail: info@hearingloss.org
www.hearingloss.org

A glimpse into the lives of 10 people; each showing how sharing insights about hearing loss helps people on the road to healing and a life well examined.
Jerry Portis, Executive Director
Brenda Battat, Assistant Executive Director

4428 Okada Hearing Ear Guide
RR 1 Box 640F
414-275-5226
Fontana, WI 53125-9714
Trains dogs to aid hearing-impaired persons.

4429 On My Own
Gallaudet University
11030 S Langley Avenue
Chicago, IL 60628-3819
800-621-2736
Fax: 800-621-8476
TTY: 888-630-9347
www.gallaudet.edu/~gupress

Book examining doorbell devices, alarm clocks, telephone amplifiers and other assistive devices for the deaf.
50 pages Teacher's Guide

4430 Oral Interpreting Selections from Papers from Kirsten Gonzales
Alexander Graham Bell Association
3417 Volta Place NW
202-337-5220
Washington, DC 20007-2737
Fax: 202-337-8270
TTY: 202-337-5220

These six easy to read articles discuss speech reading and oral interpreting. The articles answer questions that are frequently asked by professionals and the general public.
30 pages

4431 Other Side of Silence
Gallaudet University
11030 S Langley Avenue
Chicago, IL 60628-3819
800-621-2736
Fax: 800-621-8476
TTY: 888-630-9347
www.gallaudet.edu/~gupress

Explores the deaf community through interviews from across the country.
256 pages

4432 Our Forgotten Children
Alexander Graham Bell Association
3417 Volta Place NW
202-337-5220
Washington, DC 20007-2737
Fax: 202-337-8270
TTY: 202-337-5220

This simple book describes characteristics of hard-of-hearing children in the school and discusses their educational requirements, psychological and social needs and amplification options.
68 pages

4433 Our Forgotten Children: Hard of Hearing Pupils in the Schools
Julia M Davis, PhD, author
Hearing Loss Association of America
7910 Woodmont Avenue
301-657-2248
Bethesda, MD 20814-3079
Fax: 301-913-9413
TTY: 301-657-2249
e-mail: info@hearingloss.org
www.hearingloss.org

Important resource about the educational environment.
2001
Jerry Portis, Executive Director
Brenda Battat, Assistant Executive Director

4434 Outsiders in a Hearing World
Gallaudet University
11030 S Langley Avenue
Chicago, IL 60628-3819
800-621-2736
Fax: 800-621-8476
TTY: 888-630-9347
www.gallaudet.edu/~gupress

The author gives a sociologist's view of what it is like to be deaf.
240 pages

4435 Parents and Teachers: Partners in Language Development
Alexander Graham Bell Association
3417 Volta Place NW
202-337-5220
Washington, DC 20007-2737
Fax: 202-337-8270
TTY: 202-337-5220

Outlines the essential role of the teacher and parent in the development of language in the school aged child with hearing impairment.
386 pages

4436 Perigee Visual Dictionary of Signing
Harris Communications
6541 City W Parkway
612-906-1180
Eden Prairie, MN 55344-3248
Fax: 612-946-0924
An A-to-Z guide to American Sign Language vocabulary.
450 pages

4437 Perspectives Folio: Mainstreaming
Gallaudet University
11030 S Langley Avenue
Chicago, IL 60628-3819
800-621-2736
Fax: 800-621-8476
TTY: 888-630-9347
www.gallaudet.edu/~gupress

Presents 14 articles from Perspectives magazine that offer practical, experience-based advice on mainstreaming for parents and students themselves.
39 pages

4438 Perspectives on Deafness
National Association of the Deaf
8630 Fenton Street
301-587-1788
Silver Spring, MD 20910
Fax: 301-587-1791
TTY: 301-587-1789
www.nad.org

Focuses on the many perspectives which constitute diversity within the deaf community.
Paperback
Donna Morris, Publications Manager

4439 Place of Their Own: Creating the Deaf Community in America
Gallaudet University Press
11030 S Langley Avenue
Chicago, IL 60628-3819
800-621-2736
TTY: 888-630-9347
www.gallaudet.edu

Traces the history of deaf people and views deafness not from the perspective of a pathology, but of culture, not as a disease or disability to overcome or be cured, but as the distinguishing characteristic of a distinct community of individuals whose history and achievement are worthy of study.

4440   Politics of Deafness
Gallaudet University
11030 S Langley Avenue
Chicago, IL 60628   800-621-2736
                                                     Fax: 800-621-8476
                                                    TTY: 888-630-9347
                                                www.gallaudet.edu/~gupress
Embarks upon a postmodern examination of the search for identity in deafness and its relationship to the prevalent Hearing culture that has marginalized Deaf people.
June 1997 304 pages Softcover
ISBN: 1-563680-58-0

4441   Possible Dream: Mainstream Experiences of Hearing-Impaired Students
Alexander Graham Bell Association
3417 Volta Place NW   202-337-5220
Washington, DC 20007-2737   Fax: 202-337-8270
                                                    TTY: 202-337-5220
This collection highlights the experiences of auditory-oral children who are Bell Association financial aid winners and their families.
66 pages
Mildred L Oberkotter, Editor

4442   Post Milan
Gallaudet University
11030 S Langley Avenue
Chicago, IL 60628-3819   800-621-2736
                                                     Fax: 800-621-8476
                                                    TDD: 800-621-8476
                                                www.gallaudet.edu/~gupress
Timely issues covering trends in ASL and ASL/English literacy.
323 pages

4443   PreReading Strategies
Gallaudet University
11030 S Langley Avenue
Chicago, IL 60628-3819   800-621-2736
                                                     Fax: 800-621-8476
                                                    TTY: 888-630-9347
                                                www.gallaudet.edu/~gupress
Here is a wealth of good advice for preparing students to understand what they read, building comprehension and enjoyment.
65 pages

4444   Psychoeducational Assessment of Hearing-Impaired Students
Pro-Ed, Inc.
8700 Shoal Creek Boulevard   512-451-3246
Austin, TX 78757-6897   Fax: 512-451-8542
                                                e-mail: info@proedinc.com
                                                      www.proedinc.com
This book includes a comprehensive presentation of issues and procedures related to the assessment of hearing-impaired students.
251 pages Paperback
ISBN: 0-890794-55-3
Lindy Jordaan, Marketing Coordinator

4445   Reading and Deafness
Pro-Ed, Inc.
8700 Shoal Creek Boulevard   512-451-3246
Austin, TX 78757-6897   800-897-3202
                                                     Fax: 800-397-7633
                                                e-mail: info@proedinc.com
                                                      www.proedinc.com
Three areas are looked at in this book: deaf children's prereading development of real-world knowledge; cognitive abilities and linguistic skills.
422 pages Hardcover
ISBN: 0-887441-07-6
Lindy Jordaan, Marketing Coordinator

4446   Rebuilt: My Journey Back to the Hearing World
Michael Chorost, author
Hearing Loss Association of America
7910 Woodmont Avenue   301-657-2248
Bethesda, MD 20814-3079   Fax: 301-913-9413
                                                    TTY: 301-657-2249
                                                e-mail: info@hearingloss.org
                                                      www.hearingloss.org
Brimming with insight and written with charm and self-deprecating humor, Rebuilt unveils, in personal terms, the astounding possibilities of a new technological age.
240 pages Paperback
ISBN: 0-618717-60-9
Jerry Portis, Executive Director
Brenda Battat, Assistant Executive Director

4447   Say That Again, Please
Gallaudet University
11030 S Langley Avenue
Chicago, IL 60628-3819   800-621-2736
                                                     Fax: 800-621-8476
                                                    TTY: 888-630-9347
                                                www.gallaudet.edu/~gupress
This book serves to enlighten those who are interested.
370 pages

4448   Schedules of Development for Hearing Impaired Infants and their Parents
Alexander Graham Bell Association
3417 Volta Place NW   202-337-5220
Washington, DC 20007-2737   Fax: 202-337-8270
                                                    TTY: 202-337-5220
Written for parents and teachers, this assessment record of verbal learning will help to evaluate each child's language development.
1977 14 pages

4449   Science of Sound
Gallaudet University
11030 S Langley Avenue
Chicago, IL 60628-3819   800-621-2736
                                                     Fax: 800-621-8476
                                                    TTY: 888-630-9347
                                                www.gallaudet.edu/~gupress
This exciting book is carefully designed to help hearing-impaired students understand, use and enjoy the principles of sound.
32 pages

4450   Seeds of Disquiet: One Deaf Woman's Experience
Gallaudet University
11030 S Langley Avenue
Chicago, IL 60628-3819   800-621-2736
                                                     Fax: 800-621-8476
                                                    TTY: 888-630-9347
                                                www.gallaudet.edu/~gupress
This book relates to the story of how Cheryl Heppner reacted to two severe losses in her hearing.
192 pages

4451   Seeing Voices: A Journey Into the World of the Deaf
Gallaudet University
11030 S Langley Avenue
Chicago, IL 60628-3819   800-621-2736
                                                     Fax: 800-621-8476
                                                    TTY: 888-630-9347
                                                www.gallaudet.edu/~gupress
Dr. Sacks takes us into the world of deaf people.
180 pages

4452   Sign Communication: A Family Affair
Gallaudet University
11030 S Langley Avenue
Chicago, IL 60628-3819   800-621-2736
                                                     Fax: 800-621-8476
                                                    TTY: 888-630-9347
                                                www.gallaudet.edu/~gupress
Book designed to help hearing parents communicate effectively with their deaf children on issues of good health and personal growth.
132 pages

4453 Sign Language Feelings
Gallaudet University
11030 S Langley Avenue
Chicago, IL 60628-3819
800-621-2736
Fax: 800-621-8476
TTY: 888-630-9347
www.gallaudet.edu/~gupress
Worksheets teach signs for happy, sad and all of the feelings in between.

4454 Sign Language Interpreters and Interpreting
Gallaudet University
11030 S Langley Avenue
Chicago, IL 60628-3819
800-621-2736
Fax: 800-621-8476
TTY: 888-630-9347
www.gallaudet.edu/~gupress
This monograph presents articles about personal characteristics and abilities of interpreters, the effects of lag time on interpreter errors, and the interpretation of register.
161 pages

4455 Sign Language Made Simple
Gospel Publishing House
1445 N Boonville Avenue
Springfield, MO 65802-1894
417-862-2781
Fax: 417-862-7566
e-mail: jclore@ag.org
www.GospelPublishing.com
Illustrated sign language text with descriptions of the origin of selected signs and examples of how each is used. Second edition.
240 pages
Judy Clore, Promotions Coordinator

4456 Sign Language Talk
Franklin Watts Grolier
90 Old Sherman Tpke
Danbury, CT 06816-0001
203-797-3500
800-843-3749
Fax: 203-797-3197
www.grolier.com
Using 300 easy-to-follow illustrations, this book introduces the structure of sign language, shows how sentences are formed and how signed conversations differ from spoken ones.
96 pages
ISBN: 0-531105-97-0

4457 Sign Language and the Deaf Community: Essays in Honor of William Stokoe
National Association of the Deaf
8630 Fenton Street
Silver Spring, MD 20910
301-587-1788
Fax: 301-587-1791
TTY: 301-587-1789
www.nad.org
Collection of essays, written by professionals in the field of sign language research and usage, describing how information has dramatically altered society's understanding of deaf people and their culture.
267 pages Paperback
Donna Morris, Publications Manager

4458 Signed English Starter
Harris Communications
6541 City W Parkway
Eden Prairie, MN 55344-3248
612-906-1108
Fax: 612-946-0924
The first book to use when learning Signed English.
208 pages

4459 Signing Exact English
Modern Signs Press
PO Box 1181
Los Alamitos, CA 90720-1181
562-596-8548
800-572-7332
Fax: 562-795-6614
TTY: 562-493-4168
e-mail: modsigns@aol.com
www.modsigns.com
A reference manual containing manual signs representing nearly 4,000 words, plus signs for letters, numbers, prefixes and suffixes.
1993 479 pages Softcover
ISBN: 0-196708-23-3

4460 Signing Illustrated
Gallaudet University
11030 S Langley Avenue
Chicago, IL 60628-3819
800-621-2736
Fax: 800-621-8476
TTY: 888-630-9347
www.gallaudet.edu/~gupress
A guide presenting illustrations of over 1,350 signs.
85 pages

4461 Signing Naturally: Teacher's Curriculum Guide-Level 1
DawnSignPress
6130 Nancy Ridge Drive
San Diego, CA 92121-3223
619-625-0600
800-549-5350
Fax: 619-625-2336
e-mail: DawnSign@aol.com
Guide and video.
336 pages 22 minutes
ISBN: 0-915035-07-3

4462 Signs Everywhere
Modern Signs Press
PO Box 1181
Los Alamitos, CA 90720-1181
562-596-8548
800-572-7332
Fax: 562-795-6614
TTY: 562-493-4168
e-mail: modsigns@aol.com
www.modsigns.com
Includes signs for cities, towns and states through United States, Canada and Mexico. Drawings and descriptions of the signs accompany maps showing locations of states and cities.
280 pages
ISBN: 0-916708-05-5

4463 Signs for Computing Terminology
National Association of the Deaf
8630 Fenton Street
Silver Spring, MD 20910-4500
301-587-1788
Fax: 301-587-1791
TTY: 301-587-1789
www.nad.org
Contains over 600 computer related sign illustrations used by deaf and hearing computer specialists.
182 pages Paperback
ISBN: 0-913072-63-X
Donna Morris, Publications Manager

4464 Silent Alarm: On the Edge with a Deaf EMT
Gallaudet University
11030 S Langley Avenue
Chicago, IL 60628-3819
800-621-2736
Fax: 800-621-8476
TTY: 888-630-9347
www.gallaudet.edu/~gupress
Silent Alarm tells the gripping story of survival and the good that the author did as a topnotch EMT.
160 pages

4465 Silent Garden: Raising Your Deaf Child
Gallaudet University
11030 S Langley Avenue
Chicago, IL 60628
800-621-2736
Fax: 800-621-8476
TTY: 888-630-9347
www.gallaudet.edu/~gupress
Provides parents with a firm foundation for making the difficult decisions necessary for their deaf child's future. Includes information on critical concerns, communication, technological alternative, and reassurance through case studies and interviews.
304 pages Softcover
ISBN: 1-563680-58-0

4466 Simultaneous Communication, ASL and Other Communication Modes
Gallaudet University
11030 S Langley Avenue
Chicago, IL 60628-3819
800-621-2736
Fax: 800-621-8476
TTY: 888-630-9347
www.gallaudet.edu/~gupress

This monograph presents four major articles that examine issues surrounding communications in an educational environment.
236 pages

4467 Sing Praise
Sunday School Board of the Southern Baptists
127 9th Avenue N
Nashville, TN 37234-0001   800-458-2772
For use by interpreters to the deaf.

4468 Sociolinguistics in Deaf Communities
Gallaudet University
11030 S Langley Avenue
Chicago, IL 60628-3819   800-621-2736
                                    Fax: 800-621-8476
                                    TTY: 888-630-9347
                                    www.gallaudet.edu/~gupress
The first volume in a series offering assessments and up-to-date information on sign language linguistics.
280 pages

4469 Software to Go
Gallaudet University
11030 S Langley Avenue
Chicago, IL 60628-3819   800-621-2736
                                    Fax: 800-621-8476
                                    TTY: 888-630-9347
                                    www.gallaudet.edu/~gupress
Lists and describes commercial software that may be borrowed by educators of hearing impaired students.
100 pages

4470 Sound and Sign, Childhood Deafness and Mental Health
Gallaudet University
11030 S Langley Avenue
Chicago, IL 60628-3819   800-621-2736
                                    Fax: 800-621-8476
                                    TTY: 888-630-9347
                                    www.gallaudet.edu/~gupress
Presents research to support beliefs that deaf children should be educated using a combination manual and oral communication in residual hearing and speech.
265 pages

4471 Speak to Me
Gallaudet University
11030 S Langley Avenue
Chicago, IL 60628-3819   800-621-2736
                                    Fax: 800-621-8476
                                    TTY: 888-630-9347
                                    www.gallaudet.edu/~gupress
A story of a single mother confronted with the deafness of her son.
160 pages

4472 Speech and the Hearing-Impaired Child
Alexander Graham Bell Association
3417 Volta Place NW   202-337-5220
Washington, DC 20007-2737   Fax: 202-337-8270
                                    TTY: 202-337-5220
Provides a systematic approach to the teaching of speech and a challenge to all involved in the development of spoken language skills in hearing-impaired children.
402 pages

4473 Speechreading in Context
Gallaudet University
11030 S Langley Avenue
Chicago, IL 60628-3819   800-621-2736
                                    Fax: 800-621-8476
                                    TTY: 888-630-9347
                                    www.gallaudet.edu/~gupress
This useful guide for teachers and therapists approaches speechreading instruction with the help of context cues.
32 pages

4474 Speechreading: A Way to Improve Understand ing
Harriet Kaplan, author
Hearing Loss Association of America

7910 Woodmont Avenue   301-657-2248
Bethesda, MD 20814   Fax: 301-913-9413
                                    TTY: 3016572249
                                    e-mail: info@hearingloss.org
                                    www.hearingloss.org
Discusses the nature and process of speechreading, its benefits, and its limitations. This useful book clarifies commonly-held misconceptions about speechreading. The beginning chapters address difficult communication situations and problems related to the speaker, the speechreader, and the environment It then offers strategies to manage them.
160 pages Paperback
Jerry Portis, Executive Director
Brenda Battat, Assistant Executive Director

4475 Study of American Deaf Folklore
Gallaudet University
11030 S Langley Avenue
Chicago, IL 60628-3819   800-621-2736
                                    Fax: 800-621-8476
                                    TTY: 888-630-9347
                                    www.gallaudet.edu/~gupress
Presents a discussion of the different functions that folklore serves in the community.
156 pages

4476 Substance Abuse and Recovery: Empowerment of Deaf Persons
Gallaudet University
11030 S Langley Avenue
Chicago, IL 60628-3819   800-621-2736
                                    Fax: 800-621-8476
                                    TTY: 888-630-9347
                                    www.gallaudet.edu/~gupress
Professionals in the field of substance abuse and deafness present their views on abuse.
217 pages

4477 Talk with Me
Alexander Graham Bell Association
3417 Volta Place NW   202-337-5220
Washington, DC 20007-2737   Fax: 202-337-8270
                                    TTY: 202-337-5220
Written by a clinical psychologist and mother, this book educates parents and professionals about crucial early decisions that affect the speech, language, auditory, social and emotional development of children with hearing impairments.
222 pages

4478 Teaching English to the Deaf as a Second Language
Depart. of English, Gallaudet University
800 Florida Avenue NE   202-651-5000
Washington, DC 20002   e-mail: janice-johnson@gallaudet.edu
                                    eli.gallaudet.edu/
Publishes articles of practical interest to classroom teachers of hearing impaired and second language students.
Kendall Green

4479 There's a Hearing Impaired Child in my Class
Gallaudet University
11030 S Langley Avenue
Chicago, IL 60628-3819   800-621-2736
                                    Fax: 800-621-8476
                                    TTY: 888-630-9347
                                    www.gallaudet.edu/~gupress
This complete package provides basic facts about deafness, practical strategies for teaching hearing impaired children, and the question-and-answer information for all students.
44 pages

4480 Thirteen Keys to A Successful High School Experience
Alexander Graham Bell Association
3417 Volta Place NW   202-337-5220
Washington, DC 20007-2737   Fax: 202-337-8270
                                    TTY: 202-337-5220
In this booklet, three students who have profound hearing losses share their mainstream education experiences. This booklet is great for teachers of any age child and many of the suggestions to make mainstreaming easier are practical and easy to implement.
1996 28 pages

4481 Toward Effective Public School Programs for Deaf Students
Thomas N. Kluwin, Donald F. Moores, Gonter Gaustad, author

Teachers College Press
1234 Amsterdam Avenue   212-678-3929
New York, NY 10027   Fax: 212-678-4149
e-mail: tcpress@tc.columbia.edu
www.teacherscollegepress.com
Examining various options for providing effective education-including the highly controversial practice of mainstreaming-the editors base their study on one of the largest and longest-running studies ever of public school programs for the deaf.
272 pages
ISBN: 0-807731-59-5
Martha Gonter Gaustad, Editors

4482 Understanding Deafness Socially
Gallaudet University
11030 S Langley Avenue
Chicago, IL 60628-3819   800-621-2736
Fax: 800-621-8476
TTY: 888-630-9347
www.gallaudet.edu/~gupress
Articles on the social dynamics of deafness.
196 pages

4483 Understanding Ear Infections
Alexander Graham Bell Association
3417 Volta Place NW   202-337-5220
Washington, DC 20007-2737   Fax: 202-337-8270
TTY: 202-337-5220
Based on medical research, this clinical aid for medical and hearing professionals explains ear infections and their complications to patients and their families. Sturdily designed of cardboard and spiral-bound, each page has photos and diagrams that explain each topic and answer commonly asked questions about ear infections.
1993 27 pages

4484 Viewpoints on Deafness
National Association of the Deaf
8630 Fenton Street   301-587-1788
Silver Spring, MD 20910   Fax: 301-587-1791
TTY: 301-587-1789
www.nad.org
Monograph presents a collection of viewpoints on deafness.
157 pages Paperback
Donna Morris, Publications Manager

4485 Visible Speech
SRC Software Research Corporation
Box 4277, Station A
Victoria, BC, V8X 3X8,   250-727-3744
Computerized speech culture, analysis and computer-based speech training.
6 pages
AE Wright, Publisher

4486 Voyage to an Island
Gallaudet University
11030 S Langley Avenue
Chicago, IL 60628-3819   800-621-2736
Fax: 800-621-8476
TTY: 888-630-9347
www.gallaudet.edu/~gupress
This book recounts the story of how the author, a deaf woman from Finland, adjusts to moving to the exotic island of St. Lucia.
248 pages

4487 Week the World Heard Gallaudet
Gallaudet University
11030 S Langley Avenue
Chicago, IL 60628-3819   800-621-2736
Fax: 800-621-8476
TTY: 888-630-9347
www.gallaudet.edu/~gupress
This book gives the readers a day-by-day description of the Deaf President Now movement as it unfolded from March 6 to 13, 1988.
176 pages Paperback

4488 What is an Audiogram?
Gallaudet University
11030 S Langley Avenue
Chicago, IL 60628-3819   800-621-2736
Fax: 800-621-8476
TTY: 888-630-9347
www.gallaudet.edu/~gupress
Here's a cheery friend to solve the mysteries of the audiogram.
16 pages

4489 What's that Pig Outdoors? A Memoir of Deafness
Henry Kisor, author

Pengiuin Group
375 Hudson Street
New York, NY 10014-3657   800-526-0275
Fax: 212-366-2952
e-mail: ecommerce@us.penguin.com
www.us.penguin.com
Life of a journalist who is deaf and lives in a hearing world lipreading. Discusses some of the technical advances which help the deaf.
288 pages Hardcover
ISBN: 0-140148-99-2

4490 When Your Child is Deaf: A Guide for Parents
Alexander Graham Bell Association
3417 Volta Place NW   202-337-5220
Washington, DC 20007-2737   Fax: 202-337-8270
TTY: 202-337-5220
This book gives encouragement and advice to parents on their essential roles in teaching speech to their child.
182 pages

4491 When the Mind Hears
Gallaudet University
11030 S Langley Avenue
Chicago, IL 60628-3819   800-621-2736
Fax: 800-621-8476
TTY: 888-630-9347
www.gallaudet.edu/~gupress
Told largely from the vantage point of Laurent Clerc.
460 pages

4492 Who Speaks for the Deaf Community?
National Association of the Deaf
8630 Fenton Street   301-587-1788
Silver Spring, MD 20910   Fax: 301-587-1791
TTY: 301-587-1789
www.nad.org
Paperback
Donna Morris, Publications Manager

4493 Wired for Sound
Gallaudet University
11030 S Langley Avenue
Chicago, IL 60628-3819   800-621-2736
Fax: 800-621-8476
TTY: 888-630-9347
www.gallaudet.edu/~gupress
Secondary school edition of Ear Gear, this attractive workbook is designed to give older students an in-depth understanding of hearing and hearing aids.
156 pages

4494 Working with Deaf People: Accessibility and Accommodation in the Workplace
2600 S 1st Street   217-789-8980
Springfield, IL 62704-4730   Fax: 217-789-9130
e-mail: books@ccthomas.com
www.ccthomas.com
Reveals the kinds of patterns of work adjustment problems that can surface among deaf employees, including the points of view of both supervisors an deaf people.
250 pages Paperback
ISBN: 0-398061-26-2
Charles C Thomas, Publisher

4495 Working with Deaf Persons in Sunday School
Sunday School Board of the Southern Baptists

127 9th Avenue N
Nashville, TN 37234-0001   800-458-2772
Provides guidance for organizing and conducting Sunday School classes/departments for deaf children, youth and adults.

4496   Writer's Workshop
Gallaudet University
11030 S Langley Avenue
Chicago, IL 60628-3819   800-621-2736
                                Fax: 800-621-8476
                                TTY: 888-630-9347
                                www.gallaudet.edu/~gupress
Offers suggestions to teachers who are interested in turning the classroom into an environment where students learn to express themselves in writing.
95 pages

4497   You Just Don't Understand
Deborah Tannen, author
Hearing Loss Association of America
7910 Woodmont Avenue   301-657-2248
Bethesda, MD 20814-3079   Fax: 301-913-9413
                                TTY: 301-657-2249
                                e-mail: info@hearingloss.org
                                www.hearingloss.org
Studded with lively and entertaining examples of real conversations, this book gives you the tools to understand what went wrong — and to find a common language in which to strengthen relationships at work and at home. A classic in the field of interpersonal relations, this book will change forever the way you approach conversations.
Softcover
ISBN: 0-060959-62-2
Jerry Portis, Executive Director
Brenda Battat, Assistant Executive Director

4498   You and Your Deaf Child
Gallaudet University
11030 S Langley Avenue
Chicago, IL 60628-3819   800-621-2736
                                Fax: 800-621-8476
                                TTY: 888-630-9347
                                www.gallaudet.edu/~gupress
This guide for parents explores how families interact to deal with the special impact of a child who is hearing impaired.
1997 224 pages 2nd edition

Children's Books

4499   ABC's of Finger Spelling
Modern Signs Press
PO Box 1181   562-596-8548
Los Alamitos, CA 90720-1181   800-572-7332
                                Fax: 562-795-6614
                                TTY: 562-493-4168
                                e-mail: modsigns@aol.com
                                www.modsigns.com
Helps teach upper and lower case letters of the alphabet. Includes printed letters and easy-to-follow drawings of the hand shapes.
60 pages
ISBN: 0-916708-13-6

4500   Alphabet of Animal Signs
Garlic Press
605 Powers Street   541-345-0063
Eugene, OR 97402-5337   Fax: 541-345-0063
                                e-mail: garlicpress@mindspring.com
                                www.garlicpress.com
Presents animal illustrations and associated signs for each letter of the alphabet.
16 pages Paperback
ISBN: 0-931993-65-2
SH Collins, Contact

4501   Animal Signs: A First Book of Sign Language
Gallaudet University

11030 S Langley Avenue
Chicago, IL 60628-3819   800-621-2736
                                Fax: 800-621-8476
                                TTY: 888-630-9347
                                www.gallaudet.edu/~gupress
Full-color photos of animals and their signs.
16 pages Ages 1-4

4502   Another Handful of Stories
Gallaudet University
11030 S Langley Avenue
Chicago, IL 60628-3819   800-621-2736
                                Fax: 800-621-8476
                                TTY: 888-630-9347
                                www.gallaudet.edu/~gupress
Second book contains a series of 37 stories told by deaf individuals.
124 pages

4503   At Grandma's House
Modern Signs Press
PO Box 1181   562-596-8548
Los Alamitos, CA 90720-1181   800-572-7332
                                Fax: 562-795-6614
                                TTY: 562-493-4168
                                e-mail: modsigns@aol.com
                                www.modsigns.com
Pictures, signs and printed words tell the tale of April, a cuddly little rabbit who loves to play with her beloved Grandma.
28 pages

4504   Be Happy, Not Sad
Modern Signs Press
PO Box 1181   562-596-8548
Los Alamitos, CA 90720   800-572-7332
                                Fax: 562-795-6614
                                TTY: 562-493-4168
                                e-mail: modsigns@aol.com
                                www.modsigns.com
These books help children understand hard to explain emotions through signing. Includes Be Happy Not Sad coloring workbook.
2 Book Set

4505   Belonging
Gallaudet University
11030 S Langley Avenue
Chicago, IL 60628-3819   800-621-2736
                                Fax: 800-621-8476
                                TTY: 888-630-9347
                                www.gallaudet.edu/~gupress
Gustie Blaine loses her hearing after an illness and must now learn to accept her loss and understand the changes it brings.
176 pages

4506   Chris Gets Ear Tubes
Gallaudet University
11030 S Langley Avenue
Chicago, IL 60628-3819   800-621-2736
                                Fax: 800-621-8476
                                TTY: 888-630-9347
                                www.gallaudet.edu/~gupress
A helpful book for parents and children to share concerning ear tubes and hospitals.
44 pages

4507   Clerc: The Story of His Early Years
Gallaudet University
11030 S Langley Avenue
Chicago, IL 60628-3819   800-621-2736
                                Fax: 800-621-8476
                                TTY: 888-630-9347
                                www.gallaudet.edu/~gupress
A novel by Laurent Clerc, a deaf teacher who helped Gallaudet establish schools to educate deaf Americans.
208 pages

4508   Come Sign with Us: Sign Language Activities for Children
Gallaudet University

11030 S Langley Avenue
Chicago, IL 60628-3819

800-621-2736
Fax: 800-621-8476
TTY: 888-630-9347
www.gallaudet.edu/~gupress

Revised version, offering more follow-up activities, including many in context, to teach children sign language. Features more than 300 line drawings of both adults and children signing familiar words, phrases, and sentences using ASL. Shows how to form each sign exactly and also presents the origins of ASL, facts about deafness, and the deaf community.
160 pages Softcover
ISBN: 1-563680-51-3

4509   Day We Met Cindy
Gallaudet University
11030 S Langley Avenue
Chicago, IL 60628-3819

800-621-2736
Fax: 800-621-8476
TTY: 888-630-9347
www.gallaudet.edu/~gupress

A picture storybook telling the story of Cindy, the hearing impaired aunt of one of the students of a first grade class.
32 pages

4510   Finger Alphabet
Gallaudet University
11030 S Langley Avenue
Chicago, IL 60628-3819

800-621-2736
Fax: 800-621-8476
TTY: 888-630-9347
www.gallaudet.edu/~gupress

Includes activities for improving fingerspelling.
30 pages

4511   Flying Fingers Club
Gallaudet University
11030 S Langley Avenue
Chicago, IL 60628-3819

800-621-2736
Fax: 800-621-8476
TTY: 888-630-9347
www.gallaudet.edu/~gupress

Three young friends, one deaf and two hearing find they can communicate secretly in sign language.
104 pages

4512   Gift of the Girl Who Couldn't Hear
Alexander Graham Bell Association
3417 Volta Place NW
Washington, DC 20007-2737

202-337-5220
Fax: 202-337-8270
TTY: 202-337-5220

This fictional novel for middle school readers introduces Eliza, a gifted singer and Lucy, her best friend who has been deaf since birth.
79 pages

4513   Goldilocks and the Three Bears
Gallaudet University
11030 S Langley Avenue
Chicago, IL 60628-3819

800-621-2736
Fax: 800-621-8476
TTY: 888-630-9347
www.gallaudet.edu/~gupress

Offers children ages 3-8 the classic story with new words and matching signs in Signed English.
48 pages Casebound
ISBN: 1-563680-57-2

4514   Grandfather Moose
Modern Signs Press
PO Box 1181
Los Alamitos, CA 90720-1181

562-596-8548
800-572-7332
Fax: 562-795-6614
TTY: 562-493-4168
e-mail: modsigns@aol.com
www.modsigns.com

Offers exciting and beautifully illustrated rhymes, games and chants in sign language.
32 pages

4515   Handful of Stories
Gallaudet University
11030 S Langley Avenue
Chicago, IL 60628-3819

800-621-2736
Fax: 800-621-8476
TTY: 888-630-9347
www.gallaudet.edu/~gupress

Sometimes incredible, moving and amusing, these stories are based on the personal experiences of deaf storytellers.
118 pages

4516   Handmade Alphabet
Gallaudet University
11030 S Langley Avenue
Chicago, IL 60628-3819

800-621-2736
Fax: 800-621-8476
TTY: 888-630-9347
www.gallaudet.edu/~gupress

This book presents 26 beautiful color drawings showing a hand forming a letter of the manual alphabet.
26 pages

4517   Hasta Luego, San Diego
Gallaudet University
11030 S Langley Avenue
Chicago, IL 60628-3819

800-621-2736
Fax: 800-621-8476
TTY: 888-630-9347
www.gallaudet.edu/~gupress

A Flying Fingers Club mystery.
104 pages

4518   Hearing Loss
Franklin Watts Grolier
90 Old Sherman Tpke
Danbury, CT 06816-0001

203-797-3500
800-621-1115
Fax: 203-797-3197
www.grolier.com

Offers a concise explanation of how and why hearing losses occur, how the ear works and how to protect your hearing.
144 pages Grades 7-12
ISBN: 0-531125-19-0

4519   I Have a Sister, My Sister is Deaf
TJ Publishers
817 Silver Spring Avenue
Silver Spring, MD 20910-4617

301-585-4440
800-999-1168
Fax: 301-585-5930
TTY: 301-585-4441
e-mail: tjpubinc@aol.com

An emphatic, affirmative look at the relationship between siblings, as a young deaf child is affectionately described by her older sister. This Coretta Scott King honor award winner helps young children develop an understanding that deaf children share the same interests as hearing children.
1977 32 pages Softcover
ISBN: 0-064430-59-6
Angela K Thames, President
Jerald A Murphy, VP

4520   I Was So Mad!
Modern Signs Press
PO Box 1181
Los Alamitos, CA 90720-1181

562-596-8548
800-572-7332
Fax: 562-795-6614
TTY: 562-493-4168
e-mail: modsigns@aol.com
www.modsigns.com

Includes manual alphabet and glossary of signs.
40 pages
ISBN: 0-916708-16-0

4521   In Our House
Modern Signs Press
PO Box 1181
Los Alamitos, CA 90720-1181

562-596-8548
800-572-7332
Fax: 562-795-6614
TTY: 562-493-4168
e-mail: modsigns@aol.com
www.modsigns.com

This colorful picturebook tells the story of Joy and Jason helping Mom and Dad around the house. Has a 140-word vocabulary listed in an alphabetical glossary.
32 pages
ISBN: 0-191670-81-1

4522 Invisible Inc #4
Alexander Graham Bell Association
3417 Volta Place NW   202-337-5220
Washington, DC 20007-2737   Fax: 202-337-8270
                                   TTY: 202-337-5220
The intrepid trio accept an invitation to doom as they solve the mystery behind their school's haunted computer.
1996 42 pages

4523 King Midas With Selected Sentences in ASL
Gallaudet University
11030 S Langley Avenue
Chicago, IL 60628-3819   800-621-2736
                                   Fax: 800-621-8476
                                   TTY: 888-630-9347
                          www.gallaudet.edu/~gupress
Fairytale retold with full color illustrations and American Sign Language sentences.
72 pages Casebound
ISBN: 0-930323-75-0

4524 Learning to Sign in my Neighborhood
Gallaudet University
11030 S Langley Avenue
Chicago, IL 60628-3819   800-621-2736
                                   Fax: 800-621-8476
                                   TTY: 888-630-9347
                          www.gallaudet.edu/~gupress
Here are signs to learn and pictures to color, all in one friendly book.
32 pages

4525 Little Green Monsters
Modern Signs Press
PO Box 1181   562-596-8548
Los Alamitos, CA 90720-1181   800-572-7332
                                   Fax: 562-795-6614
                                   TTY: 310-493-4168
Forty-five word vocabulary in signs and printed words introduces concept of directionality. Includes manual alphabet and glossary of signs.
36 pages

4526 Little Red Riding Hood
Gallaudet University
11030 S Langley Avenue
Chicago, IL 60628-3819   800-621-2736
                                   Fax: 800-621-8476
                                   TTY: 888-630-9347
                          www.gallaudet.edu/~gupress
A beloved folktale that is told in American Sign Language format.
48 pages

4527 Living with Deafness
Franklin Watts Grolier
90 Old Sherman Tpke   203-797-3500
Danbury, CT 06816-0001   800-621-1115
                                   Fax: 203-797-3197
                                       www.grolier.com
Shows how deaf persons can overcome their disability and live happy, productive lives.
32 pages Grades 5-7
ISBN: 0-531108-42-2

4528 Mandy
Gallaudet University
11030 S Langley Avenue
Chicago, IL 60628-3819   800-621-2736
                                   Fax: 800-621-8476
                                   TTY: 888-630-9347
                          www.gallaudet.edu/~gupress
A beautiful story about a young deaf girl's relationship with her grandmother.
32 pages

4529 Matthew Pinkowski's Special Summer
Gallaudet University
11030 S Langley Avenue
Chicago, IL 60628-3819   800-621-2736
                                   Fax: 800-621-8476
                                   TTY: 888-630-9347
                          www.gallaudet.edu/~gupress
Matthew begins his special summer by moving to Minnesota, where he meets some special friends.
150 pages

4530 Messy Monsters, Jungle Joggers and Bubble Baths
Alexander Graham Bell Association
3417 Volta Place NW   202-337-5220
Washington, DC 20007-2737   Fax: 202-337-8270
                                   TTY: 202-337-5220
This child's work book is filled with poems, stories and delightful drawings that make speaking lip reading and using residual hearing fun for the elementary school aged child.
97 pages

4531 Mother Goose in Sign
Garlic Press
605 Powers Street   541-345-0063
Eugene, OR 97402-5337   Fax: 541-345-0063
                     e-mail: garlicpress@mindspring.com
                                    www.garlicpress.com
Fully illustrated Mother Goose nursery rhymes in sign language.
16 pages Paperback
ISBN: 0-931993-66-0
SH Collins, Contact

4532 My ABC Signs of Animal Friends
DawnSignPress
6130 Nancy Ridge Drive   619-625-0600
San Diego, CA 92121-3223   800-549-5350
                                   Fax: 619-625-2336
                        e-mail: DawnSign@aol.com
Sign language primer for both hearing and deaf children from birth to age five.
32 pages
ISBN: 0-915035-31-6

4533 My First Book of Sign
Gallaudet University
11030 S Langley Avenue
Chicago, IL 60628-3819   800-621-2736
                                   Fax: 800-621-8476
                                   TTY: 888-630-9347
                          www.gallaudet.edu/~gupress
This book makes signing fun for children from three to eight.
76 pages

4534 My Signing Book of Numbers
Gallaudet University
11030 S Langley Avenue
Chicago, IL 60628-3819   800-621-2736
                                   Fax: 800-621-8476
                                   TTY: 888-630-9347
                          www.gallaudet.edu/~gupress
Picture book helps children learn their numbers in sign language.
56 pages

4535 Nick's Mission
Alexander Graham Bell Association
3417 Volta Place NW   202-337-5220
Washington, DC 20007-2737   Fax: 202-337-8270
                                   TTY: 202-337-5220
Twelve-year-old Nick plans to spend his summer vacation at the lake, snorkeling and playing with Wags, his dog, not at speech therapy as his mother has planned. But the summer will embroil Nick and Wags in an exciting mystery that includes kidnapping, smuggling, stolen macaws and maybe even speech therapy.
1996 148 pages

4536 Now I Understand
Gallaudet University

11030 S Langley Avenue
Chicago, IL 60628-3819

800-621-2736
Fax: 800-621-8476
TTY: 888-630-9347
www.gallaudet.edu/~gupress

Explores what happens when a hard-of-hearing boy is mainstreamed.
56 pages

4537 Number and Letter Games
Gallaudet University
11030 S Langley Avenue
Chicago, IL 60628-3819

800-621-2736
Fax: 800-621-8476
TTY: 888-630-9347
www.gallaudet.edu/~gupress

A fascinating way to learning sign language with games, riddles and map skills for children and adults.
30 pages

4538 Nursery Rhymes from Mother Goose
Gallaudet University
11030 S Langley Avenue
Chicago, IL 60628-3819

800-621-2736
Fax: 800-621-8476
TTY: 888-630-9347
www.gallaudet.edu/~gupress

The complete nursery rhyme is presented in Signed English.
64 pages

4539 Popsicles are Cold
Modern Signs Press
PO Box 1181
Los Alamitos, CA 90720-1181

562-596-8548
800-572-7332
Fax: 562-795-6614
TTY: 562-493-4168
e-mail: modsigns@aol.com
www.modsigns.com

Colorful pictures and rhyming words highlight this storybook with a 33-word vocabulary in signs and printed words.
32 pages

4540 Season of Change
Gallaudet University
11030 S Langley Avenue
Chicago, IL 60628-3819

800-621-2736
Fax: 800-621-8476
TTY: 888-630-9347
www.gallaudet.edu/~gupress

A cheerful teenager tired of having people treat her as a problem just because she does not hear very well.
108 pages

4541 Secret Signing: A Sign Language Activity Book
Gallaudet University
11030 S Langley Avenue
Chicago, IL 60628-3819

800-621-2736
Fax: 800-621-8476
TTY: 888-630-9347
www.gallaudet.edu/~gupress

Children will enjoy this activity book with signs.
64 pages Level K-1

4542 Secret in the Dorm Attic
Gallaudet University
11030 S Langley Avenue
Chicago, IL 60628-3819

800-621-2736
Fax: 800-621-8476
TTY: 888-630-9347
www.gallaudet.edu/~gupress

Susan, Donald and Matt are back, as the Flying Fingers Club solving yet another mystery.
104 pages

4543 Sesame Street Sign Language ABC
Gallaudet University

11030 S Langley Avenue
Chicago, IL 60628-3819

800-621-2736
Fax: 800-621-8476
TTY: 888-630-9347
www.gallaudet.edu/~gupress

Muppets learn words and letters signed by Linda Bove.
30 pages

4544 Sesame Street Sign Language Fun
Gallaudet University
11030 S Langley Avenue
Chicago, IL 60628-3819

800-621-2736
Fax: 800-621-8476
TTY: 888-630-9347
www.gallaudet.edu/~gupress

This book uses the Muppets to explain concepts such as opposites, words and feelings.
62 pages

4545 Sign Numbers
Modern Signs Press
PO Box 1181
Los Alamitos, CA 90720-1181

562-596-8548
800-572-7332
Fax: 562-795-6614
TTY: 562-493-4168
e-mail: modsigns@aol.com
www.modsigns.com

A manual teaching sign language and written numbers that includes printed numbers and easy-to-follow drawings of the number hand shapes.
60 pages

4546 Sign-Me-Fine
Gallaudet University
11030 S Langley Avenue
Chicago, IL 60628-3819

800-621-2736
Fax: 800-621-8476
TTY: 888-630-9347
www.gallaudet.edu/~gupress

Written for young adults, this book introduces American Sign Language and how it differs from English.
120 pages

4547 Signed Language Coloring Books
Gallaudet University
11030 S Langley Avenue
Chicago, IL 60628-3819

800-621-2736
Fax: 800-621-8476
TTY: 888-630-9347
www.gallaudet.edu/~gupress

Six coloring books made up of easy-to-color pictures that include the printed, signed and fingerspelled words for each image.
16 pages

4548 Signing for Kids
Gallaudet University
11030 S Langley Avenue
Chicago, IL 60628-3819

800-621-2736
Fax: 800-621-8476
TTY: 888-630-9347
www.gallaudet.edu/~gupress

Contains 17 chapters dealing with special areas of interest to children like pets, family, friends and people.
142 pages

4549 Signs for Me: Basic Vocabulary for Children, Parents and Teachers
DawnSignPress
6130 Nancy Ridge Drive
San Diego, CA 92121-3223

619-625-0600
800-549-5350
Fax: 619-625-2336
e-mail: DawnSign@aol.com

ASL/English vocabulary primer filled with all the basics for preschoolers. The focus is on learning ASL signs and English words for better language development. Illustrates the meaning of the sign, the sign itself, and the English word in bold print.
112 pages
ISBN: 0-915035-27-8

4550 Silent Dances
Gallaudet University
11030 S Langley Avenue
Chicago, IL 60628-3819   800-621-2736
                                    Fax: 800-621-8476
                                    TTY: 888-630-9347
                            www.gallaudet.edu/~gupress
Space adventure story featuring a deaf graduate of Gallaudet University.
275 pages

4551 Silent Garden: Raising Your Deaf Child
Alexander Graham Bell Association
3417 Volta Place NW   202-337-5220
Washington, DC 20007-2737   Fax: 202-337-8270
                                    TTY: 202-337-5220
This book provides parents of deaf children with crucial information on the possibilities afforded their children. Ogden, deaf since birth and a professor of deaf studies offers parents the foundation for making the difficult decisions necessary to start their children on the road to realizing their full potential.
1996 313 pages

4552 Silent Observer
Gallaudet University
11030 S Langley Avenue
Chicago, IL 60628-3819   800-621-2736
                                    Fax: 800-621-8476
                                    TTY: 888-630-9347
                            www.gallaudet.edu/~gupress
Lovely illustrations tell the story of an affectionate memoir of childhood presented through the eyes of a deaf girl.
48 pages

4553 Simple Signs
Gallaudet University
11030 S Langley Avenue
Chicago, IL 60628-3819   800-621-2736
                                    Fax: 800-621-8476
                                    TTY: 888-630-9347
                            www.gallaudet.edu/~gupress
Charming, full-color pictures and hints introducing ASL to children.
32 pages

4554 Sleeping Beauty
Gallaudet University
11030 S Langley Avenue
Chicago, IL 60628-3819   800-621-2736
                                    Fax: 800-621-8476
                                    TTY: 888-630-9347
                            www.gallaudet.edu/~gupress
Classic story with full-color illustrations and line drawings of more than 30 sentences rendered in ASL, offering new dimensions of imagination while also strengthening young readers' language skills.
64 pages
ISBN: 0-930323-97-1

4555 Songs in Sign
Gallaudet University
11030 S Langley Avenue
Chicago, IL 60628-3819   800-621-2736
                                    Fax: 800-621-8476
                                    TTY: 888-630-9347
                            www.gallaudet.edu/~gupress
Fully illustrated sign English.
30 pages

4556 Very Special Sister
Gallaudet University
11030 S Langley Avenue
Chicago, IL 60628-3819   800-621-2736
                                    Fax: 800-621-8476
                                    TTY: 888-630-9347
                            www.gallaudet.edu/~gupress
Tells the story of Laura who is deaf and her delight at the fact that she will soon have a brother.
36 pages

4557 Where Is Spot?
Gallaudet University
11030 S Langley Avenue
Chicago, IL 60628-3819   800-621-2736
                                    Fax: 800-621-8476
                                    TTY: 888-630-9347
                            www.gallaudet.edu/~gupress
A Signed English edition of a childhood favorite.
20 pages

4558 Word Signs: A First Book of Sign Language
Gallaudet University
11030 S Langley Avenue
Chicago, IL 60628-3819   800-621-2736
                                    Fax: 800-621-8476
                                    TTY: 888-630-9347
                            www.gallaudet.edu/~gupress
Full-color photos of basic words and their signs.
16 pages Ages 1-4

Magazines

4559 American Annals of the Deaf
Convention of American Instructors of the Deaf
800 Florida Avenue NE   202-651-5530
Washington, DC 20002-3660   Fax: 202-651-5860
                                    TTY: 202-651-5530
                        e-mail: mary.carew@galludet.edu
                            gupress.gallaudet.edu/annals/
Scholarly journal at the forefront of research related to the education of deaf people. Annual reference Issue identifies programs and services for deaf people nationwide.
64 pages 5x Year
Donald Moores, Editor
Mary E Carew, Managing Editor

4560 American Journal of Audiology
American Speech-Language-Hearing Association
10801 Rockville Pike   301-897-5700
Rockville, MD 20852-3226   800-638-8255
                            e-mail: actioncenter@asha.org
                                    www.asha.org

Russell L Malone PhD, Editor

4561 American Journal of Speech-Language Pathology
American Speech-Language-Hearing Association
10801 Rockville Pike   301-897-5700
Rockville, MD 20852-3226   800-638-8255
Russell L Malone PhD, Editor

4562 Audiology Today
1735 N Lynn Street   703-524-1923
Arlington, VA 22209-2019   Fax: 703-524-2303
Jerry Northern PhD, Editor

4563 Auricle
Auditory-Verbal International
2121 Eisenhower Avenue   703-739-1049
Alexandria, VA 22314-4688   Fax: 703-739-0395
                                    TTY: 703-739-0874
                            e-mail: audiverb@aol.com
                                www.auditory-verbal.org
To provide the choice of listening and speaking as the way of life for children and adults who are deaf on hard of hearing.
Magazine
Sara Lake, Executive Director/CEO/Publisher
Mary Benson, Executive Assistant

4564 Deaf Life
MSM Productions
PO Box 23380   716-442-6370
Rochester, NY 14692-3380   Fax: 716-442-6371
                                    www.deaflife.com
This magazine focuses on profiles, news, controversial issues, cultural topics and more relating to the Deaf community.
50 pages Monthly
Matthew Moore, Publisher

4565 Deaf Sports Review
American Athletic Association of the Deaf
3607 Washington Boulevard 801-393-8710
Ogden, UT 84403-1737 Fax: 801-393-2263
TTY: 801-393-7916
A magazine that describes deaf athletes and past and upcoming events.
Quarterly
Shirley Platt, Editor

4566 Deaf USA
Eye Festival Communications
6917B Woodley Avenue 818-902-9800
Van Nuys, CA 91406-4844 Fax: 818-902-9840
Provides news coverage on all activities and issues of interest to deaf and hard of hearing readers as well as professionals and associates within this specialized market.
Monthly
David Rosenbaum, Editor

4567 Deaf-Blind American
American Association of the Deaf-Blind
814 Thayer Avenue
Silver Spring, MD 20910-4500 800-735-2258
Fax: 301-588-8705
TTY: 301-588-6545
e-mail: aadb@erols.com
A journal of the American Association of the Deaf-Blind with articles on new technology, legislation news affecting deaf-blind Americans, success stories on deaf-blind, conference news, and many other topics of interest to deaf-blind people.
4x Year
Jamie McNamara, Editor

4568 Hearing Health
1050 17th Street NW 209-289-5850
Washington, DC 20036 e-mail: info@hearinghealthmag.com
A publication for deaf and hard-of-hearing people, as well as hearing health care professionals, libraries, agencies, schools and organizations.
BiMonthly
Paula Bartone-Bonillas, Editor

4569 Journal of AAA
American Academy of Audiology
1735 N Lynn Street 703-524-1923
Arlington, VA 22209-2019 800-222-2336
Fax: 703-524-2303
James Jerger, Editor

4570 Journal of Speech-Language-Hearing Research
American Speech-Language-Hearing Association
10801 Rockville Pike 301-897-5700
Rockville, MD 20852-3226 800-638-8255
Russell L Malone PhD, Editor

4571 Language, Speech and Hearing Services in the Schools
American Speech-Language-Hearing Association
10801 Rockville Pike 301-897-5700
Rockville, MD 20852 800-638-8255
Professional journal for clinicians, audiologists and speech-language pathologists.

Russell L Malone PhD, Editor

4572 NADmag
National Association of the Deaf
8630 Fenton Street 301-587-1788
Silver Spring, MD 20910 Fax: 301-587-1791
TTY: 301-587-1789
www.nad.org/nadmagadrates
Each NADmag focuses on a specific theme, such as technology and telecommunications, human services, deaf culture, education, and interpreting.
32 pages Bi-Monthly
Donna Morris, Publications Manager

4573 Perspectives in Education and Deafness
Gallaudet University

11030 S Langley Avenue
Chicago, IL 60628-3819 800-621-2736
Fax: 800-621-8476
TTY: 888-630-9347
www.gallaudet.edu/~gupress
A practical, reader-friendly magazine, offering help and advice in and beyond the classroom, tuned to the needs of today's students, teachers, and families.
5x Annually
Mary Abrams Perica, Editor

4574 SHHH Journal
Self Help For Hard of Hearing People
7910 Woodmont Avenue 301-657-2248
Bethesda, MD 20814-3079 Fax: 301-913-9413
TTY: 301-657-2249
An educational journal about hearing loss for hard-of-hearing people.
BiMonthly
Barbara G Harris, Editor

4575 Silent News
1425 Jefferson Road 716-272-4900
Rochester, NY 14623-3139 Fax: 716-272-4904
TTY: 716-272-4900
Covers news and events of interest to deaf and hard-of-hearing people all over the world.
Monthly
Tom Willard, Editor

4576 Silent News Job Bulletin
1425 Jefferson Road 716-272-4900
Rochester, NY 14623-3139 Fax: 716-272-4904
TTY: 716-272-4900
Lists current job openings and career opportunities working with deaf and hard-of-hearing people.
BiAnnually

4577 Tinnitus Today
American Tinnitus Association
PO Box 5 503-248-9985
Portland, OR 97207-0005 800-634-8978
Fax: 503-248-0024
www.ata.org
A quarterly magazine published by the American Tinnitus Association.
28 pages Quarterly
ISBN: 1-530656-9 -
David P. Fagerlie, Chief Executive Officer
Terri Baltus, Chief Development Officer

4578 USA Deaf Sports Federation
3607 Washington Boulevard 801-393-8710
Ogden, UT 84403-1737 Fax: 801-393-2263
TTY: 801-393-7916
e-mail: homeoffice@usadsf.org
www.usadsf.org
A glossy magazine called Deaf Sports Review featuring articles on all deaf sports and recreation.
Dr. Bobbie Beth Scoggins, President
Valerie Kinney, Adminstrative Assistant

4579 Volta Review
Alexander Graham Bell Association
3417 Volta Place NW 202-337-5220
Washington, DC 20007-2737 Fax: 202-337-8270
TTY: 202-337-5220
A professionally reviewed journal highlighting research and studies in the field of deafness.
5x Year
Michelle Vanderhoff, Managing Editor

4580 Volta Voices
Alexander Graham Bell Association
3417 Volta Place NW 202-337-5220
Washington, DC 20007-2737 Fax: 202-337-8270
TTY: 202-337-5220
A magazine highlighting inspirational stories from parents of children who are deaf, legislative news, technology update and stories

pertaining to speech, speech reading, and the use of residual hearing.
BiMonthly
Michelle Vanderhoff, Managing Editor

4581 World Around You
Gallaudet University
11030 S Langley Avenue
Chicago, IL 60628-3819   800-621-2736
                                          Fax: 800-621-8476
                                          TTY: 888-630-9347
                                          www.gallaudet.edu/~gupress
A current events magazine directed at keeping junior high and high school deaf and hard-of-hearing students informed about deaf people and the deaf community.
5x Year
Cathryn Carroll, Editor

Newsletters

4582 AAAD Bulletin
American Athletic Association of the Deaf
3607 Washington Boulevard   801-393-8710
Ogden, UT 84403-1737   Fax: 801-393-2263
                                          TTY: 801-393-7916
A newsletter describing deaf athletes and upcoming events.
Quarterly
Shirley Platt, Editor

4583 ADARA Updated
ADARA
PO Box 251554   501-868-8850
Little Rock, AR 72225-1554   Fax: 501-868-8812
Updates readers on events, resources, legislation, information of national interest, conferences, workshops and employment opportunities. Information from and about local chapters, special interest sections, and national organizations is included in this publication.
Quarterly
Nanncy Long PhD, Editor

4584 ALDA News
Association of Late-Deafened Adults
1131 Lake Street   877-907-1738
Oak Park, IL 60301   Fax: 877-907-1738
                                          TTY: 708-358-0135
                                          www.alda.org
Marilyn Howe, Publisher

4585 Adult Bible Lessons for the Deaf
Sunday School Board of the Southern Baptists
127 9th Avenue N
Nashville, TN 37234-0001   800-458-2772
Bible study quarterly that relates to the needs of deaf and hearing impaired persons.
Quarterly

4586 Audiology Express
American Academy of Audiology
1735 N Lynn Street   703-524-1923
Arlington, VA 22209-2019   800-222-2336
                                          Fax: 703-524-2303

4587 Better Hearing News
Better Hearing Institute
5021B Backlick Road   703-642-0580
Annandale, VA 22003-6043   800-327-9355
                                          Fax: 703-750-9302
Quarterly
Jerry J Rizzo, Executive Director

4588 Canine Listener
Dogs for the Deaf

10175 Wheeler Road   541-826-9220
Central Point, OR 97502   800-990-3647
                                          Fax: 541-826-6696
                                          TTY: 541-826-9220
                                          TDD: 541-826-9220
                                          e-mail: info@dogsforthedeaf.org
                                          www.dogsforthedeaf.org
Offers information on various dogs for the deaf that are available, hotlines, support groups and articles on the newest technology for the hard of hearing person.
Quarterly
Robin Dickson, President/CEO

4589 Caption Center News
Caption Center
125 Western Avenue   617-429-9225
Boston, MA 02134-1008   Fax: 617-562-0590
Reports developments in closed captioning for persons with hearing impairments.

4590 Deaf Artists of America
302 Goodman Street N   716-244-3460
Rochester, NY 14607-1148   Fax: 716-244-3690
                                          TTY: 716-244-3460
Tom Willard, Editor

4591 Deaf Episcopalian
Episcopal Conference of the Deaf
PO Box 27459   215-247-1059
Philadelphia, PA 19118-0459   e-mail: Bmose@aol.com
                                          www.ecdeaf.com/
Rev. Virginia Nagel, Editor

4592 Deaf Work
Baptist Sunday School Board
127 9th Avenue N   615-251-2000
Nashville, TN 37234-0002
Offers information for religious workers and church educators who teach the handicapped.

4593 Deafpride Advocate
Deafpride
1350 Potomac Avenue SE   202-675-6700
Washington, DC 20003-4412

4594 Endeavor
American Society for Deaf Children
PO Box 3355   717-334-7922
Gettysburg, PA 17325-1373   800-942-2732
                                          Fax: 717-334-8808
                                          TTY: 717-334-7922
                                          e-mail: asdc1@aol.com
                                          www.deafchildren.org
Newsletter for parents of deaf children.
36 pages Quarterly
Linda Zumbrun, Operations Manager

4595 Frat
National Fraternal Society of the Deaf
1300 W NW Highway   847-392-9282
Mt Prospect, IL 60056-2217   Fax: 847-392-9298
                                          TTY: 708-392-1409
Offers fraternal insurance information and news about members.
BiMonthly
Wayne D Shook, Editor

4596 GA-SK Newsletter
Telecommunications for the Deaf
8630 Fenton Street   301-589-3786
Silver Spring, MD 20910-3822   Fax: 301-589-3797
                                          TTY: 301-589-3006
A newsletter focusing on issues for the deaf and hearing impaired person.
Quarterly
Barry Solomon, Editor
Alfred Sonnenstrahl, Manager

4597 Gallaudet Today
Galladet University

575 5th Avenue
Washington, DC 20002
212-599-0027
Fax: 212-599-0039
www.drf.org

A university publication with both general and special issues on deafness-related topics.
Quarterly
Vickie Walter, Editor

4598 Hear
Deafness Research Foundation
15 W 39th Street
New York, NY 10018-3806
212-768-1181

Offers information on the Foundation's activities and events, technical updates on assistive devices, legislative and medical information on the latest breakthroughs and laws for the hearing impaired, book reviews and resources.
Monte H Jacoby, Executive Director

4599 NTID Focus
National Technical Institute for the Deaf
52 Lomb Memorial Drive
Rochester, NY 14623-5604
716-475-6906
Fax: 716-475-5623
e-mail: ntidmc@rit.edu
www.rit.edu/ntid

A college publication featuring news and stories about NTID programs and community members.
TriAnnual
Kathryn Shwartz, Editor

4600 Newsletter of American Hearing Research
American Hearing Research Foundation
8 S Michigan Avenue
Chicago, IL 60603-4539
312-726-9670
Fax: 312-726-9695
e-mail: blederer@american-hearing.org
www.american-hearing.org

Concerned with hearing research and education.
6-8 pages 3 per year
William L Lederer, Executive Director
Sharon Parmet, Development/Communications Associate

4601 Newsline
Sertoma Foundation
1912 E Meyer Boulevard
Kansas City, MO 64132-1141
816-333-8300
Fax: 816-333-4320
e-mail: info@sertoma.org
www.sertoma.org

Reports on activities of the Sertoma Foundation in the field of speech and hearing impairments.

4602 Otoscope
EAR Foundation
1817 Patterson Street
Nashville, TN 37203
615-329-7807
800-545-4327
Fax: 615-329-7935
TTY: 615-329-7849
e-mail: ear@earfoundation.org
www.earfoundation.org

8-14 pages Quarterly
Amy Nielsen, Director Educational Progams

4603 Research at Gallaudet
Gallaudet University
11030 S Langley Avenue
Chicago, IL 60628-3819
800-621-2736
Fax: 800-621-8476
TTY: 888-630-9347
www.gallaudet.edu/~gupress
Newsletter reporting research and activities of the Institute.

4604 Speech and Deafness Newsletter
Hearing, Speech
1620 18th Avenue
Seattle, WA 98122-2798
206-323-5770
Agency newsletter for membership and community.
8 pages
Patty Tumberg, Editor

4605 Tech Talk
Caption Center

125 Western Avenue
Boston, MA 02134-1008
617-492-9225
Fax: 617-562-0590

4606 USA Deaf Sports Federation
3607 Washington Boulevard
Ogden, UT 84403-1737
801-393-8710
Fax: 801-393-2263
TTY: 801-393-7916
e-mail: homeoffice@usadsf.org
www.usadsf.org

A matte newsletter called USADSF Bulletin featuring articles on all deaf sports and recreation.
Dr. Bobbie Beth Scoggins, President
Valerie Kinney, Adminstrative Assistant

Pamphlets

4607 25 Ways to Promote Spoken Language in Your Child with a Hearing Loss
Alexander Graham Bell Association
3417 Volta Place NW
Washington, DC 20007-2737
202-337-5220
Fax: 202-337-8270
TTY: 202-337-5220

This pamphlet teaches twenty-five golden rules about preparing your child to listen and to speak.
1995 62 pages

4608 Aging and Hearing Loss: Some Commonly Asked Questions
National Information Center on Deafness
800 Florida Avenue NE
Washington, DC 20002-3660
202-651-5051
Fax: 202-651-5054
TTY: 202-651-5052

Discusses the hearing evaulation, tests used to determine type and extent of hearing loss and what an audiogram tells us.

4609 Alerting and Communication Devices for Deaf and Hard of Hearing People
National Information Center on Deafness
800 Florida Avenue NE
Washington, DC 20002
202-651-5051
Fax: 202-651-5054
TTY: 202-651-5052

Describes general communication in everyday life.

4610 Alexander Graham Bell's Life
Alexander Graham Bell Association
3417 Volta Place NW
Washington, DC 20007-2737
202-337-5220
Fax: 202-337-8270
TTY: 202-337-5220

This pamphlet highlights Alexander Gram Bell's professional and personal involvement with deafness as a teacher of the deaf; a friend of many notable persons, including Helen Keller; a scientist interested in acoustics; the inventor of the telephone; and the founder of the Bell Association.
1996

4611 All About the New Generation of Hearing Aids
National Information Center on Deafness
800 Florida Avenue NE
Washington, DC 20002-3660
202-651-5051
Fax: 202-651-5054
TTY: 202-651-5052

Explains the terms digital hearing aid, and digitally controlled hearing aid.

4612 Assistive Devices Demonstration Centers
National Information Center on Deafness
800 Florida Avenue NE
Washington, DC 20002-3660
202-651-5051
Fax: 202-651-5054
TTY: 202-651-5052

A resource list identifying demonstration centers across the United States.

4613 Books for Parents of Deaf and Hard of Hearing Children
National Information Center on Deafness
800 Florida Avenue NE
Washington, DC 20002
202-651-5051
Fax: 202-651-5054
TTY: 202-651-5052

Identifies books written for parents and everday experiences of deaf and hard of hearing children.

4614 Care of the Ears and Hearing for Health
American Hearing Research Foundation

8 S Michigan Avenue
Chicago, IL 60603-4539

312-726-9670
Fax: 312-726-9695
e-mail: blederer@american-hearing.org
www.american-hearing.org

Offers information on ear infections relating to chronic progressive deafness.
William L Lederer, Executive Director
Sharon Parmet, Development/Communications Associate

4615 Consumer's Guide to Hearing Aids
Hearing Loss Association of America
7910 Woodmont Avenue
Bethesda, MD 20814-3079

301-657-2248
Fax: 301-913-9413
TTY: 301-657-2249
e-mail: info@hearingloss.org
www.hearingloss.org

Color booklet illustrating the different styles of hearing aids and comparing different models and features. Illustrates the technology pyramid and hearing aid pricing.
2006 24 pages
Jerry Portis, Executive Director
Brenda Battat, Assistant Executive Director

4616 Deaf Culture Videotapes
National Information Center on Deafness
800 Florida Avenue NE
Washington, DC 20002-3660

202-651-5051
Fax: 202-651-5054
TTY: 202-651-5052

This list identifies deaf culture and deaf history videotapes available from the Historic Film Collection of the National Association of the Deaf.

4617 Deaf Culture: Suggested Readings
National Information Center on Deafness
800 Florida Avenue NE
Washington, DC 20002-3660

202-651-5051
Fax: 202-651-5054
TTY: 202-651-5052

A selected reading list providing annotations for 62 books highlighting the community, and history of deaf people.

4618 Deafness: A Fact Sheet
National Information Center on Deafness
800 Florida Avenue NE
Washington, DC 20002-3660

202-651-5051
Fax: 202-651-5054
TTY: 202-651-5052

4619 Developing Cognition in Young Children Who are Deaf
Hope
55 E 100 N
Logan, UT 84321-4648

435-752-9533
Fax: 435-752-9533

Presents interesting, updated information on the importance of early cognition development in young children who are deaf. Contains many ideas for ways to promote early thinking skills, especially those that promote and enhance early communication and language development.

4620 Ear and Hearing
National Information Center on Deafness
800 Florida Avenue NE
Washington, DC 20002-3660

202-651-5051
Fax: 202-651-5054
TTY: 202-651-5052

An illustrated publication of the ear and what can go wrong with it.

4621 Educating Deaf Children: An Introduction
National Information Center on Deafness
800 Florida Avenue NE
Washington, DC 20002-3660

202-651-5051
Fax: 202-651-5054
TTY: 202-651-5052

Describes the different settings in which deaf children are currently educated.

4622 Facts About Hearing Aids
Alexander Graham Bell Association
3417 Volta Place NW
Washington, DC 20007-2737

202-337-5220
Fax: 202-337-8270
TTY: 202-337-5220

This brochure describes defferent types of hearing aids, factors to consider when choosing a hearing aid, the best way to go about purchasing a hearing aid. It also addresses cost and provides information on hearing conservation.

4623 Facts and Fancies About Hearing Aids
American Hearing Research Foundation
8 S Michigan Avenue
Chicago, IL 60603-4539

312-726-9670
Fax: 312-726-9695
e-mail: blederer@american-hearing.org
www.american-hearing.org

Offers information on types of hearing aids and hearing aid evaluations.
William L Lederer, Executive Director
Sharon Parmet, Development/Communications Associate

4624 Genetics and Deafness
National Information Center on Deafness
800 Florida Avenue NE
Washington, DC 20002-3660

202-651-5051
Fax: 202-651-5054
TTY: 202-651-5052

Written for deaf people and their families who wish to learn more about the relationship between heredity and deafness.

4625 Hearing Loss: Information for Professionals in the Aging Network
National Information Center on Deafness
800 Florida Avenue NE
Washington, DC 20002-3660

202-651-5051
Fax: 202-651-5054
TTY: 202-651-5052

Introduces professionals in the aging network to the realities of hearing loss.

4626 How Does Your Child Hear and Talk?
American Speech-Language-Hearing Association
10801 Rockville Pike
Rockville, MD 20852-3226

301-897-8682
800-638-8255
e-mail: actioncenter@asha.org
www.asha.org

Offers a chart to parents on children's growth pertaining to their hearing and speech.

4627 Late-Deafened Adults: A Selected Annotated Bibliography
National Information Center on Deafness
800 Florida Avenue NE
Washington, DC 20002-3660

202-651-5051
Fax: 202-651-5054
TTY: 202-651-5052

A selected reading list of books and articles for late-deafened people and their families.

4628 Leading National Publications of and for Deaf People
National Information Center on Deafness
800 Florida Avenue NE
Washington, DC 20002

202-651-5051
Fax: 202-651-5054
TTY: 202-651-5052

Identifies publications with national circulations to deaf audiences.

4629 Making New Friends
National Information Center on Deafness
800 Florida Avenue NE
Washington, DC 20002-3660

202-651-5051
Fax: 202-651-5054
TTY: 202-651-5052

Identifies resources that offer opportunities for deaf people.

4630 Meniere's Disease: Hearing Loss & Inner Ear Blood Flow
Self Help for Hard of H
7910 Woodmont Avenue
Bethesda, MD 20814-3079

301-657-2248
Fax: 301-913-9413
TTY: 301-657-2249
e-mail: national@shhh.org
www.shhh.org

Includes a personal narrative.

4631 National Information Center on Deafness Brochure
National Information Center on Deafness
800 Florida Avenue NE
Washington, DC 20002

202-651-5051
Fax: 202-651-5054
TTY: 202-651-5052

A description of services offered by NICD.

4632 Noise Can Be Harmful to Your Health
Deafness Research Foundation
15 W 39th Street
New York, NY 10018-3806

212-768-1181

Offers information, including a chart of noise levels, low to harmful, and the effects these noise levels have on your hearing.

4633 Otitis Media
Deafness Research Foundation
15 W 39th Street   212-768-1181
New York, NY 10018-3806
Offers information on Otitis Media, prevention, causes, treatments and symptoms.

4634 Perspectives Folio: Parent-Child
Gallaudet University
11030 S Langley Avenue
Chicago, IL 60628-3819   800-621-2736
                                Fax: 800-621-8476
                                TTY: 888-630-9347
                        www.gallaudet.edu/~gupress
Seven articles emphasizing family communication while providing important information for parents about deafness and the deaf culture.
29 pages

4635 Publications from the National Information Center on Deafness
National Information Center on Deafness
800 Florida Avenue NE
Washington, DC 20002-3660   Fax: 202-651-5051
                                Fax: 202-651-5054
                                TTY: 202-651-5052
Order form and explanations of NICD publications.

4636 Questions and Answers About Employment of Deaf People
National Information Center on Deafness
800 Florida Avenue NE   202-651-5051
Washington, DC 20002-3660   Fax: 202-651-5054
                                TTY: 202-651-5052

4637 Questions and Answers on Hearing Loss
Self Help for Hard of H
7910 Woodmont Avenue   301-657-2248
Bethesda, MD 20814-3079   Fax: 301-913-9413
                                TTY: 301-657-2249
                        e-mail: national@shhh.org
                                www.shhh.org

4638 So You Have Had an Ear Operation...What Next?
American Hearing Research Foundation
8 S Washington Avenue   312-726-9670
Chicago, IL 60603-4539   Fax: 312-726-9695
                e-mail: blederer@american-hearing.org
                        www.american-hearing.org
Offers information on ear infections and surgery.
William L Lederer, Executive Director
Sharon Parmet, Development/Communications Associate

4639 Statewide Services for Deaf and Hard of Hearing People
National Information Center on Deafness
800 Florida Avenue NE   202-651-5051
Washington, DC 20002   Fax: 202-651-5054
                                TTY: 202-651-5052
A resource list of states that have established commissions and other offices to serve deaf people.

4640 Travel Resources for Deaf and Hard of Hearing People
National Information Center on Deafness
800 Florida Avenue NE   202-651-5051
Washington, DC 20002   Fax: 202-651-5054
                                TTY: 202-651-5052
A publication list of travel industry resources for deaf and hard of hearing people.

4641 What are TTY's? TDDs? TTs?
National Information Center on Deafness
800 Florida Avenue NE   202-651-5051
Washington, DC 20002-3660   Fax: 202-651-5054
                                TTY: 202-651-5052
Discusses text telephones used by deaf people.

4642 World of Sound
International Hearing Society
16880 Middlebelt Road   313-478-2610
Livonia, MI 48154-3367   Fax: 313-478-4520

The purpose of this booklet is to provide basic information for those with questions about hearing loss, hearing aids and Hearing Instrument Specialists.

4643 You Don't Have to Hate Meetings: Try Computer-Assisted Notetaking Instead
Self Help for Hard of H
7910 Woodmont Avenue   301-657-2248
Bethesda, MD 20814-3079   Fax: 301-913-9413
                                TTY: 301-657-2249
                        e-mail: national@shhh.org
                                www.shhh.org

Audio & Video

4644 ASL Poetry: Selected Works of Clayton Valli
DawnSignPress
6130 Nancy Ridge Drive   858-625-0600
San Diego, CA 92121-3223   800-549-5350
                                Fax: 858-625-2336
                                TTY: 858-625-0600
                    e-mail: comments@dawnsign.com
                                www.dawnsign.com
Twenty one original Valli poems recited by a diversity of native signers. Guided experience through the richness of poetry in another language.
105 minutes
ISBN: 0-915035-23-5
Barry Howland, Marketing Director

4645 Basic Course in American Sign Language Vid eotape Package
TJ Publishers
2544 Tarpley Road   972-416-0800
Carrollton, TX 75006   800-999-1168
                                Fax: 972-416-0944
                e-mail: customerservice@tjpublishers.com
                        www.tjpublishers.com/index.html
The A Basic Course in American Sign Language Vocabulary Videotape features four Deaf models signing each vocabulary word contained in all 22 lessons of the text plus the alphabet and numbers. The tape has captions and voice which can be turned off to sharpen visual acuity. It is ideal for classroom reinforcement and independent home study.
Angela K Thames, President
Jerald A Murphy, VP

4646 Beginning Reading and Sign Language Video
TJ Publishers
2544 Tarpley Road   972-416-0800
Carrollton, TX 75006   800-999-1168
                                Fax: 972-416-0944
                e-mail: customerservice@tjpublishers.com
                        www.tjpublishers.com/index.html
Learning sign improves reading, motor skills and visual perception and increases language acquisition abilities. For kids from 2 to 12, this video picture book features deaf actress Susan Bressler signing over a hundred words at the zoo, at home and around the community.
Video
Angela K Thames, President
Jerald A Murphy, VP

4647 Come Sign With Us
Gallaudet University
11030 S Langley Avenue
Chicago, IL 60628-3819   800-621-2736
                                Fax: 800-621-8476
                                TTY: 888-630-9347
                        www.gallaudet.edu/~gupress
Lessons including fingerspelling and signing are overviewed.
90 minutes
ISBN: 1-563680-50-5

4648 Deaf Children Signers
Harris Communications

15155 Technology Drive
Eden Prairie, MN 55344

952-906-1180
800-825-6758
Fax: 952-906-1099
TTY: 800-825-9187
e-mail: info@harriscomm.com
www.harriscomm.com/

This 5-part collection of children signers is great for children, teachers, parents and interpreters.
Robert Harris Ph.D, Founder/President/CEO

4649   Deaf Culture Autobiographies
Harris Communications
15155 Technology Drive
Eden Prairie, MN 55344

952-906-1180
800-825-6758
Fax: 952-906-1099
TTY: 800-825-9187
e-mail: info@harriscomm.com
www.harriscomm.com/

Inspiring videotapes offer encouragement and enlightenment to the hearing impaired. Total of eight videotapes.
Robert Harris Ph.D, Founder/President/CEO

4650   Deaf Culture Series
Harris Communications
15155 Technology Drive
Eden Prairie, MN 55344

952-906-1180
800-825-6758
Fax: 952-906-1099
TTY: 800-825-9187
e-mail: info@harriscomm.com
www.harriscomm.com/

Each video in this 5-part series features a variety of Deaf talent. It is an excellent resource for Deaf studies programs, Interpreter Preparation programs and Sign Language programs.
Robert Harris Ph.D, Founder/President/CEO

4651   Deaf Mosaic Series
Harris Communications
15155 Technology Drive
Eden Prairie, MN 55344

952-906-1180
800-825-6758
Fax: 952-906-1099
TTY: 800-825-9187
e-mail: info@harriscomm.com
www.harriscomm.com/

A national magazine show produced monthly by Gallaudet University, this show has been awarded nine Emmys. As the only nation-wide program about the Deaf community, these videotapes are the best of the best from the shows programs.
Robert Harris Ph.D, Founder/President/CEO

4652   Diagnosis and Treatment of Unilateral Hearing Loss
American Academy of Otolaryngology
1 Prince Street
Alexandria, VA 22314-3357

703-836-4444
Fax: 703-683-5100
www.entnet.org

This CD-ROM focuses on evaluation and treatment of unilateral hearing loss arising from skull base lesion.

4653   Do You Hear That?
Alexander Graham Bell Association
3417 Volta Place NW
Washington, DC 20007-2737

202-337-5220
Fax: 202-337-8270
TTY: 202-337-5220

This video documents auditory-verbal therapy as it is practiced at North York General Hospital in Toronto, Canada.
1992 35 minutes

4654   Fantastic Series
Gallaudet University Bookstore
800 Florida Avenue NE
Washington, DC 20002-3660

800-451-1073
Fax: 800-621-8476
TTY: 888-630-9347
www.gallaudet.edu/~gupress

Tapes designed to encourage both deaf and hearing children to use their imaginations.
Ages 6-10

4655   Fingers that Tickle and Delight
National Association of the Deaf

8630 Fenton Street
Silver Spring, MD 20910

301-587-1788
Fax: 301-587-1791
TTY: 301-587-1789
www.nad.org

One's woman's experiences from childhood, school, marriage, her career as a teacher and interpreter trainer, and her life as an entertainer. Closed captioned.
13+ 32 minutes
Bill Stark, Project Director
Donna Morris, Publications Manager

4656   Fingerspelling and Numbers Software
American Sign Language (ASL) Productions
c/o Harris Communications
Eden Prairie, MN 55344

952-906-1180
800-767-4461
Fax: 952-906-1099
TTY: 800-767-4461
e-mail: ASLProductions@harriscomm.com
www.americansignlanguageproductions.com

Fingerspelling practice partner that allows you to control the speed and vocabulary level. Requires Windows 3.1 or greater.
Robert Harris Ph.D, Founder/President-Harris Communications
Jenna Cassell, Founder ASL Productions

4657   Getting in Touch
Research Press
2612 N Mattis Avenue
Champaign, IL 61822-1053

217-352-3273
800-519-2707
Fax: 217-352-1221
e-mail: rp@researchpress.com
www.researchpress.com

Shows how to create an individualized communications system based on the abilities and needs of the child. Illustrates seven basic communication procedures that involve the use of touch cues and object cues.

4658   Gospel of Luke
Gallaudet University Bookstore
800 Florida Avenue NE
Washington, DC 20002-3660

800-451-0173
Fax: 800-621-8476
TTY: 888-630-9347
www.gallaudet.edu/~gupress

A set of five videotapes of the Gospel of Luke told in ASL.
Set of five

4659   Granny Good's Sign of Christmas
Gallaudet University Bookstore
800 Florida Avenue NE
Washington, DC 20002-3660

800-451-1073
Fax: 800-621-8476
TTY: 888-630-9347
www.gallaudet.edu/~gupress

Twas The Night Before Christmas told in American Sign Language.

4660   Hearing Loss and Rehabilitation
American Academy of Otolaryngology
1 Prince Street
Alexandria, VA 22314-3357

703-836-4444
Fax: 703-683-5100
www.entnet.org

Slides

4661   I Can Hear!
Alexander Graham Bell Association
3417 Volta Place NW
Washington, DC 20007-2737

202-337-5220
Fax: 202-337-8270
TTY: 202-337-5220

This inspirational video describes the auditory-verbal approach for developing speech and language for hearing impaired children and adults.
1992 23 minutes

4662   I Can Hear!: II
Alexander Graham Bell Association
3417 Volta Place NW
Washington, DC 20007-2737

202-337-5220
Fax: 202-337-8270
TTY: 202-337-5220

An exciting videotape that gives more examples of auditory-verbal therapy and a variety of kids who have been taught to speak using this method.
1996 19 minute video

4663 I See What You Say: Self Help Lip Reading Program
Alexander Graham Bell Association
3417 Volta Place NW
Washington, DC 20007-2737
202-337-5220
Fax: 202-337-8270
TTY: 202-337-5220
Easy to follow videotape and manual for consumers teaches visual recognition of speech sounds in single words and phrases.
1995 54 minutes

4664 Interpreters in Public Schools Kit
Sign Media
4020 Blackburn Lane
Burtonsville, MD 20866-1167
301-421-0268
800-475-4756
Fax: 301-421-0270
TTY: 301-421-4460
e-mail: signmedia@aol.com
www.signmedia.com
Videotapes individually specialized for administrators, classroom teachers and for interpreters. Provides practical insights to some of the most crucial issues and problems facing mainstreamed programs. Contains reproducible printed material.
Three videos
Barbara Olmert, Director Marketing

4665 Interview with Kirsten Gonzales
Alexander Graham Bell Association
3417 Volta Place NW
Washington, DC 20007-2737
202-337-5220
Fax: 202-337-8270
TTY: 202-337-5220
Interviews a longtime user and trainer of oral interpreters who offers techniques in articulation and natural gestures.
20 minutes

4666 It's Not Just Hearing AIDS: Deaf People and the Epidemic
National Association of the Deaf
8630 Fenton Street
Silver Spring, MD 20910
301-587-1788
Fax: 301-587-1791
TTY: 301-587-1789
www.nad.org
Straightforward and factual information on how AIDS is transmitted, who gets AIDS, procedures for an HIV test, and an interview with a person who actually has the AIDS virus.
9 - 13+ Video
Bill Stark, Project Director
Donna Morris, Publications Manager

4667 Joy of Signing
Gallaudet University Bookstore
800 Florida Avenue NE
Washington, DC 20002-3660
800-451-1073
Fax: 800-621-8476
TTY: 888-630-9347
www.gallaudet.edu/~gupress
Three tapes full of useful information to help increase skill and comfort with sign.
1 Videotape

4668 King Midas
Gallaudet University
11030 S Langley Avenue
Chicago, IL 60628-3819
800-621-2736
Fax: 800-621-8476
TTY: 888-630-9347
www.gallaudet.edu/~gupress

30 minutes
ISBN: 0-930323-71-8

4669 King Midas Videotape
Gallaudet University Bookstore
800 Florida Avenue NE
Washington, DC 20002-3660
800-451-1073
Fax: 800-621-8476
TTY: 888-630-9347
www.gallaudet.edu/~gupress
Story of King Midas told in American Sign Language.

4670 Learning to Communicate: The First Three Years Videotape
Alexander Graham Bell Association
3417 Volta Place NW
Washington, DC 20007-2737
202-337-5220
Fax: 202-337-8270
TTY: 202-337-5220
This video shows normal communication development in young children under three years of age. It discusses factors which can affect speech and language development, including anatomy and environment. Closed captioned.
11 minutes

4671 Let's Be Friends
Britannica Film Company
345 4th Street
San Francisco, CA 94107-1206
415-597-5555
The teacher left the room and asked Shelly, a hearing impaired child to be the mother. Margaret, an emotionally disturbed child, became frightened and verbally attacked Shelly. The teacher worked to get them to become friends and understand each other's problems.
Films

4672 Once Upon a Time - Children's Classics Ret old in American Sign Language
Harris Communications
15155 Technology Drive
Eden Prairie, MN 55344
952-906-1180
800-825-6758
Fax: 952-906-1099
TTY: 800-825-9187
e-mail: info@harriscomm.com
www.harriscomm.com/
Children's classics come alive on videotapes.
Robert Harris Ph.D, Founder/President/CEO

4673 Parent Sign Video Series
TJ Publishers
2544 Tarpley Road
Carrollton, TX 75006
972-416-0800
800-999-1168
Fax: 972-416-0944
e-mail: customerservice@tjpublishers.com
www.tjpublishers.com/index.html
Ten instructional videotapes specifically designed for parents of deaf children, present frequently used vocabulary and phrases. The tapes are perfect for home use and as a compliment to sign language and educational programs. Deaf and hearing parents, each having a deaf and a hearing child, reflect common communication needs of all families.
Video
Angela K Thames, President
Jerald A Murphy, VP

4674 People vs. Noise
Better Hearing Institute
5021B Backlick Road
Annandale, VA 22003-6043
703-684-3391
e-mail: mail@betterhearing.org
www.betterhearing.org

4675 Read My Lips
Alexander Graham Bell Association
3417 Volta Place NW
Washington, DC 20007-2737
202-337-5220
Fax: 202-337-8270
TTY: 202-337-5220
A six videotape series that takes adults from lip reading to basic words to complex phrases and sentences in a variety of real life situations.

4676 See What I'm Saying
Thomas Kaufman, author

Fanlight Productions
4196 Washington Street
Boston, MA 02131-1731
617-469-4999
800-937-4113
Fax: 617-469-3379
e-mail: fanlight@fanlight.com
www.fanlight.com
Follows Patricia, a deaf child from a hearing, Spanish speaking family, through her first year of elementary school. Illustrates how the acquisition of communication skills enhances a child's self-esteem, confidence and family relationships. Open captioned.
1992 31 Minutes
ISBN: 1-572950-90-0

4677 Seeing and Hearing Speech: Lessons in Lipreading and Listening
Hearing Loss Association of America
7910 Woodmont Avenue   301-657-2248
Bethesda, MD 20814-3079   Fax: 301-913-9413
                                         TTY: 301-657-2249
                                 e-mail: info@hearingloss.org
                                        www.hearingloss.org
This CD-Rom helps people with hearing loss learn to combine
what they see with what they hear to understand speech better in
difficult situations. This interactive CD-ROM contains carefully
planned lessons to improve speech understanding through
lipreading.
CD-ROM
Jerry Portis, Executive Director
Brenda Battat, Assistant Executive Director

4678 Show & Tell: Explaining Hearing Loss to Teachers
Alexander Graham Bell Association
3417 Volta Place NW   202-337-5220
Washington, DC 20007-2737   Fax: 202-337-8270
                                         TTY: 202-337-5220
This video introduces mainstreamed teachers to the challenges that
hearing impairments impose on normal communication.
20 minutes

4679 Show 'N' Tell Stories
Modern Signs Press
PO Box 1181   562-596-8548
Los Alamitos, CA 90720-1181   800-572-7332
                                         Fax: 562-795-6614
                                         TTY: 562-493-4168
                                 e-mail: modsigns@aol.com
                                        www.modsigns.com
A bilingual storytelling series for Deaf children and their families,
featuring both Signing Exact English (SEE) and American Sign
Language (ASL).
Videotape

4680 Sign-Me-A-Story
DawnSignPress
6130 Nancy Ridge Drive   858-625-0600
San Diego, CA 92121-3223   800-549-5350
                                         Fax: 858-625-2336
                                         TTY: 858-625-0600
                                 e-mail: info@dawnsign.com
                                        www.dawnsign.com
Linda Bove, the deaf actress from Sesame Street, introduces children to American Sign Language. Teaches simple signs and then
acts out fairy tales. Stories are voiced and closed captioned, accessible to all.
30 minutes
ISBN: 0-394892-32-1
Joe Dannis, Founder/Publisher/President

4681 Sleeping Beauty Videotape
Gallaudet University Bookstore
800 Florida Avenue NE
Washington, DC 20002-3660   800-451-1073
                                         Fax: 800-621-8476
                                         TTY: 888-630-9347
                                 www.gallaudet.edu/~gupress
Presents the entire story of Sleeping Beauty told in American Sign
Language.

4682 Sleeping Beauty: With Selected Sentences in ASL
Gallaudet University
11030 S Langley Avenue
Chicago, IL 60628-3819   800-621-2736
                                         Fax: 800-621-8476
                                         TTY: 888-630-9347
                                 www.gallaudet.edu/~gupress
Features the full story in ASL and includes vocabulary and sentence structure focusing on adjectives, with a voice-over throughout.
30 minutes
ISBN: 0-930323-98-X

4683 Sound Hearing
Hearing Loss Association of America

7910 Woodmont Avenue   301-657-2248
Bethesda, MD 20814-3079   Fax: 301-913-9413
                                         TTY: 301-657-2249
                                 e-mail: info@hearingloss.org
                                        www.hearingloss.org
Provides listening samples to illustrate sound, hearing, and hear-
ing loss. Listeners will hear as people who have hearing loss might,
listening to music, a story, etc.
CD-ROM, 26 mins
Jerry Portis, Executive Director
Brenda Battat, Assistant Executive Director

4684 Telecoil: Plugging Into Sound
Hearing Loss Association of America
7910 Woodmont Avenue   301-657-2248
Bethesda, MD 20814-3079   Fax: 301-913-9413
                                         TTY: 301-657-2249
                                 e-mail: info@hearingloss.org
                                        www.hearingloss.org
In The Telecoil: Plugging Into Sound, members of SHHH give ac-
counts of their experiences with using the telecoil, describing how
the telecoil makes a noticeable difference in their social and pro-
fessional lives.
Open Captioned
Jerry Portis, Executive Director
Brenda Battat, Assistant Executive Director

4685 Telecoil: Plugging into Sound
7910 Woodmont Avenue   301-657-2248
Bethesda, MD 20814-3079   Fax: 301-913-9413
                                         TTY: 301-657-2249
                                 e-mail: national@shhh.org
                                        www.shhh.org
Guide for consumers concerning why they should include a
telecoil in their hearing aid. SHHH members are featured, talking
about their experiences. Includes 50 brochures. Open-captioned.
1996 10 minutes

4686 Telling Stories
Harris Communications
15155 Technology Drive   952-906-1180
Eden Prairie, MN 55344   800-825-6758
                                         Fax: 952-906-1099
                                         TTY: 800-825-9187
                                 e-mail: info@harriscomm.com
                                        www.harriscomm.com/
This international, award winning play, now on video, uses the
symbols and myths drawn from the struggles between the world of
the deaf and the world of the hearing.
Robert Harris Ph.D, Founder/President/CEO

4687 Treasure
Gallaudet University Bookstore
800 Florida Avenue NE   773-568-1550
Washington, DC 20002-3660   Fax: 800-621-8476
                                         TTY: 888-630-9347
                                 www.gallaudet.edu/~gupress
Ella Mae Lentz, a well-known deaf poet, signs some of her poems.

4688 Unheard Voices
Hearing Loss Association of America
7910 Woodmont Avenue   301-657-2248
Bethesda, MD 20814-3079   Fax: 301-913-9413
                                         TTY: 301-657-2249
                                 e-mail: info@hearingloss.org
                                        www.hearingloss.org
Unheard Voices is a candid and compassionate portrayal of people
coping with the life-changing impact of hearing loss. Open-cap-
tioned.
23 minutes
Jerry Portis, Executive Director
Brenda Battat, Assistant Executive Director

Web Sites

4689 Alexander Graham Bell Association
                                        www.agbell.org
Information on pediatric hearing loss, and educational issues for
hearing impaired children, promotes better public understanding

of hearing loss in children and adults, provides scholarships and financial aid to families of children with hearing loss, and promotes early detection of hearing loss in infants.

4690 American Academy of Audiology

www.audiology.org

Provides professional development, education and research and provides increased public awareness of hearing disorders and audiologic services.

4691 American Academy of Otolaryngology

www.entnet.org

Advance the art and science of otalaryngology-head and neck surgury through state-of-the-art education, research, and learning; and to unite, serve, and represent the interests of its members and their patients to the public.

4692 American Society for Deaf Children

www.deafchildren.org

Provides support, encouragement, and current information about deafness to families with deaf and hard of hearing children.

4693 American Tinnitus Association

www.ata.org

Provides information about tinnitus and referrals to local contacts/support groups nationwide.

4694 Auditory-Verbal International

www.auditory-verbal.org

Promotes the Auditory-Verbal Therapy approach, which is based on the belief that the overwhelming majority of these children can hear and talk by using their residual hearing and hearing aids.

4695 Better Hearing Institute

www.betterhearing.org

Information programs on hearing loss and available medical, surgical, hearing aid, and rehabilitation assistance for millions with uncorrected hearing problems.

4696 Council on Education of the Deaf

www.deafed.net

Offers information and referral services to the hearing impaired.

4697 Deafness Research Foundation

www.drf.org

Committed to public awareness and support for basic and clinical research into deafness and hearing disabilities.

4698 EAR Foundation

www.earfoundation.org

Provides the general public support services promoting the integration of the hearing and balance impaired into mainstream society and to educate young people and adults about hearing preservation and early detection of hearing loss, enabling them to prevent at an early age hearing and balance disorders.

4699 Healing Well

www.healingwell.com

An online health resource guide to medical news, chat, information and articles, newsgroups and message boards, books, disease-related web sites, medical directories, and more for patients, friends, and family coping with disabling diseases, disorders, or chronic illnesses.

4700 Health Finder

www.healthfinder.gov

Searchable, carefully developed web site offering information on over 1000 topics. Developed by the US Department of Health and Human Services, the site can be used in both English and Spanish.

4701 Healthlink USA

www.healthlinkusa.com

Health information concerning treatment, cures, prevention, diagnosis, risk factors, research, support groups, email lists, personal stories and much more. Updated regularly.

4702 Hear Now

www.sotheworldmayhearnow.org

Committed to making technology accessible to deaf and hard of hearing individuals throughout the United States. Also raises funds to provide hearing aids, cochlear implants and related services to children and adults who have hearing losses but do not have financial resources to purchase their own devices.

4703 Hearing Education and Awareness for Rocker

www.hearnet.com

Educates the public about the real dangers of hearing loss resulting from repeated exposure to excessive noise levels.

4704 Helios Health

www.helioshealth.com

Online resource for your health information. Detailed information about specific health topics, access to expert advice from our Medical Advisory Board, and up-to-date health news.

4705 House Ear Institute

www.hei.org

A national non-profit otologic research and educational institute that provides information on hearing and balance disorders.

4706 John Tracy Clinic

www.johntracycyclinic.org

An educational facility for preschool age children who have hearing losses and their families. In addition to on-site services, worldwide correspondence courses in English and Spanish are offered to parents whose children are of preschool age and are hard of hearing, deaf, or deaf-blind.

4707 MedicineNet

www.medicinenet.com

An online resource for consumers providing easy-to-read, authoritative medical and health information.

4708 Medscape

www.medscape.com

Medscape offers specialists, primary care physicians, and other health professionals the Web's most robust and integrated medical information and educational tools.

4709 National Association of the Deaf

www.nad.org

Focus on advocacy, captioned media, deafness-related information/publications, legal assistance and more.

4710 National Captioning Institute

ncicap.org

Advocates captioned television for people who want to see, as well as hear, the dialogue of a television program. It not only enables deaf and hard-of-hearing people to understand all of a program's content, but it is also beneficial for new Americans learning English as a second language, as well as children learning to read.

4711 National Information Center on Deafness

www.gallaudet.edu

Provides information or referrals on questions about deafness, including general information, education, research, legislation, assistive devices and more. Offers a bibliography of readings available on 30 topics relating to deafness.

4712 National Information Clearinghouse on Children Who are Deaf-Blind

www.tr.wou.edu/dblink

Collects, organizes and disseminates information related to children and youth who are deaf-blind and connects consumers of deaf-blind information to sources of information about deaf-blindness, assistive technology and deaf-blind people.

4713 National Institute on Deafness and Other Communication Disorders

www.nih.gov/nidcd

A national resources center for information about hearing, balance, smell, taste, voice, speech and language.

4714 Registry of Interpreters for the Deaf

www.RID.org

Professional interpreters and translators, persons with deafness or hearing impairments and professionals in related fields.

4715 Self-Help for Hard of Hearing People

www.shhh.org/

Promotes awareness and information about hearing loss, communication, assistive devices, and alternative communication skills through publications, exhibits and presentations.

4716   USA Deaf Sports Federation

www.usadsf.org

Website published by a governing body for all deaf sports and recreation in the United States.

4717   WebMD

www.webmd.com

Information on deafness, including articles and resources.

Description

4718 Heart Disease

There is a wide range of heart (cardiac) diseases that can be divided into several major categories: heart failure; problems in electrical conduction; heart rate and rhythm; and malfunction of the heart valves. Coronary disease relates to the arteries that supply oxygen to the heart muscle itself.

Heart failure is the general inability of the heart to function effectively as the pumping mechanism to distribute oxygenated blood and nutrients to the cells and tissues. As the heart's pumping action declines, blood does not get distributed properly and normal circulation gets disrupted. As a result, the fluid accumulates, or backs up, causing swelling (edema) in the body, often noticeable in the ankles, as well as within the lungs (pulmonary edema) causing difficulty in breathing. Numerous mechanisms are responsible for heart failure so treatment is aimed at the underlying causes, improving heart contractibility (and thus pump efficiency), and removal of excess fluid through the kidneys.

Problems in the electrical conduction that makes the heart contract result in irregular heart rate and rhythm, either slower, faster, or, in life-threatening situations, absence of heart beat or ineffective heart contractions. Specific medications and procedures are used in treatment, again depending on the underlying problem.

New diagnostic (angiography) and therapeutic catheter techniques have been developed to accurately identify the rhythm problem, and in some cases, cure it bydelivering radio frequency energy to the abnormal pathway.

Malfunctions of heart valves are also common, but surgical advances enable successful repair and replacement of defective or diseased valves.

The arteries that directly supply the heart (known as coronary arteries) can also be affected by disease processes. Deposits or fatty plaques may cause narrowing of the arteries, or the arteries can become blocked by a clot that originated somewhere else in the body. Either way, the heart may be deprived of oxygenated blood and the particular muscle that is fed by the artery is injured or dies. Angina is chest pain produced when the heart is not receiving enough oxygen but no direct damage occurs. A heart attack (or myocardial infarction) occurs when the heart is deprived of its blood for a significant amount of time. The outcome of a heart attack depends on the amount of damage sustained by the affected heart muscle and the speed with which treatment is started. Immediate medical intervention has a marked effect on long-term prognosis. Administration of agents that dissolve the clot (blood thinners, antithrombotics) significantly reduce heart attack deaths when given within 6 hours of the onset of chest pain. Catheter interventions (angioplasty) can include balloons and metallic stents that are placed in coronary arteries to push obstructions against the arterial walls thereby re-opening the vessel. The most recent advance is a stent that is coated with a drug that is coated to prevent reformation of the clot.

The symptoms of heart disease are varied, but may include chest pain, difficulty breathing, fatigue, palpitations, dizziness and fainting. See also *Congenital Heart Disease.*

National Agencies & Associations

4719 American Heart Association
7272 Greenville Avenue
Dallas, TX 75231   800-242-8721
www.americanheart.org
Supports research education and community service programs with the objective of reducing premature death and disability from cardiovascular diseases and stroke; coordinates the efforts of health professionals and other engaged in the fight against heart disease.
Nancy Brown, CEO

4720 Canadian Adult Congenital Heart Network
2233 Argentia Road   905-826-6665
Mississauga, ON L5N 2-2L2   e-mail: erwin.oechslin@cachnet.org
www.cachnet.org
Was created to pool the knowledge and experience of congenital heart disease professionals in Canada to help strengthen their skills and knowledge of the discipline, and to create a community of individuals committed to caring for adults with congenital heart disease and their families.
Dr Erwin Oechslin, President
Dr Ariane Marelli, Vice-President

4721 Children's Heart Society
PO BOX 52088   780-454-7665
Edmonton, AB T6G 2-2T5   888-247-9404
Fax: 780-454-7665
e-mail: childrensheart@shaw.ca
www.childrensheart.org
Supports families of children with acquired and congenital heart disease.
Shannon Moroz, President
Tina Krieger, Vice-President

4722 National Heart, Lung and Blood Institute
National Institutes of Health
PO BOX 30105   301-592-8573
Bethesda, MD 20824   Fax: 301-592-8563
TTY: 240-629-3255
e-mail: NHLBIinfo@nhlbi.nih.gov
www.nhlbi.nih.gov
Primary responsibility of this organization is the scientific investigation of heart, blood vessel, lung and blood disorders. Oversees research, demonstration, prevention, education, control and training activities in these fields and emphasizes the prevention and control of heart diseases.
Gary H Gibbons, Director
Susan B Shurin, Deputy Director

4723 Pulmonary Hypertension Association
801 Roeder Road   301-565-3004
Silver Spring, MD 20910   800-748-7274
Fax: 301-565-3994
e-mail: pha@PHAssociation.org
www.PHAssociation.org
A nonprofit organization for pulmonary hypertension patients, families, caregivers and PH-treating medical professionals. The mission of the Pulmonary Hypertension Association (PHA) is to find ways to prevent and cure pulmonary hypertension, and to provide hope for the pulmonary hypertension community through support, education, advocacy and awareness.
Vallerie McLaughlin, MD, Chair
Rino Aldrighetti, President

Research Centers

4724 Arizona Heart Institute
2632 N 20th Street
Phoenix, AZ 85006-1300
602-266-2200
800-345-4278
Fax: 602-604-5047
e-mail: information@azheart.com
www.azheart.com
Edward Diethrich, Medical Director and Founder

4725 Baylor College of Medicine: Debakey Heart Center
Texas Medical Center
1 Baylor Plaza
Houston, TX 77030-3411
713-798-4710
Fax: 713-798-3692
e-mail: president@bcm.edu
www.bcm.tmc.edu
Research activities have an emphasis on therapeutic intervention and prevention of heart disease.
James T Hackett, Chair
Paul Klotman MD, President

4726 Bees-Stealy Research Foundation
2001 4th Avenue
San Diego, CA 92101-2303
619-235-8744
Fax: 619-234-8190
Basic cardiac research.
HD Peabody Jr, Director

4727 Bockus Research Institute Graduate Hospital
Graduate Hospital
415 S 19th Street
Philadelphia, PA 19146-1464
215-893-2000
Offers research in cardiovascular diseases with emphasis on muscle tissue studies.
Dr Robert Cox, Director

4728 Boston University, Whitaker Cardiovascular Institute
715 Albany Street
Boston, MA 02118
617-638-4887
Fax: 617-638-4066
www.bumc.bu.edu
Offers basic and clinical care research relating to cardiovascular diseases.
Gary J Balady MD, Clinical Investigator

4729 Cardiovascular Research and Training Center University of Alabama
THT Room 311
Birmingham, AL 35294-6
205-934-3624
Fax: 205-345-96
Robert C Bueourge, Director

4730 Children's Heart Institute of Texas
PO Box 3966
Corpus Christi, TX 78463-3966
512-887-4505
Fax: 512-887-0539
Offers research and statistical information on pediatric cardiology.
Laura Berlanga, Director

4731 Cleveland Clinic Lerner Research Institute
9500 Euclid Avenue
Cleveland, OH 44195
216-444-3900
Fax: 216-444-3279
e-mail: dicorlp@ccf.org
www.lerner.ccf.org
Research institute focusing on diseases of the cardiovascular system.
Paul E DiCorleto PhD, Institute Chairman
Guy M Chisolm, III, PhD, Institute Vice-Chair

4732 Columbia University Irving Center for Clinical Research Adult Unit
Presbyterian Hospital
116 Street and Broadway
New York, NY 10027
212-854-1754
Fax: 212-053-13
e-mail: askcuit@columbia.edu
www.columbia.edu
Research center focusing on pulmonary diseases.
Lee C Bollinger, President
John H Coatsworth, Provost

4733 Congenital Heart Disease Anomalies Support, Education & Resources CHASER
2112 N Wilkins Road
Swanton, OH 43558-9445
419-825-5575
Fax: 419-825-2880
e-mail: myer106w@wonder.em.cdc.gov
www.csun.edu
An organization established to meet the emotional and educational needs of parents and professionals who deal with congenital heart disease in children. Offers resource materials and support for parent to parent networking.

4734 Creighton University Cardiac Center
3006 Webster Street
Omaha, NE 68131-2137
402-280-4566
800-237-7828
Fax: 402-280-4938
thecardiaccenter.creighton.edu
Research into the clinical aspects of cardiology and heart disease.
Tami Ward, Nurse Practitioner
Kimberly Harm, Nurse Practitioner

4735 Duke University Pediatric Cardiac Catheterization Laboratory
T901/Children's Health Center
Durham, NC 27705-0001
919-681-4080
Fax: 919-681-2714
e-mail: john.rhodes@duke.edu
pediatrics.duke.edu
Research into pediatric cardiology.
Joseph St Geme, III, MD, Chair
Kay Marshall, Chief Administrator

4736 Florida Heart Research Institute
4770 Biscayne Boulevard
Miami, FL 33137
305-674-3020
Fax: 305-535-3642
e-mail: pak@floridaheart.org
www.miamiheartresearch.org
General cardiovascular research.
Kathleen T DuCasse, Chief Executive Officer

4737 Framingham Heart Study
73 Mount Wayte Avenue
Framingham, MA 01702-5828
508-935-3418
Fax: 508-626-1262
e-mail: LLehmann1@partners.org
www.framinghamheartstudy.org
Lisa Soleymani Lehmann, M.D.,, Chair

4738 General Clinical Research Center at Beth Israel Hospital
330 Brookline Avenue
Boston, MA 02215-5400
617-667-7000
800-667-5356
TDD: 800-439-0183
www.bidmc.org
Studies into cardiology pulmonary disorders and heart disease.
Stephen B Kay, Chair
Kevin Tabb, MD, President & Chief Executive Officer

4739 General Clinical Research Center: University of California at LA
Center for Health Sciences
10833 Le Conte Avenue
Los Angeles, CA 90095
310-825-7177
Fax: 310-206-5012
e-mail: lshakerirwin@mednet.ucla.edu.
www.gcrc.medsch.ucla.edu
Cardiovascular and heart disease disorders and illness research.
Isidro Salus MD, Program Director
Gerald Levey, Principal Investigator

4740 Hahnemann University Likoff Cardiovascular Institute
Broad & Vine Streets
Philadelpia, PA 19102
215-854-8100
Diseases of the heart and vessels.
William S Frankl MD, Director

4741 Harvard Throndike Laboratory Harvard Medical Center
Harvard Medical Center
330 Brookline Avenue
Boston, MA 02215-5400
617-735-3020
Fax: 617-735-4833
Dr James Morgan, Director

4742 Heart Disease Research Foundation
50 Court Street
Brooklyn, NY 11201-4801
718-649-6210
Robert A Teters, Director

4743 Heart Research Foundation of Sacramento
1007 39th Street
Sacramento, CA 95816-5502
916-456-3365
e-mail: rjfrink@pol.net
www.hrfsac.org

Dr Frink, Founder/Principal Investigator

4744 Hope Heart Institute
1380 112th Ave. NE
Bellvue, WA 98004
425-456-8700
Fax: 425-456-8701
e-mail: info@hopeheart.org
www.hopeheart.org

Heart and blood vessel research.
Dr Lester R Sauvage MD, Founder
Cherie Skager, Interim Executive Director

4745 John L McClellan Memorial Veterans' Hospital Research Office
4300 W 7th Street
Little Rock, AR 72205-5446
501-257-1000
Fax: 501-671-2510
www2.va.gov

Karl David Straub MD, Chief Staff

4746 Krannert Institute of Cardiology
1801 N Senate Boulevard
Indianapolis, IN 46202-4832
317-962-0500
800-843-2786
Fax: 317-962-0501
medicine.iupui.edu/krannert
The cardiovascular program at the Indiana University School of Medicine is recognized throughout the world for its commitment to excellence in patient care research and education. While we're known for our experience and ability to take care of the most complex cardiovascular problems we are equally focused on prevention and early detection.
Peng-Sheng Chen, MD, Division Director
Eric Williams, MD, Associate Dean

4747 Loyola University of Chicago Cardiac Transplant Program
2160 S 1st Avenue
Maywood, IL 60153-3304
708-216-9000
888-584-7888
Fax: 708-216-4918
www.loyolamedicine.org/
Loyola University Health System is committed to excellence in patient care and the education of health professionals. They believe that our Catholic heritage and Jesuit traditions of ethical behavior academic distinction and scientific research lead to new knowledge and advance our healing mission in the communities we serve.
Larry M Goldberg, President & CEO
Wendy S Leutgens, Senior Vice President and COO

4748 Medstar Georgetown University Hospital Facility
3800 Reservoir Road NW
Washington, DC 20007-2195
202-444-2000
www.georgetownuniversityhospital.org
Studies of medical sciences with particular emphasis on heart disease.
Dr Richard Goldberg, President

4749 Mount Sinai Medical Center
4300 Alton Road
Miami Beach, FL 33140-2997
305-674-2121
Fax: 305-743-09
www.msmc.com

General cardiovascular research.
Steven D Sonenreich, President & Chief Executive Officer

4750 Oklahoma Medical Research Foundation: Cardiovascular Research Program
825 NE 13th Street
Oklahoma City, OK 73104-5097
405-271-6673
800-522-0211
Fax: 405-271-3980
e-mail: contact@omrf.org
www.omrf.ouhsc.edu
The Cardiovascular Biology Research Program investigates fundamental mechanisms involved in blood coagulation inflammation and atherogenesis with special emphasis on the regulation of theses processes.
Dr Stephen M Prescott, President
Mike D Morgan, Executive Vice President & COO

4751 Pennsylvania State University Artificial Heart Research Project
Milton S Hershey Medical Center

500 University Drive
Hershey, PA 17033-2391
717-531-8407
Fax: 717-531-5011
www.psu.edu

William S Pierce MD, Director

4752 Preventive Medicine Research Institute
900 Bridgeway
Sausalito, CA 94965-2158
415-332-2525
Fax: 415-325-30
e-mail: Tandis@pmri.org
www.pmri.org

Nonprofit organization focusing on prevention and treatment of heart disease through modification of diet exercise and relaxation techniques.
Dean Ornish, MD, Founder & President
Anne Ornish, Vice President, Director of Program Deve

4753 Purdue University William A Hillenbrand Biomedical Engineering Center
AA Potter Engineering Center
206 S. Martin Jischke Drive
W Lafayette, IN 47907-2032
765-494-2995
877-598-4233
Fax: 765-494-6628
e-mail: WeldonBME@purdue.edu
engineering.purdue.edu/BME
Cardiology and heart disease research.
Brian J Knoy, Director of Development
Kathryn Copper, Secretary

4754 Rockefeller University Laboratory of Cardiac Physiology
1230 York Avenue
New York, NY 10065
212-327-8000
Fax: 212-327-7974
e-mail: pubinfo@rockefeller.edu
www.rockefeller.edu
Causes of cardiac arrhythmias and prevention of heart disease.
David Rockfeller, Honorary Chair
Russell L Carson, Chair

4755 San Francisco Heart & Vascular Institute
1900 Sullivan Avenue
Daly City, CA 94015-2200
650-991-6712
800-82H-EART
Fax: 650-755-7315
e-mail: webmaster@sfhi.com
www.sfhi.com

At Seton Medical Center we are committed to providing a full range of high quality services and state-of-the-art cardiovascular treatments for our patients. Our medical nursing and social services staff provide quality care and compassion as a coordinated team focusing on the medical emotional and spiritual needs of patients and their families.
Colman J Ryan, MD, Executive Medical Director
Michael Girolami, MD, Chief of Cardiology

4756 Specialized Center of Research in Ischemic Heart Disease
1802 6th Avenue South
Birmingham, AL 35294-0001
205-934-4011
800-822-8816
www.health.uab.edu

Coronary artery disease.
Will Ferniany, CEO
Becky Armstrong, Program Manager

4757 Texas Heart Institute St Lukes Episcopal Hospital
St Lukes Episcopal Hospital
6770 Bertner Avenue
Houston, TX 77030-0345
832-355-4011
800-292-2221
Fax: 713-791-3089
e-mail: mmattsson@heart.thi.tmc.edu
www.texasheartinstitute.org

Denton A Cooley MD, President Emeritus
James T Willerson MD, President, Medical Director

4758 University of Alabama at Birmingham: Congenital Heart Disease Center
1720 2nd Avenue South
Birmingham, AL 35294
205-934-4011
Fax: 205-934-7514
TDD: 205-934-4642
www.uab.edu

Ray L Watts, MD, President
Linda Lucas, PhD, Provost

4759 University of California San Diego General Clinical Research Center
UCSD Medical Center
200 W Arbor Drive   619-543-3102
San Diego, CA 92103-1910   858-657-7000
                                           Fax: 619-435-36
                                           www.health.ucsd.edu
General clinical research.
Paul Viviano, Chief Executive Officer and Associate Vi
Margarita Baggett, Interim Chief Operating Officer and Chie

4760 University of California: Cardiovascular Research Laboratory
Center for Health Sciences
UCLA Medical Center   310-825-6824
Los Angeles, CA 90024   Fax: 310-206-5777
Cellular and subcellular cardiac conditions.
Dr Glenn Langer, Director

4761 University of Cincinnati Department of Pathology & Laboratory Medicine
234 Goodman Street   513-584-7284
Cincinnati, OH 45219-0529   Fax: 513-584-3892
                                           e-mail: pathology@uc.edu
                                           pathology.uc.edu
Fred V Lucas, MD, Chair of Pathology
James Hill, Business Manager

4762 University of Iowa: Iowa Cardiovascular Center
College of Medicine
200 Hawkins Drive   319-335-8588
Iowa City, IA 52242   Fax: 319-335-6969
                                           www.int-med.uiowa.edu
The purpose is to coordinate the cardiovascular programs of the College into a more cohesive unit to permit us to 1) utilize our cardiovascular resources optimally 2) intensify expand and integrate basic and clinical research programs in areas related to cardiovascular research and 3) evaluate the role of new measures for prevention diagnosis and treatment of cardiovascular disease.
Barry London, MD, PhD, Director Cardiovascular Medicine

4763 University of Michigan Pulmonary and Critical Care Division
University Hospital
1500 E Medical Center Drive   734-647-9342
Ann Arbor, MI 48109   888-287-1084
                                           Fax: 734-763-4585
                     www2.med.umich.edu/healthcenters/clinic_
Kevin Michael Chan, MD, Division Director

4764 University of Michigan: Cardiovascular Med icine
325 Briarwood Circle   734-647-9000
Ann Arbor, MI 48108-0001   Fax: 734-936-0133
                     www2.med.umich.edu/departments/cvc/servi
Focuses on the diagnosis, treatment and prevention of cardiovascular and heart diseases.
Kim Allen Eagle, MD, Division Director

4765 University of Missouri Columbia Division of Cardiothoracic Surgery
School of Medicine
Columbia, MO 65212   573-882-2121
                                           Fax: 573-884-0437
                                           e-mail: AldenM@missouri.edu
                                           www.missouri.edu
Cardiac surgery research.
Mike Alden, Director
Brian Foster, Provost

4766 University of Pennsylvania Muscle Institut e
School of Medicine
700A Clinical Research Building   215-573-9758
Philadelphia, PA 19104-2646   Fax: 215-898-2653
                              e-mail: mafoster@mail.med.upenn.edu
                                           www.med.upenn.edu/pmi/
Studies in tissue science.
E. Michael Ostap, PhD, Director

4767 University of Pittsburgh: Human Energy Research Laboratory
4200 Fifth Avenue
Pittsburgh, PA 15260-0001   412-624-4141
                                           www.pitt.edu

Focuses on exercise and cardiac rehabilitation.
Mark A Nordenberg, Chancellor
Patricia E Beeson, Provost and Senior Vice Chancellor

4768 University of Rochester: Clinical Research Center
601 Elmwood Avenue   585-275-2907
Rochester, NY 14642-0001   Fax: 585-256-3805
             e-mail: germaine_reinhardt@urmc.rochester.edu
                              www.urmc.rochester.edu/crc/
Studies of normal tissue functions pertaining to heart diseases.
Thomas A Pearson, MD, MPH, PhD, Director, Principal Investigator
Giovanni Schifitto , MD, Program Director

4769 University of Southern California: Coronary Care Research
1200 N State Street   213-226-7242
Los Angeles, CA 90033-1029
Dr. L Julian Haywood, Director

4770 University of Tennessee: Division of Cardiovascular Diseases
920 Madison Avenue   901-448-5750
Memphis, TN 38163-0001   Fax: 901-448-8084
                                           www.utmem.edu\cardiology
Cardiovascular system disorders including heart disease prevention and treatment.
Karl T Weber MD, Director

4771 University of Texas Southwestern Medical Center at Dallas
University of Texas
5323 Harry Hines Boulevard   214-648-3111
Dallas, TX 75390-7208   Fax: 214-483-11
                                           www.utsouthwestern.edu
Cardiology department research.
Daniel K Podolsky, MD, President
J. Gregory Fitz, MD, Executive Vice President

4772 University of Utah: Artificial Heart Research Laboratory
50 North Medical Drive   801-581-2121
Salt Lake City, UT 84132-1414   Fax: 801-581-4044
                                           healthsciences.utah.edu
Cardiac and blood vessel research.
Allen Stephens, Associate Director

4773 University of Utah: Cardiovascular Genetic Research Clinic
420 Chipeta Way   801-581-3888
Salt Lake City, UT 84132-0001   Fax: 801-581-6862
                      www.medicine.utah.edu/internalmedicine/c
Cardiovascular genetics research.
Dr Roger Williams, Founder

4774 Urban Cardiology Research Center
2300 Garrison Boulevard   410-945-8600
Baltimore, MD 21216-2308
Causes diagnosis and treatment of cardiovascular diseases.
Arthur White MD, Director

4775 Warren Grant Magnuson Clinical Center
National Institute of Health
10 Center Drive MSC 1078   301-496-3311
Bethesda, MD 20892   800-411-1222
                                           Fax: 301-496-2390
                                           TTY: 866-411-1010
                                           e-mail: mmichael@cc.nih.gov
                         www.dnrc.nih.gov/reports/programs/ncc.as
Established in 1953 as the research hospital of the National Institutes of Health. Designed so that patient care facilities are close to research laboratories so new findings of basic and clinical scientists can be quickly applied to the treatment of patients. Upon referral by physicians, patients are admitted to NIH clinical studies.
Madeline Michael, Chief, Clinical Nutrition Services

4776 Yeshiva University General Clinical Research Center
500 West 185th Street
New York, NY 10033   212-960-5400
                                           www.yu.edu
Cardiovascular research.
Dr Henry Kressel, Chairman
Richard M Joel, President

Support Groups & Hotlines

4777 American Autoimmune Related Diseases Association
22100 Gratiot Avenue   586-776-3900
East Detroit, MI 48021   800-598-4668
                                                     Fax: 586-776-3903
                                              e-mail: aarda@aarda.org
                                                        www.aarda.org
Awareness, education, referrals for patients with any type of auto-
immune disease.
Stanley M Finger, PhD, Chairman of the Board
Virginia T Ladd, President & Executive Director

4778 Mended Hearts
8150 N. Central Expressway   214-206-9259
Dallas, TX 75206   888-432-7899
                                                     Fax: 214-295-9552
                                          e-mail: info@mendedhearts.org
                                                   www.mendedhearts.org
Mutual support for persons who have heart disease, their families,
friends, and other interested persons.
Gordon Littlefield, President of the Board
Donnette Smith, Executive Vice President

4779 Mitral Valve Prolapse Program of Cincinnati Support Group
10525 Montgomery Road   513-745-9911
Cincinnati, OH 45242   e-mail: kscordo@wright.edu
                                               www.nursing.wright.edu
Brings together persons frightened by their symptoms in order to
learn to better cope with MVP. Fosters use of non-drug therapies.
Supervised exercise sessions, diagnostic evaluations and specialized testing. Information and referrals, conferences, literature,
group meetings, MVP Hot Line, and assistance in starting groups.

4780 National Health Information Center
PO Box 1133   310-565-4167
Washington, DC 20013   800-336-4797
                                                     Fax: 301-984-4256
                                                  e-mail: info@nhic.org
                                                   www.health.gov/nhic
Offers a nationwide information referral service, produces direc-
tories and resource guides.

4781 National Society for MVP and Dysautonomia
880 Montclair Road   205-595-8229
Birmingham, AL 35213   866-595-8229
                                                     Fax: 205-595-8222
                                    e-mail: nancysawyermd@bellsouth.net
Assists individuals suffering from mitral valve prolapse syndrome
and dysautonomia to find support and understanding. Education
on symptoms and treatment. Other areas of focus are Fibromyalgia
and Sjogren's Syndrome.
Nancy Sawyer, MD

4782 Pulmonary Hypertension Association
801 Roeder Road   301-565-3004
Silver Spring, MD 20910   800-748-7274
                                                     Fax: 301-565-3994
                                       e-mail: PHCR@PHAssociation.org
                                                   www.phassociation.org
A nonprofit organization funded and for pulmonary hypertension
patients. Our mission is to seek a cure, provide hope, support, education and to promote awareness and advocate for the PH
community.
Vallerie McLaughlin, MD, Chair
Rev. Steve White, PhD, Chair-Elect

4783 Society of Mitral Valve Prolapse Syndrome
PO Box 431   630-250-9327
Itasca, IL 60143-0431   Fax: 630-773-0478
                                             e-mail: bonnie0107@aol.com
                                           www.mitralvalveprolapse.com/
Provides support and education to patients, families and friends
about mitral valve prolapse syndrome.
Jim Durante, Co-Founder
Bonnie Durante, Co-Founder

Books

4784 Advances in Cardiac and Pulmonary Rehabilitation
Haworth Press
10 Alice Street   607-722-5857
Binghamton, NY 13904-1580   800-429-6784
                                                     Fax: 607-722-0012
                                                   www.haworthpress.com
Enhance your rehabilitation program with this authoritative
volume.
74 pages Hardcover
ISBN: 0-866569-86-0

4785 Congenital Heart Disease
Northwestern University Press
625 Colfax Street   847-491-5313
Evanston, IL 60208-4210   800-621-2736
                                                   www.nupress.nwu.edu

1993 300 pages
ISBN: 1-880416-82-4

4786 Dr. Dean Ornish's Program for Reversing Heart Disease
Random House Trade Books
400 Hahn Road
Westminster, MD 21157-4663   800-733-3000
                                                     Fax: 800-659-2436

ISBN: 0-804110-38-7

4787 Expert Guide to Beating Heart Disease: What You Absolutely Must Know
Dr. Harlan M. Krumholz, author
HarperCollins
10 E. 53rd Street   212-207-7000
New York, NY 10022-5299   e-mail: orders@harpercollins.com
                                                   www.harpercollins.com
Translates key medical data into clear guidelines capturing the
highest treatment standards for heart disease. Profiles care
alternatices from supplements to stress reduction as well as treatments on the horizon.
2005 288 pages
ISBN: 0-060578-34-3

4788 Heart Disease
Franklin Watts Grolier
90 Old Sherman Turnpike   203-797-3500
Danbury, CT 06816-0001   800-621-1115
                                                     Fax: 203-797-3197
                                                        www.grolier.com
Using diagrams, this book discusses strokes and other blood vessel
disorders, as well as their treatment and prevention.
112 pages Grades 7-12
ISBN: 0-531108-84-8

4789 Heart of a Child: What Families Need to Know About Heart Disorders
Johnss Hopkins University Press
2715 N Charles Street   410-935-6900
Baltimore, MD 21218-4319   800-537-5487
                                                     Fax: 410-516-6998
                                                      www.press.jhu.edu

1993 352 pages Paperback
ISBN: 0-801866-36-7

4790 Living with Heart Disease
Franklin Watts Grolier
90 Old Sherman Turnpike   203-797-3500
Danbury, CT 06816-0001   800-621-1115
                                                     Fax: 203-797-3197
                                                        www.grolier.com
Shows how persons with heart disease can overcome their illness
and lead productive lives.
32 pages Grades 5-7
ISBN: 0-531108-45-7

4791 Mitral Valve Prolapse Syndrome/Dysautonomia Survival Guide
Society of Mitral Valve Prolapse Syndrome

PO Box 431
Itasca, IL 60143-0431

630-250-9327
Fax: 630-773-0478
e-mail: bonnie0107@aol.com
www.mitralvalveprolapse.com

Provides support and education to patients, families and friends about mitral valve prolapse syndrome.
175 pages
ISBN: 1-572243-03-1
Bonnie Durante, Vice President
Cheryl Durante, Editor

4792   What Every Woman Must Know About Heart Disease
Warner Books
1271 Avenue of the Americas
New York, NY 10020-1300

212-484-2900
Fax: 818-507-5596
e-mail: nylandimmunojobs@boxter.com
www.twbookmark.com

1996
ISBN: 0-446519-86-3

4793   Women Take Heart
Putnam Publishing Group
200 Madison Avenue
New York, NY 10016-3903

212-951-8400

1993 224 pages
ISBN: 0-399138-88-9

4794   Women and Heart Disease
Random House Trade Books
400 Hahn Road
Westminster, MD 21157-4663

800-733-3000
Fax: 800-659-2436

ISBN: 0-345386-20-5

Children's Books

4795   Village by the Sea
Franklin Watts Grolier
90 Old Sherman Turnpike
Danbury, CT 06816-0001

203-797-3500
Fax: 203-797-3197
www.grolier.com

This story focuses on the relationship between Emma and her father as he prepares to undergo bypass surgery.
Grades 5-8

Newsletters

4796   American Heart Association News
American Heart Association
7272 Greenville Avenue
Dallas, TX 75231-5129

214-706-1162
Fax: 214-696-5211

News reports and journal reports on the latest information concerning heart disease.

4797   And the Beat Goes On
Society of Mitral Valve Prolapse Syndrome
PO Box 431
Itasca, IL 60143-0431

630-250-9327
Fax: 630-773-0478
e-mail: bonnie0107@aol.com
www.mitralvalveprolapse.com

Bi-monthly newsletter. Provides support and education to patients, families and friends about mitral valve prolapse syndrome.
6 pages
Bonnie Durante, Vice President
Cheryl Durante, Editor

4798   Heartstyle
American Heart Association
7272 Greenville Avenue
Dallas, TX 75231-5129

214-706-1162
Fax: 214-696-5211

Reports on heart and blood vessel diseases and stroke.
Quarterly

4799   MVPS & Anxiety
Society of Mitral Valve Prolapse Syndrome

PO Box 431
Itasca, IL 60143-0431

630-250-9327
Fax: 630-773-0478
e-mail: bonnie0107@aol.com
www.mitralvalveprolapse.com

6 pages
Bonnie Durante, Vice President
Cheryl Durante, Editor

Pamphlets

4800   About High Blood Pressure
American Heart Association
7272 Greenville Avenue
Dallas, TX 75231-5129

214-706-1162
Fax: 214-696-5211

Offers information on what blood pressure is, risk factors and at risk persons.

4801   American Heart Association Diet
American Heart Association
7272 Greenville Avenue
Dallas, TX 75231-5129

214-706-1162
Fax: 214-696-5211

An eating plan for healthy americans.

4802   Cholesterol and Your Heart
American Heart Association
7272 Greenville Avenue
Dallas, TX 75231-5129

214-706-1162
Fax: 214-696-5211

Offers information on lowering blood cholesterol levels.

4803   Congenital Heart Defects
March of Dimes
233 Park Avenue South
New York, NY 10003

212-353-8353
Fax: 212-254-3518
e-mail: NY639@marchofdimes.com
www.marchofdimes.com

4804   E is for Exercise
American Heart Association
7272 Greenville Avenue
Dallas, TX 75231-5129

214-706-1162
Fax: 214-696-5211

Offers information on what kinds of exercise are the best and how to exercise properly.

4805   Easy Food Tips for Heart Healthy Eating
American Heart Association
7272 Greenville Avenue
Dallas, TX 75231-5129

214-706-1162
Fax: 214-696-5211

Offers food selection hints for fat-controlled meals.

4806   Eat Well, But Wisely
American Heart Association
7272 Greenville Avenue
Dallas, TX 75231-5129

214-706-1162
Fax: 214-696-5211

Offers information on good nutrition to reduce the risks of heat attacks.

4807   Exercise and Your Heart
American Heart Association
7272 Greenville Avenue
Dallas, TX 75231-5129

214-706-1162
Fax: 214-696-5211

Offers information on how to get enough exercise from daily activities, what the benefits of exercise are and what the risks of exercising are.

4808   Heart Defects
Association of Birth Defect Children
5400 Diplomat Circle
Orlando, FL 32810-5603

800-922-9234

Informational sheet on the causes, symptoms and statistics of heart defects and heart disease in children.

4809   How to Have Your Cake and Eat It Too
American Heart Association
7272 Greenville Avenue
Dallas, TX 75231-5129

214-706-1162
Fax: 214-696-5211

A guide to low-fat, low-cholesterol eating.

Web Sites

4810 American Heart Association

www.americanheart.org

Supports research, education and community service programs with the objective of reducing premature death and disability from cardiovascular diseases and stroke; coordinates the efforts of health professionals, and other engaged in the fight against heart and circulatory disease.

4811 Healing Well

www.healingwell.com

An online health resource guide to medical news, chat, information and articles, newsgroups and message boards, books, disease-related web sites, medical directories, and more for patients, friends, and family coping with disabling diseases, disorders, or chronic illnesses.

4812 Health Finder

www.healthfinder.gov

Searchable, carefully developed web site offering information on over 1000 topics. Developed by the US Department of Health and Human Services, the site can be used in both English and Spanish.

4813 Healthlink USA

www.healthlinkusa.com

Health information concerning treatment, cures, prevention, diagnosis, risk factors, research, support groups, email lists, personal stories and much more. Updated regularly.

4814 Helios Health

www.helioshealth.com

Online resource for your health information. Detailed information about specific health topics, access to expert advice from our Medical Advisory Board, and up-to-date health news.

4815 MedicineNet

www.medicinenet.com

An online resource for consumers providing easy-to-read, authoritative medical and health information.

4816 Medscape

www.medscape.com

Medscape offers specialists, primary care physicians, and other health professionals the Web's most robust and integrated medical information and educational tools.

4817 National Heart, Lung and Blood Institute

www.nhlbi.nih.gov

Primary responsibility of this organization is the scientific investigation of heart, blood vessel, lung and blood disorders. Oversees research, demonstration, prevention, education, control and training activities in these fields and emphasizes the prevention and control of heart diseases.

4818 WebMD

www.webmd.com

Information on Heart disease, including articles and resources.

Description

4819 # Hemophilia

Hemophilia is a genetic disorder that disrupts the body's normal blood clotting function because there is a deficiency of specific proteins known as clotting factors—specifically, factor VIII and factor IX. About 20,000 Americans are affected with the disorder and, currently, there is no cure.

Hemophilia is linked to the X-chromosome because that is where both factor genes are located. As a result, hemophilia affects males almost exclusively, with females being carriers, whose sons have a 50 percent chance of having the disorder.

Hemophiliacs, like anyone else, will bleed if injured, but they will bleed longer and more profusely. They may also bleed in response to injuries that are inconsequential in other people. For instance, normal daily activities may cause bleeding within a joint, leading to severe pain and swelling, and over time destroying the joint.

The severity of hemophilia varies dramatically depending on the factor VIII and IX levels, thus, affecting a person's prognosis and need for therapy. Treatment is with transfusions of the appropriate factor, and usually has to be repeated frequently. Most hemophiliacs treated with plasma concentrate in the early 1980s are infected with HIV contracted from contaminated blood and transfusions. HIV is now responsible for over half of deaths among hemophiliacs.

Most hemophiliacs are now treated at comprehensive hemophilia centers, which offer not just factor replacement but multispecialty expertise, sophisticated laboratory testing, physical therapy and psychological support. New techniques allow for identification of carrier females in these families. This is important for genetic counseling and family planning.

National Agencies & Associations

4820 **American Red Cross Blood Services**
2025 E Street, NW   202-303-5214
Washington, DC 20006   800-733-2767
e-mail: lkeefe@arlingtonredcross.org
www.redcross.org
Distributes a wide variety of plasma therapeutics to benefit people with hemophilia A and B, immune disorders and hypoalbuminemia.
Bonnie McElveen Hunter, Chairman of the Board
Gail J McGovern, President & CEO

4821 **Baxter Hyland Division**
One Baxter Parkway   224-948-2000
Deerfield, IL 60015-1900   800-422-9837
Fax: 800-568-5020
www.baxter.com
Government affairs office that monitors and selectively lobbies on issues relating to Medicare Medicaid Orphan Drugs and other subjects relating to hemophilia.
Robert L Parkinson, Jr, Chairman of the Board & CEO
David P Scharf, Corporate Vice President and General Cou

4822 **Canadian Hemophilia Society**
400-1255 University Street   514-848-0503
Montreal, Quebec, H3B3B-3B6   800-668-2686
Fax: 514-848-9661
e-mail: chs@hemophilia.ca
www.hemophilia.ca
Strives to improve the health and quality of life for all people with inherited bleeding disorders and to find a cure.
Craig Upshaw, President
David Page, National Executive Director

4823 **Hemophilia Health Services**
201 Great Circle Road   615-352-2500
Nashville, TN 37228   866-712-5200
Fax: 800-330-0756
e-mail: info@hemophiliahealth.com
www.hemophiliahealth.com
Largest homecare company devoted solely to serving people with bleeding disorders.
Ken Trader, VP of Sales and Marketing

4824 **National Hemophilia Foundation**
116 W 32nd Street   212-328-3700
New York, NY 10001   800-424-2634
Fax: 212-328-3777
e-mail: info@hemophilia.org
www.hemophilia.org
Dedicated to the treatment and the cure of hemophilia, related bleeding disorders and complications of those disorders or their treatment, including HIV infection, as well as improving the quality of life of all those affected.
Jorge de la Riva, Chair
Val Bias, Chief Executive Officer

4825 **World Federation of Hemophilia**
1425, boul. Ren-Lvesque   514-875-7944
Montreal, QB H3G1T-1T7   Fax: 514-875-8916
e-mail: wfh@wfh.org
www.wfh.org
An international not-for-profit organization to improving the lives of people with hemophilia and related bleeding disorders.
John E Bournas, CEO/Executive Director
Elizabeth Myles, Chief Operating Officer

State Agencies & Associations

Alabama

4826 **Hemophilia and Bleeding Disorders of Alaba ma, Inc.**
151 Market Place   334-277-9446
Montgomery, AL 36117-1640   855-469-4232
Fax: 334-272-9167
www.hbda.us/

Brian Ward, Chairman
Vicki Jackson, Executive Director

Arkansas

4827 **Hemophilia Foundation of Arkansas**
351 Valley Oak Lane   501-941-3109
Austin, AR 72007   888-941-4366
e-mail: angieclark1315@sbcglobal.net
www.hemophilia.org

Angie Clark, President
John Little, VP

California

4828 **Central California Chapter of the National Hemophilia Foundation**
PO Box 163689   916-448-0370
Sacramento, CA 95816   Fax: 916-489-1569
e-mail: cchfsac@yahoo.com
www.cchfsac.org
A very small and family-oriented chapter. Offers an active youth group, an annual summer camp, a men's and women's group and

various family activities for persons living in the central California valley from its center in Sacramento to the borders of Nevada.
Sean Hubbert, President
Tracey Huntington, Vice-President

4829 Hemophilia Association of San Diego County
3550 Camino Del Rio North   619-325-3570
San Diego, CA 92108   Fax: 619-325-4350
e-mail: info@hasdc.org
www.hasdc.org
Provides summer camp programs for young persons with hemophilia, sponsors educational programs for the general public, sponsors support groups for parents to help them deal with hemophilia, monitors legislation pertaining to hemophilia and related conditions.
Mike Brown, Board President
Melissa Pregill, Executive Director

4830 Hemophilia Foundation of Northern California
6400 Hollis Street   510-658-3324
Emeryville, CA 94608-3024   Fax: 510-658-3384
e-mail: merlin.wedepohl@hemofoundation.org
www.hemofoundation.org
A volunteer, nonprofit organization serving the needs of people with hemophilia and other related bleeding disorders in 35 counties in Northern California. Provides hemophilia literature, scholarships, youth programs and annual summer camps.
Merlin Wedepohl, Executive Director
Nancy Trunzo, Office Manager and Walk Manager

4831 Hemophilia Foundation of Southern California
6720 Melrose Avenue   323-525-0440
Hollywood, CA 90038   800-371-4123
Fax: 323-525-0445
e-mail: hfsc@hemosocal.org
www.hemosocal.org
Tamara Kato, President
Linda Corrente, Executive Director

Colorado

4832 Colorado Chapter National Hemphilila Foun dation
2465 Sheridan Blvd   720-626-1263
Edgewater, CO 80214   88 - 7 - 02
e-mail: info@cohemo.org
www.cohemo.org
Amy Board, Executive Director

Florida

4833 Florida Hemophilia Association
915 Middle River Drive   813-367-0050
Ft Lauderdale, FL 33304   888-880-8330
Fax: 813-367-0051
e-mail: dadamkin@floridahemophilia.org
www.floridahemophilia.org
Barbie Arrebola, President
Debbi Adamkin, Executive Director

Georgia

4834 Hemophilia Foundation of Georgia
8800 Roswelll Road   770-518-8272
Atlanta, GA 30350   Fax: 770-518-3310
e-mail: mail@hog.org
www.hog.org
Established to help Georgia residents with hemophilia lead normal and productive lives. Because this organization is comprised of patients, their friends and families, it is especially motivated to provide the best in personalized and comprehensive services.
Patricia Dominic, CEO
Andrew Maurer, Chief Governance Officer

Hawaii

4835 Hemophilia Foundation of Hawaii Kapiolani Medical Center
Kapiolani Medical Center

45-1031B. Wailele Road   808-782-5506
Kaneohe, HI 96744   Fax: 808-638-2910
e-mail: hawaiihemophiliafoundation@hotmail.com
www.hawaiihemo.org/
Cinda Hueu, President
Jennifer Chun, Executive Director

Idaho

4836 Hemophilia Foundation of Idaho
4696 Overland Road   208-344-4476
Boise, ID 83705-1622   866-453-4476
Fax: 208-344-4476
e-mail: tmagrini@hemophilia.org
www.idahoblood.org/
Shane Bell, President
Taryn Magrini, Executive Director

Illinois

4837 Hemophilia Foundation of Illinois
332 S. Michigan Avenue   312-427-1495
Chicago, IL 60604   Fax: 312-427-1602
e-mail: brobinson.hfi@mindspring.com
www.hemophiliaillinois.org
Serves as an information source referral service and advocate for persons with hemophilia and their families. The mission of this chapter is to provide counseling, educational information and support services to persons affected by hemophilia and related disorders.
Mike Toohey, President
Robert P Robinson, Executive Director

Indiana

4838 Hemophilia Foundation of Indiana
5172 E 65th Street   317-570-0039
Indianapolis, IN 46220   800-241-2873
Fax: 317-570-0058
e-mail: cfeay@hoii.org
www.hemophiliaofindiana.org
Scott Ehnes, Executive Director
Briana Vieke, Program Director

Kentucky

4839 Kentucky Hemophilia Foundation
1850 Taylor Avenue   502-456-3233
Louisville, KY 40213   800-582-2873
Fax: 502-456-3234
e-mail: info@kyhemo.org
www.kyhemo.org
Assists individuals with hemophilia and related inherited bleeding disorders through education, advocacy and support services. Services include quarterly newsletter, post secondary education scholarship, summer camp for children, seminars and support functions.
Quarterly
Eric Marcum, President
Ursela Lacer, Executive Director

Louisiana

4840 Louisiana Chapter of the National Hemophilia Foundation
3636 S Sherwood Forest   225-291-1675
Baton Rouge, LA 70816-2285   800-749-1680
Fax: 225-291-1679
e-mail: contact@lahemo.org
www.lahemo.org/
Lori Keels, Executive Director
Edgar Guedry, President

Maryland

4841 Hemophilia Foundation of Maryland
13 Class Court   410-661-2307
Parkville, MD 21234-2602   800-964-3131
                                  Fax: 410-661-2308
                       e-mail: Miller8043@comcast.net
                                   www.hfmonline.org
The Hemophilia foundation of Maryland is a private not for profit organization which devotes its efforts to improving the quality of life for persons affected with bleeding disorders and their complications.
Harvey Gates, President
Emma Miller-Clark, Executive Director

Massachusetts

4842 New England Hemophilia Association
347 Washington Street   781-326-7645
Dedham, MA 02026   Fax: 781-329-5122
                  e-mail: info@newenglandhemophilia.org
                            www.newenglandhemophilia.org
New England Hemophilia Association is dedicated to improving the quality of life for persons with bleeding disorders (hemophilia, von Willebrands, and other factor deficiencies) and their families through education, support and advocacy.
Patrick Mancini, President
Kevin R Sorge, Executive Director

Michigan

4843 Hemophilia Foundation of Michigan
1921 W Michigan Avenue   734-544-0015
Ypsilanti, MI 48197   800-482-3041
                                  Fax: 734-544-0095
                           e-mail: hfm@hfmich.org
                                      www.hfmich.org
Coordinates funding, professional education, and networking, with Hemophilia Treatment Centers in Michigan, Indiana, and Ohio. Provides educational services, including workshops, meetings, symposiums, and numerous publications.
Carrie Reaume, Executive Director
Suzanne Kapica, Regional Coordinator

Minnesota

4844 Hemophilia Foundation of Minnesota and the Dakotas
750 S Plaza Drive   651-406-8655
Mendota Heights, MN 55120   Fax: 651-406-8656
                     e-mail: hemophiliafound@visi.com
                                        www.hfmd.org
A nonprofit organization established to be a leader and a catalyst within the community to enable and inspire members to impact their own lives, with the ultimate aim of cures for both hemophilia and HIV/AIDS.
John Schulte, President/Board of Directors
James Paist, Executive Director

Mississippi

4845 Mississippi Hemophilia Foundation
PO Box 13608   601-957-2706
Jackson, MS 39236   e-mail: haleyjones80@yahoo.com
                                  www.mshemophilia.com/
Haley Jones, President
Leslee Loden, Vice-President

Missouri

4846 Gateway Hemophilia Association
14248 F Manchester Road   314-482-5973
Manchester, MO 63011   877-623-8300
                                  Fax: 314-729-7033
                  e-mail: NicFahey@gatewayhemophilia.org
                              www.gatewayhemophilia.org
Nic Fahey, President
Bridget Tyrey, Executive Director

Nebraska

4847 Nebraska Chapter of the National Hemophilia Foundation
215 Centennial Mall S   402-742-5663
Lincoln, NE 68508   Fax: 402-742-5677
                       e-mail: office@nebraskanhf.org
                                  www.nebraskanhf.org
The mission of this chapter is to provide support, education, communication and advocacy for men, women and children challenged by Hemophilia. Services provided include a toll free telephone hotline for persons seeking information on HIV and hemophilia.
Jason Everts, President
Kristi Harvey-Simi, Executive Director

Nevada

4848 Hemophilia Foundation of Nevada
7473 W. Lake Mead Blvd.   702-564-4368
Las Vegas, NV 89128   Fax: 702-446-8134
                                e-mail: Info@hfnv.org
                                        www.hfnv.org
Dennis Flynn, President Executive Committee
Kelli Walters, Executive Director

New Mexico

4849 Hemophilia Foundation of New Mexico
PO Box 51494   505-341-9321
Albuquerque, NM 87181   866-341-9321
                                  Fax: 505-292-5818
                   e-mail: sangredeoro@comcast.net
                                    www.hemophilia.org
Lori Long, President
Loretta Cordova, Executive Director

New York

4850 Hemophilia Center of Western New York
936 Delaware Ave   716-896-2470
Buffalo, NY 14209   866-434-6551
                                  Fax: 716-218-4010
                    e-mail: info@hemophiliawny.com
                                 www.hemophiliawny.com
Robert Long, Chairman
Thomas Long, President

4851 National Hemophilia Foundation: Mary M. Gooley Hemophilia Center
1415 Portland Avenue   585-922-5700
Rochester, NY 14621   Fax: 585-922-5775
              e-mail: robert.fox@rochestergeneral.org
                                    www.hemocenter.org
Robert Fox, CEO/ President
Linda Magliocco, Senior Vice President

North Carolina

4852 Hemophilia Foundation of North Carolina
260 Town Hall Dr.   919-319-0014
Morrisville, NC 27560   800-990-5557
                                  Fax: 919-319-0016
                      e-mail: info@hemophilia-nc.org
                                  www.hemophilia-nc.org
A nonprofit organization that serves as an information source for the hemophilia community of North Carolina. Supply the most up-to-date information concerning hemophilia and hemophilia related HIV/AIDS.
Steven Peretti, PhD, President
Leonard Poe, Vice President & Advocacy Chair

Ohio

4853 Central Ohio Chapter of the National Hemophilia Foundation
200 E. Campus View Blvd   614-985-3752
Columbus, OH 43235-0345   800-847-0345
                                        Fax: 614-985-3601
                    e-mail: ralexander@hemophilia.org
                                   www.nhfcentralohio.org

Jeff Stewart, President
Rob Alexander, Executive Director

4854 Northern Ohio Chapter of the National Hemophilia Foundation
One Independence Place
5000 Rockside Road   216-834-0051
Independence, OH 44131   800-554-HEMO
                                        Fax: 216-834-0055
                          e-mail: jtooley@nohf.org
                                           www.nohf.org

Marlene Piatak, President
Janet Tooley, Executive Director

4855 Northwest Ohio Hemophilia Association
2121 Hughes Drive   419-291-5882
Toledo, OH 43606   Fax: 419-479-3269
                     e-mail: carla@nwohemophilia.org
                              www.nwohemophilia.org/

Jim Knepp, President
Carla Wells, Executive Director

4856 Southwestern Ohio Chapter of the National Hemophilia Foundation
3131 S Dixie Drive   937-298-8000
Moraine, OH 45439   Fax: 937-298-8080
                     e-mail: info@swohiohemophilia.org
                              www.swohiohemophilia.org

This chapter serves persons with hemophilia and blood clotting disorders in an 11 county area. It is dedicated to offering people with hemophilia and related blood disorders and their families educational opportunities about the diseases.
Dena Shepard, President
John Gale, Executive Director

Oklahoma

4857 Oklahoma Chapter of the National Hemophilia Foundation
720 W. Wilshire Blvd   405-463-6634
Oklahoma City, OK 73116   800-735-3855
                        e-mail: tayers@okhemophilia.org
                                   www.okhemophilia.org

Tom Ayers, President
Bob Goodley, Executive Director

Oregon

4858 Hemophilia Foundation of Oregon
10940 SW Barnes Rd #129   503-297-7207
Portland, OR 97225   Fax: 503-297-0127
                     e-mail: info@hemophiliaoregon.org
                              www.hemophiliaoregon.org/

Jeremy Swanlund, President
Marita Postma, Executive Director

Pennsylvania

4859 Delaware Valley Chapter of the National Hemophilia Foundation
14 E. 6th Street   215-393-3611
Lansdale, PA 19446   Fax: 215-393-9419
                      e-mail: hemophilia@navpoint.com
                               www.hemophiliasupport.org

Thomas Galvin, President
William Widerman, Vice-President

4860 Western Pennsylvania Chapter of the National Hemophilia Foundation
20411 Rt. 19   724-741-6160
Cranberry Township, PA 16066   800-824-0016
                                        Fax: 724-741-6167
                    e-mail: info@westpennhemophilia.org
                                www.westpennhemophilia.org

Brings together and serves as a focal point for those segments of the community most concerned with hemophilia. They include medical and social service providers, people with hemophilia and their families educators and the general public.
Scott E Miller, President
Nathan Rost, Vice-President

Rhode Island

4861 Rhode Island Hemophilia Foundation
347 Washington Street   781-326-7645
Dedham, MA 02026   Fax: 781-329-5122
                    e-mail: info@newenglandhemophilia.org
                                www.newenglandhemophilia.org

Patrick Mancini, President
Kevin R Sorge, Executive Director

South Carolina

4862 Hemophilia Association of South Carolina
PO Box 3874   864-350-9941
Sumter, SC 29151   888-829-4849
        e-mail: information@hemophiliaofsouthcarolina.ne
                      www.hemophiliaofsouthcarolina.net/
Sue Martin, President

Tennessee

4863 Tennessee Hemophilia & Bleeding Disorder Foundation
1819 Ward Drive   615-900-1486
Murfreesboro, TN 37129-5281   888-703-3269
                                        Fax: 615-900-1487
                               e-mail: mary@thbdf.org
                                           www.thbdf.org

Offers a hemophilia clinic, social workers and consultants, a state hemophilia program, blood donor programs, counseling programs, genetic counseling, literature and resources, summer camp, grants, and more for the hemophilia and HIV/AIDS community.
Kent Russ, President
Mary Hord, Executive Director

Texas

4864 Lone Star Chapter of the National Hemophilia Foundation
10500 NW Freeway   713-686-6100
Houston, TX 77092   888-LSC-NHF1
                                        Fax: 832-383-4601
                     e-mail: Debbiedelariva@yahoo.com
                               www.lonestarhemophilia.org

Nick Zasowski, President

4865 Texas Central Chapter of the National Hemophilia Foundation
12700 Hillcrest Road   972-386-3865
Dallas, TX 75230   Fax: 214-654-9954
                            e-mail: mail@texcen.org
                                          www.texcen.org

A group of volunteers seeking solutions to the various aspects of the hemophilia problem. Supports blood drives sponsors a summer camp for hemophiliac children, conducts educational member meetings, arranges for genetic counseling and sponsors group support meetings.
Shannon Brush, President
Brendan Hayes, Executive Director

Utah

4866 Utah Chapter of the National Hemophilia Foundation
772 E 3300 S   801-484-0325
Salt Lake City, UT 84106   877-463-6893
                                        Fax: 801-746-2488
                                   www.hemophiliautah.org

Offers educational information, pamphlets, fundraising events and more for persons and families affected by hemophilia.
Reg Ecker, President
Scott Muir, Executive Director

Virginia

4867 Hemophilia Association of the Capital Area
10560 Main Street
Fairfax, VA 22030-1504
703-352-7641
Fax: 540-427-6589
e-mail: admin@HACAcares.org
www.hacacares.org
A nonprofit organization serving persons with bleeding disorders and their families in northern Virginia Washington DC and Montgomery and Prince George's Counties in Maryland. This chapter's mission is to improve the quality of life for persons with hemophilia.
Miriam Goldstein, President
Karen Krzmarzick, Executive Director

4868 United Virginia Chapter of the National Hemophilia Foundation
PO Box 188
Midlothian, VA 23113-8824
804-748-7896
800-266-8438
Fax: 800-266-8438
e-mail: info@vahemophilia.org
www.vahemophilia.org

Kelly Waters, Executive Director
Heather Conner, Administrative Assistant

Washington

4869 Bleeding Disorder Foundation of Washington
9639 Firdale Avenue
Edmonds, WA 98020
206-533-1660
Fax: 206-533-1686
e-mail: general@bdfwa.org
www.bdfwa.org

Caprice Sauter, President
Stephanie Simpson, Executive Director

4870 Inland Empire Bleeding Disorders
1010 Riverside Drive
W Richland, WA 99353
509-967-7417
866-710-4323
e-mail: iebd4u@verizon.net
www.hemophilia.org

Debbie Campeau, President
Jill McCary, President

Wisconsin

4871 Great Lakes Hemophilia Foundation
638 N 18th Street
Milwaukee, WI 53233
414-257-0200
888-797-GLHF
Fax: 414-257-1225
e-mail: info@glhf.org
www.glhf.org
The only Wisconsin organization that addresses the physical, emotional social and financial needs of individuals affected by hemophilia. This chapter supports high-quality cost-effective programs for patient care, education, research and public awareness.
Bill Finn, President
Danielle Leitner Baxter, Executive Director

Foundations

4872 National Hemophilia Foundation
116 West 32nd Street
New York, NY 10001
212-328-3700
800-424-2634
Fax: 212-328-3777
e-mail: info@hemophilia.org
www.hemophilia.org
The National Hemophilia Foundation is dedicated to finding better treatments and cures for bleeding and clotting disorders and to preventing the complications of these disorders through education, advocacy and research.
Jorge de la Riva, Chair
Val Bias, Chief Executive Officer

Research Centers

4873 Albany Medican Center
43 New Scotland Avenue
Albany, NY 12208-3479
518-262-3125
800-773-7080
Fax: 518-262-6320
e-mail: albanyhtc@mail.amc.edu
www.amc.edu
Providing excellence in medical education biomedical research and patient care.
Joanne Faunce, President

4874 Albert Einstein Medical Center Hemophilia Program
5501 Old York Road
Philadelphia, PA 19141
215-456-7890
Fax: 215-456-6179
www.einstein.edu
With humanity humility and honor to heal by providing exceptionally intelligent and responsive healthcare and education for as many as we can reach
Barry R Freedman, CEO/ President
John Finger, Chief Administrative Officer

4875 American Red Cross Hemophilia Center
2025 E Street, NW
Washington, DC 20006-0905
202-303-5214
800-733-2767
Fax: 608-233-8318
www.redcross.org

Greg Mandell, CEO
Sandra Fenwick, President

4876 Boston Hemophilia Center Fegan 5 Children's Hospital
Fegan 5 Children's Hospital
300 Longwood Avenue
Boston, MA 02115
617-355-6000
800-355-7944
Fax: 617-730-0152
TTY: 617-730-0152
www.childrenshospital.org
The program offers comprehensive care to people with hemophilia and their families. Our services range from medical treatment counseling and support to discounts on clotting-factor replacement and other products that people with hemophilia require.
Dr James Mandell, CEO
Sandra Fenwick, President

4877 Bowman Grey School of Medicine: Hemophilia Diagnostic Center
Wake Forest University
Department of Pediatrics
Winston Salem, NC 27157-0001
919-716-4324
Fax: 910-716-7100
Christine A MD, Director
Michael Fisher, CEO

4878 Children's Hospital Hemophilia Treatment Center
3333 Burnet Avenue
Cincinnati, OH 45229
513-636-4200
800-344-2462
Fax: 513-636-5599
TTY: 513-636-4900
www.cincinnatichildrens.org
Cincinnati Children's will improve child health and transform delivery of care through fully integrated globally recognized research education and innovation.
Ralph Gruppo Cohen MD, Medical Director

4879 Childrens Hospital of Philadelphia Hemophilia Program
Division of Hematology
34th Street and Civic Center Boulev
Philadelphia, PA 19104
215-590-3437
800-879-2467
Fax: 215-903-92
www.chop.edu
The Children's Hospital of Philadelphia the oldest hospital in the United States dedicated exclusively to pediatrics strives to be the world leader in the advancement of healthcare for children by integrating excellent patient care innovative research and quality professional education into all of its programs.
Leslie J Raffini, Physician
Char Witmer, Physician

4880 Christus Santa Rosa Health System
Children's Hospital

333 N Santa Rosa Street
San Antonio, TX 78207-3108

210-704-2011
877-ALL-KIDZ
Fax: 210-704-2396
www.christussantarosa.org

Patrick Carrier, Presidnent, CEO

4881 Comprehensive Hemophilia Diagnostic and Treatment Center
University of North Carolina
101 Manning Drive
Chapel Hill, NC 27514

919-966-4131
Fax: 919-966-3036
e-mail: lccc@med.unc.edu
www.unchealthcare.org

Multidisciplinary clinics are dedicated to patients with hemophilia (through the Comprehensive Hemophilia Diagnostic and Treatment Center) sickle cell disease brain tumors late effects of anticancer therapy as well as general hematology/oncology.
William RN

4882 Comprehensive Pediatric Hemophilia Center University of South Florida
University of South Florida
450 W Drive
Tampa, FL 33612-4742

813-974-2201

Sara Griggs Kirschke

4883 Eastern Michigan Hemophilia Center St. Joseph Hospital
St. Joseph Hospital
302 Kensington Avenue
Flint, MI 48503-2044

810-762-8656

Leslie RN

4884 Eau Claire Hemophilia Center
900 W Clairemont Avenue
Eau Claire, WI 54701

715-839-4418
Fax: 715-833-4976

Vicky Anders RN, Program Manager

4885 Fairview-University Hemophilia & Thrombosis Center
Harvard Street at E River Road
Minneapolis, MN 55455

612-626-6455
800-688-5252
Fax: 612-625-4955

Serves over 700 adults and children in Minnesota with inherited bleeding disorders. Offers access to current technologies and treatments. Special programs include patient support group family retreats and camps.
Linda Swanso Macfarlane, Director

4886 Great Plains Regional Hemophilia Center University of Iowa Hospitals
University of Iowa Hospitals
200 Howkins Drive
Iowa City, IA 52242

319-384-8442
800-777-8442
Fax: 319-567-59
www.uiowa.edu

Donald E Fahner MD

4887 Greater Grand Rapids Pediatric Hemophilia Program
DeVos at Spectrum Health Systems
100 Michigan NE
Grand Rapids, MI 49503

616-391-2033

James B Trujillo, Financial Administer
W Hoots, Medical Director

4888 Gulf States Hemophilia Diagnostic and Treatment Center
University of Texas Health Science Center Houston
6655 Travis Street
Houston, TX 77030-3005

713-500-8360
800-464-1440
Fax: 713-500-8364
www.livingwithhaemophilia.com

Marisela Thompson, Chief Executive Officer
Joan Curran, Chief Government Relations and External

4889 Gundersen Clinic Comprehensive Hemophilia Treatment Center
Gundersen Clinic
1900 S Avenue
LaCrosse, WI 54601

608-782-7300
800-362-9567
Fax: 608-775-6692
e-mail: info@GundLuth.org
www.gundersenhealth.org/

Jeffrey E Thompson, Chief Executive Officer
Julio Bird, Executive Vice President

4890 Hematology Treatment Center of the Great Lakes Hemophilia Foundation
638 North 18th Street
Milwaukee, WI 53233-2178

414-257-0200
888-797-GLHF
Fax: 414-257-1225
e-mail: info@glhf.org
www.glhf.org

Bill Finn, President
Danielle Leitner Baxter, Executive Director

4891 Hemophilia Association of the Huntington Area
Marshall University School of Medicine
1600 Medical Center Drive
Huntington, WV 25703-1518

304-691-1384
877-691-1600
Fax: 304-691-1375

McKowen, Dean, Vice President
Andrew Tendleton, Medical Director

4892 Hemophilia Center of Central Pennsylvania Penn State Milton S Hershey Medical Cent
Penn State Milton S Hershey Medical Center
500 University Drive
Hershey, PA 17033

717-531-8521
800-243-1455
Fax: 717-310-4021
TTY: 717-531-4395
www.pennstatehershey.org/

Harold L Paz, Chief Executive Officer
Alan L Brechbill, Executive Director

4893 Hemophilia Center of Rhode Island Rhode Island Hospital
Rhode Island Hospital
593 Eddy Street
Providence, RI 02903

401-444-5184
Fax: 401-444-5017
www.rirad.org

Brian Stainken, President
Terrance Healey, Vice-President

4894 Hemophilia Center of West Virginia University Health Sciences Center
University Health Sciences Center
Medical Center Drive
Morgantown, WV 26506

304-293-4229
Fax: 304-293-3793

John S Holmberg, Executive Director
Thomas Long, President

4895 Hemophilia Center of Western New York Erie County Medical Center
Erie County Medical Center
936 Delaware Ave
Buffalo, NY 14209-3021

716-896-2470
866-434-6551
Fax: 716-218-4010
www.hemophiliawny.com

The center provides a variety of services to the hemophilia and HIV/AIDS community. Included among these services are diagnostics registration outpatient treatment home care programs home visits school visits dental services and counseling services. Offers an adult unit and a pediatric unit.
Robert Long, Chairman
Thomas Long, President

4896 Hemophilia Center of the Huntington Hospital
100 W California Boulevard
Pasadena, CA 91105-3023

626-397-5000
www.huntingtonhospital.com

At Huntington our mission is to excel at the delivery of health care to our community.
Stephen Ralph, President and Chief Executive Officer
Jim Noble, Executive Vice President, COO and CFO

4897 Hemophilia Clinic: Childrens' Rehabilitation Service
1870 Pleasant Avenue
Mobile, AL 36617

334-479-8617
800-879-8163
Fax: 334-450-5037
e-mail: djackson@rehab.state.al.us
www.hemophilia.org

Dianna Jackson

4898 Hemophilia Treatment Center at Children's National Medical Center
Department of Hematology/Oncology

111 Michigan Avenue NW
Washington, DC 20010

202-884-3622
Fax: 202-884-2976
www.livingwithhaemophilia.com

Gordon L Cowen, President

4899 Los Angeles Orthopaedic Hospital
2400 S Flower Street
Los Angeles, CA 90007-2629

213-742-1000
Fax: 213-742-1103
e-mail: info@laoh.ucla.edu
www.orthohospital.org

Anthony A Scaduto, M.D, Presirdent, CEO

4900 Louisiana Comprehensive Hemophilia Care Center
1430 Tulane Avenue
New Orleans, LA 70112-2699

504-988-5433
Fax: 504-883-08
e-mail: cleissi@tulane.edu
tulane.edu

Cindy Leissinger, MD, Chief

4901 Maine Hemophilia Treatment Center
19 Bramhall Street
Portland, ME 04102

207-885-7683
Fax: 207-885-7565

Nancy Roy Langstraat, Director

4902 Mayo Comprehensive Hemophilia Center Mayo Clinic
Mayo Clinic
200 1st Street SW
Rochester, MN 55905

507-284-2511
800-660-4582
Fax: 507-284-8286
www.mayoclinic.org/hemophilia/

A World Federation of Hemophilia-designated International Hemophilia Training Center provides multidisciplinary assessment and care of persons with bleeding disorders. Offers consultation with hemotologists specializing in the care of pediatric and adult patients a special consultation laboratory testing center and more.
Harlan ARNP

4903 Miami Comprehensive Hemophilia Center Jackson Medical Towers
Jackson Medical Towers
1500 NW
Miami, FL 33136-3609

305-243-4791
Fax: 305-324-9785

Susan Schmal MD, Head Physician

4904 Michigan State University Hemophilia Comprehensive Care Clinic
Michigan State University
2900 Hannah Boulevard
E Lansing, MI 48823

517-353-9385
800-759-5595
Fax: 517-353-9421

John Penner Gioia RN

4905 Missouri Illinois Regional Hemophilia Comprehensive Treatment Center
3635 Vista Avenue & Grand Boulevard
Saint Louis, MO 63104-1003

314-268-5275
Fax: 314-268-5104

Kathleen P Crist MD, Vice President

4906 Mountain State Regional Hemophilia Center
University of Arizona Health Sciences Center
1501 N Campbell Avenue
Tucson, AZ 85724-0001

520-626-1197
Fax: 520-626-1460
e-mail: phanthourath@ahsc.arizona.edu
www.ahsc.arizona.edu

Anoma Phanthourath, Deputy & Chief of Staff

4907 Nadeene Brunini Comprehensive Hemophilia Care Center
St Michael s Medical Center
197 Route 18 South
East Brunswick, NJ 08816-2011

732-249-6000
Fax: 732-249-7999
e-mail: hemnj@comcast.net
www.hanj.org

Hemophilia and other bleeding disorder treatment center.
Louis

4908 North Dakota Comprehensive Hemophilia Center
Roger Maris Cancer Center
820 4th Street N
Fargo, ND 58122-0001

701-234-7544
800-437-4010
Fax: 701-234-7592

A treatment center for diseases of hemotosis and thrombosis which includes a clinical research program in bleeding disorders. Hemotologists are available for consultation 24 hours a day.

4909 North Dakota Hemostasis and Thrombosis Treatment Center
Roger Maris Cancer Center
820 4th Street N
Fargo, ND 58122-0001

701-234-7544
800-437-4010
Fax: 701-234-7577
www.meritcare.com

A treatment center for diseases of hemotosis and thrombosis which includes a clinical research program in bleeding disorders. Hemotologists are available for consultation 24 hours a day.
Dr Nathan Podolsky MD, President

4910 North Texas Comprehensive Pediatric Hemophilia Center
1935 Motor Street
Dallas, TX 75235-7701

214-456-2382
Fax: 214-456-6133
www.hemophiliaregion6.org

Andrea Johns Steele, President
Ann Gilbert, Director

4911 Northwest Ohio Hemophilia Treatment Center
The Toledo Hospital
2142 N Cove Boulevard
Toledo, OH 43606-3895

419-471-2291
Fax: 412-916-01
www.toledochildrens.org

4912 Oklahoma Comprehensive Hemophilia Diagnostic Treatment Center
940 NE 13th Street
Oklahoma City, OK 73126-0307

405-271-3661
800-688-5288
Fax: 405-271-3756

Beverly Stev Kasper, Hematology
Richard W Cook, Chairman, CEO

4913 Puget Sound Blood Center
921 Terry Avenue
Seattle, WA 98104-1256

206-292-6500
800-398-7888
e-mail: schedule@psbc.org
www.psbc.org

Dr. James P AuBuchon, Presirdent, CEO
David C Fennell, Chief Operating Officer and Chief Inform

4914 Regional Hemophilia Treatment Center Children's Hospital of Michigan
Children's Hospital of Michigan
1921 W. Michigan Avenue
Ypsilanti, MI 48197-2196

734-544-0015
800-482-3041
Fax: 734-544-0095
www.hfmich.org

Carrie Reaume, Executive Director
Suzanne Kapica, Regional Coordinator

4915 Richland Memorial Comprehensive Pediatric Hemophilia Center
Children's Hospital for Cancer & Blood Disorders
7 Richland Medical Park Drive
Columbia, SC 29203

803-434-3533
Fax: 803-434-4598

Daniel Fink, Chief Executive Officer & President

4916 Riley Hemophilia & Hemophilia Center Riley Hospital for Children
Riley Hospital for Children
705 Riley Hospital Drive
Indianapolis, IN 46202-5200

317-944-5000
800-248-1199
Fax: 317-278-0616
e-mail: mheiny@iupui.edu
rileychildrenshospital.com

Jeff Sperring, MD, Presirdent, CEO
Paul R Haut, MD, Chief Medical Officer

4917 SouthWestern Medical Center
University of Texas Southwestern Medical Center
5323 Harry Hines Boulevard
Dallas, TX 75390-7208

214-648-3111
www.utsouthwestern.edu

Daniel K Podolsky, MD, President
J. Gregory Fitz, MD, Executive Vice-President

4918 Southern Tier Hemophilia Center United Health Services-Wilson Hospital
United Health Services-Wilson Hospital
33-57 Harrison Street
Johnson City, NY 13790
607-763-6436
Fax: 607-763-5514
Doris Michal RN

4919 St. Joseph's Hemophilia Center
2927 N 7th Avenue
Phoenix, AZ 85013-4102
602-406-3770
Rachel Stuar MD, Director

4920 Ted R Montoya Hemophilia Program University of New Mexico
University of New Mexico
Albuquerque, NM 87131-0001
505-277-0111
800-225-5866
Fax: 505-272-6845
www.unm.edu

Prasad Mathe Barchi, President

4921 Tennessee Hemophilia and Bleeding Disorder Foundation
1819 Ward Drive
Murfreesboro, TN 37129
615-900-1486
888-703-3269
Fax: 615-900-1487
e-mail: mary@thbdf.org
www.thbdf.org

Kent Russ, President
Mary Hord, Executive Director

4922 The Vanderbilt Hemostasis Clinic
2200 Children's Way
Nashville, TN 37232-9830
615-936-1765
866-372-5663
Fax: 615-936-8400
www.mc.vanderbilt.edu/vhtc
The mission of the Vanderbilt Hemostasis-Thrombosis Clinic is to provide the highest quality compassionate care for individuals with inherited disorders of bleeding or clotting. The team emphasizes the empowerment of patients in their own care while also providing opportunities to participate in scientific advances in the diagnosis and treatment of bleeding and clotting disorders.
Anne T Neff, Director of Hemostasis Clinic
Mary G Hudson, Nurse Coordinator

4923 Thomas Jefferson University: Cardenza Foundation for Hematologic Research
1020 Walnut Street
Philadelphia, PA 19107-5005
215-955-6000
Fax: 215-955-2342
www.jefferson.edu

Robert L Abildgaard MD

4924 Tufts Medical Center
Tufts New England Medical Center
800 Washington Street
Boston, MA 02111-1526
617-636-5000
Fax: 617-636-7738
e-mail: webinfo@tuftsmedicalcenter.org
www.tuftsmedicalcenter.org
Comprehensive care for pediatric and young adult individuals with bleeding and prothrombotic disorders.
Eric Beyer, President and Chief Executive Officer
Michael Wagner, Chief Medical Officer

4925 UCD Northern Central California Hemophilia Program
PO Box 163689
Sacramento, CA 95816-2208
916-448-0370
Fax: 916-489-1569
e-mail: cchfsac@yahoo.com
www.cchfsac.org
An all-volunteer nonprofit organization dedicated to helping people with bleeding disorders.
Sean Hubbert, President
Tracey Huntington, Vice President

4926 UCSD Comprehensive Hemophilia Treatment Center
9500 Gilman Drive
La Jolla, CA 92093
619-471-0336
Fax: 858-822-6444
e-mail: kdherbst@ucsd.edu
hem-onc.ucsd.edu

Sanford J Shattil, M.D., Professor of Medicine
Edward Ball, MD, Professor of Medicine

4927 University Medical Center Hemophilia Program
1800 W Charleston Boulevard
Las Vegas, NV 89102-2329
702-383-2000
www.umcsn.com

Lawrence Weekly, Chair
Chris Giunchigliani, Vice Chair

4928 University Treatment Center of University Hospitals of Cleveland
11100 Euclid Avenue
Cleveland, OH 44106
216-844-8447
888-844-8447
Fax: 216-844-5431
www.uhhospitals.org

Thomas F Zenty III, CEO

4929 University of Cincinnati Adult Hemophilia Treatment Program
231 Bethesda Avenue
Cincinnati, OH 45267-0001
513-558-4233
Fax: 513-558-3878
Kathleen E Coleman, President

4930 University of Michigan Hemophilia Center
1500 E Medical Center Drive
Ann Arbor, MI 48109
734-764-1817
Fax: 734-635-15
www.umich.edu

Mary Sue Hord, Executive Director

4931 Vermont Regional Hemophilia Center
108 Cherry Street
Burlington, VT 05402
802-863-7200
800-464-4343
Fax: 802-865-7754
e-mail: vtadap@vdh.state.vt.us
healthvermont.gov
Provides care to persons with types of bleeding disorders. We see people from Vermont and upstate New York.
Miriam Huste Kinsaul, President, CEO
Emmett Broxson, Director Hemothology

4932 West Central Ohio Hemophilia Center Childens Medical Center
Childens Medical Center
1 Childrens Plaza
Dayton, OH 45404-1815
937-641-3000
800-228-4055
Fax: 937-641-5878
www.childrensdayton.org
The center provides complete care for individuals and families with hemophilia and related bleeding disorders. Some of the services offered include a comprehensive clinic emergency treatment network consultations diagnostic coagulation laboratory home infusion programs HIV/AIDS education and counseling and more.
Elizabeth H Ey, Chair
Deborah Feldman, President/ CEO

Support Groups & Hotlines

4933 National Health Information Center
PO Box 1133
Washington, DC 20013
310-565-4167
800-336-4797
Fax: 301-984-4256
e-mail: info@nhic.org
www.health.gov/nhic
Offers a nationwide information referral service, produces directories and resource guides.

Books

4934 Avoiding Indecision and Hesitation with Hemophilia-Related Emergencies
American Health Consultants
3525 Piedmont Road NE
Atlanta, GA 30305
800-688-2421
Provides detailed information necessary for physicians, and ED staff to deal effectively and expeditiously with hemophilia emergencies.
12 pages

4935 Federal Medicaid Drug Program
1730 E Street NW
Washington, DC 20006-5300
202-628-9292
Discusses changes in government reimbursement and its effect on plasma derived products distributed by the American Red Cross.

Includes law information, individual state billing procedures and Medicaid program coverage for the hemophilia community.

4936 Guide to Insurance Coverage for People with Hemophilia
Armour Pharmaceutical Company
500 Arcola Road   215-454-3720
Collegeville, PA 19426-3930
An educational guide designed to assist with health insurance concerns.

4937 Hemophilia Camp Directory
National Hemophilia Foundation
116 W 32nd Street   212-219-8180
New York, NY 10001-3212   800-424-2634
                              Fax: 212-328-3777
                              www.hemophilia.org
Lists camps in the United States for children with hemophilia and other coagulation disorders.
16 pages
Alan Kinniburgh, PhD, CEO

4938 Procedure Coding for Hemophilia Treatment
Armour Pharmaceutical Company
500 Arcola Road   215-454-3720
Collegeville, PA 19426-3930
Educational guide designed to facilitate the appropriate use of CPT codes for the hemophilia community.

Children's Books

4939 Adventures of Maxx
Nova Factor
1620 Century Centery Parkway   901-348-8129
Memphis, TN 38137   800-424-2634
                              Fax: 901-385-3778
An activity book for children with hemophilia, this publication is intended to be both educational and entertaining.
15 pages

4940 Children's Hemophilia Book
Porton Products Limited
30401 Agoura Road   818-879-2200
Agoura Hills, CA 91301-2006
Coloring book that discusses what hemophilia is, bleeding episodes and treatment from a child's point of view.
25 pages

4941 Harold Talks About How He Inherited Hemophilia
Kentucky Hemophilia Foundation
982 Eastern Parkway   502-634-8161
Louisville, KY 40217-1571   800-582-2873
                              Fax: 502-634-9995
                              e-mail: info@kyhemo.org
                              www.kyhemo.org
Children's brochure explaining hemophilia causes, symptoms and living a regular life.
Ursela M Lacer, Executive Director

4942 Harold's Secret: A Boy with Hemophilia
Bayer
400 Morgan Lane   203-937-2765
West Haven, CT 06516-4175
A comic book for youngsters pertaining to children with hemophilia and understanding of the illness among school friends.
16 pages

4943 Understanding Hemophilia: A Young Person's Guide
Armour Pharmaceuticals Company
500 Arcola Road
Collegeville, PA 19426-3930   800-424-2634
This publication is designed for young persons with hemophilia. Presented in very basic and accessible language, this text with colored illustrations points out what hemophilia is, how to cope and more.
91 pages

Magazines

4944 HEMALOG
Maleria Medica
101 W 23rd Street PMB 2246   212-725-5151
New York, NY 10011-2490   Fax: 212-725-2794
                              e-mail: hemalog@hotmail.com
The purpose of Hemalog is to serve as a national forum for the hemophilia community, providing current news, information, opinion and contact with others in the community. The material contained in this journal reflects the experience and opinion of a wide range of people connected with hemophilia and encourages story and art contributions.
36 pages Quarterly
Barbara Robin Slonevsky, Publisher
Janet Spencer-King, Editor-in-Chief

4945 HemAware
National Hemophilia Foundation
116 W 32nd Street   888-463-6643
New York, NY 10001-3212   800-424-2634
                              Fax: 212-328-3777
                              www.hemophilia.org
NHF magazine that offers treatment news about bleeding disorders and provides comprehensive articles on the latest developments in treatment and research as well as highlighting new programs and new resources in the field.
Bi-Monthly
Alan Kinniburgh, PhD, CEO

4946 Human Factor
Hemophilia Health Services
6820 Charlotte Pike
Nashville, TN 37209-4206   800-800-6606
This journal is provided as a free service for the purpose of informing, educating and empowering the hemophilia community.
Quarterly

Newsletters

4947 Artery
Hemophilia Foundation of Michigan
230 1 Platt Road   734-761-2535
Ann Arbor, MI 48103-2973   800-482-3041
                              Fax: 734-975-2889
                              www.hfmich.org
Offers information on the chapter's activities and events, support groups and hotlines, technical and medical updates pertaining to the hemophilia and HIV/AIDS community.
Quarterly
Susan Lerch, Editor

4948 Big Red Factor
National Hemophilia Foundation: Nebraska
215 Centennial Mall South   402-742-5663
Lincoln, NE 68508   Fax: 402-742-5677
                              e-mail: office@nebraskanhf.org
                              www.nebraskanhf.org/chapter/
Chapter newsletter offering legislative and medical updates, technology, resources, assistive devices and more for persons affected by hemophilia and other blood disorders.

4949 Bloodlines
Hemophilia Association of San Diego County
3570 Camoni del Rio N   619-325-3570
San Diego, CA 92108   Fax: 619-325-4350
                              www.hasdc.org
Updates membership on the newest techniques and technologies on the treatment of hemophilia.
Quarterly
Jessica Swann, Executive Director
Teresa Ramirez, Coordinator Member Services

4950 Concentrate
Hemophilia of North Carolina
2 Centerview Drive   919-852-4788
Greensboro, NC 27407-3708

Offers information on summer camps, resources, book reviews, parent information and articles pertaining to hemophilia.
Monthly

4951 Factor Nine News
Coalition for Hemophilia B
225 W 34th Street
New York, NY 10122
212-628-3445
Fax: 212-554-6906
e-mail: cfb@web-depot.com
www.boygenius.com/cfb
Offers information on FDA approvals, annual meetings and the latest in technology and information regarding hemophilia.
Kimberly Phelan, VP

4952 Hemophilia NewsBriefs
Great Lakes Hemophilia Foundation
638 North 18th Street
Milwaukee, WI 53233
414-257-0200
Fax: 414-257-1225
e-mail: info@glhf.org
www.glhf.org

4953 Infusion
Kentuckian Hemophilia Foundation
982 Eastern Parkway
Louisville, KY 40217-1571
510-634-8161
800-582-CURE
Fax: 510-568-6111
e-mail: officeinfo@HFNonline.org
www.hfnconline.org
Offers information on summer camps, association activities and events, national projects touching on hemophilia and HIV related disorders and articles on the newest breakthroughs and technology for fighting bleeding disorders.
Quarterly

4954 Initiatives
Quantum Health Resources
790 The City Drive S
Orange, CA 92868-4941
714-750-1610
Aimed at keeping patients and other interested individuals informed on important economic trends, legislation and medical issues.
Quarterly

4955 Linking Factor
National Hemophila Foundation: Utah Chapter
340 E 400 S
Salt Lake City, UT 84111-2909
800-800-6606
A newsletter offering chapter association news and information.
BiMonthly
Charles Hand, Executive Director
Linda Aagard, Editor

4956 New England Hemophilia Association Newsletter
180 Rustcraft Road
Dedham, MA 02026-4558
781-326-7645
800-228-6342
e-mail: neha@world.std.com
www.newenglandhemophilia.org
New England Hemophilia Association is dedicated to improving the quality of life for persons with bleeding disorders (hemophilia, von Williebrands, and other factor deficiencies) and their families through education, support and advocacy. NEHA is a chapter of the National Hemophilia Foundation.
Quarterly
Catherine I Cornell, Executive Director

4957 TN Hemo & Bleeding Disorders Foundation Newsletter
TN Hemo & Bleedin Disorders Foundation
203 Jefferson Street
Smyrna, TN 37167-5281
615-220-4868
888-703-3269
Fax: 615-220-4889
e-mail: mary@thbdf.org
www.thbdf.org

3x/year
Mary Hord, Executive Director
H Kent Russ, President

4958 Ways & Means
Quantum Health Resources
790 The City Drive S
Orange, CA 92868-4941
714-750-1610

Features pertinent health care information for hemophilia patients and their families.
Quarterly

4959 Infusion
Northern California Chapter of the NHF
7700 Edgewater Drive
Oakland, CA 94621-3023
650-568-NCHF
Informs members of medical, dental and orthopedic treatment advances and the latest research in the field. Helps to keep people with hemophilia and their families aware of relevant local and national meetings and includes important updates regarding research and treatment.
BiMonthly

Pamphlets

4960 Anyone Can Have a Bleeding Problem
Hemophilia Foundation of Michigan
411 Huronview Boulevard
Ann Arbor, MI 48103-2973
734-761-2535
800-482-3041
Offers information on Hemophilia and Von Willebrand's Disease. How persons can get it, prevention and causes of the illnesses.

4961 Article Reprint Exchange
HANDI-The National Hemophilia Foundation
116 W 32nd Street
New York, NY 10001-3212
212-219-8180
800-424-2634
Fax: 212-328-3777
Offers various reprinted articles concerning hemophilia and the newest medical technology.

4962 Basics of HIV Disease: Questions and Answers
National Hemophilia Foundation
116 W 32nd Street
New York, NY 10001-3212
888-463-6643
800-424-2634
Fax: 212-328-3777
www.hemophilia.org
This publication contains basic information about hemophilia and HIV disease.
1992 28 pages
Alan Kinniburgh, PhD, CEO

4963 Clotting Agents Are Lifesavers
Hemophilia Foundation of Michigan
411 Huronview Boulevard
Ann Arbor, MI 48103-2973
734-761-2535
Offers information on what hemophilia is, treatments, occurances, heredity, Von Willebrand's Disease, patient services and direct services for hemophiliacs and HIV/AIDS patients.

4964 Comprehensive Care
National Hemophilia Foundation
116 W 32nd Street
New York, NY 10001-3212
888-463-6643
800-424-2634
Fax: 212-328-3777
www.hemophilia.org
Discusses the nature of comprehensive care and its functions and defines the care team. Also touches upon essential resources, HIV, and the benefits of comprehensive care.
1991 12 pages
Alan Kinniburgh, PhD, CEO

4965 Comprehensive Services for Persons with Hemophilia
Hemophilia Foundation of Minnesota/Dakotas
2304 Park Avenue
Minneapolis, MN 55404-3712
612-871-3340
Fax: 612-871-1359
Offers information on what hemophilia is and information and resources for persons with hemophilia and other bleeding disorders.

4966 Consumer Bill of Rights and Responsibilities for Healthcare Service
National Hemophilia Foundation
116 W 32nd Street
New York, NY 10001-3212
888-463-6643
800-424-2634
Fax: 212-328-3777
www.hemophilia.org

Serves as a set of goals for both the provider and consumer in seeking, providing, and receiving high quality health care within a setting of honesty and respect.
1994
Alan Kinniburgh, PhD, CEO

4967 Countdown to a Cure
Louisiana Hemophilia Foundation
3636 S Sherwood Forest Boulevard 225-291-1675
Baton Rouge, LA 70816-2285 Fax: 225-291-1679
e-mail: lahemophilia@hipoint.net
www.louisianahemophilia.org/
Offers information on chapter resources and services for hemophiliacs and their families. Offers information and services to families/patients affected by bleeding disorders.
Lori Keels, Executive Director

4968 Fight Hemophilia with Facts Not Fiction
Great Lakes Hemophilia Foundation
638 North 18th Street 414-257-0200
Milwaukee, WI 53233 Fax: 414-257-1225
www.glhf.org
Offers information on what hemophilia is, research information and treatments.

4969 Get Real and Be Safe!
National Hemophilia Foundation
116 W 32nd Street 888-463-6643
New York, NY 10001-3212 800-424-2634
Fax: 212-328-3777
www.hemophilia.org
Comic book style, this pamphlet offers information to young adults on the hazards and precautions of sex. Offers an Ask The Doctor question and answer section to books and resources for young adults on safer sex and HIV/AIDS.
1991 14 pages
Alan Kinniburgh, PhD, CEO

4970 Guidelines for Finding Childcare
National Hemophilia Foundation
116 W 32nd Street 888-463-6643
New York, NY 10001-3212 800-424-2634
Fax: 212-328-3777
www.hemophilia.org
Information for parents on how to hire a good babysitter, information on daycare centers, how to tell daycare staff about hemophilia, cooperative childcare and suggested reading for parents.
1987 10 pages
Alan Kinniburgh, PhD, CEO

4971 HIV Disease in People with Hemophilia: Your Questions Answered
National Hemophilia Foundation
116 W 32nd Street 888-463-6643
New York, NY 10001-3212 800-424-2634
Fax: 212-328-3777
www.hemophilia.org
Discusses hemophilia and HIV disease, AIDS, management of HIV disease, risks to sexual partners, and issues for children with hemophilia.
1991 48 pages
Alan Kinniburgh, PhD, CEO

4972 HIV Infection and Hemophilia
Hemophilia Foundation of Illinois
332 S Michigan Avenue 312-427-1495
Chicago, IL 60604-4434
Offers information on HIV/AIDS relating to persons with hemophilia.

4973 Hemophilia: Current Medical Management
National Hemophilia Foundation
116 W 32nd Street 888-463-6643
New York, NY 10001-3212 800-424-2634
Fax: 212-328-3777
www.hemophilia.org

Provides an overview of all aspects of hemophilia treatment, including prophylaxis, home therapy, inhibitors, orthopedic solutions, surgery, and dental care.
1994 30 pages
Alan Kinniburgh, PhD, CEO

4974 How to Control Bleeds: Inspired by Vince, an 8-year-old Boy with Hemophilia
Bayer
400 Morgan Lane 203-937-2765
West Haven, CT 06516-4175
An educational comic book story by Vince about hemophilia and treatment for bleeds.
26 pages

4975 Living with HIV: Talking with Your Child
Bobbie Steinhart, author
National Hemophilia Foundation
116 W 32nd Street 888-463-6643
New York, NY 10001-3212 800-424-2634
Fax: 212-328-3777
www.hemophilia.org
A pamphlet directed at caregivers of young children living with hemophilia and HIV disease.
1990 8 pages
Alan Kinniburgh, PhD, CEO

4976 Mild Hemophilia
National Hemophilia Foundation
116 W 32nd Street 888-463-6643
New York, NY 10001-3212 800-424-2634
Fax: 212-328-3777
www.hemophilia.org
Defines mild hemophilia and details its discovery, diagnosis, inheritance, symptoms, treatment, and activity limitations.
1994 25 pages
Alan Kinniburgh, PhD, CEO

4977 Participating in a Clinical Trial: Your Life, Your Choice
National Hemophilia Foundation
116 W 32nd Street 888-463-6643
New York, NY 10001-3212 800-424-2634
Fax: 212-328-3777
www.hemophilia.org
This brochure explains what clinical trials are and what they are like for patients, describes what kinds of HIV therapies are being tested in clinical trials, and lists questions to ask before joining a trial. This publication is ideal for patients, their families, and/or healthcare personnel who counsel HIV-positive patients.
1994 6 pages
Alan Kinniburgh, PhD, CEO

4978 Physical Therapy in Hemophilia
Nationa Hemophilia Foundation
110 Greene Street 212-328-3700
New York, NY 10012-3832 800-424-2634
Fax: 212-328-3777
www.hemophilia.org
Targeted at physical therapy students or new therapists at comprehensive hemophilia care clinics. Also provides basic treatment care information for persons with hemophilia and their families.
1986 13 pages

4979 Simple & Complex: A Hemophilia Primer
Western Pennsylvania Chapter of the NHF
580 S Aiken Avenue 412-685-2231
Pittsburgh, PA 15232-1531 Fax: 412-683-2568
Offers information on what hemophilia is, explains AIDS and HIV infection, offers information on the treatments for hemophilia and what hemophilia care costs.

4980 Student with Hemophilia: A Resource for the Educator
National Hemophilia Foundation
116 W 32nd Street 888-463-6643
New York, NY 10001-3212 800-424-2634
Fax: 212-328-3777
www.hemophilia.org

Written for teachers, nurses, and other school personnel, this booklet aims to dispel the myths and fears surrounding hemophilia.
1995 16 pages
Alan Kinniburgh, PhD, CEO

4981 Treatment of Hemophilia: Current Orthopedic Management
Marvin Gilbert, Jerome Wiedel, author

National Hemophilia Foundation
116 W 32nd Street   888-463-6643
New York, NY 10001-3212   800-424-2634
                                    Fax: 212-328-3777
                                     www.hemophilia.org
Covers a wide range of orthopedic treatment issues, including hemophilic arthropathy, clinical considerations, diagnostic imaging, surgical and nonsurgical treatments, hemophilic synovitis, soft-tissue bleeding, the hemophilia pseudotumor, fracture care, other musculoskelatal problems, and HIV infections.
1995 25 pages
Alan Kinniburgh, PhD, CEO

4982 Understanding Hepatitis
Leonard Seeff, Maribel Johnson, author

National Hemophilia Foundation
116 W 32nd Street   888-463-6643
New York, NY 10001-3212   800-424-2634
                                    Fax: 212-328-3777
                                     www.hemophilia.org
Provides comprehensive information about viral hepatitis for people with bleeding disorders, their caregivers, and families. Discusses the different hepatitis viruses, viral transmissions, how the liver is affected by hepatitis, blood product concerns, prevention, diagnosis, treatment, and psychosocial issues.
1997 24 pages
Alan Kinniburgh, PhD, CEO

4983 Von Willebrand Disease: A Guide for Patients and Families
Hemophilia Health Services
6820 Charlotte Pike
Nashville, TN 37209-4206   800-800-6606
Offers information on this disease, explains the causes, treatments, prevention and offers resources and books.

4984 What Is Hemophilia?
Hemophilia Foundation of Georgia
8800 Roswell Road   770-518-8272
Atlanta, GA 30328-1689   800-866-4366
                                    Fax: 770-518-3310
                                 e-mail: hog@america.net
                                         www.hog.org
Offers information on what hemophilia is, common factors in hemophilia, the cost and treatments offered to hemophiliacs and more.

4985 What Women Should Know About HIV Infection AIDS and Hemophilia
Hemophilia Foundation of Illinois
332 S Michigan Avenue   312-427-1495
Chicago, IL 60604-4434
For spouses/partners of men with hemophilia and women with bleeding disorders. Provides information about HIV/AIDS and how it affects women in the hemophilia community.
25 pages

4986 What You Should Know About Hemophilia
National Hemophilia Foundation
116 W 32nd Street   888-463-6643
New York, NY 10001-3212   800-424-2634
                                    Fax: 212-328-3777
                                     www.hemophilia.org
Defines hemophilia, explains its effects, and provides a historical overview of treatment and treatment complications.
1991 13 pages
Alan Kinniburgh, PhD, CEO

4987 Who Will Tell Them of Your Special Needs?
MedicAlert
2323 Colorado Avenue
Turlock, CA 95382-2018   800-432-5378

Offers information on MedicAlert bracelets, personal identification medical information needed for treatment in case of emergency.

Audio & Video

4988 Song of Superman
National Hemophilia Foundation
116 W 32nd Street   888-463-6643
New York, NY 10001-3212   800-424-2634
                                    Fax: 212-328-3777
                                     www.hemophilia.org
Designed to help young people with bleeding disorders come to terms with their HIV status, sexuality, and living with HIV. The video explores issues of disclosure in relationships and safer sex through dramatic scenes and frank testimonials by young people living with hemophilia and/or HIV. The companion workbook contains group exercises that follow each of the main topics of the video and serve as a bridge to discussion.
1993 49 pages
Alan Kinnibrugh, PhD, CEO

4989 Treat Yourself to a Brighter Future - It's Time to Hit the Freedom Trail
c/o Hemophilia Association of the Capital Area
10560 Main Street   703-352-7641
Fairfax, VA 22030-7182   Fax: 703-352-2145
                              e-mail: info@hacacares.org
                          www.hacacares.org/ed_publist.html
A booklet and videotape published by the American Red Cross providing a list of required supplies and equipment for self-infusion concentrates for persons with hemophilia A. It is an instructional piece for home self-infusion and concise text and illustrations depict seven steps for self-infusion.
20 pages Video & Booklet
Keith Bushey, President
Cliff Krug Jr, Vice President

Web Sites

4990 American Red Cross Blood Services
                          www.redcross.org/services/biomed
Distributes a wide variety of plasma therapeutics to benefit people with hemophilia A and B, immune disorders and hypoalbuminemia.

4991 Healing Well
                                     www.healingwell.com
An online health resource guide to medical news, chat, information and articles, newsgroups and message boards, books, disease-related web sites, medical directories, and more for patients, friends, and family coping with disabling diseases, disorders, or chronic illnesses.

4992 Health Finder
                                      www.healthfinder.gov
Searchable, carefully developed web site offering information on over 1000 topics. Developed by the US Department of Health and Human Services, the site can be used in both English and Spanish.

4993 Healthlink USA
                                     www.healthlinkusa.com
Health information concerning treatment, cures, prevention, diagnosis, risk factors, research, support groups, email lists, personal stories and much more. Updated regularly.

4994 Helios Health
                                      www.helioshealth.com
Online resource for your health information. Detailed information about specific health topics, access to expert advice from our Medical Advisory Board, and up-to-date health news.

4995 MedicineNet
                                       www.medicinenet.com
An online resource for consumers providing easy-to-read, authoritative medical and health information.

4996 Medscape

www.medscape.com

Medscape offers specialists, primary care physicians, and other health professionals the Web's most robust and integrated medical information and educational tools.

4997 National Hemophilia Foundation

www.hemophilia.org

Information on the treatment and the cure of hemophilia, related bleeding disorders and complications of those disorders or their treatment, including HIV infection, as well as improving the quality of life of all those affected.

4998 WebMD

www.webmd.com

Information on Hemophilia, including articles and resources.

Description

4999 Hepatitis

Hepatitis, or inflammation of the liver, has multiple causes and several stages. Hepatitis is usually caused by viruses or by excess alcohol consumption. Less common causes include prescription medications, accidental poisoning, and auto-immune diseases in which the body attacks its own liver.

The severity of the disease is highly variable. At an early stage, hepatitis may cause no symptoms, vague mild symptoms, or overwhelming disease. Early symptoms include vague abdominal pain, jaundice, fever, loss of appetite and nausea. If the disease becomes chronic, it may lead to irreversible scarring, or cirrhosis, which causes weakness, fatigue and weight loss. Late stage disease includes fluid accumulation in the abdominal cavity, gastrointestinal bleeding and mental changes. Abdominal pain and liver enlargement are generally present. Advanced cirrhosis is a risk factor for cancer of the liver.

There are four major kinds of viral hepatitis. Type A is very common world-wide, is spread by contaminated food and water, and generally causes a mild to moderately severe illness that runs its course over several weeks and disappears without further damage. Type B is also very common, and is spread by bodily fluids, generally through blood transfusion, sexual intercourse, sharing of needles or contaminated items like shaving razors and tattoo needles. The disease may resolve without further consequences, but frequently becomes chronic and may lead to cirrhosis as well as chronic infections. Hepatitis C is also spread through blood transfusion and needle sharing. Although it is not usually severe at onset, it can lead to the same serious consequences as type B. Finally, there is a type D, which is spread by blood products, and only infects people who already have Type B. Type D is associated with a more severe course.

Prevention of any of these forms of viral hepatitis depends on avoiding the usual routes of transmission. In addition, there is an effective vaccine available for hepatitis B. Close family contacts of persons with this disease should receive the vaccine if they have not yet received it as part of routine childhood immunization.

Treatment of hepatitis is largely supportive, but antiviral drugs and interferon are used in certain stages of Type B and Type C infection. End-stage or overwhelming infection may necessitate liver transplantation. See also *Liver Disease*.

National Agencies & Associations

5000 American Hepatitis Association
133 E 58th Street
New York, NY 10022
212-753-8068

Conducts educational and prevention programs concerning hepatitis provides screening and vaccines and offers support groups for individuals with hepatitis.
Gerberding, MD, Director

5001 Centers for Disease Control and Prevention Hepatitis Branch
1600 Clifton Road
Atlanta, GA 30333
404-639-2709
800-232-4636
TTY: 888-232-6348
www.cdc.gov/ncidod/diseases/hepatitis
Monitors the rates of viral hepatitis in the United States; provides epidemiologic assistance for outbreaks of viral hepatitis; coordinates and implements epidemiologic studies to define the risk factors for acute and chronic viral hepatitis; provides viral hepatitis reference/diagnostic services; serves as the World Health Organization Collaborating Center for Reference and Research on Viral Hepatitis.
Julie Louise Foy, Contact
Judy Greenspan, Contact

5002 HIV/Hepatitis C in Prison (HIP) Committee
California Prison Focus
San Francisco, CA 94103
510-665-1935
e-mail: contact@prisons.org
www.prisons.org/hivin
The HIV/HCV in Prison Committee of California Prison Focus works on behalf of prisoners to fight for consistent access to quality medical care including access of all new HIV and hepatitis C medications, diagnostic testing and combination therapies.
Michelle Wexler MD, Executive Director
Diane C Peterson, Associate Director for Immunization

5003 Hepatitis Foundation International
504 Blick Drive
Silver Spring, MD 20904-2901
301-879-6891
800-891-0707
Fax: 301-879-6890
e-mail: info@hepatitisfoundation.org
www.hepfi.org
Grassroots support network for persons with viral hepatitis. Provides education about the prevention diagnosis and treatment of viral hepatitis as well as phone network support and various literature.
Thelma King Thiel, CEO
Theodore Karrison, Vice-Chairman

5004 Immunization Action Coalition
1573 Selby Avenue
Saint Paul, MN 55104
651-647-9009
Fax: 651-647-9131
e-mail: admin@immunize.org
www.immunize.org
The mission of the Immunization Action Coalition is to boost immunization rates and prevent disease. The coalition promotes physician, community and family awareness of and responsibility for appropriate immunization of all children and adults against all diseases.
Deborah L Wexler, MD, Executive Director
Litjen Tan, MS, PhD, Chief Strategy Officer

5005 Inter-Provincial Roof Consultants, Ltd.
5828 176th Street
Surrey, BC V3S 4-6J9
604-576-5740
800-616-2437
Fax: 604-576-5790
e-mail: inbox@iprc.ca
www.iprc.ca
Through partnerships and collaboration, will work to reduce the incidence of new HIV/AIDS/HEP C and other blood borne pathogens and to improve the quality of life for those infected and affected.
Sean M Lang, President/Owner/Chief Consultant/Spec Wr
Mike Kosman, Consultant/Spec Writer/Roof Observer

5006 National Hepatitis C Coalition
PO Box 5058
Hemet, CA 92544
951-766-8238
e-mail: mail@nationalhepatitis-c.org
www.nationalhepatitis-c.org
The National Hepatitis C Coalition is a 501(c)(3) tax exempt organization that relies on private donations from good folks like you in order to continue helping others with hepatitis C.
Patty Krueger, Co-Founder

Foundations

5007 Hepatitis B Foundation
3805 Old Easton Road
Doylestown, PA 18902
215-489-4900
Fax: 215-489-4313
e-mail: info@hepb.org
www.hepb.org
We are dedicated to finding a cure and improving the quality of life for those affected by hepatitis B worldwide. Our commitment includes funding focused research, promoting disease awareness, supporting immunization and treatment initiatives, and serving as the primary source of information for patients and their families, the medical and scientific community, and the general public.

Joel Rosen, Chairman, Esq
Timothy M Block, PhD, President

Libraries & Resource Centers

5008 Hepatitis Education Project
911 Western Avenue
Seattle, WA 98104
206-732-0311
Fax: 206-732-0312
e-mail: hep@scn.org
www.hepeducation.org
The mission of the Hepatitis Education Project is to help raise awareness among patients, medical personnel and the public of the facts concerning hepatitis patients and the resources available to help those who live with the disease.
Steve Graham, President
Michael Ninburg, Executive Director

Support Groups & Hotlines

5009 Christ Hospital Hepatitis C Support Group
Christ Hospital
176 Palisade Avenue
Jersey City, NJ 07306
201-795-1230
e-mail: dkatz65717@aol.com
For anyone interested in becoming advocates for increasing awareness of this illness.
Graham, President
Michael Ninburg, Executive Director

5010 Hepatitis Education Project
911 Western Avenue
Seattle, WA 98104
206-732-0311
e-mail: hepinfo@hepeducation.org
www.hepeducation.org
Helps raise awareness among patients, medical personeel and the public of the facts concerning hepatitis patients and the resources available to help those who live with the disease
Steve Graham, President
Michael Ninburg, Executive Director

5011 National Health Information Center
PO Box 1133
Washington, DC 20013
310-565-4167
800-336-4797
Fax: 301-984-4256
e-mail: info@nhic.org
www.health.gov/nhic
Offers a nationwide information referral service, produces directories and resource guides.
Borden, NE Regional Contact

Books

5012 Hepatitis B Prevention: A Resource Guide
National Digestive Diseases Info. Clearinghouse
2 Information Way
Bethesda, MD 20824
301-654-3810
800-891-5389
Fax: 301-907-8906
e-mail: nddic@info.niddk.uih.goc
www.niddk.nih.gov
Designed to assist health care and other professionals who work in planning or administering hepatitis B prevention programs.
252 pages

5013 Understanding Hepatitis
James L Achord, MD, author
University Press of Mississippi
3825 Ridgewood Road
Jackson, MS 39211-6492
601-432-6205
Fax: 601-432-6217
e-mail: kburgess@ihl.state.ms.us
www.upress.state.ms.us
For general readers a comprehensive discussion of the causes and of the treatments of hepatitis.
2002 152 pages Paperback
ISBN: 1-578064-36-8
Kathy Burgess, Advertising/Marketing Services Manager

5014 Viral Hepatitis: Scientific Basis and Clinical Management
Churchill Livingstone
PO Box 3188
Secaucus, NJ 07096-3188
201-319-9800
800-553-5426
Fax: 201-319-9659
www.harcourt-international.com/cl/
1997 800 pages Hardcover
ISBN: 0-443057-97-4

Magazines

5015 Hepatitis Magazine
Quality Publishing Services
523 N Sam Houston Parkway E
Houston, TX 77060
281-272-2744
800-310-7047
Fax: 281-847-5440
e-mail: info@hepatitismag.com
www.hepatitismag.com
Magazine for those with hepatitis. Price listed is for a one year subscription.
Quarterly
Barbara Veres, Publisher
Geoff Drushel, Editor

Newsletters

5016 American Liver Foundation: Progress Newsletter
75 Maiden Lane
New York, NY 10038-4826
212-668-1000
800-465-4837
Fax: 212-483-8179
e-mail: info@liverfoundation.org
www.liverfoundation.org
The American Liver Foundation is the nation's leading nonprofit organization promoting liver health and disease prevention. ALF provides research education and sdvocacy for those affected by liver-related diseases, including hepatitis
8 pages 2 per year
Sarah Wilson Brown, Manager Marketing/Communications

5017 B Connected
3805 Old Easton Road
Doylestown, PA 18902
215-489-4900
Fax: 215-489-4313
e-mail: info@hepb.org
www.hepb.org
Features practical health tips, frequently asked questions, and other useful information for patients and families to live well with chronic hepatitis B. Available in both print and online versions.
3x/year
Molli Conti, Chair
Timothy Block, PhD, Founder/President

5018 B-Informed Newsletter
Hepatitis B Foundation
3805 Old Easton Road
Doylestown, PA 18902
215-489-4900
Fax: 215-489-4920
e-mail: info@hepb.org
www.hepb.org
Includes a Drug Watch of approved and experimental therapies for Hepatitis B, reasearch updates, Foundation news and events, and feature articles on special topics. Available in print and online.
Molli C. Conti, Executive Director

5019 Hepatitis Alert
Hepatitis Foundation International (HFI)

30 Sunrise Terrace
Cedar Grove, NJ 07009-1423

973-239-1035
800-891-0707
Fax: 973-875-5044
e-mail: hfi@intac.com
www.hepfi.org

Provides information for the public, patients, educators, and medical professionals about the diagnosis, treatment, and prevention of viral hepatitis.

5020 Hepatitis B Coalition News
Hepatitis B Coalition
1573 Selby Avenue
Saint Paul, MN 55104-6328

651-647-9009
Fax: 651-647-9131
e-mail: admin@inmunize.org

Newsletter with brochures, articles, videotapes, audio-cassette tapes and manuals for different ethnic populations.

5021 NEEDLE TIPS & the Hepatitis B Coalition News
Hepatitis B Coalition
1573 Selby Avenue
St. Paul, MN 55104-6328

651-647-9009
Fax: 651-647-9131
e-mail: admin@immunize.org
www.immunize.org

Information on immunization for health professionals.
28 pages 2x Year
Deborah L Wexler

5022 VACCINATE ADULTS! Coalition News
Hepatitis B Coalition
1573 Selby Avenue
St. Paul, MN 55104-6328

651-647-9009
Fax: 651-647-9131
e-mail: admin@immunize.org
www.immunize.org

Information on immunization: adult medicine specialist.
12 pages 2x Year
Deborah L Wexler MD

Pamphlets

5023 Advice to Parents of Children with HBV
Hepatitis B Foundation
3805 Old Easton Road
Doylestown, PA 18902

215-489-4900
Fax: 215-489-4920
e-mail: info@hepb.org
www.hepb.org

Provides information to people affected by hepatitis B and their loved ones. Current HBV research, telephone numbers, and a medical glossary.
Molli C. Conti, Executive Director

5024 Caring for Your Liver
Hepatitis Foundation International (HFI)
30 Sunrise Terrace
Cedar Grove, NJ 07009-1423

973-239-1035
800-891-0707
Fax: 973-875-5044
e-mail: hfi@intac.com
www.hepfi.org

Information for the person with hepatitis.

5025 Caution! Treating Children with Acetaminophen
Hepatitis Foundation International (HFI)
30 Sunrise Terrace
Cedar Grove, NJ 07009-1423

973-239-1035
800-891-0707
Fax: 973-875-5044
e-mail: hfi@intac.com
www.hepfi.org

Information on hepatitis.

5026 Chronic Viral Hepatitis Backgrounder
Schering Corporation
Kenilworth, NJ 07033

908-298-4000
www.sch-plough.com

Offers information and statistics on viral hepatitis.

5027 Cirrhosis: Many Causes
American Liver Foundation

1425 Pompton Avenue
Cedar Grove, NJ 07009-1000

800-223-0179
Fax: 973-256-3214
e-mail: info@liverfoundation.org
www.liverfoundation.org

Gives basic facts about cirrhosis including causes, signs, symptoms and treatments.
Rick Smith, President & CEO
Rebecca Frank, Chief Development Officer

5028 Diagnosis and Treatment
Hepatitis Foundation International (HFI)
30 Sunrise Terrace
Cedar Grove, NJ 07009-1423

973-239-1035
800-891-0707
Fax: 973-875-5044
e-mail: hfi@intac.com
www.hepfi.org

Information for the person with hepatitis.

5029 Health Insurance
Hepatitis Foundation International (HFI)
30 Sunrise Terrace
Cedar Grove, NJ 07009-1423

973-239-1035
800-891-0707
Fax: 973-875-5044
e-mail: hfi@intac.com
www.hepfi.org

Information on hepatitis and health insurance.

5030 Helpful Tips for Carriers of HBV
Hepatitis Foundation International (HFI)
30 Sunrise Terrace
Cedar Grove, NJ 07009-1423

973-239-1035
800-891-0707
Fax: 973-875-5044
e-mail: hfi@intac.com
www.hepfi.org

Information for people with Hepatitis B.

5031 Hepatitis
National Institute of Allergy & Infectious Disease
31 Center Drive
Bethesda, MD 20892-0001

301-496-4000
www.niaid.nih.gov/default.htm

A pamphlet discussing the cause, symptoms, transmission, diagnosis, tests, prevention and the latest research on Hepatitis.

5032 Hepatitis A and B Vaccination
Hepatitis Foundation International (HFI)
30 Sunrise Terrace
Cedar Grove, NJ 07009-1423

973-239-1035
800-891-0707
Fax: 973-875-5044
e-mail: hfi@intac.com
www.hepfi.org

Information on hepatitis vaccination.

5033 Hepatitis A, B & C
Hepatitis Foundation International (HFI)
30 Sunrise Terrace
Cedar Grove, NJ 07009-1423

973-239-1035
800-891-0707
Fax: 973-875-5044
e-mail: hfi@intac.com
www.hepfi.org

Information for the person with hepatitis.

5034 Hepatitis A, B & C: Liver Disease You Should Know About
American Liver Foundation
1425 Pompton Avenue
Cedar Grove, NJ 07009

800-465-4837
Fax: 973-256-3214
e-mail: info@liverfoundation.org
www.liverfoundation.org

Explains viral hepatitis, transmission, symptoms, testing and acute chronic hepatitis.
Rick Smith, President & CEO
Rebecca Frank, Chief Development Officer

5035 Hepatitis B Prevention
National Center For Infectious Diseases
Hepatitis Branch
Atlanta, GA 30333

404-332-4555

Explains what hepatitis B is, what behaviors are risky and how to protect oneself against it.

5036   Hepatitis Fact Sheet

www.cdc.gov/ncidod/diseases/hepatitis/c
Offers information on the causes, symptoms, prevention and treatments for hepatitis.

5037   How Many Times a Day Do You Risk Being Infected with Hepatitis B?
American Liver Foundation
1425 Pompton Avenue
Cedar Grove, NJ 07009   800-465-4837
                                        Fax: 973-256-3214
                            e-mail: info@liverfoundation.org
                                    www.liverfoundation.org
A flyer emphasizing the importance of vaccination against hepatitis B.
Rick Smith, President & CEO
Rebecca Frank, Chief Development Officer

5038   Is Your Liver Giving You the Silent Treatment?
Hepatitis Foundation International (HFI)
30 Sunrise Terrace   973-239-1035
Cedar Grove, NJ 07009-1423   800-891-0707
                                        Fax: 973-875-5044
                                    e-mail: hfi@intac.com
                                            www.hepfi.org
Provides information for patients with hepatitis.

5039   Living with Hepatitis C: Self Help Tips
Hepatitis Foundation International (HFI)
30 Sunrise Terrace   973-239-1035
Cedar Grove, NJ 07009-1423   800-891-0707
                                        Fax: 973-875-5044
                                    e-mail: hfi@intac.com
                                            www.hepfi.org
Information for people with Hepatitis C.

5040   Protect Yourself and Those You Love Against HBV
Hepatitis B Foundation
3805 Old Easton Road   215-489-4900
Doylestown, PA 18902   Fax: 215-489-4920
                                    e-mail: info@hepb.org
                                            www.hepb.org
Provides information to people affected by hepatitis B and their loved ones.
Molli C. Conti, Executive Director

5041   Q and A: Hepatitis B Prevention
SmithKline Beecham Pharmaceuticals
1 Franklin Plaza   215-751-4000
Philadelphia, PA 19102-1282
Informational booklet written for healthcare personnel by the manufacturer of Engerix-B vaccine, reviews hepatitis B prevention.

5042   Someone You Know Has Hepatitis B
Hepatitis B Foundation
3805 Old Easton Road   215-489-4900
Doylestown, PA 18902   Fax: 215-489-4920
                                    e-mail: info@hepb.org
                                            www.hepb.org
Provides information to people affected by hepatitis B and their loved ones.
Molli C. Conti, Executive Director

5043   Tips on Coping with Chronic Hepatitis
Hepatitis Foundation International (HFI)
30 Sunrise Terrace   973-239-1035
Cedar Grove, NJ 07009-1423   800-891-0707
                                        Fax: 973-875-5044
                                    e-mail: hfi@intac.com
                                            www.hepfi.org
Information for people with hepatitis.

5044   Viral Hepatitis: Everybody's Problem?
American Liver Foundation
1425 Pompton Avenue
Cedar Grove, NJ 07009-1000   800-223-0179
                                        Fax: 973-256-3214
                            e-mail: info@liverfoundation.org
                                    www.liverfoundation.org

Covering a broad range of topics including: a definition of the disease, descriptions of types of infections, transmission, symptoms, treatment options and prevention of hepatitis.
Rick Smith, President & CEO
Rebecca Frank, Chief Development Officer

5045   What Health Care Workers Should Know About Hepatitis B
Channing L Bete Company
200 State Road
South Deerfield, MA 01373   800-628-7733
Presents information in easy-to-read, simple English for health care workers about hepatitis B.
15 pages

Audio & Video

5046   Hepatitis B Video
Hepatitis B Foundation
3805 Old Easton Road   215-489-4900
Doylestown, PA 18902   Fax: 215-489-4920
                                    e-mail: info@hepb.org
                                            www.hepb.org
Provides information to people affected by hepatitis B and their loved ones.
Molli C. Conti, Executive Director

5047   Hepatitis C: A Viral Mystery
Terry Strauss, Stephen Steady, author

Fanlight Productions
4196 Washington Street   617-469-4999
Boston, MA 02131-1731   800-937-4113
                                        Fax: 617-469-3379
                            e-mail: fanlight@fanlight.com
                                        www.fanlight.com
This timely video is about living with a serious, chronic illness. In addition to discussing the medical treatments available, the video also explores alternatives which appear to help some people.
2000 30 Minutes
ISBN: 1-572953-08-X

Web Sites

5048   HIV/Hepatitis C in Prison (HIP) Committee

www.prisons.org/hivin.htm
Fighting for consistent access to quality medical care including access to all new HIV and Hepatitis C medications, diagnostic testing and combination therapies.

5049   Healing Well

www.healingwell.com
An online health resource guide to medical news, chat, information and articles, newsgroups and message boards, books, disease-related web sites, medical directories, and more for patients, friends, and family coping with disabling diseases, disorders, or chronic illnesses.

5050   Health Finder

www.healthfinder.gov
Searchable, carefully developed web site offering information on over 1000 topics. Developed by the US Department of Health and Human Services, the site can be used in both English and Spanish.

5051   Healthlink USA

www.healthlinkusa.com
Health information concerning treatment, cures, prevention, diagnosis, risk factors, research, support groups, email lists, personal stories and much more. Updated regularly.

5052   Healthy Lives

www.healthylives.com/hepatitis

5053   Helios Health

www.helioshealth.com
Online resource for your health information. Detailed information about specific health topics, access to expert advice from our Medical Advisory Board, and up-to-date health news.

5054 Hepatitis B Coalition

www.immunize.org

Works to prevent transmission of hepatitis B in high-risk groups; to promote HBsAG screening for all pregnant women; to achieve vaccination of all infants, children, and adolescents; and to promote education and treatment for the person who is chronically infected with hepatitis B.

5055 Hepatitis Information Network

www.hepnet.com

5056 MedicineNet

www.medicinenet.com

An online resource for consumers providing easy-to-read, authoritative medical and health information.

5057 Medscape

www.medscape.com

Medscape offers specialists, primary care physicians, and other health professionals the Web's most robust and integrated medical information and educational tools.

5058 WebMD

www.webmd.com

Information on hepatitis, including articles and resources.

Description

5059 # Hydrocephalus

The normal brain and spinal cord are surrounded with a watery substance called cerebro-spinal fluid, CSF, which collects within the brain in several larger pools called ventricles, connected to one another through tiny channels. The CSF is formed in some of these ventricles, circulates widely and is eventually reabsorbed. If CFS production exceeds reabsorption, or if the fluid is blocked from circulating and it may build up pressure that expands the ventricles and presses on the normal brain tissue, causing hydrocephalus, or water on the brain.

Hydrocephalus can cause change in behavior, headache, visual loss, vomiting and weakness. Hydrocephalus may be congenital, that is, present from birth. If it occurs in a child whose skull bones have not yet fused together, it may cause the head to enlarge.

In adults whose brains are encased in the rigid skull, there is no room to expand and pressure builds up in the brain. Excess CSF may be in response to infection such as meningitis or to blockage of CSF movement by tumor. Treatment and outlook depend on the underlying cause. Medical therapy may cause limited temporary improvement. Surgical treatment may be able to correct the underlying cause. If it cannot, the surgeon may still give substantial relief by placing a shunt which allows extra CSF to drain from the ventricles to some other part of the body.

National Agencies & Associations

5060 **Association of Hydrocephalus Education Advocacy & Discussion (AHEAD)**
1730 Autumn Leaf Lane   215-355-4728
Huntingdon Valley, PA 19006-1515
Organized by young adults with hydrocephalus for the purpose of providing telephone support nationwide.
Lane Fischetti, Founder
Jamie Fischetti, Secretary

5061 **Guardians of Hydrocephalus Research Foundation**
2618 Avenue Z   718-743-4473
Brooklyn, NY 11235-2023   Fax: 718-743-1171
e-mail: ghrf2618@aol.com
www.ghrforg.org
Non-profit organization made up of concerned parents and dedicated volunteers. The goal is to wipe out this top ranking birth defect.
Michael Kranz, Director of Research
Pip Marks, Director of Support & Education

5062 **Hydrocephalus Association Hydrocephalus Association**
Hydrocephalus Association
4340 East West Highway   301-202-3811
Bethesda, MD 20814   888-598-3789
Fax: 301-202-3813
e-mail: info@hydroassoc.org
www.hydroassoc.org
The association provides support education and advocacy for families and professionals. The goal is to insure that families and individuals dealing with the complexities of hydrocephalus receive personal support, comprehensive educational materials and outreach.
Barrett O'Connor, Chair
Dawn Mancuso, Chief Executive Officer

5063 **Hydrocephalus Foundation**
910 Rear Broadway   781-942-1161
Saugus, MA 01906   e-mail: HyFII@netscape.net
www.hydrocephalus.org
Dedicated to providing support educational resources and networking opportunities to patients and families affected by hydrocephalus. The Foundation also promotes related research and facilitates the training of healthcare professionals to improve patient care.
Greg A Tocco, Founder & Executive Director
Michael Tocco R.Ph., M.Ed., President

5064 **National Hydrocephalus Foundation**
12413 Centralia Road   562-924-6666
Lakewood, CA 90715   888-857-3434
Fax: 562-924-6666
e-mail: debbifields@nhfonline.org
www.nhfonline.org
The foundation is a national organization with almost 30 years of history. We provide information and education along with peer-to-peer support a physician referral sheet along with patient and family comments and several different types of help sheets.
Michael Fields, President
Debbi Fields, Executive Director

5065 **Spina Bifida & Hydrocephalus Association of Nova Scotia**
15 Laura Drive   902-679-1124
Nova Scotia, B3G 1-1B6   800-304-0450
Fax: 902-679-1433
e-mail: info@sbhans.ca
www.sbhans.ca
It is a non-profit, registered charitable organization affiliated with the Spina Bifida and Hydrocephalus Association of Canada, and currently has one chapter in Cape Breton.

5066 **Spina Bifida & Hydrocephalus Association o f Ontario**
555 Richmond Street West   416-214-1056
Toronto, Ontario, M5V 3-3B1   800-387-1575
Fax: 416-214-1446
e-mail: provincial@sbhao.on.ca
www.sbhao.on.ca/
It is a non-profit registered charitable organization affiliated with the Spina Bifida and Hydrocephalus Association of Canada and currently has one chapter in Cape Breton.
Marc Garson, Chair
Joan Booth, Executive Director

5067 **The Kidney Foundation of Canada**
300-5165 Sherbrooke Street W   514-369-4806
Montreal, QC H4A 1-1T6   800-361-7494
Fax: 514-369-2472
e-mail: info@kidney.ca
www.kidney.ca
A national volunteer organization committed to reducing the burden of kidney disease through: funding and stimulating innovative research; providing education and support; promoting access to high quality healthcare; and increasing public awareness and commitment to advancing kidney health and organ donation.
Dr Julian Midgley, President
Andrew MacRitchie, Treasurer

5068 **World Hypertension League**
Medical University of Ohio   419-383-5270
Toledo, OH 43614-5809   Fax: 419-383-3120
e-mail: gmonhollen@meduohio.edu
hsc.utoledo.edu
Devoted to the advancement of hypertension prevention and control through joint efforts of all national leagues and societies.
Lloyd A Gross, Chairman
Raymond Moser, Vice Chairman

State Agencies & Associations

Maryland

5069 Hydrocephalus Association
4340 East West Highway
Bethesda, MD 20814
301-202-3811
888-598-3789
Fax: 301-202-3813
e-mail: info@hydroassoc.org
www.hydroassoc.org
Founded in 1976 this group was formed as a group of concerned families and patients with hydrocephalus to share information and experiences in dealing with this disease locally and nationwide.
Barrett O'Connor, Chair
Dawn Mancuso, Chief Executive Officer

Michigan

5070 Hydrocephalus Support Group of Michigan Children's Hospital of Michigan
Children's Hospital of Michigan
3901 Beaubien
Detroit, MI 48201
313-745-5437
Fax: 313-993-8744
Founded in 1992 this group provides information to families and gives them support.
Mary Smellie

Pennsylvania

5071 Hydrocephalus Association of Philadelphia
PO Box 2099
Boothwyn, PA 19061-8099
610-497-0375
Fax: 610-497-2836
Founded in 1992 the Association provides support information advocacy and telephone support to families in Pennsylvania New Jersey and Delaware.
Halmi, Director

Rhode Island

5072 Hydrocephalus Association of Rhode Island
PO Box 343
Valley Falls, RI 02864-0343
401-723-6065
Founded in 1993 the mission of this Association is to provide information support and advocacy for individuals with hydrocephalus and for friends and family members.
Gabriella Pike, President

Texas

5073 Hydrocephalus Association of North Texas
PO Box 670552
Dallas, TX 74637-0552
214-528-2877
http://nhfonline.org/treatment.php?id=or
Founded in 1987 the mission is to provide information and support to parents of children with hydrocephalus in the state of Texas and neighboring states.
Beverly Pozzi

Washington

5074 Children's Hydrocephalus Support Group
PO Box 1611
Woodinville, WA 98072
425-482-0479
e-mail: lpoliski@hydrosupport.org
www.hydrosupport.org
Founded in 1993 the group of Seattle provides support to individuals with hydrocephalus.
Lori Poliski, Co-Founder
Paul Gross, Co-Founder

Support Groups & Hotlines

5075 Hydrocephalus Parents Support Group
1325 Louis Street
Manville, NJ 08835
908-722-4691
Founded in 1993, the group provides support for parents of children with hydrocephalus.
Andrea

5076 National Health Information Center
PO Box 1133
Washington, DC 20013
310-565-4167
800-336-4797
Fax: 301-984-4256
e-mail: info@nhic.org
www.health.gov/nhic
Offers a nationwide information referral service, produces directories and resource guides.
Sansone, Executive Director
Mary Trifault, Executive Associate

Books

5077 Hydrocephalus: A Guide for Patients, Families, and Friends
O'Reilly and Associates
101 Morris Street
Sebastopol, CA 95472
800-998-9938
Fax: 707-829-0104
e-mail: order@oreilly.com
www.oreilly.com
Hydrocephalus: A Guide for Patients, Families, and Friends provides individuals and families with the guidance, information and support needed to make the right decisions at the right time.
350 pages Paperback
ISBN: 1-565924-10-X

5078 Spina Bifida Association of America: Insights into Spina Bifida
Spina Bifida Association of America
4590 MacArthur Boulevard NW
Washington, DC 20007-4226
202-944-3285
800-621-3141
Fax: 202-944-3295
e-mail: sbaa@sbaa.org
www.sbaa.org
News on medical, legislative and education topics relevant to individuals with spina bifida.
bi-monthly
Marybeth Leamyini, Communications Director

Children's Books

5079 Loving Ben
Delacorte
1540 Broadway
New York, NY 10036-4039
212-354-6500
This is a moving story of a sister who cares for her baby brother and tries to help him learn despite his birth defects and deteriorating health.
Grades 7-10

Newsletters

5080 Alliance of Genetic Support Groups
35 Wisconsin Circle
Chevy Chase, MD 20815
202-331-0942
800-336-4363
A coalition of voluntary genetic support groups, consumers and professionals addressing the needs of individuals and families affected by genetic disorders from a national perspective.

5081 Hydrocephalus Association Newsletter
Hydrocephalus Association
870 Market Street
San Francisco, CA 94102-2912
415-732-7040
888-598-3789
Fax: 415-732-7044
e-mail: info@hydroassoc.org
www.hydroassoc.org
Offers information on association news, conference articles, meetings, support and educational groups.
12 pages Quarterly
Dory Kranz, Executive Director
Pip Marks, Director Outreach Services

5082 Hydrocephalus Parents Support Group Newsletter
1325 Louis Street
Manville, NJ 08835
908-722-4691

Founded in 1993, the group provides support for parents of children with hydrocephalus.
Andrea Liptak, Founder

5083 Hydrocephalus Support Group Newsletter
PO Box 4236   636-532-8228
Chesterfield, MO 63005-4236   Fax: 314-995-4108
e-mail: hydrodb@earthlink.net
Founded in 1986, this group provides information, education and support to anyone dealing with hydrocephalus.
Debby Buffa, Founder/Chairman

5084 National Hydrocephalus Foundation Newsletter
12413 Centrailia Road   562-402-3523
Lakewood, CA 90715-1623   888-857-3434
Fax: 562-924-6666
e-mail: hydrobrat@earthlink.net
nhfonline.org
Founded in 1979, the foundation is a national organization whose purpose is to provide information and education, along with peer support newsletter quarterly. Group meeting quarterly in Long Beach, CA. $35 a year.
Quarterly
Debbie Fields, Executive Director

5085 New York University Medical Center Auxiliary of Tisch Hospital
560 1st Avenue
New York, NY 10016   212-263-5040
www.nyukidshealth.org
Conducts national symposiums on hydrocephalus.
Doris Farrelly, Contact

Pamphlets

5086 About Hydrocephalus: A Book for Families
Hydrocephalus Association
870 Market Street   415-732-7040
San Francisco, CA 94102-2912   888-598-3789
Fax: 415-732-7044
e-mail: info@hydroassoc.org
www.hydroassoc.org
A booklet in either English or Spanish, detailing all aspects of hydrocephalus from diagnosis and treatment to complications and follow-up care.
36 pages Paperback
Dory Kranz, Executive Director
Pip Marks, Director Outreach Services

5087 About Normal Pressure Hydrocephalus: A Book for Adults & Their Families
Hydrocephalus Association
870 Market Street   415-732-7040
San Francisco, CA 94102-2912   888-598-3789
Fax: 415-732-7044
e-mail: info@hydroassoc.org
www.hydroassoc.org
Booklet discusses the diagnosis and treatment of adult-onset normal pressure hydrocephalus.
24 pages Paperback
Dory Kranz, Executive Director
Pip Marks, Director Outreach Services

5088 Directory of Neurosurgeons Who Treat Adults
Hydrocephalus Association
870 Market Street   415-732-7040
San Francisco, CA 94102-2912   888-598-3789
Fax: 415-732-7044
e-mail: info@hydroassoc.org
www.hydroassoc.org
Names and addresses of neurosurgeons who treat adult-onset normal pressure hydrocephalus and adult-acquired hydrocephalus, listed alphabetically and geographically.
Dory Kranz, Executive Director
Pip Marks, Director Outreach Services

5089 Directory of Pediatric Neurosurgeons
Hydrocephalus Association

870 Market Street   415-732-7040
San Francisco, CA 94102-2912   888-598-3789
Fax: 415-732-7044
e-mail: info@hydroassoc.org
www.hydroassoc.org
Names and addresses of more than 200 neurosurgeons who specialize in pediatrics, listed alphabetically and geographically.
Dory Kranz, Executive Director
Pip Marks, Director Outreach Services

5090 Endoscopic Third Ventriculotomy
Hydrocephalus Association
870 Market Street   415-732-7040
San Francisco, CA 94102-2912   888-598-3789
Fax: 415-732-7044
e-mail: info@hydroassoc.org
www.hydroassoc.org
Series includes information on primary care, learning disabilities, eye problems, social skills development, headaches, endoscopic third ventriculostomy, shunts and more.
Dory Kranz, Executive Director
Pip Marks, Director Outreach Services

5091 Eye Problems Associated with Hydrocephalus in Children
Hydrocephalus Association
870 Market Street   415-732-7040
San Francisco, CA 94102-2912   888-598-3789
Fax: 415-732-7044
e-mail: info@hydroassoc.org
www.hydroassoc.org
Series includes information on primary care, learning disabilities, eye problems, social skills development, headaches, endoscopic third ventriculostomy, shunts and more.
Dory Kranz, Executive Director
Pip Marks, Director Outreach Services

5092 Fact Sheet: Hydrocephalus
Hydrocephalus Association
870 Market Street   415-732-7040
San Francisco, CA 94102-2912   888-598-3789
Fax: 415-732-7044
e-mail: info@hydroassoc.org
www.hydroassoc.org
Available in Spanish.
Dory Kranz, Executive Director
Pip Marks, Director Outreach Services

5093 Headaches and Hydrocephalus
Hydrocephalus Association
870 Market Street   415-732-7040
San Francisco, CA 94102-2912   888-598-3789
Fax: 415-732-7044
e-mail: info@hydroassoc.org
www.hydroassoc.org
Series includes information on primary care, learning disabilities, eye problems, social skills development, headaches, endoscopic third ventriculostomy, shunts and more.
Dory Kranz, Executive Director
Pip Marks, Director Outreach Services

5094 Hospitalization Tips
Hydrocephalus Association
870 Market Street   415-732-7040
San Francisco, CA 94102-2912   888-598-3789
Fax: 415-732-7044
e-mail: info@hydroassoc.org
www.hydroassoc.org
1997
Dory Kranz, Executive Director
Pip Marks, Director Outreach Services

5095 How to Be an Assertive Parent on the Treatment Team
Hydrocephalus Association
870 Market Street   415-732-7040
San Francisco, CA 94102-2912   888-598-3789
Fax: 415-732-7044
e-mail: info@hydroassoc.org
www.hydroassoc.org
Dory Kranz, Executive Director
Pip Marks, Director Outreach Services

5096 ID Card for Third Ventriculostomy Patients
Hydrocephalus Association
870 Market Street   415-732-7040
San Francisco, CA 94102-2912   888-598-3789
                              Fax: 415-732-7044
                     e-mail: info@hydroassoc.org
                              www.hydroassoc.org

Dory Kranz, Executive Director
Pip Marks, Director Outreach Services

5097 LINK Directory Information
Hydrocephalus Association
870 Market Street   415-732-7040
San Francisco, CA 94102-2912   888-598-3789
                              Fax: 415-732-7044
                     e-mail: info@hydroassoc.org
                              www.hydroassoc.org
A nationwide network of individuals listed in directory format giving members direct access to others in similar circumstances.
Dory Kranz, Executive Director
Pip Marks, Director Outreach Services

5098 Learning Disabilities in Children with Hydrocephalus
Hydrocephalus Association
870 Market Street   415-732-7040
San Francisco, CA 94102-2912   888-598-3789
                              Fax: 415-732-7044
                     e-mail: info@hydroassoc.org
                              www.hydroassoc.org
Available in Spanish.
Dory Kranz, Executive Director
Pip Marks, Director Outreach Services

5099 Nonverbal Learning Disorder Syndrome
Hydrocephalus Association
870 Market Street   415-732-7040
San Francisco, CA 94102-2912   888-598-3789
                              Fax: 415-732-7044
                     e-mail: info@hydroassoc.org
                              www.hydroassoc.org
1998
Dory Kranz, Executive Director
Pip Marks, Director Outreach Services

5100 Prenatal Hydrocephalus: A Book for Parents
Hydrocephalus Association
870 Market Street   415-732-7040
San Francisco, CA 94102-2912   888-598-3789
                              Fax: 415-732-7044
                     e-mail: info@hydroassoc.org
                              www.hydroassoc.org

Dory Kranz, Executive Director
Pip Marks, Director Outreach Services

5101 Resource Guide
Hydrocephalus Association
870 Market Street   415-732-7040
San Francisco, CA 94102-2912   888-598-3789
                              Fax: 415-732-7044
                     e-mail: info@hydroassoc.org
                              www.hydroassoc.org
A comprehensive listing of 450 articles on all aspects of hydrocephalus. Articles may be ordered from the association for a small fee.
Dory Kranz, Executive Director
Pip Marks, Director Outreach Services

5102 Resource Guide: Normal Pressure Hydrocephalus/Adult Onset
Hydrocephalus Association
870 Market Street   415-732-7040
San Francisco, CA 94102-2912   888-598-3789
                              Fax: 415-732-7044
                     e-mail: info@hydroassoc.org
                              www.hydroassoc.org

Dory Kranz, Executive Director
Pip Marks, Director Outreach Services

5103 Social Skills Development in Children with Hydrocephalus
Hydrocephalus Association

870 Market Street   415-732-7040
San Francisco, CA 94102-2912   888-598-3789
                              Fax: 415-732-7044
                     e-mail: info@hydroassoc.org
                              www.hydroassoc.org

Dory Kranz, Executive Director
Pip Marks, Director Outreach Services

5104 Survival Skills for the Family Unit
Hydrocephalus Association
870 Market Street   415-732-7040
San Francisco, CA 94102-2912   888-598-3789
                              Fax: 415-732-7044
                     e-mail: info@hydroassoc.org
                              www.hydroassoc.org

Dory Kranz, Executive Director
Pip Marks, Director Outreach Services

5105 Understanding Your Child's Education Needs/Individualized Education Program
Hydrocephalus Association
870 Market Street   415-732-7040
San Francisco, CA 94102-2912   888-598-3789
                              Fax: 415-732-7044
                     e-mail: info@hydroassoc.org
                              www.hydroassoc.org

Dory Kranz, Executive Director
Pip Marks, Director Outreach Services

Audio & Video

5106 Hydrocephalus: A Neglected Disease
Guardians of Hydrocephalus Research Foundation
2618 Avenue Z   718-743-4473
Brooklyn, NY 11235-2023   Fax: 718-743-1171
                        e-mail: ghrf2618@aol.com
                        www.homestead.com/ghrf.html

Marie Fischetti, Founder

Web Sites

5107 Healing Well
                              www.healingwell.com
An online health resource guide to medical news, chat, information and articles, newsgroups and message boards, books, disease-related web sites, medical directories, and more for patients, friends, and family coping with disabling diseases, disorders, or chronic illnesses.

5108 Health Finder
                              www.healthfinder.gov
Searchable, carefully developed web site offering information on over 1000 topics. Developed by the US Department of Health and Human Services, the site can be used in both English and Spanish.

5109 Healthlink USA
                              www.healthlinkusa.com
Health information concerning treatment, cures, prevention, diagnosis, risk factors, research, support groups, email lists, personal stories and much more. Updated regularly.

5110 Helios Health
                              www.helioshealth.com
Online resource for your health information. Detailed information about specific health topics, access to expert advice from our Medical Advisory Board, and up-to-date health news.

5111 Hydrocephalus Association
                              www.hydroassoc.org
Provides support, education and advocacy for families and professionals. The goal is to insure that families and individuals dealing with the complexities of hydrocephalus receive personal support, comprehensive educational materials and on-going medical care.

5112 Hydrocephalus Center
                              www.patientcenters.com/hydrocephalus
An online reference that was created especially as a resource for those with hydrocephalus and their families.

5113 MedicineNet

www.medicinenet.com

An online resource for consumers providing easy-to-read, authoritative medical and health information.

5114 Medscape

www.medscape.com

Medscape offers specialists, primary care physicians, and other health professionals the Web's most robust and integrated medical information and educational tools.

5115 Neurology Channel

www.neurologychannel.com

Find clearly explained, medically accurate information regarding conditions, including an overview, symptoms, causes, diagnostic procedures and treatment options. On this site it is possible to ask questions and get information from a neurologist and connect to people who have similar health interests.

5116 WebMD

www.webmd.com

Information on hydrocephalus, including articles and resources.

Description

5117 ## Hypertension

Hypertension is an abnormal elevation of blood pressure. Blood pressure is noted as a top number (systolic) over a bottom number (diastolic) with a reading of 120/80 being recognized as normal. Hypertension is defined as a systolic pressure greater than 140 and/or a diastolic pressure greater than 90. It is a common disorder that affects about 20 percent of the population. Primary, or essential, hypertension is the most common form, and it has no known cause. It is more prevalent in African-Americans, males, and those with a family history of high blood pressure. Other risk factors include obesity, diabetes, high levels of fat and cholesterol, smoking, sedentary lifestyle and psychological stress. It is a significant risk factor for coronary heart disease, heart failure, stroke, and kidney failure.

Patients with hypertension generally have no symptoms. Diagnosis is made by simple measurement with a blood pressure cuff. Several measurements are necessary at different times to establish the diagnosis.

Treatment of hypertension is done in a step-wise fashion beginning with lifestyle modifications (weight reduction, regular exercise, smoking cessation, a low salt, fat and cholesterol diet and improved stress reduction.) If medications are necessary, doctors can choose from a wide variety of effective and usually well-tolerated drugs. Therapy generally must be lifelong.

Occasionally the blood pressure may be refractory, or difficult to control with medicines. In this instance, screening is needed for unusual causes of hypertension, such as renovascular disease (narrowing of the arteries feeding the kidneys), hyperaldosteronism (a tumor or overgrowth of the adrenal gland which secretes hormones that raise the blood pressure), or aortic coarctation (a congenital malformation of the major blood vessels near the heart.) If no specifically treatable cause is identified, the patient will require combination therapy with high doses of drugs. Given a commitment to doing so, it is almost always possible to control the pressure.

National Agencies & Associations

5118 **American Society of Hypertension**
45 Main Street
Brooklyn, NY 11201
212-696-9099
Fax: 347-916-0267
e-mail: ash@ash-us.org
www.ash-us.org
To organize and conduct educational seminars, materials and products in all aspects of hypertension and other cardiovascular diseases.
William B White, President
Torry Mark Sansone, Executive Director

5119 **National Heart, Lung & Blood Institute**
PO Box 30105
Bethesda, MD 20824-0105
301-592-8573
Fax: 301-592-8563
TTY: 240-629-3255
e-mail: nhlbiinfo@nhlbi.nih.gov
www.nhlbi.nih.gov

Primary responsibility of this organization is the scientific investigation of heart, blood vessel, lung and blood disorders. Oversee research, demonstration, prevention, education and training activities in these fields and emphasizes the control of stroke.
Gary H Gibbons, MD, Director

5120 **National Hypertension Association**
324 E 39th Street
New York, NY 10016
212-889-3557
Fax: 212-447-7032
e-mail: nathypertension@aol.com
www.nathypertension.org
Conducts research on the cause of hypertension through basic laboratory and clinical studies sponsors seminars and symposia to keep the medical profession and public abreast of services and advances in the treatment of hypertension.
William M Manger, MD, PhD, Chairman

5121 **National Stroke Association**
9707 E Easter Lane
Centennial, CO 80112-3747
303-649-9299
800-787-6537
Fax: 303-649-1328
e-mail: Info@stroke.org
www.stroke.org
A national organization whose sole purpose is to reduce the incidence and impact of stroke through prevention treatment rehabilitation and research and support for stroke survivors and their families. NSA produces a variety of education materials and other support services.
Michael D Walker, MD, Chairman
James Baranski, CEO

5122 **Pulmonary Hypertension Association**
801 Roeder Road
Silver Spring, MD 20910
301-565-3004
800-748-7274
Fax: 301-565-3994
e-mail: pha@PHAssociation.org
www.PHAssociation.org
A nonprofit organization for pulmonary hypertension patients families caregivers and PH-treating medical professionals. The mission of the Pulmonary Hypertension Association (PHA) is to find ways to prevent and cure pulmonary hypertension.
Vallerie McLaughlin, MD, Chair
Rino Aldrighetti, President & CEO

5123 **Sentry Health Monitors**
200 East Randolph
Chicago, IL 60601
877-446-3743
Fax: 301-476-9388
e-mail: lcreasman@sentryhealthmonitors.com
www.lifeclinic.com
The lifeclinic.com web site was developed to provide an in-depth resource for information about prevalent, long-term health conditions and an online service to track your health over time. It also provides the information, resources and tools that can help patients and their families.
Leslie Creasman, Manager of Customer Service

Research Centers

5124 **Creighton University Midwest Hypertension Research Center**
601 N 30th Street
Omaha, NE 68131-2137
402-280-4507
Fax: 402-280-4101
Dr William PhD, Director

5125 **Hahnemann University: Division of Surgical Research**
230 N Broad Street
Philadelphia, PA 19102
215-762-7000
866-884-4HUH
Fax: 215-762-8109
www.hahnemannhospital.com
Studies hypertension and management of stress ulcers.
Teuro Matsum Carretero, Division Head
William H Beierwaltes, Scientist

5126 **Henry Ford Hospital: Hypertension and Vascular Research Division**
2799 W Grand Boulevard
Detroit, MI 48202-2689
313-972-1693
Fax: 313-876-1479
e-mail: ocarret1@hfhs.org
www.hypertensionresearch.org

Basic biomedical research seeks to understand: The role of vaso-constrictors and vasodilators (angiotensin II bradykinin nitric oxide natriuretic peptides) in the regulation of blood pressure development of hypertension and development of target organ damage (myocardial infarction heart failure vascular injury and renal disease); The generation of reactive oxygen species by blood vessels and kidney cells and how this contributes to target organ damage; and The mechanisms by which therape
William H Beierwaltes, Ph.D., Faculty
Oscar A Carretero, Faculty

5127 Indiana University: Hypertension Research Center
425 University Boulevard   317-274-4591
Indianapolis, IN 46202-0001   800-274-4862
                                              Fax: 317-278-0673
                                              www.indiana.edu/medical
The mission of the Center is to conduct research in the causes diagnosis treatment and prevention of high blood pressure and its complications.
Dr Myron Rom MPH, Director
Eric Schips, Divisional Administrator

5128 New York University General Clinical Research Center
NYU Medical Center
550 First Avenue   212-263-7300
New York, NY 10016   Fax: 212-263-8501
                                              www.med.nyu.edu
Focuses in the areas of hypertension and studies into endocrinology.
Robert I Grossman, MD, Dean & CEO
Steven B Abramson, MD, Senior Vice President and Vice Dean for

5129 University of Michigan: Division of Hypertension
1500 E Medical Center   734-615-0863
Ann Arbor, MI 48109   855-855-0863
                                              www.med.umich.edu
Excellence in medical education patient care and research.
Douglas L Stoulil, Study Coordinator

5130 University of Minnesota: Hypertensive Research Group
611 Beacon Street SE   612-624-1438
Minneapolis, MN 55455
Research pertaining to hypertension and stress disorders.
Jack Massry, Head

5131 University of Southern California: Division of Nephrology
2025 Zonal Avenue   323-442-5100
Los Angeles, CA 90033-1034   Fax: 213-226-3958
                                              www.usc.edu/health/internal/divisions/ne
Research into hypertension and sleep disorders.
Gbemisola A Adeseun, MD, MPH, Faculty
Vito M Campese, MD, Faculty

5132 University of Virginia: Hypertension and Atherosclerosis Unit
Medical Center   804-924-8470
Charlottesville, VA 22908-0001   Fax: 804-924-2581
Dr Carlos DVM, Director

5133 Wake Forest University: Arteriosclerosis Research Center
Department of Comparative Medicine
300 S Hawthorne Road   336-764-3600
Winston-Salem, NC 27103-2732   Fax: 336-764-5818
Hypertension research.
Thomas Clark

Support Groups & Hotlines

5134 National Health Information Center
PO Box 1133   310-565-4167
Washington, DC 20013   800-336-4797
                                              Fax: 301-984-4256
                                              e-mail: info@nhic.org
                                              www.health.gov/nhic
Offers a nationwide information referral service, produces directories and resource guides.

Books

5135 Courage: Poems & Positive Thoughts for Stroke Survivors
National Stroke Association
9707 E Easter Lane   303-649-9299
Englewood, CO 80112-3747   800-787-6537
                                              Fax: 303-649-1328
                                              www.stroke.org
Words of inspiration from survivors and caregivers.
83 pages
Colette Lafosse, Director Rehabilitation/Recovery Program

5136 Discovery Circles
National Stroke Association
9707 E Easter Lane   303-649-9299
Englewood, CO 80112-3747   800-787-6537
                                              Fax: 303-649-1328
                                              www.stroke.org
NSA's guide to organizing and facilitating stroke support groups. This detailed manual describes the support group structure and the facilitator's role.
213 pages
Colette Lafosse, Director Rehabilitation/Recovery Program

5137 Magic of Humor in Caregiving
National Stroke Association
9707 E Easter Lane   303-649-9299
Englewood, CO 80112-3747   800-787-6537
                                              Fax: 303-649-1328
                                              www.stroke.org
A dynamic researching tool focusing on the necessity of humor in daily caregiving interaction.
Colette Lafosse, Director Rehabilitation/Recovery Program

5138 Management of Hypertension
EMIS Medical Publishers
PO Box 1607   580-924-0643
Durant, OK 74702-1607   800-225-0694
                                              Fax: 580-924-9414

ISBN: 0-929240-62-6

5139 November Days
National Stroke Association
9707 E Easter Lane   303-649-9299
Englewood, CO 80112-3747   800-787-6537
                                              Fax: 303-649-1328
                                              www.stroke.org
A caregiver's story of her struggle with a loved one's stroke.
225 pages

5140 Ted's Stroke: The Caregiver's Story
National Stroke Association
9707 E Easter Lane   303-649-9299
Englewood, CO 80112-3747   800-787-6537
                                              Fax: 303-649-1328
                                              www.stroke.org
Personal experiences, guidance and tips for caregivers.
175 pages
ISBN: 0-962487-61-9

5141 Women in Your Life: Protect Yourself, Protect Your Family
National Stroke Association
9707 E Easter Lane   303-649-9299
Englewood, CO 80112-3747   800-787-6537
                                              Fax: 303-649-1328
                                              www.stroke.org
Valuable information about the unique toll stroke takes on women.
Colette Lafosse, Director Rehabilitation/Recovery Program

Magazines

5142 American Journal of Hypertension
American Society of Hypertension
515 Madison Avenue   212-644-0650
New York, NY 10022   Fax: 212-644-0658
                                              e-mail: ash@ash-us.org
                                              www.ash-us.org

5143 Ethnicity & Disease
International Society on Hypertension in Blacks
2045 Manchester Street NE   404-875-6263
Atlanta, GA 30324-4110   Fax: 404-875-6334
e-mail: member@ishib.org
www.ishib.org
International journal on ethnic minority population differences in diesae patterns. Provides a comprehensive source of information on the causal relationships in the etiology of common illnesses through the study of ethnic patterns of disease.
Quarterly
Christopher T Fitzpatrick, CEO
Melanie T Cockfield, Director Administration

5144 Ethnicity Disease
International Society on Hypertension in Blacks
2045 Manchester Street NE   404-875-6263
Atlanta, GA 30324-4110   Fax: 404-875-6334
e-mail: member@ishib.org
www.ishib.org
Determined to accomplish the overall mission to improving the health and life expectancy of ethnic minority populations around the world. Publishes a quarterly journal and holds an annual conference.
150 pages Quarterly
Christopher T Fitzpatrick, CEO
Melanie T Cockfield, Director Administration

5145 Magazine of the National Institute of Hypertension Studies
13217 Livernois Avenue   313-931-3427
Detroit, MI 48238-3162
Association news.

Newsletters

5146 News Report
National Hypertension Association
324 E 30th Street   212-889-3557
New York, NY 10016-8329   Fax: 212-447-7032
e-mail: nathypertension@aol.com
www.nathypertension.org
Offers information and medical updates regarding hypertension. Recent book publication: 100 Questions and Answers about Hypertension by WM Manger, MD, PhD, and RW Gifford, Jr, MT available through National Hypertension Association.
W.M. Manger MD, PhD, Chairman

Pamphlets

5147 African-Americans and Stroke
National Stroke Association
9707 E Easter Lane   303-649-9299
Englewood, CO 80112-3747   800-787-6537
Fax: 303-649-1328
www.stroke.org
Colette Lafosse, Director Rehabilitation/Recovery Program

5148 Aneurysm Answers
National Stroke Association
9707 E Easter Lane   303-649-9299
Englewood, CO 80112-3747   800-787-6537
Fax: 303-649-1328
www.stroke.org
Colette Lafosse, Director Rehabilitation/Recovery Program

5149 Check Your Pulse, America: Atrial Fibrillation
National Stroke Association
9707 E Easter Lane   303-649-9299
Englewood, CO 80112-3747   800-787-6537
Fax: 303-649-1328
www.stroke.org
Colette Lafosse, Director Rehabilitation/Recovery Program

5150 Cholesterol and Stroke
National Stroke Association

9707 E Easter Lane   303-649-9299
Englewood, CO 80112-3747   800-787-6537
Fax: 303-649-1328
www.stroke.org
Colette Lafosse, Director Rehabilitation/Recovery Program

5151 High Blood Pressure and Stroke
National Stroke Association
9707 E Easter Lane   303-649-9299
Englewood, CO 80112-3747   800-787-6537
Fax: 303-649-1328
www.stroke.org
Colette Lafosse, Director Rehabilitation/Recovery Program

5152 Mobility: Issues Facing Stroke Survivors and Their Families
National Stroke Association
9707 E Easter Lane   303-649-9299
Englewood, CO 80112-3747   800-787-6537
Fax: 303-649-1328
www.stroke.org
Colette Lafosse, Director Rehabilitation/Recovery Program

5153 Recurrent Stroke
National Stroke Association
9707 E Easter Lane   303-649-9299
Englewood, CO 80112-3747   800-787-6537
Fax: 303-649-1328
www.stroke.org
Colette Lafosse, Director Rehabilitation/Recovery Program

5154 Smoking Cessation: Be Smoke Free in 3 Minutes
National Stroke Association
9707 E Easter Lane   303-649-9299
Englewood, CO 80112-3747   800-787-6537
Fax: 303-649-1328
www.stroke.org
Colette Lafosse, Director Rehabilitation/Recovery Program

5155 Transient Ischemic Attack
National Stroke Association
9707 E Easter Lane   303-649-9299
Englewood, CO 80112-3747   800-787-6537
Fax: 303-649-1328
www.stroke.org
Colette Lafosse, Director Rehabilitation/Recovery Program

Audio & Video

5156 Stroke: Touching the Soul of Your Family
National Stroke Association
9707 E Easter Lane   303-649-9299
Englewood, CO 80112-3747   800-787-6537
Fax: 303-649-1328
www.stroke.org
Fifteen minute video chronicling three stroke survivors and their courageous struggle to overcome daily challenges and educate others about stroke.
Colette Lafosse, Director Rehabilitation/Recovery Program

Web Sites

5157 American Society of Hypertension
www.ash-us.org
To organize and conduct educational seminars, materials, and products in all aspects of hypertension and other cardiovascular diseases.

5158 Healing Well
www.healingwell.com
An online health resource guide to medical news, chat, information and articles, newsgroups and message boards, books, disease-related web sites, medical directories, and more for patients, friends, and family coping with disabling diseases, disorders, or chronic illnesses.

5159   **Health Finder**

www.healthfinder.gov

Searchable, carefully developed web site offering information on over 1000 topics. Developed by the US Department of Health and Human Services, the site can be used in both English and Spanish.

5160   **Healthlink USA**

www.healthlinkusa.com

Links to websites which may include treatment, cures, diagnosis, prevention, support groups, email lists, messageboards, personal stories, risk factors, statistics, research and more.

5161   **Helios Health**

www.helioshealth.com

Online resource for your health information. Detailed information about specific health topics, access to expert advice from our Medical Advisory Board, and up-to-date health news.

5162   **Hypertension: Journal of the American Heart Association**

hyper.ahajournals.org

Lists current issues of journals about hypertension and the American Heart Association.

5163   **Inter-American Society of Hypertension**

www.iashonline.org

Website hosted by IASH, a non-profit professional organization devoted to the understanding, prevention and control of hypertension and vascular diseases in the American population. Members from 20 different countries in the Americas as well as Europe, Australia and Asia. Stimulates research and the exchange of ideas in hypertension and vascular diseases amoung physicians and scientists. Promotes the detection, control and prevention of hypertension and other cardiovascular risk factors.

5164   **Lifeclinic.Com**

www.lifeclinic.com

Online information about blood pressure, hypertension, diabetes, cholesterol, stroke, heart failure and more. Maintains current, up-to-date and accurate information for patients to help them manage their conditions better and to improve communications between them and their doctors.

5165   **Mayo Clinic Health Oasis**

www.mayohealth.org

Mission is to empower people to manage their health, by providing useful and up-to-date information and tools that reflect the expertise and standard of excellence of the Mayo Clinic.

5166   **MedicineNet**

www.medicinenet.com

An online resource for consumers providing easy-to-read, authoritative medical and health information.

5167   **Medscape**

www.medscape.com

Medscape offers specialists, primary care physicians, and other health professionals the Web's most robust and integrated medical information and educational tools.

5168   **National Heart, Lung & Blood Institute**

www.nhlbi.nih.gov

Information on the scientific investigation of heart, blood vessel, lung and blood disorders. Oversee research, demonstration, prevention, education and training activities in these fields and emphasizes the control of stroke.

5169   **WebMD**

www.webmd.com

Information on hypertension, including articles and resources.

Description

5170 Impotence

Impotence, also called erectile dysfunction (ED), is defined as the inability of a male to achieve and maintain an erection of sufficient quality to allow sexual intercourse. ED is very common, affecting millions of American males. Although it may occur at any age, it becomes dramatically more common with advancing age. Impotence may be caused by diabetes, circulatory disturbance, genital injury, hormonal disorders, medication side effects, depression, surgery (for instance, prostate removal) and many less well-characterized physical and psychological states. Impotence may be situational, that is, involving place, time, partner and degree of self-esteem.

Few cases of impotence are completely cured, but several kinds of effective treatment exist, including correction, if possible, of underlying causes. Oral medications that increase blood flow to the penis have been effective in many instances. Psychological factors that accompany ED should be considered in every case, including behavioral therapy and counseling, as needed.

National Agencies & Associations

5171 American Urlogical Association American Foundation for Urologic Disease
American Foundation for Urologic Disease
1000 Corporate Boulevard 410-689-3700
Linthicum, MD 21090 866-746-4282
Fax: 410-689-3800
e-mail: aua@AUAnet.org
www.auafoundation.org
The American Foundation for Urologic Disease Inc. is a charitable organization established to raise funds for research lay education and patient advocacy for the prevention detection management and cure of urologic disease.
Pramod C Sogani, MD, FACS, FRCS c, President
Gopal H Badlani, MD, Secretary

5172 Impotence Institute of America
119 S Ruth Street 865-379-2154
Maryville, TN 37803 800-669-1603
e-mail: iwatenn@aol.com
A non-profit organization dedicated to education about impotence. The IIA is a division of the Impotence World Association. Provides information on the causes, impact and treatments on this topic. Also publishes a quarterly newsletter on impotence topics.

5173 Impotence Resource Center of the Geddings Osbon Sr Foundation
PO Box 1593
Augusta, GA 30903 800-433-4215
Fax: 706-821-2782
e-mail: impotence@afud.org
www.impotence.org
Offers a free medical discussion where the consumer can obtain accurate unblessed information in a confidential understanding and thoughtful manner.
Rodgers, Director

5174 National Kidney and Urologic Diseases Information Clearinghouse
31 Center Drive MSC 2560 301-496-3583
Bethesda, MD 20892-2560 800-891-5390
Fax: 301-907-8906
e-mail: nkudic@info.niddk.nih.gov
www.niddk.nih.gov

Provides information about diseases of the kidneys and urologic system to people with such afflictions and to their families, health care professionals and the public. Answers inquiries; develops, reviews and distributes publications.
Dr Griffin P Rodgers, Director
Camille M Hoover, Executive Officer

Research Centers

5175 Central New York Male Sexual Dysfunction Center
357 Genesee Street 315-363-8862
Oneida, NY 13421 888-269-6732
Fax: 315-363-5477
www.cnymsdc.com

Burman, Director

5176 Male Sexual Dysfunction Clinic
3401 N Central Avenue 800-788-2873
Chicago, IL 60634 800-788-2873
Fax: 847-231-4130
e-mail: info@msdclinic.com
www.msdclinic.com
Helping men overcome male sexual dysfunctions such as impotence since 1981.
Sheldon O MD, Director

5177 New York Male Reproductive Center: Sexual Dysfunction Unit
161 Fort Washington Avenue 212-305-0123
New York, NY 10032 Fax: 212-305-0126
e-mail: rshabsigh@urology.columbia.edu
The New York Male Reproductive Center at Columbia-Presbyterian Medical Center offers state-of-the-art diagnosis and treatment for impotence. Treatments include surgical and non-surgical procedures.
Ridwan Shabs

Support Groups & Hotlines

5178 Impotence Information Center
PO Box 9
Minneapolis, MN 55440 800-843-4315
MacKenzie, Founder

5179 Impotents Anonymous
8630 Fenton Street 301-588-5777
Silver Spring, MD 20910-3803
Serves as an educational organization providing concerned individuals with information regarding impotence.
Bruce

5180 National Health Information Center
PO Box 1133 310-565-4167
Washington, DC 20013 800-336-4797
Fax: 301-984-4256
e-mail: info@nhic.org
www.health.gov/nhic
Offers a nationwide information referral service, produces directories and resource guides.
MPA, Executive Director
John M Barry MD, President

Books

5181 Impotence: How to Overcome It
HealthProInk Publishing
562 Wind Drift Lane 313-355-3686
Spring Lake, MI 49456-2168

5182 It's Not All in Your Head
Impotence Institute of America
8201 Corporate Drive 301-577-0650
Landover, MD 20785-2230
A couple's guide to overcoming impotence.

Newsletters

5183 Impotence Worldwide
8201 Corporate Drive   301-577-0650
Landover, MD 20785-2230
Provides information from professionals and lay persons concerning impotence plus manufactured product information.
Monthly

5184 Your Sexuality & Health
Impotence Resource Center
PO Box 1593
Augusta, GA 30903-1593   800-433-4215
                                     e-mail: info@gdo.org
                                     www.impotence.org
Quarterly newsletter that features articles by medical experts and highlights current research and tidbits of healthy living advice.
Quarterly

Pamphlets

5185 Answers to the Most Asked Questions About Impotence
Impotence World Services
8201 Corporate Drive   301-577-0650
Landover, MD 20785-2230

5186 Impotence Causes and Treatments
American Medical Systems
10700 Bren Road E   952-933-4666
Minnetonka, MN 55343   800-843-4315
                                     Fax: 952-930-6157
                                     www.visitams.com
Offers information on what impotence is, physical and emotional causes, treatments, questions and answers.

5187 Male Treatment Guide
Impotence Resource Center
PO Box 1593
Augusta, GA 30903-1593   800-433-4215
                                     e-mail: info@gdo.org
                                     www.impotence.org
Explains impotence - what it is, what causes it and how it is treated.
Free

5188 Woman's Perspective
Impotence Resource Center
PO Box 1593
Augusta, GA 30903-1593   800-433-4215
                                     e-mail: info@gdo.org
                                     www.impotence.org
Talking with your partner about impotence and choosing a treatment together.
Free

Audio & Video

5189 Impotence Treatment Options
Impotence Resource Center
PO Box 1593
Augusta, GA 30903-1593   800-433-4215
                                     e-mail: info@gdo.org
                                     www.impotence.org
Actual taping of a men's sexual health seminar - presented by Gary Leach, MD.

5190 Male Treatment Guide
Impotence Resource Center
PO Box 1593
Augusta, GA 30903-1593   800-433-4215
                                     e-mail: info@gdo.org
                                     www.impotence.org
Explains impotence - what it is, what causes it and how it is treated.
Audio Tape

5191 Medical Management of Impotence
Impotence Resource Center

PO Box 1593
Augusta, GA 30903-1593   800-433-4215
                                     e-mail: info@gdo.org
                                     www.impotence.org

5192 Woman's Perspective
Impotence Resource Center
PO Box 1593
Augusta, GA 30903-1593   800-433-4215
                                     e-mail: info@gdo.org
                                     www.impotence.org
Talking with your partner about impotence and choosing a treatment together.
Audio Tape

Web Sites

5193 American Foundation for Urologic Disease
                                     www.impotence.org
Online information about impotence, provided by the Sexual Function Health Council of the American Foundation for Urologic Disease.

5194 Family Meds
                                     www.familymeds.com
A site providing information on impotence and its various treatments, including over the counter, natural, and prescription medication choices.

5195 Healing Well
                                     www.healingwell.com
An online health resource guide to medical news, chat, information and articles, newsgroups and message boards, books, disease-related web sites, medical directories, and more for patients, friends, and family coping with disabling diseases, disorders, or chronic illnesses.

5196 Health Finder
                                     www.healthfinder.gov
Searchable, carefully developed web site offering information on over 1000 topics. Developed by the US Department of Health and Human Services, the site can be used in both English and Spanish.

5197 Healthlink USA
                                     www.healthlinkusa.com
Health information concerning treatment, cures, prevention, diagnosis, risk factors, research, support groups, email lists, personal stories and much more. Updated regularly.

5198 Helios Health
                                     www.helioshealth.com
Online resource for your health information. Detailed information about specific health topics, access to expert advice from our Medical Advisory Board, and up-to-date health news.

5199 Impotence Resource Center of the Geddings Osbon Sr Foundation
                                     www.impotence.org
Offers a free medical discussion service where the consumer can obtain accurate, unbiased information in a confidential, understanding and thoughtful manner.

5200 Impotence Specialists.com
                                     www.impotencespecialists.com
Offers information on physicians in your area, treatment options, online resources and more. A guide to the nation's impotence specialists.

5201 Impotence World Association
                                     www.impotence.com
Informs and educates the public on the subject of impotence and its causes and treatments. Serving the impotence industry since 1983 by bringing total care to the treatment of impotence.

5202 MedicineNet
                                     www.medicinenet.com
An online resource for consumers providing easy-to-read, authoritative medical and health information.

5203 Medscape

www.medscape.com

Medscape offers specialists, primary care physicians, and other health professionals the Web's most robust and integrated medical information and educational tools.

5204 WebMD

www.webmd.com

Information on impotence, including articles and resources.

Description

5205 Incontinence

Urinary incontinence is the involuntary leakage of urine, whether during waking or sleeping hours. One common type is urge incontinence, resulting from involuntary bladder contractions. The person feels a sudden urge to urinate, so intense that it may not be controlled long enough to reach the toilet. Common causes of urge incontinence are urinary tract infections, spinal cord injury, and kidney stones. Stress incontinence is the instantaneous leakage of urine without bladder contractions. It manifests as loss of urine during stress events, such as coughing, sneezing, laughing, or lifting. This may occur in women due to weak bladder tone from multiple pregnancies. In men, stress incontinence can occur after prostate removal or trauma to the bladder. Overflow incontinence, in which the bladder cannot control urine output, can be caused by nerve injury, alcoholism, and some diseases. Symptoms include urgency, and having to urinate more often (frequency) and at night (nocturia).

Treatment of incontinence focuses on therapy for the underlying causes. Infections are treated with the appropriate antibiotics. Stress incontinence in women can be treated with exercises to strengthen the bladder muscles. Other therapies include biofeedback and electrical stimulation. Severe cases may require surgical repair. Urinary incontinence remains largely a neglected problem, despite the fact that it can often be successfully treated.

National Agencies & Associations

5206 International Foundation for Functional Gastrointestinal Disorders (IFFGD)
700 W. Virginia Street
Milwaukee, WI 53204-8076

414-964-1799
888-964-2001
Fax: 414-964-7176
e-mail: iffgd@iffgd.org
www.iffgd.org

Nonprofit education, support and research organization devoted to increasing awareness and understanding of functional gastrointestinal disorders including irritable bowel syndrome (IBS), constipation, diarrhea, pain and incontinence.
Nancy J Norton, Co-Founder & President
William Norton, Co-Founder

5207 Intestinal Disease Foundation
100 W Station Square Drive
Pittsburgh, PA 15219-1122

412-261-5888
877-587-9606
Fax: 412-471-2722
www.intestinalfoundation.org

Provides one-on-one telephone support, educational programs and materials and self-help groups for people with irritable bowel syndrome (IBS), diverticular disease, inflammatory bowel diseases and short bowel syndrome; sponsors educational seminars; provides educational materials.
Harriet Gibb Deng, Chairperson
Nancy Muller, Executive Director

5208 National Association for Continence
PO Box 1019
Charleston, SC 29402-1019

843-377-0900
800-BLA-DDER
Fax: 843-377-0905
e-mail: memberservices@nafc.org
www.nafc.org

Founded as Help for Incontinent People, NAFC is the foremost consumer advocacy organization dedicated to helping people who struggle with incontinence and related voiding dysfunction. Its mission is focused on public education, awareness and collaboration.
Donna Browdie, Chair
James Firman EdD, President/CEO

5209 National Council on Aging
1901 L Street NW
Washington, DC 20036

202-479-1200
800-677-1116
Fax: 202-479-0735
TTY: 202-479-6674
TDD: 202-479-6674
e-mail: info@ncoa.org
www.ncoa.org

Organizations and professionals promoting the dignity self-determination and well-being of older persons.
Richard Gartley, President/Founder
Elizabeth LaGro, Vice President, Communications & Educati

5210 Simon Foundation for Continence
PO Box 815
Wilmette, IL 60091

847-864-3913
800-237-4666
Fax: 847-864-9758
e-mail: info@simonfoundation.org
www.simonfoundation.org

Seeks to bring the topic of incontinence out of the closet and remove the associated stigma; provides educational materials to patients their families and the health care professionals who provide patient care.
Cheryle

5211 Urology Care Foundation
1000 Corporate Boulevard
Linthicum, MD 21090

410-689-3700
800-828-7866
Fax: 410-689-3998
e-mail: info@urologycarefoundation.org
www.urologyhealth.org

A charitable organization whose mission is the prevention and cure of urologic diseases through the expansion of research education and public awareness.
Sandra Vasso Norton, President

Support Groups & Hotlines

5212 Greater New York Pull-Thru Network
62 Edgewood Avenue
Wyckoff, NJ 07481

201-891-5977

National support network providing emotional support and information to patients and families of children who have had or will have a pull-thru type surgery to correct an imperforate anus or associated malformation, Hirschsprung's or other fecal incontinence problems. Support group meetings held quarterly.

5213 National Health Information Center
PO Box 1133
Washington, DC 20013

301-565-4167
800-336-4797
Fax: 301-984-4256
e-mail: info@nhic.org
www.health.gov/nhic

Offers a nationwide information referral service, produces directories and resource guides.
Gartley, Founder/President
Elizabeth LaGro, Vice President, Communications & Educati

5214 Simon Foundation Helpline for Incontinence Information
Simon Foundation for Continence
PO Box 815
Wilmette, IL 60091

847-864-3913
800-237-4666
Fax: 847-864-9758
e-mail: info@simonfoundation.org
www.simonfoundation.org

Offers information and help to persons with incontinence problems and professionals who work with them.
Cheryle Brown MD, Director

5215 **University of California at San Francisco Women's Continence Center**
2356 Sutter Street
San Francisco, CA 94115
415-885-7788
877-366-8532
coe.ucsf.edu/wcc
Offers a comprehensive array of clinical services for women with incontinence, urethal or bladder dysfuntion and pelvic support problems.
Jeanette S Vecchiarello, President/Board of Directors
Doni DeBolt, Executive Director

Books

5216 **Managing Incontinence: a Guide to Living with Loss of Bladder Control**
Simon Foundation for Incontinence
PO Box 815
Wilmette, IL 60091
847-864-3913
800-237-4666
Fax: 847-864-9768
e-mail: simoninfo@simonfoundation.org
www.simonfoundation.org
Seeks to bring the topic of incontinence out of the closet and remove the associated stigma; provides information to patients, their families and the health care professionals who provide patient care.
Quarterly
Cheryle B Gartley, President

5217 **Pocket Guide for Continence Care**
National Association for Continence
PO Box 1019
Charleston, SC 29402
843-377-0900
800-252-3337
Fax: 843-377-0905
e-mail: memberservices@nafc.org
www.nafc.org
Condensed version of the Blueprint for Continence Care, this guide is designed for a first line supervisor or any health care professional in any eldercare environment to help address any issues related to bladder health. The guide is perfect for a quick referral because it can actually fit in the healthcare professional's pocket.
Nancy Muller, Executive Director
Caryn Antos, Publicity/Publications Associate

5218 **Resource Guide: Products and Services for Incontinence**
National Association for Continence
PO Box 1019
Charleston, SC 29402
843-377-0900
800-252-3337
Fax: 843-377-0905
e-mail: memberservices@nafc.org
www.nafc.org
Complete directory of products and services available. Categories include disposable products, reusable products, skin care products, deodorizing products, pelvic organ support devices, medications to treat incontinence and others. Also includes a listing of distributors and mail/phone order companies.
Nancy Muller, Executive Director
Caryn Antos, Publicity/Publications Associate

5219 **Your Personal Guide to Bladder Health**
National Association for Continence
PO Box 1019
Charleston, SC 29402
843-377-0900
800-252-3337
Fax: 843-377-0905
e-mail: memberservices@nafc.org
www.nafc.org
Designed for residents of assisted living environments, other older individuals living independently and their involved family members. It encompasses a wide variety of informative topics, including diet and daily habits, pelvic muscle exercises odor control and more.
48 pages
Nancy Muller, Executive Director
Caryn Antos, Publicity/Publications Associate

Magazines

5220 **Digestive Health Matters**
Intl. Foundation for Gastrointestinal Disorders
PO Box 170864
Milwaukee, WI 53217-0864
414-964-1799
888-964-2001
Fax: 414-964-7176
e-mail: iffgd@iffgd.org
www.iffgd.org
Quarterly journal focuses on upper and lower gastrointestinal disorders in adults and children. Educational pamphlets and factsheets are available. Patient and professional membership.

Newsletters

5221 **Discoveries**
National Association for Continence
PO Box 1019
Charleston, SC 29402
843-377-0900
800-252-3337
Fax: 843-377-0905
e-mail: memberservices@nafc.org
www.nafc.org
Compendium comprised of the most recently released incontinence products and newly approved protocol. Includes editorial sections, authored by leading clinicians and researchers, describing new product technology and research in other medical advances related to continence care.
32 pages BiAnnual
Nancy Muller, Executive Director
Caryn Antos, Publicity/Publications Associate

5222 **Informer**
Simon Foundation for Incontinence
PO Box 815
Wilmette, IL 60091
847-864-3913
800-237-4666
Fax: 847-864-9768
e-mail: simoninfo@simonfoundation.org
www.simonfoundation.org
Seeks to bring the topic of incontinence out of the closet and remove the associated stigma; provides information to patients, their families, and the health care professionals who provide patient care.
Quarterly
Cheryle B Gartley, President

5223 **Intestinal Fortitude**
Intestinal Disease Foundation
One Station Square, Suite 525
Pittsburgh, PA 15219
412-261-5888
Fax: 412-471-2722
www.intestinalfoundation.org
Newsletter, brochures and books for Intestinal Disease Foundation members.

5224 **Participate**
IFFGD
PO Box 17864
Milwaukee, WI 53217-0864
414-964-1799
888-964-2001
Fax: 414-964-7176
e-mail: iffgd@iffgd.org
www.aboutincontinence.org
Provides information for people affected by the various forms of functional bowel disorders, including irritable bowel syndrome, constipation, diarrhea, pain and incontinence.
Quarterly

5225 **Pull-Thru Network News**
Greater New York Pull-Thru Network
62 Edgewood Avenue
Wyckoff, NJ 07481-3456
201-891-5977
www.pullthrough.org/ptnn.html
Quarterly newsletter for patients and families who have had or will have a pull-thru type surgery to correct an imperforate anus or associated malformation, Hirschsprung's or other fecal incontinence problem.

5226 **Quality Care**
National Association for Continence

PO Box 1019
Charleston, SC 29402

843-377-0900
800-252-3337
Fax: 843-377-0905
e-mail: memberservices@nafc.org
www.nafc.org

Quarterly newsletter addressing causes, symptoms, management and treatment options for incontinence and related disorders.
Quarterly
Nancy Muller, Executive Director
Caryn Antos, Publicity/Publications Associate

Pamphlets

5227 Bladder Control for Women
National Kidney and Urologic Diseases Information
3 Information Way
Bethesda, MD 20892-3580

800-891-5390
Fax: 301-907-8906
e-mail: nkudic@info.nidkk.nih.gov

Comprehensive introduction to the causes, symptoms, and treatments for bladder control problems in women.

5228 Exercising Your Pelvic Muscles
National Kidney and Urologic Diseases Information
3 Information Way
Bethesda, MD 20892-3580

800-891-5390
Fax: 301-907-8906
e-mail: nkudic@info.nidkk.nih.gov

A description of exercises for the pelvic floor muscles, called Kegel exercises, and how they can help to restore or maintain bladder control.

5229 Menopause and Bladder Control
National Kidney and Urologic Diseases Information
3 Information Way
Bethesda, MD 20892-3580

800-891-5390
Fax: 301-907-8906
e-mail: nkudic@info.nidkk.nih.gov

An introduction to the changes to your body that occur during menopause, how these changes can result in loss of bladder control, and how your health care team can help you restore or maintain bladder control.

5230 NAFC Fact Sheets
National Association for Continence
PO Box 1019
Charleston, SC 29402

843-377-0900
800-252-3337
Fax: 843-377-0905
e-mail: memberservices@nafc.org
www.nafc.org

Offering helpful tips and information on a variety of topics, the sheets provide consumers and professionals with the necessary information on managing incontinence. Some titles include medications, diet and daily habits, odor control, prostatectomy and many more.
Nancy Muller, Executive Director
Caryn Antos, Publicity/Publications Associate

5231 Pregnancy, Childbirth, and Bladder Control
National Kidney and Urologic Diseases Information
3 Information Way
Bethesda, MD 20892-3580

800-891-5390
Fax: 301-907-8906
e-mail: nkudic@info.nidkk.nih.gov

A look at the effects that pregnancy and childbearing can have on bladder control and ways you can counter those effects.

5232 Talking to Your Health Care Team About Bladder Control
National Kidney and Urologic Diseases Information
3 Information Way
Bethesda, MD 20892-3580

800-891-5390
Fax: 301-907-8906
e-mail: nkudic@info.nidkk.nih.gov

Tips for giving your health care provider the information needed to diagnose and treat your bladder control problem. Includes a questionnaire for you to fill out and take to your first appointment.

5233 Urinary Incontinence in Women
National Kidney and Urologic Diseases Information

3 Information Way
Bethesda, MD 20892-3580

800-891-5390
Fax: 301-907-8906
e-mail: nkudic@info.nidkk.nih.gov

An overview of the types, diagnosis, and treatment of urinary incontinence in women.

5234 What Your Female Patients Want to Know About Bladder Control
National Kidney and Urologic Diseases Information
3 Information Way
Bethesda, MD 20892-3580

800-891-5390
Fax: 301-907-8906
e-mail: nkudic@info.nidkk.nih.gov

Fact sheet with tips for health care providers on raising the issue of incontinence with female patients who may be reluctant to talk about their problem.

5235 Your Body's Design for Bladder Control
National Kidney and Urologic Diseases Information
3 Information Way
Bethesda, MD 20892-3580

800-891-5390
Fax: 301-907-8906
e-mail: nkudic@info.nidkk.nih.gov

An introduction to the female urinary system. Includes diagrams of the bladder and pelvic floor muscles.

5236 Your Daily Bladder Diary
National Kidney and Urologic Diseases Information
3 Information Way
Bethesda, MD 20892-3580

800-891-5390
Fax: 301-907-8906
e-mail: nkudic@info.nidkk.nih.gov

An easy-to-use form for patients to note liquid intake, trips to the bathroom, urine leaks, and other details that may help explain your incontinence.

5237 Your Medicines and Bladder Control
National Kidney and Urologic Diseases Information
3 Information Way
Bethesda, MD 20892-3580

800-891-5390
Fax: 301-907-8906
e-mail: nkudic@info.nidkk.nih.gov

Booklet describing the effects that your medications could have on bladder control, with a recommendation for discussing all your medicines with your doctor.

Audio & Video

5238 Solution Starts with You
Simon Foundation for Continence
PO Box 815
Wilmette, IL 60091

847-864-3913
800-237-4666
Fax: 847-864-9758
e-mail: cbgartley@simonfoundation.org
www.simonfoundation.org

Seeks to bring the topic of incontinence out of the closet and remove the associated stigma; provides information to patients, their families, and the health care professionals who provide patient care.
Quarterly
Cheryle Gartley, Founder/President
Jasmine Schmidt, Director of Education

Web Sites

5239 American Foundation for Urologic Disease

www.incontinence.org

Large website detailing information on incontinence, ranging from various treatment options to links and resources.

5240 Healing Well

www.healingwell.com

An online health resource guide to medical news, chat, information and articles, newsgroups and message boards, books, disease-related web sites, medical directories, and more for patients, friends, and family coping with disabling diseases, disorders, or chronic illnesses.

5241   Health Finder

www.healthfinder.gov

Searchable, carefully developed web site offering information on over 1000 topics. Developed by the US Department of Health and Human Services, the site can be used in both English and Spanish.

5242   Healthlink USA

www.healthlinkusa.com

Health information concerning treatment, cures, prevention, diagnosis, risk factors, research, support groups, email lists, personal stories and much more. Updated regularly.

5243   Helios Health

www.helioshealth.com

Online resource for your health information. Detailed information about specific health topics, access to expert advice from our Medical Advisory Board, and up-to-date health news.

5244   MedicineNet

www.medicinenet.com

An online resource for consumers providing easy-to-read, authoritative medical and health information.

5245   Medscape

www.medscape.com

Medscape offers specialists, primary care physicians, and other health professionals the Web's most robust and integrated medical information and educational tools.

5246   National Association for Continence

www.nafc.org

Interactive website packed with useful information about diagnosis, treatment options and management solutions for incontinence. The site currentlyfeatures a specialist search engine of healthcare providers who have recieved specific training in the diagnosis and treatment of incontinence to assist consumers in locating a specialist in their area. Other features include archived Quality Care articles, a message board, online database of active support groups and much more.

5247   Simon Foundation for Continence

www.simonfoundation.org

Seeks to bring the topic of incontinence out of the closet and remove the associated stigma; provides educational materials to patients, their families, and the health care professionals who provide patient care.

5248   WebMD

www.webmd.com

Information on incontinence, including articles and resources.

Description

5249 Infertility

Infertility is defined as the failure to achieve conception by couples who have not used contraception for at least one year, and affects 1 in 5 couples in the United States.

Female causes of infertility include dysfunction of the ovaries (20 percent of couples), blockage of the tubes connecting the ovaries to the uterus (30 percent), and abnormal secretions (5 percent). Infertility in males is mostly related to sperm disorders (35 percent of couples), either insufficient production of sperm, ineffective sperm, or defective delivery of sperm. Unidentified factors account for the remaining 10 percent of couples.

A variety of tests are needed to determine the exact cause of infertility and then identify the appropriate treatment options. Failure to conceive can be both an emotional and financial burden on couples. Counseling and psychological support are important parts of treatment.

National Agencies & Associations

5250 Adopt-A-Special-Kid America
8201 Edgewater Drive
Oakland, CA 94621
510-553-1748
888-680-7349
Fax: 510-553-1747
e-mail: info@aask.org
www.aask.org/

Adopt-A-Special-Kid provides information on adoption of children with special needs.
Roberto Hribek, Chair
Ken Mosesian, Executive Director

5251 American Fertility Association
315 Madison Avenue
New York, NY 10017-0004
888-917-3777
Fax: 718-601-7722
e-mail: info@theafa.org
www.theafa.org

Purpose is to educate the public about reproductive disease and support families during struggles with infertility and adoption. Exists to serve the unique needs of men and women confronting infertility issues.
Don Giudice, MD, PhD, President
Robert W Rebar MD, Executive Director

5252 American Society for Reproductive Medicine
1209 Montgomery Highway
Birmingham, AL 35216-2809
205-978-5000
Fax: 205-978-5005
e-mail: asrm@asrm.org
www.asrm.com

Purpose is to educate the public about reproductive disease and support families during struggles with infertility and adoption. Exists to serve the unique needs of men and women confronting infertility issues.
Linda C. Coffey, President

5253 Hysterectomy Educational Resources & Services (HERS) Foundation
422 Bryn Mawr Avenue
Bala Cynwyd, PA 19004
610-667-7757
888-750-4377
Fax: 610-677-8096
e-mail: HERS@hersfoundation.org
www.hersfoundation.com

A nonprofit foundation which provides information about the alternatives to hysterectomy the risks of the alternatives and the consequences of the surgery. HERS provides telephone counseling by appointment.
Nora W Berger, MD, Member of Advisory Board
Geoffrey Sher, MD, Member of Advisory Board

5254 International Council on Infertility Information Dissemination
PO Box 6836
Arlington, VA 22206
703-379-9178
Fax: 703-379-1593
e-mail: INCIIDinfo@inciid.org
www.inciid.org

Provides information on infertility pregnancy loss adoption high risk pregnancy and parenting after the above.
Gary S Collura, President/CEO
Margaret Chandler Berardelli, Director, Development

5255 RESOLVE: The National Infertility Association
1760 Old Meadow Road
McLean, VA 22102
703-556-7172
Fax: 703-506-3266
e-mail: info@resolve.org
www.resolve.org

A nationwide nonprofit consumer organization serving the unique needs of those striving to build a family. Provides compassionate and informed help to people who are experiencing the infertility crisis and strives to increase the visibility of infertility in the community.
Barbara Collura, Executive Director
Dawn Gannon, Professional Outreach Manager

State Agencies & Associations

Alabama

5256 RESOLVE of Alabama
1760 Old Meadow Road
McLean, VA 22102
703-556-7172
888-473-3062
Fax: 703-506-3266
e-mail: info@southeast.resolve.org
www.southeast.resolve.org/

Barbara Nelson, President
Denny Ceizyk, VP

Arizona

5257 RESOLVE of Valley of the Sun
PO Box 36252
Phoenix, AZ 85067-6252
602-995-3933
e-mail: resolveaz@hotmail.com
www.resolveaz.org

Tina Collura, President/CEO
Margaret Chandler Berardelli, Director, Development

Arkansas

5258 RESOLVE Affiliate of Northwest Arkansas
2230 Country Way
Fayetteville, AR 72703-4215
501-521-3763
888-895-6055
e-mail: info@southcentral.resolve.org
www.southcentral.resolve.org/

Barbara Waldron, CA/San Diego Chair

California

5259 RESOLVE of Greater Los Angeles
PO Box 12529
Newport Beach, CA 92658
310-326-2630
877-203-7771
e-mail: info@southwest.resolve.org
www.southwest.resolve.org

Mari Waldron, CA/San Diego Chair

5260 RESOLVE of Greater San Diego
PO Box 12529
Newport Beach, CA 92658-7385
310-326-2630
877-203-7771
e-mail: info@southwest.resolve.org
www.southwest.resolve.org

Mari Munoz, Northern California Coordinator

5261 RESOLVE of Northern California
312 Sutter Street
San Francisco, CA 94108
415-788-6772
888-591-6663
Fax: 415-788-6774
e-mail: info@northpacific.resolve.org
www.northpacific.resolve.org/
Volunteer-based organization that provides infertility education
adoption information advocacy and support.
Tracie Fletcher, Local Area Affiliate Chair

Colorado

5262 RESOLVE of Colorado
PO Box 260725
Littleton, CO 80163-0725
303-469-5261
888-592-4449
e-mail: info@mountain.resolve.org
www.mountain.resolve.org/
Jennifer Malave, Support Services
Maryann Post, Helpline Coordinator

Connecticut

5263 RESOLVE of Fairfield County
PO Box 930
S Norwalk, CT 06856-0930
914-686-1490
888-765-2810
Fax: 203-255-2561
e-mail: info@northeast.resolve.org
northeast.resolve.org
Anne Odeen-Lodato,, Chair
Erin Lasker, Executive Director

5264 RESOLVE of Greater Hartford
PO Box 290964
Wethersfield, CT 06129
781-890-2225
e-mail: admin@resolvenewengland.org
www.resolvenewengland.org/
Pam Bare, Regional Chair
Cindy Peterson, Volunteer Coordinator

District of Columbia

5265 RESOLVE of the Washington Metro Area
PO Box 3423
Merrifield, VA 22116-3423
202-362-5555
888-583-4441
e-mail: info@midatlantic.resolve.org
www.res.pub30.convio.net/Regions/mid-atl
Cindy Gedaro, Florida, Orlando Coordinator

Florida

5266 RESOLVE Affiliate of Central Florida
1050 W Morse Boulevard
Winter Park, FL 32789
407-637-0142
888-473-3062
e-mail: resolveofcentralflorida@gmail.com
www.southeast.resolve.org/
Susanna Witt, Florida, Tampa Coordinator
Kathy Fountain, Florida, Tampa Coordinator

5267 RESOLVE of North Florida
1929 Logging Lane
Jacksonville, FL 32221-2071
904-737-0140
888-473-3062
e-mail: Nicole@theadoptionconsultancy.com
www.southeast.resolve.org/
Nicole Linder, Cooordinator

5268 RESOLVE of South Florida
3342 SW 51 Street
Ft Lauderdale, FL 33312
954-749-9500
888-473-3062
e-mail: resolvesf@yahoo.com
www.southeast.resolve.org/
Elise Badey, Coordinator
Renee Whitley, Advocacy Chair

Georgia

5269 RESOLVE of Georgia
3904 N Druid Hills Road
Decatur, GA 30333
404-233-8443
888-473-3062
e-mail: Katie9924@hotmail.com
southeast.resolve.org
Kate Collura, President/CEO
Margaret Chandler Berardelli, Director, Development

Hawaii

5270 RESOLVE of Hawaii
PO Box 29193
Honolulu, HI 96820
808-528-8559
888-591-6663
e-mail: info@resolveofhawaii.org
www.res.pub30.convio.net/Regions/north-p
Barbara Collura, President/CEO
Margaret Chandler Berardelli, Director, Development

Illinois

5271 RESOLVE of Illinois
PO Box 56
Hinsdale, IL 60521
773-743-1623
888-255-1399
e-mail: info@greatlakes.resolve.org
www.res.pub30.convio.net/Regions/great-l
Barbara Collura, President/CEO
Margaret Chandler Berardelli, Director, Development

Indiana

5272 RESOLVE of Indiana
5155 Sandy Court
Pittsboro, IN 46167-9129
317-329-9519
888-255-1399
e-mail: info@greatlakes.resolve.org
www.res.pub30.convio.net/Regions/great-l
Barbara Collura, President/CEO
Margaret Chandler Berardelli, Director, Development

Iowa

5273 RESOLVE Affiliate of Iowa
1348 Atlantic
Dunuque, IA 52001
319-557-2763
888-959-0333
e-mail: info@midwest.resolve.org
www.res.pub30.convio.net/Regions/midwest
Barbara Verhiley, Kentucky State Coordinator

Kentucky

5274 RESOLVE of Kentucky
851 Van Dyke Mill Road
Taylorsville, KY 40071-9502
502-834-7568
888-255-1399
e-mail: kentucky@greatlakes.resolve.org
www.res.pub30.convio.net/Regions/great-l
Stephanie Collura, President/CEO
Margaret Chandler Berardelli, Director, Development

Louisiana

5275 RESOLVE of Louisiana
PO Box 55693
Metairie, LA 70055-5693
504-454-6987
888-895-6055
e-mail: info@southcentral.resolve.org
www.res.pub30.convio.net/Regions/south-c
Barbara Bare, Regional Chair
Cindy Peterson, Volunteer Coordinator

Massachusetts

5276 RESOLVE of the Bay State
395 Totten Pond Road
Waltham, MA 02451-1553
781-890-2225
Fax: 781-890-2249
e-mail: admin@resolvenewengland.org
www.resolvenewengland.org/
Information on the Massachusetts chapter of a national, nonprofit
consumer based infertility support organization. Information and a

variety of services to answer your questions about infertility, treatments, coping techniquesand insurance issues.
1,000 Homes
Pam Rollinger, Detroit, MI Area Coordinator

Michigan

5277 **RESOLVE of Michigan**
3601 W Thirteen Mile Road   586-412-8712
Royal Oak, MI 48068-9998   888-255-1399
e-mail: info@greatlakes.resolve.org
www.res.pub30.convio.net/Regions/great-l
Kathy Collura, President/CEO
Margaret Chandler Berardelli, Director, Development

Minnesota

5278 **RESOLVE of Minnesota**
1161 E Wayzata Boulevard   651-659-0333
Wayzata, MN 55391   888-959-0333
e-mail: info@midwest.resolve.org
www.res.pub30.convio.net/Regions/midwest
Barbara Myrick, Missouri Local Area Coordinator

Missouri

5279 **RESOLVE of St. Louis, Missouri**
PO Box 411072   314-567-8788
Saint Louis, MO 63141-3072   888-959-0333
e-mail: MMyrickResolveMissouri@Yahoo.com
www.res.pub30.convio.net/Regions/midwest
Melissa Isaacson, Nevada Chair

Nevada

5280 **RESOLVE of Nevada**
Barbara Greenspun Women's Care Center
8280 W Warm Springs Road   702-616-4900
Las Vegas, NV 89074   877-203-7771
e-mail: rpbooklover@cox.net
www.res.pub30.convio.net/Regions/southwe
Robyn Odeen-Lodato, Chair
Erin Lasker, Executive Director

New Hampshire

5281 **RESOLVE of New Hampshire**
131 Daniel Webster Highway   781-890-2225
Nashua, NH 03060-5224   e-mail: admin@resolvenewengland.org
www.resolvenewengland.org/
Pam Griffiths, New Jersey Coordinator

New Jersey

5282 **RESOLVE of New Jersey**
1830 Front Street   908-322-9180
Scotch Plains, NJ 07076-0335   888-RNJ-2810
e-mail: griffithskm@yahoo.com
www.res.pub30.convio.net/Regions/northea
Kim Rodriguez, New Mexico State Coordinator

New Mexico

5283 **RESOLVE of New Mexico**
PO Box 93386   505-291-5066
Albuquerque, NM 87199   888-895-6055
e-mail: nmresolve@yahoo.com
www.res.pub30.convio.net/Regions/south-c
Rachel Soto-Lugo, President Advocacy Chair
April R Simanoff, VP Outreach Coordinator

New York

5284 **RESOLVE of Long Island**
PO Box 303   631-385-5026
Long Island, NY 11714   e-mail: racchair@northeast.resolve.org
www.northeast.resolve.org

Arelys Malave, Support Services
Maryann Post, Helpline Coordinator

5285 **RESOLVE of New York City**
178 Columbus Avenue   212-799-7400
New York, NY 10023   888-765-2810
e-mail: info@northeast.resolve.org
www.res.pub30.convio.net/Regions/northea
Anne Malave, Support Services
Maryann Post, Helpline Coordinator

5286 **RESOLVE of the Capital District**
PO Box 14591   518-242-3848
Albany, NY 12212-4591   888-765-2810
e-mail: info@northeast.resolve.org
www.res.pub30.convio.net/Regions/northea
Anne Pell, North Carolina Coordinator

North Carolina

5287 **RESOLVE of North Carolina**
101 Gettysburg Drive   919-380-8497
Cary, NC 27513   888-473-3062
e-mail: resolvenc@gmail.com
www.southeast.resolve.org/
Terry Collura, President/CEO
Margaret Chandler Berardelli, Director, Development

Ohio

5288 **RESOLVE of Ohio**
3000 NW Boulevard   614-340-0905
Columbus, OH 43221   888-255-1399
Fax: 614-340-0916
e-mail: info@greatlakes.resolve.org
www.res.pub30.convio.net/Regions/great-l
Barbara Zornes, Oklahoma State Coordinator

Oklahoma

5289 **RESOLVE of Oklahoma**
PO Box 18151   405-949-8857
Oklahoma City, OK 73154-0151   888-895-6055
e-mail: christina-zornes@ouhsc.edu
www.res.pub30.convio.net/Regions/south-c
Christy Collura, President/CEO
Margaret Chandler Berardelli, Director, Development

Oregon

5290 **RESOLVE of Oregon**
PO Box 175   503-762-0449
Scappoose, OR 97056   888-591-6663
e-mail: resolve_oregon@yahoo.com
www.res.pub30.convio.net/Regions/north-p
Barbara Fries, Philadelphia Coordinator

Pennsylvania

5291 **RESOLVE of Philadelphia**
PO Box 2456   215-849-3920
Southeastern, PA 19399-2456   888-765-2810
e-mail: phillyresolve@gmail.com
www.res.pub30.convio.net/Regions/northea
Katie Collura, President/CEO
Margaret Chandler Berardelli, Director, Development

5292 **RESOLVE of Pittsburgh**
PO Box 11203   703-861-2910
Pittsburgh, PA 15238-0203   888-255-1399
e-mail: info@greatlakes.resolve.org
www.res.pub30.convio.net/Regions/great-l
Barbara

5293 **RESOLVE of Southcentral Pennsylvania**
PO Box 402   717-234-8583
Camp Hill, PA 17001-0402
Odeen-Lodato,, Chair
Erin Lasker, Executive Director

Rhode Island

5294 RESOLVE of the Ocean State
PO Box 28201   781-890-2225
Providence, RI 02908-0201 e-mail: admin@resolvenewengland.org
www.resolvenewengland.org/

Pam Collura, President/CEO
Margaret Chandler Berardelli, Director, Development

South Carolina

5295 RESOLVE of South Carolina
204 Fernbrook Circle   864-542-9092
Spartanburg, SC 29307-2966   888-473-3062
e-mail: info@southeast.resolve.org
www.southeast.resolve.org/

Barbara Myers, Tennessee Coordinator

Tennessee

5296 RESOLVE of Tennessee
4770 Riverdale Road   615-244-5582
Memphis, TN 38141-8529   888-473-3062
e-mail: resolvetn@gmail.com
www.southeast.resolve.org/

Jessica Collura, President/CEO
Margaret Chandler Berardelli, Director, Development

Texas

5297 RESOLVE of Central Texas
PO Box 49783   512-453-2171
Austin, TX 78765   888-895-6055
e-mail: info@southcentral.resolve.org
www.res.pub30.convio.net/Regions/south-c
Barbara Collura, President/CEO
Margaret Chandler Berardelli, Director, Development

5298 RESOLVE of Dallas/Fort Worth
434 N Manus Drive
Dallas, TX 77244   888-895-6055
e-mail: info@southcentral.resolve.org
www.res.pub30.convio.net/Regions/south-c
Barbara Collura, President/CEO
Margaret Chandler Berardelli, Director, Development

5299 RESOLVE of Houston
PO Box 441212   713-975-5324
Houston, TX 77244-1212   888-895-6055
e-mail: info@southcentral.resolve.org
www.res.pub30.convio.net/Regions/south-c
Barbara Collura, President/CEO
Margaret Chandler Berardelli, Director, Development

5300 RESOLVE of South Texas
PO Box 782061   210-967-6771
San Antonio, TX 78278   888-895-6055
e-mail: info@southcentral.resolve.org
www.res.pub30.convio.net/Regions/south-c
Barbara Barron, Salt Lake City Coordinator

Utah

5301 RESOLVE of Utah
PO Box 57531   801-483-4024
Salt Lake City, UT 84157-0531   888-592-4449
e-mail: resolveutah@gmail.com
www.res.pub30.convio.net/Regions/mountai
Jennifer Odeen-Lodato,, Chair
Erin Lasker, Executive Director

Vermont

5302 RESOLVE of Vermont
PO Box 1094   781-890-2225
Williston, VT 05495-1094 e-mail: admin@resolvenewengland.org
www.resolvenewengland.org/

Pam Guthrie, Chair
Carol Knoph, Chair

Wisconsin

5303 RESOLVE of Wisconsin
PO Box 13842   262-521-4590
Wauwatosa, WI 53213-0842   888-255-1399
e-mail: info@greatlakes.resolve.org
www.res.pub30.convio.net/Regions/great-l
Barbara Jansen, Executive Director
Asgerally T Fazleabas, President

5304 Society for the Study of Reproduction
1619 Monroe Street   608-256-2777
Madison, WI 53711-2063   Fax: 608-256-4610
e-mail: ssr@ssr.org
www.ssr.org

International scientific society promotes the study of reproductive biology by fostering interdisciplinary communication within the science by holding conferences and by publishing meritorious studies.
2,400 members
Susan S Suarez, President
Judith Jansen, Executive Director

Foundations

5305 Fertility Research Foundation
877 Park Avenue   212-744-5500
New York, NY 10021   888-439-2999
Fax: 212-744-6536
e-mail: info@frfbaby.com
www.frfbaby.com

Offers information on treatment and the latest research on male and female infertility.
Masood Khatamee MD, Executive Director

Libraries & Resource Centers

5306 National Women's Health Resource Center
157 Broad Street
Red Bank, NJ 07701   877-986-9472
Fax: 732-530-3347
e-mail: info@healthywomen.org
www.healthywomen.org

NWHRC provides the most current women's health care information through website articles, online mini-courses, a monthly electronic newsletter, and periodic news releases.
Eve Dryer, Chair
Elizabeth Battaglino, Chief Executive Officer

Research Centers

5307 California Center for Population Research
759 Chestnut Street
Springfield, MA 01199-1001   413-784-5252
www.tufts.edu

Dr Donald Higby, Director

5308 Fertility Clinic at the Shepherd Spinal Center
Shepherd Spinal Center
2020 Peachtree Road NW
Atlanta, GA 30309-1465   404-352-2020
www.shepherd.org

This clinic makes it possible for paralyzed men to father children.
Gary Ulicny, Chief Executive Officer

5309 Fertility and Women's Health Care Center
130 Maple Street   413-781-8220
Springfield, MA 01103-2202   Fax: 413-732-9088
Conducts basic and clinical studies of male and female infertility.
Ronald K Burke MD, Head

5310 Melpomene Institute for Women's Health Research
550 Rice Street   651-789-0140
Saint Paul, MN 55103   Fax: 651-292-9417
e-mail: shawne@melpomene.org
www.melpomene.org

Focuses on women's health including fertility issues.
Judy Mahle Lutter, President

5311 University of California: UCLA Population Research Center
4284 Public Affairs Building   310-206-7566
Los Angeles, CA 90095-2006   Fax: 310-825-8762
e-mail: stats@ccpr.ucla.edu
www.ccpr.ucla.edu
Clinical investigations of overpopulation and infertility.
Judith A Seltzer, Director
Jennie Brand, Associate Director

5312 University of Michigan Reproductive Sciences Program
1500 East Medical Center Drive   734-764-8123
Ann Arbor, MI 48109   Fax: 734-763-5992
e-mail: juckno@umich.edu
www.med.umich.edu/OBGYN/research/rsp/
Research done into reproductive medicine and infertility treatments.
Timothy R. B Johnson, Chair
Janet Hall, Clinical Department Administrator

5313 Vanderbilt University: Center for Fertility and Reproductive Research
Nashville, TN 37232-0001   615-322-6576
Fax: 615-343-4902
Reproductive biology and fertility research.

5314 Wayne State University: University Women's Care
26400 W 12 Mile Road   248-352-8200
Southfield, MI 48034   Fax: 248-356-8224
wayne.edu
Reproductive endocrine infertility and gynecologic surgery research. The research spans the woman's life cycle. Research projects include: endometriosis polycystic ovary syndrome sexual dysfunction fibroids and menopause. Additional studies pertaining to women's health and male infertility.
Elizabeth Pu MD, Associate Professor
Nancy Angel RN, Research Nurse Coordinator

Support Groups & Hotlines

5315 National Health Information Center
PO Box 1133   301-565-4167
Washington, DC 20013   800-336-4797
Fax: 301-984-4256
e-mail: info@nhic.org
www.health.gov/nhic
Offers a nationwide information referral service, produces directories and resource guides.

5316 National Infertility Network Exchange
PO Box 204   516-794-5772
East Meadow, NY 11554   Fax: 516-794-0008
e-mail: info@nine-infertility.org
www.nine-infertility.org/
The National Infertility Network Exchange (NINE) is a national, notfor profit organization for persons and couples with impaired fertility. NINE supportes the decision of legal and medical means to build families as well as the decision to remain childfree.

Books

5317 Adopt the Baby You Want
Simon & Schuster
1230 Avenue of the Americas   212-698-7000
New York, NY 10020-1586   800-223-2348
A how-to adoption book written by an attorney specializing in all areas of adoption.
272 pages

5318 Adopting After Infertility: The Decision, the Commitment, the Experience
American Society for Reproductive Medicine
1209 Montgomery Highway   205-978-5000
Birmingham, AL 35216-2809   Fax: 205-978-5018

Emphasizes the importance of communication between partners and offers several guidelines for maintaining a healthy relationship during such a stressful process.
318 pages

5319 Adoption Directory
American Society for Reproductive Medicine
1209 Montgomery Highway   205-978-5000
Birmingham, AL 35216-2809   Fax: 205-978-5018
An extensive reference text covering such specifics as state statutes, adoption agencies, exchanges and agencies.
515 pages

5320 Adoption Fact Book
American Society for Reproductive Medicine
1209 Montgomery Highway   205-978-5000
Birmingham, AL 35216-2809   Fax: 205-978-5018
A comprehensive source of statistics, regulations and facts on adoption.
277 pages

5321 Adoption Resource Book
Harper Collins
10 E 53rd Street   212-207-7000
New York, NY 10022-5299   800-242-7737
Explores and describes all types and styles of adoption and provides excellent resources for each path taken.
421 pages Third edition

5322 Baby of Your Own: New Ways to Overcome Infertility
Taylor Publishing Company
1550 W Mockingbird Lane   214-637-2800
Dallas, TX 75235-5007
Provides current information regarding the psychological aspects of infertility.
244 pages

5323 Conquering Infertility: A Guide for Couples
Prentice Hall Press
15 Columbus Circle   212-373-8000
New York, NY 10023-7707
Covers various aspects of infertility.

5324 Consumer's Guide to Insurance
American Society for Reproductive Medicine
1209 Montgomery Highway   205-978-5000
Birmingham, AL 35216-2809   Fax: 205-978-5018
A how-to book for infertile couples who are experiencing difficulty with insurance reimbursement.
106 pages

5325 Consumer's Legal Guide to Today's Health Care
American Society for Reproductive Medicine
1209 Montgomery Highway   205-978-5000
Birmingham, AL 35216-2809   Fax: 205-978-5018
Provides accurate and up-to-date information concerning patient rights and medical care.
384 pages

5326 Designs on Life
American Society for Reproductive Medicine
1209 Montgomery Highway   205-978-5000
Birmingham, AL 35216-2809   Fax: 205-978-5018
Provides real life stories regarding assisted reproductive technology.
276 pages

5327 Family Bonds: Adoption and the Politics of Parenting
American Society for Reproductive Medicine
1209 Montgomery Highway   205-978-5000
Birmingham, AL 35216-2809   Fax: 205-978-5050
A well organized book is written for people struggling with some of the issues encountered in their journey through infertility and ultimately adoption.
1993 273 pages

5328 Fertility and Pregnancy Guide for DES Daughters and Sons
American Society for Reproductive Medicine
1209 Montgomery Highway   205-978-5000
Birmingham, AL 35216-2809   Fax: 205-978-5018

Guide offering information related to the reproductive potential of individuals who have been exposed to DES in utero.
48 pages

5329 For Want of a Child: A Psychologist and His Wife Explore Infertility
Continuum Publishing Corporation
370 Lexington Avenue   212-532-3650
New York, NY 10017-6503
A psychologist and his wife go through the emotional effects and challenges of infertility.

5330 Getting Pregnant When You Thought You Couldn't
Warner Books
1271 Avenue of the Americas   www.twbookmark.com
New York, NY 10020
A concise guide to understanding infertility that covers issues from diagnosis to treatment and is useful for couples at any stage of infertility treatment.
1993 512 pages

5331 Guide for the Childless Couple
American Society for Reproductive Medicine
1209 Montgomery Highway   205-978-5000
Birmingham, AL 35216-2809   Fax: 205-978-5018
A short text which focuses on the emotional aspects of infertility, including its effects on marriage and self-esteem.
201 pages

5332 Guide to In Vitro Fertilization & Other Assisted Reproduction Methods
Pharos Books
200 Park Avenue   212-692-3700
New York, NY 10166-0005   800-221-4816
This book discusses assisted reproductive technologies from a laboratory and a patient's perspective.

5333 Having Your Baby By Donor Insemination
Houghton Mifflin Company
222 Berkeley Street
Boston, MA 02116   617-351-5000
                                      www.hmco.com
A resource guide to donor insemination which discusses the experience, traditions and techniques of donor insemination, sperm freezing, and known vs. anonymous donors.
352 pages

5334 Healing the Infertile Family
University of California Press
1445 Lower Ferry Road   205-978-5000
Ewing, NJ 08618   800-777-4726
                                      Fax: 800-999-1958
              e-mail: orders@cpfs.pupress.princeton.edu
This well-written book is dedicated to the psychological concerns of the infertile couple.
335 pages
ISBN: 0-520211-80-4

5335 Hormones
American Society for Reproductive Medicine
1209 Montgomery Highway   205-978-5000
Birmingham, AL 35216-2809   Fax: 205-978-5018
Highly recommended text for patients who are suffering from reproductive disorders.
216 pages

5336 How Can I Help?: A Handbook for Practical Suggestions for Infertility
American Society for Reproductive Medicine
1209 Montgomery Highway   205-978-5000
Birmingham, AL 35216-2809   Fax: 205-978-5018
Designed to provide greater understanding of the infertility experience.
18 pages

5337 How to Be a Successful Fertility Patient
American Society for Reproductive Medicine
1209 Montgomery Highway   205-978-5000
Birmingham, AL 35216-2809   Fax: 205-978-5018

Offers extensive interviews with dozens of male and female infertility patients.
1993 447 pages

5338 In Pursuit of Fertility
American Society for Reproductive Medicine
1209 Montgomery Highway   205-978-5000
Birmingham, AL 35216-2809   Fax: 205-978-5018
A comprehensive text which can be used as a tool for couples who want to achieve an understanding of their problem as well as treatment options.
348 pages

5339 In Vitro Fertilization
Facts on File
11 Penn Plaza   212-967-8800
New York, NY 10001   800-322-8755
                                      Fax: 800-678-3633
The A.R.T. of making babies. (Assisted Reproductive Technology) A complete and caring overview of the options available to infertile couples.
208 pages Hardcover
ISBN: 0-816032-69-6

5340 Infertility Book: A Comprehensive Medical & Emotional Guide
American Society for Reproductive Medicine
1209 Montgomery Highway   205-978-5000
Birmingham, AL 35216-2809   Fax: 205-978-5018
Enables the infertile couple to learn how to take control and educate themselves about the trials and tribulations of infertility treatment.
420 pages Softcover

5341 Infertility: A Comprehensive Text
Appleton & Lange
11 W 19th Street   203-838-4400
New York, NY 10011-4209   800-423-1359
A medical reference book.

5342 Issues in Reproductive Management
Thieme Med Publishers
381 Park Avenue S   212-683-5088
New York, NY 10016-8806   Fax: 212-779-9020
1993
ISBN: 0-865775-05-2

5343 Lethal Secrets: The Psychology of Donor Insemination
Warner Books
1271 Avenue of the Americas   www.twbookmark.com
New York, NY 10020
An interview of a cross-section of people who participated in donor insemination.
1993 277 pages
ISBN: 1-567430-20-1

5344 Lifeline: The Action Guide to Adoption Search
American Society for Reproductive Medicine
1209 Montgomery Highway   205-978-5000
Birmingham, AL 35216-2809   Fax: 205-978-5018
A very interesting text describing how an adoptee or adoptive parent may track down birth parents.
384 pages

5345 Long-Awaited Stork: A Guide to Parenting After Infertility
Jossey-Bass
350 Sansome Street   415-433-1740
San Francisco, CA 94104   Fax: 415-433-0499
                                 e-mail: webperson@jbp.com
                                      www.josseybass.com
An excellent resource for couples who are moving from being patients to being parents.
300 pages
ISBN: 0-787940-53-4

5346 Love Cycles: The Science of Intimacy
Random House
1540 Broadway   212-782-9000
New York, NY 10036   Fax: 212-302-7985
Book providing patients with refreshing, scientific concepts of rhythms and relationships between the sexes.
330 pages

5347 Loving Journeys Guide to Adoption
American Society for Reproductive Medicine
1209 Montgomery Highway   205-978-5000
Birmingham, AL 35216-2809   Fax: 205-978-5018
Describes the basic prerequisits agencies and social workers expectations of prospective adoptive parents. Part two offers a directory of state-by-state listings of public and private adoption agencies and adoption attorneys.
394 pages

5348 Male Body
Firestone Touchstone Paperbacks/Simon & Schuster
200 Old Tappan Road
Old Tappan, NJ 07675-7005   800-999-5479
An informative and reassuring reference written to meet increasing interest in male health issues. This book discusses varied aspects of health such as infections and injuries, vasectomies, the emotional aspects of sexual difficulties and preventive measures that can be taken against AIDS and other sexually transmitted diseases.
208 pages
ISBN: 0-671864-26-2

5349 Men, Women and Infertility
American Society for Reproductive Medicine
1209 Montgomery Highway   205-978-5000
Birmingham, AL 35216-2809   Fax: 205-978-5018
A helpful book offering suggestions for a positive self-image and high self-esteem through the trauma of infertility.
1993 256 pages

5350 Miscarriage Women: Sharing from the Heart
American Society for Reproductive Medicine
1209 Montgomery Highway   205-978-5000
Birmingham, AL 35216-2809   Fax: 205-978-5018
A well organized book offering help and information to benefit patients who have experienced pregnancy loss as well as professionals working with these couples.
1993 258 pages

5351 Missed Conceptions: Overcoming Infertility
McGraw-Hill
1221 Avenue of the Americas   212-512-2000
New York, NY 10020
Book about infertility and the emotional agony that goes along with it. Addresses all aspects surrounding infertility care and offers in-depth discussions of the many fertility options now available.
377 pages

5352 Motherhood: A Feminist Perspective
American Society for Reproductive Medicine
1209 Montgomery Highway   205-978-5000
Birmingham, AL 35216-2809   Fax: 205-978-5018
A compilation of papers from conference proceedings designed to define motherhood. Offers information on infertility, emotional and financial difficulties and daily living.
234 pages

5353 Mothers of Thyme: Customs and Rituals of Infertility and Miscarriage
Lida Rose Press
An organized book that offers details on rituals and misconceptions concerning infertility and miscarriage.
128 pages
ISBN: 0-962595-75-6

5354 Never to Be a Mother
Harper Collins Publishers
10 E 53rd Street   212-207-7000
New York, NY 10022-5299   800-242-7737
Offers childless women a plan for confronting their grief, anger and guilt, as well as offering alternative ways to mother and live.

5355 No-Hysterectomy Option
American Society for Reproductive Medicine
1209 Montgomery Highway   205-978-5000
Birmingham, AL 35216-2809   Fax: 205-978-5018

An excellent reference for women faced with decisions regarding hysterectomy.
265 pages

5356 One Women's Passionate Quest to Complete Her Family
Viking Penguin
375 Hudson Street   212-366-2000
New York, NY 10014-3658
The author presents a highly emotional account of the years of anguish, disappointment, and finally the joy she achieved in trying to complete her family.

5357 Overcoming Infertility
Doubleday
666 5th Avenue   212-765-6500
New York, NY 10103-0001   800-223-6834
Paints a clear picture of the medical and emotional aspects of infertility.

5358 Preventing Miscarriage: The Good News
American Society for Reproductive Medicine
1209 Montgomery Highway   205-978-5000
Birmingham, AL 35216-2809   Fax: 205-978-5018
Provides information on possible causes of miscarriages with information on infections, abnormalities and more.
240 pages Softcover

5359 Reproductive Hazards in the Workplace: Mending Jobs, Managing Pregnancies
Regina H Kenen, PhD, author
Haworth Press
10 Alice Street   607-722-5857
Binghamton, NY 13904-1580   800-429-6784
                                      Fax: 607-722-0012
                                      www.haworthpress.com
Offers information on the history and present of potential reproductive hazards. Includes pregnancy hazard hotlines, specific contact points where women can get information on working environments and more.
286 pages Hardcover
ISBN: 1-560241-54-3

5360 Resolving Infertility
RESOLVE: National Infertility Association
1310 Broadway   617-623-1156
Somerville, MA 02144-1779   888-623-0744
                                      Fax: 617-623-0252
                                 e-mail: info@resolve.org
                                      www.resolve.org
Understanding the options and choosing solutions when you want to have a baby is a definitive resource to help you sort out the options and negative through the experience with confidence. This book tells you everything you need to know about infertility treatment and exploring other family building options.
370 pages
ISBN: 0-062735-22-5
Bonny Gilbert, Executive Director

5361 Science and Babies: Private Decisions, Public Dilemmas
American Society for Reproductive Medicine
1209 Montgomery Highway   205-978-5000
Birmingham, AL 35216-2809   Fax: 205-978-5018
Offers a superb summary of key reproductive issues ranging from conception to contraception.
250 pages

5362 Silent Sorrow
Delta-Dell Publishers
666 5th Avenue   212-765-6500
New York, NY 10103-0001   800-223-6834
A book dealing with the emotional and psychological aspects of losing a child.

5363 Surrogate Motherhood: The Legal and Human Issues
Harvard University Press
79 Garden Street   617-495-2600
Cambridge, MA 02138-1423
A discussion of the psychological, legal and policy questions raised by surrogacy.

5364 Surviving Infertility
Tapestry Books
PO Box 359   908-806-6695
Ringoes, NJ 08551-0359   800-765-2367
    Fax: 732-288-2999
A valuable source of support and practical advice for coping with
the many intense feelings associated with being infertile.
389 pages

**5365 Surviving Pregnancy Loss: A Complete Sourcebook for Women
& Their Families**
American Society for Reproductive Medicine
1209 Montgomery Highway   205-978-5000
Birmingham, AL 35216-2809   Fax: 205-978-5018
Contains practical approaches to coping with the emotional and
psychological problems associated with pregnancy loss.
298 pages

5366 Sweet Grapes: How to Stop Being Infertile and Living Again
American Society for Reproductive Medicine
1209 Montgomery Highway   205-978-5000
Birmingham, AL 35216-2809   Fax: 205-978-5018
Recommended for couples nearing the end of their options or for
those who are unsure if they wish to pursue infertility therapy.

5367 To Love a Child
Addison Wesley Publishing
Route 128   781-944-3700
Reading, MA 01867   800-447-2226
A thoughtful and informative overview of alternatives to bio/ge-
netic parenting.

5368 Understanding and Infertility
Tapestry Books
PO Box 359   908-806-6695
Ringoes, NJ 08551-0359   800-765-2367
    Fax: 732-288-2999
Provides specific advice to the family on how to be supportive of
members and/or friends who suffer from infertility.
28 pages

5369 WHO Laboratory Manual
American Society for Reproductive Medicine
1209 Montgomery Highway   205-978-5000
Birmingham, AL 35216-2809   Fax: 205-978-5018
Third edition

5370 Waiting: A Diary of Loss and Hope in Pregnancy
American Society for Reproductive Medicine
1209 Montgomery Highway   205-978-5000
Birmingham, AL 35216-2809   Fax: 205-978-5018
Provides clear insight into coping with the trials and tribulations of
infertility.
121 pages

5371 Without Child
American Society for Reproductive Medicine
1209 Montgomery Highway   205-978-5000
Birmingham, AL 35216-2809   Fax: 205-978-5018
Covers topics including the doctor-patient relationship, religion
and infertility, living child-free and the adoption process for persons without children investigating their options.
226 pages

5372 Women Without Children
Pharos Books
200 Park Avenue   212-692-3700
New York, NY 10166-0005   800-221-4816
Offers women without children support through their struggle and
decision making.

Children's Books

**5373 Mommy, Did I Grow in Your Tummy? Where Some Babies Come
From**
American Society for Reproductive Medicine
1209 Montgomery Highway   205-978-5000
Birmingham, AL 35216-2809   Fax: 205-978-5018

Illustrated book that helps parents explain the different ways children can come into the world, including IVF, surrogacy, game donation and adoption.
28 pages Ages 4-8

Magazines

**5374 American Society for Reproductive Medicine: Clinic Specific
Annual Report**
1209 Montgomery Highway   205-978-5000
Birmingham, AL 35216-2809   Fax: 205-978-5005
    e-mail: asrm@asrm.com
    www.asrm.com
Gives the success rates of treatment for fertility centers around the
country.

5375 Biology of Reproduction
1603 Monroe Street   608-256-2777
Madison, WI 53711-2021   Fax: 608-256-4610
    e-mail: bor@ssr.org
    www.biolreprod.org
A monthly, peer-reviewed journal.
250 pages Monthly

5376 Family Building Magazine
RESOLVE: National Infertility Association
1310 Broadway   617-623-1156
Somerville, MA 02144-1779   888-623-0744
    Fax: 617-623-0252
    e-mail: info@resolve.org
    www.resolve.org
Offers various information on the newest technology and advances
in infertility treatments, support groups, helplines, centers and in
depth articles written by professionals in the field.
15-18 pages Quarterly
Bonny Gilbert, Executive Director

5377 Infertility and Adoption
RESOLVE: National Infertility Association
1310 Broadway   617-623-1156
Somerville, MA 02144-1779   888-623-0744
    Fax: 617-623-0252
    e-mail: info@resolve.org
    www.resolve.org
Published by RESOLVE: The National Infertility Association.
Bonny Gilbert, Executive Director

5378 Journal of Occupational & Environmental Medicine
Williams & Wilkins
351 W Camden Street   301-528-4000
Baltimore, MD 21201-7912   800-638-0672

Newsletters

5379 Hers Newsletter
Hysterectomy Educational Resources & Services
422 Bryn Mawr Avenue   610-667-7757
Bala Cynwyd, PA 19004-2708   800-777-4377
    Fax: 610-667-8096
    e-mail: hersfdn@aol.com
    www.hersfoundation.com
Offers information and support for women who have had or are go-
ing through hysterectomies.
Quarterly
Nora W Coffey, President

5380 RESOLVE of the Bay State
PO Box 541553   781-647-1614
Waltham, MA 02454-1553   Fax: 781-899-7207
    e-mail: admin@resolveofthebaystate.org
    www.resolveofthebaystate.org
Information on the Massachusetts chapter of a national, nonprofit,
consumer based infertility support organization. Information on a
variety of services to answer your questions about infertility, treatments, coping techniques, insurance issues and family building
options.

Pamphlets

5381 ART-Assisted Reproductive Technologies
Serono Symposia USA
100 Longwater Circle
Norwell, MA 02061-1616   800-283-8088

5382 Abnormal Uterine Bleeding
American Society for Reproductive Medicine
1209 Montgomery Highway   205-978-5000
Birmingham, AL 35216-2809   Fax: 205-978-5018
                                 e-mail: asrm@asrm.com

1996

5383 Adoption
American Society for Reproductive Medicine
1209 Montgomery Highway   205-978-5000
Birmingham, AL 35216-2809   Fax: 205-978-5018
                                 e-mail: asrm@asrm.com

1990

5384 Affording Your Infertility
Serono Symposia USA
100 Longwater Circle
Norwell, MA 02061-1616   800-283-8088

5385 Age and Fertility
American Society for Reproductive Medicine
1209 Montgomery Highway   205-978-5000
Birmingham, AL 35216-2809   Fax: 205-978-5018
                                 e-mail: asrm@asrm.com

1996

5386 Bibliography
RESOLVE: National Infertility Association
1310 Broadway   617-623-1156
Somerville, MA 02144-1779   888-623-0744
                                     Fax: 617-623-0252
                                 e-mail: info@resolve.org
                                        www.resolve.org
Annotated guide to books and articles on medical and emotional
aspects of infertility.
Bonny Gilbert, Executive Director

5387 Birth Defects of the Female Reproductive System
American Society for Reproductive Medicine
1209 Montgomery Highway   205-978-5000
Birmingham, AL 35216-2809   Fax: 205-978-5018
                                 e-mail: asrm@asrm.com

1993

5388 Coping with the Holidays
RESOLVE
1310 Broadway   781-643-0744
Somerville, MA 02144-1779

5389 Donor Insemination
American Society for Reproductive Medicine
1209 Montgomery Highway   205-978-5000
Birmingham, AL 35216-2809   Fax: 205-978-5018
                                 e-mail: asrm@asrm.com

1995

5390 Early Menopause (Premature Ovarian Failure)
American Society for Reproductive Medicine
1209 Montgomery Highway   205-978-5000
Birmingham, AL 35216-2809   Fax: 205-978-5018
                                 e-mail: asrm@asrm.com

1996

5391 Ectopic Pregnancy
American Society for Reproductive Medicine
1209 Montgomery Highway   205-978-5000
Birmingham, AL 35216-2809   Fax: 205-978-5018
                                 e-mail: asrm@asrm.com

1996

5392 Emotional Aspects of Infertility
RESOLVE: National Infertility Association
1310 Broadway   617-623-1156
Somerville, MA 02144-1779   888-623-0744
                                     Fax: 617-623-0252
                                 e-mail: info@resolve.org
                                        www.resolve.org
Published by RESOLVE: The National Infertility Association.
Bonny Gilbert, Executive Director

5393 Ending Infertility Treatment
RESOLVE: National Infertility Association
1310 Broadway   617-623-1156
Somerville, MA 02144-1779   888-623-0744
                                     Fax: 617-623-0252
                                 e-mail: info@resolve.org
                                        www.resolve.org
Published by RESOLVE: The National Infertility Association.
Bonny Gilbert, Executive Director

5394 Endometriosis
American Society for Reproductive Medicine
1209 Montgomery Highway   205-978-5000
Birmingham, AL 35216-2809   Fax: 205-978-5018
                                 e-mail: asrm@asrm.com

Available in Spanish.
1994

5395 Environmental Toxins and Fertility
RESOLVE: National Infertility Association
1310 Broadway   617-623-1156
Somerville, MA 02144-1779   888-623-0744
                                     Fax: 617-623-0252
                                 e-mail: info@resolve.org
                                        www.resolve.org
Published by the National Infertility Association (RESOLVE).
Bonny Gilbert, Executive Director

5396 Fertility After Cancer Treatment
American Society for Reproductive Medicine
1209 Montgomery Highway   205-978-5000
Birmingham, AL 35216-2809   Fax: 205-978-5018
                                 e-mail: asrm@asrm.com

1995

5397 Getting Started: How Do I Know If I'm Infertile?
RESOLVE
1310 Broadway   781-643-0744
Somerville, MA 02144-1779

5398 Hirsutism and Polycystic Ovarian Syndrome
American Society for Reproductive Medicine
1209 Montgomery Highway   205-978-5000
Birmingham, AL 35216-2809   Fax: 205-978-5018
                                 e-mail: asrm@asrm.com

1995

5399 Husband Insemination
American Society for Reproductive Medicine
1209 Montgomery Highway   205-978-5000
Birmingham, AL 35216-2809   Fax: 205-978-5018
                                 e-mail: asrm@asrm.com

1995

5400 IVF & GIFT: A Guide to Assisted Reproductive Technologies
American Society for Reproductive Medicine
1209 Montgomery Highway   205-978-5000
Birmingham, AL 35216-2809   Fax: 205-978-5018
                                 e-mail: asrm@asrm.com

Available in Spanish.
1995

5401 If You are Having Trouble Conceiving
American Society for Reproductive Medicine
1209 Montgomery Highway   205-978-5000
Birmingham, AL 35216-2809   Fax: 205-978-5018

5402 Infertility Insurance
Serono Symposia USA
100 Longwater Circle
Norwell, MA 02061-1616   800-283-8088

5403 Infertility: An Overview
American Society for Reproductive Medicine
1209 Montgomery Highway   205-978-5000
Birmingham, AL 35216-2809   Fax: 205-978-5018
      e-mail: asrm@asrm.com
Available in Spanish.
1994

5404 Infertility: Causes and Treatment
American College/Obstetricians and Gynecologists
409 12th Street SW   www.acog.com
Washington, DC 20024
To obtain a free copy of this publication, please send a self-addressed stamped #10 envelope and request by title. (#AP002)

5405 Infertility: Coping and Decision Making
American Society for Reproductive Medicine
1209 Montgomery Highway   205-978-5000
Birmingham, AL 35216-2809   Fax: 205-978-5018
      e-mail: asrm@asrm.com

1995

5406 Infertility: The Emotional Roller Coaster
Serono Symposia USA
100 Longwater Circle
Norwell, MA 02061-1616   800-283-8088

5407 Insights Into Infertility
Serono Symposia USA
100 Longwater Circle
Norwell, MA 02061-1616   800-283-8088

5408 Introduction to Infertility: The First Steps
RESOLVE: National Infertility Association
1310 Broadway   617-623-1156
Somerville, MA 02144-1779   888-623-0744
      Fax: 617-623-0252
      e-mail: info@resolve.org
      www.resolve.org
Published by RESOLVE: The National Infertility Association.
Bonny Gilbert, Executive Director

5409 Laparoscopy and Hysteroscopy
American Society for Reproductive Medicine
1209 Montgomery Highway   205-978-5000
Birmingham, AL 35216-2809   Fax: 205-978-5018
      e-mail: asrm@asrm.com

1995

5410 Male Infertility
Serono Symposia USA
100 Longwater Circle
Norwell, MA 02061-1616   800-283-8088

5411 Male Infertility and Vasectomy Reversal
American Society for Reproductive Medicine
1209 Montgomery Highway   205-978-5000
Birmingham, AL 35216-2809   Fax: 205-978-5018
      e-mail: asrm@asrm.com

1995

5412 Managing Family & Friends
RESOLVE
1310 Broadway   781-643-0744
Somerville, MA 02144-1779

5413 Miscarriage
American Society for Reproductive Medicine
1209 Montgomery Highway   205-978-5000
Birmingham, AL 35216-2809   Fax: 205-978-5018
      e-mail: asrm@asrm.com

1995

5414 Myths & Facts
RESOLVE
1310 Broadway   781-643-0744
Somerville, MA 02144-1779

5415 Ovulation Detection
American Society for Reproductive Medicine

1209 Montgomery Highway   205-978-5000
Birmingham, AL 35216-2809   Fax: 205-978-5018
      e-mail: asrm@asrm.com
1995

5416 Ovulation Drugs
American Society for Reproductive Medicine
1209 Montgomery Highway   205-978-5000
Birmingham, AL 35216-2809   Fax: 205-978-5018
      e-mail: asrm@asrm.com

1995

5417 Patient Information Series Publications
American Society for Reproductive Medicine
1209 Montgomery Highway   205-978-5000
Birmingham, AL 35216-2809   Fax: 205-978-5018
      e-mail: asrm@asrm.com

Offers a set of 20 various brochures ranging from artificial insemination to male infertility problems.

5418 Pelvic Pain
American Society for Reproductive Medicine
1209 Montgomery Highway   205-978-5000
Birmingham, AL 35216-2809   Fax: 205-978-5018
      e-mail: asrm@asrm.com

1997

5419 Pregnancy After Infertility
American Society for Reproductive Medicine
1209 Montgomery Highway   205-978-5000
Birmingham, AL 35216-2809   Fax: 205-978-5018
      e-mail: asrm@asrm.com

1997

5420 Premenstrual Syndrome (PMS)
American Society for Reproductive Medicine
1209 Montgomery Highway   205-978-5000
Birmingham, AL 35216-2809   Fax: 205-978-5018
      e-mail: asrm@asrm.com

1997

5421 Third Party Reproduction (Donor Eggs, Donor Sperm, Donor Embryos, & Surrogacy)
American Society for Reproductive Medicine
1209 Montgomery Highway   205-978-5000
Birmingham, AL 35216-2809   Fax: 205-978-5018
      e-mail: asrm@asrm.com

1996

5422 Tubal Factor Infertility
American Society for Reproductive Medicine
1209 Montgomery Highway   205-978-5000
Birmingham, AL 35216-2809   Fax: 205-978-5018
      e-mail: asrm@asrm.com

1995

5423 Understanding: A Guide to Impaired Fertility for Family and Friends
American Society for Reproductive Medicine
1209 Montgomery Highway   205-978-5000
Birmingham, AL 35216-2809   Fax: 205-978-5018
A pamphlet designed for families of patients with infertility and for distribution to individuals who may want to become involved in the counseling and support of these couples.
28 pages

5424 Unexplained Infertility
American Society for Reproductive Medicine
1209 Montgomery Highway   205-978-5000
Birmingham, AL 35216-2809   Fax: 205-978-5018
      e-mail: asrm@asrm.com

1997

5425 Uterine Fibroids
American Society for Reproductive Medicine
1209 Montgomery Highway   205-978-5000
Birmingham, AL 35216-2809   Fax: 205-978-5018
      e-mail: asrm@asrm.com

1997

Audio & Video

5426 Candid Talk About Loss in Adoption
Mary Martin Mason
4505 York Avenue S   612-922-1136
Minneapolis, MN 55410-1422
Discusses losses incurred by the adopted persons and adoptive persons issues for children adopted into different race families.
Videotape

5427 Coping with Infertility
Distributed By UC Video
425 Ontario Street SE
Minneapolis, MN 55414-3002   612-627-4444
Features five couples talking about their infertility experiences.
Odessa Flores

5428 Infertility: Exploring the Male Factor
American Society for Reproductive Medicine
1209 Montgomery Highway   205-978-5000
Birmingham, AL 35216-2809   Fax: 205-978-5018
A well-orchestrated video discussing male factor infertility, including the infertility workup, physical exam, semen analysis, and surgical options available.
1993 47 minutes

5429 One, Two, Three, Zero: Infertility
Filmmaker's Library
133 E 58th Street   212-355-6545
New York, NY 10022-1236
Videotape

5430 Six Phases of Infertility Treatment: Medical & Emotional Aspects
RESOLVE of Maryland
PO Box 19049   410-243-0235
Baltimore, MD 21284-9049
Gives an overview of infertility treatment, addressing the medical and emotional aspects.
Videotape

5431 So You're Going to Adopt
Mary Martin Mason
4505 York Avenue S   612-922-1136
Minneapolis, MN 55410-1422
This video prepares adoptive parents for pre and post adoption issues.
Videotape

Web Sites

5432 Adopt-A-Special-Kid America
www.adoptaspecialkid.org
Adopt-A-Special-Kid provides information on adoption of children with special needs.

5433 American Society for Reproductive Medicine
www.asrm.com
Devoted to advancing the knowledge, understanding and expertise in all phases of reproductive medicine and biology. Offers patient education brochures, recommended readings and support.

5434 Center for Disease Control
www.cdc.gov
Reproductive health information source. Also a resource for the Society of Reproductive Technology. Invitro fertilization data reports and men's reproductive health. Interesting well balanced site.

5435 Fertilethoughts.com
www.fertilethoughts.com
A support sytem concerned with helping reach a goal of finding the perfect doctor, the diagnosis, as well as the treatment.

5436 Healing Well
www.healingwell.com
An online health resource guide to medical news, chat, information and articles, newsgroups and message boards, books, disease-related web sites, medical directories, and more for patients, friends, and family coping with disabling diseases, disorders, or chronic illnesses.

5437 Health Finder
www.healthfinder.gov
Searchable, carefully developed web site offering information on over 1000 topics. Developed by the US Department of Health and Human Services, the site can be used in both English and Spanish.

5438 Healthlink USA
www.healthlinkusa.com
Health information concerning treatment, cures, prevention, diagnosis, risk factors, research, support groups, email lists, personal stories and much more. Updated regularly.

5439 Helios Health
www.helioshealth.com
Online resource for your health information. Detailed information about specific health topics, access to expert advice from our Medical Advisory Board, and up-to-date health news.

5440 Infertility Books
www.infertilitybooks.com
Nonprofit site includes book titles regarding infertility and a short explanation of each book and how to get it.

5441 International Council on Infertility Information Dissemination
www.inciid.org
A nonprofit organization that helps individuals and couples explore their family-building options.

5442 Internet Health Resources
www.ihr.com/infertility
This web site provides extensive information about IVF, ICSI, infertility clinics, donor egg and surrogacy services, sperm banks, pharmacies, infertility books and videotapes, sperm testing, infertility newsgroups and support organizations, and drugs and medications.

5443 Ivf.com
www.ivf.com
Goal is to provide the latest women's healthcare innovations to address infertility, polycystic ovaries, endometriosis, and pelvic pain treatment.

5444 MedicineNet
www.medicinenet.com
An online resource for consumers providing easy-to-read, authoritative medical and health information.

5445 Medscape
www.medscape.com
Medscape offers specialists, primary care physicians, and other health professionals the Web's most robust and integrated medical information and educational tools.

5446 National Institutes of Health
www.medlineplus.gov
Information regarding all aspects of infertility. Some of the topics include: Latest news, overview of anatomy and physiology, clinical trails, diagnoses and symptoms, treatment, genetics, plus lots of links to other sites. Type infertility into the search engine.

5447 RESOLVE
www.resolve.org
Provides help to people who are experiencing the infertility crisis and strives to increase the visibility of infertility issues via concerted advocacy and public education.

5448 Uterine Artery Embolization
www.uterinearteryembolization.com
Provides information on Uterine Artery Embolization, or Uterine Fibroid Embolization as an alternative to hysterectomy or myomectomy as a treatment for uterine fibroids.

5449 WebMD
www.webmd.com
Information on infertility, including articles and resources.

Description

5450 Kidney Disease

The diseases that affect the kidney can be divided into diseases of the kidney itself, such as nephritis, polycystic kidney disease, kidney infections and stones, and diseases of other body systems that cause damage to the kidneys, such as diabetes, high blood pressure and lupus. In either instance, disruption of kidney function results in failure to remove excess fluids and wastes from the blood. This may lead to end stage kidney, or renal, failure.

Symptoms of kidney disease and their severity, depend on the underlying cause. If there is damage or disease in the urinary tract, there can be pain when urinating, blood in the urine, or changes in frequency and urgency of urination. If excess fluid cannot be removed, there may be swelling around the eyes and ankles. When the kidney is damaged directly, back or flank tenderness may be present. In many cases, kidney disease causes no symptoms until the advanced stages, although it may be detected much earlier through tests of blood or urine.

Treatment is directed to the cause, and may include antibiotics for infections, removal of kidney stones by surgery or ultrasound waves, management of the systemic disease such as diabetes, dietary modification, especially of salt and protein intake, and close monitoring and correction of fluids and electrolytes. Treatment may also include control of high blood pressure, which can be caused by kidney disease and further damage the kidney. The most severe cases of kidney failure require either dialysis, in which the blood's toxins are mechanically filtered and removed, or a kidney transplant.

National Agencies & Associations

5451 Alabama Kidney Foundation
31 Center Drive MSC 2560
Bethesda, MD 20892-3580

301-496-6325
800-891-5390
Fax: 301-480-3510
e-mail: starr@mail.nih.gov
www.niddk.nih.gov

Strives to increase knowledge and understanding about diseases of the kidneys and urologic system among people with these conditions their families health care professionals and the general public.
Dr Robert Star, Director

5452 American Association of Kidney Patients
2701 N Rocky Point Drive
Tampa, FL 33607-1796

813-636-8100
800-749-2257
Fax: 813-636-8122
e-mail: info@aakp.org
www.aakp.org

Serves the needs and interests of all kidney patients and their families. Founded in 1969 by kidney patients, for kidney patients, the purpose of this association is to help patients and their families cope with the emotional, physical and social impact of kidney disease.
Sam Pederson, President
Paul T Conway, Vice-President

5453 National Diabetes Information Clearinghous e
11921 Rockville Pike
Rockville, MD 20852

301-881-3052
800-638-8299
Fax: 301-881-0898
e-mail: patientservice@kidneyfund.org
www.akfinc.org

A nonprofit national health organization providing direct financial assistance to thousands of Americans who suffer from kidney disease.
John P Butler, Chair
LaVarne A Burton, President/ CEO

5454 National Institute of Diabetes & Digestive & Kidney Diseases
National Institutes of Health
1 Information Way
Bethesda, MD 20892-2560

301-496-4000
800-860-8747
Fax: 703-738-4929
TTY: 866-569-1162
e-mail: ndic@info.niddk.nih.gov
www.diabetes.niddk.nih.gov

Conducts and supports research on many of the most serious diseases affecting public health. The Institute supports much of the clinical research on the diseases of internal medicine and related subspecialty fields as well as many basic science disciplines.
Dr Griffin Rodgers, Acting Director

5455 National Kidney Foundation
30 E 33rd Street
New York, NY 10016

212-889-2210
800-622-9010
Fax: 212-689-9261
e-mail: info@kidney.org
www.kidney.org

A major voluntary health organization dedicated to preventing kidney and urinary tract diseases improving the health and well-being of individuals and families affected by these diseases and increasing the availability of all organs for transplantation.
Bruce Skyer, Chief Executive Officer
Joseph Vassalotti, MD, Chief Medical Officer

State Agencies & Associations

Alabama

5456 Alabama Chapter of the American Association of Kidney Patients
PO BOX 12505
Birmingham, AL 35202-2238

205-934-2111
800-750-3331
Fax: 205-975-6682
e-mail: jack@alkidney.org
www.alkidney.org

Gwen Deierhoi, President
E.W. Jackson III, Executive Director

Arizona

5457 Arizona Kidney Foundation
4203 E Indian School Road
Phoenix, AZ 85018

602-840-1644
Fax: 602-840-2360
www.azkidney.org

Leonard J McDonald, Chair
Jeffrey D Neff, Chief Executive Officer

5458 Central Arizona Chapter of the American Association of Kidney Patients
4401 W Hatcher Road
Glendale, AZ 85302-3821

602-939-7248

Dale A Ester, President

Arkansas

5459 National Kidney Foundation of Arkansas
1818 N Taylor Street
Little Rock, AR 72207

501-664-4343
800-622-9010
Fax: 816-221-7984
e-mail: nkfar@kidney.org
www.kidney.org

Nonprofit health organization. Our mission is to prevent kidney and urinary tract disease improve the health and well being of indi-

viduals and families affected by these diseases and increase the availability of all organs for transplantation.
R D Todd Baur, Member of the Board of Directors
Derek E Bruce, Member of the Board of Directors

California

5460 Harbor-South Bay Orange County Chapter of the American Assoc. of Kidney Patients
PO Box 8
Seal Beach, CA 90740
714-527-8009
e-mail: delrita@aol.com
www.aakp.org

Rita McQuire, President

5461 Los Angeles Chapter of the American Association of Kidney Patients
9854 National Boulevard
Los Angeles, CA 90034
310-364-1807
e-mail: aakpla@yahoo.com
www.aakp.org

Robin Siegal, President

5462 National Kidney Foundation of Northern California
131 Steuart Street
San Francisco, CA 94105
415-543-3303
888-427-5653
Fax: 415-543-3331
e-mail: infopacific@kidney.org
www.kidney.org/site/503/index.cfm
Work with kidney patients both pre ESRD dialysis and transplant. Financial assistance educational workshops scholarships children's and family camps transplant games information and referral.
Brad J Small, Division President
Connie M Nieri, Division Director of Finance/Operations

5463 National Kidney Foundation of Southern California
15490 Ventura Boulevard
Sherman Oaks, CA 91403
818-783-8153
800-747-5527
Fax: 818-783-8160
e-mail: nkfsca@kidney.org
www.kidney.org

Pier Merone, Division President
Natalie Kanooni, Division Program Manager

5464 Redding Chapter of the American Association of Kidney Patients
790 Pioneer Drive
Redding, CA 96001-0258
530-241-6451
e-mail: teamward@c-zone.net
www.aakp.org

5465 Sacramento Valley Chapter of the American Association of Kidney Patients
565 Morrison Avenue
Sacramento, CA 95838
916-924-1996

Colorado

5466 Colorado Chapter of the American Association of Kidney Patients
PO Box 8442
Denver, CO 80201
303-758-8610

5467 National Kidney Foundation of Colorado: Idaho, Montana, and Wyoming
650 South Cherry Street
Denver, CO 80246
720-748-9991
800-596-7943
Fax: 720-748-1273
e-mail: nkfcmw@kidney.org
www.kidney.org/site/505/
Brandi Krause, State Director
Stacey Lux, Development Director

5468 Western Slope Chapter of the American Association of Kidney Patients
1539 Ptarmigan Ridge
Grand Junction, CO 81056
970-244-9196
Vicki Hathaway, CEO
Donna Sciacca, Director of Patient Programs/Services

Connecticut

5469 National Kidney Foundation of Connecticut
1463 Highland Avenue
Cheshire, CT 06410
203-439-7912
800-441-1280
Fax: 203-439-7934
e-mail: nkfct@kidney.org
www.kidney.org/site/102/index.cfm

Marcia Hilditch, Program Manager
Deb Ramada, Development Coordinator

District of Columbia

5470 Georgetown University Center for Hypertension and Renal Disease Research
3800 Reservoir Road NW
Washington, DC 20007
202-687-9183
Fax: 202-687-7893
e-mail: wilcoxch@qunet.georgetown.edu
www.georgetown.edu/research/hrdrc
International institute for basic and clinical investigation education and clinical practice in hypertension and renal disease.
Christopher Englert, Jr. CAE, President/CEO

5471 National Kidney Foundation of the National Capital Area
5335 Wisconsin Avenue NW
Washington, DC 20015-2030
202-244-7900
Fax: 202-244-7405
e-mail: infowdc@kidney.org
www.kidney.org/site/203/index.cfm

Pamela D Gatz, Division President
Sherrita Lancaster, Division Office Manager

Florida

5472 American Association of Kidney Patients
2701 N Rocky Point Drive
Tampa, FL 33607
813-636-8100
800-749-2257
Fax: 813-636-8122
e-mail: info@aakp.org
www.aakp.org

Sam Pederson, President
Paul T Conway, Vice-President

5473 Kidney Association of South Florida
6801 Lake Worth Road
Lake Worth, FL 33467
561-434-4559
e-mail: jansym@bellsouth.net
www.aakp.org

Jan Symonette, President

5474 National Kidney Foundation of Florida
1040 Woodcock Road
Orlando, FL 32803
407-894-7325
800-927-9659
Fax: 407-895-0051
e-mail: nkf@kidneyfla.org
www.kidney.org/site/204/index.cfm

Andrew Helfan, President
Stephanie Hutchinson, CEO

5475 South Florida Chapter of the American Association of Kidney Patients
5217 Northlake Boulevard
Palm Beach Gardens, FL 33418
561-471-2588
e-mail: diazgray@aol.com
www.aakp.org

Robert Kirby, President

5476 Sunshine Chapter of the American Association of Kidney Patients
PO Box 4716
Hialeah, FL 33014-0716
305-821-4827
Elaine Printup

Georgia

5477 Atlanta Georgia Chapter of the American Association of Kidney Patients
6409 Lakeview Drive
Buford, GA 30518
404-932-1100
Pamela Sachs, Division President
Tracy Jenny, Division Program Director

5478 National Kidney Foundation of Georgia
2951 Flowers Road S
Atlanta, GA 30341
770-452-1539
800-633-2339
Fax: 770-452-7564
e-mail: nkfga@kidney.org
www.kidney.org

Barbara McDowell, President

5479 Rome Georgia Chapter of the American Association of Kidney Patients
118 Woodcrest Drive
Rome, GA 30161
706-232-8989
Hazel Hayashida, Chief Executive Officer
Diana Pinard, Director of Organization Planning

Hawaii

5480 National Kidney Foundation of Hawaii
1314 S King Street
Honolulu, HI 96814
808-593-1515
800-488-2277
Fax: 808-589-5993
e-mail: Glen@kidneyhi.org
www.kidneyhi.org
Hawaii's leading voluntary health agency to the education prevention and treatment of kidney and urinary tract diseases and increase the availability of all organs for transplantation in Hawaii.
Aileen Utterdyke, President
Glen Hayashida, CEO

Idaho

5481 National Kidney Foundation of Colorado, Idaho, Montana, and Wyoming
650 South Cherry Street
Denver, CO 80246
720-748-9991
800-596-7943
Fax: 720-748-1273
e-mail: nkfcmw@kidney.org
www.kidney.org/site/505/
Brandi Krause, State Director
Stacey Lux, Development Director

Illinois

5482 Chicagoland Chapter of the American Association of Kidney Patients
70 Lincoln Oaks Drive
Chicago, IL 60514
708-325-3475
Gloria Lang, Chief Executive Officer
Kate Grubbs O'Connor, Chief Operating Officer

5483 National Kidney Foundation of Illinois
215 W Illinois
Chicago, IL 60654
312-321-1500
Fax: 312-321-1505
e-mail: kidney@nkfi.org
www.nkfi.org

Mark L Schwartz, President
Kate Grubbs O'Connor, Chief Executive Officer

Indiana

5484 National Kidney Foundation of Indiana
911 E 86th Street
Indianapolis, IN 46240-1840
317-722-5640
800-382-9971
Fax: 317-722-5650
e-mail: nkfi@kidneyindiana.org
www.kidney.org/site/303/index.cfm
The mission of the NKFI is to prevent kidney and urinary tract disease improve the health and well-being of individuals and family affected by these disease and increase the availability of all organs for transplantation.
Margie Evans Fort, Chief Executive Officer
Heather Gallagher, Communications Director

Iowa

5485 Iowa Chapter of the Association of Kidney Patients
2203 75th Place
Davenport, IA 52806-1107
319-391-1194
Dave Hagarty, Executive Director
Lori Donald, Accounting Coordinator

Kansas

5486 National Kidney Foundation of Kansas and Western Missouri
6405 Metcalf Avenue
Overland Park, KS 66202
913-262-1551
800-596-7943
Fax: 913-722-4841
e-mail: nkfkswmo@kidney.org
www.kidney.org/site/305/index.cfm
Sherri Denny, Regional Administrative Assistant
Alexandra Wilson, Special Events Manager

Kentucky

5487 National Kidney Foundation of Kentucky
250 E Liberty Street
Louisville, KY 40202
502-585-5433
800-737-5433
Fax: 502-585-1445
e-mail: infonkfk@kidney.org
www.nkfk.org

April Enix, Director of Development
Nital Desai, Community Outreach Manager

Louisiana

5488 Bayou Area Chapter of the American Association of Kidney Patients
PO Box 400
Lockport, LA 70374
504-532-3542
Louisiana Kranze, Chief Executive Officer
Tracey Eldridge, Director of Special Events

5489 National Kidney Foundation of Louisiana
8200 Hampson Street
New Orleans, LA 70118
504-861-4500
800-462-3694
Fax: 504-861-1976
e-mail: info@kidneyla.org
www.kidneyla.org

Shawn Donelon, Chairman
Torie Kranze, Chief Executive Officer

Maine

5490 National Kidney Foundation of Maine
85 Astor Avenue
Norwood, ME 02062
781-278-0222
800-542-4001
Fax: 781-278-0333
e-mail: nkfofmrnv@kidneyhealth.org
www.kidney.org/site/105/index.cfm
Andrea Savisky RN CNN, Division Program Director
Mark Daley, Division Donor Records Director/User Ser

Maryland

5491 National Kidney Foundation of Maryland
Heaver Plaza, 1301 York Road
Lutherville, MD 21093-2136
410-494-8545
800-671-5369
Fax: 410-494-8549
e-mail: cshafer@kidneymd.org
www.kidneymd.org
Also covers the Harrisburg area of Pennsylvania and portions of Virginia and West Virginia.
Cassie Shafer, President/CEO
Christie Vera, Vice President of Development and Market

Massachusetts

5492 National Kidney Foundation of MA/RI/NH/VT
85 Astor Avenue   781-278-0222
Norwood, MA 02062   800-542-4001
                                    Fax: 781-278-0333
e-mail: nkfofmrnv@kidneyhealth.org
www.kidney.org/site/105/index.cfm
Andrea Savisky RN CNN, Division Program Director
Mark Daley, Division Donor Records Director/User Ser

Michigan

5493 Michigan Kidney Foundation
1169 Oak Valley Drive   734-222-9800
Ann Arbor, MI 48108   800-482-1455
                                    Fax: 734-222-9801
e-mail: info@nkfm.org
www.nkfm.org

Andrew Boschma, Chairman
Daniel M Carney, President/CEO

Minnesota

5494 National Kidney Foundation of Minnesota
1970 Oakcrest Avenue   651-636-7300
Saint Paul, MN 55113   800-596-7943
                                    Fax: 651-636-9700
e-mail: jille@kidney.org
www.kidney.org/site/313/index.cfm
Also covers North Dakota and South Dakota.
Jill Evenocheck, Division President
Amy Busack, Regional Vice-President

Mississippi

5495 National Kidney Foundation of Mississippi
3000 Old Canton Road   601-981-3611
Jackson, MS 39216   800-232-1592
                                    Fax: 601-981-3612
e-mail: gail@kidneyms.org
www.kidneyms.org

Paul Howell, President
Lee Parrott, Vice President

Missouri

5496 National Kidney Foundation of Eastern Missouri and Metro East
1001 Craig Road   314-961-2828
Creve Coeur, MO 63146   800-489-9585
                                    Fax: 314-961-0888
e-mail: nkfemo@kidney.org
www.kidney.org/site/308/index.cfm
Chad Iseman, State Director
Alayna Tatum, Special Events Manager

Montana

5497 National Kidney Foundation of Colorado/Idaho/Montana/Wyoming
650 South Cherry Street   720-748-9991
Denver, CO 80246   800-596-7943
                                    Fax: 720-748-1273
e-mail: nkfcmw@kidney.org
www.kidney.org/site/505/
Brandi Krause, State Director
Stacey Lux, Development Director

Nebraska

5498 Nebraska Kidney Association
11725 Arbor Street   402-932-7200
Omaha, NE 68144-2116   800-642-1255
                                    Fax: 402-933-0087
e-mail: nkfnoffice@kidneyne.org
www.kidneyne.org
Improve the lives of all Nebraskans through advocacy, education, early disease detection and patient services.

New Hampshire

5499 National Kidney Foundation of MA/RI/NH/VT
85 Astor Avenue   781-278-0222
Norwood, MA 02062   800-542-4001
                                    Fax: 781-278-0333
e-mail: nkfofmrnv@kidneyhealth.org
www.kidney.org/site/105/index.cfm
Andrea Savisky RN CNN, Division Program Director
Mark Daley, Division Donor Records Director/User Ser

New Jersey

5500 Garrett Mountain Chapter of the American Association of Kidney Patients
PO Box 8496   973-523-3959
Haledon, NJ 07538
Hurwitz, President

5501 Meadowlands Chapter of the American Association of Kidney Patients
PO Box 3032   201-471-5674
Clifton, NJ 07012-3032
Howard

5502 Northern New Jersey Chapter of the American Association of Kidney Patients
1095 Stone Street   732-382-1092
Rahway, NJ 07065-1913
Burnett

New Mexico

5503 National Kidney Foundation of New Mexico
3167 San Mateo Boulevard NE   505-830-3542
Albuquerque, NM 87110   800-282-0190
                                    Fax: 816-221-7984
e-mail: nkfnm@kidney.org
www.kidney.org

Connie Giarrusso, President
Shirley Baer, Executive Director

New York

5504 Kidney & Urology Foundation of America
2 West 47th Street   212-629-9770
New York, NY 10036   800-633-6628
                                    Fax: 212-629-5652
e-mail: info@kidneyurology.org
www.kidneyurology.org

Sam Giarrusso, President
Kerri Shapiro, Director of Operations/Administration

5505 Long Island Chapter of the American Association of Kidney Patients
2 Maplewood Avenue   516-756-9126
Farmingdale, NY 11735
Margie Ng Makhuli, Chief Executive Officer
Laura Squadrito, Director of Programs and Services

5506 National Kidney Foundation of Central New York
731 James Street   315-476-0311
Syracuse, NY 13203   877-8KI-DNEY
                                    Fax: 315-476-3707
e-mail: info@cnykidney.org
www.kidney.org/site/110/index.cfm
Nannette Carbone, Chief Executive Officer
Susan Burns, Director of Administration

5507 National Kidney Foundation of Northeast New York
1971 Western Avenue   518-458-9697
Albany, NY 12203   800-622-9010
                                    Fax: 518-458-9690
e-mail: info@nkfneny.org
www.kidney.org/about/local_info.cfm?sear
Carol MS Ed CFRE, Executive Director
Mary Jones, Division Development Director

5508 National Kidney Foundation of Western New York
310 Packetts Landing   585-598-3963
Fairport, NY 14450   800-724-9421
                                                Fax: 585-598-3966
                                    e-mail: infoupny@kidney.org
                                    www.kidney.org/site/109/index.cfm

Nonprofit health organization.
Joanne Spink, Division President
Megan Alchowiak, Community Outreach Manager

5509 New York Chapter of the American Association of Kidney Patients
450 Clarkson Avenue   718-270-1548
Brooklyn, NY 11203   e-mail: linda.cohen@downstate.edu
                                                www.aakp.org

Linda Welch, Kidney Early Evaluation Program Contact

North Carolina

5510 National Kidney Foundation of North Carolina
5950 Fairview Road   704-552-1351
Charlotte, NC 28210   800-356-5362
                                                Fax: 704-552-7870
                                                www.nkfnc.org

Kenya Welch, Kidney Early Evaluation Program Contact

Ohio

5511 Miami Valley Ohio Chapter of the American Association of Kidney Patients
4511 W State Route   513-698-5847
W Milton, OH 45383
Bob B Gold, Division President
Danielle Estep, Division Program Director

5512 National Kidney Foundation of Ohio
2800 Corporate Exchange Drive   614-882-6184
Columbus, OH 43231-2804   800-242-2133
                                                Fax: 614-882-6564
                                    e-mail: nkfoh@kidney.org
                                                www.nkfofohio.org

Patti V.B. Gold, Division President
Danielle Estep, Division Program Director

Oklahoma

5513 American Association of Kidney Patients: Tulsa Chapter
911 North Woodland Drive   918-241-3969
Sand Springs, OK 74063   800-749-2257
                                    e-mail: jasonmikles@hotmail.com
Jason Tallent, CEO

5514 National Kidney Foundation of Oklahoma
10600 S Pennsylvania Avenue   816-221-9559
Oklahoma City, OK 73170   800-622-9010
                                                Fax: 816-221-7984
                                    e-mail: nkfok@kidney.org
                                    www.kidney.org/about/local_info.cfm?sear

Jeff Baumgardner, CEO
Glenda McClure, Operations Manager

Pennsylvania

5515 Lehigh Valley Chapter of the American Association of Kidney Patients
1242 N 19th Street   610-776-1091
Allentown, PA 18104-3058   e-mail: info@aakp.org
                                                www.aakp.org

Jill Spink, Division President
Mary Reilly, Development Director

5516 National Kidney Foundation of Delaware Valley
111 S Independence Mall E   215-923-8611
Philadelphia, PA 19106   800-697-7007
                                                Fax: 215-923-2199
                                    e-mail: nkfdv@kidney.org
                                    www.kidney.org/site/112/index.cfm

Also covers Delaware and Southern New Jersey.
Joseph Mullen, Chairman
Joanne Spink, Division President

5517 National Kidney Foundation of Western Pennsylvania
3109 Forbes Avenue   412-261-4115
Pittsburgh, PA 15213   800-261-4115
                                                Fax: 412-261-1405
                                    e-mail: info@kidneyall.org
                                    www.kidney.org/site/113/index.cfm

Also covers Northern West Virginia.
James Sullivan, Chairman
David Vanella, Vice Chairman

Rhode Island

5518 National Kidney Foundation of MA/RI/NH/VT
85 Astor Avenue   781-278-0222
Norwood, MA 02062   800-542-4001
                                                Fax: 781-278-0333
                                    e-mail: nkfofmrnv@kidneyhealth.org
                                    www.kidney.org/site/105/index.cfm

Andrea Savisky RN CNN, Division Program Director
Mark Daley, Division Donor Records Director/User Ser

South Carolina

5519 National Kidney Foundation of South Carolina
508 Hampton Street   803-798-3870
Columbia, SC 29201   800-488-2277
                                                Fax: 803-799-3871
                                    e-mail: karen.bailey@kidney.org
                                    www.kidney.org/site/209/index.cfm

Beth Irick, Division President
Karen Bailey, Division Senior Administrative Assistant

South Dakota

5520 National Kidney Foundation Serving Minneso ta, Dakotas & Iowa Division Office
1970 Oakcrest Avenue   651-636-7300
Saint Paul, MN 55113   800-596-7943
                                                Fax: 651-636-9700
                                    e-mail: jille@kidney.org
                                    www.kidney.org/site/313/index.cfm

Jill Evenocheck, Division President
Amy Busack, Regional Vice President

Tennessee

5521 National Kidney Foundation of East Tennessee
5201 Kingston Pike   865-688-5481
Knoxville, TN 37919-1523   800-242-2133
                                                Fax: 865-688-5495
                                    e-mail: nkfetn@kidney.org
                                    www.kidney.org/about/local_info.cfm?sear
The National Kidney Foundation of East Tennessee works to prevent kidney and urinary tract diseases improve the health and well-being of individuals and family members affected by these diseases and increase the availability of all organs for transplantation.
Helen

5522 National Kidney Foundation of West Tennessee
857 Mount Moriah Road   901-683-6185
Memphis, TN 38117   800-273-3869
                                                Fax: 901-683-6189
                                    www.kidney.org/about/local_info.cfm?sear
Bruce Skyer, Chief Executive Officer
Joseph Vassalotti, MD, Chief Medical Officer

5523 National Kidney Foundation of West Texas
5429 Lyndon B Johnson Fwy   214-351-2393
Dallas, TX 75240   877-543-6397
                                                Fax: 214-351-3797
                                    e-mail: texasinfo@kidney.org
                                    www.kidney.org/site/406/index.cfm

Marrie Collins, President
Mark Edwards, Division Program Director

5524 Tennessee Kidney Foundation
95 White Bridge Road   615-383-3887
Nashville, TN 37205-2613   800-380-3887
Fax: 615-383-2647
e-mail: info@tennesseekidneyfoundation.org
www.tennesseekidneyfoundation.org

Ron Carter, President
Bob Horton, First Vice President

Texas

5525 American Association of Kidney Patients: Piney Woods Chapter
PO Box 1012   903-537-7031
Mount Vernon, TX 75457   800-749-2257
e-mail: edwinhargraves@webtv.net

Edwin Wager, President

5526 Lone Star Chapter of the American Association of Kidney Patients
10042 Sugarloaf Drive
San Antonio, TX 78245   210-523-1605
www.aakp.org

Robert Eaton, CEO
Cameron Hernholm, Director of Development

5527 National Kidney Foundation of North Texas
5429 Lyndon B Johnson Freeway   214-351-2393
Dallas, TX 75240   877-543-6397
Fax: 214-351-3797
e-mail: texasinfo@kidney.org
www.kidney.org/site/406/index.cfm
Public and professional education about kidney and urinary tract diseases. Peer mentoring medical emergency identification jewelry kidney early evaluation program Camp Reynal transplant games.
Marrie Collins, President
Mark Edwards, Division Program Director

5528 National Kidney Foundation of Southeast Texas
5429 Lyndon B Johnson Freeway   214-351-2393
Dallas, TX 75240   877-543-6397
Fax: 214-351-3797
e-mail: texasinfo@kidney.org
www.kidney.org/site/406/index.cfm
Provides services for people who suffer with kidney and urinary tract diseases.
Marrie Collins, President
Mark Edwards, Division Program Director

5529 National Kidney Foundation of Texas
5429 Lyndon B Johnson Fwy   214-351-2393
Dallas, TX 75240   877-543-6397
Fax: 214-351-3797
e-mail: texasinfo@kidney.org
www.kidney.org/site/406/index.cfm
Marie Collins, Division President
Mark Edwards, Divisional Program Director

5530 National Kidney Foundation of the Texas Coastal Bend
PO Box 9172   361-884-5892
Corpus Christi, TX 78469   Fax: 361-884-2332
e-mail: info@coastalbendkidneyfoundation.org
www.coastalbendkidneyfoundation.org

Bess Stone, President
Becky Gardner, Executive Director

Utah

5531 National Kidney Foundation of Utah
3707 N Canyon Road   801-226-5111
Provo, UT 84604-4585   800-869-5277
Fax: 801-226-8278
e-mail: NKFU@KidneyUT.org
www.kidneyut.org
Serving kidney dialysis and transplant patients through out Utah providing patient service and support programs medical research and public and patient education regarding kidney disease and its treatment and prevention and the promotion of organ donations.
E.J. Garn, Chairman
Deen Vetterli, Chief Executive Officer

Vermont

5532 National Kidney Foundation of MA/RI/NH/VT
85 Astor Avenue   781-278-0222
Norwood, MA 02062   800-542-4001
Fax: 781-278-0333
e-mail: nkfofmrnv@kidneyhealth.org
www.kidney.org/site/105/index.cfm
Andrea Savisky RN CNN, Division Program Director
Mark Daley, Division Donor Records Director/User Ser

Virginia

5533 National Kidney Foundation of Virginia
1622 East Parham Road   804-288-8342
Richmond, VA 23228   800-543-6398
Fax: 804-282-7835
e-mail: eleanor.myers@kidney.org
www.kidney.org/site/203/index.cfm
An affiliate of the National Kidney Foundation it serves kidney patients and their families in Virginia and portions of West Virginia. Mission includes professional and public education prevention and working to increase the availability of all organs for donation.
Eleanor Myers, Regional Program Director
Liz King, Community Outreach Manager

Wisconsin

5534 National Kidney Foundation of Wisconsin
16655 W Bluemound Road   262-821-0705
Brookfield, WI 53005-5935   800-543-6393
Fax: 262-821-5641
e-mail: nkfw@kidneywi.org
www.kidneywi.org
Offers prevention detection and education programs for those at risk for kidney disease. The National Kidney Foundation of Wisconsin is making life's better through its programs and services. Brochures are offered at no charge.
Mary Braband, Chair
Cindy Huber, Chief Executive Officer

Wyoming

5535 National Kidney Foundation of Colorado/Idaho/Montana/Wyoming
650 South Cherry Street   720-748-9991
Denver, CO 80246   800-596-7943
Fax: 720-748-1273
e-mail: nkfcmw@kidney.org
www.kidney.org/site/505/

Brandi Krause, State Director
Stacey Lux, Development Director

Research Centers

5536 Kidney Disease Institute
Wadsworth Center for Laboratories and Research
Empire State Plaza   518-474-7354
Albany, NY 12237   Fax: 518-737-71
e-mail: dohweb@health.state.ny.us
www.nyhealth.gov
An information and referral organization for polycystic kidney disease autoimmune kidney disease and transplantation.
Andrew M Cuomo, Governor
Nirav R Shah, Commissioner

5537 Lovelace Medical Foundation
2425 Ridgecrest Drive SE   505-348-9400
Albuquerque, NM 87108-5127   Fax: 505-348-8567
e-mail: info@lrri.org
www.lrri.org

Jackie Lovelace Johnson, Director
Frank Bond, Director

5538 Lovelace Respiratory Research Institute
615 S Preston Street   502-852-7350
Louisville, KY 40202-0001   Fax: 502-852-7643
e-mail: cbrown@kdp.louisville.edu
kdpnet.kdp.louisville.edu

Educates residents and patients regarding kidney diseases and offers a dialysis clinic for people afflicted with kidney disease.
George R Ottensmeyer, President

5539 Nevada Kidney Disease & Hypertension Cente rs
210 S Desplaines Street   312-654-2720
Chicago, IL 60661   Fax: 312-654-0118
                       e-mail: charlotte.chapple@ainmd.com
                                           www.ainmd.com/
A medical group practicing nephrology in the Chicago metropolitan area and it suburbs. Includes 21 nephrologists with expertise in many areas in the field of nephrology including hypertension chronic and acute renal failure hemodialysis and peritoneal dialysis glomerulonephritis acid base disturbances fluid and electrolytes management. Provides personal high quality care to patients with kidney diseases.
Eduardo Kantor MD, Founder

5540 PKD Foundation Polycystic Kidney Disease Foundation
Polycystic Kidney Disease Foundation
9221 Ward Parkway   816-931-2600
Kansas City, MO 64114-3367   800-PKD-CURE
                                           Fax: 816-931-8655
                               e-mail: pkdcure@pkdcure.org
                                           www.pkdcure.org
The foundation exists to win the war with PKD. Their mission is to promote research into the treatment and cure of polycystic kidney disease by raising financial support for peer approved biomedical research projects and fostering public awareness among medical professionals patients and the general public.
Frank Condella, Jr, Chair
Michelle Davis, Interim CEO and Chief Development Office

5541 University of Kansas Kidney and Urology Research Center
3901 Rainbow Boulevard   913-588-5000
Kansas City, KS 66160   Fax: 913-588-3995
                                           TTY: 913-588-7963
                                           www.kumc.edu

Jared J Brosius, Chief
Joseph Messana, Professor/ Service Chief

5542 University of Michigan Nephrology Division
University of Michigan Health System
1500 E Medical Center Drive   734-936-5645
Ann Arbor, MI 48109   Fax: 734-763-4151
                       www.med.umich.edu/intmed/nephrology
Focuses on kidney research.
Eric Mullen, Division Administrator
Susan Geisser, Financial Consultant

5543 University of Rochester: Nephrology Research Program
601 Elmwood Avenue   585-275-3660
Rochester, NY 14642-0001   Fax: 716-442-9201
                                           www.urmc.rochester.edu
Focuses on kidney disorders.
David A Bushinsky, MD, Division Chief

5544 Warren Grant Magnuson Clinical Center
National Institute of Health
10 Center Drive MSC 1078   301-496-3311
Bethesda, MD 20892   800-411-1222
                                           Fax: 301-496-2390
                                           TTY: 866-411-1010
                               e-mail: mmichael@cc.nih.gov
                       www.dnrc.nih.gov/reports/programs/ncc.as
Established in 1953 as the research hospital of the National Institutes of Health. Designed so that patient care facilities are close to research laboratories so new findings of basic and clinical scientists can be quickly applied to the treatment of patients. Upon referral by physicians, patients are admitted to NIH clinical studies.
John Slatopolsky, Director

5545 Washington University Chromalloy American Kidney Center
One Barnes-Jewish Hospital Plaza   314-362-7209
Saint Louis, MO 63110-1036   Fax: 314-747-3743
                                           renal.wustl.edu
Offers a dialysis unit for people afflicted with kidney disease.
Dr Eduardo Lanning RN/JD, President Board of Directors
Sean Tully, Vice President Board of Directors

Support Groups & Hotlines

5546 Kidneeds
Greater Cedar Rapids Community Foundation
200 First Street Southwest   319-366-2862
Cedar Rapids, IA 52404   Fax: 319-386-0431
                             e-mail: kidneedsmpgn@yahoo.com
                               www.medicine.uiowa.edu/kidneeds/
Primary mission of kidneeds is to fund research on membranoproliferative giomerulonephritis type 2 (MPON type 2, aka, dense deposit disease). Phone support and annual newsletter availiable. No computerized version availiable. No mailing list availble.
Lynne

5547 National Health Information Center
PO Box 1133   310-565-4167
Washington, DC 20013   800-336-4797
                                           Fax: 301-984-4256
                                           e-mail: info@nhic.org
                                           www.health.gov/nhic

Offers a nationwide information referral service, produces directories and resource guides.
Cathcart, Executive Director

Books

5548 Family and ADPKD: A Guide for Children and Parents
Polycystic Kidney Disease Foundation
9221 Ward Parkway   816-931-2600
Kansas City, MO 64114   800-753-2873
                                           Fax: 816-931-8655
                               e-mail: pkdcure@pkdcure.org
                                           www.pkdcure.org
This book focuses on the questions most commonly asked by children and parents about ADPKD. It is divided into two sections: one for children and one for parents.
48 pages
ISBN: 0-961456-75-2
Dave Switzer, National Director, Educational Programs

5549 Kidney Beginnings: A Patient's Guide to Li ving with Reduced Kidney Function
American Association of Kidney Patients
3505 E Frontage Road   813-636-8100
Tampa, FL 33607   800-749-2257
                                           Fax: 813-636-8122
                                           e-mail: info@aakp.org
                                           www.aakp.org
Provides patients with the information they need to take control of their healthcare and do what is necessary to preserve and protect their kidney function. The book addresses concerns of those at risk for kidney disease and their family members; featuring information about the workings of the kidneys, common medications, hypertention, testing, and answers to health, diet and lifestyle questions.
62 pages
Kim Buettner, Executive Director

5550 Kidney Cooking
National Kidney Foundation of Georgia
1639 Tullie Circle NE   404-248-1315
Atlanta, GA 30329-2304
A unique cookbook with over one hundred recipes that have been analyzed for sodium, potassium and protein content.

5551 Nutrition & the Kidney
Little Brown & Company
34 Beacon Street   617-227-0730
Boston, MA 02108-1415   Fax: 617-227-4633
1993 480 pages
ISBN: 0-316575-00-3

5552 PKD Patient's Manual
Polycystic Kidney Disease Foundation

9221 Ward Parkway
Kansas City, MO 64114

816-931-2600
800-753-2873
Fax: 816-931-8655
e-mail: pkdcure@pkdcure.org
www.pkdcure.org

Covers everything from cysts to how persons can be active if they have ARPKD.
Dave Switzer, National Director, Educational Programs

5553 Q&A on PKD
Polycystic Kidney Disease Foundation
9221 Ward Parkway
Kansas City, MO 64114

816-931-2600
800-753-2873
Fax: 816-931-8655
e-mail: pkdcure@pkdcure.org
www.pkdcure.org

A goldmine of information for the PKD patient and physician. Includes 88 pages of PKD questions and answers by the scientific advisers of the PKR Foundation.
88 pages Paperback
ISBN: 0-961456-72-8
Dave Switzer, National Director, Educational Programs

5554 Real Lifestyles Manual
R&D Laboratories
4204 Glencoe Avenue
Marina Del Rey, CA 90292-5612

800-338-9066

A complete renal guide including diets for hemodialysis and CAPD patients. Delicious menus, ADA exchange lists, gourmet recipes with nutritional analysis for renal patients and exercises.

5555 Your Child, Your Family & ARPKD
Polycystic Kidney Disease Foundation
9221 Ward Parkway
Kansas City, MO 64114

816-931-2600
800-753-2873
Fax: 816-931-8655
e-mail: pkdcure@pkdcure.org
www.pkdcure.org

This second edition book focuses on the questions most commonly asked about ARPKD in order to help families understand more about the disease.
Dave Switzer, National Director, Educational Programs

5556 Your Child, Your Family and Autosomal Recessive Polycystic Kidney Disease
Polycystic Kidney Disease Foundation
9221 Ward Parkway
Kansas City, MO 64114

816-931-2600
800-753-2873
Fax: 816-931-8655
e-mail: pkdcure@pkdcure.org
www.pkdcure.org

This secong edition book focuses on the questions most commonly asked about autosomal recessive PKD in order to help families understand more about the disease.
26 pages Paperback
Dave Switzer, National Director, Educational Programs

Magazines

5557 Kindey Beginnings: The Magazine
American Association of Kidney Patients
3505 E Frantage Road
Tampa, FL 33607

813-636-8100
800-749-2257
Fax: 813-636-8122
e-mail: info@aakp.org
www.aakp.org

This quarterly member magazine provides articles, news items and information of interest to those at risk or recently diagnosed with kidney disease, their famliy, and healthcare professionals.
Kmi Buettner, Executive Director

5558 aakpRENALIFE
American Association of Kidney Patients
35052 E Frantage Road
Tampa, FL 33607

813-636-8100
800-749-2257
Fax: 813-636-8122
e-mail: info@aakp.org
www.aakp.org

The official publication for AAKP members, offering articles, news and health care information for kidney patients,and health care professionals.
BiMonthly
Kim Buettner, Executive Director

Newsletters

5559 Family Focus
National Kidney Foundation
30 E 33rd Street
New York, NY 10016-5337

212-889-2210
800-622-9010
Fax: 212-689-9261
www.kidney.org

A patient and family newspaper targeted toward dialysis populations.
Quarterly

5560 PKD Progress
PKD Foundation
4901 Main Street
Kansas City, MO 64112-2634

816-931-2600
800-753-2873
Fax: 816-931-8655
e-mail: pkdcure@pkdcure.org
www.pkdcure.org

Offers information and updated medical news for persons and professionals with an interest in kidney disorders.
Monthly
Dave Switzer, Marketing/Public Relations Director

5561 Renal Recipes Quarterly
R&D Laboratories
4204 Glencoe Avenue
Marina Del Rey, CA 90292-5612

800-338-9066

Features timely holiday and ethnic food menus and recipes, shopping and food tips, analysis of nutrients and calculation of food exchanges.
Quarterly

5562 Transplant Chronicles
National Kidney Foundation
30 E 33rd Street
New York, NY 10016

212-889-2210
800-622-9010
Fax: 212-689-9261
www.kidney.org

A patient and family newsletter targeted towards transplant recipients.
Quarterly

Pamphlets

5563 About Kidney Stones
National Kidney Foundation
30 E 33rd Street
New York, NY 10016

212-889-2210
800-622-9010
Fax: 212-689-9261
www.kidney.org

Discusses causes, treatment and prevention of kidney stones.

5564 Advance Directives: A Guide for Patients and Their Families
National Kidney Foundation
30 E 33rd Street
New York, NY 10016-5337

212-889-2210
800-622-9010
Fax: 212-689-9261
www.kidney.org

Everyone has the right to make an advance directive, which is a legal document stating how you want decisions made concerning your medical care when your no longer able to make them yourself. This booklet describes the different types of advance directives and the medical decisions they cover.
12 pages Package

5565 American Kidney Fund Helps When Nobody Else Will
American Kidney Fund

6110 Executive Boulevard
Rockville, MD 20852-3915

301-881-3052
800-638-8299
Fax: 301-881-0898
e-mail: helpline@AFINC.org
www.kidneyfund.org

Focuses on the services and programs offered by the American Kidney Fund.

5566 At Home with AAKP
American Association of Kidney Patients
3505 E Frantage Road
Tampa, FL 33607

813-636-8100
800-749-2257
Fax: 813-636-8122
e-mail: info@aakp.org
www.aakp.org

A free publication, this was developed to address the growing need for information about home dialysis treatment options.
Kim Buettner, Executive Director

5567 Children and Kidney Disease
American Kidney Fund
6110 Executive Boulevard
Rockville, MD 20852-3915

301-881-3052
800-638-8299
Fax: 301-881-0898
www.arbon.com/kidney/

5568 Choosing a Treatment for Kidney Failure
National Kidney Foundation
30 E 33rd Street
New York, NY 10016

212-889-2210
800-622-9010
Fax: 212-689-9261
www.kidney.org

Introduces treatment options for kidney failure and explains the pros and cons of each.
16 pages

5569 Diabetes and Kidney Disease
National Kidney Foundation
30 E 33rd Street
New York, NY 10016-5337

212-889-2210
800-622-9010
Fax: 212-689-9261
www.kidney.org

Explains the connection between diabetes and kidney disease covering prevention, recognition and treatments.
12 pages Pkg. of 100

5570 Dialysis Patient: An Informative Guide for the Dentist
American Kidney Fund
6110 Executive Boulevard
Rockville, MD 20852-3915

301-881-3052
800-638-8299
Fax: 301-881-0898
www.arbon.com/kidney/

5571 Diet Guide for the CAPD Patient
American Kidney Fund
6110 Executive Boulevard
Rockville, MD 20852-3915

301-881-3052
800-638-8299
Fax: 301-881-0898
www.arbon.com/kidney/

5572 Diet Guide for the Hemodialysis Patient
American Kidney Fund
6110 Executive Boulevard
Rockville, MD 20852-3915

301-881-3052
800-638-8299
Fax: 301-881-0898
www.arbon.com/kidney/

5573 Facts About Kidney Diseases and Their Treatment
American Kidney Fund
6110 Executive Boulevard
Rockville, MD 20852-3915

301-881-3052
800-638-8299
Fax: 301-881-0898
www.arbon.com/kidney/

Offers information about what kidneys are and their functions, diagnosis and treatment of kidney disease.

5574 Facts About Kidney Stones
American Kidney Fund

6110 Executive Boulevard
Rockville, MD 20852-3915

301-881-3052
800-638-8299
Fax: 301-881-0898
www.arbon.com/kidney/

5575 Glomerulonephritis
National Kidney Foundation
30 E 33rd Street
New York, NY 10016-5337

212-889-2210
800-622-9010
Fax: 212-689-9261
www.kidney.org

Defines the types of Glomerulonephritis, signs, causes and symptoms.
8 pages Pkg. of 100

5576 Hemodialysis
National Kidney Foundation
30 E 33rd Street
New York, NY 10016

212-889-2210
800-622-9010
Fax: 212-689-9261
www.kidney.org

Introduces and explains the hemodialysis treatment process.
12 pages Pkg. of 100

5577 High Blood Pressure and Your Kidneys
National Kidney Foundation
30 E 33rd Street
New York, NY 10016-5337

212-889-2210
800-622-9010
Fax: 212-689-9261
www.kidney.org

Offers a description of hypertension, including symptoms, detection, causes and effects. Also available in Spanish.
8 pages Pkg. of 100

5578 High Blood Pressure and its Effects on the Kidneys
American Kidney Fund
6110 Executive Boulevard
Rockville, MD 20852

301-881-3052
800-638-8299
Fax: 301-881-0898
www.arbon.com/kidney/

5579 Kid
American Kidney Fund
6110 Executive Boulevard
Rockville, MD 20852-3915

301-881-3052
800-638-8299
Fax: 301-881-0898
www.arbon.com/kidney/

5580 Kidney Disease: A Guide for Patients and Their Families
American Kidney Fund
6110 Executive Boulevard
Rockville, MD 20852

301-881-3052
800-638-8299
Fax: 301-881-0898
www.arbon.com/kidney/

Offers information on how the kidneys work, symptoms of kidney disease, kidney failure and treatment alternatives.

5581 Kidney Transplant: A New Lease on Life
National Kidney Foundation
30 E 33rd Street
New York, NY 10016

212-889-2210
800-622-9010
Fax: 212-689-9261
www.kidney.org

A brochure that answers common questions about transplants, such as patient expectations, drug therapy, complications including rejection and recovery.
10 pages Pkg. of 100

5582 Kidneys for Kids
American Kidney Fund
6110 Executive Boulevard
Rockville, MD 20852-3915

301-881-3052
800-638-8299
Fax: 301-881-0898
www.arbon.com/kidney/

5583 Nutrition and Changing Kidney Function
National Kidney Foundation
30 E 33rd Street
New York, NY 10016-5337

212-889-2210
800-622-9010
Fax: 212-689-9261
www.kidney.org

Explains how to slow the progression of kidney disease by controlling the intake of vitamins, minerals, fluids, calories and proteins.
12 pages Pkg. of 100

5584 Organ Donor Program
National Kidney Foundation
30 E 33rd Street   212-889-2210
New York, NY 10016-5337   800-622-9010
                                     Fax: 212-689-9261
                                          www.kidney.org
A comprehensive description of the organ donor program that explains organ and tissue donation, brain death, routine inquiry and becoming an organ donor.
12 pages Pkg. of 100

5585 Peritoneal Dialysis
National Kidney Foundation
30 E 33rd Street   212-889-2210
New York, NY 10016   800-622-9010
                                     Fax: 212-689-9261
                                          www.kidney.org
Introduces and explains the peritoneal dialysis treatment process
8 pages

5586 Understanding Nephrotic Syndrome
American Kidney Fund
6110 Executive Boulevard   301-881-3052
Rockville, MD 20852-3915   800-638-8299
                                     Fax: 301-881-0898
                                     www.arbon.com/kidney/

5587 Urinary Tract Infections
National Kidney Foundation
30 E 33rd Street   212-889-2210
New York, NY 10016-5337   800-622-9010
                                     Fax: 212-689-9261
                                          www.kidney.org
Defines urinary tract infections, its symptoms, causes and treatments.
10 pages Pkg. of 100

5588 Warning Signs of Kidney Disease
National Kidney Foundation
30 E 33rd Street   212-889-2210
New York, NY 10016-5337   800-622-9010
                                     Fax: 212-689-9261
                                          www.kidney.org
A one-panel leaflet that numbers and lists the six early warning signs of kidney disease.
Pkg. of 100

5589 Winning the Fight Against Silent Killers
National Kidney Foundation
30 E 33rd Street   212-889-2210
New York, NY 10016-5337   800-622-9010
                                     Fax: 212-689-9261
                                          www.kidney.org
Written for the African-American community, this brochure discusses the increased risk of high blood pressure and diabetes in this population.
12 pages Pkg. of 100

5590 Your Kidneys: Master Chemists of the Body
National Kidney Foundation
30 E 33rd Street   212-889-2210
New York, NY 10016-5337   800-622-9010
                                     Fax: 212-689-9261
                                          www.kidney.org
Offers an overview of kidneys and urinary system, describing the kidneys' filtering system, hereditary, congenital and acquired kidney diseases.
12 pages Pkg. of 100

Audio & Video

5591 It's Just Part of My Life
National Kidney Foundation
30 E 33rd Street   212-889-2210
New York, NY 10016-5337   800-622-9010
                                     Fax: 212-689-9261
                                          www.kidney.org
A 15-minute program for adolescent dialysis patients and their families.

5592 People Like Us
National Kidney Foundation
30 E 33rd Street   212-889-2210
New York, NY 10016-5337   800-622-9010
                                     Fax: 212-689-9261
                                          www.kidney.org
A seven-part video series targeted toward the newly-diagnosed chronic kidney disease patient.

Web Sites

5593 American Association of Kidney Patients
                                          www.aakp.org
Serves the needs and interests of kidney patients, for kidney patients, the purpose of this Association is to help patients and their families cope with the emotional, physical and social impact of kidney disease.

5594 American Kidney Fund
                                          www.akfinc.org/
A nonprofit, national health organization providing direct financial assistance to thousands of Americans who suffer from kidney disease.

5595 Healing Well
                                          www.healingwell.com
An online health resource guide to medical news, chat, information and articles, newsgroups and message boards, books, disease-related web sites, medical directories, and more for patients, friends, and family coping with disabling diseases, disorders, or chronic illnesses.

5596 Health Finder
                                          www.healthfinder.gov
Searchable, carefully developed web site offering information on over 1000 topics. Developed by the US Department of Health and Human Services, the site can be used in both English and Spanish.

5597 Healthlink USA
                                          www.healthlinkusa.com
Links to websites which may include treatment, cures, diagnosis, prevention, support groups, email lists, messageboards, personal stories, risk factors, statistics, research and more.

5598 Helios Health
                                          www.helioshealth.com
Online resource for your health information. Detailed information about specific health topics, access to expert advice from our Medical Advisory Board, and up-to-date health news.

5599 MedicineNet
                                          www.medicinenet.com
An online resource for consumers providing easy-to-read, authoritative medical and health information.

5600 Medscape
                                          www.medscape.com
Medscape offers specialists, primary care physicians, and other health professionals the Web's most robust and integrated medical information and educational tools.

5601 Polycystic Kidney Research Foundation
                                          www.pkdcure.org
Provide information on research into the cause, treatment, and cure of polycystic kidney disease by raising financial support for peer approved biomedical research projects and fostering public awareness among medical professionals, patients and the general public.

5602 WebMD
                                          www.webmd.com
Information on kidney disease, including articles and resources.

Description

5603 Liver Disease

Liver disease covers a wide range of disorders that can result in chronic liver damage, such as scarring (fibrosis) or the development of cirrhosis. An estimated 43,000 Americans die each year from liver disease.

Specific liver diseases that damage the liver include infection (e.g., viral hepatitis), chronic alcoholism or drug abuse, medications and certain systemic illnesses. Severe disease can permanently damage the liver, causing it to fail totally.

Common signs of liver damage are fatigue, loss of appetite, nausea and tea-colored urine. Yellowing of the skin and the whites of the eye (jaundice) is seen in 50 percent of cases. Other symptoms include liver enlargement and tenderness, and fluid collection in the abdominal cavity. A shriveling liver indicates more chronic and severe damage.

Treatment for liver disease depends on the underlying cause. In less severe injury, due to its remarkable capacity to heal itself, the liver can completely recover. Liver transplantation is accepted as appropriate treatment for end-stage liver dysfunction. See also *Hepatitis*.

National Agencies & Associations

5604 American Association for the Study of Liver Diseases
1001 North Fairfax Street
Alexandria, VA 22314
703-299-9766
Fax: 703-299-9622
e-mail: aasld@aasld.org
www.aasld.org
Physicians, researchers, and allied hepatology health professionals.
J. Gregory Fitz, MD, President
Nellie Sarkissian, COO

5605 American Liver Foundation
39 Broadway
New York, NY 10006
212-668-1000
800-GOL-IVER
Fax: 212-483-8179
e-mail: info@liverfoundation.org
www.liverfoundation.org
National, nonprofit organization dedicated to the prevention treatment and cure of hepatitis and other liver diseases through research and advocacy. The ALF offers information, physician referrals, a 24-hour, 7 day-a-week national helpline and support groups.
Thomas F Nealon III, Chairman
David Ticker, Chief Financial Officer

State Agencies & Associations

Arizona

5606 American Liver Foundation Arizona Chapter
4545 E Shea Boulevard
Phoenix, AZ 85028
602-953-1800
866-953-1800
Fax: 602-953-1806
e-mail: mmcracken@liverfoundation.org
www.liverfoundation.org
Melissa McCracken, Executive Director
Ashley Drew, Events Manager

California

5607 American Liver Foundation Greater Los Angeles Chapter
5777 Century Boulevard
Los Angeles, CA 90045
310-670-4624
Fax: 310-670-4672
e-mail: tfantini@liverfoundation.org
www.liverfoundation.org
Taly Fantini, Executive Director

5608 American Liver Foundation Northern CA Chapter
870 Market Street
San Francisco, CA 94102
415-248-1060
800-292-9099
Fax: 415-248-1066
e-mail: gmartin@liverfoundation.org
www.liverfoundation.org
Greg Martin, Executive Director

5609 American Liver Foundation San Diego Chapte r
2515 Camino del Rio S
San Diego, CA 92108
619-291-5483
800-749-2630
Fax: 619-295-7181
e-mail: mdemotto@liverfoundation.org
www.liverfoundation.org
Michele De Motto, Executive Director

Colorado

5610 American Liver Foundation Rocky Mountain Division
1660 S Albion Street
Denver, CO 80222
303-988-4388
Fax: 303-988-4398
e-mail: jmccormack@liverfoundation.org
www.liverfoundation.org
Joe McCormack, Executive Director

Connecticut

5611 American Liver Foundation: Connecticut Chapter
127 Washington Avenue
N Haven, CT 06473
203-234-2022
Fax: 203-234-1386
e-mail: jthompson@liverfoundation.org
www.liverfoundation.org
Offers support for patients and families provides educational meetings and conferences raising vital liver research dollars; encouraging the beautifully unselfish gift of organ donation and the medical miracle of organ transplantation.
12 pages Quarterly
JoAnn Thompson, Executive Director

Florida

5612 American Liver Foundation Gulf Coast Chapter
202 S 22nd Street
Ybor City, FL 33605
813-248-3337
Fax: 813-248-3340
e-mail: jbourgeois@liverfoundation.org
www.liverfoundation.org
Jennifer Nillias, Executive Director

Illinois

5613 American Liver Foundation Illinois Chapter
67 East Madison Street
Chicago, IL 60603
312-377-9030
Fax: 312-377-9035
e-mail: info@illinois-liver.org
www.illinois-liver.org
Kevin Sutton, Executive Director
Kristin Gray, Development Coordinator

Indiana

5614 American Liver Foundation Indiana Chapter
PO BOX 36085
Indianapolis, IN 46236
317-635-5074
877-548-3730
Fax: 317-635-5075
e-mail: dsparksunsworth@liverfoundation.org
www.liverfoundation.org
Katrina Marshall, Executive Director

Michigan

5615 **American Liver Foundation Michigan Chapter**
21886 Farmington Road
Farmington, MI 48336
248-615-5768
888-MYL-IVER
Fax: 248-615-5778
e-mail: michigan@liverfoundation.org
www.liverfoundation.org

Jennifer L Stibbe, Executive Director
Meghan Likes, Community Events Coordinator

Minnesota

5616 **American Liver Foundation Minnesota Chapte r**
2626 E 82nd Street
Bloomington, MN 55425
952-854-6181
Fax: 952-854-6956
e-mail: dgirard@liverfoundation.org
www.liverfoundation.org

Dee Girard, Executive Director

Missouri

5617 **American Liver Foundation Greater Kansas City Chapter**
16 Hampton Village Plaza
St. Louis, MO 63109
314-352-7377
866-455-4837
Fax: 612-892-8442
e-mail: rmattler@liverfoundation.org
www.liverfoundation.org

Richard Mattler, Executive Director

New York

5618 **American Liver Foundation Greater New York Chapter**
39 Broadway
New York, NY 10006
212-943-1059
877-307-7507
Fax: 212-943-1314
e-mail: greaterny@liverfoundation.org
www.liverfoundation.org

Randa Adib, Director, Development
Stephanie Paul, Gala Director

5619 **American Liver Foundation Western New York Chapter**
25 Canterbury Road
Rochester, NY 14607
585-271-2859
Fax: 585-271-8642
e-mail: nkoris@liverfoundation.org
www.liverfoundation.org

Nancy Rodwa MNO, Executive Director

Pennsylvania

5620 **American Liver Foundation Delaware Valley Chapter**
1341 North Delaware Avenue
Philadelphia, PA 19125
215-425-8080
Fax: 215-425-8181
e-mail: iallison@liverfoundation.org
www.liverfoundation.org

Ivory Allison, Executive Director

5621 **American Liver Foundation Western Pennsylv ania**
100 W Station Square Drive
Pittsburgh, PA 15219
412-434-7044
Fax: 412-434-7040
e-mail: samasartis@liverfoundation.org
www.liverfoundation.org

Suzanna Masartis, Executive Director

Tennessee

5622 **American Liver Foundation Midsouth Chapter**
PO BOX 486
Ellendale, TN 38029
901-766-7668
866-756-7668
Fax: 901-881-3842
e-mail: midsouth@liverfoundation.org
www.liverfoundation.org

Winn Stephenson, Division Founder
Tina Sandoval, Board Chair

Washington

5623 **American Liver Foundation Pacific Northwest Chapter**
PO BOX 22108
Seattle, WA 98122
212-668-1000
800-465-4837
Fax: 206-443-1511
www.liverfoundation.org

Dr. Stephen Corrigan Rayhill, MD, Director
Dr. Andrew Precht, MD, Director

Wisconsin

5624 **American Liver Foundation Wisconsin Chapter**
1845 N Farwell Avenue
Milwaukee, WI 53202
414-763-3435
Fax: 414-961-7288
e-mail: dgirard@liverfoundation.org
www.liverfoundation.org

Dee Girard, Executive Director

Research Centers

5625 **Clinical Research Center: Pediatrics Children's Hospital Research Foundation**
Children's Hospital Research Foundation
Elland & Bethesda Avenues
Cincinnati, OH 45229
513-559-4412
Fax: 513-559-7431
Studies of pediatric acquired diseases including liver disease and Reye's Syndrome.
Dr James G Redeker, Co-director

5626 **University of California Liver Research Unit**
7601 E Imperial Highway
Downey, CA 90242
562-940-8961
Fax: 562-940-6628
Dr Allan Lee MD Facp, Professor InteRNal Medicine / Director

5627 **University of Texas Southwestern Medical Center**
5323 Harry Hines Boulevard
Dallas, TX 75390-9151
214-645-8300
Fax: 214-645-7999
www.utsouthwestern.edu

Daniel K Podolsky, MD, President
J. Gregory Fitz, Executive Vice President

5628 **University of Texas Southwestern Medical**
5323 Harry Hines Boulevard
Dallas, TX 75390
214-645-8300
Fax: 214-645-7999
e-mail: news@utsouthwestern.edu
www.utsouthwestern.edu

Daniel K Podolsky, MD, President
J. Gregory Fitz, Executive Vice President

5629 **Yeshiva University Marion Bessin Liver Research Center**
Albert Einstein College of Medicine
1300 Morris Park Avenue
Bronx, NY 10461-1975
718-430-2000
Fax: 718-918-0857
www.einstein.yu.edu/centers/liver-resear
Liver disease research and therapy.
Allan W Wolkoff, MD, Director
David A Shafritz, MD, Associate Director

Support Groups & Hotlines

5630 **Children's Liver Association for Support S ervices**
25379 Wayne Mills Place
Valencia, CA 91355
661-263-9099
877-679-8256
Fax: 661-263-9099
e-mail: admin@classkids.org
www.classkids.org

Dedicated to addressing the emotional, educational, and financial needs of families with children with liver disease or liver transplantation. Telephone hotline, newsletter, parent matching, literature and financial assistance. supports research and educates public about organ donations.
Mark Sumner, Co-Founder
Diane Sumner, Co-Founder

5631 National Gaucher Foundation (NGF)
2227 Idlewood Road
Tucker, GA 30084   800-504-3189
                                                              Fax: 770-934-2911
                                              e-mail: ngf@gaucherdisease.org
                                                  www.gaucherdisease.org/
The National Gaucher Foundation (NGF), established in 1984,
supports and promotes research into the causes of, and a cure for
Gaucher Disease. NGF provides information and assistance for
those affected by Gaucher disease in addition to education and out-
reach to increase public awareness. NGF operates the Gaucher
Disease Family Support Network.
Brian E Berman, President
Rhonda P Buyers, CEO/Executive Director

5632 National Health Information Center
PO Box 1133   310-565-4167
Washington, DC 20013   800-336-4797
                                                              Fax: 301-984-4256
                                                   e-mail: info@nhic.org
                                                   www.health.gov/nhic
Offers a nationwide information referral service, produces direc-
tories and resource guides.
Freudenberger, President
Larry Lasky, Vice President

5633 National Reye's Syndrome Foundation
426 N Lewis Street   419-636-2679
Bryan, OH 43506   800-233-7393
                                                              Fax: 419-636-9897
                                              e-mail: nrsf@reyesyndrome.org
                                                  www.reyessyndrome.org
Devoted to conquering Reye's syndrome, primarily a children's
disease affecting the liver and brain, but can affect all ages. Provides support, information and referrals. Encourages research.
John Symonds, Executive Director

5634 Wilson's Disease Association
5572 North Diversey Boulevard   414-961-0533
Milwaukee, WI 53217   866-961-0533
                                                              Fax: 330-264-0974
                                              e-mail: info@wilsonsdisease.org
                                                  www.wilsonsdisease.org
Serves as a communications support network for individuals affected by Wilson's disease; distributes information to profession-
als and the public; makes referrals; and holds meetings.
8 pages
Mary L Graper, President
Stefanie F Kaplan, Vice-President

Books

5635 Liver Cancer
Churchill Livingstone
PO Box 3188   201-319-9800
Secaucus, NJ 07096-3188   800-553-5426
                                                              Fax: 201-319-9659
                                                   www.churchillmed.com
1997 640 pages Hardcover
ISBN: 0-443054-81-9

5636 Liver Disease in Children
Mosby Year Book
11830 Westline Industrial Drive   314-872-8370
Saint Louis, MO 63146-3313   800-325-4177
1993 800 pages
ISBN: 1-556443-77-2

Magazines

5637 American Association for the Study of Liver Diseases
1729 King Street   703-299-9766
Alexandria, VA 22314   Fax: 703-299-9622
                                                   e-mail: aasld@aasld.org
                                                   www.aasld.org

Information for professionals interested in disease of the liver and
biliary tract.
Sherrie H Cathcart, Executive Director

5638 Hepatology
American Assoc. for the Study of Liver Disease
1729 King Street   703-299-9766
Alexandria, VA 22314   Fax: 703-299-9622
                                                   e-mail: aasld@aasld.org
                                                   www.aasld.org
Information for professionals interested in disease of the liver and
biliary tract.
Sherrie H Cathcart, Executive Director

Newsletters

5639 Children's Liver Association for Support S ervices Newsletter
25379 Wayne Mills Place   661-263-9099
Valencia, CA 91355   877-679-8256
                                                              Fax: 661-263-9099
                                              e-mail: SupportSrv@aol.com
                                                   www.classkids.org
Dedicated to addressing the emotional, educational, and financial
needs of families with children with liver disease or liver transplantation. Telephone hotline, newsletter, parent matching, litera-
ture and financial assistance. supports research and educates
public about organ donations.
Yearly
Diane Summer, President Board of Directors
Ann Whitehead RN/JD, Vice President Board of Directors

5640 Liver Update
American Liver Foundation
1425 Pompton Avenue
Cedar Grove, NJ 07009-1000   800-465-4837
                                                              Fax: 973-256-3214
                                              e-mail: info@liverfoundation.org
                                                   www.liverfoundation.org
Clinical newsletter for physicians.
BiAnnually
Rick Smith, President & CEO
Rebecca Frank, Chief Development Officer

5641 LiverLink
Alagille Syndrome Alliance
10630 SW Garden Park Place   503-639-6217
Tigard, OR 97223-3832
Newsletter for Alagille Syndrome.

5642 Progress
American Liver Foundation
1425 Pompton Avenue
Cedar Grove, NJ 07009-1000   800-465-4837
                                                              Fax: 973-256-3214
                                              e-mail: info@liverfoundation.org
                                                   www.liverfoundation.org
Newsletter about liver disease and ALF.
TriAnnually
Rick Smith, President & CEO
Rebecca Frank, Chief Development Officer

Pamphlets

5643 Alcohol and the Liver: Myth vs. Facts
American Liver Foundation
1425 Pompton Avenue   973-256-2550
Cedar Grove, NJ 07009-1000   800-223-0179
                                              e-mail: info@liverfoudation.org
                                                   www.liverfoundation.org
Rick Smith, President & CEO
Rebecca Frank, Chief Development Officer

5644 Biliary Atresia
American Liver Foundation

1425 Pompton Avenue
Cedar Grove, NJ 07009-1000

973-857-2626
800-223-0179
e-mail: info@liverfoundation.org
www.liverfoundation.org

Rick Smith, President & CEO
Rebecca Frank, Chief Development Officer

5645   Diet and Your Liver
American Liver Foundation
1425 Pompton Avenue
Cedar Grove, NJ 07009-1000

800-223-0179
Fax: 973-256-3214
e-mail: info@liverfoundation.org
www.liverfoundation.org

Rick Smith, President & CEO
Rebecca Frank, Chief Development Officer

5646   Facts on Liver Transplantation
American Liver Foundation
1425 Pompton Avenue
Cedar Grove, NJ 07009-1000

800-223-0179
Fax: 973-256-3214
e-mail: info@liverfoundation.org
www.liverfoundation.org

Rick Smith, President & CEO
Rebecca Frank, Chief Development Officer

5647   Fatty Liver
American Liver Foundation
1425 Pompton Avenue
Cedar Grove, NJ 07009-1000

800-223-0179
Fax: 987-256-3214
e-mail: info@liverfoundation.org
www.liverfoundation.org

Rick Smith, President & CEO
Rebecca Frank, Chief Development Officer

5648   Gallstones
American Liver Foundation
1425 Pompton Avenue
Cedar Grove, NJ 07009-1000

800-223-0179
Fax: 973-256-3214
e-mail: info@liverfoundation.org
www.liverfoundation.org

Rick Smith, President & CEO
Rebecca Frank, Chief Development Officer

5649   Getting Help to Hepatitis
American Liver Foundation
1425 Pompton Avenue
Cedar Grove, NJ 07009-1000

800-223-0179
Fax: 973-256-3214
e-mail: info@liverfoundation.org
www.liverfoundation.org

Rick Smith, President & CEO

5650   Hemochromatosis
American Liver Foundation
1425 Pompton Avenue
Cedar Grove, NJ 07009-1000

800-223-0179
Fax: 973-256-3214
e-mail: info@liverfoundation.org
www.liverfoundation.org

Rick Smith, President & CEO

5651   Hepatitis A, B & C
American Liver Foundation
1425 Pompton Avenue
Cedar Grove, NJ 07009-1000

800-223-0179
Fax: 973-256-3214
e-mail: info@liverfoundation.org
www.liverfoundation.org

Rick Smith, President & CEO

5652   Hepatitis B: Your Child at Risk
American Liver Foundation

1425 Pompton Avenue
Cedar Grove, NJ 07009-1000

800-223-0179
Fax: 973-256-3214
e-mail: info@liverfoundation.org
www.liverfoundation.org

Rick Smith, President & CEO

5653   How Can You Love Me
American Liver Foundation
1425 Pompton Avenue
Cedar Grove, NJ 07009-1000

973-857-2626
800-223-0179
Fax: 973-256-3214
e-mail: info@liverfoundation.org
www.liverfoundation.org

Rick Smith, President & CEO

5654   Liver Function Tests
American Liver Foundation
1425 Pompton Avenue
Cedar Grove, NJ 07009-1000

973-256-2550
800-223-0179
Fax: 973-256-3214
e-mail: info@liverfoundation.org
www.liverfoundation.org

Rick Smith, President & CEO

5655   Liver Transplant Fund
American Liver Foundation
1425 Pompton Avenue
Cedar Grove, NJ 07009-1000

973-256-2550
800-223-0179
Fax: 973-256-3214
e-mail: info@liverfoundation.org
www.liverfoundation.org

Rick Smith, President & CEO

5656   Liver Transplantation
American Liver Foundation
1425 Pompton Avenue
Cedar Grove, NJ 07009-1000

973-857-2626
800-223-0179
Fax: 973-256-3214
e-mail: info@liverfoundation.org
www.liverfoundation.org

Rick Smith, President & CEO

5657   Viral Hepatitis
American Liver Foundation
1425 Pompton Avenue
Cedar Grove, NJ 07009-1000

973-256-2550
800-223-0179
Fax: 973-256-3214
e-mail: info@liverfoundation.org
www.liverfoundation.org

Rick Smith, President & CEO

5658   Your Liver Lets You Live
American Liver Foundation
1425 Pompton Avenue
Cedar Grove, NJ 07009-1000

973-256-2550
800-223-0179
Fax: 973-256-3214
e-mail: info@liverfoundation.org
www.liverfoundation.org

Rick Smith, President & CEO

Web Sites

5659   American Association for the Study of Liver Diseases

www.aasld.org/

Conducts symposia and educational courses for professionals interested in disease of the liver and biliary tract. The leading organization for advancing the science and practice of hepatology.

5660   Children's Liver Alliance

www.liverkids.org.au/

Empowering the hearts and minds of children with liver disease, their families and the medical professionals who care for them.

5661   Healing Well

www.healingwell.com

An online health resource guide to medical news, chat, information and articles, newsgroups and message boards, books, disease-related web sites, medical directories, and more for patients, friends, and family coping with disabling diseases, disorders, or chronic illnesses.

5662 Health Finder

www.healthfinder.gov

Searchable, carefully developed web site offering information on over 1000 topics. Developed by the US Department of Health and Human Services, the site can be used in both English and Spanish.

5663 Healthlink USA

www.healthlinkusa.com

Health information concerning treatment, cures, prevention, diagnosis, risk factors, research, support groups, email lists, personal stories and much more. Updated regularly.

5664 Helios Health

www.helioshealth.com

Online resource for your health information. Detailed information about specific health topics, access to expert advice from our Medical Advisory Board, and up-to-date health news.

5665 Liver Support

www.liversupport.com

Information about the world's safest, most powerful liver-protecting supplement, milk thistle. Specifically facts about the safe, yet highly potent, Phytosome form.

5666 MedicineNet

www.medicinenet.com

An online resource for consumers providing easy-to-read, authoritative medical and health information.

5667 Medscape

www.medscape.com

Medscape offers specialists, primary care physicians, and other health professionals the Web's most robust and integrated medical information and educational tools.

5668 WebMD

www.webmd.com

Information on liver disease, including articles and resources.

Description

5669 ## Lung Disease

The lungs are in intimate contact with a person's environment, so they may be damaged by scores of agents, including dusts, gases and micro-organisms. The majority of lung, or pulmonary, diseases are related to exposure to external irritants, such as cigarette smoke, asbestos, bacteria and viruses. The most common chronic lung diseases of this type are emphysema and chronic bronchitis; both are part of the class of diseases called Chronic Obstructive Pulmonary Disease, or COPD. Most cases are associated with tobacco usage. High-risk occupations for lung disease include mining, farming, building construction and certain types of manufacturing. Lung cancer may be primary (originating in the lung) or secondary (spread, or metastasized, from another area). Bronchogenic cancer accounts for more than 90 percent of all lung tumors; cigarette smoking is the principal cause. Lung cancer is usually seen in people with COPD, because the two conditions have similar causes. Other lung disorders are secondary to clots originating from other sites in the body, systemic illness, and skeletal abnormalities that interfere with chest expansion during breathing.

Symptoms of lung disease may include coughing, sputum production, breathlessness, and sometimes fever or chest pain. In advanced cases, breathlessness is constant, and cyanosis (a bluish discoloration of the lips and fingernails) may occur.

Diagnosis of pulmonary disorders depends on a very careful history, physical examination, chest x-ray and pulmonary function testing, or spirometry. These measures are also important in following disease progression and response to treatment. Other chest imaging techniques, such as computed tomography (CT) scans and MRIs, and examination of fluid in the lung and lung tissue help establish a diagnosis. Recent research indicates that PET (positron emission tomography) scans may be helpful in the earlier diagnosis and treatment of lung cancer. Treatment of lung disease depends on the underlying cause. Management of COPD includes avoiding tobacco or other environmental exposure, antibiotics to control heavy sputum production and drugs to open up the narrowed airways. In advanced cases, breathing oxygen directly by nasal prongs improves quality of life and survival. Lung transplantation has occasionally been attempted, usually when COPD is due to a genetic disorder. Early screening for lung cancer has been disappointing; quitting smoking early is the only meaningful way of reducing one's risk of dying of the disease. Treatment may include surgery, radiation, or chemotherapy; success depends on the stage of the tumor and its precise type as determined by tissue biopsy.

Severe Acute Respiratory Syndrome, known as SARS, is an infectious disease that first appeared in China in 2002. SARS is caused by a corona-virus, which is related to the virus behind the common cold. The symptoms of SARS are a fever, greater than 100.4 degrees, fatigue, headache and chills. It is also accompanied by a dry cough and difficulty breathing, owing to the inflamed lungs. Until effective treatment or a vaccine is developed, prevention in SARS-infected areas includes isolating patients, wearing protective surgical masks, and restricting travel.

National Agencies & Associations

5670 **American Association for Respiratory Care**
9425 N MacArthur Boulevard
Irving, TX 75063-4706
972-243-2272
Fax: 972-484-2720
e-mail: info@aarc.org
www.aarc.org
Committed to enhancing professionalism as a respiratory care practitioner improving your performance on the job and helping to broaden the scope essential for success.
Michael T Amato, Chair
Neil MacIntyre, Vice-Chair

5671 **American Lung Association**
1301 Pennsylvania Avenue NW
Washington, DC 20004
202-785-3355
800-LUN-GUSA
e-mail: lungdc@lung.org
www.lung.org
The mission of the American Lung Association is to prevent lung disease and promote lung health. Founded in 1904 to fight tuberculosis the American Lung Association today fights disease in all its forms with special emphasis on asthma and tobacco control.
Ross P Lanzafame, Chairman
Harold P Wimmer, President & CEO

5672 **Coalition for Pulmonary Fibrosis**
10866 W. Washington Boulevard
Culver City, CA 90232
888-222-8541
Fax: 408-266-3289
e-mail: info@coalitionforpf.org
www.coalitionforpf.org
Founded to further education patient support and research efforts for pulmonary fibrosis specifically idiopathic pulmonary fibrosis.
Marvin I Schwarz, MD, Chairman
Gregory Tino, MD, Vice-Chairman

5673 **National Jewish Medical and Research Center**
1400 Jackson Street
Denver, CO 80206
303-398-1565
877-225-5654
e-mail: allstetterw@njhealth.org
www.nationaljewish.org
Offers comprehensive diagnosis treatment and rehabilitation of people with chronic obstructive pulmonary disease asthma allergies and other respiratory and immune diseases.
Rich Schierburg, Chair
Michael Salem, MD, President & CEO

5674 **Pulmonary Fibrosis Association**
230 East Ohio Street
Chicago, IL 60611-0004
888-733-6741
Fax: 866-587-9158
e-mail: info@pulmonaryfibrosis.org
www.pulmonaryfibrosis.org
Dedicated to finding a cure for and raising awareness of pulmonary fibrosis an often fatal lung disease.
Daniel M Rose, Chief Executive Officer and Chairman of
Patti Tuomey, President and Chief Operating Officer

5675 **Pulmonary Fibrosis Foundation**
230 East Ohio Street
Chicago, IL 60611
888-733-6741
Fax: 866-587-9158
e-mail: info@pulmonaryfibrosis.org
www.pulmonaryfibrosis.org
A non-profit corporation founded in the state of Colorado in 2000 by Albert Rose and Michael Rosenzweig, both of whom were diagnosed with Pulmonary Fibrosis (IPF).
Daniel M Rose, Chief Executive Officer and Chairman of
Patti Tuomey, President and Chief Operating Officer

5676 Pulmonary Hypertension Association
801 Roeder Road
Silver Spring, MD 20910
301-565-3004
800-748-7274
Fax: 301-565-3994
e-mail: pha@PHAssociation.org
www.PHAssociation.org

A nonprofit organization for pulmonary hypertension patients, families, caregivers and PH-treating medical professionals. The mission of the Pulmonary Hypertension Association (PHA) is to find ways to prevent and cure pulmonary hypertension.
Vallerie McLaughlin, MD, Chair
Rino Aldrighetti, President & CEO

5677 US Environmental Protection Agency: Indoor Environments Division
1200 Pennsylvania Avenue NW
Washington, DC 20460
202-343-9370
Fax: 202-343-2392
e-mail: iaqinfo@aol.com
www.epa.gov/iaq

Responsible for implementing EPA's Indoor Environments Program, a voluntary (non-regulatory) program to address indoor air pollution.
Gina McCarthy, Administrator
Bob Perciasepe, Deputy Administrator

5678 White Lung Association
PO Box 1483
Baltimore, MD 21203-1483
410-243-5864
e-mail: jfite@whitelung.org
www.whitelung.org

A national nonprofit organization dedicated to the education of the public to the hazards of asbestos exposure. The association developed programs of public education and consults with victims of asbestos exposure, school boards, building owners and government representatives.
Jim Perry, Director of Development

State Agencies & Associations

Alabama

5679 American Lung Association of Alabama
PO BOX 2178
Ridgeland, AL 35244
601-206-5810
Fax: 202-452-1805
e-mail: inquiries@breathehealthy.org
www.lung.org/associations/states/alabama

Robin Robinson, Chair
Sara Dreiling, Chief Executive Officer

Alaska

5680 American Lung Association of Alaska
500 W International Airport Road
Anchorage, AK 99518-1105
907-276-5864
800-LUN-GUSA
Fax: 907-565-5587
e-mail: mstoneking@aklung.org
www.lung.org/associations/states/alaska/

Marge Pfeifer, President/CEO

Arizona

5681 American Lung Association of Arizona
102 W McDowell Road
Phoenix, AZ 85003-1299
602-258-7505
800-LUN-GUSA
Fax: 602-258-7507
e-mail: calexander@lungarizona.org
www.lung.org/associations/states/arizona

Through research education and advocacy the American Lung Association of Arizona works to prevent lung disease and promote lung health. Our areas of focus are asthma air quality and tobacco control.
Terry Daane, Chair
Stacey Mortenson, Executive Director

Arkansas

5682 American Lung Association of Arkansas
211 Natural Resources Drive
Little Rock, AR 72205-1539
501-224-5864
800-880-5864
Fax: 501-224-5654
e-mail: klackey@lungark.org
www.lungark.org

Karen S Abate, President/CEO
Sylvia Goodin, Secretary

California

5683 American Lung Association of California
424 Pendleton Way
Oakland, CA 94621-2189
510-638-5864
Fax: 510-638-8984
e-mail: cainfo@lung.org
www.lung.org/associations/states/califor

A.Linda Hinojosa, Chair
Jane Warner, President/CEO

Colorado

5684 American Lung Association of Colorado
5600 Greenwood Plaza Boulevard
Greenwood Village, CO 80111
303-388-4327
800-LUN-GUSA
Fax: 303-377-1102
e-mail: info@lungcolorado.org
http://www.lung.org/associations/states/

Curt Huber, Executive Director
Connor Michael, Communications Manager

Connecticut

5685 American Lung Association of Connecticut
45 Ash Street
E Hartford, CT 06108-3272
860-289-5401
800-586-4872
Fax: 860-289-5405
e-mail: bcase@alact.org
www.alact.org

Part of the American Lung Association the oldest voluntary health agency dedicated to fighting a single disease. Highest priorities are asthma tobacco control and clean air.
Lisa Brown, VP Community Outreach
Susan DeNardo, Development Director

Delaware

5686 American Lung Association of Delaware
630 Churchmans Road
Wilmington, DE 19702-3280
302-737-6414
800-LUN-GUSA
Fax: 888-415-5757
e-mail: llyons@lunginfo.org
www.lung.org/associations/charters/mid-a

Christopher Carney, Chair
Deborah Brown, CEO

District of Columbia

5687 American Lung Association of the District of Columbia
1301 Pennsylvania Avenue NW
Washington, DC 20004-2617
202-785-3355
e-mail: lungdc@lung.org
www.lung.org/associations/charters/distr

Resource for information and programs in the area of lung health, including asthma, tobacco control, air quality, sarcoidosis, and turberculosis.
Dennis C Alexander, Regional Executive Director
Marc Ittelson, Regional Development Director

Florida

5688 American Lung Association of Florida
6852 Belfort Oaks Place
Jacksonville, FL 32216-5216
904-743-2933
800-940-2933
Fax: 904-743-2916
e-mail: alaf@lungfla.org
www.lung.org/associations/states/florida

Works for the prevention and control of lung disease through education, advocacy and research.
Marcia Williams, Chairwoman
Martha C Bogdan, President/CEO

5689 Goodwill Industries-Suncoast
Goodwill Industries-Suncoast
10596 Gandy Boulevard   727-523-1512
St. Petersburg, FL 33702   888-279-1988
                                      Fax: 727-563-9300
e-mail: gw.marketing@goodwill-suncoast.com
www.goodwill-suncoast.org
A non-profit community based organization whose purpose is to improve the quality of life for people who are disabled, disadvantaged and/or aged. This mission is accomplished through a staff of over 1,200 employees providing independent living skills, affordable housing, career assessment and planning, job skills, training, placement, and job retention assistance with useful employment. Annually, Goodwill Industries-Suncoast serves over 30,000 people in Citrus, Hernando, Levy, Marion and more.
Oscar J Horton, Chair
Deborah A Passerini, President/CEO

Georgia

5690 American Lung Association of Georgia
2452 Spring Road   770-434-5864
Smyrna, GA 30080-3862   Fax: 770-319-0349
e-mail: alaga@lungga.org
www.lung.org/associations/states/georgia
Marcia Williams, Chairwoman of the Board
Martha C Bogdan, President/CEO

Hawaii

5691 American Lung Association of Hawaii
650 Iwilei Road   808-537-5966
Honolulu, HI 96817   Fax: 808-537-5971
e-mail: lleslie@ala-hawaii.org
www.lung.org/associations/states/hawaii
Lorraine Leslie, Hawaii Director
Debbie Apolo, Tobacco Control Manager

Idaho

5692 American Lung Association of Idaho
1412 W Idaho   208-345-5864
Boise, ID 83702   800-LUN-GUSA
                                      Fax: 208-345-5896
e-mail: jflynn@lungmtpacific.org
www.lung.org/associations/states/idaho/
Wimmer, CEO
Kim Streib, Vice President Finance

Illinois

5693 American Lung Association of Illinois
55 West Wacker Drive   312-781-1100
Chicago, IL 60601   800-LUN-GUSA
                                      Fax: 318-781-9250
e-mail: info@lungil.org
www.lung.org/associations/states/illinoi
Frank Keldermans, Chair
Lewis Bartfield, President/CEO

Indiana

5694 American Lung Association of Indiana
115 W Washington Street   317-819-1181
Indianapolis, IN 46204-1470   800-LUN-GUSA
                                      Fax: 317-819-1187
e-mail: info@lungin.org
www.lung.org/associations/states/indiana
Alan D Rowe, Chair
Lewis Bartfield, President/CEO

Iowa

5695 American Lung Association of Iowa
2530 73rd Street   515-309-9507
Des Moines, IA 50322-1800   800-LUN-GUSA
                                      Fax: 515-334-9564
e-mail: info@lungia.org
www.lung.org/associations/states/iowa/
Alan D Rowe, Chair
Lewis Bartfield, President/CEO

Kansas

5696 American Lung Association of Kansas
6701 W. 64th Street   913-912- 719
Overland Park, KS 66202-2419   800-LUN-GUSA
                                      Fax: 913-912-7206
e-mail: inquiries@breathehealthy.org
www.lung.org/associations/charters/plain
Robin Robinson, Chair
Veena B Antony, Director

Kentucky

5697 American Lung Association of Kentucky
4100 Churchman Avenue   502-363-2652
Louisville, KY 40215-0067   800-LUN-GUSA
                                      Fax: 502-363-0222
e-mail: bgottschalk@midlandlung.org
www.lung.org/associations/states/kentuck
Barry Gottschalk, President/CEO
Robert Singletary, Vice President - Finance & Administratio

Louisiana

5698 American Lung Association of Louisiana
2325 Severn Avenue   504-828-5864
Metairie, LA 70001-6918   800-586-4872
                                      Fax: 504-828-5867
e-mail: inquiries@breathehealthy.org
www.lung.org/associations/charters/plain
Robin Robinson, Chair
Veena B Antony, Director

Maine

5699 American Lung Association of Maine
122 State Street   207-622-6394
Augusta, ME 04330   888-241-6566
                                      Fax: 207-626-2919
e-mail: info@lungne.org
www.lung.org/associations/states/maine/
Ross P Lanzafame, Chairman of the Board
John F Emanuel, Secretary/ Treasurer

Maryland

5700 American Lung Association of Maryland
211 East Lombard Street   443-451-4950
Baltimore, MD 21202   800-LUN-GUSA
                                      Fax: 410-560-0829
e-mail: lungmd@lungusa.org
www.lung.org/associations/states/marylan
Dennis C Alexander, Regional Executive Director
Marc Ittelson, Regional Development Director

Massachusetts

5701 American Lung Association of Massachusetts
5 Mountain Road   781-272-2866
Burlington, MA 01903
Adams, CEO
Nicole Crumpton, Executive Office Manager

Michigan

5702 American Lung Association of Michigan
1475 E 12 Mile Road
Madison Heights, MI 48071
248-784-2000
800-543-LUNG
Fax: 248-784-2008
e-mail: midland@midlandlung.org
www.lung.org/associations/states/michiga
Barry Gottschalk, President/CEO
Robert Singletary, Vice President-Finance & Administration

Minnesota

5703 American Lung Association of Minnesota
490 Concordia Avenue
Saint Paul, MN 55103-2441
651-227-8014
800-LUN-GUSA
Fax: 651-227-5459
e-mail: info@lungmn.org
www.lung.org/associations/states/minneso
Angie Carlson, PhD, Chair
Lewis Bartfield, President/CEO

Mississippi

5704 American Lung Association of Mississippi
PO Box 2178
Ridgeland, MS 39158
601-206-5810
Fax: 601-206-5813
e-mail: inquiries@breathehealthy.org
www.lung.org/associations/charters/plain
Robin Robinson, Chair
Veena B Antony, Director

5705 American Lung Association of Missouri
6701 W. 64th Street
Overland Park, KS 66202
913-912- 719
Fax: 913-912-7206
e-mail: inquiries@breathehealthy.org
www.lung.org/associations/charters/plain
Robin Robinson, Chair
Veena B Antony, Director

Missouri

5706 American Lung Association of Eastern Missouri
1118 Hampton Avenue
Saint Louis, MO 63139-3196
314-645-5505
Fax: 314-645-7128
www.lungusa2.org/missouri/index.html

5707 American Lung Association: Kansas City Office
2400 Troost
Kansas City, MO 64108
816-842-5242
Fax: 816-842-5470
e-mail: qnimrod@breathehealthy.org
www.lungusa2.org/missouri/index.html
National health association dedicated to promoting lung health
and preventing lung disease.

Montana

5708 American Lung Association of Northern Rockies
825 Helena Avenue
Helena, MT 59601-3459
406-442-6556
Fax: 406-442-2346
e-mail: ala-nr@ala-nr.org
www.lungusa.org

Nebraska

5709 American Lung Association of Nebraska
8990 West Dodge
Omaha, NE 68114
402-502-4950
800-LUN-GUSA
Fax: 402-502-3112
e-mail: inquiries@breathehealthy.org
www.lung.org/associations/charters/plain
Robin Robinson, Chair
Veena B Antony, Director

Nevada

5710 American Lung Association of Nevada
10615 Double R Boulevard
Reno, NV 89521
775-829-LUNG
800-LUN-GUSA
Fax: 775-829-5850
e-mail: lgenasci@lungnevada.org
www.lungusa.org
Lisa Genasci, Executive Director
Heather Lunsford, Development & Program Manager

New Hampshire

5711 American Lung Association of New Hampshire
1800 Elm Street
Manchester, NH 03104
603-369-3977
800-83L-UNGS
Fax: 603-369-3978
e-mail: info@lungne.org
www.lung.org/associations/states/new-ham
Ross P Lanzafame, Chairman of the Board
John F Emanuel, Secretary/ Treasurer

New Jersey

5712 American Lung Association of New Jersey
1031 Route 22 West
Bridgewater, NJ 08807-3410
908-685-8040
Fax: 888-415-5757
e-mail: jgrinwald@lunginfo.org
www.lung.org/associations/charters/mid-a
Christopher Carney, Chair
Deborah Brown, CEO

New Mexico

5713 American Lung Association of New Mexico
5911 Jefferson Street NE
Albuquerque, NM 87109
505-265-0732
800-LUN-GUSA
Fax: 505-260-1739
e-mail: info@lungnewmexico.org
www.lung.org/associations/states/new-mex
Support group for adults with lung disease. Also offers lung health
education.
Deborah Hoffman, Executive Director
JoAnna DeMaria, Director of Programs

New York

5714 American Lung Association of New York State
418 Broadway
Albany, NY 12207-2804
518-465-2013
800-499-LUNG
Fax: 781-890-4280
e-mail: info@lungne.org
www.lung.org/associations/charters/north
Brian Simonds, Chair
Jeff Seyler, President/CEO

North Carolina

5715 American Lung Association of North Carolina
514 Daniels Street
Raleigh, NC 27605
919-424-6069
800-586-4872
Fax: 919-856-8530
e-mail: lungnc@lungusa.org
www.lungnc.org
Better breathing clubs for chronic lung disease patients.
Dennis C Alexander, Regional Executive Director
Marc Ittelson, Regional Development Director

North Dakota

5716 American Lung Association of North Dakota
212 N. 2nd Street
Bismarck, ND 58501
701-223-5613
800-252-6325
Fax: 701-223-5727
e-mail: info@lungnd.org
http://www.lung.org/associations/states/
A voluntary health agency whose objective is the conquest of lung
disease and the promotion of lung health. We sponsor Super
Asthma Saturday and open airways for schools events to educate

asthmatics and their families and Dakota Superkids Asthma Camp for kids 8-15 with asthma. Smoking cessation classes for adults and youth.
Alan D Rowe, Chair
Lewis Bartfield, President/CEO

Ohio

5717 **American Lung Association of Ohio**
1950 Arlingate Lane   614-279-1700
Columbus, OH 43228-4102   800-LUN-GUSA
                                              Fax: 614-279-4940
                              e-mail: alao@ohiolung.org
                       www.lung.org/associations/states/ohio/in
Barry Gottschalk, President/CEO
Robert Singletary, Vice President - Finance & Administratio

Oklahoma

5718 **American Lung Association of Oklahoma**
11212 N May Avenue   405-748-4674
Oklahoma City, OK 73120   800-LUN-GUSA
                                              Fax: 405-748-6274
                          e-mail: inquiries@breathehealthy.org
                      www.lung.org/associations/charters/plain
Robin Robinson, Chair
Veena B Antony, Director

Oregon

5719 **American Lung Association of Oregon**
7420 SW Bridgeport Road   503-924-4094
Tigard, OR 97224-7790   800-LUN-GUSA
                                              Fax: 503-924-4120
                           e-mail: info@lungmtpacific.org
                       www.lung.org/associations/states/oregon/

Pennsylvania

5720 **American Respiratory Alliance of Western Pennsylvania**
201 Smith Drive   724-772-1750
Cranberry Township, PA 16066   800-220-1990
                                              Fax: 724-772-1180
                            e-mail: info@healthylungs.org
                            www.healthylungs.org
Dedicated to the prevention and control of lung disease through education training, direct services, research funding and advocacy since 1904.
Christine R Cavan, Director
Robert Petix, Chair/Executive Committee

5721 **Breathe Pennsylvania**
3001 Old Gettysburg Road   717-541-5864
Camp Hill, PA 17011   800-932-0903
                                              Fax: 888-415-5757
                             e-mail: dbrown@lunginfo.org
                       www.lung.org/associations/charters/mid-a
Provide education, research and information on lung disease and lung health, including asthma, tobacco prevention and cessation, chronic obstructive pulmonary disease, indoor and outdoor air quality, children's summer camps, support groups and specialty programs.
Christopher Carney, Chair
Deborah Brown, CEO

Rhode Island

5722 **American Lung Association of Rhode Island**
260 W Exchange Street   401-421-6487
Providence, RI 02903-3700   800-586-4872
                                              Fax: 401-331-5266
                               e-mail: info@lungne.org
                       www.lung.org/associations/charters/north
Brian Simonds, Chair
Jeff Seyler, President/CEO

South Carolina

5723 **American Lung Association of South Carolina**
44-A Markfield Drive   843-556-8451
Charleston, SC 29407-2344   800-849-5864
                                              Fax: 843-766-3294
                            e-mail: alasc1@lungsc.org
                       www.lung.org/associations/states/south-c
Marcia Williams, Chairwoman of the Board
William R Cook, Chair-Elect

South Dakota

5724 **American Lung Association of South Dakota**
401 East 8th Street   605-336-7222
Sioux Falls, SD 57103-0233   800-873-5864
                                              Fax: 605-336-7227
                               e-mail: info@lungsd.org
                       www.lung.org/associations/states/south-d
Alan D Rowe, Chair
Lewis Bartfield, President/CEO

Tennessee

5725 **American Lung Association of Tennessee**
1 Vantage Way   615-329-1151
Nashville, TN 37228   800-LUN-GUSA
                                              Fax: 615-329-1723
                            e-mail: gbost@midlandlung.org
                       www.lung.org/associations/states/tenness
A statewide organization the oldest national health agency in the US. Our mission is to prevent lung disease and to promote lung health. Our program priorities include environmental health asthma education tobacco control for children and finding a cure.
Dr Steven Coulter, Chairman
Barry Gottschalk, President/CEO

Texas

5726 **American Lung Association of Texas**
5926 Balcones Drive   512-467-6753
Austin, TX 78731   800-252-LUNG
                                              Fax: 512-467-7621
                          e-mail: inquiries@breathehealthy.org
                              www.texaslung.org
Robin Robinson, Chair
Veena B Antony, Director

Utah

5727 **American Lung Association of Utah**
1930 S 1100 E   801-484-4456
Salt Lake City, UT 84106-2317   800-548-8252
                                              Fax: 801-484-5461
                               e-mail: info@lungutah.org
                       www.lung.org/associations/states/utah/
Troy Neerings, Chair
W. Glenn Lanham, Executive Director

Virginia

5728 **American Lung Association of Virginia**
9702 Gayton Road   804-955-4910
Richmond, VA 23238   800-345-5864
                                              Fax: 804-267-5634
                             e-mail: lungva@lungusa.org
                              www.lungva.org
Dennis C Alexander, Regional Executive Director
Marc Ittelson, Regional Development Director

Washington

5729 American Lung Association of Washington
822 John Street
Seattle, WA 98109   206-441-5100
    800-732-9339
    Fax: 206-441-3277
    e-mail: info@alaw.org
    www.lung.org/associations/states/washing
Marina Crickenberger, Executive Director
Chantal Fields, Assistant Executive Director

West Virginia

5730 American Lung Association of West Virginia
2102 Kanawha Blvd   304-342-6600
East Charleston, WV 25311   800-LUN-GUSA
    Fax: 888-415-5757
    e-mail: cfields@lunginfo.org
    www.lung.org/associations/charters/mid-a
Christopher Carney, Chair
Deborah Brown, CEO

Wisconsin

5731 American Lung Association of Wisconsin
13100 W Lisbon Road   262-703-4200
Brookfield, WI 53005-2508   800-LUN-GUSA
    Fax: 262-781-5180
    e-mail: info@lungwi.org
    www.lung.org/associations/states/wiscons
Alan D Rowe, Chair
Lewis Bartfield, President/CEO

Research Centers

5732 Enzymology Research Laboratory Dept. of Veterans Affairs Medical Center
Dept. of Veterans Affairs Medical Center
150 Muir Road   925-228-6800
Martinez, CA 94553
Studies affecting emphysema in mankind.
Michael C Gaussig, President

5733 National Jewish Center for Immunology
1400 Jackson Street   303-388-4461
Denver, CO 80206   877-225-5654
    www.nationaljewish.org
Offers basic and clinical research into the causes and treatments of various lung diseases and respiratory problems.
Rafeul Alam, Division Chief

5734 University of Utah Rocky Mountain Center for Occupational & Environmental Health
University of Utah
391 Chipeta Way   801-581-4800
Salt Lake City, UT 84108   Fax: 801-817-24
    TTY: 801-581-7224
    e-mail: rmoser@rmcoeh.utah.edu
    medicine.utah.edu/rmcoeh/
Provides graduate and continuing education programs in occupational medicine occupational health nursing ergonomics and safety industrial hygiene and hazardous materials. Additionally provides clinical evaluations and consultations in the listed areas.
Dennis Lloyd, Chair
Sen Karen Mayne, Advisory Member

5735 Warren Grant Magnuson Clinical Center
National Institute of Health
10 Center Drive MSC 1078   301-496-3311
Bethesda, MD 20892   800-411-1222
    Fax: 301-496-2390
    TTY: 866-411-1010
    e-mail: mmichael@cc.nih.gov
    www.clinicalcenter.nih.gov
Established in 1953 as the research hospital of the National Institutes of Health. Designed so that patient care facilities are close to research laboratories so new findings of basic and clinical scientists can be quickly applied to the treatment of patients. Upon referral by physicians, patients are admitted to NIH clinical studies.
John Mark, Lung Help Line Director

Support Groups & Hotlines

5736 American Lung Association Help Line
American Lung Association
3000 Kelly Lane   217-787-5864
Springfield, IL 62711   800-586-4872
    Fax: 217-787-5916
    www.helpline.org
Provides information for the lung association of the state in which you make the call. Offers support group referrals.
Michael Salem MD, President/CEO
William Allstetter, Public Affairs/Media

5737 Lung Facts
National Jewish Center for Immunology
1400 Jackson Street   303-388-4461
Denver, CO 80206   877-225-5654
    Fax: 303-270-2220
    e-mail: allstetterw@njc.org
    www.nationaljewish.org
An automated information service with recorded health messages developed by Lung Line Information Service. The information provided on this system offers help and support, as well as medical updates for persons suffering from lung diseases.
Michael

5738 National Health Information Center
PO Box 1133   310-565-4167
Washington, DC 20013   800-336-4797
    Fax: 301-984-4256
    e-mail: info@nhic.org
    www.health.gov/nhic
Offers a nationwide information referral service, produces directories and resource guides.
Austin, PhD

Books

5739 American Lung Association Family Guide to Asthma and Allergies
American Lung Association
1740 Broadway   212-315-8700
New York, NY 10019-4315   e-mail: info@lungusa.org
    www.lungusa.org

5740 Health Consequences of Smoking: Cancer & Chronic Lung Disease in the Workplace
DIANE Publishing Company
330 Pusey Avenue, Unit #3 Rear   610-461-6200
Darby, PA 19023   800-782-3833
    Fax: 610-461-6130
    e-mail: dianepublishing@gmail.com
    www.dianepublishing.net
Examines the relationship between cigarette smoking and occupational exposures. Establishes that in order to protect the workers fully, forces of labor, management, insurers and government must become as engaged in attempts to reduce the prevalence of cigarette smoking as they are in occupational exposure. Tables and figure. Extensive bibliography, index.
542 pages Paperback
ISBN: 0-788123-11-4
Herman Baron, Publisher

5741 Management of Acute Exacerbations of Chronic Obstructive Pulmonary Disease
DIANE Publishing Company
330 Pusey Avenue, Unit #3 Rear   610-461-6200
Darby, PA 19023   800-782-3833
    Fax: 610-461-6130
    e-mail: dianepublishing@gmail.com
    www.dianepublishing.net
This report describes evidence about the clinical assessment and management of patients presenting with acute exacerbation of

chronic obstructive pulmonary disease, a frequent cause of health care utilization, morality and decreased quality of life.
256 pages Paperback
ISBN: 0-756721-99-7
Herman Baron, Publisher

5742 Seven Steps to a Smoke-Free Life
American Lung Association
1740 Broadway   212-315-8700
New York, NY 10019-4315   e-mail: info@lungusa.org
                                                            www.lungusa.org

Pamphlets

5743 Around the Clock with COPD
American Lung Association
1740 Broadway   212-315-8700
New York, NY 10019-4315   800-586-4872
                                                     e-mail: info@lungusa.org
                                                            www.lungusa.org
A booklet with non-medical helpful hints written by persons living with a chronic lung disease for others.

5744 Asbestos in Your Home
American Lung Association
1740 Broadway   212-315-8700
New York, NY 10019-4315   800-586-4872
Offers information on asbestos.

5745 Black Lung
National Jewish Center for Immunology
1400 Jackson Street   303-388-4461
Denver, CO 80206-2762   800-222-5864
Offers information on black lung and the respiratory system.

5746 Emphysema
American Lung Association of Connecticut
45 Ash Street   860-289-5401
East Hartford, CT 06108-3294   800-586-4872
                                                     Fax: 860-289-5405
                                                            www.alact.org
Offers information on who gets emphysema, how it attacks, causes, effects, prevention and treatment.
John E Zinn, President/CEO

5747 Exercise Guidelines for the Person with Lung Disease
American Lung Association of Connecticut
45 Ash Street   860-289-5401
East Hartford, CT 06108-3294   800-586-4872
                                                     Fax: 860-289-5405
                                                            www.alact.org
Offers exercise information and illustrations for persons with lung disease.
John E Zinn, President/CEO

5748 Facts About AAT Deficiency-Related Emphysema
American Lung Association
1740 Broadway   212-315-8700
New York, NY 10019-4315
Offers information on this type of emphysema, risk factors, development, symptoms and early detection.

5749 Facts About Asbestos
American Lung Association
1740 Broadway   212-315-8700
New York, NY 10019-4315
Offers information on lung hazards on the job and what employers can do to protect themselves and the people that work for them.

5750 Facts About Asthma
American Lung Association
1740 Broadway   212-315-8700
New York, NY 10019-4315   800-586-4872

5751 Steps to a Better Understanding of Lung Cancer: A Patient and Family Guide
American Lung Association

1740 Broadway   212-315-8700
New York, NY 10019-4315   800-586-4872
                                                     e-mail: info@lungusa.org
                                                            www.lungusa.org
A booklet with non-medical helpful hints written by persons living with a chronic lung disease for others.

5752 Understanding Emphysema
National Jewish Center for Immunology
1400 Jackson Street   303-388-4461
Denver, CO 80206-2762   800-222-5864
Offers information on emphysema, causes, treatments, symptoms and prevention.

Audio & Video

5753 Keeping the Balance
Fanlight Productions
4196 Washington Street   617-469-4999
Boston, MA 02131-1731   800-937-4113
                                                     Fax: 617-469-3379
                                                  e-mail: fanlight@fanlight.com
                                                            www.fanlight.com
Siblings of children with serious lung disease share their experiences of being the normal child, exploring the frequent conflict between their feelings of love and concern and their resentment over the attention denied to them because of the sibling's illness. Offers advice on how parents can keep the balance between the needs of all of their children.
1993 23 Minutes
ISBN: 1-572950-89-7

5754 Sickle Cell Disease: Faces of Our Children
Fanlight Productions
4196 Washington Street   617-469-4999
Boston, MA 02131-1731   800-937-4113
                                                     Fax: 617-469-3379
                                                  e-mail: fanlight@fanlight.com
                                                            www.fanlight.com
This program examines the devastating impact of sickle cell disease on these young people and their families and caregivers. It will be an important tool for increasing awareness in the community and among healthcare and social service providers in community clinics, hospitals, and other settings.
1999 14 Minutes
ISBN: 1-572953-05-5

Web Sites

5755 American Lung Association
                                                            www.lungusa.org
Offers research, medical updates, fund-raising, educational materials and public awareness campaigns relating to lung disease causes.

5756 Healing Well
                                                            www.healingwell.com
An online health resource guide to medical news, chat, information and articles, newsgroups and message boards, books, disease-related web sites, medical directories, and more for patients, friends, and family coping with disabling diseases, disorders, or chronic illnesses.

5757 Health Central
                                                            www.healthcenter.com
Provides support group and diagnostic information regarding lung disease.

5758 Health Finder
                                                            www.healthfinder.gov
Searchable, carefully developed web site offering information on over 1000 topics. Developed by the US Department of Health and Human Services, the site can be used in both English and Spanish.

5759 Healthlink USA
                                                            www.healthlinkusa.com

429

Health information concerning treatment, cures, prevention, diagnosis, risk factors, research, support groups, email lists, personal stories and much more. Updated regularly.

5760 Helios Health

www.helioshealth.com

Online resource for your health information. Detailed information about specific health topics, access to expert advice from our Medical Advisory Board, and up-to-date health news.

5761 Lung Disease

www.lungusa.org

The American Lung Association's website, including information on diseases A to Z, living with lung disease, tobacco control, air quality, data, statistics, research, and more.

5762 MedicineNet

www.medicinenet.com

An online resource for consumers providing easy-to-read, authoritative medical and health information.

5763 Medscape

www.medscape.com

Medscape offers specialists, primary care physicians, and other health professionals the Web's most robust and integrated medical information and educational tools.

5764 National Heart, Lung & Blood Institute

www.nhlbi.nih.gov

A website maintained by the National Institute of Health offering general information regarding the heart, lungs, and blood.

5765 WebMD

www.webmd.com

Information on lung disease, including articles and resources.

Description

5766 Lupus Erythematosus

Lupus erythematosus refers to two distinct but overlapping conditions. Systemic lupus erythematosus, SLE, is a chronic multi-organ inflammatory illness that may involve the brain, skin, kidneys, joints, bowel, and eyes. Discoid lupus erythematosus, DLE, is a much less serious disease that is limited to the skin. In DLE, patches of skin may turn red and develop white scales, followed by thinning and scarring. About 10 percent of patients with DLE will go on to develop SLE; roughly 25 percent of patients with SLE also have the manifestations of DLE.

Of SLE cases, 90 percent are women, and the disease usually begins during the child-bearing years. Although the cause is unclear, SLE causes its damage through auto-immune mechanisms. The body's own immune system, designed to fight off invasion from micro-organisms, turns against its own tissues, evidence of which can be measured in the blood. Almost any organ system can be affected, and symptoms include fatigue, fever, loss of appetite, skin rash, sensitivity to light (photophobia), joint pain, headaches, personality change, eye irritation, and inflammation of the kidney.

In general, the course of SLE is chronic and relapsing, often with long periods (years) of remission. It may only be mild or progress towards more serious illness and death from infection, kidney failure, or neurologic damage. Survival has improved markedly in the past two decades because, for most patients with SLE, the disease can be controlled with large, prolonged doses of steroids, and other drugs that affect the immune system. Some of these therapies may be associated with long-term complications.

National Agencies & Associations

5767 American Juvenile Arthritis Organization (AJAO)
1330 West Peachtree Street
Atlanta, GA 30309
404-872-7100
800-283-7800
Fax: 440-872-9559
e-mail: help@arthritis.org
www.arthritis.org
A council of the Arthritis Foundation devoted to serving the special needs of children, teens and young adults with childhood rheumatic diseases (including systemic lupus erythematosus) and their families. Provides support groups, information, advocacy, research updates, and conferences.
Daniel T McGowan, Chair
John H Klippel, President & CEO

5768 American Juvenile Arthritis Organization
1330 W Peachtree Street
Atlanta, GA 30309
404-872-7100
800-283-7800
Fax: 440-872-9559
e-mail: help@arthritis.org
www.arthritis.org
A council of the Arthritis Foundation devoted to serving the special needs of children teens and young adults with childhood rheumatic diseases (including systemic lupus erythematosus) and their families. Provides support groups, information and advocacy.
Daniel T McGowan, Chair
John H Klippel, President & CEO

5769 Autoimmune Diseases Association
22100 Gratiot Avenue
E Detroit, MI 48021
586-776-3900
Fax: 586-776-3903
e-mail: aarda@aarda.org
www.aarda.org
Provides mutual support and education for patients with any type of autoimmune disease. Support includes advocacy referral to support groups literature and conferences.
Stanley M Finger, Chair
Virginia T Ladd, President & CEO

5770 Lupus Foundation of America
2000 L Street NW
Washington, DC 20036
202-349-1155
800-558-0121
Fax: 202-349-1156
e-mail: info@lupus.org
www.lupus.org
The Lupus Foundation of America is the nation's leading non-profit voluntary health organization dedicated to finding the causes and cure for lupus. Our mission is to improve the diagnosis and treatment of lupus and support individuals and families affected by this disease.
Peter M Schwab, Chair
Sandra C Raymond, President & CEO

5771 Lupus Network
230 Ranch Drive
Bridgeport, CT 06606
203-372-5795
Seeks to foster better understanding of the disease among patients and the general public educators and professionals through the distribution of educational materials.

State Agencies & Associations

Alaska

5772 Lupus Foundation of America: Alaska Chapter
PO Box 240628
Anchorage, AK 99524
907-338-6332
800-307-5878
Fax: 907-345-0695
e-mail: LFA_Alaska@hotmail.com
www.lupus.org/webmodules/webarticlesnet/
Judy Powell, Chair of the Board
Anna Tillman, Executive Director

Arizona

5773 Lupus Foundation of America: Greater Arizona Chapter
2001 West Camelback Road
Phoenix, AZ 85015-4908
480-201-5334
e-mail: juliano@lupus.org
www.lupus.org/webmodules/webarticlesnet/
David Juliano, Outreach Development Manager

5774 Lupus Foundation of America: Southern Arizona Chapter
2583 North 1st Avenue
Tucson, AZ 85719
480-201-5334
e-mail: juliano@lupus.org
www.lupus.org/webmodules/webarticlesnet/
David Juliano, Outreach Development Manager

Arkansas

5775 Lupus Foundation of America: Arkansas Chapter
220 Mockingbird
Hot Springs, AR 71913
501-525-9380
800-294-8878
Fax: 501-525-9380
e-mail: lupusarkhs@direclynx.net
www.lupus-arkansas.com
Jamesetta Smith, President

California

5776 Bay Area LE Foundation
2635 N 1st Street
San Jose, CA 95134
408-954-8600
800-523-3363
Chapter of the Lupus Foundation of America.

5777 **Lupus Foundation of America: California Chapter**
18000 Studebaker Road   562-467-8994
Cerritos, CA 90703   800-558-0121
                                         Fax: 916-973-8124
                                         e-mail: gray@lupus.org
                           www.lupus.org/webmodules/webarticlesnet/
Laurie Gray, National Manager of Walk Development
Luz Maria Hernandez, Health Educator

Colorado

5778 **Lupus Foundation of Colorado**
1211 S Parker Road   303-597-4050
Denver, CO 80231   800-858-1292
                                         Fax: 303-597-4054
                                         e-mail: info@lupuscolorado.org
                                         www.lupuscolorado.org
Chapter of the Lupus Foundation of America.
Carol Wright, Chair
Debbie Lynch, Chief Executive Officer

Connecticut

5779 **Lupus Foundation of America: Connecticut Chapter**
270 Farmington Avenue   860-269-6240
Farmington, CT 06032-2402   800-699-6967
                                         Fax: 860-269-6243
                                         e-mail: office@lupusct.org
                           www.lupus.org/webmodules/webarticlesnet/
A non-profit organization and a National Health Agency established for the purpose of enlightening the public by focusing professional and public attention on Lupus Erythematosus promotes research by providing financial assistance and serves as the support bond for patients and their families.
Ron Marek, Chair
Michael Tommasi, President & CEO

Delaware

5780 **Lupus Foundation of America: Delaware Chapter**
100 West 10th Street   302-622-8700
Wilmington, DE 19801   800-880-8686
                           www.lupus.org/webmodules/webarticlesnet/
Debra L Riegel Jepson, Chair
James Stewart, Treasurer

Florida

5781 **Lupus Foundation of America: Northeast Florida Chapter**
PO Box 10486   904-645-8398
Jacksonville, FL 32247-0486   800-853-8398
Lee, President
Jon Kagan, Vice President

5782 **Lupus Foundation of America: Northwest Florida Chapter**
PO Box 17841   904-444-7070
Pensacola, FL 32522-7841   800-458-8211
                                         e-mail: info@lupus.pensacola.com
                                         www.lupus.pensacola.com
Brenda Barto, Executive Director
Kathleen Laca, Director of Operations

5783 **Lupus Foundation of America: Southeast Florida Chapter**
2300 High Ridge Road   561-279-8606
Boynton Beach, FL 33426   855-905-8787
                                         Fax: 561-935-1435
                                         e-mail: info@lupusfl.org
                                         www.lupusfl.com
John Apgar, Chair
Amy Kelly-Yalden, President & CEO

5784 **Lupus Foundation of America: Suncoast Chapter**
3637 4th Street N   727-447-7075
St Petersburg, FL 33704-7485   800-684-9276
                                         Fax: 727-447-8925
                                         e-mail: info@lupusflorida.org
                                         www.lupusfl.com

5785 **Lupus Foundation of America: Tampa Area Chapter**
Dibbs Plaza

4119-20A Gunn Highway   813-960-3992
Tampa, FL 33624   800-330-3992
                                         www.milupus.org/southeast.htm

5786 **Lupus Foundation of Florida**
535 Central Avenue   727-447-7075
St. Petersburg, FL 33701   800-684-9276
                                         Fax: 727-447-7075
                                         e-mail: rmccolllum@lupusflorida.org
                                         www.hstrial-lupusfoundati.intuitwebsites
Chapter of the Lupus Foundation of America.
Maggi McQueen, Chairman
Rick McCollum, President & CEO

Georgia

5787 **Lupus Foundation of America: Columbus Chapter**
233 12th Street
Columbus, GA 31901   706-571-8950
                                         www.milupus.org/southeast.htm

5788 **Lupus Foundation of America: Greater Atlanta Chapter**
1850 Lake Park Drive   770-333-5930
Smyrna, GA 30080-2203   800-800-4532
                                         Fax: 770-333-5932
                                         e-mail: info@lgaga.org
                           www.lupus.org/webmodules/webarticlesnet/
Maria Myler, President & CEO
Teri Emond, Program Director

Hawaii

5789 **Hawaii Lupus Foundation**
1200 College Walk   808-538-1522
Honolulu, HI 96817   800-201-1522
Chapter of the Lupus Foundation of America.

Illinois

5790 **Lupus Foundation of America: Illinois Chapter**
525 W. Monroe Street   312-542-0002
Chicago, IL 60661   800-258-7872
                                         Fax: 312-255-8020
                                         e-mail: charles@lupusil.org
                           www.lupus.org/webmodules/webarticlesnet/
Offers support to individuals and families affected by Lupus, and looks to improve the diagnosis of and treatment of Lupus.
Charles Brummell, President & CEO
Mary Dollear, Vice-President

Indiana

5791 **Lupus Foundation of America: Northeast Indiana Chapter**
5401 Keystone Drive   219-482-8205
Fort Wayne, IN 46825
Largent, Director

5792 **Lupus Foundation of America: Northwest Indiana Lupus Chapter**
PO Box 2763   219-762-6575
Portage, IN 46368   800-948-8806
                                         e-mail: lupusnwichapter@aol.com
                                         www.lupusnwichapter.org
Tammie

5793 **Lupus Foundation of Indiana**
9302 N. Meridian Street   317-225-4400
Indianapolis, IN 46260   800-948-8806
                                         e-mail: info@lupusindiana.org
                           www.lupus.org/webmodules/webarticlesnet/
Chapter of the Lupus Foundation of America.
Matthew Johnson, Chair
Jan Ferris, Chief Executive Officer

Iowa

5794 Lupus Foundation of America: Iowa Chapter
3839 Merle Hay Road   515-279-3048
Des Moines, IA 50310-1044   888-279-3048
e-mail: info@lupusia.org
www.lupus.org/webmodules/webarticlesnet/
Barb Logue, President
Marilyn Rumsey, Treasurer

Kansas

5795 Lupus Foundation of America: Heartland Chapter
PO Box 12204   316-262-6180
Wichita, KS 67277   e-mail: ruth@lupus.org
www.lupus.org/webmodules/webarticlesnet/
Ruth Busch, Board Chair
Sandy Blaylock, Recording Secretary

Kentucky

5796 Lupus Foundation of Kentuckiana
4004 Hillsboro Pike   615-298-2273
Nashville, TN 37215   877-865-8787
Fax: 615-292-0520
e-mail: info@lupusmidsouth.org
www.lupus.org/webmodules/webarticlesnet/
Chapter of the Lupus Foundation of America.
Tanisha Hall, Chair
Mike Singer, President & CEO

Louisiana

5797 Louisiana Lupus Foundation
7732 Goodwood Boulevard   225-927-8052
Baton Rouge, LA 70806   800-355-7473
www.louisianalupusfoundation.org/
Chapter of the Lupus Foundation of America.
Linda B Perkins, President
Carolyn M Bajoie, Board Member

Maine

5798 Lupus Group of Maine
PO Box 8168
Portland, ME 04104   207-878-8104
www.milupus.org/northeast.htm
Chapter of the Lupus Foundation of America.
Watson, Executive Director
Jessica Gilbart, Health Education Coordinator

Maryland

5799 Lupus Foundation of America: DC, Maryland and Central & Northern Virginia
2000 L Street NW   202-787-5380
Washington, DC 20036   888-787-5380
Fax: 202-787-5399
e-mail: info@lupusgw.org
www.lupus.org/webmodules/webarticlesnet/
Chapter of the Lupus Foundation of America.
Marguerete A Luter, Chair
Jessica Gilbart, President & CEO

Massachusetts

5800 Lupus Foundation of America: Massachusetts Chapter
425 Watertown Street   617-332-9014
Newton, MA 02158   e-mail: info@lupusne.org
www.lupusmass.org

Michigan

5801 Lupus Foundation of America: Michigan Lupus Foundation
26507 Harper Avenue   586-775-8310
Saint Clair Shores, MI 48081   800-705-6677
Fax: 586-775-8494
e-mail: info@milupus.org
www.milupus.org
Judith A Sova, President
Frank Mortl, III, Executive Director

Minnesota

5802 Lupus Foundation of America: Minnesota Chapter
2626 E 82nd Street   952-746-5151
Bloomington, MN 55425   800-645-1131
Fax: 942-746-5155
e-mail: info@lupusmn.org
www.lupusmn.org
Scott Brown, Chair
Jennifer Monroe, President

Mississippi

5803 Lupus Foundation of America: Mississippi Chapter
PO Box 24292   601-366-5655
Jackson, MS 39225-4292   800-866-9606
www.milupus.org/southeast.htm

Missouri

5804 Lupus Foundation of America: Kansas City
4640 Shenandoah Avenue
St Louis, MO 63110   800-958-7876
e-mail: info@LFAheartland.org
www.lupus.org/webmodules/webarticlesnet/
Kevin Cheung, Chair of the Board
Amy Ondr, President & CEO

5805 Lupus Foundation of America: Ozarks Chapter
3150 W Marty Street
Springfield, MO 65807   417-887-1560
www.lupus.org

Montana

5806 Lupus Foundation of America: Montana Chapter
29 1/2 Alderson
Billings, MT 59102   406-254-2082
www.lupus.org

Nebraska

5807 Lupus Foundation of America: Omaha Chapter
Community Health Plaza
7101 Newport Avenue
Omaha, NE 68152   402-572-3150
www.milupus.org/midwest.htm

5808 Lupus Foundation of America: Western Nebraska Chapter
HCR 72 Box 58   308-764-2474
Sutherland, NE 69165

New Hampshire

5809 New Hampshire Lupus Foundation
PO Box 444
Nashua, NH 03061-0444   603-424-0111
www.milupus.org
Chapter of the Lupus Foundation of America.
Beck-Clemens, Interim President and CEO
Adam Gold, Development Associate

New Jersey

5810 Lupus Foundation of America: New Jersey Chapter
150 Morris Avenue, Suite 102 973-379-3226
Springfield, NJ 07081 800-322-5816
Fax: 973-379-1053
e-mail: info@lupusnj.org
www.lupus.org/webmodules/webarticlesnet/
Ranit C Shriky, Chairman
Leonard J Andriuzzi, President & CEO

5811 Lupus Foundation of America: South Jersey Chapter
One Greentree Center 856-988-5444
Marlton, NJ 08053 Fax: 856-596-8359
e-mail: lupusinfo@sjlupus.org
www.sjlupus.org

New Mexico

5812 Lupus Foundation of America: New Mexico Chapter
PO Box 9125 505-999-1981
Albuquerque, NM 87119 800-843-9081
e-mail: info@lupusnm.org
www.lupus.org/webmodules/webarticlesnet/
Quinn, Executive Director
Nancy Beder, Director of Resources

New York

5813 Lupus Alliance of America LIQ Affiliate
2255 Centre Avenue 516-783-3370
Bellmore, NY 11710 800-850-9000
Fax: 516-826-2058
e-mail: info@lupusliqueens.org
www.lupusliqueens.org
Carol Goldklang, President
Kate Anastasia, Executive Director

5814 Lupus Alliance of Upstate New York
3871 Harlem Road 716-835-7161
Cheektowaga, NY 14215 800-300-4198
Fax: 716-835-7251
e-mail: info@lupusupstateny.org
www.lupusupstateny.org
Lynn Szubinski, President
Honi Kurzeja, Executive Director

5815 Lupus Foundation of America: Bronx Chapter
PO Box 1117
Bronx, NY 10462 718-822-6542
www.milupus.org/northeast.htm

5816 Lupus Foundation of America: Central New York Chapter
Pickard Office Building
5858 E Molloy Road 315-454-9886
Syracuse, NY 13211 e-mail: cnylupus@dreamscape.com
www.milupus.org/northeast.htm
Aman, President/CEO
Bob Stewart, Chairperson

5817 Lupus Foundation of America: Genessee Valley Chapter
500 Helendale Road 585-288-2910
Rochester, NY 14609 Fax: 585-288-1608
e-mail: lupusgvc@frontiernet.net
www.lupusgvc.org
Eileen M Arntsen, President/CEO
James E Mitchell Jr, Vice President

5818 Lupus Foundation of America: Westchester
100 S Bedford Road 914-948-1032
Mt Kisco, NY 10549 888-57L-UPUS
e-mail: pguidice@stellarishealth.org
www.lupushudsonvalley.org

5819 Lupus Foundation of Mid and Northern New York
PO Box 139 315-829-4272
Utica, NY 13503-4303 866-258-7874
Fax: 315-829-4272
e-mail: lupusmidny@aol.com
www.nolupus.org
David L Arntsen, Chairman
Kathleen A Arntsen, President/CEO

5820 SLE Foundation
330 Seventh Avenue 212-685-4118
New York, NY 10001 800-74L-UPUS
Fax: 212-545-1843
e-mail: lupus@lupusny.org
www.lupusny.org
Chapter of the Lupus Foundation of America.
Bruce Cronstein, Chairman
Richard K DeScherer, President

North Carolina

5821 Lupus Foundation of America: Winston-Triad Lupus Chapter NCLF
2841 Foxwood Lane 910-768-1493
Winston Salem, NC 27103
Ruth John, President/CEO
Ginger Dickerson, Chairman of the Board

5822 Lupus Foundation of America: North Carolin a Chapter
4530 Park Road 704-716-5640
Charlotte, NC 28209 877-849-8271
Fax: 704-716-5641
e-mail: info@lupuslinks.org
www.lupus.org/webmodules/webarticlesnet/
Christine John-Fuller, President/CEO
Lorna Denton, Administrative Assistant

Ohio

5823 Lupus Foundation of America: Greater Ohio Chapter
12930 Chippewa Road 440-717-0183
Brecksville, OH 44141 888-665-8787
Fax: 440-717-0186
e-mail: suzanne@lupusgreaterohio.org
www.lupuscleveland.org
John Sheldon, Chairman
Suzanne Tierney, President & CEO

Oklahoma

5824 Oklahoma Lupus Association
4100 N Lincoln Boulevard 405-427-8787
Oklahoma City, OK 73105 Fax: 405-427-8778
e-mail: oklupus@flash.net
www.oklupus.com
Chapter of the Lupus Foundation of America.
Katherine

Pennsylvania

5825 Lupus Foundation of America: Central Pennsylvania Chapter
Old Liberty Square
4813 Jonestown Road 717-671-9515
Harrisburg, PA 17109 800-800-5776
e-mail: hbginfo@lupuspa.org
www.lupuspa.org
Cheston M Berlin, Branch Council
Douglas C Berlin, Branch Council

5826 Lupus Foundation of America: Northeast Pennsylvania Chapter
615 Jefferson Avenue 570-558-2008
Scranton, PA 18510 800-800-5776
Fax: 570-558-2009
e-mail: neinfo@lupuspa.org
www.lupuspa.org
Marilyn Deutsch, PhD, Branch Council
Devon Fawcett, Branch Council

5827 **Lupus Foundation of America: Northwestern Pennsylvania Chapter**
PO Box 885
Erie, PA 16512-0885
724-962-0368
800-800-5776
Fax: 724-962-0368
e-mail: erieinfo@lupuspa.org
www.lupuspa.org

Jane Lippinc Myarick, CEO

5828 **Lupus Foundation of America: Western Pennsylvania Chapter**
Landmarks Building
100 West Station Square Drive
Pittsburgh, PA 15219
412-261-5886
800-800-5776
Fax: 412-261-5365
e-mail: info@lupuspa.org
www.lupuspa.org

Deborah Nigro, Executive Director
Shelly Tonti, Branch Director

5829 **Lupus Foundation of Philadelphia**
500 Old York Road
Jenkintown, PA 19046
215-517-5070
866-517-5070
Fax: 215-517-8483
e-mail: info@lupustristate.org
www.lupus.org/webmodules/webarticlesnet/
Chapter of the Lupus Foundation of America.
Debra L Riegel Jepson, Chair
Annette Myarick, CEO

Rhode Island

5830 **Lupus Foundation of America: Rhode Island Chapter**
#8 Fallon Avenue
Providence, RI 02908
401-421-7227
www.milupus.org

South Carolina

5831 **Lupus Foundation of America: South Carolina Chapter**
L.E. Support Club
8039 Nova Court
Charleston, SC 29420-8934
843-764-1769
e-mail: hmeisic@awod.com
www.galaxymall.com/commerce/lupus

Nelson, Executive Director

Tennessee

5832 **Lupus Foundation of America Memphis Area Chapter**
3181 Poplar Avenue
Memphis, TN 38111
901-458-5302
888-915-8787
Fax: 901-217-3193
e-mail: info@memphislupus.org
www.lupus.org/webmodules/webarticlesnet/
To educate and support those affected by lupus and to assist in finsing its cure. The goal is to unite and provide moral support and group strength for those individuals who are suspected of or diagnosed victims of Systemic Lupus Erythematosus and related disorders.
Yvonne D

5833 **Lupus Foundation of America: East Tennessee Chapter**
5612 Kingston Pike
Knoxville, TN 37919
615-584-5215
e-mail: lupustn@aol.com
www.lupus.org/chapters/southeastern.html

Hammond, Executive Director
Renee Levay Stewart, President

5834 **Lupus Foundation of America: Mid-South Area Chapter**
4004 Hillsboro Pike
Nashville, TN 37215
615-298-2273
877-865-8787
Fax: 615-292-0520
e-mail: info@lupusmidsouth.org
www.lupus.org/webmodules/webarticlesnet/

Tanisha Hall, Chair
Mike Singer, President & CEO

Texas

5835 **Lupus Foundation of America: North Texas Chapter**
15660 North Dallas Parkway
Dallas, TX 75248
469-374-0590
866-205-2369
Fax: 469-374-0794
e-mail: tessie@lupus-northtexas.org
www.lupus.org/webmodules/webarticlesnet/

Saundra Finley, Chair
Tessie Holloway, President & CEO

5836 **Lupus Foundation of America: South Central Texas Chapter**
9330 Corporate Drive
Selma, TX 78154
210-651-9480
866-205-2369
e-mail: salupus@texas.net
www.lupus.org/webmodules/webarticlesnet/

Sylvia Arcos, Chair
Amy Humphrey, Treasurer

5837 **Lupus Foundation of America: Texas Gulf Coast Chapter**
3701 Kirby Drive
Houston, TX 77098
713-529-0126
800-458-7870
Fax: 713-529-0780
e-mail: info@lupustexas.org
www.lupus.org/webmodules/webarticlesnet/

Tamara Atkins, Chair
Rebecca Kramer, President & CEO

5838 **Lupus Foundation of America: West Texas Chapter**
1717 Avenue K
Lubbock, TX 79401
806-744-6666
800-580-5878
e-mail: lfawesttx@juno.com
www.milupus.org/southwest.htm

Reymond, Executive Director
Katie Fillnow, President

Utah

5839 **Lupus Foundation of America Utah Chapter**
352 S Denver Street
Salt Lake City, UT 84111
801-364-0366
800-657-6398
e-mail: info@utahlupus.org
www.lupus.org/webmodules/webarticlesnet/

Noelle Reymond, President & CEO
Annette Lee, Development Director

Vermont

5840 **Lupus Foundation of America: Vermont Chapter**
57 S Main Street
Waterbury, VT 05676
802-244-5988
877-735-8787
e-mail: lupusvermont@myfairpoint.net
www.lupus.org/webmodules/webarticlesnet/

Virginia

5841 **Lupus Foundation of America: Eastern Virginia Chapter**
Pembroke One
281 Independence Boulevard
Virginia Beach, VA 23462
757-490-2793
www.lupus.org/webmodules/webarticlesnet/

Fletcher, President
Sarah Guy, Executive Assistant

Washington

5842 **Lupus Foundation of America: Pacific Northwest Chapter**
800 5th Avenue
Seattle, WA 98104
877-774-2992
Fax: 206-546-8946
e-mail: info@lupuspnw.org
www.lupus.org/webmodules/webarticlesnet/

Kristi Thomsen, President
Celia Y Weisman, CEO

5843 **Lupus Foundation of America: Wisconsin Chapter**
1109 N Mayfair Road
Milwaukee, WI 53226

414-443-6400
866-LUP-USWI
Fax: 414-443-6400
e-mail: lupuswi@lupuswi.org
www.lupus.org/webmodules/webarticlesnet/
Mary E Cronin, MD, Chairperson
Dawn T Thomas-Semanko, Executive Director

Foundations

5844 **SLE Lupus Foundation**
330 Seventh Avenue
New York, NY 10001

212-685-4118
800-74L-UPUS
Fax: 212-545-1843
e-mail: lupus@lupusny.org
www.lupusny.org

The Foundation helps people with lupus, as well as their families and friends, cope with the anxieties and frustrations that often accompany daily living with a chronic illness. Sharing information and networking among patients and their families further helps dispel myths and provides daily support to those learning to live with lupus.
Bruce Cronstein, MD, Chairman
Richard K DeScherer, President

Research Centers

5845 **Alliance for Lupus Research**
28 W 44th Street
New York, NY 10036

212-218-2840
800-867-1743
e-mail: info@lupusresearch.org
www.lupusresearch.org

Research foundation dedicated to providing information about lupus.
Robert Wood Johnson IV, Chairman
Ira Akselrad, Director

5846 **Hahnemann University Lupus Study Center Hahnemann University Medical Center**
Hahnemann University Medical Center
Broad and Vine Street
Philadelphia, PA 19102

215-762-7000
866-884-4HUH
Fax: 215-762-8109
www.hahnemannhospital.com

Raphael J Gotthelf, President

5847 **Terri Gotthelf Lupus Research Institute**
3 Duke Place
S Norwalk, CT 06854

800-828-87
Fax: 203-852-9720

Founded to help millions of lupus victims in the world and to encourage coordinate and direct future progress in the etiology diagnosis and treatment of this disease.
Theodore

Support Groups & Hotlines

5848 **National Health Information Center**
PO Box 1133
Washington, DC 20013

310-565-4167
800-336-4797
Fax: 301-984-4256
e-mail: info@nhic.org
www.health.gov/nhic

Offers a nationwide information referral service, produces directories and resource guides.

Books

5849 **Coping with Lupus**
Lupus Foundation of America
1300 Piccard Drive
Rockville, MD 20850-4303

301-670-9292
800-558-0121
www.lupus.org

A practicing psychologist offers sound, meaningful and compassionate advice to individuals who must deal with lupus.
276 pages Paperback
ISBN: 0-895294-75-3

5850 **Disability Workbook for Social Security Disability Applicants**
Lupus Foundation of America
1300 Piccard Drive
Rockville, MD 20850-4303

301-670-9292
800-558-0121
www.lupus.org

Helps people get their disability benefits promptly, without unnecessary appeals. Tells what you have to prove and how to prove it.
137 pages

5851 **Get to Sleep! How to Sleep Well...Despite Lupus**
Lupus Foundation of America
1300 Piccard Drive
Rockville, MD 20850-4303

301-670-9292
800-558-0121

Written in a simple, straightforward style, this easy-to-follow action guide teaches you the most effective strategies for enabling you to get the sleep you want and need!
17 pages

5852 **Lupus Book**
Lupus Foundation of America
1300 Piccard Drive
Rockville, MD 20850-4303

301-670-9292
800-558-0121

Packed with useful, easy-to-understand information and practical guidance for people with lupus, their family members, friends and physicians. This hardcover book explains virtually every aspect of the disease and will help people better manage their day-to-day fight with lupus.

ISBN: 0-195084-43-8

5853 **Lupus Erythematosus: A Handbook for Physicians, Patients & Families**
Lupus Foundation of America
1300 Piccard Drive
Rockville, MD 20850-4303

301-670-9292
800-558-0121
www.lupus.org

Written for physicians, people with lupus, their families and friends, this is LFA's most popular publication. The handbook provides a brief, but detailed, overview of the disease and guide for living well with lupus.
60 pages

5854 **Lupus: Everything You Need to Know**
Lupus Foundation of America
1300 Piccard Drive
Rockville, MD 20850-4303

301-670-9292
800-558-0121
e-mail: lupusinfo@aol.com
www.lupus.org

Resource written for patients that want to learn more about lupus than what their doctors may or may not tell them.
236 pages

5855 **Sick and Tired of Feeling Sick and Tired**
Lupus Foundation of America
1300 Piccard Drive
Rockville, MD 20850-4303

301-670-9292
800-558-0121
www.lupus.org

Written in simple terms, the authors offer all readers- people with invisible chronic illness (ICI's), spouses, friends, family members, employers or health care providers, both understanding and practical guidance. This is a very useful resource for all those who live with ICI's and those who care for and about them.
288 pages

5856 **We Are Not Alone: Learning to Live with Chronic Illness**
Lupus Foundation of America
1300 Piccard Drive
Rockville, MD 20850-4303

301-670-9292
800-558-0121
www.lupus.org

Complete and comprehensive, this book is about redesigning your life... about how to live better, not just differently.
335 pages

Children's Books

5857 **Embracing the Wolf: A Lupus Victim and Her Family Learn to Live**
Cherokee Publishing Company
PO Box 1730   770-438-7366
Marietta, GA 30061-1730   800-653-3952
This book gives a very detailed account of the effects of the disease that include emotions and moods for the victim and the way in which these attributes affect loved ones.
192 pages Hardcover
ISBN: 0-877971-66-8
Kenneth W Boyd, Publisher

5858 **In Search of the Sun: A Woman's Courageous Victory Over Lupus**
Scribner
866 3rd Avenue   212-702-2000
New York, NY 10022-6221   800-257-5755
This book is a revision of Henrietta Aladjem's book, The Sun Is My Enemy. In this book, with Peter Schur she discusses her fight with this deadly and widespread disease.
Grades 10-12

5859 **When Mom Gets Sick**
Lupus Foundation of America
1300 Piccard Drive   301-670-9292
Rockville, MD 20850-4303   800-558-0121
                                               www.lupus.org
Written and illustrated by a 9-year-old, this is a compelling story based on the experiences of a sensitive and insightful young girl who makes the best from what could be a devastating situation.
27 pages

Newsletters

5860 **Heliogram**
Lupus Network
230 Ranch Drive   203-372-5795
Bridgeport, CT 06606-1747
Includes book reviews, medical abstracts and resource listings of physicians.
Quarterly
ISBN: 0-887168-0 -
Linda Rosinsky, Editor

5861 **Informer**
Simon Foundation
PO Box 815   847-864-3913
Wilmette, IL 60091-0815   Fax: 847-864-9758
Offers information and the latest updates concerning incontinence treatments, cures, medical aspects, resources and more.
Quarterly

5862 **Lupus Foundation of America Memphis Area Chapter Newsletter**
Lupus Foundation of America Memphis Area Chapter
3181 Poplar Avenue   901-458-5320
Memphis, TN 38111   888-915-8787
                                               Fax: 901-217-3193
                                       e-mail: info@memphislupus.org
                                               memphislupus.org
Monthly
Yvonne D Nelson, Executive Director

5863 **Lupus Informer**
Lupus Foundation of America: Arkansas Chapter
220 Mockingbird   501-525-9380
Hot Springs, AR 71913   800-294-8878
                                               Fax: 501-525-9380
                                 e-mail: lupusarkhs@direclynx.net
                                       www.lupus-arkansas.com
Lupus Chapter membership dues annually
Jamesetta Smith, President/CEO

5864 **Lupus News**
Lupus Foundation of America

1300 Piccard Drive   301-670-9292
Rockville, MD 20850-4303   800-558-0121
Provides detailed news for physicians, patients, their families and friends on lupus.
Quarterly

5865 **Pennsylvania Lupus News**
Lupus Foundation of Pennsylvania
Landmarks Building   412-261-5886
Pittsburgh, PA 15219   Fax: 412-261-5365
                                       e-mail: info@lupuspa.org
                                               www.lupuspa.org
Deborah Nigro, Executive Director
Marian Belotti RN, Patient Services Director

5866 **The Loop**
SLE Lupus Foundation
330 Seventh Avenue   212-685-4118
New York, NY 10001   Fax: 212-545-1843
                                       e-mail: lupus@lupusny.org
                                               www.lupusny.org
Richard K DeScherer, President
Margaret G Dowd, Executive Director

Pamphlets

5867 **Control Your Pain!**
Lupus Foundation of America
1300 Piccard Drive   301-670-9292
Rockville, MD 20850-4303   800-558-0121
                                               www.lupus.org
This easy to read booklet offers 144 concrete strategies for reducing and managing the pain of lupus.
48 pages

5868 **Facts About Lupus**
Lupus Foundation of America
1300 Piccard Drive   301-670-9292
Rockville, MD 20850-4303   800-558-0121
A series of brochures on a wide range of lupus-related topics including lab tests, medications, joint and muscle involvement, skin involvement, lupus and the kidneys, central nervous system involvement, lupus in men, pregnancy, well/coping, etc.
21 Brochures

5869 **Handout on Health: Systemic Lupus Erythematosus**
NAMSIC/National Institutes of Health
1 AMS Circle   301-495-4484
Bethesda, MD 20892-0001   877-226-4267
                                               Fax: 301-718-6366
                                               TTY: 301-565-2966
                                   e-mail: niamsinfo@mail.nih.gov
                                               www.nih.gov/niams

5870 **Living Well, Despite Lupus!**
Lupus Foundation of America
1300 Piccard Drive   301-670-9292
Rockville, MD 20850   800-558-0121
This booklet offers 204 sure-fire strategies for taking charge of your life to enable you to live well.
1996 50 pages
ISBN: 0-895294-75-3

5871 **Lupus Eritematoso (Spanish Booklet)**
Lupus Foundation of America
1300 Piccard Drive   301-670-9292
Rockville, MD 20850-4303   800-558-0121
                                               www.lupus.org
Written for physicians, people with lupus, their families and friends, this is LFA's most popular publication. The handbook provides a brief, but detailed, overview of the disease and guide for living well with lupus.

5872 **Lupus Erythematosus**
Lupus Foundation of America
1300 Piccard Drive   301-670-9292
Rockville, MD 20850-4303   800-558-0121
                                               www.lupus.org/lupus

This booklet is intended to help patients understand what lupus is, how it may affect their lives and what they can do to help themselves and their physician in the management of the illness.

5873 Lupus Information Package
NAMSIC/National Institutes of Health
1 AMS Circle   301-495-4484
Bethesda, MD 20892-0001   877-226-4267
                                                         Fax: 301-718-6366
                                                         TTY: 301-565-2966
                                            e-mail: niamsinfo@mail.nih.gov
                                                         www.nih.gov/niams

5874 Many Shades of Lupus: Information for Multicultural Communities
NAMSIC/National Institutes of Health
1 AMS Circle   301-495-4484
Bethesda, MD 20892-0001   877-226-4267
                                                         Fax: 301-587-4352
                                                         TTY: 301-565-2966
                                            e-mail: niamsinfo@mail.nih.gov
                                                         www.nih.gov/niams

Audio & Video

5875 For Life: More Stories of Lupus
Marcia Urbin Raymond, author

Fanlight Productions
4196 Washington Street   617-469-4999
Boston, MA 02131   800-937-4113
                                                         Fax: 617-469-3349
                                            e-mail: fanlight@fanlight.com
                                                         www.fanlight.com
Three years after 'Stories of Lupus', the filmmaker revisits five people from the earlier film, to explore the day-to-day challenges and gifts that come to people living with a chronic illness as it evolves over time.
2002 53 Minutes
ISBN: 1-572954-17-5
Nicole Johnson, Publicity Coordinator

5876 Stories of Lupus
Fanlight Productions
4196 Washington Street   617-469-4999
Boston, MA 02131   800-937-4113
                                                         Fax: 617-469-3379
                                            e-mail: fanlight@fanlight.com
                                                         www.fanlight.com
Recently diagnosed with lupus, the filmmakers go on the road to interview others enduring the precarious roller coaster of symptoms, treatment, flare-ups and recoveries which characterize this complex, mysterious, and often life-threatening disease.
1999 27 Minutes
ISBN: 1-572954-16-7
Nicole Johnson, Publicity Coordinator

Web Sites

5877 Healing Well
                                                         www.healingwell.com
An online health resource guide to medical news, chat, information and articles, newsgroups and message boards, books, disease-related web sites, medical directories, and more for patients, friends, and family coping with disabling diseases, disorders, or chronic illnesses.

5878 Health Finder
                                                         www.healthfinder.gov
Searchable, carefully developed web site offering information on over 1000 topics. Developed by the US Department of Health and Human Services, the site can be used in both English and Spanish.

5879 Healthlink USA
                                                         www.healthlinkusa.com
Health information concerning treatment, cures, prevention, diagnosis, risk factors, research, support groups, email lists, personal stories and much more. Updated regularly.

5880 Helios Health
                                                         www.helioshealth.com
Online resource for your health information. Detailed information about specific health topics, access to expert advice from our Medical Advisory Board, and up-to-date health news.

5881 Lupus Foundation of America
                                                         www.lupus.org
The LFA mission is to assist local chapters in their efforts to provide supportive services to individuals living with lupus, educate the public about lupus, and supports research into the cause and cure of lupus.

5882 MedicineNet
                                                         www.medicinenet.com
An online resource for consumers providing easy-to-read, authoritative medical and health information.

5883 Medscape
                                                         www.medscape.com
Medscape offers specialists, primary care physicians, and other health professionals the Web's most robust and integrated medical information and educational tools.

5884 WebMD
                                                         www.webmd.com
Information on Lupus Erythematosus, including articles and resources.

Description

5885 Mental Illness/General

Mental illness includes disorders of mood, thinking and behavior, with psychiatry being the branch of medicine responsible for their study, diagnosis, treatment, and prevention. Mental illness may be determined by genetic, physical, chemical, psychological, and social factors. Mental or emotional illness includes such conditions as major depression, schizophrenia, bipolar disorder (i.e., manic depression), panic and other anxiety disorders, substance abuse and dependence, and dementia and other cognitive disorders.

Psychiatric diagnoses generally are based on criteria outlined in *Diagnostic and Statistical Manual of Mental Disorders* (DSM-5), published by the American Psychiatric Association. Depending on the specific diagnosis, treatment can include medication, counseling, behavior modification, psychotherapy, and modification of the patient's environment. See also *Mental Illness/Depression* and *Mental Illness/Schizophrenia*.

National Agencies & Associations

5886 Action Autonomie
3958 Rue Dandurand
Montreal, Quebec, H1X 1-2H2   Fax: 514-525-5580
514-525-5060
e-mail: lecollectif@actionautonomie.qc.ca
www.actionautonomie.qc.ca
Community organization set up by people living or having lived with mental health problems who believed in the necessity of uniting their efforts collectively in order to defend their rights.
Hendren, President

5887 American Academy of Child & Adolescent Psychiatry
3615 Wisconsin Avenue NW   202-966-7300
Washington, DC 20016   Fax: 202-966-2891
e-mail: communications@aacap.org
www.aacap.org
A professional organization that represents 7 500 child and adolescent psychiatrists that actively research diagnose and treat psychiatric and mental illness disorders in children and adolescents.
Martin J Drell, MD, President
Kristin Kroeger Ptakowski, Director & Sr. Deputy Executive Director

5888 American Association of Children's Residential Centers
11700 W Lake Park Drive   877-332-2272
Milwaukee, WI 53224   Fax: 877-36A-ACRC
e-mail: info@aacrc-dc.org
www.aacrc-dc.org
Brings professionals together to advance the frontiers of knowledge pertaining to the spectrum of therapeutic living environments for adolescents with behavioral health disorders.
Christopher Bellonci, M.D., President
Kari Sisson, Director

5889 American Association on Intellectual and D evelopmental Disabilities
501 3rd Street NW   202-387-1968
Washington, DC 20001-1512   800-424-3688
Fax: 202-387-2193
e-mail: mnygren@aaidd.org
www.aamr.org
Promotes progressive policies sound research effective practices and universal human rights for people with intellectual and developmental disabilities.
Marc J Tasse, PhD, President
Margaret A Nygren, EdD, Executive Director & CEO

5890 American Psychiatric Association
1000 Wilson Boulevard   703-907-7300
Arlington, VA 22209-3901   888-357-7924
e-mail: apa@psych.org
www.psych.org
Works to promote the best interest of patients and those actually or potentially making use of psychiatric services.
Bray, President

5891 American Psychological Association
750 1st Street NE   202-336-5500
Washington, DC 20002-4242   800-374-2721
TTY: 202-336-6123
TDD: 202-336-6123
e-mail: practice@apa.org
www.apa.org
A scientific and professional organization the represents psychology in the United States. The largest association of psychologists worldwide.
Donald N Bersoff, PhD, JD, President
Norman B Anderson, PhD, Chief Executive Officer and Executive Vi

5892 Calgary Association of Self Help
1019-7th Avenue SW   403-266-8711
Calgary, Alberta, T2P 1-1A8   Fax: 403-266-2478
e-mail: info@calgaryselfhelp.com
www.calgaryselfhelp.com
Calgary Association of Self Help have been assisting people with a mental illness to live full lives within our community since 1973.
Samuel Peter Mckenzie, Chairperson
Marian McGrath, Chief Executive Officer

5893 Canadian Federation of Mental Health Nurse s
1 Concorde Gate   416-426-7029
Toronto, Ontario, M3C 3-3C6   Fax: 416-426-7280
e-mail: info@cfmhn.ca
www.cfmhn.ca
A national voice for psychiatric and mental health (PMH) nursing.
Lorelei Faulkner-Gibson, President
Joanna Lynch, Director of Communication

5894 Canadian Mental Health Association
1110-151 Slater Street   416-484-7750
Ottawa, Ontario, K1P 5-1Z8   Fax: 613-745-5522
e-mail: info@cmha.ca
www.cmha.ca
Promotes the mental health of all and supports the resilience and recovery of people experiencing mental illness.
David Copus, Chair
Peter Coleridge, Chief Executive Officer

5895 Center for Mental Health Services: Knowledge Exchange Network
PO Box 42557
Washington, DC 20015   800-789-2647
Fax: 240-221-4295
TTY: 866-889-2647
TDD: 866-889-2647
e-mail: ken@mentalhealth.org
www.mentalhealth.org
Goal is to provide the treatment and support services needed by adults with mental disorders and children with serious emotional problems.
A Kathryn PsyD, Past President
Donna Colonna, Vice President

5896 Community Access
2 Washington Street   212-780-1400
New York, NY 10004   Fax: 212-780-1412
e-mail: info@communityaccess.org
www.cairn.org
A nonprofit agency providing housing and advocacy for people with psychiatric disabilities.
Stephen H Chase, President
Steve Coe, Chief Executive Officer

5897 **Federation of Families for Children's Mental Health**
9605 Medical Center Drive 240-403-1901
Rockville, MD 20850 Fax: 240-403-1909
e-mail: ffcmh@ffchm.org
www.ffcmh.org
Provides leadership to develop and sustain a nationwide network
of family-run organizations.
Teka Dempson, President
Sandra Spencer, Executive Director

5898 **Mental Health America**
2000 N Beauregard Street 703-684-7722
Alexandria, VA 22311 800-969-6642
Fax: 703-684-5968
TTY: 800-433-5959
e-mail: info@mentalhealthamerica.net
www.mentalhealthamerica.net
Mental Health America (formerly National Mental Health Association) is dedicated to helping all people live mentally healthier
lives. With our more than 320 affiliates nationwide, we represent a
growing movement of Americans who promote mental health.
340+ Members
Ann Boughtin, Chair of the Board
Eric Ashton, Vice-Chair

5899 **Mental Health America Resource Center**
2000 North Beauregard Street 703-684-7722
Alexandria, VA 22311 800-969-6642
Fax: 703-684-5968
TTY: 800-433-5959
e-mail: info@mentalhealthamerica.net
www.mentalhealthamerica.net
The NMHA publishes pamphlets and booklets on many aspects of
mental health and mental illnesses. Topics include children and
families, recovery, doctor/patient communication, mental health
policy, culturally competent services, teen suicide, coping,
schizphrenia, stress, depression and many others.
340+ Members
Ann Boughtin, Chair of the Board
Eric Ashton, Vice-Chair

5900 **National Alliance for Hispanic Health**
1501 16th Street NW 202-387-5000
Washington, DC 20036 Fax: 202-797-4353
e-mail: alliance@hispanichealth.org
www.hispanichealth.org
Members are Spanish-speaking mental health professionals and
patients and those interested in the special emotional needs of
Hispanics.
Augustine C Baca, Chairperson
Jane L Delgado, PhD, President & CEO

5901 **National Alliance for the Mentally Ill**
Colonial Place Three
3803 N. Fairfax Drive 703-524-7600
Arlington, VA 22203-3042 800-950-6264
Fax: 703-524-9094
TDD: 703-516-7227
e-mail: bbc@naimi.org
www.nami.org
The leading self-help organization for families and friends of those
suffering from serious mental illnesses and those persons themselves. Over 900 affiliate groups nationwide offer support to members, advocate better lives for their loved ones, support research
efforts and educate the public to reduce the stigma attached to
serious mental illnesses.
Keris Jan Myrick, President
Jim Payne, Vice President

5902 **National Association of State Mental Health Program Directors**
66 Canal Center Plaza 703-739-9333
Alexandria, VA 22314 Fax: 703-548-9517
e-mail: webmaster@nasmhpd.org
www.nasmhpd.org
Offers referrals to state mental health programs services and physicians for persons with mental illness.
Robert W Glover, PhD, Executive Director
Shina Animasahun, Network Manager

5903 **National Association of Therapeutic Wilderness Camps**
437 William Avenue Suite 5
Davis, WV 26260 e-mail: natwc@gcol.net
www.natwc
Represents nearly fifty therapeutic wilderness camps located all
over the US. We believe therapeutic wilderness camps represent
the most effective method to help troubled young people change
the way they deal with their parents, school and other authorities.
Rick MSW CSW, President/ CEO
Jeannie Campbell, Executive Vice President

5904 **National Council for Community Behavior Healthcare**
1701 K Street NW 202-684-7457
Washington, DC 20006 Fax: 301-881-7159
e-mail: lindar@thenationalcouncil.org
www.thenationalcouncil.org
Represents community mental health centers working on Capitol
Hill to ensure funding for community mental health services. Offers technical support and guidance and serves as a liaison with
state organizations and other mental health related organizations.
Linda Rosenb Delgado PhD, President
Adolph Falcon, Vice President for Science and Policy

5905 **National Institute of Mental Health**
6001 Executive Boulevard 301-443-4513
Bethesda, MD 20892-9663 866-615-6464
Fax: 301-443-4279
TTY: 301-443-8431
e-mail: nimhinfo@nih.gov
www.nimh.nih.gov
A federal agency that supports research nationwide on mental illness and mental health. The Institute provides research, demonstrations and technical assistance concerning the housing and
service needs of the homeless mentally ill population.
Thomas R Power MEd, Director
Edward B Searle, Deputy Director

5906 **National Mental Health Services Knowledge Exchange Network**
PO Box 42557
Washington, DC 20015 800-789-2647
Fax: 240-747-5470
TTY: 866-889-2647
TDD: 866-889-2647
e-mail: nmhic-info@samhsa.hhs.gov
www.mentalhealth.org
The National Mental Health Information Center was developed for
users of mental health services and their families, the general pub-
lic, policy makers, providers and the media.
A Kathryn Muise, President
Joan Edwards-Karmazyn, VP

5907 **Obsessive Compulsive Information Center Dean Foundation**
Dean Foundation
7617 Mineral Point Road 608-827-2470
Madison, WI 53717-1914 Fax: 608-827-2479
e-mail: mim@miminc.org
www.miminc.org
Provides access to published literature on obsessive compulsive
disorder certain obsessive compulsive spectrum disorders and
their treatments.

5908 **Option Istitute Learning and Training Center**
2080 S. Undermountain Road 413-229-2100
Sheffield, MA 01257 800-714-2779
Fax: 413-229-8931
e-mail: happiness@option.org
www.option.org
As the worldwide teaching center for the Option Process(R). The
Option Institute offers empowering personal growth programs and
seminars using life-changing experiential learning techniques that
help people overcome adversity, maximize their success and happiness and greatly improve their health, career, relationships and
quality of life.
Barry Neils Kaufman, Co-Founder/ Co-Director
Samahria Lyte Kaufman, Co-Founder/ Co-Director

5909 Texas Mining and Reclamation Association
100 Congress Avenue   512-236-2325
Austin, TX 78701   Fax: 512-236-2002
e-mail: information@tmra.com
www.tmra.com

Serves as a unified voice for mental health patients in consumer social and political affairs. Helps members to live outside a hospital setting by providing assistance in the areas of resocialization, employment and housing.
Greg Shurbet, Chair
Trey G Powers, Executive Director

5910 The Coalition of Behavioral Health Agencies
90 Broad Street   212-742-1600
New York, NY 10004   Fax: 212-742-2080
e-mail: kkrampitz@coalitionny.org
www.coalitionny.org

An umbrella advocacy organization of New York's mental health community representing over 100 non-profit community health agencies that serve more than 300 000 clients in the five boroughs of New York City and its environs.
Tino Hernandez, President
Phillip A Saperia, Chief Executive Officer

5911 World Federation for Mental Health
PO Box 807   703-494-6515
Occoquan, VA 22125   Fax: 703-490-6926
e-mail: info@wfmh.com
www.wfmh.com

WFMH is an international membership organization founded in 1948 to advance among all peoples and nations the prevention of mental and emotional disorders the proper treatment and care of those with such disorders and the promotion of mental health.
Deborah Wan, President
Helen Millar, Treasurer

State Agencies & Associations

Alabama

5912 National Alliance on Mental Illness of Alabama: NAMI Alabama
1401 I-85 Parkway   334-396-4797
Montgomery, AL 36106-1902   800-626-4199
Fax: 334-396-4794
e-mail: wlaird@namialabama.org
www.namialabama.org

Will O'Rear, President
Sue Guffey, 1st Vice President

Alaska

5913 National Alliance on Mental Illness of Alaska
144 W 15th Avenue   907-277-1300
Anchorage, AK 99501-5106   800-478-4462
Fax: 907-277-1400
e-mail: trishmcd@nami.org
www.nami.org/sites/alaska

Scott Owens, Co-President
Pat Dobbins, Co-President

Arizona

5914 Mentally Ill Kids In Distress
2642 E Thomas Road   602-253-1240
Phoenix, AZ 85016-2723   800-35M-IKID
Fax: 602-253-1250
e-mail: Phoenix@MIKID.org
www.mikid.org

Steve Carter, President
Vicki L Johnson, Executive Director

5915 National Alliance on Mental Illness of Arizona
5025 E. Washington Street   602-244-8166
Phoenix, AZ 85034-1604   Fax: 602-252-1349
e-mail: namiaz@namiaz.org
www.namiaz.org

Provides emotional support education and advocacy to persons of all ages who are affected by serious mental illnesses. Supports research to find a cure.
Robert McCabe

5916 Navaho Nation K'E Project: Tuba City Children & Families Advocacy Corp
PO Box 3937   520-283-5415
Tuba City, AZ 86045   Fax: 520-283-5413
Rueben Clark

5917 Navaho Nation K'E Project: Winslow Children & Families Advocacy Corp
HC 63 Box E   520-657-3234
Winslow, AZ 86047   Fax: 520-657-3207
Jayne

Arkansas

5918 Arkansas FFCMH Jane Burgan
Jane Burgan
PO Box 56667   501-374-7218
Little Rock, AR 72115-4023   Fax: 501-374-2711
e-mail: pammarshall7218@sbcglobal.net
www.affcmh.org/

Billie Denney, Board Member
James Wilson, Board Member

5919 NAMI Arkansas
1012 Autumn Road   501-661-1548
Little Rock, AR 72211-2222   800-844-0381
Fax: 501-312-7540
e-mail: nami-ar@namiarkansas.org
www.nami.org

Grassroots organization that focuses on improving mental health services. The mission is three prong: Support, Education, and Advocacy. Support Group meetings are held at 11 locations across the state.
Rick Scott, First Vice President
Karen H Henry, President

California

5920 NAMI California
1851 Heritage Lane   916-567-0163
Sacramento, CA 95815-3218   Fax: 916-567-1757
e-mail: nami.california@namicalifornia.org
www.namicalifornia.org

Dorothy Hendrickson, President
Jessica Cruz, Executive Director

5921 United Advocates for Children of California
2035 Hurley Way   916-643-1530
Sacramento, CA 95825   866-643-1530
Fax: 916-643-1592
e-mail: info@uacf4hope.org
www.uacf4hope.org

Carmen Diaz, President
Mary Jane Gross, Treasurer

Colorado

5922 Colorado FFCMH
2950 Tennyson Street   303-572-0302
Denver, CO 80212   888-569-7500
Fax: 303-433-1605
e-mail: tdillingham@coloradofederation.org
www.coloradofederation.org

5923 FFCMH: Denver/Aurora Chapter
12485 E 13th Avenue   303-343-1019
Aurora, CO 80011   Fax: 720-859-9367
e-mail: **ffcmhda@comcast.net

Carmen Mohr, President
Carol Reynolds, Executive Director

5924 National Alliance for the Mentally Ill of Colorado
2280 S Albion Street   303-321-3104
Denver, CO 80222-3334   888-566-6264
                                                    Fax: 303-321-0912
                            e-mail: admin@namicolorado.org
                                        www.namicolorado.org
The National Alliance for the Mentally Ill Of Colorado is a statewide, grassroots, nonprofit organization whose mission is; To give strength and hope to individuals with mental illness and their families.
Greg C Coleman, President
Scott Glaser, Executive Director

5925 No. Colorado FFCMH
2950 Tennyson Street   303-572-0302
Denver, CO 80212   888-569-7500
                                                    Fax: 303-433-1605
                                e-mail: thefeds@attbi.com
                                    www.coloradofederation.org
Meltz

Connecticut

5926 Families United For CMH, Inc.
PO Box 151   860-537-6125
New London, CT 06320   Fax: 860-537-6130
                                        www.familiesunited.org
Morgan Correll, President
Sheila King, Executive Director

5927 National Alliance for the Mentally Ill of Connecticut
576 Farmington Avenue   860-882-0236
Hartford, CT 06105   800-215-3021
                                                    Fax: 860-882-0240
                            e-mail: membership@namict.org
                                            www.namict.org
Kate Mattias, Executive Director

Delaware

5928 Alliance for the Mentally Ill in Delaware (AMID)
2400 W 4th Street   302-427-0787
Wilmington, DE 19805-3306   888-427-2643
                                                    Fax: 302-427-2075
                                e-mail: namide@namide.org
                                            www.namide.org
Mary Berger, President
John P Smoots, Treasurer

5929 Delaware FFMCH
19 Baltusrol Court   302-730-0325
Dover, DE 19904   866-994-0000
                                                    Fax: 302-730-8952
                                e-mail: marags1@aol.com
                                            www.ffcmh.org
Earline McArthur, Director Development/Communications

5930 Mental Health Association of Delaware
100 W 10th Street   302-654-6833
Wilmington, DE 19801   800-287-6423
                                                    Fax: 302-654-6838
                                e-mail: jlafferty@mhainde.org
                                            www.mhainde.org
Janet M Brown, President
James Lafferty, Executive Director

District of Columbia

5931 DC Threshold Alliance for the Mentally Ill
422 8th Street SE   202-546-0646
Washington, DC 20003-2832   Fax: 202-546-6817
                                e-mail: namidc@juno.com
                        www.nami.org/MSTemplate.cfm?MicrositeID=
Lois Fitzgerald, President
Mary J DiPietro, Secretary

5932 Family Advocacy and Support Association
PO Box 74884   202-234-2325
Washington, DC 20056   Fax: 202-576-7154
Lynne M Gladysz, Chair
R Lee Waits, President

Florida

5933 Florida Alliance for the Mentally Ill
1030 E. Lafayette Street   850-671-4445
Tallahassee, FL 32301-2646   877-626-4352
                                                    Fax: 850-671-5272
                            e-mail: Info@namiflorida.org
                                        www.namiflorida.org
James Sleeper, President
Judith Evans, Executive Director

5934 Florida FFCMH: Tampa Chapter
13301 Bruce B Downs Boulevard   813-974-7930
Tampa, FL 33612   Fax: 813-974-7712
                                e-mail: ffcmh@earthlink.net
                                    www.federationoffamilies.org
Linda M Gladysz, Chair
R Lee Waits, President/CEO

Georgia

5935 Georgia Alliance for the Mentally Ill
3050 Presidential Drive   770-234-0855
Atlanta, GA 30340-3916   800-728-1052
                                                    Fax: 770-234-0237
                            e-mail: namigeorgia@namiga.org
                                            www.namiga.org
Bill Kissel, President
Eric Spencer, Executive Director

Hawaii

5936 NAMI: The Local Affiliate of the National Alliance for the Mentally Ill
770 Kapiolani Boulevard   808-591-1297
Honolulu, HI 96813-2025   Fax: 808-591-2058
                            e-mail: info@namihawaii.org
                                            namihawaii.org
Members include consumers families health professionals and interested persons/organizations. Programs include advocacy support and education and are free and open to the public. Office has lending library of books and videos. Newsletter is published.
6 pages Quarterly
Carol Kozlovich, President
Kathleen Hasegawa, Executive Director

Idaho

5937 FFCMH: Idaho Chapter
704 North 7th Street   208-433-8845
Boise, ID 83702   800-905-3436
                                                    Fax: 208-433-8337
                            e-mail: info@idahofederation.org
                                        www.idahofederation.org
Stephen Graci, Executive Director
Cindy Shotton, Administrative Assistant

5938 Idaho Alliance for the Mentally Ill
4097 Bottle Bay Road   208-242-7430
Sagle, ID 83860-0068   800-572-9940
                                                    Fax: 208-673-6685
                            e-mail: namiidaho@yahoo.com
                        www.nami.org/MSTemplate.cfm?MicrositeID=
Douglas McKnight, President
Tom Hanson, Vice President

Illinois

5939 Illinois Alliance for the Mentally Ill
218 W Lawrence Avenue   217-522-1403
Springfield, IL 62704-2612   800-346-4572
                                    Fax: 217-522-3598
                            e-mail: namiil@sbcglobal.net
                                            il.nami.org

Hugh Brady, President
Brian Allen, Vice President

5940 Illinois Federation of Families
PO Box 413   847-265-0500
McHenry, IL 60051   800-871-8400
                                    Fax: 847-265-0501
                              e-mail: iffcmh@msn.com
                                        www.iffcmh.net

Cynthia Hamilton

Indiana

5941 FFCMH: Indiana Chapter
2205 Costello Drive   765-622-0601
Anderson, IN 46011   866-247-8547
                                    Fax: 765-622-0643
                      e-mail: indianafedfam@comcast.net
                          www.indianafamilies.org/page4.php

Brenda Hamilton

5942 Family Action Network
PO Box 322   765-643-4357
Winnetka, IN 60093-2206 e-mail: info@familyactionnetwork.net
                              www.familyactionnetwork.net

Susan Rooney, Co-Chair
Lonnie Stonitsch, Co-Chair

5943 NAMI Indiana
PO Box 22697   317-925-9399
Indianapolis, IN 46222-0697   800-677-6442
                                    Fax: 317-925-9398
                           e-mail: info@namiindiana.org
                                   www.namiindiana.org/
Grass roots advocacy support and educational group for families
affected by severe and persistent mental illnesses.
Joshua G Sprunger, Executive Director
Joanne Abbott, Program Director

Iowa

5944 FFCMH: Iowa Chapter
106 S Booth   319-462-2187
Anamosa, IA 52205   888-400-6302
                                    Fax: 319-462-6789
                              e-mail: help@iffcmh.org
                                        www.iffcmh.org

Lori Reynolds, Executive Director
Heidi Reynolds, Program Director

5945 NAMI Iowa: National Alliance on Mental Illness
5911 Meredith Drive   515-254-0417
Des Moines, IA 50322-1903   800-417-0417
                                    Fax: 515-254-1103
                           e-mail: info@namiiowa.com
                                      www.namiiowa.com

Dawn Adams

Kansas

5946 Keys for Networking: Kansas FFCMH
900 South Kansas Avenue   785-233-8732
Topeka, KS 66612   800-499-8732
                                    Fax: 785-235-8732
                              e-mail: jadams@keys.org
                                          www.keys.org

Mary Ellen Conlee, President
Greg Whittaker, Treasurer

5947 NAMI Kansas: Kansas' Voice on Mental Illness
610 SW 10th Ave   785-233-0755
Topeka, KS 66612-0675   800-539-2660
                                    Fax: 785-233-4804
                           e-mail: info@namikansas.org
                  www.nami.org/MSTemplate.cfm?Site=NAMI_Ka
John Brennan, President
Mr Richard D Cagan, Executive Director

Kentucky

5948 KY Partnership For Families and Children
207 Holmes Street   502-875-1320
Frankfort, KY 40601   800-369-0533
                                    Fax: 502-875-1399
                          e-mail: kpfc@kypartnership.org
                                   www.kypartnership.org

Carol W Cecil, Executive Director
Joy Varney, Associate Director

5949 Kentucky Alliance for the Mentally Ill
808 Monticello Street   606-451-6935
Somerset, KY 42501-1277   800-257-5081
                                    Fax: 606-677-4052
                             e-mail: namiky@nami.org
               www.nami.org/MSTemplate.cfm?micrositeID=
Wendy Morris, Chair
Bertha Diaz-Story, 1st Vice Chair

Louisiana

5950 Louisiana Alliance for the Mentally Ill
5534 Galeria Drive   225-291-6262
Baton Rouge, LA 70816-2398   800-437-0303
                                    Fax: 225-926-8773
                        e-mail: info@namilouisiana.org
                                 www.namilouisiana.org

Stephanie Boyd, President
Mitch Bergeron, Vice President

Maine

5951 Maine Alliance for the Mentally Ill
1 Bangor Street   207-622-5767
Augusta, ME 04330-4701   800-464-5767
                                    Fax: 207-621-8430
                            e-mail: info@namimaine.org
                                     www.namimaine.org

Valerie Gamache, President
Cathy Kidman, Interim Executive Director

5952 United Families for Children's Mental Health
PO Box 2107   207-622-3309
Augusta, ME 04338-2107   Fax: 207-622-1661
Pat Bellack, Executive Director
Dana Lefko

Maryland

5953 National Alliance for the Mentally Ill: Maryland
10630 Little Patuxent Parkway   410-884-8691
Columbia, MD 21044-4486   877-878-2371
                                    Fax: 410-884-8695
                              e-mail: amimd@aol.com
                                           md.nami.org

Chris Griffin, President
Kate Farinholt, Executive Director

5954 Parents Supporting Parents of MD
PO Box 30
Kensington, MD 20895-0030   800-498-5551
                     e-mail: Marge_Samels@umail.umd.edu

Marge Sagalyn, President
Toby Fisher, Director of Public Policy

Massachusetts

5955 Massachusetts Alliance for the Mentally Ill
400 W Cummings Park 781-938-4048
Woburn, MA 01801-6528 800-370-9085
Fax: 781-938-4069
e-mail: helpline@namimass.org
www.namimass.org

Lynda Cutrell, President
Laurie Martinelli, Executive Director

Michigan

5956 Association for Children's Mental Health
6017 W Street Joseph Highway 517-372-4016
Lansing, MI 48917 888-226-4543
Fax: 517-372-4032
e-mail: acmhjane@sbcglobal.net
www.acmh-mi.org

Jane Shank, Interim Executive Director
Mary Porter, Business Manager

5957 JIMHO Affiliated Centers (Justice in Mental Health Organization)
520 Cherry Street 517-371-2221
Lansing, MI 48933 800-831-8035
Fax: 517-371-5770
e-mail: brwellwood@aol.com
www.jimho.org

JIMHO advocates for the rights and dignity that all people suffering from mental or emotional illness deserve.
Huebl, President
Sharon Solomon, Executive Director

5958 Michigan Alliance for the Mentally Ill
921 N Washington Avenue 517-485-4049
Lansing, MI 48906-5137 800-331-4264
Fax: 517-485-2333
e-mail: namimichigan@acd.net
mi.nami.org

Hubert Lloyd, President
Sue Abderholden, Executive Director

Minnesota

5959 Minnesota Alliance for the Mentally Ill
800 Transfer Road 651-645-2948
Saint Paul, MN 55114-1146 888-NAM-IHEL
Fax: 651-645-7379
e-mail: namihelps@namimn.org
www.namihelps.org

Barb Lindberg, President
Sue Abderholden, Executive Director

5960 Minnesota Association for Children's Mental Health
165 Western Avenue 651-644-7333
Saint Paul, MN 55102 800-528-4511
Fax: 651-644-7391
e-mail: info@macmh.org
www.macmh.org

Joel V Oberstar, MD, President
Deborah Saxhaug, Executive Director

Mississippi

5961 Mississippi Alliance for the Mentally Ill
411 Briarwood Drive 601-899-9058
Jackson, MS 39206-3058 800-357-0388
Fax: 601-956-6380
e-mail: stateoffice@namims.org
www.namims.org/

Debbie Waller, President
Hank Rainer, Vice President

5962 Mississippi Families as Allies
5166 Keele Street 601-355-0915
Jackson, MS 39206 800-833-9671
Fax: 601-355-0919
e-mail: info@msfaacmh.org
www.msfaacmh.org

Joy Hogge, PhD, Executive Director
Cynthia Moore-Hardy, MS, Director of Respite Services

Missouri

5963 MO-SPAN
440 Rue Saint Francois 314-972-0600
Florissant, MO 63031 Fax: 314-972-0606
www.mo-span.org

Donna Dittrich, Executive Director
Tina VarVera, Administrative Assistant

5964 Missouri Coalition Alliance for the Mentally Ill
230 W Dunklin Street 573-634-7727
Jefferson City, MO 65101-3260 800-374-2138
Fax: 573-761-5636
e-mail: Keele@aol.com

Keele, Executive Director
Karren Jones, President

5965 NAMI of Missouri
1001 SW Boulevard 573-634-7727
Jefferson City, MO 65109-2501 800-374-2138
Fax: 573-761-5636
e-mail: namimosjf@yahoo.com
www.nami.org/MSTemplate.cfm?MicrositeID=

A nonprofit education adudcacy, referal and support organization serving people with mental illness and their families.
12 pages newsletter
Cinda Holloway, President and Chairman
Cindi Keele, Executive Director

Montana

5966 Family Support Network
1002 10th Street W 406-256-7783
Billings, MT 59102 877-376-4850
Fax: 406-256-9879
e-mail: info@mtfamilysupport.org
www.mtfamilysupport.org

Barbara Milhelish, President
Matt Kuntz, Executive Director

5967 Montana Alliance for the Mentally Ill Mihelish's Residence
Mihelish's Residence
616 Helena Avenue 406-443-7871
Helena, MT 59601-6946 888-280-6264
Fax: 406-862-6352
e-mail: info@namimt.org
www.namimt.org

Matt Kuntz, Executive Director
Carole Denton, President

Nebraska

5968 National Alliance for the Mentally Ill: Nebraska (NAMI)
415 South 25th Avenue 402-345-8101
Omaha, NE 68131-2986 877-463-6264
Fax: 402-346-4070
e-mail: nami.nebraska@nami.org
www.nami.org/sites/ne

NAMI is a nonprofit organization dedicated to providing support, education and advocacy to and for anyone whose life has been touched by a mental illness.
Tim Cuddigan, President
Steve Spelic, Vice President

Nevada

5969 Nevada Alliance for the Mentally Ill
2251 N Rampart Boulevard
Las Vegas, NV 89128
702-310-5764
Fax: 775-329-1618
e-mail: joetyler@sdi.net
www.nami-nevada.org

Joe Abate

New Hampshire

5970 Granite State FFCMH
940 Mammoth Road
Manchester, NH 03104
603-296-0692
e-mail: gsffcmh@aol.com
www.ffcmh.org

Kathleen Cohen, Executive Director
Win Saltmarsh, Development Director

5971 National Alliance for the Mentally Ill: New Hampshire
85 North State Street
Concord, NH 03301-4020
603-225-5359
800-242-6264
Fax: 603-228-8848
e-mail: info@naminh.org
www.naminh.org

Family support and advocacy for consumers and family members.
Michele Grennon, President
Ken Norton, Executive Director

New Jersey

5972 All Access Mental Health
Information
819 Alexander Road
Princeton, NJ 08540
609-452-2088
Fax: 609-452-0627
e-mail: info@aamh.org
www.aamh.org

This organization was founded to create a permanent community support system for mentally ill and developmentally disabled adults and their families living in the Greater Mercer County area of New Jersey.
Cynthia Murphy, President
Lauren Murphy, Vice-President

5973 Community Mental Health Foundation
610 Industrial Avenue
Paramus, NJ 07652
201-986-5070
Fax: 201-265-3543
e-mail: staff@cmhf.org
www.cmhf.org

Perrin, President
Sylvia Axelrod, Executive Director

5974 New Jersey Alliance for the Mentally Ill
1562 Route 130
N Brunswick, NJ 08902-3004
732-940-0991
Fax: 732-940-0355
e-mail: info@naminj.org
www.naminj.org

Mark Perrin, MD, President
Sylvia Axelrod, Executive Director

New Mexico

5975 Navaho Nation K'E Project Children and Families Advocacy Corp
PO Box 309
Tohatchi, NM 87325
505-733-2474
Fax: 505-733-2444
Vera Balwin

5976 Navajo Nation K'E Project: Shiprock Children & Families Advocacy Corp
PO Box 1240
Shiprock, NM 87420
505-368-4479
Fax: 505-368-5582
Evelyn Beckett, President
Elaine Jones, Executive Director

5977 New Mexico Alliance for the Mentally Ill
8015 Mountain Rd NE
Albuquerque, NM 87110-3086
505-260-0154
Fax: 505-260-0342
e-mail: naminm@aol.com
www.nami.org/MSTemplate.cfm?MicrositeID=
Patricia D Romero, President

New York

5978 Children's Mental Health Coalition of WNY, Inc.
814 Kenmore Avenue
Buffalo, NY 14216
716-871-8997
Fax: 716-871-8656
e-mail: mtskorupa@aol.com
www.raisingminds.org

Mary Pierce, Executive Director
Joan Cullen, Program Director/Family Specialist

5979 Families Together in New York State
737 Madison Avenue
Albany, NY 12209
518-432-0333
888-326-8644
Fax: 518-434-6478
e-mail: info@ftnys.org
www.ftnys.org

Vicky McCarthy, President
Paige Pierce, Executive Director

5980 New York Alliance for the Mentally Ill
99 Pine Street
Albany, NY 12207
518-462-2000
800-950-3228
Fax: 518-462-3811
e-mail: info@naminys.org
www.naminys.org

Thomas Easterly, President
Paul A Capofari, 1st Vice President

5981 Parents United Network: Parsons Child Family Center
60 Academy Road
Albany, NY 12208
518-426-2600
Fax: 518-447-5234
e-mail: communications@parsonscenter.org
www.parsonscenter.org

Rose Mary Bailly, President
John Henley, Chief Executive Officer

North Dakota

5982 North Dakota Alliance for the Mentally Ill
PO Box 3215
Minot, ND 58702-6016
701-770-8063
Fax: 701-725-4334
e-mail: l.lund8@hotmail.com
www.namind.org/

Linda Lund, President

5983 North Dakota FFCMH
PO Box 3061
Bismarck, ND 58502-3061
701-222-3310
800-484-2263
Fax: 701-222-3310
e-mail: carlottamccleary@bis.midco.nrt
www.ndffcmh.org/

Carlotta McCleary, Executive Director
Deb Jendro, Parent Coordinator

Ohio

5984 1st Capital FFCMH
394 Chestnut Street
Chillicothe, OH 45601
740-775-2674
Fax: 740-775-7834
e-mail: rmh1@adelphia.net

Rosemary Snider, President
Jim Mauro, Executive Director

5985 Ohio Alliance for the Mentally Ill
1225 Dublin Road
Columbus, OH 43215
614-224-2700
800-686-2646
Fax: 614-224-5400
TTY: 866-924-1478
e-mail: namiohio@namiohio.org
www.namiohio.org

Bob Spada, President
Terry Russell, Executive Director

Oklahoma

5986 Oklahoma Alliance for the Mentally Ill
4200 Perimeter Drive
Oklahoma City, OK 73112-6200
405-230-1900
800-583-1264
Fax: 405-230-1903
e-mail: namiok@coxinet.net
www.namioklahoma.org/

Paula Walker, President
Traci Cook, Executive Director

5987 Tulsa Unified FFCMH
1022 N Howard
Tulsa, OK 74115
918-838-8033
e-mail: sherryscoobydoo@aol.com
www.ffcmh.org

Sherry Gorger, Education Program Director
Cora Palazzolo, Communications Coordinator

Oregon

5988 NAMI-Oregon
4701 SE 24th Avenue
Portland, OR 97202-1552
503-230-8009
800-343-6264
Fax: 503-230-2751
e-mail: namioregon@namior.org
www.nami.org/MSTemplate.cfm?Site=NAMI_Or
Providing support education and advocacy for people with biological mental illness and their families. The in-state 800 phone number is Oregon's NAMI-Line. Callers to this line are provided with information about mental illnesses and referrals to support and treatment services.
Chris Bouneff, Executive Director
Michelle Madison, Events Manager/Outreach Coordinator

5989 Oregon Family Support Network
1300 Broadway Street
Salem, OR 97301
503-363-8068
800-323-8521
Fax: 503-390-3161
e-mail: ofsn@ofsn.org
www.ofsn.org

David De Fiebre, Board President
Sandy Bumpus, Executive Director

Pennsylvania

5990 Parents Involved Network
1211 Chestnut Street
Philadelphia, PA 19107
215-751-1800
800-688-4226
e-mail: pin@pinofpa.org
www.pinofpa.org

Janet Jordan Jr, Executive Director
Jyoti Shah, President

5991 Pennsylvania Alliance for the Mentally Ill
2149 N 2nd Street
Harrisburg, PA 17011-1005
717-238-1514
800-223-0500
Fax: 717-238-4390
TTY: 800-890-6093
e-mail: nami-pa@nami-pa.org
www.nami-pa.org/

Suzanne Vogel-Scibilia, M.D, President
James W Jordan, Jr, Executive Director

Rhode Island

5992 National Alliance for the Mentally Ill of Rhode Island (NAMI)
154 Waterman Street
Providence, RI 02906-4312
401-331-3060
800-749-3197
Fax: 401-274-3020
e-mail: chaznami@cox.net
www.namirhodeisland.org

Marcia Boyd, Esq, President
Chaz J Gross, Executive Director

South Carolina

5993 NAMI-SC: National Alliance on Mental Illness: South Carolina
PO BOX 1267
Columbia, SC 29202-1267
803-733-9592
800-788-5131
Fax: 803-733-9593
e-mail: namisc@namisc.org
www.namisc.org

Advocacy, Education and Support
Joan Herbert, MS, President
Bill Lindsey, Executive Director

South Dakota

5994 NAMI South Dakota
PO Box 88808
Sioux Falls, SD 57109-1204
605-271-1871
800-551-2531
Fax: 605-271-1871
e-mail: namisd@midconetwork.com
www.nami.org/sites/NAMISouthDakota

Shelly Jablonski, President
Sita Diehl, Executive Director

Tennessee

5995 Tennessee Alliance for the Mentally Ill
1101 Kermit Drive
Nashville, TN 37217-2126
615-361-6608
800-467-3589
Fax: 615-361-6698
e-mail: rpbaxter@comcast.net
www.namitn.org

Dick Baxter, President
Jeff Fladen, Executive Director

Texas

5996 Central Texas FFCMH
6814 Orange Blossom
Austin, TX 78744
512-282-7126
Fax: 512-282-5817
e-mail: mattie_dixon@hotmail.com

Mattie Owens

5997 North Texas FFCMH
722 E Summitt
Sherman, TX 75090
e-mail: patoadv@msn.com
Pat Nazaroff

5998 San Antonio Bexar County FFCMH
2516 Bandara
San Antonio, TX 78238
210-523-2351
Fax: 210-523-2352
e-mail: ideasjn@aol.com

Joseph Peyson, Executive Director
Donna Fisher, President

5999 Texas Alliance for the Mentally Ill
Foundtain Park Plaza III
Austin, TX 78704
512-693-2000
800-633-3760
Fax: 512-693-8000
e-mail: kjeschke@namitexas.org
www.namitexas.org

Andrea Hazlitt, Board President
Ed Dickey, Vice President

6000 Texas FFCMH
7800 Shoal Creek Road
Austin, TX 78752
512-407-8844
866-893-3264
Fax: 512-407-8266
e-mail: PattiDerr@txffcmh.org
www.txffcmh.org

Patti Muller, President
Sherri Wittwer, Executive Director

6001 Utah Alliance for the Mentally Ill
1600 West 2200 South   801-323-9900
West Valley City, UT 84119-1701   877-230-6264
     Fax: 801-323-9799
     e-mail: rebecca@namiut.org
     www.namiut.org

Zara Juillerat, President
Rebecca Glathar, Executive Director

Vermont

6002 Vermont Alliance for the Mentally Ill
162 S Main Street   802-244-1396
Waterbury, VT 05676-1519   800-639-6480
     Fax: 802-244-1405
     e-mail: info@namivt.org
     www.nami.org/MSTemplate.cfm?Site=NAMI_Ve
Karen Kelley, Chair
Wendy Beinner, President/CEO

6003 Vermont FFCMH
600 Blair Park Road   802-876-7021
Williston, VT 05495-0607   800-639-6071
     Fax: 802-329-2135
     e-mail: vffcmh@vffcmh.org
     www.vffcmh.org

Ted Tighe, President
Kathy Holsopple, Executive Director

Virginia

6004 Virginia Alliance for the Mentally Ill
PO Box 8260   804-285-8264
Richmond, VA 23226-1903   888-486-8264
     Fax: 804-285-8464
     e-mail: namiva@verizon.net
     www.namivirginia.org/

Robert Cluck, President
Mira Signer, Executive Director

Washington

6005 NAMI Washington (National Alliance for the Mentally Ill of Washington)
7500 Greenwood Avenue North   206-783-4288
Seattle, WA 98103-5580   800-782-9264
     e-mail: office@namiwa.org
     www.namiwa.org/
Advocacy, support and education for the mentally ill, their families and friends.
Gordon Bopp, President
Jim Bloss, Vice President

6006 Washington FFCMH
801 E 141 Street   253-537-2145
Tacoma, WA 98445-2768   Fax: 253-537-2162
     e-mail: acvmarge@comcast.net
     www.ffcmh.org/

Marge Coleman, President
Terrie Isaly, Fast Track Program Director

West Virginia

6007 Mountain State/Parents/Children/ Adolescents Network
1201 Garfield Street   304-233-5399
McMechen, WV 26040   800-CHI-LD35
     Fax: 304-233-3847
     e-mail: ttoothman@mcpcan.org
     www.mspcan.org

Joyce Floyd, President
Hope Coleman, Vice President

6008 NAMI West Virginia
PO Box 2706   304-342-0497
Charleston, WV 25330-2706   800-598-5653
     Fax: 304-342-0499
     e-mail: namiwv@aol.com
     www.namiwv.org

Educational advocacy and support for families consumers and friends of people with mental illnesses.
Randal Rutkowski, Co-President
Terence Schnapp, Interim Executive Director

Wisconsin

6009 Wisconsin Alliance for the Mentally Ill
4233 W Beltline Highway   608-268-6000
Madison, WI 53711-3814   800-236-2988
     Fax: 608-268-6004
     e-mail: nami@namiwisconsin.org
     www.namiwisconsin.org

Jim Connors, President
Julianne Carbin, Executive Director

6010 Wisconsin Family Ties
16 N Carroll Street   608-267-6888
Madison, WI 53703   800-422-7145
     Fax: 608-267-6801
     e-mail: info@wifamilyties.org
     www.wifamilyties.org

Hugh Johnson, President
Deion Hagemeister, Vice-President

Wyoming

6011 Wyoming Alliance for the Mentally Ill
133 W 6th Street   307-265-2573
Casper, WY 82601-3124   888-882-4968
     Fax: 307-234-0440
     e-mail: coem@tctwest.net
     www.namiwyoming.org/

Marty Coe, President
Tammy Noel, Executive Director

Libraries & Resource Centers

6012 Alta Bates Summit Medical Center
2001 Dwight Way
Berkeley, CA 94704-2608   510-204-4444
     www.altabatessummit.org/
Alta Bates Summit Medical Center has made community healthcare a priority. We are proud of our many areas of clinical excellence including cardiovascular, behavioral health, women and infants, orthopedics, rehabilitation, and oncology care.
Carolyn McGee, Medical Librarian

6013 Central Louisiana State Hospital Medical and Professional Library
242 West Shamrock Street   318-484-6363
Pineville, LA 71360   Fax: 318-484-6284
     e-mail: bentonmcgee@hotmail.com
     www.clmlc.org
The Consortium was established to increase and better utilize the health information resources of Central Louisiana. Information offered on psychiatry, psychology and mental health.
Carol Rogers, Director

6014 National Mental Health Consumer's Self-Help Clearinghouse
1211 Chestnut Street   267-507-3810
Philadelphia, PA 19107   800-553-4539
     Fax: 215-636-6312
     e-mail: info@mhselfhelp.org
     www.mhselfhelp.org
The National Mental Health Consumers' Self-Help Clearinghouse, the nation's first national consumer technical assistance center, has played a major role in the development of the mental health consumer movement. The consumer movement strives for dignity, respect, and opportunity for those with mental illnesses.
Joseph Rogers, Executive Director
Susan Rogers, Director

6015 National Mental Health Consumers' Self- Help Clearinghouse
1211 Chestnut Street   267-507-3810
Philadelphia, PA 19107   800-553-4539
     Fax: 215-636-6312
     e-mail: info@mhselfhelp.org
     www.mhselfhelp.org

The National Mental Health Consumers' Self-Help Clearinghouse, the nation's first national consumer technical assistance center, has played a major role in the development of the mental health consumer movement. The consumer movement strives for dignity, respect, and opportunity for those with mental illnesses. Consumers—those who receive or have received mental health services—continue to reject the label of 'those who cannot help themselves.'

Joseph Rogers, Executive Director
Susan Rogers, Director

Research Centers

6016 Anxiety Disorders Center University of Wisconsin
University of Wisconsin
Department of Psychiatry
Madison, WI 53719-0001 608-263-6100
www.psychiatry.wisc.edu/uwpFacilities.ht
Provides evaluation and treatment for individuals suffering from anxiety disorders as well as training and education for clinicians.
Andy Alexander, PhD, Professor
Ruth Benca, MD, PhD, Professor

6017 Institute of Psychiatry and Human Behavior: University of Maryland
655 West Baltimore Street 410-706-7410
Baltimore, MD 21201-1542 Fax: 410-706-0235
e-mail: alehman@psych.umaryland.edu
www.medschool.umaryland.edu
Studies in psychiatric disorders.
Anthony Lehm MD, Director
Craig Vantyke, Chief Executive Officer

6018 Jane & Terry Semel Institute for Neuroscie nce & Human Behavior
Neuropsychiatric Institute
760 Westwood Plaza 310-825-2631
Los Angeles, CA 90095 800-825-9989
www.semel.ucla.edu
Studies behavior disorders and psychosocial adaptation and the future.
Peter Whybrow, Director
Fawzy Fawzy, Associate Director

6019 Langley Porter Psychiatric Institute University of California
University of California
401 Parnassus Avenue
San Francisco, CA 94143-9911 415-476-7365
www.universityofcalifornia.edu
Conducts clinical studies of psychiatric disorders.
Samuel Barno Faucher, Director

6020 Medical College of Pennsylvania: Eastern Psychiatric Institute
3200 Henry Avenue 215-842-6990
Philadelphia, PA 19129-1137
Offers research into all aspects of mental illness.
Michael Spohn, Director

6021 Menninger Clinic: Department of Research
12301 S. Main Street 713-275-5140
Houston, TX 77035-0829 800-351-9058
Fax: 785-350-5392
www.menningerclinic.com/
Focuses research on mental illness and mental health issues.
B. Christoph Frueh, PhD, Director of Clinical Research
Chris Fowler, PhD, Associate Director of Clinical Research

6022 Mental Illness Research and Education Institute
Eastern State Hospital
PO Box 800
Medical Lake, WA 99022-800 509-299-3121
Fax: 509-997-15
Governmental organization focusing on mental illness research.
Harold David, Director

6023 NIH Clinical Center
National Institute of Health

9000 Rockville Pike 301-496-4000
Bethesda, MD 20892 800-411-1222
Fax: 301-402-2984
TTY: 866-411-1010
e-mail: prpl@mail.cc.nih.gov
www.cc.nih.gov
Established in 1953 as the research hospital of the National Institutes of Health. Designed so that patient care facilities are close to research laboratories so new findings of basic and clinical scientists can be quickly applied to the treatment of patients. Upon referral by physicians patients are admitted to NIH clinical studies.
John I Gallin, MD, Clinical Center Director
David Henderson, MD, Deputy Director for Clinical Care

6024 State University of New York At Stony Brook: Mental Health Research
450 Clarkson Avenue
Brooklyn, NY 11203-2056 718-270-1270
www.stonybrook.edu
Benjamin S Hsiao, Phd, Vice President for Research

6025 Thresholds Psychiatric Rehabilitation
2700 N Ravenswood Avenue 773-281-3800
Chicago, IL 60614-1894 Fax: 773-818-90
e-mail: thresholds@thresholds.org
www.luc.edu
A psychosocial rehabilitation agency serving persons with severe and persistent mental illness.
Tom MD, Director
Peter Whybrow, Director

6026 University of Michigan: Mental Health Research Institute
205 Washtenaw Place 734-763-1817
Ann Arbor, MI 48109 e-mail: UMresearch@umich.edu
www.umich.edu
Focuses on the diagnosis treatment and prevention of mental illnesses and disorders.
Dr Bernard Schulz, Chair of Psychiatry

6027 University of Minnesota Department of Psychiatry
420 Delaware Street SE 612-624-2430
Minneapolis, MN 55455-374 Fax: 612-265-91
www.umn.edu
Behavior and mental illness research.
S Charles PhD, Director

6028 University of Missouri: Columbia Missouri Institute of Mental Health
5247 Fyler Avenue 573-634-8787
Saint Louis, MO 63139-1300 Fax: 314-644-8834
Mental health policy and ethics studies.
Danny Weddin MD, Director

6029 University of Pittsburgh: Western Psychiatric Institute & Clinic
3811 Ohara Street 412-246-6356
Pittsburgh, PA 15213-2593 Fax: 412-246-6350
e-mail: reitzpm@msx.upmc.edu
www.pitt.edu
Advancement of basic and clinical knowledge in mental health and psychiatric care.
Thomas Detre Camarata, Acting Director

6030 Vanderbilt Kennedy Center
Vanderbilt University
110 Magnolia Center 615-322-8240
Nashville, TN 37203-5701 Fax: 615-228-36
e-mail: kc@vanderbilt.edu
www.kc.vanderbilt.edu
Mental health research.
Donna G Eskind, Chair
Cathy S Brown, Past Chair

6031 Veterans Medical Center: Mental Health Clinical Research Center
3801 Miranda Avenue
Palo Alto, CA 94304-1207 650-858-3941
www.va.gov
Jerome Gallin, Director
David Henderson, Deputy Director for Clinical Care

6032 Yeshiva University: Soundview-Throgs Neck Community Mental Health Center
2527 Glebe Avenue 718-904-4400
Bronx, NY 10461-3109 Fax: 718-931-7307
Mental health mental illness and recovery from mental illness research.
Dr Itamar

Support Groups & Hotlines

6033 National Health Information Center
PO Box 1133 310-565-4167
Washington, DC 20013 800-336-4797
  Fax: 301-984-4256
  e-mail: info@nhic.org
  www.health.gov/nhic
Offers a nationwide information referral service, produces directories and resource guides.
Rivers, Federal Program Coordinator

Alabama

6034 Alabama Education of Homeless Children and Youth Program
Alabama State Department of Education
5348 Gordon Persons Building 334-242-8199
Montgomery, AL 36130-3901 Fax: 334-420-9633
  e-mail: mrivers@alsde.edu
  www.alsde.edu/html/home.asp
The major responsibilities of the Federal Programs Section are to administer all federally funded education programs and to provide technical assistance to local education agencies and schools. These responsibilities include promoting, supervising, and coordinating statewide educational programs with federal programs in addition to assisting schools in developing, revising, and implementing their school wide plans.
Maggie McDonald, Program/Education Director
Augusta Reimer, Leadership Project Coordinator

Alaska

6035 National Alliance for the Mentally Ill (NA MI) Alaska
144 West 15th Avenue 907-227-1300
Anchorage, AK 99501-5106 800-478-4462
  Fax: 907-227-1400
  e-mail: info@nami-alaska.org
  www.nami.org/sites/alaska
NAMI Alaska is a grassroots, 501(c)(3) nonprofit, support, educational and advocacy organization of consumers, families, and friends of people with severe brain disorders such as schizophrenia, schizo-affective disorder, bipolar disorder, major depressive disorder, obsessive-compulsive disorder, panic and anxiety disorders, and attention deficit/hyperactivity disorder. In addition, NAMI provides information and referral services and works with local media on stories about mental illness.
Scott Owens, Co-President
Pat Dobbins, Co-President

Arizona

6036 Navajo Nation Office of Special Education & Rehabilitation Services (OSERS)
PO Box 1420 928-871-6338
Window Rock, AZ 86515 866-341-9918
  Fax: 928-871-7865
  e-mail: osers@navajo.org
  www.osers.navajo-nsn.gov/
Navajo OSERS is a program within the Division of DINE Education, which offers vocational rehabilitation to people with disabilities. Vocational Rehabilitation includes an array of services, which are funded by a grant to the Navajo Nation from the U.S. Department of Education. The goal of vocational rehabilitation is to assist people with disabilities to obtain or maintain employment.
Treva M Roanhorse, Director
Paula S Seanez, Assistant Director

Colorado

6037 Laradon Services for Children and Adults w ith Developmental Disabilities
5100 Lincoln Street 303-296-2400
Denver, CO 80216 866-381-2163
  Fax: 303-296-4012
  TDD: 7209746821
  www.laradon.org/
Laradon specializes in services to children and adults with developmental disabilities, operating 15 programs that are designed to help each individual develop to his or her fullest potential and maximize self-sufficiency.
John Galvin, Chairman
Frank Lucero, PhD, Executive Director

Florida

6038 Florida Institute for Family Involvement (FIFI)
3927 Spring Creek Highway 305-293-7626
Crawfordville, FL 32327 877-926-3514
  Fax: 863-582-9358
  e-mail: HewFLMOM@aol.com
  www.fifionline.org
Florida Institute for Family Involvement (FIFI), an affiliate of Federation of Families for Children's Mental Health (FFCMH), enhances, facilitates, and supports family and consumer involvement in the development of responsive, family centered, and community based systems of care. FIFI works in collaboration with state, federal, and private programs to develop a resource and training information center to enable individuals to advocate for appropriate services and make wise service choices.
Connie Hawke, Co-Director
Tara Bremer, Co-Director

6039 Parent Education Network (PEN) Project Health
Family Network on Disabilities of Florida
2735 Whitney Road 727-523-1130
Clearwater, FL 33760 800-825-5736
  Fax: 727-523-8687
  e-mail: wilbur@fndfl.org
  www.fndfl.org/programs/pen-parent-educat
The PEN Project provides: information on specific disabilities; individual assistance by telephone, email, and in-person; referrals to local, state, and national resources; opportunities for youths with disabilities to be involved in training to parents and students; and, collaboration with Family Network on Disabilities Heart and Hope annual statewide conference for families.
Wilbur Smith, Co-Chief Executive Officer
Anna M McLaughlin, Co-Chief Executive Officer

Georgia

6040 Georgia Parent Support Network (GPSN)
1381 Metropolitan Parkway 404-758-4500
Atlanta, GA 30310 Fax: 404-758-6833
  e-mail: rheba.smith@gpsn.org
  www.gpsn.org/
Georgia Parent Support Network (GPNS) provides support, education, and advocacy for children and youth with mental illness, emotional disturbances, and behavioral differences and their families.
Kathy Dennis, Board President
Sue L Smith, Ed.D, Chief Executive Officer

Hawaii

6041 Hawaii Families As Allies (HFAA)
99-209 Moanalua Road 808-487-8785
Aiea, HI 96701 866-361-8825
  Fax: 808-487-0514
  e-mail: hfaa@hfaa.net
  www.hfaa.net/
Hawaii Families as Allies (HFAA) is a statewide parent-controlled family network organization that provides support, services and information for families of children and adolescents with emotional and/or behavioral challenges. HFAA is the Hawaii state chapter of the Federation of Families for Children's Mental

Health, a national organization that advocates for service system change so that families are valued and treated as true partners.
Linda Machado, Executive Director
Charlene Daraban, Family Resource Specialist

Illinois

6042 CANDU Parent Group
24W 681 Woodcrest Drive   630-983-9027
Naperville, IL 60540
Cathy Dennis

6043 KALEIDOSCOPE
1340 S. Damen Avenue   773-278-7200
Chicago, IL 60608   Fax: 773-278-5663
TTY: 773-292-4086
e-mail: info@kaleidoscope4kids.org
www.kaleidoscope4kids.org

William J Binder, Chair
Ivy Walker, Vice Chairman-Secretary

6044 Parents Information Network FFCMH
1926 1700th Avenue   217-735-1662
Lincoln, IL 62656
Bridget Van Gogh, President

Indiana

6045 NAMI Indiana - National Alliance on Mental Illness
PO Box 22697   317-925-9399
Indianapolis, IN 46222-0697   800-677-6442
Fax: 317-925-9398
e-mail: info@namiindiana.org
www.namiindiana.org

NAMI Indiana is a non-profit grassroots organization dedicated to improving the lives of people afflicted by serious and persistent mental illness. NAMI Indiana consists of families, consumers, and professionals that are dedicated to helping families through a network of support, education, advocacy, and promotion of research. NAMI Indiana is affiliated with the National Alliance on Mental Illness (NAMI), which is located in Arlington, Virginia.
Joshua G Sprunger, Executive Director
Joanne Abbott, Program Director

Iowa

6046 Iowa Federaion of Families for Children's Mental Health (FFCMH)
106 South Booth   319-462-2187
Anamosa, IA 52205   888-400-6302
Fax: 319-462-6789
e-mail: help@iffcmh.org
www.iffcmh.org
The mission of Iowa Federation of Families for Children's Mental Health is to link families to community, county and state partners for needed supports and services; and to promote systems change that will enable families to live in a safe, stable and respectful environment.
Lori Reynolds, Executive Director
Heidi Reynolds, Program Director

Kentucky

6047 Kentucky IMPACT
275 E Main Street   502-564-7610
Frankfort, KY 40621
Sandra Welles, Executive Director

Massachusetts

6048 Parent Professional Advocacy League
45 Bromfield Street   617-542-7860
Boston, MA 02108   866-815-8122
Fax: 617-542-7832
e-mail: info@ppal.net
www.ppal.net

Earl N Stuck, Chair
Lisa Lambert, Executive Director

Minnesota

6049 Emotional Health Anonymous
PO Box 4245   651-647-9712
St Paul, MN 55104-0245   Fax: 651-647-1593
e-mail: info2gh99jsd@emotionsanonymous.org
www.emotionsanonymous.org
A twelve-step organization, similar to Alcoholics Anonymous. Compsed of people who come together in weekly meetings for the purpose of working toward recovery from emotional difficulties.
Karen Mead, Executive Director

6050 PACER Center
8161 Normandale Boulevard   952-838-9000
Bloomington, MN 55437-1044   800-537-2237
Fax: 952-838-0199
TTY: 952-838-0190
e-mail: pacer@pacer.org
www.pacer.org

Paula F Goldberg, Executive Director
Mary Schrock, Chief Operating and Development Officer

Missouri

6051 MO-SPAN Southwest Region
210 W Vine Street   660-679-5767
Butler, MO 64730
Eldonna Dittrich, Executive Director
Tina Vervara, Administrative Assistant

6052 MOSPAN Northwest Region
440 Rue Street Franois   314-972-0600
Jefferson City, MO 63031   Fax: 314-720-06
e-mail: mospan2@fid.net.com
www.mospan.org

Donna Taycher, Executive Director

Nevada

6053 Nevada PEP
2101 S. Jones Boulevard   702-388-8899
Las Vegas, NV 89146   800-216-5188
Fax: 702-388-2966
e-mail: KTaycher@nvpep.org
www.nvpep.org
A statewide non-profit helping families who have children with disabilities, and the professionals who work with them. Support groups, training, workshops, lending resource library. Services are provided at no cost.
Karen Taycher, Executive Director
Stephanie Vrsnik, Community Development Director

New Hampshire

6054 National Alliance for the Mentally Ill: New Hampshire
85 North State Street   603-225-5359
Concord, NH 03301   800-242-6264
Fax: 603-228-8848
e-mail: info@naminh.org
www.naminh.org
Family support and advocacy for consumers and family members.
Michele Grennon, President
Ken Norton, Executive Director

New Mexico

6055 Navajo Nation Office Special Education & R ehabilitation Services
IHS PO Box 1337   505-722-1454
Gallup, NM 87301   Fax: 505-722-1554
e-mail: osers@navajo.org
www.osers.navajo-nsn.gov/
Navajo OSERS is a program within the Division of DINE Education, which offers vocational rehabilitation to people with disabilities. Vocational Rehabilitation includes an array of services, which are funded by a grant to the Navajo Nation from the U.S. Department of Education. The goal of vocational rehabilitation is to assist people with disabilities to obtain or maintain employment.
Treva M Roanhorse, Director
Paula S Seanez, Assistant Director

6056   Mental Health Association in Dutchess Coun ty
253 Mansion Street   845-473-2500
Poughkeepsie, NY 12601   Fax: 845-473-4870
                                     e-mail: mhadc@hvc.rr.com
                                              www.mhadc.com/
The Mental Health Association in Dutchess County promotes mental well-being and advances the recovery from mental illness, provides rehabilitation programs and support services for adults with a history of mental illness and their families.
Joseph Ellman, President
Andrew O'Grady, Executive Director

6057   Mental Health Association in Orange County
Mental Health Association of Orange County
73 James P. Kelly Way   845-342-2400
Middletown, NY 10940-1906   800-832-1200
                                                  Fax: 845-343-9665
                                     e-mail: mha@mhaorangeny.com
                                              www.mhaorangeny.com/
Mental Health Association of Orange County/MHA is a private, not-for-profit organization seeking to promote the mental health and emotional well being of Orange County residents. Under the leadership of a volunteer Board of Directors, MHA's staff members, consultants and volunteers provide free mental health services to thousands of Orange County residents each year. Several volunteers answer several hotlines, provide companionship, public education, direct services and assist with fundraisers.
David Goggins, President
Nadia Allen, Executive Director

6058   ND FFCMH Region II
PO Box 3061   701-222-1223
Bismarck, ND 58502-3061   Fax: 701-250-8835
                                     e-mail: carlottamccleary@bis.midco.nrt
                                                         www.ffcmh.org

Carlotta Jendro, Executive Director

6059   ND Region V FFCMH Chapter-Federation of Fa milies for Children's Mental Health
1104 2nd Avenue South   701-235-9923
Fargo, ND 58103   Fax: 701-235-9923
                                     e-mail: ndffrgv@nbinternet.com
                                              www.ffcmh.org/who_chapters.php
The FFCMH, a national family-run organization serves to: provide advocacy at the national level for the rights of children and youth with emotional, behavioral and mental health challenges and their families; provide leadership and technical assistance to a nation-wide network of family run organizations; and, collaborate with family run and other child serving organizations to transform mental health care in America.
Deborah Sevart, Executive Director

6060   ND Region VII FFCMH-Federation of Families for Children's Mental Health
2252 La Corte Loop   701-258-1628
Bismarck, ND 58503   Fax: 701-258-1628
                                     e-mail: ndffrg7@btinet.net
                                              www.ffcmh.org/who_chapters.php
The FFCMH, a national family-run organization serves to: provide advocacy at the national level for the rights of children and youth with emotional, behavioral and mental health challenges and their families; provide leadership and technical assistance to a nation-wide network of family run organizations; and, collaborate with family run and other child serving organizations to transform mental health care in America.
Becky Beale Psy.D, Group Programs Director
David J Coleman Ph.D, Director of Psychological Services

6061   Child & Adolescent Behavioral Health
919 2nd Street NE   330-454-7917
Canton, OH 44704   Fax: 330-452-8860
                                     e-mail: bsnyder@casrv.org
                                              www.childandadolescent.org/

The Child and Adolescent Service Center (CASC) was founded and incorporated in 1976 by a standing committee of the Stark County Mental Health Foundation. CASC provides dynamic leadership through innovative service, training and evaluation and is committed to providing culturally-sensitive programs and services throughout the community.
Lisa Warburton-Gregory, President
Michael Johnson, Chief Executive Officer

6062   First Ohio Chapter: FFCMH
4505 Quaker Court   330-726-9570
Canfield, OH 44406-9131   Fax: 330-726-9031
                                     e-mail: xuparents@aol.com OR ffcmh@ffcmh.org
                                              www.ffcmh.org/who_chapters.php
The Federation of Families for Children's Mental Health (FFCMH) is a national organization dedicated exclusively to helping children with mental health needs and their families achieve a better quality of life.
Chrysanne Cianon, Executive Director
Brenda Alego, Assistant Director

6063   Parent Support Network of Rhode Island
1395 Atwood Avenue   401-467-6855
Johnston, RI 02919   800-483-8844
                                                  Fax: 401-467-6903
                                     e-mail: c.ciano@psnri.org
                                                         www.psnri.org
Family-run organization whose mission is to provide support, education and advocacy to parents of children at risk for or who have emotional, behavioral, and/or mental health challenges.
Linda Winfield, Board President
Cathy Ciano, Executive Director

6064   Federation of Families of South Carolina
810 Dutch Square Boulevard   803-772-5210
Columbia, SC 29210-2344   866-779-0402
                                                  Fax: 803-772-5212
                                     e-mail: FedFamSC@yahoo.com
                                              www.fedfamsc.org/

Kathleen Scharer, President
Roxann McKinnon, Vice President

6065   Tennessee Voices for Children
701 Bradford Avenue   615-269-7751
Nashville, TN 37204   800-670-9882
                                                  Fax: 615-269-8914
                                     e-mail: tvc@tnvoices.org
                                                         www.tnvoices.org

Michele Johnson, President
Paula Sandidge, M.D, Board Secretary

6066   Harris County FFCMH
431 Breeze Park Drive   713-455-8962
Houston, TX 77015   e-mail: annn@flash.net
Elizabeth Cerar, Executive Director
Karen Greenwell, Community Education Coordinator

6067   Allies with Families
505 East 200 South   801-433-2595
Salt Lake City, UT 84102-2979   877-477-0764
                                                  Fax: 801-521-0872
                                     e-mail: Allies@AlliesWithFamilies.org
                                              www.allieswithfamilies.org
Allies with Families was created in 1991 to offer practical support and resources for parents and their children and youth who face serious emotional, behavioral and mental health challenges. It was created to support all families in the state of Utah.
Lori Cerar, Executive Director
Karen Greenwell, Project Director and Newsletter Editor

Vermont

6068 Vermont FFCMH
PO Box 1577 802-244-1955
Williston, VT 05495-0507 800-639-6071
Fax: 802-329-2135
e-mail: vffcmh@vffcmh.org
www.ffcmh.org/find-local-chapter
The Federation of Families for Children's Mental Health (FFCMH) is a national organization dedicated exclusively to helping children with mental health needs and their families achieve a better quality of life,
Kathleen Holsopple

Virginia

6069 PACCT
8032 Mechanicsville Turnpike 804-559-6833
Mechancsville, VA 23111 Fax: 804-559-6835
Joyce Scheibe

6070 PACCT of Roanoke Valley
PO Box 21112 703-989-5042
Roanoke, VA 24018 Fax: 703-989-5675
e-mail: scheibe.p@worldnet.att.net
Sue Critchlow, Director
Sandra Spencer, Executive Director Corporate Office (MD)

Washington

6071 Common Voice for Pierce County Parents
10402 Kline Street 253-537-2145
Lakewood, WA 98445-2768 Fax: 253-537-2162
e-mail: nrascon@dadsmove.org
www.ffcmh.org/find-local-chapter
A Common Voice for Pierce County Parents is affiliated with the Federation of Families for Children's Mental Health (FFCMH), a national organization dedicated exclusively to helping children with mental health needs and their families achieve a better quality of life.
Sherry Lyons

Wisconsin

6072 We Are the Children's Hope/Support Group
First Love Outreach Ministries
PO Box 06204 414-263-1323
Milwaukee, WI 53206 Fax: 414-263-1148
e-mail: zelodius@aol.com
www.firstlovelifecoaching.com

Pr Zelodius Gerlosky

Wyoming

6073 Concerned Parent Coalition
1125 Sioux Avenue 307-682-6684
Gillette, WY 82718-6529
Michelle Nikkel, Executive Director
Carla Schroeder, Deputy Director

6074 Uplift
200 W 17th Street 307-778-8686
Cheyenne, WY 82003 888-875-4383
Fax: 307-778-8681
e-mail: uplift@upliftwy.org
www.upliftwy.org

Peggy Logan, President
Richard Yep, Executive Director

Books

6075 Anatomy of a Psychiatric Illness
American Psychiatric Press
1400 K Street NW 202-682-6268
Washington, DC 20005-2403 Fax: 202-789-2648
Answers questions, provides clinical anecdotes, explains what medical science does and does not know about mental illnesses and discusses compassion and hard scientific facts surrounding the psychiatric profession.
230 pages
ISBN: 0-880485-21-3

6076 Assessing Psychopathology and Behavior Problems: Mentally Ill Persons
National Clearinghouse for Alcohol and Drug Abuse
PO Box 2345
Rockville, MD 20857-0001 800-729-6686
www.health.org

239 pages

6077 Caring for People with Severe Mental Disorders: A National Plan
Superintendent of Documents
PO Box 371954 202-512-2250
Pittsburgh, PA 15250-7954
This report offers, from three panels of expert consultants, recommendations for strengthening both services research and research resources that should lead to improvement of the standard and provision of care for persons who have severe mental disorders.
80 pages

6078 Complete Mental Health Directory
Grey House Publishing
4919 Route 22 518-789-8700
Amenia, NY 12501 800-562-2139
Fax: 518-789-0545
e-mail: books@greyhouse.com
www.greyhouse.com

Offers critical and comprehensive information on disorders, support groups, clinical management, government agencies, professional conferences, research centers and training.
687 pages
ISBN: 1-930956-06-1
Leslie Mackenzie, Publisher

6079 Creating New Options
Bazelon Center for Mental Health Law
1101 15th Street NW 202-467-5730
Washington, DC 20005-5002 Fax: 202-223-0409
TDD: 202-467-4342
e-mail: pubs@bazelon.org
www.bazelon.org

Training for corrections administrators and staff on access to federal benefits for people with mental illnesses who are leacing jail or prison. Available as a manual ($7.50), a PowerPoint presentation on CD ($5), or both ($11).
2008
Lee Carly, Communications Director

6080 Creating a Circle of Learning: The Church and the Mentally Ill
National Alliance for the Mentally Ill
PO Box 753 301-524-7600
Waldorf, MD 20604-0753 Fax: 301-843-0159
www.NAMI.org

A curriculum designed to sensitize adults in the church to the plight of people with severe mental illnesses and their families. Leaders can teach the study as 12 one-hour lessons or six two-hour lessons. The teaching sessions build on a Biblical-based theological reflection calling congregations to minister to their brothers and sisters with mental illnesses.
1997

6081 Culture and the Restructuring of Community Mental Health
William A Vega, author

Greenwood Publishing Group, Inc.
PO Box 6926
Portsmouth, NH 03802-6926 800-225-5800
Fax: 877-231-6980
e-mail: service@greenwood.com
www.greenwood.com

Examines treatment, organizational planning and research issues and offers a critique of the theoretical and programmatic aspects of providing mental health services to traditionally underserved populations.
168 pages
ISBN: 0-313268-87-8

6082 Dealing with Mental Incapacity
Center for Public Representation
PO Box 260049   608-251-4008
Madison, WI 53726-0049   800-369-0388
                                       Fax: 608-251-1263
This manual contains a comprehensive introduction to the problem of guardianship as well as chapters of financial and health care planning tools, guardianship under Wisconsin law, protective placement and Watts reviews.
Training Manual

6083 Design of Rehabilitation Services in Psychiatric Hospital Settings
American Occupational Therapy Association
PO Box 1725   301-948-9626
Rockville, MD 20849-1725   800-729-2082
Presents a design for constructing a rehabilitation system that will ensure the delivery of quality services to patients in a psychiatric hospital setting.
130 pages
Jeanette Bair, Executive Director

6084 Dimensions of State Mental Health Policy
Greenwood Publishing Group, Inc/Praeger Publishers
PO Box 6926
Portsmouth, NH 03802-6926   800-225-5800
                                Fax: 877-231-6980
                        e-mail: service@greenwood.com
                                www.greenwood.com
Introduces students to the emerging field of state mental health policy.
320 pages
ISBN: 0-275932-52-4

6085 Dual Diagnosis of Major Mental Illness and Substance Disorder
National Alliance for the Mentally Ill
PO Box 753   703-524-7600
Waldorf, MD 20604-0753   Fax: 703-524-9094
                                       www.NAMI.org
Written for professionals, readable for families including descriptions of model programs.

6086 Educating Patients and Families About Mental Illness: A Practical Guide
Aspen Publishers
7201 McKinney Circle
Frederick, MD 21704-8356   800-638-8437
Introducing the manual to specifically address educating your patients and their families about mental illness.
496 pages

6087 Elderly with Chronic Mental Illness
Springer Publishing Company
536 Broadway   212-431-4370
New York, NY 10012-3955   877-687-7476
                                  Fax: 212-941-7842
                   e-mail: marketing@springerpub.com
                                   www.springerpub.com

384 pages Hardcover
ISBN: 0-826172-80-6
Annette Imperati, Marketing Director

6088 Elders Assert Their Rights
Bazelon Center for Mental Health Law
1101 15th Street NW   202-467-5730
Washington, DC 20005-5002   Fax: 202-223-0409
                                       TDD: 202-467-4342
                          e-mail: pubs@bazelon.org
                                   www.bazelon.org
A guide for residents, family members and advocates to the legal rights of elderly people with mental disabilities in nursing homes.
Paperback
Lee Carly, Communications Director

6089 Encyclopedia of Mental Health
Facts on File
11 Penn Plaza   212-967-8800
New York, NY 10001   800-322-8755
                                  Fax: 800-678-3633

Here, readers will find incisive definitions of theories, syndromes, symptons, treatments, and contemporary issues in easy-to-understand language.
480 pages Hardcover

6090 Encyclopedia of Phobias, Fears, and Anxieties
Facts on File
11 Penn Plaza   212-967-8800
New York, NY 10001   800-322-8755
                                  Fax: 800-678-3633

500 pages Hardcover

6091 Evaluation and Treatment of the Psychogeriatric Patient
Diane Gibson, MS, author
Haworth Press
10 Alice Street   607-722-5857
Binghamton, NY 13904-1580   800-429-6784
                                  Fax: 607-722-0012
                                   www.haworthpress.com
This pertinent book assists occupational therapists and other health care providers in developing up-to-date psychogeriatric programs.
111 pages Hardcover
ISBN: 1-560240-52-1

6092 Family Caregiving in Mental Illness
National Alliance for the Mentally Ill
PO Box 753   301-524-7600
Waldorf, MD 20604-0753   Fax: 301-843-0159
                                       www.NAMI.org
Examines patients' rights and treatment needs from the point of view of all those involved. Focuses on family burden and research and theoretical perspectives that influence mental health professionals.
1996

6093 Federal Law of the Mentally Handicapped
William Hein & Company
1285 Main Street   716-882-2600
Buffalo, NY 14209-1987
Chronological compilation of all relevant federal laws dealing with the mentally handicapped along with supporting documentation necessary to create a complete legislative history.
42 volumes/set

6094 Focal Group Psychotherapy for Mental Health Professionals
New Harbinger Publications
5674 Shattuck Avenue
Oakland, CA 94609-1662   800-748-6273
                                  Fax: 510-652-5472
                                   www.newharbinger.com
Definitive guide to leading brief, theme-based groups. This book offers an extensive week-by-week description of the basic concepts and interventions for 14 theme or focal groups.
544 pages

6095 Handbook of Mental Health and Mental Disor der Among Black Americans
Greenwood Publishing Group, Inc.
PO Box 6926
Portsmouth, NH 03802-6926   800-225-5800
                                  Fax: 877-231-6980
                        e-mail: service@greenwood.com
                                   www.greenwood.com
In addition to providing a wealth of new data on the mental health status of black communities, this handbook presents analyses of specific social, structural, and cultural conditions that affect the lives of individual black Americans.
352 pages
ISBN: 0-313263-30-2

6096 How to Live with a Mentally Ill Person: A Handbook of Day-to-Day Strategies
National Alliance for the Mentally Ill
PO Box 753   301-524-7600
Waldorf, MD 20604-0753   Fax: 301-843-0159
                                       www.NAMI.org

Offers self-help-styled advice to caregivers. Includes personal experiences, education, stigma, coping, and the mental health system.
1996

6097 Last in Line
Bazelon Center for Mental Health Law
1101 15th Street NW   202-467-5730
Washington, DC 20005-5002   Fax: 202-223-0409
                                    TDD: 202-467-4342
                              e-mail: pubs@bazelon.org
                                    www.bazelon.org
discusses barriers to community integration of older adults with mental illnesses, and recommendations for change.
2006 72 pages
Lee Carly, Communications Director

6098 Living with Mental Handicaps
Jessica Kingsley Publishers
118 Pentonville Road   071-833-2307
London, England,   Fax: 071-837-2917
The focus of this book lies in its insistence that mentally handicapped people make transitions like the rest of us from youth to old age.
176 pages

6099 Madness in the Streets
Free Press
866 3rd Avenue
New York, NY 10022-6221   800-323-7445
                                Fax: 800-943-9831
                                  www.simonsays.com
How psychiatry and the law abandoned the mentally ill.
436 pages
ISBN: 0-029153-80-8

6100 Making Child Welfare Work
Bazelon Center for Mental Health Law
1101 15th Street NW   202-467-5730
Washington, DC 20005-5002   Fax: 202-223-0409
                                    TDD: 202-467-4342
                              e-mail: pubs@bazelon.org
                                    www.bazelon.org
How the RC lawsuit forged new partnership to protect children and sustain families. The story of systems reform from the bottom up and the rededication of a burocracy to focus on the children and families it is meant to serve.
1998 126 pages
Lee Carly, Communications Director

6101 Managed Mental Health Care
American Psychiatric Press
1400 K Street NW   202-682-6268
Washington, DC 20005-2403   Fax: 202-789-2648
This text presents the collective wisdom of 40 experts experienced in clinical and managerial issues in managed care.
425 pages Hardcover
ISBN: 0-880483-55-5

6102 Managing Managed Care: A Mental Health Practitioner's Survival Guide
American Psychiatric Press
1400 K Street NW   202-682-6268
Washington, DC 20005-2403   Fax: 202-789-2648
Provides an easy-to-learn system for communicating with external reviewers and documenting quality of care.
200 pages Hardcover
ISBN: 0-880483-69-5

6103 Manic Depressive Illness
National Alliance for the Mentally Ill
PO Box 753
Waldorf, MD 20604-0753   703-524-7600
                                Fax: 703-524-9094
                                      www.NAMI.org
A definitive overview of bipolar disorder.

6104 Medicare Rx Consumer Workbook
Mental Health America

2000 North Beauragard Street   703-684-7722
Alexandria, VA 22311   800-969-6642
                                  Fax: 703-684-5968
                                  TTY: 800-433-5959
                           www.mentalhealthamerica.net
This workbook is designed to help you as a mental health consumer to get educated about and get enrolled in the new Medicare prescription drug program. Designed as a pocket folder, the workbook includes basic language explanations, tips for enrollment preparation, questions you should ask regarding plan options, worksheets, and definitions.

6105 Membership Directory
Natl. Council for Community Behavioral Healthcare
12300 Twinbrook Parkway   301-984-6200
Rockville, MD 20852

6106 Mental Disability Law: A Primer
Commission on The Mentally Disabled
1800 M Street NW   202-331-2240
Washington, DC 20036-5802
An updated and expanded version of the 1984 edition. Addresses the considerations involved in representing clients with mental disabilities.

6107 Mental Health Care in Prisons and Jails
Vance Bibliographies
PO Box 229   217-762-3831
Monticello, IL 61856-0229
A bibliography regarding health care in prisons.
30 pages
ISBN: 0-792006-94-1

6108 Mental Health Concepts and Techniques for the Occupational Therapy Assistant
Raven Press
1185 Avenue of the Americas   212-930-9500
New York, NY 10036-2601   800-777-2295
This text offers clear and easily understood explanations of the various theoretical and practice health models. Second edition.
344 pages
ISBN: 0-781700-74-4

6109 Mental Health Law Reporter
Business Publishers, Inc.
PO Box 17592
Baltimore, MD 21297   800-274-6737
                         e-mail: custserv@bpinews.com
                                    www.bpinews.com
Brings you the most timely, focused and thorough information on the legal issues that concern you in mental health litigation.
monthly
Leonard Eiserer, Publisher

6110 Mental Health: Counseling Services
Vance Bibliographies
PO Box 229   217-762-3831
Monticello, IL 61856-0229
Selected annotated bibliography on counseling services for the mentally handicapped from a black perspective.
23 pages
ISBN: 1-555903-76-2

6111 Mental Illness-Opposing Viewpoints Series
Greenhaven Press
Thomson Gale
Farmington Hills, MI 48333-9187   800-877-4253
                                Fax: 800-414-5043
                 e-mail: gale.customerservice@thomson.com
                           www.gale.com/greenhaven
In-depth overview of the topic written for upper elementary and junior/senior high school students.
2006
ISBN: 1-560061-68-5

6112 Mental and Physical Disability Law Report
American Bar Association
1800 M Street NW   202-331-2240
Washington, DC 20036-5802

Covers case law, legislative and regulatory developments that affect persons with mental or physical disabilities.

6113 Mentally Ill Individuals
Mainstream
1030 5th Street NW   202-898-1400
Washington, DC 20001-2504
Mainstreaming mentally ill individuals into the workplace.
12 pages

6114 Mood Apart: Depression, Mania, and Other Afflictions of the Self
National Alliance for the Mentally Ill
PO Box 753   301-524-7600
Waldorf, MD 20604-0753   Fax: 301-843-0159
                                                       www.NAMI.org
Discussion of depression and mania includes the symptoms, human costs, biological underpinnings, and therapies. Uses case histories, appendices, and historical references.
1997

6115 National Plan for Research on Child and Adolescent Mental Disorders
Superintendent of Documents
PO Box 371954   202-512-2250
Pittsburgh, PA 15250-7954
Summarizes the current knowledge about the prevalence and causes of mental disorders among children, identifies the possible treatments and prevention strategies and notes promising areas of research.
64 pages

6116 Occupational Therapy Practice Guidelines for Adults with Mood Disorders
American Occupational Therapy Association
4720 Montgomery Lane   301-652-2682
Bethesda, MD 20824-1220   Fax: 301-652-7711
                                                    TDD: 800-377-8555
                                                       www.aota.org
27 pages
ISBN: 1-569001-10-3

6117 Playing Cure
Jason Aronson
PO Box 15100
York, PA 17405-7100   800-782-0015
                                                     www.aronson.com
400 pages Hardcover
ISBN: 0-765700-21-2

6118 Protection and Advocacy Program for the Mentally Ill
US Department of Health and Human Services
5600 Fishers Lane   301-443-3667
Rockville, MD 20857-0001
Federal formula grant program to protect and advocate the rights of people with mental illnesses who are in residential facilities and to investigate abuse and neglect in such facilities.
Natalie Reatia, Chief

6119 Somatization Disorder in the Medical Setting
Superintendent of Documents
PO Box 371954   202-512-2250
Pittsburgh, PA 15250-7954
Somatization is a process in which psychological distress is expressed in multiple physical symptoms that have no discernible medical cause.
98 pages

6120 Strengthening the Role of Families in States' Early Intervention Systems
CEC, Department K00757   703-471-9543
Herdon, VA 22091
Policy guide for procedural safeguards for infants and toddlers under Part H of the Individuals with Disabilities Education Act.
213 pages Report

6121 Surviving Mental Illness
National Alliance for the Mentally Ill
PO Box 753   703-524-7600
Waldorf, MD 20604-0753   Fax: 703-524-9094
                                                       www.NAMI.org

The subjective experiences of people with multiple diagnoses including schizophrenia, bipolar disorder and manic depression.

6122 Teaching Adults with Mental Handicaps
Sunday School Board of the Southern Baptists
127 9th Avenue N
Nashville, TN 37234-0001   800-458-BSSB
Offers guidelines in methods of teaching adults with mental handicaps, their needs, outreach ideas, curriculum resources, adaptation procedures, and ministry suggestions.

6123 Troubled Journey
National Alliance for the Mentally Ill
PO Box 753   301-524-7600
Waldorf, MD 20604-0753   Fax: 301-843-0159
                                                       www.NAMI.org
Long associated with NAMI's former Siblings and Adult Children Network, the authors use their years of listening to stories - plus Marsh's professional experience - to provide a book that offers support to siblings and a caring and heartfelt approach to healing.
1997

6124 Turning Point
American Psychiatric Press
1400 K Street NW   202-682-6268
Washington, DC 20005-2403   Fax: 202-789-2648
The first comprehensive chronicle of the contributions made by conscientious objectors who volunteered for service in America's mental hospitals and state institutions for the developmentally disabled.
314 pages Hardcover
ISBN: 0-880485-60-4

6125 Understanding Depression
Patricia Ainsworth, MD, author

University Press of Mississippi
3825 Ridgewood Road   601-432-6205
Jackson, MS 39211-6492   Fax: 601-432-6217
                                          e-mail: kburgess@ihl.state.ms.us
                                                  www.upress.state.ms.us
A clear explanation for those who know the illness personally and for those who want to understand them.
2000 120 pages Paperback
ISBN: 1-578061-69-5
Kathy Burgess, Advertising/Marketing Services Manager

6126 Understanding Mental Retardation
Patricia Ainsworth, MD; Pamela C Baker, PhD, author

University Press of Mississippi
3825 Ridgewood Road   601-432-6205
Jackson, MS 39211-6492   Fax: 601-432-6217
                                          e-mail: kburgess@ihl.state.ms.us
                                                  www.upress.state.ms.us
A resource for parents, caregivers, and counselors.
2004 192 pages Paperback
ISBN: 1-578066-47-6
Kathy Burgess, Advertising/Marketing Services Manager

6127 Understanding Panic and Other Anxiety Disorders
Benjamin Root, MD, author

University Press of Mississippi
3825 Ridgewood Road   601-432-6205
Jackson, MS 39211-6492   Fax: 601-432-6217
                                          e-mail: kburgess@ihl.state.ms.us
                                                  www.upress.state.ms.us
A patients guide to panic disorders, panic attacks, and other stress-related maladies.
2000 128 pages Paperback
ISBN: 1-578062-45-4
Kathy Burgess, Advertising/Marketing Services Manager

6128 Victims of Dementia
Haworth Press
10 Alice Street   607-722-5857
Binghamton, NY 13904-1580   800-429-6784
                                             Fax: 607-722-0012
                                          www.haworthpress.com

Provides an in-depth look at the concept, construction and operation of Wesley Hall, a special living area at the Chelsea United Methodist retirement home in Michigan.
1993 155 pages Hardcover
ISBN: 1-560242-64-0

6129 Way to Go: School Success for Children wit h Mental Health Care Needs
Bazelon Center for Mental Health Law
1101 15th Street NW   202-467-5730
Washington, DC 20005-5002   Fax: 202-223-0409
                                                TDD: 202-467-4342
                                       e-mail: pubs@bazelon.org
                                              www.bazelon.org
A report and fact sheets that document how states and school districts have successfully combined school-wide positive behavior support (PBS) with effective mental health services to foster a school environment that is conducive to learning, and improves children's lives. Order book and fact sheets sheets seperately or together. Pricing according to volume begins at $25 per book, $10 per fact sheet, or $29 for the combination.
1998
Lee Carly, Communications Director

6130 What

6131 What Fair Housing Means for People with Disabilities
Bazelon Center for Mental Health Law
1101 15th Street NW   202-467-5730
Washington, DC 20005-5002   Fax: 202-223-0409
                                                TDD: 202-467-4342
                                       e-mail: pubs@bazelon.org
                                              www.bazelon.org
Explains in plain language how three federal laws protect the housing rights of people with mental or physical disabilities. 2003 edition available as pdf download.
2006 56 pages
Lee Carly, Communications Director

6132 When Madness Comes Home
National Alliance for the Mentally Ill
PO Box 753   301-524-7600
Waldorf, MD 20604-0753   Fax: 301-843-0159
                                                www.NAMI.org
Personal accounts offer first-hand, day-to-day experiences with mental illness of a sibling (mostly) and partner/spouse (briefly) and discuss the effects of growing up in a family whose energies are focused on an ill family member.
1997

6133 When Someone You Love Has a Mental Illness
National Alliance for the Mentally Ill
PO Box 753   703-524-7600
Waldorf, MD 20604-0753   Fax: 703-524-9094
                                                www.NAMI.org
Excellent for families recently stricken with severe mental illness.

Children's Books

6134 Compassion Books, Inc.
7036 State Highway 80 South   828-675-5909
Burnsville, NC 28714-7569   800-970-4220
                                                Fax: 828-675-9687
                          e-mail: orders@compassionbooks.com
                                         www.compassionbooks.com
Hand picked resources to help people through loss, grief and changes of all kinds. Carry over 400 books and videos on death and dying, bereavement and change, comfort and healing, hope and much more.
Bruce Greene, VP

Magazines

6135 AJMR
American Association on Mental Retardation

444 N Capitol Street NW   202-387-1968
Washington, DC 20001-1508   800-424-3688
                                                Fax: 202-387-2193
                                 e-mail: AAMR@access.digex.net
                                              www.aamr.org
Provides information on the latest program advances, current research, and information on products and services in the developmental disabilities field.
BiMonthly

6136 American Journal of Psychiatry
American Psychiatric Association
1400 K Street NW   202-682-6220
Washington, DC 20005-2492
Professional papers on topics in psychiatry.
Monthly
Public Affairs, Division

6137 American Psychologist
American Psychological Association
750 First Street NE   202-336-5510
Washington, DC 20002-4242   800-374-2721
                                                Fax: 202-336-5502
                                                TDD: 202-336-6123
                                        e-mail: books@apa.org
                                               www.apa.org
Articles on current issues in psychology as well as empirical, theoretical and practical articles on broad aspects of psychology.
9x a year

6138 Journal of Clinical Psychology
Clinical Psychology Publishing Company
4 Conant Square   802-247-6877
Brandon, VT 05733-1018
Scholarly research reports in the field of psychology.

6139 Mental Retardation
American Association on Mental Retardation
444 N Capitol Street NW   202-387-1968
Washington, DC 20001-1508   800-424-3688
                                                Fax: 202-387-2193
                                 e-mail: AAMR@access.digex.net
                                              www.aamr.org
Provides information on the latest program advances, current research, and information on products and services in the developmental disabilities field.
BiMonthly

6140 Psychopharmacology Bulletin
Superintendent of Documents/NIMH Journal
PO Box 371954   202-512-2250
Pittsburgh, PA 15250-7954
Emphasizes rapid, informal dissemination of recent research findings that have not previously appeared in the more formal literature.
Quarterly

6141 Psychosocial Rehabilitation Journal
Int'l Assoc. of Psychosocial Rehab. Services
730 Commonwealth Avenue   617-353-3549
Boston, MA 02215-1209
Discusses issues, programs and research on psychiatric rehabilitation.

Newsletters

6142 ACMH Newsletter
Association for Children's Mental Health
1705 Coolidge Road   517-336-7222
East Lansing, MI 48823-1735   800-782-0883
Offers the latest information, including unmet needs and notices of relevant agency and legislative activities, hearings, public meetings and other opportunities for promoting children's mental health.
Quarterly
Gail Allen, Director
Marla Holle, Parent Advocate

6143 Advocate
National Alliance for the Mentally Ill
200 N Glebe Road   703-524-7600
Arlington, VA 22203-3754   Fax: 703-524-9094
Offers reviews of books, medical information, legislative information and Alliance activities for persons with mental illness, their families and professionals who work with them.
Quarterly

6144 Mental Health Law News
Interwood Publications
PO Box 20241   513-221-3715
Cincinnati, OH 45220-0241
Mental health case law summaries.
6 pages Monthly
ISBN: 0-889017-0 -
Frank J Bardack, Editor

6145 News & Notes
American Association on Mental Retardation
444 N Capitol Street NW   202-387-1968
Washington, DC 20001-1508   800-424-3688
                                     Fax: 202-387-2193
                                     e-mail: AAMR@access.digex.net
                                     www.aamr.org
Covers legislative, program, and research developments of interest to the field, as well as international news, Association activities, job ads and other classifieds, and upcoming events.
BiMonthly

Pamphlets

6146 14 Worst Myths About Recovered Mental Patients
National Institutes of Health
5600 Fishers Lane   301-496-4000
Rockville, MD 20857-0001   e-mail: NIHInfo@nih.gov
                                     www.nih.gov
Refutes false beliefs that stigmatize recovered mental patients and suggests ways that the public can help advance the truth.

6147 Bipolar Disorder
National Institutes of Health
5600 Fishers Lane   301-443-3706
Rockville, MD 20857-0001   Fax: 301-443-6349
A short booklet offering a concise description of this disorder, which is also called manic-depressive illness.

6148 Coping with Mental Illness in the Family
National Alliance for the Mentally Ill
PO Box 753   703-524-7600
Waldorf, MD 20604-0753   Fax: 703-524-9094
                                     www.NAMI.org
A handbook for families.

6149 Dual Diagnosis: Substance Abuse and Mental Illness
National Alliance for the Mentally Ill
PO Box 753   703-524-7600
Waldorf, MD 20604-0753   Fax: 703-524-9094
                                     www.NAMI.org
A booklet for families and consumers.

6150 Helping Families Understand PTSD
National Veterans Services Fund
PO Box 2465   203-656-0003
Darien, CT 06820-0465   Fax: 203-656-1957
                                     e-mail: NatVetSvc@aol.com
Pamphlet

6151 Let's Talk Facts About Childhood Disorders
American Psychiatric Association
1400 K Street NW   202-682-6220
Washington, DC 20005-2492
Offers information on depression and depressive disorders including the causes, symptoms, treatments, anxiety, and various other phobias.
Public Affairs, Division

6152 Mental Health Problems of Vietnam Veterans
National Veterans Services Fund

PO Box 2465   203-656-0003
Darien, CT 06820-0465   Fax: 203-656-1957
                                     e-mail: NatVetSvc@aol.com
Pamphlet

6153 Minority Advocacy Notebook
Bazelon Center for Mental Health Law
1101 15th Street NW   202-467-5730
Washington, DC 20005-5002   Fax: 202-223-0409
                                     TDD: 202-467-4342
                                     e-mail: pubs@bazelon.org
                                     www.bazelon.org
Selected materials and models from our manual on outreach and advocacy for African Americans and Latinos with mental disabilities; includes Impediments to Services and Advocacy for Black and Hispanic People with Mental Illness.
1998
Lee Carly, Communications Director

6154 New Challenge: Responding to Families
Federation for Children with Special Needs
95 Berkeley Street   617-482-2915
Boston, MA 02116-6230   800-331-0688
Addresses the needs of children with emotional, behavioral and mental disorders and their families.

6155 PTSD and the Family: Secondary Traumatization
National Veterans Services Fund
PO Box 2465   203-656-0003
Darien, CT 06820-0465   Fax: 203-656-1957
                                     e-mail: NatVetSvc@aol.com
Pamphlet

6156 Plain Talk About...Dealing with the Angry Child
Superintendent of Documents
PO Box 371954   202-512-2250
Pittsburgh, PA 15250-7954
A flyer that offers suggestions for helping children cope with their anger in a healthy and constructive way.

6157 Plain Talk About...Handling Stress
Superintendent of Documents
PO Box 371954   202-512-2250
Pittsburgh, PA 15250-7954
Information on stress and how you can make it work for you rather than against you.

6158 Psychotherapy with Traumatized Vietnam Combatants
National Veterans Services Fund
PO Box 2465   203-656-0003
Darien, CT 06820-0465   Fax: 203-656-1957
                                     e-mail: NatVetSvc@aol.com
Pamphlet

6159 Triumph Over Fear
National Alliance for the Mentally Ill
PO Box 753   703-524-7600
Waldorf, MD 20604-0753   Fax: 703-524-9094
                                     www.NAMI.org
Step-by-step treatment plans for the many faces of phobias, panic disorder, obsessive-compulsive disorder, and post-traumatic stress. Includes case histories.
1994 Softcover

Audio & Video

6160 And After Tomorrow
G. Allan Roeher Institute
4700 Keele Street   416-661-9611
Downsview, ON, M3J 1P3,
A film about lives of people with a mental handicap and their families, in which parents and friends speak candidly about their personal experiences.
Films

6161 With a Little Help from My Friends
L'institut Roeher Institute
York University, 4700 Keele Street   416-661-9611
North York, ON, M3J 1P3,   Fax: 416-661-5701

This three-part video provides insight into inclusive education for people with mental handicaps.

Web Sites

6162 American Psychological Association

www.apa.org

Mission is to advance psychology as a science and professional organization that represents psychology in the United States.

6163 Coalition of Voluntary Mental Health Agencies

www.cvmha.org/

An umbrella advocacy organization of New York's mental health community, representing over 100 non-profit community based mental health agencies that serve more than 300,000 clients in the five boroughs of New York City and its environs.

6164 Community Access

www.cairn.org/

A nonprofit agency providing housing and advocacy for people with psychiatric disabilities.

6165 Federation of Families for Children's Mental Health

www.ffcmh.org/

Providing leadership to develop and sustain a nationwide network of family-run organizations.

6166 Healing Well

www.healingwell.com

An online health resource guide to medical news, chat, information and articles, newsgroups and message boards, books, disease-related web sites, medical directories, and more for patients, friends, and family coping with disabling diseases, disorders, or chronic illnesses.

6167 Health Finder

www.healthfinder.gov

Searchable, carefully developed web site offering information on over 1000 topics. Developed by the US Department of Health and Human Services, the site can be used in both English and Spanish.

6168 Healthlink USA

www.healthlinkusa.com

Health information concerning treatment, cures, prevention, diagnosis, risk factors, research, support groups, email lists, personal stories and much more. Updated regularly.

6169 Helios Health

www.helioshealth.com

Online resource for your health information. Detailed information about specific health topics, access to expert advice from our Medical Advisory Board, and up-to-date health news.

6170 Internet Mental Health

www.mentalhealth.com

A site whose goal is to improve understanding, diagnosis, and treatment of mental illness throughout the world. Includes information on specific disorders, medications, diagnosis, research, news, and other internet links.

6171 MedicineNet

www.medicinenet.com

An online resource for consumers providing easy-to-read, authoritative medical and health information.

6172 Medscape

www.medscape.com

Medscape offers specialists, primary care physicians, and other health professionals the Web's most robust and integrated medical information and educational tools.

6173 Mental Health America (formerly NMHA) Information Center

www.mentalhealthamerica.net

Provides informational materials, lobbies for Federal mental health legislation, stimulates funding of research on the causes and treatment of mental illnesses.

6174 National Alliance for the Mentally Ill

www.nami.org

Over 900 affiliate groups nationwide offer support to members, advocate better lives for their loved ones, support research efforts and educate the public to reduce the stigma attached to serious mental illnesses.

6175 National Mental Health Services Knowledge Exchange Network

www.mentalhealth.org

Leading the national system that delivers mental health services. Provides the treatment and support services neede by adults with mental disorders and children with serious emotional problems.

6176 WebMD

www.webmd.com

Information on mental illness, including articles and resources.

6177 World Federation for Mental Health

www.wfmh.com

Mission is to promote, among all people and nations, the highest possible level of mental health in its broadest biological, medical, educational, and social aspects.

Description

6178 Mental Illness/Depression

Depression is a mood disorder that can cause marked impairment of physical and social function and work capacity. It differs from normal grief which occurs in response to a significant separation or loss. It affects twice as many women as men and is more common in people with a family history of depression.

Research is gathering evidence of the relationship between depression and chemical imbalances in the brain. Clinical depression can also be associated with medication or other physical illnesses.

Common symptoms associated with depression include irritability, sleeping problems, changes in appetite, sadness, apathy, loss of interest in previously enjoyed activities and anxiety. Depression frequently disrupts a person's relationship with friends, family members and colleagues. It is also associated with alcohol and substance abuse. Suicide is the cause of death in approximately 15 percent of untreated patients.

Treatment must be tailored to the individual and can include talk therapy and/or medication. Newer groups of antidepressant medications have markedly improved the success of treatment. Patient and family education can play a crucial role. See also *Mental Illness/General and Mental Illness/Schizophrenia.*

National Agencies & Associations

6179 American Counseling Association
5999 Stevenson Avenue
Alexandria, VA 22304
800-347-6647
Fax: 800-473-2329
e-mail: webmaster@counseling.org
www.counseling.org
The American Counseling Association is a non-profit professional and educational organization that is dedicated to the growth and enhancement of the counseling profession. Founded in 1952 ACA is the world's largest such association.
Cirecie A West, President
Robert L Smith, President Elect

6180 American Psychiatric Association
1000 Wilson Boulevard
Arlington, VA 22209-3901
703-907-7300
888-357-7924
e-mail: apa@psych.org
www.psychiatry.org
The American Psychiatric Association is a medical specialty society recognized world wide. Its over 35,000 U.S. and international member physicians work together to ensure humane care and effective treatment for all persons with mental disorders.
Jeffrey Lieberman, MD, President

6181 Anxiety Disorders Association of America
8701 Georgia Avenue
Silver Spring, MD 20910
240-485-1001
Fax: 240-485-1035
e-mail: information@adaa.org
www.adaa.org
The Anxiety Disorders Association (ADAA) is a non profit organization whose mission is to promote the prevention treatment and cure of anxiety disorders and to improve the lives of all people who suffer from them.
Terence M Keane, PhD, President
Alies Muskin, Executive Director

6182 Brain & Behavior Research Foundation
60 Cutter Miller Road
Great Neck, NY 11021-3104
516-829-0091
800-829-8289
Fax: 516-487-6930
e-mail: info@bbrfoundation.org
www.bbrfoundation.org/
NARSAD Information and helpline staff is available to answer basic questions about the symptoms, causes and treatments of psychiatric illnesses. Information on support groups and other mental health organizations can also be provided.
Steve Lieber, Chairman of the Board
Jeffrey Borenstein, M.D., President & CEO

6183 Mental Health America
PO Box 17598
Baltimore, MD 21297-2257
800-239-1265
Fax: 443-782-0739
e-mail: info@ifred.org
www.ifred.org
Founded in 1983 to correct the myths and misconceptions surrounding the illness and help reverse the devastating effects depression has on the individual and our society. NAFDI's purpose is to educate the public and primary health care providers.
Kathryn Goetzke, Founder
Tom Dean, Chairman of the Board

6184 National Alliance On Mental Illness
3803 N. Fairfax Drive
Arlington, VA 22203
703-524-7600
800-950-6264
Fax: 703-524-9094
TDD: 703-516-7227
www.nami.org
Membership organization with over 858 affiliates in 50 states, offers newsletters, a mail-order bookstore and many programs, conferences, symposia and groups meetings for family members and patients.
Keris Jan Myrick, President
Jim Payne, Vice President

6185 National Anxiety Foundation
3135 Custer Drive
Lexington, KY 40517-4001
606-272-7166
www.lexington-on-line.com/naf.html
Offers information and help to persons with panic disorders manic and depressive disorders and mental illness.
Stephen Cox, President
Linda Vernon Blair, Vice-President

6186 National Mental Health Association
2000 N Beauregard Street
Alexandria, VA 22311
703-684-7722
800-969-6642
Fax: 703-684-5968
TTY: 800-433-5959
e-mail: infoctr@nmha.org
www.mentalhealthamerica.net
Serves over 700 affiliates nationally providing information publications and other services.
Ann Boughtin, Chair of the Board
Eric Ashton, Vice-Chair

6187 National Mental Health Information Center
2000 N Beauregard Street
Alexandria, VA 22311
703-684-7722
800-969-6642
Fax: 703-684-5968
TTY: 866-889-2647
TDD: 866-889-2647
e-mail: nmhic-info@samhsa.hhs.gov
www.mentalhealthamerica.net
The Center for Mental Health Services (CMHS) is charged with leading the national system that delivers mental health services. The goal of this system is to provide the treatment and support services needed by adults and children with mental disorders.
Ann Boughtin, Chair of the Board
Eric Ashton, Vice-Chair

6188 Option Institute
2080 S Undermountain Road   413-229-2100
Sheffield, MA 01257   800-714-2779
Fax: 413-229-8931
e-mail: participantsupport@option.org
www.option.org
Self-defeating beliefs, along with attitudes and judgments can lead to depression and a host of physical and psychological challenges. The Option Institute offers programs designed to help uproot self-defeating beliefs and remove roadblocks to happiness.
Barry Neils Kaufman, Co-Founder/ Co-Director
Samahria Lyte Kaufman, Co-Founder/ Co-Director

6189 Screening For Mental Health
Screening For Mental Health
One Washington Street   781-239-0071
Wellesley Hills, MA 02481   Fax: 781-431-7447
e-mail: smhinfo@mentalhealthscreening.org
www.mentalhealthscreening.org
Screening for Mental Health (SHM) is the non-profit organization that first introduced the concept of large-scale mental health screenings with its flagship program National Depression Screening Day in 1991. SHM programs now include both in-person and online.
Douglas George Jacobs, President & Medical Director
Effie Malley, Executive Director

Research Centers

6190 University of Pennsylvania: Depression Research Unit
School of Medicine
Department of Psychiatry   215-662-3462
Philadelphia, PA 19104   Fax: 215-662-6443
Focuses on mental health and depression.
Jay D MD, Chairman
Alex Cabrera, Clinic Manager

6191 University of Texas Mental Health Clinical Research Center
University of Texas
5323 Harry Hines Boulevard   214-645-8300
Dallas, TX 75390   Fax: 214-645-7999
e-mail: news@utsouthwester.edu
www.utsouthweseRN.edu
Research activity of major and atypical depression.
Daniel K Podolsky, MD, President
J. Gregory Fitz, Executive Vice President

6192 Yale University: Behavioral Medicine Clinic
Yale School of Medicine
333 Cedar Street
New Haven, CT 06510   203-432-7960
www.medicine.yale.edu
Focuses on mental disorders including schizophrenia and depression.
Peter Salovey, President
Richard Belitsky, Deputy Dean for Education

6193 Yale University: Ribicoff Research Facilities/CT Mental Health Center
34 Park Street   203-789-7300
New Haven, CT 06511   Fax: 203-562-7079
Clinical research in the areas of schizophrenia depression and mental disorders.
George Henin Ashenden, President

Support Groups & Hotlines

6194 Depression and Bipolar Support Alliance
730 N Franklin Street   312-642-0049
Chicago, IL 60654   800-826-3632
Fax: 312-642-7243
e-mail: adoederlein@dbsalliance.org
www.dbsalliance.org

Consists of approximately 900 patient groups providing support and direct services to persons with clinical depression and/or bipolar disorder.
Lucinda Jewell, Chair
Allen Doederlein, President

6195 National Health Information Center
PO Box 1133   310-565-4167
Washington, DC 20013   800-336-4797
Fax: 301-984-4256
e-mail: info@nhic.org
www.health.gov/nhic
Offers a nationwide information referral service, produces directories and resource guides.
Steele, President
Paul F Dell PhD, President-Elect

Books

6196 Columbia University Complete Home Guide to Mental Health
Henry Holt & Company
115 W 18th Street   212-886-9200
New York, NY 10011-4113   Fax: 212-633-0748
A compendium of information on all aspects of mental health; written primarily for the lay reader.
476 pages

6197 Coping with Depression and Mood Disorders
Rosen Publishing Group
29 E 21st Street   212-777-3017
New York, NY 10010   800-237-9932
Fax: 888-436-4643
e-mail: customerservice@rosenpub.com
www.rosenpublishing.com
With an emphasis on life's myriad difficulties, the authors help teens find practical ways to cope with depression.

ISBN: 0-823929-73-6
Lawrence Clayton PhD, Author
Sharon Carter, Author

6198 Depression Sourcebook
Brian P. Quinn, author
McGraw-Hill Companies
Returns Department
Dubuque, IA 52002   877-833-5524
Fax: 614-759-3749
e-mail: pbg.ecommerce_custserv@mcgrw-hill.com
www.mcgraw-hill.com
Everything anyone afflicted with a depressive disorder - or the people who care about them - need to know about unipolar and bipolar depression.
2000 288 pages
ISBN: 0-737303-79-4

6199 Depression and its Treatment
Warner Books
1271 Avenue of the Americas   212-522-7200
New York, NY 10020-1300
A layman's guide to help one understand and cope with America's #1 mental health problem.
157 pages

6200 Depressive Illnesses: Treatments Bring New Hope
Superintendent of Documents
PO Box 371954   202-512-2250
Pittsburgh, PA 15250-7954
Offers the general public an overview of the various depressive illnesses. Topics include causes, symptoms and types of depression, clinical evaluation and treatment, helpful suggestions for family and friends, and other sources of information.
28 pages

6201 Encyclopedia of Depression
Facts on File
11 Penn Plaza   212-967-8800
New York, NY 10001   800-322-8755
Fax: 800-678-3633

This volume defines and explains all terms and topics relating to depression.
170 pages Hardcover

6202 Essential Guide to Psychiatric Drugs
St. Martin's Press
175 5th Avenue   212-674-5151
New York, NY 10010-7848   800-221-7945
                                       Fax: 212-420-9314
Basic information on 123 drugs used for depression, anxiety and bipolar illness.

6203 Everything You Need to Know About Depression
Rosen Publishing Group
29 E 21st Street   212-777-3017
New York, NY 10010   800-237-9932
                                       Fax: 888-436-4643
                   e-mail: customerservice@rosenpub.com
                              www.rosenpublishing.com
An important resource for teens who are looking for help with depression.
Grades 7-12
ISBN: 0-823934-39-X
Elanor H Ayer, Author

6204 Inside Manic Depression
Sunnyside Press
PO Box 1717   619-424-3348
San Marcos, CA 92079-1717
The true story of one victim's triumph over despair. A first person account.
176 pages

6205 Medical Management of Depression
EMIS Medical Publishers
PO Box 1607   580-924-0643
Durant, OK 74702-1607   800-225-0694
                                       Fax: 580-924-9414

ISBN: 0-929240-62-6

6206 Mood Apart
Basic Books
10 E 53rd Street   212-207-7057
New York, NY 10022-5244
An overview of the depression and manic depression and the available treatments for them.
363 pages

6207 Overcoming Depression
Harper & Row
10 E 53rd Street   212-207-7000
New York, NY 10022-5299
318 pages Paperback

6208 Panic Disorder in the Medical Setting
Superintendent of Documents
PO Box 371954   202-512-2250
Pittsburgh, PA 15250-7954
This book serves the primary care physicians as a helpful guide in recognizing and treating panic disorder in patients and in identifying those who need psychiatric consultation or rerferrals.
1993 135 pages

6209 Pastoral Care of Depression
The Haworth Press
10 Alice Street   607-722-5857
Binghamton, NY 13904-1580   800-429-6784
                                       Fax: 607-895-0582
                       e-mail: getinfo@haworth.com
                                  www.haworth.com
Helps caregivers by overcoming the simplistic myths about depressive disorders and probing the real issues.
Paperback
ISBN: 0-789002-65-5

6210 Prozac Nation: Young & Depressed in America: A Memoir
Houghton Mifflin Company
Wayside Road
Burlington, MA 01803   800-225-3362

Struck with depression at 11, now 27, Wurtzel chronicles her struggle with the illness. Witty, terrifying and sometimes funny, it tells the story of a young life almost destroyed by depression.
317 pages

6211 Psychotherapy of Severe and Mild Depression
Jason Aronson
PO Box 15100
York, PA 17405-7100   800-782-0015
                                       Fax: 201-840-7242
                                          www.aronson.com

464 pages Softcover
ISBN: 1-568211-46-5

6212 Questions & Answers About Depression & Its Treatment
Ivan K Goldberg, MD, author

Charles Press Publishers
PO Box 15715   215-561-2786
Philadelphia, PA 19103-0715   Fax: 215-561-0191
                  e-mail: mailbox@charlespresspub.com
                              www.charlespresspub.com
All the questions you'd like to ask, asked and answered.
139 pages
ISBN: 0-914783-68-8

6213 Report of the Secretary's Task Force on Youth Suicide, Volume 1
Superintendent of Documents
PO Box 371954   202-512-2250
Pittsburgh, PA 15250-7954
A comprehensive review of information about youth suicide. The task force recommendations are presented in Volume 1.
110 pages

6214 Touched with Fire:- Manic Depressive Illness & the Artistic Temperment
Free Press
866 3rd Avenue
New York, NY 10022-6221   Fax: 800-943-9831
                                        www.simonsays.com
Describing and discussing the markedly increased rates of severe mood disorders and suicides among the artistically creative and the reasons why.
370 pages

6215 Winter Blues
Norman E Rosenthal, author

Guilford Press
72 Spring Street
New York, NY 10012-4019   800-265-7006
                                       Fax: 212-966-6708
                            e-mail: info@guilford.com
                                    www.guilford.com
Complete information about Seasonal Affective Disorder and its treatment.
2005
ISBN: 1-593852-14-2

6216 Women and Depression
Springer Publishing Company
536 Broadway   212-431-4370
New York, NY 10012-3955   877-687-7476
                                       Fax: 212-941-7842
                     e-mail: marketing@springerpub.com
                                 www.springerpub.com
This volume examines depression in women within a developmental context. It ranges from issues in childhood and adolescence through premenstrual syndrome and postpartum depression to issues of menopause and aging.
328 pages Hardcover
ISBN: 0-826151-40-X
Annette Imperati, Marketing Director

6217 Yesterday's Tomorrow
Hazelden
15251 Pleasant Valley Road   651-257-4010
Center City, MN 55012-9640   800-328-9000
                                       Fax: 651-213-4426
                                       www.hazelden.org

A meditation book that shows why and how recovery works, from the author's own experiences.
432 pages Paperback
ISBN: 1-568381-60-3

Children's Books

6218   Compassion Books, Inc.
7036 State Highway 80 South   828-675-5909
Burnsville, NC 28714-7569   800-970-4220
                                            Fax: 828-675-9687
e-mail: orders@compassionbooks.com
www.compassionbooks.com
Hand picked resources to help people through loss, grief and changes of all kinds. Carry over 400 books and videos on death and dying, bereavement and change, comfort and healing, hope and much more.
Bruce Greene, VP

Newsletters

6219   NFDI Newsletter
National Foundation for Depressive Illness
PO Box 2257   212-268-4260
New York, NY 10116-2257   800-248-4344
                                            Fax: 212-268-4434
e-mail: pross@att.net
www.depression.org
To correct the myths and misconceptions surrounding the illness and help reverse the devastating effects depression has on the individual and our society and to inform the public, primary health care providers, other healthcare professionals and corporations about depression and manic depression and to provide the information about correct diagnosis and treatment and the availability of qualified doctors and support groups.
4 pages Quarterly

Pamphlets

6220   Depression is a Treatable Illness: A Patients Guide
Department of Health & Human Services
2101 E Jefferson Street   301-217-1245
Rockville, MD 20852-4908
Tells about major depressive disorder, which is only one form of depressive illness. This booklet answers important questions regarding this disorder and gives information on where to go for more help.

6221   If You're Over 65 and Feeling Depressed...
National Institutes on Mental Health
5600 Fishers Lane   301-443-3706
Rockville, MD 20857-0001   Fax: 301-443-6349
Many older people believe that their age alone is responsible for feelings of exhaustion, helplessness and worthlessness. This brochure discusses the causes of depression in the older years, symptoms, types of treatment and where to go for help.
12 pages

6222   Let's Talk About Depression
Superintendent of Documents
PO Box 371954   202-512-2250
Pittsburgh, PA 15250-7954
Targeted especially for inner-city youth. The colorful design will capture attention and focus on depression in a way that young people will understand and identify with.

6223   Lithium and Manic Depression
Lithium Info. Center-Dean Foundation for Health
8000 Excelsior Drive   608-836-8070
Madison, WI 53717-1972
A guidebook about lithium and its effects on bipolar affective disorders and manic depression.
1992 32 pages

6224   Living Without Depression & Manic Depression: A Workbook
National Alliance for the Mentally Ill

PO Box 753
Waldorf, MD 20604-0753   703-524-7600
www.NAMI.org
Workbook offering checklists and helpful advice targeted for individuals whose depressive illness is stabilized.
1994

6225   Panic Disorder
National Institutes of Health
5600 Fishers Lane   301-443-3706
Rockville, MD 20857-0001   Fax: 301-443-6349
Written for the lay public, this pamphlet contains a description of panic disorder, gives the symptoms, describes treatment methods, and encourages the person who has the symptoms to seek treatment.

6226   Plain Talk About Depression
Superintendent of Documents
PO Box 371954   202-512-2250
Pittsburgh, PA 15250-7954
A flyer discussing types of depression, major depression, symptoms and causes.

6227   Understanding Panic Disorder
National Institutes of Health
5600 Fishers Lane   301-443-3706
Rockville, MD 20857-0001   Fax: 301-443-6349
Offers information on what an panic disorder is, symptoms, causes, treatment, medications and therapy.

6228   Useful Information on Phobias and Panic
Superintendent of Documents
PO Box 371954   202-512-2250
Pittsburgh, PA 15250-7954
This booklet provides information on both phobias and panic. Symptoms, causes and treatments of these disorders are referred to. If you know someone who is excessively fearful, this booklet will be of great help to them in understanding their problem.
40 pages 50 copies

6229   What to Do When a Friend is Depressed: Guide for Students
Superintendent of Documents
PO Box 371954   202-512-2250
Pittsburgh, PA 15250-7954
Offers information on depression and its symptoms and suggests things a young person can do to guide a depressed friend in finding help.

6230   What to Do When an Employee is Depressed: A Guide for Supervisors
Superintendent of Documents
PO Box 371954   202-512-2250
Pittsburgh, PA 15250-7954
A D/ART program brochure that will enable an employer to recognize the symptoms of depression in an employee and offers suggestions on what to say to the employee to encourage him or her to seek help.

Audio & Video

6231   Four Lives: A Portrait of Manic Depression
Fanlight Productions
4196 Washington Street   617-469-4999
Boston, MA 02131-1731   800-937-4113
                                            Fax: 617-469-3379
e-mail: fanlight@fanlight.com
www.fanlight.com
Four patients, families and psychiatrists share their perspectives on living with manic depression.
1987 60 Minutes
ISBN: 1-572950-29-3

6232   Taking Control of Depression

                                                 800-228-2495

Dramatic program offering new hope in the understanding and treatment of depression, with actor Ed Asner and Alan Xenakis, M.D.

6233 When Someone You Love Suffers from Depression
Medcom/Trainex

800-320-1444

Helping family and friends identify depression in a loved one - offers ways to help stop the suffering and get appropriate treatment.

Web Sites

6234 Healing Well

www.healingwell.com

An online health resource guide to medical news, chat, information and articles, newsgroups and message boards, books, disease-related web sites, medical directories, and more for patients, friends, and family coping with disabling diseases, disorders, or chronic illnesses.

6235 Health Finder

www.healthfinder.gov

Searchable, carefully developed web site offering information on over 1000 topics. Developed by the US Department of Health and Human Services, the site can be used in both English and Spanish.

6236 Healthlink USA

www.healthlinkusa.com

Health information concerning treatment, cures, prevention, diagnosis, risk factors, research, support groups, email lists, personal stories and much more. Updated regularly.

6237 Helios Health

www.helioshealth.com

Online resource for your health information. Detailed information about specific health topics, access to expert advice from our Medical Advisory Board, and up-to-date health news.

6238 MedicineNet

www.medicinenet.com

An online resource for consumers providing easy-to-read, authoritative medical and health information.

6239 Medscape

www.medscape.com

Medscape offers specialists, primary care physicians, and other health professionals the Web's most robust and integrated medical information and educational tools.

6240 National Anxiety Foundation

www.lexington-on-line.com/naf.html

Offers information and help to persons with panic disorders, manic and depressive disorders and mental illness.

6241 National Foundation for Depressive Illness

www.depression.org

Provide the information about correct diagnosis and treatment and the availability of qualified doctors and support groups.

6242 WebMD

www.webmd.com

Information on depression, including articles and resources.

Description

6243 Mental Illness/Schizophrenia

Schizophrenia is a chronic mental illness that is characterized by disturbances of thinking, feeling, and behavior. It usually begins in late adolescence or early adult life, with a lifetime prevalence between 0.2 to 1 percent. Despite its literal translation of split mind, schizophrenia is not the same as split personality. Although its specific cause is unknown, most cases of schizophrenia are believed to result from a complex interaction between biologic, inherited and environmental factors.

Symptoms of schizophrenia vary in type and severity and may include delusions and auditory hallucinations (hearing voices), incoherent thought patterns, catatonic behavior, and a flat or grossly inappropriate emotional state.

Drug treatment is the cornerstone of managing schizophrenia. When treated early, patients tend to respond quickly and more fully. Effective drugs have been available for several decades, and have revolutionized treatment of the disease. However, these drug treatments may be limited by side effects (especially movement disorders resembling Parkinsons disease) and by the patient's failure or refusal to stay on treatment. Patient non-compliance is sometimes addressed with long-acting injectable medications. A new class of drugs, lacking the Parkinson-like side effects, and sometimes dramatically more effective than previously used drugs, became available during the 1990s. Their use is limited by high costs and the threat of serious blood-related side effects. Treatment includes counseling, social support, rehabilitation, and skills retraining. Poor outcome frequently leads to extensive and long-term disability. Psychological and educational interventions can reduce the rate of relapse. People close to persons with schizophrenia are often very affected by the disease and can be helped by support and advocacy groups. See also *Mental Illness/General and Mental Illness/Depression.*

National Agencies & Associations

6244 International Society for the Study of Dissociation
8400 Westpark Drive
McLean, VA 22102
703-610-9037
Fax: 703-610-0234
e-mail: info@isst-d.org
www.issd.org
A nonprofit professional association that promotes research and training in the identification of treatment of multiple personality, provides professional and public education about multiple personality and initiates international communication among clinicians.
Joan Turkus, President
Philip J Kinsler, PhD, President-Elect

6245 NARSAD: Mental Health Research Association
60 Cutter Miller Road
Great Neck, NY 11021-3104
516-829-0091
800-829-8289
Fax: 516-487-6930
e-mail: info@bbrfoundation.org
www.bbrfoundation.org/
NARSAD Information and helpline staff is available to answer basic questions about the symptoms, causes and treatments of psychi-

atric illnesses. Information on support groups and other mental health organizations can also be provided.
Steve Lieber, Chairman of the Board
Jeffrey Borenstein, M.D., President & CEO

6246 National Alliance for the Mentally Ill
Colonial Place Three
2107 Wilson Boulevard
Arlington, VA 22201-3042
703-524-7600
800-950-6264
Fax: 703-524-9094
TDD: 703-516-7227
e-mail: membership@naminyc.org
www.nami-nyc-metro.org
Nonprofit, self-help, volunteer organization that offers practical support, useful education, advocacy, comfort and understanding to those in the greater New York area who suffer or have family members suffering from mental illnesses. Chapter of the National Alliance for the Mentally Ill and the New York State Alliance for the Mentally Ill.
Charolette Hoffer, MD PhD, President
Elizabeth Plante, Director, Huxley Institute

Research Centers

6247 Huxley Insititute-American Schizophrenic Association
86-B Dorchester Drive
Lakewood, NJ 08701
www.schizohprenia.org
The ASA works to bring effective, low-cost treatment to patients woth schizophrenia and help them in a cooperative effort to cope with the disorder.
Abram Carpenter Jr, Director
Vito J Seskunas, Deputy Director for Administration

6248 Maryland Psychiatric Research Center
655 W. Baltimore Street
Baltimore, MD 21201
410-402-7666
Fax: 410-788-3837
www.mprc.umaryland.edu/default.asp
Providing treatment to patients with schizophrenia and related disorders educating professionals and consumers about schizophrenia and conducting basic and translational research into the manifestations causes and treatment of schizophrenia.
Robert Buchanan, MD, Interim Director
Vito J Seskunas, Deputy Director for Administration

6249 National Alliance for Research on Schizophrenia and Depression
Grants Office
60 Cutter Mill Road
Great Neck, NY 11021
516-829-0091
800-829-8289
Fax: 516-487-6930
e-mail: info@bbrfoundation.org
www.bbrfoundation.org/
Research focusing on varieties of mental illness and mental disorders.
Steve Lieber, Chairman of the Board
Jeffrey Borenstein, M.D., President & CEO

6250 Schizophrenia Research Branch: Division of Clinical and Treatment Research
5600 Fisher Lane, Parklawn Building
Rockville, MD 20857
301-443-4707
Fax: 301-443-6000
Plans, supports, and conducts programs of research, research training, and resource development of schizophrenia and related disorders. Reviews and evaluates research developments in the field and recommends new program directors. Collaborates with organizations in and outside of the National Institue of Mental Health (NIMH) to stimulate work in the field through conferences and workshops.

6251 Tennessee Neuropsychiatric Institute Middle Tennessee Mental Health Institute
Middle Tennessee Mental Health Institute
221 Stewarts Ferry Pike
Nashville, TN 37217
615-902-7535
Michael Eber Andreassen MD, Director

6252 University of Iowa Mental Health Clinical Research Center
University of Iowa Hospitals & Clinics

200 Hawkins Drive
Iowa City, IA 52242

319-356-1553
877-575-2864
Fax: 319-353-8300
www.iowa-mhcrc.psychiatry.uiowa.edu

Schizophrenia studies and other cognitive disorder research.
Nancy C

Support Groups & Hotlines

6253 National Health Information Center
PO Box 1133
Washington, DC 20013

310-565-4167
800-336-4797
Fax: 301-984-4256
e-mail: info@nhic.org
www.health.gov/nhic

Offers a nationwide information referral service, produces directories and resource guides.
Rydell, Executive Director & CEO
Stephen M Sergay, President

Books

6254 Encyclopedia of Schizophrenia and the Psychotic Disorders
Facts on File
11 Penn Plaza
New York, NY 10001

212-967-8800
800-322-8755
Fax: 800-678-3633

This volume details recent theories and research findings on schizophrenia and psychotic disorders, together with a complete overview of the field's history.
368 pages Hardcover

6255 Experiences of Schizophrenia
Guilford Press
72 Spring Street
New York, NY 10012

800-365-7006
Fax: 212-966-6708
e-mail: info@guilford.com
www.guilford.com

This authoritative book presents new information on seasonal affective disorder. It includes remedies such as recent advances in light box therapy,research on the effectiveness of antidepressants, and new recipes to counterbalance unhealthy winter food cravings. This book also helps distinguish various degrees of the disorder ranging from winter blues to full blown SAD, and provides a self test that readers can use to evalutate their own seasonal mood changes.
2005 372 pages
ISBN: 1-593852-14-2

6256 Occupational Therapy Practice Guidelines for Adults with Schizophrenia
American Occupational Therapy Association
4720 Montgomery Lane
Bethesda, MD 20824-1220

301-652-2682
Fax: 301-652-7711
TDD: 800-377-8555
www.aota.org

24 pages
ISBN: 1-569001-53-7

6257 Return from Madness
Jason Aronson
PO Box 15100
York, PA 17405-7100

800-783-0015
www.aronson.com

256 pages Hardcover
ISBN: 1-568216-25-4

6258 Schizophrenia and Primitive Mental States
Jason Aronson
PO Box 15100
York, PA 17405-7100

800-782-0015
Fax: 201-840-7242
www.aronson.com

288 pages Softcover
ISBN: 0-765700-27-1

6259 Schizophrenia: From Mind to Molecule
American Psychiatric Press
1400 K Street NW
Washington, DC 20005-2403

202-682-6268
Fax: 202-789-2648

Presents a change in the scientific understanding and outlook regarding the devastating disorder of schizophrenia. It provides a thorough, up-to-date look at schizophrenia that includes neural behavioral studies, technologies and medical treatments.
274 pages Hardcover
ISBN: 0-880489-50-2

Children's Books

6260 Year it Rained
MacMillan Publishing Company
866 3rd Avenue
New York, NY 10022-6221

212-702-2000
www.mcp.com

The story of a girl traumatized by an alcoholic father and her desire to commit suicide. Hospitalized for schizophrenia, Elizabeth reaches a catharsis and, with the help of a poet, discovers that her talent and therapy may be in writing.
Grades 7-10

Magazines

6261 Dissociation
ISSMP&D
5700 Old Orchard Road
Skokie, IL 60077-1036

847-966-4322
Fax: 847-966-9418

A professional journal offering the latest information about the issues and research into multiple personalities and related disorders.

6262 Schizophrenia Bulletin
Superintendent of Documents/NIMH Journal
PO Box 371954
Pittsburgh, PA 15250-7954

202-512-2250

Serves as a forum for multidisciplinary exchange of information about schizophrenia and is exclusively devoted to the exploration of this severe disorder.
Quarterly

Newsletters

6263 ISSD News
Int'l Society for the Study of Dissociation
60 Revere Drive
Northbrook, IL 60062

847-480-0899
Fax: 847-480-9282
e-mail: issd@issd.org
www.issd.org

Includes current news from other onzations of interest to members, information about recent articles and books, news from US and international affiliates and the latest issues concerning multiple personality/dissociative states.
17 pages 6 times a year
Julie A Theander, Administrative Director
Richard Koepke, Executive Director

Pamphlets

6264 Schizophrenia
National Alliance for the Mentally Ill
200 N Glebe Road
Arlington, VA 22203-3754

703-524-7600
Fax: 703-524-9094

Part of the NAMI medical information series offering information on the causes, symptoms and treatments of Schizophrenia.

Web Sites

6265 Healing Well

www.healingwell.com

An online health resource guide to medical news, chat, information and articles, newsgroups and message boards, books, disease-related web sites, medical directories, and more for patients, friends, and family coping with disabling diseases, disorders, or chronic illnesses.

6266 Health Finder

www.healthfinder.gov

Searchable, carefully developed web site offering information on over 1000 topics. Developed by the US Department of Health and Human Services, the site can be used in both English and Spanish.

6267 Healthlink USA

www.healthlinkusa.com

Health information concerning treatment, cures, prevention, diagnosis, risk factors, research, support groups, email lists, personal stories and much more. Updated regularly.

6268 Helios Health

www.helioshealth.com

Online resource for your health information. Detailed information about specific health topics, access to expert advice from our Medical Advisory Board, and up-to-date health news.

6269 International Society for the Study of Dissociation

www.issd.org

Association that promotes research and training in the identification of treatment of multiple personality.

6270 MedicineNet

www.medicinenet.com

An online resource for consumers providing easy-to-read, authoritative medical and health information.

6271 Medscape

www.medscape.com

Medscape offers specialists, primary care physicians, and other health professionals the Web's most robust and integrated medical information and educational tools.

6272 National Alliance for the Mentally Ill

www.nami-nyc-metro.org

Organization that offers practical support, useful education, advocacy, comfort, and understanding to those in the greater New York area who suffer or have family members suffering from neurobiologically based disorders.

6273 Schizophrenia Therapy Online Resource Center

www.schizophreniatherapy.com

A website which provides effective and lasting alternatives to traditional treatment for individuals suffering with schizophrenia. Offers an effective and full continium of services ranging from psychopharmacology to individual and group psychotherapy to social rehabilitation, supported work experience, assertive community training and supported housing.

6274 WebMD

www.webmd.com

Information on schizophrenia, including articles and resources.

Description

6275 Migraine

Roughly 45 million Americans suffer from chronic headaches, the most disabling of which is migraine. Classified as a vascular headache, migraine headaches are caused by intracranial vasospasm, that is, alternating swelling and constricting of blood vessels on the surface of the brain. The swelling phase brings on intense pain and nausea, while the constricting phase may cause neurologic symptoms such as focal loss of vision or numbness involving one side of the body. Another theory is that migraines are due to a different dysfunction of the neurovascular system that results in the release of a substance that leads to migraine. More than 50 percent of patients have a family history of migraine. They also appear to have a hormonal component, being more common in women and often affected by menstrual cycles or pregnancy.

Management of migraine begins with careful observation for triggering agents like foods, alcohol, or irregular sleep patterns. Acute treatment to stop a migraine involves a class of drugs which antagonize the action of the 5-HT that aggravates the migraine process. They block inflammation and can abort migraine in about 70 percent of patients. Sumatriptan, the prototype, is available in oral and subcutaneous injection forms. Ergot drugs, also available in oral and injectable forms, work by helping the swollen blood vessels constrict down to normal size. If headaches become very frequent, doctors may recommend preventive therapy, which requires daily drug administration. Drugs used in this way include beta-blockers and calcium-channel blockers, which were originally developed for hypertension and heart disease, and certain medicines ordinarily used for depression or seizures.

Pain medication should be used sparingly. Nonsteroidal anti-inflammatory drugs, such as ibuprofen are best for mild to moderate headaches. Narcotic medications should be avoided except under special circumstances and with strict guidelines. Most migraine sufferers can be satisfactorily managed by their primary care physician or a neurologist, but in refractory cases a multi-disciplinary headache center may be of help.

Tension is the other common cause of disabling headaches. They are not migraine and are not considered vascular headache, but are mentioned here because they are so common. Some of the resources listed in this section may be helpful for persons with tension headache.

National Agencies & Associations

6276 American Academy of Neurology
201 Chicago Avenue
Minneapolis, MN 55415-2311
612-928-6000
800-879-1960
Fax: 612-454-2746
e-mail: memberservices@aan.com
www.aan.com

A professional organization representing neurologists worldwide.
Timothy A Pedley, President
Catherine M Rydell, Executive Director & CEO

6277 American Council for Headache Education
19 Mantua Road
Mount Royal, NJ 08061
856-423-0043
800-255-2243
Fax: 856-423-0082
e-mail: achehq@talley.com
www.achenet.com

A not-for-profit alliance of headache sufferers and physicians who are working together to improve the quality of care and the quality of information available to people with chronic or severe headache conditions.
Paul Winner, Chair
Dawn C Buse, PhD, Member of Committee

6278 American Headache Society
19 Mantua Road
Mount Royal, NJ 08061
856-423-0043
Fax: 856-423-0082
e-mail: ahshq@talley.com
www.americanheadachesociety.org/

Professional society of health care providers who study and treat headache and face pain. AHS brings physicians from various fields and specialties together to share concepts and developments about headache and related conditions.
Linda Lucas BA, Director

6279 Help for Headaches
515 Richmond Street
London, Ontario, N6A 5-5M3
519-434-0008
e-mail: brent@helpforheadaches.org
www.headache-help.org

A non-profit organization, and a registered Canadian charity that is committed to educational services for those suffering from and treating headaches.
G Brent Lucas, BA, Director

6280 Migraine Association of Canada
356 Bloor Street E
Toronto Ontario, M4W
416-920-4916
800-663-3557
Fax: 416-920-3677
www.migraine.ca

A registered charity funded through memberships. Activities include a 24 hour telephone information access line the development of materials and assistance for those who start community self-help groups, workplace seminars and awareness programs.
Coleman, President
Terri Miller Burchfield, Exec VP & Legislative Director

6281 Migraine Awareness Group: A National Understanding for Migraineurs
100 N Union Street
Alexandria, VA 22314
703-349-1929
Fax: 703-739-2432
e-mail: comments@migraines.org
www.migraines.org

Works to bring public awareness utilizing the electronic print and artistic mediums to the fact that migraine is a true organic neurological disease.
Michael John Coleman, President & Executive Director
Terri Miller Burchfield, Executive VP & Legislative Director

6282 National Headache Foundation
820 N Orleans
Chicago, IL 60610-3132
312-274-2650
888-NHF-5552
Fax: 312-640-9049
e-mail: info@headaches.org
www.headaches.org

A nonprofit organization established in 1970 dedicated to serve as an information resource to headache sufferers, their families and the healthcare providers who treat them. Promotes research into potential headache causes and treatments.
Seymour Diamond, MD, Founder & Executive Chairman
Arthur H Elkind, MD, President

Research Centers

6283 Baltimore Headache Institute
11 E Chase Street
Baltimore, MD 21202
Brian E Goldstein, Director

410-547-0200

6284 San Francisco Clinical Research Center
909 Hyde Street
San Francisco, CA 94109

415-673-4600
Fax: 415-673-9352
e-mail: SFHACLIN@aol.com
www.sfcrc.com

This research center also specializes in diagnosis of Alzheimer's related dementia in addition to migraine headaches.
Jerome Goldstein, M.D., Director
Guy Engelmann, M.D., Team Member

Support Groups & Hotlines

6285 National Health Information Center
PO Box 1133
Washington, DC 20013

310-565-4167
800-336-4797
Fax: 301-984-4256
e-mail: info@nhic.org
www.health.gov/nhic

Offers a nationwide information referral service, produces directories and resource guides.

Books

6286 Conquering Headache
Alan Rapoport, MD, author
B.C Decker, Inc.
50 King Street E, Floor 2 PO Box620
Ontario, Canada L8N 3K7,

905-522-7017
800-568-7281
Fax: 905-522-7839
e-mail: info@bcdecker.com
www.bcdecker.com

2003 128 pages Paperback
ISBN: 1-550092-33-2

6287 Freedom from Headaches
Simon & Schuster Order Department
200 Old Tappan Road
Old Tappan, NJ 07675-7095

800-999-5479

ISBN: 0-671254-04-9

6288 Handbook of Headache Disorders
Essential Medical Information Systems
PO Box 1607
Durant, OK 74702-1607

580-924-0643
800-225-0694
Fax: 580-924-9414

1993 Paperback
ISBN: 0-929240-62-6

6289 Handbook of Headache Management: A Practic al Guide to Diagnosis & Treatment
Williams & Wilkins
351 W Camden Street
Baltimore, MD 21201-7912

301-528-4000
800-638-0672
www.wwilkins.com

1993 224 pages
ISBN: 0-683058-01-0

6290 Migraine and Other Headaches: Vascular Mechanisms
Raven Press
1185 Avenue of the Americas
New York, NY 10036-2601

212-930-9500
800-777-2295
www.raven.com

Leading international experts present new concepts on the mechanisms of migraine and other vascular headaches and detail the latest strategies for diagnosis and treatment of migraine with and without aura, tension-type headaches, cluster headaches and other vascular disorders.
368 pages
ISBN: 0-881677-95-7

6291 Migraine: The Complete Guide
American Council for Headache Education
19 Mantua Road
Mount Royal, NJ 08061

856-423-0258
800-255-2243
Fax: 856-423-0082
e-mail: achehq@talley.com
www.achenet.org

A comprehensive resource book for people with migraine, their families and physicians (updated in 1999) by Lynne M Constantine, Suzanne Scott and ACHE.

6292 Overcoming Headaches & Migraines
Longmeadow Press
PO Box 10218
Stamford, CT 06904-1469
1993 128 pages Paperback
ISBN: 0-681417-92-7

203-352-2110

6293 Understanding Migrain and Other Headaches
Stewart J Tepper, MD, author
University Press of Mississippi
3825 Ridgewood Road
Jackson, MS 39211-6492

601-432-6205
Fax: 601-432-6217
e-mail: kburgess@ihl.state.ms.us
www.upress.state.ms.us

A comprehensive overview of causes, diagnoses, and treatments.
2004 112 pages Paperback
ISBN: 1-578065-92-5
Kathy Burgess, Advertising/Marketing Services Manager

6294 Wolff's Headaches & Other Head Pain
Oxford University Press
2001 Evans Road
Cary, NC 27513-2010

212-726-6000
800-451-7556
Fax: 919-677-1303
www.oup-usa.org

1993
ISBN: 0-195082-50-8

Newsletters

6295 Headache
American Council for Headache Education
19 Mantua Road
Mount Royal, NJ 08061

856-423-0258
800-255-2243
Fax: 856-423-0082
e-mail: achehq@talley.com
www.achenet.org

The ACHE 12 page quarterly newsletter provides valuable and current information on new treatments, as well as time proven headache management strategies. All articles are written or reviewed by headache experts from the American Headache Society (AHS). Recent issues have included articles by headache experts on drug and nondrug treatment options and information on new treatments and research is regularly included.
Quarterly

6296 NHF Head Lines
National Headache Foundation
820 N Orleans
Chicago, IL 60610-3132

312-640-5399
888-643-5552
Fax: 312-640-9049
e-mail: nhf1970@headaches.org
www.headaches.org

Offers the latest information on headaches, causes and treatments. Contains news on drugs and medical forums, in depth discussions of headaches and preventions and a question and answer section in which physicians respond to reader inquiries and support group information.
16 pages Quarterly

Pamphlets

6297 52 Proven Stress Reducers
National Headache Foundation

820 N Orleans
Chicago, IL 60610
888-643-5552
Fax: 312-640-9049
e-mail: nhf1970@headaches.org
www.headaches.org
Members only.
Suzanne Simons, Executive Director

6298   About Headaches
National Headache Foundation
820 N Orleans
Chicago, IL 60610
888-643-5552
Fax: 312-640-9049
e-mail: nhf1970@headaches.org
www.headaches.org
Contains an in depth look at headaches, tips on when to seek medical advice, methods of treatment and more.
16 pages
Suzanne Simons, Executive Director

6299   Analgesic Rebound Headaches: Fact Sheet
National Headache Foundation
820 N Orleans
Chicago, IL 60610
888-643-5552
Fax: 312-640-9049
e-mail: nhf1970@headaches.org
www.headaches.org
Offers information on analgesic agents or drugs used to control pain including migraine and other types of headaches.
Suzanne Simons, Executive Director

6300   Cluster Headache: Fact Sheet
National Headache Foundation
820 N Orleans
Chicago, IL 60610
888-643-5552
Fax: 312-640-9049
e-mail: nhf1970@headaches.org
www.headaches.org
Offers information on cluster headaches and the treatment available for them. This information sheet can be downloaded from the web site.
Suzanne Simons, Executive Director

6301   Diet and Headache: Fact Sheet
National Headache Foundation
820 N Orleans
Chicago, IL 60610
888-643-5552
Fax: 312-640-9049
e-mail: nhf1970@headaches.org
www.headaches.org
Offers information on what foods should be avoided and what foods trigger headaches in all migraine sufferers. This information sheet can be dowloaded from the web site.
Suzanne Simons, Executive Director

6302   Headache Facts: What Everyone Should Know
American Council for Headache Education
19 Mantua Road
Mount Royal, NJ 08061
856-423-0258
800-255-2243
Fax: 856-423-0082
e-mail: achehq@talley.com
www.achenet.org

6303   Headache Handbook
National Headache Foundation
820 N Orleans
Chicago, IL 60610
888-643-5552
Fax: 312-640-9049
e-mail: nhf1970@headaches.org
www.headaches.org
Gives information on causes and types of headaches as well as treatments available.
8 pages

6304   Headache in Children: Fact Sheet
National Headache Foundation

820 N Orleans
Chicago, IL 60610
888-643-5552
Fax: 312-640-9049
e-mail: nhf1970@headaches.org
www.headaches.org
Offers information on vascular headaches, tension-type headaches, traction and inflammatory headaches and treatment. This information sheet can be downloaded from the web site.
Suzanne Simons, Executive Director

6305   Hormones and Migraines: Fact Sheet
National Headache Foundation
820 N Orleans
Chicago, IL 60610
888-643-5552
Fax: 312-640-9049
e-mail: nhf1970@headaches.org
www.headaches.org
Offers information on the link between hormones and migraines.
Suzanne Simons, Executive Director

6306   How to Talk to Your Doctor About Headaches
National Headache Foundation
820 N Orleans
Chicago, IL 60610
888-643-5552
Fax: 312-640-9049
e-mail: nhf1970@headaches.org
www.headaches.org
Learn how to keep a headache diary to pinpoint symptoms and effective diagnosis.
Suzanne Simons, Executive Director

6307   Impact of Migraine: A Disabling and Costly Condition
American Council for Headache Education
19 Mantua Road
Mount Royal, NJ 08061
856-423-0258
800-255-2243
Fax: 856-423-0082
e-mail: achehq@talley.com
www.achenet.org

6308   Migraine and Coexisting Conditions: Other Illnesses That May Affect Migraine
American Council for Headache Education
19 Mantua Road
Mount Royal, NJ 08061
856-423-0258
800-255-2243
Fax: 856-423-0082
e-mail: achehq@talley.com
www.achenet.org

6309   Migraine: Fact Sheet
National Headache Foundation
820 N Orleans
Chicago, IL 60610
888-643-5552
Fax: 312-640-9049
e-mail: nhf1970@headaches.org
www.headaches.org
Offers information on migraines and treatments.
Suzanne Simons, Executive Director

6310   Tap the Best Resource
National Headache Foundation
820 N Orleans
Chicago, IL 60610
888-643-5552
Fax: 312-640-9049
e-mail: nhf1970@headaches.org
www.headaches.org
Informational brochure offering facts and statistics on headaches. Everything from muscle contraction, vascular headaches, sinus headaches, TMJ and much more.
Suzanne Simons, Executive Director

6311   Tension-Type Headache: Fact Sheet
National Headache Foundation
820 N Orleans
Chicago, IL 60610
888-643-5552
Fax: 312-640-9049
e-mail: nhf1970@headaches.org
www.headaches.org
Offers information on the least known type of headache, chronic tension-type headaches. This information sheet can be downloaded from the web site.

6312 **What's the Best Medicine for My Headaches?**
American Council for Headache Education
19 Mantua Road
Mount Royal, NJ 08061
856-423-0258
800-255-2243
Fax: 856-423-0082
e-mail: achehq@talley.com
www.achenet.org

Audio & Video

6313 **Relaxation Tape**
National Headache Foundation
820 N Orleans
Chicago, IL 60610
888-643-5552
Fax: 312-640-9049
e-mail: nhf1970@headaches.org
www.headaches.org
Contains techniques to assist the listener in experiencing greater self control and relaxation.
Audio Tape
Suzanne Simons, Executive Director

6314 **Stretch and Relax Tape**
National Headache Foundation
820 N Orleans
Chicago, IL 60610
888-643-5552
Fax: 312-640-9049
e-mail: nhf1970@headaches.org
www.headaches.org
Based on a series of progressive relaxation techniques which involve the tightening and relaxing of specific muscle groups.
Audio Tape
Suzanne Simons, Executive Director

Web Sites

6315 **American Academy of Neurology**
www.aan.com/
A professional organization representing neurologists worldwide.

6316 **American Council for Headache Education (ACHE)**
www.achenet.org
The ACHE website offers an extensive library of headache information, including a searchable database of past articles from our newsletter, discussion forums that provide virtual contact with leading headache specialists and fellow headache sufferers, a searchable database of physicians to find a specialist in your area and more.

6317 **American Headache Society**
www.ahsnet.org
The AHS website offers clinically oriented information on headache, as well as information on AHS programs and activities.

6318 **American Medical Association**
Journal of the American Medical Association
www.ama-assn.org/
An organized web site focusing on treatment options, education and support available to those suffering from migraine headaches.

6319 **Cluster Headaches**
www.clusterheadaches.com
A web site devoted completely and exclusively to those that suffer from cluster headaches.

6320 **Healing Well**
www.healingwell.com
An online health resource guide to medical news, chat, information and articles, newsgroups and message boards, books, disease-related web sites, medical directories, and more for patients, friends, and family coping with disabling diseases, disorders, or chronic illnesses.

6321 **Health Finder**
www.healthfinder.gov
Searchable, carefully developed web site offering information on over 1000 topics. Developed by the US Department of Health and Human Services, the site can be used in both English and Spanish.

6322 **Healthlink USA**
www.healthlinkusa.com
Health information concerning treatment, cures, prevention, diagnosis, risk factors, research, support groups, email lists, personal stories and much more. Updated regularly.

6323 **Helios Health**
www.helioshealth.com
Online resource for your health information. Detailed information about specific health topics, access to expert advice from our Medical Advisory Board, and up-to-date health news.

6324 **MedicineNet**
www.medicinenet.com
An online resource for consumers providing easy-to-read, authoritative medical and health information.

6325 **Medscape**
www.medscape.com
Medscape offers specialists, primary care physicians, and other health professionals the Web's most robust and integrated medical information and educational tools.

6326 **Medsupport**
www.medsupport.com
An up-to-date website dedicated towards giving the headache sufferer some important insights through the eyes of those who treat headache disorders.

6327 **Migraine Awareness Group: A National Understanding for Migraineurs**
www.migraines.org/
Works to bring public awareness, utilizing the electronic, print, and artistic mediums, to the fact that migraine is a true organic neurological disease.

6328 **National Headache Foundation**
www.headaches.org
Information for headache sufferers, their families, and the physicians who treat them.

6329 **Neurology Channel**
www.neurologychannel.com
Find clearly explained, medically accurate information regarding conditions, including an overview, symptoms, causes, diagnostic procedures and treatment options. On this site it is possible to ask questions and get information from a neurologist and connect to people who have similar health interests.

6330 **WebMD**
www.webmd.com
Information on migraine, including articles and resources.

Description

6331 Multiple Sclerosis

Multiple sclerosis, MS, is a chronic disease that affects the central nervous system and impairs many of its functions. Over 300,000 Americans have MS. Although its cause is unknown, an immunologic abnormality is suspected. There also appear to be both genetic and environmental factors involved. Interestingly, the incidence of MS increases the further one lives from the equator.

Age of onset is typically between 20 and 40 years, and women are affected somewhat more than men. MS destroys the protective myelin sheath that surrounds nerve fibers. This special sheath normally allows passage of electrical signals through the brain, spinal cord, and nerves of the body. The disease is characterized by remissions and recurring exacerbations. The clinical signs vary depending on the area of demyelination and can include: generalized or focal weakness; difficulty walking; clumsiness; slurred speech; easy fatigability; numbness and tingling; visual loss; incontinence (loss of bladder and bowel control); loss of sexual function; and problems with short-term memory, judgment, or reason.

Significant strides are being made in both treating and understanding MS. Currently there is no curative treatment, but corticosteroids, interferon and other new medications may shorten or prevent relapses.

Supportive treatment includes medications to control muscle spasticity, fatigue and pain. Maintaining a normal lifestyle is recommended, avoiding fatigue and exposure to excessive heat. Physical therapy may also be helpful. Because of the debilitating nature of MS, counseling, psychiatric support, and antidepressant medication may be warranted.

National Agencies & Associations

6332 Multiple Sclerosis Association of America
706 Haddonfield Road   856-488-4500
Cherry Hill, NJ 08002-2652   800-532-7667
                                           Fax: 856-661-9797
                            e-mail: webmaster@mymsaa.org
                                           www.mymsaa.org/
A national nonprofit organization dedicated to enriching the quality of life for everyone affected by multiple sclerosis.
Robert Manley, Chair
Sue Rehmus, Vice Chair

6333 Multiple Sclerosis Foundation
6350 N Andrews Avenue   954-776-6805
Fort Lauderdale, FL 33309   888-225-6495
                                           Fax: 954-938-8708
                               e-mail: admin@msfocus.org
                                           www.msfocus.org
Dedicated to helping create a brighter tomorrow for those with MS the foundation offers a wide array of free services including: national toll-free support, educational programs, homecare, support groups, assistive technology and publications.
Jules Kuperberg, Executive Director
Alan Segaloff, Executive Director

6334 National Institute of Neurological Disorders and Stroke
NIH Neurological Institute   301-496-5751
Bethesda, MD 20824   800-352-9424
                                           Fax: 301-402-2186
                                           TTY: 301-468-5981
                                           www.ninds.nih.gov
The mission of NINDS is to reduce the burden of neurological disease - a burden borne by every age group, by every segment of society, by people all over the world.
Story C Landis, PhD, Director
Walter J Koroshetz, M.D., Deputy Director

6335 National Multiple Sclerosis Society
733 3rd Avenue   212-986-3240
New York, NY 10017-3288   800-344-4867
                                           Fax: 212-986-7981
                                     e-mail: nat@nmss.org
                              www.nationalmssociety.org/
Serves persons with MS, their families, health professionals and the interested public. The Society provides funding for research, public and professional education, advocacy and the design of rehabilitative and psychosocial programs. Direct services to MS persons are provided through local chapters and branches. Among the services offered are counseling, referral, equipment loan and other support activities.
Eli Rubenstein, Chairman of the Board
Cynthia Zagieboylo, President & CEO

6336 Toronto Parents of Multiple Births Associa tion
790 Bay Street   416-760-3944
Toronto, Ontario, M5G 1-1N9   e-mail: info@tpomba.org
                                           www.tpomba.org
A not-for-profit self-help and support organization in Canada for parents of twins, triplets, and more.
Laura Daniel, Chapter President
Taylor Lander, Development Manager

State Agencies & Associations

Alabama

6337 National Multiple Sclerosis Society: Alabama Chapter
813 Shades Creek Parkway   205-879-8881
Birmingham, AL 35209   800-FIG-HTMS
                                           Fax: 205-879-8869
                                     e-mail: alc@nmss.org
                           www.nationalmssociety.org/alc
Dedicated to serving people with MS and their families by providing programs and services designed to enhance quality of life.
Frank D McPhillips, Chairman
Jan Bell, Chapter President

Alaska

6338 National Multiple Sclerosis Society: Alaska Chapter
511 W 41st Avenue   907-563-1115
Anchorage, AK 99503-6643   800-344-4867
                                           Fax: 907-562-6673
                                     e-mail: aka@nmss.org
                           www.nationalmssociety.org/aka
Nonprofit organization providing equipment loan, information and referral, leading library, self-help groups, advocacy, education, training, newsletter, educational programs, volunteer opportunities, exercise/aquatics, newly diagnosed support and educational material.
Gary Wells, Regional Development Manager
Pam McElrath, President, All American Chapter

Arizona

6339 National Multiple Sclerosis Society Desert Southwest Chapter
National Multiple Sclerosis Society
5025 E. Washington Street   480-968-2488
Phoenix, AZ 85034-2343   800-344-4867
                                           Fax: 602-966-4049
                                e-mail: info@aza.nmss.org
                               www.nationalmssociety.org
Serves Central and Northern Arizona.

Arkansas

6340 National Multiple Sclerosis Society: Arkansas Chapter
Evergreen Place
1100 N University Avenue   501-663-8104
Little Rock, AR 72207-6367   800-344-4867
                                            Fax: 501-666-4355
                                        e-mail: arr@nmss.org
                                    www.nationalmssociety.org/arr

Rick Selig, Division Manager

California

6341 Central California Chapter National Multiple Sclerosis Society
National Multiple Sclerosis Society
334 Shaw Avenue   209-325-9293
Clovis, CA 93612-3839   Fax: 209-325-9295
                                    www.nationalmssociety.org

Dan Dietrich, Development Director
Karen Nunn, Service Director

6342 National Multiple Sclerosis Society: Southern California Chapter
2440 S Sepulveda Boulevard   310-479-4456
Los Angeles, CA 90064   800-344-4867
                                            Fax: 310-479-4436
                                    e-mail: ms@cal.nmss.org
                                    www.nationalmssociety.org

Leon A LeBuffe, President

6343 National Multiple Sclerosis Society Channel Islands Chapter
14 W Valerio Street   805-682-8783
Santa Barbara, CA 93101   800-344-4867
                                            Fax: 805-563-1489
                                    e-mail: can_info@nmss.org
                                    www.nationalmssociety.org

Joan Young, Chapter President

6344 National Multiple Sclerosis Society: Silicon Valley Chapter
2589 Scott Boulevard   408-988-7557
Santa Clara, CA 95050-2508   800-344-4867
                                            Fax: 408-988-1816
                                    e-mail: cau@nmss.org
                                    www.nationalmssociety.org
Funds, researches and supports people with MS and their families
to end the devastating effects of multiple sclerosis.
Carla Hines, Chapter President
Michelle Spam-Allen, Program Director

6345 Northern California Chapter National Multiple Sclerosis Society
National Multiple Sclerosis Society
1700 Owens Street   415-230-6678
San Francisco, CA 94158   800-344-4867
                                            Fax: 415-230-6652
                                    e-mail: can_info@nmss.org
                                    www.nationalmssociety.org

David Hartman, Chapter President
Denise Casey, Director of Chapter Programs

6346 Orange County Chapter National Multiple Sclerosis Society
National Multiple Sclerosis Society
5950 La Place Court   760-448-8400
Carlsbad, CA 92008-5677   800-344-4867
                                            Fax: 949-833-3104
                                    e-mail: msinfo@mspacific.org
                                    www.nationalmssociety.org
Richard V Israel, Chapter President
Karen Hooper, Vice President Programs & Services

6347 San Diego Area Chapter National Multiple Sclerosis Society
National Multiple Sclerosis Society
12121 Scripps Summit Dr   619-974-8640
San Diego, CA 92131-1498   800-486-6762
                                            Fax: 760-804-9266
                                    e-mail: msinfo@mspacific.org
                                    www.nationalmssociety.org

Allan Shaw, Chapter President
Karen Barton, Service Director

Colorado

6348 National MS Society: Colorado Chapter
900 S Broadway   303-698-7400
Denver, CO 80209-3442   800-344-4867
                                            Fax: 303-698-7421
                                e-mail: co-wyreceptionist@nmss.org
                                www.nationalmssociety.org/chapters/COC/i
Carrie Nolan, President
Mary Ann Peters, Executive Assistant

Connecticut

6349 National MS Society: Greater Connecticut Chapter
659 Tower Avenue   860-913-2550
Hartford, CT 06112   800-344-4867
                                            Fax: 860-761-2466
                                e-mail: info@ctfightsMS.org
                                www.nationalmssociety.org/chapters/CTN/i
Lisa Gerrol, President and Chief Professional Officer
Cheryl Donati, Executive Vice President

Delaware

6350 National MS Society: Delaware Chapter
2 Mill Road   302-655-5610
Wilmington, DE 19806-2175   800-344-4867
                                            Fax: 302-655-0993
                                e-mail: kate.cowperthwait@msdelaware.org
                                www.nationalmssociety.org/chapters/DED/i
Provides the encouragement, materials and skills needed to
achieve and maintain a productive lifestyle with multiple sclerosis. The organization is a voluntary, nonprofit entity.
1100 members
Kate Cowperthwait, Chapter President
Helen Serbu, Director of Finance

District of Columbia

6351 National MS Society: National Capital Chapter
1800 M Street   202-296-5363
Washington, DC 20036-1003   800-344-4867
                                            Fax: 202-296-3425
                                e-mail: INFORMATION@MSandYOU.ORG
                                www.nationalmssociety.org/chapters/DCW/i
J Christophe Broullire, Chapter President
Kevin Dougherty, Vice President Programs and Services

Florida

6352 Central Florida Chapter
2701 Maitland Center Parkway   407-478-8880
Orlando, FL 32751-6726   800-344-4867
                                            Fax: 407-478-8893
                                e-mail: INFO@FLC.NMSS.ORG
                                www.nationalmssociety.org/chapters/FLC/i

Tami Caesar, President
Ryan Bumgardner, Bike MS Manager

6353 Florida Gulf Coast Chapter National Multiple Sclerosis Society
National Multiple Sclerosis Society
4919 Memorial Highway   813-889-8303
Tampa, FL 33634-3540   800-344-4867
                                            Fax: 813-889-8313
                                www.nationalmssociety.org/chapters/FLC/i
Judy Wilkinson, Service Director
Tim Hanke, Chairman

6354 Goodwill Industries-Suncoast
Goodwill Industries-Suncoast
10596 Gandy Boulevard   727-523-1512
St. Petersburg, FL 33733   Fax: 727-577-2749
                                    www.goodwill-suncoast.org
A nonprofit community based organization whose purpose is to improve the quality of life for people who are disabled, disadvantaged and/or aged. This mission is accomplished through a staff of
over 1,200 employees providing independent living skills, affordable housing, career assessment and planning, job skills, training,
placement, and job retention assistance with useful employment.

Annually, Goodwill Industries-Suncoast serves over 30,000 people in Citrus, Hernando, Levy, Marion and more.
Jay Mc Cloe, Director Resource Development

6355   National Multiple Sclerosis Society: North Florida Chapter
4237 Salisbury Road   904-332-6810
Jacksonville, FL 32216-8171   800-344-4867
                                                                             Fax: 904-332-0898
                                                                             TDD: 800-955-8770
                                                              e-mail: msnorfla@fln.nmss.org
                                                              www.nationalmssociety.org/fln

Jennifer Lee, Chapter President
Sabrah Witkamp, Client Program Director

6356   South Florida Chapter National Multiple Sclerosis Society
National Multiple Sclerosis Society
3201 W Commercial Boulevard   954-731-4224
Fort Lauderdale, FL 33309-6350   800-344-4867
                                                                             Fax: 954-739-1398
                                                                             e-mail: fls@nmss.org
                                                                             fls.nationalmssociety.org

Karen Dresbach, Chapter President
Fred Zuckerman, Chairman

Georgia

6357   National MS Society: Georgia Chapter
1117 Perimeter Center W   678-672-1000
Atlanta, GA 30338-3097   800-344-4867
                                                                             Fax: 678-672-1015
                                                              e-mail: gaa.mailbox@nmss.org
                                                              www.nationalmssociety.org/chapters/GAA/i
Roy A Rangel, Chapter President
Nicole Hill, Director of Finance & Administrative

Hawaii

6358   National MS Society: Hawaii Chapter
418 Kuwili Street   808-532-0806
Honolulu, HI 96817   800-344-4867
                                                                             Fax: 808-532-0814
                                                              e-mail: HIH@NMSS.ORG
                                                              www.nationalmssociety.org/chapters/HIH/i
Jeffrey D Peier, Chairman
Pam McElrath, President

Idaho

6359   National MS Society: Idaho Division
6901 W Emerald Street   208-388-4253
Boise, ID 83704   800-344-4867
                                                                             Fax: 208-388-1907
                                                              e-mail: idi@nmss.org
                                                              www.nationalmssociety.org/chapters/IDI/i
Pam McElrath, Chapter President
Suzanne Bland, Executive Vice President

Illinois

6360   National MS Society: Chicago, Greater Illinois Chapter
525 West Monroe Street   312-922-8000
Chicago, IL 60661-3814   800-344-4867
                                                                             Fax: 312-922-2752
                                                              e-mail: cgic@ild.nmss.org
                                                              www.nationalmssociety.org
The Greater Illnois Chapter is comprised of all the Illinoisans whohave chosen to fight MS and the work that they do through the National Multiple Sclerosis Society Volunteers, staff, healthcare workers, researchers, donors, advocated, and partners together represent the Greater Illinoisans Chapter, and all the many ways it's possible to join the fight against multiple sclerosis.
Steven Pratapous, Chapter President

Indiana

6361   National MS Society: Indiana State Chapter
3500 DePauw Blvd.   317-870-2500
Indianapolis, IN 46268   800-344-4867
                                                                             Fax: 317-870-2520
                                                              e-mail: Indiana@nmss.org
                                                              www.nationalmssociety.org/chapters/INI/i
Tiffany Bogard, Chapter President
Lisa Coffman, Director of Chapter Programs

Iowa

6362   National MS Society: Iowa Chapter
8187 University Boulevard   515-270-6337
Clive, IA 50325   800-344-4867
                                                                             Fax: 515-270-0337
                                                              e-mail: mark.davis@nmss.org
                                                              www.nationalmssociety.org/chapters/NTH/a
Brett Ridge, Chapter President
Mark Davis, Area Director

Kansas

6363   National MS Society: Mid-America Chapter
7611 State Line   913-432-3926
Kansas City, KS 64114-2915   800-344-4867
                                                                             Fax: 816-361-2369
                                                              e-mail: info@nmsskc.org
                                                              www.nationalmssociety.org/chapters/KSG/i
The National Multiple Sclerosis Society is a not-for-profit organization serving people with MS in every state. The Mid-America Chapter serves the 25,000 people who are affected by MS in eastern Kansas and western Missouri.
Kay Julian, Chapter President
Amy Goldstein, Program Director

6364   National MS Society: South Central & West Kansas Division
9415 E Harry Street   316-264-7043
Wichita, KS 67211-1515   800-344-4867
                                                                             Fax: 316-264-5436
                                                              e-mail: KSS@NMSS.ORG
                                                              www.nationalmssociety.org/chapters/KSS/i
Cammy Mathews, Donor Relations Coordinator
Becky Kimbell, Regional Programs and Services Manager

Kentucky

6365   National MS Society: Kentucky Chapter
1201 Story Avenue   502-451-0014
Louisville, KY 40206   800-344-4867
                                                                             Fax: 502-581-1010
                                                              e-mail: KYW@NMSS.ORG
                                                              www.nationalmssociety.org
Jeff Hamilton, Chairman
Stacy Funk, Chapter President

Louisiana

6366   National Multiple Sclerosis Society: Louisiana
4613 Fairfield Street   504-832-4013
Metairie, LA 70006   800-344-4867
                                                                             Fax: 504-831-7188
                                                              e-mail: louisianachapter@lam.nmss.org
                                                              www.nationalmssociety.org/chapters/LAM/i
Brian Berrigon, Chapter President
Crystal Smith, Director of Programs and Services

Maine

6367   National MS Society: Maine Chapter
170 US Route One   800-344-4867
Falmouth, ME 04105   800-344-4867
                                                                             Fax: 207-781-7961
                                                              e-mail: info@msmaine.org
                                                              www.nationalmssociety.org/chapters/MEM/i
The National Multiple Sclerosis Societ is dedicated to enind the devastating the devastating effects of multiple sciersis, a chronic,

disease of the central nervous system often diagnosed in young adults
Robin Doughty, Director of Finance & Operations
Denise Clavette, Chapter President

Maryland

6368 **National MS Society: Maryland Chapter Hunt Valley Business Center**
Hunt Valley Business Center
2219 York Road.   443-641-1200
Timonium, MD 21093   800-344-4867
                          Fax: 443-641-1201
                  e-mail: INFO@NMSS-MD.ORG
        www.nationalmssociety.org/chapters/MDM/i
Mark Roeder, Chapter President
Nicole Weedon, Executive Assistant/Office Manager

Massachusetts

6369 **National MS Society: Massachusetts Chapter**
101A 1st Avenue   781-890-4990
Waltham, MA 02451-1160   800-344-4867
                          Fax: 781-890-2089
              e-mail: CommunicationsGNE@nmss.org
        www.nationalmssociety.org/chapters/MAM/i
Linda Guiod, Executive Vice President
Arlyn White, Chapter President & CEO

Michigan

6370 **National MS Society: Michigan Chapter**
21311 Civic Center Drive   248-351-2190
Southfield, MI 48076   800-344-4867
                           Fax: 248-350-0029
                   e-mail: info@mig.nmss.org
              www.nationalmssociety.org/mig
Offer a variety of programs and services benefiting people with multiple sclerosis and their family members. Programs include educational seminars, information and referrals, peer support, advocacy, free legal clinic, financial assistance for medical equipment, medical transportation, home care, technical assistance and much more
Elana Sullivan, Chapter President
Melissa Ryan, Executive Administrative Assistant

Minnesota

6371 **National MS Society: Minnesota Chapter**
200 12th Avenue S   612-335-7900
Minneapolis, MN 55415   800-344-4867
                           Fax: 612-335-7997
              e-mail: INFO@MSSOCIETY.ORG
        www.nationalmssociety.org/chapters/MNM/i

Mississippi

6372 **National Multiple Sclerosis Society: Alaba ma-Mississippi Chapter**
145 Executive Drive   601-856-5831
Madison, MS 39110-9198   800-344-4867
                           Fax: 601-856-7173
                   e-mail: alc@nmss.org
              www.nationalmssociety.org/alc
Angie Jackson, Area Director
Andi Agnew, Programs and Services Coordinator

Missouri

6373 **National MS Society: Gateway Area Chapter**
1867 Lackland Hill Parkway   314-781-9020
Saint Louis, MO 63146-3545   800-344-4867
                             Fax: 314-781-1440
                   e-mail: info@mos.nmss.org
        www.nationalmssociety.org/chapters/MOS/i

Sponsors research and offers educational programs, counseling, lending library, referral services, independent living aids, legislative advocacy and therapeutic recreation for people with MS.
Phyllis Robsham, Chapter President
Kathi Taylor, Executive Assistant

Montana

6374 **National MS Society: Montana Division**
1629 Avenue D   406-252-5927
Billings, MT 59102   800-344-4867
                           Fax: 406-252-5956
                   e-mail: MTT@NMSS.ORG
        www.nationalmssociety.org/chapters/MTT/i
Rebecca Wiehe, Regional Programs and Services Manager
Heather Ohs, Regional DevelopmentManager

Nebraska

6375 **National MS Society: Midlands Chapter Community Health Plaza**
Community Health Plaza
328 S 72nd Street   402-505-4000
Omaha, NE 68114-2153   800-344-4867
                           Fax: 402-572-3002
                   e-mail: NEN@NMSS.ORG
        www.nationalmssociety.org/chapters/NEN/i
Lisa Brink, Chapter President
Milton Trabal, Director of Finance

Nevada

6376 **Natioanl Multiple Sclerosis Society Desert Southwest Chapter**
National Multiple Sclerosis Society
6000 S Eastern Avenue   702-736-1478
Las Vegas, NV 89119-3157   800-344-4867
                           Fax: 702-736-2487
                   e-mail: NVL@NMSS.ORG
        www.nationalmssociety.org/chapters/NVL/i
Serves southern Nevada & northwest Arizona.
Nicole Rainey, Development Coordinator Special Events
Linda Nowell, Programs and Services Coordinator

6377 **National MS Society: Great Basin Sierra Chapter**
4600 Keitzke Lane   702-329-7180
Reno, NV 89502   800-344-4867
                           Fax: 775-827-3167
                   e-mail: nvn@nvn.nmss.org
        www.nationalmssociety.org/chapters/NVN/i
Linda Lott, Regional Development Manager
Danielle Lutzow, Programs and Services Coordinator

New Hampshire

6378 **National MS Society: Central New England Chapter**
101A First Avenue   781-890-4990
Waltham, MA 02451-1115   800-493-9255
                           Fax: 781-490-2089
              e-mail: CommunicationsGNE@nmss.org
                   www.nationalmssociety.org
Serving people with MS in Massachusetts and New Hampshire.
Judy Cotton, Director Chapter Services
Arlyn White, Chapter President & CEO

New Jersey

6379 **National MS Society: Greater North Jersey Chapter**
1 Kalisa Way   201-967-5599
Paramus, NJ 07652-3550   800-344-4867
                           Fax: 201-967-7085
                   e-mail: Njminfo@nmss.org
        www.nationalmssociety.org/chapters/NJM/i
Michael Elkow, Chapter President
Marianne Maddocks, Vice President of Operations

6380 National MS Society: Mid-Jersey Chapter
246 Monmouth Road   732-660-1005
Oakhurst, NJ 07755   800-344-4867
                                       Fax: 732-660-1388
                            e-mail: Njminfo@nmss.org
                  www.nationalmssociety.org/chapters/NJM/i
The National Multiple Sclerosis Society is the only voluntary
health agency that supports an international program of scientific
research designed to cure, prevent and treat MS.
Michael Elkow, Chapter President
Marianne Maddocks, Vice President of Operations

New Mexico

6381 National MS Society: Rio Grande Division
4125-A Carlisle Boulevard NE   505-243-2792
Albuquerque, NM 87107   800-344-4867
                                       Fax: 505-244-0629
                            e-mail: NMX@NMSS.ORG
                  www.nationalmssociety.org/chapters/NMX/i
Maggie Schold, Development Coordinator Special Events
Sheri Wharton, Programs and Services Coordinator

New York

6382 National MS Society: Long Island Chapter
40 Marcus Drive   631-864-8337
Melville, NY 11747   800-344-4867
                                       Fax: 631-864-8342
                        e-mail: PMASTROTA@NMSSLI.ORG
                  www.nationalmssociety.org/chapters/NYH/i
The National Multiple Sclerosis Society, Long Island Chapter, is
dedicated to helping people with MS and their families live useful
and fulfilling lives by opening their minds to opportunities and
providing the tools to live with dignity.
Pamela Jones Mastrota, President & CEO
Barbara Travis, Vice President of Donor Development

6383 National MS Society: New York City Chapter
733 Third Avenue   212-463-7787
New York, NY 10017-2098   800-344-4867
                                       Fax: 212-989-4362
                            e-mail: INFO@MSNYC.ORG
                  www.nationalmssociety.org/chapters/NYN/i
Committed to providing comprehensive support services to help
people with MS and their families cope with the consequences of
the disease. The goal is to empower people with MS and their loved
ones so that they can better control their lives.
Ruth Brenner, Chapter President
Robin Einbinder, Executive Vice President Programs

6384 National MS Society: Northeastern New York Chapter
421 New Karner Road   585-271-0801
Albany, NY 12205-5156   800-344-4867
                                       Fax: 518-464-1232
                        e-mail: chapter@msupstateny.org
                  www.nationalmssociety.org/chapters/NYR/i
Barbara R Milano, Chapter President
Elliey Kiale-Ingalsb, Chapter Chair

6385 National MS Society: Southern New York Chapter
2 Gannett Drive   914-694-1655
White Plains, NY 10604-2145   800-344-4867
                                       Fax: 914-345-3504
                            e-mail: NYV@NMSS.ORG
                  www.nationalmssociety.org/chapters/NYV/i
The mission of the National MS Society is to end the devastating
effects of multiple sclerosis. The Southern NY Chapter is commit-
ted to helping people with MS to live independently.
Andrea Maloney, Interim Chapter President
Christina Szeliga, Administrative Coordinator

6386 National MS Society: Upstate New York Chapter
457 State Street   585-271-0801
Binghamton, NY 13901-2341   800-344-4867
                                       Fax: 607-722-1485
                        e-mail: chapter@msupstateny.org
                  www.nationalmssociety.org/chapters/NYR/i
James Ahearn, Chapter President
Jonathan Smith, Program Coordinator

**6387 National MS Society: Western New York/ Northwestern
Pennsylvania Chapter**
4245 Union Road   585-271-0801
Buffalo, NY 14225-5040   800-344-4867
                                       Fax: 716-634-2979
                        e-mail: chapter@msupstateny.org
                  www.nationalmssociety.org/chapters/NYR/i
Arthur V Cardella, Chapter President
Betsy Farkas, Director Chapter Programs

6388 National Multiple Sclerosis: Upstate New York Chapter
National Multiple Sclerosis Society
1650 S Avenue   716-271-0801
Rochester, NY 14620-3901   800-344-4867
                                       Fax: 716-442-2817
                    e-mail: CHAPTER@MSUPSTATENY.ORG
                  www.nationalmssociety.org/chapters/NYR/i
Randal A Simonetti, President& CEO
Stephanie Mincer, Senior Vice President of Programs

North Carolina

6389 National MS Society: Central North Carolina Chapter
2211 W Meadowview Road   336-299-4136
Greensboro, NC 27407-3400   800-344-4867
                                       Fax: 336-855-3039
                            e-mail: NCC@NMSS.ORG
                  www.nationalmssociety.org/chapters/NCC/i
Elizabeth Green, Chapter President
Davishia Baldwin, Volunteer Coordinator

6390 National MS Society: Eastern North Carolina Chapter
3101 Industrial Drive   919-834-0678
Raleigh, NC 27609-7577   800-344-4867
                                       Fax: 919-834-9822
                            e-mail: NCT@NMSS.ORG
                  www.nationalmssociety.org/chapters/NCT/i
Craig Robertson, Interim Chapter President
Debbie Hoffman, Vice President Operations

6391 National Multiple Sclerosis Society
9801-I Southern Pine Boulevard   704-525-2955
Charlotte, NC 28273-5561   800-344-4867
                                       Fax: 704-527-0406
                            e-mail: mac@nmss.org
                        www.nationalmssociety.org/mac
The Mid-Atlantic chapter of the National MS Society serves
80,000 people with multiple sclerosis in South Carolina and western North Carolina. The Chapter is dedicated to helping people
with MS learn to manage and understand their disease and to
achieve maximum independence.
Allison Mertens, Chair Board of Trustees
Jennifer Lee, Chapter President

North Dakota

6392 National MS Society: Dakota Chapter
5990 14th Street S   701-235-2678
Fargo, ND 58104   800-344-4867
                                       Fax: 701-235-6358
                  www.nationalmssociety.org/chapters/NTH/i
Kelly Boeddeker, Senior Development Manager
Amanda Noce, Programs Manager

Ohio

6393 Columbus Center of the National Multiple Sclerosis Society
National Multiple Sclerosis Society
651 G Lakeview Plaza Boulevard   614-880-2290
Worthington, OH 43229-3626   800-344-4867
                                       Fax: 614-880-2296
                        www.nationalmssociety.org
Stacey Wilko LSW, Program Coordinator
Tony Bernard LSW, Program Coordinator

**6394 National MS Soceity: Western Ohio Chapter The Woolpert
Building**
The Woolpert Building

409 E Monument Avenue
Dayton, OH 45402-1261

937-461-5232
800-344-4867
Fax: 937-461-3500
e-mail: donnasimpson@ohm.nmss.org
www.nationalmssociety.org

Providing accurate, up-to-date information to individuals with MS, their families and healthcare providers is central to our mission.
12 pages
Karen Joseph, Program Director
Judy LaMusga, Chapter Chair

6395 National MS Society: Southwestern Ohio/Northern Kentucky
4440 Lake Forest Drive
Cincinnati, OH 45242-3755

513-769-4400
800-344-4867
Fax: 513-769-6019
e-mail: OHGinfo@nmss.org
www.nationalmssociety.org

Tena Bunnell, Chapter President
Becky Wiehe, Service Director

6396 National MS Society: Northeast Ohio Chapter
The Hanna Building
6155 Rockside Road
Independence, OH 44131-1901

216-696-8220
800-344-4867
Fax: 216-696-2817
e-mail: WEBMASTER@NMSSOHA.ORG
www.nationalmssociety.org

Janet Kramer, Chapter President
Greg Kovach, Director of Services

6397 National MS Society: Northwest Ohio Chapter
401 Tomahawk Drive
Maumee, OH 43537-1633

419-897-9533
800-344-4867
Fax: 419-897-9733
e-mail: Maureen.Mohney@nmss.org
www.nationalmssociety.org/chapters/OHO/i

Jacque Pratt, Chapter Program Coordinator
Tonya Scherf, Program Director

Oklahoma

6398 National MS Society: Oklahoma Chapter
4604 E 67th Street
Tulsa, OK 74136-4946

918-488-0882
800-344-4867
Fax: 918-488-0913
e-mail: LISA.GRAY@OKE.NMSS.ORG
www.nationalmssociety.org/chapters/OKE/i

Paula Cortner, Chapter President
Denise Allen, Finance/HR Manager

Oregon

6399 National MS Society: Oregon Chapter
5331 SW Macadam Avenue
Portland, OR 97239

503-223-9511
800-344-4867
Fax: 503-223-2912
e-mail: INFO@DEFEATMS.COM
www.nationalmssociety.org/chapters/ORC/i

The Pregon Chapter is aggressively pursuing the mission to end the devastating effects of MS by providing programs designed to enhance the families throughout Oregon and Clark County, Washington.
Wendy Allison, Office Coordinator
Sally Alworth, Director of Finance

Pennsylvania

6400 National MS Society: Central Pennsylvania Chapter
2040 Linglestown Road
Harrisburg, PA 17110-1095

717-652-2108
800-344-4867
Fax: 717-652-2590
e-mail: PAC@NMSS.ORG
www.nationalmssociety.org/chapters/PAC/i

Margie Adelmann, President
Debbie Rios, Executive Vice President

6401 National MS Society: Greater Delaware Valley Chapter
30 South 17th Street
Philadelphia, PA 19103-5519

215-271-1500
800-344-4867
Fax: 215-271-6122
e-mail: PAE@NMSS.ORG
www.nationalmssociety.org/chapters/PAE/i

John H Scott, President
Randee Forstein, VP Programs & Community Outreach

Rhode Island

6402 National MS Society: Rhode Island Chapter
205 Hallene Road
Warwick, RI 02886-2452

401-738-8383
800-344-4867
Fax: 401-738-8469
e-mail: christina.roche@nmss.org
www.nationalmssociety.org/chapters/RIR/i

Provides local programs and services to people with MS and their families. These services include information and referral, equipment loans, purchase assistance, programs for the newly diagnosed and education and support groups.
3M Members
Kathy Mechnig, Chapter President
Catie Dussault, Director of Special Events

South Carolina

6403 National MS Society: South Carolina Branch
2711 Middleburg Drive
Columbia, SC 29204-2413

803-799-7848
800-344-4867
www.nationalmssociety.org/chapters/NCP/i

Tennessee

6404 National MS Society: Southeast Tennessee/North Georgia Chapte
5720 Uptain Road
Chattanooga, TN 37411-5642

423-954-9700
800-344-4867
Fax: 423-855-9667
e-mail: questions@msmidsouth.org
www.nationalmssociety.org

Jeanne Brice, Services Manager

6405 National MS Society: Mid-South Chapter
3100 Walnut Grove Road
Memphis, TN 38111-3530

901-755-4900
800-344-4867
Fax: 901-324-9668
www.nationalmssociety.org

The mission of the National Multiple Sclerosis Society is to end the devastating effects of MS.
Dee Blake, Chapter President
Sherree Wilson, Services Director

6406 National MS Society: Mid-South Chapter, Nashville Office
4219 Hillsboro Road
Nashville, TN 37215-3332

615-269-9055
800-344-4867
Fax: 615-269-9470
e-mail: TNS@NMSS.ORG
www.nationalmssociety.org/chapters/TNS/i

Jim Ward, Chapter President
Beth Smith, Vice President of Client Programs

Texas

6407 National MS Society: North Central Texas Chapter
4086 Sandshell Drive
Fort Worth, TX 76137

817-306-7003
800-344-4867
Fax: 817-877-1205
www.nationalmssociety.org/chapters/TXH/i

Educational programs, self-help groups, and information and referral for persons and families diagnosed with multiple sclerosis.
12 pages Quarterly
Justin Martin, Coordinator Development
Lynette Jarvis-Barre, Senior Manager Programs & Services

6408 National MS Society: Panhandle Chapter
6222 Canyon Drive   806-468-8005
Amarillo, TX 79109-6730   800-344-4867
Fax: 806-468-8022
e-mail: TXP@NMSS.ORG
www.nationalmssociety.org/chapters/TXP/i
Gail Lindsey, Programs and Services Coordinator
April Brownlee, Development Coordinator Special Events

6409 National MS Society: Southern Texas
8111 N Stadium Drive   713-526-8967
Houston, TX 77054   800-344-4867
Fax: 713-394-7422
e-mail: TXH@NMSS.ORG
www.nationalmssociety.org/chapters/TXH/i
Mark Neagli, Chapter President
Deborah Pope, VP - Operations

6410 National MS Society: West Texas Division
1031 Andrews Highway   432-522-2143
Midland, TX 79701-4636   800-344-4867
Fax: 432-694-7970
e-mail: TXQ@NMSS.ORG
www.nationalmssociety.org/chapters/TXQ/i
Sharon Rader, Regional Development Manager
Rona Bowerman, Regional Programs and Services Manager

6411 National MS Socisty: Southeast Texas Chapter
8111 N Stadium Drive   713-526-8967
Houston, TX 77054-4051   800-344-4867
Fax: 713-394-7422
e-mail: TXH@NMSS.ORG
www.nationalmssociety.org
Mark Neagli, Chapter President
Jim Tidwell, Chairman

Utah

6412 National MS Society: Utah State Chapter
1440 Foothill Drive   801-493-0113
Salt Lake City, UT 84108-3537   800-527-8116
Fax: 801-493-0122
e-mail: utah.idaho@nmss.org
www.nationalmssociety.org
Our mission is to end the devastating effects of MS. Serving individuals with MS and their families through programs, research, awareness and education.
Annette Royle, Chapter President
Dee Dee Fox, Director of Client Programs and Services

Vermont

6413 National MS Society: Vermont Division
75 Talcott Road   802-864-6356
Williston, VT 05495   800-344-4867
Fax: 802-864-6509
e-mail: VTN@NMSS.ORG
www.nationalmssociety.org/chapters/VTN/i
Committed to ending the devastating effects of MS.
Christine Newberr, Programs and Services Coordinator
Lindsay Going, Development Coordinator Special Events

Virginia

6414 National MS Society: Blue Ridge Chapter
1020 Carrington Place   804-971-8010
Charlottesville, VA 22901   800-344-4867
Fax: 804-979-4475
e-mail: VAB@NMSS.ORG
www.nationalmssociety.org/chapters/VAB/i
Faith Painter, Chapter President
Delton Hanson, Operations Director

6415 National MS Society: Central Virginia Chapter
2112 W Laburnum Avenue   804-353-5008
Richmond, VA 23227   800-344-4867
Fax: 804-353-5595
e-mail: JUDY.GRIFFIN@NMSS.ORG
www.nationalmssociety.org/chapters/VAR/i
Sherri Ellis, Chapter President
Andy Page, Director of Community Development

6416 National MS Society: Hampton Roads Chapter
760 Lynnhaven Parkway   757-490-9627
Virginia Beach, VA 23452-6311   800-344-4867
Fax: 757-490-1617
e-mail: info@fightms.com
www.nationalmssociety.org/chapters/VAX/i
Sharon Grossman, Chapter President
Michelle Derr, Vice President Finance/Administration

Washington

6417 National MS Society: Greater Washington Chapter
192 Nickerson Street   206-284-4254
Seattle, WA 98109   800-344-4867
Fax: 206-284-4972
e-mail: MSnorthwest@nmsswas.org
www.nationalmssociety.org/chapters/WAS/i
Patricia Shepherd-Ba, Chapter President
Erin Poznanski, Vice President Chapter Programs

6418 National MS Society: Inland Northwest Chapter
818 E Sharp Avenue   509-482-2022
Spokane, WA 99202-1935   800-344-4867
Fax: 509-483-1077
e-mail: WAI@NMSS.ORG
www.nationalmssociety.org/chapters/WAI/i
Robert Hansen, Chapter President
Patty Mathias, Office Manager

Wisconsin

6419 National MS Society: Wisconsin Chapter
1120 James Drive   262-369-4400
Hartland, WI 53029   800-344-4867
Fax: 262-369-4410
e-mail: info.wisms@nmss.org
www.nationalmssociety.org/chapters/WIG/i
Colleen Kalt, President & CEO
Melissa Palfery, Executive Assistant

Wyoming

6420 National MS Society: Wyoming Chapter
525 Randall Avenue   307-433-9590
Cheyenne, WY 82001-1627   800-344-4867
Fax: 307-433-8657
e-mail: WYY@NMSS.ORG
www.nationalmssociety.org/chapters/WYY/i
Cheryl Seaberg, Programs and Services Coordinator
Stephanie Batson, Development Coordinator Special Events

Libraries & Resource Centers

6421 Information Resource Center and Library
National Multiple Sclerosis Society
733 Third Avenue   866-675-4787
New York, NY 10017   800-344-4867
www.nationalmssociety.org
The primary venue for educating the community about multiple sclerosis.Offers the latest information about MS information and provides referrals to local MS care centers, physicians and service providers.
Weyman T Johnson, Jr, Chairman
Joyce M Nelson, President/CEO

6422 St. Agnes Hospital Medical: Health Science Library
305 North Street   914-681-4500
White Plains, NY 10605   Fax: 914-328-6408
Labe C Scheinberg MD, Director

Research Centers

6423 Brigham and Women's Hospital: Center for Neurologic Diseases
LMRC Building
75 Francis Street   617-732-5500
Boston, MA 02115   800-294-9999
                                     TTY: 617-732-6458
                                     www.brighamandwomens.org
Offers research relating to Multiple Sclerosis and other autoimmune diseases.
Dennis J. Selkoe, Co-Director
Howard L. Weiner, Co-Director

6424 Center for Neuroimmunology: University of Alabama at Birmingham
1720 7th Ave S   205-934-0683
Birmingham, AL 35294   Fax: 205-996-4039
                                     www.main.uab.edu/neurology
Evaluate and treat acute and chronic neurological and neuromuscular diseases which are caused by autoimmune mechanisms or linked to presumed abnormalities affecting the immune system.
Khurram Bashir, Director

6425 Jimmie Heuga Center
27 Main Street   970-926-1290
Edwards, CO 81632   800-367-3101
                                     Fax: 970-926-1295
                                     e-mail: info@mscando.org
                                     www.mscando.org
Conducts research and studies on multiple sclerosis patients.
Kim Lennox Sharkey, Chief Executive Officer
Carrie Van Beek, Office Coordinator

6426 Neuromuscular Treatment Center: Univ. of Texas Southwestern Medical Center
Department of Neurology
Dallas, TX 75390   214-648-3111
                                     www.utsouthwestern.edu
Basic and clinical studies of myasthenia gravis.
Daniel K Podolsky MD, President
Diane Jeffries, Director

6427 Rush University Multiple Sclerosis Center
1653 W. Congress Parkway   312-942-5000
Chicago, IL 60612   888-352-RUSH
                                     TTY: 312-942-2207
                                     e-mail: complaint@jointcommission.org
                                     www.rush.edu
The Multiple Sclerosis Center combines comprehensive treatment with clinical and laboratory research to provide the highest quality patient care.
Floyd A Davis, Director

Support Groups & Hotlines

6428 MS Toll-Free Information Line
National Multiple Sclerosis Society
733 3rd Avenue
New York, NY 10017-3288   800-344-4867
Offers public and professional information, brochures and referrals to MS patients, their families and health care professionals.

6429 MSWorld
1943 Morrill Street   415-701-1117
Sarasota, FL 34236   877-710-0302
                                     e-mail: msworld@msworld.org
                                     www.msworld.org/
MSWorld is for people with multiple sclerosis their families and friends, offer support via chat, e-mail, message boards, magazines.
Kathleen Wilson, Founder/President

6430 Multiple Sclerosis Action Group
National Multiple Sclerosis Society

733 3rd Avenue   409-883-2282
New York, NY 10017   800-344-4867
                                     e-mail: msag@erasems.com
                                     www.nationalmssociety.org/index.aspx
Richard J Mengel, Treasurer
Fred J Lublin, Director

6431 National Health Information Center
PO Box 1133   310-565-4167
Washington, DC 20013   800-336-4797
                                     Fax: 301-984-4256
                                     e-mail: info@nhic.org
                                     www.health.gov/nhic
Offers a nationwide information referral service, produces directories and resource guides.

6432 Traditional Tibetan Healing
13 Harrison Street   617-666-8635
Sommerville, MA 2143-6504   866-628-6504
                                     e-mail: Kelob@gte.net
                                     www.tibetanherbalhealing.com/
To rid mankind from chronic illnesses using alternative methods.
Keyzon Bhutti, Chief Physician

Books

6433 300 Tips for Making Life with Multiple Sclerosis Easier
Demos Medical Publishing
386 Park Avenue S   212-683-0072
New York, NY 10016   Fax: 212-683-0118
                                     e-mail: orderdept@demospub.com
                                     www.demosmedpub.com
Techniques for better living.
109 pages
ISBN: 1-888799-23-4
Dr. Diana M Schneider

6434 Alternative Medicine and Multiple Sclerosis
Demos Medical Publishing
386 Park Avenue S   212-683-0072
New York, NY 10016   Fax: 212-683-0118
                                     e-mail: orderdept@demospub.com
                                     www.demosmedpub.com
272 pages
ISBN: 1-888799-52-8
Dr. Diana M Schneider

6435 Fall Down Seven Times Get Up Eight
Miramar Communications
PO Box 8987
Malibu, CA 90265-8987   800-543-4116
The second in Dr. Wolf's series on MS management: including chapters on stress and fatigue, planning for serious disability and lots more.
211 pages

6436 Living with Multiple Sclerosis
Demos Medical Publishing
386 Park Avenue S   212-683-0072
New York, NY 10016   Fax: 212-683-0118
                                     e-mail: orderdept@demospub.com
                                     www.demosmedpub.com
ISBN: 1-888799-26-9
Dr. Diana M Schneider

6437 Living with Multiple Sclerosis: A Wellness Approach
Demos Vermande
386 Park Avenue S   212-683-0072
New York, NY 10016-8804   800-532-8663
112 pages
ISBN: 1-888799-00-5

6438 Meeting the Challenge of Progressive Multiple Sclerosis
Demos Medical Publishing

386 Park Avenue S
New York, NY 10016

212-683-0072
Fax: 212-683-0118
e-mail: orderdept@demospub.com
www.demosmedpub.com

128 pages
ISBN: 1-888799-46-3
Dr. Diana M Schneider

6439 Multiple Sclerosis
Demos Medical Publishing
386 Park Avenue S
New York, NY 10016

212-683-0072
800-532-8663
Fax: 212-683-0118
e-mail: orderdept@demospub.com
www.demosmedpub.com

A consistent bestseller in multiple sclerosis management.
224 pages
ISBN: 1-888799-54-4
Dr. Diana M Schneider

6440 Multiple Sclerosis, The Questions you Have Answers You Need
Demos Medical Publishing
386 Park Avenue S
New York, NY 10016

212-683-0072
Fax: 212-683-0118
e-mail: orderdept@demospub.com
www.demosmedpub.com

592 pages
ISBN: 1-888799-43-9
Dr. Diana M Schneider

6441 Multiple Sclerosis: A Guide for Families
Demos Medical Publishing
386 Park Avenue S
New York, NY 10016-8804

212-683-0072
800-532-8663
Fax: 212-683-0118
e-mail: orderdept@demospub.com
www.demosmedpub.com

With its complex and unpredictable course, MS affects every area of family life. This book covers a broad range of medical, psychological, social, vocational, economic and legal problems.
1997 207 pages Paperback
ISBN: 1-888799-14-5
Dr. Diana M Schneider, President

6442 Multiple Sclerosis: A Guide for Patients and Their Families
Raven Press
1185 Avenue of the Americas
New York, NY 10036-2601

212-930-9500
800-777-2295

Second edition.
288 pages Paperback
ISBN: 0-881672-55-6

6443 Multiple Sclerosis: A Personal Exploration
Demos Vermande
386 Park Avenue S
New York, NY 10016-8804

212-683-0072
800-532-8663
Fax: 212-683-0118

1993 192 pages
ISBN: 0-285650-18-1

6444 Multiple Sclerosis: Your Legal Rights
Demos Medical Publishing
386 Park Avenue S
New York, NY 10016

212-683-0072
Fax: 212-683-0118
e-mail: orderdept@demospub.com
www.demosmedpub.com

156 pages
ISBN: 1-888799-31-5
Dr. Diana M Schneider

6445 The Comfort of Home Multiple Sclerosis Edi tion: A Guide for Caregivers
Marie M. Meyer and Paula Derr, RN, author

CareTrust Publications
PO Box 10283
Portland, OR 97296-0283

800-565-1533
Fax: 415-673-2005
e-mail: sales@comfortofhome.com
www.comfortofhome.com

Reviews caregiving options and discusses the financial and legal decisions you may encounterr. Readers will learn how to set up a safe and comfortable home for the person whose needs are changing and abilities declining. Comfort offers guidance through every caregiving stage and most decisions one will face in daily living, as well as in avoiding caregiver burnout. Valuable for the caregiver and the patient.
324 pages
ISBN: 0-966476-76-X

6446 Understanding Multiple Sclerosis
Melissa Stauffer, author

University Press of Mississippi
3825 Ridgewood Road
Jackson, MS 39211-6492

601-432-6205
Fax: 601-432-6217
e-mail: kburgess@ihl.state.ms.us
www.upress.state.ms.us

For patients and companions, an overview of all aspects of MS.
2006 144 pages Paperback
ISBN: 1-578068-03-7
Kathy Burgess, Advertising/Marketing Services Manager

Magazines

6447 Inside MS
National Multiple Sclerosis Society
733 3rd Avenue
New York, NY 10017-3288

212-986-3240
800-344-4867
Fax: 212-986-7981
www.nmss.org

Full color quarterly magazine on living well with mutiple sclerosis. Articles by people with MS; daily living, achievments, news, treatments, research, advocacy, humor, travel, helpful resources, large type. The magazine is a benefit of membership.
64 pages 4x Year

Newsletters

6448 Inside MS Bulletin
National Multiple Sclerosis Society
733 3rd Avenue
New York, NY 10017-3288

212-986-3240
800-344-4867
Fax: 212-986-7981

Newsletter offering information on the organization activities. Profiles of donors, and reports on MS research programs.

6449 MS Connection
National Multiple Sclerosis Society
9801-I Southern Pine Boulevard
Charlotte, NC 28273

704-525-2955
Fax: 704-527-0406
e-mail: mac@nmss.org
www.nationalmssociety.org/mac

Provides education, support and information about Chapter activities for people living with multiple sclerosis in South Carolina and western North Carolina.
Quarterly
Allison Mertens, Chair, Board of Trustees
Jennifer Lee, Chapter President

6450 Motivator
Multiple Sclerosis Foundation
6350 N Andrews Avenue
Fort Lauderdale, FL 33309-2130

954-776-6805
800-441-7055
e-mail: msfacts@icanect.net
www.msfacts.org

Reports on the latest advancements regarding medical treatments/therapies for MS, inspirational feature stories, coping skills, correspondence from readers, and ongoing MSAA programs, services, and activities.
BiMonthly

6451 Multiple Sclerosis Quarterly Report
Demos Vermande
386 Park Avenue S
New York, NY 10016-8804

212-683-0072
800-532-8663
Fax: 212-683-0118

This is the definitive newsletter for everyone who has MS, with feature articles, research updates, book reviews, and more. It is developed with the sponsorship of the Eastern Paralyzed Veterans of America and the National Multiple Sclerosis Society. The MSQR will keep you informed of new developments in the management of MS and strategies for living successfully with the disease.
1997 Quarterly

6452   National Multiple Sclerosis Society: Allegheny District Chapter
1040 5th Avenue   412-261-6347
Pittsburgh, PA 15219-6220   800-544-5250
                                             Fax: 412-232-1461
                                         e-mail: pa@nmss.org
                                            www.nmss-pgh.org

12 pages 4 per year
Colleen McGuire, Chapter President

Pamphlets

6453   ADA and People with MS
National Multiple Sclerosis Society
733 3rd Avenue   212-986-3240
New York, NY 10017-3288   800-344-4867
                                             Fax: 212-986-7981
What the Americans with Disabilities Act means in employment, public accommodations, transportation, and telecommunications.
24 pages

6454   At Home with MS: Adapting Your Environment
National Multiple Sclerosis Society
733 3rd Avenue   212-986-3240
New York, NY 10017-3288   800-344-4867
                                             Fax: 212-986-7981
Modify a house or apartment to save energy, compensate for reduced vision or mobility, and live comfortably. Many do-it-yourself changes.
28 pages

6455   At Our House
National Multiple Sclerosis Society
733 3rd Avenue   212-986-3240
New York, NY 10017-3288   800-344-4867
                                             Fax: 212-986-7981
A coloring book for children, ages 5-8, about a Mama Bear with MS. contains some very basic facts with an afterword for parents on how to talk to young children about MS.
20 pages

6456   Chapter Services at a Glance
National Multiple Sclerosis Society
733 3rd Avenue   212-986-3240
New York, NY 10017-3288   800-344-4867
                                             Fax: 212-986-7981
A summary of services offerred by local chapters. Contains membership form.

6457   Check Your Multiple Sclerosis Facts
National Multiple Sclerosis Society
733 3rd Avenue   212-986-3240
New York, NY 10017-3288   800-344-4867
                                             Fax: 212-986-7981
A brief checklist of MS basics - definition, symptoms, and outlook.

6458   Choosing a Pharmacy Service
National Multiple Sclerosis Society
733 3rd Avenue   212-986-3240
New York, NY 10017-3288   800-344-4867
                                             Fax: 212-986-7981
What to look for when choosing a prescription drug provider.
20 pages

6459   Clear Thinking About Alternative Therapies
National Multiple Sclerosis Society
733 3rd Avenue   212-986-3240
New York, NY 10017-3288   800-344-4867
                                             Fax: 212-986-7981
Highlights facts and common misconceptions, compares alternative and conventional medicine, and suggests ways to evaluate benefits and risks.

6460   Controlling Spasticity
National Multiple Sclerosis Society
733 3rd Avenue   212-986-3240
New York, NY 10017-3288   800-344-4867
                                             Fax: 212-986-7981
An overview of ways to control this common and sometimes disabling MS symtpom. Includes roles of self-help, medications, physical therapists, nurses, and physicians.

6461   Food for Thought: MS and Nutrition
National Multiple Sclerosis Society
733 3rd Avenue   212-986-3240
New York, NY 10017-3288   800-344-4867
                                             Fax: 212-986-7981
A guide to healthy eating and coping with symptoms that may affect eating habits.
20 pages

6462   Getting a Grip on Gait
National Multiple Sclerosis Society
733 3rd Avenue   212-986-3240
New York, NY 10017-3288   800-344-4867
                                             Fax: 212-986-7981
Walking problems and how they can be addressed.

6463   Hiring Help at Home?
National Multiple Sclerosis Society
733 3rd Avenue   212-986-3240
New York, NY 10017-3288   800-344-4867
                                             Fax: 212-986-7981
Checklists and worksheets for people who need help at home. Forms for needs assessment, job description, and employment contract.

6464   Insight Into Eyesight
National Multiple Sclerosis Society
733 3rd Avenue   212-986-3240
New York, NY 10017-3288   800-344-4867
                                             Fax: 212-986-7981
Current therapy for MS-related eye disorders. Discusses low-vision aids.

6465   Living with MS
National Multiple Sclerosis Society
733 3rd Avenue   212-986-3240
New York, NY 10017-3288   800-344-4867
                                             Fax: 212-986-7981
Answers to 28 questions most often asked when the diagnosis is MS - from possible causes to advice on coping.
20 pages

6466   Moving with Multiple Sclerosis
National Multiple Sclerosis Society
733 3rd Avenue   212-986-3240
New York, NY 10017-3288   800-344-4867
                                             Fax: 212-986-7981
Step-by-step illustrations of passive and active stretching, balance, and conditioning exercises.
30 pages

6467   Multiple Sclerosis and Your Emotions
National Multiple Sclerosis Society
733 3rd Avenue   212-986-3240
New York, NY 10017-3288   800-344-4867
                                             Fax: 212-986-7981
How to manage some of the emotional challenges created by MS.
32 pages

6468   On the Question of Pregnancy
National Multiple Sclerosis Society
733 3rd Avenue   212-986-3240
New York, NY 10017-3288   800-344-4867
                                             Fax: 212-986-7981
Reassuring answers on pregnancy, delivery, and nursing.

6469   On: Alternative Therapies
National Multiple Sclerosis Society
733 3rd Avenue   212-986-3240
New York, NY 10017-3288   800-344-4867
                                             Fax: 212-986-7981
Checklist for people who are considering an alternative treatment.

6470 On: Diagnosis...Putting the Pieces Together
National Multiple Sclerosis Society
733 3rd Avenue   212-986-3240
New York, NY 10017-3288   800-344-4867
                                          Fax: 212-986-7981
Explains usual steps and tests. Includes how to prepare for an MRI.

6471 On: Energy Management
National Multiple Sclerosis Society
733 3rd Avenue   212-986-3240
New York, NY 10017-3288   800-344-4867
                                          Fax: 212-986-7981
Guidelines for budgeting your energy when it's limited by fatigue through prioritizing, delegating, and simplifying tasks.

6472 On: Fatigue
National Multiple Sclerosis Society
733 3rd Avenue   212-986-3240
New York, NY 10017-3288   800-344-4867
                                          Fax: 212-986-7981
The mystery of MS fatigue, practical tips for coping, and the medications sometimes prescribed.

6473 On: Genes
National Multiple Sclerosis Society
733 3rd Avenue   212-986-3240
New York, NY 10017-3288   800-344-4867
                                          Fax: 212-986-7981
Recent information on MS and heredity.

6474 On: Pain
National Multiple Sclerosis Society
733 3rd Avenue   212-986-3240
New York, NY 10017-3288   800-344-4867
                                          Fax: 212-986-7981
Myths and facts about MS pain. Covers types of pain and possible treatment.

6475 Plaintalk: A Booklet About MS for Families
National Multiple Sclerosis Society
733 3rd Avenue   212-986-3240
New York, NY 10017-3288   800-344-4867
                                          Fax: 212-986-7981
Discusses some of the more difficult physical and emotional problems families may face.
32 pages

6476 Rehab Outlook
National Multiple Sclerosis Society
733 3rd Avenue   212-986-3240
New York, NY 10017-3288   800-344-4867
                                          Fax: 212-986-7981
What rehabilitation can do for mobility, fatigue, driving, speech, memory, bowel or bladder problems, sexuality, and more.
24 pages

6477 Research Directions in Multiple Sclerosis
National Multiple Sclerosis Society
733 3rd Avenue   212-986-3240
New York, NY 10017-3288   800-344-4867
                                          Fax: 212-986-7981
An overview of current research on key areas of immunology, genetics, virology, and cell biology explained for nonscientists.
16 pages

6478 Sexual Problems Your Doctor Didn't Mention
National Multiple Sclerosis Society
733 3rd Avenue   212-986-3240
New York, NY 10017-3288   800-344-4867
                                          Fax: 212-986-7981
How MS may affect sexuality and what can be done.

6479 Solving Cognitive Problems
National Multiple Sclerosis Society
733 3rd Avenue   212-986-3240
New York, NY 10017-3288   800-344-4867
                                          Fax: 212-986-7981
Mental functions most likely to be affected by MS. Suggestions for self-help and information about cognitive rehabiitation.
20 pages

6480 Someone You Know Has MS: A Book for Families
National Multiple Sclerosis Society
733 3rd Avenue   212-986-3240
New York, NY 10017-3288   800-344-4867
                                          Fax: 212-986-7981
For children ages 6-12 who have a parent with MS. Provides facts and explores children's fears and concerns.
32 pages

6481 Taking Care: A Guide for Well Partners
National Multiple Sclerosis Society
733 3rd Avenue   212-986-3240
New York, NY 10017-3288   800-344-4867
                                          Fax: 212-986-7981
Introduces the concept of carepartnering to balance both partners' needs. Includes practical suggestions about getting and giving help.
16 pages

6482 Taming Stress in Multiple Sclerosis
National Multiple Sclerosis Society
733 3rd Avenue   212-986-3240
New York, NY 10017-3288   800-344-4867
                                          Fax: 212-986-7981
Stress and depression, and how both relate to MS. Tips on simplifying daily life. Instructions on muscle relaxation, deep breathing, and visualization relaxation.
36 pages

6483 Things I Wish Someone Had Told Me
National Multiple Sclerosis Society
733 3rd Avenue   212-986-3240
New York, NY 10017-3288   800-344-4867
                                          Fax: 212-986-7981
First-person story. A positive and practical approach to adjusting to life with MS.
20 pages

6484 Understanding Bladder Problems in Multiple Sclerosis
National Multiple Sclerosis Society
733 3rd Avenue   212-986-3240
New York, NY 10017-3288   800-344-4867
                                          Fax: 212-986-7981
The three main types of bladder dysfunction explained. Guidelines for management.
12 pages

6485 Understanding Bowel Problems in MS
National Multiple Sclerosis Society
733 3rd Avenue   212-986-3240
New York, NY 10017-3288   800-344-4867
                                          Fax: 212-986-7981
An exploration of ways to manage bowel problems in MS.
24 pages

6486 What Everyone Should Know About Multiple Sclerosis
National Multiple Sclerosis Society
733 3rd Avenue   212-986-3240
New York, NY 10017-3288   800-344-4867
                                          Fax: 212-986-7981
Overview of MS, suitable for the whole family.
16 pages

6487 What Is Multiple Sclerosis?
National Multiple Sclerosis Society
733 3rd Avenue   212-986-3240
New York, NY 10017-3288   800-344-4867
                                          Fax: 212-986-7981
For the newly diagnosed and others who need an overview of symptoms, disease patterns, diagnosis, prognosis, treatment, and research efforts.

6488 When a Parent Has MS: A Teenager's Guide
National Multiple Sclerosis Society
733 3rd Avenue   212-986-3240
New York, NY 10017-3288   800-344-4867
                                          Fax: 212-986-7981
For older children and teenagers who have a parent with MS. Discusses issues brought up by real kids.
24 pages

6489 Win-Win Approach to Reasonable Accommodations
National Multiple Sclerosis Society
733 3rd Avenue   212-986-3240
New York, NY 10017-3288   800-344-4867
                                    Fax: 212-986-7981
A practical guide to obtaining workplace accommodations.
20 pages

Audio & Video

6490 Aqua Exercises for Multiple Sclerosis
National Multiple Sclerosis Society
733 3rd Avenue   212-986-3240
New York, NY 10017-3288   800-344-4867
                                    Fax: 212-986-7981
A workout that cools and supports the body, with exercises to reduce spasticity, build muscles, and improve posture. With waterproof chart.
20 minutes

6491 Clinical Trials in Multiple Sclerosis: Searching for New Therapies
National Multiple Sclerosis Society
733 3rd Avenue   212-986-3240
New York, NY 10017   800-344-4867
                                    Fax: 212-986-7981
Describes studies to determine the safety and efficacy of new drugs to treat MS. Why studies are essential, how they are conducted, and the role of participants.
20 minutes

6492 Now, More Than Ever: Progress in Multiple Sclerosis Research
National Multiple Sclerosis Society
733 3rd Avenue   212-986-3240
New York, NY 10017-3288   800-344-4867
                                    Fax: 212-986-7981
Traces the National Multiple Sclerosis Society's historic role in propelling MS research and explains current approaches for nonscientists.
10 minutes

Web Sites

6493 Healing Well
                          www.healingwell.com
An online health resource guide to medical news, chat, information and articles, newsgroups and message boards, books, disease-related web sites, medical directories, and more for patients, friends, and family coping with disabling diseases, disorders, or chronic illnesses.

6494 Health Finder
                          www.healthfinder.gov
Searchable, carefully developed web site offering information on over 1000 topics. Developed by the US Department of Health and Human Services, the site can be used in both English and Spanish.

6495 Healthlink USA
                          www.healthlinkusa.com
Health information concerning treatment, cures, prevention, diagnosis, risk factors, research, support groups, email lists, personal stories and much more. Updated regularly.

6496 Helios Health
                          www.helioshealth.com
Online resource for your health information. Detailed information about specific health topics, access to expert advice from our Medical Advisory Board, and up-to-date health news.

6497 MedicineNet
                          www.medicinenet.com
An online resource for consumers providing easy-to-read, authoritative medical and health information.

6498 Medscape
                          www.medscape.com
Medscape offers specialists, primary care physicians, and other health professionals the Web's most robust and integrated medical information and educational tools.

6499 Multiple Sclerosis Foundation
                          www.msfocus.org
Dedicated to helping create a brighter tomorrow for those with MS, the foundation offers a wide array of free services including: national toll-free support, educational programs, homecare, support groups, assitive technology, publications, a comprehensive website and more to improve the quality of life for those affected by MS.

6500 National Multiple Sclerosis Society
                          www.nmss.org
Provides research, public and professional education, advocacy and the design of rehabilitative and psychosocial programs.

6501 Neurology Channel
                          www.neurologychannel.com
Find clearly explained, medically accurate information regarding conditions, including an overview, symptoms, causes, diagnostic procedures and treatment options. On this site it is possible to ask questions and get information from a neurologist and connect to people who have similar health interests.

6502 WebMD
                          www.webmd.com
Information on Multiple Sclerosis, including articles and resources.

Description

6503 Muscular Dystrophy

Muscular dystrophy is a group of genetic disorders marked by progressive weakness and degeneration of the skeletal, or voluntary, muscles that control movement. The muscles of the heart and other involuntary muscles may also affected in some forms of muscular dystrophy, and a few forms of the disease involve other organs as well.

Muscular dystrophy can affect people of all ages. The most common form, Duchenne, appears in childhood, but others may not appear until middle age or later.

Duchenne muscular dystrophy affects males almost exclusively. By age five, those with Duchenne experience progressive weakness and difficulty in climbing, jumping and hopping. By ages eight to ten, leg braces are often required, and eventually walking is impossible. Duchenne is also associated with heart problems, although without symptoms, and intellectual impairment that affects verbal ability more than performance. Death usually occurs in the third decade of life, often as a result of pneumonia.

No specific treatment exists. Daily prednisone provides significant benefit but owing to the medication's numerous side effects, it should be reserved for patients with major functional decline. Other treatment includes physical therapy, which can help minimize the shortening of the muscles that occurs around joints; assistive devices; and avoidance of prolonged immobility. There are now techniques available to detect female carriers of the defective gene, enabling genetic counseling for families and couples considering conception.

Other forms of muscular dystrophy are myotonic, Becker, limb-girdle and facioscapulohumeral. Information about when and where muscle weakness first occurred, and its severity, is very helpful in classifying the type of muscular dystrophy. Studying a small piece of muscle tissue can indicate whether the disorder is muscular dystrophy and which form of the disease it is.

National Agencies & Associations

6504 Muscular Dystrophy Association
3300 E Sunrise Drive
Tucson, AZ 85718-3299
520-529-2000
800-572-1717
e-mail: mda@mdausa.org
www.mda.org
Primary objective of MDA is the support of scientific investigators seeking the causes of and effective treatments for muscular dystrophy and related neuromuscular disorders. The worldwide research program supports over 400 scientific investigations annually.
Robert Ross, President/CEO

6505 Muscular Dystrophy Canada
2345 Yonge Street
Toronto, Ontario, M4P-2E5
866-687-2538
Fax: 416-488-7523
e-mail: info@muscle.ca
www.muscle.ca
Since 1954, Muscular Dystrophy Canada has been committed to improving the quality of life for the tens of thousands of Canadians

with neuromuscular disorders and funding leading research for the discovery of therapies and cures for neuromuscular disorders.

6506 Parent Project: Muscular Dystrophy
401 Hackensack Avenue
Hackensack, NJ 07601
201-250-8440
800-714-5437
Fax: 201-250-8435
e-mail: info@parentprojectmd.org
www.parentprojectmd.org
Organization of families around the world who have children diagnosed with DMD/BMD. Our goal is to invest significant amounts of money raised into medical research with clinical application.
Patricia Furlong, President
Kimberly Galberaith, Executive Vice President

6507 Society for Muscular Dystrophy Information International
PO Box 7490
Bridgewater, Nova Scotia, B4V-2X6
902-685-3961
Fax: 902-685-3962
e-mail: smdi@auracom.com
users.auracom.com
A registered Canadian charity founded in 1983 by us, to provide a non-technical worldwide information links via publications and now this web site, for neuromuscular disorders.

Research Centers

6508 Baylor College of Medicine: Jerry Lewis Neuromuscular Disease Research
Methodist Neurological Institute
Department of Neurology
Houston, TX 77030
713-798-4333
Fax: 713-798-3854
e-mail: neurochair@bcm.edu
www.bcm.edu/neurology
Offers research into biochemistry molecular genetics and neuromuscular disorders.
Eli M. Mizrahi, M.D., Chair, Department of Neurology
Travis G. Corwin, Department Administrator

6509 Columbia Presbyterian Medical Center Neurological Institute
Columbia University
710 W 168th Street
New York, NY 10032
212-305-2700
Fax: 212-058-98
www.cumc.columbia.edu
Neuromuscular clinical research center.
Hiroshi Mits MD, Division Head Neuromuscular Division

6510 Columbia University Clinical Research Center for Muscular Dystrophy
College of Physicians & Surgeons
116th and Broadway
New York, NY 10027
212-854-1754
Fax: 212-305-1343
www.columbia.edu
Salvatore DiMauro, Co Director

6511 Hospital of the University of Pennsylvania University of Pennsylvania
University of Pennsylvania
3400 Spruce Street
Philadelphia, PA 19104
215-662-4000
800-789-PENN
Fax: 215-903-09
e-mail: pleasure@email.chop.edu
www.pennhealth.com
Research program centering its efforts on finding better ways to prevent and treat neuromuscular disorders.
David E Pleasure MD, Director

6512 Mayo Clinic and Foundation Mayo Foundation
Mayo Foundation
201 W Center Street
Rochester, MN 55905
507-284-2511
Fax: 507-284-0161
TTY: 507-284-9786
www.mayo.edu
Neuromuscular clinical research center with a primary research interest in neuropathies.
Peter J Dyck MD, Director Nerve Studies
Andrew G Engel MD, Director Muscle Studies

6513 Muscular Dystrophy Association
3300 E Sunrise Drive
Tucson, AZ 85718-3299
520-529-2000
800-572-1717
Fax: 520-529-5300
e-mail: mda@mdausa.org
www.MDausa.org
Fights neuromuscular disease including all muscular dystrophies. Conducts extensive programs of research services and public education including 230 clinics.
Robert Ross, President/CEO

6514 University of Utah Utah Genome Depot University of Utah
University of Utah
20 S 2030 E
Salt Lake City, UT 84112
801-585-7606
Fax: 801-857-7177
e-mail: bob.weiss@genetics.utah.edu
www.genome.utah.edu
Focuses research on human muscular dystrophies.
Robert Weiss, Principal Investigator
Jackie Tyce, Program Coordinator

Support Groups & Hotlines

6515 Facioscapulohumeral Muscular Dystrophy Soc iety (FSH Society)
450 Bedford Street
Lexington, MA 02420
781-860-0501
Fax: 781-860-0599
e-mail: solvefshd@fshsociety.org
www.fshsociety.org
The Facioscapulohumeral Muscular Dystrophy Society (FSH Society) serves as a resource for individuals and families with FSHD, representing them and advocating on their behalf. Purposes of the organization are to accumulate, disseminate and encourage the exchange of information about FSHD, including educating the general public, relevant governmental bodies, and the medical and scientific professions about the existence, diagnosis and treatment of FSHD.
Daniel Paul Perez, President/CEO
June Kinoshita, Executive Director

6516 National Health Information Center
PO Box 1133
Washington, DC 20013
310-565-4167
800-336-4797
Fax: 301-984-4256
e-mail: info@nhic.org
www.health.gov/nhic
Offers a nationwide information referral service, produces directories and resource guides.

Books

6517 Clinical Evaluation and Diagnostic Tests for Neuromuscular Disorders
Butterworth-Heinemann Medical
200 Wheeler Road
Burlington, MA 01803
781-221-2212
Fax: 781-221-1615
e-mail: custserv.bh@elsevier.com
www.bh.com
Expert advice from leading authorities on how and when to use the numerous evaluation tests now available for diagnosis and management of neuromuscular disorders.
2002

6518 Everyday Life with ALS: A Practical Guide
Muscular Dystrophy Association
3300 E Sunrise Drive
Tucson, AZ 85718-3299
520-529-2000
800-572-1717
Fax: 520-529-5383
e-mail: publications@mdausa.org
www.mda.org
Advice and information addressing degrees of affliction of those with ALS. Ways to conserve energy, to modifying your home space, to medical devices and equipment. Consider using the Guide with your care team.
2005
Christina Medvescek, Director of Editorial Services

6519 Journey of Love: Parent's Guide to Duchenne Muscular Dystrophy
Muscular Dystrophy Association
3300 E Sunrise Drive
Tucson, AZ 85718-3299
520-529-2000
800-572-1717
Fax: 520-529-5383
e-mail: publications@mdausa.org
www.mda.org
Complete guide for parents with children diagnosed with DMD. Information includes explanation of the disease, treatments, research, services provided by MDA, guides to finding assistance and more.
170 pages Paperback
Bob Mackle, Director Public Information
Christina Medvescek, Director of Editorial Services

6520 MDA ALS Caregiver's Guide
Muscular Dystrophy Association
3300 E Sunrise Drive
Tucson, AZ 85718-3299
520-529-2000
800-572-1717
e-mail: publication@mdusa.org
www.mda.org
A comprehensive guide to caring for a person with ALS at home. Covers everything from physical care to psychological and emotional concerns to getting financial assistance. Companion to Everyday Life with ALS: A Practical Guide.
2008 58 pages Paperback
Bob Mackle, Director Public Information
Christina Medvescek, Director of Editorial Services

6521 Moonrise: One Family, Genetic Identity, & Muscular Dystrophy
St. Martin's Press
175 5th Avenue
New York, NY 10010
212-674-5151
Fax: 212-420-9314
www.stmartins.com
A mother writes about her teen-age son who has Duchenne muscular dystrophy, the life he leads, and the one he can look forward to.
2003

6522 Muscular Dystrophy & Other Neuromuscular Diseases: Psychological Issues
Leon Charash, Robert Lovelace, author
Haworth Press
10 Alice Street
Binghamton, NY 13904
607-722-5857
800-429-6784
Fax: 607-722-0012
www.haworthpress.com
Thoughtful book from professionals who assist people with neuromuscular disorders to help them adapt to lifestyle changes accompanying these disorders.
250 pages Hardcover
ISBN: 1-560240-77-0

6523 Muscular Dystrophy in Children: Guide for Families
Demos Medical Publishing
386 Park Avenue S
New York, NY 10015
800-532-8663
Fax: 212-683-0118
e-mail: orderdept@demospub.com
www.demosmedpub.com
Addresses emotional as well as physical challenges that families and caregivers will have to face and gives readers information on muscular dystrophy, how to adapt to a child's needs, and present research being conducted. In addition, it gives parents and caregivers sources for additional support and suggestions for further reading.
1999

6524 Neuromuscular Dis. of Infancy, Childhood & Adolesesce: A Clinician's Approach
Butterworth-Heinemann Medical
200 Wheeler Road
Burlington, MA 01803
781-221-2212
Fax: 781-221-1615
e-mail: custserv.bh@elsevier.com
www.bh.com
Explains how childhood neuromuscular diseases differ from those in adult patients, and provides clinicians with all the knowledge they need to successfully diagnose and treat pediatric patients.
2003

6525 Noninvasive Mechanical Ventilation
John Bach, MD, author
Elsevier
Book Customer Service Department
St. Louis, MO 63146
800-545-2522
Fax: 800-535-9935
e-mail: usbkinfo@elsevier.com
www.elsevier.com
Describes the use of inspiratory and expiratory muscle aids to prevent the pulmonary complications of lung disease and conditions with muscle weakness. It also describes treatment and rehabilitation interventions specific for patients with these conditions. This book is unique in presenting the use of entirely noninvasive management alternatives to eliminate respiratory morbidity and avoid the need to resort to tracheostomy for the majority of patients with lung or neuromuscular disease.
2002 348 pages Paperback
ISBN: 1-560535-49-0

6526 Physical Medicine & Rehabilitation
WB Saunders/Elsevier Science/Harcourt
200 Wheeler Road
Burlington, MA 01803
781-221-2212
Fax: 781-221-1615
e-mail: custserv.bh@elsevier.com
www.us.elsevierhealth.com
Current aspects of physical medicine and rehabilitation in a single, readable volume. Completely updated and revised edition includes all the latest advances and techniques.
2001

Children's Books

6527 Abby & the South Seas Adventure Series
Tyndale House Publishers
PO Box 80
Wheaton, IL 60189
630-668-8300
Fax: 630-668-3245
www.tyndalecatalog.com
Delightful new series, focusing on the travels of Abby Kendall, who has muscular dystrophy, is a sure-fire hit for 8 to 12 year old girls. Lots of surprises will keep them coming back for each new Abby title.
2000

6528 Heartsongs, Journey Through Heartsongs, Hope Through Heartsongs, Celebrate
Hyperion Books
1344 Crossman Avenue
Sunnyvale, CA 94089
408-744-9500
Fax: 408-744-0400
www.hyperion.com
By the 2002-2003 National Goodwill Ambassador for the Muscular Dystrophy Association. The first two books of inspiring poems were both on the New York Times bestseller list. Mattie's struggle with muscular dystrophy has never kept him from feeling deep love for his family, friends, country and faith — heartfelt emotions that are reflected throughout these pages by a precociously brilliant boy.
2001-2003
Carol Sowell, Director Publications

6529 Muscular Dystrophy
Enslow Publishers
40 Industrial Road
Berkeley Heights, NJ 07922-0398
800-398-2504
Fax: 908-771-0925
e-mail: info@enslow.com
www.enslow.com
Written for children, this book follows two families with muscular dystrophy and describes various forms of the disease, who gets it, and how to learn to live with it.
2000

Magazines

6530 Quest Magazine
Muscular Dystrophy Association
3300 E Sunrise Drive
Tucson, AZ 85718-3299
520-529-2000
800-572-1717
Fax: 520-529-5300
e-mail: publications@mdusa.org
www.mda.org
Quarterly magazine. Contains stories about vital concerns of people with neuromuscular diseases and their community. Find tips, hobbies, resources, treatments, findings, and products. Available online.
30 pages Paperback
Bob Mackle, Director Public Information
Christina Medvescek, Director of Editorial Services

Pamphlets

6531 Breathe Easy: Respiratory Care with Muscular Dystrophy
Muscular Dystrophy Association
3300 E Sunrise Drive
Tucson, AZ 85718-3299
520-529-2000
800-572-1717
Fax: 520-529-5383
e-mail: publications@mdausa.org
www.mda.org
Members of a respiratory care team describe how muscular dystrophy can affect breathing, maintaining respiratory health and types of therapies. Also available in Spanish.
2006
Christina Medvescek, Director of Editorial Services

6532 Everybody's Different Nobody's Perfect
Muscular Dystrophy Association
3300 E Sunrise Drive
Tucson, AZ 85718-3299
520-529-2000
800-572-1717
Fax: 520-529-5300
e-mail: publications@mdausa.org
www.mda.org
Children's Book. Explains how muscular dystrophy affects children and describes how people are different from each other in many ways. Emphasizing fun, friendship and caring, this booklet is ideal for heightening awareness and encouraging understanding of persons with disabilities. Also available in Spanish.
1999 11 pages Paperback
Bob Mackle, Director Public Information
Christina Medvescek, Director of Editorial Services

6533 Facts About Charcot-Marie-Tooth Disease
Muscular Dystrophy Association
3300 E Sunrise Drive
Tucson, AZ 85718-3299
520-529-2000
800-572-1717
Fax: 520-529-5383
e-mail: publications@mdausa.org
www.mda.org
Covers the forms of the disease and outlines the characteristics and genetic patterns of the CMTs. Research efforts aimed at finding the causes, treatments and cures are also described. Also available in Spanish.
15 pages
Christina Medvescek, Director of Editorial Services

6534 Facts About Duchenne & Becker Muscular Dystrophies
Muscular Dystrophy Association
3300 E Sunrise Drive
Tucson, AZ 85718-3299
520-529-2000
800-572-1717
Fax: 520-529-5383
e-mail: publications@mdausa.org
www.mda.org
Introductory booklet describes the two disorders, testing, inheritance and treatments. Also available in Spanish.
Christina Medvescek, Director of Editorial Services

6535 Facts About Facioscapulohumeral Muscular Dystrophy
Muscular Dystrophy Association
3300 E Sunrise Drive
Tucson, AZ 85718-3299
520-529-2000
800-572-1717
Fax: 520-529-5383
e-mail: publications@mdausa.org
www.mda.org

Introductory booklet describes FSHD in easy-to-understand terms and answers commonly asked questions about the disease. Also available in Spanish.
Christina Medvescek, Director of Editorial Services

6536　Facts About Friedreich's Ataxia
Muscular Dystrophy Association
3300 E Sunrise Drive
Tucson, AZ 85718-3299
520-529-2000
800-572-1717
Fax: 520-529-5300
e-mail: publications@mdusa.org
www.mda.org
Explains Friedreich's ataxia in layman's terms and answers commonly asked questions about the disease. Also available in Spanish.
15 pages Paperback
Bob Mackle, Director Public Information
Christina Medvescek, Director of Editorial Services

6537　Facts About Limb-Girdle Muscular Dystrophy
Muscular Dystrophy Association
3300 E Sunrise Drive
Tucson, AZ 85718-3299
520-529-2000
800-572-1717
Fax: 520-529-5383
e-mail: publications@mdausa.org
www.mda.org
Introductory booklet provides basic facts about LGMD and contains information regarding the many forms, diagnostic tests and current treatments. Also available in Spanish.
Christina Medvescek, Director of Editorial Services

6538　Facts About Metabolic Diseases of Muscle
Muscular Dystrophy Association
3300 E Sunrise Drive
Tucson, AZ 85718-3299
520-529-2000
800-572-1717
Fax: 520-529-5300
e-mail: publications@mdusa.org
www.mda.org
Provides an overview of the 11 inheritable metabolic diseases of muscle encompassed by MDA's program. Addresses commonly asked questions and highlights MDA's research efforts aimed at finding the causes of and effective treatments for these disorders. Also available in Spanish.
20 pages Paperback
Bob Mackle, Director Public Information
Christina Medvescek, Director of Editorial Services

6539　Facts About Mitochondrial Myopathies
Muscular Dystrophy Association
3300 E Sunrise Drive
Tucson, AZ 85718-3299
520-529-2000
800-572-1717
Fax: 520-529-5300
e-mail: publications@mdusa.org
www.mda.org
Explains mitochondrial myopathies in layman's terms and answers the most frequently asked questions about this disease. Also available in Spanish.
24 pages Paperback
Bob Mackle, Director Public Information
Christina Medvescek, Director of Editorial Services

6540　Facts About Myasthenia Gravis
Muscular Dystrophy Association
3300 E Sunrise Drive
Tucson, AZ 85718-3299
520-529-2000
800-572-1717
Fax: 520-529-5300
e-mail: publications@mdusa.org
www.mda.org
Explains myasthenia gravis and Lambert-Eaton syndrome in layman's terms and answers the most frequently asked questions about these diseases. Also available in Spanish.
19 pages Paperback
Bob Mackle, Director Public Information
Carol Sowall, Director Publications

6541　Facts About Myopathies
Muscular Dystrophy Association

3300 E Sunrise Drive
Tucson, AZ 85718-3299
520-529-2000
800-572-1717
Fax: 520-529-5300
e-mail: publications@mdusa.org
www.mda.org
Overview of the myopathies encompassed by MDA's program. Addresses commonly asked questions and highlights MDA's research efforts aimed at finding the causes of and effective treatments for these disorders. Also available in Spanish.
18 pages Paperback
Bob Mackle, Director Public Information
Christina Medvescek, Director of Editorial Services

6542　Facts About Myotonic Muscular Dystrophy
Muscular Dystrophy Association
3300 E Sunrise Drive
Tucson, AZ 85718-3299
520-529-2000
800-572-1717
Fax: 520-529-5383
e-mail: publications@mdausa.org
www.mda.org
Introductory booklet provides basic facts about the disorder and explains the causes and effects, as well as tests used to diagnose and MDA's search for treatments and cures. Also available in Spanish.
Christina Medvescek, Director of Editorial Services

6543　Facts About Plasmapheresis
Muscular Dystrophy Association
3300 E Sunrise Drive
Tucson, AZ 85718-3299
520-529-2000
800-572-1717
Fax: 520-529-5300
e-mail: publications@mdusa.org
www.mda.org
Describes plasmapheresis, a plasma exchange procedure often utilized as a treatment for autoimmune disease such as myasthenia gravis and Lambert-Eaton syndrome.
Paperback
Bob Mackle, Director Public Information
Christina Medvescek, Director of Editorial Services

6544　Facts About Polymyostis/Dermatomyositis
Muscular Dystrophy Association
3300 E Sunrise Drive
Tucson, AZ 85718-3299
520-529-2000
800-572-1717
Fax: 520-529-5300
e-mail: publications@mdusa.org
www.mda.org
Outlines these two front forms of inflammatory myopathy. Current approaches to treatment and MDA's efforts in continued research are described. Also available in Spanish.
13 pages Paperback
Bob Mackle, Director Public Information
Christina Medvescek, Director of Editorial Services

6545　Facts About Rare Muscular Dsytrophies
Muscular Dystrophy Association
3300 E Sunrise Drive
Tucson, AZ 85718-3299
520-529-2000
800-572-1717
Fax: 520-529-5300
e-mail: publications@mdusa.org
www.mda.org
This brochure gives basic facts about four forms of muscular dystrophy (Congenital, Distal, Emery-Dreifuss and Oculopharyngeal) and addresses commonly asked questions. Also available in Spanish.
28 pages Paperback
Bob Mackle, Director Public Information
Christina Medvescek, Director of Editorial Services

6546　Facts About Spinal Muscular Atrophy
Muscular Dystrophy Association
3300 E Sunrise Drive
Tucson, AZ 85718-3299
520-529-2000
800-572-1717
Fax: 520-529-5300
e-mail: publications@mdusa.org
www.mda.org
Covers the four forms of the disease and outlines the characteristics and genetic patterns of the SMAs. Research efforts aimed at

finding the causes, treatments and cures are also described. Also available in Spanish.
15 pages Paperback
Bob Mackle, Director Public Information
Christina Medvescek, Director of Editorial Services

6547   Genetics and Neuromuscular Diseases
Muscular Dystrophy Association
3300 E Sunrise Drive   520-529-2000
Tucson, AZ 85718-3299   800-572-1717
                                                                          Fax: 520-529-5383
                                                            e-mail: publications@mdausa.org
                                                                                www.mda.org
Booklet describes what a genetic disorder is and explains how genetic testing and counseling can help people understand how disorders that may affect them or their children are inherited. Also available in Spanish.
Christina Medvescek, Director of Editorial Services

6548   Hey, I'm Here Too
Muscular Dystrophy Association
3300 E Sunrise Drive   520-529-2000
Tucson, AZ 85718-3299   800-572-1717
                                                                          Fax: 520-529-5383
                                                            e-mail: publications@mdausa.org
                                                                                www.mda.org
Help for siblings of boys with Duchenne muscular dystrophy. Explores how they feel about themselves, their brothers and their families. Also provides specific answers to some questions that siblings may wonder about. Also available in Spanish.
28 pages
Bob Mackle, Director Public Information
Christina Medvescek, Director of Editorial Services

6549   Learning to Live with Neuromuscular Desease: A Message to Parents
Muscular Dystrophy Association
3300 E Sunrise Drive   520-529-2000
Tucson, AZ 85718-3299   800-572-1717
                                                                          Fax: 520-529-5383
                                                            e-mail: publications@mdausa.org
                                                                                www.mda.org
Helps parents and families cope with the fact that their child has a neuromuscular disease and with the impact the disease will have on everyday life. Also available in Spanish.
Christina Medvescek, Director of Editorial Services

6550   MDA Camp: A Special Place
Muscular Dystrophy Association
3300 E Sunrise Drive   520-529-2000
Tucson, AZ 85718-3299   800-572-1717
                                                                          Fax: 520-529-5300
                                                            e-mail: publications@mdausa.org
                                                                                www.mdusa.org
Highlights the activities of MDA dummer camps for youngsters diagnosed with one of the more than 40 diseases in MDA's program. Shares camper and volunteer reactions. Also available in Spanish.
Paperback
Bob Mackle, Director Public Information
Carol Sowall, Director Publications

6551   MDA Fact Sheet
Muscular Dystrophy Association
3300 E Sunrise Drive   520-529-2000
Tucson, AZ 85718-3299   800-572-1717
                                                                          Fax: 520-529-5383
                                                            e-mail: publications@mdausa.org
                                                                                www.mda.org
Basic information on MDA's origins and purposes; the more than 40 neuromuscular diseases in MDA's program, and brief symptom descriptions by category. Also available in Spanish.
Christina Medvescek, Director of Editorial Services

6552   MDA Services for the Individual, Family and Community
Muscular Dystrophy Association
3300 E Sunrise Drive   520-529-2000
Tucson, AZ 85718-3299   800-572-1717
                                                                          Fax: 520-529-5383
                                                            e-mail: publications@mdausa.org
                                                                                www.mda.org

Lists the diseases covered by MDA as well as eligibility criteria for MDA's services program, a list of MDA-sponsored clinics nationwide, and the services available through local MDA offices. Also available in Spanish.
Christina Medvescek, Director of Editorial Services

6553   Teacher's Guide to Neuromuscular Disease
Muscular Dystrophy Association
3300 E Sunrise Drive   520-529-2000
Tucson, AZ 85718-3299   Fax: 520-529-5383
                                                            e-mail: publications@mdausa.org
                                                                                www.mda.org
This publication provides a source of guidance and information to teachers, giving details about neuromuscular diseases, how they affect school participation, and ways that teachers can help meet the needs of students affected by these disorders.
2005
Christina Medvescek, Director of Editorial Services

6554   Travis, I Got Lots of Neat Stuff Children Living with Muscular Dystrophy
Muscular Dystrophy Association
3300 E Sunrise Drive   520-529-2000
Tucson, AZ 85718-3299   800-572-1717
                                                                          Fax: 520-529-5383
                                                            e-mail: publications@mdausa.org
                                                                                www.mda.org
Booklet illustrates that a child with muscular dystrophy can do many things. Adapted for MDA's Hop-a-Thon program, the booklet heightens awareness and understanding of people with disabilities. It's suitable for youngsters in elementary school. Also available in Spanish.
24 pages
Christina Medvescek, Director of Editorial Services

Audio & Video

6555   Muscular Dystrophy
Films for the Humanities & Sciences
Box 2053   609-419-8000
Princeton, NJ 08543-2053   800-257-5126
                                                                          Fax: 609-275-3767
Video deals with how Muscular Dystrophy sufferers deal with the disease that has no cure. Three life stories dealing with surgery, medicine, therapy and bracing as a means to survive. Dr. Betty Banke discusses the need to find a cure while Richard Nordgren from the Dartmouth-Hitchcock Medical Center discusses treatment.
20 Minutes

Web Sites

6556   Healing Well
                                                                          www.healingwell.com
An online health resource guide to medical news, chat, information and articles, newsgroups and message boards, books, disease-related web sites, medical directories, and more for patients, friends, and family coping with disabling diseases, disorders, or chronic illnesses.

6557   Health Finder
                                                                          www.healthfinder.gov
Searchable, carefully developed web site offering information on over 1000 topics. Developed by the US Department of Health and Human Services, the site can be used in both English and Spanish.

6558   Healthlink USA
                                                                          www.healthlinkusa.com
Health information concerning treatment, cures, prevention, diagnosis, risk factors, research, support groups, email lists, personal stories and much more. Updated regularly.

6559   Helios Health
                                                                          www.helioshealth.com
Online resource for your health information. Detailed information about specific health topics, access to expert advice from our Medical Advisory Board, and up-to-date health news.

6560   MedicineNet

www.medicinenet.com

An online resource for consumers providing easy-to-read, authoritative medical and health information.

6561   Medscape

www.medscape.com

Medscape offers specialists, primary care physicians, and other health professionals the Web's most robust and integrated medical information and educational tools.

6562   Muscular Dystrophy Association

www.mdausa.org

Information on effective treatments for muscular dystrophy, related neuromuscular disorders and research programs. In addition, MDA offers a comprehensive program of patient and community services, with access to over 230 MDA-supported clinics nationwide.

6563   Parent Project: Muscular Dystrophy

www.parentdmd.org

Organization of families around the world who have children diagnosed with DMD/BMD. Our goal is to invest significant amounts of money raised into medical research with clinical application.

6564   WebMD

www.webmd.com

Information on Muscular Dystrophy, including articles and resources.

Description

6565 # Myasthenia Gravis

Myasthenia gravis is a disease of the neuromuscular junction - the structure which carries the nerve's chemical signal that tells the muscle to contract. Circulating antibodies attack this junction, leading to weakness of voluntary muscles and muscle fatigue after exercise. Any muscle may be involved, but muscles in the face and throat are especially susceptible. The disease therefore especially affects chewing, swallowing, coughing and facial expressions. These manifestations fluctuate in intensity over hours to days.

Because this disease is caused by an overactive immune system, most treatments target this system. These include corticosteroids, immunosuppressive drugs such as azathioprine, plasmapheresis (filtration of the blood with retention of the cells and removal of the plasma), intravenous immunoglobulins and surgical removal of the thymus gland. In addition, anticholinesterase drugs like pyridostigmine increase the level of the messenger chemical at the neuromuscular junction, thereby increasing muscle strength.

Because of the progressive weakness associated with this disease, physical therapy and assistive devices are generally required.

National Agencies & Associations

6566 **Myasthenia Gravis Association of BC**
2805 Kingsway
Vancouver, BC, V5R-5H9   640-451-5511
e-mail: mgabc@centreforability.bc.ca
www.myasthenia.org
Informs members about new treatment thods and research concerning myasthenia gravis.

6567 **Myasthenia Gravis Foundation**
29234 Piney Way   218-562-4594
Breezy Point, MN 56472   800-541-5454
Fax: 651-917-1835
e-mail: minnesota@myasthenia.org
www.myasthenia.org
The mission of the Foundation is to facilitate the timely diagnosis end optimal care of individuals affected by myasthenia gravis and closely related disorders and to improve their lives through programs of patient services, public information and medical reports.
Marcia Lorimer, Executive Committee
Sam Schulhof, Chair

State Agencies & Associations

Alabama

6568 **Alabama Chapter of the Myasthenia Gravis Foundation of America**
PO Box 530623   205-868-1210
Birmingham, AL 35253   866-749-0844
Fax: 205-868-1211
e-mail: alabama@myasthenia.org
www.myasthenia.org

Michael Greene, President
Joyce Wood, Vice President

Arizona

6569 **Jim L Walker: Arizona Chapter of the Myasthenia Gravis Foundation of America**
PO Box 34173   480-451-3060
Phoenix, AZ 85067-1136   877-347-7905
Fax: 623-321-9032
e-mail: azmgfa@myastheniagravisfoundation.phxcox
www.azmgfa.org

Jim LoVecchio, Chairman
Stephane Borsk, Vice Chairman

Arkansas

6570 **Arkansas Chapter of the Myasthenia Gravis Foundation of America**
5204 Crystal Hill Road   501-753-5974
N Little Rock, AR 72118   877-455-4442
Fax: 501-753-5978
e-mail: mgfoundationar@sbcglobal.net
www.myasthenia.org

Connecticut

6571 **Connecticut Chapter of the Myasthenia Gravis Foundation of America**
PO Box 91   203-556-5012
Clinton, CT 06413-4511   866-329-8784
e-mail: conn@myasthenia.org
www.myasthenia.org

Irving Beck ED

Delaware

6572 **MD/DC/Delaware Chapter of Myasthenia Gravis Foundation of America**
PO Box 186   410-437-1157
Pasedena, MD 21123-0186   866-437-2881
e-mail: maryland@myasthenia.org
www.myasthenia.org/LivingwithMG/MGFAChap

District of Columbia

6573 **MD/DC/Delaware Chapter of Myasthenia Gravis Foundation of America**
PO Box 186   410-437-1157
Pasedena, MD 21113-0186   866-437-2881
e-mail: maryland@myasthenia.org
www.myasthenia.org/LivingwithMG/MGFAChap

Florida

6574 **East Central Florida Chapter of the Myasthenia Gravis Foundation of America**
14502 87 Avenue N   727-596-1491
Seminole, FL 33776-0623   877-596-1491
Fax: 727-596-1491
e-mail: wcflorida@myasthenia.org
www.myasthenia.org

6575 **South Florida Gold Coast Chapter of the Myasthenia Gravis Foundation of America**
6185 Winding Brook Way   561-638-2636
Delray Beach, FL 33484   e-mail: oldjack@gateway.net
www.4-mga.org/?

Jack Moore, Chairman
Loise Cororan, Vice Chairman

6576 **West Central Florida Chapter of the Myasthenia Gravis Foundation of America**
13540 Andova Drive   727-596-1491
Largo, FL 33774-4633   e-mail: mpeters@aol.com
www.4-mga.org/?

Marie Peters, Chairman

Georgia

6577 Georgia Chapter of the Myasthenia Gravis Foundation of America
PO Box 93604   770-973-3269
Atlanta, GA 30318   800-743-4339
Fax: 770-973-3269
e-mail: gachapter_mgfa@hotmail.com
www.ga-mgfa.or

Indiana

6578 Greater Indianapolis Chapter of the Myasthenia Gravis Foundation of America
8922 Haverstick Road   317-846-1462
Indianapolis, IN 46240   e-mail: Spknke@aol.com
www.4-mga.org/?

Earl Zimmerman, Chair

Kentucky

6579 Kentucky Chapter of the Myasthenia Gravis Foundation of America
2628 Rush Trail   270-684-4555
Owensboro, KY 42303   Fax: 270-926-2234
e-mail: shlane@bellsouth.net
www.myasthenia.org

Maryland

6580 MD/DC/Delaware Chapter of Myasthenia Gravis Foundation of America
PO Box 186   410-437-1157
Pasadena, MD 21123-0186   866-437-2881
e-mail: maryland@myasthenia.org
www.myasthenia.org

Massachusetts

6581 Mass./New Hampshire Chapter of the Myasthenia Gravis Foundation of America
5 Alcott Drive   978-562-4570
Northboro, MA 01532   e-mail: djemery@juno.com

6582 Massachusetts Chapter of the MG Foundation
5 Alcott Drive   508-393-1403
Northboro, MA 01532   Fax: 508-393-1403
e-mail: djemery@juno.com
www.4-mga.org/?

6583 Myasthenia Gravis: Massachusetts Chapter
28 Bayview Road
Wellesley, MA 02181   508-851-3218
www.4-mga.org/?

Michelle Ronchetti

Michigan

6584 Great Lakes Chapter of the Myasthenia Gravis Foundation of America
2660 Horizon Drive SE   616-956-0622
Grand Rapids, MI 49546   800-224-9180
Fax: 616-956-9234
e-mail: myasthenia.info@gmail.com
www.myasthenia-mi.org
Autoimmune, neuromuscular disease manifest in weakness of voluntary muscles; arms, legs, eyes, facial expressions, severe cases of breathing.
Susan Richards, Executive Director
Paulus Heule, President

6585 Myasthenia Gravis Association
1000 John R   248-591-4419
Troy, MI 48083   Fax: 248-591-4423
e-mail: mgadetroit1@hotmail.com
www.mgadetroit-easternmi.org

Agnes Wisner, Executive Director
Taylor Bleibtrey, Board Member

Minnesota

6586 Minnesota State Chapter of the Myasthenia Gravis Foundation of America
29234 Piney Way   218-562-4594
Breezy Point, MN 56472-1715   e-mail: minnesota@myasthenia.org
www.myasthenia.org

New Hampshire

6587 Mass./New Hampshire Chapter of the Myasthenia Gravis Foundation of America
460 S River Street   508-435-3808
Marshfield, MA 02050   e-mail: massachusetts@myasthenia.org
www.ma-nhmgfa.org

Marilyn Buckner, Chair
Virginia Pierce, RN, Treasurer

New Jersey

6588 Garden State Chapter of the Myasthenia Gravis Foundation of America
PO Box 4258   973-633-6900
Wayne, NJ 07474-1362   800-437-4949
Fax: 973-633-6908
e-mail: gsmg@webspan.net
www.mgnj.org

Robert Allen, Chairman
Kelley DeVincentis, Executive Director

New Mexico

6589 New Mexico Chapter of the Myasthenia Gravis Foundation of America
PO Box 34173   480-451-3060
Phoenix, AZ 85067-6873   877-347-7905
Fax: 623-321-9032
e-mail: azmgfa@myastheniagravisfoundation.phxcox
www.azmgfa.org

Jim LoVecchio, Chairman
Stephane Borsk, Vice Chairman

New York

6590 Metro New York Chapter of Myasthenia Gravis Foundation of America
PO Box 40   516-538-0738
Stony Brook, NY 11790   800-667-9807
e-mail: MetroNY@myasthenia.org
www.metronymgfa.org

Cindie Killeen, Chairperson
Debbie Thompsen, Vice Chairperson

6591 Myasthenia Gravis Support Group: Long Island
N Shore University Hospital   516-785-7538
Manhasset, NY   e-mail: KARKENN@SPEC.NET
limger.tripod.com/limgsupport.html?

6592 Upstate NY Chapter of the Myasthenia Gravis Foundation of America
355 Lexington Ave   212-297-2156
New York, NY 10017   800-581-5377
Fax: 518-439-8783
e-mail: upstatenewyork@myasthenia.org
www.myasthenia.org

Barry Levine, President/Chair

North Carolina

6593 Carolinas Chapter of the Myasthenia Gravis Foundation of America
506 E Forest Hills Boulevard   919-966-4131
Durham, NC 27707-1801   800-842-8711
Fax: 919-489-7564
e-mail: tvassar56@aol.com
www.med.unc.edu/mgfa/mgnc-hom.htm

Ohio

6594 Mahoning-Shenango Chapter of the Myasthenia Gravis Foundation of America
PO Box 282   330-539-5582
Girard, OH 44420-0282

6595 Ohio Chapter of the Myasthenia Gravis Foundation of America
2907 B Lincoln Way E   513-242-7442
Massillon, OH 44646   Fax: 330-834-9067
                        e-mail: ohiochaptermgf@att.net
                                www.mgfohio.org

Sharon Meyer, Local Contact
Jack Paas, Local Contact

Oklahoma

6596 Oklahoma Chapter of the Myasthenia Gravis Foundation of America
4606 E 67th St S   918-494-4951
Tulsa, OK 74136   Fax: 918-494-4951
                        e-mail: oklahoma@myasthenia.org
                                www.myasthenia.org

Peggy Foust, Executive Director
Margret Feller, Vice-President/Treasurer

Pennsylvania

6597 Myasthenia Gravis Association of Western Pennsylvania
490 EN Avenue   412-566-1545
Pittsburgh, PA 15212   Fax: 412-566-1550
                        e-mail: mgaoffice@mgawpa.org
                                www.mgawpa.org

A neuromuscular disorder with no known cause or cure. The mission is to provide access to superior medical treatment and medications at reasonable cost providing those patients and their families adequate social and psychological support and education.
Maree Gallagher, Executive Director
Alan Weidman, LPN, Patient Care Coordinator

6598 Pennsylvania Chapter of the Myasthenia Gravis Foundation of America
2665 Pinewood Road   717-581-1271
Lancaster, PA 17601   e-mail: PennaMGFA@aol.com
                                www.myasthenia.org

South Carolina

6599 Carolinas Chapter of the Myasthenia Gravis Foundation of America
506 E Forest Hills Boulevard   919-490-2937
Durham, NC 27707-1801   800-842-8711
                                 Fax: 919-489-7564
                        e-mail: tvassar56@aol.com
                                www.myasthenia.org

Texas

6600 Greater South Texas Chapter of the Myasthenia Gravis Foundation of America
10592 Fuqua Street #A   281-987-9393
Houston, TX 77089-1402   Fax: 281-328-2430
                        e-mail: gowens@accesscomm.net
                                www.myasthenia.org

6601 Northwest Texas Chapter of the Myasthenia Gravis Foundation of America
3406 Manioca Road   806-749-3126
Lubbock, TX 79403   Fax: 915-554-7044
                        e-mail: nwtexas@myasthenia.org
                                www.nwtcmg.org

Lowell McBroom, Vice-Chairperson

Utah

6602 Utah State Intermountain Chapter of the Myasthenia Gravis Foundation of America
8717 South 910 East   801-816-2204
Sandy, UT 84094-1831   Fax: 801-572-1787
                e-mail: dawnascheib@waterfordschool.org
                                www.myasthenia.org

Virginia

6603 Virginia Chapter of the Myasthenia Gravis Foundation of America
PO Box 71193   804-308-1674
Richmond, VA 23255   800-728-4405
                                 Fax: 804-308-1674
                        e-mail: va-wvchapmgfa@comcast.net
                                www.myasthenia.org

Georgiann C Davis, President
Anita Steele, VP

Washington

6604 Pacific Northwest Chapter of the Myasthenia Gravis Foundation of America
PO Box 58785   425-235-1435
Renton, WA 98058-6562   877-252-0677
                                 Fax: 425-204-2070
                        e-mail: washington@myasthenia.org
                                www.myasthenia.org

Wisconsin

6605 Wisconsin Chapter of the Myasthenia Gravis Foundation of America
2474 S 96 Street   262-938-9800
W Allis, WI 53227   800-541-5454
                                 Fax: 262-789-3363
                        e-mail: wisconsin@myasthenia.org
                                www.myasthenia.org

The Myasthenia Gravis Foundation of America is the only national volunteer health agency dedicated solely to fight against myasthenoia gravis.
Patricia Lamp, Chairperson
Ellie Burbach, Vice-Chairperson

Support Groups & Hotlines

6606 Myasthenia Gravis Association of Colorado
POB 390083   303-360-7080
Denver, CO 80239   Fax: 303-360-7080
                        e-mail: 4mga@4-mga.org
                                www.4-mga.org/?

Sharon Leahy, Chairperson

6607 Myasthenia Gravis Support Group
4606 E 67th St S   918-494-4951
Tulsa, OK 74136-7808   Fax: 918-494-4951
                        e-mail: oklahoma@myasthenia.org
                                www.myasthenia.org

Provides education and patient services to improve the lives of all people affected by MG and to promote awareness of the disease myasthenia gravis.
Peggy Foust, Executive Director/President

6608 Myasthenia Gravis Support Group East Central Illinois
Myasthenia Gravis Foundation of Illinois
310 W Lake Street   630-835-0153
Elmhurst, IL 60126   800-888-6208
                        e-mail: myastheniaill@aol.org
                                www.myasthenia.org

To facilitate the timely diagnosis and optimal care of individuals affected by myasthenia gravis and to improve their lives through programs of patient services, public awareness, medical research, professional education, advocacy and patient care

6609 Myasthenia Gravis Support Group of Wiscons in
2474 S 96 Street
West Allis, WI 53227-2204   262-938-9800
Fax: 262-789-3363
e-mail: wisconsin@myasthenia.org
www.myasthenia.org
Serves patients and their families throughout the state of Wisconsin. The goal is to help achieve the conquest of Myasthenia Gravis through research, education, public awareness, anf fundraising.

6610 Myasthenia Gravis Support Group: Virginia/ West Virginia
PO Box 71193
Richmond, VA 23255   804-308-1674
Fax: 804-308-1647
e-mail: va-wvchapmgfa@comcast.net
www.myasthenia.org
To facilitate the timely diagnosis and optimal care of individuals affected by MG and closely related disorders and to improve their lives with programs of patient services, public information, medical research, professional education, advocacy and patient care.
Georgiann Davis, President

6611 National Health Information Center
US Department of Health and Human Services
PO Box 1133
Washington, DC 20013-1133   301-565-4167
800-336-4797
Fax: 301-984-4256
e-mail: info@nhic.org
www.health.gov/nhic
Offers a nationwide referral service, produces directories and resource guides.

Books

6612 Myasthenia Gravis
CRC Press
2000 NW Corporate Boulevard
Boca Raton, FL 33431-7385   561-994-0555
Fax: 561-994-3625
1993
ISBN: 0-849363-43-8

Newsletters

6613 Alabama Chapter of the Myasthenia Gravis Foundation of America
Alabama Chapter of the Myasthenia Gravis Found
300 Office Park Drive
Birmingham, AL 35223   205-868-1210
Fax: 205-868-1211
e-mail: alchaptermgfa@aol.com
Three to four newsletters per year. Support Group Information, articles about MG and it's treatment, information about chapters operations.

6614 Connecticut Nutmeg
Myasthenia Gravis Foundation
113 Folly Brook Boulevard
Wethersfield, CT 06109   860-529-8784
Fax: 860-529-8784

6615 Conquer
Myasthenia Gravis Foundation of Illinois
2411 New Street
Blue Island, IL 60406-2328   708-385-3888
800-888-6208
Fax: 708-385-0447
e-mail: mystheniaill@aol.com
myastheniagravis.org
A quarterly newsletter containing articles and stories relating to myasthenia gravis.
16 pages Quarterly
Gerald Tarka, Executive Director

6616 East Central Florida Chapter of the Myasthenia Gravis Foundation of America
PO Box 623
Ormond Beach, FL 32175-0623   904-672-2635
Published bi-monthly, and contains information about latest research. area meetings, and topics of concern for our readers.

6617 Facts About Myasthenia Gravis for Patients and Families
Myasthenia Gravis Foundation of America

5841 Cedar Lake Road
Minneapolis, MN 55416   952-545-9438
800-541-5454
Fax: 952-646-2028
e-mail: mystheniagravis@msn.com
www.myasthenia.org
Offers information on the history, clinical symptoms and features, causes, diagnosis, treatment and prognosis of Myasthenia Gravis.
16 pages 4 per year
Debora K Boelz, CEO
Jennifer Heidelberger, Chapter Relations Manager

6618 MG Communicator
Great Lakes Chapter of the Myasthenia Gravis Found
2680 Horizon Drive SE
Grand Rapids, MI 49546   616-956-0622
800-224-9180
Fax: 616-956-9234
e-mail: myasthenia.info@gmail.com
www.myasthenia-mi.org
3x/year
Susan Richards, Executive Director
Paulus Heule, President

6619 Myasthenia Gravis Association
2300 E Meyer Boulevard
Kansas City, MO 64132-1199   816-276-4585
Fax: 816-276-4569
e-mail: mga@planetkc.org
A nonprofit, United Way agency offering a variety of programs. The programs include; individualized education and advocacy, specialized outpatient clinics, patient support group meetings and newsletters.
Carole Bowe Thompson, Executive Director
Danna Garabedian, Administrative Assistant

6620 Myasthenia Gravis Association: Detroit Chapter
17117 W Nine Mile Road
Southfield, MI 48075   248-423-9700
A quarterly newslatter containing medical articles, personal stories relating to myasthenia gravis.

6621 Myasthenia Gravis Foundation: Geater South Texas
10592 A Fuqua
Houston, TX 77089-1402   281-987-9393
Fax: 281-328-2430
e-mail: gowens@accesscomm.net
Six issues per year. Support Group Information, articles about MG and it's treatment, information about Chapter operations.
Gary Owens, Chair

6622 Myasthenia Gravis Foundation: Northwest Texas Chapter
281 County Road 135
Ovalo, TX 79541   e-mail: nwtxmg@hotmail.com
A quarterly newsletter containing articles and stories relating myasthenia gravis.
Jenne McVicker, Editor

6623 Myasthenia Gravis Foundation: Ohio Chapter
PO Box 6392
Canton, OH 44706   330-477-7727
e-mail: ohiochaptermgf@nci2000,net

6624 Puget Sound Chapter Newsletter
PO Box 587853
Renton, WA 98058-1785   206-235-1435
Fax: 206-204-2070
A quarterly newsletter containing the latest articles and stories relating to myasthenia gravis.

Web Sites

6625 Healing Well
www.healingwell.com
An online health resource guide to medical news, chat, information and articles, newsgroups and message boards, books, disease-related web sites, medical directories, and more for patients, friends, and family coping with disabling diseases, disorders, or chronic illnesses.

6626 Health Finder
www.healthfinder.gov
Searchable, carefully developed web site offering information on over 1000 topics. Developed by the US Department of Health and Human Services, the site can be used in both English and Spanish.

6627   Healthlink USA

www.healthlinkusa.com

Health information concerning treatment, cures, prevention, diagnosis, risk factors, research, support groups, email lists, personal stories and much more. Updated regularly.

6628   Helios Health

www.helioshealth.com

Online resource for your health information. Detailed information about specific health topics, access to expert advice from our Medical Advisory Board, and up-to-date health news.

6629   MedicineNet

www.medicinenet.com

An online resource for consumers providing easy-to-read, authoritative medical and health information.

6630   Medscape

www.medscape.com

Medscape offers specialists, primary care physicians, and other health professionals the Web's most robust and integrated medical information and educational tools.

6631   Myasthenia Gravis Foundation of America

www.myasthenia.org

Dedicated to the conquest of the disease through research, education, information and patient services. Offers over 54 chapters and over 100 support groups across the country as well as 8 international chapters.

6632   Neurology Channel

www.neurologychannel.com

Find clearly explained, medically accurate information regarding conditions, including an overview, symptoms, causes, diagnostic procedures and treatment options. On this site it is possible to ask questions and get information from a neurologist and connect to people who have similar health interests.

6633   WebMD

www.webmd.com

Information on Myasthenia Gravis, including articles and resources.

Description

6634 Neurofibromatosis

Neurofibromatosis, or von Recklinghausen disease, named after a German pathologist, is an inherited genetic disorder. The more common form occurs once in 4,000 births. The skin and the nervous system are the primary target organs. Characteristic skin lesions are large, flat brown freckles, called cafe au lait spots, owing to their light coffee color. They are apparent at birth or in infancy in more than 90 percent of patients. Flesh-colored tumors appear in late childhood. Abnormal growths may be detectable in the brain, perhaps accounting for the seizures and learning difficulties commonly seen in this syndrome. Tumors may appear on the nerves from the eyes or the ears, sometimes causing hearing loss or visual disturbance.

There is no specific therapy for this condition, but tumors that produce severe symptoms can be surgically removed or irradiated. Genetic counseling is important for the entire family.

National Agencies & Associations

6635 Association for the Neurologically Disable d of Canada
59 Clement Road
Etobicoke, Ontario, M9R-1Y5
416-244-1992
Fax: 416-244-4099
e-mail: info@and.ca
www.and.ca
Provides functional rehabilitation programs to individuals with neurological disabilities.
Basil Ziv, Executive Director
Dr John Unruh, Director of Rehabilitation

6636 BC Centre for Ability
2805 Kingsway
Vancouver, BC, V5R-5H9
604-451-5511
Fax: 604-451-5651
e-mail: home@centreforability.bc.ca
www.centreforability.bc.ca
Founded in 1969 by families who desired alternatives to hospital or institutional-based services. The centre provides education and promotes the rights of individuals with disabilities to participate as valued members of their communities.
Angie Kwok, Executive Director
Moses Gabriel, Director of Resource Development

6637 Children's Tumor Foundation
95 Pine Street
New York, NY 10005
212-344-6633
800-323-7938
Fax: 212-747-0004
e-mail: info@ctf.org
www.ctf.org
Dedicated to health and well being of individuals and families affected by the neurofibromatoses (NF).
Allison Walsh, Communications Officer
John Risner, President

6638 NF Canada
PO Box 5055
Victoria, BC V8R 6-2R7
888-986-3876
e-mail: infocanada@nfcanada.ca
www.nfcanada.ca
To ensure that all Canadians living with neurofibromatosis benefit from support, understanding, appropriate medical treatment and the hope that a cure is on the horizon.
Inara Kundzins, President

6639 Neurofibromatosis
Po Box 18246
Minneapolis, MN 55418
651-225-1720
800-942-6825
Fax: 301-918-0009
e-mail: info@nfinc.org
www.nfnetwork.org
A national nonprofit organization with independent and regional chapters that provides support and services to NF families. Simulates funds and encourages participation in NF research. Works closely with clinical and research professionals.
Miguel Lessing, President
Rosemary Anderson, Vice President

6640 Neurofibromatosis Society of Ontario
2004 Underhill Court
Pickering, Ontario, L1X 2-3T2
905-683-0811
Fax: 705-685-1409
e-mail: info@nfon.ca
www.nfon.ca
Support individuals and families affected by NF, to educate its members, professionals, and the general public about NF, and support NF research.
Lynne Leyland, Director
Gladys Hamilton, Director

6641 Neurological Science Federation
7015 Macleod Trail SW
Calgary, AB, T2H-2K6
403-229-9544
Fax: 403-229-1661
e-mail: info@cnsfederation.org
www.ccns.org
To promote and encourage all aspects of neurology, including research, education, assessment and accreditation.

State Agencies & Associations

Alabama

6642 NNFF Alabama Affiliate
1205 Branchwater Lane
Birmingham, AL 35216
205-529-8006
e-mail: info@ctf.org
www.ctf.org
Jeff Albright, Chairperson

Arizona

6643 Neurofibromatosis Association of Arizona
Po Box 2718
Chandler, AZ 85244
480-945-9650
Fax: 480-945-9650
e-mail: info@nfaz.org
www.nfaz.org
Nicole Hicks, Executive Director
Michael Sheedy, President

Arkansas

6644 NNFF Arkansas Affilaite
139 Rainbow Lne
Bigelow, AR 72016
501-759-2710
e-mail: info@ctf.org
www.ctf.org
Lesley Oslica, Information and Support

Colorado

6645 NNFF Colorado Chapter
70 N Ranch Road
Littleton, CO 80127
303-734-9942
e-mail: info@ctf.org
www.ctf.org
Mark Ebel, Chapter President

Connecticut

6646 NNFF Connecticut Chapter
8 S Barn Hill Road
Bloomfield, CT 06002-1622
860-286-2705
Fax: 860-286-2705
TTY: 860-286-2705
TDD: 860-286-2705
e-mail: StevenSand@aol.com
Steve Sandler, Chapter President

Florida

6647 **NNFF Florida Chapter**
PO Box 410684 321-253-1622
Melbourne, FL 32941 800-540-5721
e-mail: info@ctf.org
www.ctf.org
Suzanne Earle, Chapter President

Georgia

6648 **NNFF Georgia Affiliate**
5 Ardmore Circle 678-428-9711
Cartersville, GA 30120 e-mail: info@ctf.org
www.ctf.org
Randy Watkins, Chairman

Idaho

6649 **NNFF Idaho Chapter**
4419 E Linden Street 208-459-6022
Caldwell, ID 83605-8037
Suzy Crici, Chapter President

Illinois

6650 **Illinois Midwest Neurofibromatosis**
Neurofibromatosis
473 Dunham Rd 630-945-3562
St. Charles, IL 60174 800-322-6363
Fax: 630-932-8119
e-mail: info@nfmidwest.org
nfmidwest.org
Diana Haberkamp, Executive Director
Jenny Perkins, Development Director/ Great Steps

6651 **NF Center: North Broward Medical Center Neurofibromatosis**
Neurofibromatosis
213 S. Wheaton Ave. 630-510-1115
Wheaton, IL 60187-3502 800-942-6825
Fax: 630-510-8508
e-mail: admin@nfnetwork.org
www.nfnetwork.org

6652 **NNFF Illinois Chapter: Chicago Area**
5604 W Henderson 3 W
Chicago, IL 60634 e-mail: info@ctf.org
www.ctf.org
Debbi Callahan, Vice President

6653 **NNFF Illinois Chapter: Silvis Area**
513 16th Street 309-792-4195
Silvis, IL 61282 e-mail: nfquadcities@juno.com
Sue Rockwell, Patient Information and Support

6654 **NNFF Illinois Chapter: Springfield Area**
5 Twilight Lane 217-529-0834
Springfield, IL 62712 e-mail: info@ctf.org
www.ctf.org
Marcia Miller, Treasurer

6655 **NNFF Illinois Chapter:Peoria Region**
PO Box 213 217-732-8568
Emden, IL 62635 e-mail: info@ctf.org
www.ctf.org
Paul Beach, President

Indiana

6656 **NNFF Indiana Chapter**
1173 Hague Court 317-736-7577
Franklinolis, IN 46131 e-mail: info@ctf.org
www.ctf.org
Dottie Whitehurst, Chapter President

Iowa

6657 **NNFF Iowa Chapter**
321 Glenview Drive 515-277-8494
De Moines, IA 50312 e-mail: info@ctf.org
www.ctf.org
Sheila Drevyanko, Chapter President

Kansas

6658 **NNFF Kansas Affiliate**
12606 E 49th Terrace 816-737-8378
Independence, MO 64055 e-mail: info@ctf.org
www.ctf.org
Annette Novak, Chairperson

6659 **Neurofibromatosis Kansas and Central Plains**
Neurofibromatosis
9218 Metcalf 620-669-8453
Overland Park, KS 66212-1792 800-942-6825
e-mail: nprieb@sbcglobal.net
www.nfnetwork.org

Louisiana

6660 **NNFF Louisiana Chapter**
PO Box 499 225-665-3547
Baton Rouge, LA 70821 e-mail: info@ctf.org
www.ctf.org
Debbie Bouy, Chairperson

Maryland

6661 **Neurofibromatosis: Mid-Atlantic**
Neurofibromatosis
2 Village Square. 443-423-0535
Baltimore, MD 21210-2924 800-942-6825
Fax: 301-577-0016
e-mail: info@nfmidatlantic.org
www.nfmidatlantic.org

Mid-Atlantic Chapter serves the following states: Maryland Virginia District of Columbia Delaware New Jersey Pennsylvania West Virginia and North Carolina.
Barbra Levin, Executive Director
Beverly B Dobson, President

Massachusetts

6662 **Neurofibromatosis: New England**
Neurofibromatosis
9 Bedford Street 781-272-9936
Burlington, MA 01803-3702 Fax: 781-272-9937
e-mail: info@nfincne.org
www.nfincne.org
Karen Peluso, Executive Director
Dr Paul Epstein, President

Minnesota

6663 **Neurofibromatosis: Minnesota**
Neurofibromatosis
PO Box 18246 651-225-1720
Minneapolis, MN 55418 e-mail: JohnE@cipmn.org
www.nfincmn.org
John Everett, President
Steven Schutts, Vice-President

Nevada

6664 **NNFF Nevada Affiliate: Reno Area**
8065 White Falls Drive 775-972-1882
Reno, NV 89506 e-mail: info@ctf.org
www.ctf.org
David Rice, Chairperson

Oregon

6665 **NNFF Oregon Affiliate Kaiser Permanente Northwest**
Kaiser Permanente Northwest

2806 SW Troy   503-331-6325
Portland, OR 97227   Fax: 503-331-6320
                                      e-mail: info@ctf.org
                                      www.ctf.org
Katie Crow, Genetic Counselor

South Carolina

6666   NNFF South Carolina Chapter
111 Oakview Drive   843-393-9672
Darlington, SC 29532   e-mail: info@ctf.org
                                      www.ctf.org
Pat Chrisely, Chairperson

Wisconsin

6667   NNFF Wisconsin Chapter
6562 W Glenbrook Road   414-362-0211
Brown Deer, WI 53223   e-mail: info@ctf.org
                                      www.ctf.org
Elaine Pankow, President

Support Groups & Hotlines

6668   Children's Tumor Foundation
95 Pine Street   212-344-6633
New York, NY 10005   800-323-7938
                                      Fax: 212-747-0004
                                      e-mail: info@ctf.org
                                      www.ctf.org
Sponsors critical research, public awareness and patient support
services.
Allison Walsh, Communications Officer

6669   NF Support Group of West Michigan
Spectrum Health
PO Box 6026   616-451-3699
Grand Rapids, MI 49516   e-mail: nfwestmich@aol.com
                                      www.nfsupport.org
Rose Mary Anderson, Patient Advocate

6670   National Health Information Center
PO Box 1133   310-565-4167
Washington, DC 20013   800-336-4797
                                      Fax: 301-984-4256
                                      e-mail: info@nhic.org
                                      www.health.gov/nhic
Offers a nationwide information referral service, produces direc-
tories and resource guides.

6671   Neurofibromatosis
9320 Annapolis Road   301-918-4600
Lanham, MD 20706-3123   800-942-6825
                                      Fax: 301-918-0009
                                      e-mail: nfinfo@nfinc.com
                                      www.nfnetwork.org
Dedicated to individuals and families affected by the
neurofibromatosis through educational, support, clinical and re-
search programs.
Miguell Lessing, President
Rosemary Anderson, Vice President

6672   Neurofibromatosis Foundation: Colorado
2505 18th Street, Denver   303-433-8383
Denver, CO 80211   800-323-7938
                                      e-mail: UsRKids@aol.com
                                      www.unitedwaydenver.org
Offers a support group to persons affected by neurofibromatosis.
Offers panel discussion, sharing, fundraising, and fun activities.
Also provides new patient information.
Charles Taylor
Jane Cahn

6673   Neurofibromatosis Support Network
Parents Helping Parents
1400 Parkmoor Avenue   408-727-5775
San Jose, CA 95126   855-727-5775
                                      Fax: 408-286-1116
                                      www.php.com

Helping children with special needs receive the resources, love,
hope, respect, health care, education and other services they need
to achieve their full potential by providing them with strong families and dedicated professionals to serve them.
Sheri Sobrato, MA/MFC

6674   Neuroscience Institute at Mercy Hospital
4120N W Memorial Road
Oklahoma City, OK 73120   800-996-3729
                                      Fax: 405-752-3977
                                      www.okmercy.net
Mike Patt, Chief Executive Officer

6675   Texas Neurofibromatosis Foundation
3030 Olive Street   972-868-794
Dallas, TX 75219   Fax: 972-868-7626
                                      www.texasnf.org
Cindy Hahn, Executive Director
Emily Deutscher, Development Coordinator

Newsletters

6676   Neurofibromatosis
9320 Annapolis Road   301-918-4600
Lanham, MD 20706-3123   800-942-6825
                                      Fax: 301-918-0009
                                      e-mail: nfinfo@nfinc.org
                                      www.nfinc.org
Provides a variety of resources for NF families, professionals and
researchers.
SemiAnnual
Gwen Charest, Executive Director

Pamphlets

6677   Child with Neurofibromatosis 1
Children's Tumor Foundation
95 Pine Street   212-344-NNFF
New York, NY 10005-1703   800-323-7938
                                      e-mail: info@ctf.org
                                      www.ctf.org
Offers information on the prognosis, management, complications,
genetic implications, and sources of support for children with
neurofibromatosis 1.
Allison Walsh, Communications Officer

6678   Guide for Teens
Children's Tumor Foundation
95 Pine Street   212-344-NNFF
New York, NY 10005-1703   800-323-7938
                                      e-mail: info@ctf.org
                                      www.ctf.org
Offers information for teenagers on how to face neurofibromatosis
on a daily basis.
Allison Walsh, Communications Officer

6679   How NF-1 Affects the Body
Neurofibromatosis
9320 Annapolis Road   301-918-4600
Lanham, MD 20706-3123   800-942-6825
                                      Fax: 301-918-0009
                                      e-mail: nfinfo@nfinc.org
                                      www.nfinc.org
A graphic showing the parts of the body where symptoms of NF-1
can occur.
Gwen Charest, Executive Director

6680   How NF-2 Affects the Body
Neurofibromatosis
9320 Annapolis Road   301-918-4600
Lanham, MD 20706-3123   800-942-6825
                                      Fax: 301-918-0009
                                      e-mail: nfinfo@nfinc.org
                                      www.nfinc.org
A graphic showing the parts of the body where symptoms of NF-2
can occur.
Gwen Charest, Executive Director

6681 National NF Medical Resource Listing
Neurofibromatosis
9320 Annapolis Road   301-918-4600
Lanham, MD 20706-3123   800-942-6825
                                        Fax: 301-918-0009
                                    e-mail: nfinfo@nfinc.org
                                              www.nfinc.org
A listing of medical centers in the US where geneticists and NF experts are located.
Gwen Charest, Executive Director

6682 Neurofibromatosis
March of Dimes
233 Park Avenue South   212-353-8353
New York, NY 10003   Fax: 212-254-3518
                             e-mail: NY639@marchofdimes.com
                                      www.marchofdimes.com
Located on the website.

6683 Neurofibromatosis Type 2: Information for Patients and Families
Children's Tumor Foundation
95 Pine Street   212-344-6633
New York, NY 10005-1703   800-323-7938
                                      e-mail: info@ctf.org
                                              www.ctf.org
Offers extensive information on what NF2 is and answers the most asked about questions regarding the illness.
Allison Walsh, Communications Officer

6684 Understanding Neurofibromatosis
9320 Annapolis Road   301-918-4600
Lanham, MD 20706-3123   800-942-6825
                                        Fax: 301-918-0009
                                    e-mail: nfinfo@nfinc.org
                                              www.nfinc.org
A handbook specifically designed for the newly diagnosed NF families.
Gwen Charest, Executive Director

Web Sites

6685 Healing Well
                                        www.healingwell.com
An online health resource guide to medical news, chat, information and articles, newsgroups and message boards, books, disease-related web sites, medical directories, and more for patients, friends, and family coping with disabling diseases, disorders, or chronic illnesses.

6686 Health Finder
                                         www.healthfinder.gov
Searchable, carefully developed web site offering information on over 1000 topics. Developed by the US Department of Health and Human Services, the site can be used in both English and Spanish.

6687 Healthlink USA
                                        www.healthlinkusa.com
Health information concerning treatment, cures, prevention, diagnosis, risk factors, research, support groups, email lists, personal stories and much more. Updated regularly.

6688 Helios Health
                                         www.helioshealth.com
Online resource for your health information. Detailed information about specific health topics, access to expert advice from our Medical Advisory Board, and up-to-date health news.

6689 MGH Neurology
                                          www.mgh.harvard.edu
Provides both unmonderated message boards and chat rooms for specific neurological disorders including: amyloidosis, arachnoiditis, cerebellar ataxia, congenital fiber type disproportion, CFS leak, DeMorsiers syndrome, erythromealgia, Lewy body disease, meningitis, meralgia paresthetic, Norrie disease, periodic paralysis, phantom limb pain, Romberg disorder, Syndenhams chorea, tethered cord syndrome, and thoracic outlet syndrome.

6690 MedicineNet
                                          www.medicinenet.com

An online resource for consumers providing easy-to-read, authoritative medical and health information.

6691 Medscape
                                          www.medscape.com
Medscape offers specialists, primary care physicians, and other health professionals the Web's most robust and integrated medical information and educational tools.

6692 Neurology Channel
                                      www.neurologychannel.com
Find clearly explained, medically accurate information regarding conditions, including an overview, symptoms, causes, diagnostic procedures and treatment options. On this site it is possible to ask questions and get information from a neurologist and connect to people who have similar health interests.

6693 WebMD
                                              www.webmd.com
Information on Neurofibromatosis, including articles and resources.

Description

6694 **Obesity**

Obesity refers to a condition in which there is an excessive accumulation of fat in subcutaneous and other tissues of the body. Being obese and being overweight are not necessarily synonymous, as people who are overweight may have increased body size as a result of increased muscle or skeletal tissue mass. Obesity may develop at any age, but peak development periods occur during the first 12 months of life, between the ages of five and six years, and during the adolescent years in children. In adults, obesity may develop at any time, but many people may find that weight gain progresses through the 3rd-6th decade. It is clear from numerous medial, public health and sociologic studies that obesity in the United States occurs in a staggering proportion of the population and many consider it to be an epidemic.

Obesity may result from an increase in the actual number of fat cells or from an increase in the size of the individual fat cells. Researchers believe that fat cells increase in number in proportion to caloric intake increase and that this increase is particularly evident in the first 12 months of life. As children grow, increases in fat cell populations continue at a slower rate. Because the number of fat cells cannot be decreased, except surgically, later weight loss must result from the reduction of fat in individual cells.

Obesity usually results when caloric intake exceeds the energy demands of the body, thus increasing the storage of body fat. Fat accumulation is usually a progressive process, resulting from repeated episodes of food intake exceeding the body's demand for energy (calories). Many factors may influence appetite or obesity. Such factors may include environmental influences; psychosocial disturbances that may be induced by stress or emotional upset or trauma; brain lesions that may involve certain area of the brain such as the hypothalamus or the pituitary gland (both essential to hormone production); an overabundance of insulin in the body (hyperinsulinism); and genetic influences. In addition, in rare instances, obesity may be a feature of certain genetic disorders (see *Prader-Willi syndrome*). the most common cause in North America however, is the excessive intake of calories, particularly those from fats and sugars, and the concomitant lack of physical exercise and activity that uses calories.

Complications of obesity in the child and the adult may include respiratory difficulties such as shortness of breath and increased cardiovascular risk factors such as high blood pressure, elevated total cholesterol levels as well as increased bad or LDL cholesterol and decreased good or HDL cholesterol, and increased levels of fatty acid and glycerol compounds (triglycerides). These are risk factors for the development of coronary artery disease, one of the leading causes of morbidity and the mortality in North America. In addition, obesity may be associated with a resistance to the hormone insulin that aids in the metabolism of glucose, fats, carbohydrates, and proteins. This resistance may lead to excessive levels of circulating insulin in the body (hyperinsulinism); however, the body is not able to appropriately use insulin and high blood sugar (hyperglycemia) may occur. This condition is known as Type II Diabetes Mellitus and its incidence in the population is also increasing dramatically in both children and adults. The diagnosis of obesity in children, adolescents and adults is usually determined through the use of certain screening methods such as measurement of the body mass index (BMI) as well as the triceps skinfold thickness.

Patterns of behavior that may lead to obesity may be established as early as infancy. For example, if parents or caregivers persistently use a bottle to pacify a crying baby, the baby may learn that food is equivalent to relief of stress. Treatment for obesity should include the cooperation and support of the entire family and may be directed toward psychological considerations, as well as proper exercise and nutrition to psychological and emotional needs may include behavior modification, as well as individual and family counseling. See also *Eating Disorders.*

National Agencies & Associations

6695 **Active Healthy Kids Canada**
77 Bloor Street West 416-913-0238
Toronto, Ontario, M5S 1-3C6 888-446-7432
Fax: 416-913-1541
e-mail: info@activehealthykids.ca
www.activehealthykids.ca
Established in 1994 to advocate the importance of quality, accessible, and enjoyable physical activity participation experiences for children and youth.
Stacie Smith, Communications Manager
Jennifer Crowie-Bonne, Director of Development/Programs

6696 **American Obesity Association**
1250 24th Street NW 202-776-7711
Washington, DC 20037 Fax: 202-776-7712
e-mail: executive@obesity.org
obesity1.tempdomainname.com
AOA provides obesity awareness and prevention information.
Morgan Downey, Executive Director
Richard L Atkinson, President

6697 **Canadian Obesity Network**
10240 Kingsway Avenue 780-735-6764
Edmonton, AB T5H 3-2X2 Fax: 780-735-6763
e-mail: info@obesitynetwork.ca
www.obesitynetwork.ca
Focuses the expertise and deciation of more than 1,000 member researchers, clinicans, allied health care providers and other professionals with an interest in obesity in a unified effort to reduce the mental, physical and economic burden of obesity in Canadians.
Dr. Arya M. Sharma, Scientific Director & CEO
Ximena Ramos Salas, Managing Director

6698 **National Association to Advance Fat Acceptance**
PO Box 4662 916-558-6880
Foster City, CA 94404 Fax: 916-558-6881
e-mail: naafa@naafa.org
www.naafaonline.com/dev2/
NAAFA provides educational information a newsletter and hosts a national conference.
Carole Cullum, Co-Chair
Kara Brewer Allen, Co-Chair

6699 **Overeaters Anonymous World Service Office**
World Service Office

PO Box 44020
Rio Rancho, NM 87174-4020

505-891-2664
Fax: 505-891-4320
e-mail: info@oa.org
www.oa.org

A fellowship of men and women from all walks of life who meet in order to help solve a common problem - compulsive overeating.
Naomi, Managing Director, Board Administrator

6700 Research Chair on Obesity
2725 Chemin Sainte-Foy
Quebec, Canada, G1V

418-656-8711
Fax: 418-656-4929
e-mail: obesite.chair@crhl.ulaval.ca
http://obesity.chair.ulaval.ca

Provides understanding of the pathophysiology of obesity. Promotes communication and interaction among basic scientists and clinicians, involved in nutrition, energy metabolism, obesity, lipid metabolism and cardiovascular research., Provides continuing education about the best possible knowledge on obesity to health professionals, physicians and to the public at large regarding the causes, the complications and the treatment of obesity.
Paul Boisvert, Coordinator
Denis Richard, Ph. D., Chair

Libraries & Resource Centers

6701 Weight-control Information Network
1 WIN Way
Bethesda, MD 20892-3665

202-828-1025
877-946-4627
Fax: 202-828-1028
e-mail: win@info.niddk.nih.gov
http://win.niddk.nih.gov/

WIN addresses the health information needs of individuals through the production and dissemination of educational materials. In addition, WIN is developing communication strategies for a pilot program to encourage at-risk individuals to achieve and maintain a healthy weight by making changes in their lifestyle.

Research Centers

6702 Harvard Clinical Nutrition Research Center
Harvard Medical School
Boston, MA 02215

617-998-8803
Fax: 617-998-8804
e-mail: allan_walker@hms.harvard.edu
nutrition.med.harvard.edu

Mission is to derive the benefit of continuity in assessing the effectiveness of the Center from year to year while still allowing flexibility for new insights as the Center's activities evolve.
W Allan Walker, Director
George Blackburn, Associate Director

6703 Minnesota Obesity Center
1334 Eckles Avenue
St Paul, MN 55108

763-807-0559
e-mail: mnoc@tc.umn.edu
www.mnoc.umn.edu

Mission is to find ways to prevent weight gain obesity and its complications. The Center incorporates 46 Participating Investigators who are studying the causes and treatments of obesity. Provides the general public with a source of information on the happenings of the Center and on the current developments in the field of obesity.
Catherine C Welch, Program Coordinator

6704 New York Obesity/Nutrition Research Center
31 Center Drive MSC 2560
Bethesda, MD 20892-2560

301-496-3583
www2.niddk.nih.gov

Griffin P Rodgers, Director

6705 Obesity Research Center St. Luke's-Roosevelt Hospital
St. Luke's-Roosevelt Hospital
1090 Amsterdam Avenue
New York, NY 10025

212-523-4196
Fax: 212-523-3416
e-mail: dg108@columbia.edu
www.nyorc.org

The mission of the New York Obesity Research Center is to help reduce the incidence of obesity and related diseases through leadership in basic research clinical research epidemiology and public health patient care and public education.
Dr Xavier Pi-Sunyer, Director
Janet Crane, Dietitians

Support Groups & Hotlines

6706 Greater New York Metro Intergroup of Overeaters Anonymous
Madison Square Station
New York, NY 10159-1235

212-946-4599
e-mail: office@oanyc.org
www.oanyc.org

Tom M, Chairman
Raina M, Vice chairman

6707 Office of Chronic Disease Prevention and Nutrition Services
Obesity Prevention Program
150 N. 18th Avenue
Phoenix, AZ 85007

602-542-1025
Fax: 602-542-0883
www.azdhs.gov/search/index.htm

Mission is to improve the health and quality of life of Arizona residents by reducing the incidence and severity of chronic disease and obesity through physical activity and nutrition interventions.
Renae Cunnien, Program Manager

Books

6708 An Atlas of Obesity and Weight Control
George A. Bray, author

212-216-7800
Fax: 212-564-7854
www.taylorandfrancisgroup.com

This informative guide is a clearly written, beautifully illustrated color atlas on obesity, including its etiology, development and treatment. Contains nearly 150 clinical pictures of obesity and its related conditions, as well as many pertinent clinical guidelines and up-to-the-minute data on assessment and treatment.
135 pages

6709 Dietary Guidelines for Americans 2005
U.S. Government Printing Office
200 Independence Avenue, S.W.
Washington, DC 20201

202-619-0257
877-696-6775
www.health.gov/dietaryguidelines

80 pages
Tommy G. Thompson, HHS-Secretary
Ann M. Veneman, USDA-Secretary

6710 Encyclopedia of Obesity and Eating Disorders
Facts on File
11 Penn Plaza
New York, NY 10001

212-967-8800
800-322-8755
Fax: 800-678-3633

From abdominoplasty to Zung Rating Scale, this volume defines and explains these disorders, along with medical and other problems associated with them.
272 pages Hardcover

6711 Handbook of Obesity Treatment
Guilford Press
72 Spring Street
New York, NY 10012

800-365-7006
Fax: 212-966-6708
e-mail: info@guilford.com
www.guilford.com

This comprehensive handbook guides mental, medical, and allied health professionals through the process of planning and delivering individualized treatment services for those seeking help for Obesity.
2001 624 pages Hardcover
ISBN: 1-572307-22-6

6712 Obesity
National Academies Press
500 Fifth Street, NW
Washington, DC 20055

202-334-3313
888-624-8373
Fax: 202-334-2451
www.nap.edu

A ground breaking report on childhood obesity providing indepth background and instructive case studies that illustrate just how serious and widespread the problem is; gives honest, authorative, based advice that consitute our best weapons in this critical battle.
280 pages

6713   Overeaters Anonymous
World Service Office
117 W 26th Street   505-891-2664
New York, NY 10001-6807   Fax: 505-891-4320
                                              www.overeatersanonymous.org
World Service Office offers literature, provides information or meetings world wide.
204 pages Hardcover

6714   Preventing Childhood Obesity: Health in the Balance
National Academies Press
500 Fifth Street NW   202-334-3313
Washington, DC 20055   888-624-8373
                                                   Fax: 202-334-2451
                                                         www.nap.edu
Provides a broad-based examination of the nature, extent, and consequences of obesity. Also explores the underlying causes of this serious health problem and the actions needed to initiate support, and sustain the societal and lifestyle changes that can reverse the trend among our children and youth.
436 pages
ISBN: 0-309091-96-9

6715   Shape Up America!
6707 Democracy Boulevard   www.shapeup.org
Bethesda, MD 20817
A high profile national initiative to promote healthy weight and increased physical activity in America. Involves a broad based coalition of industry, medical/health, nutrition, physical fitness, and related organizations and experts.
C. Everett Koop, Founder
Barbara J. Moore, President And CEO

6716   Understanding Childhood Obesity
J Clinton Smith, MD, author

University Press of Mississippi
3825 Ridgewood Road
Jackson, MS 39211-6492   601-432-6205
                                                   Fax: 601-432-6217
                                       e-mail: press@ihl.state.ms.us
                                                 www.upress.state.ms.us
A clear explanation of causes, diagnosis, and treatment of childhood obesity.
1999 120 pages Paperback
ISBN: 1-578061-34-2
Kathy Burgess, Advertising/Marketing Services Manager

6717   Understanding Obesity: The Five Medical Causes
Lance Levy, author

Firefly Books Ltd
66 Leek Crescent   416-499-8412
Richmond Hill, Ontario, L4B-1H1   Fax: 416-499-1142
                                                 www.fireflybooks.com
An authoritative book that focuses on the causes of, and the treatment for, obesity. Obesity is usually related to other health problems and treatment for them is the first step.
200 pages

Children's Books

6718   I Was a Fifteen-Year-Old Blimp
Harper & Row
10 E 53rd Street   212-207-7000
New York, NY 10022-5299
This story focuses on Gabby, a teenage girl who overhears others discuss her weight and takes radical steps to become popular.
Grades 6-9

Magazines

6719   CheckUp
Medical University of South Carolina

135 Cannon Street   843-792-1414
Charleston, SC 29425   800-424-6872
                                              www.muschealth.com/weight
Provides health information about screenings, treatments, medical advances and services available through MUSC, as well as advice about nutrition and prevention.
Susan Kammeraad-Campbell, Managing Editor
Damon Simmons, Art Director

6720   Official Journal of NAASO
NAASO
Boston Med. Center, 650 Albany St.   617-638-7107
Boston, MA 02118   Fax: 617-638-6630
                                             e-mail: teffk!niddk.nih.gov
                                                         www.naaso.org
Promotes research, education and advocacy to better understand, prevent and treat obesity and improve the lives of those affected.
Barbara E. Corkey, Editor-In-Chief
Deborah Moskowitz, Managing Editor

6721   Progress Notes
Medical University of South Carolina
135 Cannon Street   843-792-2200
Charleston, SC 29425   800-922-5250
                                              www.muschealth.com/weight
Designed to inform the medical community developments at the Medical University of South Carolina and as a continuing medical education resource for practicing physicians and faculty.
Susan Kammeraad-Campbell, Managing Editor
Lynne Barber Associate Editor, Alex Sargent, Associate Editor

Newsletters

6722   Trim & Fit
Obesity Foundation
5600 S Quebec Street   303-850-0328
Englewood, CO 80111-2202
Offers nutrition facts and articles, low-fat recipes, medical information on heart disease and cancer relating to nutrition and more.
James F Merker CAE, Editor

Pamphlets

6723   About Overeaters Anonymous
Metro Intergroup of Overeaters Anonymous
117 W 26th Street   212-206-8621
New York, NY 10001-6807

6724   An Inside View
Metro Intergroup of Overeaters Anonymous
117 W 26th Street   212-206-8621
New York, NY 10001-6807

6725   Anonymity
Metro Intergroup of Overeaters Anonymous
117 W 26th Street   212-206-8621
New York, NY 10001-6807

6726   Before You Take That First...
Metro Intergroup of Overeaters Anonymous
117 W 26th Street   212-206-8621
New York, NY 10001-6807

6727   Compulsive Overeaters in the Military
Metro Intergroup of Overeaters Anonymous
117 W 26th Street   212-206-8621
New York, NY 10001-6807

6728   Compulsive Overeating & Overeaters Anonymous
Metro Intergroup of Overeaters Anonymous
117 W 26th Street   212-206-8621
New York, NY 10001-6807

6729   For the Obese Employee
Metro Intergroup of Overeaters Anonymous
117 W 26th Street   212-206-8621
New York, NY 10001-6807

6730   Guide to the 12 Steps for You
Metro Intergroup of Overeaters Anonymous
117 W 26th Street   212-206-8621
New York, NY 10001-6807

6731   Hazelden Step Pamphlets for Overeaters
Hazelden
15251 Pleasant Valley Road   651-257-4010
Center City, MN 55012-9640   800-328-9000
                                    Fax: 651-213-4426
                                       www.hazelden.org
A 12 pamphlet collection that offers one person's interpretation of
the Twelve Steps for overeaters.

6732   If God Spoke to Overeaters Anonymous
Metro Intergroup of Overeaters Anonymous
117 W 26th Street   212-206-8621
New York, NY 10001-6807

6733   Many Symptoms, One Disease
Metro Intergroup of Overeaters Anonymous
117 W 26th Street   212-206-8621
New York, NY 10001-6807

6734   Members in Relapse
Metro Intergroup of Overeaters Anonymous
117 W 26th Street   212-206-8621
New York, NY 10001-6807

6735   One Day at a Time
Metro Intergroup of Overeaters Anonymous
117 W 26th Street   212-206-8621
New York, NY 10001-6807

6736   Overeaters Anonymous Cares
Metro Intergroup of Overeaters Anonymous
117 W 26th Street   212-206-8621
New York, NY 10001-6807

6737   Overeaters Anonymous is Not a Diet Club
Metro Intergroup of Overeaters Anonymous
117 W 26th Street   212-206-8621
New York, NY 10001-6807

6738   Person to Person
Metro Intergroup of Overeaters Anonymous
117 W 26th Street   212-206-8621
New York, NY 10001-6807

6739   Program of Recovery
Metro Intergroup of Overeaters Anonymous
117 W 26th Street   212-206-8621
New York, NY 10001-6807

6740   Questions and Answers
Metro Intergroup of Overeaters Anonymous
117 W 26th Street   212-206-8621
New York, NY 10001-6807

6741   So You've Reached Goal Weight
Metro Intergroup of Overeaters Anonymous
117 W 26th Street   212-206-8621
New York, NY 10001-6807

6742   Think First...
Metro Intergroup of Overeaters Anonymous
117 W 26th Street   212-206-8621
New York, NY 10001-6807

6743   To the Family
Metro Intergroup of Overeaters Anonymous
117 W 26th Street   212-206-8621
New York, NY 10001-6807

6744   To the Man
Metro Intergroup of Overeaters Anonymous
117 W 26th Street   212-206-8621
New York, NY 10001-6807

6745   To the Newcomer
Metro Intergroup of Overeaters Anonymous
117 W 26th Street   212-206-8621
New York, NY 10001-6807

6746   To the Teen
Metro Intergroup of Overeaters Anonymous
117 W 26th Street   212-206-8621
New York, NY 10001-6807

6747   Tools of Recovery
Metro Intergroup of Overeaters Anonymous
117 W 26th Street   212-206-8621
New York, NY 10001-6807

6748   Twelve Traditions of Overeaters Anonymous
Metro Intergroup of Overeaters Anonymous
117 W 26th Street   212-206-8621
New York, NY 10001-6807

6749   Welcome Back
Metro Intergroup of Overeaters Anonymous
117 W 26th Street   212-206-8621
New York, NY 10001-6807

Audio & Video

6750   Obesity Online
NAASO
                                             301-563-6526
Educational resource for clinicians, researchers and educators
with an interest in obesity and its related disorders.
Samuel Klein, Editor
Christie M. Ballantyne, Editor

Web Sites

6751   Boston Obesity Nutrition Research Center (BONRC)
                                             www.bmc.org
Provides resources and support for studies in the area of obesity
and nutrition. Comprised of four research cores located within the
Boston area. In the areas of adipocytes, epidemiology and statistics, body composition, energy expenditure and genetic analyses,
and transgenic animal models.

6752   Center for Human Nutrition
                                      www.uchsc.edu/nutrition
A interdisciplinary team encompassing basic and clinical research,
post-graduate training and career development of nutrition professionals, and commuity outreach. The research conducted at the
CHN focuses on obesity prevention and treatment, nutrient metabolism, and micronutrient status in children. Activities conducted
aim to improve the quallity of life by promoting physical activity
and nutritional awareness.

6753   Clinical Nutrition Research Unit (CNRU)
                                http://depts.washington.edu/uwcnru
Promotes and enhances the interdisciplinary nutrition research
and education at the Univeristy of Washington. By providing a
number of Core Facilities, the CNRU attempts to integrate and coordinate the abundant ongoing activities with the goals of fostering new interdiscilinary research collaborations, stimulating new
research activities, improving nutrition education at multiple levels, and facilitating the nutritional management of patients.

6754   MedicineNet
                                        www.medicinenet.com
An online resource for consumers providing easy-to-read, authoritative medical and health information.

6755   New York Obesity/Nutrition Research Center (ONRC)
                                www.niddk.nih.gov/fund/other/centers.htm
Funded by the National Institute of Diabetes and Digestive and
Kidney Diseases (NIDDK). A combined effort of Columbia ane
Cornell Universities. Provides participating investigators of
funded projects relevant to obesity research with valuable laboratory, technical, and educational services that otherwise would not
be available to them, thereby improving the productivity an
efficiency of their operations.

6756   North American Association for the Study of Obesity
                                             www.naaso.org
The leading scientific society dedicated to the study of obesity.
Committed to encouraging research on the causes and treatment of

obesity, and to keeping the medical community and public informed of new advances.

6757 Research Chair on Obesity
2725 Chemin Sainte Foy   418-656-8711
Quebec,Canada,   e-mail: obesite.chair@crhl.ulaval.ca
                                       http://obesity.chair.ulaval.ca
Expand our understanding of the pathophysiology of obesity, through scientific research program, to promote communication and interaction among basic scientists and clinicians, involved in nutrition, energy metabolism, obesity, lipid metabolism and cardiovascular research, and to provide continuing education about the best possible knowledge on obesity to health professionals, physicians and to the public at large regarding the causes, the complications and the treatment of obesity.

6758 University of Pittsburgh Obesity/Nutrition Research Center
                                          www.pitt.edu/~onrc
Goal is to develop more effective interventions for the prevention and treatment of obesity. Exists to support research functions for investigators studying the broad areas of obesity and nutrition. Focuses on behavioral aspects of obesity and behavioral treatment of this disease.

6759 Vanderbilt Clinical Nutrition Research Unit (CNRU)
                                 www.vanderbilt.edu/nutrition/index.html
A core center grant funded by the National Institute of Diabetes and Digestive and Kidney Diseases (NIDDK). Nutrition research is carried out by faculty members i most academic departments and extends from basic laboratory research to clinical and applied research. Maintains service facilities to support both basic and clinical research. Supports research cores that bring nutrition investigators together to discuss their work.

6760 Weight-control Information Network
                                 www.niddk.nih.gov/health/nutrit/win.htm
WIN addresses the health information needs of individuals through the production and dissemination of educational materials. In addition, WIN is developing communication strategies for a pilot program to encourage at-risk individuals to achieve and maintain a healthy weight by making changes in their lifestyle.

Description

6761 ## Osteogenesis Imperfecta

Osteogenesis imperfecta, OI, often called "brittle bone" disease, is actually is a group of serious genetic disorders that are characterized by abnormally fragile bones that break or fracture easily. There are at least four distinct forms of the disorder, with neonatal (congenital) being the most severe. A person with OI has either less collagen, the major protein of the connective tissue, including bone, or a poorer quality collagen. Infants born with OI may have multiple bone fractures and hearing loss, and routine vaginal delivery may lead to significant bone fracture, hemorrhage into the brain and other major problems. Survivors develop shortened extremities and other bony abnormalities. If no injury to the brain occurs then mental and intellectual function should be unaffected. Hearing loss may occur.

At present, there is no effective treatment for this disorder. Careful handling of these infants is essential. Gentle exercise and physical therapy are directed at preventing fractures and increasing function. Surgical implants can provide stability to the skeletal structure. Genetic counseling is also important.

National Agencies & Associations

6762 **NIH Osteoporosis and Related Bone Diseases - National Resource Center**
2 AMS Circle   301-496-8190
Bethesda, MD 20892-3676   877-226-4267
Fax: 301-480-2814
TTY: 301-565-2966
e-mail: niamsboneinfo@mail.nih.gov
www.niams.nih.gov
Provides patients, health professionals and the public with an important link to resources and information on osteoporosis, Paget's disease of bone, osteogenesis imperfecta, and other metabolic bone diseases. The National Resource Center's mission is to expand awareness and enhance knowledge and understanding of the prevention, early detection, and treatment of these diseases.

6763 **National Institute of Child Health and Human Development**
National Institutes of Health
31 Center Drive   301-496-5133
Bethesda, MD 20892-0001   Fax: 301-496-7107
Supports several basic and clinical research projects on osteogenesis imperfecta.
Duane Alexander, Director

6764 **Osteogenesis Imperfecta Foundation**
804 W Diamond Avenue   301-947-0083
Gaithersburg, MD 20878-1414   800-981-2663
Fax: 301-947-0456
TTY: 202-466-4315
TDD: 202-466-4315
e-mail: BoneLink@oif.org
www.oif.org
Support and resources for families and medical professionals dealing with osteogeneis imperfecta.
Mary Beth Huber, Information/Resource Director
Tracy Smith Hart, CEO

Libraries & Resource Centers

6765 **NIH Osteoporosis and Related Bone Diseases - National Resource Center**
2 AMS Circle   202-223-0344
Bethesda, MD 20892-3676   800-624-2663
Fax: 202-293-2356
TTY: 202-466-4315
e-mail: niamsboneinfo@mail.nih.gov
www.osteo.org
Provides patients, health professionals and the public with an important link to resources and information on osteoporosis, Paget's disease of bone, osteogenesis imperfecta, and other metabolic bone diseases. The National Resource Center's mission is to expand awareness and enhance knowledge and understanding of the prevention, early detection, and treatment of these diseases.

Research Centers

6766 **American Society for Bone and Mineral Research**
2025 M Street NW   202-367-1161
Washington, DC 20036-3309   Fax: 202-672-2161
e-mail: asbmr@asbmr.org
www.asbmr.org
The mission of the ASBMR is to be the premier society in the field of bone and mineral metabolism through promoting excellence in bone and mineral research fostering integration of clinical and basic science and facilitating the translation of that science to health care and clinical practice.
Ann Elderkin, Executive Director
Douglas Fesler, Associate Executive Director

6767 **Children's Brittle Bone Foundation**
7701 95th Street   773-236-2223
Pleasant Pride, WI 53158   866-694-2223
Fax: 262-947-0724
e-mail: info@cbbf.org
www.cbbf.org
The mission of the Children's Brittle Bone Foundation is to provide for research into the causes diagnosis treatment prevention a eventual cure for Osteogenesis Imperfecta (OI) while supporting programs which improve the quality of life for people afflicted.

Support Groups & Hotlines

6768 **National Health Information Center**
PO Box 1133   310-565-4167
Washington, DC 20013   800-336-4797
Fax: 301-984-4256
e-mail: info@nhic.org
www.health.gov/nhic
Offers a nationwide information referral service, produces directories and resource guides.

6769 **Osteogenesis Imperfecta Foundation**
804 W Diamond Avenue   301-947-0083
Gaithersburg, MD 20878   800-981-2663
Fax: 301-947-0456
TDD: 202-466-4315
e-mail: BoneLink@oif.org
www.oif.org
Support and resources for families and medical professional dealing with osteogeneis imperfecta.
Marybeth Huber, Information Resource Director
Bill Bradner, Director Communication/Events

Books

6770 **Children with Ostegogenesis Imperfecta: St raties to Enhance Performance**
Holly Lea Cintas, Lynn Gerber, author

Osteogenesis Imperfecta Foundation

804 W Diamond Avenue
Gaithersburg, MD 20878

301-947-0083
800-981-2663
Fax: 301-947-0456
e-mail: BoneLink@oif.org
www.oif.org

This guide covers the same issues, but has been written especially for elementary school readers.
252 pages Paperback
ISBN: 0-964218-95-X
Mary Beth Huber, Information/Resource Director

6771   Growing Up with OI: A Guide for Children
Ellen Painter Dollar, author

Osteogenesis Imperfecta Foundation
804 W Diamond Avenue
Gaithersburg, MD 20878

301-947-0083
800-981-2663
Fax: 301-947-0456
e-mail: bonelink@oif.org
www.oif.org

This guide covers the same issues as the adult book, Growing Up with OI: A Guide for Families and Caregivers, but has been written especially for elementary school readers.
122 pages Paperback
ISBN: 0-964218-92-5
Mary Beth Huber, Information/Resource Director

6772   Growing Up with OI: A Guide for Families a nd Caregivers
Ellen Painter Dollar, author

Osteogenesis Imperfecta Foundation
804 W Diamond Avenue
Gaithersburg, MD 20878-1414

301-947-0083
800-981-2663
Fax: 301-947-0456
e-mail: BoneLink@oif.org
www.oif.org

This guide covers common questions parents, family members and caregivers have about raising a child with OI. The focus is onmaximizing abilities and proactive problem solving. Chapters cover medical, financial, emotional and school related issues.
295 pages Paperback
ISBN: 0-964218-91-7
Mary Beth Huber, Information/Resource Director

6773   Managing Osteogenesis Imperfecta: A Medical Manual
Priscilla Wacaster, MD, author

Osteogenesis Imperfecta Foundation
804 W Diamond Avenue
Gaithersburg, MD 20878-1414

301-947-0083
800-981-2663
Fax: 301-947-0456
e-mail: BoneLink@oif.org
www.oif.org

The manual is designed for physicians, physical and occupational therapists, orthopedic technologists, early intervention providers and others who come in contact with persons with OI. It covers a broad range of topics including genetics, diagnosis, pregnancy, arthritis, osteoperosis and rodding.
Mary Beth Huber, Information/Resource Director

6774   Therapeutic Strategies: A Guide for Occupational & Physical Therapists
Ellen Painter Dollar, author

Osteogenesis Imperfecta Foundation
804 W Diamond Avenue
Gaithersburg, MD 20878-1414

301-947-0083
800-981-2663
Fax: 301-947-0456
e-mail: BoneLink@oif.org
www.oif.org

This booklet is intended for medical professionals, or for families to use as a resource while working with a medical professional.
14 pages
Mary Beth Huber, Information/Resource Director

Newsletters

6775   Breakthrough
Osteogenesis Imperfecta Foundation

804 W Diamond Avenue
Gaithersburg, MD 20878-1414

301-947-0083
800-981-2663
Fax: 301-947-0456
e-mail: BoneLink@oif.org
www.oif.org

Newsletter of the Osteogenesis Imperfecta Foundation that provides information on current research and OIF fundraising activities as well as support features.
15 pages Quarterly
Mary Beth Huber, Information/Resource Director

Pamphlets

6776   Caring for Infants and Children with Osteogenesis Imperfecta
Osteogenesis Imperfecta Foundation
804 W Diamond Avenue
Gaithersburg, MD 20878-1414

301-947-0083
800-981-2663
Fax: 301-947-0456
e-mail: BoneLink@oif.org
www.oif.org

A companion to the videotape You Are Not Alone. Presents some basic information and unique tips on caring for a baby with OI. Available in Spanish.
24 pages
Mary Beth Huber, Information/Resource Director

6777   Osteogenesis Imperfecta: A Guide for Medic al Professionals, Individuals & Families
Osteogenesis Imperfecta Foundation
804 W Diamond Avenue
Gaithersburg, MD 20878-1414

301-947-0083
800-981-2663
Fax: 301-947-0456
e-mail: BoneLink@oif.org
www.oif.org

This pamphlet contains basic information about the types of OI, inheritance factors, diagnosis and treatment.
10 pages Paperback
Mary Beth Huber, Information/Resource Director

Audio & Video

6778   Going Places and Plan for Success: An Educ ator's Guide to Students with OI
Osteogenesis Imperfecta Foundation
804 W Diamond Avenue
Gaithersburg, MD 20878-1414

301-947-0083
800-981-2663
Fax: 301-947-0456
e-mail: BoneLink@oif.org
www.oif.org

A 15-minute video with booklet that guides educators and parents through planning steps that will help children with OI fully participate in school activities.
Mary Beth Huber, Information/Resource Director

6779   Within Reach
Osteogenesis Imperfecta Foundation
804 W Diamond Avenue
Gaithersburg, MD 20878-1414

301-947-0083
800-981-2663
Fax: 301-947-0456
TDD: 202-466-4315
e-mail: BoneLink@oif.org
www.oif.org

This 50-minute video features in-depth interviews with adults living with OI. They talk candidly about how they have achieved independent and satisfying lives, addressing such issues as travel, career, marriage and family.
VHS/DVD
Mary Beth Huber, Information/Resource Director

6780   You Are Not Alone
Osteogenesis Imperfecta Foundation
804 W Diamond Avenue
Gaithersburg, MD 20878-1414

301-947-0083
800-981-2663
Fax: 301-947-0456
TDD: 202-466-4315
e-mail: BoneLink@oif.org
www.oif.org

Explores the emotional turmoil of dealing with the diagnosis of OI and offers practical and uplifting solutions for caring for infants with Type II to severe Type III OI. Also valuable for new families with the more mild forms of OI. Available open captioned or with Spanish subtitles (specify if needed). Add $5.00 per video for Canadian orders and $11.00 per video for overseas orders.
Mary Beth Huber, Information/Resource Director

Web Sites

6781 Healing Well

www.healingwell.com

An online health resource guide to medical news, chat, information and articles, newsgroups and message boards, books, disease-related web sites, medical directories, and more for patients, friends, and family coping with disabling diseases, disorders, or chronic illnesses.

6782 Health Finder

www.healthfinder.gov

Searchable, carefully developed web site offering information on over 1000 topics. Developed by the US Department of Health and Human Services, the site can be used in both English and Spanish.

6783 Healthlink USA

www.healthlinkusa.com

Health information concerning treatment, cures, prevention, diagnosis, risk factors, research, support groups, email lists, personal stories and much more. Updated regularly.

6784 Helios Health

www.helioshealth.com

Online resource for your health information. Detailed information about specific health topics, access to expert advice from our Medical Advisory Board, and up-to-date health news.

6785 MedicineNet

www.medicinenet.com

An online resource for consumers providing easy-to-read, authoritative medical and health information.

6786 Medscape

www.medscape.com

Medscape offers specialists, primary care physicians, and other health professionals the Web's most robust and integrated medical information and educational tools.

6787 Osteogenesis Imperfecta Foundation

www.oif.org

A website for those who want to learn more about Osteogenesis Imperfecta, the OI Foundation, and what they do.

6788 Osteoporosis and Related Bone Diseases: National Resource Center (NIGH)

www.osteo.org

Provides patients, health professionals and the public with an important link to resources and information on osteoporosis and other metabolic bone diseases.

6789 WebMD

www.webmd.com

Information on Osteogenesis Imperfecta, including articles and resources.

Description

6790 Osteoporosis

Osteoporosis is a general term for many conditions which result in a reduction in bone mass. Most cases occur in post-menopausal women because estrogen loss is associated with decreased bone mass. These women are at risk for fractures of the wrist, spine and hip. Post-menopausal osteoporosis may also cause marked reduction in a woman's height, as multiple vertebral bodies in the spine compress downwards over the years. Risk factors for osteoporosis include white race, cigarette smoking, thin body build and early menopause. Men can develop a similar condition, but it is generally much less severe. Excessive activity of the adrenal glands (Cushing's syndrome), the thyroid gland (thyrotoxicosis), the parathyroid glands (hyperparathyroidism), and the pituitary gland (hyperprolactinemia) cause bones to thin, as does underactivity of the testes or ovaries. Anorexia nervosa and prolonged administration of cortisone or heparin will also thin the bones.

Treatment is in part nonspecific, and can include surgery or other immobilization to treat fractures of the hip or wrist, control of pain with medications and physical therapy to encourage return to pre-fracture function. Specific therapy includes calcium and Vitamin D supplementation and weight-bearing exercises. Biphosphonates, such as alendronate, have been approved for osteoporosis and other new therapies are being developed.

National Agencies & Associations

6791 National Osteoporosis Foundation
1232 22nd Street NW
Washington, DC 20037-1292
202-223-2226
800-223-9994
Fax: 202-223-2237
e-mail: communications@nof.org
www.nof.org
The nation's leading resource for people seeking up-to-date medically sound information on the causes prevention detection and treatment of osteoporosis.
Leo Schargorodski, Executive Director
Ethel Siris, President

6792 Osteoporosis Canada
1090 Don Mills Road
Toronto, Ontario, M3C-3R6
416-696-2663
800-463-6842
Fax: 416-696-2673
e-mail: info@osteoporosis.ca
www.osteoporosis.ca
A registered charity, is the only national organization serving people who have, or are at risk for, osteoporosis.
Cheryl Baldwin, Chairman
Emliy Bartens, Vice chairman

Libraries & Resource Centers

6793 NIH Osteoporosis and Related Bone Diseases - National Resource Center
2 AMS Circle
Bethesda, MD 20892-3676
202-223-0344
800-624-2663
Fax: 202-293-2356
TTY: 202-466-4315
e-mail: niamsboneinfo@mail.nih.gov
www.osteo.org
Provides patients, health professionals and the public with an important link to resources and information on osteoporosis, Paget's disease of bone, osteogenesis imperfecta, and other metabolic bone diseases. The National Resource Center's mission is to expand awareness and enhance knowledge and understanding of the prevention, early detection, and treatment of these diseases.

Research Centers

6794 Medical College of Pennsylvania Center for the Mature Woman
3300 Henry Avenue
Philadelphia, PA 19129
215-842-6000
our purpose is to provide consumers information to help them get high quality services and products at the best possible prices.
Jon Schneider,MD, Director

6795 Osteoporosis Center Memorial Hospital/Advanced Medical Diagn
Memorial Hospital/Advanced Medical Diagnostic
1700 Coffee Road
Modesto, CA 95355
209-526-4500
www.memorialmedicalcenter.org
Memorial Medical Center is part of Memorial Hospitals Association a not-for-profit organization that exists to maintain and improve the health status of citizens in the greater Stanislaus County.
David Benn, Director
Bev Finley, Director

6796 Regional Bone Center Helen Hayes Hospital
Helen Hayes Hospital
51-55 Route 9W
W Haverstraw, NY 10993
845-786-4000
1 8-8 7- 734
Fax: 845-947-3097
TTY: 845-947-3187
e-mail: info@helenhayeshospital.org
www.helenhayeshospital.org
The mission of the Regional Bone conduct a broad-based research program focused on the elucidation of cellular mechanisms underlying metabolic bone disease and the development of new treatments for bone disease.
David W Dempster PhD, Director
Adrienne Tewksbury, Grants Administrator

6797 University of Connecticut Osteoporosis Center
263 Farmington Avenue
Farmington, CT 06030
860-679-2000
800-535-6232
Fax: 860-679-1258
www.uchc.edu
Jay R Lieberman, Director

Support Groups & Hotlines

6798 National Health Information Center
PO Box 1133
Washington, DC 20013
310-565-4167
800-336-4797
Fax: 301-984-4256
e-mail: info@nhic.org
www.health.gov/nhic
Offers a nationwide information referral service, produces directories and resource guides.

6799 National Osteoporosis Foundation (NOF)
1232 22nd Street NW
Washington, DC 20037-1292
202-223-2226
Fax: 202-223-2237
e-mail: webmaster@nof.org
www.nof.org
Dedicated to reducing the widespread prevalence of osteoporosis through programs of research, education and advocacy. Provides

referrals to existing support groups, as well as free resources, training and materials to assist people to start groups.
Amy Porter, Executive Director& CEO
Robert R Recker, Chairman of the Board

Books

6800   One-Hundred-Fifty Most Asked Questions About Osteoporosis
Hearst Books
1350 Avenue of the Americas   212-261-6500
New York, NY 10016   Fax: 212-261-6595
1993
ISBN: 0-688123-34-1

6801   Preventing & Reversing Osteoporosis: Every Woman's Guide
Prima Publishing
PO Box 1260
Rocklin, CA 95677-1260   916-624-5718
                                               www.primapub.com
1993 275 pages
ISBN: 1-559582-98-7

6802   Preventing and Managing Osteoporosis
Springer Publishing Company
536 Broadway   212-431-4370
New York, NY 10012-3955   877-687-7476
                                               Fax: 212-941-7842
                                               e-mail: springer@springerpub.com
                                               www.springerpub.com
This book will raise awareness and inform health professionals about this often preventable and treatable disease. Written by a team of authors from medicine, nursing, nutrition, exercise physiology, and physical therapy, the book provides an overview of the disease process.
216 pages Hardcover
ISBN: 0-826113-18-4
M Susan Burke MD, Editor
Helen Wright PhD, Editor

Newsletters

6803   Osteoporosis Report
National Osteoporosis Foundation
1232 22nd Street NW   202-223-2226
Washington, DC 20037-1292   800-223-9994
                                               Fax: 202-223-2237
                                               e-mail: communications@nof.org
                                               www.nof.org
A benefit to members of the National Osteoporosis Foundation (NOF), the Osteoporosis Report includes updates on recent research, strategies for bone health and other information. NOF is the only nonprofit, voluntary health organization dedicated to reducing the widespread prevalence of osteoporosis through programs of research, education and advocacy. Contact the foundation for membership information.
Quarterly

Pamphlets

6804   Boning Up on Osteoporosis
National Osteoporosis Foundation
1232 22nd Street NW   202-223-2226
Washington, DC 20037-1292   800-223-9994
                                               Fax: 202-223-2237
                                               e-mail: communications@nof.org
                                               www.nof.org
Risk factor card.

6805   How Strong Are Your Bones?
1232 22nd Street NW   202-223-2226
Washington, DC 20037-1292   800-223-9994
                                               Fax: 202-223-2237
                                               e-mail: communications@nof.org
                                               www.nof.org

Describes the various methods for determining bone mass, including types of equipment and how bone density testing is used in the diagnosis and treatment of osteoporosis.
12 pages

6806   Living with Osteoporosis
1232 22nd Street NW   202-223-2226
Washington, DC 20037-1292   800-223-9994
                                               Fax: 202-223-2237
                                               e-mail: communications@nof.org
                                               www.nof.org
A guide to preventing falls in the home and to protecting yourself from injury during your daily routine.

6807   Medications and Bone Loss
1232 22nd Street NW   202-223-2226
Washington, DC 20037-1292   800-223-9994
                                               Fax: 202-223-2237
                                               e-mail: communications@nof.org
Designed for women dealing with menopause, this brochure provides information of estrogen replacement therapy and its relationship to bone health and osteoporosis prevention and treatment.

6808   Men with Osteoporosis: In Their Own Words
1232 22nd Street NW   202-223-2226
Washington, DC 20037-1292   800-223-9994
                                               Fax: 202-223-2237
                                               e-mail: communications@nof.org
                                               www.nof.org

6809   Official Prevention Month Poster
1232 22nd Street NW   202-223-2226
Washington, DC 20037-1292   800-223-9994
                                               Fax: 202-223-2237
                                               e-mail: communications@nof.org
                                               www.nof.org
Poster promotes public awareness about osteoporosis. It can be used as a compliment to the education kit, or by itself for exhibits, health fairs or community programs.

6810   Official Prevention Week Poster
1232 22nd Street NW   202-223-2226
Washington, DC 20037-1292   800-223-9994
                                               Fax: 202-223-2237
                                               e-mail: communications@nof.org
                                               www.nof.org
Poster promotes public awareness about osteoporosis. It can be used as a compliment to the education kit, or by itself for exhibits, health fairs or community programs.

6811   Osteoporosis Education Kit
1232 22nd Street NW   202-223-2226
Washington, DC 20037-1292   800-223-9994
                                               Fax: 202-223-2237
                                               e-mail: communications@nof.org
                                               www.nof.org
This kit is designed for preparing public and patient education programs. Updated annually and includes age-targeted materials, nutrition information and osteoporosis fact sheets that are easily duplicated.

6812   Osteoporosis Education Poster
1232 22nd Street NW   202-223-2226
Washington, DC 20037-1292   800-223-9994
                                               Fax: 202-223-2237
                                               e-mail: communications@nof.org
                                               www.nof.org
Ideal for health care settings, the poster clearly illustrates the effect of osteoporosis on bone tissue and common fracture sites.

6813   Osteoporosis Information Package
NAMSIC/National Institutes of Health
1 AMS Circle   301-495-4484
Bethesda, MD 20892-0001   877-226-4267
                                               Fax: 301-718-6366
                                               TTY: 301-565-2966
                                               e-mail: niamsinfo@mail.nih.gov
                                               www.nih.gov/niams
19 pages

6814 Osteoporosis International
1232 22nd Street NW
Washington, DC 20037-1292
202-223-2226
800-223-9994
Fax: 202-223-2237
e-mail: communications@nof.org
www.nof.org

An international multidisciplinary, clinically oriented journal for the exchange of ideas concerning osteoporosis.

6815 Osteoporosis in Men Information Package
NAMSIC/National Institutes of Health
1 AMS Circle
Bethesda, MD 20892-0001
301-495-4484
877-226-4267
Fax: 301-715-6366
TTY: 301-565-2966
e-mail: niamsinfo@mail.nih.gov
www.nih.gov/niams

19 pages

6816 Osteoporosis: Clinical Updates
1232 22nd Street NW
Washington, DC 20037-1292
202-223-2226
800-223-9994
Fax: 202-223-2237
e-mail: communications@nof.org
www.nof.org

NOF's health profession newsletter provides an in depth focus on varying clinical topics.

6817 Osteoporosis: The Silent Disease-Slide Lecture Presentation
1232 22nd Street NW
Washington, DC 20037-1292
202-223-2226
800-223-9994
Fax: 202-223-2237
e-mail: communications@nof.org
www.nof.org

This 42-slide presentation is ideal for community, patient and worksite education progams. It covers basic bone biology, osteoporosis risk factors, diagnosis, prevention and treatment and concludes with a patient case history. A question and answer document is also provided to assist the presenter with audience questions.
Slide set

6818 Patient Education Sample Pack
1232 22nd Street NW
Washington, DC 20037-1292
202-223-2226
800-223-9994
Fax: 202-223-2237
e-mail: communications@nof.org
www.nof.org

This pack contains one of each of NOF's patient education brochures and a catalog; health professionals can select the brochures appropriate for their audience.
Ten brochures

6819 Risk Factor Card: Can It Happen to You?
National Osteoporosis Foundation
1232 22nd Street NW
Washington, DC 20037-1292
202-223-2226
800-223-9994
Fax: 202-223-2237
e-mail: communications@nof.org
www.nof.org

Explains osteoporosis, the causes, symptoms and preventions and high risk persons.

6820 Stand Up to Osteoporosis
National Osteoporosis Foundation
1232 22nd Street NW
Washington, DC 20037-1292
202-223-2226
800-223-9994
Fax: 202-223-2237
e-mail: communications@nof.org
www.nof.org

One of 25 educational brochures on all aspects of this chronic and debilitating disease. The National Osteoporosis Foundation (NOF) is the nation's only private, nonprofit organization dedicated to education, advocacy and public services. Memberships are available to health professionals and public. Quarterly newsletter and physician's guide.

6821 Strategies for People with Osteoporosis
1232 22nd Street NW
Washington, DC 20037-1292
202-223-2226
800-223-9994
Fax: 202-223-2237
e-mail: communications@nof.org
www.nof.org

This series of articles from NOF's newsletter helps patients learn how to cope with osteoporosis. Articles cover hip, vertebrae and wrist fracture recovery, fall-proofing your home, finding the right doctor, what to do after you've been diagnosed and more.

Audio & Video

6822 Be BoneWise: Exercise
National Osteoperosis Foundation
1232 22nd Street NW
Washington, DC 20037-1292
202-223-2226
800-223-9994
Fax: 202-223-2237
e-mail: communications@nof.org
www.nof.org

Take steps toward better bones, health, flexibility and balance with the offical weight bearing and strength training exercise video.

6823 Osteoperosis: The Silent Disease
National Osteoperosis Foundation
1232 22nd Street NW
Washington, DC 20037-1292
202-223-2226
800-223-9994
Fax: 202-223-2237
e-mail: communications@nof.org
www.nof.org

A scripted, visual presentation covers basic bone biology, osteoperosis risk factors, diagnosis, prevention and treatment. Available as a slide presentation or power point CD Rom.

6824 Patient Education Video
National Osteoperosis Foundation
1232 22nd Street NW
Washington, DC 20037-1292
202-223-2226
800-223-9994
Fax: 202-223-2237
e-mail: communications@nof.org
www.nof.org

Discusses treatment, exercise, nutrition and coping strategies for those already diagnoses with osteoporosis.
15 minutes

Web Sites

6825 Healing Well
www.healingwell.com
An online health resource guide to medical news, chat, information and articles, newsgroups and message boards, books, disease-related web sites, medical directories, and more for patients, friends, and family coping with disabling diseases, disorders, or chronic illnesses.

6826 Health Finder
www.healthfinder.gov
Searchable, carefully developed web site offering information on over 1000 topics. Developed by the US Department of Health and Human Services, the site can be used in both English and Spanish.

6827 Healthlink USA
www.healthlinkusa.com
Health information concerning treatment, cures, prevention, diagnosis, risk factors, research, support groups, email lists, personal stories and much more. Updated regularly.

6828 Helios Health
www.helioshealth.com
Online resource for your health information. Detailed information about specific health topics, access to expert advice from our Medical Advisory Board, and up-to-date health news.

6829 MedicineNet
www.medicinenet.com
An online resource for consumers providing easy-to-read, authoritative medical and health information.

6830 **Medscape**

www.medscape.com

Medscape offers specialists, primary care physicians, and other health professionals the Web's most robust and integrated medical information and educational tools.

6831 **NIH Osteoporosis and Related Bone Disease**

www.osteo.org

Information on prevention, early detection, and treatment of these diseases is also available. The Resource Center is operated by the National Osteoporosis Foundation, in collaboration with The Paget Foundation and the Osteogenesis Imperfecta Foundation.

6832 **National Osteoporosis Foundation**

www.nof.org

The nation's leading resource for people seeking up-to-date, medically sound information on the causes, prevention, detection and treatment of osteoporosis.

6833 **WebMD**

www.webmd.com

Information on osteoporosis, including articles and resources.

Description

6834 Paget's Disease

Paget's disease is a disorder of the bone, which typically results in enlarged and deformed bones in one or more regions of the skeleton. Excessive bone breakdown and formation cause new bone to be dense but fragile. Paget's disease occurs most frequently in the spine, skull, pelvis, and legs.

Early symptoms of Paget's disease include bone and joint pain and fatigability, as well as headaches and hearing loss, when the skull is affected. Deformities of bone such as enlargement of the forehead, bowing of a limb, and curvature of the spine may occur as the disease progresses.

The cause of Paget's disease is unknown. It is sometimes familial, but a specific genetic pattern is unclear.

The course of the disease varies greatly and may range from complete stability to rapid progression. Generally, symptoms progress slowly in affected bones with usually no spread to normal ones.

Although there is no cure for Paget's disease at the present, treatments include drugs that suppress disease activity. Orthopedic surgery for joint replacement or stabilization may also be beneficial.

National Agencies & Associations

6835 Arthritis Foundation
1330 W Peachtree Street
Atlanta, GA 30309
404-872-7100
800-283-7800
Fax: 404-872-0457
e-mail: help@arthritis.org
www.arthritis.org
A nonprofit organization that depends on volunteers to provide services to help people with arthritis. Supports research to find ways to cure and prevent arthritis and provides services to improve the quality of life for those affected by arthritis.
Daniel T. McGowen, Chair
John H Klippel MD, President and CEO

6836 Paget Foundation for Paget's Disease of Bone & Related Disorders
120 Wall Street
New York, NY 10005-4001
212-509-5335
800-237-2438
Fax: 212-509-8492
e-mail: PagetFdn@aol.com
www.paget.org
Private voluntary health agency that provides information to patients and health professionals on several bone disorders including: Paget's disease of bone, primary hyperparathyroidism, fibrous dysplasia, osteoporosis (not osteoporosis) and complications of these conditions.
Teresa A. Guise, Chair
Christal Sumpter, Administrator & Web Manager

Support Groups & Hotlines

6837 National Health Information Center
PO Box 1133
Washington, DC 20013
310-565-4167
800-336-4797
Fax: 301-984-4256
e-mail: info@nhic.org
www.health.gov/nhic

Offers a nationwide information referral service, produces directories and resource guides.

Newsletters

6838 Update
Paget Foundation
120 Wall Street
New York, NY 10005-4001
212-509-5335
800-237-2438
Fax: 212-509-8492
e-mail: PagetFdn@aol.com
www.paget.org
Provides information for consumers and health professionals on the following disorders: paget's disease of bone, primary hyperparathyroidism, fibrous dysplasia, osteopetrosis (not osteoporosis) and the complications of breast and prostate cancer metastic to the bone.
3 per year
Charlene Waldman, Executive Director

Pamphlets

6839 Questions & Answers About Paget's Disease of Bone
Paget Foundation
120 Wall Street
New York, NY 10005-4001
212-509-5335
800-237-2438
Fax: 212-509-8492
e-mail: pagetfdn@aol.com
www.paget.org
The Paget Foundation provides this and other question and answer booklets and fact sheets on Paget's disease of bone, primary hyperparathyroidism,, fibrous dysplasia, osteopetrosis (not osteoporosis) and breast and prostate cancer metastic to bone. These publications are available on the foundation websit and in print.
Charlene Waldman, Executive Director

Web Sites

6840 Healing Well
www.healingwell.com
An online health resource guide to medical news, chat, information and articles, newsgroups and message boards, books, disease-related web sites, medical directories, and more for patients, friends, and family coping with disabling diseases, disorders, or chronic illnesses.

6841 Health Finder
www.healthfinder.gov
Searchable, carefully developed web site offering information on over 1000 topics. Developed by the US Department of Health and Human Services, the site can be used in both English and Spanish.

6842 Healthlink USA
www.healthlinkusa.com
Health information concerning treatment, cures, prevention, diagnosis, risk factors, research, support groups, email lists, personal stories and much more. Updated regularly.

6843 Helios Health
www.helioshealth.com
Online resource for your health information. Detailed information about specific health topics, access to expert advice from our Medical Advisory Board, and up-to-date health news.

6844 MedicineNet
www.medicinenet.com
An online resource for consumers providing easy-to-read, authoritative medical and health information.

6845 Medscape
www.medscape.com
Medscape offers specialists, primary care physicians, and other health professionals the Web's most robust and integrated medical information and educational tools.

6846   Paget Foundation for Paget's Disease of Bone & Related Disorders

www.paget.org

Includes information for patients and health professionals on Paget's disease of bone, primary hyperparathyroidism, fibrous dysplasia, osteopetrosis (not osteoporosis) and the complications of certain cancers on the skeleton.

6847   WebMD

www.webmd.com

Information on Paget's disease, including articles and resources.

Description

6848 Parkinson Disease

Parkinson disease is a neurological condition characterized by slow and decreased movement. It affects about 1 percent of those over age 65. The cause of Parkinson disease is unknown, but both genetic and environmental factors may play a role. In a minority of cases, Parkinson disease develops after repeated head trauma, carbon monoxide poisoning, drug use, or viral infections that affect the brain.

In about 50 percent to 80 percent of patients, Parkinson disease begins with a slight tremor in the hands, resembling "pill-rolling." With fatigue and stress, the tremor becomes more pronounced. As the disease progresses, voluntary movements, such as walking and eating, become more and more difficult. Rigidity and postural instability (difficulty standing up) develop. Dementia affects approximately one third of patients with advanced Parkinson disease.

Because Parkinson disease is characterized by reduced levels of neurotransmitter chemicals, notably dopamine, in certain parts of the brain, therapy has focused on restoring these levels to normal. Monoamine oxidase type B inhibitors given early in the disease, may protect the cells that secrete these chemicals, and thus delay the need for other therapy. When it is necessary to directly manipulate the chemical levels because of progression of the disease, levodopa, related to dopamine, is the mainstay of treatment and is associated with improvement of all Parkinson symptoms. Anticholinergic medications are especially helpful in treating tremor.

Parkinson disease is the subject of intense research, and experimental surgical or drug treatments are frequently available to patients whose response to standard therapy has been unsatisfactory. General supportive care should not be neglected, and includes physical therapy and an exercise program to help optimize mobility.

National Agencies & Associations

6849 American Parkinson Disease Association

135 Parkinson Avenue 718-981-8001
Staten Island, NY 10305-1943 800-223-2732
Fax: 718-981-4399
e-mail: apda@apdaparkinson.org
www.apdaparkinson.org
Funds research towards finding the cause(s) and cure for Parkinson's Disease, patient education, information, support groups nationwide.
Lesli A. Chambers, President&CEO
Fred Greene, Chairman of the Board

6850 Michael J. Fox Foundation for Parkinson's Research

Grand Central Station
New York, NY 10163 800-708-7644
www.michaeljfox.org
The Michael J. Fox Foundation is dedicated to ensuring the development of a cure for Parkinson's disease within this lifetime through an aggressively funded research center.
Deborah W Brooks, Co-Founder
Todd Sherer, CEO

6851 National Health Information Center

PO Box 1133 310-565-4167
Washington, DC 20013 800-336-4797
Fax: 301-984-4256
e-mail: info@nhic.org
www.health.gov/nhic
Offers a nationwide information referral service, produces directories and resource guides.

6852 National Institute of Neurological Disorders and Stroke

NIH Neurological Institute 301-496-5751
Bethesda, MD 20824 800-352-9424
Fax: 301-402-2186
TTY: 301-468-5981
www.ninds.nih.gov
The mission of NINDS is to reduce the burden of neurological disease - a burden borne by every age group, by every segment of society, by people all over the world.
Story C Landis PhD, Director
Walter J Koroshetz, Deputy Director

6853 National Parkinson Foundation

1501 NW 9th Avenue 305-243-6666
Miami, FL 33136-1407 800-327-4545
Fax: 305-243-6073
e-mail: contact@parkinson.org
www.parkinson.org
A nonprofit organization dedicated to research, diagnosis, treatment and care for men and women suffering from Parkinson's and other related neurological diseases. The Foundation also supports the Bob Hope research and rehabilitation center.
Bernard J. Fogel, Chairman
Joyce A Oberdorf, President and Chief Executive Officer

6854 Parkinson Society Canada

4211 Yonge Street 416-227-9700
Toronto, Ontario, M2P-2A9 800-565-3000
Fax: 416-227-9600
e-mail: info@parkinson.ca
www.parkinson.ca
A not-for-profit, national charitable organization. The Society raises money through corporate sponsorships, public donations, and planned gifts. Finding the cause and cure for Parkinson's disease remains our mission.
Bruce Ireland, President/CEO
Jean Pascal Souque, Vice President

6855 Parkinson's Action Network (PAN)

1025 Vermont Avenue NW 202-638-4101
Washington, DC 20005 800-850-4726
Fax: 202-638-7257
e-mail: info@parkinsonaction.org
www.parkinsonsaction.org
The Parkinson's Action Network is the unified voice of the Parkinson's disease community-advocating for more than one million Americans and their families.
Ronald H Galowich, Chair
Ed Weidenfield, Vice Chair

6856 Parkinson's Institute

675 Almanor Avenue 408-734-2800
Sunnyvale, CA 94085-1605 800-655-2273
Fax: 408-734-8455
e-mail: info@thepi.org
www.thepi.org
The mission of the Parkinson's Institute is to find the cause(s) and a cure for Parkinson's Disease and provide the best possible treatment to those afflicted with the disease.
Thomas D Follet, Chair
Thomas E Bailard, Secretory of Board

6857 WE MOVE

5731 Mosholu Avenue 212-875-8312
New York, NY 10471 e-mail: wemove@wemove.org
www.wemove.org
WE MOVE's mission is to raise awareness of neurologic movement disorder among healthcare professionals, patients and families and the public.
Susan B Bressman, President
Mo Moadeli, Vice President

State Agencies & Associations

Arizona

6858 **Arizona Chapter of the National Parkinson Foundation**
20280 N 59th Avenue   480-607-1960
Glendale, AZ 85308-6182   866-637-8772
                                        Fax: 480-607-1957
                                        e-mail: info@aznpf.org
                                        www.aznpf.org
Affiliate chapter of The National Parkinson Foundation Inc.
Alan Marks, President
Kenneth Larkin, Vice President

California

6859 **Los Angeles Alliance Against Parkinson's Disease**
3251 Oakley Drive   323-851-3230
Los Angeles, CA 90068-1315   e-mail: Millard@millardtipp.com
                             www.parkinson.org/chapters.htm#
Affiliate of the National Parkinson Foundation.

6860 **National Parkinson Foundation: California Office**
4929 Wilshire Boulevard   323-442-8434
Los Angeles, CA 90010-3899

6861 **National Parkinson Foundation: Orange County Chapter**
PO Box 2207   949-945-6200
Newport Beach, CA 92659   Fax: 949-548-4624
                                        e-mail: info@yahoo.com
                                        www.npfocc.org
Affiliate of The National Parkinson Foundation.
George Strickland, President
Janet Buell, Vice president

6862 **Northstate Parkinson's Chapter**
1003 Yuba Street
Redding, CA 96001
                                        530-229-0878
                                        www.parkinson.org
Affiliate of The National Parkinson Foundation, Inc.
Craig Boyer

6863 **Parkinson Association of the Sacramento Valley**
900 Fulton Avenue   916-534-7279
Sacramento, CA 96825-4502   800-473-4636
                                        Fax: 916-489-0241
                                        e-mail: parkanc@sbcglobal.net
                                        www.parkinsonsacramento.org
Bernardine Ford, President
George Johnston, 2nd Vice President

6864 **Parkinson Network of Mount Diablo**
Po Box 3127   925-284-2189
Walnut Creek, CA 94598-0127   e-mail: mmhansell@hotmail.com
                                        www.parkinson.org
Affiliate of the National Parkinson Foundation.
Mary Hansell

Colorado

6865 **Colorado Parkinson Foundation**
1155 Kelly Johnson Boulevard   719-884-0103
Colorado Springs, CO 90920-1494   800-327-4545
                                        Fax: 719-495-909
                                        e-mail: rpfarrer@msn.com
                                        colorado.parkinson.org
The mission of the National Parkinson Foundation if to find the cause of the cure for Parkinson disease through research. To improve the quality if life for persons with Parkinson and their caregivers. To also educate persons with Parkinson their carecar
Ric Pfarrer, Chairperson

Florida

6866 **Alzheimer/Parkinson Association of Indian River County**
2300 5th Avenue   772-563-0505
Vero Beach, FL 32960   e-mail: alzsupport@fastmail.fm
                                        www.parkinson.org
Toni Teresi, Chairperson

6867 **Goodwill Industries-Suncoast**
Goodwill Industries-Suncoast
10596 Gandy Boulevard   727-523-1512
St. Petersburg, FL 37023   888-279-1988
                                        Fax: 727-563-9300
                                        e-mail: gw.marketing@goodwill-suncoast.org
                                        www.goodwill-suncoast.org
A nonprofit community based organization whose purpose is to improve the quality of life for people who are disabled, disadvantaged and/or aged. This mission is accomplished through a staff of over 1,200 employees providing independent living skills, affordable housing, career assessment and planning, job skills, training, placement, and job retention assistance with useful employment. Annually, Goodwill Industries-Suncoast serves over 30,000 people in Citrus, Hernando, Levy, Marion and more.
R Lee Waits, President/CEO
Martin W Gladysz, Chair

6868 **Parkinson Association of Greater Daytona Beach**
111 North Frederick Avenue   386-252-8959
Daytona Beach, FL 32114   e-mail: goatie@cfl.rr.com
                                        www.parkinson.org
Nancy Dawson, Chairperson

6869 **Parkinson Association of Southwest Florida**
1048 Goodlette-Frank Road   239-417-3465
Naples, FL 34102   Fax: 239-417-3469
                                        e-mail: pasfi@aol.com
                                        www.pasfi.org
Affiliate of the National Parkinson Foundation.
Scott Leamon, Chair
Chris Spine, Executive Director

6870 **South Palm Beach County Chapter of NFP**
PO Box 880145
Boca Raton, FL 33433-0145   561-482-2867
                                        www.parkinson.org
Irving Layton, Chairperson

6871 **Southeast Parkinson Disease Association**
6530 Metrowest Boulevard   407-489-4124
Orlando, FL 32835-6520   e-mail: srh_pres@sepda.org
                                        www.sepda.org
Steve Hochberger, Chairperson

Georgia

6872 **Northwest Georgia Parkinson Disease Association**
708 Glen Milner Boulevard   706-235-3164
Rome, GA 30161   e-mail: webmaster@gaparkinsons.org
                                        www.gaparkinsons.org
James Trussel, Chairperson

Hawaii

6873 **Hawaii Parkinson Association Gwendolyn A Montibon President**
Gwendolyn A Montibon, President
3375 Koapaka St.,   808-734-9398
Honolulu, HI 96817   Fax: 808-528-1897
                                        e-mail: kekim@hawaii.edu
                                        www.parkinson.org
Affiliate of The National Parkinson Foundation.

Kansas

6874 **Northeast Kansas Parkinson Association**
PO Box 251
Topeka, KS 66601   785-228-1337
                                        www.parkinson.org
Mary Hatke, Chairperson

6875 **Parkinson Association of Greater Kansas City**
8900 State Line Road   913-341-8828
Leawood, KS 66206   Fax: 913-341-8885
                                        e-mail: meg@parkinsonheartland.org
                                        www.parkinsonheartland.org
Affiliate of The National Parkinson Foundation.
Kirk Gutekunst, President
Mary Lee Shucart, Secretary

Louisiana

6876 Eljay Foundation for Parkinson Syndrome Awareness
715 Ryan Street   337-310-0083
Lake Charles, LA 70601   e-mail: info@eljayfd.org
                                                      www.eljayfd.org

Eligha Guillory, President
Anna C. Drake, Secretary

Massachusetts

6877 Cape Cod Chapter National Parkinson Foundation
33 Ships Way   508-385-2333
Buzzards Bay, MA 02532-0584   e-mail: meacapecod@yahoo.com
                                                      www.parkinson.org
Affiliate of The National Parkinson Foundation.
Joseph Wimbrow, President

6878 National Parkinson Foundation:Cape Cod Chapter
33 Ships Way   508-385-2333
Buzzards Bay, MA 02532-0584   e-mail: meacapecod@yahoo.com
                                                      www.parkinson.org
Garland Smith, Chairperson

6879 Northeast Parkinson's and Caregivers
27 Sutcliffe Road   508-756-7721
Brimfield, MA 01010   e-mail: rstake@northeastparkinsons.com
                                                www.northeastparkinsons.com
Richard Stake, Chairperson

Minnesota

6880 Parkinson Association of Minnesota
5905 Golden Valley Road,   763-545-1272
Golden Valley, MN 55422-4602   800-327-4545
                                                e-mail: info@parkinsonmn.org
                                                      www.parkinsonmn.org
Affiliate of The National Parkinson Foundation.
Paul Blom, President
Collen Crane, Therapy Representative

New Jersey

6881 Parkinson Alliance
PO Box 308   609-688-0870
Kingston, NJ 08528   800-579-8440
                                                      Fax: 609-688-0875
                                          e-mail: admin@parkinsonalliance.net
                                                www.parkinsonalliance.net
The Princeton-New Jersey based Parkinson Alliance is a National
nonprofit organization dedicated to raising funds to help finance
the most promising research to find the cause and curefor Parkin-
son's disease.
Martin Tuchman, Chairman
Margaret Tuchman, President

New York

6882 National Parkinson Foundation: New York Office
122 E 42nd Street
New York, NY 10017-5622
                                                      800-457-6676
                                                      www.parkinson.org/

6883 Parkinsons Wellness Group of Western New York
5140 Main Street   716-218-1027
Depew, NY 14221   e-mail: coach71395@aol.com
                                                http://www.npfwny.org/
Site changed
Robert J Plunket, President
Gary Kurdziel, Vice President

Oklahoma

6884 Parkinson Foundation of the Heartland Oklahoma Branch
1000 W Wilshire   405-810-0695
Oklahoma City, OK 73116   e-mail: jimk@parkinsonheartland.org
                                                      www.parkinson.org
Satellite office of the Kansas Chapter
Jim Keating, Chairperson

Oregon

6885 Parkinsons Resources of Oregon
3975 Mercantile Drive   503-594-0901
Lake Oswego, OR 97035   800-426-6806
                                                      Fax: 503-594-0547
                                          e-mail: info@parkinsonsresources.org
                                                www.parkinsonsresources.org
Holly Chaimov, Executive Director

Pennsylvania

6886 Parkinson Chapter of Greater Pittsburgh
6507 Wilkins Avenue   412-365-2086
Pittsburgh, PA 15217   e-mail: info@pfwpa.org.
                                                www.parkinsonpittsburgh.org

Doreen Grasso, Chairperson
Maggie Schmidt, Executive Director

6887 Parkinson Council
111 Presidential Boulevard   610-668-4292
Bala Cynwyd, PA 19004   Fax: 610-668-4275
                                          e-mail: info@theparkinsoncouncil.org
                                                www.theparkinsoncouncil.org
The Parkinson Council is dedicated to promoting research initiat-
ing to find the causes and cure for Parkinson Disease educating patients their caregivers healthcare professionals and the general
public about Parkinson's and improving the quality of lif
Jeff Keefer, President
Jo Ann Zoll, Vice President

South Dakota

6888 Parkinson Association of South Dakota
PO Box 87952   605-328-4227
Sioux Falls, SD 57109-9938   Fax: 605-328-7150
                                                e-mail: info@parkinsonsd.org
                                                      www.parkinsonsd.org
Affiliate of The National Parkinson Foundation.
Elaine Spader, President
Lori Jones, Vice President

Virginia

6889 Parkinson Foundation of the National Capitol Area
7700 Leesburg Pike,   703-734-1017
Falls church, VA 22043-4201   Fax: 703-734-1241
                                          e-mail: pfnca@parkinsonfoundation.org
                                                www.parkinsonfoundation.org
Daniel M Lewis, Chairperson
Donna Schena, Vice Chairman

Wisconsin

6890 Wisconsin Parkinson Association
945 N 12th Street   414-219-7061
Milwaukee, WI 53233   800-972-5455
                                                      Fax: 414-219-6564
                                                      www.wiparkinson.org
Chapter of The National Parkinson Foundation.
Keith Brewer, President

Foundations

6891 Parkinsons Disease Foundation
1359 Broadway   212-923-4700
New York, NY 10018   800-457-6676
                                                      Fax: 212-923-4778
                                                      e-mail: info@pdf.org
                                                      www.pdf.org
The foundation has been one of teh leaders in subsidizing research
into Parkinson's Disease. Offers many services including The
Summer Fellowship Program, The Postdoctoral Fellowship Pro-
gram, support groups nationwide, grants for clinical and laboratory studies, public awareness and government promotion of the
disease.
Howard D. Morgan, chair/Co Preident
Constance Woodruff atwell, Vice Chair

Libraries & Resource Centers

6892 Parkinson's Resource Organization
74090 El Paseo   760-773-5628
Palm Desert, CA 92260-4135   877-775-4111
                                                  Fax: 760-773-9803
                                  e-mail: info@parkinsonsresource.org
                                           www.parkinsonsresource.org
Our mission is to help families affected by Parkinson's forge through the journey of the disease's progression with as much quality as life can provide. Working so no one is isolated because of Parkinson's
Jo Rosen, Visionary, President, Founder
William R Remery, Treasurer

Research Centers

6893 California Institute for Medical Research
2260 Clove Drive   408-998-4554
San Jose, CA 95128   Fax: 408-998-2723
                                            e-mail: admin@clmr.org
                                                        www.cimr.org
Medical research including infectious diseases stroke and cancer specializing in Parkinson's Disease related studies.
David A Stevens, President
John Hotson, Vice President

6894 Texas Tech University Tarbox Parkinson's Disease Institute
3601 4th Street
Lubbock, TX 79430   806-743-1000
                                                        www.ttuhsc.edu
The current objectives of the Tarbox Institute are to provide services for Parkinson's disease patients and their families in the underserved West Texas area; to maintain a Parkinson's Disease Information and Referral Center to enable both healthcare professionals and affected families to obtain the latest information on services available new developments in research support groups and educational literature.
Tedd L Mitchell, President
Pureza Martinez, Chief of Staff

6895 University of Alabama at Birmingham Parkinsons Disease Center
1720 7th Avenue S   205-934-9100
Birmingham, AL 35294   Fax: 205-346-78
                                            e-mail: apda@uab.edu
                                                        www.uab.edu
Offers educational emotional and political support to Parkinson disease patients and their families.
Ray Watts, Interim CEO
David G Standaert, Director

6896 William T Gossett Parkinson's Disease Center
Henry Ford Hospital
Department of Neurology   313-972-1693
Detroit, MI 48202
Jay M Gorell MD, Director

Support Groups & Hotlines

California

6897 Parkinson's Disease Association of San Die go (PDASD)
8555 Areo Drive   858-273-6763
San Diego, CA 92123-1746   877-737-7576
                                                  Fax: 858-273-6764
                                             e-mail: info@pdasd.org
                                                        www.pdasd.org
Information and referral research center for Parkinson's disease patients and their families.
Jerry Henberger, Executive Director
Rick Brydges, President

Florida

6898 Greater Daytona Area Parkinson Support Group
Bishop's Glen Retirement Center   904-322-4748
Daytona, FL   e-mail: boba@n-jcenter.com
                                                        www.parkinson.org
Affiliate of the National Parkinson Foundation.

6899 National Parkinson Foundation Hotline
National Parkinson Foundation
1501 NW 9th Avenue Bob Hope Road   305-243-6666
Miami, FL 33136   800-327-4545
                                                  Fax: 305-243-5595
                                                        www.parkinson.org
Offers support and emergency information for persons with Parkinson's and their families.
Jose Garcia Pebrosa, Director

6900 Pembroke Pines Parkinson Support Group
Century Village, Club House
Pembroke Pines, FL 33027   954-433-0947
                                                        www.parkinson.org
Affiliate of the National Parkinson Foundation.

Hawaii

6901 Kuakini Parkinson Disease (PD) Information & Referral
Kuakini Medical Center
347 North Kuakini Street   808-536-2236
Honolulu, HI 96817   800-570-1101
                                                  Fax: 808-528-1897
                                            e-mail: pr@kuakini.org
                                             www.kuakini.org/SiteMap.asp
The Kuakini Parkinson Disease (PD) Information & Referral Office provides referrals to neurologists and other special services for Parkinson disease patients; provides information about community services to assist PD patients and their caregivers in finding optimal care; distributes educational materials; conducts educational conferences and other activities; and assists with support groups for PD patients and caregivers.
Gary K Kajiwara, President/Chief Executive Officer
Gregg Oishi, SVP/Chief Operating Officer

Illinois

6902 Rockford Parkinson's Support Group
5415 Watson Road   815-654-0614
Rockford, IL 61108   800-972-5455
Affiliate of The National Parkinson Foundation, Inc.

Maryland

6903 Parkinson Support Groups of America
11376 Cherry Hill Road   301-937-1545
Beltsville, MD 20705
Offers support networks and groups for persons with Parkinson's disease, families, friends and professionals.

Missouri

6904 APDA Center for Advanced Parkinson Disease Research
Washington University School of Medicine
660 South Euclid   314-362-6909
St Louis, MO 63110   Fax: 314-362-0168
                                         e-mail: joel@npg.wustl.edu
                                            www.neuro.wustl.edu/parkinson/
Information and referral research center for Parkinson's disease patients and their families.
David m Holtzman, Chairman
Brad a Racette, Vice Chairman

6905 Ozarks Parkinson Support Group
Po Box 50595
Springfield, MO 65805   417-885-9595
                                            www.parkinson.org/shell/areacode.pl
Affiliate of the National Parkinson Foundation.
Monty Montgomery, Contact

6906   New Jersey Parkinson's Disease Information Center
Robert Wood Johnson University Hospital
One Robert Wood Johnson Place   732-828-3000
New Brunswick, NJ 08901   Fax: 732-745-3114
e-mail: elizabeth.schaaf@rwjuh.edu
www.rwjuh.edu/medical_services/
The New Jersey Parkinson's Disease Information and Referral
Center reaches out to persons affected by Parkinson's disease, including patients, families and healthcare professionals. This Information and Referral Center is committed to providing community
education and information as well as support groups for caregivers
and persons with Parkinson's disease.
Elizabeth Schaaf, Parkinson's Disease Center Coordinator

6907   American Parkinson Disease Association Hotline
1250 Hylan Boulevard
Staten Island, NY 10305   800-908-2732
Fax: 718-981-4399
www.attaparkinson.org
Offers information and physician referrals to patients and their
families.
Joel Gerstel, Director

6908   New York College of Osteopathic Medicine
PO Box 8000   516-686-3747
Old Westbury, NY 11568-8000   800-345-6948
Fax: 516-686-7613
e-mail: Barbara
http://www.nyit.edu/medicine/
Information and referral research center for Parkinson's disease
patients and their families.
Rosslee , Vice President

6909   Parkinson's Support Group of Upstate New York
PO Box 23204
Rochester, NY 14692-3204   716-377-6718
www.parkinson.org/upstate.htm
Affiliate of The National Parkinson Foundation, Inc.
David Look, President

6910   St. John's Episcopal Hospital
327 Beach 19th street
Smithtown, NY 11691   718-869-7000
www.ehs.org
Information and referral research center for Parkinson's disease
patients and their families.
Nelson toebbe, Chief Executive Officer
Richard A Brown, Chief Operating Officer

6911   University of Rochester
500 Wilson Boulevard   585-275-3221
Rochester, NY 14627   888-822-2256
www.rochester.edu/
Information and referral research center for Parkinson's disease
patients and their families.

6912   Oregon Health Sciences University
3181 SW Sam Jackson Park Road   503-494-5285
Portland, OR 97239   888-222-6478
www.ohsu.edu
Information and referral research center for Parkinson's disease
patients and their families.

6913   University of Pittsburgh
4200 Fifth avenue   412-624-4141
Pittsburgh, PA 15260   Fax: 412-383-2264
e-mail: webmaster@pitt.edu
www.pitt.edu
Information and referral research center for Parkinson's disease
patients and their families.
Patricia E. Beeson, Vice Chancellor
John P Elliott, Director of Internal Affairs

6914   Presbyterian Hospital of Dallas
612 E. Lamar Boulevard
Arlington, TX 76011   214-345-6789
www.texashealth.org
Information and referral research center for Parkinson's disease
patients and their families.
Phillip Moroneso, Chair
Brock Campton, Vice Chair

6915   University of Texas HSC at San Antonio
7703 Floyd Curl Drive
San Antonio, TX 78229-3900   210-567-7000
www.uthscsa.edu/
Information and referral research center for Parkinson's disease
patients and their families.

6916   University of Washington
Box 355840   206-543-5369
Seattle, WA 98195-5840   e-mail: uwvic@u.washington.edu
www.washington.edu/
Information and referral research center for Parkinson's disease
patients and their families.

Books

6917   Coping with Parkinson's Disease
American Parkinson's Disease Association
1250 Hylan Boulevard
Staten Island, NY 10305-1944   800-223-2732
88 pages

6918   Living with Parkinson's Disease
Demos Medical Publishing
386 Park Avenue S   212-683-0072
New York, NY 10016-8804   800-532-8663
Fax: 212-683-0118
e-mail: orderdept@demospub.com
www.demospub.com
Written specifically for anyone who has been diagnosed with Par-
kinson's disease, as well as family members and friends.
1996 150 pages
ISBN: 1-888799-10-2
Dr. Diana M Schneider, President

6919   Parkinson's - A Personal Story of Acceptance
Branden Publishing Company
17 Station Street Box 843   617-734-2045
Brookline Village, MA 02147   Fax: 617-734-2046
www.branden.com
1993 162 pages Paperback
ISBN: 0-828319-49-9

6920   Parkinson's Disease & Movement Disorders
Williams & Wilkins
351 W Camden Street   301-528-4000
Baltimore, MD 21201-7912   800-638-0672
1993 640 pages
ISBN: 0-683043-80-3

6921   Parkinson's Disease Handbook
National Parkinson Foundation
1501 NW 9th Avenue   305-547-6666
Miami, FL 33136-1407   800-327-4545
Fax: 305-548-4403
www.parkinson.org
A guide for patients and their families regarding the illness of Par-
kinson's.
Paperback

6922   Parkinson's Disease: A Guide for Patient and Family
Raven Press
1185 Avenue of the Americas   212-930-9500
New York, NY 10036-2601   800-777-2295
Recommended by patients, the medical community and the leading
medical journals, this guide offers information on the most recent

medical advances in the field of Parkinson's disease and answers the patients most frequently asked questions about the illness.
224 pages Hardcover
ISBN: 0-781703-12-3

6923 Parkinsonian Syndromes
John H Dekker & Sons
2941 Clydon Avenue SW   616-538-5160
Grand Rapids, MI 49509-2403   Fax: 616-538-0720
1993 584 pages
ISBN: 0-824788-38-9

6924 The Comfort of Home for Parkinson Disease: A Guide for Caregivers
Marie Meyer & Paula Derr, RN with Susa Imke, RN/MS, author
CareTrust Publications
PO Box 10283
Portland, OR 97296-0283   800-565-1533
                                         Fax: 415-673-2005
                          e-mail: sales@comfortofhome.com
                                    www.comfortofhome.com
Comfort will help caregivers be equipped with information about everything from the importance of and noticing wearing off signs to making difficult decisions to travel, equipment options, therapies and dietary guidelines. It offers caregivers mental and emotional support in coping with their challenging role, as well.
2007 298 pages
ISBN: 0-966476-77-8

Children's Books

6925 Journey to Almost There
Clarion Books
215 Park Avenue S   212-420-5800
New York, NY 10003-1603
An interesting tale that surrounds the relationship of Alison and her Granfather O'Brien when Alison's mother feels that he should enter an elderly home.
Grades 6-9

Newsletters

6926 APDA Newsletter
American Parkinson Disease Association
135 Parkinson Avenue   718-981-8001
Staten Island, NY 10305-1943   800-223-2732
                                         Fax: 718-981-4399
                          e-mail: apda@apdaparkinson.org
                                    www.apdaparkinson.org
Current information on matters of interest for PD patients and families.
Joel A Miele, President
Joel Gerste, Executive Director

6927 American Parkinson Disease Association Newsletter
60 Bay Street   718-981-8001
Staten Island, NY 10301-2514   800-223-2732
Offers information on the association activities and events, convention and legislative information, medical updates and research reports for the Parkinson's patient and their families.
Quarterly

6928 News & Review
Parkinsons Disease Foundation
1359 Broadway   212-923-4700
New York, NY 10018   800-457-6676
                                         Fax: 212-923-4778
                                    e-mail: info@pdf.org
                                         www.pdf.org
In each issue we include reports on scientific research and discoveries, treatments and therapies, commentary from physicians and insight from Parkinson's specialists. We also provide practical

suggestions, tips and articles from people who live with the disease and wish to share their experiences.
Quarterly
Lewis P Rowland, MD, President
Robin A Elliott, Executive Director

6929 Parkinson Report
National Parkinson Foundation
1501 NW 9th Avenue   305-547-6666
Miami, FL 33136-1407   800-327-4545
                                         Fax: 305-548-4403
                                         www.parkinson.org
Offers association news and events, conference and symposia news, legislative and medical updates, research reports and more for the Parkinson's patient, their families and the general public.
Quarterly

6930 Parkinson's Disease Foundation Newsletter
Parkinson's Disease Foundation
650 W 168th Street   212-923-4700
New York, NY 10032-3702   800-457-6676
Provides information on Parkinson's Disease Foundation events, news stories of research findings, and technical advances in the field of patient care.

Pamphlets

6931 A One-Stop Shop for Parkinson's Informatio n
Parkinsons Disease Foundation
1359 Broadway   212-923-4700
New York, NY 10018   800-457-6676
                                         Fax: 212-923-4778
                                    e-mail: info@pdf.org
                                         www.pdf.org
An explanation of PDF's services and resources that are available to answer your most important questions about Parkinson's disease. These services include a toll-free helpline, our Ask the Expert web service and print/video materials.
Lewis P Rowland, MD, President
Robin A Elliott, Executive Director

6932 Adjustment, Adaptation and Accomodation: Psychological Approaches
National Parkinson Foundation
1501 NW 9th Avenue   305-547-6666
Miami, FL 33136-1407   800-327-4545
                                         Fax: 305-548-4403
                                         www.parkinson.org
Coping strategies for Parkinson's disease.

6933 Akathisia in Parkinson's Disease
Parkinson United Foundation
833 W Washington Boulevard   312-733-1893
Chicago, IL 60607
1990

6934 Answering Your Questions About PROPATH
525 Middlefield Road
Menlo Park, CA 94025-3447   800-776-7284
This brochure explains and offers an introduction to PROPATH, a program for Parkinson's disease patients.

6935 Autonomic Failure and Parkinson's Disease
United Parkinson Foundation
833 W Washington Boulevard   312-733-1893
Chicago, IL 60607-2316
1990

6936 Balance Disturbances and Parkinson's Disease
United Parkinson Foundation
833 W Washington Boulevard   312-733-1893
Chicago, IL 60607-2316
1990

6937 Basic Information About Parkinson's Disease
American Parkinson's Disease Association
1250 Hylan Boulevard
Staten Island, NY 10305-1944   800-223-2732
Offers information on the illness, incidence, treatments, education and support for both patients and professionals.

6938 Deep Brain Stimulation for Parkinson's Disease
Parkinsons Disease Foundation
1359 Broadway   212-923-4700
New York, NY 10018   800-457-6676
                                            Fax: 212-923-4778
                                        e-mail: info@pdf.org
                                                www.pdf.org
This booklet addresses the newest area of surgical options in the
treatment of PD symptoms _ deep brain stimulation (or DBS) sur-
gery _ while also describing older surgical approaches used to treat
PD.
Lewis P Rowland, MD, President
Robin A Elliott, Executive Director

6939 Dental Care for the Patient with Parkinson's Disease
United Parkinson Foundation
833 W Washington Boulevard   312-733-1893
Chicago, IL 60607-2316
1987

6940 Depression and Dementia in Parkinson's Disease
United Parkinson Foundation
833 W Washington Boulevard   312-733-1893
Chicago, IL 60607-2316
1993

6941 Diagnosis Parkinson's Disease: You Are Not Alone
Parkinsons Disease Foundation
1359 Broadway   212-923-4700
New York, NY 10018   800-457-6676
                                            Fax: 212-923-4778
                                        e-mail: info@pdf.org
                                                www.pdf.org
Designed for the person newly diagnosed with Parkinson's, this in-
formational booklet serves as a reference for the many questions
that may arise. It shares resources, medical expert testimony and
the experiences of people who have dealt with the diagnosis of
Parkinson's disease.
Booklet
Lewis P Rowland, MD, President
Robin A Elliott, Executive Director

6942 Dietary Considerations for Parkinson's Disease Patients
United Parkinson Foundation
833 W Washington Boulevard   312-733-1893
Chicago, IL 60607-2316

6943 Differential Diagnosis of Parkinsonism
United Parkinson Foundation
833 W Washington Boulevard   312-733-1893
Chicago, IL 60607-2316
1984

**6944 Driving and the Parkinson's Disease Patient: Some
Considerations**
United Parkinson Foundation
833 W Washington Boulevard   312-733-1893
Chicago, IL 60607-2316
1994

6945 Efficacy of Antiparkinson Medications
United Parkinson Foundation
833 W Washington Boulevard   312-733-1893
Chicago, IL 60607-2316
1983

6946 Equipment and Suggestions for Persons with Parkinson's Disease
American Parkinson's Disease Association
1250 Hylan Boulevard
Staten Island, NY 10305-1944   800-223-2732
19 pages

6947 Eyes and Parkinson's Disease
United Parkinson Foundation
833 W Washington Boulevard   312-733-1893
Chicago, IL 60607-2316
1986

6948 Fighting Back Against PD: One Women's Story
National Parkinson Foundation

1501 NW 9th Avenue   305-547-6666
Miami, FL 33136-1407   800-327-4545
                                            Fax: 305-548-4403
                                                www.parkinson.org
One woman's battle against Parkinson's disease.

**6949 Fulfilling the Hope: Our Commitment to the Parkinson's
Community**
Parkinsons Disease Foundation
1359 Broadway   212-923-4700
New York, NY 10018   800-457-6676
                                            Fax: 212-923-4778
                                        e-mail: info@pdf.org
                                                www.pdf.org
This brochure provides an overview of Parkinsons Disease Foun-
dations services and programs.
Lewis P Rowland, MD, President
Robin A Elliott, Executive Director

6950 Good Nutrition in Parkinson's Disease
American Parkinson Disease Association
60 Bay Street
Staten Island, NY 10301-2514   800-223-2732
Offers information on diet, nutrients, proteins and recipes for peo-
ple with Parkinson's disease.

6951 How to Start a Parkinson's Disease Support Group
American Parkinson's Disease Association
1250 Hylan Boulevard
Staten Island, NY 10305-1944   800-223-2732
42 pages

6952 MR Imaging in Parkinson's Disease
United Parkinson Foundation
833 W Washington Boulevard   312-733-1893
Chicago, IL 60607-2316
1990

6953 Micrographia
United Parkinson Foundation
833 W Washington Boulevard   312-733-1893
Chicago, IL 60607-2316
1991

6954 Neuropsychology and Parkinson's Disease
United Parkinson Foundation
833 W Washington Boulevard   312-733-1893
Chicago, IL 60607-2316
1992

6955 Neurotrophic Factors in Parkinson's Disease
United Parkinson Foundation
833 W Washington Boulevard   312-733-1893
Chicago, IL 60607-2316
1992

6956 One Step at a Time Brochure
United Parkinson Foundationon
833 W Washington Boulevard   312-733-1893
Chicago, IL 60607-2316
An exercise manual for the Parkinsonian patient.
1985

6957 Pain Syndromes and Parkinson's Disease
United Parkinson Foundation
833 W Washington Boulevard   312-733-1893
Chicago, IL 60607-2316
1990

6958 Parkinson Handbook: A Guide for Patients and Their Families
National Parkinson Foundation
1501 NW 9th Avenue   305-547-6666
Miami, FL 33136-1407   800-327-4545
                                            Fax: 305-548-4403
                                                www.parkinson.org
Offers informative, up-to-date information on exercises, hobbies,
treatments, speech impairments and psychological aspects.

6959 Parkinson's Advocacy: The Keys to Empowerment
Parkinsons Disease Foundation

1359 Broadway
New York, NY 10018

212-923-4700
800-457-6676
Fax: 212-923-4778
e-mail: info@pdf.org
www.pdf.org

Use this informational brochure to learn how to harness your power as a person living with Parkinson's and join the fight for a cure.
Lewis P Rowland, MD, President
Robin A Elliott, Executive Director

6960 Parkinson's Disease Handbook
American Parkinson's Disease Association
1250 Hylan Boulevard
Staten Island, NY 10305-1944   800-223-2732
40 pages

6961 Parkinson's Disease Q&A: A Guide for Patients
Parkinsons Disease Foundation
1359 Broadway
New York, NY 10018

212-923-4700
800-457-6676
Fax: 212-923-4778
e-mail: info@pdf.org
www.pdf.org

This booklet answers the most frequently asked questions about Parkinson's disease. Movement disorder specialists from the Columbia University Medical Center address topics ranging from signs of Parkinson's to treatment options to daily living issues.
Booklet
Lewis P Rowland, MD, President
Robin A Elliott, Executive Director

6962 Parkinson's Disease and the Menstrual Cycle
United Parkinson Foundation
833 W Washington Boulevard   312-733-1893
Chicago, IL 60607-2316
1990

6963 Parkinson's Disease: The Patient Experience
United Parkinson Foundation
833 W Washington Boulevard   312-733-1893
Chicago, IL 60607-2316
Booklet designed for patients with Parkinson's disease and their families to explain medical terminology and offer suggestions on how to deal with the disease more easily.
1986

6964 Parkinson's Patient: What You and Your Family Should Know
National Parkinson Foundation
1501 NW 9th Avenue   305-547-6666
Miami, FL 33136-1407   800-327-4545
Fax: 305-548-4403
www.parkinson.org

Offers a brief overview of Parkinson's Disease causes, symptoms and treatments as well as offering an insight into statistical information on the illness.

6965 Patient Perspectives on Parkinson's
National Parkinson Foundation
1501 NW 9th Avenue   305-547-6666
Miami, FL 33136-1407   800-327-4545
Fax: 305-548-4403
www.parkinson.org

Offers a brief overview of Parkinson's disease, the onset of the illness, depression, sexuality, exercise, sleep and nutrition information for daily living.
45 pages

6966 Perioperative Management of Parkinson's Disease
United Parkinson Foundation
833 W Washington Boulevard   312-733-1893
Chicago, IL 60607-2316
1989

6967 Pet Scans: A New Look at Parkinson's Disease
United Parkinson Foundation
833 W Washington Boulevard   312-733-1893
Chicago, IL 60607-2316
1989

6968 Podiatry and Parkinson's Disease
United Parkinson Foundation
833 W Washington Boulevard   312-733-1893
Chicago, IL 60607-2316
1983

6969 Postural Hypotension
United Parkinson Foundation
833 W Washington Boulevard   312-733-1893
Chicago, IL 60607-2316
1988

6970 Practical Pointers for Parkinson Patients
National Parkinson Foundation
1501 NW 9th Avenue   305-547-6666
Miami, FL 33136-1407   800-327-4545
Fax: 305-548-4403
www.parkinson.org

6971 Role of Physical Therapy in Parkinson's Disease
United Parkinson Foundation
833 W Washington Boulevard   312-733-1893
Chicago, IL 60607-2316
1985

6972 Sexual and Bladder Difficulties in Parkinson's Disease
United Parkinson Foundation
833 W Washington Boulevard   312-733-1893
Chicago, IL 60607-2316
1988

6973 Sleep Problems with Parkinson's Disease
United Parkinson Foundation
833 W Washington Boulevard   312-733-1893
Chicago, IL 60607-2316
1992

6974 Speech & Swallowing Problems for Parkinsonians
National Parkinson Foundation
1501 NW 9th Avenue   305-547-6666
Miami, FL 33136-1407   800-327-4545
Fax: 305-548-4403
www.parkinson.org

6975 Speech Problems & Swallowing Problems in Parkinson's Disease
American Parkinson Disease Association
60 Bay Street
Staten Island, NY 10301-2514   800-223-2732
Offers information on speech problems, swallowing problems, hearing impairments and facial mobility for the person with Parkinson's.

6976 Speech and Voice Impairment
United Parkinson Foundation
833 W Washington Boulevard   312-733-1893
Chicago, IL 60607-2316
1983

6977 Stages of Parkinson's Disease
United Parkinson Foundation
833 W Washington Boulevard   312-733-1893
Chicago, IL 60607-2316
1983

6978 Suggested Exercise Program for People with Parkinson's Disease
American Parkinson Disease Association
60 Bay Street
Staten Island, NY 10301-2514   800-223-2732
Exercise program pamphlet with full illustrations explaining each exercise.
23 pages

6979 Treatment of Parkinson's Disease with Carbidopa-Levodopa
National Parkinson Foundation
1501 NW 9th Avenue   305-547-6666
Miami, FL 33136-1407   800-327-4545
Fax: 305-548-4403
www.parkinson.org

Offers information on treating Parkinson's Disease.

Audio & Video

6980 Diagnosis Parkinson's Disease: You Are Not Alone
Parkinsons Disease Foundation
1359 Broadway   212-923-4700
New York, NY 10018   800-457-6676
                              Fax: 212-923-4778
                         e-mail: info@pdf.org
                                 www.pdf.org
Designed for the person newly diagnosed with Parkinson's, this informational booklet and video serve as a reference for the many questions that may arise. It shares resources, medical expert testimony and the experiences of people who have dealt with the diagnosis of Parkinson's disease.
Video & Booklet
Lewis P Rowland, MD, President
Robin A Elliott, Executive Director

6981 Motivating Moves for People with Parkinson's
Parkinsons Disease Foundation
1359 Broadway   212-923-4700
New York, NY 10018   800-457-6676
                              Fax: 212-923-4778
                         e-mail: info@pdf.org
                                 www.pdf.org
Motivating Moves is a unique program of 24 seated exercises designed especially for people with Parkinson's. Exercises address typical Parkinson's symptoms such as stability, flexibility, posture, vocal range and facial expressivity. The video is divided into three sections, How to Do Motivating Moves (45 minutes), The Exercise Class (36 minutes) and Practical Tips for Daily Living (4 minutes).
Video
Lewis P Rowland, MD, President
Robin A Elliott, Executive Director

6982 PDF Exercise Program
Parkinsons Disease Foundation
1359 Broadway   212-923-4700
New York, NY 10018   800-457-6676
                              Fax: 212-923-4778
                         e-mail: info@pdf.org
                                 www.pdf.org
This program consists of three sets of exercises specifically designed for PD patients. Each exercise is clearly illustrated in a 3-ring binder with flip-chart pages and includes two cassette tapes, which provide verbal cues and music for timing.
Cassettes
Lewis P Rowland, MD, President
Robin A Elliott, Executive Director

6983 Parkingson's: Lynda's Story
David Tucker, author
Fanlight Productions
4196 Washington Street   617-469-4999
Boston, MA 02131   800-937-4113
                              Fax: 617-469-3379
                     e-mail: fanlight@fanlight.com
                                www.fanlight.com
Parkingson's disease is robbing Lynda McKenzie of normal coordination and movement. She's prepared to participate in a clinical study of surgery to transplant fetal cells directly into her brain, but she will have to live for a year not knowing whether she has received the actual cells or a placebo.
1999 46 Minutes
ISBN: 1-572954-22-1
Nicole Johnson, Publicity Coordinator

Web Sites

6984 Healing Well
                            www.healingwell.com
An online health resource guide to medical news, chat, information and articles, newsgroups and message boards, books, disease-related web sites, medical directories, and more for patients, friends, and family coping with disabling diseases, disorders, or chronic illnesses.

6985 Health Finder
                            www.healthfinder.gov
Searchable, carefully developed web site offering information on over 1000 topics. Developed by the US Department of Health and Human Services, the site can be used in both English and Spanish.

6986 Healthlink USA
                            www.healthlinkusa.com
Health information concerning treatment, cures, prevention, diagnosis, risk factors, research, support groups, email lists, personal stories and much more. Updated regularly.

6987 Helios Health
                            www.helioshealth.com
Online resource for your health information. Detailed information about specific health topics, access to expert advice from our Medical Advisory Board, and up-to-date health news.

6988 MedicineNet
                            www.medicinenet.com
An online resource for consumers providing easy-to-read, authoritative medical and health information.

6989 Medscape
                            www.medscape.com
Medscape offers specialists, primary care physicians, and other health professionals the Web's most robust and integrated medical information and educational tools.

6990 National Parkinson Foundation
                            www.parkinson.org
Information on research, diagnosis, treatment and care for men and women suffering from parkinson's and other related neurological diseases.

6991 Neurology Channel
                            www.neurologychannel.com
Find clearly explained, medically accurate information regarding conditions, including an overview, symptoms, causes, diagnostic procedures and treatment options. On this site it is possible to ask questions and get information from a neurologist and connect to people who have similar health interests.

6992 WebMD
                            www.webmd.com
Information on Parkinson's disease, including articles and resources.

Description

6993 Post-Polio Syndrome

Post-Polio syndrome, PPS, also known as the late effects of polio or post polio sequelae, is characterized by new symptoms that occur in people with a history of polio after a long period of stability during which whatever strength they had recovered remained unchanged. PPS affects approximately 60 percent of polio survivors, 20 to 40 years after the initial episode. The hallmark of PPS is new weakness. Other symptoms include fatigue, pain, difficulty breathing and swallowing, intolerance to cold, and new muscle atrophy.

While the cause of PPS is not clearly understood, two theories exist. One suggests that it is caused by normal muscle loss that accompanies aging. The other is that PPS is caused by the repeated over use of muscle groups. In both cases, muscle groups not previously known to have been affected by polio are weakened, and it is this weakness that is the major indicator of PPS. A polio survivor with an affected leg may find that his or her arms are newly affected. Whether the arm problems are a result of undetected muscle damage that occurred at the time of the original polio or newer damage resulting from the over use of the remaining good muscles, or a combination of the two, is not clearly understood.

PPS is frequently emotionally difficult for polio survivors. Many feel they have triumphed over their initial polio, or have come to terms with their resulting disabilities. To think that the polio is coming back is often terrifying. These emotional issues are frequently made more difficult by the fact that PPS is often mis-diagnosed as other conditions or normal aging. Also, patients are often given misinformation about PPS.

Post-polio syndrome, like most diseases classified as syndromes, does not have a specific diagnostic test, but a diagnosis of exclusion. This means that other medical conditions that may present with symptoms similar to those found in PPS should be considered and excluded, if possible. Once diagnosis of PPS is determined, treatment is individualized by primary symptoms and may include medications, supervised therapy, injections and, in some cases, surgery.

National Agencies & Associations

6994 Post Polio Awareness and Support Society o f British Columbia
#2-2630 Ross Lane
Victoria, BC, V8T-5L5
250-477-8244
Fax: 250-477-8287
e-mail: ppass@ppass.bc.ca
www.ppass.bc.ca
A non-profit society that links area groups, through our board and our provincial office in Victoria.
Joan Toone, President

Support Groups & Hotlines

6995 PostPolio Health International
4207 Lindell Boulevard
Saint Louis, MO 63108-2915
314-534-0475
Fax: 314-534-5070
e-mail: info@postpolio.org
www.post-polio.org/
Post-Polio Health International's mission is to enhance the lives and independence of polio survivors and home ventilator users through education, advocacy, research and networking.
Willism G Stothers, President
Saul J Morse, Legal counsel

Books

6996 Managing Post-Polio: A Guide for Polio Survivors and Their Families
Yale University Press
PO Box 209040
New Haven, CT 06520-9040
203-732-0960
Fax: 203-432-0948
Diagnosis and management of polio-related health problems . Essential resources for polio survivors, their families and health care providers.

6997 Managing Post-Polio: A Guide to Living Well with Post-Polio Syndrome
ABI Professional Publications
PO Box 5243
Arlington, VA 22205
703-525-5488
Fax: 703-524-4105
Practical information resulting from a combination of professional knowledge and personal experience. A comprehensive array of topics are addressed: the diagnostic process, finding expert medical care, energy conservation, psychosocial aspects of disability, support groups, vocational strategies, managed care concerns, Social Security benefits, and internet resources.
256 pages

Newsletters

6998 Polio Network News
Post-Polio Health International
4207 Lindell Boulevard
St. Louis, MO 63108-2915
314-534-0475
Fax: 314-534-5070
e-mail: ventinfo@post-polio.org
www.post-polio.org/IVUN

Joan Headley, Executive Director

6999 Post-Polio Health
Post-Polio Health International
4207 Lindell Boulevard
Saint Louis, MO 63108-2915
314-534-0475
Fax: 314-534-5070
e-mail: ventinfo@post-polio.org
www.post-polio.org/IVUN

12 pages Quarterly
Joan Headley, Executive Director

7000 Post-Polio Health International
Joan L Headley, author
4207 Lindell Boulevard
St. Louis, MO 63108-2915
314-534-0475
Fax: 314-534-5070
e-mail: info@post-polio.org
www.post-polio.org

Provides educational materials, advocacy, networking and support research to enhance the lives and independence of polio survivors and users of home mechanical ventilators. Minimum $25.00 with membership.
12 pages
Joan Headley, Executive Director

7001 Ventilator-Assisted Living
Joan L Headley, author
4207 Lindell Boulevard
St. Louis, MO 63108-2915
314-534-0475
Fax: 314-534-5070
e-mail: info@post-polio.org
www.post-polio.org

Provides educational materials, advocacy, networking and support research to enhance the lives and independence of polio survivors and users of home mechanical ventilators. Minimum $25.00 with membership.
12 pages
Joan Headley, Executive Director

7002 **Ventilator: Assisted Living**
Post-Polio Health International
4207 Lindell Boulevard
St. Louis, MO 63108-2915   314-534-0475
                                             Fax: 314-534-5070
                                 e-mail: ventinfo@post-polio.org
                                      www.post-polio.org/IVUN

The newsletter of the International Ventilator Users Network, an affiliate of Post-Polio Health International.
12 pages Newsletter
Joan Headley, Executive Director

Pamphlets

7003 **Guidelines for People Who Have Had Polio**
March of Dimes
PO Box 1657   717-820-8104
Wilkes-Barre, PA 18703   800-367-6630
                                             Fax: 570-825-1987
Located on website as a PDF file. Information based on March of Dimes International Conference on Post-Polio Syndrome.

7004 **Post-Polio Syndrome: Identifying Best Practices in Diagnosis and Care**
March of Dimes
233 Park Avenue South   212-353-8353
New York, NY 10003   Fax: 212-254-3518
                             e-mail: NY639@marchofdimes.com
                                        www.marchofdimes.com
Located on website as PDF file.

Web Sites

7005 **EMedicine**
                              www.emedicine.com/pmr/topic110.htm
EMedicine was launched in 1996 and is the largest and most current clinical knowledge base available to physicians and health professionals.

7006 **International Rehabilitation Center for Polio**
                                             www.polioclinic.org
International Rehabilitation Center for Polio (IRCP) at Spaulding Rehabilitation HOspital website offers information about PPS and resources for polio survivors and others with an interest in post-polio syndrome.

7007 **MedicineNet**
                                            www.medicinenet.com
An online resource for consumers providing easy-to-read, authoritative medical and health information.

7008 **Polio Experience Network**
                                               www.polionet.org
The Polio Experience Network offers information, inspiration, ideas and resources for polio survivors and those seeking information on post-polio syndrome.

7009 **Social Security Administration**
                                          www.ssa.gov/disability
The Social Security Administration website on disability benefits includes information about how to apply for benefits.

Description

7010 Prader-Willi Syndrome

Prader-Willi syndrome, PWS, is a group of abnormalities first described by Drs. Prader, Labart, and Willi in 1956. This uncommon condition occurs in about one in every 20,000 births. In about 50 percent of PWS patients, there is a missing piece (deletion) of part of chromosome 15.

PWS is characterized by obesity, short stature, small penis and testicles (hypogonadism), small hands and feet, mental retardation and decreased muscle tone. During the toddler years, many patients begin to overeat. Some persons with PWS may show signs of obsessive-compulsive disorder, apart from their obsessions with food. In addition to insatiable hunger, other behavioral features include emotional highs and lows, poor motor skills and cognitive impairment. Sexual development is halted, and facial and skeletal abnormalities develop.

Therapies for PWS are aimed at symptoms with an emphasis on specialized diets and customized exercise programs and support.

National Agencies & Associations

7011 National Institute of Child Health and Human Development
9000 Rockville Pike
Bethesda, MD 20892
301-496-5133
Fax: 301-496-7101
www.nih.gov
Offers reprints, articles and various information on Prader-Willi Syndrome in children and adults.
Dr Francis Collin, Director

7012 Prader-Willi Syndrome Association (USA)
Prader-Willi Syndrome Association (USA)
17777 S. W. 285 Street
Homestead, FL 33030
305-245-6484
800-926-4797
Fax: 941-312-0142
e-mail: webmaster1@pwsausa.org
www.pwsausa.org
Provides to parents and professionals a national and international network of information, support services and research endeavors to expressly meet the needs of affected children and adults and their families. Offers 31 state chapters and published materials.
Janalee Heinemann, Executive Director

State Agencies & Associations

Arizona

7013 Prader-Willi Syndrome Arizona Association: Phoenix Area
Prader-Willi Syndrome Association
3920 East Bronco Trail
Phoenix, AZ 85044
602-481-5314
e-mail: shemc@netzero.net
www.pwsausa.org

Sheila McMahon, President

7014 Prader-Willi Syndrome Arizona Association
Prader-Willi Syndrome Association
13839 N Bentwater Drive
Tucson, AZ 85737
602-481-5314
e-mail: p.penta@comcast.net
www.pwsausa.org

Tammie Penta, President

Arkansas

7015 Prader-Willi Arkansas Association Prader-Willi Syndrome Association
Prader-Willi Syndrome Association

107 Jessica Drive
Sherwood, AR 72120-4245
501-920-6768
e-mail: jpattpnlr@msn.com
www.pwsausa.org
Jim Patton, President

California

7016 Prader-Willi California Foundation
514 N Prospect Avenue
Redondo Beach, CA 90277
310-372-5053
800-400-9994
Fax: 310-372-4329
e-mail: PWCF1@aol.com
www.pwsausa.org

Lisa Graziano, Executive Director

Colorado

7017 Prader-Willi Colorado Association
Prader-Willi Syndrome Association
8290 S Yukon Way
Littleton, CO 80128
303-973-4780
e-mail: hosler@dynamicsolutions.com
www.pwsausa.org

Lynette Hosler, President

Connecticut

7018 Prader-Willi Connecticut Association
Prader-Willi Syndrome Association
129 Way Road
Salem, CT 06420-3306
203-239-9902
e-mail: pwsactchapter@yahoo.com
www.pwsausa.org

Vicki Knoph, President

Delaware

7019 Prader-Willi Delaware Association
Prader-Willi Syndrome Association
300 Bethel Circle Millwood
Middletown, DE 19709
302-378-7385
e-mail: swede455@aol.com
www.pwsausa.org

Karen Swanson, President

Florida

7020 Prader-Willi Florida Associaton
Prader-Willi Syndrome Association
17777 S W 285 Street
Homestead, FL 33030
305-245-6484
e-mail: pwfa2000@aol.com
www.pwsausa.org

Debbie Stallings, Co-President
John Stallings, Co-President

Georgia

7021 Prader-Willi Georgia Association
Prader-Willi Syndrome Association
562 Lakeland Plaza
Cumming, GA 30040
770-886-2334
877-866-2334
Fax: 770-886-2335
e-mail: pwsaga@earthlink.net
www.pwsausa.org

Debbie Lang, Executive Director
Greg Talley, President

Hawaii

7022 Prader-Willi Hawaii Association
Prader-Willi Syndrome Association
269 Kaha Street
Hailua, HI 96734
808-263-8177
e-mail: susanlundh@yahoo.com
www.pwsausa.org

Susan Lundh, President

Idaho

7023 Prader-Willi Idaho Association
Prader-Willi Syndrome Association

550 Lodgepole Road
Athol, ID 83801

208-683-2993
e-mail: idaho4ts@aol.com
www.pwsausa.org

Susan Lundh, President
Gene Todhunter, Local Contact

1465 S Grand Boulevard Missouri Str
Louis, MO 63104

314-268-4027
Fax: 314-935-7461
e-mail: national@pwsausa.org
www.pwsausa.org

Barbara Whitman, President

Illinois

7024 Prader-Willi Illinois Association
Prader-Willi Syndrome Association
2128 N Sedgwick Street
Chicago, IL 60614

773-281-9170
e-mail: illinois@pwsausa.org
www.pwsausa.org

Jeffrey Fender, President

Indiana

7025 Prader-Willi Indiana Association
Prader-Willi Syndrome Association
7536 Moonbeam Drive
Indianapolis, IN 46259

317-527-9173
e-mail: pwsain@yahoo.com
www.pwsausa.org

Jacque McGuire, President

Iowa

7026 Prader-Willi Iowa Association
Prader-Willi Syndrome Association
15130 Holcomb Avenue
Clive, IA 50325-9695

515-987-0288
e-mail: ktcaedav@netins.net
www.pwsausa.org

Tammi Davis, President
Edie Bogaczyk, President

Kentucky

7027 Prader-Willi Kentucky Association
Prader-Willi Syndrome Association
9213 Reigate Court
Louisville, KY 40222

502-339-7872
e-mail: national@pwsausa.org
www.pwsausa.org

Frank Beckles, President
Rick Settles

Massachusetts

7028 Prader-Willi New England Association
Prader-Willi Syndrome Association
Andover, MA 01757

978-475-5570
e-mail: pwsane@aol.com
www.pwsausa.org

Eileen Rullo, President

Michigan

7029 Prader-Willi Michigan Association
2155 Ascot Rd
Ann Arbor, MI 48103

734-998-3507
e-mail: chrishendrick@cablespeed.com
www.pwsausa.org

Jon Hendrick, Co-Chairperson
Chris Hendrick, Co-Chairperson

Minnesota

7030 Prader-Willi Minnesota Association
Prader-Willi Syndrome Association
7209 Oaklawn Avenue
Woodbury, MN 55105

952-893-9318
e-mail: national@pwsausa.org
www.pwsausa.org

Jey Behnken, President

Missouri

7031 Prader-Willi Missouri Association
Prader-Willi Syndrome Association

Nebraska

7032 Prader-Willi Nebraska Association
Prader-Willi Syndrome Association
302 S 49th Avenue
Omaha, NE 68132

402-551-9168
e-mail: national@pwsausa.org
www.pwsausa.org

Jennifer Varner, Local Contact

New Jersey

7033 Prader-Willi New Jersey Association
Prader-Willi Syndrome Association
514 Gatewod Road
Cherry Hill, NJ 08003

856-795-4229
e-mail: national@pwsausa.org
www.pwsausa.org

Sybil Cohen, President
Judy Livny, Vice-President

New York

7034 Prader-Willi New York Association
Prader-Willi Syndrome Association
PO Box 1114
Niagara Falls, NY 14304

716-276-2211
800-442-1655
e-mail: alliance@prader-willi.org
www.prader-willi.org

Nina Roberto, Executive Director
Amy McDougall, President

North Carolina

7035 Prader-Willi North Carolina Association
Prader-Willi Syndrome Association
1404 Sutton Drive
Kinston, NC 28501

252-527-1813
e-mail: national@pwsausa.org
www.pwsausa.org

Becky Smith, President

North Dakota

7036 Prader-Willi North Dakota Association
Prader-Willi Syndrome Association
2902 S University Drive
Fargo, ND 58103-6032

701-232-3301
Fax: 701-237-5775
e-mail: fraser@fraserltd.org
www.fraserltd.org

Sandra leyland, Executive Director
Michael Kirk, Vice President

Ohio

7037 Prader-Willi Ohio Association
Prader-Willi Syndrome Association
4075 W 226 Street
Fairview Park, OH 44126

440-716-0552
e-mail: pwsaohio@aol.com
www.pwsausa.org

Jennifer Bolander, President

Oklahoma

7038 Prader-Willi Oklahoma Association
Prader-Willi Syndrome Association
3816 SE 89th Street
Oklahoma City, OK 74135-6222

405-677-8089
e-mail: national@pwsausa.org
www.pwsausa.org

Daphne Mosley, President

Oregon

7039 Prader-Willi Oregon Association
Prader-Willi Syndrome Association

303 E Historic Columbia
Troutdale, OR 97060   503-669-7191
e-mail: national@pwsausa.org
www.pwsausa.org

Lennae Elkington, President

Pennsylvania

7040 Prader-Willi Pennsylvania Association
Prader-Willi Syndrome Association
104 Persimmon Place   724-779-4415
Cranberry Township, PA 16066   e-mail: national@pwsausa.org
www.pwsausa.org

Debbie Fabio, President

South Carolina

7041 Prader-Willi South Carolina Association
Prader-Willi Syndrome Association
912 Lake Spur Lane   803-345-1379
Chapin, SC 29036   e-mail: national@pwsausa.org
www.pwsausa.org

Rhett Eleazer, Local Contact

Tennessee

7042 Prader-Willi Tennessee Association
Prader-Willi Syndrome Association
1200 Villa Place   615-790-6659
Nashville, TN 37212   e-mail: national@pwsausa.org
www.pwsausa.org

Misti Love, President

Texas

7043 Prader-Willi Texas Association
Prader-Willi Syndrome Association
14427 Perchin Drive   210-946-6789
San Antonio, TX 78247   e-mail: national@pwsausa.org
www.pwsausa.org

Amber Robenson, President

Utah

7044 Prader-Willi Utah Association
Prader-Willi Syndrome Association
2652 Nottingham Way   801-582-0998
Salt Lake City, UT 84108   Fax: 801-768-3924
e-mail: national@pwsausa.org
www.pwsausa.org

Lisa Thornton, President

Washington

7045 Prader-Willi Washington Association
Prader-Willi Syndrome Association
16208 SE 46th Place   206-285-7679
Bellevue, WA 98006   e-mail: jlubderwood@juno.com
www.pwsausa.org

Joanne Underwood, Co-President
Susan Lundh, Co-President

Wisconsin

7046 Prader-Willi Wisconsin Association
Prader-Willi Syndrome Association
2701 N Alexander Street   920-882-6371
Appleton, WI 54911-2512   866-797-2947
e-mail: wisconsion@pwsausa.org
www.pwsausa.org

Mary Lynn Larson, Program Director
Mike Larson, President

Support Groups & Hotlines

7047 National Health Information Center
PO Box 1133   310-565-4167
Washington, DC 20013   800-336-4797
Fax: 301-984-4256
e-mail: info@nhic.org
www.health.gov/nhic
Offers a nationwide information referral service, produces directories and resource guides.

7048 PraderWilli Syndrome Association
PraderWilli Syndrome Association
5700 Midnight Pass Road   941-312-0400
Sarasota, FL 34242   800-926-4797
Fax: 941-312-0142
e-mail: pwsuasa@aol.com
www.pwsausa.org

John Heybatch, Co-Chair
Julie Doherty, Secretary

Books

7049 Child with Prader-Willi Syndrome: Birth to Three
Prader-Willi Syndrome Association (USA)
8588 Potter Park Drive   941-312-0400
Sarasota, FL 34238   800-926-4797
Fax: 941-312-0142
e-mail: info@pwsausa.com
www.pwsausa.org
Discusses the common concerns of the first three years and offers specific recommendations for early intervention strategies. A helpful and positive resource for families, physicians, early intervention workers and other care providers. Booklet
2004 34 pages
Craig Pulhemus, Executive Director

7050 Early Years
Prader-Willi Syndrome Association (USA)
8588 Potter Park Drive   941-312-0400
Sarasota, FL 34238   800-926-4797
Fax: 941-312-0142
e-mail: info@pwsausa.org
www.pwsausa.org
Collection of articles regarding young children with PWS — many from a parent's perspective.
1998 37 pages
Craig Polhemus, Executive Director

7051 Growing Up with Prader-Willi Syndrome: Personal Reflections of a Mother
Prader-Willi Syndrome Association (USA)
8588 Potter Park Drive   941-312-0400
Sarasota, FL 34238   800-926-4797
Fax: 941-312-0142
e-mail: info@pwsausa.com
www.pwsausa.org
Collection of 15 articles. Tips for managing family life on a practical level. Booklet
2003 37 pages
Craig Polhemus, Executive Director

7052 Growth Hormone & Prader-Willi Syndrome: A Reference for Familes & Care Providers
Linda S. Keder, author
Prader-Willi Syndrome Association (USA)
8588 Potter Park Drive   941-312-0400
Sarasota, FL 34238   800-926-4797
Fax: 941-312-0142
e-mail: info@pwsausa.com
www.pwsausa.org
Reference for families and care providers.
2001 52 pages
Craig Polhemus, Executive Director

525

7053 Handbook for Parents
Shirley Neason, author

Prader-Willi Syndrome Association (USA)
8588 Potter Park Drive   941-312-0400
Sarasota, FL 34238   800-926-4797
                                  Fax: 941-312-0142
                          e-mail: info@pwsausa.com
                                    www.pwsausa.org
Parent-to-Parent handbook for understanding and managing issues related to PWS, from birth to adulthood.
1999 75 pages
Craig Polhemus, Executive Director

7054 Nutrition Care for Children with PWS: Infants and Toddlers
J. Hovasi & D. Doorlag, with J. Loker & C. Loker, author

Prader-Willi Syndrome Association (USA)
8588 Potter Park Drive   941-312-0400
Sarasota, FL 34238   800-926-4797
                                  Fax: 941-312-0142
                          e-mail: info@pwsausa.com
                                    www.pwsausa.org
Provides answers to frequently asked questions about nutrition and feeding infants and toddlers with PWS.
2004 62 pages
Craig Polhemus, Executive Director

7055 Sometimes I'm Mad, Sometimes I'm Glad - A Sibling Booklet
Sarah Heinemann, author

Prader-Willi Syndrome Association (USA)
8588 Potter Park Drive   941-312-0400
Sarasota, FL 34238   800-926-4797
                                  Fax: 941-312-0142
                          e-mail: info@pwsausa.com
                                    www.pwsausa.org
Explains sibling relationships and how they are affected by Prader-Willi syndrome. Written in the voice of a sibling of someone with PWS. Ages 5-13
32 pages
Craig Polhemus, Executive Director

7056 Supporting Adults with Prader-Willi Syndro me in a Residential Setting
B.J. Goff, Ed.D, author

Prader-Willi Syndrome Association (USA)
8588 Potter Pass Drive   941-312-0400
Sarasota, FL 34238   800-926-4797
                                  Fax: 941-312-0142
                          e-mail: info@pwsausa.com
                                    www.pwsausa.org
Filling a large gap for care givers of those with Prader-Willi Sydrome, this is an extensive manual covering residential care issues; including management strategies, specifics for phase of life, and a number of additional ideas.
2002 121 pages
Craig Polhemus, Executive Director

Newsletters

7057 Gathered View
Prader-Willi Syndrome Association (USA)
8588 Potter Park Drive   941-312-0400
Sarasota, FL 34238   800-926-4797
                                  Fax: 941-312-0142
                          e-mail: info@pwsausa.com
                                    www.pwsausa.org
The official newsletter of PWSA, mailed 6 time/year to members. Offers current research findings, behavior and weight management techniques, educational news, articles and more.
BiMonthly
Craig Polhemus, Executive Director

Pamphlets

7058 An Early Prader-Willi Syndrome Diagnosis & How to Make it Easier on Parents
Prader-Willi Foundation
40 Holly Lane   516-944-8136
Roslyn Hts, NY 11577-1533   800-253-7993
                                  Fax: 516-944-3173
              e-mail: foundation@prader-willi.inter.net
                                   www.prader-willi.org
A parent of a child with PWS and an advocate for others with the afflication speaks.

7059 Behavior Management: Collection of Articless
Prader-Willi Syndrome Association (USA)
8588 Potter Park Drive   941-312-0400
Sarasota, FL 34238   800-926-4797
                                  Fax: 941-312-0142
                          e-mail: info@pwsausa.com
                                    www.pwsausa.org
Includes general articles of behavior concerns, use of psychotropic medications, skin picking and teaching social skills.
2003 49 pages
Craig Polhemus, Executive Director

7060 Educational Choices for Children with PWS
Prader-Willi Foundation
40 Holly Lane   516-944-8136
Roslyn Hts, NY 11577-1533   800-253-7993
                                  Fax: 516-944-3173
              e-mail: foundation@prader-willi.inter.net
                                   www.prader-willi.org
Parents of young children with Prader-Willi syndrome discuss their individual philosophies of educational choice - inclusion vs. specialized setting.

7061 Nutrition Care for Adolescents and Adults with PWS
Karenn H. Borgie, MA, RD, author

Prader-Willi Syndrome Association (USA)
8588 Potter Park Drive   941-312-0400
Sarasota, FL 34238   800-926-4797
                                  Fax: 941-312-0142
                          e-mail: info@pwsausa.com
                                    www.pwsausa.org
covers essential diet information for families, caregivers, and residential service providers.
Craig Polhemus, Executive Director

7062 Nutrition Care for Children with PWS, Ages 3-9
Karen H. Borgie, MA, RD, author

Prader-Willi Syndrome Association (USA)
8588 Potter Park Drive   941-312-0400
Sarasota, FL 34238   800-926-4797
                                  Fax: 941-312-0142
                          e-mail: info@pwsausa.com
                                    www.pwsausa.org
Discusses calorie needs, supplements, diet planning, food management, and exchange lists. Softvcover.
Craig Polhemus, Executive Director

7063 What Educators Should Know About Prader-Willi Syndrome
Prader-Willi Syndrome Association (USA)
8588 Potter Park Drive   941-312-0400
Sarasota, FL 34238   800-926-4797
                                  Fax: 941-312-0142
                          e-mail: info@pwsausa.com
                                    www.pwsausa.org
Offers guidelines and strategies for helping the student with PWS stay focused, develop skills and knowledge, and minimize problems associated with the syndrome in the school setting.
Craig Polhemus, Executive Director

Audio & Video

7064 Prader-Willi Syndrome: An Overview for Health Professionals
Prader-Willi Syndrome Association

5700 Midnight Pass Road 941-312-0400
Sarasota, FL 34242-3000 800-926-4797
Fax: 941-312-0142
e-mail: national@pwsausa.org
www.pwsausa.org

Essential viewing for all health care professionals who are not experts on prader-willi syndrome. It deals with all major genetics and health care issues of the child with PWS.
2002

7065 Prader-Willi Syndrome: the Early Years
Prader-Willi Syndrome Association
5700 Midnight Pass Road 941-312-0400
Sarasota, FL 34242-3000 800-926-4797
Fax: 941-312-0142
e-mail: national@pwsausa.org
www.pwsausa.org

Offers help and practical suggestions for those families with a young child newly diagnosed with PWS. Genetics, medical, early intervention and family issues are presented, personalized with family interviews. Although focusing on young children, this video is a wonderful resource for schools and families with children of all ages.
2002

Web Sites

7066 Healthlink USA
www.healthlinkusa.com

Health information concerning treatment, cures, prevention, diagnosis, risk factors, research, support groups, email lists, personal stories and much more. Updated regularly.

7067 MedicineNet
www.medicinenet.com

An online resource for consumers providing easy-to-read, authoritative medical and health information.

7068 Medscape
www.medscape.com

Medscape offers specialists, primary care physicians, and other health professionals the Web's most robust and integrated medical information and educational tools.

Description

7069 Raynaud's Disease

Raynaud's disease is the spasm of blood vessels to fingers and toes, resulting in restricted blood supply in response to cold or emotional upset. Symptoms include tingling and numbness. During an episode, which can last from minutes to hours, the arteries contract briefly and the skin, deprived of oxygen, turns pale and then blue. As arteries relax and blood begins to flow, reddening, tingling, or swelling may occur. While hands and feet are most commonly affected, the nose and ears can also be subject to Raynaud's.

Raynaud's most commonly affects women under 40, accounting for perhaps 90 percent of all cases. When the classic symptoms are present, without other complaints, the condition is referred to as Raynaud's disease (primary Raynaud's), and generally results in no serious consequences. The second form, Raynaud's phenomenon (secondary Raynaud's), is the result of other underlying medical conditions, including scleroderma, vascular disease, rheumatoid arthritis and lupus.

Certain drugs can also trigger Raynaud's, including ergotamine and a number of beta-blocking drugs that are used in the treatment of heart disease. About 10 percent of Raynaud's cases are related to specific repetitive stress activities such as the operation of pneumatic drills and other hand-held vibrating machinery. In most Raynaud's cases, symptoms are discomforting but not serious. In extreme cases, Raynaud's can result in tissue atrophy and gangrene. Preventative measures include protection from cold, even when taking food out of the refrigerator or freezer, and avoiding behavior that disrupts bloodflow, for instance, smoking cigarettes.

Medical treatment of Raynaud's is directed toward improving blood flow to the extremities. In many cases, simple exercises are prescribed, and relaxation techniques, such as biofeedback, teach the body to ignore trivial or transient signals of cold. In other cases, vasodilator drugs which are designed to relax and open blood vessels to improve blood flow are prescribed. In the most extreme cases, surgery may be performed to cut nerves that may be inappropriately triggering the contraction of arteries, although relief may last only 1 to 2 years. Herbal remedies have been used in the treatment of Raynaud's and other circulatory conditions, especially the Chinese herb Dong quai. There is also evidence that foods rich in vitamin E, and fish oils, may help to reduce or moderate the vascular spasms that produce Raynaud's symptoms.

National Agencies & Associations

7070 Arthritis Foundation
1330 W Peachtree Street
Atlanta, GA 30309

404-872-7100
800-283-7800
Fax: 404-872-0457
e-mail: help@arthritis.org
www.arthritis.org

A nonprofit organization that depends on volunteers to provide services to help people with arthritis. Supports research to find ways to cure and prevent arthritis and provides services to improve the quality of life for those affected by arthritis.
Daniel T Mcgowen, Chair
Rowland W chang, Vice Chair

7071 Raynaud's Foundation
11 Topstone Road
Redding, CT 06896-6176

773-622-9220
Fax: 773-622-9221
www.raynauds.org

The Raynaud's Foundation is a non-profit dedicated to the promotion of education and research Raynaud's Phenomenon and related diseases, both autoimmune and non-autoimmune.
Ida Therese Jablanovec, Executive Director

7072 United Scleroderma Foundation
300 Rosewood Drive
Danvers, MA 01923-0350

978-463-5843
800-722-4673
Fax: 978-463-5809
www.scleroderma.org

Offers materials and referrals conducts workshops and support groups for those with Raynaud's and their families.
Mary Ann Berman, Office Assistant
Liz Dorsett, Communications Manager

Libraries & Resource Centers

7073 Arizona Telemedicine Program
University of Arizona, Health Science Center
PO Box 245105
Tucson, AZ 85724-5105

520-626-2493
Fax: 520-626-4774
e-mail: kerps@email.arizona.edu
www.telemedicine.arizona.edu/index.html

The Arizona Telemedicine Program is a large, multidisciplinary, university-based program that provides telemedicine services, distance learning, informatics training, and telemedicine technology assessment capabilities to communities throughout Arizona, the sixth largest state in the United States, in square miles.
Ronald S Weinstein, MD, Director
Ana Maria Lopez, Medical Director

Support Groups & Hotlines

7074 National Health Information Center
PO Box 1133
Washington, DC 20013

310-565-4167
800-336-4797
Fax: 301-984-4256
e-mail: info@nhic.org
www.health.gov/nhic

Offers a nationwide information referral service, produces directories and resource guides.

Books

7075 Raynaud's Phenomenon
Oxford University Press
This is a detailed and technical work on the physiology finger circulation, and on diagnosis and treatment of Raynaud's Phenomenon and Raynaud's Disease. Includes a chapter on Acrocyanosis and Livedo reticularis.
186 pages
ISBN: 0-195057-56-2

Pamphlets

7076 Raynaud's Phenomenon
Arthritis Foundation
PO Box 7669
Atlanta, GA 30357-0669

404-872-7100
800-283-7800
Fax: 404-872-0457

Web Sites

7077   Health Finder

www.healthfinder.gov

Searchable, carefully developed web site offering information on over 1000 topics. Developed by the US Department of Health and Human Services, the site can be used in both English and Spanish.

7078   MedicineNet

www.medicinenet.com

An online resource for consumers providing easy-to-read, authoritative medical and health information.

7079   United Scleroderma Foundation

www.scleroderma.org

Offers materials and referrals, conducts workshops and support groups for those with Raynaud's and their families.

Description

7080 Sarcoidosis

Sarcoidosis is a chronic disease that can affect almost any part of the body. It is characterized by the deposit of small masses of tissue (granulomas) in multiple organs. The cause is unknown, although it is speculated to be related to an immunologic defect or infection. Incidence varies widely between countries. In the United States, sarcoidosis is 10- to 18-fold higher in African Americans than in whites. Most cases start between the ages of 30 and 50 years.

Clinical features vary considerably, depending on the site and extent of involvement. Systemic symptoms may include fatigue, weight loss, loss of appetite and fever. Local symptoms may involve any organ, but the most commonly affected are the lungs, skin, eyes and lymph nodes. If the disease becomes severe and life-threatening, it is usually because of lung involvement. Patients develop cough, wheeze, chest pain and difficulty breathing.

Both the severity and the long-term outlook are extremely variable. In most patients, the disease regresses within 2 years and does not recur. In approximately 25 percent of patients, the disease progresses and causes serious disability. If progressive symptoms require treatment, corticosteroids are usually given. If these are not effective or tolerated, immuno suppressive drugs such as methotrexate or azathioprine may be tried. Approximately 5 percent of patients die of respiratory failure.

National Agencies & Associations

7081 National Sarcoidosis Family Aid and Research Foundation
1400 Parkmoor Avenue   www.php.com
San Jose, CA 95126
Provides information on a rare disease involving inflammation in lymph nodes and other body tissues, usually in young adults.
Suzanne Cistulli, Board Chair
Joyce Uggla, Board Secretary

7082 National Sarcoidosis Resource Center
PO Box 1593   732-463-0497
Piscataway, NJ 08855-1593   Fax: 732-463-0467
                                        www.nsrc-global.net
The center provides a national computer database with statistical information and studies, telephone support for patients, subscriptions to national magazines and newsletters and public information provided by mail.
Sandra Conroy, President

Research Centers

7083 Sarcoidosis Center
6005 Park Avenue   901-761-5877
Memphis, TN 38119   866-727-2643
                                        Fax: 901-761-2280
                            e-mail: sarcoid@sarcoidcenter.com
                                        www.sarcoidcenter.com
A nonprofit tax exempt organization dedicated to increasing knowledge of the disease sarcoidosis. This broad goal encompasses three main areas: Disseminating information to professionals who assist with treatment of the disease obtaining and dispersing funds to assist with investigation into the cause and

treatment of the disease and providing support for individuals afflicted with the disease.

7084 Sarcoidosis Treatment and Research Center Thomas Jefferson University Hospital
Thomas Jefferson University Hospital
111 S 11th Street   215-955-6840
Philadelphia, PA 19107-5092   Fax: 215-923-5828
                                        www.jeffersonhospital.org
Stephen K klasko, President/CEO
Sergio Jimen MD, Professor

Support Groups & Hotlines

7085 Better Breather's Clubs
American Lung Association of Virginia
1301 Pennsylvania Ave.   202-785-3355
Richmond, Dc 20004   Fax: 202-452-1805
                                e-mail: chamm@lungva.org
                                        www.lungusa.org
Support Groups for those suffering from chronic obstructive pulmonary disease (COPD) such as emphysema, chronic bronchitis and asthma. In these meetings members give and receive support, and learn more about chronic lung disease from health care professionals who share trends in therapy, medication and other topics, or simply answer members' questions.
Catherine G Hamm, President/Chief Excutive Officer
Michelle LaRose, Development Director

7086 Let's Breathe Sarcoidosis Support Group
2225 Foster Street   708-328-9410
Evanston, IL 60201-3353   e-mail: bharris354@aol.com
Brenda Harris, Facilitator

7087 Middle Tennessee Sarcoidosis Support Group
PO Box 1342
Cookesville, TN 38503   931-528-7826
                    www.tennesseesarcoidosisawareness.org
Becky Robertson, Group Leader

7088 Mount Sinai Sarcoidosis Support Group
One Gustave L. Levy Place   212-241-6500
New York, NY 10029   86- 67- 372
                                        www.mountsinai.org

7089 National Health Information Center
PO Box 1133   310-565-4167
Washington, DC 20013   800-336-4797
                                   Fax: 301-984-4256
                                e-mail: info@nhic.org
                                        www.health.gov/nhic
Offers a nationwide information referral service, produces directories and resource guides.

7090 Pacific NW Support Group
Providence Hospital
PO Box 58785   42- 2-5 14
Renton, WA 98058   877- 25- 067
                                    Fax: 42- 2-4 20
                        e-mail: washington@myasthenia.org
                                        www.myasthenia.org
Ed Girvan, Facilitator

7091 Sarcoidosis HelpNet
PO Box 022642   732-463-0497
Brooklyn, NY 11202   Fax: 732-463-0467
                                        www.nsrc-gllobal.net
Soneni B Smith, Contact

7092 Sarcoidosis Research Institute (SRI)
3475 Central Avenue   901-766-6951
Memphis, TN 38111   Fax: 901-774-7294
                            e-mail: sarcoid@sarcoidcenter.com
                                www.sarcoidcenter.com/saradd.htm
The Sarcoidosis Research Institute is a non-profit, tax-exempt organization dedicated to increasing knowledge of the disease sarcoidosis. This broad goal encompasses three main areas: Disseminating information to professionals who assist with treatment of the disease; Obtaining and dispersing funds to assist with inves-

tigation into the cause and treatment of the disease; and, providing support for individuals afflicted with the disease.
Paula Yette Polite, Board of Directors President
Wayne Crook, Vice President Board of Directors

7093 **Sarcoidosis Self-Help Group: New York**
Nassau County Medical Center
2201 Hempstead Turnpike   516-483-2666
East Meadow, NY 11554
Robert Schoenfeld, Facilitator

7094 **Sarcoidosis Self-Help Group: Virginia**
American Lung Association of Northern Virginia
9735 Main Street   703-591-4131
Fairfax, VA 22031
Carolyn Thomas, Facilitator

7095 **Sarcoidosis Support Group Delaware**
American Lung Association of Delaware
1021 Gilpin Avenue   302-655-7258
Wilmington, DE 19806   800-548-8252
                                          Fax: 302-655-8546
                                     e-mail: dbrown@alade.org
                                               www.alade.org

Peter Shanley, Chairman
Harold P. Wimmer, President/CEO

7096 **Sarcoidosis Support Group: New Jersey**
268 Dr. ML King Boulevard   201-374-7570
Newark, NJ 07106
Jean Curlin-Miller, Facilitator

7097 **Sarcoidosis Support Group: Washington DC**
110 Irving Street   202-877-6286
Washington, DC 20010   Fax: 202-877-5779

7098 **Triangle Area Sarcoidosis Support Group**
Soapstone UM Church
12837 Norwood Road   919-676-6498
Raleigh, NC 27613   e-mail: fairleyl@bellsouth.net
Priscilla Fairley, Facilitator

7099 **Understanding Sarcoidosis Self-Help Group**
2112 Highland Avenue   412-652-6089
New Castle, PA 16105

7100 **University of North Carolina Sarcoidosis Support Group**
UNC Chapel Hill Healthcare
130 Mason Farm Road   919-966-2531
Chapel Hill, NC 27599   e-mail: sharikia_burt@med.unc.edu
Sharikia Burt, Clinical Coordinator

7101 **West Tennessee Sarcoidosis Support Group**
1670 McLemoresville Road
Huntington, TN 38344   731-986-9832
                            www.tennesseesarcoidosisawareness.org
Patricia Coleman, Group Leader

Books

7102 **Sarcoidosis Resource Guide and Directory**
PC Publications
PO Box 1593   732-699-0733
Piscataway, NJ 08855-1593   Fax: 732-699-0882
1993 304 pages Paperback
ISBN: 0-963122-25-8

Newsletters

7103 **Online Sarcoidosis Newsletter**
National Sarcoidosis Resource Center
PO Box 1593   732-699-0733
Piscataway, NJ 08855-1593   Fax: 732-699-0882
Offers information on the center's activities and events, medical and legislative updates for the patients and their families.
Quarterly

Pamphlets

7104 **Anemia of Sarcoidosis**
PC Publications
PO Box 1593   732-699-0733
Piscataway, NJ 08855-1593   800-223-6429
                                          Fax: 732-699-0882

7105 **Bronchoalveolar Lymphocytes in Sarcoidosis**
PC Publications
PO Box 1593   732-699-0733
Piscataway, NJ 08855-1593   800-223-6429
                                          Fax: 732-699-0882

7106 **Case Report: MR Imaging of Myocardial Sarcoidosis**
PC Publications
PO Box 1593   732-699-0733
Piscataway, NJ 08855-1593   800-223-6429
                                          Fax: 732-699-0882

7107 **Case Report: Osseous Sarcoidosis and Chronic Polyarthritis**
PC Publications
PO Box 1593   732-699-0733
Piscataway, NJ 08855-1593   800-223-6429
                                          Fax: 732-699-0882

7108 **Case Report: Overlap of Granulomatous Vasculitis and Sarcoidosis**
PC Publications
PO Box 1593   732-699-0733
Piscataway, NJ 08855-1593   800-223-6429
                                          Fax: 732-699-0882

7109 **Case Report: Rapidly Dev. Confusion, Impaired Memory and Unsteady Gait**
PC Publications
PO Box 1593   732-699-0733
Piscataway, NJ 08855-1593   800-223-6429
                                          Fax: 732-699-0882

7110 **Coping with Sarcoidosis**
National Sarcoidosis Resource Center
PO Box 1593   732-699-0733
Piscataway, NJ 08855-1593   800-223-6429
                                          Fax: 732-699-0882
A pamphlet offering information on how to manage and live with sarcoidosis.

7111 **Disability Law: A Legal Primer**
PC Publications
PO Box 1593   732-699-0733
Piscataway, NJ 08855-1593   800-223-6429
                                          Fax: 732-699-0882

7112 **Drugs That Have Been Used for the Treatment of Sarcoidosis**
PC Publications
PO Box 1593   732-699-0733
Piscataway, NJ 08855-1593   800-223-6429
                                          Fax: 732-699-0882

7113 **Effect of Corticosteroid or Methotrexate Therapy on Lung Lymphocytes**
PC Publications
PO Box 1593   732-699-0733
Piscataway, NJ 08855-1593   800-223-6429
                                          Fax: 732-699-0882

7114 **Effects of Sarcoid and Steroids on Angiotensin-Converting Enzyme**
PC Publications
PO Box 1593   732-699-0733
Piscataway, NJ 08855-1593   800-223-6429
                                          Fax: 732-699-0882

7115 **Evaluation of the Efficacy and Toxicity of the Cyclosporine**
PC Publications
PO Box 1593   732-699-0733
Piscataway, NJ 08855-1593   800-223-6429
                                          Fax: 732-699-0882

7116 **Gastrointestinal Presentation of Churg Strauss Syndrome**
PC Publications

PO Box 1593
Piscataway, NJ 08855-1593

732-699-0733
800-223-6429
Fax: 732-699-0882

7117 Governor New Jersey Proclamation: Sarcoidosis Awareness Day
PC Publications
PO Box 1593
Piscataway, NJ 08855-1593

732-699-0733
800-223-6429
Fax: 732-699-0882

7118 How to Get the Most Out of Your Doctor: A Neurologist's Perspective
PC Publications
PO Box 1593
Piscataway, NJ 08855-1593

732-699-0733
800-223-6429
Fax: 732-699-0882

7119 Ideas and Considerations for Starting a Self-Help Mutual Aid Group
PC Publications
PO Box 1593
Piscataway, NJ 08855-1593

732-699-0733
800-223-6429
Fax: 732-699-0882

7120 Masqueraders of Sarcoidosis
PC Publications
PO Box 1593
Piscataway, NJ 08855-1593

732-699-0733
800-223-6429
Fax: 732-699-0882

7121 Mayor Piscataway, NJ Proclamation: Sarcoidosis Awareness Day
PC Publications
PO Box 1593
Piscataway, NJ 08855-1593

732-699-0733
800-223-6429
Fax: 732-699-0882

7122 Multidisciplinary Clinico-Pathologic Conference
PC Publications
PO Box 1593
Piscataway, NJ 08855-1593

732-699-0733
800-223-6429
Fax: 732-699-0882

7123 National Sarcoidosis Resource Center
PC Publications
PO Box 1593
Piscataway, NJ 08855-1593

732-699-0733
Fax: 732-699-0882
www.nsrc-global.net

A booklet offering a brief introduction to the illness and offers information on the role of the Center in finding a cure and educating the public on Sarcoidosis.

7124 Neurosarcoidosis
PC Publications
PO Box 1593
Piscataway, NJ 08855-1593

732-699-0733
800-223-6429
Fax: 732-699-0882

7125 Neurosarcoidosis or Multiple Sclerosis?
National Sarcoidosis Resource Center
PO Box 1593
Piscataway, NJ 08855-1593

732-699-0733
800-223-6429
Fax: 732-699-0882

7126 Paranoid Psychosis Due to Neurosarcoidosis
PC Publications
PO Box 1593
Piscataway, NJ 08855-1593

732-699-0733
800-223-6429
Fax: 732-699-0882

7127 Patient Information Package
National Sarcoidosis Resource Center
PO Box 1593
Piscataway, NJ 08855-1593

732-699-0733
800-223-6429
Fax: 732-699-0882

Contains various brochures and pamphlets offering information about Sarcoidosis.

7128 Physician Listings
PC Publications
PO Box 1593
Piscataway, NJ 08855-1593

732-699-0733
800-223-6429
Fax: 732-699-0882

7129 Possible Association of Rheumatoid Arthritis & Sarcoidosis
PC Publications
PO Box 1593
Piscataway, NJ 08855-1593

732-699-0733
800-223-6429
Fax: 732-699-0882

7130 Presidential Proclamation - National Sarcoidosis Awareness Day
PC Publications
PO Box 1593
Piscataway, NJ 08855-1593

732-699-0733
800-223-6429
Fax: 732-699-0882

7131 Psychological Factors in Sarcoidosis
PC Publications
PO Box 1593
Piscataway, NJ 08855-1593

732-699-0733
800-223-6429
Fax: 732-699-0882

7132 Public Law 102-94
PC Publications
PO Box 1593
Piscataway, NJ 08855-1593

732-699-0733
800-223-6429
Fax: 732-699-0882

7133 Pulmonary Sarcoidosis: Evaluation with High Resolution
PC Publications
PO Box 1593
Piscataway, NJ 08855-1593

732-699-0733
800-223-6429
Fax: 732-699-0882

7134 Pulmonary Sarcoidosis: What We Are Learning
PC Publications
PO Box 1593
Piscataway, NJ 08855-1593

732-699-0733
800-223-6429
Fax: 732-699-0882

7135 Questionnaire Responses for Demographics and Symptoms from 1000 Patients
PC Publications
PO Box 1593
Piscataway, NJ 08855-1593

732-699-0733
800-223-6429
Fax: 732-699-0882

7136 Right & Left Ventricular Function at Rest in Patients with Sarcoidosis
PC Publications
PO Box 1593
Piscataway, NJ 08855-1593

732-699-0733
800-223-6429
Fax: 732-699-0882

7137 Role of Magnetic Resonance Imaging in Neurosarcoidosis
PC Publications
PO Box 1593
Piscataway, NJ 08855-1593

732-699-0733
800-223-6429
Fax: 732-699-0882

7138 Sarcoidosis
PC Publications
PO Box 1593
Piscataway, NJ 08855-1593

732-699-0733
800-223-6429
Fax: 732-699-0882

Offers information on the illness, causes, symptoms and treatments.

7139 Sarcoidosis Diagnosed in a Patient with Known HIV Infection
PC Publications
PO Box 1593
Piscataway, NJ 08855-1593

732-699-0733
800-223-6429
Fax: 732-699-0882

7140 Sarcoidosis Patient Questionnaire
PC Publications
PO Box 1593
Piscataway, NJ 08855-1593

732-699-0733
800-223-6429
Fax: 732-699-0882

7141 Sarcoidosis Questionnaire: Demographics and Symptomatology-The Patients Respond
PC Publications
PO Box 1593
Piscataway, NJ 08855-1593

732-699-0733
800-223-6429
Fax: 732-699-0882

7142 **Sarcoidosis and Pregnancy: Clinical Observation**
PC Publications
PO Box 1593   732-699-0733
Piscataway, NJ 08855-1593   800-223-6429
                                      Fax: 732-699-0882

7143 **Sarcoidosis and You: A Listing of Possible Symptoms**
PC Publications
PO Box 1593   732-699-0733
Piscataway, NJ 08855-1593   800-223-6429
                                      Fax: 732-699-0882

7144 **Sarcoidosis in India: A Review of 125 Biopsy-Proven Cases from India**
PC Publications
PO Box 1593   732-699-0733
Piscataway, NJ 08855-1593   800-223-6429
                                      Fax: 732-699-0882

7145 **Sarcoidosis of the Liver**
PC Publications
PO Box 1593   732-699-0733
Piscataway, NJ 08855-1593   800-223-6429
                                      Fax: 732-699-0882

7146 **Sarcoidosis: A Multisystem Disease**
PC Publications
PO Box 1593   732-699-0733
Piscataway, NJ 08855-1593   800-223-6429
                                      Fax: 732-699-0882
Explains the effects of the illness on the lungs and joints.

7147 **Sarcoidosis: International Review**
PC Publications
PO Box 1593   732-699-0733
Piscataway, NJ 08855-1593   800-223-6429
                                      Fax: 732-699-0882

7148 **Sarcoidosis: Pleural Involvement Mimicking a Coin Lesson**
PC Publications
PO Box 1593   732-699-0733
Piscataway, NJ 08855-1593   800-223-6429
                                      Fax: 732-699-0882

7149 **Sarcoidosis: Usual and Unusual Manifestations**
PC Publications
PO Box 1593   732-699-0733
Piscataway, NJ 08855-1593   800-223-6429
                                      Fax: 732-699-0882

7150 **Seasonal Clustering of Sarcoidosis**
National Sarcoidosis Resource Center
PO Box 1593   732-699-0733
Piscataway, NJ 08855-1593   800-223-6429
                                      Fax: 732-699-0882

7151 **Successful Treatment of Myocardial Sarcoidosis with Steriods**
PC Publications
PO Box 1593   732-699-0733
Piscataway, NJ 08855-1593   800-223-6429
                                      Fax: 732-699-0882

7152 **Support Group Listing**
PC Publications
PO Box 1593   732-699-0733
Piscataway, NJ 08855-1593   800-223-6429
                                      Fax: 732-699-0882

7153 **Use of Low Dose Methotrexate in Refractory Sarcoidosis**
PC Publications
PO Box 1593   732-699-0733
Piscataway, NJ 08855-1593   800-223-6429
                                      Fax: 732-699-0882

7154 **World Association Sarcoidosi Other Granulatomous**
PC Publications
PO Box 1593   732-699-0733
Piscataway, NJ 08855-1593   800-223-6429
                                      Fax: 732-699-0882

Audio & Video

7155 **Dialogue with Doris**
PC Publications
PO Box 1593   732-699-0733
Piscataway, NJ 08855-1593   800-223-6429
                                      Fax: 732-699-0882

7156 **Help with a Hidden Disease Update**
PC Publications
PO Box 1593   732-699-0733
Piscataway, NJ 08855-1593   800-223-6429
                                      Fax: 732-699-0882

7157 **Of Their Own: Person to Person Show**
PC Publications
PO Box 1593   732-699-0733
Piscataway, NJ 08855-1593   800-223-6429
                                      Fax: 732-699-0882

7158 **Sarcoidosis Conference 2**
PC Publications
PO Box 1593   732-699-0733
Piscataway, NJ 08855-1593   800-223-6429
                                      Fax: 732-699-0882

7159 **Sarcoidosis Conference 3**
PC Publications
PO Box 1593   732-699-0733
Piscataway, NJ 08855-1593   800-223-6429
                                      Fax: 732-699-0882

7160 **Sarcoidosis and Lyme Disease**
PC Publications
PO Box 1593   732-699-0733
Piscataway, NJ 08855-1593   800-223-6429
                                      Fax: 732-699-0882

7161 **Sarcoidosis: What's That?**
PC Publications
PO Box 1593   732-699-0733
Piscataway, NJ 08855-1593   800-223-6429
                                      Fax: 732-699-0882

7162 **XIV International World Conference on Sarcoidosis: Patient Symposium**
PC Publications
PO Box 1593   732-699-0733
Piscataway, NJ 08855-1593   800-223-6429
                                      Fax: 732-699-0882
Cassette.

Web Sites

7163 **Healing Well**
                                      www.healingwell.com
An online health resource guide to medical news, chat, information and articles, newsgroups and message boards, books, disease-related web sites, medical directories, and more for patients, friends, and family coping with disabling diseases, disorders, or chronic illnesses.

7164 **Health Finder**
                                      www.healthfinder.gov
Searchable, carefully developed web site offering information on over 1000 topics. Developed by the US Department of Health and Human Services, the site can be used in both English and Spanish.

7165 **Healthlink USA**
                                      www.healthlinkusa.com
Health information concerning treatment, cures, prevention, diagnosis, risk factors, research, support groups, email lists, personal stories and much more. Updated regularly.

7166 **Helios Health**
                                      www.helioshealth.com
Online resource for your health information. Detailed information about specific health topics, access to expert advice from our Medical Advisory Board, and up-to-date health news.

7167 MedicineNet

www.medicinenet.com

An online resource for consumers providing easy-to-read, authoritative medical and health information.

7168 Medscape

www.medscape.com

Medscape offers specialists, primary care physicians, and other health professionals the Web's most robust and integrated medical information and educational tools.

7169 National Sarcoidosis Resource Center

www.nsrc-global.net

Provides the general public with sarcoidosis information, for patients to obtain medical and emotional help and to provide government officials with the information they need.

7170 WebMD

www.webmd.com

Information on sarcoidosis, including articles and resources.

Description

7171 Scleroderma

Scleroderma, literally 'hard skin', is a form of systemic sclerosis, a generalized disturbance of connective and vascular tissue which leads to scarring (sclerosis). Scleroderma is a rare disease, with about 5,000 new cases in the United States each year. Women are 3 or 4 times as likely as men to get the disease, which typically begins between the ages of 30 and 50 years. It is comparatively rare in children. The cause of the disease is unknown.

Since almost any organ may be involved, the list of possible symptoms is extensive. Important ones include weakness, fatigue, stiffness, weight loss, shortness of breath, abdominal bloating and pain, diarrhea and irritation of the eyes. Kidney involvement usually causes abrupt acceleration of high blood pressure. A very characteristic symptom, although not unique to this disease, is Raynaud's phenomenon. On exposure to cold, the arteries of the patient's hands and feet contract, causing the skin color to change from red, to white (blanch), to blue (cyanosis), accompanied by pain and numbness.

If the disease is limited to the skin the outlook is good, but involvement of lung and kidney in the systemic form may be fatal. Use of the ACE inhibitor class of anti-hypertensive drugs has helped preserve kidney function. Many immunosuppressive drugs have been tried without clear success. Clinical trials of new agents are often available to patients. When end-stage kidney disease cannot be prevented, dialysis and transplant can be used, although the death rate remains high.

National Agencies & Associations

7172 Canadian Dermatology Association

1385 Bank Street
Ottawa, Ontario, K1H-8N4

613-738-1748
800-267-3376
Fax: 613-738-4695
e-mail: contact.cda@dermatology.ca
www.dermatology.ca

Ensure the Canadian public has equal access to timely and exemplary dermatologic care, by advocating on dermatologic issues, providing leadership in continuing medical and public education, and promoting and disseminating dermatologic knowledge and research.
Dr Richard Langley, President of the Board
Chantal Courchesne, Executive Director

7173 Scleroderma Foundation

462 Boston Street
Topsfield, MA 01983

978-887-0658
800-722-4673
Fax: 978-463-5809
e-mail: newengland@scleroderma.org
www.scleroderma.org

A national nonprofit organization serving the interests of persons with Scleroderma. The Foundation's 26 chapters and 135 support groups nationwide help to carry out its three-fold mission of support, education and research.
Joseph Camerino, Chair
Carol Feghali-Bostwi, Vice Chair

7174 Scleroderma Society of Ontario

393 University Avenue
Toronto, Ontario, M5G-1E6

905-544-0343
Fax: 416-979-8366
www.sclerodermaontario.ca

Committed to promoting increased public awareness, advancing patient wellness and supporting research in scleroderma.
Brian Hinchey, Treasurer
Maureen Sauve, President of the Board

State Agencies & Associations

Arizona

7175 Scleroderma Foundation: Arizona Chapter

18402 N 19th Avenue
Phoenix, AZ 85023

623-847-3757
e-mail: carolnader@cox.net
www.scleroderma.org

Local chapter of the national Scleroderma Foundation in Byfield, Massachusetts. Please contact this group for information on area support groups.
Carol Nader, President

California

7176 Scleroderma Foundation: Greater San Diego Chapter

PO Box 502948
San Diego, CA 92150

619-655-4342
e-mail: kellyd.sclerosd@gmail.com
www.scleroderma.org

Local chapter of the national Scleroderma Foundation in Byfield, Massachusetts. Please contact this group for information on area support groups.
Fletcher Diehl, President
Carol Ireland, Vice President

7177 Scleroderma Foundation: Northern California Chapter

PO Box 601313
Sacramento, CA 95860

916-832-1102
e-mail: NoCAchapter@scleroderma.org
www.scleroderma.org

Local chapter of the national Scleroderma Foundation in Byfield, Massachusetts. Please contact this group for information on area support groups.
Cathy Eddy, President
Cheryl George, Vice President

7178 Scleroderma Foundation: Southern California Chapter

10319 Jefferson Blvd.
Culver City, CA 90232

310-287-0793
877-443-5755
Fax: 310-477-8774
e-mail: SoCAchapter@scleroderma.org
www.scleroderma.org

Local chapter of the national Scleroderma Foundation in Byfield, Massachusetts. Please contact this group for information on area support groups.
Brian Ross Adams, Executive Director
Dan Furst, President

Colorado

7179 Scleroderma Foundation: Colorado Chapter

2280 S Albion Street
Denver, CO 80222-0940

303-806-6686
e-mail: COchapter@scleroderma.org
www.scleroderma.org

Local chapter of the national Scleroderma Foundation in Danvers, Massachusetts. Please contact this group for information on area support groups.
Rita Miller, President
Fran Penk, Vice President

District of Columbia

7180 Scleroderma Foundation: Greater Washington DC Chapter

2010 Corporate Ridge
McLean, VA 22102

202-999-4562
888-233-4779
e-mail: GWDCchapter@scleroderma.org
www.scleroderma.org

Local chapter of the national Scleroderma Foundation in Byfield, Massachusetts. Please contact this group for information on area support groups.
Carol Sodetz, President

Florida

7181 Scleroderma Foundation: Southeast Florida Chapter
3930 Oaks Clubhouse Drive   954-798-1854
Pompano Beach, FL 33069-3913   Fax: 954-255-8081
e-mail: sclerodermasefl@gmail.com
www.scleroderma.org
Local chapter of the national Scleroderma Foundation in Byfield, Massachusetts. Please contact this group for information on area support groups.
Berna Falkoff, President
Ruth Greenspan, Vice - Chair

Georgia

7182 Scleroderma Foundation: Georgia Chapter Scleroderma Foundation
Scleroderma Foundation
PO Box 522   770-925-7037
Liburn, GA 30048   800-722-4673
e-mail: GAchapter@scleroderma.org
www.scleroderma.org
Local chapter of the national Scleroderma Foundation in Byfield, Massachusetts. Call the national office for contact information on the Georgia Chapter. Please contact this group for information on area support groups.
Stacy Wright, Contact
Mary Haulk, Contact

Illinois

7183 Scleroderma Foundation: Greater Chicago Chapter
134 N. LaSalle St.   312-660-1131
Chicago, IL 60602   Fax: 312-660-1133
e-mail: GCchapter@scleroderma.org
www.scleroderma.org
Local chapter of the national Scleroderma Foundation. Please contact group for information on area support groups.
Mike Robbins, President

Maine

7184 Scleroderma Foundation: New England Chapter
462 Boston Street   978-887-0658
Topsfield, MA 01983   888-525-0658
Fax: 978-887-0659
e-mail: newengland@scleroderma.com
www.scleroderma.org
Local chapter of the national Scleroderma Foundation in Byfield, Massachusetts. Please contact this group for information on area support groups. Includes MA, ME, NH, VT, & RI.
Marie Coyle, President
Peter L. Hart, Treasurer

Massachusetts

7185 Scleroderma Foundation: New England Chapter
462 Boston Street   978-887-0658
Topsfield, MA 01983   888-525-0658
Fax: 978-887-0659
e-mail: newengland@scleroderma.com
www.scleroderma.org
Local chapter of the national Scleroderma Foundation in Byfield, Massachusetts. Please contact this group for information on area support groups.
Marie Coyle, President
Peter L. Hart, Treasurer

Michigan

7186 Scleroderma Foundation: Michigan Chapter
23999 Telegraph   248-595-8526
Southfield, MI 48033   800-716-6554
Fax: 248-595-8586
e-mail: MIchapter@scleroderma.org
www.scleroderma.org
Local chapter of the national Scleroderma Foundation in Danvers, Massachusetts. Please contact this group for information on area

support groups, medical referrals, confrence dates and fund raising activities.
Duane Maladecki, President
Paul Rybicki, Vice President

Minnesota

7187 Scleroderma Foundation: Minnesota Chapter
PO Box 385246   877-794-0347
Bloomington, MN 55438   877-794-0347
e-mail: MNChapter@scleroderma.org
www.scleroderma.org
Local chapter of the national Scleroderma Foundation in Byfield, Massachusetts. Please contact this group for information on area support groups.
Bonnie Handmacher, President
Jordana Schmidt, Vice President

Missouri

7188 Scleroderma Foundation: Missouri Chapter
PO Box 4123   417-887-3269
Springfield, MO 65808   e-mail: MOchapter@scleroderma.org
www.scleroderma.org
Local chapter of the national Scleroderma Foundation in Byfield, Massachusetts. Please contact this group for information on area support groups.
Mary Blades, President
Rhonda Costa, Vice President

Nevada

7189 Scleroderma Foundation: Nevada Chapter
6760 Surrey Street   702-368-1572
Las Vegas, NV 89119   e-mail: NVchapter@scleroderma.org
www.scleroderma.org
Local chapter of the national Scleroderma Foundation in Byfield, Massachusetts. Please contact this group for information on area support groups.
Barbara Dempsey, President
Sheila Gray, VP Support Group

New Hampshire

7190 Scleroderma Foundation: New England Chapter
462 Boston Street   978-887-0658
Topsfield, MA 01983   888-525-0658
Fax: 978-887-0659
e-mail: newengland@scleroderma.com
www.scleroderma.org
Local chapter of the national Scleroderma Foundation in Byfield, Massachusetts. Please contact this group for information on area support groups.
Marie Coyle, President
Peter L. Hart, Treasurer

New York

7191 Scleroderma Foundation: Tri-State Chapter
59 Front Street   800-867-0885
Binghamton, NY 13905   800-867-0885
Fax: 607-723-2039
e-mail: chribar@scleroderma.org
www.scleroderma.org
Local chapter of the national Scleroderma Foundation in Byfield, Massachusetts. Please contact this group for information on area support groups.
Jeff Mace, President
Bruce Cowen, Vice President

7192 Scleroderma Foundation: Western New York Chapter
PO Box 708   716-627-2283
Hamburg, NY 14075   877-969-2478
e-mail: wnychpt@aol.com
www.scleroderma.org
Local chapter of the national Scleroderma Foundation in Byfield, Massachusetts. Please contact this group for information on area support groups.
Laura Henry, Co-President

Ohio

7193 **Scleroderma Foundation: Ohio Chapter**
PO Box 105   614-334-0846
Worthington, OH 43085-0846   866-849-9030
                    e-mail: OHchapter@scleroderma.org
                                www.scleroderma.org
Local chapter of the national Scleroderma Foundation in Byfield,
Massachusetts. Please contact this group for information on area
support groups.
Debbie Metz, President
Garry Lazenby, Vice President

Oregon

7194 **Scleroderma Foundation: Oregon Chapter**
PO Box 19296   503-245-4588
Portland, OR 97280-0296   e-mail: ORchapter@scleroderma.org
                                www.scleroderma.org
Local chapter of the national Scleroderma Foundation in Byfield,
Massachusetts. Please contact this group for information on area
support groups.
Liz Orem-Bedel, President
Richard Bates, Vice President

Pennsylvania

7195 **Scleroderma Foundation: Western Pennsylvania Chapter**
3500 Terrace Street   800-603-8960
Pittsburgh, PA 15261   800-722-4673
                    e-mail: WPAchapter@scleroderma.org
                                www.scleroderma.org
Local chapter of the national Scleroderma Foundation in Byfield,
Massachusetts. Please contact this group for information on area
support groups.
Betty Aquino, President
Thomas A Medsger Jr, Treasurer

Rhode Island

7196 **Scleroderma Foundation: New England Chapter**
462 Boston Street   978-887-0658
Topsfield, MA 01983   888-525-0658
                                    Fax: 978-887-0659
                    e-mail: newengland@scleroderma.com
                                www.scleroderma.org
Local chapter of the national Scleroderma Foundation in Byfield,
Massachusetts. Please contact this group for information on area
support groups.
Marie Coyle, President
Peter L. Hart, Treasurer

South Carolina

7197 **Scleroderma Foundation: South Carolina Chapter**
713-D east Greenvile Street   864-617-0237
Anderson, SC 29621   866-557-3729
                    e-mail: SCchapter@scleroderma.org
                                www.scleroderma.org
Local chapter of the national Scleroderma Foundation in Byfield.
Massachusetts. Please contact this group for information on area
support groups.
Susan Melvin, President
Karen Kemper, Vice President

Tennessee

7198 **Scleroderma Foundation: Tennessee Chapter**
PO Box 281977   615-792-4610
Nashville, TN 37228   800-497-5193
                                    Fax: 615-792-4610
                    e-mail: TNchapter@scleroderma.org
                                www.scleroderma.org
Local chapter of the national Scleroderma Foundation in Byfield,
Massachusetts. Please contact this group for information on area
support groups.
April Simpkins, President
Charles Cowell, Vice President

Texas

7199 **Scleroderma Foundation: Bluebonnet Chapter**
PO Box 1836   972-396-9400
Allen, TX 75013-1894   866-532-7673
                                    Fax: 972-649-7910
                    e-mail: TXchapter@scleroderma.org
                                www.scleroderma.org
Local chapter of the national Scleroderma Foundation in Byfield,
Massachusetts. Please contact this group for information on area
support groups.
Cindi Brannum, President
Peggy Brown, Vice President

Vermont

7200 **Scleroderma Foundation: New England Chapter**
462 Boston Street   978-887-0658
Topsfield, MA 01983   888-525-0658
                                    Fax: 978-887-0659
                    e-mail: newengland@scleroderma.com
                                www.scleroderma.org
Local chapter of the national Scleroderma Foundation in Byfield,
Massachusetts. Please contact this group for information on area
support groups.
Marie Coyle, President
Peter L. Hart, Treasurer

Virginia

7201 **Scleroderma Foundation: Greater Washington DC Chapter**
2010 Corporate Ridge   202-999-4562
McLean, VA 22102   888-233-4779
                    e-mail: GWDCchapter@scleroderma.org
                                www.scleroderma.org
Local chapter of the national Scleroderma Foundation in Byfield,
Massachusetts. Please contact this group for information on area
support groups.
Carol Sodetz, President
Solomon reed, Treasurer

Washington

7202 **Scleroderma Foundation: Evergreen Chapter**
PO Box 84506   206-285-9822
Seattle, WA 98124-5806   e-mail: WAchapter@scleroderma.org
                                www.scleroderma.org
Local chapter of the national Scleroderma Foundation in Byfield,
Massachusetts. Please contact this group for information on area
support groups.
Bunny Garthe, President
Nic Evans, Vice President

Foundations

7203 **Juvenile Scleroderma Network**
1204 W 13th Street   310-519-9511
San Pedro, CA 90731   866-338-5892
                    e-mail: OutreachJSDN@jsdn.org
                                www.jsdn.org
Organization that is working to provide educational programs
about JSD, and to help children and their families to gain a better
understanding.
Jerry Gaither, Chairman
Kathy Gaither, President

Research Centers

7204 **Boston University University Medical Center**
University Medical Center
One Boston Medical Center Place
Boston, MA 02118   617-638-8000
                                        www.bmc.org
Ongoing clinical trials and studies in scleroderma. Office hours by
appointment.
Kate Walsh, President/CEO
Melynn Nuite RN, Clinical Trails Contact

7205 Center for Rheumatology
1367 Washington Avenue
Albany, NY 12206   518-489-4471
                        e-mail: cbarr@joint-docs.com
                        www.joint-docs.com
This is a committed research facility as well as a medical practice.
Our research practice is made up of seven physicians a certified
physician's assistant and four research coordinators. We may have
as many as 20 ongoing trails at a time in various indications within
the study of rheumatology. Investigational treatment of interstitial
lung disease associated with systemic sclerosis.
Norman R Romanoff, Practitioner
Joel M Kremer, Practitioner

7206 Georgetown University Hospital: Department of Rheumatology
3800 Reservoir Road NW   202-444-8233
Washington, DC 20007   Fax: 202-444-7584
                        www.medicine.georgetown.edu
Research is based on clinical trials and special interest in
scleroderma and kidney pulmonary hypertension pregnancy epi-
demiology and natural history of scleroderma subsets.
Sherry Magrudar, Executive Assistant
Ann Nichols, Senior Adminstrator

7207 Johns Hopkins University: Scleroderma Center
Johns Hopkins Bayview Medical Center
5501 Hopkins Bayview Circle   410-550-7715
Baltimore, MD 21224   Fax: 410-550-1363
                        www.scleroderma.jhmi.edu
Specializes in the management of systemic sclerosis (scleroderma)
Raynaud's phenomenon and related disorders. In addition to pa-
tient care the center is involved in both basic and clinical research
projects.
Frederick M Wigley MD, Director
Sheila Friend, medical office coordinator

7208 Mayo Clinic Scottsdale Center for Scleroderma Care & Research
Mayo Clinic
13400 E Shea Boulevard   480-301-8000
Scottsdale, AZ 85259   800-446-2279
                        Fax: 480-301-7006
                        e-mail: newsbureau@mayo.edu
                        www.mayoclinic.org/rheumatology
Integrates multiple medical as well as surgical specialties under
the direction of the Division of Rheumatology to provide coordi-
nated and comprehensive evaluations and treatment. New clinical
trails are in development.
John H. Noseworthy MD, President/CEO
April Chang-Miller, Assistant Professor of Medicine

7209 Medical University of South Carolina Medical University of South Carolina
Medical University of South Carolina
171 Ashley Avenue   843-792-1414
Charleston, SC 29425   800-424-6872
                        Fax: 843-792-2601
                        e-mail: wickman@musc.edu
                        www.musc.edu
Actively engaged in basic and clinical research of scleroderma.
Raymond S Greenburg, President
Dr. Mark Sothman, Vice President

7210 Scleroderma Clinical & Research Center State University of New York at Stonybro
State University of New York at Stonybrook
26 Research Way   631-444-0580
E Setauket, NY 01173-9260   Fax: 631-444-0562
                        www.scleroderma.org
Ongoing research of scleroderma.
Joseph Camerino, chair
Carol Feghali-Bostwick, Vce Chair

7211 Scleroderma Research Foundation
220 Montgomery Street   415-834-9444
San Francisco, CA 94104   800-637-4005
                        Fax: 415-834-9177
                        e-mail: info@sclerodermaresearch.org
                        www.srfcure.org
Mission is to find a cure for scleroderma a life threatening and degenerative illness by funding and facilitating the most promising

highest quality research and placing the disease and its need for a
cure in the public eye.
Alex Gonzalez, Director of Development
Amy Hewitt, Executive Director

7212 Thomas Jefferson University Hospital
111 S 11th Street   215-955-6840
Philadelphia, PA 19107   Fax: 215-923-5828
                        www.jeffersonhospital.org
Provides diagnostic evaluations treatment and access to the latest
research studies for more than one thousand patients with
scleroderma and related diseases.
Stephen K klasko, President/CEO
Sergio Jimen MD, Professor

7213 University of Alabama Birmingham
1720 second Av Soyth
Birmingham, AL 35294   205-934-4011
                        www.uab.edu
Located in the Clinical Immunology and Rheumatology depart-
ment Oral Type 1 Collagen in Scleroderma is studied.
Carol Garrison, President
William Ferniany, CEO

7214 University of Chicago Center for Advanced Medicine Duchossis Center
University of Chicago hospital
5841 S Maryland Avenue   773-702-1000
Chicago, IL 60637   888-824-0200
                        Fax: 773-028-02
                        e-mail: orogers@medicine.bsd.uchicago.edu
                        www.uchospitals.com
Scleroderma clinic.
Michael Ellm MD, Clinic Contact
Ornery Rogers, Clinic Contact

7215 University of Illinois at Chicago Medical Center Outpatient Clinical Center
University of Illinois
600 S Hoyne Avenue   312-996-7000
Chicago, IL 60612   800-842-1002
                        Fax: 312-633-3434
                        TTY: 312-413-0123
                        e-mail: info@iMDc.org
                        www.uic.edu
Scleroderma clinic held on the first and third Thursdays of every
month.
Paula Allen Meares, Chancellor
Lon S. Kauffman, Vice Chancellor

7216 University of Pittsburgh
4200 Fifth avenue   412-624-4141
Pittsburgh, PA 15260   Fax: 412-383-2264
                        e-mail: webmaster@pitt.edu
                        www.pitt.edu
Clinic and research of scleroderma.
Patricia E. Beeson, Vice Chancellor
John P Elliott, Director of Internal Affairs

7217 University of Tennessee Medical Group
956 Court Avenue   901-866-8383
Memphis, TN 38103   Fax: 901-866-8380
                        www.utmedicalgroup.com
Ongoing research protocols.
Charles E. Woeppel MD, CEO

7218 University of Texas Health Science Center
7000 Fannin   713-500-4472
Houston, TX 77030   Fax: 713-500-3026
                        e-mail: sclerodermaregister@uth.tmc.edu
                        www.uthouston.edu
Clinic research and clinical trials concerning scleroderma.
Giuseppe N. Colasurdo, President

Support Groups & Hotlines

7219 National Health Information Center
PO Box 1133
Washington, DC 20013
310-565-4167
800-336-4797
Fax: 301-984-4256
e-mail: info@nhic.org
www.health.gov/nhic
Offers a nationwide information referral service, produces directories and resource guides.

7220 Rhode Island Scleroderma Support Group
18 Talbot Manor
Cranston, RI 02905
401-781-5013
e-mail: scleroderma@hotmail.com
www.angelfire.com/ri/scleroderma
Meets on the fourth Wednsday of every month at Roger Williams Hospital.
Carole Cowell, President

7221 Scleroderma Support Groups
Scleroderma Foundation
12 Kent Way
Byfield, MA 01922
978-463-5843
800-722-4633
Fax: 978-463-5809
e-mail: sfinfo@scleroderma.org
www.scleroderma.org
Please contact the Scleroderma Foundation or visit our web site for a listing of support groups in your area.

Books

7222 Best of the Beacon
Scleroderma Foundation
12 Kent Way
Byfield, MA 01922
978-463-5843
800-722-4673
Fax: 978-463-5809
e-mail: sfinfo@scleroderma.org
www.scleroderma.org/store.html#books
Interesting, readable and highly practical collection of articles of particular interest to those living with scleroderma. This mini encyclopedia includes 11 medical articles, 358 most frequently asked questions, 34 sharing stories, 62 articles of special interest on a variety of useful topics and a glossary that defines 240 words you may encounter when reading about scleroderma.
Marie Coyle, Editor

7223 Handout on Health: Scleroderma
NAMSIC/National Institutes of Health
1 AMS Circle
Bethesda, MD 20892-0001
301-495-4484
877-226-4267
Fax: 301-718-6366
TTY: 301-565-2966
e-mail: niamsinfo@mail.nih.gov
www.nih.gov/niams

143 pages

7224 Helpful Hints for Living with Scleroderma
Scleroderma Foundation
12 Kent Way
Byfield, MA 01922
978-463-5843
800-722-4673
Fax: 978-463-5809
e-mail: sfinfo@scleroderma.org
www.scleroderma.org/store.html#books
Booklet of helpful suggestions from our chapters and members, for the comfort and convienience of others who share the same challenges.
57 pages

7225 Perspectives on Living with Scleroderma
Scleroderma Foundation
12 Kent Way
Byfield, MA 01922
978-463-5843
800-722-4673
Fax: 978-463-5809
e-mail: sfinfo@scleroderma.org
www.scleroderma.org/store.html#books

Insightful articles on coping with scleroderma come from not only from Dr. Flapan's counseling and volunteer work, but also from his personal experience as a scleroderma patient.
233 pages

7226 Scleroderma Book
Scleroderma Foundation
12 Kent Way
Byfield, MA 01922
978-463-5843
800-722-4673
Fax: 978-463-5809
e-mail: sfinfo@scleroderma.org
www.scleroderma.org/store.html#books
Definitive guide to scleroderma for patients and their families, with easy to understand explanations.
182 pages

7227 Scleroderma: Surviving a Seventeen-Year Itch
Scleroderma Foundation
978-463-5809
800-722-4673
Fax: 978-463-5809
e-mail: sfinfo@scleroderma.org
www.scleroderma.org
Self-help manual including history, diagnosis, daily routines and exercise programs for persons with scleroderma.

7228 Scleroderma: a New Role for Patients and Families
Scleroderma Foundation
12 Kent Way
Byfield, MA 01922
978-463-5843
800-722-4673
Fax: 978-463-5809
e-mail: sfinfo@scleroderma.org
www.scleroderma.org/store.html#books
Provides an overview of key issues and offers resources that enable patients and their families to find more resources on thier own.
168 pages

7229 Understanding & Managing Scleroderma
Scleroderma Foundation
12 Kent Way
Byfield, MA 01923
978-463-5843
800-722-4633
Fax: 978-463-5809
e-mail: sfinfo@scleroderma.org
www.scleroderma.org
Booklet intended to help persons with scleroderma, their families and others interested in scleroderma to better understand what scleroderma is, what effects it may have, and what those with scleroderma can do to help themselves and their physicians manage the disease. It answers some of the most frequently asked questions about scleroderma.

Magazines

7230 Scleroderma Voice
Scleroderma Foundation
12 Kent Way
Byfield, MA 01922
978-463-5843
800-722-4673
Fax: 978-463-5809
e-mail: sfinfo@scleroderma.org
www.scleroderma.org
Feautures the latest information available on scleroderma treatments and research. Subscription to the Voice includes a one-year membership in the Scleroderma Foundation.
Quarterly

Pamphlets

7231 If You Have Scleroderma You Need Not Feel Alone
Scleroderma Foundation
12 Kent Way
Byfield, MA 01922
978-463-5843
800-722-4673
Fax: 978-463-5809
e-mail: sfinfo@scleroderma.org
www.scleroderma.org/store.html#brochures
Scleroderma Foundation's membership brochure. Free of charge, also available in Spanish.

7232 Scleroderma: an Overview
Scleroderma Foundation
12 Kent Way
Byfield, MA 01922
978-463-5843
Fax: 978-463-5809
e-mail: sfinfo@scleroderma.org
www.scleroderma.org/store.html#brochures
Concise genral overview of sytemic scleroderma. Also available in Spanish, and downloadable in Portugese.

7233 What Causes Scleroderma?
Scleroderma Foundation
12 Kent Way
Byfield, MA 01922
978-463-5843
800-722-4673
Fax: 978-463-5809
e-mail: sfinfo@scleroderma.org
www.scleroderma.org/store.html#brochures
Discusses the puzzling nature of scleroderma. Also available in Spanish, and downloadable in Portugese.

Web Sites

7234 Healing Well
www.healingwell.com
An online health resource guide to medical news, chat, information and articles, newsgroups and message boards, books, disease-related web sites, medical directories, and more for patients, friends, and family coping with disabling diseases, disorders, or chronic illnesses.

7235 Health Finder
www.healthfinder.gov
Searchable, carefully developed web site offering information on over 1000 topics. Developed by the US Department of Health and Human Services, the site can be used in both English and Spanish.

7236 Healthlink USA
www.healthlinkusa.com
Health information concerning treatment, cures, prevention, diagnosis, risk factors, research, support groups, email lists, personal stories and much more. Updated regularly.

7237 Helios Health
www.helioshealth.com
Online resource for your health information. Detailed information about specific health topics, access to expert advice from our Medical Advisory Board, and up-to-date health news.

7238 MedicineNet
www.medicinenet.com
An online resource for consumers providing easy-to-read, authoritative medical and health information.

7239 Medscape
www.medscape.com
Medscape offers specialists, primary care physicians, and other health professionals the Web's most robust and integrated medical information and educational tools.

7240 Scleroderma Foundation
www.scleroderma.org
501 (c)3 national nonprofit organization serving the interests of persons with scleroderma. The Foundation's 26 chapters and 135 support groups nationwide help to carry out its three-fold mission of support, education and research. The Scleroderma Foundation is a leading nonprofit supporter of scleroderma research — funding over $1 million of new grants each year to find the cause and cure of scleroderma.

7241 WebMD
www.webmd.com
Information on scleroderma, including articles and resources.

Description

7242 **Scoliosis**

Scoliosis is a lateral curvature of the spine, with 60 to 80 percent of the cases occurring in girls. It may first be suspected when one of the teenager's shoulders appears higher than the other or clothes don't hang straight. The spinal curve is more pronounced when the adolescent bends forward. More than 80 percent of scoliosis is idiopathic, that is, there is no known cause.

Symptoms include prominent shoulder blades, uneven hip levels, and fatigue in the lower back after sitting or standing for prolonged periods of time. In many cases there are no symptoms unless the scoliosis is severe.

The prognosis depends on the site and severity of the curve, and the age of onset of symptoms. Early detection through school screening provides more treatment options, and prompt referral to an orthopedist is indicated. The majority of cases require only observation for progression. Approximately 20 percent of those with scoliosis will require an orthopedic brace or spinal fusion surgery.

National Agencies & Associations

7243 **American Academy of Orthopaedic Surgeons**
6300 N River Road
Rosemont, IL 60018-4238
847-823-7186
800-346-2267
Fax: 847-823-8125
e-mail: custserv@aaos.org
www.aaos.org
The American Academy of Orthopaedic Surgeons provides education and practice management services for orthopaedic surgeons and allied health professionals. The Academy also serves as an advocate for improved patient care and informs the public.
Joshua J. Jacobs, President
Andrew N. Pollack, Treasurer

7244 **International Federation of Spine Associations**
Howard M Shulman
9908 Cape Scott Court
Raleigh, NC 27614-9025
919-846-2204
www.scoliosisrx.com
IFOSA is a federation of various national Spine Associations from countries in North America Europe and Australia. These organizations principally represent the spine patients and their families.

7245 **National Scoliosis Foundation**
5 Cabot Place
Stoughton, MA 02072
781-341-6333
800-673-6922
Fax: 781-341-8333
e-mail: NSF@scoliosis.org
www.scoliosis.org
Promotes school screening offers public awareness materials to promote public education maintains a resource center for professional information conducts scoliosis conferences and offers support groups to people affected by the disease.
Joseph P O'Brien, President/CEO
Dennis J Fusco, Treasurer

7246 **Scoliosis Association**
PO Box 811705
Boca Raton, FL 33481-1705
561-994-4435
800-800-0669
Fax: 561-994-2455
e-mail: normlipin@aol.com
www.scoliosis-assoc.org
Sponsors and encourages spinal screening programs. Disseminates information throughout the country and raises funds for

scoliosis research. Membership fee includes subscription to newsletter. Videos and printed information available.

Research Centers

7247 **Scoliosis Research Society**
555 E Wells Street
Milwaukee, WI 53202
414-289-9107
Fax: 414-276-3349
e-mail: info@srs.org
www.srs.org
This society provides an international forum for those interested in the management of spinal deformities. It holds a yearly meeting at which health professionals meet to share observations and results and to explore new avenues of research.
Kamal N. Ibrahim, President
Hubert Labelle, Treasurer

7248 **Shriners Hospital for Crippled Children Chicago Unit**
Chicago Unit
2211 N Oak Park Avenue
Chicago, IL 60707
813-281-0300
Fax: 773-855-88
www.shrinershospitalsforchildren.org
A 60-bed orthopedic hospital providing comprehensive spinal cord injury care to children. Provides care for spinal deformities Cerebral Palsy Osteoeneisis Imperfecta and Scoliosis as well as others.
John A. Cinotto, Chairman
Diether Sturm, Chief of Staff

Support Groups & Hotlines

7249 **National Health Information Center**
PO Box 1133
Washington, DC 20013
310-565-4167
800-336-4797
Fax: 301-984-4256
e-mail: info@nhic.org
www.health.gov/nhic
Offers a nationwide information referral service, produces directories and resource guides.

Books

7250 **Adult Scoliosis Surgery...It Can Be Done**
St. Luke's Spine Center
11311 Shaker Boulevard
Cleveland, OH 44104-3805
216-368-7000
Describes various types of surgery and procedures used in adult scoliosis patients.
21 pages

7251 **Coalition Index**
American School Health Association
PO Box 708
Kent, OH 44240
330-678-1601
800-445-2742
Fax: 330-678-4526
e-mail: asha@ashaweb.org
www.ashaweb.org
A professional membership organization dedicated to promoting the health and well being of children and youth through coordinated school health programs.
Susan Wooley, Executive Director

7252 **Getting Ready, Getting Well**
National Scoliosis Foundation
5 Cabot Place
Stoughton, MA 02072
781-341-6333
800-673-6922
Fax: 781-341-8333
e-mail: NSF@scoliosis.org
www.scoliosis.org
Guide for those anticipating surgery. Divided into three sections: Making up Your Mind, Taking Charge, and Home Again.
73 pages
Joseph P O'Brien, President/CEO

7253 **Handbook of Scoliosis**
Scoliosis Research Society

555 East Wells Street
Milwaukee, WI 53202

414-289-9107
Fax: 414-276-3349
www.srs.org

Tressa Goulding, Executive Director

7254 Stopping Scoliosis
National Scoliosis Foundation
5 Cabot Place
Stoughton, MA 02072

781-341-6333
800-673-6922
Fax: 781-341-8333
e-mail: NSF@scoliosis.org
www.scoliosis.org

Filled with accurate, currently researched information for adults concerned with their condition or that of a young person.
Joseph P O'Brien, President/CEO

7255 Twenty Years at Hull House
New American Library
375 Hudson Street
New York, NY 10014

212-366-2000

Book dealing with Scoliosis.
Grades 7-12

Children's Books

7256 Deenie
Bradbury Press
866 3rd Avenue
New York, NY 10022-6221

212-702-2000
800-257-5755

Deenie, a beautiful thirteen-year-old girl, had a mother who was pushing her to become a model. The agency representatives told Deenie she had the looks but walked differently. Deenie's main wish was to become a cheerleader. Her close friend, Janet, made the cheerleading squad but Deenie didn't make the finalist list. After this her gym teacher noticed her posture and called her family. After seeing therapists, the diagnosis of adolescent idiopathic scoliosis was made.
159 pages Hardcover
ISBN: 0-027110-20-6

7257 Tina's Story...Scoliosis and Me
Alfred I DuPont Institute
PO Box 269
Wilmington, DE 19801

302-651-4000

Suggested for parents of children anticipating surgery. This outstanding book, written as an eighth grade project by a gifted thirteen year old writer and scoliosis patient, relates her experiences and emotions while wearing a brace for three years prior to surgery.

7258 What Young People and Parents Need to Know about Scoliosis
American Physical Therapy Association
1111 N Fairfax Street
Alexandria, VA 22314

703-684-2782

A physical therapist's perspective.

Newsletters

7259 Backtalk
Scoliosis Association
PO Box 811705
Boca Raton, FL 33481-1705

561-994-4435
800-800-0669
Fax: 561-994-2455
e-mail: scolioassn@aol.com
www.scoliosis.org

Information for families, patients and health care professionals.

Pamphlets

7260 1 in Every 10 Persons Has Scoliosis
National Scoliosis Foundation
5 Cabot Place
Stoughton, MA 02072

781-341-6333
800-673-6922
Fax: 781-341-8333
e-mail: NSF@scoliosis.org
www.scoliosis.org

Explains what scoliosis is and illustrates how to screen for it. It also contains facts about the Foundation.
Joseph P O'Brien, President/CEO

7261 Adolescent Idiopathic Scoliosis: Prevelance, Natural History, Treatments
National Scoliosis Foundation
5 Cabot Place
Stoughton, MA 02072

781-341-6333
800-673-6922
Fax: 781-341-8333
e-mail: NSF@scoliosis.org
www.scoliosis.org

Expert overview of a condition that affects many young people.
Joseph P O'Brien, President/CEO

7262 Boston Bracing System for Idiopathic Scoliosis
National Scoliosis Foundation
5 Cabot Place
Stoughton, MA 02072

781-341-6333
800-673-6922
Fax: 781-341-8333
e-mail: NSF@scoliosis.org
www.scoliosis.org

Explaination of an available option.
Joseph P O'Brien, President/CEO

7263 Brace & Her Brace is No Handicap
National Scoliosis Foundation
5 Cabot Place
Stoughton, MA 02072

781-341-6333
800-673-6922
Fax: 781-341-8333
e-mail: NSF@scoliosis.org
www.scoliosis.org

Contains two illustrated short stories, each about a teenage girl coping successfully with scoliosis.
Joseph P O'Brien, President/CEO

7264 Getting a Second Opinion
National Scoliosis Foundation
5 Cabot Place
Stoughton, MA 02072

781-341-6333
800-673-6922
Fax: 781-341-8333
e-mail: NSF@scoliosis.org
www.scoliosis.org

Reprinted from Health Tips.
Joseph P O'Brien, President/CEO

7265 Going Home
University Hospital Spine Center
2074 Abington Road
Cleveland, OH 44106

216-844-1616

Instructions for pediatric and adult patients who have had a spinal fusion.

7266 Medical Update Column
National Scoliosis Foundation
5 Cabot Place
Stoughton, MA 02072

781-341-6333
800-673-6922
Fax: 781-341-8333
e-mail: NSF@scoliosis.org
www.scoliosis.org

Reprints from past issues of the Spinal Connections Medical Update Column available on various topics.
Joseph P O'Brien, President/CEO

7267 NSF Packets
National Scoliosis Foundation
5 Cabot Place
Stoughton, MA 02072

781-341-6333
800-673-6922
Fax: 781-341-8333
e-mail: NSF@scoliosis.org
www.scoliosis.org

Packet contains information for parents and young people, adults, and healthcare professionals.
Joseph P O'Brien, President/CEO

7268 Patient with Scoliosis
Educational Services, Division of AJV Company
555 W 57th Street
New York, NY 10019-2925

212-996-6473

A reprint from the American Journal of nursin.

7269 Postural Screening Program
National Scoliosis Foundation
5 Cabot Place   781-341-6333
Stoughton, MA 02072   800-673-6922
                                                  Fax: 781-341-8333
                                           e-mail: NSF@scoliosis.org
                                                   www.scoliosis.org
Guidelines for physicians and school nurses.
Joseph P O'Brien, President/CEO

7270 Questions Most Often Asked the NSF
National Scoliosis Foundation
5 Cabot Place   781-341-6333
Stoughton, MA 02072   800-673-6922
                                                  Fax: 781-341-8333
                                           e-mail: NSF@scoliosis.org
                                                   www.scoliosis.org
Answers the most frequently asked questions about scoliosis and
the foundation in general.
Joseph P O'Brien, President/CEO

7271 Scoliosis
Scoliosis Research Society
611 E Wells Street   414-289-9107
Milwaukee, WI 53202   Fax: 414-276-3349
                                                          www.srs.org
Brochure describing scoliosis, kyphosis, lordosis; causes, preven-
tion, treatment and adult scoliosis.
Tressa Goulding, Executive Director

7272 Scoliosis Patient Becomes a Model
National Scoliosis Foundation
5 Cabot Place   781-341-6333
Stoughton, MA 02072   800-673-6922
                                                  Fax: 781-341-8333
                                           e-mail: NSF@scoliosis.org
                                                   www.scoliosis.org
Reprinted from Children's Today.
Joesph P O'Brien, President/CEO

7273 Scoliosis Road Map
University Hospital Spine Center
2074 Abington Road   216-844-1616
Cleveland, OH 44106
Written for teenagers affected by this illness.

7274 Scoliosis Screening: The Carlsbad Program
National Scoliosis Foundation
5 Cabot Place   781-341-6333
Stoughton, MA 02072   800-673-6922
                                                  Fax: 781-341-8333
                                           e-mail: NSF@scoliosis.org
                                                   www.scoliosis.org
Exceptional scoliosis screening program.
Joseph P O'Brien, President/CEO

7275 Scoliosis Surgery, What's It All About?
University Hospital Spine Center
2074 Abington Road   216-844-1616
Cleveland, OH 44106
This pamphlet answers many of the questions patients ask before
having surgery.

7276 Scoliosis and Kyphosis
Scoliosis Research Society
555 East Wells Street   414-289-9107
Milwaukee, WI 53202   Fax: 414-276-3349
                                                          www.srs.org
Information and advice from parents.
Tressa Goulding, Executive Director

7277 Scoliosis, Me?
North Dallas Scoliosis Center
1910 N Collins Boulevard   972-644-1930
Richardson, TX 75080-3525
Detailed answers to questions most asked by parents and teens.

7278 Scoliosis... Now it Can Be Treated in Adults as Well as Children
National Scoliosis Foundation

5 Cabot Place   781-341-6333
Stoughton, MA 02072   800-673-6922
                                                  Fax: 781-341-8333
                                           e-mail: NSF@scoliosis.org
                                                   www.scoliosis.org
Reprinted from Cleveland Magazine.
Joseph P O'Brien, President/CEO

7279 Scoliosis: Handbook for Patients
National Scoliosis Foundation
5 Cabot Place   781-341-6333
Stoughton, MA 02072   800-673-6922
                                                  Fax: 781-341-8333
                                           e-mail: NSF@scoliosis.org
                                                   www.scoliosis.org
Information on detection and treatment of adolescent scoliosis,
kyphosis and lordosis and adult scoliosis.
Joseph P O'Brien, President/CEO

7280 Screening Procedure Guidelines for Spinal Deformity
Scoliosis Research Society
555 East Wells Street   414-289-9107
Milwaukee, WI 53202   Fax: 414-276-3349
                                                          www.srs.org
Seven page brochure covers reasons, organizations and procedures for spinal screening. Signs of spinal deformity, as seen in
both standing and forward bending positions are illustrated and
discussed. Includes sample screening form.
7 pages
Tressa Goulding, Executive Director

7281 Spinal Deformity: Congenital Scoliosis and Kyphosis
Scoliosis Research Society
555 East Wells Street   414-289-9107
Milwaukee, WI 53202   Fax: 414-276-3349
                                                          www.srs.org
Discusses signs and causes of congenital spinal deformities, asso-
ciated conditions, treatment options and a glossary of terms.
12 pages
Tressa Goulding, Executive Director

7282 Spinal Deformity: Scoliosis and Kyphosis
Scoliosis Research Society
555 East Wells Street   414-289-9107
Milwaukee, WI 53202   Fax: 414-276-3349
                                                          www.srs.org
Twelve page brochure discusses signs and causes of scoliosis and
kyphosis, indications for treatment, treatment options, commonly
asked questions and a glossary of terms.
12 pages
Tressa Goulding, Executive Director

**7283 What Young People & Their Parents Need to Know About
Scoliosis**
American Physical Therapy Association
1111 N Fairfax Street   703-684-2782
Alexandria, VA 22314-1488
A physical therapists' perspective.

7284 What if You Need an Operation for Scoliosis?
St. Luke's Spine Center
11311 Shaker Boulevard   216-368-7000
Cleveland, OH 44104-3805

7285 When the Spine Curves
National Scoliosis Foundation
5 Cabot Place   781-341-6333
Stoughton, MA 02072   800-673-6922
                                                  Fax: 781-341-8333
                                           e-mail: NSF@scoliosis.org
                                                   www.scoliosis.org

Joseph P O'Brien, President/CEO

7286 You and Your Brace
University Hospital Spine Center
2074 Abington Road   216-844-1616
Cleveland, OH 44106

Audio & Video

7287 Cutting Edge Medical Report
National Scoliosis Foundation
5 Cabot Place   781-341-6333
Stoughton, MA 02072   800-673-6922
                                  Fax: 781-341-8333
                            e-mail: NSF@scoliosis.org
                                    www.scoliosis.org
As seen on the Discovery Channel, this video is an indepth exami-
nation of the latest developments in the diagnosis and treatment of
scoliosis.
Joseph P O'Brien, President/CEO

7288 Growing Straighter and Stronger
National Scoliosis Foundation
5 Cabot Place   781-341-6333
Stoughton, MA 02072   800-673-6922
                                  Fax: 781-341-8333
                            e-mail: NSF@scoliosis.org
                                    www.scoliosis.org
Fifteen-minute presentation available in VHS video format, for the
pre-screening education of students in grades 5 through 7.
Videotape
Joseph P O'Brien, President/CEO

**7289 Preparing Yourself for Spinal Surgery for Teenagers with Severe
Scoliosis**
National Scoliosis Foundation
5 Cabot Place   781-341-6333
Stoughton, MA 02072   800-673-6922
                                  Fax: 781-341-8333
                            e-mail: NSF@scoliosis.org
                                    www.scoliosis.org
Patient education video helping to reduce anxiety for teenagers
facing surgery by giving a sense of what to expect before, during,
and after surgery.
Joseph P O'Brien, President/CEO

7290 School Screening with Dr. Robert Keller
National Scoliosis Foundation
5 Cabot Place   781-341-6333
Stoughton, MA 02072   800-673-6922
                                  Fax: 781-341-8333
                            e-mail: NSF@scoliosis.org
                                    www.scoliosis.org
Training video that teaches the proper technique for doing spinal
screening. Defines scoliosis and kyphosis. Four teenagers, three
with curves and one without, are examined and the findings
explained.
Videotape
Joseph P O'Brien, President/CEO

7291 Scoliosis: An Adult Perspective
National Scoliosis Foundation
5 Cabot Place   781-341-6333
Stoughton, MA 02072   800-673-6922
                                  Fax: 781-341-8333
                            e-mail: NSF@scoliosis.org
                                    www.scoliosis.org
Dr. Blackman and five women patients provide an overall perspec-
tive of what scoliosis is, who gets it, the types of devices, myths
about the disorder, and options for treatment.
Joseph P O'Brien, President/CEO

7292 Sharing Scoliosis: You're Not Alone
National Scoliosis Foundation
5 Cabot Place   781-341-6333
Stoughton, MA 02072   800-673-6922
                                  Fax: 781-341-8333
                            e-mail: NSF@scoliosis.org
                                    www.scoliosis.org
The Missouri chapter of the NSF, shares their experience with
scoliosis including diagnosis, wearing a brace, surgery, and recovery. It is a good source of support for patients of all ages and their
families.
Joseph P O'Brien, President/CEO

7293 Spinal Screening Program
Scoliosis Research Society

555 East Wells Street   414-289-9107
Milwaukee, WI 53202   Fax: 414-276-3349
                                          www.srs.com
Twenty minute videotape designed to instruct screeners in the spi-
nal screening program. It demonstrates methods of screening,
showing adolescents with normal and abnormal spines. Includes
sample screening form.
VHS Video Tape
Tressa Goulding, Executive Director

7294 Taking the Mystery Out of Spinal Deformities
Children's Hospital of LA, Div. of Orthopaedics
4650 Sunset Boulevard   213-660-2450
Los Angeles, CA 90027   800-841-7439
                         e-mail: RWETZEL@chla.usc.edu
Answers questions most often asked by screeners, patients and
parents.
Videotape

7295 Understanding Scoliosis
National Scoliosis Foundation
5 Cabot Place   781-341-6333
Stoughton, MA 02072   800-673-6922
                                  Fax: 781-341-8333
                            e-mail: NSF@scoliosis.org
                                    www.scoliosis.org
Kaiser Permanente's educational video clearly and positively ad-
dresses the patient community. In this video four teenagers at vari-
ous stages of treatment talk about their life with scoliosis.
Joseph P O'Brien, President/CEO

7296 What's This Thing Called Scoliosis
National Scoliosis Foundation
5 Cabot Place   781-341-6333
Stoughton, MA 02072   800-673-6922
                                  Fax: 781-341-8333
                            e-mail: NSF@scoliosis.org
                                    www.scoliosis.org
Comprehensive overview of scoliosis using the latest computer
technology. The anatomical spine and animated model work together to truly show the 3D aspects of scoliosis and the corresponding impact on the patient.
Joseph P O'Brien, President/CEO

7297 You Are Not Alone
Minnesota Spine Center
606 24th Avenue S   612-332-3843
Minneapolis, MN 55454-1438
A video presenting two women's experiences with surgery. Per-
sonal life, concerns, hospital experience, recovery and improved
lifestyle are openly discussed.
Videotape

Web Sites

7298 American Association of Neurological Surgeons
                              www.neurosurgery.org/
Official web site of the American Association of Neurological Surgeons and Congress of Neurological Surgeons. Whether you are a
patient, physician, health care professional, or member of the media, this site is your online resource for neurosurgical information.

7299 British Scoliosis Research Society
                                www.ndos.ox.ac.uk/pzs/
This site contains: background to the meeting, Scoliosis Research
Society review papers on the aetiology of idiopathic scoliosis, a
list of participants, abstracts classified by discussion group and the
chairman's conclusions for each group.

7300 Healing Well
                                    www.healingwell.com
An online health resource guide to medical news, chat, information and articles, newsgroups and message boards, books, disease-related web sites, medical directories, and more for patients,
friends, and family coping with disabling diseases, disorders, or
chronic illnesses.

7301 Health Finder
                                    www.healthfinder.gov

Searchable, carefully developed web site offering information on over 1000 topics. Developed by the US Department of Health and Human Services, the site can be used in both English and Spanish.

7302 Healthlink USA

www.healthlinkusa.com

Health information concerning treatment, cures, prevention, diagnosis, risk factors, research, support groups, email lists, personal stories and much more. Updated regularly.

7303 Helios Health

www.helioshealth.com

Online resource for your health information. Detailed information about specific health topics, access to expert advice from our Medical Advisory Board, and up-to-date health news.

7304 MedicineNet

www.medicinenet.com

An online resource for consumers providing easy-to-read, authoritative medical and health information.

7305 Medscape

www.medscape.com

Medscape offers specialists, primary care physicians, and other health professionals the Web's most robust and integrated medical information and educational tools.

7306 Patients Rate Their Scoliosis Doctors

This web site is a free internet service for communicating subjective impressions of medical doctor (MD) reputations among scoliosis patients. Please use this system to learn some of the subjective impressions of the treatment other patients have received from their doctors.

7307 Scoliosis Association

www.sauk.org.uk/

The Scoliosis Association (UK) was founded in 1981. It is the only independent support group for scoliosis in the UK. SAUK aims to provide information about scoliosis, eliminate fear and stigma, and offer contacts for shared experiences.

7308 WebMD

www.webmd.com

Information on scoliosis, including articles and resources.

Description

7309 Seizure Disorders

There are two types of seizure disorders: an isolated, nonrecurring attack, such as may occur with high fevers in children, head trauma, or from other diseases (metabolic abnormalities or brain tumor) and epilepsy, which is characterized by recurrent, sudden, rapid changes in brain function caused by abnormalities in the electrical activity of the brain. Roughly 2 million Americans suffer from epilepsy, with half of the cases found in children and adolescents.

Seizures can be classified as generalized, affecting the whole brain at once, or partial, affecting a part of the brain. Absence (petit mal) attacks are generalized seizures in which there is only a brief (10-30 second) loss of consciousness, with eye and muscle fluttering but no loss of muscle tone. A generalized tonic-clonic seizure (grand mal) usually lasts 1-2 minutes, and includes loss of consciousness, falling, and involuntary contractions of the arms and legs. Some patients report that they see flashing lights and experience a heightened sense of taste and smell (known as an aura) that indicates they are about to have a seizure.

In many cases there is no apparent cause of the disorder, and it is therefore called idiopathic epilepsy.

Treatment aims primarily to control seizures. Causative or precipitating factors should be eliminated. Drug treatment is the mainstay of therapy for most types of seizures. In order to limit toxic effects, an attempt is made to use only a single drug. Some patients may need to take more than one drug. In most cases, acceptable control can be achieved with medications alone. Rarely, seizures will not respond to drugs, and surgery on the brain will be recommended. In this procedure, the surgeon tries to identify and destroy the part of the brain that is triggering the seizures.

National Agencies & Associations

7310 American Epilepsy Society
342 N Main Street 860-586-7505
W Hartford, CT 06117-2500 Fax: 860-568-7550
e-mail: ctubby@aesnet.org
www.aesnet.org
Fosters treatment of epilepsy in its biological clinical and social phases.
M Suzanne C Berry, Executive Director
Cheryl-Ann Tubby, Assistant Executive Director

7311 Epilepsy Foundation
8301 Professional Place 866-330-2718
Landover, MD 20785 800-332-1000
Fax: 301-459-1569
e-mail: postmaster@efa.org
www.epilepsyfoundation.org
A national charitable nonprofit volunteer agency in the US dedicated to the welfare of people with epilepsy. Its goals are the prevention and cure of seizure disorders, the alleviation of their effects and the promotion of independence.
Lee Gaston, CFO
Phil Gattone, President & CEO

7312 National Association of Epilepsy Centers
5775 Wayzata Boulevard 202-484-1100
Minneapolis, MN 55416-1222 888-525-6232
Fax: 202-484-1244
e-mail: info@naec-epilepsy.org
www.naec-epilepsy.org
A nonprofit organization that encourages and supports professional and technical education in the treatment of epilepsy. Over 50 centers nationwide are members of the trade association which will make referrals to its member centers.
David M. Labiner, President
Nathan B. Fountain, VP

7313 National Institute of Neurological Disorders and Stroke
NIH Neurological Institute 301-496-5751
Bethesda, MD 20824 800-352-9424
Fax: 301-402-2186
TTY: 301-468-5981
www.ninds.nih.gov
The mission of NINDS is to reduce the burden of neurological disease - a burden borne by every age group, by every segment of society, by people all over the world.
Story C Landis PhD, Director
Walter J Koroshetz, Deputy Director

State Agencies & Associations

California

7314 Epilepsy Foundation of Northern California
5700 Stoneridge Mall Road 415-677-4011
Pleasanton, CA 94588-2824 800-632-3532
Fax: 415-677-4190
e-mail: efnca@epilepsynorcal.org
www.epilepsynorcal.org
Nonprofit organization serving families affected by epilepsy.
Katherine Keene, President & CEO
Mary Lee Cascino, Programme Manager

Florida

7315 Epilepsy Association of Big Bend
1215 Lee Avenue 850-222-1777
Tallahassee, FL 32303-2651 Fax: 850-222-7440
e-mail: epilepsyassoc@embarqmail.com
www.epilepsyassoc.org
Services include: Case management, prevention education, counseling and advocacy, information and referral.

7316 Epilepsy Foundation of South Florida
7300 N Kendall Drive 305-670-4949
Miami, FL 33156-7840 Fax: 305-670-0904
e-mail: information@epilepsysofla.org
www.epilepsyfound.org
A twenty five year old nonprofit community based organization dedicated to enhancing the personal and social adjustments of individuals with seizure disorders and their families.
Karen Basha Egozi, Executive Director
Ana Alfonso, Executive Administrator

7317 Epilepsy Services Foundation
4618 N Armenia Avenue 813-374-8907
Tampa, FL 33603-2706 Fax: 813-443-5546
e-mail: info@epilepsysf.org
www.epilepsysf.org
Information on medical and supportive services for persons affected by epilepsy living in West Central Florida. Raise funds to provide medical and supportive services and to build an endowment to make a difference in the lives of generations to come.
Thomas Orth, Executive Director

7318 Epilepsy Services of North Central Florida
11200 NW 8th Avenue 352-392-6449
Gainesville, FL 32601-4946 800-330-9746
Fax: 352-392-5792
e-mail: jlyons@college.med.ufl.edu
www.floridaepilepsy.org/northcentral.htm
Jim Lyons, Program Director
Mike Dorsey, PE Coordinator

7319 Epilepsy Services of Northeast Florida
5209 San Jose Boulevard   904-731-3751
Jacksonville, FL 32207-2267   e-mail: epilepsy@bellsouth.net
Services include: Program case management, program prevention
and education, employment services, children's summer camp,
counseling and advocacy, and information and referrals.

7320 Epilepsy Services of Southwest Florida
1900 Main Street   941-953-5988
Sarasota, FL 34236   Fax: 941-366-5890
                                 www.epilepsyservicesofswfl.org
Dedicated to providing case management and medical services for
individuals with seizure disorders who meet eligibility criteria.
Provides employment education for individuals and families af-
fected by seizure disorders and prevention education to the com
Thomas Garrity, Executive Director

7321 Manattee County Office Epilepsy Services of Southwest Florida
1701 14th Street W   941-746-6488
Bradenton, FL 34205-7132   Fax: 941-746-8382
                                 e-mail: bardentonep@aol.com

Brian Larocque, Social Worker

New Jersey

7322 Epilepsy Foundation of New Jersey
429 River View Plaza   800-336-5843
Trenton, NJ 08611-3420   800-336-5843
                                      Fax: 609-392-5621
                                      TTY: 800-852-7899
                                      TDD: 800-852-7899
                                 e-mail: efnj@efnj.com
                                           www.efnj.com

Robert L. D'Avanzo, President
Michael P. Rinaldo, Chairman of the Board

New York

7323 Epilepsy Foundation of Long Island
506 Stewart Avenue   516-739-7733
Garden City, NY 11530-4700   888-672-7154
                                      Fax: 516-794-2180
                                 e-mail: info@epil.org
                                           www.efli.org

Jeffrey L. Nagel, President
Henry Klosowski, Vice President

Pennsylvania

7324 Epilepsy Foundation of Western Pennsylvania
1323 Forbes Avenue   412-261-5880
Pittsburgh, PA 15219-4725   Fax: 412-261-5361
                                 e-mail: staff@efwp.org
                                           www.efwp.org

Judith K. Painter, Executive Director
Peggy Beem, Associate Director

Washington

7325 Epilepsy Foundation of North West Washington
2311 N 45th Street   206-547-4551
Seattle, WA 98103   800-752-3509
                                      Fax: 206-547-4557
                                 e-mail: mail@epilepsynw.org
                                           www.epilepsyfoundation.org

Brent Herrmann, President/CEO
Alta C Hancock, Associate Director

Research Centers

7326 Baylor College of Medicine: Epilepsy Research Center
Texas Medical Center
6550 Fannin   713-798-4333
Houston, TX 77030   Fax: 713-798-7533
                                 e-mail: neurochair@bcm.edu
                                           www.bcm.edu/neurology

The clinical program at Baylor College of Medicine for the comprehensive evaluation of those with epilepsy or those suspected of
having seizures or epilepsy.
Eli Mizrahi MD, Director

7327 Duke University Center for the Advanced Study of Epilepsy
Duke Neuroscience Clinic
200 Trent Drive   919-668-7600
Durham, NC 27710   888-ASK-DUKE
                                           www.dukehealth.org
Clinical and research unit that experiments in limbic epilepsy.
James McNama MD, Director
William B Gallentine

7328 Neurology Research Center Helen Hayes Hospital
Helen Hayes Hospital
53-55 Route 9W   845-786-4535
W Haverstraw, NY 10993   888-70R-EHAB
                                      Fax: 845-947-3097
                                 e-mail: info@helenhayeshospital.org
                                           www.helenhayeshospital.org
Robert Linds MD, Chief Internal medicine
Jason P Greenberg, Assistant Clinical Professor of Neurolog

7329 University of Illinois at Chicago Consultation Clinic for Epilepsy
912 S Wood Street   312-996-7000
Chicago, IL 60612-7330   800-842-1002
                                      Fax: 312-633-3434
                                      TTY: 312-413-0123
                                 e-mail: neu50@uic.edu
                                           www.uic.edu

Paula Allen Meares, Chancellor
Lon S. Kauffman, Vice Chancellor

7330 University of Tennessee: Center for Neuroscience
875 Monroe Avenue   901-448-5960
Memphis, TN 38163-0001   Fax: 901-448-4685
                                           www.uthsc.edu/neuroscience/
Epilepsy research and studies.
William E Armstrong, Director
Anton J Reiner, Co-Director

7331 University of Wisconsin Madison Neurophysiology Laboratory
UW Hospital and Clinics
600 Highland Avenue   608-263-6400
Madison, WI 53792   800-323-8942
                                      Fax: 608-265-5512
                                           www.uwhealth.org
Epilepsy research.
Thomas P Sutula, Chairman of Neurology
Paul A Rutecki, Vice Chairman of Neurology

Support Groups & Hotlines

7332 Epilepsy Foundation of America Helpline
Epilepsy Foundation of America
4351 Garden City Drive   866-330-1000
Landover, MD 20785-7223   800-332-1000
                                      Fax: 301-459-1569
                                 e-mail: postmaster@esa.org
                                           www.epilepsyfoundation.org
A toll free information and referral service staffed by specially
trained people who will answer questions and discuss concerns
about seizure disorders and their treatment. Staff will direct callers
to local affiliates of the EFA and tell about a broad range of medical
services that respond to the needs of people with seizure disorders.
Phil Gattone, Chief Executive Officer

7333 National Health Information Center
PO Box 1133   310-565-4167
Washington, DC 20013   800-336-4797
                                      Fax: 301-984-4256
                                 e-mail: info@nhic.org
                                           www.health.gov/nhic
Offers a nationwide information referral service, produces direc-
tories and resource guides.

Books

7334 Americans with Disabilities Act
Epilepsy Foundation of America
4351 Garden City Drive   301-459-3700
Landover, MD 20785-2267   800-332-1000
                                            Fax: 301-577-9056
Learn how the Americans With Disabilities Act of 1990 can benifit you. Excellent comprehensive resource for individuals with seizure disorders.
46 pages Softcover
ISBN: 0-802774-65-2

7335 Bomb in the Brain: A Heroic Tale of Science, Surgery and Survival
MacMillan Publishing Company
866 3rd Avenue   212-702-2000
New York, NY 10022
The autobiographical account of this author's struggle with epilepsy and the debilitating effects it has on health, emotions, and mental stability.
Grades 10-12

7336 Brainstorms: Epilepsy in Our Words
4351 Garden City Drive   301-459-3700
Landover, MD 20785-2267   800-332-1000
                                            Fax: 301-577-9056
Patients describe their experiences with seizures. Sixty-eight in-depth personal accounts of actual seizures are followed by a short section on how epilepsy affects the lives of the patients.
197 pages Paperback
ISBN: 0-802774-65-2

7337 Children with Epilepsy
Epilepsy Foundation of America
4351 Garden City Drive   301-459-3700
Landover, MD 20785-2267   800-332-1000
                                            Fax: 301-577-9056
Offers direction and support to parents of a child with epilepsy, by first educating them about epilepsy and then helping them cope with the effects this disorder will have on their child and family.
314 pages Paperback
ISBN: 0-933149-19-0

7338 Does Your Child Have Epilepsy?
4351 Garden City Drive   301-459-3700
Landover, MD 20785-2267   800-332-1000
                                            Fax: 301-577-9056
This book establishes Ten Basic Rules for parents of children with epilepsy.
201 pages Softcover

7339 Embrace the Dawn
Epilepsy Foundation of America
4351 Garden City Drive   301-459-3700
Landover, MD 20785-2267   800-332-1000
                                            Fax: 301-577-9056
A moving biographical account of one person's lifelong experience with epilepsy.
127 pages Softcover

7340 Epilepsy A to Z
4351 Garden City Drive   301-459-3700
Landover, MD 20785-2267   800-332-1000
                                            Fax: 301-577-9056
This book is designed to give health-care personnel a convenient way to find brief answers to questions about epilepsy. It includes definitions of terms, ranging all the way from abdominal epilepsy to Zonisimide.
322 pages Softcover

7341 Epilepsy Diet Treatment: An Introduction to the Ketogenic Diet
Epilepsy Foundation of America
4351 Garden City Drive   301-459-3700
Landover, MD 20785-2267   800-332-1000
                                            Fax: 301-577-9056
The only book devoted exclusively to the ketogenic diet - a rigid, mathematically calculated, doctor-supervised diet that is high in fat and low in carbohydrate and protein with strictly limited calories and liquid intake. Gives all the facts about the diet, plus quotes from parents showing what the experience is really like and 30 sample recipes.
1996 200 pages
ISBN: 0-939957-86-8

7342 Epilepsy Surgery
Raven Press
1185 Avenue of the Americas   212-930-9500
New York, NY 10036-2601
The most complete and current references on surgical treatments of the epilepsies.
880 pages
ISBN: 0-881678-21-0

7343 Epilepsy and the Family: A New Guide
Harvard University Press
79 Garden Street
Cambridge, MA 02138   800-448-2242
                        www.hup.harvard.edu/catalog/LECEPF.html

ISBN: 0-674258-97-5

7344 Epilepsy: 199 Answers
Demos Medical Publishing
386 Park Avenue S   212-683-0072
New York, NY 10016-8804   800-532-8663
                                        Fax: 212-683-0118
                            e-mail: orderdept@demosmed.com
                                       www.demosmedpub.com
Addresses the needs of everyone with epilepsy. A helpful guide to the most common questions asked by people with epilepsy and will help the reader to work with his physician and take charge of the epilepsy.
1996 152 pages
ISBN: 1-888799-09-9
Dr. Diana M Schneider, President

7345 Epilepsy: A Behavior Medicine Approach to Assessment & Treatment in Children
Hogrefe & Huber Publications
PO Box 51   716-282-1610
Lewiston, NY 14092-0051   Fax: 716-484-4200
1993 200 pages
ISBN: 0-889371-06-7

7346 Epilepsy: Current Approaches to Diagnosis and Treatment
Raven Press
1185 Avenue of the Americas   212-930-9500
New York, NY 10036-2601
288 pages
ISBN: 0-881676-15-2

7347 Epilepsy: I Can Live with That
4351 Garden City Drive   301-459-3700
Landover, MD 20785-2267   800-332-1000
                                            Fax: 301-577-9056

The experience of epilepsy as recorded by a group of ordinary men and women living in Australia. Each story focuses on personal growth, triumph over disability and emphasizes individual courage and hope.
Softcover
ISBN: 0-802774-65-2

7348 Epilepsy: Models, Mechanisms & Concepts
Cambridge University Press
40 W 20th Street   212-924-3900
New York, NY 10011-4211   800-221-4512
                                        Fax: 212-691-3239
                          e-mail: customerservice@cup.org
                                               www.cup.org

1993 400 pages
ISBN: 0-521392-98-5
Alice Ra, Assistant Marketing Manager

7349 Epilepsy: Patient and Family Guide
O Devinsky, MD, author

FA Davis Company

1915 Arch Street   215-568-2172
Philadelphia, PA 19103   800-523-4049
Fax: 215-568-5065
e-mail: mrt@fadavis.com
www.fadavis.com

Epilepsy expert Dr. Orrin Devinsky provides an easy-to-read guide to understanding the disease so that patients can achieve — and maintain — a higher quality of life. This book will educate recently-diagnosed patients, as well as those who have been living with epilepsy for years.

434 pages Paperback
ISBN: 0-803604-98-X
Michael Torso, Marketing Manager

7350 Equal Partners
Epilepsy Foundation of America
4351 Garden City Drive   301-459-3700
Landover, MD 20785-2267   800-332-1000
Fax: 301-577-9056

This book tells the story of a young Harvard-trained doctor whose experiences with seizures, brain surgery and subsequent epilepsy turns her from physician to patient.

257 pages Hardcover
ISBN: 0-802774-65-2

7351 Guide to Understanding and Living with Epilepsy
4351 Garden City Drive   301-459-3700
Landover, MD 20785-2267   800-332-1000
Fax: 301-577-9056

Easy-to-understand resource for people with epilepsy and their families. Covers a wide range of medical, social and legal issues. Topics include expanation of seizures and epilepsy; information about medication, side effects and risks; and getting the best medical care.

7352 Ketogenic Diet: A Treatment for Epilepsy
Demos Medical Publishing
386 Park Avenue S   212-683-0072
New York, NY 10016   Fax: 212-683-0118
e-mail: orderdept@demopub.com
www.demosmedpub.com

256 pages
ISBN: 1-888799-39-0
Dr. Diana M Schneider

7353 Living Well with Epilepsy
Epilepsy Foundation of America
4351 Garden City Drive   301-459-3700
Landover, MD 20785-2267   800-332-1000
Fax: 301-577-9056

Designed to help both health-care professionals and patients to understand all aspects of diagnosis and of pharmacologic and surgical management; to enable patients to participate more knowledgeably in interactions with their health care team and to help steer them toward a more normal, fulfilling life.

166 pages Softcover
ISBN: 1-888799-11-0

7354 Managing Seizure Disorder
Epilepsy Foundation of America
4351 Garden City Drive   301-459-3700
Landover, MD 20785-2267   800-332-1000
Fax: 301-577-9056

Provides health professionals with detailed information, on a variety of subjects, designed to help them help people with epilepsy live the kind of life they desire.

276 pages Softcover
ISBN: 0-802774-65-2

7355 Miles to Go Before I Sleep
Epilepsy Foundation of America
4351 Garden City Drive   301-459-3700
Landover, MD 20785-2267   800-332-1000
Fax: 301-577-9056

This book tells the story of a hijacking in which the author sustained a severe brain injury that, among other things, affected her vision, her memory, and left her with epilepsy.

230 pages Hardcover
ISBN: 0-802774-65-2

7356 Students with Seizures: A Manual for School Nurses
Epilepsy Foundation of America
4351 Garden City Drive   301-459-3700
Landover, MD 20785-2267   800-332-1000
Fax: 301-577-9056

A professional text with the sole purpose of creating a more accepting and understanding school environment for children with seizure disorders.

131 pages Paperback

Children's Books

7357 Dotty the Dalmatian has Epilepsy
Epilepsy Foundation of America
4351 Garden City Drive   301-459-3700
Landover, MD 20785-2267   800-332-1000
Fax: 301-577-9056

This is the story of Dotty the Dalmatian who discovers she has epilepsy.

16 pages Softcover
ISBN: 0-802774-65-2

7358 Epilepsy
Franklin Watts Grolier
90 Old Sherman Tpke   203-797-3500
Danbury, CT 06816-0001   800-621-1115
Fax: 203-797-3197
www.grolier.com

This book explains what epilepsy is, causes of epileptic seizures, diagnosis and treatments.

96 pages Grades 7-12
ISBN: 0-531108-07-4

7359 Lee the Rabbit with Epilepsy
4351 Garden City Drive   301-459-3700
Landover, MD 20785-2267   800-332-1000
Fax: 301-577-9056

Written for children ages 3-6, this illustrated picture book follows the adventures of a small rabbit who has seizures during a fishing trip with her Grandpa.

23 pages Hardcover

7360 Season of Secrets
Little, Brown & Company
3 Center Plz   617-227-0730
Boston, MA 02108   800-759-0190
Fax: 800-286-9471

Grades 4-6

Newsletters

7361 Epilepsia: Journal of the International League Against Epilepsy
Blackwell Publishing, Inc.
Commerce Place   781-388-8200
Malden, MA 02148   800-862-6657
Fax: 781-388-8210
www.blackwellpublishing.com

The leading international journal on the epilepsies for more than 30 years, Epilepsia provides comprehensive coverage of current clinical and research results.

7362 Epilepsy Services Foundation Newsletter
4618 N Armenia Avenue   813-870-3414
Tampa, FL 33603-2706   Fax: 813-870-1321
e-mail: eswcf@epilepsyservices.com
www.epilepsyservices.com

Information on medical and supportive services for persons affected by epilepsy living in West Central Florida. Raise funds to provide medical and supportive services to build and endowment to make a difference in the lives of generations to come.

2 pages 2-3 x/year
Thomas Orth, Executive Director

Pamphlets

7363 Child with Epilepsy at Camp
Epilepsy Foundation of America
4351 Garden City Drive   301-459-3700
Landover, MD 20785-2267   800-332-1000
Fax: 301-577-9056
Helps to explain why the child with epilepsy should be included in the camping experience.
14 pages Pamphlet

7364 Children and Seizures: Information for Babysitters
Epilepsy Foundation of America
4351 Garden City Drive   301-459-3700
Landover, MD 20785-2267   800-332-1000
Fax: 301-577-9056
Explains seizures, routine and special care, emergency aid and first aid to babysitters. Also offers a graph to write down important information about the child with seizure disorders for a quick reference.

7365 Epilepsy Medicines and Dental Care
Epilepsy Foundation of America
4351 Garden City Drive   301-459-3700
Landover, MD 20785-2267   800-332-1000
Fax: 301-577-9056
Explains dental care and includes instructions for brushing and flossing.

7366 Epilepsy: Legal Rights, Legal Issues
Epilepsy Foundation of America
4351 Garden City Drive   301-459-3700
Landover, MD 20785-2267   800-332-1000
Fax: 301-577-9056
Offers persons diagnosed with epilepsy information on their legal rights in employment, education, insurance and general disability benefits.
9 pages

7367 Epilepsy: Part of Your Life Series
Epilepsy Foundation of America
4351 Garden City Drive   301-459-3700
Landover, MD 20785-2267   800-332-1000
Fax: 301-577-9056
Provides information for staying healthy, describes various tests and diagnostic procedures, includes information for parents of children with epilepsy and provides general answers to questions about epilepsy.
Series of 4

7368 Epilepsy: You and Your Child, a Guide for Parents
Epilepsy Foundation of America
4351 Garden City Drive   301-459-3700
Landover, MD 20785-2267   800-332-1000
Fax: 301-577-9056
This instructional booklet offers information on emotional aspects of epilepsy, how to handle seizures, medication, diet and nutrition, and offers referral organizations for parents.

7369 Epilepsy: You and Your Treatment
Epilepsy Foundation of America
4351 Garden City Drive   301-459-3700
Landover, MD 20785-2267   800-332-1000
Fax: 301-577-9056
Reviews medical tests and diagnostic procedures used by physicians in diagnosing epilepsy.

7370 Facts About Epilepsy
Epilepsy Foundation of America
4351 Garden City Drive   301-459-3700
Landover, MD 20785-2267   800-332-1000
Fax: 301-577-9056
Designed for use by physicians and other health professionals with an interest in or who deal with the problems of people with epilepsy.
16 pages Softcover

7371 Finding Out About Seizures: A Guide to Medical Tests
Epilepsy Foundation of America
4351 Garden City Drive   301-459-3700
Landover, MD 20785-2267   800-332-1000
Fax: 301-577-9056
Introduces adults and children with epilepsy to the types of tests they may have to undergo.

7372 Kits for Adults with Epilepsy
Epilepsy Foundation of America
4351 Garden City Drive   301-459-3700
Landover, MD 20785-2267   800-332-1000
Fax: 301-577-9056
A variety of informative pamphlets for persons with epilepsy or seizure disorders.

7373 Management by Common Sense
Epilepsy Foundation of America
4351 Garden City Drive   301-459-3700
Landover, MD 20785-2267   800-332-1000
Fax: 301-577-9056
Promotes the employability of people with seizure disorders. Provides employers with information about epilepsy, customer/client reactions, workers' compensation issues, side effects of medication and other information relevant to employing a person with epilepsy.
46 pages Paperback
ISBN: 0-802774-65-2

7374 Me and My World Packet for Children
Epilepsy Foundation of America
4351 Garden City Drive   301-459-3700
Landover, MD 20785-2267   800-332-1000
Fax: 301-577-9056
Collection of pamphlets designed for children with epilepsy.

7375 Medicines for Epilepsy
Epilepsy Foundation of America
4351 Garden City Drive   301-459-3700
Landover, MD 20785-2267   800-332-1000
Fax: 301-577-9056
Offers information on medication and treatments, generic drugs, side effects, drug abuse and more. Contains a color chart with picyures of the most common medications for epilepsy.

7376 Mom I Have a Staring Problem
Epilepsy Foundation of America
4351 Garden City Drive   301-459-3700
Landover, MD 20785-2267   800-332-1000
Fax: 301-577-9056
Tiffany, a seven-year-old, describes her experience with petit mal seizures; her feelings, wishes and fears. Written to help adults recognize a hidden problem that could be occuring with a child who has learning problems.
24 pages Softcover
ISBN: 0-802774-65-2

7377 My Brother Matthew
Woodbine House
4351 Garden City Drive   301-459-3700
Landover, MD 20785-2267   800-332-1000
Fax: 301-577-9056
A picture and text book for children who have a brother or sister with developmental delay.
25 pages Harcoverr
ISBN: 0-802774-65-2

7378 My Friend Emily
Epilepsy Foundation of America
4351 Garden City Drive   301-459-3700
Landover, MD 20785-2267   800-332-1000
Fax: 301-577-9056
A story about Emily and her best friend Katy. Emily, a self confident child who enjoys life, shows that kids with epilepsy are just like other kids.
35 pages Softcover
ISBN: 0-802774-65-2

7379 Patient's Guide to Everyday Life
Epilepsy Foundation of America
4351 Garden City Drive   301-459-3700
Landover, MD 20785-2267   800-332-1000
Fax: 301-577-9056

Provides information for the newly diagnosed individual with epilepsy.

7380 Preventing Epilepsy
Epilepsy Foundation of America
4351 Garden City Drive   301-459-3700
Landover, MD 20785-2267   800-332-1000
                                     Fax: 301-577-9056
Examines some known causes of seizures and suggests precautionary measures which may prevent the occurrence of epilepsy.
16 pages

7381 Recognizing the Signs of Childhood Seizures
Epilepsy Foundation of America
4351 Garden City Drive   301-459-3700
Landover, MD 20785-2267   800-332-1000
                                     Fax: 301-577-9056
Explains what seizures are and what to look for in your child.

7382 Seizure Recognition and First Aid
Epilepsy Foundation of America
4351 Garden City Drive   301-459-3700
Landover, MD 20785-2267   800-332-1000
                                     Fax: 301-577-9056
Helps you recognize a seizure when it happens and give basic first aid.

7383 Surgery for Epilepsy
Epilepsy Foundation of America
4351 Garden City Drive   301-459-3700
Landover, MD 20785-2267   800-332-1000
                                     Fax: 301-577-9056
Describes current surgical treatment and the testing that precedes it.
12 pages

7384 Talking to Your Doctor About Seizure Disorders
Epilepsy Foundation of America
4351 Garden City Drive   301-459-3700
Landover, MD 20785-2267   800-332-1000
                                     Fax: 301-577-9056
Designed to help the patient talk with medical personnel about treatment of epilepsy.
Pamphlet

7385 Teacher's Role, A Guide for School Personnel
Epilepsy Foundation of America
4351 Garden City Drive   301-459-3700
Landover, MD 20785-2267   800-332-1000
                                     Fax: 301-577-9056
Provides tips on recognizing seizures and handling a seizure in the classroom.
14 pages

Audio & Video

7386 Comprehensive Clinical Management of the Epilepsies
Epilepsy Foundation of America
4351 Garden City Drive   301-459-3700
Landover, MD 20785-2267   800-332-1000
                                     Fax: 301-577-9056
Excellent reference on the treatment of epilepsy.
17 minutes

7387 How to Recognize and Classify Seizures
Epilepsy Foundation of America
4351 Garden City Drive   301-459-3700
Landover, MD 20785-2267   800-332-1000
                                     Fax: 301-577-9056
Discusses the classification of seizures and epileptic syndromes.
25 minutes

7388 Just Like You and Me
TASH
1025 Vermont Avenue   202-263-5600
Washington, DC 20005   Fax: 202-637-0138
                             e-mail: btrader@tash.org
                             www.tash.org/index.html

A video/print package on successful living with epilepsy.
Lu Zeph, Executive of Board Operating Committee
Barbara A Trader, Human Resources Director

7389 Meeting the Challenge: Employment Issues and Epilepsy
Epilepsy Foundation of America
4351 Garden City Drive   301-459-3700
Landover, MD 20785-2267   800-332-1000
                                     Fax: 301-577-2684
This video answers the fquestions most often asked by emloyers. It covers issues such as driving, absenteeism, productivity, accidents and first aid, and emphasized that most people with epilepsy can be gainfully employed.
9 minutes

7390 Rest of the Family
Epilepsy Foundation of America
4351 Garden City Drive   301-459-3700
Landover, MD 20785-2267   800-332-1000
                                     Fax: 301-577-9056
Presents the feelings and concerns of other family members including siblings, of children with epilepsy.
Video cassette

7391 Seizure First Aid
Epilepsy Foundation of America
4351 Garden City Drive   301-459-3700
Landover, MD 20785-2267   800-332-1000
                                     Fax: 301-577-9056
This video combines footage of real seizures with reenactments to demonstrate proper first aid procedures. In addition, people with epilepsy talk about how they feel when they have a seizure, discuss how they would like friends, family and the general public to react when a seizure occurs.
10 minutes

7392 Understanding Seizure Disorders
Epilepsy Foundation of America
4351 Garden City Drive   301-459-3700
Landover, MD 20785-2267   800-332-1000
                                     Fax: 301-577-9056
Provides an explanation of seizure disorders in everyday language and dispels many misconceptions about epilepsy with medically accurate information.
Video cassette

7393 Voices from the Workplace
Epilepsy Foundation of America
Epilepsy Foundation of America   301-459-3700
4351 Garden City Drive, MD 20785   800-332-1000
                                     Fax: 301-577-2684
Inspirational tape to help people with epilepsy cope with employment challenges. Individuals with epilepsy describe personal and social challenges in the workplace. They explain how they cope with their seizures and the reactions of co-workers and the public.

Web Sites

7394 American Epilepsy Society
                                     www.aesnet.org
Fosters treatment of epilepsy in its biological, clinical and social phases.

7395 Epilepsy Foundation of America
                                     www.efa.org
Information on the prevention and cure of seizure disorders, the alleviation of their effects, and the promotion of independence and optimal quality of life for people who have these disorders.

7396 Healing Well
                                     www.healingwell.com
An online health resource guide to medical news, chat, information and articles, newsgroups and message boards, books, disease-related web sites, medical directories, and more for patients, friends, and family coping with disabling diseases, disorders, or chronic illnesses.

7397 Health Finder
                                     www.healthfinder.gov

Searchable, carefully developed web site offering information on over 1000 topics. Developed by the US Department of Health and Human Services, the site can be used in both English and Spanish.

7398   Healthlink USA

www.healthlinkusa.com

Health information concerning treatment, cures, prevention, diagnosis, risk factors, research, support groups, email lists, personal stories and much more. Updated regularly.

7399   Helios Health

www.helioshealth.com

Online resource for your health information. Detailed information about specific health topics, access to expert advice from our Medical Advisory Board, and up-to-date health news.

7400   MedicineNet

www.medicinenet.com

An online resource for consumers providing easy-to-read, authoritative medical and health information.

7401   Medscape

www.medscape.com

Medscape offers specialists, primary care physicians, and other health professionals the Web's most robust and integrated medical information and educational tools.

7402   National Institute of Neurological Disorders and Stroke

www.ninds.nih.gov

The mission of NINDS is to reduce the burden of neurological disease - a burden borne by every age group, by every segment of society, by people all over the world.

7403   Neurology Channel

www.neurologychannel.com

Find clearly explained, medically accurate information regarding conditions, including an overview, symptoms, causes, diagnostic procedures and treatment options. On this site it is possible to ask questions and get information from a neurologist and connect to people who have similar health interests.

7404   WebMD

www.webmd.com

Information on seizure disorders, including articles and resources.

Description

7405 Sexually Transmitted Diseases

Sexually transmitted diseases, STDs, are among the most common infectious diseases in the U.S. More than 20 STDs have been identified, and roughly 13 million persons are affected. Fortunately, most STDs are curable with prompt treatment, and do not become chronic. These include bacterial vaginosis, gonorrhea, syphilis, trichomoniasis and chlamydia. People who suffer from these diseases over long periods almost always do so because of re-infection rather than treatment failure. HIV and hepatitis B are commonly transmitted through sexual intercourse; see also *AIDS* and *Hepatitis*.

Fortunately, behavioral changes in sexual practices can drastically reduce the risk of STDs. Abstinence from intercourse or having a long-term mutually faithful monogamous relationship with an uninfected partner give essentially complete protection. Risk rises with multiple partners, unprotected intercourse between males, anonymous sex and contact with high-risk individuals, such as prostitutes. Barrier methods, notably condoms, give significant but not complete protection.

Until recently, no vaccines were available for any common STD except hepatitis B. However, researchers developed a vaccine for human papilloma virus (HPV) that is, amazingly, 100 percent effective. The vaccine is such a critical discovery because one specific type of HPV causes cervical cancer. Common STDs which may become chronic despite treatment are described below.

Genital herpes is a virus of the herpes family characterized by blisters (vesicles) in the genital area. The appearance of the blisters is often preceded by low-grade fever and by burning pain in the affected area. The first episode is often the most painful. Specific anti-viral therapy will shorten the duration and intensity of an attack. Herpes infections are self-limited but recurrent because the virus chronically infects nerves that radiate from the spinal column. Under certain conditions, such as febrile illness and physical or emotional stress, the virus reactivates and causes another outbreak. People with frequent recurrences can lower the risk of repeat attacks by taking a low dose of the anti-viral medication every day.

Genital warts are caused by the human papilloma virus (HPV.) There are roughly 750,000 new cases each year in the United States. The warts may appear anywhere in the genital and rectal area, making transmission difficult to prevent with a condom. Genital warts in the male, unless quite large, are often just a cosmetic nuisance, although a wart inside the urinary passage may cause discomfort. Women with genital warts not only need to have the warts removed, but to be observed for pre-cancerous changes in the cervix. Warts are generally destroyed by application of chemicals, but doctors have also used laser beams, freezing and electrical currents to

destroy them. Recurrence after treatment is common, even in the absence of re-infection.

Pelvic inflammatory disease (PID) is not always sexually transmitted, but it is included here because chlamydia and gonorrhea, which are sexually transmitted, are commonly the cause of PID. In this condition, the sensitive pelvic reproductive organs are attacked, leading to fever and lower abdominal pain and occasionally collection of pus in a pelvic abscess. Even after the attack is treated with high doses of antibiotics, residual scarring may lead to chronic pelvic pain, pain with intercourse, infertility and ectopic pregnancy, in which the fertilized egg implants in other pelvic structures outside the uterus. Prompt recognition and vigorous treatment of the acute attack of PID are important.

National Agencies & Associations

7406 American Foundation for the Prevention of Venereal Disease
799 Broadway
New York, NY 10003   212-759-2069
                                          www.chclibrary.org
Encourages every individual to assume responsible sexual relations and proper personal hygiene.
Mary O'Connell, Secretary

7407 American Social Health Association
PO Box 13827   919-361-8400
Research Triangle Park, NC 27709-3827   800-227-8922
                                          Fax: 919-361-8425
                                             www.ashastd.org
Provides resources to local communities to improve STD control programs through citizen action.
Lynn Barclay, President CEO
Deborah Arrindell, Vice President Health Policy

7408 American Venereal Disease Association
PO Box 1753
Baltimore, MD 21203-1753   301-955-3150
                                  www.alternativemedicine.com
Primary interest of this organization is in the reduction of the prevalence of the diseases.
Edward Hook III MD, Secretary

7409 Centers for Disease Control and Prevention
1600 Clifton Road   404-639-3534
Atlanta, GA 30333   800-232-4636
                                          TTY: 888-232-6348
                                       e-mail: cdcinfo@cdc.gov
                                                  www.cdc.gov
An information awareness resource produced by the Division of Adolescent and School Health. The database offers descriptions of various educational resources for professionals relevant to the education of children and youth about HIV infection and AIDS.
Thomas R. Frieden, Director
Ileana Arias, Principal Deputy Director

7410 Citizens Alliance for VD Awareness
5002 W Madison   773-379-1000
Chicago, IL 60644   Fax: 773-379-1342
                                       e-mail: info@cfhcn.org
                                       www.circlefamilycare.org
Seeks to increase commitment of health professionals to venereal disease and AIDS control.
Bruce Peoples, President/CEO
Patrick C Nwaezeigwe, CFO

7411 Herpes Resource Center
PO Box 13827   919-361-8400
Research Triangle Park, NC 27709-3827   800-227-8922
                                          Fax: 919-361-8425
                                             www.ashastd.org

Gives emotional support to individuals and provides information to the public about herpes.
Carolyn Mabry, Coordinator
Lynn Barclay, President CEO

7412 National Institute of Allergy and Infectious Diseases
6610 Rockledge Drive   301-496-5717
Bethesda, MD 20892-6612   866-284-4107
                                        Fax: 301-402-3573
                                        www.niaid.nih.gov
Dr. Anthony Fauci, Director

Research Centers

7413 Herpes Resource Center
PO Box 13827   919-361-8400
Research Triangle Park, NC 27709   800-227-8922
                                        Fax: 919-361-8425
                                        www.ashastd.org
Offers information and referrals for persons affected by herpes and other sexually transmitted disease prevention.
Lynn Barclay, President and Chief Executive Officer
Deborah Arrindell, Vice President Health Policy

7414 International Union Against Venereal Diseases
New York Hospital - Cornell Medical Center
1153 York Avenue   212-746-1200
New York, NY 10021   Fax: 212-746-1202
                                        e-mail: ajacobso@myp.org
Encourages campaigns medical and social against venereal disease.
Lewis Drusin MD, Director

7415 University of Chicago Committee on Virology
Marjorie B Kovler Viral Oncology Laboratories
910 E 58th Street   773-702-1620
Chicago, IL 60637   Fax: 773-702-1631
                                        mgcb.bsd.uchicago.edu
Focuses research into the area of sexually transmitted disease.
Bernard Roizman, Chairman
Olaf Schneewind, Professor and Chairman

Support Groups & Hotlines

7416 National Health Information Center
PO Box 1133   310-565-4167
Washington, DC 20013   800-336-4797
                                        Fax: 301-984-4256
                                        e-mail: info@nhic.org
                                        www.health.gov/nhic
Offers a nationwide information referral service, produces directories and resource guides.

Books

7417 Herpes and Papilloma Viruses Volume I & II
Raven Press
1185 Avenue of the Americas   212-930-9500
New York, NY 10036-2601
382 pages
ISBN: 0-881671-95-9

7418 Sexually Transmitted Diseases
Raven Press
1185 Avenue of the Americas   212-930-9500
New York, NY 10036-2601
Focuses on the clinically important subject of the immune response to sexually transmitted diseases.
350 pages
ISBN: 0-881678-82-1

7419 Understanding Helps
University Press of Mississippi

3825 Ridgewood Road   601-432-6205
Jackson, MS 39211-6492   800-737-7788
                                        Fax: 601-432-6217
                                        e-mail: press@ihl.state.ms.us
                                        www.upress.state.ms.us
This book is for people who wish to learn about herpes simplex viruses, two remarkably complex microbes capable of causing a wide variety of infections. These include genital herpes, a very common chronic sexually transmitted disease.
120 pages Hardcover
ISBN: 1-578060-40-0
Kathy Burgess, Advertising Manager/Marketing Assistant

7420 Understanding Herpes: Revised Second Edition
Lawrence R Stanberry, MD; PhD, author
University Press of Mississippi
3825 Ridgewood Road   601-432-6205
Jackson, MS 39211-6492   Fax: 601-432-6217
                                        e-mail: kburgess@ihl.state.ms.us
                                        www.upress.state.ms.us
A concise overview of advances and resources.
2006 144 pages Paperback
ISBN: 1-578068-68-1
Kathy Burgess, Advertising/Marketing Services Manager

7421 Women at Risk
Bristol Publishing
PO Box 1737   415-895-4461
San Leandro, CA 94577-0811   Fax: 415-895-4459
1993 159 pages
ISBN: 0-917851-62-5

Children's Books

7422 Teen Guide to Safe Sex
Franklin Watts Grolier
90 Old Sherman Tpke   203-797-3500
Danbury, CT 06816-0001   800-621-1115
                                        Fax: 203-797-3197
                                        www.grolier.com
A basic book about sexually transmitted diseases. Describes what they are, what causes them, how to recognize them and how teenagers can protect against them.
64 pages Grades 9-12
ISBN: 0-531105-92-0

Newsletters

7423 Sexually Transmitted Diseases: Journal
Julius Schachter, PhD, author
Lippincott Wiliiams & Wilkins
PO Box 1600
Hagerstown, MD 21741-1600   800-638-3030
                                        Fax: 301-223-2400
                                        e-mail: orders@lww.com
                                        www.lww.com
This timely, scholarly journal publishes original, peer-reviewed articles on clinical, laboratory, immunologic, epidemiologic, sociologic, and historical topics pertaining to sexually transmitted diseases and related fields.
Monthly

7424 Step Perspective
Seattle Treatment Education Project
127 Broadway E   206-329-4857
Seattle, WA 98102-5711   800-869-7837
A publication of the Seattle Treatment Education Project. Published three times a year.
Michael Auch, Executive Director

Pamphlets

7425 AIDS...What We Need To Know Pamphlet
March of Dimes

233 Park Avenue South
New York, NY 10003
212-353-8353
Fax: 212-254-3518
e-mail: NY639@marchofdimes.com
www.marchofdimes.com
Discusses the facts about HIVinfection and AIDS and how you can reduce your risk.
Pkg of 50
ISBN: 0-923500- -

7426 Chlamydial Infection
National Institute of Allergy/Infectious Diseases
National Institutes of Health   301-496-5717
Bethesda, MD 20892-0001
Offers information on diagnosis, treatment, effects, prevention and research.

7427 Genital Herpes
National Institute of Allergy/Infectious Diseases
National Institutes of Health   301-496-5717
Bethesda, MD 20892-0001
Offers information on symptoms, causes, diagnosis and reccurences.

7428 Genital Herpes Fact Sheet
March of Dimes
233 Park Avenue South
New York, NY 10003
212-353-8353
Fax: 212-254-3518
e-mail: NY639@marchofdimes.com
www.marchofdimes.com
Fact Sheets: one to two page review written for the general public.

7429 Gonorrhea
National Institute of Allergy/Infectious Diseases
National Institutes of Health   301-496-5717
Bethesda, MD 20892-0001
Offers information on the symptoms, diagnosis, treatment, complications, prevention and research.

7430 Human Papillomavirus and Genital Warts
National Institute of Allergy/Infectious Diseases
National Institutes of Health   301-496-5717
Bethesda, MD 20892-0001
Offers information on diagnosis, treatment, complications and prevention of the diseases.

7431 Introduction to Sexually Transmitted Diseases
National Institute of Allergy/Infectious Diseases
National Institutes of Health   301-496-5717
Bethesda, MD 20892-0001
Offers information on STDs, various types and symptoms, research, and referral services.

7432 Other Important STD's
National Institute of Allergy/Infectious Diseases
National Institutes of Health   301-496-5717
Bethesda, MD 20892-0001
Lists over ten of the most common sexually transmitted diseases. Offers information on what they are, the causes and treatments, research being done in these areas and referral numbers of where to call for more information on the diseases.

7433 Pelvic Inflammatory Disease
National Institute of Allergy/Infectious Diseases
National Institutes of Health   301-496-5717
Bethesda, MD 20892-0001
Offers information on the causes, symptoms, risk factors, diagnosis, treatment, and prevention.

7434 Syphilis
National Institute of Allergy/Infectious Diseases
National Institutes of Health   301-496-5717
Bethesda, MD 20892-0001
Offers information on what syphilis is, the symptoms, complications, diagnosis, prevention and treatment methods available.

7435 Vaginal Infections
National Institute of Allergy/Infectious Diseases
National Institutes of Health   301-496-5717
Bethesda, MD 20892-0001
Lists three specific types of vaginitis, with information on their symptoms, prevention, complications and treatments.

Web Sites

7436 American Social Health Association
sunsite.unc.edu/asha
Provides resources to local communities to improve STD control programs through citizen action.

7437 Centers for Disease Control
www.cdc.gov
Offers reprints, reports, public awareness and educational materials and research on sexually transmitted diseases.

7438 Healing Well
www.healingwell.com
An online health resource guide to medical news, chat, information and articles, newsgroups and message boards, books, disease-related web sites, medical directories, and more for patients, friends, and family coping with disabling diseases, disorders, or chronic illnesses.

7439 Health Finder
www.healthfinder.gov
Searchable, carefully developed web site offering information on over 1000 topics. Developed by the US Department of Health and Human Services, the site can be used in both English and Spanish.

7440 Healthlink USA
www.healthlinkusa.com
Health information concerning treatment, cures, prevention, diagnosis, risk factors, research, support groups, email lists, personal stories and much more. Updated regularly.

7441 Helios Health
www.helioshealth.com
Online resource for your health information. Detailed information about specific health topics, access to expert advice from our Medical Advisory Board, and up-to-date health news.

7442 MedicineNet
www.medicinenet.com
An online resource for consumers providing easy-to-read, authoritative medical and health information.

7443 Medscape
www.medscape.com
Medscape offers specialists, primary care physicians, and other health professionals the Web's most robust and integrated medical information and educational tools.

7444 WebMD
www.webmd.com
Information on sexually transmitted diseases, including articles and resources.

Description

7445 Sickle Cell Disease

Sickle cell disease (also called sickle cell anemia) is an inherited defect of hemoglobin, the oxygen-carrying element in the blood. Under some circumstances, the normally disc-shaped red blood cell takes on a crescent or sickle shape. It then becomes lodged in small capillaries and prevents normal oxygen flow to the tissues. This oxygen deprivation can cause sickle cell crises, with symptoms of severe pain in the back, joints, hands, and feet, and may even include neurologic changes. Severe abdominal pain and vomiting may also occur.

Sickle cell anemia occurs almost exclusively in African Americans. There are approximately 55,000 people in the United States with this condition. These children have sickle cell trait, occurring when one receives a copy of the sickle cell gene from only one parent. Only if a child receives a copy of the defective gene from both parents will the full-blown disease develop.

Therapy for sickle cell disease is aimed at preventing and treating infections, maintaining an adequate diet and fluid intake, and managing acute attacks with painkillers, oxygen, antibiotics and blood transfusion. Hydroxyurea has been shown to reduce the number of attacks by 50 percent as well as the need for transfusion. In the past, death typically occurred because of overwhelming infection or from organ destruction brought about by multiple sickling crises. Modern therapy has improved life expectancy dramatically, but some level of disability is common. Geneticcounseling is important for the patient and all family members.

National Agencies & Associations

7446 American Sickle Cell Anemia

10300 Carnegie Avenue
Cleveland, OH 44106-0171
216-229-8600
Fax: 216-229-4500
e-mail: irabragg@ascaa.org
www.ascaa.org

Provides education testing counseling and supportive services for sickle cell anemia and its hemoglobinopathy variants.
Ira Bragg-Grant, Executive Director
Leslie Carter, Newborn Screening Coordinator

7447 Comprehensive Sickle Cell Center

80 Jesse Hill Jr Drive SE
Atlanta, GA 30303
404-616-3572
Fax: 404-616-5998
e-mail: aplatt@emory.edu
www.scinfo.org

The mission of Sickle Cell Information Center is to provide sickle cell patient and professional education, news, research updates and world wide sickle cell resources, as well as world class compassionate care.
James R Eckman, Medical Director
Lewis Hsu, Interim Director

7448 Sickle Cell Anemia Foundation

503 S Center Street
Statesville, NC 28687
704-878-0732

This program is designed to provide information about sickle cell disease symptoms available treatments and service facilities by distributing literature and dispatching foundation members to address organizations church or school groups.
Priscilla Dudley

7449 Sickle Cell Association of Ontario

3199 Bathurst Street
Toronto, Ontario, M6A-2B2
416-789-2855
Fax: 416-789-1903
e-mail: sicklecell@look.ca
www.sicklecellontario.com

A voluntary, non-profit, charitable organization which is funded by donations from individuals, organizations and employee charitable funds.
John Kirya, President

7450 Sickle Cell Disease Association of America

231 E Baltimore Street
Baltimore, MD 21202
410-528-1555
800-421-8453
Fax: 410-528-1495
e-mail: scdaa@sicklecelldisease.org
www.sicklecelldisease.org

Purpose is to promote leadership on a national level in order to create awareness in all circles of the impact of sickle cell disease on emotional and economic well-being of families and the individual.
Christopher Hollins, Chair
Jeannine Knight, Executive Assistant to the President/COO

7451 Sickle Cell Information Center Grady Memorial Hospital

Grady Memorial Hospital
80 Jesse Hill Jr Drive SE
Atlanta, GA 30303
404-616-3572
Fax: 404-616-5998
e-mail: aplatt@emory.edu
www.SCInfo.org

Our mission is to provide sickle cell patient and professional education news research updates and world wide sickle cell resources. It is the mission of our organizations to provide world class compassionate care.
James R Eckman, Medical Director
Lewis Hsu, Interim Director

Foundations

7452 James R Clark Memorial Sickle Cell Foundation

1420 Gregg Street
Columbia, SC 29201
803-765-9916
800-506-1273
Fax: 803-799-6471
e-mail: sicklecell@sc.rr.com

Genetic Blood Disorder Disease.
Melodie A Hunnicutt, Executive Director
Saundra Kidwell, Director Finance

7453 Northeast Louisiana Sickle Cell Anemia Foundation

1604 Winnsboro Road
Monroe, LA 71202
318-322-0896
Fax: 318-387-4740
e-mail: sickle@bayou.com

The Foundation is a community-based non-profit, tax-exempt organization whose purpose is to provide services to sickle cell patients and their families, as well as be a resource in the communities we serve (12 northeast parishes) We provide education, trait counseling, patient assistance and social services. Our services are free.
Lasandre R Starks, Executive Director
Cheryl Minor, Registered Social Worker

7454 Sickle Cell Foundation of Georgia

2391 Benjamin E Mays Drive
Atlanta, GA 30311
404-755-1641
800-326-5287
Fax: 404-755-7955
e-mail: n_nichols@sicklecellatlaga.org
www.sicklecellatlaga.org

Our mission is dedicated to providing education, screening and counseling programs for Sickle Cell and other abnormal hemoglobin.
D Jean Brannan, President
Nesby Gibson, Project Director

7455 Sickle Cell Foundation of Greater Montgomery

3180 US Highway 8 West
Montgomery, AL 36108
334-286-9122
800-742-5534
e-mail: sicklec2@aol.com
www.scfgm.org

The main objectives of the Foundation are to give accurate information about sickle cell disease and related hemoglobinpathies, to provide testing and diagnostic services to interested persons, to

counsel individuals with positive test results so they can make in-formed decisions about their lives and to provide supportive ser-vices for clients and their family members.
Willie Owens, Executive Director

Research Centers

7456 Boston Sickle Cell Center Boston Medical Center
Boston Medical Center
88 E Newton Street   617-414-1020
Boston, MA 02118-2999   Fax: 617-414-1021
                                                 e-mail: mhsteinb@bu.edu
                                                       www.bu.edu/sicklecel
The treatment facility of choice for Boston-area patients with sickle cell disease. The Center also promotes interactive basic and clinical research and patient and professional educational activities.
Martin Steinberg, Director
Shawn H Eung, Program Manager

7457 Columbia University: Comprehensive Sickle Cell Center
Harlem Hospital
506 Lenox Avenue
New York, NY 10037-1000   212-939-1426
                           www.nyc.gov/html/hhc/html/facilities/har
Research into sickle cell disease.
Dr Jeanne Smith, Director

7458 Comprehensive Sickle Cell Center Children's Hospital Research Foundation
Children's Hospital Research Foundation
3333 Burnet Avenue   513-636-4541
Cincinnati, OH 45229   800-344-2462
                                                          Fax: 513-636-5562
                                                 e-mail: blood@cchmc.org
                                                 www.cincinnatichildrens.org
Offers research and statistical information in the area of sickle cell disease.
Clinton Joiner, Director
Karen Kalinyak, Clinical Director

7459 Howard University Center for Sickle Cell Disease
1840 7th Street NW   202-865-8284
Washington, DC 20001   Fax: 202-232-6719
                                            e-mail: sicklecell@howard.edu
                                                 www.sicklecell.howard.edu

Victor R Gordeuk, Director
Catherine Nwokolo, Clinical Staff Member

7460 Medical College of Georgia: Sickle Cell Center
1521 Pope Avenue   706-721-2171
Augusta, GA 30912-0002   Fax: 706-721-4575
                                            www.mcg.edu/centers/sicklecel
Offers research into sickle cell disease.
Abdullah Kutlar, Director
Kavita Natarajan

7461 Philadelphia Biomedical Research Institute
100 Ross and Royal Road   610-962-0615
King of Prussia, PA 19406   Fax: 610-254-9332
                                            e-mail: stohmishi@aol.com
                                        members.aol.com/stohinishi/phila_biomed
Study on the management of sickle cell anemia through nutrition.
S Tsuyoshi Ohinishi PhD, Director

7462 SUNY Health Science Center at Brooklyn Sickle Cell Center
450 Clarkson Avenue   718-270-1000
Brooklyn, NY 11203   Fax: 718-270-7592
                                                       www.hscbklyn.edu

John C LaRosa, President
Paul J Davis, Interim Chief Financial Officer

7463 Sickle Cell Anemia Research Foundation
2625 3rd Street   913-588-5000
Alexandria, VA 71309   877-722-7370
                                                          Fax: 318-487-9990
                                        e-mail: scarf@sicklecelldisease.org
                                                                www.kumc.edu

The Sickle Cell Anemia Research Foundation provides a compre-hensive program on Sickle Cell Disease. We offer education train-ing counseling and help with prescriptions.

7464 Sickle Cell Association of the Texas Gulf Coast
2626 S Loop W   713-666-0300
Houston, TX 77054-2649   Fax: 713-660-17
Rebecca Jasso, Executive Director

7465 University of California Northern Comprehensive Sickle Cell Center
Childrens Hospital Research Center
747 50 2nd Street   510-428-3651
Oakland, OK 94609-3594
Sickle cell disease research.
Elliot Vichinsky, Director

7466 University of Southern California: Comprehensive Sickle Cell Center
2025 Zonal Avenue   213-342-1259
Los Angeles, CA 90033-1034
Dr Cage S Johnson, Director

7467 University of Texas Southwestern Medical Center/Sickle Cell Management
Southwestern Medical Center
1935 Medical District Drive   214-456-7000
Dallas, TX 75235-7701   Fax: 214-648-3122
                                      e-mail: jsquires@childmed.dallas.tx.us
                                                             www.childrens.com
Focuses on the prevention of disease complications and manage-ment using the newest treatment strategies including hydroxyurea chronic transfusions stem cell (bone marrow) transplantation and state-of-the-art approaches to infection prevention pain manage-ment and treatment of specific organ-related complications (chest syndrome priapism avascular necrosis of the femoral head etc.).
George Bucha MD, Director
James F Amatruda

7468 Wayne State University: Comprehensive Sickle Cell Center
Curricular Affairs Office
Scott Hall   313-577-2424
Detroit, MI 48201   Fax: 313-577-8777
                                                                     wayne.edu

Charles F Whitten MD, President

Support Groups & Hotlines

7469 Keon Paschal Perry Sickle Cell Anemia Disease Awareness
7510 Granby Street, Perry Building
Norfolk, VA 23505   888-406-5111
                                            e-mail: keon4u@aol.com
International Sickle Cell Anemia Disease Awareness Campaign.
Roy L Perry-Bey, CEO/Executive Director

7470 Lehigh Valley Sickle Cell Support Group
PO Box 1711   610-706-0636
Allentown, PA 18105-1711   e-mail: SororW@aol.com
                                            www.members.aol.com/SororW/index.html
Anyone affected/effected by Sickle Cell and all interested persons. Our mission is to educate the local community about Sickle Cell.

7471 National Health Information Center
PO Box 1133   310-565-4167
Washington, DC 20013   800-336-4797
                                                          Fax: 301-984-4256
                                                       e-mail: info@nhic.org
                                                       www.health.gov/nhic
Offers a nationwide information referral service, produces direc-tories and resource guides.

7472 Sickle Cell Anemia Association of Austin: Marc Thomas Chapter
PO Box 201092   512-335-2306
Austin, TX 78720-1092   e-mail: llthomas@austin.cc.tx.us
                                                          www.tdh.state.tx.us
To raise awareness, resources and support for clients with sickle cell disease.
Linda L Thomas

7473 Sickle Cell Disease Association of America Philadelphia/Delaware Valley Chapter
4601 Market Street   215-471-8686
Philadelphia, PA 19139   Fax: 215-471-7441
e-mail: scdaa.pdvc@verizon.net
www.sicklecelldisorder.com
The Philadelphia/Delaware Valley Chapter of the Sickle Cell Disease Association of America (SCDAA/PDVC) assists the sickle cell community by serving as a vehicle and resource center for the psycho-social and social service needs of those individuals affected by the disease through the following services: case management; counseling; hospital/clinic visits; advocacy; career/vocational assistance; newborn screening follow-up; transportation; and outreach/community education.
Stanley A Simpkins, Executive Director
Karin Darius, Program Director

Pamphlets

7474 Sickle Cell Disease
March of Dimes
233 Park Avenue South   212-353-8353
New York, NY 10003   Fax: 212-254-3518
e-mail: NY639@marchofdimes.com
www.marchofdimes.com
Fact Sheets: one to two page review written for the general public.

Web Sites

7475 American Sickle Cell Anemia
www.ascaa.org
Provides education, testing, counseling and supportive services for sickle cell anemia and its hemoglobinopathies variants.

7476 Healing Well
www.healingwell.com
An online health resource guide to medical news, chat, information and articles, newsgroups and message boards, books, disease-related web sites, medical directories, and more for patients, friends, and family coping with disabling diseases, disorders, or chronic illnesses.

7477 Health Finder
www.healthfinder.gov
Searchable, carefully developed web site offering information on over 1000 topics. Developed by the US Department of Health and Human Services, the site can be used in both English and Spanish.

7478 Healthlink USA
www.healthlinkusa.com
Health information concerning treatment, cures, prevention, diagnosis, risk factors, research, support groups, email lists, personal stories and much more. Updated regularly.

7479 Helios Health
www.helioshealth.com
Online resource for your health information. Detailed information about specific health topics, access to expert advice from our Medical Advisory Board, and up-to-date health news.

7480 MedicineNet
www.medicinenet.com
An online resource for consumers providing easy-to-read, authoritative medical and health information.

7481 Medscape
www.medscape.com
Medscape offers specialists, primary care physicians, and other health professionals the Web's most robust and integrated medical information and educational tools.

7482 Sickle Cell Disease Association of America
sicklecelldisease.org
Purpose is to promote leadership on a national level in order to create awareness in all circles of the impact of sickle cell disease on emotional and economic well-being of families and the individual.

7483 WebMD
www.webmd.com
Information on Sickle Cell disease, including articles and resources.

Description

7484 Sjogren's Syndrome

Sjogren's syndrome (also called sicca syndrome) is an autoimmune disorder characterized by dryness of the mouth, eyes and mucous membranes. Variable enlargement of the lacrimal (tear) or salivary gland can occur. The disorder has no known cause, but many researchers believe that it has a genetic basis. Sjogren's syndrome is divided into primary (affecting only the eyes and mouth) and secondary (generalized) forms which may be associated with connective tissue diseases such as rheumatoid arthritis, systemic lupus erythematosus, polymyositis or scleroderma.

Patients who suffer from Sjogren's syndrome often complain initially of a gritty sensation in the eyes or severe dryness of the mouth. Patients may develop kidney, skin, neurologic, pulmonary or joint problems.

Treatment for Sjogren's is mainly symptomatic in the form of artificial tears, sipping fluids throughout the day, chewing gum and using special mouthwash. Pilocarpine may be used to stimulate saliva production. Severe cases, especially if they affect parts of the body outside of the glands, may require corticosteroid therapy. Dental caries (cavities) are a complication of dry mouth, so close dental follow-up is important.

National Agencies & Associations

7485 National Sjogren's Syndrome Foundation NSSA
NSSA
5815 N Blk Canyon Highway
Phoenix, AZ 85015-2200
301-530-4420
800-395-6772
Fax: 301-530-4415
e-mail: NSSA@aol.com
www.sjogrens.org
Provides educational materials to members about medical developments and research concerning SS nationally and internationally. Membership also includes assorted discounts on additional materials and events.
S. Lance Forstot, Chairman
Sheriese DeFruscio, Vice President of Development

7486 Sjogren's Syndrome Foundation
6707 Democracy Boulevard
Bethesda, MD 20817-2025
301-530-4420
800-475-6473
Fax: 301-530-4415
e-mail: tms@sjogrens.org
www.sjogrens.org
A non-profit voluntary health organization whose purposes are to educate patients and their families about Sjogren's syndrome and help them cope with the problems and frustrations of living with Sjogren's syndrome and to increase public and medical awareness.
Philip C Fox, President
Steven Taylor, CEO

Support Groups & Hotlines

7487 National Health Information Center
PO Box 1133
Washington, DC 20013
310-565-4167
800-336-4797
Fax: 301-984-4256
e-mail: info@nhic.org
www.health.gov/nhic
Offers a nationwide information referral service, produces directories and resource guides.

Books

7488 New Sjogren's Syndrome Handbook
Sjogren's Syndrome Foundation
366 N Broadway
Jericho, NY 11753-2025
516-933-6365
800-475-4736
Fax: 516-933-6368
www.sjogrens.org
An authoritative guide for patients and health care providers on the many aspects of Sjogren's syndrome written by renowned experts, plus practical suggestions for living more comfortably with this chronic illness.
Hardcover
ISBN: 0-195117-24-7
Steven Carsons MD, Editor
Elaine K Harris, Editor

Newsletters

7489 Moisture Seekers Newsletter
Sjogren's Syndrome Foundation
366 N Broadway
Jericho, NY 11753-2025
516-933-6365
800-475-4736
Fax: 516-933-6368
www.sjogrens.org
Contains up-to-date information on Sjogren's syndrome including new treatments, new products, and clinical trails; also features articles on the ways members cope with this chronic disease.
9x Year
Linda Saslow, Editor

Pamphlets

7490 Dry Eyes? Dry Mouth? Dry Nose? Arthritis? If Two or More: Sjogren's Syndrome
Sjogren's Syndrome Foundation
382 Main Street
Port Washington, NY 11050-3136
516-767-2866
Fax: 516-767-7156
Offers a brief overview of what the illness is, a history, statistical information, causes, symptoms and treatments.

7491 Sjogren's Syndrome
NAMSIC/National Institutes of Health
1 AMS Circle
Bethesda, MD 20892-0001
301-495-4484
Fax: 301-587-4352
TTY: 301-565-2966
www.nih.gov/niams/

14 pages

Audio & Video

7492 SjoGren's Syndrome Survival Guide
6707 Democracy Boulevard
Bethesda, MD 20817
301-530-4420
800-475-6473
Fax: 301-530-4415
e-mail: staylor@sjogrens.org
www.sjogrens.org
A complete resource for Sjogren's sufferers providing the newest medical information, research results, and treatment methods available, as well as the most effective and practical self-help strategies. Sjogren's syndrome is an autoimmune disease in which the body's immune system mistakenly attacks its own moisture producing glands.
Steven Taylor, Chief Executive Officer
Sheriese DeFruscio, Vice President of Development

Web Sites

7493 Healing Well
www.healingwell.com
An online health resource guide to medical news, chat, information and articles, newsgroups and message boards, books, disease-related web sites, medical directories, and more for patients,

friends, and family coping with disabling diseases, disorders, or chronic illnesses.

7494   Health Finder

www.healthfinder.gov

Searchable, carefully developed web site offering information on over 1000 topics. Developed by the US Department of Health and Human Services, the site can be used in both English and Spanish.

7495   Healthlink USA

www.healthlinkusa.com

Health information concerning treatment, cures, prevention, diagnosis, risk factors, research, support groups, email lists, personal stories and much more. Updated regularly.

7496   Helios Health

www.helioshealth.com

Online resource for your health information. Detailed information about specific health topics, access to expert advice from our Medical Advisory Board, and up-to-date health news.

7497   MedicineNet

www.medicinenet.com

An online resource for consumers providing easy-to-read, authoritative medical and health information.

7498   Medscape

www.medscape.com

Medscape offers specialists, primary care physicians, and other health professionals the Web's most robust and integrated medical information and educational tools.

7499   National Sjogren's Syndrome Association

www.sjogrens.org

Provides educational materials to members about medical developments and research concerning SS nationally and internationally. Membership also includes assorted discounts on additional materials and events.

7500   Sjogren's Syndrome Foundation

www.sjogrens.org

Information on Sjogren's Syndrome, the SS Foundation, and links to other related sites.

7501   WebMD

www.webmd.com

Information on Sjogren's Syndrome, including articles and resources.

Description

7502 Skin Disorders

The three most common chronic skin disorders are acne, psoriasis and eczema. Although these conditions do not shorten one's life, or cause significant disability, they can have a profound effect on one's quality of life and self-esteem.

Acne is probably the most common skin disorder, and can affect all age groups. It typically occurs in adolescents and young adults. Acne involves the sebaceous glands - glands that produce sebum, a substance that preserves the skin's natural oiliness. In acne, the glands' pores become plugged, trapping the sebum and bacteria. Inflammation follows, resulting in small red tender bumps with a corresponding blackhead or whitehead. These lesions can become pus-filled or even cystic ranging from 1 mm to 5 mm. Acne is seen most commonly on the face, neck, back and shoulders. Treatment starts with keeping affected areas clean. Locally-applied creams include retinoic acid, benzoyl peroxide and various antibiotics. Oral antibiotics (tetracycline) are especially effective for large, deep pimples. Oral tretinoin (Accutane) is very affective, but causes birth defects and other side effects and should be used only as a last resort and in consultation with a dermatologist. Oral contraceptives are often helpful in young women.

Psoriasis usually begins in early adult life, and affects 2 to 4 percent of the white population. A family history is common. The disease is characterized by scaly patches, some as small rain drop, others a few inches in diameer. Typical locations are the scalp, knees and elbows, but any part of the body may be affected. The patches are extremely itchy, and compulsive scratching may further damage the skin. In roughly 10 percent there is an associated arthritis. Milder cases are treated with steroid creams applied to skin and tar preparations or oral psoralen drugs, is effective in more severe cases. The most severe cases may require immunomodulating drugs like methotrexate or cyclosporine.

Eczema is a catchall term for many diseases which involve skin inflammation in response to some irritant. The irritant may be a direct one, such as contact dermatitis from the metal in a belt buckle, or an indirect one, as in atopic dermatitis triggered by various environmental agents (inhalants) and factors (certain foods). Atopic dermatitis is frequently associated with a personal or family history of allergic disorders (hay fever, asthma). For either situation, treatment consists of identifying and eliminating the offending agent(if possible) and local application of corticosteroid creams or nonspecific soothing and hydrating substances. Topical tacrolimus, approved by the FDA in 2000, is an immunosuppressive ointment effective for severe eczema without damaging the skin in the way that long-term topical steroids sometimes do.

National Agencies & Associations

7503 American Academy of Dermatology
PO Box 4014
Schaumburg, IL 60168-4014
847-240-1280
866-503-7546
Fax: 847-240-1859
e-mail: volunteer@aad.org
www.aad.org

The largest, most influential dermatologic association in the world. The Academy is committed to the highest quality standards in continuing medical education and plays a major role in formulating socioeconomic solutions.
Cyndi Del Boccio, Board of Director
Barbara Greenan, Advisory Board

7504 American Board of Dermatology American Society for Dermatologic Surger
American Society for Dermatologic Surgery
5550 Meadowbrook Drive
Rolling Meadows, IL 60008
847-956-0900
Fax: 847-956-0999
e-mail: info@asds.net
www.asds.net

Sole mission is to ensure competence for patients with cutaneous diseases through board representation.
Timothy Flynn, President
Debra Kennedy, Associate Executive Director

7505 American Dermatological Association University of Iowa Hospital and Clinics
University of Iowa Hospital and Clinics
5550 Meadowbrook Drive
Rolling Meadows, IL 60008
847-956-0900
Fax: 847-956-0999
e-mail: info@asds.net
www.asds-net.org

Professional society of physicians specializing in dermatology. Promotes teaching, practice, public education and research into dermatology.
Katherine J Svedman, Executive Director
Debra Kennedy, Associate Executive Director

7506 American Society for Dermatologic Surgery
5550 Meadowbrook Drive
Rolling Meadows, IL 60008-2005
847-956-0900
Fax: 847-956-0999
e-mail: info@asds.net
www.asds.net

Seeks to improve the quality of abnormal skin conditions especially the structural changes produced by skin cancer and other disease.
Katherine J Svedman, Executive Director
Robert A Weiss, President

7507 American Society of Plastic and Reconstructive Surgeons
444 E Algonquin Road
Arlington Heights, IL 60005-4654
847-228-9900
800-475-2784
e-mail: media@plasticsurgery.org
www.plasticsurgery.org

This Society sends free information about various surgical procedures and also provides the names of board certified plastic surgeons in a patient's area.
Dr.Gregory evans, President

7508 Dermatology Foundation
1560 Sherman Avenue
Evanston, IL 60201-4808
847-328-2256
Fax: 847-328-0509
e-mail: dfgen@dermatologyfoundation.org
www.dermfnd.org

Raises funds for the control of skin diseases through research improved education and better patient care. Supports basic clinical investigations.
Michael D tharp, President
Bruce U Wintroub, Chairman

7509 Eczema Association for Science and Education
4460 Redwood Highway
San Rafael, CA 94903
415-499-3474
800-818-7546
Fax: 415-472-5345
e-mail: info@nationaleczema.org
www.nationaleczema.org

Offers research and information to persons with eczema and other skin disorders.
Susan Tofte, Secretary
jamie Huber, Chair

7510 International Society of Dermatology
2323 N State Street   386-437-4405
Bunnell, FL 32110-0001   Fax: 386-437-4427
                                      e-mail: info@intsocderm.org
                                              www.intsocderm.org
Promotes interest education and research in dermatology.
Sigfrid A Muller MD, President
Mark Davis, Vice President

**7511 National Arthritis and Musculoskeletal & Skin Diseases
Information Clearinghouse**
National Institutes of Health
1 AMS Circle   301-495-4484
Bethesda, MD 20892-2350   Fax: 301-718-6366
                                         TTY: 301-565-2966
                                      e-mail: niamsinfo@mail.nih.gov
                                              www.niams.nih.gov
Our mission is to support research into the causes, treatment and prevention of arthritis and musculoskeletal and skin diseases, the training of basic and clinical scientists to carry out this research and the dissemination of information on research.
Stephen I Katz MD PhD, Director

**7512 National Institute of Arthritis and Musculoskeletal and Skin
Disease (NIAMS)**
1 AMS Circle   301-495-4484
Bethesda, MD 20892   877-226-4267
                                        Fax: 301-718-6366
                                        TTY: 301-565-2966
                                      e-mail: niamsinfo@mail.nih.gov
                                              www.niams.nih.gov
The NIAMS Information Clearinghouse provides free information about various forms of arthritis and rheumatic disease and bone, muscle and skin diseases. It distributes patient and professional education materials and refers people to other sources of information.
Stephen I Katz MD PhD, Director

Foundations

7513 National Psoriasis Foundation
6600 SW 92nd Avenue   503-244-7404
Portland, OR 97223-7195   800-723-9166
                                        Fax: 503-245-0626
                                      e-mail: getinfo@psoriasis.org
                                              www.psoriasis.org
Misson: To find a cure for psoriasis arthritis and to eliminate their devastating effects through research, advocacy, and education. Provides: patient services; public and professional education; community services; government affairs; research.
Randy Beranek, President/CEO
Bill Cardmon, Chief Field Operations

Research Centers

7514 Agromedicine Program Medical University of South Carolina
Medical University of South Carolina
171 Ashley Av.   843-792-1414
Charleston, SC 29425-0100   Fax: 843-792-1798
                                              www.musc.edu
Does research into the effects of pesticides on humans including epidemiology and skin diseases.
Dr Stanley Schuman, Director
W Stuart Smith, Vice President for Clinical Operations a

7515 Duke University Plastic Surgery Research Laboratories
Medical Center
Box 3974   919-681-8555
Durham, NC 27710-1   e-mail: elizabeth.yundt@duke.edu
                                    plastic.surgery.duke.edu

Conducts studies on skin cancer and aging skin.
Gregory Georgiade, Chief Division of Plastic and Reconstru
Detlev Erdmann, Associate Professor of Surgery

**7516 Laboratory of Dermatology Research Memorial Sloane-Kettering
Cancer Center**
Memorial Sloane-Kettering Cancer Center
1275 York Avenue   212-639-2000
New York, NY 10065-6007   Fax: 212-717-3363
                                              www.mskcc.org/mskcc
Specific studies on the identification of skin disorders and dermatology.
Allan C Halpern, Chief Dermatology Service

**7517 Massachusetts General Hospital: Harvard Cutaneous Biology
Research Center**
Massachusetts General Hospital
55 Fruit Street   617-726-5254
Boston, MA 02114   Fax: 617-726-1875
                                        TTY: 617-724-8800
                                              www.massgeneral.org
Dermatology research.
Peter L Flavin, President
John R Hinghman, Secretary

7518 Orentreich Foundation for the Advancement of Science
855 Route 301   212-606-0836
Cold Spring, NY 10516-4155   Fax: 845-265-4210
                                      e-mail: ofas@orentreich.org
                                       http://www.orentreich.org/team
Conducts biomedical research on dermatology.
Norman Orentreich, Founder and Co-Director
David S Orentreich, Co-Director

7519 Psoriasis Research Institute
6600 SW 92nd Avenue   503-244-7404
Portland, OR 97223   800-723-9166
                                        Fax: 503-245-0626
                                      e-mail: getinfo@psoriasis.org
                                              www.psoriasis.org
Studies the causes symptoms and treatments of psoriasis.
Randy Beranek, President/CEO
Bill Cardmon, Chief Field Operations

7520 Rockefeller University Laboratory for Investigative Dermatology
Rockefeller University
1230 York Avenue   212-327-7458
New York, NY 10021-6399   Fax: 212-570-8232
                                              www.rockefeller.edu
Research into skin disorders and the whole specialty of dermatology in general.
D Martin Carter MD, PhD, Head

7521 Rockefeller University, Laboratory for Investigative Dermatology
1230 York Avenue   212-327-7458
New York, NY 10021-6399   Fax: 212-570-8232
                                              www.rockefeller.edu

D Martin Carter MD, PhD, Head

**7522 Scripps Clinic and Research Foundation: Autoimmune Disease
Center**
10550 N Torrey Pines Road   858-784-1000
La Jolla, CA 92037-1092   Fax: 619-554-6805
                                              www.scripps.edu
Research into dermatomyostis and polymyositis.
Eng Tan, Professor Emeritus

7523 Sulzberger Institute for Dermatologic Education
PO Box 94020   847-330-0230
Palatine, IL 60094-4020   Fax: 847-330-0050
                                       http://www.aad.org/
A nonprofit research center whose sole goal is to enhance patient care through the development and promotion of quality educational programs on the care and disorders of the skin, hair, nails and mucous membranes.
Dirk M. Elston, President
Lisa A. Garner, Vice president

7524 Sulzberger Institute for Dermatologic Educ
PO Box 94020   847-330-0230
Palatine, IL 60094   Fax: 847-330-0050
                                http://www.aad.org/
A nonprofit research center whose sole goal is to enhance patient care through the development and promotion of quality educational programs on the care and disorders of the skin hair nails and mucous membranes.
Dirk M. Elston, President
Lisa A. Garner, Vice president

7525 University of California: San Francisco Dermatology Drug Research
515 Spruce   415-476-2001
San Francisco, CA 94143-0001   Fax: 415-221-4751
                                www.ucsf.edu
Conducts clinical testing of new or existing pharmalogic agents used in the treatment of skin disorders.
John Koo MD, Director
Susan Desmond, Chancellor

7526 University of Texas: Southwestern Medical Center at Dallas, Immunodermatology
5323 Harry Hines Boulevard   214-648-3111
Dallas, TX 75390-7208   Fax: 214-688-8275
                                www.utsouthwestern.edu
Provides a focus for research into the causes prevention and management of diseases such as immune deficiencies and infections. Studies are aimed at increasing basic-level understanding of immunologic skin diseases.
Daniel K Podolsky MD, President
Diane Jeffries, Director

Support Groups & Hotlines

7527 National Health Information Center
PO Box 1133   310-565-4167
Washington, DC 20013   800-336-4797
                                Fax: 301-984-4256
                                e-mail: info@nhic.org
                                www.health.gov/nhic
Offers a nationwide information referral service, produces directories and resource guides.

Books

7528 Managing Your Psoriasis
MasterMedia
33 Beecker Street   212-260-5600
New York, NY 10012   800-334-8232
1993 Paperback
ISBN: 0-942361-83-0

7529 Psoriasis and Psoriatic Arthritis Pocket Guide
National Psoriasis Foundation
6600 SW 92nd Avenue   503-244-7404
Portland, OR 97223-7195   800-723-9166
                                Fax: 503-245-0626
                                e-mail: getinfo@psoriasis.org
                                www.psoriasis.org
The Pocket Guide includes algorithms for therapy_including combination and biologic treatments_based on patient types. This second edition was revised to provide guidance for managing patients with severe psoriasis and to put the roll of new biologics into perspective.
2005 79 pages

7530 Q&A's About Psoriasis
NAMSIC/National Institutes of Health
1 AMS Circle   301-495-4484
Bethesda, MD 20892-0001   877-226-4267
                                Fax: 301-718-6366
                                TTY: 301-565-2966
                                e-mail: niamsinfo@mail.nih.gov
                                www.nih.gov/niams

Offers various information for the psoriasis patient and their family regarding treatments, risks, nutrition and more.
24 pages

7531 Therapy of Moderate-to-Severe Psoriasis
National Psoriasis Foundation
6600 SW 92nd Avenue   503-244-7404
Portland, OR 97223-7195   800-723-9166
                                Fax: 503-245-0626
                                e-mail: getinfo@psoriasis.org
                                www.psoriasis.org
Edited by Gerald D. Weinstein, MD, and Alice Gottlieb, MD, PhD, this book includes information on state-of-the-art clinical management through contributions from national experts on psoriasis.
2002
Gail M Zimmerman, President/CEO
Paula Fasano, Director Marketing/Communications

7532 Treatment Guide for the Health Insurance Industry
National Psoriasis Foundation
6600 SW 92nd Avenue   503-244-7404
Portland, OR 97223-7195   800-723-9166
                                Fax: 503-245-0626
                                e-mail: getinfo@psoriasis.org
                                www.psoriasis.org
This easy-to-read general overview is a valuable tool for the insurer or any health professional interested in detailed information about psoriasis and psoriatic arthritis, patient quality of life issues, and many available treatments.
Gail M Zimmerman, President/CEO
Paula Fasano, Director Marketing/Communications

Magazines

7533 International Journal of Dermatology
International Society of Dermatology
200 1st Street SW   507-284-3736
Rochester, MN 55905-0001
Focuses on information for dermatologists and the whole specialty of dermatology research and education.
10x Year

7534 Journal of Dermatologic Surgery and Oncology
International Society for Dermatologic Surgery
930 N Meachan Road   847-330-9830
Schaumburg, IL 60173   Fax: 847-330-1135
Focuses on medical updates and information on dermatology.
Monthly

7535 Journal of the Academy of Dermatology
American Academy of Dermatology
PO Box 94020   847-330-0230
Palatine, IL 60094-4020   Fax: 847-330-0050
A scientific publication serving the clinical needs of the specialty and provides a wide selection of articles on various topics important to continuing medical education of Academy members and the international dermatologic community.
Monthly

7536 Psoriasis Advance
National Psoriasis Foundation
6600 SW 92nd Avenue   503-244-7404
Portland, OR 97223-7195   800-723-9166
                                Fax: 503-245-0626
                                e-mail: getinfo@npfusa.org
                                www.psoriasis.org
Written especially for the psoriatis community four times a year. Provides current articles to keep you up to date with treatmetnt and research information, pave the way to empowerment, and connect you with others.
40 pages BiMonthly
Sheri Decker, Director Communication

7537 Psoriasis Forum
National Psoriasis Foundation

6600 SW 92nd Avenue
Portland, OR 97223-7195

503-244-7404
800-723-9166
Fax: 503-245-0626
e-mail: getinfo@psoriasis.org
www.psoriasis.org

Dedicated to providing up-to-date and practical information to health care providers on the frontline of psoriasis treatment. Professional Members only.
Quarterly
Gail M Zimmerman, President/CEO
Paula Fasano, Director Marketing/Communications

Newsletters

7538 Dermatology Focus
Dermatology Foundation
1560 Sherman Avenue
Evanston, IL 60201-4808

847-328-2256
Fax: 847-328-0509
e-mail: dfgen@dermatologyfoundation.org
www.dermfnd.org

Designed to communicate to practitioners the latest advances in medical and surgical dermatology. The publication also serves as the Foundation's newsletter, recognizing the accomplishments and activities of the many dermatologists who give not only their monetary support, but countless hours to develop the research and teaching careers of future leaders throughout the specialty.
Quarterly
Sandra Rahn Benz, Executive Director

7539 Dermatology Focus
Dermatology Foundation
1560 Sherman Avenue
Evanston, IL 60201-4808

847-328-2256
Fax: 847-328-0509
e-mail: dfgen@dermatologyfoundation.org
www.dermfnd.org

Designed to communicate to practitioners the latest advances in medical and surgical dermatology. The publication also serves as the Foundation's newsletter recognizing the accomplishments and activities of the many dermatologists who give not only their monetary support, but countless hours to develop the research and teaching careers of future leaders throughout the specialty.
Quarterly
Sandra Rahn Benz, Executive Director

7540 Dermatology World
American Academy of Dermatology
PO Box 94020
Palatine, IL 60094-4020

847-330-0230
Fax: 847-330-0050

Offers Academy members information outside the clinical realm. It carries news of government actions, reports of socioeconomic issues, societal trends and other events which impinge on the practice of dermatology.
Monthly

7541 Progress in Dermatology
Dermatology Foundation
1560 Sherman Avenue
Evanston, IL 60201-4808

847-328-2256
Fax: 847-328-0509
e-mail: dfgen@dermatologyfoundation.org
www.dermfnd.org

The journal provides in-depth coverage of clinically relevant topics as well as basic scientific advances affecting all of dermatology. Distributed exclusively to members of the Foundation.
Quarterly
Sandra Rahn Benz, Executive Director

7542 Psoriasis Newsletter
Psoriasis Research Institute
600 Town & Country Center
Palo Alto, CA 94301

650-326-1848
Fax: 650-326-1262
e-mail: emfpri@aol.com

Offers information and medical updates on the disease of psoriasis, events, fundraising and more.
4 pages Quarterly

Pamphlets

7543 Acne
American Academy of Dermatology
PO Box 4014
Schaumburg, IL 60168-4014

847-330-0230
Fax: 847-330-0050

Explains the causes of acne. Treatments are explored, including diet, medications, antibiotics, and sun exposure. Available in Spanish.
1996

7544 Allergic Contact Rashes
American Academy of Dermatology
PO Box 4014
Schaumburg, IL 60168-4014

847-330-0230
Fax: 847-330-0050

Lists the common causes of skin rashes, including jewelry and hidden ingredients in fabrics and household products.
1997

7545 Athlete's Foot
American Academy of Dermatology
PO Box 4014
Schaumburg, IL 60168-4014

847-330-0230
Fax: 847-330-0050

This common fungal infection is not only a problem for athletics. Discusses what causes it and how to treat it.
1994

7546 Black Skin
American Academy of Dermatology
PO Box 4014
Schaumburg, IL 60168-4014

847-330-0230
Fax: 847-330-0050

Explains the skin diseases common with black skin and how they are diagnosed and treated.
1996

7547 Conception, Pregnancy & Psoriasis
National Psoriasis Foundation
6600 SW 92nd Avenue
Portland, OR 97223-7195

503-244-7404
800-723-9166
Fax: 503-245-0626
e-mail: getinfo@npfusa.org
www.psoriasis.org

Explains pregnancy factors for persons with psoriasis.

7548 Cosmetics & Skin Care
American Academy of Dermatology
PO Box 4014
Schaumburg, IL 60168-4014

847-330-0230
Fax: 847-330-0050

Discusses skin reactions to fragrances, makeup, and bath and body care products.
1994

7549 Darker Side of Tanning
American Academy of Dermatology
PO Box 4014
Schaumburg, IL 60168-4014

847-330-0230
Fax: 847-330-0050

Discusses the dangers of ultraviolet radiation from the sun, tanning beds, and sun lamps. Includes descriptions of the different skin types and tips to help minimize the sun's damage to the skin and eyes.
1996

7550 Eczema/Atopic Dermatitis
American Academy of Dermatology
PO Box 4014
Schaumburg, IL 60168-4014

847-330-0230
Fax: 847-330-0050

Explains how to recognize and treat dermatitis.
1995

7551 For Parents
National Psoriasis Foundation
6600 SW 92nd Avenue
Portland, OR 97223-7195

503-244-7404
800-723-9166
Fax: 503-245-0626
e-mail: getinfo@npfusa.org
www.psoriasis.org

Offers advice and resources on how to educate yourself about psoriasis and your child, as well as treatment information and summer camps.

7552 Genital Psoriasis
National Psoriasis Foundation
6600 SW 92nd Avenue   503-244-7404
Portland, OR 97223-7195   800-723-9166
                                          Fax: 503-245-0626
                               e-mail: getinfo@npfusa.org
                                            www.psoriasis.org
Introduces the reader to the basics of genital psoriasis, and treatment options.

7553 Hand Eczema
American Academy of Dermatology
PO Box 4014   847-330-0230
Schaumburg, IL 60168-4014   Fax: 847-330-0050
Shows examples of hand rashes, explains causes, lists protective measures and treatments.
1993

7554 Hives
American Academy of Allergy, Asthma and Immunology
611 E Wells Street   414-272-6071
Milwaukee, WI 53202-3889   800-822-2762
                                          Fax: 414-272-6070
                                                 www.aaaai.org
This brochure offers information on what causes hives, what is Angioedema, and how hives can be treated.

7555 Home Phototherapy
National Psoriasis Foundation
6600 SW 92nd Avenue   503-244-7404
Portland, OR 97223-7195   800-723-9166
                                          Fax: 503-245-0626
                               e-mail: getinfo@npfusa.org
                                            www.psoriasis.org
Talks about the use of a home UVB unit to treat psoriasis.

7556 Methotrexate (MTX)
National Psoriasis Foundation
6600 SW 92nd Avenue   503-244-7404
Portland, OR 97223-7195   800-723-9166
                                          Fax: 503-245-0626
                               e-mail: getinfo@npfusa.org
                                            www.psoriasis.org
An introductions to MTX treatment.

7557 Oral Retinoid Therapy (Soriatane)
National Psoriasis Foundation
6600 SW 92nd Avenue   503-244-7404
Portland, OR 97223-7195   800-723-9166
                                          Fax: 503-245-0626
                               e-mail: getinfo@npfusa.org
                                            www.psoriasis.org
Explains Soriatane treatment options.

7558 PUVA (Psoralen Plus Ultraviolet Light A)
National Psoriasis Foundation
6600 SW 92nd Avenue   503-244-7404
Portland, OR 97223-7195   800-723-9166
                                          Fax: 503-245-0626
                               e-mail: getinfo@npfusa.org
                                            www.psoriasis.org
Explains PUVA treatment options, pros, cons, and potential side-effects.

7559 Pityriasis Rosea
American Academy of Dermatology
PO Box 4014   847-330-0230
Schaumburg, IL 60168-4014   Fax: 847-330-0050
Discusses the appearance, symptoms, and causes of this common rash. Diagnosis and treatment are also explained.
1996

7560 Psoriasis on Specific Skin Sites
National Psoriasis Foundation
6600 SW 92nd Avenue   503-244-7404
Portland, OR 97223-7195   800-723-9166
                                          Fax: 503-245-0626
                               e-mail: getinfo@npfusa.org
                                            www.psoriasis.org
Including nails, ears, eyelids, face, mouth and lips, hands and feet.

7561 Psoriasis: How It Makes You Feel
National Psoriasis Foundation
6600 SW 92nd Avenue   503-244-7404
Portland, OR 97223-7195   800-723-9166
                                          Fax: 503-245-0626
                               e-mail: getinfo@npfusa.org
                                            www.psoriasis.org

7562 Psoriatic Arthritis
National Psoriasis Foundation
6600 SW 92nd Avenue   503-244-7404
Portland, OR 97223-7195   800-723-9166
                                          Fax: 503-245-0626
                               e-mail: getinfo@npfusa.org
                                            www.psoriasis.org

7563 Rosacea
American Academy of Dermatology
PO Box 4014   847-330-0230
Schaumburg, IL 60168-4014   Fax: 847-330-0050
The condition, do's and don'ts for rosacea patients, and treatment are explained.
1995

7564 Scabies
American Academy of Dermatology
PO Box 4014   847-330-0230
Schaumburg, IL 60168-4014   Fax: 847-330-0050
Explains the nature of the scabies parasite, symptoms, at-risk groups, individual and large group treatments. Available in Spanish.
1997

7565 Scalp Psoriasis
National Psoriasis Foundation
6600 SW 92nd Avenue   503-244-7404
Portland, OR 97223-7195   800-723-9166
                                          Fax: 503-245-0626
                               e-mail: getinfo@npfusa.org
                                            www.psoriasis.org

7566 Seborrheic Dermatitis
American Academy of Dermatology
PO Box 4014   847-330-0230
Schaumburg, IL 60168-4014   Fax: 847-330-0050
Answers the most frequently asked questions about this common, easily treatable skin condition.
1995

7567 Seborrheic Keratoses
American Academy of Dermatology
PO Box 4014   847-330-0230
Schaumburg, IL 60168-4014   Fax: 847-330-0050
Describes seborrheic keratosis growths, causes, and treatments.
1997

7568 Skin Cancer
American Academy of Dermatology
PO Box 4014   847-330-0230
Schaumburg, IL 60168-4014   Fax: 847-330-0050
Warning signs and how to perform self-examinations are discussed.
1994

7569 Skin Conditions Related to AIDS
American Academy of Dermatology
PO Box 4014   847-330-0230
Schaumburg, IL 60168-4014   Fax: 847-330-0050
What AIDS is, who's at risk, and other important information about this major health problem are discussed.
1997

7570 Specific Forms of Psoriasis
National Psoriasis Foundation
6600 SW 92nd Avenue   503-244-7404
Portland, OR 97223-7195   800-723-9166
                                          Fax: 503-245-0626
                               e-mail: getinfo@npfusa.org
                                            www.psoriasis.org
Pustular, Guttate, Inverse, and Erythrodermic.

7571 Spider Veins, Varicose Vein Therapy
American Academy of Dermatology
PO Box 4014   847-330-0230
Schaumburg, IL 60168-4014   Fax: 847-330-0050
Discusses the latest methods for removing unsightly and unwanted blood vessels that appear mostly on the legs.
1995

7572 Sun & Water Therapy
National Psoriasis Foundation
6600 SW 92nd Avenue   503-244-7404
Portland, OR 97223-7195   800-723-9166
                                                    Fax: 503-245-0626
                                     e-mail: getinfo@npfusa.org
                                                       www.psoriasis.org

7573 Sun Protection for Children
American Academy of Dermatology
PO Box 4014   847-330-0230
Schaumburg, IL 60168-4014   Fax: 847-330-0050
Teaches parents how to protect their children from the sun's harmful rays.
1996

7574 Sun and Your Skin
American Academy of Dermatology
PO Box 4014   847-330-0230
Schaumburg, IL 60168-4014   Fax: 847-330-0050
Information on acute sunburn, premature aging of the skin, allergies, and skin cancer. Tips on how to be sun smart.
1994

7575 Sunlight, Ultraviolet Radiation and the Skin
National Cancer Institute
Building 31
Bethesda, MD 20892-0001   800-422-6237

7576 Tinea Versicolor
American Academy of Dermatology
PO Box 4014   847-330-0230
Schaumburg, IL 60168-4014   Fax: 847-330-0050
Discusses the symptoms, diagnosis, and treatment of this often misunderstood fungal infection.
1995

7577 Treatment Overview
National Psoriasis Foundation
6600 SW 92nd Avenue   503-244-7404
Portland, OR 97223-7195   800-723-9166
                                                    Fax: 503-245-0626
                                     e-mail: getinfo@npfusa.org
                                                       www.psoriasis.org
Discusses a number of available psoriasis treatments, what is considered by the doctor when developing a treatment plan, and treatment resources.

7578 Vascular Birthmarks
American Academy of Dermatology
PO Box 4014   847-330-0230
Schaumburg, IL 60168-4014   Fax: 847-330-0050
Includes descriptions and treatments for most common types of vascular birthmarks - macular stains, hemangiomas, and port-wine stains.
1997

7579 Vitiligo
American Academy of Dermatology
PO Box 4014   847-330-0230
Schaumburg, IL 60168-4014   Fax: 847-330-0050
Discusses lost skin pigmentation and what can be done about it, including repigmentation therapy.
1994

7580 Young People and Psoriasis
National Psoriasis Foundation
6600 SW 92nd Avenue   503-244-7404
Portland, OR 97223-7195   800-723-9166
                                                    Fax: 503-245-0626
                                     e-mail: getinfo@npfusa.org
                                                       www.psoriasis.org
Infancy through adolescence.

7581 Your Diet & Psoriasis
National Psoriasis Foundation
6600 SW 92nd Avenue   503-244-7404
Portland, OR 97223-7195   800-723-9166
                                                    Fax: 503-245-0626
                                     e-mail: getinfo@npfusa.org
                                                       www.psoriasis.org
A discussion of particular diets, foods and supplements and the effect they have on psoriasis.

7582 Your Skin and Your Dermatologist
American Academy of Dermatology
PO Box 4014   847-330-0230
Schaumburg, IL 60168-4014   Fax: 847-330-0050
Explains why a dermatologist is the appropriate specialist for the care of diseases of the skin, hair, nails, and mucous membranes.
1997

Audio & Video

7583 Allergic Skin Reactions
American Academy of Allergy, Asthma and Immunology
611 E Wells Street   414-272-6071
Milwaukee, WI 53202-3889   800-822-2762
                                                    Fax: 414-272-6070
                                                             www.aaaai.org
In some people, allergy symptoms include itching redness, rashes, or hives. This video describes the symptoms, triggers, and treatment for common skin reactions such as dermatitis, hives and angioedema.
10-13 minutes

7584 Basic Science Series
American Academy of Dermatology
PO Box 4014   847-330-0230
Schaumburg, IL 60168-4014   Fax: 847-330-0050
Combines high-quality 35mm slides and accompanying narration on audiocassette and features topics that underline and support clinical dermatology. The series is useful for residents in training as well as practicing dermatologists.
Slides

7585 CME Video Library
American Academy of Dermatology
PO Box 4014   847-330-0230
Schaumburg, IL 60168-4014   Fax: 847-330-0050
A series of video programs developed by AAD experts recognized for their continued efforts in dermatologic advancement.
Videotapes

7586 Facts About Acne
American Academy of Dermatology
PO Box 4014   847-330-0230
Schaumburg, IL 60168-4014   Fax: 847-330-0050
The etiology of acne and treatment choices are explained by consultants, with patient encounters.
13 minutes

7587 Mystery of Contact Dermatitis
American Academy of Dermatology
PO Box 4014   847-330-0230
Schaumburg, IL 60168-4014   Fax: 847-330-0050
The causes and treatment of some common forms of contact dermatitis are shown with consultation and commentary.
10 minutes

7588 National Library of Dermatologic Teaching Slides
American Academy Of Dermatology
PO Box 94020   847-330-0230
Palatine, IL 60094-4020   Fax: 847-330-0050
A collection of dermatologic teaching slides offering the most comprehensive series ever assembled. Each set offers a realistic presentation of classic clinical skin conditions encountered by the dermatologist.

7589 Skin Cancer: The Undeclared Epidemic
American Academy of Dermatology
PO Box 4014   847-330-0230
Schaumburg, IL 60168-4014   Fax: 847-330-0050

Examples of skin cancer lesions, interviews with patients at screenings, and comments from Academy members.
9 minutes

7590   Skin Care Under the Sun
American Academy of Dermatology
PO Box 4014   847-330-0230
Schaumburg, IL 60168-4014   Fax: 847-330-0050
Dramatization of the dangers of overexposure to the sun, providing explanations of the effects of ultraviolet radiation on the skin.
7 minutes

Web Sites

7591   American Academy of Dermatology
www.aad.org
Promotes and advances the science and art of medicine and surgery related to the skin, promotes the highest possible standards in clinical practice, education and research.

7592   American Society of Plastic and Reconstructive Surgeons
www.plasticsurgery.org
This Society sends free information about various surgical procedures and also provides the names of board certified plastic surgeons in a patient's area.

7593   Derma Doctor
www.dermadoctor.com
The most informative skin care site on the Web. An extensive library of newsletters to help answer your questions.

7594   Dermatology Foundation
www.dermfnd.org
Raises funds for the control of skin diseases through research, improved education and better patient care. Supports basic clinical investigations.

7595   Healing Well
www.healingwell.com
An online health resource guide to medical news, chat, information and articles, newsgroups and message boards, books, disease-related web sites, medical directories, and more for patients, friends, and family coping with disabling diseases, disorders, or chronic illnesses.

7596   Health Finder
www.healthfinder.gov
Searchable, carefully developed web site offering information on over 1000 topics. Developed by the US Department of Health and Human Services, the site can be used in both English and Spanish.

7597   Healthlink USA
www.healthlinkusa.com
Health information concerning treatment, cures, prevention, diagnosis, risk factors, research, support groups, email lists, personal stories and much more. Updated regularly.

7598   Helios Health
www.helioshealth.com
Online resource for your health information. Detailed information about specific health topics, access to expert advice from our Medical Advisory Board, and up-to-date health news.

7599   MedicineNet
www.medicinenet.com
An online resource for consumers providing easy-to-read, authoritative medical and health information.

7600   Medscape
www.medscape.com
Medscape offers specialists, primary care physicians, and other health professionals the Web's most robust and integrated medical information and educational tools.

7601   Nat'l Arthritis and Musculoskeletal Skin
www.niams.nih.gov
Supports and provides clinical and public information and research to increase understanding of the many skin diseases and related disorders. Also provides lists and order forms for their resources and materials.

7602   Nat'l Institute of Arthritis
www.nih.gov
Handles inquiries on the following - arthritis, bone diseases and skin diseases. Consumer and professional education materials are available.

7603   National Psoriasis Foundation
www.psoriasis.org
Offers information, support and referrals for victims of psoriasis and their families.

7604   Skin Store
www.skinstore.com
Carries over 500 of the finest skincare products, available at the lowest prices, delivered immediately to your home.

7605   WebMD
www.webmd.com
Information on skin disorders, including articles and resources.

Description

7606 Sleep Disorders

Sleep disorders are defined as disturbances that affect the ability to fall or stay asleep, that involve sleeping too much, or that result in abnormal sleep-related behavior. They can be categorized into primary sleep disorders; sleep disorders related to another mental disorder or a general medical condition; and substance induced sleep disorder. The two conditions discussed here, narcolepsy and obstructive sleep apnea, are both primary sleep disorders.

Narcolepsy is a rare disorder of abnormal and irresistible daytime drowsiness. Excessive daytime sleepiness with involuntary daytime sleep episodes, disturbed nighttime sleep, and cataplexy (sudden weakness or loss of muscle tone, often triggered by emotion), are the most common symptoms of narcolepsy. Generally, symptoms appear between the onset of puberty and age 25, and worsen as the patient ages. There are 100,000 people in the US with this condition.

Although the exact cause of narcolepsy is unknown, there appears to be a genetic link.

Oral medication, including stimulant agents, as well as specific sleep schedules and other forms of behavioral therapy are also prescribed.

Obstructive sleep apnea is a serious and common sleep disorder that features heavy snoring and breathing irregularities. It is chronic and relapsing, and varies in severity from mild to lethal. Almost 90 percent of the estimated 12 million sleep apnea sufferers are male. Obstructive sleep apnea is biomechanical and usually occurs when tissues in the back of the throat collapse and close the breathing passage. Sufferers experience heavy snoring, periods during sleep when breathing halts for 10 seconds or more, and many short awakenings which they do not remember. In the worst cases, sufferers may cease breathing for more than half of total sleeping time, which can result in daytime fatigue, oxygen deprivation and hypertension.

Signs of sleep apnea or a related sleeping disorder include loud, habitual snoring, fatigue on waking, daytime sleepiness, and choking, gasping or holding one's breath while asleep. Overweight persons and smokers are more prone to develop this disorder. Heavy eating, late-night snacking, sedative use, and alcohol consumption are often contributing factors.

The diagnosis of sleep apnea often requires a polysomnography, or sleep study, which monitors brain waves, muscle tension, eye movement, respiration and blood-oxygen levels. Obviously, a partner can easily help to confirm these symptoms; single people can arrange for sleep observation in a hospital or clinic setting. Behavior modification is frequently sufficient to reduce or eliminate many snoring problems, as is sleep-

ing on one's side and/or without a pillow. In addition to behavioral changes, mild cases are often responsive to oral devices that help to keep airways open by bringing the jaw forward, elevating the soft palate, or repositioning the tongue. More severe cases can be treated with a C-PAP (continuous positive airway pressure) machine, or a Bi-Level (Bi-PAP) machine, both of which blow air into the patient's airways in a regulated manner. Surgery is sometimes indicated, when facial or oral irregularities, such as jaw irregularities, small throat openings, enlarged tonsils, a large tongue or other tissue in front of the airway, or a deviated septum, impede proper airflow.

National Agencies & Associations

7607 American Narcolepsy Association
129 Waterwheel Lane
North Kingstown, RI 02852-6230   800-222-6085
http://www.narcolepsynetwork.org/
Offers help and information to persons with narcolepsy and their families.

7608 American Sleep Apnea Association
6856 E Avenue   202-293-3650
Washington, DC 20012   Fax: 202-293-3656
e-mail: asaa@sleepapnea.org
www.sleepapnea.org
Offers help and information to persons with sleep apnea and their families.
Michael P Coppola MD, President and Chief Medical Officer
Nancy Rothstein, Secretary

7609 Association of Professional Sleep Societies
One Westbrook Corporate Center   708-492-0930
Westchester, IL 60154   Fax: 708-273-9354
www.apss.org
Works to facilitate the research and development of sleep disorders medically by encouraging exchange of information among members.
Jerome A Barrett, Executive Director
Jennifer Markkanen, Assistant Executive Director

7610 Lung Association
6856 E Avenue   202-293-3650
Washington, DC 20012-6K2   Fax: 202-293-3656
e-mail: asaa@sleepapnea.org
www.sleep-apnea-ab.ca
The Lung Association - Sleep Apnea (LASA) is a patient and professional coalition providing support through improved care for patients with respiratory disorders of sleep.

7611 NIH/National Institute of Neurological Disorders and Stroke
PO Box 5801   301-496-5751
Bethesda, MD 20824   800-352-9424
TTY: 301-468-5981
www.ninds.nih.gov
Mission is to reduce the burden of neurological disease, a burden borne by every age group, by every segment of society, by people all over the world.
Story C Landis, Director
Walter J Koroshetz, Deputy Director

7612 Narcolepsy Institute/Montefiore Medical Center
111 E 210th Street   718-920-6799
Bronx, NY 10467-2490   Fax: 718-654-9580
e-mail: MGoswami@aol.com
www.montefiore.org
Offers services such as screening, information on narcolepsy, counseling and referrals for individuals and their families with problems arising as a consequence of narcolepsy, and adult and teenage support groups to help individuals develop positive self-images.
Dr Meeta Goswami, Director

7613 National Sleep Foundation
1522 K Street NW   202-347-3471
Washington, DC 20005-1253   Fax: 202-347-3472
e-mail: nsf@sleepfoundation.org
www.sleepfoundation.org
The National Sleep Foundation (NSF) is an independent nonprofit organization dedicated to improving public health and safety by achieving understanding of sleep and sleep disorders and by supporting education sleep-related research and advocacy.
Meir H Kryger, Chairman
Thomas J Balkin, Vice Chairman

7614 Sleep Research Society American Academy of Sleep Medicine
American Academy of Sleep Medicine
One Westbrook Corporate Center   708-492-1093
Westchester, IL 60154   Fax: 708-492-0943
e-mail: ncekosh@srsnet.org
www.sleepresearchsociety.org
Facilitates communication among research workers in this field but does not sponsor research investigations on its own.
Michael V Vitiello, President
Ronald Szymusiak, Secretary/Treasurer

Research Centers

7615 Baylor College of Medicine: Sleep Disorder and Research Center
6620 Main St   713-798-1000
Houston, TX 77030-3498   800-229-5671
Fax: 713-796-9718
e-mail: baylorclinicweb@bcm.edu
www.baylorclinic.com
Internal unit of the College that focuses on research into sleep and sexual dysfunction in males.
Shyam Subramanian, Medical Director
Charlie Lan, Assistant Professor of Medicine

7616 Capital Regional Sleep-Wake Disorders Center
St. Peter's Hospital and Albany Medical Center
25 Hackett Boulevard   518-436-9253
Albany, NY 12208-3420
Cheryl Carlu MD

7617 Center for Narcolepsy Research at the University of Illinois at Chicago
University of Illinois
845 S Damen Avenue   312-996-5176
Chicago, IL 60612-7350   Fax: 312-996-7008
e-mail: CNSHR@listserv.uic.edu
www.uic.edu/depts/cnr
Provides information to health professionals and people with sleep disorders regarding diagnosis and treatment. Maintain national network with sleep professionals throughout the US.
6-8 pages 2 per year
David W Carley, Director
Julie Law, Center Administrator

7618 Center for Research in Sleep Disorders Affiliated with Mercy Hospital
Mercy Hospital of Hamilton/Fairfield
1275 E Kemper Road   513-671-3101
Cincinnati, OH 45246
Martin Schar PhD

7619 Center for Sleep & Wake Disorders: Miami Valley Hospital
One Wyoming Street
Dayton, OH 45409-2722   937-208-8000
www.miamivalleyhospital.org
Offering the largest variety of sleep disorder testing available in the area it also offers comprehensive sleep care and care of related issues with a sleep lab clinical treatment pulmonary treatment and behavioral treatment in the same facility.
Kevin Huban, Director
Amy Cline, Administrative Director

7620 Center for Sleep Medicine of the Mount Sinai Medical Center
One Gustave L.Levy Place   212-241-6500
New York, NY 10029-6500   Fax: 212-875-84
www.mountsinai.org

The Center for Sleep Medicine at The Mount Sinai Medical Center is a comprehensive program dedicated to the diagnosis and treatment of all aspects of sleep pathology including breathing related sleep disorders periodic limb movements in sleep insomnia and narcolepsy. Mechanical (CPAP BiPAP ventilator) surgical dental and pharmacologic therapies are available.
E Neil Schachter, Professor
Gwen S Skloot, Associates Professor

7621 Geisinger Wyoming Valley Medical Center: Sleep Disorders Center
1000 E Mountain Drive
Wilkes-Barre, PA 18711   570-819-5770
www.geisinger.org
Our dedicated sleep team operates service sleep centers and laboratories to diagnose and treat a broad range of sleep disorders. Geisinger sleep centers are conveniently located in Danville Bloomsburg Shamokin Wilkes-Barre and Mt. Pocono.
Andrew Paul Matragrano, Director
Stephanie Schaefer, Nurse Practitioner

7622 Johns Hopkins University: Sleep Disorders Francis Scott Key Medical Center
Francis Scott Key Medical Center
601 N Caroline Street
Baltimore, MD 21287   410-550-0545
www.hopkinshospital.org
The Johns Hopkins University Sleep Disorders Center is a tertiary care center for patients with sleep/wake disorders and medical disorders associated with sleep.
Phillip L Smith, Director

7623 Knollwoodpark Hospital Sleep Disorders Center
5600 Girby Road   251-660-5120
Mobile, AL 36693-3398   Fax: 251-660-5245
e-mail: 71054.2530@compuserve.com
www.southalabama.edu/usakph

7624 Knollwoodpark Hospital Sleep Disorders Cen
5600 Girby Road   251-660-5120
Mobile, AL 36693   Fax: 251-660-5245
e-mail: 71054.2530@compuserve.com
www.southalabama.edu/usakph

7625 Loma Linda University Sleep Disorders Clinic
VA Hospital Medical Services Center
11201 Benton Street   909-825-7084
Loma Linda, CA 92357-1   800-741-8387
Fax: 909-963-64
www.lom.med.va.gov

Ralph Downey III MD, Director

7626 Methodist Hospital Sleep Center Winona Memorial Hospital
Rehab Centers
6565 Fannin Street   713-441-7854
Houston, TX 77030-8126   Fax: 713-790-2612
www.methodisthealth.com

Marc L Boom, President & CEO
David M Underwood, Vice Chairman

7627 MidWest Medical Center: Sleep Disorders Center
Winona Memorial Hospital
Indianapolis, IN 46208-4688   317-927-2100
Fax: 317-927-2914

7628 Northwest Ohio Sleep Disorders Center Toledo Hospital
Toledo Hospital
2142 N Cove Boulevard   419-471-5629
Toledo, OH 43606-3896
Frank O Horton III MD, Director

7629 Ohio Sleep Medicine Institute
4975 Bradenton Avenue   614-766-0773
Dublin, OH 43017-3521   Fax: 614-766-2599
e-mail: info@sleepmedicine.com
www.sleepmedicine.com
A comprehensive accredited sleep disorders center that is dedicated to excellence in sleep medicine care. Offer evaluation, diagnosis and treatment for adults and children with sleep apnea, insomnia, restless legs syndrome, narcolepsy, parasomnias, circa-

569

dian rhythms disorders, shift work, fatigue and other sleep problems.
Betty Palmer, Director

7630 Penn Center for Sleep Disorders: Hospital of the University of Pennsylvania
3400 Spruce Street   215-662-7772
Philadelphia, PA 19104-4204   Fax: 215-349-8038
Joanne Getsy MD, Director

7631 Presbyterian-University Hospital: Pulmonary Sleep Evaluation Center
DeSoto At O'Hara Street   412-647-3475
Pittsburgh, PA 15213
Mark Sanders MD, Director

7632 Scripps Clinic Sleep Disorders Center Scripps Clinic
Scripps Clinic
10666 N Torrey Pines Road   858-455-9100
La Jolla, CA 92037-1027   Fax: 858-828-64
e-mail: malcoRN@scrippsclinic.com
www.scripps.org
The Scripps Clinic Sleep Center provides evaluation diagnosis and treatment of a full range of sleep disorders such as Circadian rhythm disorders Insomnia Narcolepsy Night terror Nightmares Restless legs syndrome Sleep apnea Sleepwalking and Snoring.
Dan Dworsky MD, Medical Director
Merrill M Mitler MD, Scientific Director

7633 Sleep Alertness Center: Lafayette Home Hospital
2400 S Street   765-447-6811
Lafayette, IN 47904-3027   e-mail: glenda.eberhard@glhsi.org
Frederick Ro MD

7634 Sleep Center: Community General Hospital
750 East Adams Street
Syracuse, NY 13210-5100   315-464-5540
www.cgh.org
The Sleep Center at Community General Hospital is a specialized facility providing accurate diagnosis and recommending treatment of sleep-related problems.
Robert Westl MD, Medical Director
Antonio Cule MD, Neurology Consultant

7635 Sleep Disorders Center Bethesda Oak Hospital
619 Oak Street
Cincinnati, OH 45206-1613   513-569-5400
www.trihealth.com

Milton Krame MD

7636 Sleep Disorders Center Columbia Presbyterian Medical Center
The University Hospital of Columbia & Cornell
161 Fort Washington Avenue   212-305-1860
New York, NY 10032   Fax: 212-305-5496
e-mail: inquire@sleepNYP.com
www.sleepnyp.com
A Highly specialized outpatient facility for the evaluation and treatment of patients with problems related to sleep and wakefulness.
Neil B Kavey, Medical Director
Andrew Tucker, Director

7637 Sleep Disorders Center Dartmouth Hitchcock Medical Center
Darthmouth Hitchcock medical Center
One Rope Ferry Road   603-650-1200
Hanover, NH 03755-1   877-367-1797
Fax: 603-650-1202
e-mail: Joanne.MacQuarrie@dartmouth.edu
dms.dartmouth.edu
Provides consultation and testing for all varieties of sleep-related disturbances including snoring sleep apnea narcolepsy restless legs syndrome periodic limb movement disorder insomnia parasomnias and circadian rhythm disorders.
Glen Greenough, Fellowship Director
Michael Sate MD, Director

7638 Sleep Disorders Center Lankenau Hospital
100 E Lancaster Avenue   610-645-3400
Wynnewood, PA 19096-3498   Fax: 610-645-2291

7639 Sleep Disorders Center Ohio State University Medical Center
410 W.10th Ave   614-257-2500
Columbus, OH 43210-1228   800-293-5123
Fax: 614-257-2551
e-mail: webmaster@osumc.edu
medicalcenter.osu.edu
Ulysses J Magalang MD, Medical Director

7640 Sleep Disorders Center at California: Pacific Medical Center
2340 Clay Street   415-923-3336
San Francisco, CA 94115-1932   Fax: 415-923-3584
e-mail: 76307.2221@compuserve.com

7641 Sleep Disorders Center at California: Paci
2340 Clay Street   415-923-3336
San Francisco, CA 94115   Fax: 415-923-3584
e-mail: 76307.2221@compuserve.com

7642 Sleep Disorders Center of Metropolitan Toronto
500 Alden Road   905-475-5155
Markham Ontario, CA M6B-4H6   888-401-5155
Fax: 647-436-7607
e-mail: sleep@compuserve.com
www.sdc.ca

Jeffrey Lips MD, Director

7643 Sleep Disorders Center of Rochester: St. Mary's Hospital
2110 Clinton Avenue S   716-442-4141
Rochester, NY 14618-2616
Donald Green MD

7644 Sleep Disorders Center of Western New York Millard Fillmore Hospital
726 Exchange Street   716-859-5600
Buffalo, NY 14210-1120   Fax: 716-887-5332
gates.kaleidahealth.org

Daniel Rifkin, Director

7645 Sleep Disorders Center: Cleveland Clinic Foundation
9500 Euclid Avenue   216-636-5860
Cleveland, OH 44195-0001   800-223-2273
Fax: 216-445-1022
TTY: 216-444-0261
my.clevelandclinic.org
Accredited by the American Academy of Sleep Medicine the Cleveland Clinic Sleep Disorders Center is staffed by physicians specializing in sleep disorders from a variety of disciplines including adult and child neurology pulmonary and critical care medicine psychology psychiatry otolaryngology and dentistry.
Nancy Foldva Schaefer DO, Director
Petra Podmor RPSGT, Laboratory Manager

7646 Sleep Disorders Center: Community Medical Center
1822 Mulberry Street   717-969-8931
Scranton, PA 18510-2375
John Goodnow, Director

7647 Sleep Disorders Center: Crozer-Chester Medical Center
Sleep Disorders Center
175 E Chester Pike
Ridley Park, PA 19078-3975   610-447-2689
www.crozer.org
A multidisciplinary facility for the investigation and treatment of sleep problems
Calvin Staff MD, Medical Director

7648 Sleep Disorders Center: Good Samaritan Medical Center
1020 Franklin Street   814-533-1661
Johnstown, PA 15905-4109
Richard Parc DO, Director

7649 Sleep Disorders Center: Kettering Medical Center
3935 Southern Boulevard   937-395-8805
Kettering, OH 45439-1295   Fax: 937-395-8821
www.kmcnetwork.org

Donna Arand PhD, Clinical Director
George G Burton MD, Medical Director

7650 **Sleep Disorders Center: Medical College of Pennsylvania**
3200 Henry Avenue   215-842-4250
Philadelphia, PA 19129-1137
June M Fry MD PhD, Director

7651 **Sleep Disorders Center: Newark Beth Israel Medical Center**
201 Lyons Avenue at Osborne Terrace
Newark, NJ 07112-2027   973-926-2973
                                     www.sbhcs.com
Evaluates a wide range of disorders including sleep apnea snoring insomnia narcolepsy sleep-wake schedule disorders and male impotency. The center also provides board-certified consultants in sleep medicine neurology urology endocrinology psychiatry cardiology and ear nose and throat surgery in addition to certified sleep technologists.
Monroe S Karetzky MD

7652 **Sleep Disorders Center: Rhode Island Hospital**
70 Catamore Boulevard   401-431-5420
E Providence, RI 02914   Fax: 401-431-5429
                                     www.lifespan.org

Richard Mill MD, Director

7653 **Sleep Disorders Center: St. Vincent Medical Center**
2213 Cherry Street   419-321-4980
Toledo, OH 43608-2691
Joseph Schaf PhD, Director

7654 **Sleep Disorders Center: University Hospital, SUNY at Stony Brook**
240 Middle Country Road   631-444-2500
Smithtown, NY 11787-0001   Fax: 631-444-2580
                uhmc-xweb1.uhmc.sunysb.edu/sleepdisorder
Wallace Mend MD

7655 **Sleep Disorders Center: Winthrop, University Hospital**
259 First Street
Mineola, NY 11501-3808   516-663-0333
                                     www.winthrop.org

Steven H Feinsilver MD

7656 **Sleep Disorders Unit Beth Israel Deaconess Medical Center**
330 Brookline Avenue
Boston, MA 02215-5400   617-667-3237
                                     www.bidmc.org

Jean K Matheson MD

7657 **Sleep Laboratory St Joseph's Hospital**
St Joseph's Hospital
301 Prospect Ave   315-703-2138
Syracuse, NY 13203   888-785-6371
                                Fax: 315-755-77
                                     www.sjhsyr.org
The Sleep Lab focuses on diagnosing and treating Obstructive Sleep Apnea and sleep-related breathing disorders and has the largest number of sleep-credentialed physicians and registered sleep technologists of any sleep lab in the area.
Edward T Downing, Director

7658 **Sleep Laboratory, Maine Medical Center**
22 Bramhall Street   207-871-2279
Portland, ME 04102-3134

7659 **Sleep Medicine Associates of Texas**
5477 Glen Lakes Drive   214-750-7776
Dallas, TX 13210-4353   Fax: 214-750-4621
                         e-mail: smat@sleepmed.com
                                     www.sleepmed.com
First largest and longest standing accredited sleep center in North Texas.
Philipp Becker, President and Founding Partner
Andrew O Jamieson MD, Chairman of the Board and Founding Partn

7660 **Sleep Research Foundation**
170 Morton Street   617-522-9270
Boston, MA 02130-3735
Ernest Hartm MD, Director

7661 **Sleep Wake Disorders Center Montefiore Sleep Disorders Center**
111 E 210th Street   718-920-4321
Bronx, NY 10467-2401   Fax: 718-798-4352
                                     www.montefiore.org
Provide outstanding clinical care for patients with disorders that affect the sleep-wake cycle and are committed to performing high quality research and to making outstanding contributions to the areas of clinical research that includes the entire spectrum of sleep medicine.
Michael J Thorpy MD, Director
Karen Ballab MD, Associate Director

7662 **Sleep and Chronobiology Center: Western Psychiatric Institute and Clinic**
3811 Ohara Street   412-624-2246
Pittsburgh, PA 15213-2593
Charles F Reynolds III MD, Director

7663 **Sleep-Wake Disorders Center: New York Hospital-Cornell Medical Center**
520 E 70th Street   212-746-2623
New York, NY 10021-1504   Fax: 212-746-5509
                                     www.weillcornell.org

Charles Poll MD, Director

7664 **Sleep/Wake Disorders Center: Community Hospitals of Indianapolis**
1500 N Ritter Avenue   317-355-4275
Indianapolis, IN 46219-3027   Fax: 317-351-2785
                         e-mail: mevollmer@pol.net
Marvin E Vollmer MD

7665 **Sleep/Wake Disorders Center: Hampstead Hospital**
E Road   603-329-5311
Hampstead, NH 03841
Deborah Sewi PhD

7666 **Stanford University Center for Narcolepsy Dept of Psychiatry & Behavioral Sciences**
450 Broadway Street   650-725-6517
Redwood City, CA 94063-5102   Fax: 650-498-7761
                          e-mail: jck@stanford.edu
                                     med.stanford.edu

Dr Emanuel Mignot, Director
Marlene Iry, Admin Associate

7667 **Thomas Jefferson University: Sleep Disorders Center**
Jefferson Medical College
1020 Walnut Street   215-955-6000
Philadelphia, PA 19107-5083   800-JEF-FNOW
                                Fax: 215-955-9783
                                     www.jefferson.edu
A comprehensive clinical research and educational program in sleep and sleep disorders medicine.
Karl Doghram MD, Medical Director

7668 **University of Texas Sleep/Wake Disorders Center**
Southwestern Medical Center
5323 Harry Hines Boulevard   214-648-7350
Dallas, TX 75390-9070   Fax: 214-487-59
Studies sleep/wake disorders including insomnia apnea and narcolepsy.
Howard Roffw MD, Director

Support Groups & Hotlines

7669 **Narcolepsy Institute/Montefiore Medical Center**
111 E 210th Street   718-920-6799
Bronx, NY 10467-2490   Fax: 718-654-9580
                         e-mail: MGoswami@aol.com
                                     www.narcolepsyinstitute.org
The Narcolepsy Institute provides psychosocial support services for narcolepsy.
Dr. Meeta Goswami, Director

7670   Narcolepsy Network
129 Waterwheel Lane
North Kingstown, RI 02852

401-667-2523
888-292-6522
Fax: 401-633-6567
e-mail: narnet@narcolepsynetwork.org
www.narcolepsynetwork.org

Provides advocacy and education, supports research. Newsletter, conferences, phone support and group development guidelines.
Patricia Higgins, President
Eveline V. Honig, Md, MPh, Executive Director

7671   National Health Information Center
PO Box 1133
Washington, DC 20013

310-565-4167
800-336-4797
Fax: 301-984-4256
e-mail: info@nhic.org
www.health.gov/nhic

Offers a nationwide information referral service, produces directories and resource guides.

Books

7672   ABC of ZZZs
National Sleep Foundation
1522 K Street NW
Washington, DC 20005-1235

202-347-3471
Fax: 202-347-3472
www.sleepfoundation.org

A primer on sleep basics, including getting enough sleep, why sleep is important, and ' sleep stealers.'
Emerson Darbonne, Communications Coordinator

7673   Doctor, I Can't Sleep: Insomnia Training Manual
Narcolepsy Network
PO Box 42460
Cincinnati, OH 45242-0460

513-891-3522
Fax: 513-891-9936
e-mail: narnet@aol.com

Comprehensive course manual for primary care physicians and the public. Outlines basic facts about epidemiology, sleep hygiene, relaxation techniques, diagnosis, and treatment.
100+ pages

7674   International Classification of Sleep Disorders
American Academy of Sleep Medicine
One Westbrook Corporate Center
Westchester, IL 60154

708-492-0930
Fax: 708-492-0943
www.aasmnet.org

A comprehensive manual for physicians and other healthcare professionals containing information on 84 sleep disorders. The extensive text describes the diagnostic features of each disorder and includes specific diagnostic and severity criteria for each disorder.
396 pages Paperback

7675   Living with Narcolepsy
National Sleep Foundation
1522 K Street
Washington, DC 20005-1235

202-347-3471
Fax: 202-347-3472
www.sleepfoundation.org

Defines and describes narcolepsy and what can be expected after diagnosis, including effects on education, career, social and family life.
Emerson Darbonne, Communications Coordinator

7676   Melatonin: The Basic Facts
National Sleep Foundation
1522 K Street
Washington, DC 20005-1235

202-347-3471
Fax: 202-347-3472
www.sleepfoundation.org

If you're curious about melatonin, it's not suprising. There has been a lot of attention paid to the hormone in popular magazines and books, scholarly journals, and advertisements. You may habe heard claims that malatonin cures everything from jet lag to insomnia to aging.
Emerson Darbonne, Communications Coordinator

7677   Narcolepsy Primer
Meeta Goswami, Michael Thorpy, author
Narcolepsy Institute/Montefiore Medical Center

111 E 210th Street
Bronx, NY 10467-2401

718-920-6799
Fax: 718-654-9580
e-mail: MGsowami@aol.com
narcolepsyinstitute.org

A guide for physicians, patients and their families on the affects, causes and prevention of narcolepsy.
Dr. Meeta Goswami, Director

7678   Narcolepsy Primer Package
Meeta Goswami, Michael Thorpy, author
Narcolepsy Institute/Montefiore Medical Center
111 E 210th Street
Bronx, NY 10467-2401

718-920-6799
Fax: 718-654-9580
e-mail: MGsowami@aol.com
narcolepsyinstitute.org

The package includes: Narcolepsy Primer; Manuel on Narcolepsy and A Counseling Service for Narcolepsy: A Sociomedical Model.
Dr. Meeta Goswami, Director

7679   Pain and Sleep
National Sleep Foundation
1522 K Street NW
Washington, DC 20005-1235

202-347-3471
Fax: 202-347-3472
www.sleepfoundation.org

Whether pain results from headache, backache, arthritis, or other conditions, it frequently occurs with sleep difficulty. This overview of the pain and sleep connection describes behavioral and pharmacological approaches to pain management.
Emerson Darbonne, Communications Coordinator

7680   Sleep Aids: Everything You Wanted To Know But Were Too Tired To Ask
National Sleep Foundation
1522 K Street NW
Washington, DC 20005-1235

202-347-3471
Fax: 202-347-3472
www.sleepfoundation.org

If you have trouble falling or staying asleep, or you wake up feeling unrefreshed, you may be suffering from insomnia. Insomnia is a symptom. It may be caused by stress, anxiety, depression, disease, pain, medications, sleep disorders or poor sleep habits.
Emerson Darbonne, Communications Coordinator

7681   Sleep Apnea
National Sleep Foundation
1522 K Street, NW
Washington, DC 20005-1235

202-347-3471
Fax: 202-347-3472
www.sleepfoundation.org

A brochure about sleep apnea, a breathing disorder characterized by brief interruptions of breathing during sleep. Brochure explains what it is, who gets it, and how it is diagnosed and treated.
Emerson Darbonne, Communications Coordinator

7682   Snoring and Sleep Apnea
Demos Medical Publishing
386 Park Avenue S
New York, NY 10016

212-683-0072
Fax: 212-683-0118
e-mail: orderdept@demopub.com
www.demosmedpub.com

A straightforward, jargon-free approach to dealing with snoring and sleep problems.
222 pages
ISBN: 1-888799-29-3
Dr. Diana M Schneider, President

7683   You Don't LOOK Sick!: Living Well with Invisible Chronic Illness
Joy Selak, Steven Overman, author
Haworth Press
10 Alice Street
Binghamton, NY 13904-1580

607-722-5857
800-429-6784
Fax: 607-722-0012
www.haworthpress.com

Chronicles a patient's true-life stories and her physician's compassionate commentary as they take a journey through the three stages of chronic illness - Getting Sick, Being Sick, and Living Well.
Hardcover $29.95 (ISBN): 978-0-7890-2488-0, Paperback $14.95 (ISBN): 978-0-7890-2499-7.
145 pages Hrdcover/Ppbck

Magazines

7684 SleepMatters
National Sleep Foundation
1522 K Street NW
Washington, DC 20005-1235
202-347-3471
Fax: 202-347-3472
www.sleepfoundation.org
Covering hot sleep news, profiles, advice from experts and much more!
Quarterly
Cameron Darbonne, Communications Coordinator

Newsletters

7685 Eye Opener
American Narcolepsy Association
425 California Street, Suite 201
San Francisco, CA 94126-6230
415-788-4793
Offers information on sleep disorders including a question and answer column for persons suffering from disorders.

7686 Narcolepsy Institute/Montefiore Medical Center
Meeta Goswami, author

Narcolepsy Institute
111 E 210th Street
Bronx, NY 10467-2490
718-920-6799
Fax: 718-654-9580
e-mail: MGsowami@aol.com
narcolepsyinstitute.org
The Narcolepsy Institute provides psychosocial support services for narcolepsy and has a newsletter, a video, and a primer on narcolepsy.
8 pages Bi-Annual
Dr. Meeta Goswami, Director

7687 Sleep Medicine Alert
Nationa Sleep Foundation
1522 K Street NW
Washington, DC 20005-1235
202-347-3471
Fax: 202-347-3472
www.sleepfoundation.org
This quearterly newsletter is for healthcare professionals. It offers updates on sleep research and its clinical implications, information on diagnosing and treating a variety of sleep disorders.

7688 Wake-Up Call
American Sleep Apnea Association
6856 E Avenue
Washington, DC 20012
202-293-3650
Fax: 202-293-3656
e-mail: asaa@sleepapnea.org
www.sleepapnea.org
Contains information of interest to APNEA patients and their families.
Quarterly
Michael P Coppola MD, President and Chief Medical Officer
Nancy Rothstein, Secretary

Pamphlets

7689 Get the Facts About Sleep Apnea
American Sleep Apnea Association
1424 K Street NW
Washington, DC 20005
202-293-3650
Fax: 202-293-3656
e-mail: asaa@sleepapnea.org
www.sleepapnea.org

7690 Helping Yourself to a Good Night's Sleep
Nantional Sleep Foundation
1522 K Street NW
Washington, DC 20005-1253
202-347-3471
Fax: 202-347-3472
www.sleepfoundation.org
About half of Americans report sleep difficulty at least occasionally, according to National Sleep Foundation surveys. These woescalled insomnia by doctors-have far reaching effects. This brochure details the many things you can do to improve your sleep.

7691 Narcolepsy
American Academy of Sleep Medicine

One Westbrook Corporate Center
Westchester, IL 60154
708-492-0930
Fax: 708-492-0943
www.aasmnet.org
Describes the causes, symptoms and treatments of a disorder characterized by excessive sleepiness.
Lot of 50

7692 Sleep Diary
National Sleep Foundation
1522 K Street, NW
Washington, DC 20005-1235
202-347-3471
Fax: 202-347-3472
www.sleepfoundation.org
It includes sections on sleep schedules, quality and quantity of sleep, sleep disturbances, sleep hygiene and daytime sleepiness. It enables people to identify their sleep and health habits and note any sleep problems they may have.
Emerson Darbonne, Communications Coordinator

7693 Sleep Strategies for Shift Workers
National Sleep Foundation
1522 K Street NN
Washington, DC 20005-1235
202-347-3471
Fax: 202-347-3472
www.sleepfoundation.org
This brochure outlines the common effects of shift work on health, workplace alertness and productivity and offers tips about diet, sleep environment, medications, light therapy and sleep hygiene.
Cameron Darbonne, Communications Coordinator

7694 Wake Up! Brochure
National Sleep Foundation
1522 K Street NW
Washington, DC 20005-1235
202-347-3471
Fax: 202-347-3472
www.sleepfoundation.org
A blooklet dedicated to the drowsy driving problem, including the risks, the myths, the danger signals and recommendations.
Cameron Darbonne, Communications Coordinator

7695 When You Can't Sleep
Narcolepsy Network
Po Box 294
Pleasantville, NY 10570-0460
401-667-2523
888-292-6522
Fax: 401-633-6567
e-mail: narnet@aol.com
A primer on sleep basics, including getting enough sleep, why sleep is important, and sleep stealers. Plus a sleep quotient quiz.

7696 Women and Sleep
National Sleep Foundation
1522 K Street NW
Washington, DC 20005-1235
202-347-3471
Fax: 202-347-3472
www.sleepfoundation.org
A brochure dealing with the effects of sleep on women which explores reasons for tiredness, increased accidents, problems concentrating, and poor performance on the job and in school, and possible increased sickness.
Cameron Darbonne, Communications Coordinator

Audio & Video

7697 Narcolepsy
American Academy of Sleep Medicine
One Westbrook Corporate Center
Westchester, IL 60154
708-492-0930
Fax: 708-492-0943
www.aasmnet.org
Addresses the etiology, pathophysiology, diagnosis and management of narcolepsy.
58 slides

7698 Narcolepsy: Fanlight Productions
Jason Margolis, author

Fanlight Productions
4196 Washington Street
Boston, MA 02131-1731
617-469-4999
800-937-4113
Fax: 617-469-3379
e-mail: fanlight@fanlight.com
www.fanlight.com

This remarkable film presents the experiences of three individuals whose lives and relationships have been disrupted by narcolepsy.
2000 25 Minutes
ISBN: 1-572953-23-2

7699 Video on Narcolepsy
Narcolepsy Institute/Montefiore Medical Center
111 E 210th Street   718-920-6799
Bronx, NY 10467   Fax: 718-654-9580
e-mail: MGsowami@aol.com
www.narcolepsyinstitute.org
Clinical symptoms, genetics, diagnosis, effects of Narcolepsy, support groups.
Dr. Meeta Goswami, Director

Web Sites

7700 American Sleep Apnea Association
www.sleeppapnea.org
The ASAA is a 501(c)(3) organization dedicated to reducing injuiry, disability, and depth from sleep apnea and to enhancing the well-being of those affected by this common disorder. The ASAA promotes education and awareness, the ASAA A.W.A.K.E. network of voluntary mutual support groups, research, and continuous improvement of care.

7701 American Sleep Disorders Association
Provides full diagnostic and treatment services to improve the quality of care for patients with all types of sleep disorders.

7702 Healing Well
www.healingwell.com
An online health resource guide to medical news, chat, information and articles, newsgroups and message boards, books, disease-related web sites, medical directories, and more for patients, friends, and family coping with disabling diseases, disorders, or chronic illnesses.

7703 Health Finder
www.healthfinder.gov
Searchable, carefully developed web site offering information on over 1000 topics. Developed by the US Department of Health and Human Services, the site can be used in both English and Spanish.

7704 Healthlink USA
www.healthlinkusa.com
Health information concerning treatment, cures, prevention, diagnosis, risk factors, research, support groups, email lists, personal stories and much more. Updated regularly.

7705 Helios Health
www.helioshealth.com
Online resource for your health information. Detailed information about specific health topics, access to expert advice from our Medical Advisory Board, and up-to-date health news.

7706 MGH Neurology WebForums
Online. Provides both unmoderated message boards and chat rooms for specific neurological disorders.

7707 MedicineNet
www.medicinenet.com
An online resource for consumers providing easy-to-read, authoritative medical and health information.

7708 Medscape
www.medscape.com
Medscape offers specialists, primary care physicians, and other health professionals the Web's most robust and integrated medical information and educational tools.

7709 National Sleep Foundation
www.sleepfoundation.org
Information for millions of Americans who suffer from sleep disorders, and to prevent the catastrophic accidents that are related to poor or disordered sleep through research, education and the dissemination of information.

7710 Neurology Channel
www.neurologychannel.com

Find clearly explained, medically accurate information regarding conditions, including an overview, symptoms, causes, diagnostic procedures and treatment options. On this site it is possible to ask questions and get information from a neurologist and connect to people who have similar health interests.

7711 Sleep Research Society
www.sleepresearchsociety.org
Facilitates communication among research workers in this field, but does not sponsor research investigations on its own.

7712 WebMD
www.webmd.com
Information on Narcolepsy, including articles and resources.

Description

7713 ## Spina Bifida

Spina bifida refers to conditions which result in an incomplete closure of the spinal column during fetal development. It is the most serious of a group of disorders called neural tube defects. The severity of spina bifida ranges from mild to severe.

Spina bifida occulta is an opening in one or more vertebrae without damage to the spinal cord. Meningocele is when the protective covering around the spinal cord (meninges) has protruded into the vertebrae, with little, if any, damage. Myelomeningocele, the most severe form of spina bifida, is when part of the actual spinal cord pushes through the back and exposes nerves and tissues.

The effects of spina bifida, in its most extreme state, are serious. They can include paralysis, loss of bowel and bladder control and hydrocephalus. Other inherited abnormalities may be present. Open spina bifida can be diagnosed in utero by finding elevations of a specific protein in maternal amniotic fluid. Prevention involves supplementation with folic acid. Treatments for spina bifida require a united effort by a team of specialists, and depend on the severity of the defects. With proper care, many children with spina bifida live fairly normal lives. See also *Birth Defects*.

National Agencies & Associations

7714 **Canadian & American Spinal Research Organi zation**
120 Newkirk Road
Richmond Hill, ON, L4C-9S7
905-508-4000
800-361-4004
Fax: 905-508-4002
e-mail: info@csro.com
www.csro.com
Dedicated to the improvement of the physical quality of life for persons with a spinal cord injury and those with related neurological deficits, through targeted medical and scientific research.
Barry Munro, Chair
Dave Lostchuk, Treasurer

7715 **Easter Seals**
233 South Wacker Drive
Chicago, IL 60606-4703
312-726-6200
800-221-6827
Fax: 312-726-1494
TTY: 312-726-4258
e-mail: info@easter-seals.org
www.easter-seals.org
Provides serves to children and adults with disabilities as well as support to their families.
Reenie Kavalar, VP Medical/Rehabilitation Services

7716 **March of Dimes Birth Defects Foundation**
1275 Mamaroneck Avenue
White Plains, NY 10605
914-949-7166
www.marchofdimes.com
Our mission is to improve the health of babies by preventing birth defects premature birth and infant mortality. The March of Dimes carries out this mission through programs of research community services education and advocacy to save babies' lives.

7717 **Spina Bifida Association of America**
4590 Macarthur Boulevard NW
Washington, DC 20007-4226
202-944-3285
800-621-3141
Fax: 202-944-3295
e-mail: sbaa@sbaa.org
www.sbaa.org

The association works for people with spina bifida and their families through education advocacy research and service. There is also an annual conference and publications available.
Cindy Brownstein, CEO
Maya House, Resource Center Manager

7718 **Spina Bifida and Hydrocephalus Association of Canada**
#977-167 Lombard Avenue
Winnipeg, Manitoba, R3B-0V3
204-925-3650
800-565-9488
Fax: 204-925-3654
e-mail: spinab@mts.net
www.sbhac.ca

To improve the quality of life of all individuals with spina bifida and/or hydrocephalus and their families, through awareness, education, research, and advocacy, and to reduce the incidence of neural tube defects.
Lorelei Fletcher, President
Gene Layton, VP

State Agencies & Associations

Alabama

7719 **Spina Bifida Association of Alabama**
PO Box 13254
Birmingham, AL 35202-0538
256-617-1414
e-mail: info@sbaofal.org
www.sbaofal.org

Betsy Hopson, President
Steven Horne, Vice President

Arizona

7720 **Spina Bifida Association of Arizona**
1001 E Fairmount Avenue
Phoenix, AZ 85014-4806
602-274-3323
Fax: 602-274-7632
e-mail: office@sbglobal.net
www.sbaaz.org

Benjaman D Scanlan, President
Ron Whiteside, Treasurer

California

7721 **Spina Bifida Association of Greater San Diego**
PO Box 232272
San Diego, CA 92193-2272
619-491-9018
Fax: 619-275-3361
e-mail: sbaofgsd@hotmail.com
www.spinabifidasandiego.com

Erika Jorquera, President

Colorado

7722 **Spina Bifida Association of Colorado**
PO Box 22994
Denver, CO 80222-0994
303-797-7870
Fax: 303-730-8032
e-mail: sbacolorado@gmail.com
www.coloradospinabifida.org

Chris Mestas, Chairman
Lavon Birney, Executive Director

Connecticut

7723 **Spina Bifida Association of Connecticut**
370 Osgood Avenue
New Britain, CT 06053-2545
860-839-0115
800-574-6274
Fax: 860-832-6260
e-mail: sbac@sbac.org
www.sbac.org

Mary Attardo, President
Kiley J Carlson, Executive Director

Delaware

7724 **Spina Bifida Association of Delaware**
PO Box 807
Wilmington, DE 19899-0807
302-478-4805
e-mail: kbasar@aol.com
www.angelfire.com/de/sbaofde/

Blake Heath, Vice President
Andy Anderso Jr, Treasurer

Florida

7725 Spina Bifida Association of Florida Space Coast
100 W Lucerne Circle
Orlando, FL 32801-2549
407-248-9210
Fax: 321-454-9737
e-mail: sbafscearthlink.com
www.sbacentralflorida.org

Rob Roy, Chairman
Melisa Portnoy, Secretary

7726 Spina Bifida Association of Jacksonville
807 Childrens Way
Jacksonville, FL 32207-8426
904-697-3686
800-722-6355
Fax: 904-390-3466
e-mail: sbaj@sbaj.org
www.sbaj.org

Michael Erhard, Chairperson

7727 Spina Bifida Association of Tampa
100 W Lucerne Circle
Orlando, FL 32801-1038
407-248-9210
Fax: 813-872-9845
e-mail: sbatampabay@aol.com
www.sbatampabay.org

Dianne Gore, President

Georgia

7728 Spina Bifida Association of Georgia
1448 Mclendon Drive
Decatur, GA 30033
770-939-1044
Fax: 770-939-1049
e-mail: info@spinabifidaga.org
www.spinabifidaofgeorgia.org
Provides referrals, evaluation, treatment and therapeutic activities for children and teens afflicted with spina bifida. The goal of this center is to help children or teenagers prepare for life.
William Turnispeed, President
Judy Thibadeau, Vice President

Illinois

7729 Illinois Spina Bifida Association
8765 W Higgins Road
Chicago, IL 60631-1693
773-444-0305
800-969-4722
Fax: 630-637-1066
e-mail: info@i-sba.org
www.sbail.org

Dedicated to improving the quality of life of people with spina bifida through direct services, information and referral and public awareness. Direct services include a residential summer camp for children with spina bifida over the age of seven.
Scott J Munkvold, President
Amy Maggio, CEO

Indiana

7730 Spina Bifida Association of Central Indiana
PO Box 19814
Indianapolis, IN 46279-0814
317-592-1630
Fax: 317-351-2010
e-mail: pres@sbaci.org
www.sbaci.org

James Zetzl, President

Iowa

7731 Spina Bifida Association of Iowa
8525 Douglas Avenue
Urbandale, IA 50322-1456
515-278-7013
e-mail: contact@sbaia.org
www.spinabifidaia.com

Rod Tressel, President

Kentucky

7732 Spina Bifida Association of Kentucky
Kosair Charities Center

982 Eastern Parkway
Louisville, KY 40217-1568
502-637-7363
866-340-7225
Fax: 502-637-1010
e-mail: sbak@sbak.org
www.sbak.org

Angela Cosby, President
Patty Dissell, Executive Director

Louisiana

7733 Spina Bifida Association of Greater New Orleans
PO Box 1346
Kenner, LA 70063-1346
504-737-5181
Fax: 504-538-9046
e-mail: sbagno@sbagno.com
www.sbagno.com

Al Hitt, President
Judy Otto, Vice-President

Maryland

7734 Spina Bifida Association of Maryland
2416 Lampost Lane
Baltimore, MD 21234-1460
410-665-1543
Fax: 410-833-1700
e-mail: sbamaryland@comcast.net
www.home.comcast.net/~sbamaryland

7735 Spina Bifida Association of the Eastern Shore
316 Prospect Avenue
Easton, MD 21601-4046
410-822-8609
Fax: 410-822-5455
www.spinabifidaassociation.org

Massachusetts

7736 Spina Bifida Association of Massachusetts
321 Fortune Boulevard
Milford, MA 01757-2741
617-742-2574
888-479-1900
Fax: 978-649-8725
e-mail: bsullivan@sbaMass.org
www.msbaweb.org

Brendan Sullivan, President
Cara Packard, Vice President

Michigan

7737 Spina Bifida Association of Grand Rapids
235 Wealthy Street SE
Grand Rapids, MI 49503-5299
616-240-9672
Fax: 616-222-1541
e-mail: WMiSBA@hotmail.com
www.spinabifida.org

Carol Carpenter, President

7738 Spina Bifida Association of Upper Peninsula Michigan
1220 N 3rd Street
Ishpeming, MI 44849-1108
906-485-5127
Fax: 906-225-7230
e-mail: cbengson@nmu.edu
www.sba-up.8m.com

Lois Bengson, President

7739 Spina Bifida and Hydrocephalus Association of Southwestern Michigan
PO Box 212
Mattawan, MI 49071-0212
269-385-3959
Fax: 269-392-9765
e-mail: marenhorkness@yahoo.com

Richard Benthnin, President

Minnesota

7740 Spina Bifida Association of Minnesota
PO Box 29323
Minneapolis, MN 55429-0212
651-222-6395
Fax: 952-591-0246
e-mail: sbamn@hotmail.com
www.sbamn.com

Wendy Swanson, President
Jim Thayer, Executive Director

Missouri

7741 Spina Bifida Association of Greater St. Louis
8050 Watson Road
Saint Louis, MO 63119-2000
314-843-2244
800-784-0983
Fax: 314-353-1446
e-mail: sbastl@charter.net
www.sbstl.com

Mark Abbott, President

Nebraska

7742 Spina Bifida Association of Nebraska
7612 Maple Street
Omaha, NE 68134-2153
402-932-5826
Fax: 402-572-3002
www.spinabifidanebraska.org

LeAnn Karman, President

New Jersey

7743 Spina Bifida Association of the Tri-State Region
84 Park Avenue
Flemington, NJ 08822-1174
908-782-7475
877-722-8774
Fax: 908-782-6102
e-mail: info@thesbrn.org
www.sbatsr.org
Serves New Jersey, New York Metro Area and Southern Connecticut.
Jane Horowitz, Executive Director and President
K David Holmes, Chairman of the Board

New Mexico

7744 Spina Bifida Association of New Mexico
1127 University Boulevard NE
Albuquerque, NM 87102-1740
505-242-1184
www.sbanm.com

Rey Garduno, Executive Director
Ann Beddingfield, Interim Treasurer

New York

7745 Spina Bifida Association of Albany/Capital District
100 Spring
Scotia, NY 12302-3312
518-399-9151
e-mail: sbaalbany102@aol.com
www.abaalbany.org

Kevin Chamberlain, Co-President
Vanessa Chamberlain, Co-President

7746 Spina Bifida Association of Greater Rochester
PO Box 3
Fairport, NY 14450-0003
585-381-5471
Fax: 585-264-9547
e-mail: jarmst4459@aol.com

JoAnn Armstrong, President

7747 Spina Bifida Association of Nassau County
12 Hampton Road
Sound Beach, NY 11789
631-821-9028
e-mail: kid3418@optonline.net
www.spinabifidaassociation.org

Leslieann Sussman, President

North Carolina

7748 Spina Bifida Association of North Carolina
3915 Grace Court
Indian Trail, NC 28079
704-882-0988
800-847-2262
Fax: 704-882-0988
e-mail: sbanc@mindspring.com
www.spinabifidaassociation.org

Julie Yindra, President
Kin Gates, Executive Director

Ohio

7749 Spina Bifida Association of Canton
S Cherokee Trail
Malvern, OH 44644
330-863-2531
Fax: 330-863-1172
e-mail: cmgriffin@nero.rr.com
www.spinabifidasupport.com

Connie Griffin, President

7750 Spina Bifida Association of Central Ohio
7239 Upper Cambridge Way
Westerville, OH 43082
614-818-3840
e-mail: sbaco@sbaco.net
www.sbaco.net

Laurie Schulze, Treasurer
Chrissy Zepfel, President

7751 Spina Bifida Association of Cincinnati
644 Linn Street
Cincinnati, OH 45203-0152
513-923-1378
e-mail: sbacincy@sbacincy.org
www.sbacincy.org

Brady Sellet, President
Diane Burns, Executive Director

7752 Spina Bifida Association of Greater Dayton
4801 Springfield Street
Dayton, OH 45431
937-236-1122
Fax: 937-434-4899
e-mail: mvspinabifida@yahoo.com
www.sbadayton.org

David Skinner, President
Lisa Maas, Vice President

7753 Spina Bifida Association of Northwest Ohio
302 Conant St
Maumee, OH 43537
419-794-0561
Fax: 419-533-3952
e-mail: sba@sbaofnorthwestohio.org
www.sbaofnorthwestohio.org

Ginnette Clark, President
Julie Harley, Vice President

Pennsylvania

7754 Spina Bifida Association of Central Pennsylvania
209 E State Street
Quarryville, PA 17566-1242
717-786-9280
888-770-SBPA
Fax: 717-786-8821
e-mail: SBAofPA@aol.com
www.geocities.com/sbaofgpa

Patricia Fulvio, President
Amy Graver, Chairman

7755 Spina Bifida Association of Delaware Valley
Havertown, PA 19083-0289
610-584-5530
800-223-0222
Fax: 215-412-9396
e-mail: info@sbadv.org
www.sbadv.org
Spina Bifida is the most common permanently disabling birth defect in the United States. An average of 8 babies every day are born with Spina Bifida or a similar birth defect of the brain and spine. There are over 60 million women in the U.S. who could become pregnant and each one is at risk of having a baby born with Spina Bifida. The mission of the Spina Bifida Association of Delaware Valley is to promote the prevention of Spina Bifida and to enhance the lives of all affected.
Marilyn Lieb, President
Keri Mascaro, Executive Director

7756 Spina Bifida Association of Greater Pennsylvania
209 E State Street
Quarryville, PA 17566-9614
717-786-9280
Fax: 717-786-8821
e-mail: sbaofpa@aol.com
www.spinabifidaresource.weebly.com
The Spina Bifida Resource was started in the 1970's, when a group of Moms met while their children had therapy.

As the needs and issues were discussed, the group decided to band together for support. Thus the Spina Bifida Association of Lancaster County was born. Our first public meeting had 45 parents and concerned professionals in attendance.

After about 20 years, the Board felt the need to change our name to reflect all those we served in and around Pennsylvania. Thus we became the Spina

Amy Graver, President
Patricia Fulvio, Executive Director

Rhode Island

7757 Spina Bifida Association of Rhode Island
Warwick, RI 02887-6948
401-732-7862
Fax: 401-732-7862
www.spinabifidaassociation.org

Tennessee

7758 Spina Bifida Association of Tennessee
Nashville, TN 37202-5529
615-791-8117
Fax: 615-791-1518
e-mail: lynnhess56@comcast.net
www.spinabifidasupport.com

Lynn Cook, President

Texas

7759 Spina Bifida Association of Austin
9301 Bradner Drive
Austin, TX 78748
512-292-6317
Fax: 512-479-3845
e-mail: austinspinabifida@yahoo.com
www.spinabifidasupport.com

Kelley Hively, President

7760 Spina Bifida Association of Dallas
705 W Avenue B
Garland, TX 75040
972-238-8755
Fax: 972-414-3772
e-mail: sbdal@aol.com
www.sbdallas.org

Robin Lee, President
Ryan McCoy, Vice President

7761 Spina Bifida Association of Texas, Gulf Coast
440 Benmar
Houston, TX 77060-2460
281-447-2707
Fax: 281-997-2278
e-mail: fandfsports@sbcglobal.net
www.sbahgc.org
The mission of Spina Bifida Houston Gulf Coast is to promote public awareness and enrich the lives of individuals and families living with spina bifida.
Jennifer Franklin, Vice President
Joan Peck, Treasurer

Washington

7762 Spina Bifida Association of Washington State
611 2nd Street
Snohomish, WA 98290
253-589-3700
888-289-3702
Fax: 775-766-1654
e-mail: sbaws@yahoo.com
www.sbaws.org
The Spina Bifida Association of Washington State is an affiliated chapter of the national Spina Bifida Association.
Jason Lane, Chair
Ryan Callaway, Director

Wisconsin

7763 Spina Bifida Association of Northern Wisconsin
Schofield, WI 54476-0421
715-798-3944
e-mail: dtackley@chegnet.net

David Blanchard, President

7764 Spina Bifida Association of Southeastern Wisconsin
830 N 109th Street
Wauwatosa, WI 53226
414-607-9061
Fax: 414-607-9602
e-mail: sbawi@sbawi.org
www.sbawi.org

Spina Bifida occurs when the spine of the baby fails to close. This creates an opening, or lesion, on the spinal column. Because of the opening on the spinal column, the nerves in the spinal column may be damaged and not work properly. This results in some degree of paralysis. The higher the lesion is on the spinal column, the greater the likelihood of increased paralysis. Surgery to close the spine is generally done within hours after birth. The surgery helps reduce the risk of infection and pr
Karen Drzewiecki, President
David G. Tucker, MSW, Executive Director

7765 Spina Bifida Association of the Greater Fox Valley
325 N John Street
Kimberly, WI 54136
920-687-0801
e-mail: fus1234@athenet.net
www.spinabifidasupport.com

Kelly Richard, President

Support Groups & Hotlines

7766 National Health Information Center
Washington, DC 20013
310-565-4167
800-336-4797
Fax: 301-984-4256
e-mail: info@nhic.org
www.health.gov/nhic
Offers a nationwide information referral service, produces directories and resource guides.

Books

7767 Answering Your Questions About Spina Bifida
Spina Bifida Association of America
4590 Macarthur Boulevard NW
Washington, DC 20007-4226
202-944-3285
800-621-3141
Fax: 202-944-3295
e-mail: sbaa@sbaa.org
www.sbaa.org
Provides information to help people understand the basic medical, educational and social issues which commonly affect people with Spina Bifida.

7768 Bowel Continence and Spina Bifida
Spina Bifida Association of America
4590 Macarthur Boulevard NW
Washington, DC 20007-4226
202-944-3285
800-621-3141
Fax: 202-944-3295
e-mail: sbaa@sbaa.org
www.sbaa.org
An excellent book aimed at anyone (infant or adult) trying to attain bowel continence. Focuses on continence programs, bowel management development and techniques.

7769 Clinic Directory
Spina Bifida Association of America
4590 Macarthur Boulevard NW
Washington, DC 20007-4226
202-944-3285
800-621-3141
Fax: 202-944-3295
e-mail: sbaa@sbaa.org
www.sbaa.org
A directory of health care clinics throughout the United States for children and adults with spina bifida.
200 pages 3-Ring Binder

7770 Complete IEP Guide: How to Advocate for Your Special Ed Child
Spina Bifida Association
4590 Macarthur Boulevard NW
Washington, DC 20007-4226
202-944-3285
800-621-3141
e-mail: sbaa@sbaa.org
www.sbaa.org
This all-in-one guide will help you understand special education law, identify your child's needs, prepare for meetings, develop the IEP and resolve disputes.

7771 Confronting the Challenges of Spina Bifida
Spina Bifida Association of America

4590 Macarthur Boulevard NW
Washington, DC 20007-4226

202-944-3285
800-621-3141
Fax: 202-944-3295
e-mail: sbaa@sbaa.org
www.sbaa.org

A group curriculum addressing self-care, self-esteem, and social skills in 8 to 13 year olds.

7772 Healthcare Guidelines
Spina Bifida Association of America
4590 Macarthur Boulevard NW
Washington, DC 20007-4226

202-944-3285
800-621-3141
Fax: 202-944-3295
e-mail: sbaa@sbaa.org
www.sbaa.org

7773 Learning Disabilities and the Person with Spina Bifida
Spina Bifida Association of America
4590 Macarthur Boulevard NW
Washington, DC 20007-4226

202-944-3285
800-621-3141
Fax: 202-944-3295
e-mail: sbaa@sbaa.org
www.sbaa.org

7774 Negotiating the Special Education Maze: A Guide for Parents and Teachers
Spina Bifida Association
4590 Macarthur Boulevard NW
Washington, DC 20007-4226

202-944-3285
800-621-3141
e-mail: sbaa@sbaa.org
www.sbaa.org

An excellent aid for the development of an effective special education program.

7775 New Language of Toys: Teaching Communication Skills to Children...
Spina Bifida Association
4590 Macarthur Boulevard NW
Washington, DC 20007-4226

202-944-3285
800-621-3141
e-mail: sbaa@sbaa.org
www.sbaa.org

A guide for parents and teachers, this reader-friendly resource guide provides a wealth of information on how play activities affect a child's language development (with a focus on special needs) and where to get the toys and materials to use in these activities.

7776 Nick Joins In
Spina Bifida Association
4590 Macarthur Boulevard NW
Washington, DC 20007-4226

202-944-3285
800-621-3141
e-mail: sbaa@sbaa.org
www.sbaa.org

When Nick, who is in a wheelchair, enters a regular classroom, for the first time he realizes that he has much to contribute.

7777 Princess Pooh
Spina Bifida Association
4590 Macarthur Boulevard NW
Washington, DC 20007-4226

202-944-3285
800-621-3141
e-mail: sbaa@sbaa.org
www.sbaa.org

Jealous of her disabled sister's royal treatment as she sits on her throne with wheels, Patty Jean borrows it and discovers that life in a wheelchair isn't so easy.

7778 SBAA General Information Packet
Spina Bifida Association of America
4590 Macarthur Boulevard NW
Washington, DC 20007-4226

202-944-3285
800-621-3141
Fax: 202-944-3295
e-mail: sbaa@sbaa.org
www.sbaa.org

7779 Sexuality and the Person with Spina Bifida
Spina Bifida Association of America
4590 Macarthur Boulevard NW
Washington, DC 20007-4226

202-944-3285
800-621-3141
Fax: 202-944-3295
e-mail: sbaa@sbaa.org
www.sbaa.org

Focuses on sexuality, sexual development, sexual activity, and other important issues.

7780 Social Development and the Person with Spina Bifida
Spina Bifida Association of America
4590 Macarthur Boulevard NW
Washington, DC 20007-4226

202-944-3285
800-621-3141
Fax: 202-944-3295
e-mail: sbaa@sbaa.org
www.sbaa.org

7781 Steps to Independence: Teaching Everyday Skills to Children with Special Needs
Spina Bifida Association
4590 Macarthur Boulevard NW
Washington, DC 20007-4226

202-944-3285
800-621-3141
e-mail: sbaa@sbaa.org
www.sbaa.org

A guide to help parents teach life skills to their disabled child.

7782 Taking Charge
Spina Bifida Association of America
4590 Macarthur Boulevard NW
Washington, DC 20007-4226

202-944-3285
800-621-3141
Fax: 202-944-3295
e-mail: sbaa@sbaa.org
www.sbaa.org

Teenagers talk about life and physical disabilities.

7783 Unlocking Potential: College and Other Choices for People with LD and AD/HD
Spina Bifida Association
4590 Macarthur Boulevard NW
Washington, DC 20007-4226

202-944-3285
800-621-3141
e-mail: sbaa@sbaa.org
www.sbaa.org

An indispensible tool for high school students with learning disabilities and AD/HD. Includes a comprehensive listing of resources.

Children's Books

7784 Margaret's Moves
Dutton Children's Books
375 Hudson Street
New York, NY 10014-3658

212-366-2000

This story deals with all the nuances and impairments that children afflicted with spina bifida must encounter and succeed in overcoming.
Grades 4-6

7785 Rolling Along with Goldilocks and the Three Bears
Spina Bifida Association
4590 Macarthur Boulevard NW
Washington, DC 20007-4226

202-944-3285
800-621-3141
e-mail: sbaa@sbaa.org
www.sbaa.org

The familiar folktale with a special-needs twist.

7786 Views from Our Shoes: Growing Up with a Brother or Sister with Special Needs
Spina Bifida Association
4590 Macarthur Boulevard NW
Washington, DC 20007-4226

202-944-3285
800-621-3141
e-mail: sbaa@sbaa.org
www.sbaa.org

A balanced view of the positives and negatives of living with a disabled sibling. Written for siblings ages nine and up.

Newsletters

7787 Insights Into Spina Bifida
Spina Bifida Association of America
4590 Macarthur Boulevard NW
Washington, DC 20007-4226

202-944-3285
800-621-3141
Fax: 202-944-3295
e-mail: sbaa@sbaa.org
www.sbaa.org

Includes articles on the latest research, the latest up-dates on legislation, features and emotional aspects specific to Spina Bifida, educational information and information on the Association's national conference.
BiMonthly

7788 NASS News
222 S Prospect Avenue   847-698-1628
Park Ridge, IL 60068-4037
Association activities newsletter.

Pamphlets

7789 Educational Issues Among Children with Spina Bifida
Spina Bifida Association of America
4590 Macarthur Boulevard NW   202-944-3285
Washington, DC 20007-4226   800-621-3141
Fax: 202-944-3295
e-mail: sbaa@sbaa.org
www.sbaa.org
1995

7790 Learning Among Children with Spina Bifida
Spina Bifida Association of America
4590 Macarthur Boulevard NW   202-944-3285
Washington, DC 20007-4226   800-621-3141
Fax: 202-944-3295
e-mail: sbaa@sbaa.org
www.sbaa.org
1995

7791 Monetary Allowance, Health Care and Vocational Training
National Veterans Services Fund
PO Box 2465   203-656-0003
Darien, CT 06820-0465   Fax: 203-656-1957
e-mail: NatVetSvc@aol.com
Monetary allowance, health care and vocational training and rehabilitation for Vietnam Veterans' children with spine bifida.
Pamphlet

7792 Sexual Issues in Spina Bifida
Spina Bifida Association of America
4590 Macarthur Boulevard NW   202-944-3285
Washington, DC 20007-4226   800-621-3141
Fax: 202-944-3295
e-mail: sbaa@sbaa.org
www.sbaa.org
1993

7793 Urologic Care of the Child with Spina Bifida
Spina Bifida Association of America
4590 Macarthur Boulevard NW   202-944-3285
Washington, DC 20007-4226   800-621-3141
Fax: 202-944-3295
e-mail: sbaa@sbaa.org
www.sbaa.org
1994

Audio & Video

7794 Protecting Against Latex Allergy
Spina Bifida Association of America
4590 Macarthur Boulevard NW   202-944-3285
Washington, DC 20007-4226   800-621-3141
Fax: 202-944-3295
e-mail: sbaa@sbaa.org
www.sbaa.org
Audio-visual resource focusing on the awareness of latex allergies.
Audio-Visual
Cindy Brownstein, Chief Executive Officer
Caroline Alston, Program Director

7795 Raising a Child with Spina Bifida: An Introduction
Ajn Company
New York, NY 10019   212-582-8820
800-226-6256
Fax: 212-586-5462

Offers information parents need when their child is born with spina bifida. Uses clear explanations to define spina bifida and discuss its implications for the child. Covers procedures the child may face, such as a ventricular shunt. Emphasizes the importance of early intervention and contains footage of happy and healthy children and interviews with parents.
29 minutes

7796 The Challenge
Spina Bifida Association of America
4590 Macarthur Boulevard NW   202-944-3285
Washington, DC 20007-4226   800-621-3141
Fax: 202-944-3295
e-mail: sbaa@sbaa.org
www.sbaa.org
A human look of how people come to grips with and overcome the challenges related to living with Spina Bifida.
14 minutes
Cindy Brownstein, Chief Executive Officer
Caroline Alston, Program Director

Web Sites

7797 Healing Well
www.healingwell.com
An online health resource guide to medical news, chat, information and articles, newsgroups and message boards, books, disease-related web sites, medical directories, and more for patients, friends, and family coping with disabling diseases, disorders, or chronic illnesses.

7798 Health Finder
www.healthfinder.gov
Searchable, carefully developed web site offering information on over 1000 topics. Developed by the US Department of Health and Human Services, the site can be used in both English and Spanish.

7799 Healthlink USA
www.healthlinkusa.com
Health information concerning treatment, cures, prevention, diagnosis, risk factors, research, support groups, email lists, personal stories and much more. Updated regularly.

7800 Helios Health
www.helioshealth.com
Online resource for your health information. Detailed information about specific health topics, access to expert advice from our Medical Advisory Board, and up-to-date health news.

7801 March of Dimes Birth Defects Foundation
www.modimes.org
Information on the treatment and prevention of birth defects, including spina bifida.

7802 MedicineNet
www.medicinenet.com
An online resource for consumers providing easy-to-read, authoritative medical and health information.

7803 Medscape
www.medscape.com
Medscape offers specialists, primary care physicians, and other health professionals the Web's most robust and integrated medical information and educational tools.

7804 Spina Bifida Association of America
www.sbaa.org
Represents approximately 60 chapters of parents and other members of families having children born with spina bifida, individuals with spina bifida, and health professionals who work with them.

7805 WebMD
www.webmd.com
Information on Spina Bifida, including articles and resources.

Description

7806 ## Spinal Cord Injuries

Spinal cord injury results from trauma to or disease of the spinal cord. Depending on where the spinal cord was injured, paraplegia (paralysis affecting the legs and lower part of the body) or quadriplegia (paralysis affecting all muscles below the neck and therefore all four limbs), may occur. Bladder and/or sexual function may be damaged. Each year, 12,000 people, mostly teenage males, sustain a spinal cord injury as a result of motor vehicle or sports-related accidents, or violent crimes.

Modern medical and surgical care has dramatically increased both long-term survival and quality of life in victims of spinal cord injury. This improvement reflects intensive medical care and appropriate surgical stabilization at the time of the injury, and in later years, attention to preventing the complications, such as skin breakdown, bladder infection and lung dysfunction. One of the greatest challenges is helping persons with spinal cord injuries to live as productive and independent a life as possible. Rehabilitation should begin as soon as possible after the injury. It usually starts with several weeks at a specialized inpatient facility, then transitions to family-assisted or independent living, depending on the extent of the disability. The multidisciplinary team provides education, emotional support, physical and occupational therapy, assistive devices, braces, and beds, and helps arrange special vans or modifications to the patient's home. Many voluntary societies and government agencies can help with the transition to life in the community.

National Agencies & Associations

7807 **American Association of Spinal Cord Injury Nurses**
801 18th Street NW 202-416-7704
Washington, DC 20006 Fax: 202-416-7641
e-mail: aascin@pva.org
www.aascin.org
Comprised of nurses who specialize in spinal cord research nursing and education.
Maurice L Jordan, Acting Executive Director
Sara Lerman MPH, Program Manager

7808 **American Paraplegic Society**
801 18th Street NW 202-416-7704
Washington, DC 20006-1131 Fax: 202-416-7641
e-mail: aps@pva.org
www.apssci.org
A professional membership organization for physicians scientists and allied health care professionals.
Maurice L Jordan, Acting Executive Director
Brenda Finkel, Administrative Assistant

7809 **American Spinal Cord Injury Association**
2020 Peachtree Road NW 404-355-9772
Atlanta, GA 30309 Fax: 404-355-1826
e-mail: ASIA_Office@shepherd.org
www.asia-spinalinjury.org
Promotes and establishes standards of excellence for all aspects of health care of individuals with spinal cord injury from onset throughout life.
Michael Haak, M.D, President
Mary . Jane Mulcahey, PhD., O.T, President-Elect

7810 **American Spinal Injury Association (ASIA)**
2020 Peachtree Road NW 404-355-9772
Atlanta, GA 30309 Fax: 404-355-1826
e-mail: ASIA_Office@shepherd.org
www.asia-spinalinjury.org
Promotes and establishes standards of excellence for all aspects of health care of individuals with spinal cord injury from onset throughout life.
Michael Haak, M.D, President
Mary . Jane Mulcahey, PhD., O.T, President-Elect

7811 **Association of Spinal Cord Injury Psychologists and Social Workers**
801 18th Street NW 202-416-7704
Washington, DC 20006-1131 Fax: 202-416-7641
e-mail: aascipsw@epua.org
www.aascipsw.org
Formed in 1986 to provide a forum for the exchange of ideas and information with assistance of the Eastern Paralyzed Veterans Association.
Maurice L Jordan, Acting Executive Director
Brenda Finkel, Administrative Assistant

7812 **Christopher & Dana Reeve Foundation Paralysis Resource Center**
636 Morris Turnpike 973-467-8270
Short Hills, NJ 07078 800-225-0292
e-mail: info@paralysis.org
www.christopherreeve.org
The Reeve Foundation is dedicated to curing spinal cord injury by funding innovative research, and improving the quality of life for people living with paralysis through grants, information and advocacy.
John M. Hughes, Chairman
John E. McConnell, Vice Chairman

7813 **Eastern Paralyzed Veterans Association of America**
7520 Astoria Boulevard 718-803-3782
E Elmhurst, NY 11370-1177 800-444-0120
Fax: 718-803-0414
Dedicated to serving veterans with a spinal cord injury or disease in New York New Jersey Connecticut or Pennsylvania. Based in New York City EPVA is the leader in funding SCI research and care.
Angela Wu, Director of Library Information

7814 **FES Information Center WO Walker Industrial Rehabilitation Cent**
WO Walker Industrial Rehabilitation Center
11000 Cedar Avenue
Cleveland, OH 44106-3052 800-666-2353
FES offers technology to persons with neuromuscular disorders resulting from spinal cord injury, head injury or stroke. The most widely known use of FES in the spinal community is for exercise.

7815 **International Medical Society of Paralegia: US Office**
T Giles
1333 Moursend Avenue 713-797-5910
Houston, TX 77030 Fax: 713-799-7017
National non-profit organization offers information resources and research for people with spinal cord injury or dysfunction. Professional organization for physicians.

7816 **International Spinal Cord Regeneration Center**
PO Box 451 619-463-5350
Bonita, CA 91908 Fax: 619-460-2699
e-mail: spinal@mailutopia.net
www.spinal.siteutopia.net
Specializes in spinal cord regeneration as well as Embryonic Cell Transplant Therapy.
Fernando C Ramirez del Rio, Medical Director
Wolfram W Kuhnau, Associate

7817 **Kent Waldrep National Paralysis Foundation Main Office**
Main Office
16415 Addison Road 972-248-7100
Addison, TX 75001 800-925-2873
Fax: 972-248-7313

National non-profit organization offers information referral resources and research for people with spinal cord injury their family members or service providers.

7818 National Spinal Cord Injury Association: Metropolitan Washington Chapter

6701 Democracy Boulevard
Bethesdae, MD 20817

301-214-4006
800-962-9629
Fax: 301-881-9817
e-mail: stevetowle@cs.com

The mission of the National Spinal Cord Injury Association is to enable people with spinal cord injury and disease to achieve their highest level of indepedence, health, and personal fulfillment by providing resources, services, and peer support.
Harley Thomas, President

7819 National Spinal Cord Injury Statistical Center

University of Alabama, Dept. of Physical Medicine
1717 6th Ave South
Birmingham, AL 35233

205-934-3342
Fax: 205-975-4691
TDD: 205-934-4642
e-mail: nscisc@uab.edu
www.nscisc.uab.edu

The UAB Department of Physical Medicine and Rehabilitation is funded by the National Institute on Disability and Rehabilitation Research (NIDRR) to operate the National Spinal Cord Injury Statistical Center (NSCISC). NSCISC supports and directs the collection, management and analysis of the world's largest and longest spinal cord injury research database. Organizationally, NSCISC is currently at the hub of a network of 14 NIDRR-sponsored and 5 subcontract-funded Spinal Cord Injury Model Systems
Yuying Chen, MD, PhD, Director
Pam Mott, Director Research Services

7820 Paralyzed Veterans of America

801 18th Street NW
Washington, DC 20006-3517

202-872-1300
800-424-8200
Fax: 202-785-4452
TTY: 800-795-4327
e-mail: info@pva.org
www.pva.org

For more than 67 years, Paralyzed Veterans of America has been on a mission to change lives and build brighter futures for our seriously injured heroes-to empower these brave men and women with what they need to achieve the things they fought for: freedom and independence.
Bill Lawson, National President
Al Kovach, Jr., National Senior Vice President

7821 Rick Hansen Foundation

300-3820 Cessna Drive
Richmond, BC V7B 0-1A1

604-295-8149
800-213-2131
Fax: 604-295-8159
e-mail: info@rickhansen.com
www.rickhansen.com

The Rick Hansen Foundation unifies organizations and leaders to work in partnership towards positive change for a healthy and inclusive world, with a key focus of improving the lives of those with spinal cord injuries.

Through Rick's leadership, the Foundation has leveraged the $26 million raised during the original Tour to more than $280 million in investments toward SCI research, rehabilitation and quality of life initiatives.

Doramy Ehling, Executive Vice President
Colin Ewart, Vice President of Strategic Relations

7822 Spinal Cord Injury Network International

3911 Princeton Drive
Santa Rosa, CA 95405-7013

707-577-8796
800-548-2673
Fax: 707-577-0605
e-mail: spinal@sonic.net
www.spinalcordinjury.org

Spinal Cord Injury Network International was founded in 1986 by Lennice Ambrose after her son suffered a spinal cord injury in a car accident. She soon came to the realization that there was a lack of collected resources for those seeking help. Starting the organization at her home in Santa Rosa, California; the organization has grown to be recognized internationally for being dedicated to helping injured persons and their families reach the best possible care and knowledgable information. Our o
Lennice Ambrose, Executive Director
Sharon E Hunt, Medical Librarian

7823 Spinal Cord Society

19051 County Highway 1
Fergus Falls, MN 56537

218-739-5252
Fax: 218-739-5262
www.scsus.org

Funds research for spinal cord injuries and provides physician referrals.

State Agencies & Associations

Arizona

7824 Arizona Spinal Cord Injury Association

Samaritan Rehab Institute R-2
5025 E Washington St
Phoenix, AZ 85034

602-507-4209
888-889-2185
Fax: 602-507-4214
e-mail: info@azspinal.org
www.azspinal.org

The Arizona Spinal Cord Injury Association is a nonprofit organization dedicated to enhancing the lives of individuals with spinal cord injuries. We also offer support and education to family members, professionals, and community members.
Don Price, President
Donna Powers, Vice President

California

7825 National Spinal Cord Injury Association: San Diego County Chapter

6645 Alvarado Road
San Diego, CA 92120

619-229-7001
e-mail: rehabdsg@gte.net
www.users.erols.com

Organization dedicated to improving the quality of life for persons with spinal cord injury and related disorders and their families. Seeks to fufill this mission by raising awareness about spinal cord injury through education, injury prevention, improvement of medical, rehabilitative and supportive services, research and public policy formulation.
Royce Hamrick

7826 National Spinal Cord Injury Association: Los Angeles Chapter

311 Robertson Boulevard
Beverly Hills, CA 90211

310-553-4833
Fax: 310-659-5040
www.users.erols.com

Organization dedicated to improving the quality of life for persons with spinal cord injury and related disorders and their families. Seeks to fufill this mission by raising awareness about spinal cord injury through education, injury prevention, improvement of medical, rehabilitative and supportive services, research and public policy formulation.
Paul Berns MD, President

Connecticut

7827 National Spinal Cord Injury Association: Connecticut Chapter

Wallingford, CT 06492

203-284-1045
e-mail: nscia@sciact.org
www.users.erols.com

Organization dedicated to improving the quality of life for persons with spinal cord injury and related disorders and their families. Seeks to fufill this mission by raising awareness about spinal cord injury through education, injury prevention, improvement of medical, rehabilitative and supportive services, research and public policy formulation.
Bill Mancini, President
Liza Ethier, Contact

Florida

7828 Goodwill Industries-Suncoast
Goodwill Industries-Suncoast
10596 Gandy Boulevard   727-523-1512
Saint Petersburg, FL 33702   888-279-1988
                                          Fax: 727-579-0850
                                          TTY: 727-579-1068
e-mail: gw.marketing@goodwill-suncoast.com
www.goodwill-suncoast.org
Goodwill-Suncoast was founded in October 1954 in downtown St. Petersburg. We began by assisting a handful of people with disabilities to gain work skills and paychecks. Now we help thousands of people overcome a variety of barriers to employment through employment programs, five subsidized apartment buildings, work activities centers for adults with developmental disabilities, as well as rehabilitative community corrections facilities. To support these services, Goodwill-Suncoast operates 15 ret
Oscar J. Horton, Chair
Martin W. Gladysz, Sr. Vice Chair

Georgia

7829 Shepherd Center
2020 Peachtree Road NW   404-352-2020
Atlanta, GA 30309   e-mail: admissions@shepherd.org
www.shepherd.org
Shepherd Center is a 152-bed facility. Last year Shepherd had 965 admissions to its inpatient programs and 571 to its day patient programs. In addition, Shepherd sees more than 6,600 people annually on an outpatient basis.
Gary R. Ulicny, Ph.D, President/CEO
Brock K Bowman, Assistant Medical Director

Illinois

7830 Spinal Cord Injury Association of Illinois
1032 S LaGrange Road   708-352-6223
LaGrange, IL 60525   877-373-0301
                                          Fax: 708-352-9065
e-mail: sciinjury@aol.com
www.sci-illinois.org
Spinal Cord Injury Association of Illinois (formerly NSCIA, Illinois Chapter) is a 501(c)3 non-profit organization providing information and support resources for people paralyzed by trauma and medical conditions, family members, and health care and related professionals that serve the SCI community. Our office is located in LaGrange, IL, a suburb of Chicago, but we serve the entire state.
Kim Eberhardt Muir, MS, OTR, President
Vic Myers, Vice President

Indiana

7831 National Spinal Cord Injury Association: Central Indiana Chapter
2109 Cleveland Street   219-944-8037
Garyanapolis, IN 46404   Fax: 317-329-2530
e-mail: rjackson@ci.gary.in.us
Organization dedicated to improving the quality of life for persons with spinal cord injury and related disorders and their families. Seeks to fulfill this mission by raising awareness about spinal cord injury through education, injury prevention, improvement of medical, rehabilitative and supportive services, research and public policy formulation.
Lucille Hightower

Kentucky

7832 National Spinal Cord Injury Association: Derby City Area Chapter
Center for Accessible Living
305 W. Broadway   502-588-8574
Louisville, KY 40202   e-mail: dallgood@calky.org
www.derbycityspinalcord.org
Derby City Area Spinal Cord Injury Association, the Louisville Kentucky Chapter of the (N.S.C.I.A.) National Spinal Cord Injury Association. Derby City Area Spinal Cord Injury Association is a organization for individuals with spinal cord injuries, their families, and health professionals across Kentucky. Founded in 1984 as

a Charter Member of the N.S.C.I.A., it was incorporated under IRS Section 501 (c) 3 as a not for profit organization.
David Allgood, President
Adam Ford, Vice President

Louisiana

7833 National Spinal Cord Injury Association: Louisiana Chapter
3650 18th Street   504-455-1178
Metairie, LA 70002   Fax: 504-455-7315
Organization dedicated to improving the quality of life for persons with spinal cord injury and related disorders and their families. Seeks to fulfill this mission by raising awareness about spinal cord injury through education, injury prevention, improvement of medical, rehabilitative and supportive services, research and public policy formulation.
Yadi Mark

Massachusetts

7834 National Spinal Cord Injury Association
545 Concord Avenue   301-588-6959
Cambridge, MA 02138-1173   800-962-9629
                                          Fax: 301-588-9414
e-mail: nscia2@aol.com
www.spinalcord.org
Organization dedicated to improving the quality of life for persons with spinal cord injury and related disorders and their families. Seeks to fulfill this mission by raising awareness about spinal cord injury through education, injury prevention, improvement of medical, rehabilitative and supportive services, research and public policy formulation.

7835 National Spinal Cord Injury Association: Greater Boston Chapter
New England Rehabilitation Hospital
Two Rehabilitation Way   781-933-8666
Woburn, MA 01801   Fax: 781-933-0043
e-mail: sciboston@aol.com
www.sciboston.com
Organization dedicated to improving the quality of life for persons with spinal cord injury and related disorders and their families. Seeks to fulfill this mission by raising awareness about spinal cord injury through education and injury prevention.
Dave Estrada, Director
Kevin Gibson, Coordinator

New Hampshire

7836 New Hampshire Chapter NSCIA
Northeast Rehabilitation Hospital
21 Chenell Drive   603-479-0560
Concord, NH 03301-3974   800-826-3700
                                          Fax: 928-438-9607
e-mail: debbie@gsil.org
www.spinalcord.org

Lisa Thompson, President

New York

7837 Greater Rochester Area Chapter NSCIA
Rochester, NY 14602-0076   585-234-3269
e-mail: rochesternscia@yahoo.com
www.spinalcord.org

Karen Genet, Contact
Cathy Flanagan, Contact

7838 National Spinal Cord Injury Association
75-20 Astoria Blvd   718-803-3782
Jackson Heights, NY 11370   800-962-9629
                                          Fax: 301-990-0445
e-mail: nscia2@aol.com
www.spinalcord.org
National Spinal Cord Injury Association, the membership division of United Spinal, was founded in 1948 to improve the lives of all paralyzed Americans. Our mission is to improve the quality of life of all people living with a spinal cord injury or disease. We provide active-lifestyle information, peer support and advocacy that em-

power individuals to achieve their highest potential in all facets of life
Steven A Towle, Contact

Pennsylvania

7839 Shriners Hospital for Children
3551 N Broad Street 215-430-4000
Philadelphia, PA 19140 800-281-4050
Fax: 215-430-4079
e-mail: tdiamond@shrinenet.org
www.shrinershospitalsforchildren.org
Studies and research done on children with spinal cord injuries.
Scott . Kozin, M.D, Chief of Staff
Terry Diamond, Development Officer

7840 Spinal Cord Injury Program at Harmarville Rehabilitation Center
Pittsburgh, PA 15238 412-828-1300
800-624-4673
Most comprehensive center for the treatment of spinal cord injury and disease.

Texas

7841 Rio Grande Chapter: NSCIA Rio Vista Rehabilitation Hospital
Rio Vista Rehabilitation Hospital
1395 George Dieter 915-298-7241
El Paso, TX 79936-2901 e-mail: riograndenscia@aol.com
www.spinalcord.org

Sukie Armendariz, Contact
Ron Prieto, Contact

Virginia

7842 Old Dominion Area Chapter: NSCIA
5206 Markel Road 804-726-4990
Richmond, VA 23226 Fax: 888-752-7857
e-mail: info@odcnscia.org
www.odcnscia.org
Our mission is to enable people with spinal cord injuries and disease to achieve their highest level of health, independence and quality of life. We educate public officials, community leaders, and citizens to the needs of persons with spinal cord injury and disease, and the importance of creating an environment of greater independence for all. We offer a variety of services and a wealth of knowledge towards unlocking the door for active living with SCI.
Steve Fetrow, President
Craig Fabian, Vice President

Wisconsin

7843 Southeastern Wisconsin Chapter of the Nati onal Spinal Cord Injury Association
Sacred Heart Rehabilitation Hospital
540 South 1st Street 414-384-4022
Milwaukee, WI 53204-1993 Fax: 414-384-7820
e-mail: office@spinalcordwi.org
www.spinalcord.org
The mission of the NSCIA-SWC is to assist people who have some degree of paralysis through injury or disease with a goal of returning them to a life of dignity, self-confidence and independence in a community that is all inclusive.
John Dzicwa, President

Research Centers

7844 Miami Project to Cure Paralysis
1095 NW 14th Terrace 305-243-6001
Miami, FL 33101 800-STA-NDUP
Fax: 205-243-6017
e-mail: miamiproject@med.miami.edu
www.miamiproject.miami.edu
In 1985, Barth A. Green, M.D. and NFL Hall of Fame linebacker Nick Buoniconti helped found TheMiami Projectto Cure Paralysis after Nick's son, Marc, sustained a spinal cord injury during a college football game. Today, The Miami Project is the world's most comprehensive spinal cord injury research center, and is a desig-

nated Center of Excellence at the University of Miami Miller School of Medicine. The Miami Project's international team is housed in the Lois Pope LIFE Center and includes more t
Barth A. Green, M.D., Co-Founder and Chairman
Marc A Buoniconti, President

7845 Pushin On: RRTC on Secondary Conditions of Spinal
UAB Office of Research Services
1717 6th Avenue South 205-934-3283
Birmingham, AL 35249-7330 Fax: 205-975-4691
TDD: 205-934-4642
e-mail: sciweb@uab.edu
www.spinalcord.uab.edu
Pushin' On is an enewsletter published to provide persons with SCI and their families with information of interest. The newsletter is offered 2 times per year and sent electronically to subscribers to the UAB-SCIMS Email List, and it is posted online for our follows on facebook and twitter.
8 pages 2 per year
Amie B McLain, MD., Program Director
Phil Klebine, Editor

7846 RRTC on Aging with a Disability Los Amigos Research and Education Instit
Los Amigos Research and Education Institute
7601 E Imperial Highway 562-401-7402
Downey, CA 90242-3456 Fax: 562-401-7011
e-mail: lcarrothers@agingwithdisability.org
www.agingwithdisability.org
A federally funded rehabilitation research and training center.
Bryan Kemp PhD, Director
Leanne Carro Pt PhD, Training Director

Support Groups & Hotlines

7847 Georgia National Spinal Cord Injury Association Support Group Network
Columbus, GA 31920
800-422-3352
Support group dedicated to improving the quality of life for persons with spinal cord injury and related disorders and their families. Seeks to fufill this mission by raising awareness about spinal cord injury through rehabilitative and supportive services, research and public policy formulation.
Andy Harp

7848 HEALTHSOUTH Rehabilitation Hospital of Tal lahassee
1675 Riggins Road 850-656-4800
Tallahassee, FL 32308 Fax: 850-656-4809
www.healthsouthtallahassee.com
Our hospital provides a wide range of physical rehabilitation services, a vast network of highly-skilled, independent private practice physicians and HealthSouth therapists and nurses, and the most innovative equipment and rehabilitation technology, ensuring that all patients have access to the highest quality care. Designed with our patient's care in mind, HealthSouth Rehabilitation Hospital of Tallahassee offers semi-private rooms, which promote social interaction and support throughout the re
Dale Neely, Chief Executive Officer
Robert Rowland, M.D., Medical Director

7849 Maryland National Spinal Cord Injury Association Support Group Network
Kerman Hospital
2200 Kerman Drive 410-448-6307
Baltimore, MD 21207 800-962-9629
e-mail: mhenley@kernan.umm.edu
www.spinalcord.org
Open group for all caregivers and does not focus on a specific disability, disease or condition.

7850 National Health Information Center
Washington, DC 20013 310-565-4167
800-336-4797
Fax: 301-984-4256
e-mail: info@nhic.org
www.health.gov/nhic
Offers a nationwide information referral service, produces directories and resource guides.

7851 National Spinal Cord Injury Support Goups
Florida Rehabilitation and Sports Medicine
5165 Adanson Street　　　　　407-895-7991
Orlando, FL 32804
Support group dedicated to improving the quality of life for persons with spinal cord injury and related disorders and their families. Seeks to fufill this mission by raising awareness about spinal cord injury through rehabilitative and supportive services, research and public policy formulation.

7852 VIVA!
Health Enhancement Learning Programs
Dallas, TX 75354-3065　　　　972-986-2977
　　　　　　　　　　　　　　800-334-4403
A computer-based patient education system on spinal cord injury.

7853 National Spinal Cord Injury Support Groups
Healthsouth Central Georgia Rehab Hospital
3351 Northside Drive　　　　478-201-6500
Macon, GA 31210　　　　　　800-491-3550
　　　　　　　　　Fax: 478-633-5134
　　　e-mail: tamboli.sara@mccg.org
　　　　www.centralgarehab.com/
Support group dedicated to improving the quality of life for persons with spinal cord injury and related disorders and their families. Seeks to fufill this mission by raising awareness about spinal cord injury through rehabilitative and supportive services, research and public policy formulation.
Kathy Parks Combs RN, SCI Support Group Coordinator

7854 National Spinal Cord Injury Support Groups
HEALTHSOUTH, Sea Pines Rehabilitation Hospital
101 E Florida Avenue　　　　407-984-4600
Melbourne, FL 32901　　e-mail: laura.leitz@healthsouth.com
　　　　　　　　　　　www.spinalcord.org
In a support group, members provide each other with various types of help for shared purposes. The help can take the form of providing and evaluating relevant information, relating personal experiences, listening to and accepting others' experiences, educating and guiding, or for providing sympathetic understanding and establishing social networks. Support Groups may each have their own way of accomplishing their mission but all of them share the same goal of improving the lives of participants.

7855 National Spinal Cord Injury Support Groups
115 Alpine Street　　　　　334-456-1768
Chickasaw, AL 36611
Support group dedicated to improving the quality of life for persons with spinal cord injury and related disorders and their families. Seeks to fufill this mission by raising awareness about spinal cord injury through rehabilitative and supportive services, research and public policy formulation.

Books

7856 Body Silent: An Anthropologist Embarks into the World of the Disabled
WW Norton Publishing
500 Fifth Avenue　　　　　212-354-5500
New York, NY 10110　　　　Fax: 212-869-0856
　　　　　　　　　　　www.wwnorton.com
Diagnosed at midlife in the early 1980s with an inoperable (and, at the time, untreatable) ependymona of the spine, an anthropologist frankly discusses his progressive disability.

ISBN: 0-393307-02-6

7857 Climbing Back
Miramar Communications
PO Box 8987
Malibu, CA 90265-8987　　　800-543-4116
The author broke his back after a climbing fall. With his sights at the top of the mountain he climbs back in this inspiring story.
256 pages Hardcover

7858 Occupational Therapy Practice Guidelines for Adults with Spinal Cord Injury
American Occupational Therapy Association

4720 Montgomery Lane　　　301-652-2682
Bethesda, MD 20824-1220　　Fax: 301-652-7711
　　　　　　　　　　　TDD: 800-377-8555
　　　　　　　　　　　www.aota.org
31 pages
ISBN: 1-569001-54-5

7859 Options: Spinal Cord Injury and the Future
National Spinal Cord Injury Association
8300 Colesville Road　　　　301-588-6959
Silver Spring, MD 20910-3243　800-962-9629
　　　　　　　　　　　Fax: 301-588-9414
　　　　　　　e-mail: nscia2@aol.com
　　　　　　　www.spinalcord.org
A collection of conversations with people who have had spinal cord injuries who share some of their experiences and emotions.
150 pages

7860 Spinal Cord Injury Home Care Manual
Santa Clara Valley Medical Center
751 S Bascom Avenue
San Jose, CA 95128-2699　　408-885-5000
　　　　　　　　　　　www.scvmed.org
Provides people with spinal cord injury, their families and professionals with information about physical care, independent living, psychosocial issues, attendant care and supplies.

7861 Spinal Network
Miramar Communications
PO Box 8987
Malibu, CA 90265　　　　　800-543-4116
Total wheelchair resource book.

Children's Books

7862 Follow Your Dreams
National Spinal Cord Injury Association
8300 Colesville Road　　　　301-588-6959
Silver Spring, MD 20910-3243　800-962-9629
　　　　　　　　　　　Fax: 301-588-9414
　　　　　　　e-mail: nscia2@aol.com
　　　　　　　www.spinalcord.org
JT, born with spina bifida, goes on an adventure. Written for and by children with SCI, for children ages 9-12.
30 pages

7863 Tell it Like it is
National Spinal Cord Injury Association
8300 Colesville Road　　　　301-588-6959
Silver Spring, MD 20910-3243　800-962-9629
　　　　　　　　　　　Fax: 301-588-9414
　　　　　　　e-mail: nscia2@aol.com
　　　　　　　www.spinalcord.org
Written by teenagers with SCI for teenagers with SCI.

Magazines

7864 SCI Life
National Spinal Cord Injury Association
8300 Colesville Road　　　　301-588-6959
Silver Spring, MD 20910-3243　800-962-9629
　　　　　　　　　　　Fax: 301-588-9414
　　　　　　　e-mail: nscia2@aol.com
　　　　　　　www.spinalcord.org
Official magazine of NSCIA. Updates on topics such as research, medical issues, prevention, new products, books, and Association activities.
Quarterly

7865 Spinal Column
Shepherd Spinal Center
2020 Peachtree Road NW　　404-352-2020
Atlanta, GA 30309-1465
This quarterly magazine from the spinal center offers information on the newest treatments, therapies, referral centers, assistive devices and much more for persons living with spina bifida, multiple sclerosis and other chronic physical ailments.
Quarterly

Newsletters

7866 Progress in Research
American Paralysis Association
500 Morris Avenue 973-379-2690
Springfield, NJ 07081-1020 800-225-0292
Fax: 973-912-9433
Offers information on the association, news, reviews, books, and information on the latest medical and technological advances in spinal cord injury research.
Quarterly
Susan P Howley, Research Director
Mitchell R Stoller, President/CEO

7867 Pushing on: University of Alabama
Christopher Reeve Association
500 Morris Avenue 973-379-2690
Springfield, NJ 07081 800-225-0292
Fax: 973-912-9433
A research newsletter regarding spinal cord injuries.
Quarterly
Mitchell R Stoller, President/CEO

7868 Spinal Cord Society Newsletter
Spinal Cord Society
19051 County Highway 1 218-739-5252
Fergus Falls, MN 56537 Fax: 218-739-5262
www.members.aol.com/scsweb
Offers medical reports, articles, convention news, chapter news and more for persons with spinal cord injury.
Monthly

7869 Walking Tomorrow: University of Alabama
Christopher Reeve Association
500 Morris Avenue 973-379-2690
Springfield, NJ 07081-1020 800-225-0292
Fax: 973-912-9433
A research newsletter regarding spinal cord injuries.
Quarterly
Mitchell R Stoller, President/CEO

Pamphlets

7870 Autonomic Dysreflexia
National Spinal Cord Injury Association
8300 Colesville Road 301-588-6959
Silver Spring, MD 20910-3243 800-962-9629
Fax: 301-588-9414
e-mail: nscia2@aol.com
www.spinalcord.org

7871 Choosing A Spinal Cord Injury Rehabilitation Program
National Spinal Cord Injury Association
8300 Colesville Road 301-588-6959
Silver Spring, MD 20910-3243 800-962-9629
Fax: 301-588-9414
e-mail: nscia2@aol.com
www.spinalcord.org
Includes a listing of programs accredited by CARF & Model Centers designated by NIDRR.

7872 Fun and Games
National Spinal Cord Injury Association
8300 Colesville Road 301-588-6959
Silver Spring, MD 20910-3243 800-962-9629
Fax: 301-588-9414
e-mail: nscia2@aol.com
www.spinalcord.org

7873 Functional Electrical Stimulation: Clinical Applications
National Spinal Cord Injury Association
8300 Colesville Road 301-588-6959
Silver Spring, MD 20910-3243 800-962-9629
Fax: 301-588-9414
e-mail: nscia2@aol.com
www.spinalcord.org

7874 Importance of Basic Science in Research
National Spinal Cord Injury Association

8300 Colesville Road 301-588-6959
Silver Spring, MD 20910-3243 800-962-9629
Fax: 301-588-9414
e-mail: nscia2@aol.com
www.spinalcord.org

7875 Male Reproductive Function After Spinal Cord Injury
National Spinal Cord Injury Association
8300 Colesville Road 301-588-6959
Silver Spring, MD 20910-3243 800-962-9629
Fax: 301-588-9414
e-mail: nscia2@aol.com
www.spinalcord.org

7876 Medical Facilities and Resources for Ventilator Users
National Spinal Cord Injury Association
8300 Colesville Road 301-588-6959
Silver Spring, MD 20910-3243 800-962-9629
Fax: 301-588-9414
e-mail: nscia2@aol.com
www.spinalcord.org

7877 Reading Resources on Spinal Cord Injury
National Spinal Cord Injury Association
8300 Colesville Road 301-588-6959
Silver Spring, MD 20910-3243 800-962-9629
Fax: 301-588-9414
e-mail: nscia2@aol.com
www.spinalcord.org

7878 Sexuality After Spinal Cord Injury
National Spinal Cord Injury Association
8300 Colesville Road 301-588-6959
Silver Spring, MD 20910-3243 800-962-9629
Fax: 301-588-9414
e-mail: nscia2@aol.com
www.spinalcord.org

7879 Spinal Cord Injury Awareness
National Spinal Cord Injury Association
8300 Colesville Road 301-588-6959
Silver Spring, MD 20910-3243 800-962-9629
Fax: 301-588-9414
e-mail: nscia2@aol.com
www.spinalcord.org
Understanding the importance of language and images.

7880 Spinal Cord Injury: Statistical Information
National Spinal Cord Injury Association
8300 Colesville Road 301-588-6959
Silver Spring, MD 20910-3243 800-962-9629
Fax: 301-588-9414
e-mail: nscia2@aol.com
www.spinalcord.org

7881 Starting a Support Group
National Spinal Cord Injury Association
8300 Colesville Road 301-588-6959
Silver Spring, MD 20910-3243 800-962-9629
Fax: 301-588-9414
e-mail: nscia2@aol.com
www.spinalcord.org

7882 Tendon Transfer Surgery
National Spinal Cord Injury Association
8300 Colesville Road 301-588-6959
Silver Spring, MD 20910-3243 800-962-9629
Fax: 301-588-9414
e-mail: nscia2@aol.com
www.spinalcord.org

7883 Travel After Spinal Cord Injury
National Spinal Cord Injury Association
8300 Colesville Road 301-588-6959
Silver Spring, MD 20910-3243 800-962-9629
Fax: 301-588-9414
e-mail: nscia2@aol.com
www.spinalcord.org

7884 Understanding Spinal Muscular Atrophy
Families of Spinal Muscular Atrophy

PO Box 196
Libertyville, IL 60048-0196

847-367-7620
800-886-1762
Fax: 847-367-7623
e-mail: info@fsma.org
www.curesma.com

Offers a brief overview of Spinal Muscular Atrophy, causes, treatments, symptoms and unknowns.
Kenneth Hobby, Executive Director

7885   What is Spinal Cord Injury?
National Spinal Cord Injury Association
8300 Colesville Road
Silver Spring, MD 20910-3243

301-588-6959
800-962-9629
Fax: 301-588-9414
e-mail: nscia2@aol.com
www.spinalcord.org

7886   What is a Physiatrist?
National Spinal Cord Injury Association
8300 Colesville Road
Silver Spring, MD 20910-3243

301-588-6959
800-962-9629
Fax: 301-588-9414
e-mail: nscia2@aol.com
www.spinalcord.org

7887   What's New in Spinal Cord Injury Research?
National Spinal Cord Injury Association
8300 Colesville Road
Silver Spring, MD 20910-3243

301-588-6959
800-962-9629
Fax: 301-588-9414
e-mail: nscia2@aol.com
www.spinalcord.org

Audio & Video

7888   Living with Spinal Cord Injury
Barry Corbet, author

Fanlight Productions
4196 Washington Street
Boston, MA 02131-1731

617-469-4999
800-937-4113
Fax: 617-469-3379
e-mail: fanlight@fanlight.com
www.fanlight.com

A series of three videos produced by an individual who has experienced spinal cord injury himself. Changes is about coming to terms with spinal cord injury and beginning rehabilitation. Outside looks at the life-long process by which some injured people have created active and rewarding lives. Survivors explores the problems of growing old with a disability.
1973 84 Minutes

7889   SCI and Lower Extremity Orthoses
Health Enhancement Learning Programs
PO Box 543065
Dallas, TX 75354-3065

214-902-8277
800-334-4403

A video presenting an overview of indications and use of HKAFO, KAFO and AFO. Perfect resource for medical presentations and professional workshops.

7890   Spinal Cord Injury Video Access
Spinal Cord Injury Access International
39111 Princeton Drive
Santa Rosa, CA 95405

800-548-2673

Offers informational videotapes on spinal cord injury.

7891   Spinal Injury Slide Series
Health Enhancement Learning Programs
PO Box 543065
Dallas, TX 75354-3065

214-902-8277
800-334-4403

A slide series based on the VIVA program, a patient education system on spinal cord injury.

Web Sites

7892   American Association of Spinal Cord Injury Nurses
www.aascin.org
Comprised of nurses who specialize in spinal cord research, nursing and education.

7893   American Paraplegic Society
www.apssci.org
A professional membership organization for physicians, scientists and allied health care professionals.

7894   Christopher Reeve Paralysis Foundation
www.apacure.com
Dedicated to finding a cure for paralysis caused by spinal cord injury, head injury and stroke. A network of chapters across the country formed to provide comfort to the paralyzed but primarily to help raise funds to find a paralysis cure.

7895   Healing Well
www.healingwell.com
An online health resource guide to medical news, chat, information and articles, newsgroups and message boards, books, disease-related web sites, medical directories, and more for patients, friends, and family coping with disabling diseases, disorders, or chronic illnesses.

7896   Health Finder
www.healthfinder.gov
Searchable, carefully developed web site offering information on over 1000 topics. Developed by the US Department of Health and Human Services, the site can be used in both English and Spanish.

7897   Healthlink USA
www.healthlinkusa.com
Health information concerning treatment, cures, prevention, diagnosis, risk factors, research, support groups, email lists, personal stories and much more. Updated regularly.

7898   Helios Health
www.helioshealth.com
Online resource for your health information. Detailed information about specific health topics, access to expert advice from our Medical Advisory Board, and up-to-date health news.

7899   MedicineNet
www.medicinenet.com
An online resource for consumers providing easy-to-read, authoritative medical and health information.

7900   Medscape
www.medscape.com
Medscape offers specialists, primary care physicians, and other health professionals the Web's most robust and integrated medical information and educational tools.

7901   Miami Project to Cure Paralysis
www.miamiproject.miami.edu
Science and clinical research to restore function after spinal cord injury. The primary emphasis is on basic science research, under the direction of Dr. Richard Bunge, an eminent researcher.

7902   Sexual Health Network
www.sexualhealth.com
Informative site dealing with disability, sexuality and fertility.

7903   Spinal Cord Injury Information Network Center
www.spinalcord.uab.edu
Supervises and directs the collection, management and analysis of an extensive spinal cord injury database.

7904   Spinal Cord Injury Network International
www.sonic.net/~spinal
A non-profit organization that provides information and referral services and lends videos.

7905   University of Alabama, (UAB)
www.spinalcord.uab.edu
Up-to-date statistical information as well as extensive fact sheets on many aspects of Spinal Cord Injury.

7906   WebMD
www.webmd.com
Information on spinal cord injuries, including articles and resources.

Description

7907 Stroke

Strokes are caused by an interruption of blood flow in the brain, and usually — 80 percent of cases — are the result of a blocked blood vessel. The incidence increases with age, is higher in men than in women, and is higher in blacks than in whites. Depending on the severity and location of the damage, symptoms of stroke may include sudden weakness or paralysis (especially on one side of the body), blurred vision, difficulty speaking, slurred speech, dizziness and falling, extreme headache, stiff neck, altered level of alertness, and loss of bladder control. High blood pressure, atherosclerosis (fatty deposits), heart disease, diabetes, cigarette smoking, and heavy alcohol use are the major risk factors predisposing someone to stroke.

Preventive therapy is aimed at treatment of high blood pressure, heart disease, and diabetes. If someone has had a stroke they may be treated with blood thinning agents and/or other medication to prevent brain swelling. Research has shown that patients who are given one of these agents within three hours of stroke symptoms may have some or total restoration of neurologic function. To that end, the Golden Hour program was developed in which emergency medical personnel can initiate therapy in certain patients on the way to the hospital. Rehabilitation after the stroke involves physical and occupational therapy. Many stroke survivors experience depression and difficulty regaining independence, so it is important to provide emotional support for both survivors and their families.

National Agencies & Associations

7908 American Heart Association
7272 Greenville Avenue
Dallas, TX 75231

214-373-6300
800-242-8721
www.heart.org

The American Heart Association is the nation's oldest, largest voluntary organization devoted to fighting cardiovascular diseases and stroke. Founded by six cardiologists in 1924, our organization now includes more than 22.5 million volunteers and supporters working tirelessly to eliminate these diseases. We fund innovative research, fight for stronger public health policies and provide life-saving tools and information to save and improve lives.
Bernie Dennis, Chairman
Mariell Jessup, President

7909 American Stroke Association
7272 Greenville Avenue
Dallas, TX 75231

888-478-7653
www.heart.org

Created in 1997, the American Stroke Association is dedicated to prevention, diagnosis and treatment to save lives from stroke - America's No. 4 killer and a leading cause of serious disability. We fund scientific research, help people better understand and avoid stroke, encourage government support, guide healthcare professionals and provide information to enhance the quality of life for stroke survivors. To learn more, call 1-888-4-STROKE or browse strokeassociation.org.
Gordon F. Tomaselli, President

7910 Heart and Stroke Foundation of Canada
222 Queen Street
Ottawa, Ontario, ON K1P 5-5V9

613-569-4361
Fax: 613-569-3278
www.heartandstroke.com

The Foundation's health promotion and advocacy programs across the country are saving lives every day. Working together, our employees, volunteers, donors and world-class researchers have made the Heart and Stroke Foundation what we are today: Canada's most widely recognized and trusted authority on cardiovascular health. Our mission is to create healthy lives free of heart disease and stroke. Together, we will make it happen.
Douglas B. Clement, CM, MD, Chair
Mark R. Andrews, Director

7911 National Heart, Lung & Blood Institute
PO Box 301051
Bethesda, MD 20824

301-592-8573
Fax: 301-592-8563
TTY: 240-629-3255
e-mail: nhlbiinfo@nhlbi.nih.gov
www.nhlbi.nih.gov

The NHLBI stimulates basic discoveries about the causes of disease, enables the translation of basic discoveries into clinical practice, fosters training and mentoring of emerging scientists and physicians, and communicates research advances to the public. It creates and supports a robust, collaborative research infrastructure in partnership with private and public organizations, including academic institutions, industry, and other government agencies. The Institute collaborates with patients, f
Gary H. Gibbons, MD, Director
Susan B. Shurin, MD, Chief of Staff

7912 National Institute of Neurological Disorders and Stroke
PO Box 5081
Bethesda, MD 20824

301-496-5751
800-352-9424
Fax: 301-402-2186
TTY: 301-468-5981
e-mail: webManagers@ninds.nih.gov
www.ninds.nih.gov

The mission of NINDS is to reduce the burden of neurological disease - a burden borne by every age group, by every segment of society, by people all over the world.
Story C Landis PhD, Director
Walter J Koroshetz, Deputy Director

7913 National Institute of Neurological Disorde rs and Stroke
PO Box 5801
Bethesda, MD 20824

301-496-5751
800-352-9424
Fax: 301-402-2186
TTY: 301-468-5981
e-mail: webManagers@ninds.nih.gov
www.ninds.nih.gov

The mission of NINDS is to reduce the burden of neurological disease - a burden borne by every age group, by every segment of society, by people all over the world.
Story C Landis PhD, Director
Walter J Koroshetz, Deputy Director

7914 National Stroke Association
9707 E Easter Lane
Centennial, CO 80112-3747

303-649-9299
800-787-6537
Fax: 303-649-1328
e-mail: Info@stroke.org
www.stroke.org

A national organization whose sole purpose is to reduce the incidence and impact of stroke through prevention treatment rehabilitation and research and support for stroke survivors and their families.
Jamie Charbonneau, Director, Corporate Alliances
James Baranski, Chief Executive Officer

7915 Stroke Recovery Canada
10 Overlea Boulevard
Toronto, Ontario, ON M4H 1-1A4

416-425-3463
800-263-3463
Fax: 416-425-1920
e-mail: info@marchofdimes.ca
www.marchofdimes.ca

Stroke Recovery Canadar is a national service offering support, education and community programs for stroke survivors, their caregivers and families. Stroke Recovery Canada will connect you with a network of support that can help you reclaim your independence, your sense of community and your ability to thrive.
Andria Spindel, President/Chief Executive Officer
Jerry Lucas, Vice President, Programs

Foundations

7916   American Stroke Foundation
5916 Dearborn   913-649-1776
Mission, KS 66202   866-549-1776
                                              Fax: 913-649-6661
                                          www.americanstroke.org
The vision of the American Stroke Foundation is to reach out to
stroke survivors and their families across America and empower
them to reclaim hope for life after stroke
Joan McDowd, Executive Director
Jen Creed, Director of Programs and Outreach

Research Centers

7917   Bowman Gray School of Medicine
Medical Center Boulevard   919-716-7461
Winston Salem, NC 27157-0001   Fax: 919-716-5639
                                              www.web.bgsm.edu

James Toole MD, Professor

**7918   Cerebral Blood Flow Laboratories Veterans Administration
Medical Center**
Veterans Administration Medical Center
2002 Holcombe Boulevard   713-795-5807
Houston, TX 77030-4211   Fax: 713-957-01
Offers research in cerebrovascular disorders and risk factors for
stroke.
John S Meyer MD, Director

**7919   Comprehensive Stroke Center of Oregon University of Oregon
Health Sciences Cen**
University of Oregon Health Sciences Center
3181 SW Sam Jackson Park Road
Portland, OR 97239-3098   503-494-7225
                                                  www.ohsu.edu
The Oregon Stroke Center (OSC) was established over 20 years
ago to provide comprehensive treatment and prevention services
to stroke patients throughout the Northwest. Recognized as a national leader in acute stroke treatment, the OSC mobile stroke team
provides novel stroke treatments to multiple Portland hospitals. In
addition to clinical care, the OSC is actively involved in clinical
and basic research and provides extensive stroke related education
to the public and providers. Quick action
Wayne Clark, M.D., Professor
Helmi Lutsep, M.D., Professor

**7920   Departments of Neurology & Neurosurgery: University of
California, San Francisco**
UCSF Medical Center
505 Parnassus Avenue   415-476-1537
San Francisco, CA 94143   Fax: 415-476-0616
                              e-mail: bill.dillon@radiology.ucsf.edu
                                          www.radiology.ucsf.edu
The Department of Radiology & Biomedical Imaging at the Uni-
versity of California, San Francisco combines clinical excellence,
trailblazing research, and outstanding education in a leading academic health sciences institution. Our faculty includes some of the
foremost names in diagnostic and interventional radiology today.
Dr. Ronald Arenson, Chairman
Catherine Garzio, Director of Administration

7921   Hospital of the University of Pennsylvania
3400 Spruce Street   215-662-4000
Philadelphia, PA 19104   800-789-PENN
                                               Fax: 215-903-09
                              e-mail: pleasure@email.chop.edu
                                          www.pennmedicine.org
The Hospital of the University of Pennsylvania (HUP) is world-renowned for its clinical and research excellence, forging the way
for newer and better ways to diagnose and treat illnesses and disorders. The world-class faculty and staff of the Hospital of the University of Pennsylvania are dedicated to superior patient care,
education and research for a better, healthier future. Their significant and groundbreaking contributions to medicine are recognized
both nationally and internationally. The
David E Pleasure MD, Director

**7922   Massachusetts General Departments of Neurology and
Neurosurgery**
Massachusetts General Hospital
55 Fruit Street
Boston, MA 02114   617-726-2000
                                          www.massgeneral.org
Guided by the needs of our patients, our mission is to be the preem-
inent academic neurology department in the US by: providing outstanding clinical care while rapidly discovering new treatments to
reduce and eliminate the devastating impact of neurological disorders; training the very best neurologists and scientists of the future, and improving the health and well-being of the diverse
communities we serve.
Peter Slavin, Director
Robert Ackerman, Doctor

7923   Stroke Research and Treatment Center UAB Medical Center
Medical Center
1530 3rd Ave S   205-934-9999
Birmingham, AL 35294-7   800-822-6478
                                              Fax: 205-996-4039
                                          www.main.uab.edu/neurology
The nationally-ranked UAB Department of Neurology is home to
eight comprehensive divisions and seven centers offering an array
of clinical activities. Over 26,000 patients are cared for annually
through state-of-the-art subspecialty care and innovative treatments. Our residents have the opportunity to work in various neurology fields with 50 clinical and research faculty members.
Andrei V Alexandrov MD, Director and Professor
*Andrei V. Alexandrov, M.D., Director, Comprehensive Stroke Re-
search*

7924   University of Iowa College of Medicine
451 Newton Road   319-335-6707
Iowa City, IA 52242   e-mail: webmaster@mail.medicine.uiowa.edu
                                          www.medicine.uiowa.edu
The Roy J. and Lucille A. Carver College of Medicine is a highly
ranked medical school where students learn to become accomplished clinicians and top-flight researchers and educators. Students come to Iowa to study medicine in a program that uses
case-based learning as the basis of their education. With its emphasis on problem-solving skills, early exposure to patients, and enhanced community-based experiences, UI medical students
typically earn impressive scores on Step 1 of the U.S. Medical Li
Debra A. Schwinn, MD, Dean
Donna L. Hammond, PhD, Executive Associate Dean

**7925   University of Maryland Center for Studies of Cerebrovascular
Disease & Stroke**
16 S Utah Street   410-328-4323
Baltimore, MD 21201   Fax: 410-328-1149
Thomas R Price MD, Principal Investor

**7926   University of Miami School of Medicine Department of
Neurology**
1120 NW 14th Street   305-243-6732
Miami, FL 33136   877-243-4340
                                              Fax: 305-243-1632
                              e-mail: RSacco@med.miami.edu
                                          www.med.miami.edu
Ralph L Sacco MD, Chairman-Department of Neurology
Myron D Ginsberg MD, Professor

7927   Wake Forest University: Cerebrovascular Research Center
Department of Neurology
300 S Hawthorne Road   336-748-2338
Winston-Salem, NC 27103-2732   Fax: 336-748-5477
Cerebrovascular research.
Dr James Toole, Director

7928   Washington University School of Medicine
660 S Euclid Avenue   314-362-5000
Saint Louis, MO 63110-1016   e-mail: web@medicine.wustl.edu
                                          www.medicine.wustl.edu
Washington University School of Medicine is a leader in improving human health throughout the world. As noted leaders in patient
care, research and education, our outstanding faculty members
have contributed many discoveries and innovations to the field of
science since the founding of the School of Medicine in 1891. The

School of Medicine is one of seven schools of Washington University in St. Louis.
Larry J. Shapiro, M.D, Executive Vice Chancellor for Medical Af

Support Groups & Hotlines

7929 National Health Information Center
Washington, DC 20013
310-565-4167
800-336-4797
Fax: 301-984-4256
e-mail: info@nhic.org
www.health.gov/nhic
Offers a nationwide information referral service, produces directories and resource guides.

7930 Stroke Clubs International
805 12th Street
Galveston, TX 77550
409-762-1022
e-mail: strokeclubs@earthlink.net
www.ninds.nih.gov
Organization of persons who have experienced strokes, their families and friends for the purpose of mutual support, education, social and recreational activities. Provides information and assistance to Stroke Clubs (which are usually sponsored by local organizations).
Ellis Williamson

Books

7931 Alzheimer's, Stroke and 29 Other Neurological Disorders Sourcebook
Omnigraphics
615 Griswold Street
Detroit, MI 48226-3993
313-961-1340
800-234-1340
Fax: 800-875-1340
www.omnigraphics.com
Provides vital information for the nontechnical reader focusing on Alzheimer's disease, stroke and various neurological disorders. Answers thousands of questions related to afflications of the central nervous system with each chapter reviwing a particular disorder and offers in-depth discussions.

7932 Courage: Poems & Positive Thoughts for Stroke Survivors
National Stroke Association
9707 E Easter Lane
Englewood, CO 80112-3747
303-649-9299
800-787-6537
Fax: 303-649-1328
www.stroke.org
Words of inspiration from survivors and caregivers.
83 pages
Colette Lafosse, Director Rehabilitation/Recovery Program

7933 Discovery Circles
National Stroke Association
9707 E Easter Lane
Englewood, CO 80112-3747
303-649-9299
800-787-6537
Fax: 303-649-1328
www.stroke.org
NSA's guide to organizing and facilitating stroke support groups. This detailed manual describes the support group structure and the facilitator's role.
213 pages
Colette Lafosse, Director Rehabilitation/Recovery Program

7934 Magic of Humor in Caregiving
National Stroke Association
9707 E Easter Lane
Englewood, CO 80112-3747
303-649-9299
800-787-6537
Fax: 303-649-1328
www.stroke.org
A dynamic researching tool focusing on the necessity of humor in daily caregiving interaction.
Colette Lafosse, Director Rehabilitation/Recovery Program

7935 November Days
National Stroke Association
9707 E Easter Lane
Englewood, CO 80112-3747
303-649-9299
800-787-6537
Fax: 303-649-1328
www.stroke.org
A caregiver's story of her struggle with a loved one's stroke.
225 pages

7936 Occupational Therapy Practice Guidelines for Adults with Stroke
American Occupational Therapy Association
4720 Montgomery Lane
Bethesda, MD 20824-1220
301-652-2682
Fax: 301-652-7711
TDD: 800-377-8555
www.aota.org
15 pages
ISBN: 1-569001-55-3

7937 Stroke Book
William Morrow & Company
1350 Avenue of the Americas
New York, NY 10019-4702
212-261-6500
1993
ISBN: 0-688090-55-9

7938 Stroke: A Clinical Approach
Butterworth-Heinemann
225 Wildwood Avenue
Woburn, MA 01801-2079
617-928-2500
800-366-2665
1993 584 pages
ISBN: 0-750691-81-6

7939 Stroke: A Guide for Patient and Family
Raven Press
1185 Avenue of the Americas
New York, NY 10036-2601
212-930-9500
224 pages
ISBN: 0-881672-79-3

7940 Stroke: Your Complete Exercise Guide
Human Kinetics Publishers
PO Box 5076
Champaign, IL 61825-5076
217-351-1549
800-747-4457
Fax: 217-351-5076
Part of the Cooper Clinic and Research Institute Fitness Series providing exercise rehabilitation for persons suffering from strokes.
126 pages Paperback
ISBN: 0-873224-28-0

7941 Ted's Stroke: The Caregiver's Story
National Stroke Association
9707 E Easter Lane
Englewood, CO 80112-3747
303-649-9299
800-787-6537
Fax: 303-649-1328
www.stroke.org
Personal experiences, guidance and tips for caregivers.
175 pages
ISBN: 0-962487-61-9

7942 The Comfort of Home for Stroke: A Guide fo r Caregivers
Marie Meyer & Paula Derr, RN with Jon Caswell, author
CareTrust Publications
PO Box 10283
Portland, OR 97296-0283
800-565-1533
Fax: 415-673-2005
e-mail: sales@comfortofhome.com
www.comfortofhome.com
Comfort guides readers through every caregiving stage, from understanding personality changes, preparing the home, equipment, the healthcare team, and the activities of daily living. It helps take the fear out of home care and assists caregivers in maintaining peace of mind.
2007 344 pages
ISBN: 0-966476-78-6

7943 Women in Your Life: Protect Yourself, Protect Your Family
National Stroke Association
9707 E Easter Lane
Englewood, CO 80112-3747
303-649-9299
800-787-6537
Fax: 303-649-1328
www.stroke.org

Valuable information about the unique toll stroke takes on women.
Colette Lafosse, Director Rehabilitation/Recovery Program

Magazines

7944 **Stroke Connection**
American Stroke Foundation
8700 Lamar   913-649-1776
Overland Park, KS 66207   Fax: 913-649-6661
www.americanstroke.org
Official magazine of the American Stroke Foundation. Supports stroke survivors, their families, caregivers and friends by providing resources, services, education and information that improves the quality of life.

Pamphlets

7945 **African-Americans and Stroke**
National Stroke Association
9707 E Easter Lane   303-649-9299
Englewood, CO 80112-3747   800-787-6537
Fax: 303-649-1328
www.stroke.org
Colette Lafosse, Director Rehabilitation/Recovery Program

7946 **Aneurysm Answers**
National Stroke Association
9707 E Easter Lane   303-649-9299
Englewood, CO 80112-3747   800-787-6537
Fax: 303-649-1328
www.stroke.org
Colette Lafosse, Director Rehabilitation/Recovery Program

7947 **Check Your Pulse, America: Atrial Fibrillation**
National Stroke Association
9707 E Easter Lane   303-649-9299
Englewood, CO 80112-3747   800-787-6537
Fax: 303-649-1328
www.stroke.org
Colette Lafosse, Director Rehabilitation/Recovery Program

7948 **Cholesterol and Stroke**
National Stroke Association
9707 E Easter Lane   303-649-9299
Englewood, CO 80112-3747   800-787-6537
Fax: 303-649-1328
www.stroke.org
Colette Lafosse, Director Rehabilitation/Recovery Program

7949 **Facts on Heart Disease, Heart Attack, Stroke and Risk Factors**
American Heart Association
7272 Greenville Avenue   214-373-6300
Dallas, TX 75231-5129   Fax: 214-706-1341
Offers information on how to recognize a heart attack or stroke, recovery and rehabilitation techniques and risk factors.

7950 **High Blood Pressure and Stroke**
National Stroke Association
9707 E Easter Lane   303-649-9299
Englewood, CO 80112-3747   800-787-6537
Fax: 303-649-1328
www.stroke.org
Colette Lafosse, Director Rehabilitation/Recovery Program

7951 **Mobility: Issues Facing Stroke Survivors and Their Families**
National Stroke Association
9707 E Easter Lane   303-649-9299
Englewood, CO 80112-3747   800-787-6537
Fax: 303-649-1328
www.stroke.org
Colette Lafosse, Director Rehabilitation/Recovery Program

7952 **Recurrent Stroke**
National Stroke Association

9707 E Easter Lane   303-649-9299
Englewood, CO 80112-3747   800-787-6537
Fax: 303-649-1328
www.stroke.org
Colette Lafosse, Director Rehabilitation/Recovery Program

7953 **Smoking Cessation: Be Smoke Free in 3 Minutes**
National Stroke Association
9707 E Easter Lane   303-649-9299
Englewood, CO 80112-3747   800-787-6537
Fax: 303-649-1328
www.stroke.org
Colette Lafosse, Director Rehabilitation/Recovery Program

7954 **Stroke: Hope Through Research**
Office of Scientific & Health Reports
Building 31   301-496-5751
Bethesda, MD 20892-0001   800-352-9424
Offers information on stroke, research and advances in treatments and rehabilitation programs to help patients.

7955 **Transient Ischemic Attack**
National Stroke Association
9707 E Easter Lane   303-649-9299
Englewood, CO 80112-3747   800-787-6537
Fax: 303-649-1328
www.stroke.org
Colette Lafosse, Director Rehabilitation/Recovery Program

Audio & Video

7956 **Secret Life of the Brain**
PBS Home Video
PO Box 751089
Charlotte, NC 28275   877-727-7467
Fax: 703-739-8131
www.pbs.org/wnet/brain/about.html
Reveals the facinating processes involved in brain development across a lifetime. The five-part series informs viewers of exciting new information in the brain sciences, introduces the foremost researchers in the field, and utilizes dynamic visual imagry and compelling human stories to help a general audience understand otherwise difficult scientific concepts.
5 Tapes
Paula Kerger, President/CEO
Wayne Godwin, Chief Operating Officer

7957 **Stroke: Touching the Soul of Your Family**
National Stroke Association
9707 E Easter Lane   303-649-9299
Englewood, CO 80112-3747   800-787-6537
Fax: 303-649-1328
www.stroke.org
Fifteen minute video chronicling three stroke survivors and their courageous struggle to overcome daily challenges and educate others about stroke.
Colette Lafosse, Director Rehabilitation/Recovery Program

Web Sites

7958 **American Heart Association**
www.americanheart.org
A national organization whose primary concern is the reduction of death and disability due to cardiovascular diseases and stroke.

7959 **Healing Well**
www.healingwell.com
An online health resource guide to medical news, chat, information and articles, newsgroups and message boards, books, disease-related web sites, medical directories, and more for patients, friends, and family coping with disabling diseases, disorders, or chronic illnesses.

7960 **Health Finder**
www.healthfinder.gov
Searchable, carefully developed web site offering information on over 1000 topics. Developed by the US Department of Health and Human Services, the site can be used in both English and Spanish.

7961 Healthlink USA

www.healthlinkusa.com

Health information concerning treatment, cures, prevention, diagnosis, risk factors, research, support groups, email lists, personal stories and much more. Updated regularly.

7962 Helios Health

www.helioshealth.com

Online resource for your health information. Detailed information about specific health topics, access to expert advice from our Medical Advisory Board, and up-to-date health news.

7963 MedicineNet

www.medicinenet.com

An online resource for consumers providing easy-to-read, authoritative medical and health information.

7964 Medscape

www.medscape.com

Medscape offers specialists, primary care physicians, and other health professionals the Web's most robust and integrated medical information and educational tools.

7965 National Heart, Lung & Blood Institute

www.nhlbi.nih.gov/nhlbi/nhlbi.htm

Primary responsibility of this organization is the scientific investigation of heart, blood vessel, lung and blood disorders. Oversee research, demonstration, prevention, education and training activities in these fields and emphasizes the control of stroke.

7966 National Institute of Neurological Disorders and Stroke

www.ninds.nih.gov

The mission of NINDS is to reduce the burden of neurological disease - a burden borne by every age group, by every segment of society, by people all over the world.

7967 National Stroke Association

www.stroke.org

A national organization whose sole purpose is to reduce the incidence and impact of stroke through prevention, treatment, rehabilitation and research, and support for stroke survivors and their families. Educational resources on all aspects of stroke available on website.

7968 Neurology Channel

www.neurologychannel.com

Find clearly explained, medically accurate information regarding conditions, including an overview, symptoms, causes, diagnostic procedures and treatment options. On this site it is possible to ask questions and get information from a neurologist and connect to people who have similar health interests.

7969 WebMD

www.webmd.com

Information on stroke, including articles and resources.

Description

7970 **Substance Abuse**

Substance abuse is a broad term that refers to any illegal, dangerous or destructive use of some substance. This use may be legal (binge drinking by an adult) or illegal (smoking marijuana). Abused substances include alcohol, nicotine, marijuana, heroin, prescription painkillers and tranquilizers, stimulants such as amphetamines and cocaine, and hallucinogens such as LSD. The abuse may be a danger to the user, family members, business associates, close friends or even total strangers. Substance dependence refers to a state of strong compulsion to use the substance, in many cases accompanied by physical withdrawal symptoms if the substance is not regularly available.

The cause of substance abuse is very complex, and involves an interplay between the individual's behavioral choices, their genetic background and past and present social environment. Some substance abusers also have a definable psychiatric disorder such as depression or schizophrenia; treatment of these dual-disorder patients is especially challenging.

The consequences of substance abuse are well-known, and include job loss, arrest, family breakup, automobile and other accidents, birth defects (fetal alcohol syndrome), direct toxic effects (cirrhosis of the liver from alcohol or lung cancer from smoking), and infections (HIV or hepatitis B from sharing needles). Substance abuse, unless it occurs in extremely isolated persons, greatly affects family members and loved ones. Family members often deny the reality of the abuse, and may help, or enable, the abuser to cover up the problem and avoid its consequences.

There is no quick and universally effective treatment for substance abuse. Options range from inexpensive peer-based organizations such as Alcoholics Anonymous to very expensive long-term inpatient programs. Some peer-based programs appeal to a niche defined by sex, race, age or religious affiliation. Treatment is much more likely to succeed if it is freely chosen by the individual rather than mandated by a court. Dropout during treatment and relapse after initial success are common, but many people do achieve life-long cures with abstinence from further substance abuse. Family members should look for education and support through groups like Al-Anon, which bring them together with people facing similar situations.

National Agencies & Associations

7971 **AAA Foundation for Traffic Safety**
607 14th Street NW
Washington, DC 20005-6001
202-638-5944
Fax: 202-638-5943
e-mail: info@aaafoundation.org
www.aaafoundation.org
This national organization publishes drinking and traffic safety programs for K-6 and junior high students. Courses offered are taught by school district teachers who have participated in two-hour in-service training seminars.
J Peter Kissinger, President
Kristin Backstrom, Senior Manager Development

7972 **African American Family Services**
2616 Nicollet Avenue
Minneapolis, MN 55408
612-871-7878
Fax: 612-871-2567
e-mail: contact@aafs.net
www.aafs.net
African American Family Services works with individuals, families and communities affected by addiction and mental illness. From our holistic standpoint, we provide culturally-specific chemical and mental health services that impact family preservation and promote community-based change and wellness.
Terry J Ticey, Chairman of the Board
Thomas Adams, PhD (ABD), MSW, Chief Executive Officer

7973 **Al-Anon Family Group Headquarters**
1600 Corporate Landing Parkway
Virginia Beach, VA 23454-5617
757-563-1600
888-425-2666
Fax: 757-563-1655
e-mail: wso@al-anon.org
www.al-anon.alateen.org
At Al-Anon Family Group meetings, the friends and family members of problem drinkers share their experiences and learn how to apply the principles of the Al-Anon program to their individual situations.
Robert Schneider, Director of Communications

7974 **Alateen Al-Anon Family Group Headquarters**
Al-Anon Family Group Headquarters
1600 Corporate Landing Parkway
Virginia Beach, VA 23454-5617
757-563-1600
800-425-2666
Fax: 757-563-1655
e-mail: wso@al-anon.org
www.al-anon.alateen.org
A part of the Al-Anon program Alateen is for teenagers who have been affected by someone else's drinking whether it be a family member or a friend.
Robert Schneider, Director Communications

7975 **Alcoholics Anonymous General Service Office/Grand Central Sta**
General Service Office/Grand Central Station
Grand Central Station
New York, NY 10163-0459
212-870-3400
Fax: 212-870-3003
e-mail: international@aa.org
www.aa.org
Alcoholics Anonymousr is a fellowship of men and women who share their experience, strength and hope with each other that they may solve their common problem and help others to recover from alcoholism. The only requirement for membership is a desire to stop drinking. There are no dues or fees for AA membership; we are self-supporting through our own contributions.

7976 **American Council for Drug Education**
50 Jay Street
Brooklyn, NY 11201-2301
718-222-6641
877-769-9698
Fax: 212-595-2553
e-mail: hlozada@phoenixhouse.org
www.phoenixhouse.org
The Career Academy guides clients as they work toward their personal and professional goals. Residents live, learn, and work in an environment specifically tailored to meet their needs. Our specialized programs provide training in such high-demand fields as building maintenance and repairs and culinary arts.
J David Hawkins, Director
Herman Lozada, Contact

7977 **American Council on Alcohol Problems**
1000 E Indian School Road
Phoenix, AZ 85014
602-264-7897
800-527-5344
Fax: 602-264-7403
e-mail: info@aca-usa.com
www.aca-usa.com
The American Council on Alcoholism (ACA) is a national non-profit 501(c)3 health organization dedicated to educating the public about the effects of alcohol, alcoholism and alcohol abuse,

and the need for prompt, effective, readily-available, and afford-able alcoholism treatment.

Lloyd R. Vocovsky, Chairman
Jeff Becker, Vice Chairman

7978   American Dental Association Department of Library Services
Department of Library Services
211 E Chicago Avenue   312-440-2500
Chicago, IL 60611-2637   Fax: 312-440-2822
                                    e-mail: affiliates@ada.org
                                    www.ada.org
Founded in 1859, the not-for-profit ADA is the nation's largest dental association, representing 157,000 dentist members. Since then, the ADA has grown to become the leading source of oral health related information for dentists and their patients. Learn more about the ADA's mission and vision, and our commitment to the public's oral health, ethics, science and professional advance-ment and access to care for all Americans.

Linda Kittel MS RN, Manager
Brandon R Maddox, Representative

7979   Associate Administrator for Alcohol Prevention and Treatment Policy
Substance Abuse & Mental Health Services Offices
200 Independance Avenue   301-443-8956
Washington, DC 20201-0001   e-mail: info@samhsa.gov
                                    www.samhsa.gov
Promotes monitors evaluates and coordinates programs for the prevention and treatment of alcoholism and alcohol abuse.

7980   Association of Halfway House Alcoholism Programs of North America
401 E Sangamon Avenue   217-523-0527
Springfield, IL 62702   Fax: 217-698-8234
                                    e-mail: president@ahhap.org
                                    www.ahhap.org
Acts as a clearinghouse of the latest literature on alcoholism assists chemical dependency counselors in placing post treatment indi-viduals in halfway houses and helps in setting up halfway houses.

Olivia Howard, President
David Logan, Vice President

7981   BACCHUS of the US
PO Box 938   303-871-0901
Littleton, CO 80160   Fax: 303-871-0907
                                    e-mail: admin@bacchusnetwork.org
                                    www.bacchusnetwork.org
BACCHUS develops cutting edge tools for campuses consisting of student-friendly training programs, resource manuals, posters, and pamphlets. Currently there are 120 educational resources and training materials offered by our organization. In addition, each af-filiate group receives health issue campaigns that, when used in combination, lay the foundation for a year-round prevention program.

Janet Cox, MA, President/CEO
Ann . Quinn-Zobeck, Ph.D, Director of Education and Training

7982   CSAP State Liason Program CSAP Division of Communications Programs
CSAP Division of Communications Programs
7200 Wisconsin Avenue
Bethesda, MD 20857-0001   301-941-8500
                                    www.covesoft.com/csap.html
This program is designed to support alcohol and other drug abuse prevention efforts in the States.

7983   Center for Substance Abuse Prevention
Substance Abuse and Mental Health Services Admin.
PO Box 2345
Rockville, MD 20847-2345   800-279-6686
                                    TTY: 800-487-4886
                                    TDD: 800-487-4886
                                    e-mail: info@health.org.
                                    www.ncadi.samhsa.gov
This organization's goal is to connect people and resources with innovative ideas strategies and programs designed to encourage creative and effective efforts aimed at reducing and eliminating al-cohol tobacco and other drug problems in our society.

7984   Chemical People Project Public Television Outreach Alliance
Public Television Outreach Alliance

4802 5th Avenue   412-391-0900
Pittsburgh, PA 15213-2957
The project supplies information in the form of tapes literature and seminars.

7985   Cocaine Anonymous: World Service Office
3740 Overland Avenue   310-559-5833
Los Angeles, CA 90049-6337   800-999-9951
                                    Fax: 310-559-2554
                                    e-mail: webservant@ca.org
                                    www.ca.org
The best way to reach someone is to speak to them on a common level. The members of C.A. are all recovering addicts who main-tain their individual sobriety by working with others. We come from various social, ethnic, economic and religious backgrounds, but what we have in common is addiction.

7986   Drug Abuse Resistance Education of America
PO Box 512090   310-215-0575
Los Angeles, CA 90051-0090   800-223-3273
                                    Fax: 310-215-0180
                                    www.dare.com
Provides information, resources, tips, warning signs and other in-formation for parents and kids to help keep children off drugs.

Francisco X Pegueros, President/CEO
Thomas Hazelton, President of Development

7987   Drugs Anonymous
PO Box 473   212-874-0700
New York, NY 10023
A twelve-step program that holds more than 30 meetings for drug addicts in the Greater New York Area including several in hospi-tals and institutions.

7988   Families Anonymous
PO Box 3475   310-815-8010
Culver City, CA 90231-3475   800-736-9805
                                    Fax: 310-815-9682
                                    e-mail: famanon@familiesanonymous.org
                                    www.familiesanonymous.org
Addresses the needs of families who are concerned about a relative with a drug problem and with related behavioral problems. Offers informational packets meetings and support networks for these families.

7989   Families in Action National Drug Information Center
2957 Clairmont Road NE   404-248-9676
Atlanta, GA 30333   Fax: 404-248-1312
                                    e-mail: nfia@nationalfamilies.org
                                    www.nationalfamilies.org
National Families in Action is a 501 (c) (3) nonprofit organization that was founded in Atlanta, Georgia in 1977. The organization ob-tained the nation's first state laws banning the sale of drug para-phernalia. It led a national effort to help parents replicate Georgia's laws in other states to prevent the marketing of drugs and drug use to children and helped them form parent groups to protect children's health.

Sue Rusche, President
Carol S. Reeder, Treasurer

7990   Hazelden
PO Box 11   651-213-4200
Center City, MN 55012-0011   800-257-7810
                                    Fax: 651-213-4411
                                    e-mail: info@hazeldon.org
                                    www.hazelden.com
Hazelden helps individuals, families, and communities struggling with alcohol abuse, substance abuse, and drug addiction transform their lives. Our locations across the United States help people at all stages of the treatment and recovery process, supporting them with our Twelve Step-based model that is the modern standard for ad-diction treatment and recovery services.

Mark Mishek, President/CEO
Ann Bray, General Counsel/Vice President of Strate

7991   Indian Health Service
801 Thompson Avenue
Rockville, MD 20852-1627   605-226-7456
                                    www.ihs.gov

Charged with providing a comprehensive program of alcoholism and substance abuse prevention and treatment for Native Americans and Alaskan natives.

7992   Lawyers Concerned for Lawyers
2550 University Avenue W   651-646-5590
Saint Paul, MN 55114-4127   866-525-6466
                                            Fax: 651-646-2364
                                            e-mail: help@mnlcl.org
                                            www.mnlcl.org

A nonprofit organization of recovering lawyers and judges and concerned others. Educates lawyers and judges about the disease of chemical dependency assists in assessments and arranging interventions and offers lawyer-only AA meetings.
Joan Bibelhausen, Executive Director
Ellen Murphy-Fritsch, Case Manager

7993   Marijuana Anonymous: World Services
Marijuana Anonymous World Services
PO Box 7807
Terrance, CA 90504-2318   800-766-6779
                         e-mail: office@marijuana-anonymous.org
                                    www.marijuana-anonymous.org

A fellowship of men and women who share our experience strength and hope with each other that we may solve our common problem and help others to recover from marijuana addiction.

7994   Mothers Against Drunk Driving (MADD)
511 E John Carpenter Freeway   214-744-6233
Irving, TX 75062   877-275-6233
                                            Fax: 972-869-2206
                                            www.madd.org

Founded by a small group of mothers and has turned into one of the largest crime victims organizations in the world.
Janet Withers, President
Debbie Wier, CEO

7995   Narcotics Anonymous World Service Office
World Service Office
PO Box 9999
Van Nuys, CA 91409-9099   818-773-9999
                                            Fax: 818-700-0700
                                            e-mail: fsmail@na.org
                                            www.na.org

Similar to Alcoholics Anonymous this program is a fellowship of men and women who meet to help one another with their drug dependency problems.

7996   National Association for Children of Alcoholics
11426 Rockville Pike   301-468-0985
Rockville, MD 20852-3007   888-554-2627
                                            Fax: 301-468-0987
                                            e-mail: nacoa@nacoa.org
                                            www.nacoa.org

Advocates for all children and families affected by alcohol and other drug dependencies.
Sis Wenger, President/CEO
Judy Galloway, Coordinator-Affiliate Services

7997   National Association for Native American Children of Alcoholics
Seattle Indian Health Board
1402 Third Avenue   206-467-7686
Seattle, WA 98114-3364   800-322-5601
                                            Fax: 206-467-7689
                                            e-mail: nanacoa@aol.com

Formed to facilitate positive change in individuals and communities in order to break the intergenerational cycle of addiction among Native Americans.

7998   National Association of Alcoholism and Drug Abuse Counselors
1001 N Fairfax Street   703-741-7686
Alexandria, VA 22314   800-548-0497
                                            Fax: 703-741-7698
                                            e-mail: naadac2@naadac.org
                                            www.naadac.org

Largest membership organization serving addiction counselors educators and other addiction-focused health care professionals who specialize in addiction prevention treatment and education.
Cynthia Tuhoy, Executive Director
Shirley Mikell, Director of Certification and Education

7999   National Association on Drug Abuse Problems
Director of Corporate and Community Services
355 Lexington Avenue   212-986-1170
New York, NY 10017   Fax: 212-697-2939
                                            e-mail: info@nadap.org
                                            www.nadap.org

Provides skills evaluation job training and job placement to recovering drug addicts in the metropolitan New York area.
John A Darin, President/CEO
Gary Stankowski, Senior Vice President

8000   National Clearinghouse for Alcohol and Drug Information
11420 Rockville Pike   301-468-2600
Rockville, MD 20847-2345   800-729-6686
                                            Fax: 240-221-4292
                                            TTY: 800-487-4889
                                            TDD: 800-487-4889
                                            e-mail: webmaster@health.org
                                            www.health.org

Nation's one-stop resource for information about substance abuse prevention and addiction treatment.

8001   National Council on Alcoholism and Drug Dependence
217 Broadway   212-269-7797
New York, NY 10007-3128   800-622-2255
                                            Fax: 212-269-7510
                                            e-mail: national@ncadd.org
                                            www.ncadd.org

The National Council on Alcoholism and Drug Dependence, Inc and it's Affiliate Network is a voluntary health organization dedicated to fighting the Nation's #1 health problem-alcholism, drug addiction and the devestating consequences of alcohol and other drugs on individuals, families and communities.
Robert Lindsey, President
Leah Brock, Director of Affiliate Relations

8002   National Crime Prevention Council
2001 Jefferson Davis Highway   202-466-6272
Arlington, VA 22202   Fax: 202-296-1356
                                            www.ncpc.org

This organization works to prevent crime and drug use in many ways including developing materials for parents and children.
Alfonso E Lenhardt, President/CEO
David A Dean, Executive Committee Chair

8003   National Families in Action
2957 Clairmont Rd   404-248-9676
Atlanta, GA 30329   Fax: 404-248-1312
                                            e-mail: nfia@nationalfmailies.org
                                            www.nationalfamilies.org

Mission is to help families and communities prevent drug use among children by promoting policies based on science.
William F. Carter, Chairman
Sue Rusche, President & CEO

8004   National Organization on Fetal Alcohol Syndrome
1200 Eton Court NW   202-785-4585
Washington, DC 20007   800-666-6327
                                            Fax: 202-466-6456
                                            e-mail: information@nofas.org
                                            www.nofas.org

Dedicated to eliminating birth defects caused by alcohol consumption during pregnancy and to improving the quality of life for those affected individuals and families.
Kate Boyce, Chair
Tom Donaldson, President

8005   Office of Applied Studies Substance Abuse & Mental Health Services
Substance Abuse & Mental Health Services Offices
5600 Fishers Lane
Rockville, MD 20857-0001   301-443-8956
                                            www.samhsa.gov

Provides the leadership needed for collecting data on mental illness and substance abuse including incidence and prevalence studies.

8006 Office of Substance Abuse Prevention
5600 Fishers Lane
Rockville, MD 20857-0001　　　301-443-0373
　　　　　　　　　　　　　　www.samhsa.gov
Reviews the government's alcohol and drug abuse policy operates a grant program supports development of model programs and conducts prevention workshops.

8007 Office of Women's Services Substance Abuse & Mental Health Services
Substance Abuse & Mental Health Services Offices
5600 Fishers Lane　　　　　　301-443-8956
Rockville, MD 20857-0001
Provides leadership and guidance in creating and maintaining an agency-wide focus for addressing the substance abuse and mental health needs of women.

8008 Office on Smoking and Health: CDCP
Centers for Disease Control And Prevention
1600 Clifton Road　　　　　　404-639-3311
Atlanta, GA 30333　　　　　　800-232-4636
　　　　　　　　　　　　　TTY: 888-232-6348
　　　　　　　　　e-mail: tobaccoinfo@cdc.gov
　　　　　　　　　　　　www.cdc.gov/tobacco
Offers reference services to researchers through the Technical Information Center. Publishes and distributes a number of titles in the field of smoking and health.

8009 PRIDE Youth Programs
707 West Main Street　　　　　231-924-1662
Fermont, MI 49412　　　　　　800-668-9277
　　　　　　　　　　　　　Fax: 231-924-5663
　　　　　　　e-mail: info@prideyouthprograms.org
　　　　　　　　　www.prideyouthprograms.org
A provider of prevention services in the area of alcohol and other drugs. Mission is to build a drug-free America.
Jay Dewispelaere, President/CEO
Lou Anne Wheater, Membership Coordinator

8010 Partnership for a Drug-Free America
352 Park Avenue South　　　　212-922-1560
New York, NY 10010-0002　　Fax: 212-922-1570
　　　　　　　　　　　　　　www.drugfree.org
Non-profit coalition of communication health medical and educational professionals working to reduce illicit drug use and help people live health drug-free lives.
Stephen J Pasierb, President & CEO
Robert Caruso, CFO

8011 Remove Intoxicated Drivers (RID-USA)
Schenectady, NY 12301　　　518-372-0034
　　　　　　　　　　　　　877-823-9235
　　　　　　　　　　　　　Fax: 518-310-4917
　　　　　　　　　e-mail: dwi@rid-usa.org
　　　　　　　　　　　　　rid-usa.org
Volunteers working to deter impaired driving, to help its victims obtain justice, restitution and peace of mind when faced with the maze of criminal justice systems, and to curb the alcohol abuse which leads to drunken driving.
Doris Aiken, Founder/President
Bill Aiken, VP/Manager

8012 Safe Homes
4 Mann Street　　　　　　　　508-755-0333
Worcester, MA 01602-0702　Fax: 508-836-5560
　　　　　　　e-mail: safehomes@thebridgecm.org
　　　　　　　　　　　www.safehomesma.org
This national organization encourages parents to sign a contract stipulating that when parties are held in one another's homes they will adhere to a strict no-alcohol/no-drug-use rule.
Laura Farnsworth, Director of Safe Homes & Worcester PFLAG
Michael S Petracca, Clinician

8013 Students Against Destructive Decisions
255 Main Street　　　　　　　508-481-3568
Marlborough, MA 01752　　　877-723-3462
　　　　　　　　　　　　　Fax: 508-481-5759
　　　　　　　　　　e-mail: info@sadd.org
　　　　　　　　　　　　www.sadd.org

To provide students with the best prevention tools possible to deal with the issues of underage drinking, other drug use, risky and impaired driving, and other destructive decisions.
Larry Bailin, Founder/CEO
Ovidio B. Bermudez MD, Chairman/Chief Medical Officer

8014 Substance Abuse and Mental Health Services Administration
1 Choke Cherry Road　　　　877-726-4727
Rockville, MD 20857-0001　　877-696-6775
　　　　　　　　　　　　　TTY: 800-487-4889
　　　　　　　　　　　　　　www.samhsa.gov
The goal of this organization is to reduce incidence and prevalence of mental disorders and substance abuse and improve treatment outcomes for persons suffering from addictive and mental health problems and disorders.

8015 Workplace Program CSAP Division of Communication Programs
CSAP Division of Communication Programs
5600 Fishers Lane　　　　　　301-443-9936
Rockville, MD 20857-0001
This program sets standards for drug testing in workplace settings.

State Agencies & Associations

Alabama

8016 Division of Mental Illness and Substance Abuse Community Programs
Department of Mental Health
Montgomery, AL 36130-1410　　334-242-3454
　　　　　　　　　　　　　　800-367-0955
　　　　　　　　　　　　　Fax: 334-242-0725
　　　　　　　e-mail: Alabama.DMH@mh.alabama.gov
　　　　　　　　　　　　www.mh.alabama.gov
Kent Hunt, Associate Commissioner Substance Abuse
Susan P Chambers, Associate Commissioner Mental Illness

Alaska

8017 Office of Alcohol and Substance Abuse Department of Health and Social Services
Department of Health and Social Services
350 Main Street　　　　　　　907-465-3030
Juneau, AK 99811　　　　　　800-465-4828
　　　　　　　　　　　　　Fax: 907-465-3068
　　　　　　　e-mail: Stacy.Toner@Alaska.gov
　　　　　　　dhss.alaska.gov/Pages/default.aspx
William J. Streuss, Commissioner
Tara Horton, Special Assistant

Arizona

8018 Alcoholism and Drug Abuse: Office of Community Behavioral Health
Department of Health Services
150 N 18th Avenue　　　　　602-364-4558
Phoenix, AZ 85007-3228　　Fax: 602-364-4570
　　　　　　　　e-mail: cancerlr@azdhs.gov
　　　　　　　　　　　　www.azdhs.gov
The Arizona Department of Health Services promotes and protects the health of Arizona's children and adults. Its mission is to set the standard for personal and community health through direct care, science, public policy, and leadership.
January Contreras, Acting Director

Arkansas

8019 Office of Alcohol and Drug Abuse Prevention
305 South Palm Street　　　　501-686-9866
Little Rock, AR 72205　　　　877-726-4727
　　　　　　　　　　　　　Fax: 501-686-9035
　　　　　　　e-mail: linda.baker@arkansas.gov
　　　　　www.captus.samhsa.gov/grantee-organizati
SAMHSA's mission is to reduce the impact of substance abuse and mental illness on America's communities.

California

8020 **California Women's Commission on Alcohol and Drug Dependencies**
14622 Victory Boulevard   818-376-0470
Van Nuys, CA 91411
Dedicated to improving the quality and increasing the quantity of services to women with alcohol-related problems.

8021 **Department of Alcohol and Drug Programs**
1700 K Street   916-445-0834
Sacramento, CA 95811-4037   800-879-2772
                                      Fax: 916-323-1270
                e-mail: resourcecenter@adp.state.ca.us
                               www.colorado.gov/CDHS
Kathryn P Jett, Director

Colorado

8022 **Alcohol and Drug Abuse Division Department of Human Services**
Department of Human Services
4055 S Lowell Boulevard   303-866-7480
Denver, CO 80236-3120   Fax: 303-866-7481
                  e-mail: jaqueline.enriques@state.co.us
                                  www.cdhs.state.co.us
Janet Wood, Director
Mary McCann, Acting Manager

Connecticut

8023 **Connecticut Alcohol and Drug Abuse Commission**
410 Capitol Avenue   860-418-7000
Hartford, CT 06134   800-446-7348
                                      Fax: 860-418-6780
                                      TTY: 860-418-6707
                  e-mail: ronna.keil@pa.state.ct.us
                                  www.dmhas.state.ct.us
The mission of the Department of Mental Health and Addiction Services is to improve the quality of life of the people of Connecticut by providing an integrated network of comprehensive, effective and efficient mental health and addiction services that foster self-sufficiency, dignity and respect.
Patricia Rehmer, Commissioner

Delaware

8024 **Delaware Division of Alcoholism, Drug Abuse and Mental Health**
Alcohol And Drug Services
1901 North DuPont Highway   302-255-9399
New Castle, DE 19720   Fax: 302-255-4427
                      e-mail: DHSSInfor@state.de.us
                                  www.dhss.delware.gov
Our mission is to promote health and recovery by ensuring that Delawareans have access to quality prevention and treatment for mental health, substance use, and gambling conditions.
Renata J. Henry, Director

District of Columbia

8025 **Health Planning and Development**
825 N Capitol Street NE   202-727-8473
Washington, DC 20002   Fax: 202-727-8411
                                  e-mail: doh@dc.gov
                    doh.dc.gov/service/doh-substance-abuse

Florida

8026 **Alcohol and Drug Abuse Program Department Of Children And Families**
Department Of Children And Families
1317 Winewood Boulevard   850-487-2920
Tallahassee, FL 32399-6570   Fax: 850-414-7474
                        www.dcf.state.fl.us/mentalhealth/sa
The Substance Abuse and Mental Health (SAMH) Program, within the Florida Department of Children and Families, is the single state authority on substance abuse and mental health as designated by the federal Substance Abuse and Mental Health Services Administration (SAMHSA). The Department's SAMH Program oversees a statewide system of care for the prevention, treatment, and recovery of children and adults with serious mental illnesses and/or substance abuse disorders.
Cynthea Panzarino, Director

Georgia

8027 **Alcohol and Drug Services Addictive Diseases Program**
Addictive Diseases Program
Two Peachtree Street NW   404-657-2331
Atlanta, GA 30303-3171   Fax: 404-657-2160
                              www.mhddad.dhr.georgia.gov
DBHDD contracts with providers in all 6 regions to provide outpatient and residential substance abuse treatment to men and women who are struggling with the disease of addiction
Frank Berry, Commissioner

Hawaii

8028 **Alcohol and Drug Abuse Division Department of Health**
Department of Health
601 Kamokila Boulevard   808-692-7506
Kapoleiu, HI 96707   Fax: 808-692-7521
                      e-mail: ATRINFO@doh.hawaii.gov
                                  www.hawaii.gov/health
The mission of the Department of Health is to protect and improve the health and environment for all people in Hawai'i .
Loretta J. Fuddy, Director
Keith Yamamoto, Asst. Director

Idaho

8029 **Department of Health and Welfare Department Of Health And Welfare**
Department Of Health And Welfare
1720 Westgate Drive   208-334-6747
Boise, ID 83704-0036   800-926-2588
                                      Fax: 208-334-6738
                          e-mail: rossil@dhw.idaho.gov
                          www.healthandwelfare.idaho.gov
Landis Rossi, Regional Director
Richard Armstrong, Director

Illinois

8030 **Department of Alcoholism and Substance Abuse**
Department Of Human Services
100 W Randolph Street   312-814-3840
Chicago, IL 60601   800-843-6154
                                      Fax: 312-814-2419
                                      TTY: 800-447-6404
                      e-mail: dhsas16@dhs.state.il.us
                                  www.dhs.state.il.us
Theodora Binion-Tayl, Director

8031 **Illinois Church Action on Alcohol Problems**
1132 W Jefferson Street   217-546-6871
Springfields, IL 62702   Fax: 217-546-2814
                      e-mail: ilcaaap@sbcglobal.net
                                  www.ilcaaap.org
An interdenominational Christian agency representing church groups in Illinois. Works to prevent alcohol and other drug-related problems through education legislative action and public awareness.

8032 **Parkside Medical Services Corporation**
205 W Touhy Avenue   847-698-9866
Park Ridge, IL 60068-4256   800-727-5723
This establishment offers treatment and hope for the alcoholic/substance abuser. A resource center that provides information books and resources pertaining to substance abuse and offers treatment facilities in various states across the country.

Indiana

8033 **Division of Addiction Services Department of Mental Health**
Department of Mental Health

402 W Washington Street
Indianapolis, IN 46204-3614

317-232-7800
800-662-4357
Fax: 317-233-3472
www.in.gov/fssa

Gina Eckart, Director
Alma Burrus, Operations Manager

Iowa

8034 Department of Public Health: Division of Substance Abuse and Health
Lucas State Office Building
321 E 12th Street
Des Moines, IA 50319-0075

515-281-7689
866-227-9878
Fax: 515-281-4535
e-mail: jzwick@idphstate.ia.us
www.idph.state.ia.us

The Iowa Department of Public Health (IDPH) partners with local public health, policymakers, health care providers, business and many others to fulfill our mission of promoting and protecting the health of Iowans.
Kathy Stone, Director

Kansas

8035 Alcohol and Drug Abuse Services
915 Harrison Street
Topeka, KS 66612

785-296-3959
800-586-3690
Fax: 785-296-7275
TTY: 785-296-1491
e-mail: dxmd@srskansas.org
www.srskansas.org

Don Jordan, Secretary
Laura Howard, Deputy Secretary/CFO

Kentucky

8036 Division of Substance Abuse: Department of Mental Health
Department For MH/MR Services
100 Fair Oaks Lane
Frankfort, KY 40621

502-564-2880
Fax: 502-564-7152
TTY: 502-564-5777
www.mhmr.ky.gov

Louisiana

8037 Office of Human Services: Division of Alcohol and Drug Abuse
628 N 4th Street
Baton Rouge, LA 70802-2790

225-342-9500
855-229-6848
Fax: 225-342-3875
TTY: 225-342-5568
e-mail: dhhwebinfo@la.gov
www.dhh.louisiana.gov

Maine

8038 Office of Alcohol and Drug Abuse Prevention
Ofice Of Substance Abuse
AMHI Complex, Marquardt Building
Augusta, ME 04333-0159

207-289-2595
Fax: 207-287-4334
e-mail: osa.ircosa@state.me.us
www.maine.gov/dhhs/samhs/osa/

Kimberly A. Johnson, Director

Maryland

8039 Maryland State Alcohol and Drug Abuse Administration
55 Wade Avenue
Catonsville, MD 21228

410-402-8600
Fax: 410-402-8601
e-mail: adaainfo@dhmh.state.md.us
www.maryland-adaa.org

The Alcohol and Drug Abuse Administration is committed to providing access to a quality and effective substance abuse prevention, intervention and treatment service system for the citizens of Maryland.
Kathleen Rebbert-Fra, Acting Director
Steve Bocian, Acting Deputy Director

Massachusetts

8040 Division of Substance Abuse
250 Washington Street
Boston, MA 02108-4619

617-624-5111
800-327-5050
Fax: 617-624-5185
TTY: 888-448-8321
e-mail: bsas.questions@state.ma.us
www.mass.gov/eohhs/gov/departments/dph/p

Michael Botticelli, Director

Michigan

8041 Office of Substance Abuse Services Department of Public Health
Department of Public Health
320 S Walnut Street
Lansing, MI 48913

517-373-4700
888-736-0253
Fax: 517-335-2121
TTY: 517-373-3573
www.michigan.gov/mdch

Yvonne Blackmond, Director

Minnesota

8042 Chemical Dependency Program Division Department of Human Services
Department of Human Services
Saint Paul, MN 55164-3899

651-431-2460
800-627-3529
Fax: 651-582-1865
e-mail: dhs.info@state.mn.us
mn.gov/dhs/about-dhs/

The Minnesota Department of Human Services, working with many others, helps people meet their basic needs so they can live in dignity and achieve their highest potential.

8043 Dentists Concerned for Dentists
450 N Syndicate
Saint Paul, MN 55104

651-641-0730
www.medhelp.org/amshc/amshc53.htm

A nonprofit organization for chemically dependent Minnesota dentists and concerned others.

Mississippi

8044 Division of Alcohol & Drug Abuse: Mississippi
Department of Mental Health
1101 Robert E Lee Building
Jackson, MS 39201

601-359-1288
877-210-8513
Fax: 601-359-6295
TTY: 601-359-6230
www.dmh.state.ms.us

Supporting a better tomorrow by making a difference in the lives of Mississippians with mental illness, substance abuse problems and intellectual/developmental disabilities one person at a time.
Rose Roberts, Chair
Jim Herzog, Vice Chair

8045 Division of Alcohol & Drug Abuse: South Department of Mental Health
1101 Robert E Lee Building
Jackson, MS 39201

601-359-1288
877-210-8513
Fax: 601-359-6295
TTY: 601-359-6230
www.dmh.state.ms.us

Supporting a better tomorrow by making a difference in the lives of Mississippians with mental illness, substance abuse problems and intellectual/developmental disabilities one person at a time.
Rose Roberts, Chair
Jim Herzog, Vice Chair

Missouri

8046 Missouri Division of Alcohol and Drug Abuse
Department of Mental Health

1706 E Elm Street
Jefferson City, MO 65102

573-751-4942
800-575-7480
Fax: 573-751-8224
TTY: 573-526-1201
e-mail: dmhmail@dmh.mo.gov
dmh.mo.gov/ada/

Keith Schafer, Director
Heidi DiBiaso, Administrative Assistant

Montana

8047   Department of Institutions, Alcohol and Drug Abuse Division
Helena, MT 59620-2905

406-444-3964
Fax: 406-444-9389
e-mail: jcassidy@mt. gov
www.dphhs.st.mt.us

Nebraska

8048   Department of Public Instruction: Division of Alcoholism and Drug Abuse
Division Of Behavioral Health
Lincoln, NE 68509-8925

402-471-7818
800-648-4444
Fax: 402-479-5162
e-mail: richard.deliberty@hhss.ne.gov
www.hhs.state.ne.us

Scot Adams, Director
GibsonBlaine Shaffer, CEO

Nevada

8049   Alcohol and Drug Abuse Bureau: Department of Human Resources
4126 Technology Way
Carson City, NV 89706

775-684-5943
Fax: 775-684-5964
e-mail: MHDS@MHDS.NV.GOV
www.mhds.nv.gov

Maria Canfield, Chief

New Hampshire

8050   Office of Alcohol and Drug Abuse Prevention
State Office Park South
129 Pleasant Street
Concord, NH 03301-3852

800-804-0909
Fax: 603-271-6105
e-mail: rosemary.shannon@dhhs.sate.nh.us
www.dhhs.state.nh.us

New Jersey

8051   Department of Health
120 S Stockton Street
Trenton, NJ 08625-0362

609-292-7837
800-367-6543
Fax: 609-292-3816
e-mail: georgene.rhodunda@dhs.state.nj.us
www.state.nj.us

Heather Howard, Commissioner
Mary E O'Dowd, Chief of Staff

8052   Division of Narcotic and Drug Abuse Control
120 S Stockton Street
Trenton, NJ 08625-0362

609-292-5760
800-238-2333
Fax: 609-292-3816
www.state.nj.us/humanservices

Jeffers, Director

New Mexico

8053   Substance Abuse Bureau
1190 Saint Francis Drive
Santa Fe, NM 87502

505-827-2601
800-362-2013
Fax: 505-827-0097
www.nmcares.org

New York

8054   Division of Substance Abuse Services
Substance Abuse Services
1450 Western Avenue
Albany, NY 12203-3526

518-473-3460
877-846-7369
Fax: 518-457-5474
e-mail: communications@oasas.ny.gov
www.oasas.ny.gov

Karen M Carpenter-Palumbo, Commissioner
Kathleen Caggiano-Si, Executive Deputy Commissioner

North Carolina

8055   Alcohol and Drug Abuse Section
Division of Mental Health & Mental Retardation
2001 Mail Service Center
Raleigh, NC 27699-3007

919-733-7011
800-662-7030
Fax: 919-508-0951
www.dhhs.state.nc.us

Leza Wainwright, Director
Michael S Lancaster, Director

North Dakota

8056   Division of Alcoholism & Drug Abuse: Department of Human Services
Department Of Human Services
1237 W Divide Avenue
Bismarck, ND 58501

701-328-8920
800-755-2719
Fax: 701-328-8969
e-mail: dhsmhsas@nd.gov
www.nd.gov/dhs/services/mentalhealth/

The Mental Health and Substance Abuse Services Division provides leadership for the planning, development, and oversight of a system of care for children, adults, and families with severe emotional disorders, mental illness, and/or substance abuse issues.

Ohio

8057   Bureau on Alcohol Abuse and Recovery Ohio Department of Health
Ohio Department of Health
30 East Broad Street
Columbus, OH 43215-2550

614-466-3445
Fax: 614-752-8645
e-mail: info@ada.ohio.gov
www.odadas.state.oh.us

The mission of the Ohio Department of Mental Health and Addiction Services (OhioMHAS) is to provide statewide leadership of a high-quality mental health and addiction prevention, treatment and recovery system that is effective and valued by all Ohioans.
Tracy J. Plouck, Director
Orman Hall, Director of the Governor's Cabinet Opiat

8058   Bureau on Drug Abuse: Ohio Department of Health
Ohio Department of Health
30 East Broad Street
Columbus, OH 43215

614-466-3445
Fax: 614-752-8645
e-mail: info@ada.ohio.gov
www.odadas.state.oh.us

The mission of the Ohio Department of Mental Health and Addiction Services (OhioMHAS) is to provide statewide leadership of a high-quality mental health and addiction prevention, treatment and recovery system that is effective and valued by all Ohioans.
Tracy J. Plouck, Director
Orman Hall, Director of the Governor's Cabinet Opiat

Oklahoma

8059   Oklahoma Department of Mental Health and Substance Abuse Services
Substance Abuse Program

1200 NE 13th Street
Oklahoma City, OK 73117-3277

405-522-3908
800-522-9054
Fax: 405-522-3650
TTY: 405-522-3851
e-mail: jglover@odmhsas.org
www.odmhsas.org

J. Andy Sullivan, Chairperson
Larry McCauley, Vice Chair

Oregon

8060 Office of Alcohol and Drug Abuse Programs
500 Summer Street NE
Salem, OR 97301-1118

503-945-5763
Fax: 503-378-8467
TTY: 800-375-2863
e-mail: omhas.web@state.or.us
www.oregon.gov/DHS/addiction/index.shtml

Pennsylvania

8061 Drug and Alcohol Programs Department Of Health
Department Of Health
02 Kline Plaza
Harrisburg, PA 17104-0090

717-783-8200
877-724-3258
Fax: 717-787-6285
e-mail: rkauffman@state.pa.us
www.ddap.pa.gov

Gary Tennis, Secretary
Kim Bowman, Deputy Secretary

Rhode Island

8062 Division of Substance Abuse: Department of Mental Health and Hospitals
Department Of Mental Health And Retardation
14 Harrington Road
Cranston, RI 02920-0944

401-462-2339
800-622-7422
Fax: 401-462-3204
e-mail: CStenning@bhddh.ri.gov
www.mhrh.state.ri.us

Committed to assuring access to quality services and supports for Rhode Islanders with developmental disabilities, mental health and substance abuse issues, and chronic long term medical and psychiatric conditions. Our mission includes addressing the stigma attached to these disabilities as well as planning for the development of new services and prevention activities.
Craig S Stenning, Executive Director

South Carolina

8063 South Carolina Commission on Alcohol and Drug Abuse
Department Of Alcohol And Drug Abuse Services
2414 Bull Street
Columbia, SC 29201-9498

803-896-5555
Fax: 803-896-5557
www.daodas.org

The department's mission is to ensure the provision of quality services to prevent or reduce the negative consequences of substance use and addictions.
Bob Toomey, Director
Kaitlin Blanco-Silva, Project Manager

South Dakota

8064 Division of Alcohol & Drug Abuse: South Dakota
Department Of Human Services
3800 E Highway 34
Pierre, SD 57501-5070

605-773-5990
800-265-9684
Fax: 605-773-5483
TTY: 605-773-6412
e-mail: infodhs@state.sd.us
www.dhs.sd.gov

Gilbert Sudbeck, Director

Tennessee

8065 Department of Mental Health and Mental Retardation, Alcohol & Drug Service
Bureau Of Alcohol And Drug Abuse Services

601 Mainstream Drive
Nashville, TN 37243-4401

615-532-6500
800-560-5767
Fax: 615-532-2419
e-mail: oca.mhdd@tn.gov
www.state.tn.us

Michael A. Rabin, Director and Meida Contact
Lorene Lambert, Publications & Web Management

Texas

8066 Texas Commission on Alcohol and Drug Abuse Department Of State Health
Department Of State Health
Austin, TX 78714

512-206-5000
866-378-8440
Fax: 512-458-7477
TTY: 800-735-2989
TDD: 800-735-2989
e-mail: web.master@dshs.state.tx.us
www.dshs.state.tx.us/mhsa/

Mission is to improve health and well-being in Texas.
David L. Lakey, Commissioner

Utah

8067 Department of Social Services: Division of Substance Abuse
Department Of Human Services
195 North 1950 West
Salt Lake City, UT 84116

801-538-3939
Fax: 801-538-9892
e-mail: jemarrott@utah.gov
www.hsdsa.utah.gov

The Utah Division of Substance Abuse and Mental Health is the State agency responsible for ensuring that prevention and treatment services for substance abuse and mental health are available statewide. If you, a friend, or family member is struggling with a mental health problem or a problem with alcohol, tobacco, or other drugs there is help available. Hope and recovery are possible.
Paula Bell, Chairperson
Darryl Wagner, Vice Chairman

Vermont

8068 Alcohol and Drug Abuse Programs of Vermont Department Of Health
Department Of Health
108 Cherry Street
Burlington, VT 05402-1531

802-651-1550
Fax: 802-651-1573
e-mail: vtadap@vdh.state.vt.us
www.healthvermont.gov

Virginia

8069 Substance Abuse Services Office of Virginia
Department of Mental Health & Mental Retardation
1220 Bank Street
Richmond, VA 23218-1797

804-786-3921
800-451-5544
Fax: 804-371-6638
TTY: 804-371-8977
e-mail: wglover@co.dmhmrsas.virginia.gov
www.dmhmrsas.virginia.gov

Available to citizens statewide, Virginia's public mental health, intellectual disability and substance abuse services system is comprised of 16 state-operated facilities and 40 locally-run community services boards (CSBs) The CSBs and facilities serve children and adults who have-or who are at risk of-mental illness, serious emotional disturbance, intellectual disabilities, or substance abuse disorders.
Jim Stewart, Commissioner
Olivia Garland, Deputy Commissioner

Washington

8070 Washington Department of Social and Health Services, Alcohol and Drug Prog.
Department Of Social And Health Services

Olympia, WA 98504-5330

877-301-4557
800-737-0617
Fax: 360-438-8078
TTY: 877-301-4557
e-mail: starkkd@dshs.wa.gov
www1.dshs.wa.gov

West Virginia

8071 West Virginia Division of Alcohol & Drug Abuse
Department Of Health And Human Resources
350 Capitol Street   304-356-4811
Charleston, WV 25304-3702   Fax: 304-558-1008
e-mail: obhs@wvdhhr.org
www.dhhr.wv.gov

The Division on Alcoholism and Drug Abuse, an operating division of the Bureau for Behavioral Health and Health Facilities (BBHHF) within the West Virginia Division of Health and Human Services is charged in code with being the Single State Authority (SSA) primarily responsible for prevention, control, treatment, rehabilitation, educational research and planning for substance abuse related services
Craig A. Richards, Deputy Commissioner

Wisconsin

8072 Office of Alcohol and Other Drug Abuse
1 W Wilson Street   608-266-1865
Madison, WI 53703-7851   Fax: 608-266-1533
TTY: 608-267-7371
e-mail: dhswebmaster@wisconsin.gov
www.dhfs.state.wi.us

John Easterday, Administrator
Susan Gadacz, Contact

Wyoming

8073 Alcohol & Drug Abuse Programs of Wyoming Department Of Health
Department Of Health
401 Hathaway Building   307-777-7656
Cheyenne, WY 82002-0480   866-571-0944
Fax: 307-777-7439
e-mail: aburde@state.wy.us
health.wyo.gov/default.aspx

Thomas O. Forslund, Director
Lee Clabots, Deputy Director

Libraries & Resource Centers

8074 National Clearinghouse for Alcohol and Drug Information
Rockville, MD 20847-2345   240-221-4019
800-729-6686
Fax: 240-221-4292
TDD: 800-487-4889
e-mail: info@health.org
www.ncadi.samhsa.gov

A resource for alcohol and other drug information. It carries a wide variety of publications dealing with alcohol and other drug abuse.
John Noble, Director

8075 Parents Resource Institute for Drug Education
160 Vanderbilt Court
Bowling Green, KY 42103   800-279-6361
Fax: 270-746-9598
e-mail: info@pridesurveys.com
www.pridesurveys.com

Offers national information and educational materials pertaining to alcohol and drug dependency.
Thomas J Gleaton, EdD, President
Janie Pitcock, President

Research Centers

8076 Alcohol Disease Foundation
33 Eglantine Avenue   609-737-0088
Pennington, NJ 08534-2308

Founded in 1988 to promote research on testing systems that could diagnose the metabolic aspects of alcoholism. Seeks to educate the public on the validity of the disease concept of alcoholism.

8077 Alcohol Research Group Public Health Institute
Public Health Institute
6475 Christie Avenue   510-597-3440
Emeryville, CA 94608-1324   Fax: 510-985-6459
e-mail: info@arg.org
www.arg.org

The Alcohol Research Group (ARG) of the Public Health Institute was established in 1959 to conduct and disseminate high-quality research in epidemiology of alcohol consumption and problems including alcohol use disorders, alcohol-related health services research, and analyses of alcohol policy and its impacts.
Dominique La MPH, Executive Director
Thomas K. Greenfield, Scientific Director

8078 Boston University Laboratory of Neuropsychology
Dept of Behavioral Neuroscience
80 E Concord Street M9   617-638-4803
Boston, MA 02118   Fax: 617-638-4806
www.bu.edu

Offers research and studies into the effects of Alcoholism pertaining to aphasia apraxia dementia memory disorders and various other neurological malfunctions.
Marlene Osca Berman PhD, Director

8079 Center for Alcohol & Addiction Studies Brown University
Brown University
121 South Main Street   401-863-6600
Providence, RI 02903-0001   Fax: 401-863-6697
e-mail: caas@brown.edu
www.caas.brown.edu

The Center for Alcohol and Addiction Studies through its affiliation with the Brown Medical School occupies a unique position within the University. The Center brings together more that 90 faculty and professional staff members from 11 University departments and eight affiliated hospitals to promote the identification prevention and effective treatment of alcohol and other substance abuse.
Peter M Monti PhD, Center Director
Suzanne Colby Ph. D, Associate Director

8080 Cornerstone Medical Arts Center Hospital
Medical Arts Center Hospital
159-05 Union Turnpike   718-906-6700
Fresh Meadows, NY 11366-2802   800-233-9999
Fax: 718-906-6840
e-mail: admin@cornerstoneny.com
www.cornerstoneny.com

Offers a complete integrated program for alcohol assessment alcohol and drug rehabilitation continuing care community education and comprehensive family recovery.
Norine Hurtado, Senior Vice President of Human Resources

8081 Do it Now Foundation
PO Box 27658   480-736-0599
Tempe, AZ 85285-7658   Fax: 480-736-0599
e-mail: info@dci-dcitnaw.com
www.doitnow.org

An information clearinghouse for service providers that publishes well-written pamphlets booklets and materials on chemical dependency and recovery.

8082 Dorothea Dix Hospital Clinical Research Unit
809 Ruggles Drive   919-733-5227
Raleigh, NC 27603   866-349-5627
Fax: 919-733-5351
www.med.unc.edu

Researches the biological risk factors of alcoholism using young adults without the disease but with history of familial alcoholism.
Terry Spell, Director
William L Roper, CEO

8083 Ernest Gallo Clinic and Research Center
5858 Horton Street   510-985-3100
Emeryville, CA 94608   Fax: 510-985-3101
e-mail: ngreen@gallo.ucsf.edu
www.galloresearch.org

Alcoholism studies with a special emphasis on genetics.
John A. De Luca PHD, Chairman of the Board/President
Joseph E Gallo, President/Chief Executive Officer

8084   Families in Action National Drug Abuse Center
National Drug Abuse Center
PO Box 3553   252-237-1242
Wilson, NC 27895   Fax: 252-237-6544
e-mail: phil@familiesinaction.org
www.familiesinaction.org
Publish prevention materials and serves as an information clear-
inghouse for families with a member suffering from a drug or alco-
hol addiction.
Phillip A Mooring, Executive Director
Anna Godwin, Coordinator

8085   Friends Medical Science Research Center
1229 West Mount Royal Avenue   410-752-4218
Baltimore, MD 21217   Fax: 310-477-9601
www.wellness.com
Studies narcotic addictions.
John Valenty, President
Rob Greenstein, President

8086   Hahnemann University Laboratory of Human Pharmacology
Department of Pharmacology
Broad and Vine   215-762-7000
Philadelphia, PA 19102   Fax: 215-762-8109
www.hahnemannhospital.com
Hahnemann University hospital is committed to providing quality
patient care in an academic setting.
Benjamin Cal MD, Director

8087   Harvard Cocaine Recovery Project
1493 Cambridge Street   617-498-1000
Cambridge, MA 02139-1099   Fax: 617-642-58
Six-year study of relapse and recovery in cocaine addicts.
William McAu MD, Principal Investigator

8088   Interdisciplinary Program in Cell and Molecular Pharmacology
Medical University of South Carolina
173 Ashley Avenue BSB 358   843-792-8975
Charleston, SC 29425   Fax: 843-792-0481
www.musc.edu/pharm
Research into pharmacology and toxicology.
Kenneth D Tew, Ph.D., D.Sc., Professor and Chairman
Michelle Shorter, Administrative Coordinator

8089   Johns Hopkins University: Behavioral Pharmacology Research Unit
John Hopkins Bay View Campus
5510 Nathan Shock Drive   410-955-5000
Baltimore, MD 21224-2735   Fax: 410-550-0030
e-mail: bigelow@jhmi.edu
www.hopkinsmedicine.org
An internationally recognized center of excellence in research on
psychoactive drugs. As the name implies BPRU's orientation is behavioral and pharmacological emphasizing a behavioral analysis
of drug action.
George E Bigelow PhD, Scientific Director
Eric C Strain MD, Medical Director

8090   Kettering-Scott Magnetic Resonance Laboratory
Wright State University, School of Medicine
PO Box 927
Dayton, OH 45435-0927   937-775-2934
www.med.wright.edu
No information found on the website.
Marjorie Bowman, MD and Dean
Betty Kangas, Assistant to the dean

8091   Marin Institute
24 Belvedere Street   415-456-5692
San Rafael, CA 94901-4817   Fax: 415-456-0491
www.marinInstitute.org
The mission of this Institute is to reduce the toll of alcohol and
other drug problems on Marin County and society in general. The
Institute fulfills this mission by developing implementing evaluat-

ing and disseminating innovative approaches to prevention locally
nationally and internationally.
Bruce Lee Livingston MPP, Executive Director
Michele Simo JD MPH, Research & Policy Director

8092   Narcotic and Drug Research
11 Beach Street   212-966-8700
New York, NY 10013-2429   Fax: 212-334-8058
Nonprofit organization that is devoted to drug abuse education
treatment and prevention.
Douglas S Lipton PhD, Director

8093   National Center on Addiction and Substance Abuse
Columbia University
633 3rd Avenue   212-841-5200
New York, NY 10017-6706   800-622-4357
Fax: 212-956-8020
www.casacolumbia.org
The only nation-wide organization that brings together under one
roof all the professional disciplines needed to study and combat
abuse of all substances - alcohol nicotine as well as illegal prescription and performance enhancing drugs - in all sectors of
society.
Lee C. Bollinger, President
Ursula M. Burns, Chairman and CEO

8094   National Prevention Resource Center CSAP Division of Communications Programs
CSAP Division of Communications Programs
5600 Fishers Lane   301-443-9936
Rockville, MD 20857-0001
Supports an array of prevention program evaluation approaches
including individual grantee evaluations program evaluations and
a National Evaluation Project. Also offers a National Data Base to
provide information on programs for prevention of substance
abuse.

8095   National Treatment Consortium for Alcohol and Other Drugs
PO Box 1294
Washington, DC 20013   202-434-4780
www.ntc-usa.org

8096   National Volunteer Training Center for Substance Abuse Prevention
CSAP Division of Communications Programs
5600 Fishers Lane   301-443-9936
Rockville, MD 20857
Volunteers are always on hand to provide answers, information, referrals and resources pertaining to alcohol, drugs and substance
abuse.

8097   National Volunteer Training Center for Sub CSAP Division of Communications Programs
5600 Fishers Lane   301-443-9936
Rockville, MD 20857
Volunteers are always on hand to provide answers information referrals and resources pertaining to alcohol drugs and substance
abuse.

8098   Ohio State University Clinical Pharmacology Division
College of Medicine
370 Western 9th Avenue   614-292-2220
Columbus, OH 43210-1239   800-252-3636
Fax: 614-292-4293
e-mail: medicine@osu.ede
www.medicine.osu.edu
Substance abuse and alcohol related research.
Robert Bornstein PHD, Vice dean for academic affairs
Glen Apsloss, Director

8099   RADAR Network National Clearinghouse for Alcohol & Dru
National Clearinghouse for Alcohol & Drug Info
PO Box 2345   301-468-2600
Rockville, MD 20847-2345   800-729-6686
Fax: 240-221-4292
TTY: 800-487-4889
TDD: 800-487-4889
ncadi.samhsa.gov
Consists of state clearinghouses specialized information centers
of national organizations and the Department of Education Re-

gional Training Centers. Each RADAR member can offer the public a variety of information services.
John Noble, Director

8100 **Research Institute on Alcoholism State University of New York at Buffalo**
State University of New York at Buffalo
1021 Main Street 716-887-2566
Buffalo, NY 14203 Fax: 716-872-52
e-mail: connors@ria.buffalo.edu
www.ria.buffalo.edu
Integral part of the New York State Division of Alcoholism and Alcohol Abuse.
Kenneth E Leonard, PhD, Director
Kimberly S Walitzer, PhD, Deputy Director

8101 **Rockefeller University Laboratory of Biology**
1230 York Avenue 212-327-8000
New York, NY 10065 Fax: 212-327-7974
www.rockefeller.edu

Marc Tessier Lavigne, President

8102 **Rutgers University Center of Alcohol Studies**
Busch Campus
607 Allison Road 732-445-2190
Piscataway, NJ 08854 Fax: 732-445-3500
e-mail: alclib@rci.rutgers.edu
alcoholstudies.rutgers.edu
Causes and treatment of alcoholism.
Robert Pandi PhD, Director

8103 **Rutgers University: Controlled Drug- Delivery Research Center**
College of Pharmacy
PO Box 789 732-932-3834
Piscataway, NJ 08855-0789 Fax: 732-932-5767
Yie W Chien, Director

8104 **Ruth E Golding Clinical Pharmacokinetics Laboratory**
College of Pharmacy
1703 E Mabel 520-626-1938
Tucson, AZ 85721-1427 e-mail: webmaster@pharmacy.arizona.edu
www.pharmacy.arizona.edu
Conducts studies of drugs in humans and animals.
Michael Maye MD, Head

8105 **Southern California Research Institute**
7065 Hayvenhurst Avenue 310-390-8481
Van Nuys, CA 90066 Fax: 310-390-8482
www.scri.org

Effects of alcohol and drugs on behavior studies.
Dary Fiorent PhD, Executive Director
Bergetta Die BA, Research Associate

8106 **Stanford Center for Research in Disease Prevention**
Stanford University School of Medicine
1070 Arastradero Road 650-723-6254
Palo Alto, CA 94304 Fax: 650-723-6254
prevention.stanford.edu
Prevention and control of alcohol and drug abuse related disorders.
John P.A Loannidis, MD, DSc, Director

8107 **State University of New York at Buffalo Toxicology Research Center**
3435 Main Street 716-831-2125
Buffalo, NY 14214 Fax: 716-829-2806
www.smbs.buffalo.edu
Toxicology-related research and services including the development of tests to evaluate toxins chemicals and drugs.
Michale E. Cain, Director
Dr James R Olson, Assistant Director

8108 **University of California: Los Angeles Alcohol Research Center**
405 Hilgard Ave 310-825-4321
Los Angeles, CA 90095-8353 Fax: 310-206-7309
www.ucla.edu

Causes of alcoholism including genetics.
Dr Ernest Noble, Director

8109 **University of Michigan: Alcohol Research Center**
400 E Eisenhower Parkway 734-764-1817
Ann Arbor, MI 48108-3318 Fax: 734-998-7994
www.umich.edu
Alcohol abuse studies among the elderly including the relationship between alcohol and aged disorders.
Robert A Zucker PhD, Contact

8110 **University of Michigan: Psychiatric Center**
4250 Plymouth road 734-936-5900
Ann Arbor, MI 48109-0001 Fax: 734-936-9761
www.umich.edu
Psychiatric disease research pertaining to the effects of alcoholism and drug abuse.
Gregory W Dalack, MD

8111 **University of Minnesota: Program on Alcohol/Drug Control**
Stadium Gate 27 612-624-6861
Minneapolis, MN 55455
Alcohol tobacco and drug research.
Dr James Schaefer, Director

8112 **University of Missouri: Kansas City Drug Information Service**
2464 Charlotte 816-235-5490
Kansas City, MO 64108-2640 Fax: 816-235-5491
e-mail: umkcdruginformation@umkc.edu
dic.umkc.edu
Literature research and evaluation of clinical drug problems and questions.
Pat Bryant PhD, Director
Heather A Pace PhD, Assistant Director

8113 **University of Tennessee Drug Information Center**
875 Monroe Avenue 901-528-5555
Memphis, TN 38163-1 Fax: 901-448-5419
e-mail: utdic@utmem.edu
dop.utmem.edu/dic

Katie Suda, Director
Camille Thornton, Assistant Professor

8114 **University of Texas Health Science Center Neurophysiology Research Center**
Speech & Hearing Institute
7000 Fannin 713-500-4472
Houston, TX 77030-3405 Fax: 713-792-4513
Conducts clinical and animal studies aimed at combating alcohol drug and tobacco dependence.
Giuseppe N Colasurdo, Director

8115 **University of Texas at Austin: Drug Synamics Institute**
1 University Station 512-475-9746
Austin, TX 78712 Fax: 512-471-2746
www.utexas.edu

Pharmaceutical and drug research.
Janet C Walkow PhD, Director
Carla Van Den Berg PhD, Associate Professor

8116 **University of Utah: Center for Human Toxicology**
30 South 2000 East 801-581-6731
Salt Lake City, UT 84112-1210 Fax: 801-581-3716
e-mail: dwilkins@alanine.pharm.utah.edu
www.pharmacy.utah.edu
Clinical forensic and toxicology research.
Chris M . Ireland PHd, Dean
Dennis Crouch, Director

8117 **University of Wisconsin Milwaukee Medicinal Chemistry Group**
University of Wisconsin
PO Box 413
Milwaukee, WI 53201-413 414-229-1122
www4.uwm.edu
Research on drugs including studies of valium receptors.
Michael R. Lovell, Chancellor

Support Groups & Hotlines

8118 Al-Anon Alateen Family Group Hotline
1600 Corporate Landing Parkway   757-563-1600
Virginia Beach, VA 23454-970   888-425-2666
Fax: 757-563-1655
e-mail: wso@alanon.org
www.al-anon.alateen.org
A mutual peer-to-peer support program with groups meeting worldwide to provide hope and help to the families of alcoholics. Although a seperate entity from Alcoholics Anonymous, our program is based upon the Twelve Steps.
Ric Buchanan, Executive Director

8119 Alcohol Drug Treatment Referral
1316 South Coast Highway
Laguna Beach, CA 92651-3118   800-454-8966
Fax: 949-281-1933
National Help and Referral Network, a nonprofit organization available 24 hours a day to assist people troubled by drug or alcohol abuse. Here to provide information on addiction treatment and support services and to help save lives and mend broken dreams.
Mike Cohan, Director

8120 Alcoholics Anonymous World Services
PO Box 459   212-870-3400
New York, NY 10163-4059   Fax: 212-870-3003
www.aa.org
Alcoholics Anonymous is a fellowship of men and women who share their experience, strength and hope with each other that they may solve their common problem and help others to recover from alcoholism. The only requirement for membership is a desire to stop drinking. There are no dues or fees for AA membership; they are self-supporting through their own contributions.
Greg M, General Manager

8121 Drug Free Workplace Hotline
Division of Workplace Programs
Samhsa Diagonal CSAP 1 Choke Cherry   240-276-2612
Rockville, MD 20857   877-726-4727
Fax: 240-276-1210
TDD: 800-457-4889
e-mail: webmaster@samhsa.hhs.gov
www.drugfreeworkplace.gov
A hotline for businesses to obtain information on a wide range of drug abuse related problems, issues and services.
Robert Stephenson II, Director

8122 Friday Night Live
California Dept of Drug & Alcohol Programs
1700 K Street   916-445-7456
Sacramento, CA 95814   Fax: 916-230-59
e-mail: laura@tcoe.org
www.communitycounseling.org/fnl
These groups, located in California, are all run by students with a faculty adviser. They arrange local alcohol and drug free events, from dances and movies to visiting hospitalized children. Students not only have fun but they learn to have fun sober.
Jim Kooler, Administrator
Laura Purcellabuzo, Project Coordinator

8123 Images Within: A Child's View of Parental Alcoholism
Children of Alcoholics Foundation
PO Box 4185   212-595-5810
New York, NY 10163-4185   800-359-2623
e-mail: coaf@phoenixhouse.org
www.coaf.org
An innovative program designed to teach all children about family alcoholism. Middle-school-aged children learn how to get help for themselves or give help to their friends.

8124 International Lawyers in Alcoholics Anonymous
39 Smith Neck Road   860-529-7474
Old Lyme, CT 6371   e-mail: bert@bertwitehead.com
www.ilaa.org

Provides 40 independent local groups.
Scoot Huyghebaert, Chairman

8125 National Health Information Center
PO Box 1133   310-565-4167
Washington, DC 20013   800-336-4797
Fax: 301-984-4256
e-mail: info@nhic.org
www.health.gov/nhic
Offers a nationwide information referral service, produces directories and resource guides.

8126 ToughLove International
PO Box 1069   215-348-7090
Doylestown, PA 18901-0019   800-333-1069
www.toughlove.org
This national self-help group for parents, children and communities emphasizes cooperation, personal initiative and action. Publishes books, brochures and promotional information and holds workshops and seminars across the country.

8127 WFS' New Life Program
Women for Sobriety
PO Box 618   215-536-8026
Quakertown, PA 18951-0618   Fax: 215-538-9026
e-mail: newlife@nni.com
www.womenforsobriety.org
A self-help program for women that can be used independent from AA or with AA. Groups are in many states in the United States. Donations suggested.
Rebecca M Fenner, Director

Books

8128 AA Comes of Age
Alcoholics Anonymous
PO Box 459   212-870-3400
New York, NY 10163-0459   Fax: 212-870-3137
Tells how AA was started, how the Steps and Traditions evolved and how the AA Fellowship grew and spread overseas.

8129 AA in Prison: Inmate to Inmate
Alcoholics Anonymous
PO Box 459   212-870-3400
New York, NY 10163-0459   Fax: 212-870-3137
Thirty-two stories that share the experience of men and women who found AA while in prison.
128 pages

8130 Accepting Ourselves & Others
Hazelden
15251 Pleasant Valley Road   651-257-4010
Center City, MN 55012-9640   800-328-9000
Fax: 651-213-4426
www.hazelden.org
Fully revised and expanded second edition. Examines recovery as it affects the gay, lesbian, and bisexual community, as well as their friends, family, and therapists. Addresses the relationship between substance abuse and being a sexual minority, and discusses the impact of other issues such as anxiety, depression, sexual abuse, and learning disabilities.
379 pages Paperback
ISBN: 1-568381-20-4

8131 Addiction and Responsibility
The Crossroad Publishing Company
370 Lexington Avenue   212-532-3650
New York, NY 10017-6503   800-395-0690
Fax: 212-532-4922
Anyone who has wrestled with such basic questions about addiction such as: Is drug addiction a behavior disorder or a character flaw? Is it genetic or learned? What is it like to be addicted? will find welcome answers in this groundbreaking philosophical inquiry into the addictive mind. The author helps readers understand addiction.
192 pages
ISBN: 0-824513-65-7

8132 Addictions Counseling
The Crossroad Publishing Company

370 Lexington Avenue   212-532-3650
New York, NY 10017-6503   800-395-0690
    Fax: 212-532-4922
A practical guide to counseling people with chemical and other addictions.
144 pages Paperback
ISBN: 0-824513-86-0

8133 Addictive Personality
Hazelden
15251 Pleasant Valley Road   651-257-4010
Center City, MN 55012-9640   800-328-9000
    Fax: 651-213-4426
    www.hazelden.org
Understanding how an individual becomes an addict through examination of addiction's causes, stages of development, and consequences. Second edition further refines these ideas and includes the most recent information on the addictive process, cultural influences on addictive behaviors, recovery, genetic factors in addiction, mental health issues, and new research findings.
130 pages Paperback
ISBN: 1-568381-29-8

8134 Addictive Thinking Understanding Self-Deception
Hazelden
15251 Pleasant Valley Road   651-257-4010
Center City, MN 55012-9640   800-328-9000
    Fax: 651-213-4426
    www.hazelden.org
Illustrates the irrational perspective and complicated, contradictory thinking patterns of addictive thinking, and demonstrates how they lead to low self-esteen, addiction, and relapse. Revised edition includes expanded information on depression and affective disorders, the relationship between addictive thinking and relapse, and the new research related to the origins of addictive thinking.
140 pages Paperback
ISBN: 1-568381-38-7

8135 Adult Children of Alcoholics
Hazelden
15251 Pleasant Valley Road   651-257-4010
Center City, MN 55012-9640   800-328-9000
    Fax: 651-213-4426
    www.hazelden.org
Written to and for adult children of dysfunctional families.
138 pages Paperback

8136 Al-Anon Family Groups
Al-Anon Family Group Headquarters
1600 Corporate Landing Parkway   757-563-1600
Virginia Beach, VA 23454-5617   800-425-2666
    Fax: 757-563-1655
    e-mail: wso@al-anon.org
    www.al-anon.alateen.org
Basic book that explains the purpose of fellowship, how it works and how it is held in unity. Includes real life stories by husbands, wives, parents and children of those who suffer from alcoholism.
177 pages
ISBN: 0-910034-54-0
Caryn Johnson, Director Communications

8137 Al-Anon's Twelve Steps and Twelve Traditions
Al-Anon Family Group Headquarters
1600 Corporate Landing Parkway   757-563-1600
Virginia Beach, VA 23454-5617   800-425-2666
    Fax: 757-563-1655
    e-mail: wso@al-anon.org
    www.al-anon.alateen.org
Written for people whose lives have been affected by alcoholism.
142 pages Hardcover
ISBN: 0-910034-24-9
Caryn Johnson, Director Communications

8138 Alateen: A Day at a Time
Al-Anon Family Group Headquarters
1600 Corporate Landing Parkway   757-563-1600
Virginia Beach, VA 23454-5617   800-425-2666
    Fax: 757-563-1655
    e-mail: wso@al-anon.org
    www.al-anon.alateen.org

A collection of positive, daily sharings written by teenagers around the world.
384 pages
ISBN: 0-910034-53-2
Caryn Johnson, Director Communications

8139 Alateen: Hope for Children of Alcoholics
Al-Anon Family Group Headquarters
1600 Corporate Landing Parkway   757-563-1600
Virginia Beach, VA 23454-5617   800-425-2666
    Fax: 757-563-1655
    e-mail: wso@al-anon.org
    www.al-anon.alateen.org
A gold mine of information written by Alateens themselves. It covers the history of Alateen, understanding alcoholism and personal stories.
115 pages
ISBN: 0-910034-20-6
Caryn Johnson, Director Communications

8140 Alcohol and Other Drug Services: Dir. of California's Community Services
Department of Alcohol and Drug Programs
1700 K Street   916-445-0834
Sacramento, CA 95814-4022
A directory listing agencies, alcohol and drug providers, county 504 coordinators and county program administrators for the state of California.
136 pages

8141 Alcohol, Drug and Other Addictions: A Directory of Treatment Centers
Oryx Press
4041 N Central Avenue   602-265-2651
Phoenix, AZ 85012-3397   800-279-4663
Lists 18,000 federal, state and local addiction treatment regimens that include public and private centers.

8142 Alcohol, Tobacco and Other Drugs May Harm the Unborn
National Clearinghouse for Alcohol and Drug Info.
PO Box 2345
Rockville, MD 20847-2345   800-729-6686
Presents the most recent findings of basic research and clinical studies conducted on the effects of alcohol, drugs and tobacco on the unborn.

8143 Alcoholics Anonymous
Alcoholics Anonymous
PO Box 459   212-870-3400
New York, NY 10163-0459   Fax: 212-870-3137
Third edition of the Big Book, basic text of AA. Chapters describe the AA recovery program and personal histories have been added.

8144 Alcoholics Anonymous: The Big Book
Hazelden
15251 Pleasant Valley Road   651-257-4010
Center City, MN 55012-9640   800-328-9000
    Fax: 651-213-4426
    www.hazelden.org
Classic text that guides Alcoholics Anonymous programs and describes how millions of men and women have recovered from alcoholism.
575 pages Paperback

8145 American Academy of Psychiatrists in Alcoholism and Addiction Directory
Box 376   301-220-0951
Greenbelt, MD 20768   Fax: 301-220-0941
Lists 900 member professionals who are concerned with drug and alcohol abuse.

8146 An Annotated Bibliography of Recent Empirical Research In Methadone
National Clearinghouse for Alcohol and Drug Info.
PO Box 2345
Rockville, MD 20847-2345   800-729-6686
Provides guidelines and suggestions to investigators engaged in the demanding and essential task of followup research on intravenous drug users who have contracted AIDS.
97 pages

8147   As Bill Sees It
Alcoholics Anonymous
PO Box 459   212-870-3400
New York, NY 10163-0459   Fax: 212-870-3137
This collection of Bill W's writings offers a daily source of comfort and inspiration.

8148   As We Understood...
Al-Anon Family Group Headquarters
1600 Corporate Landing Parkway   757-563-1600
Virginia Beach, VA 23454-5617   800-425-2666
                                                     Fax: 757-563-1655
                                              e-mail: wso@al-anon.org
                                              www.al-anon.alateen.org
Al-Anon members share their understanding of a higher power, fellowship, spiritual awakening, prayer, meditation and letting go.
269 pages
ISBN: 0-910034-56-7
Caryn Johnson, Director Communications

8149   Black, Beautiful and Recovering
African American Family Services
2616 Nicollet Avenue S   612-871-7878
Minneapolis, MN 55408
A helpful guide for Black people who are in the process of recovering from alcohol or other substance abuse problems.
10 pages

8150   Body, Mind, and Spirit
Hazelden
15251 Pleasant Valley Road   651-257-4010
Center City, MN 55012-9640   800-328-9000
                                                     Fax: 651-213-4426
                                                     www.hazelden.org
Addressing such issues as self-esteem, fear, anger, and spirituality, these 366 daily meditations and affirmations integrate the physical, mental, and spiritual aspects of healing from addiction.
410 pages Paperback
ISBN: 1-568380-77-1

8151   Came to Believe
Alcoholics Anonymous
PO Box 459   212-870-3400
New York, NY 10163-0459   Fax: 212-870-3137
A collection of stories by AA members who write about what the phrase spiritual awakening means to them.
120 pages

8152   Chemically Dependent Older Adults
Hazelden
15251 Pleasant Valley Road   651-257-4010
Center City, MN 55012-9640   800-328-9000
                                                     Fax: 651-213-4426
                                                     www.hazelden.org
Reviews the importance of considering the older adult's health, living conditions and social and economic resources when developing treatment and aftercare plans.
136 pages Paperback

8153   Childhood and Adolescent Drug Abuse: A Physician's Guide
American Council on Drug Education
204 Monroe Street
Rockville, MD 20850-4425   800-488-3784
A scientific monograph which educates and sensitizes doctors to the dimensions of drug problems.
68 pages

8154   Circle of Hope
Hazelden
15251 Pleasant Valley Road   651-257-4010
Center City, MN 55012-9640   800-328-9000
                                                     Fax: 651-213-4426
                                                     www.hazelden.org
Spirituality, acceptance, and living one day at a time are show through personal stories of individuals living with HIV and AIDS and dealing with adiction and recovery.
364 pages Paperback
ISBN: 0-894866-10-9

8155   Citizen's Alcohol and Other Drug Prevention Directory
National Clearinghouse for Alcohol and Drug Info.
PO Box 2345
Rockville, MD 20847-2345   800-729-6686
National directory of over 3,000 state, local and government agencies dealing with alcohol and other drug-related topics.
276 pages

8156   Cocaine Today
American Council on Drug Education
204 Monroe Street
Rockville, MD 20850-4425   800-488-3784
A recent revision of this popular book. Cocaine Today takes a new look at cocaine and its derivative, crack.

8157   Codependent No More
Hazelden
15251 Pleasant Valley Road   651-257-4010
Center City, MN 55012-9640   800-328-9000
                                                                 Fax: 651-213-4426
                                                                 www.hazelden.org
Explains codependent behaviors in clear, simple terms.
208 pages Paperback

8158   Color of Light
Hazelden
15251 Pleasant Valley Road   651-257-4010
Center City, MN 55012-9640   800-328-9000
                                                                 Fax: 651-213-4426
                                                                 www.hazelden.org
These 366 meditations speak to both the practical and spiritual journey of living with HIV/AIDS, and demonstrate how to integrate personal values with those offered in chemical dependency recovery and the Twelve Steps.
400 pages Paperback
ISBN: 0-894865-11-0

8159   Confusion is a State of Grace
Hazelden
15251 Pleasant Valley Road   651-257-4010
Center City, MN 55012   800-328-9000
                                                                 Fax: 651-213-4426
                                                                 www.hazelden.org
Compilation of quotes that captures the wisdom, humor, and healing found in Al-Anon and other Twelve Step groups.
153 pages Paperback
ISBN: 1-568380-89-5

8160   Courage to Be Me: Living with Alcoholism
Al-Anon Family Group Headquarters
1600 Corporate Landing Parkway   757-563-1600
Virginia Beach, VA 23454-5617   800-425-2666
                                                                 Fax: 757-563-1655
                                                          e-mail: wso@al-anon.org
                                                          www.al-anon.alateen.org
Written for and by Alateens of all ages who will treasure the honesty and strength of recovery shown.
326 pages
ISBN: 0-910034-30-3
Caryn Johnson, Director Communications

8161   Daily Reflections: A Book of Reflections by AA Members for AA Members
Alcoholics Anonymous
PO Box 459   212-870-3400
New York, NY 10163-0459   Fax: 212-870-3137
AAs reflect on favorite quotations from A.A. literature. A reading for each day of the year.

8162   Day at a Time: Daily Reflections for Recovering People
Hazelden
15251 Pleasant Valley Road   651-257-4010
Center City, MN 55012-9640   800-328-9000
                                                                 Fax: 651-213-4426
                                                                 www.hazelden.org
Offers inspiration and hope for people recovering from chemical dependency or other addictions. Each daily passage reinforces the message of Twelve Step recovery.
384 pages Paperback
ISBN: 1-568380-36-4

8163 Day by Day
Hazelden
15251 Pleasant Valley Road   651-257-4010
Center City, MN 55012   800-328-9000
                                              Fax: 651-213-4426
                                                www.hazelden.org
A book of daily meditations for recovering addicts that reinforce
Narcotics Anonymous principles and objectives.
400 pages Paperback

8164 Days of Healing, Days of Joy
Hazelden
15251 Pleasant Valley Road   651-257-4010
Center City, MN 55012-9640   800-328-9000
                                              Fax: 651-213-4426
                                                www.hazelden.org
Three hundred and sixty-six daily quotes, meditations and affirmations to help adult children in their search for serenity.
400 pages Paperback

8165 Developing Chemical Dependency Services for Black People
African American Family Services
2616 Nicollet Avenue S   612-871-7878
Minneapolis, MN 55408
This manual has been developed to address many of the questions
asked by new or expanding programs as they establish new culturally specific initiatives for African-American clients.
78 pages

8166 Dilemma of the Alcoholic Marriage
Al-Anon Family Group Headquarters
1600 Corporate Landing Parkway   757-563-1600
Virginia Beach, VA 23454-5617   800-425-2666
                                              Fax: 757-563-1655
                                           e-mail: wso@al-anon.org
                                             www.al-anon.alateen.org
This book explores the problem of alcoholism in marriage and in-
cludes questions for applying the twelve steps to relationships.
100 pages
ISBN: 0-910034-18-4
Caryn Johnson, Director Communications

8167 Dr. Bob and the Good Oldtimers
Alcoholics Anonymous
PO Box 459   212-870-3400
New York, NY 10163-0459   Fax: 212-870-3137
The life story of the fellowship's co-founder, interwoven wth rec-
ollections of early AA in the Midwest.

8168 Drug Abuse and Addiction Information/Treatment Programs
American Business Directories
5711 S 86th Circle   402-593-4600
Omaha, NE 68127-4146   Fax: 402-331-1505
Number of entries is 9,425.

**8169 Drug Use Among American High School Seniors, College
Students & Youth**
National Clearinghouse for Alcohol and Drug Info.
PO Box 2345
Rockville, MD 20847-2345   800-729-6686
Comprehensive reports presenting the results of the 16th national
survey of the drug use and related attitudes of American high
school seniors.
199 pages Volumes I & II

8170 Drugs and Pregnancy: It's Not Worth the Risk
American Council on Drug Education
204 Monroe Street
Rockville, MD 20850   800-488-3784
A scientific monograph for health care providers which teaches
them to identify alcohol and drug problems in their patients.
48 pages

8171 Dual Diagnosis
Hazelden
15251 Pleasant Valley Road   651-257-4010
Center City, MN 55012-9640   800-328-9000
                                              Fax: 651-213-4426
                                                www.hazelden.org

Focuses on the issues surrounding the treatment of clients with coexisting chemical dependency and psychiatric conditions.
191 pages Paperback

8172 Dual Disorders
Hazelden
15251 Pleasant Valley Road   651-257-4010
Center City, MN 55012-9640   800-328-9000
                                              Fax: 651-213-4426
                                                www.hazelden.org
Presents case histories and analyses of psychiatric disorders.
140 pages Paperback

8173 Dual Disorders Recovery Book
Hazelden
15251 Pleasant Valley Road   651-257-4010
Center City, MN 55012-9640   800-328-9000
                                              Fax: 651-213-4426
                                                www.hazelden.org
Helps individuals with dual disorders develop a plan for daily liv-
ing through a specially-designed Twelve-Step program.
242 pages Paperback
ISBN: 1-568380-34-8

8174 Each Day a New Beginning
Hazelden
15251 Pleasant Valley Road   651-257-4010
Center City, MN 55012-9640   800-328-9000
                                              Fax: 651-213-4426
                                                www.hazelden.org
Promotes the development of a significant spiritual core for recovery that can be enhanced throughout the rest of life.
400 pages Paperback

8175 Elephant in the Living Room: A Leader's Guide
Hazelden
15251 Pleasant Valley Road   651-257-4010
Center City, MN 55012-9640   800-328-9000
                                              Fax: 651-213-4426
                                                www.hazelden.org
The adult companion to the classic children's book. Caretakers
learn how to explain addiction and its effect on the family to small
children who's parents or siblings are chemically dependent.
129 pages Paperback
ISBN: 1-568380-34-8

8176 Encyclopedia of Drug Abuse
Facts on File
11 Penn Plaza   212-967-8800
New York, NY 10001   800-322-8755
                                              Fax: 800-678-3633
More that 500 entries explore: specific drugs, countries, organizations, treatment programs, laws, medical terms, and psychosocial
concepts.
496 pages Hardcover

8177 Ethics for Addiction Professionals
Hazelden
15251 Pleasant Valley Road   651-257-4010
Center City, MN 55012-9640   800-328-9000
                                              Fax: 651-213-4426
                                                www.hazelden.org
Probes crucial, complex ethical issues including counselor relapse, paid referrals and discrimination.
60 pages

**8178 Extent and Adequacy of Insurance Coverage for Substance
Abuse I & II**
National Clearinghouse for Alcohol and Drug Info.
PO Box 2345
Rockville, MD 20847-2345   800-729-6686
These volumes examine the extent to which the cost of alcohol and
other drug treatments is covered by private insurance, public fi-
nancing and other sources.

8179 Eye Opener
Hazelden
15251 Pleasant Valley Road   651-257-4010
Center City, MN 55012-9640   800-328-9000
                                              Fax: 651-213-4426
                                                www.hazelden.org

Daily meditations about understanding the Alcoholics Anonymous program, writen by a favorite early AA member and author.
380 pages Cloth
ISBN: 0-894860-23-2

8180   Fact Is...Hispanic Parents Can Help Their Children Avoid Alcohol/Drugs
National Clearinghouse for Alcohol and Drug Info.
PO Box 2345
Rockville, MD 20847-2345   800-729-6686

8181   Feeding the Hungry Heart, the Experience of Compulsive Eating
Gurze Books
PO Box 2238
Carlsbad, CA 92018-2238   800-756-7533
                                             Fax: 760-434-5476
                                             e-mail: gzcatl@aol.com
                                             www.bulimia.com
This is a widely respected, extremely readable book from Ms. Roth and the many participants of early breaking free workshops. It is an intimate, vulnerable sharing of experiences which continues to touch and change lives.
212 pages Paperback

8182   Food for Thought: Daily Meditations for Overeaters
Hazelden
15251 Pleasant Valley Road   651-257-4010
Center City, MN 55012-9640   800-328-9000
                                             Fax: 651-213-4426
                                             www.hazelden.org
Offers guidance in the early days of living a Twelve Step program.
400 pages Paperback
ISBN: 0-894860-90-9

8183   Forum Favorites: Volumes 1, 2, 3 & 4
Al-Anon Family Group Headquarters
1600 Corporate Landing Parkway   757-563-1600
Virginia Beach, VA 23454-5617   800-425-2666
                                             Fax: 757-563-1655
                                             e-mail: wso@al-anon.org
                                             www.al-anon.alateen.org
Personal sharings show how the fundamentals of the Al-Anon programs are applied to everyday situations.
428 pages Set of 4
ISBN: 0-910034-51-6
Caryn Johnson, Director Communications

8184   Freedom from Smoking at Work Program
American Lung Association
1740 Broadway
New York, NY 10017   212-315-8700
                                             www.lungusa.org
ALA program for organizations interested in creating a healthier workplace environment through a comprehensive, multicomponent smoking education, cessation and policy development program designed for the workplace.

8185   Future by Design/A Community Framework
National Clearinghouse for Alcohol and Drug Info.
PO Box 2345
Rockville, MD 20847-2345   800-729-6686
Provides communities with a manageable framework for getting involved in alcohol and other drug prevention.
234 pages

8186   Gentle Path Through the Twelve Steps
Hazelden
15251 Pleasant Valley Road   651-257-4010
Center City, MN 55012-9640   800-328-9000
                                             Fax: 651-213-4426
                                             www.hazelden.org
This workbook provides a unique set of structured forms and exercises to help recoving people integrate the Twelve Steps in all aspects of their lives.
224 pages Paperback
ISBN: 1-568380-58-5

8187   Getting Started in AA
Hazelden

15251 Pleasant Valley Road   651-257-4010
Center City, MN 55012-9640   800-328-9000
                                             Fax: 651-213-4426
                                             www.hazelden.org
Practical suggestions for staying sober, summaries of AA principles, concepts, and slogans, and a historical overview to help the reader understand the spirit of the program.
211 pages Paperback
ISBN: 1-568380-91-7

8188   Getting Tough on Gateway Drugs: A Guide for the Family
American Council On Drug Education
204 Monroe Street
Rockville, MD 20850-4425   800-488-3784
Gateway drugs including marijuana, alcohol and tobacco are those which open doors into all drug abuse. This family survival guide helps parents understand the consequences of drug dependence and suggests actions the family can take to prevent and solve drug problems.
332 pages

8189   Getting it Together: Promoting Drug Free Communities
National Clearinghouse for Alcohol and Drug Info.
PO Box 2345
Rockville, MD 20847   800-729-6686
Provides resources and step-by-step information on how local communities and organizations can work effectively with young people who are committed to preventing alcohol and other drug abuse.
71 pages

8190   God Grant Me the Laughter: A Treasury of Twelve Step Humor
Hazelden
15251 Pleasant Valley Road   651-257-4010
Center City, MN 55012-9640   800-328-9000
                                             Fax: 651-213-4426
                                             www.hazelden.org
Hearty cartoons and humorous anecdotes clearly demonstrate how readers' lives today contrast with their drinking and drug using in the past.
200 pages Paperback
ISBN: 1-568380-38-0

8191   Good First Step
Hazelden
15251 Pleasant Valley Road   651-257-4010
Center City, MN 55012-9640   800-328-9000
                                             Fax: 651-213-4426
                                             www.hazelden.org
Features a structured format and emphasis on the meaning of the First Step to help build a solid foundation for recovery.
60 pages Paperback
ISBN: 1-568381-13-1

8192   Goodbye Hangovers, Hello Life
Women for Sobriety
PO Box 618   215-536-8026
Quakertown, PA 18951-0618   Fax: 215-536-8026
                                             e-mail: NewLife@nni.com
                                             www.womenforsobriety.org
A book about recovery - how it happens, what problems arise and how to overcome these problems.
250 pages Paperback

8193   Grateful to Have Been There
Hazelden
15251 Pleasant Valley Road   651-257-4010
Center City, MN 55012   800-328-9000
                                             Fax: 651-213-4426
                                             www.hazelden.org
Aide and executive secretary to AA's co-founder Bill W. for 20 years, Wing shares her memories and impressions of 42 years of involvement with the Fellowship.
150 pages Paperback
ISBN: 0-942421-44-2

8194   Growing Up Drug Free: A Parent's Guide to Prevention
National Clearinghouse for Alcohol and Drug Info.
PO Box 2345
Rockville, MD 20852   800-729-6686

Offers information on what parents can do to prevent their child from becoming a substance abuser/alcoholic. Focuses on counseling, peer pressure issues, education, school-parent cooperation and offers an introduction to each drug, symptoms and how to spot the warning signs of drug addiction.
47 pages

8195   Handle with Care
Hazelden
15251 Pleasant Valley Road   651-257-4010
Center City, MN 55012-9640   800-328-9000
                                            Fax: 651-213-4426
                                              www.hazelden.org
A comprehensive look at how parents, teachers and other care givers of children ages 10 and younger can identify and meet their special needs.

8196   Help for Helpers: Daily Meditations for Counselors
Hazelden
15251 Pleasant Valley Road   651-257-4010
Center City, MN 55012-9640   800-328-9000
                                            Fax: 651-213-4426
                                              www.hazelden.org
Written by addiction treatment center staff members from across the country, these daily meditations encourage, comfort, and challenge helpers to understand others and themselves.
400 pages Paperback
ISBN: 1-568380-61-5

8197   Helping Homeless People with Alcohol and Other Drug Problems
National Clearinghouse for Alcohol and Drug Info.
PO Box 2345
Rockville, MD 20847   800-729-6686
Developed by professionals who work directly with homeless people, this manual provides basic information about homeless people with AOD problems.
50 pages

8198   Helping Your Students Say No Teacher's Guide
National Clearinghouse for Alcohol and Drug Info.
PO Box 2345
Rockville, MD 20847-2345   800-729-6686
Explains the effects of alcohol on the body, why children start to drink, how teachers can help their students refuse alcohol and deal with the first signs of drinking.
13 pages

8199   How to Manage Your Drug-Free Workplace Programs
American Council on Drug Education
204 Monroe Street
Rockville, MD 20850-4425   800-488-3784
Step-by-step process for introducing and managing a drug awareness program that includes a variety of additional tips to complement messages in the drug awareness pamphlet series.
48 pages

8200   I'm Black and I'm Sober
Hazelden
15251 Pleasant Valley Road   651-257-4010
Center City, MN 55012-9640   800-328-9000
                                            Fax: 651-213-4426
                                              www.hazelden.org
An autobiography written by a recovering African American woman who discusses the impact of discrimination and the obstacles faced through the journey back to sobriety.
279 pages Paperback
ISBN: 1-568380-71-2

8201   If Only I Could Quit
Hazelden
15251 Pleasant Valley Road   651-257-4010
Center City, MN 55012-9640   800-328-9000
                                            Fax: 651-213-4426
                                              www.hazelden.org
Promotes the Twelve Step process for recovery from nicotine addiction.
320 pages Paperback

8202   In God's Care
Hazelden

15251 Pleasant Valley Road   651-257-4010
Center City, MN 55012-9640   800-328-9000
                                            Fax: 651-213-4426
                                              www.hazelden.org
Excellent relaxation and education tool for clients working on their Second and Third Steps.
400 pages Paperback

8203   Keep Quit
Hazelden
15251 Pleasant Valley Road   651-257-4010
Center City, MN 55012-9640   800-328-9000
                                            Fax: 651-213-4426
                                              www.hazelden.org
Daily motivational guide to help the new nonsmoker understand the craving for nicotine and learn how to break the rituals and patterns associated with relapse.
300 pages Paperback
ISBN: 1-568381-04-2

8204   Keep it Simple
Hazelden
15251 Pleasant Valley Road   651-257-4010
Center City, MN 55012-9640   800-328-9000
                                            Fax: 651-213-4426
                                              www.hazelden.org
Daily prayers that help clients learn to ask for help and to turn their self-will over to a Higher Power.
400 pages Paperback

8205   Learning to Live Drug Free: A Curriculum Model for Prevention
National Clearinghouse for Alcohol and Drug Info.
PO Box 2345
Rockville, MD 20847-2345   800-729-6686
Provides a flexible framework for classroom-based prevention efforts for kindergarten through grade 12.
52 pages

8206   Let's Talk About Alcohol Abuse
Rosen Publishing Group's PowerKids Press
29 E 21st Street   212-777-3017
New York, NY 10010   800-237-9932
                                            Fax: 888-436-4643
        e-mail: customerservice@rosenpub.com
                                         www.rosenpublishing.com
In gentle and sensitive terms this book talks about when a parent drinks and what alcohol can do to the body. Kids are told about the illegality of drinking as minors. Recommended for grade K-4.

ISBN: 0-823923-03-7
Marianne Johnston, Author

8207   Life of My Own: Daily Meditations on Hope and Acceptance
Hazelden
15251 Pleasant Valley Road   651-257-4010
Center City, MN 55012-9640   800-328-9000
                                            Fax: 651-213-4426
                                              www.hazelden.org
Offers daily access to strength, serenity, and insight in our relationships with chemically dependent people.
400 pages Paperback
ISBN: 0-894868-63-2

8208   Little Red Book
Hazelden
15251 Pleasant Valley Road   651-257-4010
Center City, MN 55012-9640   800-328-9000
                                            Fax: 651-213-4426
                                              www.hazelden.org
A primer for members of Alcoholics Anonymous. Each page acts as a study guide to the Big Book and its teachings.
164 pages Paperback
ISBN: 0-894869-85-X

8209   Living Sober
Hazelden
15251 Pleasant Valley Road   651-257-4010
Center City, MN 55012-9640   800-328-9000
                                            Fax: 651-213-4426
                                              www.hazelden.org

Offers clients sound advice about how to stay sober.
88 pages Paperback

8210 Lois Remembers
Al-Anon Family Group Headquarters
1600 Corporate Landing Parkway   757-563-1600
Virginia Beach, VA 23454-5617   800-425-2666
                                   Fax: 757-563-1655
                              e-mail: wso@al-anon.org
                              www.al-anon.alateen.org
The memoirs of a co-founder of Al-Anon. Lois tells her personal
story and recalls the eventful years before and after the founding of
AA and Al-Anon.
204 pages
ISBN: 0-910034-23-0
Caryn Johnson, Director Communications

8211 Marijuana
Branden Publishing Company
17 Station Street   617-734-2045
Brookline Village, MA 02147   Fax: 617-734-2046
                                        www.branden.com
Paperback
ISBN: 0-828319-49-9

8212 Marijuana Smoking Prevention Program for Schools
American Lung Association
1740 Broadway   212-315-8700
New York, NY 10017
Cast of the TV show FAME enlivens highly motivational program
to inform parents about the dangers of pot and discourages 9-11
year olds from using it.

8213 Marijuana Today
American Council on Drug Education
204 Monroe Street
Rockville, MD 20850-4425   800-488-3784
A revision of the long time bestseller, this book examines the history of marijuana, its use, the risks associated with use and the
short and long-term effects of use.

8214 Marijuana and Reproduction
American Council on Drug Education
204 Monroe Street
Rockville, MD 20850-4425   800-488-3784
A scientific monograph for physicians which describes marijuana,
profiles the users and discusses the effects on the reproductive
system.
30 pages

8215 Marketing Booze to Blacks
African American Family Services
2616 Nicollet Avenue S   612-871-7878
Minneapolis, MN 55408
This controversial book details how liquor industries target the
black population with its advertising.
55 pages

8216 Mistaken Beliefs About Relapse
Hazelden
15251 Pleasant Valley Road   651-257-4010
Center City, MN 55012-9640   800-328-9000
                                   Fax: 651-213-4426
                                       www.hazelden.org
Examines mistaken beliefs people have about relapse.
30 pages Paperback

8217 My Mind is Out to Get Me: Humor and Wisdom in Recovery
Hazelden
15251 Pleasant Valley Road   651-257-4010
Center City, MN 55012   800-328-9000
                                   Fax: 651-213-4426
                                       www.hazelden.org
Five hundred inspirational sayings and slogans that reflect both
the lighter side of living a sober life and the profound wisdom of-
fered in recovery. Each quote has been drawn from the wisdom of
Alcoholics Anonymous.
180 pages Paperback
ISBN: 1-568380-10-0

8218 Narcotics Anonymous
Hazelden
15251 Pleasant Valley Road   651-257-4010
Center City, MN 55012-9640   800-328-9000
                                   Fax: 651-213-4426
                                       www.hazelden.org
Men and women describe the N.A. program and how it works.
289 pages Paperback

8219 National Conference on Drug Abuse Researcg & Practice
National Clearinghouse for Alcohol and Drug Info.
PO Box 2345
Rockville, MD 20847   800-729-6686
Offers summaries of workshops, forums, dinner speeches and ses-
sions presented at the National Conference on Drug Abuse Re-
search and Practice.
275 pages

8220 National Directory of Drug Abuse and Alcoholism Treatment and Programs
US National Institute On Drug Abuse
5600 Fishers Lane
Rockville, MD 20857   202-625-8400
                                        www.nida.nih.gov
Eleven thousand listings of agencies that administer treatment and
services on the federal, state and local levels.

8221 Night Light: A Book of Nighttime Meditations
Hazelden
15251 Pleasant Valley Road   651-257-4010
Center City, MN 55012-9640   800-328-9000
                                   Fax: 651-213-4426
                                       www.hazelden.org
Three hundred and sixty-six meditations designed to help relax
and encourage prayer. Reminds readers to look to their Higher
Power for strength, reassurance, comfort, and guidance.
400 pages Paperback
ISBN: 0-894863-81-9

8222 Not God: A History of Alcoholics Anonymous
Hazelden
15251 Pleasant Valley Road   651-257-4010
Center City, MN 55012-9640   800-328-9000
                                   Fax: 651-213-4426
                                       www.hazelden.org
Documenting AA's philosophical and social development within
the larger context of American culture, this book follows the remarkable story of the evolution of a small group of Depression-era
alcoholics into a worldwide movement.
436 pages Paperback
ISBN: 0-894860-65-8

8223 Occupational Therapy Practice Guidelines for Adults with Substance Use Disorders
American Occupational Therapy Association
4720 Montgomery Lane   301-652-2682
Bethesda, MD 20824-1220   Fax: 301-652-7711
                                    TDD: 800-377-8555
                                          www.aota.org
22 pages
ISBN: 1-569001-60-X

8224 Of Course You're Angry
Hazelden
15251 Pleasant Valley Road   651-257-4010
Center City, MN 55012-9640   800-328-9000
                                   Fax: 651-213-4426
                                       www.hazelden.org
Revised edition dealing with the nature and resolution of anger.
Demonstrates how to make anger work in a positive and effective
way that can ease, rather than exacerbate, the challenges of early
recovery.
120 pages Paperback
ISBN: 1-568381-41-7

8225 One Day at a Time in Al-Anon
Al-Anon Family Group Headquarters

1600 Corporate Landing Parkway
Virginia Beach, VA 23454-5617
757-563-1600
800-425-2666
Fax: 757-563-1655
e-mail: wso@al-anon.org
www.al-anon.alateen.org
Inspirational daily readings cover various aspects of the Al-Anon philosopha and relate it to everyday situations.
376 pages
ISBN: 0-910034-21-4
Caryn Johnson, Director Communications

8226   Operation PAR
National Clearinghouse for Alcohol and Drug Info.
PO Box 2345
Rockville, MD 20847-2345
800-729-6686
Describes successful community alcohol and other drug abuse prevention and treatment programs.
40 pages

8227   Parent Training is Prevention
National Clearinghouse for Alcohol and Drug Info.
PO Box 2345
Rockville, MD 20847-2345
800-729-6686
Contains information to help communities identify and carry out programs on parenting.
184 pages

8228   Pass it On
Alcoholics Anonymous
World Services
New York, NY 10163
212-870-3400
Fax: 212-870-3137
The story of Bill Wilson, the co-founder of AA and the development of the Fellowship.

8229   Passages Through Recovery
Hazelden
15251 Pleasant Valley Road
Center City, MN 55012-9640
651-257-4010
800-328-9000
Fax: 651-213-4426
www.hazelden.org
Guides clients through the six stages of recovery.
130 pages Paperback

8230   Peer Pressure Reversal
Human Resource Development Press
22 Amherst Road
Amherst, MA 01002-9730
413-253-3488

8231   Pregnancy and Exposure to Alcohol and Other Drug Use
National Clearinghouse for Alcohol and Drug Info.
PO Box 2345
Rockville, MD 20847-2345
800-729-6686
www.health.org
This report is for health care professionals presenting the state-of-the-art information about preventing ATOD use among women of childbearing age.

8232   Preparing for the Drug-Free Years: A Family Activity Book
Developmental Research and Programs
130 Nickerson Street
Seattle, WA 98145-1746
206-286-1805
800-736-2630
Fax: 206-286-1462
www.drp.org

8233   Presence at the Center
Hazelden
15251 Pleasant Valley Road
Center City, MN 55012-9640
651-257-4010
800-328-9000
Fax: 651-213-4426
www.hazelden.org
About a new way of life that addresses transformation, change, the presence of a Higher Power, letting go of reluctance and fear, and the freedom commitment can bring.
76 pages Paperback
ISBN: 1-568380-01-1

8234   Prevention Plus II: Tools for Creating & Sustaining a Drug-Free Community
National Clearinghouse for Alcohol and Drug Info.

PO Box 2345
Rockville, MD 20847-2345
800-729-6686
www.health.org
Provides a framework for organizing or expanding community alcohol and other drug problem prevention activities for youth into a coordinated, complimentary system.
541 pages

8235   Prevention Plus III: Assessing Alcohol & Other Prevention Programs
National Clearinghouse for Alcohol and Drug Info.
PO Box 2345
Rockville, MD 20847-2345
800-729-6686
www.health.org
Provides tools and techniques for alcohol and other drug prevention, planning and implementation.
470 pages

8236   Prevention Resource Guide: Alcohol and Other Drug Related Periodicals
National Clearinghouse for Alcohol and Drug Info.
PO Box 2345
Rockville, MD 20847-2345
800-729-6686
www.health.org
Provides a concise annotated bibliography of journals, newsletters and other publications related to the AOD prevention field.
12 pages

8237   Prevention Resource Guide: American Indian/Native Alaskans
National Clearinghouse for Alcohol and Drug Info.
PO Box 2345
Rockville, MD 20847-2345
800-729-6686
www.health.org
This resource guide is a survey of current data on alcohol abuse among American Indians and Native Alaskans.
24 pages

8238   Prevention Resource Guide: Asian and Pacific Islander Americans
National Clearinghouse for Alcohol and Drug Info.
PO Box 2345
Rockville, MD 20847-2345
800-729-6686
www.health.org
Contains facts and figures about Asian and Pacific Islander Americans and alcohol and other drug prevention.
13 pages

8239   Prevention Resource Guide: Elementary Youth
National Clearinghouse for Alcohol and Drug Info.
PO Box 2345
Rockville, MD 20847-2345
800-729-6686
www.health.org
This resource guide includes materials specifically developed for youth that may be used in an elementary school setting.
23 pages

8240   Prevention Resource Guide: Pregnant Postpartum Women and Their Infants
National Clearinghouse for Alcohol and Drug Info.
PO Box 2345
Rockville, MD 20847-2345
800-729-6686
www.health.org
This resource guide targets health care providers, prevention program planners and counselors of pregnant and postpartum women between the ages of 15 and 44.
30 pages

8241   Prevention Resource Guide: Secondary School Students
National Clearinghouse for Alcohol and Drug Info.
PO Box 2345
Rockville, MD 20847-2345
800-729-6686
www.health.org
This resource guide targets teachers, administrators and program leaders who come in contact with secondary school youth.
27 pages

8242   Prevention Resource Guide: Women
National Clearinghouse for Alcohol and Drug Info.

PO Box 2345
Rockville, MD 20847-2345   800-729-6686
www.health.org
This resource guide provides the latest information about the effects of drugs and alcohol on women.
32 pages

8243 Prevention in Action
National Clearinghouse for Alcohol and Drug Info.
PO Box 2345
Rockville, MD 20847-2345   800-729-6686
Provides descriptions selected by representatives of national organizations and State alcohol and drug agency representatives.
20 pages

8244 Program for You
Hazelden
15251 Pleasant Valley Road   651-257-4010
Center City, MN 55012-9640   800-328-9000
Fax: 651-213-4426
www.hazelden.org
Study guide interpreting the original AA program as described in Alcoholics Anonymous and helps apply the wisdom to everyday life.
183 pages Paperback
ISBN: 0-894867-41-5

8245 Promise of a New Day: A Book of Daily Meditations
Hazelden
15251 Pleasant Valley Road   651-257-4010
Center City, MN 55012-9640   800-328-9000
Fax: 651-213-4426
www.hazelden.org
Simple, inspiring wisdom about creating and maintaining inner peace. Each of the 366 daily meditations expresses the essence of Twelve Step spirituality without the program jargon.
400 pages Paperback
ISBN: 0-894862-03-0

8246 Quit & Stay Quit: A Personal Program to Stop Smoking
Hazelden
15251 Pleasant Valley Road   651-257-4010
Center City, MN 55012-9640   800-328-9000
Fax: 651-213-4426
www.hazelden.org
Guide to nicotine recovery offerring an effective long-term program to quit by showing readers how smoking has subtly shaped their values, attitudes, and lives.
196 pages Paperback
ISBN: 1-568381-09-3

8247 Quit Smoking Manual
American Lung Association
1740 Broadway   212-315-8700
New York, NY 10019-4315
Original self-help smoking cessation manual showing the public how to quit smoking in 20 days.
64 pages

8248 Recovery Journal for Exploring Who I Am
Hazelden
15251 Pleasant Valley Road   651-257-4010
Center City, MN 55012-9640   800-328-9000
Fax: 651-213-4426
www.hazelden.org
Introduces clients to journal writing as an effective therapeutic adjunct for addiction recovery.
48 pages

8249 School Answers Back: Responding to Student Drug Use
American Council on Drug Education
204 Monroe Street
Rockville, MD 20850   800-488-3784
Provides teachers, counselors, administrators and parents with a model for schools to use in confronting drug and alcohol abuse.
145 pages

8250 Search for Serenity
Hazelden

15251 Pleasant Valley Road   651-257-4010
Center City, MN 55012-9640   800-328-9000
Fax: 651-213-4426
www.hazelden.org
Provides clients with practical inspiration to change their feelings toward people and situations.
152 pages Paperback

8251 Shame Faced
Hazelden
15251 Pleasant Valley Road   651-257-4010
Center City, MN 55012-9640   800-328-9000
Fax: 651-213-4426
www.hazelden.org
Discusses the relationship between shame and chemical dependency.
28 pages

8252 Skeptic's Guide to the 12 Steps
Hazelden
15251 Pleasant Valley Road   651-257-4010
Center City, MN 55012-9640   800-328-9000
Fax: 651-213-4426
www.hazelden.org
Investigates each of the 12 steps to gain a deeper understanding of a Higher Power.
241 pages Paperback

8253 Smoking and Pregnancy Kit for Health Care Providers
American Lung Association
1740 Broadway   212-315-8700
New York, NY 10019-4315
A program kit for health care providers designed to educate pregnant women not to smoke and to help them kick the habit.

8254 Smoking, Drinking & Illicit Drug Use
National Clearinghouse for Alcohol and Drug Info.
PO Box 2345
Rockville, MD 20847-2345   800-729-6686
Comprehensive reports representing the results of the 12th national survey on drug use and analyzing data collected from young Americans from 1975-1991.

8255 Sober But Stuck
Hazelden
15251 Pleasant Valley Road   651-257-4010
Center City, MN 55012-9640   800-328-9000
Fax: 651-213-4426
www.hazelden.org
Collection of personal stories by men and women who are long-time members of Alcoholics Anonymous. Each story shares the anecdotes and resources which helped members break through the barriers that limited their enjoyment of a sober life.
215 pages Paperback
ISBN: 1-568380-78-X

8256 Social Policy Prevention Handbook
African American Family Services
2616 Nicollet Avenue S   612-871-7878
Minneapolis, MN 55408
A manual that details IBCA's community based approach to the development of alcohol and drug abuse prevention strategies.
24 pages

8257 Staying Clean
Hazelden
15251 Pleasant Valley Road   651-257-4010
Center City, MN 55012-9640   800-328-9000
Fax: 651-213-4426
www.hazelden.org
Each section focuses on one of 33 proven ideas for staying drug-free, such as professional help, prayer, support groups and meditation.
76 pages Paperback

8258 Staying Sober
Hazelden
15251 Pleasant Valley Road   651-257-4010
Center City, MN 55012-9640   800-328-9000
Fax: 651-213-4426
www.hazelden.org

Discusses addictive diseases and its physical, psychological and social effects.
228 pages Paperback

8259   Step Zero: Getting to Recovery
Hazelden
15251 Pleasant Valley Road
Center City, MN 55012-9640
651-257-4010
800-328-9000
Fax: 651-213-4426
www.hazelden.org
Explains the concepts of Step Zero, when clients drop their defenses, begin to face themselves and start to assess their behavior and the reasons for it.
170 pages Paperback

8260   Stools and Bottles
Hazelden
15251 Pleasant Valley Road
Center City, MN 55012-9640
651-257-4010
800-328-9000
Fax: 651-213-4426
www.hazelden.org
Depicts the first Three steps using a three-legged stool and eight whiskey bottles representing character defects revealed when working Step Four.
160 pages Hardcover

8261   Substance Abuse and Physical Disability
Allen Heinemann, PhD, author
Haworth Press
10 Alice Street
Binghamton, NY 13904-1580
607-722-5857
800-429-6784
Fax: 607-722-0012
www.haworthpress.com
This book offers information on alcohol and drug abuse being a contributing factor in traumatic and disabling injuries.
1993 289 pages Hardcover
ISBN: 1-560242-89-3

8262   Success Stories from Drug-Free Schools
National Clearinghouse for Alcohol and Drug Info.
PO Box 2345
Rockville, MD 20847-2345
800-729-6686
www.health.org
Salutes the 107 schools honored by the US Department of Education's Drug-Free Recognition Program.
59 pages

8263   Tackling Alcohol Problems on Campus: Tools for Media Advocacy
National Clearinghouse for Alcohol and Drug Info.
PO Box 2345
Rockville, MD 20847-2345
800-729-6686
Reviews the role of alcohol on campus and shows how to use the media to get attention and support.
38 pages

8264   Team Up for Drug Prevention with America's Young Athletes
Drug Enforcement Administration, Demand Reduction
1405 I Street NW
Washington, DC 20537-0001
202-307-5550
www.usdoj.gov/dea/programs/demand.htm

8265   Ten Steps to Help Your Child Say No: A Parent's Guide
National Clearinghouse for Alcohol and Drug Info.
PO Box 2345
Rockville, MD 20847-2345
800-729-6686

8266   Things My Sponsors Taught Me
Hazelden
15251 Pleasant Valley Road
Center City, MN 55012-9640
651-257-4010
800-328-9000
Fax: 651-213-4426
www.hazelden.org
Features AA philosophy, quotes, slogans and refreshing reminders.
76 pages Paperback

8267   Today I Will Do One Thing: Daily Readings for Awareness & Hope
Hazelden

15251 Pleasant Valley Road
Center City, MN 55012-9640
651-257-4010
800-328-9000
Fax: 651-213-4426
www.hazelden.org
Specially designed to integrate recovery from addiction with the treatment of emotional or psychiatric illness. Each meditation focuses on a task or goal to be completed each day.
400 pages Paperback
ISBN: 1-568380-83-6

8268   Today's Gift
Hazelden
15251 Pleasant Valley Road
Center City, MN 55012-9640
651-257-4010
800-328-9000
Fax: 651-213-4426
www.hazelden.org
Inspiring meditations bringing families together and strengthening family bonds.
400 pages Paperback

8269   Touchstones
Hazelden
15251 Pleasant Valley Road
Center City, MN 55012-9640
651-257-4010
800-328-9000
Fax: 651-213-4426
www.hazelden.org
A book of daily meditations for men in the Twelve-Step program.
400 pages Paperback

8270   Turnabout
Women for Sobriety
PO Box 618
Quakertown, PA 18951-0618
215-536-8026
Fax: 215-536-8026
e-mail: WFSobriey@aol.com
www.mediapulse.com/wfs/
This is the story of the founder of Women for Sobriety and her struggle to quit drinking.
183 pages

8271   Turning Awareness Into Action: What Your Community Can Do About Drug Use
National Clearinghouse for Alcohol and Drug Info.
PO Box 2345
Rockville, MD 20847-2345
800-729-6686
www.health.org
This bilingual booklet is designed to show leaders at the grassroots level how to make the most of their talents and their community's resources.
73 pages

8272   Twelve Step Sponsorship: How it Works
Hazelden
15251 Pleasant Valley Road
Center City, MN 55012-9640
651-257-4010
800-328-9000
Fax: 651-213-4426
www.hazelden.org
Complete handbook for working with a newcomer. Based on Twelve Step traditions and knowledge passed orally through the generations, this working manual defines the sponsorship role and guides sponsors through the rewards and pitfalls of reaching out to help new program members.
260 pages Paperback
ISBN: 1-568381-22-0

8273   Twelve Steps and Traditions
Hazelden
15251 Pleasant Valley Road
Center City, MN 55012-9640
651-257-4010
800-328-9000
Fax: 651-213-4426
www.hazelden.org
Outlines the core principles by which AA members recover and by which the fellowship functions.
192 pages Paperback

8274   Twelve Steps and Twelve Traditions
Alcoholics Anonymous
PO Box 459
New York, NY 10163-0459
212-870-3400
Fax: 212-870-3137
Twenty-four essays on the Steps and Traditions that discuss the principles of individual recovery and group unity.

8275 Twelve Steps and Twelve Traditions for Alateen
Al-Anon Family Group Headquarters
1600 Corporate Landing Parkway   757-563-1600
Virginia Beach, VA 23454-5617   800-425-2666
                                        Fax: 757-563-1655
                                    e-mail: wso@al-anon.org
                                    www.al-anon.alateen.org
Questions, discussions and personal reflections of Alateen members.
60 pages
Caryn Johnson, Director Communications

8276 Twelve Steps for Everyone...Who Really Wants Them
Hazelden
15251 Pleasant Valley Road   651-257-4010
Center City, MN 55012-9640   800-328-9000
                                     Fax: 651-213-4426
                                     www.hazelden.org
A basic primer outlining how spiritual and emotional health can be found by working and living the Twelve Steps. Emphasizes that the Twelve Steps are for anyone who wants to change.
208 pages Paperback
ISBN: 1-568380-47-X

8277 Twelve Steps of Alcoholics Anonymous
Hazelden
15251 Pleasant Valley Road   651-257-4010
Center City, MN 55012-9640   800-328-9000
                                     Fax: 651-213-4426
                                     www.hazelden.org
A series of short discussions that interpret each of the Twelve Steps, from admission of individual powerlessness outlined in Step One to the moral inventory of Step Four and the spiritual awakening of Step Twelve.
130 pages Paperback
ISBN: 0-894869-04-3

8278 Twenty Four Hours a Day
Hazelden
15251 Pleasant Valley Road   651-257-4010
Center City, MN 55012-9640   800-328-9000
                                     Fax: 651-213-4426
                                     www.hazelden.org
Offers a resource that serves as a solid foundation in a spiritual program. Simple, yet effective resource that helps clients relate to the Twelve-Step program.
400 pages Paperback

8279 Walk in Dry Places
Hazelden
15251 Pleasant Valley Road   651-257-4010
Center City, MN 55012-9640   800-328-9000
                                     Fax: 651-213-4426
                                     www.hazelden.org
Core-recovery book filled with practical spiritual advice and time-honored Twelve Step philosophy. Insightful explorations of the deeper issues of living in recovery address the daily concerns of those new to life without alcoholism, as well as those with long-term sobriety.
400 pages Paperback
ISBN: 1-568381-27-1

8280 Wasted Tales of a Gen X Drunk
Hazelden
15251 Pleasant Valley Road   651-257-4010
Center City, MN 55012-9640   800-328-9000
                                     Fax: 651-213-4426
                                     www.hazelden.org
Cynicism and black humor underscore this hard-edged memoir of a young journalist's alcoholism and subsequent recovery. Captures the ethos of a generation often suspicious and alienated by the Twelve-Step approach.
250 pages Cloth
ISBN: 1-568381-42-5

8281 What Works: Schools Without Drugs
National Clearinghouse for Alcohol and Drug Info.
PO Box 2345
Rockville, MD 20847-2345   800-729-6686

8282 What You Can Do About Drug Use in America
National Clearinghouse for Alcohol and Drug Info.
PO Box 2345   301-468-2600
Rockville, MD 20847-2345   800-729-6686
                                     www.health.org
Offers information on what parents and professionals can do to prevent drug use in America.

8283 Why Am I Afraid to Tell You Who I Am?
Hazelden
15251 Pleasant Valley Road   651-257-4010
Center City, MN 55012-9640   800-328-9000
                                     Fax: 651-213-4426
                                     www.hazelden.org
Outlines types of interpersonal relationships.

8284 Woman's Way Through the Twelve Steps
Hazelden
15251 Pleasant Valley Road   651-257-4010
Center City, MN 55012-9640   800-328-9000
                                     Fax: 651-213-4426
                                     www.hazelden.org
How women understnad and work the Twelve Steps of AA, including reflections of spirituality, powerlessness, and the emergence of a sense of the feminine soul.
228 pages Paperback
ISBN: 0-894869-93-0

8285 Young Teens: Who They Are and How to Talk to Them About Alcohol & Drugs
National Clearinghouse for Alcohol and Drug Info.
PO Box 2345
Rockville, MD 20847-2345   800-729-6686
Offers information on how parents, educators and concerned citizens can work together to help youngsters avoid alcohol and other drugs by understanding the risks and dangers.
57 pages

Children's Books

8286 Alcoholism
Franklin Watts Grolier
90 Old Sherman Tpke   203-797-3500
Danbury, CT 06816-0001   800-621-1115
                                     Fax: 203-797-3197
                                     www.grolier.com
This comprehensive overview describes the different types of alcoholism, the addictive personality and the warning signs.
112 pages Grades 7-12
ISBN: 0-531108-79-1

8287 Alcoholism and the Family
Franklin Watts Grolier
90 Old Sherman Tpke   203-797-3500
Danbury, CT 06816-0001   800-621-1115
                                     Fax: 203-797-3197
                                     www.grolier.com
This book, after discussing what alcoholism is, its effects on health and behavior modifications through alcohol, starts addressing one of the most important aspects of alcoholism, the effects on the family.
32 pages Grades 3-5
ISBN: 0-531125-48-3

8288 America's War on Drugs
Franklin Watts Grolier
90 Old Sherman Tpke   203-797-3500
Danbury, CT 06816   800-621-1115
                                     Fax: 203-797-3197
                                     www.grolier.com
An overview of the United States' attempts to combat illegal drugs on the supply side, from stopping the supply of drugs into the country.
160 pages Grades 7-12
ISBN: 0-531109-54-2

8289 Buzzy's Rebound
National Clearinghouse for Alcohol and Drug Info.

PO Box 2345
Rockville, MD 20847-2345   800-729-6686
A Fat Albert comic book that describes the pressure on a new kid in town to drink.
18 pages

8290 Caffeine and Nicotine
Hazelden
15251 Pleasant Valley Road   651-257-4010
Center City, MN 55012-9640   800-328-9000
                                        Fax: 651-213-4426
                                        www.hazelden.org
Simple, clear, and accurate presentation of nicotine and caffeine dependency. How to avoid these addictions, and why teens ought to do so.
64 pages Paperback
ISBN: 1-568381-68-9

8291 Christy's Chance
Crestridge Corporate Center
10155 York Road   410-628-0390
Hunt Valley, MD 21030   Fax: 410-628-0398
                          e-mail: cboyce@networkpub.com
                                        www.networkpub.com
A story geared to younger teens that allows the reader to make a nonuse decision about marijuana.

8292 Cocaine
Hazelden
15251 Pleasant Valley Road   651-257-4010
Center City, MN 55012-9640   800-328-9000
                                        Fax: 651-213-4426
                                        www.hazelden.org
The information that teens need to stay drug-free, promoting understanding of the ramifications, both social and personal.
64 pages Paperback
ISBN: 1-568381-64-6

8293 Coping with Codependency
Hazelden
15251 Pleasant Valley Road   651-257-4010
Center City, MN 55012-9640   800-328-9000
                                        Fax: 651-213-4426
                                        www.hazelden.org
Explains the cycle of codependency, describes its destructive effects on all involved, and suggests ways to break free and live in more healthy relationships.
64 pages Paperback
ISBN: 1-568381-85-9

8294 Coping with Depression
Hazelden
15251 Pleasant Valley Road   651-257-4010
Center City, MN 55012-9640   800-328-9000
                                        Fax: 651-213-4426
                                        www.hazelden.org
Practical ways to cope with depression. Provides clear suggestions for handling life's downers, and encourages readers to seek professional help when they feel they can't deal with problems themselves.
64 pages Paperback
ISBN: 1-568381-79-4

8295 Coping with Drinking and Driving
Hazelden
15251 Pleasant Valley Road   651-257-4010
Center City, MN 55012-9640   800-328-9000
                                        Fax: 651-213-4426
                                        www.hazelden.org
Addressing teens' illusion of invulnerability, the author describes exactly how alcohol affects the body and one's driving skills, emphasizing that teens are not immune to alcohol's effects.
64 pages Paperback
ISBN: 1-568381-80-8

8296 Coping with Peer Pressure
Hazelden

15251 Pleasant Valley Road   651-257-4010
Center City, MN 55012-9640   800-328-9000
                                        Fax: 651-213-4426
                                        www.hazelden.org
Discussion of the positive and negative effects that members of a peer group can have on each other and explores ways teens can handle the pressure they face.
64 pages Paperback
ISBN: 1-568381-83-2

8297 Coping with Stress
Hazelden
15251 Pleasant Valley Road   651-257-4010
Center City, MN 55012-9640   800-328-9000
                                        Fax: 651-213-4426
                                        www.hazelden.org
Outlines positive strategies to help teens learn to cope more effectively with stress, rather than turning to destructive outlets such as drugs and even suicide.
64 pages Paperback
ISBN: 1-568381-76-X

8298 Coping with a Drug-Abusing Parent
Hazelden
15251 Pleasant Valley Road   651-257-4010
Center City, MN 55012-9640   800-328-9000
                                        Fax: 651-213-4426
                                        www.hazelden.org
Describes steps that teens, powerless to stop a drug-abusing parent from continuing on that destructive path, can take to to learn to take better care of themselves. Includes coping strategies and who to call for help.
64 pages Paperback
ISBN: 1-568381-78-6

8299 Crack Down on Drugs
National Clearinghouse for Alcohol and Drug Info.
PO Box 2345
Rockville, MD 20847   800-729-6686
Coloring book for children featuring McGruff, the crime dog, that teaches young children the importance of refusing alcohol and drug abuse.
Ages 5-8

8300 Different Like Me: A Book for Teens Who Worry About Their Parents' Using
Johnson Institute
Ohms Lane   612-831-1630
Edina, MN
Provides support and information for teens who are concerned, confused, scared and angry because their parents abuse alcohol and other drugs.
110 pages

8301 Drug Abuse: The Impact on Society
Franklin Watts Grolier
90 Old Sherman Tpke   203-797-3500
Danbury, CT 06816   800-621-1115
                                        Fax: 203-797-3197
                                        www.grolier.com
Discusses all major aspects of illegal drug usage and the health and personality effects they cause.
144 pages Grades 7-12
ISBN: 0-531105-79-2

8302 Drugs and AIDS
Hazelden
15251 Pleasant Valley Road   651-257-4010
Center City, MN 55012-9640   800-328-9000
                                        Fax: 651-213-4426
                                        www.hazelden.org
Covers many topics through case studies, including the effects of the disease on the body, transmission, homosexuality, condom use, drug treatment, and peer pressure.
64 pages Paperback
ISBN: 1-568381-72-7

8303 Drugs and Anger
Hazelden

15251 Pleasant Valley Road
Center City, MN 55012-9640

651-257-4010
800-328-9000
Fax: 651-213-4426
www.hazelden.org

True-to-life scenarios and practical techniques found here can help teens cope constructively with their anger.
64 pages Paperback
ISBN: 1-568381-73-5

8304 Drugs and Depression
Hazelden
15251 Pleasant Valley Road
Center City, MN 55012-9640

651-257-4010
800-328-9000
Fax: 651-213-4426
www.hazelden.org

Describes positive ways of handling depression, as well as suggesting resources for receiving assistance.
64 pages Paperback
ISBN: 1-568381-74-3

8305 Drugs and Domestic Violence
Hazelden
15251 Pleasant Valley Road
Center City, MN 55012-9640

651-257-4010
800-328-9000
Fax: 651-213-4426
www.hazelden.org

Describes valuable coping tactics that can help teens stay safe in situations involving domestic violence and drug use.
64 pages Paperback
ISBN: 1-568381-75-1

8306 Drugs and Your Friends
Hazelden
15251 Pleasant Valley Road
Center City, MN 55012-9640

651-257-4010
800-328-9000
Fax: 651-213-4426
www.hazelden.org

Helps teens make sound decisions on vital choices and provides many suggestions for resisting peer pressure.
64 pages Paperback
ISBN: 1-568381-70-0

8307 Drugs and Your Parents
Hazelden
15251 Pleasant Valley Road
Center City, MN 55012-9640

651-257-4010
800-328-9000
Fax: 651-213-4426
www.hazelden.org

Practical advice for teenage children of parents addicted to alcohol or other drugs. How to cope initially with the situation as well as long-term survival strategies.
64 pages Paperback
ISBN: 1-568381-71-9

8308 Drugs in the Body: Effects of Abuse
Franklin Watts Grolier
90 Old Sherman Tpke
Danbury, CT 06816

203-797-3500
800-621-1115
Fax: 203-797-3197
www.grolier.com

Traces the effects of cocaine and crack, opium, morphine, heroine, marijuana and hashish, LSD and PCP in a person's system. Special emphasis is placed on long-term adverse effects in the body.
144 pages Grades 7-12
ISBN: 0-531125-07-6

8309 Elephant in the Living Room: The Children's Book
Hazelden
15251 Pleasant Valley Road
Center City, MN 55012-9640

651-257-4010
800-328-9000
Fax: 651-213-4426
www.hazelden.org

An activity book to help children understand and cope with the problem of chemical dependency in the family.
88 pages Paperback
ISBN: 1-568380-35-6

8310 Facts on Alcohol
Franklin Watts Grolier

90 Old Sherman Tpke
Danbury, CT 06816

203-797-3500
800-621-1115
Fax: 203-797-3197
www.grolier.com

Offers various information on alcohol so young children can have an opportunity to form their own opinions and the ability to make their own decisions when it comes to alcoholism.
32 pages Grades 5-7
ISBN: 0-531108-21-0

8311 Facts on the Crack and Cocaine Epidemic
Franklin Watts Grolier
90 Old Sherman Tpke
Danbury, CT 06816

203-797-3500
800-621-1115
Fax: 203-797-3197
www.grolier.com

Offers young children information on these deadly drugs to help them become informed.
32 pages Grades 5-7
ISBN: 0-531108-22-8

8312 Feed Your Head
Hazelden
15251 Pleasant Valley Road
Center City, MN 55012-9640

651-257-4010
800-328-9000
Fax: 651-213-4426
www.hazelden.org

Offers practical guidance for young people.
137 pages Paperback

8313 Gangs and Drugs
Hazelden
15251 Pleasant Valley Road
Center City, MN 55012-9640

651-257-4010
800-328-9000
Fax: 651-213-4426
www.hazelden.org

Encouraging and helpful message that goes beyond Just say no.
240 pages Paperback
ISBN: 1-568381-35-2

8314 How to Say No and Keep Your Friends
Hazelden
15251 Pleasant Valley Road
Center City, MN 55012-9640

651-257-4010
800-328-9000
Fax: 651-213-4426
www.hazelden.org

Ideas to help teens deal with negative peer pressure.
112 pages

8315 I Can Talk About What Hurts
Hazelden
15251 Pleasant Valley Road
Center City, MN 55012-9640

651-257-4010
800-328-9000
Fax: 651-213-4426
www.hazelden.org

Written and illustrated for children whose lives have been affected by someone else's chemical dependency.
56 pages Paperback

8316 I Wish Daddy Didn't Drink So Much
Judith Vigna, author

Albert Whitman & Company
6340 Oakton Street
Morton Grove, IL 60053-2723

847-581-0033
800-255-7675
Fax: 847-581-0039
e-mail: mail@awhitmanco.com
www.albertwhitman.com

A young girl shres her feelings and frustrations about her alcoholic father's behavior.
1993 32 pages Grades P-3
ISBN: 0-807535-23-0
Pat McPartland, Sales
Joe Campbell, Customer Service

8317 If Drugs Are So Bad, Why Do So Many People Use Them?
Hazelden
15251 Pleasant Valley Road
Center City, MN 55012-9640

651-257-4010
800-328-9000
Fax: 651-213-4426
www.hazelden.org

Uses direct language to explain drugs and their effects.
29 pages Grades 5-9

8318 In a Perfect World
Hazelden
15251 Pleasant Valley Road
Center City, MN 55012-9640

651-257-4010
800-328-9000
Fax: 651-213-4426
www.hazelden.org

Kevin thinks his world will be perfect when his father stops drinking, but Kevin is in for a few surprises.
160 pages Softcover

8319 Inhalants
Hazelden
15251 Pleasant Valley Road
Center City, MN 55012-9640

651-257-4010
800-328-9000
Fax: 651-213-4426
www.hazelden.org

Clear, straightforward explanation of the dangers and consequences of using seemingly harmless chemicals, such as model airplane glue, hair spray, whipping cream, and cleaning and lighter fluids, as well as sources of help for those who need it.
64 pages Paperback
ISBN: 1-568381-69-7

8320 Inside Out
Hazelden
15251 Pleasant Valley Road
Center City, MN 55012-9640

651-257-4010
800-328-9000
Fax: 651-213-4426
www.hazelden.org

Offers open-ended sentences for readers to fill in their responses.
97 pages Paperback

8321 Kids and Alcohol: Get High on Life
Health Communications
1721 Blount Road
Pompano Beach, FL 33069

954-360-0909

A workbook designed to help children make important decisions in their lives and feel good about themselves.
Ages 11-14

8322 Let's Talk About Drug Abuse
Rosen Publishing Group's PowerKids Press
29 E 21st Street
New York, NY 10010

212-777-3017
800-237-9932
Fax: 888-436-4643
e-mail: customerservice@rosenpub.com
www.rosenpublishing.com

A first step in a child's education about the dangers of drugs. Recommended for grade K-4.

ISBN: 0-823923-02-9
Anna Kreiner, Author

8323 McGruff's Surprise Party
National Clearinghouse for Alcohol and Drug Info.
PO Box 2345
Rockville, MD 20847-2345

800-729-6686

A comic book that helps children understand the importance of refusing alcohol and other drugs.
14 pages Ages 8-10

8324 My Body is My House
Hazelden
15251 Pleasant Valley Road
Center City, MN 55012

651-257-4010
800-328-9000
Fax: 651-213-4426
www.hazelden.org

A coloring book about alcohol, drugs and health.
16 pages

8325 Sad Story of Mary Wanna or How Marijuana Harms You
Woodmere Press
PO Box 20, for children that contains pictures of the damage that
New York, NY 10025 book
40 pages Grades 1-4

8326 Should Drugs Be Legalized?
Franklin Watts Grolier

90 Old Sherman Tpke
Danbury, CT 06816-0001

203-797-3500
800-621-1115
Fax: 203-797-3197
www.grolier.com

Presents a discussion of this controversial subject.
160 pages Grades 7-12

8327 Smoking-At Issues Series
Greenhaven Press
Thomson Gale
Farmington Hills, MI 48333-9187

800-877-4253
Fax: 800-414-5043
e-mail: gale.customerservice@thomson.com
www.gale.com/greenhaven

Written in a straightforward manner, this book answers questions most young adults are asking regarding smoking and health.

ISBN: 0-737701-57-9

8328 Stand Strong
African American Family Services
2616 Nicollet Avenue S
Minneapolis, MN 55408

612-871-7878

Comic book prevention for young adults. Profiles two African-American teens as they go through the hazards and risks of drug use and sexual behavior.
16 pages

8329 Summer of Sassy Jo
Houghton Mifflin
Wayside Road
Burlington, MA 01803

800-225-3362

A story of a thirteen-year-old girl faced with reconciliation with her recovered alcoholic mother after eight years of abandonment.
192 pages Grades 7+
ISBN: 0-395669-56-1

8330 Teen Alcoholism-Teen Issues
Lucent Books
Thomson Gale
San Diego, CA 48333-9187

800-877-4253
Fax: 800-414-5043
e-mail: gale.customerservice@thomson.com
www.gale.com/lucent

Offers readable interviews for reports and answers the most frequently asked questions about alcohol.

ISBN: 1-590185-01-3

8331 Teen Guide to Pregnancy, Drugs and Smoking
Franklin Watts Grolier
90 Old Sherman Tpke
Danbury, CT 06816-0001

203-797-3500
800-621-1115
Fax: 203-797-3197
www.grolier.com

Outlines the risks of smoking and drug taking while pregnant and answers teenagers' questions about the use of legal, illegal and prescription drugs.
64 pages Grades 9-12
ISBN: 0-531108-35-0

8332 Understanding Drugs
Franklin Watts Grolier
90 Old Sherman Tpke
Danbury, CT 06816-0001

203-797-3500
800-621-1115
Fax: 203-797-3197
www.grolier.com

This series of books explains the current drug phenomenon at a high-interest, low-vocabulary level. Gives in-depth information about all aspects of commonly abused substances, including their negative mental, physical and social effects. Each book features photographs, diagrams, a glossary, an index and list of addresses for futher information and help. Set of seven volumes.
Grades 5-7

8333 Violence and Drugs
Franklin Watts Grolier

90 Old Sherman Tpke
Danbury, CT 06816-0001

203-797-3500
800-621-1115
Fax: 203-797-3197
www.grolier.com

This informative book studies the fascinating link between drug use and violent behavior.
112 pages Grades 9-12
ISBN: 0-531108-18-0

8334 What's Drunk Mama?
Al-Anon Family Group Headquarters
1600 Corporate Landing Parkway
Virginia Beach, VA 23454-5617

757-563-1600
800-425-2666
Fax: 757-563-1655
e-mail: wso@al-anon.org
www.al-anon.alateen.org

Large print illustrated booklet for use as a shared reading experience to help younger children understand alcoholism.
32 pages
Caryn Johnson, Director Communications

8335 Whiskers Says No to Drugs
Weekly Reader Skills Books
245 Long Hill Road
Middletown, CT 06457-4063

860-346-7157
www.weeklyreader.com

This book contains stories and follow-up activities for students to provide information and form attitudes before they face peer pressure to experiment.
Grades 2-3

8336 Why Do People Drink Alcohol?
Franklin Watts Grolier
90 Old Sherman Tpke
Danbury, CT 06816-0001

203-797-3500
800-621-1115
Fax: 203-797-3197
www.grolier.com

Answers young children's questions about alcoholism.
32 pages Grades 3-5
ISBN: 0-531171-34-5

8337 Why Do People Smoke?
Franklin Watts Grolier
90 Old Sherman Tpke
Danbury, CT 06816-0001

203-797-3500
800-621-1115
Fax: 203-797-3197
www.grolier.com

Raises and answers questions of specific interest to seven-to-ten year olds about smoking.
32 pages Grades 3-5
ISBN: 0-531171-92-2

8338 Why Do People Take Drugs?
Franklin Watts Grolier
90 Old Sherman Tpke
Danbury, CT 06816-0001

203-797-3500
800-621-1115
Fax: 203-797-3197
www.grolier.com

Raises important questions and offers some answers for young children on the aspects and everyday living with a drug addiction.
32 pages Grades 3-5
ISBN: 0-531171-13-2

8339 Winning the Battle Against Drugs: Rehabilitation Programs
Franklin Watts Grolier
90 Old Sherman Tpke
Danbury, CT 06816-0001

203-797-3500
800-621-1115
Fax: 203-797-3197
www.grolier.com

Programs contained in this book will help adolescents see that drug and alcohol addiction can be successfully treated.
160 pages Grades 7-12
ISBN: 0-531110-63-0

8340 Young Person's Guide to the Twelve Steps
Hazelden
15251 Pleasant Valley Road
Center City, MN 55012-9640

651-257-4010
800-328-9000
Fax: 651-213-4426
www.hazelden.org

Explains the Twelve Steps in the best way young people can understand: in their own language.
168 pages Paperback

8341 Young, Sober & Free
Hazelden
15251 Pleasant Valley Road
Center City, MN 55012-9640

651-257-4010
800-328-9000
Fax: 651-213-4426
www.hazelden.org

Features young peoples' personal experiences of living with addiction.
137 pages Paperback

Magazines

8342 ACAP Recap
American Council on Alcohol Problems
3426 Bridgeland Drive
Bridgeton, MO 63044-2603

314-739-5944
Fax: 314-739-0848

Offers information on organization activities and events, updates on resources and publications and legislative information for affiliate executives.
Monthly

8343 American Issue
American Council on Alcohol Problems
3426 Bridgeland Drive
Bridgeton, MO 63044-2603

314-739-5944
Fax: 314-739-0848

Offered to contributors of the organization.
Monthly

8344 Drug Abuse Update
2296 Henderson Mill Road
Atlanta, GA 30345-2739

770-934-6364

A journal of news and information for persons interested in drug prevention.
Quarterly

8345 Forum Magazine
Al-Anon Alateen Family Group Headquarters
1600 Corporate Landing Parkway
Virginia Beach, VA 10018-970

757-563-1600
888-425-2666
Fax: 757-563-1655
e-mail: wso@alanon.org
www.al-anon.alateen.org

Contains many personal stories of inspiration, some of which are maade available each month on the Internet by authorization of Al-Anon Family Group Headquarters, Inc.
Ric Buchanan, Executive Director

8346 Lead Line
Grapevine
PO Box 1980
New York, NY 10163-1980

212-870-3400
Fax: 212-870-3301

AA members all over the world communicate with each other through the pages of this magazine. It contains: insight into how AAs stay sober; readers' views; old-timers corner, beginners meeting, youth enjoying sobriety, and spotlight on service.
Monthly

Newsletters

8347 ADPA Professional
Alcohol/Drug Problems Association of North America
307 N Main Street
St. Charles, MO 63301

314-589-6702
Fax: 314-940-2358

Offers information to members on events, conferences and activities, reviews the newest resources and technology pertaining to alcoholism and drug addiction.

8348 Drug-Free Workplace Educator
American Council on Drug Education
204 Monroe Street
Rockville, MD 20850-4425

800-488-3784

Offers continuing education for employers and their supervisors responsible for substance abuse prevention. Practical articles fea-

ture information to help employers design, implement and maintain a drug-free workplace.
BiMonthly

8349 **Just Say Notes**
Just Say No International
2101 Webster Street 510-451-6666
Oakland, CA 94612-3065 800-258-2766
Offers information on the organizations, activities, programs, conferences and events.
BiMonthly

8350 **RID-USA Newsletter**
Remove Intoxicated Drivers (RID-USA)
PO Box 520 518-393-4357
Schenectady, NY 12301-0520 Fax: 518-370-4917
Membership news.
3x Year
Doris Aiken, President & CEO

8351 **Sobering Thoughts**
Women for Sobriety
PO Box 618 215-536-8026
Quakertown, PA 18951-0618 800-333-1606
Fax: 215-536-8026
e-mail: NewLife@nni.comcom
wwww.womenforsobriety.com
A monthly membership newsletter for women with an addiction problem who wish for recovery and start a new life.
16 pages Monthly
Rebecca Fenner, Director

8352 **Substance Abuse Funding News**
CD Publications
8204 Fenton Street 301-588-6380
Silver Spring, MD 20910-4571 800-666-6380
Fax: 301-588-6385
e-mail: chf@cdpublications.com
www.cdpublications.com
Detailed coverage of private and federal funding opportunities for alcohol, tobacco and drug abuse programs. Plus advice on successful grantseeking strategies and news affecting your programs.
18 pages BiWeekly
Mike Gerecht, Publisher
Amy Bernstein, Editor

Pamphlets

8353 **AA Member: Medications and Other Drugs**
Alcoholics Anonymous
PO Box 459 212-870-3400
New York, NY 10163-0459 Fax: 212-870-3137
Report from a group of doctors in Alcoholics Anonymous.

8354 **AA Service Manual: Twelve Concepts for World Service**
Alcoholics Anonymous
PO Box 459 212-870-3400
New York, NY 10163-0459 Fax: 212-870-3137
This manual opens with a history of AA services.

8355 **AA and the Armed Services**
Alcoholics Anonymous
PO Box 459 212-870-3400
New York, NY 10163-0459 Fax: 212-870-3137
Personal stories tell how men and women in the military can beat a drinking problem.

8356 **AA and the Gay/Lesbian Alcoholic**
Alcoholics Anonymous
PO Box 459 212-870-3400
New York, NY 10163-0459 Fax: 212-870-3137
Excerpts from experience, strength and hope of sober gay and lesbian alcoholics.

8357 **AA as a Resource for Health Care Professionals**
Alcoholics Anonymous
PO Box 459 212-870-3400
New York, NY 10163-0459 Fax: 212-870-3137

Information about the Fellowship and describes some approaches that health care professionals use in referring problem drinkers to AA.

8358 **AA for the Native North American**
Alcoholics Anonymous
PO Box 459 212-870-3400
New York, NY 10163-0459 Fax: 212-870-3137
Addressed to and contains stories by Native American AA members.

8359 **AA for the Woman**
Alcoholics Anonymous
PO Box 459 212-870-3400
New York, NY 10163-0459 Fax: 212-870-3137
Relates the experiences of alcoholic women, all ages and from all walks of life.

8360 **AA in Correctional Facilities**
Alcoholics Anonymous
PO Box 459 212-870-3400
New York, NY 10163-0459 Fax: 212-870-3137
Experience based on the functioning of AA groups in prisons, with institutional opinions recommending AA as a helpful ally.

8361 **AA in Treatment Facilities**
Alcoholics Anonymous
PO Box 459 212-870-3400
New York, NY 10163-0459 Fax: 212-870-3137
Shares experiences of treatment facility administrators and of AA's who have carried the message into these facilities.

8362 **Acceptance**
Hazelden
15251 Pleasant Valley Road 651-257-4010
Center City, MN 55012-9640 800-328-9000
Fax: 651-213-4426
www.hazelden.org
Addresses issues such as facing life, the kindness of God, suffering and contentment.

8363 **Adult Children of Alcoholics Newcomer Packet**
Al-Anon Family Group Headquarters
1600 Corporate Landing Parkway 757-563-1600
Virginia Beach, VA 23454-5617 800-425-2666
Fax: 757-563-1655
e-mail: wso@al-anon.org
www.al-anon.alateen.org
For those who have grown up with parental alcoholism, this is a loving introduction to Al-Anon and the twelve steps.
9 pieces
Caryn Johnson, Director Communications

8364 **African Americans in Treatment**
Hazelden
15251 Pleasant Valley Road 651-257-4010
Center City, MN 55012 800-328-9000
Fax: 651-213-4426
www.hazelden.org
Helps African American clients understand treatment from a cultural standpoint.
23 pages

8365 **Al-Anon Newcomers Packet**
Al-Anon Family Group Headquarters
1600 Corporate Landing Parkway 757-563-1600
Virginia Beach, VA 23454-5617 800-425-2666
Fax: 757-563-1655
e-mail: wso@al-anon.org
www.al-anon.alateen.org
Material specifically for the newcomer to Al-Anon packed in a handsome sleeve.
8 pieces
Caryn Johnson, Director Communications

8366 **Al-Anon Spoken Here**
Al-Anon Family Group Headquarters

1600 Corporate Landing Parkway
Virginia Beach, VA 23454-5617
757-563-1600
800-425-2666
Fax: 757-563-1655
e-mail: wso@al-anon.org
www.al-anon.alateen.org

Why are Al-Anon meetings the way they are? Questions and answers that lead to a better understanding of the importance of keeping Al-Anon principles.
8 pages
Caryn Johnson, Director Communications

8367 Al-Anon is for Men
Al-Anon Family Group Headquarters
1600 Corporate Landing Parkway
Virginia Beach, VA 23454-5617
757-563-1600
800-425-2666
Fax: 757-563-1655
e-mail: wso@al-anon.org
www.al-anon.alateen.org

Straight forward questions to help men identify their reactions to alcoholism in another person.
6 pages
Caryn Johnson, Director Communications

8368 Al-Anon, You and the Alcoholic
Al-Anon Family Group Headquarters
1600 Corporate Landing Parkway
Virginia Beach, VA 23454-5617
757-563-1600
800-425-2666
Fax: 757-563-1655
e-mail: wso@al-anon.org
www.al-anon.alateen.org

Answers the most frequently asked questions about Al-Anon and how it helps families deal with problems brought about by alcoholism.
12 pages
Caryn Johnson, Director Communications

8369 Alateen Newcomer Packet
Al-Anon Family Group Headquarters
1600 Corporate Landing Parkway
Virginia Beach, VA 23454-5617
757-563-1600
800-425-2666
Fax: 757-563-1655
e-mail: wso@al-anon.org
www.al-anon.alateen.org

Helpful leaflets assembled in a sleeve ready to give to the new young member.
13 pieces
Caryn Johnson, Director Communications

8370 Alateen Talk
Al-Anon Family Group Headquarters
1600 Corporate Landing Parkway
Virginia Beach, VA 23454-5617
757-563-1600
800-425-2666
Fax: 757-563-1655
e-mail: wso@al-anon.org
www.al-anon.alateen.org
Robert Schneider, Director Communications

8371 Alcohol Alert #11: Estimating the Cost of Alcohol Abuse
National Clearinghouse for Alcohol and Drug Info.
PO Box 2345
Rockville, MD 20847-2345
800-729-6686
www.health.org

Discusses the various problems of estimating the cost of alcohol abuse.

8372 Alcohol Alert #15: Alcohol and AIDS
National Clearinghouse for Alcohol and Drug Info.
PO Box 2345
Rockville, MD 20847-2345
800-729-6686
www.health.org

Discusses the relationship between alcohol consumption and HIV infection and AIDS.

8373 Alcohol Alert #16: Moderate Drinking
National Clearinghouse for Alcohol and Drug Info.
PO Box 2345
Rockville, MD 20847-2345
800-729-6686
www.health.org

Defines moderate drinking and explores the benefits and risks associated with moderate drinking.

8374 Alcohol Alert #17: Treatment Outcome Research
National Clearinghouse for Alcohol and Drug Info.
PO Box 2345
Rockville, MD 20847-2345
800-729-6686
www.health.org

Discusses purpose, methodology, randomization, blinding, followup and what treatment outcome research reveals.

8375 Alcohol Alert #18: The Genetics of Alcoholism
National Clearinghouse for Alcohol and Drug Info.
PO Box 2345
Rockville, MD 20847-2345
800-729-6686
www.health.org

Presents the results of studies that investigate the role of genes and the environment in the development of alcoholism.

8376 Alcohol Alert #21: Alcohol and Cancer
National Clearinghouse for Alcohol and Drug Info.
PO Box 2345
Rockville, MD 20847-2345
800-729-6686
www.health.org

8377 Alcohol Alert #23: Alcohol and Minorities
National Clearinghouse for Alcohol and Drug Info.
PO Box 2345
Rockville, MD 20847-2345
800-729-6686
www.health.org

8378 Alcohol Alert #24: Animal Models in Alcohol Research
National Clearinghouse for Alcohol and Drug Info.
PO Box 2345
Rockville, MD 20847-2345
800-729-6686
www.health.org

8379 Alcohol Alert #25: Alcohol-Related Impairment
National Clearinghouse for Alcohol and Drug Info.
PO Box 2345
Rockville, MD 20847-2345
800-729-6686
www.health.org

8380 Alcohol Alert #26: Alcohol and Hormones
National Clearinghouse for Alcohol and Drug Info.
PO Box 2345
Rockville, MD 20847-2345
800-729-6686
www.health.org

8381 Alcohol Alert #27: Alcohol Medication Interactions
National Clearinghouse for Alcohol and Drug Info.
PO Box 2345
Rockville, MD 20847-2345
800-729-6686
www.health.org

8382 Alcohol and Drug Abuse in Black America: A Guide for Community Action
African American Family Services
2616 Nicollet Avenue S
Minneapolis, MN 55408
612-871-7878

A booklet giving a description of the history and the current manifestations of alcohol and drug problems in Black America with a discussion of strategies for fundamental change.
24 pages

8383 Alcohol and Pregnancy
March of Dimes
233 Park Avenue South
New York, NY 10003
212-353-8353
Fax: 212-254-3518
e-mail: NY639@marchofdimes.com
www.marchofdimes.com

8384 Alcoholics Anonymous and Employee Assistance Program
Alcoholics Anonymous
PO Box 459
New York, NY 10163-0459
212-870-3400
Fax: 212-870-3137

Of interest to management and union officials, this pamphlet gives concise descriptions of the help AA can offer to the alcoholic employee.

8385 Alcoholism Tends to Run in Families
National Clearinghouse for Alcohol and Drug Info.
PO Box 2345
Rockville, MD 20847-2345
800-729-6686
www.health.org

Provides answers and questions about how to help children of alcoholics and where to find resources for additional information.

8386 Alcoholism: A Merry-Go-Round Named Denial
Al-Anon Family Group Headquarters
1600 Corporate Landing Parkway   757-563-1600
Virginia Beach, VA 23454-5617   800-425-2666
                                      Fax: 757-563-1655
                              e-mail: wso@al-anon.org
                              www.al-anon.alateen.org
Dramatic explanations that help family members and friends see the roles they play in the problems of alcoholism.
18 pages
Caryn Johnson, Director Communications

8387 Alcoholism: The Family Disease
Al-Anon Family Group Headquarters
1600 Corporate Landing Parkway   757-563-1600
Virginia Beach, VA 23454-5617   800-425-2666
                                      Fax: 757-563-1655
                              e-mail: wso@al-anon.org
                              www.al-anon.alateen.org
A treasury of information and inspiration with the purpose of the Al-Anon program, actual stories of people who found serenity in Al-Anon, questions/answers, slogans, evaluations and thoughts to live by.
48 pages
Caryn Johnson, Director Communications

8388 Anabolic Steroids: A Threat to Body and Mind
National Clearinghouse for Alcohol and Drug Info.
PO Box 2345
Rockville, MD 20847   800-729-6686
Summarizes the findings of recent studies on the use of anabolic steroids in the United States.
11 pages

8389 Anonymity
Al-Anon Family Group Headquarters
1600 Corporate Landing Parkway   757-563-1600
Virginia Beach, VA 23454-5617   800-425-2666
                                      Fax: 757-563-1655
                              e-mail: wso@al-anon.org
                              www.al-anon.alateen.org
Offers information on Al-Anon and Alateen traditions and what a big factor anonymity plays for members.
6 pages
Caryn Johnson, Director Communications

8390 Are You Concerned About Someone's Drinking
Al-Anon Family Group Headquarters
1600 Corporate Landing Parkway   757-563-1600
Virginia Beach, VA 23454-5617   800-425-2666
                                      Fax: 757-563-1655
                              e-mail: wso@al-anon.org
                              www.al-anon.alateen.org

12 pages
Caryn Johnson, Director Communications

8391 Be Kind to Nonsmokers
American Lung Association
1740 Broadway   212-315-8700
New York, NY 10019-4315
Explains why smoke hurts nonsmokers.

8392 Best of Public Outreach
Al-Anon Family Group Headquarters
1600 Corporate Landing Parkway   757-563-1600
Virginia Beach, VA 23454-5617   800-425-2666
                                      Fax: 757-563-1655
                              e-mail: wso@al-anon.org
                              www.al-anon.alateen.org
Helps groups, committees and individuals carry out their PI institutions and CPC activities; includes suggested activities and open letters to various professionals.
24 pages
Caryn Johnson, Director Communications

8393 Black, Beautiful and Recovering
Hazelden

15251 Pleasant Valley Road   651-257-4010
Center City, MN 55012-9640   800-328-9000
                                      Fax: 651-213-4426
                                      www.hazelden.org
20 pages

8394 Chemical Dependency and the African American
Hazelden
15251 Pleasant Valley Road   651-257-4010
Center City, MN 55012-9640   800-328-9000
                                      Fax: 651-213-4426
                                      www.hazelden.org
Reviews the impact alcohol and other drug abuse has on African American communities.
66 pages

8395 Chemical Dependency: An Acceptable Disease
Hazelden
15251 Pleasant Valley Road   651-257-4010
Center City, MN 55012-9640   800-328-9000
                                      Fax: 651-213-4426
                                      www.hazelden.org
Help persons identify and acknowledge their chemical dependency.
14 pages

8396 Chew or Snuff is Real Bad Stuff
National Cancer Institute
Building 31   301-496-4000
Bethesda, MD 20892
A pamphlet describing the hazards of using smokeless tobacco.
8 pages

8397 Cigarette Smoking
American Lung Association
1740 Broadway   212-315-8700
New York, NY 10019-4315
Leaflet presenting the facts about how cigarette smoke is related to lung disease.

8398 Communication Skills
Hazelden
15251 Pleasant Valley Road   651-257-4010
Center City, MN 55012-9640   800-328-9000
                                      Fax: 651-213-4426
                                      www.hazelden.org
Helps clients discover how to become better listeners.

8399 Community Campaign Brochure
National Clearinghouse for Alcohol and Drug Info.
PO Box 2345
Rockville, MD 20847-2345   800-729-6686
Information and promotional brochure discusses key prevention concepts and messages and details how to plan campaign events.

8400 Crack
Hazelden
15251 Pleasant Valley Road   651-257-4010
Center City, MN 55012-9640   800-328-9000
                                      Fax: 651-213-4426
                                      www.hazelden.org
Explains history, use and effects of crack cocaine.

8401 Crack Cocaine: The Big Lie
National Clearinghouse for Alcohol and Drug Info.
PO Box 2345
Rockville, MD 20847-2345   800-729-6686
                                          www.health.org
Offers information on what crack and cocaine are, how strong the addictions are from these drugs, how they affect the body and other risks in taking cocaine and crack.

8402 Crossing the Line Between Social Drinking and Alcoholism
Hazelden
15251 Pleasant Valley Road   651-257-4010
Center City, MN 55012-9640   800-328-9000
                                      Fax: 651-213-4426
                                      www.hazelden.org
20 pages

8403 Denial
Hazelden
15251 Pleasant Valley Road 651-257-4010
Center City, MN 55012-9640 800-328-9000
Fax: 651-213-4426
www.hazelden.org
Describes denial and its role in the five-stage acceptance process.

8404 Depression and Recovery from Chemical Dependency
Hazelden
15251 Pleasant Valley Road 651-257-4010
Center City, MN 55012-9640 800-328-9000
Fax: 651-213-4426
www.hazelden.org
Outlines depression's warning signs.

8405 Detaching with Love
Hazelden
15251 Pleasant Valley Road 651-257-4010
Center City, MN 55012-9640 800-328-9000
Fax: 651-213-4426
www.hazelden.org
Addresses the essential recovery tools clients need to cope with addiction and detach from the problem.

8406 Detachment
Al-Anon Family Group Headquarters
1600 Corporate Landing Parkway 757-563-1600
Virginia Beach, VA 23454-5617 800-425-2666
Fax: 757-563-1655
e-mail: wso@al-anon.org
www.al-anon.alateen.org
Everything you always wanted to know about detachment in an easy-to-use leaflet.
Caryn Johnson, Director Communications

8407 Did You Grow Up with a Problem Drinker?
Al-Anon Family Group Headquarters
1600 Corporate Landing Parkway 757-563-1600
Virginia Beach, VA 23454-5617 800-425-2666
Fax: 757-563-1655
e-mail: wso@al-anon.org
www.al-anon.alateen.org
Twenty personal questions help individuals decide if they can benefit from Al-Anon.
Caryn Johnson, Director Communications

8408 Do You Think You're Different?
Alcoholics Anonymous
PO Box 459 212-870-3400
New York, NY 10163-0459 Fax: 212-870-3137
Speaks to newcomers who may wonder how AA can work for someone different.

8409 Don't Let Your Dreams Go Up in Smoke
American Lung Association
1740 Broadway 212-315-8700
New York, NY 10019-4315
Photos, testimonials and clear language to deliver the message that everyone can and should stop smoking.

8410 Don't Lose a Friend to Drugs
National Crime Prevention Council
1000 Connecticut Avenue NW 202-466-6272
Washington, DC 20036-3802 Fax: 202-296-1356
www.ncpc.org
Offers practical advice to teenagers on how to say no to drugs, how to help a friend who uses drugs and how to initiate community efforts to prevent drug use.

8411 Drinking Alcohol During Pregnancy
March of Dimes
233 Park Avenue South 212-353-8353
New York, NY 10003 Fax: 212-254-3518
e-mail: NY639@marchofdimes.com
www.marchofdimes.com
Fact Sheets: one to two page review written for the general public. Also available electronically from the website www.marchofdimes.com

8412 Drug Free Zones: A Manual
African American Family Services
2616 Nicollet Avenue S 612-871-7878
Minneapolis, MN 55408
This booklet describes a variety of strategies concerned citizens are using to reclaim their neighborhoods from rampant drug abuse and dealing.
24 pages

8413 Drugs and Pregnancy
March of Dimes
233 Park Avenue South 212-353-8353
New York, NY 10003 Fax: 212-254-3518
e-mail: NY639@marchofdimes.com
www.marchofdimes.com
Brochures: 3 panel color brochures written for the general public.
pkg 50

8414 Employer's Guide to Dealing with Substance Abuse
National Clearinghouse for Alcohol and Drug Info.
PO Box 2345
Rockville, MD 20847-2345 800-729-6686
www.health.org
Instructs employers in setting up comprehensive alcohol and other drug programs in the workplace.
18 pages

8415 Enabling
Hazelden
15251 Pleasant Valley Road 651-257-4010
Center City, MN 55012-9640 800-328-9000
Fax: 651-213-4426
www.hazelden.org
Describes problems families encounter when they focus their lives on their chemically dependent family member.

8416 Facts About Alateen
Al-Anon Family Group Headquarters
1600 Corporate Landing Parkway 757-563-1600
Virginia Beach, VA 23454-5617 800-425-2666
Fax: 757-563-1655
e-mail: wso@al-anon.org
www.al-anon.alateen.org
Offers information on Alateen member services.
4 pages
Caryn Johnson, Director Communications

8417 Facts About Alcohol Abuse
Medical Arts Center Hospital
57 W 57th Street 212-838-2169
New York, NY 10019-2802 Fax: 212-755-0200
A question and answer pamphlet that offers information on alcohol abuse and the effects the abuse has on the family unit.

8418 Family Denial
Hazelden
15251 Pleasant Valley Road 651-257-4010
Center City, MN 55012-9640 800-328-9000
Fax: 651-213-4426
www.hazelden.org
Describes ways for families to recognize denial, examine common fears that cause denial and develop methods for overcoming it.

8419 Fetal Alcohol Syndrome
Hazelden
15251 Pleasant Valley Road 651-257-4010
Center City, MN 55012-9640 800-328-9000
Fax: 651-213-4426
www.hazelden.org
A source of information about the effects of drinking while pregnant.

8420 Fight Drug Abuse at Home, Work, School and in the Community
American Council for Drug Education
204 Monroe Street
Rockville, MD 20850-4425 800-488-3784
A catalog of print and video materials pertaining to substance abuse, alcoholism and drugs.

8421 For a Strong and Healthy Baby
National Clearinghouse for Alcohol and Drug Info.

PO Box 2345
Rockville, MD 20847-2345   800-729-6686
                                        www.health.org
Recommends that women not drink or use other drugs if pregnant
or planning to become pregnant.

8422   Free to Care
Hazelden
15251 Pleasant Valley Road   651-257-4010
Center City, MN 55012-9640   800-328-9000
                                        Fax: 651-213-4426
                                        www.hazelden.org
Explores today's definition of family and new attitudes about gen-
der, technology, single-parents, relatives and friends.

8423   Freedom from Despair
Al-Anon Family Group Headquarters
1600 Corporate Landing Parkway   757-563-1600
Virginia Beach, VA 23454-5617   800-425-2666
                                        Fax: 757-563-1655
                                        e-mail: wso@al-anon.org
                                        www.al-anon.alateen.org
A message of hope for those faced with a problem they can't solve
alone.
4 pages
Caryn Johnson, Director Communications

8424   Freedom from Smoking Flyer
American Lung Association
1740 Broadway   212-315-8700
New York, NY 10019-4315
4 color flyer describing all FFS programs.

8425   Getting in Touch with Al-Anon/Alateen
Al-Anon Family Group Headquarters
1600 Corporate Landing Parkway   757-563-1600
Virginia Beach, VA 23454-5617   800-425-2666
                                        Fax: 757-563-1655
                                        e-mail: wso@al-anon.org
                                        www.al-anon.alateen.org
A listing of Al-Anon information services throughout the world.
Helps members, the public and professionals located nearby
Al-Anon or Alateen groups.
Caryn Johnson, Director Communications

8426   Grieving
Hazelden
15251 Pleasant Valley Road   651-257-4010
Center City, MN 55012-9640   800-328-9000
                                        Fax: 651-213-4426
                                        www.hazelden.org
Outlines the five-phase grieving process for clients and the signifi-
cance of each.

8427   Guidance on Our Journeys
Hazelden
15251 Pleasant Valley Road   651-257-4010
Center City, MN 55012-9640   800-328-9000
                                        Fax: 651-213-4426
                                        www.hazelden.org
Examines the relationship between the recovering person and his
or her sponsor.

8428   Guide for the Family of the Alcoholic
Al-Anon Family Group Headquarters
1600 Corporate Landing Parkway   757-563-1600
Virginia Beach, VA 23454-5617   800-425-2666
                                        Fax: 757-563-1655
                                        e-mail: wso@al-anon.org
                                        www.al-anon.alateen.org
A clear and realistic look at alcoholism, problems encountered by
those close to the alcoholic and choices available to the family.
16 pages
Caryn Johnson, Director Communications

8429   Have Fun! Figure Out the Smoking Puzzle
American Lung Association
1740 Broadway   212-315-8700
New York, NY 10019-4315
Crossword puzzles make stimulating points on the effects of smok-
ing.

8430   Healthy Beginning, Promotional Flyers
American Lung Association
1740 Broadway   212-315-8700
New York, NY 10019-4315
Flyer offers tips to help protect newborn and young children from
the harmful effects of passive smoking.

8431   Help a Friend to Stop Smoking
American Lung Association
1740 Broadway   212-315-8700
New York, NY 10019-4315
This original guide to helping family members and friends support
a smoker who is trying to quit smoking.
12 pages

8432   Helping Smokers Get Ready to Quit
American Lung Association
1740 Broadway   212-315-8700
New York, NY 10019-4315
Offers suggestions on how to get smokers to think about quitting
and how to open up a dialogue on the issue.

8433   Helping Your Child Say No: A Parent's Guide
National Clearinghouse for Alcohol and Drug Info.
PO Box 2345
Rockville, MD 20847-2345   800-729-6686
Explains to parents how alcohol affects the body, how to tell if your
child has been drinking and why children start to drink.

8434   Homeward Bound
Al-Anon Family Group Headquarters
1600 Corporate Landing Parkway   757-563-1600
Virginia Beach, VA 23454-5617   800-425-2666
                                        Fax: 757-563-1655
                                        e-mail: wso@al-anon.org
                                        www.al-anon.alateen.org
A booklet designed to help beginners make the transition from the
family treatment setting to Al-Anon. Contains forty members' personal sharings, a basic glossary of Al-Anon terms, brief explanations of Al-Anon slogans and helpful suggestions for newcomers.
48 pages
Caryn Johnson, Director Communications

8435   How Can I Help My Children?
Al-Anon Family Group Headquarters
1600 Corporate Landing Parkway   757-563-1600
Virginia Beach, VA 23454-5617   800-425-2666
                                        Fax: 757-563-1655
                                        e-mail: wso@al-anon.org
                                        www.al-anon.alateen.org
Parents can help their children achieve a healthier attitude. Im-
proving our own attitudes and behavior will help the entire family.
20 pages
Caryn Johnson, Director Communications

8436   How Drug Abuse Takes Profit Out of Business
National Clearinghouse for Alcohol and Drug Info.
PO Box 2345
Rockville, MD 20847-2345   800-729-6686
Answers employers questions about substance abuse in the work-
place.

8437   How to Get the Most Out of Group Therapy
Hazelden
15251 Pleasant Valley Road   651-257-4010
Center City, MN 55012-9640   800-328-9000
                                        Fax: 651-213-4426
                                        www.hazelden.org
Answers clients' questions about going to and getting help from
group therapy.

8438   How to Help a Friend Quit Smoking
American Lung Association
1740 Broadway   212-315-8700
New York, NY 10019-4315
Discusses how friends, family and co-workers can assist smokers
with their concerns about quitting smoking.

8439   How to Take Care of Your Baby Before Birth
National Clearinghouse for Alcohol and Drug Info.

623

PO Box 2345
Rockville, MD 20847-2345   800-729-6686
                                   www.health.org
A low-literacy brochure aimed at pregnant women that describes what they should and should not do during pregnancy.

8440   I Can't Be Addicted Because...
Hazelden
15251 Pleasant Valley Road   651-257-4010
Center City, MN 55012-9640   800-328-9000
                                   Fax: 651-213-4426
                                   www.hazelden.org
Focuses on denial and elaborates on its most common forms.

8441   Ice Storm
Hazelden
15251 Pleasant Valley Road   651-257-4010
Center City, MN 55012-9640   800-328-9000
                                   Fax: 651-213-4426
                                   www.hazelden.org
Prepares treatment professionals for the complications of one of the most recently synthesized drugs - ice.

8442   If Someone Close to You Has a Problem with Alcohol or Other Drugs
National Clearinghouse for Alcohol and Drug Info.
PO Box 2345
Rockville, MD 20847-2345   800-729-6686
                                   www.health.org
This booklet is aimed at the general public and gives support and suggestions on coping with someone close who has an alcohol or drug problem.

8443   If You Are a Professional, AA Wants to Work with You
Alcoholics Anonymous
PO Box 459   212-870-3400
New York, NY 10163-0459   Fax: 212-870-3137
Directed at professionals of all types who deal with alcoholics.

8444   If Your Parents Drink Too Much
Al-Anon Family Group Headquarters
1600 Corporate Landing Parkway   757-563-1600
Virginia Beach, VA 23454-5617   800-425-2666
                                   Fax: 757-563-1655
                                   e-mail: wso@al-anon.org
                                   www.al-anon.alateen.org
Alateen's cartoon booklet.
24 pages
Caryn Johnson, Director Communications

8445   Illicit Drug Use During Pregnancy
March of Dimes
233 Park Avenue South   212-353-8353
New York, NY 10003   Fax: 212-254-3518
                                   e-mail: NY639@marchofdimes.com
                                   www.marchofdimes.com
Fact Sheets: one to two page review for the general public. Also available electronically from the website www.marchofdimes.com

8446   Index to Alcoholics Anonymous
Hazelden
15251 Pleasant Valley Road   651-257-4010
Center City, MN 55012-9640   800-328-9000
                                   Fax: 651-213-4426
Features page and line references to the topics discussed in Alcoholics Anonymous, the Big Book.

8447   Is AA for Me?
Alcoholics Anonymous
PO Box 459   212-870-3400
New York, NY 10163-0459   Fax: 212-870-3137
An illustrated easy to read version of the 12 questions in Is AA for You? pamphlet.
32 pages

8448   Is AA for You?
Alcoholics Anonymous
PO Box 459   212-870-3400
New York, NY 10163-0459   Fax: 212-870-3137
Symptoms of alcoholism are summed up in 12 questions most AA's had answered to identify themselves as alcoholics.

8449   Is There a Safe Tobacco?
American Lung Association
1740 Broadway   212-315-8700
New York, NY 10019-4315
Offers information on the health risks of cigarette smoking, pipes and cigars.

8450   Is There an Alcoholic in Your Life?
Alcoholics Anonymous
PO Box 459   212-870-3400
New York, NY 10163-0459   Fax: 212-870-3137
Explains the AA program as it affects anyone close to an alcoholic.

8451   It Happened to Alice
Alcoholics Anonymous
PO Box 459   212-870-3400
New York, NY 10163-0459   Fax: 212-870-3137
Easy to read comic-book style format for women alcoholics.

8452   It Sure Beats Sitting in a Cell
Alcoholics Anonymous
PO Box 459   212-870-3400
New York, NY 10163-0459   Fax: 212-870-3137
An illustrated pamphlet which presents the experience of seven inmates who found AA while in prison. It also offers suggested dos and don'ts for staying sober after release.

8453   Kids and Drugs: A Handbook for Parents & Professionals
PANDAA Press
4111 Watkins Trl   703-750-9285
Annandale, VA 22003-2051

8454   Let's Solve the Smokeword Puzzle
American Lung Association
1740 Broadway   212-315-8700
New York, NY 10019-4315
Fifth graders will love getting an antismoking message through solving a crossword puzzle.

8455   Let's Talk
Hazelden
15251 Pleasant Valley Road   651-257-4010
Center City, MN 55012-9640   800-328-9000
                                   Fax: 651-213-4426
                                   www.hazelden.org
Offers 12 guidelines to promote effective communication between parent and child.

8456   Letter to a Woman Alcoholic
Alcoholics Anonymous
PO Box 459   212-870-3400
New York, NY 10163-0459   Fax: 212-870-3137
Describes with sensitive understanding the problem of the alcoholic woman.

8457   Letting Go of the Need to Control
Hazelden
15251 Pleasant Valley Road   651-257-4010
Center City, MN 55012-9640   800-328-9000
                                   Fax: 651-213-4426
                                   www.hazelden.org
Discusses how control issues are common among chemically dependent people.

8458   Lifetime of Freedom from Smoking: Maintenance Manual
American Lung Association
1740 Broadway   212-315-8700
New York, NY 10019-4315
Companion manual helps persons stay quit once they have stopped smoking.
28 pages

8459   Little More About Alcohol
Alcohol Research Information Service
1120 E Oakland Avenue   517-485-9900
Lansing, MI 48906-5513   Fax: 517-485-1928
                                   e-mail: alcoholisadrugtoo@yoyoger.net
A cartoon character explains the facts about alcohol and its effects on the body.

8460 Living Sober
Alcoholics Anonymous
PO Box 459   212-870-3400
New York, NY 10163-0459   Fax: 212-870-3137
Practical book demonstrating through simple examples, how AA members throughout the world live and stay sober one day at a time.
88 pages

8461 Living in a Shelter?
Al-Anon Family Group Headquarters
1600 Corporate Landing Parkway   757-563-1600
Virginia Beach, VA 23454-5617   800-425-2666
                                        Fax: 757-563-1655
                                        e-mail: wso@al-anon.org
                                        www.al-anon.alateen.org
100 pieces
Caryn Johnson, Director Communications

8462 Look at Cross-Addiction
Hazelden
15251 Pleasant Valley Road   651-257-4010
Center City, MN 55012-9640   800-328-9000
                                        Fax: 651-213-4426
Discusses cross-addiction, denial, coping skills and avoidance.

8463 Look at Relapse
Hazelden
15251 Pleasant Valley Road   651-257-4010
Center City, MN 55012-9640   800-328-9000
                                        Fax: 651-213-4426
Addresses emotional consequences of relapse, such as decreased feelings of self-esteem and self-confidence.

8464 Managing Cocaine Cravings
Hazelden
15251 Pleasant Valley Road   651-257-4010
Center City, MN 55012-9640   800-328-9000
                                        Fax: 651-213-4426
                                        www.hazelden.org
Offers clients hands-on plan to help them stay away from cocaine.

8465 Marijuana
Hazelden
15251 Pleasant Valley Road   651-257-4010
Center City, MN 55012-9640   800-328-9000
                                        Fax: 651-213-4426
                                        www.hazelden.org
Outlines the physical and psychological effects of marijuana unique to episodic and chronic use.
65 pages

8466 Media Kit
Al-Anon Family Group Headquarters
1600 Corporate Landing Parkway   757-563-1600
Virginia Beach, VA 23454-5617   800-425-2666
                                        Fax: 757-563-1655
                                        e-mail: wso@al-anon.org
                                        www.al-anon.alateen.org
An attractive silver folder containing information necessary to work with radio and TV stations.
Caryn Johnson, Director Communications

8467 Member's Eye View of Alcoholics Anonymous
Alcoholics Anonymous
PO Box 459   212-870-3400
New York, NY 10163-0459   Fax: 212-870-3137
Designed to explain to people in the helping professionals how AA works.
30 pages

8468 Members of the Clergy Ask About Alcoholics Anonymous
Alcoholics Anonymous
PO Box 459   212-870-3400
New York, NY 10163-0459   Fax: 212-870-3137
Introduction to AA for members of the clergy unfamiliar with the Fellowship.

8469 Memo to an Inmate Who May Be an Alcoholic
Alcoholics Anonymous

PO Box 459   212-870-3400
New York, NY 10163-0459   Fax: 212-870-3137
A message from AA's who have themselves been inmates. Their personal stories offer a new outlook to inmate alcholics who want to know who AA can help.

8470 Men Newcomer Packet
Al-Anon Family Group Headquarters
1600 Corporate Landing Parkway   757-563-1600
Virginia Beach, VA 23454-5617   800-425-2666
                                        Fax: 757-563-1655
                                        e-mail: wso@al-anon.org
                                        www.al-anon.alateen.org
For men who are not sure Al-Anon is for them, this collection offers a realistic look at alcoholism and straight forward answers to frequently asked questions.
8 pieces
Caryn Johnson, Director Communications

8471 Message to Correctional Facilities Administrators
Alcoholics Anonymous
PO Box 459   212-870-3400
New York, NY 10163-0459   Fax: 212-870-3137
Information about what AA is and can do, and how groups function in correctional facilities.

8472 Message to Teenagers
Alcoholics Anonymous
PO Box 459   212-870-3400
New York, NY 10163-0459   Fax: 212-870-3137
This brochure offers a simple, 12-question quiz designed to help teenagers decide when drinking is becoming a problem in their lives.

8473 Military Packet
Al-Anon Family Group Headquarters
1600 Corporate Landing Parkway   757-563-1600
Virginia Beach, VA 23454-5617   800-425-2666
                                        Fax: 757-563-1655
                                        e-mail: wso@al-anon.org
                                        www.al-anon.alateen.org
For those in the armed services with loved ones or colleagues who are alcoholic, here's a collection that says, Al-Anon can help.
7 pieces
Caryn Johnson, Director Communications

8474 Moment to Reflect on Codependency
Hazelden
15251 Pleasant Valley Road   651-257-4010
Center City, MN 55012-9640   800-328-9000
                                        Fax: 651-213-4426
A collection of four booklets offering meditations that emphasize and reinforce self-esteem for young people recovering from addiction.

8475 Moment to Reflect on Self-Esteem
Hazelden
15251 Pleasant Valley Road   651-257-4010
Center City, MN 55012-9640   800-328-9000
                                        Fax: 651-213-4426
Focuses on the fundamental recovery issue of self-esteem.
4 Booklets

8476 Moving On! From Alateen to Al-Anon
Al-Anon Family Group Headquarters
1600 Corporate Landing Parkway   757-563-1600
Virginia Beach, VA 23454-5617   800-425-2666
                                        Fax: 757-563-1655
                                        e-mail: wso@al-anon.org
                                        www.al-anon.alateen.org
Former Alateen members experience the joy of continued recovery in Al-Anon.
12 pages
Caryn Johnson, Director Communications

8477 NIDA Capsules
National Clearinghouse for Alcohol and Drug Info.
PO Box 2345
Rockville, MD 20847-2345   800-729-6686
                                        www.health.org

8478 Newcomer Asks
Alcoholics Anonymous
PO Box 459   212-870-3400
New York, NY 10163-0459   Fax: 212-870-3137
Gives straightforward answers on 15 points that once puzzled many of us.

8479 Nicotine Addiction and Cigarettes
American Lung Association
1740 Broadway   212-315-8700
New York, NY 10019-4315
Offers information on nicotine and cigarette smoking.

8480 No Smoking Coloring Book
American Lung Association
1740 Broadway   212-315-8700
New York, NY 10019-4315
Preschool and primary grade children will enjoy drawing and coloring while getting an antismoking message.

8481 No Smoking: Lungs At Work
American Lung Association
1740 Broadway   212-315-8700
New York, NY 10019-4315
Describes how lungs work and how they are affected by smoking.

8482 Now What Do I Do for Fun?
Hazelden
15251 Pleasant Valley Road   651-257-4010
Center City, MN 55012-9640   800-328-9000
                                            Fax: 651-213-4426
                                            www.hazelden.org
Explores the dilemma of finding new interests in recovery after completing treatment.

8483 Older Adults After Treatment
Hazelden
15251 Pleasant Valley Road   651-257-4010
Center City, MN 55012-9640   800-328-9000
                                            Fax: 651-213-4426
                                            www.hazelden.org
Discusses aftercare issues, such as family relations, health, medication and relapse.

8484 Older Adults in Treatment
Hazelden
15251 Pleasant Valley Road   651-257-4010
Center City, MN 55012-9640   800-328-9000
                                            Fax: 651-213-4426
                                            www.hazelden.org
Examines past beliefs about addiction and defines chemical dependency as a disease.

8485 On the Air: A Guide to Creating A Smoke-Free Workplace
American Lung Association
1740 Broadway   212-315-8700
New York, NY 10019-4315
A step-by-step guide for organizations interested in developing and implementing a successful workplace smoking control policy.
24 pages

8486 Parents Newcomer Packet
Al-Anon Family Group Headquarters
1600 Corporate Landing Parkway   757-563-1600
Virginia Beach, VA 23454-5617   800-425-2666
                                            Fax: 757-563-1655
                                            e-mail: wso@al-anon.org
                                            www.al-anon.alateen.org
For parents who realize their child is an alcoholic, this is a compassionate and reassuring welcome to Al-Anon.
9 pieces
Caryn Johnson, Director Communications

8487 Points for Parents Perplexed About Drugs
Hazelden
15251 Pleasant Valley Road   651-257-4010
Center City, MN 55012-9640   800-328-9000
                                            Fax: 651-213-4426
                                            www.hazelden.org

Clear guidelines to help adults recognize, evaluate and deal with adolescent drug abuse.
16 pages

8488 Preventing Relapse
Hazelden
15251 Pleasant Valley Road   651-257-4010
Center City, MN 55012-9640   800-328-9000
                                            Fax: 651-213-4426
                                            www.hazelden.org
Offers practical information and personal stories to help clients better understand the relapse process.
28 pages

8489 Program Booklet
Women for Sobriety
PO Box 618   215-536-8026
Quakertown, PA 18951-0618   Fax: 215-536-8026
                                            e-mail: WFSobriety@aol.com
                                            www.womenforsobriety.org
Purse size booklet that explains the Thirteen Statements of Dr. Kirkpatrick's New Life program, statement by statement.

8490 Put on the Brakes Bulletin: Take a Look at College Drinking
National Clearinghouse for Alcohol and Drug Info.
PO Box 2345
Rockville, MD 20847-2345   800-729-6686
                                            www.health.org
This second edition continues CSAP's campaign to raise awareness about the problems of college drinking.

8491 Q&A About Smoking and Health
American Lung Association
1740 Broadway   212-315-8700
New York, NY 10019-4315
Gives fact-crammed answers to questions on smoking and health.

8492 Quick List to Build Pride in Your Communities
National Clearinghouse for Alcohol and Drug Info.
PO Box 2345
Rockville, MD 20847-2345   800-729-6686
This parent guide is an adaptation of CSAP's Be Smart! Quick List: 10 Steps to Help Your Child Say No.

8493 Reducing the Health Risks of Secondhand Smoke
American Lung Association
1740 Broadway   212-315-8700
New York, NY 10019-4315
What a person can do at home, work and in public places to reduce the health risks of secondhand smoke.

8494 Relapse and the Addict
Hazelden
15251 Pleasant Valley Road   651-257-4010
Center City, MN 55012-9640   800-328-9000
                                            Fax: 651-213-4426
                                            www.hazelden.org
Identifies specific stages and triggers of relapse.

8495 Releasing Anger
Hazelden
15251 Pleasant Valley Road   651-257-4010
Center City, MN 55012-9640   800-328-9000
                                            Fax: 651-213-4426
                                            www.hazelden.org
Discusses anger as a normal feeling and how anger can endanger recovery.

8496 Research on Drugs and the Workplace
National Clearinghouse for Alcohol and Drug Info.
PO Box 2345
Rockville, MD 20847-2345   800-729-6686
Discusses prevalence and costs to society of drug use in the workplace, along with information on employee assistance programs, drug testing, grants and additional resources.

8497 Secondhand Smoke
American Lung Association
1740 Broadway   212-315-8700
New York, NY 10019-4315
Documents the effects of tobacco smoke on nonsmokers.

8498 Seven Reasons Not to Use Drugs and Alcohol
American Council On Drug Education
204 Monroe Street
Rockville, MD 20850-4425   800-488-3784
A series of five pamphlets offering information on the hazards of
alcohol, crack, cocaine, steroids and tobacco products.
Grades 4-6

8499 Sexual Intimacy and the Alcoholic Relationship
Al-Anon Family Group Headquarters
1600 Corporate Landing Parkway   757-563-1600
Virginia Beach, VA 23454-5617   800-425-2666
                                       Fax: 757-563-1655
                                  e-mail: wso@al-anon.org
                                     www.al-anon.alateen.org
Sex and alcohol? Al-Anon members face this personal problem
when they apply to the Al-Anon program indexed.
48 pages
Caryn Johnson, Director Communications

8500 Should Tobacco Advertising and Promotion Be Banned?
American Lung Association
1740 Broadway   212-315-8700
New York, NY 10019-4315
Answers many questions about tobacco advertising and promo-
tion, and explains how ads are targeted to vulnerable populations.

8501 Smoke Free Family Promotional Leaflet
American Lung Association
1740 Broadway   212-315-8700
New York, NY 10019-4315
Leaflet and order form describe an entire range of ALA's smok-
ing-related materials.

8502 Smokeless Tobacco: No Way
American Lung Association
1740 Broadway   212-315-8700
New York, NY 10019-4315
Written for junior and senior high school students, this booklet
presents the facts about health risks of smokeless tobacco use.

8503 Smoking and Pregnancy
American Lung Association
1740 Broadway   212-315-8700
New York, NY 10019-4315
Written in a question/answer format, this pamphlet discusses many
issues relating to smoking and pregnancy.

8504 Stop Smoking, Stay Trim
American Lung Association
1740 Broadway   212-315-8700
New York, NY 10019-4315
Outlines how to avoid gaining weight while quitting smoking.

8505 Stop Smoking: A Guide to Your Options
American Lung Association
1740 Broadway   212-315-8700
New York, NY 10019-4315
Describes a variety of approaches to smoking cessation. Offers
guidance on how to choose a program.

8506 Straight Back Home
Hazelden
15251 Pleasant Valley Road   651-257-4010
Center City, MN 55012-9640   800-328-9000
                                       Fax: 651-213-4426
                                          www.hazelden.org
Written for adolescents completing inpatient treatment and return-
ing home.

8507 Stress in Recovery
Hazelden
15251 Pleasant Valley Road   651-257-4010
Center City, MN 55012-9640   800-328-9000
                                       Fax: 651-213-4426
                                          www.hazelden.org
Outlines methods for clients to overcome stress in their daily lives.

8508 This Is AA
Alcoholics Anonymous
PO Box 459   212-870-3400
New York, NY 10163-0459   Fax: 212-870-3137
A pamphlet offering an introduction to the AA recovery program.

8509 Three Talks to Medical Societies
Alcoholics Anonymous
PO Box 459   212-870-3400
New York, NY 10163-0459   Fax: 212-870-3137
Contains Bill Wilson's, the co-founder of AA, principles borrowed
from medicine and religion and a summary of AA's first 23 years.

8510 Time to Start Living
Alcoholics Anonymous
PO Box 459   212-870-3400
New York, NY 10163-0459   Fax: 212-870-3137
Addresses the older alcoholic, with nine stories of men and women
who came to AA after the age of 60 (large print edition is also avail-
able).

**8511 Too Many Young People Drink and Know Too Little About the
Consequences**
National Clearinghouse for Alcohol and Drug Info.
PO Box 2345
Rockville, MD 20847-2345   800-729-6686
Provides up-to-date resources and statistics on the widespread use
of alcohol by youth under 21 years of age.

8512 Too Young?
Alcoholics Anonymous
PO Box 459   212-870-3400
New York, NY 10163-0459   Fax: 212-870-3137
This cartoon pamphlet speaks to teenagers in their own language,
telling the varied drinking stories of six youn people (13 to 18).

8513 Treating Nicotine Addiction
Hazelden
15251 Pleasant Valley Road   651-257-4010
Center City, MN 55012-9640   800-328-9000
                                       Fax: 651-213-4426
                                          www.hazelden.org
Describes the success of one chemical dependency treatment cen-
ter that began treating nicotine as an addiction.

8514 Twelve Steps Illustrated
Alcoholics Anonymous
PO Box 459   212-870-3400
New York, NY 10163-0459   Fax: 212-870-3137
An easy-to-read version of AA's twelve steps.

8515 Twelve Steps for Tobacco Users
Hazelden
15251 Pleasant Valley Road   651-257-4010
Center City, MN 55012-9640   800-328-9000
                                       Fax: 651-213-4426
                                          www.hazelden.org
Presents the Surgeon General's findings that classify nicotine as an
addictive substance.
25 pages

8516 Understanding Depression and Addiction
Hazelden
15251 Pleasant Valley Road   651-257-4010
Center City, MN 55012-9640   800-328-9000
                                       Fax: 651-213-4426
                                          www.hazelden.org
29 pages

8517 Understanding Major Anxiety Disorders and Addiction
Hazelden
15251 Pleasant Valley Road   651-257-4010
Center City, MN 55012-9640   800-328-9000
                                       Fax: 651-213-4426
                                          www.hazelden.org
36 pages

8518 Understanding Ourselves and Alcoholism
Al-Anon Family Group Headquarters

1600 Corporate Landing Parkway
Virginia Beach, VA 23454-5617

757-563-1600
800-425-2666
Fax: 757-563-1655
e-mail: wso@al-anon.org
www.al-anon.alateen.org

Explains how compulsion, obsession and denial affect those close to an alcoholic as well as the alcoholic.
6 pages
Caryn Johnson, Director Communications

8519 Understanding Personality Problems and Addiction
Hazelden
15251 Pleasant Valley Road
Center City, MN 55012-9640

651-257-4010
800-328-9000
Fax: 651-213-4426
www.hazelden.org

Describes common features of personality problems, such as self-centeredness and setting boundaries.
28 pages

8520 Understanding Post-Traumatic Stress Disorder and Addiction
Hazelden
15251 Pleasant Valley Road
Center City, MN 55012-9640

651-257-4010
800-328-9000
Fax: 651-213-4426
www.hazelden.org

17 pages

8521 Unpuffables Promotional Brochure
American Lung Association
1740 Broadway
New York, NY 10019-4315

212-315-8700

Describes the ALA Unpuffables program.

8522 What Are the Signs of Alcoholism?
Hazelden
15251 Pleasant Valley Road
Center City, MN 55012-9640

651-257-4010
800-328-9000
Fax: 651-213-4426
www.hazelden.org

Self-test for clients to review the role of alcohol in their lives.

8523 What Happened to Joe?
Alcoholics Anonymous
PO Box 459
New York, NY 10163-0459

212-870-3400
Fax: 212-870-3137

Dramatic story of a young construction worker and his drinking problem, told in brightly colored comic book style.

8524 What Happens After Treatment?
Al-Anon Family Group Headquarters
1600 Corporate Landing Parkway
Virginia Beach, VA 23454-5617

757-563-1600
800-425-2666
Fax: 757-563-1655
e-mail: wso@al-anon.org
www.al-anon.alateen.org

100 pieces
Caryn Johnson, Director Communications

8525 What is AA?
Hazelden
15251 Pleasant Valley Road
Center City, MN 55012-9640

651-257-4010
800-328-9000
Fax: 651-213-4426
www.hazelden.org

Answers the basic questions about Alcoholics Anonymous.

8526 What is NA?
Hazelden
15251 Pleasant Valley Road
Center City, MN 55012-9640

651-257-4010
800-328-9000
Fax: 651-213-4426
www.hazelden.org

Helps clients evaluate their addiction to narcotics and answers their questions about N.A.

8527 What's Your Cigarette Smoking IQ?
American Lung Association
1740 Broadway
New York, NY 10019-4315

212-315-8700

Brief true-or-false quiz that tests a person's knowledge of the effects of smoking.

8528 When You Go Back to Work
Hazelden
15251 Pleasant Valley Road
Center City, MN 55012-9640

651-257-4010
800-328-9000
Fax: 651-213-4426
www.hazelden.org

Stories demonstrating co-workers' attitudes clients may face upon their return to work.

8529 When Your Teen is in Treatment
Hazelden
15251 Pleasant Valley Road
Center City, MN 55012-9640

651-257-4010
800-328-9000
Fax: 651-213-4426
www.hazelden.org

A guide for parents.

8530 Where Do I Go from Here?
Alcoholics Anonymous
PO Box 459
New York, NY 10163-0459

212-870-3400
Fax: 212-870-3137

For people leaving treatment facilities, single-sheet flyer tells of continuing help offered by outside AAs.

8531 Why Anonymity in Al-Anon?
Al-Anon Family Group
1600 Corporate Landing Parkway
Virginia Beach, VA 23454-5617

757-563-1600
800-425-2666
Fax: 757-563-1655
e-mail: wso@al-anon.org
www.al-anon.alateen.org

12 pages
Caryn Johnson, Director Communications

8532 Workers at Risk: Drugs and Alcohol on the Job
National Clearinghouse for Alcohol and Drug Info.
PO Box 2345
Rockville, MD 20847-2345

800-729-6686

Gives facts about drugs in the workplace and suggests appropriate behavior for employees who are confronted with a coworker's use of alcohol or other drugs.

8533 You Can Help Your Community Get Rid of Drugs
National Clearinghouse for Alcohol and Drug Info.
PO Box 2345
Rockville, MD 20847-2345

800-729-6686

Supports drug abuse treatment and explains how drug use can create problems for your community.

8534 Young Children and Drugs: What Parents Can Do
Wisconsin Clearinghouse
1964 E. Washington Avenue
Madison, WI 53704-5275

8535 Youth and the Alcoholic Parent
Al-Anon Family Group Headquarters
1600 Corporate Landing Parkway
Virginia Beach, VA 23454-5617

757-563-1600
800-425-2666
Fax: 757-563-1655
e-mail: wso@al-anon.org
www.al-anon.alateen.org

Questions and suggestions to help young people improve their own lives.
12 pages
Caryn Johnson, Director Communications

Audio & Video

8536 AA: Rap with Us
Alcoholics Anonymous
PO Box 459
New York, NY 10163-0459

212-870-3400
Fax: 212-870-3137

Features four anonymous young AA members. Rap music and lyrics bridge these four young people's stories of alcoholic despair and A.A. recovery.
16 minutes

8537 Al-Anon Video
Al-Anon Family Group Headquarters
1600 Corporate Landing Parkway   757-563-1600
Virginia Beach, VA 23454-5617   800-425-2666
                                      Fax: 757-563-1655
                                      e-mail: wso@al-anon.org
                                      www.al-anon.alateen.org
12 pages
Caryn Johnson, Director Communications

8538 Al-Anon is for African Americans...and All People of Color
Al-Anon Family Group Headquarters
1600 Corporate Landing Parkway   757-563-1600
Virginia Beach, VA 23454-5617   800-425-2666
                                      Fax: 757-563-1655
                                      e-mail: wso@al-anon.org
                                      www.al-anon.alateen.org
12 pages
Caryn Johnson, Director Communications

8539 Al-Anon's Path to Recovery: Al-Anon is for Americans/Aboriginals
Al-Anon Family Group Headquarters
1600 Corporate Landing Parkway   757-563-1600
Virginia Beach, VA 23454-5617   800-425-2666
                                      Fax: 757-563-1655
                                      e-mail: wso@al-anon.org
                                      www.al-anon.alateen.org
12 pages
Caryn Johnson, Director Communications

8540 Alcoholics Anonymous: An Inside View
Alcoholics Anonymous
PO Box 459   212-870-3400
New York, NY 10163-0459   Fax: 212-870-3137
Depicts alcoholics, recovering in A.A., going about their daily lives, attending A.A. meetings, and other gatherings.
28 minutes

8541 Art of Living with Change: Turning Your Good Intentions Into Progress...
Hazelden
15251 Pleasant Valley Road   651-213-4030
Center City, MN 55012-9640   800-328-0094
                                      Fax: 651-213-4426
                                      www.hazelden.org
45 minutes
ISBN: 0-894868-40-3

8542 Bill Discusses the Twelve Traditions
Alcoholics Anonymous
PO Box 459   212-870-3400
New York, NY 10163-0459   Fax: 212-870-3137
Bill W. tells how the principles safe-guarding A.A. unity developed.
60 minutes

8543 Bill's Own Story
Alcoholics Anonymous
PO Box 459   212-870-3400
New York, NY 10163-0459   Fax: 212-870-3137
Co-founder Bill W. tells of his drinking and recovery.
60 minutes

8544 Caring for Ourselves: Hope for Healthy Relationships
Hazelden
15251 Pleasant Valley Road   651-213-4030
Center City, MN 55012-9640   800-328-0094
                                      Fax: 651-213-4426
                                      www.hazelden.org
50 minutes
ISBN: 0-894866-38-9

8545 Hope: Alcoholics Anonymous
Alcoholics Anonymous
PO Box 459   212-870-3400
New York, NY 10163-0459   Fax: 212-870-3137
Explains the principles of AA: what it is, steps, traditions, sponsorship, and basic recovery tools.
15 minutes

8546 It Sure Beats Sitting in a Cell
Alcoholics Anonymous
PO Box 459   212-870-3400
New York, NY 10163-0459   Fax: 212-870-3137
Filmed inside correctional facilities in the United States and Canada, this film tells the story of four young AA's who were in prison as a result of drinking, yet today are sober.
17 minutes

8547 Markings on the Journey
Alcoholics Anonymous
PO Box 459   212-870-3400
New York, NY 10163-0459   Fax: 212-870-3137
Videocassette depicts 45 years of AA history, using rare materials from our archives.
35 minutes

8548 Men's Work: How to Stop the Violence that Tears Our Lives Apart
Hazelden
15251 Pleasant Valley Road   651-213-4030
Center City, MN 55012-9640   800-328-0094
                                      Fax: 651-213-4426
                                      www.hazelden.org
50 minutes
ISBN: 0-894868-28-4

8549 Secret to a Satisfied Life: The Way You Encounter Life Can Bring Happiness...
Hazelden
15251 Pleasant Valley Road   651-213-4030
Center City, MN 55012-9640   800-328-0094
                                      Fax: 651-213-4426
                                      www.hazelden.org
45 minutes
ISBN: 0-894868-17-9

8550 Women: Coming Out of the Shadows
Elyse A Williams, author
Fanlight Productions
4196 Washington Street   617-469-4999
Boston, MA 02131-1731   800-937-4113
                                      Fax: 617-469-3379
                                      e-mail: fanlight@fanlight.com
                                      www.fanlight.com
Ten women share their personal stories of addiction and recovery.
1991 27 Minutes
ISBN: 1-572950-84-6

8551 Young People and AA
Alcoholics Anonymous
PO Box 459   212-870-3400
New York, NY 10163-0459   Fax: 212-870-3137
Four young AA members describe what it is like drinking, what happened to bring them to AA, and what their lives are like sober today.
28 minutes

Web Sites

8552 AAA Foundation for Traffic Safety
                                      www.aaafts.org
This national organization publishes drinking and traffic safety programs for K-6 and junior high students.

8553 Al-Anon
                                      www.al-anon.alateen.org
The single purpose of this organization is to help families and friends of alcoholics, whether the alcoholic is still drinking or not.

8554 Alateen
A part of the Al-Anon program, Alateen is for teenagers who have been affected by someone else's drinking, whether it be a family member or a friend.

8555 American Council for Drug Education
                                      www.acde.org/
This organization provides information on drug use, publishes books and offers films and curriculum materials for prevention.

8556 CSAP State Liason Program

www.samhsa.gov/centers/csap/csap.html

This program is designed to support alcohol and other drug abuse prevention efforts in the States.

8557 Center for Substance Abuse Prevention

www.samhsa.gov/centers/csap/csap.html

This organization's goal is to connect people and resources with innovative ideas, strategies and programs designed to encourage creative and effective efforts aimed at reducing and eliminating alcohol, tobacco and other drug problems in our society.

8558 Cocaine Anonymous

www.ca.org

A support group based on the twelve steps of Alcoholics Anonymous that focuses specifically on problems of cocaine addiction.

8559 Dentists Concerned for Dentists

www.medhelp.org/amshc/amshc53.htm

A nonprofit organization for chemically dependent Minnesota dentists and concerned others.

8560 Families Anonymous

www.familiesanonymous.org/

Addresses the needs of families who are concerned about a relative with a drug problem and with related behavioral problems.

8561 Hazelden

www.hazelden.com

Organization dedicated to providing quality rehabilitation, education and professional services for chemical dependency and related addictive behaviors.

8562 Healing Well

www.healingwell.com

An online health resource guide to medical news, chat, information and articles, newsgroups and message boards, books, disease-related web sites, medical directories, and more for patients, friends, and family coping with disabling diseases, disorders, or chronic illnesses.

8563 Health Finder

www.healthfinder.gov

Searchable, carefully developed web site offering information on over 1000 topics. Developed by the US Department of Health and Human Services, the site can be used in both English and Spanish.

8564 Healthlink USA

www.healthlinkusa.com

Health information concerning treatment, cures, prevention, diagnosis, risk factors, research, support groups, email lists, personal stories and much more. Updated regularly.

8565 Helios Health

www.helioshealth.com

Online resource for your health information. Detailed information about specific health topics, access to expert advice from our Medical Advisory Board, and up-to-date health news.

8566 Indian Health Service

www.ihs.gov

Charged with providing a comprehensive program of alcoholism and substance abuse prevention and treatment for Native Americans and Alaskan natives.

8567 Lawyers Concerned for Lawyers

www.mnlcl.org/

Organization of recovering lawyers and judges and concerned others. Educates lawyers and judges about the disease of chemical dependency, assists in assessments and arranging interventions and offers lawyer-only AA meetings.

8568 MedicineNet

www.medicinenet.com

An online resource for consumers providing easy-to-read, authoritative medical and health information.

8569 Medscape

www.medscape.com

Medscape offers specialists, primary care physicians, and other health professionals the Web's most robust and integrated medical information and educational tools.

8570 National Clearinghouse for Alcohol and Drug Information

www.health.org

8571 National Council on Alcoholism and Drug Dependence

www.ncadd.org

Provides education, information, help and hope in the fight against addictions. Nationwide network of affiliates, advocates prevention, intervention and treatment, and is committed to ridding the disease of its stigma and its sufferers of their denial and shame.

8572 National Crime Prevention Council

www.ncpc.org

This organization works to prevent crime and drug use in many ways, including developing materials for parents and children.

8573 Office on Smoking and Health

www.cdc.gov/tobacco/

Offers reference services to researchers through the Technical Information Center. Publishes and distributes a number of titles in the field of smoking and health.

8574 Safe Homes

www.yescap.org/safehomes/safehomes.htm

This national organization encourages parents to sign a contract stipulating that when parties are held in one another's homes they will adhere to a strict no-alcohol/no-drug-use rule.

8575 Substance Abuse and Mental Health Services Administration

www.samhsa.gov

The goal of this organization is to reduce incidence and prevalence of mental disorders and substance abuse and improve treatment outcomes for persons suffering from addictive and mental health problems and disorders.

8576 WebMD

www.webmd.com

Information on substance abuse, including articles and resources.

Description

8577 ### Sudden Infant Death Syndrome

Sudden Infant Death Syndrome, SIDS, is the sudden death of an infant or young child that is unexpected and for which there is no demonstrable cause. It is the most common cause of death in children between 1 and 12 months of age, with a peak incidence between the second and fourth month of life. Almost all SIDS deaths occur when the infant is thought to be sleeping.

Despite extensive research, no cause for SIDS has been found, although evidence suggests that it may be related to malfunction of the mechanisms that control the heart function and breathing process. The diagnosis cannot be made without an adequate investigation of the infant after its death. The incidence of SIDS is greater in babies born to mothers who are young, unwed, smoke, have had many births, did not complete high school and have had poor prenatal care. Other possible factors include exposure to cigarette smoke, cold months, soft bedding (lamb's wool), waterbed mattresses, an overheated environment, and being a sibling of a SIDS victim.

Recent studies have indicated that having babies sleep on their backs reduces the risks of SIDS. The American Academy of Pediatrics recommends that infants be placed on their back for sleep. It further advises to avoid overwrapping the infant, remove soft bedding, and avoid smoking during and after pregnancy. In 1994, the Back to Sleep Campaign was launched, a national campaign that encourages that infants be placed to sleep on their backs. Between 1992 and 1996,the rate of SIDS dropped 38 percent and has continued to decrease since then.

Parents who lose a child to SIDS are grief-stricken and, because no definitive cause can be found for their seemingly healthy baby's death, usually have excessive guilt feelings. Bereavement support is necessary not only during the days immediately following the infant's death, but also for at least several months.

National Agencies & Associations

8578 **American SIDS Institute**
509 Augusta Drive
Marietta, GA 30067-8657
770-426-8746
800-232-7437
Fax: 770-426-1369
e-mail: prevent@sids.org
www.sids.org
Dedicated to the prevention of sudden infant death and the promotion of infant health through research clinical services education and family support.
Betty McEnti PhD, Executive Director
Marc Peterzell, Chairman

8579 **Center for Research for Mothers & Children**
National Institute of Child Health & Development
PO Box 3006
Rockville, MD 20847
800-370-5947
800-370-2943
Fax: 866-760-5947
TTY: 888-320-6942
e-mail: NICHDinformationresourcecenter@mail.nih
www.nichd.nih.gov
Mission is to ensure that every person is born healthy and wanted, that women suffer no harmful effects from reproductive processes,

and that all children have the chance to achieve their full potential for healthy and productive lives free from disease.
Duane F Alexander, Director
Christine Ma Banks, Secretary

8580 **Compassionate Friends**
PO Box 3696
Oak Brook, IL 60522
630-990-0010
877-969-0010
Fax: 630-990-0246
e-mail: nationaloffice@compassionatefriends.org
www.compassionatefriends.org
A national organization that offers 600 local chapters that give support to parents and siblings who have experienced the death of a child. Offers monthly support meetings to get through the difficult times and learn how to cope.
Patricia Loder, Executive Director

8581 **National Center for Education in Maternal and Child Health**
Georgetown University
Box 571272
Washington, DC 20057-1272
202-784-9770
Fax: 202-784-9777
e-mail: mchlibrary@ncemch.org
www.ncemch.org
Provides national leadership to the maternal and child health community in three key areas—program development education and state-of-the-art knowledge—to improve the health and well-being of the nation's children and families.
Rochelle Mayer Ed. D, Director

8582 **National Organization for Rare Disorders (NORD)**
55 Kenosia Avenue
Danbury, CT 06810-1968
203-744-0100
800-999-6673
Fax: 203-798-2291
TDD: 203-797-9590
e-mail: orphan@rarediseases.org
www.rarediseases.org
The NORD is a unique federation of voluntary health organizations dedicated to helping people with rare orphan diseases and assisting the organizations that serve them.
E Michael D. Scott, Chair
Carolyn Asbury, PhD, Vice Chair

8583 **Parent Care**
9041 Colgate Street
Indianapolis, IN 46268-1210
Fax: 317-872-5464
This organization was formed in 1982 to improve the neonatal intensive care experience for families and care providers. Provides leadership to promote the development of effective parent support services at the local level.
Sarah Killion, Administrative Director

8584 **Share Pregnancy and Infant Loss Support, Inc.**
The National Share Office
402 Jackson Street
St. Charles, MO 63301
636-947-6164
800-821-6819
Fax: 636-947-7486
e-mail: info@nationalshare.org
www.nationalshare.org
Offers support, resources and education on miscarriage, stillborn and newborn death.
Meridith Byers, MD
Rose Carlson, Program Director

8585 **Sudden Infant Death Syndrome (SIDS) Network**
PO Box 520
Ledyard, CT 06339
86 -89 -704
Fax: 860-887-7309
e-mail: sidsnet1@sids-network.org
www.sids-network.org
Dedicated to eliminate Sudden Infant Death Syndrome through the support of SIDS research projects. Provides support for those who have been touched by the tragedy of Sudden Infant Death Syndrome and to raise public awareness of this event.
Chuck Mihalko, Co-founder and President

8586 **Sudden Infant Death Syndrome Alliance**
2105 Laurel Bush Road
Baltimore, MD 21015-6605
443-640-1049
800-221-7437
Fax: 410-653-8709
e-mail: info@firstcandle.org
www.sidsalliance.org

The purpose of the Alliance is to help parents educate the community about SIDS and to support SIDS research. The Alliance assists parents to organize local chapters and provides services including a newsletter and other literature.
Marian Sokol, President
Deborah Boyd, Executive Director

State Agencies & Associations

Alabama

8587 Bureau of Family Health Services: Alabama Department of Public Health
19 South Jackson Street
201 Monroe Street   334-206-5300
Montgomery, AL 36104   800-252-1818
                                                Fax: 334-269-5200
                                         e-mail: llee@aap.net
                                                   www.adph.org

Linda P Lee, Executive Director

Alaska

8588 SIDS Information and Counseling Program: Alaska Department of Health
350 Main Street, Room 404   907-465-3030
Juneau, AK 99811-3553   Fax: 907-465-3068
                         e-mail: william.hogan@alaska.gov
                                            www.dhss.alaska.gov
Alaska Pioneer Homes assist older Alaskans to have the highest quality of life by providing assisted living in a safe home setting which promotes positive relationships, meaningful activities, physical, emotional and spiritual growth.
William J Streur, Commissioner
Jay Butler, Chief Medical Officer

Arizona

8589 Arizona SIDS Founation
PO Box 1111   520-297-6013
Phoenix, AZ 85001   800-597-7437
                                         e-mail: info@azsidf.org
                                                   www.azsidf.org

Vanessa Seaney, President

8590 Office of Womens And Childrens Health: Alabama Department of Health
State Dapartment of Healths Services
150 N 18th Avenue   602-542-1025
Phoenix, AZ 85007-2602   Fax: 602-542-0883
                                       e-mail: newbers@azdhs.gov
                                                   www.azdhs.gov
The Arizona Department of Health Services promotes and protects the health of Arizona's children and adults. Its mission is to set the standard for personal and community health through direct care, science, public policy, and leadership.
Susan Newber RN, Manager

Arkansas

8591 Arkansas Department of Health: SIDS Information & Counseling Program
4815 W Markham Street
Little Rock, AR 72205-3866   501-661-2000
                                        www.healthyarkansas.com
To protect and improve the health and well-being of allArkansans
Nathaniel Smith, MD, MPH
Dawn Graziani

California

8592 California SIDS Program
11344 Coloma Road   916-851-7437
Gold River, CA 95670-6052   800-369-7437
                                                Fax: 916-851-5937
                                  e-mail: info@californiasids.com
                                            www.californiasids.com

IT is designed to serve the many individuals affected by a SIDS death, and to educate the public about SIDS.
Gwen Edelstein RN,PNP,MPA, Program Director
Cheryl McBride, Program Manager

8593 SIDS Alliance Of Northern California
1547 Palos Verdes Mall   925-274-1109
Walnut Creek, CA 94597   877-938-7437
                                         e-mail: info@sidsnc.org
                                                   www.sidsnc.org
A non-profit, completely volunteer group of SIDS parents and professionals dedicated to family support and community education regarding SIDS.
Lorie Gehrke, President

8594 SIDS Foundation of Southern California
10811 Washington Boulevard   310-558-4511
Culver City, CA 90232   Fax: 310-558-7075
                                      e-mail: sidsfsc@aol.com
                              sidsfoundationofsoutherncalifornia.org
Margot Stern Bennett, Executive Director

Colorado

8595 Colorado SIDS Program
425 S Cherry Street   303-320-7771
Denver, CO 80224   888-285-7437
                                                Fax: 303-320-7827
                                       e-mail: rlouie@hrsa.gov
                                               www.coloradosids.org

Tena Saltzman, Executive Director

8596 Colordao Department of Health and Environment
4300 Cherry Creek Drive S   303-692-2000
Denver, CO 80246-1530   800-886-7689
                                                Fax: 303-782-5576
                                                TTY: 303-691-7700
                        e-mail: cdphe.information@state.co.us
                                               www.cdphe.state.co.us

Martha Rudolph, Director
Karin McGowan, Interim Executive Director

Connecticut

8597 Connecticut SIDS Alliance
PO Box 486   860-626-1542
Torrington, CT 06790   866-574-7437
                                                Fax: 860-496-9919
                                         e-mail: ctsids@aol.com
                                                   www.ctsids.org

Shannon Strandberg, Secretary

8598 SIDS Program: Connecticut Department of Health
410 Capitol Avenue   860-509-8074
Hartford, CT 06134   Fax: 860-509-7720
                             e-mail: marilyn.binns@po.state.ct.us
                              sidsfoundationofsoutherncalifornia.org
Marilyn Binns, Program Coordinator

Delaware

8599 SIDS Information & Counseling: Division of Public Health
1901 N DuPont Highway   302-255-9040
New Castle, DE 19720   Fax: 302-255-4429
                                 e-mail: dhssinfo@state/de/us
                                               www.dhss.delaware.gov
To improve the quality of life for Delaware's citizens by promoting health and well-being, fostering self-sufficiency, and protecting vulnerable populations.
Elaine Marke LCSW BCD, Program Coordinator

District of Columbia

8600 DC Department of Health Maternal and Family Health Administration
Maternal And Family Health Administration

899 North Capitol Street NE
Washington, DC 20002

202-442-5955
Fax: 202-442-4795
TTY: 711
e-mail: doh@dc.gov
www.dchealth.dc.gov

The Mission of the Department of Health is to promote and protect the health, safety and quality of life of residents, visitors and those doing business in the District of Columbia.
Saul M. Levin, M.D., M.P.A., Interim Director
Rosie McLaren, Program Manager

8601 Department of Health and Human Services
200 Independence Avenue SW
Washington, DC 20201

919-715-8430
877-696-6775
e-mail: april.ellis@ncmail.net
www.hhs.gov

The Department of Health and Human Services (HHS) is the United States government's principal agency for protecting the health of all Americans and providing essential human services, especially for those who are least able to help themselves.
April Ellis, SIDS Program Manager

8602 Region III Office Program: Consultants for Maternal and Child Health
Public Ledger Building
2115 Wisconsin Avenue NW
Washington, DC 20007-3309

202-784-9771
Fax: 202-784-9777
e-mail: OHRCinfo@georgetown.edu
www.mchoralhealth.org

The purpose of the National Maternal and Child Oral Health Resource Center (OHRC) is to respond to the needs of states and communities in addressing current and emerging public oral health issues. OHRC supports health professionals, program administrators, educators, policymakers, and others with the goal of improving oral health services for infants, children, adolescents, and their families.
Jolene Bertness, Health Education Specialist
Katrina Holt, Director

8603 Region IV Office Program Consultants for Maternal and Child Health
2115 Wisconsin Avenue
Washington, DC 20007-8909

202-784-9771
Fax: 202-784-9777
e-mail: OHRCinfo@georgetown.edu
www.mchoralhealth.org

The purpose of the National Maternal and Child Oral Health Resource Center (OHRC) is to respond to the needs of states and communities in addressing current and emerging public oral health issues.
E Joseph Alderman DDS MPH, Oral Health Consultant

8604 Region IX Office Program Consultants for Maternal and Child Health
2115 Wisconsin
Washington, DC 94103

202-784-9771
Fax: 202-784-9777
e-mail: OHRCinfo@georgetown.edu
www.mchoralhealth.org

Katrina Holt, Director

8605 Region VIII Office Program Consultants for Maternal and Child Health
2115 Wisconsin Avenue
Washington, DC 80294-1961

202-784-9771
Fax: 202-784-9777
e-mail: OHRCinfo@georgetown.edu
www.mchoralhealth.org

The purpose of the National Maternal and Child Oral Health Resource Center (OHRC) is to respond to the needs of states and communities in addressing current and emerging public oral health issues
Valerie Orla RDH BS, Oral Health Consultant

Florida

8606 Children's Medical Services Program: Florida SIDS Program
4052 Bald Cypress Way
Tallahassee, FL 32399

850-245-4444
Fax: 904-488-2341
e-mail: Health@doh.state.fl.us
www.doh.state.fl.us

To protect, promote & improve the health of all people in Florida through integrated state, county, & community efforts.
Susan Potts, Coordinator

8607 Florida Department of Health
4052 Bald Cypress Way
Tallahassee, FL 32399

850-245-4444
Fax: 850-245-4047
e-mail: Health@doh.state.fl.us
www.doh.state.fl.us

To protect, promote & improve the health of all people in Florida through integrated state, county, & community efforts.
Susan Potts, Coordinator

8608 Florida SIDS Alliance
4044 W Lake Mary Boulevard
Lake Mary, FL 32746

305-232-1640
800-SID-SFLA
Fax: 407-444-5208
e-mail: sidsfla@yahoo.com
www.flasids.com

Steve Bonwit, Officer
Roy Bagley, President

Georgia

8609 Georgia Department of Human Resources: Center for Family Resource Planning
2 Peach Tree Street NW
Atlanta, GA 30303

404-657-3550
Fax: 404-463-6729
e-mail: kotto@dhr.state.ga.us

Provides grief support for parents.
Katherine Ottoel, Coordinator

8610 Georgia Department of Human Resources: Inf ant and Child Health
2 Peach Tree Street NW
Atlanta, GA 30303

404-651-7371
Fax: 404-463-6729
e-mail: kotto@dhr.state.ga.us

Katherine Otto, Coordinator

8611 Georgia SIDS Project
4112-2 E Ponce De Leon Avenue
Clarkston, GA 30021

678-342-3360
Fax: 404-296-7211
e-mail: gasids@mindspring.com
www.sidsga.org

Sudden Infant Death Syndrome is the sudden death of an infant under one year of age which remains unexplained after a thorough case investigation.
Diane Manheim, Director

Hawaii

8612 Hawaii Department of Health: Family Health Division
Child Wellness Program
1250 Punchbowl Street
Honolulu, HI 96813

808-586-4400
Fax: 808-733-9032
e-mail: gwen.palmer@fshd.health.state.hi.us
ww.hawaii.gov/health

Gwen Palmer, Coordinator

Idaho

8613 Idaho Department of Health and Welfare
590 W Washington Street
Boise, ID 83720

208-334-4000
800-632-8000
Fax: 208-334-4015
e-mail: gainord@idhw.state.id.us
www.healthandwelfare.idaho.gov

We offer programs that deal with complex social, economic and individual issues, often helping people in crisis situations. Our programs are designed to strengthen families and promote self-reliance.
Richard Armstrong, Director

Illinois

8614 SIDS of Illinois
6010 Route 53
Lisle, IL 60532
630-541-3901
Fax: 630-541-8246
e-mail: pam@sidsillinois.org
www.sidsillinois.org

Marsha Cooper, President
Anita L. Jordan Johnson, Vice President

8615 Statewide SIDS Program: Illinois Department of Public Health
500 E Monroe Street
Springfield, IL 62761
217-557-2931
Fax: 217-524-2831
e-mail: bbreiden@idph.state.il.us

Babara Breidenbaugh, Program Specialist

Indiana

8616 Indiana State Department of Health Maternal And Child Health Services
Maternal And Child Health Services
2 N Meridian Street
Indianapolis, IN 46204
317-233-1325
800-457-8283
Fax: 317-233-1300
e-mail: bmjohnso@isdh.state.in.us
www.in.gov/hpb

Beth Johnson, Nurse Consultant

8617 SIDS Center of Indiana
1810 Broad Ripple Avenue
Indianapolis, IN 46220
317-254-9255
Fax: 317-254-9266
e-mail: sidscenter@insids.org

Our mission is to be a resource center that supports parents, families and friends in communities across the state whose lives are touched by sudden, unexpected infant death.
John Schutt, Chairperson

Iowa

8618 Iowa SIDS Alliance
406 SW School Street
Ankeny, IA 50023
515-965-7655
866-480-4741
Fax: 515-964-7506
e-mail: info@iowasids.org
www.iowasids.org

The Iowa Sudden Infant Death Syndrome Foundation is a statewide, non-profit, voluntary health organization dedicated to providing emotional support to SIDS and SUID familiesresidingin Iowa, educating professionals and the general public about SIDS and risk reduction, and funding medical research into the causes of SIDS.
Patty Keeley, Executive Director
Jennifer Atzen, President

8619 Iowa SIDS Program Iowa Department of Public Health
Iowa Department of Public Health
321 E 12th Street
Des Moines, IA 50319-0075
515-281-7689
866-227-9878
www.idph.state.ia.us

Promoting and protecting the health of Iowans
Jane Borst, Bureau Chief
Sally Clausen

Kansas

8620 Kansas Department of Health & Environment Bureau of Family Health
Bureau Of Children, Youth And Families
1000 SW Jackson Street
Topeka, KS 66612-1274
786-296-1500
800-332-6262
Fax: 785-296-6553
e-mail: info@kdheks.gov
www.kdheks.gov

To protect and improve the health and environment of all Kansans.
Robert Moser, Director
Kobi Gomel, Administrative Specialist

8621 SIDS Network of Kansas
1148 S Hillside
Wichita, KS 67211
316-682-1301
866-399-7437
Fax: 316-682-1274
e-mail: info@sidsks.org
www.kidsks.org

Christy Schunn, LSCSW, Executive Director
Amanda Yoder, Communications Assistant

Kentucky

8622 Department of Public Health: Adult and Child Health Division
275 E Main Street
Frankfort, KY 40621
502-564-3236
800-372-2973
Fax: 502-564-8389
TTY: 800-627-4702
e-mail: marcia.burkow@ky.gov

Marcia Burkow, SIDS Coordinator

8623 SIDS Network of Kentucky
PO Box 186
Caneyville, KY 42721-3555
800-928-7437
Fax: 859-245-0717
e-mail: info@sidsky.org
www.sidsky.org

Supporting family members and others who have been touched by the tragedy of a sids or other infants death.
Adrienne Grizzell, Executive Director

Louisiana

8624 Office of Public Health
628 N 4th Street
Baton Rouge, LA 70802
225-342-9500
Fax: 225-342-5568
e-mail: hhwebadmin@la.gov
www.dhh.louisiana.gov/offices/?ID=79

Tracy Hubbard, Coordinator

8625 Public Health Services of Louisiana
628 N 4th Street
Baton Rouge, LA 70802-0629
225-342-9500
Fax: 225-342-5568
e-mail: dhhwebadmin@la.gov
www.dhh.state.la.us/

The mission of the Department of Health and Hospitals is to protect and promote health and to ensure access to medical, preventive and rehabilitative services for all citizens of the State of Louisiana.
Jamie Roques RNC, SIDS Coordinator
Courtney Phillips, Deputy Secretary

Maine

8626 Department of Human Services
221 State Street
Augusta, ME 04333-0001
207-287-3707
Fax: 207-287-3005
TTY: 800-606-0215
www.state.me.us/dhs/

Brenda Harvey, Commissioner

8627 Maine SIDS Foundation
14 Charlonate Drive
Gray, ME 04039
207-657-2220
Fax: 207-657-3737
e-mail: roybagley@aol.com
www.sidsalliance.org

Roy Bagley, Chairperson

8628 Maine SIDS Program Department Of Human Services
Department Of Human Services
200 Main Street
Lewiston, ME 04240
207-795-4450
Fax: 207-795-4445
e-mail: luanne.crinion@maine.gov

Luanne Crinion, Program Coordinator

Maryland

8629 First Candle
2105 Laurel Bush Road
Bel Air, MD 21015
Fax: 651-310-2106
TTY: 800-221-7437
e-mail: info@firstcandle.org
www.sidsalliance.org

First Candle is a leading national nonprofit organization dedicated to safe pregnancies and the survival of babies through the first years of life. Current priorities are to eliminate Stillbirth, Sudden Infant Death Syndrome (SIDS) and other Sudden Unexpected Infant Deaths (SUID) with programs of research, education and advocacy
Michael J. Schaffer, President
Kelly Neal Mariotti, Chief Executive Officer

8630 Maryland SIDS Information & Counseling Program
22 S Green Street   410-328-8667
Baltimore, MD 21201   800-492-5538
                                     TTY: 410-328-9600
                                     TDD: 410-328-9600
                        e-mail: webmaster@umm.edu
                               www.marylandsids.com
UMMC exists to serve the state and region as a tertiary/quaternary care center, to serve the local community with a full range of care options, to educate and train the next generation of health care providers, and to be a site for world-class clinical research.
Jeffrey A Rivest, President and Chief Executive Officer
R Keith Allen, Senior Vice President

Massachusetts

8631 Region I Office Program: Consultants for Maternal and Child Health
John F Kennedy Building   617-899-1355
Boston, MA 02203   Fax: 202-833-8288
                        e-mail: Mary.Foley@mcphs.edu
                               www.mchoralhealth.org
Mary Foley RDH MPH, Oral Health Consultant

Michigan

8632 Apnea Identification Program Children's Hospital of Michigan
Children's Hospital of Michigan
3901 Beaubien Street   313-745-5437
Detroit, MI 48201-2196   888-DMC-2500
                               www.childrensdmc.org
To provide the highest quality of care for children, to inform that care through research innovations, and to ensure that children have access to the care they need.
Karen Branif RN MSW, Nurse Specialist

8633 Genesee County Health Department
630 S Saignaw Street   810-257-3612
Flint, MI 48502-3915   Fax: 810-257-3147
                        e-mail: gchd-info@gchd.us
                                        www.gchd.us

Kay Doerr, Chairperson
Brenda Clack, Vice-Chairperson

8634 Kent County Health Department
300 Monroe Avenue NE
Grand Rapids, MI 49503-1996   616-632-7590
                               www.accesskent.com
The mission of Kent County government is to be an effective and efficient steward in delivering quality services for our diverse community. Our priority is to provide mandated services, which may be enhanced and supplemented by additional services to improve the quality of life for all our citizens within the constraints of sound fiscal policy.
Colleen Jill RN, SIDs Coordinator
David Kraker

8635 Michigan Department of Community Health
3423 MLK Boulevard   517-373-1820
Lansing, MI 48909   Fax: 517-373-2129
                        e-mail: lauberc@michigan.gov
                                        www.michigan.gov

Cheryl Lauber, Coordinator

8636 Oakland County Health Division: SIDS Project
1200 N Telegraph   248-858-1280
Pontiac, MI 48341-0482   800-774-4542
                                     Fax: 248-858-0178
                                     TTY: 248-452-2247
                                     TDD: 248-452-2247
                        e-mail: oakllbph@oakland.lib.mi.us
                                        www.oakgov.com

David Conklin, Librarian
George J Miller Jr MA, Director

8637 SIDS LEAD: Children's Special Health Care Services
Michigan Department of Public Health
201 Townsend Street   517-373-3740
Lansing, MI 48913-2934   TTY: 517-373-3573
                                     TDD: 517-373-3573
                        e-mail: norris@michigan.gov
                               www.michigan.gov/mdch
Improving the experience of care, improving the health of populations, and reducing per capita costs of health care
Janet Olszewski, Director
Ed Dore, Chief Deputy Director

Minnesota

8638 Minnesota Sudden Infant Death Center Minneapolis Children's Medical Center
Minneapolis Children's Medical Center
2525 Chicago Avenue   612-813-6000
Minneapolis, MN 55404-4518   Fax: 612-813-7344
                e-mail: kathleen.fernbach@childreansHC.org
                        www.childrensmn.org/Communities/SIDs.asp
Sara Schumacher, Project Coordinator

Mississippi

8639 Mississippi SIDS Alliance
5454 I-55 North
Jackson, MS 39211-2170   877-471-7437
                        e-mail: mssids@jam.rr.com
                               www.sidsalliance.org

Scott Parrish, President
Brian Roach, Vice President

8640 Mississippi State Department of Health and Child Health Services
570 E Woodrow Wilson   601-576-7400
Jackson, MS 39216   866-458-4948
                                     Fax: 601-576-7498
                e-mail: Linda.Proctor@msdh.state.ms.us
                               www.msdh.state.ms.us

Linda Proctor, Coordinator

Missouri

8641 Region VII Office Program: Consultants for Maternal and Child Health
Federal Building
10031 Perry Drive   913-888-1377
Overland Park, KS 66212-2826   Fax: 816-426-3633
                        e-mail: lwalker17@kc.rr.com
                               www.mchoralhealth.org
Lawrence Wal DDS MPH, Oral Health Consultant

8642 SIDS Resources
1120 S Sixth Street   314-822-2323
Saint Louis, MO 63104   800-421-3511
                                     Fax: 314-588-0850
                        e-mail: lahrens@sidsresources.org
                               www.sidsresources.org
The mission of SIDS Resources, Inc. is to promote safe practices which reduce the risk of infant death and to provide bereavement support for families who have lost babies.
Lori Behrens, Executive Director
Ellen Reynolds, Program Coordinator

635

8643 Western Region SIDS Resources
4051 Broadway
Kansas City, MO 64111
816-569-6956
Fax: 816-753-6906
e-mail: slogan@sidsresources.org
www.sidsalliance.org
Provides free supportive services and education to those affected by the sudden and unexpected death of an infant - birth through 12 months. Provides education and support to professionals and communities regarding healthy and safe infant care practices and safe sleep for infants
Shay Logan, Program Coordinator

Montana

8644 Department of Public Health and Human Services
1400 Broadway
Helena, MT 59620
406-444-3565
800-232-4636
Fax: 406-444-2606
e-mail: WMcGraw@state.mt.us
www.dphhs.mt.gov

Richard H. Opper, Director
Peggy Baker, Administrative Aide

Nebraska

8645 Nebraska Department of Health Perinatal Child and Adolescent Health
301 Centennial Mall South
Lincoln, NE 68509
402-471-0165
Fax: 402-471-7049
e-mail: jan.heusinkvelt@hhss.ne.gov
Jan Heusinkvelt, RN, BSN, Community Health Nurse

8646 Nebraska SIDS Foundation University of Nebraska Medical Center
University of Nebraska Medical Center
PO Box 460905
Papillion, NE 68046
402-431-8076
e-mail: board@nesids.org
www.nesids.com

Nevada

8647 Nevada State Health Division Bureau of Family Health Services
Bureau Of Family Health Services
3427 Goni Road
Carson City, NV 89706
775-684-4285
Fax: 775-684-4245
e-mail: chuth@nvhd.state.nv.us
www.health2k.state.nv.us
Cynthia Huthht, Health Program Specialist

New Hampshire

8648 New Hampshire SIDS Program
New Hampshire Division of Public Health Services
29 Hazen Drive
Concord, NH 03301
603-271-4536
Fax: 603-271-4519
e-mail: sidsnet1@sids-network.org
www.sids-network.org

Audrey Knigh MSN CPNP, SIDS Coordinator

New Jersey

8649 New Jersey Department of Health: Child Health Program
PO Box 360
Trenton, NJ 08625
609-292-7837
800-367-6543
e-mail: lindajones@doh.state.nj.us
www.state.nj.us/health
The mission of the department of health is to improve health through leadership and innovation.
Linda Jones Hicks, Director
Shirley White-Walker, Chair

8650 New Jersey SIDS Alliance
15 Meadowbrook Road
Boonton Township, NJ 07005
973-299-6523
e-mail: njsids@yahoo.com
www.sidsalliance.org

Genny Elias-Warren, Chairperson

8651 SIDS Center of New Jersey
1 Robert Wood Johnson Place
New Brunswick, NJ 08903-1766
732-249-2160
800-704-7437
Fax: 732-235-6609
e-mail: hegyith@umdnj.edu
www2.umdnj.edu/sids
Provide public health education to reduce the risk of sudden infant death
Thomas Hegyi MD, Co-Medical Director
Barbara Ostf PhD, Program Director

New Mexico

8652 New Mexico SIDS Information and Counseling Program
University of New Mexico School of Medicine
2500 Marble NE
Albuquerque, NM 87131
505-277-3053
Fax: 505-272-3601
e-mail: sidsnet1@sids-network.org
www.sids-network.org

Beverly Whit RN MS, Director

New York

8653 NYS Center for Sudden Infant Death: Eastern Satellite Office
Albany Medical College
47 New Scotland Avenue
Albany, NY 12208
518-262-5918
Fax: 518-262-7237
e-mail: whittrm@mail.amc.edu
Mary Whittredge, Regional Coordinator

8654 New York City Center for SIDS
New York City Satellite Office
520 1st Avenue
New York, NY 10016
212-686-8854
800-522-5006
Fax: 212-532-6564
e-mail: evelyne.longchamp@sids1.ssw.sunysb.edu
Judith Gaine CSW PhD, SIDS Program Director

8655 New York State Center for SIDS: School of Social Welfare
Stony Brook University
101 Nicolls Road
Stony Brook, NY 11794-0001
631-444-4000
800-336-7437
Fax: 631-444-6475
e-mail: marie.chandick@stonybrook.edu
www.hsc.stonybrook.edu
Stony Brook Medicine expresses our shared mission of research, clinical care and education - a mission embraced by our faculty, staff, researchers, and students. It is the embodiment of everything we do on behalf of the health of patients - not only here in our community, but also in the region and worldwide.
Marie Chandi CSW, Associate Project Director

8656 Region II Office Program: Consultants for Maternal and Child Health
345 E 24th Street
New York, NY 10010-0004
212-998-9654
Fax: 212-995-4364
e-mail: ngh1@nyu.edu
www.mchoralhealth.org

Neal Herman DDS, Oral Health Consultant

8657 WNYS Center for SIDS
3580 Harlem Road
Buffalo, NY 14215
716-837-5189
Fax: 716-836-1578
e-mail: jwalkden@palliativecare.org
www.sidsalliance.org

Jan Walkden, Family Service Coordinator

North Carolina

8658 SIDS Alliance of the Carolinas
306 Lucas Park Drive
Greensboro, NC 27455
336-545-3348
e-mail: sandylkennedy@hotmail.com
www.sidsalliance.org

Sandy Kennedy, Chairperson

North Dakota

8659 North Dakota SIDS Alliance
128 Apollo Avenue
Bismarck, ND 58503

701-530-2507
Fax: 701-223-0440
e-mail: ndsids@btinet.net
www.sidsalliance.org

Barb Delvo, Chairperson

8660 North Dakota SIDS Management Program
Division of Maternal and Child Health
600 E Boulevard Avenue
Bismarck, ND 58505-0200

701-328-2372
800-472-2286
Fax: 701-328-4727
e-mail: kchintz@nd.gov
www.ndhealth.gov

Provides support education and follow-up to parents/caregivers family and childcare providers suffering a sudden infant death
Kjersti Hintz, Program Director
Terry Dwelle, MD

Ohio

8661 District Board of Health: Mahoning County
50 Westchester Drive
Youngstown, OH 44515

330-270-2855
800-873-MCHD
Fax: 330-270-2860
TTY: 800-750-0750
e-mail: mchealth@cboss.com
www.mahoning-health.org

The mission of the District Board of Health is to promote and protect the health of individuals and communities, to create a safer, healthier environment, and to improve quality of life
Lisa Weiss MD, Forum Health
Bev Fisher, Manager

8662 Ohio Department of Health
Child Fatality Review
246 N High Street
Columbus, OH 43215

614-466-3543
866-634-7654
Fax: 614-564-2433
e-mail: SmkInfo@odh.ohio.gov
www.odh.ohio.gov

Theodore E. Wymyslo, Director
Frances Veverka, RS MPH, Ohio Health Commissioners

8663 SIDS Network of Ohio
421 Graham Road
Cuyahoga Falls, OH 44221

800-477-7437
Fax: 330-929-0593
e-mail: SIDNetwork@sidsohio.org
www.sidsohio.org

The SID Network of Ohio promotes infant safety in an effort to reduce the rate of SIDS and Sudden Unexpected Infant Death (SUID). We accomplish this through the promotion of infant health and wellness, community education and medical research. We also provide supportive services to those who have been affected by the sudden loss of a child age 2 and under.
Leslie Redd, Executive Director
Jennifer Connolly, Development Coordinator

Oklahoma

8664 Oklahoma State Department of Health: Maternal and Child Health Services
1000 NE 10th Street
Oklahoma City, OK 73117-1207

405-524-3468
800-955-3468
Fax: 405-271-9202
e-mail: paulaw@health.ok.gov
www.ok.gov

As the official Internet gateway of Oklahoma, we are committed to providing citizens and businesses with efficient online access to government.
Paula Wood, Executive Assistant
Suzanna Dooley

Oregon

8665 Oregon Department of Human Services
500 Summer Street NE
Salem, OR 97301

503-945-5944
Fax: 503-378-2897
TTY: 503-945-6214
e-mail: dhs.info@state.or.us
www.oregon.gov

Joyce Edmonds, Public Nurse Consultant

Pennsylvania

8666 Pennsylvania Department of Health Bureau of Family Health
Bureau of Family Health
625 Forster Street
Harrisburg, PA 17120

717-772-2762
877-PAH-EALT
Fax: 717-772-0323
e-mail: bcaboot@state.pa.us
www.dsf.health.state.pa.us

Robert Torres, Deputy Secretary for Administration
Michael Wolf, Secretary

8667 SIDS of Pennsylvania
810 River Avenue
Pittsburgh, PA 15212

412-322-5680
800-721-7437
Fax: 412-481-5968
e-mail: sidspa@aol.com
www.cribsforkids.org

Cribs for Kidsr has been making an impact on the rates of babies dying of accidental death due to unsafe sleeping environmentsby educating parents on the importance of safe sleep practices and by providing Graco Pack 'n Play portable cribs to families who, otherwise, cannot otherwise afford a safe place for their babies to sleep.
Judith A Bannon, Executive Director
Joseph T Dominick, RN, Chairman

Rhode Island

8668 Rhode Island Department of Health
3 Capitol Hill
Providence, RI 02908

401-222-5960
800-942-7434
Fax: 401-222-6548
TTY: 711
e-mail: DOH@health.ri.gov
www.health.state.ri.us

David R Gifford MD MPH, Director
Donald L Carcieri, Governor

South Carolina

8669 Division of Perinatal Systems Mills Jarret Complex
Mills Jarret Complex
Box 101106
Columbia, SC 29211

803-898-0734
Fax: 803-898-2065
e-mail: swansokm@dhec.sc.gov

Kathy Swanson, State FIMR Director

South Dakota

8670 South Dakota Department of Health
Health Building
600 E Capitol Avenue
Pierre, SD 57501

605-773-3361
800-738-2301
Fax: 605-773-5509
e-mail: DOH.info@state.sd.us
www.doh.sd.gov

Nancy Shoup, Program Coordinator

Tennessee

8671 Tenessee Department of Health
Division of Maternal & Child Health
425 5th Avenue N
Nashville, TN 37243-4701

615-741-3111
Fax: 615-741-1063
e-mail: tn.health@tn.gov
health.state.tn.us

The Department of Health works to promote, protect and improve the health and well-being of Tennesseans
John J. Dreyzehner, MD, MPH, Commissioner

8672 Tennessee SIDS Alliance
373 Woodcrest Drive
Kingsport, TN 37663
423- 23- 821
e-mail: lisasids@cs.com
ww.sidsalliance.org

The SID Alliance of TN's mission is as a volunteer. non-profit organization dedicated to the support and service of all Tennessee SIDS families and friends.
Lisa Hunt, Chairperson

Texas

8673 Department of State Health Offices
Title V And Health Resources
100 West 49th Street
Austin, TX 78756
512-776-7111
888-963-7111
Fax: 512-458-7650
e-mail: chan.mcdermott@dshs.state.tx.us
www.dshs.state.tx.us

To improve health and well-being in Texas
David L. Lakey, MD

8674 Greater Houston Chapter SIDS Alliance
916 Satsuma Street
Pasadena, TX 77506
713-924-1419
Fax: 281-541-5340
e-mail: anita.carmona@us.rhodia.com
www.sidsalliance.org

Anita Carmona, Chairperson

8675 Harris County Public Health and Environmental Services
2223 W Lop S
Houston, TX 77027
713-439-6000
e-mail: publicinfo@hd.co.harris.tx.us
www.hcphes.org

Promoting a Healthy and Safe Community.
Herminia Palacio, Executive Director

8676 Region VI Office Program Consultants for Maternal and Child Health
1301 Young Street
Dallas, TX 75202-4325
214-767-3003
Fax: 214-767-3038
e-mail: geurink@zeecon.com
www.mchoralhealth.org

Kathy Geurin RDH BS MA, Oral Health Consultant

8677 Southwest SIDS Research Institute
Brazosport Memorial Hospital
230 Parking Way
Lake Jackson, TX 77566
979-297-2101
www.swsids.com

Our mission is to end unexpected infant mortality through education, support, medical servicesandresearch.

ISBN: 9-792992-81-4
Richard A. Hardoin, MD
Judith A. Henslee, LMSW, Executive Director

Utah

8678 Utah Department of Health
Child Adolescent & School Health Program
288 N 1460 W
Salt Lake City, UT 84116-3231
801-538-6003
Fax: 801-538-6200
www.health.utah.gov

The mission of the Utah Department of Health is to protect the public's health through preventing avoidable illness, injury, disability and premature death; assuring access to affordable, quality health care; and promoting healthy lifestyles.
David Sundwa MD, Executive Director
A Richard Melton, Deputy Director

8679 Utah SIDS Alliance
1760 American Park Circle
W Valley City, UT 84119
801-487-7800
Fax: 801-487-4477
e-mail: lisa.hughes@fnwmail.com
www.sidsalliance.org

Lisa Hughes, President
Troy Hughes, Co-President

Vermont

8680 Vermont Department of Health: SIDS Information and Counseling Program
108 Cherry Street
Burlington, VT 05402
802-652-2000
Fax: 802-652-2005
TTY: 800-253-0191
e-mail: kkelehe@vdh.state.vt.us
healthvermont.gov

Kathy Keleher, Assistant Director Public Health

Virginia

8681 SIDS Mid-Atlantic
PO Box 799
Haymarket, VA 20168
703-955-6899
Fax: 703-933-9101
e-mail: bconnal@aol.com
www.sidsma.org

Betty Connal, Executive Director

8682 Virginia SIDS Alliance
PO Box 752
Mechanicsville, VA 23111
Fax: 757-548-7074
e-mail: mail@vasids.org
www.vasids.org

Terri Newman, President
Mark Ferraro, Vice President

8683 Virginia SIDS Program: Virginia Department of Health
Virginia Department of Health
109 Governor Street
Richmond, VA 23219
804-846-7772
Fax: 804-973-9498
e-mail: WomensAndInfantsHealth@vdh.virginia.gov
www.vdh.virginia.gov

Virginia Health Information' is a resource for patients and consumers looking to learn about and compare options on everything from obstetrical services, to heart care, to pricing information on commonly performed medical procedures.
Robert Stroube, Commissioner
Rosanne Kolesar, Deputy Commissioner Public Health

Washington

8684 Region X Office Program Consultants for Maternal and Child Health
2201 Sixth Avenue
Seattle, WA 98121-1857
206-615-2518
Fax: 206-615-2500
e-mail: rslayton@acf.hhs.gov
www.mchoralhealth.org

Rebecca Slay DDS PhD, Oral Health Consultant

8685 SIDS Foundation of Washington
4649 Sunnyside Avenue N
Seattle, WA 98103
206-548-9290
800-533-0376
Fax: 206-548-9445
e-mail: info@nwsids.org
www.nisa-sids.org

The Northwest Infant Survival & SIDS Alliance is dedicated to reducing the risk of sudden unexpected infant death through education and supporting research while providing bereavement services.
Krista Cossa Sandberg, Executive Director
Lindsey Hulet, Office Administrator

8686 SIDS Northwest Regional Center
Washington Department of Health
111 Israel Rd SE
Olympia, WA 98501-7880
360-236-3502
800-533-0376
Fax: 360-236-2323
e-mail: mch.support@doh.wa.gov
www.doh.wa.gov

The Department of Health works to protect and improve the health of people in Washington State.
Lorrie Grevstad

West Virginia

8687 Office of Maternal, Child & Family Health
Bureau For Public Health

350 Capitol Street
Charelston, WV 25301   304-558-7997
     Fax: 304-558-3510
     e-mail: annmunson@wvdhhr.org
Ann Munson, SIDS Coordinator

Wisconsin

8688   **Infant Death Center of Wisconsin**
Childrens Hospital Of Wisconsin
620 S. 76th St   414-292-4000
Milwaukee, WI 53214   Fax: 414-213-4952
     e-mail: aharvieux@chw.org
     www.idcw.org

Karen Ordinana, Executive Director
Matt Crespin, Associate Director

Wyoming

8689   **Wyoming Department of Health**
Community & Family Health Section
401 Hathaway Building   307-777-7656
Cheyenne, WY 82002   Fax: 307-777-7439
     e-mail: mirandie.peterson@health.wyo.gov
     wdh.state.wy.us
Our mission is to promote, protect, and enhance the health of all Wyoming citizens. The Wyoming Department of Health is the primary state agency for providing health and human services. We administer programs maintaining the health and safety of all citizens of Wyoming and our primary approach in solving health problems is prevention.
Thomas O. Forslund, Director
Heather Babbitt, Senior Administrator

Research Centers

8690   **Massachusetts Sudden Infant Death Syndrome Boston City Hospital**
Boston City Hospital
1 Boston Medical Center Place   617-638-8000
Boston, MA 02118   Fax: 617-534-5555
     www.bmc.org
A joint program of Boston City Hospital and Children's Hospital. Services provided include around-the-clock availability for consultation to health professionals and families counseling of families parent group meetings and supportive home visits.

8691   **Pediatric Pulmonary Unit Massachusetts General Hospital**
Massachusetts General Hospital
55 Fruit Street   617-726-2000
Boston, MA 02114   Fax: 617-242-03
     TTY: 617-724-8800
     www.massgeneral.org
Sudden infant death syndrome and childhood disorders research.
Paul S Russell, MD

8692   **Sudden Infant Death Syndrome Institute of the University of Maryland**
22 S Green Street   410-538-3363
Baltimore, MD 21201   800-492-5538
     www.umm.edu

Dr M John O'Brien MB, Director
Jeffrey A Rivest, FACHE, President and Chief Executive Officer

8693   **USC: Neonatology Research Units**
1240 Mission Road   213-226-3408
Los Angeles, CA 90033   Fax: 213-226-3440
Focuses on clinical problems of the newborn and premature infant.
Paul YK Wu MD, Director

Support Groups & Hotlines

8694   **National Center for the Prevention of SIDS**
1314 Bedford Avenue
Baltimore, MD 21208-6605   800-638-7437
Offers medical updates and information on prevention of SIDS and other disorders to parents and professionals.

8695   **National Health Information Center**
PO Box 1133   310-565-4167
Washington, DC 20013   800-336-4797
     Fax: 301-984-4256
     e-mail: info@nhic.org
     www.health.gov/nhic
Offers a nationwide information referral service, produces directories and resource guides.

8696   **Parents Helping Parents A Family Resource Center**
1400 Parkmoor Avenue   408-727-5775
San Jose, CA 95126   855-727-5775
     Fax: 408-286-1116
     www.php.com
A group of parents and professionals committed to alleviating some of the problems, hardships and concerns of families with children having special needs.
Mary Ellen Peterson, Director

8697   **SIDS Information and Referral Hotline**
SIDS Alliance
2105 Laurel Bush Road   443-640-1049
Baltimore, MD 21015   800-221-7437
     Fax: 410-653-8709
     www.firstcandle.org
Twenty-four hour information and referral line for parents who wish to discuss their concerns with a SIDS counselor, request additional information about SIDS and to receive referrals to the local SIDS affiliate in their area.
Deborah Boyd, Director

8698   **SIDS Support Group**
Massachusetts Center for SIDS
Boston Medical Center   617-638-8000
Boston, MA 02118   800-641-7437
     www.bmc.org
Aids in the resolution of the early trauma of grief experienced by parents following the sudden unexpected death of their infant. The purposes are to provide a safe environemnt for parents to express their feelings, to provide contact with others who share their grief and are at various stages of resolution, to provide a reliable source of information about SIDS and to provide the opportunity to go on to help others.

Books

8699   **Apparent Life-Threatening Event and Sudden Infant Death Syndrome**
National Maternal and Child Health Clearinghouse
2070 Chain Bridge Road   703-442-9051
Vienna, VA 22182-2588   888-275-4772
     Fax: 703-821-2098
     e-mail: ask@hrsa.gov
     www.ask.hrsa.gov
Provides information about ALTE and its relationship to SIDS.

8700   **Hospice Care for Children**
Oxford University Press
2001 Evans Road   212-726-6000
Cary, NC 27513-2010   800-451-7556
     Fax: 919-677-1303
     www.oup-usa.org
A comprehensive book offering the most inclusive and up-to-date information about caring for terminally ill children and their families.
304 pages
ISBN: 0-195073-12-6
Ann Armstrong-Dailey, Editor

8701   **Professional's Role in Sudden Infant Death Syndrome**
National Maternal and Child Health Clearinghouse
2070 Chain Bridge Road   703-442-9051
Vienna, VA 22182-2588   888-275-4772
     Fax: 703-821-2098
     e-mail: ask@hrsa.gov
     www.ask.hrsa.gov
Contains abstracts of articles on the role of professionals in SIDS.

8702 Smoking and Sudden Infant Death Syndrome
National Maternal and Child Health Clearinghouse
2070 Chain Bridge Road 703-442-9051
Vienna, VA 22182-2588 888-275-4772
Fax: 703-821-2098
e-mail: ask@hrsa.gov
www.ask.hrsa.gov
Contains abstracts of materials about tobacco use, its relationship to SIDS and the dangers to the unborn and the newly born from passive and secondary smoking.

Newsletters

8703 Newsletter: SIDS
Massachusetts Center For SIDS
1 Boston Medical Center Place
Boston, MA 02118-2905 617-414-8504
www.bmc.org/program/sids/
Offers information on SIDS, articles pertaining to the latest information available on the mystery condition, latest research and fund-raising news and professional resources available.
Monthly

8704 Parent Care News Brief
Parent Care
303 Watts Branch Parkway 301-294-9338
Rockville, MD 20850-1210 Fax: 301-294-8848
e-mail: drscott@parentcare.com
www.parentcare.com
Features articles and medical updates pertaining to the care of the critically ill child.
Quarterly

Pamphlets

8705 Crib Death: The Sudden Infant Death Syndrome
US Department Of Health & Human Services
202 Independence Avenue SW 202-619-0257
Washington, DC 20201-0001 877-696-6775
e-mail: hhsmail@os.dhhs.gov
www.os.dhhs.gov
Offers information on the most frequently asked questions pertaining to SIDS and crib death.
Kristen Brett
Kathy McKnight

8706 Developmental Delays and Developmental Disorders
National Maternal and Child Health Clearinghouse
2070 Chain Bridge Road 703-442-9051
Vienna, VA 22182-2588 888-275-4772
Fax: 703-821-2098
e-mail: ask@hrsa.gov
www.ask.hrsa.gov
Contains abstracts of selected articles on developmental delays and developmental disorders and the relationship to SIDS.
1997

8707 Facts About SIDS
Sudden Infant Death Syndrome Alliance
1314 Bedford Avenue 410-653-8226
Baltimore, MD 21208-6605 800-221-7437
Fax: 410-653-8709
Offers information on basic facts, answers to the most frequently asked questions about SIDS and information on numbers to call and referral centers for more help.

8708 Grief of Children After the Loss of a Sibling or Friend
National Maternal and Child Health Clearinghouse
2070 Chain Bridge Road 703-442-9051
Vienna, VA 22182-2588 888-275-4772
Fax: 703-821-2098
e-mail: ask@hrsa.gov
www.ask.hrsa.gov
Discusses some of the common expressions of childrens grief and offers ways adults can help during the grieving process.
1995

8709 Infant Positioning and Sudden Infant Death Syndrome
National Maternal and Child Health Clearinghouse
2070 Chain Bridge Road 703-442-9051
Vienna, VA 22182-2588 888-275-4772
Fax: 703-821-2098
e-mail: ask@hrsa.gov
www.ask.hrsa.gov
Contains abstracts of selected articles on the topic of sleep position and SIDS.
1994

8710 Nationwide Survey of Sudden Infant Death Syndrome (SIDS) Service
National Maternal and Child Health Clearinghouse
2070 Chain Bridge Road 703-442-9051
Vienna, VA 22182-2588 888-275-4772
Fax: 703-821-2098
e-mail: ask@hrsa.gov
www.ask.hrsa.gov
Analysis of availability of SIDS services.
1994

8711 Parents and the Grieving Process
National Maternal and Child Health Clearinghouse
2070 Chain Bridge Road 703-442-9051
Vienna, VA 22182-2588 888-275-4772
Fax: 703-821-2098
e-mail: ask@hrsa.gov
www.ask.hrsa.gov
Defines grief, presents common reactions and emotions expressed by the bereaved.
1992

8712 SIDS Information for the EMT
National Maternal and Child Health Clearinghouse
2070 Chain Bridge Road 703-442-9051
Vienna, VA 22182-2588 888-275-4772
Fax: 703-821-2098
e-mail: ask@hrsa.gov
www.ask.hrsa.gov
Provides suggestions for first response of emergency medical technicians and others at the time of sudden infant death.
1983

8713 SIDS Research: An Analysis in Three Parts
National Maternal and Child Health Clearinghouse
2070 Chain Bridge Road 703-442-9051
Vienna, VA 22182-2588 888-275-4772
Fax: 703-821-2098
e-mail: ask@hrsa.gov
www.ask.hrsa.gov
Contains articles from a three part series on SIDS research.
1993

8714 SIDS: Toward Prevention and Improved Infant Health
American SIDS Institute
2480 Windy Hill Road SE 770-612-1030
Marietta, GA 30067-8657 800-232-7437
Fax: 770-612-8277
e-mail: prevent@sids.org
www.sids.org
A practical guide for those planning a pregnancy, for parents to be and for new parents.
Betty McEntire PhD, Executive Director

8715 Selected Book on Sudden Infant Death Syndrome
National Maternal and Child Health Clearinghouse
2070 Chain Bridge Road 703-442-9051
Vienna, VA 22182-2588 888-275-4772
Fax: 703-821-2098
e-mail: ask@hrsa.gov
www.ask.hrsa.gov
Provides a list of selected titles on SIDS covering topics such as research, support information and the professionals role.
1993

8716 Selected Resources for Children Grieving the Loss of Another Child
National Maternal and Child Health Clearinghouse

2070 Chain Bridge Road
Vienna, VA 22182-2588
703-442-9051
888-275-4772
Fax: 703-821-2098
e-mail: ask@hrsa.gov
www.ask.hrsa.gov
Provides a list of materials suitable for grieving children and teenagers.
1995

8717 Sudden Infant Death Syndrome and Risk Reduction
National Maternal and Child Health Clearinghouse
2070 Chain Bridge Road
Vienna, VA 22182-2588
703-442-9051
888-275-4772
Fax: 703-821-2098
e-mail: ask@hrsa.gov
www.ask.hrsa.gov
Contains abstracts of selected articles on risk reduction.
1997

8718 What Every Parent Should Know About SIDS
SIDS Alliance
1314 Bedford Avenue
Baltimore, MD 21208-6605
410-653-8226
800-221-7437
Fax: 410-653-8709
Pamphlet offering information on what SIDS is, causes, prevention techniques and what parents can do.

8719 What is SIDS?
National Maternal and Child Health Clearinghouse
2070 Chain Bridge Road
Vienna, VA 22182-2588
703-442-9051
888-275-4772
Fax: 703-821-2098
e-mail: ask@hrsa.gov
www.ask.hrsa.gov
Provides basic facts about SIDS and answers some of the most commonly asked questions.
1993

8720 When Sudden Infant Death Syndrome Occurs in Childcare Settings
National Maternal and Child Health Clearinghouse
2070 Chain Bridge Road
Vienna, VA 22182-2588
703-442-9051
888-275-4772
Fax: 703-821-2098
e-mail: ask@hrsa.gov
www.ask.hrsa.gov
Presents information about SIDS for child care providers.
1993

Web Sites

8721 American SIDS Institute
sids.org/
Dedicated to the prevention of sudden infant death and the promotion of infant health through research, clinical services, education and family support.

8722 Center for Research for Mothers & Children
cdrwww.who.ch/
Mission is to make sure everyone is born healthy and wanted, that women suffer no harmful effects from reproductive processes, and that all children have the chance to achieve their full potential for healthy and productive lives, free from disease or disability, and to ensure the health, productivity, independence, and well-being of all people through optimal rehabilitation.

8723 Compassionate Friends
www.compassionatefriends.org
A national organization that offers 600 local chapters that give support to parents and siblings who have experienced the death of a child.

8724 Healing Well
www.healingwell.com
An online health resource guide to medical news, chat, information and articles, newsgroups and message boards, books, disease-related web sites, medical directories, and more for patients, friends, and family coping with disabling diseases, disorders, or chronic illnesses.

8725 Healthlink USA
www.healthlinkusa.com
Health information concerning treatment, cures, prevention, diagnosis, risk factors, research, support groups, email lists, personal stories and much more. Updated regularly.

8726 Helios Health
www.helioshealth.com
Online resource for your health information. Detailed information about specific health topics, access to expert advice from our Medical Advisory Board, and up-to-date health news.

8727 MedicineNet
www.medicinenet.com
An online resource for consumers providing easy-to-read, authoritative medical and health information.

8728 Medscape
www.medscape.com
Medscape offers specialists, primary care physicians, and other health professionals the Web's most robust and integrated medical information and educational tools.

8729 National Center for Education in Maternal and Child Health
www.ncemch.org
The National Center for Education in Maternal and Child Health provides national leadership to the maternal and child health community in three key areas - program development, policy analysis and education, and state-of-the-art knowledge to improve the health and well-being of the nation's children and families.

8730 WebMD
www.webmd.com
Information on Sudden Infant Death Syndrome, including articles and resources.

Description

8731 Tay-Sachs Disease

Tay-Sachs disease results from an absence of an enzyme (hexosaminidase A) which leads to an accumulation of fat (lipid) in the specific brain tissues (cerebral neurons). The disease is genetic and is autosomal recessive; if two carriers have children, the disease would have a 1 in 4 chance of being passed on. The disease is most prevalent in those of Jewish families, particularly those of Eastern European (Ashkenazi) background.

Symptoms usually present between 3-6 months of age. Early symptoms include mild muscle weakness, muscle spasms, and feeding difficulties. As the disease progresses, the patient may experience vision loss, seizures and eventually paralysis. Death usually occurs by the age of 4 years.

Treatment for Tay-Sachs disease is supportive and there is no cure. Genetic and premarital counseling is important to those at high risk.

National Agencies & Associations

8732 National Foundation for Jewish Genetic Diseases
One Gustave L.   212-241-6500
New York, NY 10029   Fax: 212-241-6947
www.mssm.edu/jewish_genetics
Offers information and support for persons suffering from Tay-Sachs Disease as well as their families and professionals working with them. The Foundation supports research into all areas of genetic disorders.
R J Desnick PhD MD, Center Director

8733 National Institute of Child Health and Human Development
31 Center Drive   301-496-5133
Bethesda, MD 20892   800-370-2943
Fax: 866-760-5947
TTY: 888-320-6942
e-mail: NICHDInformationResourceCenter@mail.nih.
www.nichd.nih.gov
Offers reprints, articles and various information on Tay-Sachs Disease for patients and professionals.
Duane Alexan MD, Director
John McGrath, Coordinator

8734 National Institute of Neurological Disorders and Stroke
NIH Neurological Institute   301-496-5751
Bethesda, MD 20824   800-352-9424
Fax: 301-402-2186
TTY: 301-468-5981
www.ninds.nih.gov
The mission of NINDS is to reduce the burden of neurological disease - a burden borne by every age group, by every segment of society, by people all over the world.
Story C Landis PhD, Director
Walter J Koroshetz, Deputy Director

8735 National Organization for Rare Disorders
55 Kenosia Avenue   203-744-0100
Danbury, CT 06813-1968   800-999-6673
Fax: 203-798-2291
TDD: 203-797-9590
e-mail: orphan@rarediseases.org
www.rarediseases.org
Serves as a clearinghouse for information about rare disorders and brings together families with similar disorders for mutual support; fosters communication among rare disease voluntary agencies, Government agencies, industry scientific researchers and academia.
E. Michael D Scott, Chair
Carolyn Asbury, PhD, Vice Chair

8736 National Tay-Sachs and Allied Diseases Association (NTSAD)
2001 Beacon Street   617-277-4463
Brighton, MA 02135   800-906-8723
Fax: 617-277-0134
e-mail: info@ntsad.org
www.ntstad.org
Offers programs of public and professional education prevention services testing research and family services and promotion of TSD genetic screening programs nationally.
Fran Berkwits, MS, Director
Kevin Romer, President

Foundations

8737 National Tay-Sachs and Allied Diseases Association (NTSAD)
2001 Beacon Street   617-277-4463
Brighton, MA 02135   800-906-8723
Fax: 617-277-0134
e-mail: info@ntsad.org
www.ntsad.org
Dedicated to the treatment and preventin of Tay Sachs, Canavan, and related diseases, and to provide information and support services to individuals and families affected by these diseases, as well as the public at large.
Fran Berkwits, MS, Director
Kevin Romer, President

Support Groups & Hotlines

8738 National Health Information Center
PO Box 1133   310-565-4167
Washington, DC 20013   800-336-4797
Fax: 301-984-4256
e-mail: info@nhic.org
www.health.gov/nhic
Offers a nationwide information referral service, produces directories and resource guides.

8739 National Tay-Sachs Association: Delaware Valley (NTSAD-DV)
720 Greenwood Avenue   215-887-0877
Jenkintown, PA 19046   877-599-9293
Fax: 215-887-1931
e-mail: NTSAD@aol.com
www.tay-sachs.org

Rebecca Tantala, Executive Director

8740 National TaySachs & Allied Diseases
2001 Beacon Street   617-277-4463
Boston, MA 2135   800-906-8723
Fax: 617-277-0134
e-mail: info@ntsad.org
www.ntsad.org
A mutual support group coordinated by staff and volunteers who are parents of affected children or affected adults. One of several programs supported and sponsored by the association.
Fran Berkwits, MS, Director
Kevin Romer, President

Books

8741 Home Care Book
National Tay-Sachs and Allied Diseases Association
2001 Beacon Street
Brighton, MA 02135   800-906-8723
Fax: 617-277-0134
e-mail: info@ntsad.org
www.ntsad.org
Written by parents for parents and professionals, the Home Care Book is a guide to caring for children with progressive neurological disorders at home.
John F Crowley MBA, JD, President

8742 **Home-Care Book**
National Tay-Sachs and Allied Diseases Association
2001 Beacon Street
Brookline, MA 02146   800-906-8723
A guide for caring for children with progressive neurological diseases.

8743 **Late Onset Tay-Sachs Disease Medical Bibliography**
National Tay-Sachs and Allied Diseases Association
2001 Beacon Street
Brookline, MA 02146   800-906-8723

8744 **Lifting of Canavan's Carrier Testing Facilities**
National Tay-Sachs and Allied Diseases Association
2001 Beacon Street
Brookline, MA 02146   800-906-8723

8745 **Monograph on Canavan's Disease**
National Tay-Sachs and Allied Diseases Association
2001 Beacon Street
Brookline, MA 02146   800-906-8723

8746 **Tay-Sachs Carrier Testing Directory**
National Tay-Sachs and Allied Diseases Association
2001 Beacon Street
Brookline, MA 02146   800-906-8723

8747 **Tay-Sachs: The Dreaded Inheritance**
National Tay-Sachs and Allied Diseases Assocation
2001 Beacon Street
Brighton, MA 02135   800-906-8723
                              Fax: 617-277-0134
                 e-mail: NTSAD-Boston@worldnet.att.net
                                    www.ntsad.org
Descriptive narrative on caring for a child with Tay-Sachs Disease.

8748 **There is Only One Child**
National Tay-Sachs and Allied Diseases Association
2001 Beacon Street
Brookline, MA 02146   800-906-8723

8749 **What Every Family Should Know Sixth Edition**
National Tay-Sachs & Allied Diseases Association
2001 Beacon Street
Brighton, MA 02135   800-906-8723
                              Fax: 617-277-0134
                          e-mail: info@ntsad.org
                                    www.ntsad.org
Detailing lysosomal storage and leukodystrophy disorders, with sections on Tay-Sachs, Sandhoff, Niemann-Pick, Gaucher, Canavan, Fabry, Pompe, therapeutic approaches and unique disease table.
50 pages
John F Crowley MBA. JD, President

Newsletters

8750 **Breakthrough**
National Tay-Sachs and Allied Diseases Association
2001 Beacon Street
Boston, MA 02135   800-906-8723
                              Fax: 617-277-0134
                          e-mail: info@ntsad.org
                                    www.ntsad.org
Each year NTSAD publishes a newsletter for friends and supporters that focuses on the latest advances in research, profiles of families and individuals helped by NTSAD and disease profiles.
Annual
John F Crowley MBA, JD, President

8751 **Late Onset Community Newsletter**
National Tay-Sachs and Allied Diseases Association
2001 Beacon Street
Brighton, MA 02135   800-906-8723
                              Fax: 617-277-0134
                          e-mail: info@ntsad.org
                                    www.ntsad.org
PSG members dealing with chronic forms of the allied diseases receive this newsletter focused specifically on the issues and per-

spectives unique to adults struggling with long-term disability issues. Public editions of the newsletter are also available.
Bi-Monthly
John F Crowley MBA, JD, President

8752 **Lifeline**
National Tay-Sachs and Allied Diseases Association
2001 Beacon Street
Brighton, MA 02135   800-906-8723
                              Fax: 617-277-0134
                          e-mail: info@ntsad.org
                                    www.ntsad.org
The editorial content is wide ranging: symptom management and home health care; new product reviews; guidance in benefits and services advocacy for families and affected individuals of all ages; science and medical research updates; coverage of NTSAD events, fundraising, programs and administrative activities. Members only.
Quarterly
John F Crowley MBA, JD, President

Pamphlets

8753 **Late Onset Tay-Sachs Fact Sheet**
National Tay-Sachs and Allied Diseases Association
2001 Beacon Street
Brighton, MA 02135   800-906-8723
                              Fax: 617-277-0134
                          e-mail: info@ntsad.org
                                    www.ntsad.org
This quick reference information sheet on the chronic or late onset form of Tay-Sachs is available for no charge.
John F Crowley MBA, JD, President

8754 **Services to Families**
National Tay-Sachs and Allied Diseases Association
2001 Beacon Street
Brookline, MA 02146   800-906-8723
Offers information on the Association parent peer groups, referrals and advocacy services to families and patients.

8755 **Tay-Sachs Information Sheet**
March of Dimes
233 Park Avenue South   212-353-8353
New York, NY 10003   Fax: 212-254-3518
                 e-mail: NY639@marchofdimes.com
                                www.marchofdimes.com
Offers a brief overview of the illness, causes, symptoms and treatments are covered. Availabe electronically on the website: www.marchofdimes.com

8756 **Tay-Sachs is**
National Tay-Sachs and Allied Diseases Association
2001 Beacon Street
Brookline, MA 02146   800-906-8723
Information on the history of the disease, what a victim of the disease should know and what they can do as far as resources and referrals.

8757 **Understanding Lysosomal Storage Diseases**
National Tay-Sachs and Allied Diseases Association
2001 Beacon Street
Brookline, MA 02146   800-906-8723

8758 **What is Canavan Disease?**
National Tay-Sachs and Allied Diseases Association
2001 Beacon Street
Brighton, MA 02135   800-906-8723
                              Fax: 617-277-0134
                          e-mail: info@ntsad.org
                                    www.ntsad.org
The educational pamphlet describing Canavan Disease.
John F Crowley MBA, JD, President

8759 **What is Tay-Sachs? Russian Translation**
National Tay-Sachs and Allied Diseases Association

2001 Beacon Street
Brighton, MA 02135

800-906-8723
Fax: 617-277-0134
e-mail: info@ntsad.org
www.ntsad.org

This informative educational pamphlet describing Infantile Tay-Sachs, its inheritance and prevention is available for no charge.

John F Crowley MBA, JD, President

Audio & Video

8760 For My Sister, Elyssa
National Tay-Sachs & Allied Diseases Assocation
2001 Beacon Street
Brighton, MA 02135

800-906-8723
Fax: 617-277-0134
e-mail: NTSAD-Boston@worldnet.att.net
www.ntsad.org

Moving and informative 15 minute presentation told by a teenager who baby siter died from Tay-Sachs Disease. Contains information on Tay-Sachs Disease and simple steps each individual can take to prevent the tragedy of Tay-Sachs.

Web Sites

8761 Healing Well

www.healingwell.com

An online health resource guide to medical news, chat, information and articles, newsgroups and message boards, books, disease-related web sites, medical directories, and more for patients, friends, and family coping with disabling diseases, disorders, or chronic illnesses.

8762 Health Finder

www.healthfinder.gov

Searchable, carefully developed web site offering information on over 1000 topics. Developed by the US Department of Health and Human Services, the site can be used in both English and Spanish.

8763 Healthlink USA

www.healthlinkusa.com

Health information concerning treatment, cures, prevention, diagnosis, risk factors, research, support groups, email lists, personal stories and much more. Updated regularly.

8764 Helios Health

www.helioshealth.com

Online resource for your health information. Detailed information about specific health topics, access to expert advice from our Medical Advisory Board, and up-to-date health news.

8765 MedicineNet

www.medicinenet.com

An online resource for consumers providing easy-to-read, authoritative medical and health information.

8766 Medscape

www.medscape.com

Medscape offers specialists, primary care physicians, and other health professionals the Web's most robust and integrated medical information and educational tools.

8767 WebMD

www.webmd.com

Information on Tay-Sachs disease, including articles and resources.

Description

8768 **Thyroid Disease**

Thyroid Disease refers to a number of conditions that affect the thyroid, a small, butterfly-shaped gland located in the middle of the lower neck. Hormones T3 and T4, produced by the thyroid, deliver energy to cells of the body, thus controlling the body's metabolism. Conditions that result from an imbalance of these hormones are Hypothyroidism — not enough hormones that results in the body using energy slower than it should, and Hyperthyroidism — too much hormones that results in the body using energy faser than it should. These conditions can be caused by an inflammation of the thyroid gland, too much or too little iodine (used to produce thyroid hormones), or autoimmune disease, in which antibodies gradually either destroy the thyroid gland or speed up its function. Other thyroid conditions are Goiter — an enlarged thyroid; Thyroid Nodules — cysts, lumps, bumps and tumors that can be cancerous or benign; and Thyroiditis — inflammation of the thyroid gland. More than 20 million Americans have thyroid disease, and it affects many more women than men. Treatment includes synthetic hormone medication to replace missing hormones, radioactive iodine to deactivate the thyroid, and surgery for some goiters and cancerous nodules. Early diagnosis is often the key in prescribing treatment even before the onset of symptoms. Although thyroid disease is a chronic condition, careful disease management allows affected individuals to live healthy, normal lives.

National Agencies & Associations

8769 **American Thyroid Association**
6066 Leesburg Pike 703-998-8890
Falls Church, VA 22041 800-479-7634
Fax: 703-998-8893
e-mail: thyroid@thyroid.org
www.thyroid.org
Promotes excellence and innovation in clinical care research education and public policy.
Barbara R. Smith, CAE, Executive Director

8770 **National Women's Health Resource Center**
157 Broad Street 877-986-9472
Red Bank, NJ 07701 877-986-9472
Fax: 732-530-3347
e-mail: snelson@healthwomen.org
www.healthywomen.org
NWHRC develops and distributes up-to-date and objective women's health information based on the latest advances in medical research and practice.
JoAnn V. Pinkerton, Director
Elizabeth Ba Cahill, Executive Director

8771 **Thyroid Federation International**
797 Princess Street 613-544-8364
Kingston, Ontario, K7L-1G1 Fax: 613-544-9731
e-mail: tfi@on.aibn.com
www.thyroid-fed.org
Aims to work for the benefit of those affected by thyroid disorders throughout the world.
Yvonne Andersson, President, Board of Directors
Peter Lakwijk, VP, Board of Directors

8772 **Thyroid Foundation of Canada**
797 Princess Street 613-544-8364
Kingston, Ontario, K7L-1G1 800-267-8822
Fax: 613-544-9731
www.thyroid.ca
Thyroid Foundation of Canada is a registered charity.
Katherine Keen, National Office Coordinator

Books

8773 **Autoimmune Connection: Essential Informati on for Women on Diagnosis, Treatment**
National Women's Health Resource Center
157 Broad Street 877-986-9472
Red Bank, NJ 07701 Fax: 732-530-3347
e-mail: info@healthywomen.org
www.healthywomen.org
Readers learn about the recent groundbreaking discovery of the links between the different autoimmune diseases and why women are more likely to develop them.
Elizabeth Battaglino Cahill, Executive Director

8774 **The Thyroid Gland**
Joel I Hamburger MD & Michael M Kaplan, author
Thyroid Foundation of Canada
797 Princess Street 613-544-8364
Kingston, Ontario, K7L-1G1 800-267-8822
Fax: 613-544-9731
www.thyroid.ca
Provides material for the patient to study at home, and to review at subsequent visits to the physician.

8775 **Thyroid Balance**
National Women's Health Resource Center
157 Broad Street 877-986-9472
Red Bank, NJ 07701 Fax: 732-530-3347
e-mail: info@healthywomen.org
www.healthywomen.org
An authoritative guide to treating thyroid issues-using both traditional and alternative methods.
Elizabeth Battaglino Cahill, Executive Director

8776 **Thyroid Disease: The Facts**
RIS Bayliss & WMG Tunbridge MD, author
Thyroid Foundation of Canada
797 Princess Street 613-544-8364
Kingston, Ontario, K7L-1G1 800-267-8822
Fax: 613-544-9731
www.thyroid.ca
Provides patients, their friends, and relatives with an up-to-date, readable account of disorders of the thyroid and the treatments which are now available.

8777 **Thyroid Power: Ten Steps to Total Health**
Richard Shames & Karilee H Shames, author
National Women's Health Resource Center
157 Broad Street 877-986-9472
Red Bank, NJ 07701 Fax: 732-530-3347
e-mail: snelson@healthwomen.org
www.healthywomen.org
Discusses the labyrinth of diagnostic and treatment issues a patient must endure.

8778 **Thyroid Solution: A Mind-Body Program for Beating Depression and Regaining Health**
National Women's Health Resource Center
157 Broad Street 877-986-9472
Red Bank, NJ 07701 Fax: 732-530-3347
e-mail: info@healthywomen.org
www.healthywomen.org
This book explains the link between stress and thyroid imbalance; how thyroid imbalance affects your emotions, sex life, and relationships; and how to cope with the effects of this imbalance.
Elizabeth Battaglino Cahill, Executive Director

8779 **Thyroid Sourcebook**
Thyroid Foundation of Canada

797 Princess Street
Kingston, Ontario, K7L-1G1

613-544-8364
800-267-8822
Fax: 613-544-9731
www.thyroid.ca

Provides the guidance, reassurance, and important information you need to manage your health and make informed decisions.

8780 Your Thyroid: A Home Reference

Lawrence Wood MD & David S Cooper MD, author

Thyroid Foundation of Canada
797 Princess Street
Kingston, Ontario, K7L-1G1

613-544-8364
800-267-8822
Fax: 613-544-9731
www.thyroid.ca

Explains the latest scientific advances can mean to you.

Magazines

8781 Clinical Thyroidology

American Thyroid Association
6066 Leesburg Pike
Falls Church, VA 12041

703-998-8890
800-849-7634
Fax: 703-998-8893
e-mail: editorclinthy@thyroid.org
www.thyroid.org

An online publication, available monthly, this is a broad-ranging look at clinical and preclinical thyroid literature. The Editor searches the world literature for excellent thyroid studies and then summarizes them along side his expert commentary.
Ernest L. Mazzaferri, MD, Editor

8782 THYROID

American Thyroid Association
6066 Leesburg Pike
Falls Church, VA 12041

703-998-8890
800-849-7643
Fax: 703-998-8893
e-mail: thyroideditor@umassmed.edu
www.thyroid.org

The Associations monthly journal that touches on topics from the molecular biology of the thyroid gland to clinical management of thyroid disorders. All Association members receive a suvscription, and it is available to non-members.

8783 Clinical Thyroidology for Patients

American Thyroid Association
6066 Leesburg Pike
Falls Church, VA 12041

703-998-8890
800-849-7634
Fax: 703-998-8893
e-mail: editorclinthy@thyroid.org
www.thyroid.org

A collection of summaries of recently published articles fromt the medical literature that covers the broad spectrum of thryroid disorders. Notes descxribing published research studies were prepared by THYROID Editor, Ernest Mazzaferri, MD.

Newsletters

8784 SIGNAL

American Thyroid Association
6066 Leesburg Pike
Falls Church, VA 12041

703-998-8890
800-849-7643
Fax: 703-998-8893
e-mail: thyroid@thyroid.org
www.thyroid.org

Covers Association news, meetings, policies, leaders, and important thyroid-related issues.

Pamphlets

8785 Hypothyroidism Web Booklet

American Thyroid Association
6066 Leesburg Pike
Falls Church, VA 12041

703-998-8890
800-489-7643
Fax: 703-998-8893
e-mail: thyroid@thyroid.org
www.thyroid.org

This online booklet introduces the thryoid and hypothyroidism to the reader, explains symptoms, treatments, causes, who's at risk, and more.
2003 25 pages

Web Sites

8786 American Thyroid Association

www.thyroid.com

Promotes excellence and innovation in clinical care, research, education, and public policy.
David S Cooper MD, President
Gregory A Brent MD, Secretary

8787 MedicineNet

www.medicinenet.com

An online resource for consumers providing easy-to-read, authoritative medical and health information.

8788 National Women's Health Resource Center

www.healthywomen.org

NWHRC developes and distributes up-to-date and objective women's health information based on the latest advances in medical research and practice.
Elizabeth Battaglino Cahill, RN, Executive Director
Maria Bushee, Director of Marketing & Communications

8789 Thyroid Federation International

www.thyroid-fed.org

Aims to work for the benefit of those affected by thyroid disorders throughout the world.

8790 Thyroid Foundation of Canada

www.thyroid.ca

Thyroid Foundation of Canada is a registered charity.

Description

8791 Tick-Borne Disease

Ticks transmit disease to humans by being carriers for a variety of microorganismns. The most common tick-borne illness is Lyme disease, first recognized and so named in 1975 because of a cluster of cases found in Lyme, Connecticut. It is a bacterial infection spread by the bite of an infected deer tick. The disease in its earliest stages causes an expanding red rash in at least 75 percent of patients. Flu-like symptoms—headaches, fever, fatigue—are common. The rash may be followed by progressive joint pain and swelling. Dysfunction of the heart (8 percent) and nervous system (15 percent) develop weeks to months later. Further progression causes arthritis and more serious neurologic problems.

Although only one third of patients remember a tick bite, greater than 60 percent do develop the tell-tale rash. Diagnosis requires a blood test to confirm the physical symptoms.

Oral antibiotics may be sufficient for the disease caught in the early stages. Long-standing, disseminated disease responds best to intravenous antibiotics.

Rocky Mountain spotted fever, also known as tick fever, is transmitted by a bite from either a dog tick or wood tick, depending on the part of the country. Like Lyme disease, it begin with flu-like symptoms — chills, fever and loss of appetite. A rash of small, reddish bumps, which gives the disease its name, begins on the wrist and ankle and spreads to the rest of the body. Aggressive antibotic treatment should begin as early as possible. If left untreated, Rocky Mountain spotted fever has a mortality rate of 10 to 80 percent.

Prevention of tick-borne disease requires avoidance of tick bites, by using insect repellants and protective clothing, plus daily checks for ticks during periods of exposure. A vaccine may provide partial protection from Lyme disease for those regularly engaged in high-risk activities (i.e. property maintenance), although other conditions may complicate this treatment.

National Agencies & Associations

8792 Lyme Disease Foundation
PO Box332   860-870-0070
Tolland, CT 06084-0332   800-886-5963
                                        Fax: 860-870-0080
                                    e-mail: info@lyme.org
                                            www.lyme.org
Provides a wide range of services including information and referral network on Lyme Disease, distribution of educational videos to state libraries, educational materials for public and professionals, national public forums and training for community education.
John F Anderson, Board of Director
Willy Burgdorfer, Board of Director

Libraries & Resource Centers

8793 California Lyme Disease Association
PO Box 1352
Chico, CA 95927   e-mail: info@lymedisease.org
                                        www.lymedisease.org
The California Lyme Disease Association (CALDA) is an affiliate of the Lyme Disease Association, Inc. CALDA, a non-profit organization, was originally founded in 1990 as The Lyme Disease Resource Center (LDRC). We provide services for Lyme disease patients, their families and friends; provide a forum for physicians and health professionals for the exchange of ideas and information about symptoms, diagnosis, and treatment of Lyme disease.
Marilynn Barkley, Board of Directors
Barbara Barsoschinni, Board of Directors

Research Centers

8794 Ball State University Public Health Entomology Laboratory
2000 University Avenue   765-289-1241
Muncie, IN 47306   800-382-8540
                                                   TTY: 7
                                               www.bsu.edu
Offers information on mosquitoes and mosquito-born diseases specializing in Lyme Disease.
Bob Pinger, Director
Jeffrey Clark, Department Chair and Professor

8795 Centers for Disease Control Division of Vector Borne Infectious Diseases
US Public Health Service
1600 Clifton Rd.   800-232-4636
Atlanta, GA 30333   Fax: 970-216-76
                                        TDD: 888-232-6348
                                              www.cdc.gov
Research done into lyme disease tularemia bubonic plague and all vector-borne infectious diseases — including west nile virus.
Dr.Tom Frieden, Director

Support Groups & Hotlines

8796 Advocates 4 Health: Tick-borne Disease Self-Help Group
PALS
PO Box 1271   805-544-0984
San Luis Obispo, CA 93406 e-mail: advocates4heatlh@yahoo.com
Advocacy and support group increasing awareness, education and understanding of tick-borne disorders and other zoonotic diseases. This group fosters a supportive network between human/animal sufferers, caregivers, health care professionals and the general community.
Sheryl Glidden

8797 American Lyme Disease Foundation
2518 Ridge Court   785-248-3504
Lawrence, CT 66046   e-mail: Inquire@aldf.com
                                              www.aldf.com
Supports research and plays a key role in providing reliable and scientifically accurate information to the public and health care providers.
David L Weld, Executive Director
Jeffery Black, Partner

8798 Lyme Alliance
PO Box 454
Concord, MI 49237   517-563-3582
                                        www.lymealliance.org
Lyme Alliance volunteers will address your questions concerning the newsletter, website, or questions about doctor referrals, medical treatment options, or information about Lyme disease.

8799 Lyme Disease Network
43 Winton Road   651-644-7239
East Brunswick, NJ 08816
Lynn M Olivier

8800 **Lyme Disease Network Support Group of Alabama: Mobile Chapter**
Mobile, AL 35758   256-772-6482
e-mail: alabamalyme@usa.com
www.lymnet.org/supportgroups
Support information, and referrals for victims of Lyme disease and their families.
Kara Tyson

8801 **Lyme Disease Network of New Jersey**
43 Winton Road
East Brunswick, NJ 08816   e-mail: carol@lymenet.org
www.lymenet.org
Support information, and referrals for victims of Lyme disease and their families. Maintains comuter information system.
Bill Stolow, President

8802 **Lyme Disease Network of South Carolina**
Po Box 6634   803-798-5963
Columbia, SC 29260-6634   e-mail: lyme@sc-lyme.org
www.sc-lyme.org

Sue Fox

8803 **National Health Information Center**
PO Box 1133   240-453-8280
Washington, DC 20013   800-336-4797
Fax: 240-453-8282
e-mail: info@nhic.org
www.health.gov/nhic
Offers a nationwide information referral service, produces directories and resource guides.

Books

8804 **Coping with Lyme Disease: A Practical Guide**
Henry Holt & Company
115 W 18th Street   212-886-9200
New York, NY 10011-4113   Fax: 212-633-0748
1993 288 pages Paperback
ISBN: 0-805026-50-9

8805 **Ecology & Environment Management of Lyme Disease**
Rutgers University Press
109 Church Street   201-932-7762
New Brunswick, NJ 08901-1242
1993 224 pages
ISBN: 0-813519-28-4

8806 **Everything You Need to Know About Lyme Disease**
John Wiley & Sons Publishing
605 3rd Avenue   212-850-6000
New York, NY 10158-0012   800-225-5945
Fax: 212-850-6088
www.wiley.com

237 pages
ISBN: 0-471160-61-X

8807 **Let's Talk About Having Lyme Disease**
Rosen Publishing Group's PowerKids Press
29 E 21st Street   212-777-3017
New York, NY 10010   800-237-9932
Fax: 888-436-4643
e-mail: customerservice@rosenpub.com
www.rosenpublishing.com
Kids are taught to take precautions when walking in the woods and how to inspect themselves for ticks. The illness and recovery are also explained.
Grades K-4
ISBN: 0-823950-29-8
Elizabeth Weitzman, Author

Children's Books

8808 **Lyme Disease**
Franklin Watts Grolier

90 Old Sherman Tpke   203-797-3500
Danbury, CT 06816-0001   800-621-1115
Fax: 203-797-3197
www.grolier.com
This book discusses the symptoms, prevention, treatments and the role of the tick. This source will not only help readers become aware of Lyme Disease, it will help them become informed.
64 pages Grades 5-7
ISBN: 0-531109-31-3

8809 **Lyme Disease and Other Pest-Borne Illnesses**
Franklin Watts Grolier
90 Old Sherman Turnpike   203-797-3500
Danbury, CT 06816-0001   800-621-1115
Fax: 203-797-3197
www.grolier.com
Scientific, without being technical, this book explains what Lyme Disease is, symptoms, causes and what a person can do if they contract it.
112 pages Grades 7-12
ISBN: 0-531125-23-8

Magazines

8810 **Vector Borne & Zoonotic Diseases**
Mary Ann Liebert
Two Madison Avenue   914-834-3100
Larchmont, NY 10538-1961   800-654-3238
Fax: 914-834-1388
www.liebertpub.com/vbz
Essential multidisiplinary journal dedicated to all aspects of human diseases that occur as zoonoses or are transmitted by invertibrate vectors.
Quarterly

Newsletters

8811 **Lymelight Newsletter**
Lyme Disease Foundation
1 Financial Plaza   860-525-2000
Hartford, CT 06103-2608   800-886-5963
Fax: 860-525-8425
Newsletter offering up to date information on Lyme Disease and related disorders, Foundation activities, conference and fund-raising information and resources.
4x Year

Pamphlets

8812 **Frequently Asked Questions**
Lyme Disease Foundation
1 Financial Plaza   860-525-2000
Hartford, CT 06103-2608   800-886-5963
Fax: 860-525-8425
Overview of testing, treatment, transmission, and pregnancy.

8813 **Guide to Lyme Disease**
Lyme Disease Foundation
1 Financial Plaza   860-525-2000
Hartford, CT 06103-2608   800-886-5963
Fax: 860-525-8425
Detailed information about Lyme disease and the LDF.

8814 **Guide to Tick Spread Diseases**
Lyme Disease Foundation
1 Financial Plaza   860-525-2000
Hartford, CT 06103-2608   800-886-5963
Fax: 860-525-8425
www.lyme.org
Symptoms, diagnosis and treatment for a variety of diseases.
16 pages

8815 **Guide to Tick-Borne Disorders**
Lyme Disease Foundation

1 Financial Plaza   860-525-2000
Hartford, CT 06103-2608   800-886-5963
  Fax: 860-525-8425
Symptoms, diagnosis, and treatment for a variety of diseases.

8816   LD Alert Card
Lyme Disease Foundation
1 Financial Plaza   860-525-2000
Hartford, CT 06103-2608   800-886-5963
  Fax: 860-525-8425

LD symptoms and prevention information.

8817   LD Awareness Packet
Lyme Disease Foundation
1 Financial Plaza   860-525-2000
Hartford, CT 06103-2608   800-886-5963
  Fax: 860-525-8425

Educational letter-size posters, brochures listed above, case counts, Spanish information, insurance problem information, General Diagnostic poster, & more.

8818   Lyme Disease & Pets
Lyme Disease Foundation
1 Financial Plaza   860-525-2000
Hartford, CT 06103-2608   800-886-5963
  Fax: 860-525-8425
  e-mail: lymefna@aol.com
  www.lyme.org

Offers information on Lyme Disease and other tick-borne disorders, through pets and animal transmission.
T Forchaser, Executive Director

8819   Quick Guide to Lyme Disease
American Lyme Disease Foundation
293 Route 100   914-277-6970
Somers, NY 10589   Fax: 914-277-6974
  e-mail: inquire@aldf.com
  www.aldf.com

Epidemiology, the cause of the disease, recognizing the symptoms, what to do if you are bitten, treatment, vaccine and other tick-borne diseases are all covered. One free copy, quantity prices vary.

8820   Self-Help (S-H) Program
Lyme Disease Foundation
1 Financial Plaza   860-525-2000
Hartford, CT 06103-2608   800-886-5963
  Fax: 860-525-8425

How to establish and conduct a S-H Group. Video, instruction manual, brochure masters, posters, and more.
28 minutes

8821   Understanding Lyme Disease: Entendiendo Lyme Disease
American Lyme Disease Foundation
293 Route 100   914-277-6970
Somers, NY 10589   Fax: 914-277-6974
  e-mail: inquire@aldf.com
  www.aldf.com

Only available in Spanish, this brochure is for children ages 10-15 years old. Includes a basic desription of Lyme disease, symptoms, diagnosis, prevention and proper tick removal. One free copy, quantity prices vary.

8822   Understanding Ticks and Lyme Disease
American Lyme Disease Foundation
293 Route 100   914-277-6970
Somers, NY 10589   Fax: 914-277-6974
  e-mail: inquire@aldf.com
  www.aldf.com

For children 10-15 years old, basic description of Lyme disease, symptoms, diagnosis, prevention and proper tick removal. One free copy, quantity prices vary.

Audio & Video

8823   Case of the Great Imitator
American Lyme Disease Foundation

293 Route 100   914-277-6970
Somers, NY 10589   Fax: 914-277-6974
  e-mail: inquire@aldf.com
  www.aldf.com
For children ages 9-14 years old. Educational video made in cooperation with the Centers for Disease Control and Prevention.

8824   LD: Diagnosis & Treatment
Lyme Disease Foundation
1 Financial Plaza   860-525-2000
Hartford, CT 06103-2608   800-886-5963
  Fax: 860-525-8425

Physicians discuss the challenges of diagnosing and treating LD.
60 minutes

8825   LD: Facts for Kids
Lyme Disease Foundation
1 Financial Plaza   860-525-2000
Hartford, CT 06103-2608   800-886-5963
  Fax: 860-525-8425

Targeted toward kindergarten to fourth grade children, these videos educate youngsters about Lyme Disease and ticks.

8826   Lyme Disease: What You Should Know
Lyme Disease Foundation
1 Financial Plaza   860-525-2000
Hartford, CT 06103-2608   800-886-5963
  Fax: 860-525-8425

Diagnosis, treatment, transmission, prevention, and research. Interviews with patients, doctors, school officials, researchers, and health department officials.
60 minutes

8827   Tick Talk
American Lyme Disease Foundation
293 Route 100   914-277-6970
Somers, NY 10589   Fax: 914-277-6974
  e-mail: inquire@aldf.com
  www.aldf.com
For children ages 5-8 years old. Educational video made in cooperation with the Centers for Disease Control and Prevention.

Web Sites

8828   America's Doctor Online Consulting
  www.americasdoctor.com
Provides pharmaceutical and biotech companies and contract research organizations an exclusive source for conducting phase II-IV clinical research.

8829   American Lyme Disease Foundation
  www.aldf.com
Provides a wide range of information, both in English and in Spanish, on the diagnosis, treatment, prevention and control of lyme disease and other tick-borne infections.

8830   CDC Intro to Lyme Disease
  www.cdc.gov/ncidod/dvbid/lyme/incex.htm
Accurate, evidence based information on symptoms, diagnosis, treatment and prevention of Lyme disease and other tick-borne illnesses. Includes vaccine information, late-braking news, frequently asked questions and related links.

8831   Healing Well
  www.healingwell.com
An online health resource guide to medical news, chat, information and articles, newsgroups and message boards, books, disease-related web sites, medical directories, and more for patients, friends, and family coping with disabling diseases, disorders, or chronic illnesses.

8832   Health Finder
  www.healthfinder.gov
Searchable, carefully developed web site offering information on over 1000 topics. Developed by the US Department of Health and Human Services, the site can be used in both English and Spanish.

8833   Healthlink USA
  www.healthlinkusa.com

Health information concerning treatment, cures, prevention, diagnosis, risk factors, research, support groups, email lists, personal stories and much more. Updated regularly.

8834 Helios Health

www.helioshealth.com

Online resource for your health information. Detailed information about specific health topics, access to expert advice from our Medical Advisory Board, and up-to-date health news.

8835 Lyme Disease Foundation

www.lyme.org

Provides a wide range of services including information and referral network on Lyme disease.

8836 MGH Neurology WebForums

Provides both unmoderated message board and chat rooms for specific neurological disorders including: amyloidosis, asachnoiditis, cerebellar ataxia, congenital fiber type disproportion, CFS leak, DeMorsiers syndrome, erythomelalgia, Lewy body disease, meningitis, meralgia paresthetic, Norrie disease, periodic paralysis, phantom limb pain, Romber disorder, Syndenhams chorea, tethered cord syndrome, and thoracic outlet syndrome.

8837 MedicineNet

www.medicinenet.com

An online resource for consumers providing easy-to-read, authoritative medical and health information.

8838 Medscape

www.medscape.com

Medscape offers specialists, primary care physicians, and other health professionals the Web's most robust and integrated medical information and educational tools.

8839 Neurology Channel

www.neurologychannel.com

Find clearly explained, medically accurate information regarding conditions, including an overview, symptoms, causes, diagnostic procedures and treatment options. On this site it is possible to ask questions and get information from a neurologist and connect to people who have similar health interests.

8840 Pubmed

www.ncbi.nlm.nih.gov/PubMed

National institutes of Health search engine for published medical and scientific research.

8841 University of Rhode Island Tick Research Laboratory

www.riaes.org/resources/ticklab

Pictures of ticks and tick-borne disease information.

8842 WebMD

www.webmd.com

Information on Lyme disease, including articles and resources.

Description

8843 Tourette Syndrome

Tourette syndrome, TS, is a neurological disorder characterized by tics - involuntary, rapid, sudden movements or vocalizations that occur repeatedly in the same way. Onset of the disorder occurs before 18 years of age, and usually before the age of 12. Roughly one person in 2000 will demonstrate this behavior at some time in his life. Boys are 3 or 4 times as likely as girls to develop TS.

Multiple motor and vocal tics can appear separately or simultaneously as part of the syndrome. Tics may occur many times daily, or intermittently, with periodic changes in their number, frequency, type and location. Sometimes they may disappear for weeks.

Over time, symptoms can range from hand jerking and throat clearing in the syndrome's early stages to jumping and vocalizing socially unacceptable phrases. Movements may also occur in combination with each other.

Although the cause of TS is unknown, researchers have identified factors which may be involved in producing the disease. Persons with TS may show subtle abnormalities in the structure of certain parts of the brain. The disease may reflect abnormal metabolism of a neurotransmitter (a chemical that brain cells use to signal one another) called dopamine; drugs affecting dopamine levels may reduce symptoms. Relatives of affected persons have an increased risk of disease, suggesting a genetic component. Finally, in some cases the brain's function may be affected by antibodies triggered by infection with a bacterium called Group A Strep. Children who are not bothered by their tics should not be treated with drugs. Medications are reserved for those whose tics lead to symptoms which impair behavioral, physiologic or social function. Simple tics respond to benzodiazepines (tranquilizers). For more severe cases, haloperidol, an antipsychotic, may be used, but should be started slowly. Unfortunately, it sometimes causes other movement disorders after prolonged use. Whether drug treatment is used or not, patients and their families may need counseling to deal with the disease's secondary effects, which may include bullying at school or conflict within the family. Fortunately, the condition often becomes much less severe, without any treatment, after 10 or 15 years.

National Agencies & Associations

8844 American Academy of Neurology: Tourette Syndrome
201 Chicago Avenue 800-879-1960
Minneapolis, MN 55415-2311 800-879-1960
Fax: 612-454-2746
e-mail: memberservices@aan.com
www.aan.com
A medical specialty society established to advance the art and science of neurology and thereby promote the best possible care for patients wit neurological disorders.
Catherine Rydell, Executive Director

8845 National Institute of Neurological Disorders and Stroke
NIH Neurological Institute 301-496-5751
Bethesda, MD 20824 800-352-9424
Fax: 301-402-2186
TTY: 301-468-5981
www.ninds.nih.gov
The mission of NINDS is to reduce the burden of neurological disease - a burden borne by every age group, by every segment of society, by people all over the world.
Story C Landis PhD, Director
Walter J Koroshetz, Deputy Director

8846 Tourette Syndrome Association
42-40 Bell Boulevard 718-224-2999
Bayside, NY 11361 888-486-8738
Fax: 718-279-9596
e-mail: grantadministrator@tsa-usa.org
www.tsa-usa.org
The only national organization exclusively devoted to the research, diagnosis, education and treatments for persons with Tourette Syndrome.
Judit Ungar, President
Sue Levi-Pearl, VP Meical & Scientific Programs

8847 Tourette Syndrome Foundation of Canada
5945 Airport Rd 905-673-2255
Mississauga, Ontario, L4 1R9-2B7 800-361-3120
Fax: 800-387-0120
e-mail: tsfc@tourette.ca
www.tourette.ca
National voluntary organization dedicated to improving the quality of life for those with or affected by Tourette Syndrome through programs of education, advocacy, self-help and the promotion of research.
Rosie Wartecker, Executive Director

Research Centers

8848 Tourette Syndrome Clinic Yale Child Study Center
Yale Child Study Center
300 George St. 203-785-6396
New Haven, CT 06511 Fax: 203-785-6196
www.medicine.yale.edu
Clinical care center offering research solely into the causes symptoms and treatments for persons with Tourette Syndrome.
Diane B Findley, Associate Research Scientist and Clinic
Robert King, Medical Director

Support Groups & Hotlines

8849 National Health Information Center
PO Box 1133 310-565-4167
Washington, DC 20013 800-336-4797
Fax: 301-984-4256
e-mail: info@nhic.org
www.health.gov/nhic
Offers a nationwide information referral service, produces directories and resource guides.

Books

8850 Children with Tourette Syndrome
Woodbine House
6510 Bells Mill Road
Bethesda, MD 20817-1636 800-843-7323
This book offers parents information on Tourette Syndrome, causes, symptoms and medications, as well as the other disorders which are commonly linked with it. Other chapters include information on family life, education, advocacy and legal rights.
340 pages Paperback
ISBN: 0-933149-44-1

8851 Children with Tourette Syndrome: A Parent's Guide
Adam Ward Seligman, Echolalia Press

35158 Annapolis Road
Annapolis, CA 95412-9713

707-886-1972
e-mail: seligman@sonic.net
www.sonic.net/echolaliapress/

8852 Living with Tourette Syndrome
Simon & Schuster
611 W Bay Street
Tampa, FL 33606-2703   800-999-5479
Provides valuable advice for children and adults with TS, their families, co-workers, teachers and friends. Describes the symptoms and related disorders, exposes many myths surrounding the disease, and advises adults on business and personal relationships.
256 pages
ISBN: 0-684811-60-0

8853 Ryan: A Mother's Story of her TS/ADHD Child
Adam Ward Seligman, Echolalia Press
35158 Annapolis Road   707-886-1972
Annapolis, CA 95412-9713
Available in hardcover.
Softcover

8854 Teaching the Tiger: An Educator's Guide to TS/OCD/ADHD
Adam Ward Seligman, Echolalia Press
35158 Annapolis Road   707-886-1972
Annapolis, CA 95412-9713
Workbook

8855 Tourette Syndrome and Human Behavior
Adam Ward Seligman, Echolalia Press
35158 Annapolis Road   707-886-1972
Annapolis, CA 95412-9713
Available in hardcover.
Softcover

8856 Tourette Syndrome: Advances in Neurology
Tourette Syndrome Association
42-40 Bell Boulevard   718-224-2999
Bayside, NY 11361-2861   888-480-8737
Fax: 718-279-9596
In this single-volume reference, more than 90 of the foremost research and clinical leaders in the field review the current state of knowledge about this disorder.
400 pages
Thomas N Chase MD, Editor
Arnold J Friedhoff MD, Editor

8857 What Makes Ryan Tic?
Adam Ward Seligman, Echolalia Press
35158 Annapolis Road   707-886-1972
Annapolis, CA 95412-9713
Softcover

Children's Books

8858 Adam and the Magic Marble
Adam Ward Seligman, Echolalia Press
35158 Annapolis Road   707-886-1972
Annapolis, CA 95412-9713

8859 Hi! I'm Adam!
Adam Ward Seligman, Echolalia Press
35158 Annapolis Road   707-886-1972
Annapolis, CA 95412-9713

8860 Matthew and the Tics
Tourette Syndrome Association
42-40 Bell Boulevard   718-224-2999
Bayside, NY 11361-2861   888-480-8738
Fax: 718-279-9596
A story for young children with TS and their peers.
2 pages

Newsletters

8861 Tourette Syndrome Association Newsletter
42-40 Bell Boulevard   718-224-2999
Bayside, NY 11361   888-480-8738
Fax: 718-279-9596
e-mail: ts@tsa-usa.org
www.tsa-usa.org/
Offers information, articles and news on the latest technology and advancements for persons with Tourette Syndrome.
Quarterly

Pamphlets

8862 Commentary on Alternative Therapies for TS
Tourette Syndrome Association
42-40 Bell Boulevard   718-224-2999
Bayside, NY 11361-2861   888-480-8738
Fax: 718-279-9596
Summarizes physician/patient reports of symptom management through non-pharmacological interventions.
2 pages

8863 Consumer's Guide to TS Medications
Tourette Syndrome Association
42-40 Bell Boulevard   718-224-2999
Bayside, NY 11361-2861   888-480-8738
Fax: 718-279-9596
Covers common medications used for the control of TS motor and vocal ties as well as those traditionally prescribed for associated behaviors.
1992 12 pages

8864 Coping with TS in the Classroom
Tourette Syndrome Association
42-40 Bell Boulevard   718-224-2999
Bayside, NY 11361-2820   Fax: 718-279-9596
Includes practical guidelines for education developed from a study about cognitive effects on learning.
18 pages

8865 Coping with TS, A Parent's Viewpoint
Tourette Syndrome Association
42-40 Bell Boulevard   718-224-2999
Bayside, NY 11361-2861   888-480-8738
Fax: 718-279-9596
An accalaimed medical writer and mother of three children with TS, the author sensitively addresses common concerns and feelings of parents.
1994 23 pages

8866 Coping with Tourette Syndrome in Early Adulthood
Tourette Syndrome Association
42-40 Bell Boulevard   718-224-2999
Bayside, NY 11361-2861   888-480-8738
Fax: 718-279-9596
Focuses on two fundamental challenges facing adults with TS: employment and interpersonal relationships. Provides specific techniques for overcoming barriers.

8867 Current Pharmacology of TS
Tourette Syndrome Association
42-40 Bell Boulevard   718-224-2999
Bayside, NY 11361-2861   888-480-8738
Fax: 718-279-9596
Covers all current medications used to treat TS with specific information about clinical evaluations and diagnosis.
12 pages

8868 Dental Treatment of Patients with Gilles de la Tourette Syndrome
Tourette Syndrome Association
42-40 Bell Boulevard   718-224-2999
Bayside, NY 11361-2861   888-480-8738
Fax: 718-279-9596
Discusses TS movements and possible adverse interactions of dentistry and TS medications.
5 pages

8869 Development of Behavioral and Emotional Problems in TS
Tourette Syndrome Association
42-40 Bell Boulevard
Bayside, NY 11361-2861

718-224-2999
888-480-8738
Fax: 718-279-9596

Using the Child Behavior Checklist, 78 male children were assessed for a variety of behavioral problems. Relation to tic severity covered.
1989 3 pages

8870 Discipline and the Child with TS
Tourette Syndrome Association
42-40 Bell Boulevard
Bayside, NY 11361

718-224-2999
888-480-8738
Fax: 718-279-9596

Helps children redirect impulses and compulsions through teaching cause and effect relationships.
15 pages

8871 Educator's Guide to Tourette Syndrome
Tourette Syndrome Association
42-40 Bell Boulevard
Bayside, NY 11361-2861

718-224-2999
888-480-8738
Fax: 718-279-9596

Covers symptoms, treatments and techniques for classroom management, attentional, writing and language problems.
16 pages

8872 Genetics of Tourette's Syndrome: Who it Affects and How it Occurs in Families
Tourette Syndrome Association
42-40 Bell Boulevard
Bayside, NY 11361-2861

718-224-2999
888-480-8738
Fax: 718-279-9596

10 pages

8873 Getting Into College: Strategies for the Student with TS
Tourette Syndrome Association
42-40 Bell Boulevard
Bayside, NY 11361

718-224-2999
888-480-8738
Fax: 718-279-9596

10 pages

8874 Gift of Hope
Tourette Syndrome Association
42-40 Bell Boulevard
Bayside, NY 11361-2861

718-224-2999
888-480-8738
Fax: 718-279-9596

TSA Brain Bank Program registration information. Includes donor cards.

8875 Grandparents Club
Tourette Syndrome Association
42-40 Bell Boulevard
Bayside, NY 11361-2861

718-224-2999
888-480-8738
Fax: 718-279-9596

A flyer describing how to join with other grandparents to support TS research to benefit future generations.

8876 Guide to Diagnosis & Treatment
Tourette Syndrome Association
42-40 Bell Boulevard
Bayside, NY 11361-2861

718-224-2999
888-480-8738
Fax: 718-279-9596

Covers symptoms, pharmacology and clinical assessments.
30 pages

8877 Guide to Housing for Adults with TS
Tourette Syndrome Association
42-40 Bell Boulevard
Bayside, NY 11361-2861

718-224-2999
888-480-8738
Fax: 718-279-9596

A guide to finding housing, housing laws that help people with TS and ways to maximize living environments.
1991 16 pages

8878 Health Insurance & Tourette Syndrome
Tourette Syndrome Association
42-40 Bell Boulevard
Bayside, NY 11361-2861

718-224-2999
888-480-8738
Fax: 718-279-9596

Detailed, up-to-date packet of medical information for obtaining health insurance as well as information for submission to insurance carriers.

8879 Helpful Techniques to Aid the Student with TS
Tourette Syndrome Association
42-40 Bell Boulevard
Bayside, NY 11361-2861

718-224-2999
888-480-8738
Fax: 718-279-9596

Helpful hints for teacher with specific suggestions for test taking, math computation, and note taking.
1 pages

8880 Learning Problems & the Child with TS
Tourette Syndrome Association
42-40 Bell Boulevard
Bayside, NY 11361-2861

718-224-2999
888-480-8738
Fax: 718-279-9596

Report on learning problems identified through a study of 200 children with TS.
1 pages

8881 Need to Know
Tourette Syndrome Association
42-40 Bell Boulevard
Bayside, NY 11361-2861

718-224-2999
888-480-8738
Fax: 718-279-9596

Recollections of a young woman who was diagnosed with TS in her 20s.
4 pages

8882 Neuropsychological Performance in Adults with TS
Tourette Syndrome Association
42-40 Bell Boulevard
Bayside, NY 11361-2861

718-224-2999
888-480-8738
Fax: 718-279-9596

Describes clinical and neuropsychological testing on learning and memory with TS adults.
7 pages

8883 Peer Problems in Tourette's Disorder
Tourette Syndrome Association
42-40 Bell Boulevard
Bayside, NY 11361-2861

718-224-2999
888-480-8738
Fax: 718-279-9596

Detailed research findings of peer problems in children with TS. Includes statistical results obtained from these studies.
1991 7 pages

8884 Pharmacotherapy of TS and Associated Disorders
Tourette Syndrome Association
42-40 Bell Boulevard
Bayside, NY 11361-2861

718-224-2999
888-480-8738
Fax: 718-279-9596

Overview with emphasis on the complexities of prescribing TS medications.
19 pages

8885 Problem Behaviors & TS
Tourette Syndrome Association
42-40 Bell Boulevard
Bayside, NY 11361-2861

718-224-2999
888-480-8738
Fax: 718-279-9596

Describes recent research and what is now known about the relationship of a variety of behaviors and TS.
21 pages

8886 Recognizing TS in the Classroom
Tourette Syndrome Association
42-40 Bell Boulevard
Bayside, NY 11361-2861

718-224-2999
888-480-8738
Fax: 718-279-9596

Provides an overview offering detailed symptoms checklist, post-diagnosis advice and covers special education needs.
4 pages

8887 Risperidone as a Treatment for TS
Tourette Syndrome Association

42-40 Bell Boulevard

Bayside, NY 11361-2861

718-224-2999

888-480-8738

Fax: 718-279-9596

6 pages

8888 Specific Classroom Strategies and Techniques for Students with TS

Tourette Syndrome Association

42-40 Bell Boulevard

Bayside, NY 11361-2861

718-224-2999

888-480-8738

Fax: 718-279-9596

An educator with TS spells out concrete methods for managing students with TS. She outlines many valuable classroom interventions to help youngsters deal with tic symptons, ADHD, visual motor and fine motor integration, and behavioral difficulties.

1994 2 pages

8889 TS and Other Tic Disorders

Tourette Syndrome Association

42-40 Bell Boulevard

Bayside, NY 11361-2861

718-224-2999

888-480-8738

Fax: 718-279-9596

Comprehensive overview of the complexities of TS. Includes tic syndrome classifications, epidemiology, genetics, behavioral aspects, and summary.

17 pages

8890 TS and the School Nurse

Tourette Syndrome Association

42-40 Bell Boulevard

Bayside, NY 11361-2861

718-224-2999

888-480-8738

Fax: 718-279-9596

Comprehensive professional guide to educational, social and medical implications.

19 pages

8891 TS and the School Psychologist

Tourette Syndrome Association

42-40 Bell Boulevard

Bayside, NY 11361-2861

718-224-2999

888-480-8738

Fax: 718-279-9596

The role of the school psychologist is covered including testing procedures, counseling strategies and social implications.

1993 (rev.) 14 pages

8892 TS: A Look at the Interface Between TS & the Law

Tourette Syndrome Association

42-40 Bell Boulevard

Bayside, NY 11361-2861

718-224-2999

888-480-8738

Fax: 718-279-9596

Summarizes important legislation protecting the rights of students with TS. Also covers resources and hints about how to prepare for dealing successfully with educators and school systems.

1 pages

8893 TSA Medical Letters

Tourette Syndrome Association

42-40 Bell Boulevard

Bayside, NY 11361-2861

718-224-2999

888-480-8738

Fax: 718-279-9596

Annual publication of TSA's Medical Committe covering recent, significant findings from scientific articles.

16 pages

8894 Teens and Tourette Syndrome

Tourette Syndrome Association

42-40 Bell Boulevard

Bayside, NY 11361-2820

718-224-2999

Fax: 718-279-9596

e-mail: ts@tsa-usa.org

www.tsa-usa.org/

Covers self esteem, friends, dating, drugs and alcohol, stress, depression, academic and vocational planning, sibling relationships and medication.

16 pages

8895 Tourette Syndrome and the School Nurse

Tourette Syndrome Association

42-40 Bell Boulevard

Bayside, NY 11361-2820

718-224-2999

Fax: 718-279-9596

e-mail: ts@tsa-usa.org

http://tsa-usa.org

Includes symptoms, epidemiology, associated beviors, developmental consequences, causes, treatments, role of the school nurse and additional resources.

20 pages

8896 Tourette: The Man and His Times

Tourette Syndrome Association

42-40 Bell Boulevard

Bayside, NY 11361-2861

718-224-2999

888-480-8738

Fax: 718-279-9596

Rare historical biography of the famous French neurologist G. Gilles De La Tourette.

9 pages

8897 What School Bus Drivers Need to Know About Students with Tourette Syndrome

Tourette Syndrome Association

42-40 Bell Boulevard

Bayside, NY 11361-2820

718-224-2999

Fax: 718-279-9596

e-mail: ts@tsa-usa.org

http://tsa-usa.org

Includes a description of the disorder, as well as related disorders and suggestions as to what school bus drivers can do for students with TS.

1 pages

Audio & Video

8898 A Regular Kid That's Me: Inservice Film for Educators

Tourette Syndrome Association

42-40 Bell Boulevard

Bayside, NY 11361

718-224-2999

888-480-8738

Fax: 718-279-9596

e-mail: ts@tsa-usa.org

http://tsa-usa.org

Nineteen students with TS (ages 7-17) along with several educators are seen interacting in classroom settings. Includes the basic criteria for diagnosis, discussions of common associated behaviors, e.g. ADD with or without hyperactivity, obsessive compulsive symptoms and specific learning disabilities. Professionals describe the impact of having TS on educational placement and specific classroom strategies are presented. 45 minutes. May be purchased as part of a curriculum or separately. #AV-2

VHS 1/2 inch

8899 After the Diagnosis...the Next Steps

42-40 Bell Boulevard

Bayside, NY 11361

718-224-2999

888-480-8738

Fax: 718-279-9596

e-mail: ts@tsa-usa.org

http://tsa-usa.org

When the diagnosis is Tourette Syndrome, what do you do first? How do you sort out the complexities of the disorder? Whose advice do you follow? What steps do you take to lead a normal life? Six people with TS—as different as any six people can be—relate the sometimes difficult, but finally triumphant path each took to lead the rich, fulfilling life they now enjoy. Narrated by Academy Award-winning actor, Richard Dreyfuss, the stories are blends of poignancy, fact and inspiration.

8900 Clinical Counseling: Towards a Better Understanding of TS

Tourette Syndrome Association

42-40 Bell Boulevard

Bayside, NY 11361

718-224-2999

888-480-8738

Fax: 718-279-9596

e-mail: ts@tsa-usa.org

http://tsa-usa.org

Targeted to counselors, social workers, educators, psychologists and families, this video features expert physicians, allied professionals and several families summarizing key issues that can arise when counseling families with TS. 15 minutes. #AV-10A

8901 Complexities of TS Treatment: A Physician's Round Table

Tourette Syndrome Association

42-40 Bell Boulevard

Bayside, NY 11361

718-224-2999

888-480-8738

Fax: 718-279-9596

e-mail: ts@tsa-usa.org

http://tsa-usa.org

Three internationally recognized TS experts provide colleagues with valuable information about the complexities of treating and advising families with TS. Emphasis is on different clinical approaches to patients with a broad range of symptom severity. Co-morbid and associated conditions are covered. 15 minutes. #AV-10

8902 **Educator's In-Service Program**
Tourette Syndrome Association
42-40 Bell Boulevard   718-224-2999
Bayside, NY 11361   888-480-8738
Fax: 718-279-9596

A curriculum designed to train educators to recognize and understand TS and guide students with TS and associated disorders in a classroom setting. Developed by the Tourette Syndrome Association for the training of all educational personnel. Includes 2 videos, a particpant's guide, a set of 20 transparencies, 2 scripted curriculum modules and a comprehensive teacher's guide. Discounted for members.

8903 **Gift of Hope**
Tourette Syndrome Association
42-40 Bell Boulevard   718-224-2999
Bayside, NY 11361   888-480-8738
Fax: 718-279-9596
e-mail: ts@tsa-usa.org
http://tsa-usa.org

The cause of TS lies in the brain. Because their are no animal models to study this disorder, human brain tissue is of vital importance for progress in research. Increased brain bank registration is a prime objective of the TSA. VHS 1/2 inch. 14 minutes. Available for shipping cost only. #AV- 7

8904 **Guide to Diagnosis**
Tourette Syndrome Association
42-40 Bell Boulevard   718-224-2999
Bayside, NY 11361-2861   888-480-8738
Fax: 718-279-9596

A video and companion guide for interested medical professionals who have not seen a substantial number of TS patients.
30 minutes

8905 **I'm a Person Too**
Tourette Syndrome Association
42-40 Bell Boulevard   718-224-2999
Bayside, NY 11361   888-480-8738
Fax: 718-279-9596
e-mail: ts@tsa-usa.org
http://tsa-usa.org

Narrated by Cliff Robertson, this video features 5 people with TS; 2 elementary school students and 3 adults from diverse social backgrounds. They talk about a broad variety of symptoms and their personal experiences living with the disorder. VHS 1/2 inch. 22 minutes. #AV1

8906 **Panel of Experts**
Tourette Syndrome Association
42-40 Bell Boulevard   718-224-2999
Bayside, NY 11361-2861   888-480-8738
Fax: 718-279-9596

Five leading authorities bring their in-depth knowledge and experience to bear in a wide-ranging discussion that covers current strategies in TS diagnosis, and medication.
30 minutes

8907 **Parent's Perspective: Diplomacy in Action**
Tourette Syndrome Association
42-40 Bell Boulevard   718-224-2999
Bayside, NY 11361-2861   888-480-8738
Fax: 718-279-9596

The child with TS faces a set of special problems in school. The level of achievement reached in large measure is dependent on the attitude of teachers and administrators. Therefore, educating the educators becomes a high priority with the parent.
45 minutes

8908 **Stop It!... I Can't!**
Tourette Syndrome Association

42-40 Bell Boulevard   718-224-2999
Bayside, NY 11361   888-480-8738
Fax: 718-279-9596
e-mail: ts@tsa-usa.org
http://tsa-usa.org

Narrated by William Shatner, this video promotes sensitivity, education, acceptance and confidence for children with TS. Produced in the 1970's, but provides a valuable and classic message. VHS 1/2 inch. 13 minutes.

8909 **TS-The Parent's Perspective: Diplomacy in Action**
Tourette Syndrome Association
42-40 Bell Boulevard   718-224-2999
Bayside, NY 11361   888-480-8738
Fax: 718-279-9596
e-mail: ts@tsa-usa.org
http://tsa-usa.org

The child with TS faces a set of special problems in school. The level of achievement reached in large measure is dependent on the attitude of teachers and administrators. Therefore educating the educators becomes a high priority for the parent. Special education professionals provide firm guidance to famililies on school advocacy issues. Concrete suggestions are offered to smooth the road to success in school for the student with TS. VHS 1/2 inch. 45 minutes. #AV-6

8910 **TS: A Panel of Experts**
Tourette Syndrome Association
42-40 Bell Boulevard   718-224-2999
Bayside, NY 11361   888-480-8738
Fax: 718-279-9596
e-mail: ts@tsa-usa.org
http://tsa-usa.org

Five leading authorities bring their in-depth knowledge and experience to bear in a wide-ranging discussion that covers current strategies in TS diagnosis and medication, behavioral problems, predicted course and other aspects of this disorder. VHS 1/2 inch. 30 minutes. # AV-5

8911 **Talking About Tourette Syndrome**
Tourette Syndrome Association
42-40 Bell Boulevard   718-224-2999
Bayside, NY 11361   888-480-8738
Fax: 718-279-9596
e-mail: ts@tsa-usa.org
http://tsa-usa.org

When the professional is also the patient, a unique perspective emerges. A psychiatrist leads a candid probing discussion with a brother and sister- all have Tourette syndrome. This free-wheeling exchange brings to the viewer many instructive and often surprising observations about TS and obsessive compulsive symptoms. VHS 1/2 inch. 45 minutes. #AV-8

8912 **Tourette Syndrome: Guide to Diagnosis**
Tourette Syndrome Association
42-40 Bell Boulevard   718-224-2999
Bayside, NY 11361   888-480-8738
Fax: 718-279-9596
e-mail: ts@tsa-usa.org
http://tsa-usa.org

Video for interested medical professionals who have not seen substantial numbers of TS patients. Presents 7 patients with TS who exhibit the full range of movements, vocalizations and behavioral patterns associated with the disorder. Descriptions and demonstrations of other movement disorders are also presented for the purpose of differential diagnosis. VHS 1/2 inch. 30 minutes. A 29 page companion piece by Drs. Ruth Brunn, Donald Cohen and James Leckman is available at $6.00/3.50 shipping.#AV4

8913 **Family Life with Tourette Syndrome... Personal Stories: Professor Peter**
Tourette Syndrome Association
42-40 Bell Boulevard   718-224-2999
Bayside, NY 11361   888-480-8738
Fax: 718-279-9596
e-mail: ts@tsa-usa.org
tsa-usa.org

Now a world class scientific research expert and a professor of biology at Harvard and Purdue, Professor Hollenbeck talks about growing up positively with TS, never hesitating to have children, and offering good advice for newly diagnosed families. 7 minutes, 27 seconds. If purchased together, the six videos in this series are $50.00. #AV-11A

8914 Family Life with Tourette Syndrome... Personal Stories: Reverend Mike
Tourette Syndrome Association
42-40 Bell Boulevard
Bayside, NY 11361
718-224-2999
888-480-8738
Fax: 718-279-9596
e-mail: ts@tsa-usa.org
tsa-usa.org

Mike Higgins did not receive a diagnosis of TS until he was in the army! Mike overcame significant symptoms and childhood teasing. Reverend Mike talks about the value of strong family life, faith, support groups and acceptance of the person, and not the disorder as a good way to live positively with TS. If purchased together, the six videos in this series are $50.00. #AV-11B

8915 Family Life with Tourette Syndrome... Personal Stories: Rachel
Tourette Syndrome Association
42-40 Bell Boulevard
Bayside, NY 11361
718-224-2999
888-480-8738
Fax: 718-279-9596
e-mail: ts@tsa-usa.org
http://tsa-usa.org

Challenged by TS, ADHD and OCD Rachel and her family endured difficult reactions, behavioral episodes, and at times, a great loss of hope. Now seventeen years old, Rachel and family overcame stresses and strains by sticking together through the highs and lows to find Rachel today a confident and happy teen. 10 minutes. If purchased together, the six videos in this series are $50.00. #AV-11C

8916 Family Life with Tourette Syndrome... Personal Stories: The Turners
Tourette Syndrome Association
42-40 Bell Boulevard
Bayside, NY 11361
718-224-2999
888-480-8738
Fax: 718-279-9596
e-mail: ts@tsa-usa.org
http://tsa-usa.org

Three of the four Turner daughters have TS in varying degrees. The family wondered how their symptoms came to be, how to dispense attention fairly, what to say to teachers and friends. They learned how to deal with sibling issues and low self esteem among the sisters. This determined family never gave up! 12 minutes. If purchased together, the six videos in this series are $50.00. #AV-11D

8917 Family Life with Tourette Syndrome... Personal Stories: Ryan
Tourette Syndrome Association
42-40 Bell Boulevard
Bayside, NY 11361
718-224-2999
888-480-8738
Fax: 718-279-9596
e-mail: ts@tsa-usa.org
http://tsa-usa.org

Ryan's family first thought his behavior was a deliberate way to get attention. A school principal was harshly critical. The family soon learned to educate themselves and others about Ryan's TS. Things turned around as a result. A good teacher took a great interest, friends began to seek him out and Ryan grew into a young man with a positive outlook. 11 minutes, 28 seconds. If purchased together, the six videos in this series are $50.00. #AV-11E

8918 Family Life with Tourette Syndrome... Personal Stories: Dakota
Tourette Syndrome Association
42-40 Bell Boulevard
Bayside, NY 11361
718-224-2999
888-480-8738
Fax: 718-279-9596
e-mail: ts@tsa-usa.org
http://tsa-usa.org

A happy 11 year old baseball playing, video game whiz, Dakota was initially diagnosed as having a brain tumor! He was actually affected by TS and AHD. This is a story of a child who developed a strong confidence and a good attitude, learning to believe in himself. He says the love of his grandparents was a special help! 7 minutes, 12 seconds. If purchased together, the 6 videos in this series are $50.00. #AV-11F

Web Sites

8919 American Academy of Neurology: Tourette Syndrome
www.aan.com
The American Academy of Neurology (AAN) is a worldwide professional association of more than 17,000 neurologists and neuroscience professionals dedicating to providing the best possible care for patients with neurological disorders.

8920 Healing Well
www.healingwell.com
An online health resource guide to medical news, chat, information and articles, newsgroups and message boards, books, disease-related web sites, medical directories, and more for patients, friends, and family coping with disabling diseases, disorders, or chronic illnesses.

8921 Health Finder
www.healthfinder.gov
Searchable, carefully developed web site offering information on over 1000 topics. Developed by the US Department of Health and Human Services, the site can be used in both English and Spanish.

8922 Healthlink USA
www.healthlinkusa.com
Health information concerning treatment, cures, prevention, diagnosis, risk factors, research, support groups, email lists, personal stories and much more. Updated regularly.

8923 Helios Health
www.helioshealth.com
Online resource for your health information. Detailed information about specific health topics, access to expert advice from our Medical Advisory Board, and up-to-date health news.

8924 MedicineNet
www.medicinenet.com
An online resource for consumers providing easy-to-read, authoritative medical and health information.

8925 Medscape
www.medscape.com
Medscape offers specialists, primary care physicians, and other health professionals the Web's most robust and integrated medical information and educational tools.

8926 National Institute of Neurological Disorders and Stroke
www.ninds.nih.gov
The mission of NINDS is to reduce the burden of neurological disease - a burden borne by every age group, by every segment of society, by people all over the world.

8927 WebMD
www.webmd.com
Information on Tourette Syndrome, including articles and resources.

Description

8928 ## Transplant-Related Conditions

In recent decades, transplantation of solid organs (heart, liver, lung, kidney), bone marrow and stem cells has become an established part of medical care for advanced diseases in many patients who otherwise face end-organ failure and poor prognosis. While on one hand, transplantation may serve to cure the underlying disease it nonetheless often entails chronic medical therapy that will likely include the use of immunosuppressants, complications from chronic medications, frequent and long-term medical follow-up and diagnostic testing which may be invasive.

A number of clinical management protocols are utilized in the care of post-transplantation patient, and these vary depending on the type of transplant undertaken, the extent of the tissue match between donor and recipient, and the experience of the given transplantation center. In general however, most patients who receive a transplanted organ or cells will require some chronic therapy (short or long-term) with immunosuppressive medications. These can be several or many and are given in an effort to control the patient's own immunologic response to receiving an organ or cells from another person. The body's natural response after recognizing such an exposure is to "fight" these cells and tissues with its own defense cells, which are designed to attack and kill foreign material. The immunosuppressive medications help modulate this response so that the transplanted organ is not damaged, injured or "rejected" by the recipient who needs the organ or cells to function in a healthier manner. Immunosuppressive therapy and protection of the transplanted organ must be balanced against the adverse creation of an immunocompromised state in the patient placing him at greater risk for contracting infections that can be serious and even life threatening. Given these circumstances, transplant patients require close working relationships with their medical team along with a true commitment to be compliant with these potentially difficult and complicated medical regimens.

In addition to the medical therapy for patients who have received transplants, one must also consider the significant psychological and social aspects of having undergone such procedures. Strong social support systems and close attention to a healthy emotional and psychological status are important for successful management of these patients. Many transplant centers have extensive support services available to patients from which they and their families can benefit.

National Agencies & Associations

8929 **American Society of Transplantation (AST)**
15000 Commerce Parkway   856-439-9986
Mount Laurel, NJ 08054   Fax: 856-439-9982
                                  e-mail: ast@ahint.com
                                        www.a-s-t.org
The American Society of Transplantation is an international organization of transplant professionals dedicated to advancing the field of transplantation through the promotion of research education advocacy and organ donation to improve patient care.
Libby McDannell, CAE, Executive Director
Susan J Nelson, Executive Vice President

8930 **Association of Organ Procurement Organizations (AOPO)**
8500 Leesburg Pike   703-556-4242
Vienna, VA 22182   Fax: 703-556-4852
                                  e-mail: aopo@aopo.org
                                        www.aopo.org
Organization involved in helping people find and obtain the organs they need for transplantation.
Elling Eidbo, Executive Director
Sue Dunn, President/CEO

8931 **Children's Organ Transplant Association (COTA)**
2501 COTA Drive   700-366-2682
Bloomington, IN 47403   800-366-2682
                                  Fax: 812-336-8885
                                  e-mail: cota@cota.org
                                        www.cota.org
Not-for-profit national chairty dedicated to helping families and communities raise the necessary funds for transplant expenses.
Rick Lofgren, President/CEO
Lisa Fulkerson, VP/CFO

8932 **Donate Life America**
700 N Fourth Street   804-782-4920
Richmond, VA 23219   Fax: 804-782-4643
                          e-mail: coalition@donatelife.net
                                        www.donatelife.net
A not-for-profit alliance of national organizations and local coalitions across the United States that have joined forces to educate the public about organ, eye and tissue donation, correcting misconceptions about donation and creating a greater willingness to donate.
Sara Pace Jones, Chairwoman
Bruce Wilson, Director of Organ Procurement

8933 **Health Resources and Services Administration (HRSA)**
5600 Fishers Lane   301-443-7577
Rockville, MD 20857   e-mail: comments@hrsa.gov
                                        www.hrsa.gov
Envisions optimal health for all, supported by a health care system that assures access to comprehensive, culturally competant, quality care. Provides national leadership, program resources and services needed to improve access to culturally competant, quality health care.
Elizabeth M Duke PhD, Administrator
Dennis P Williams PhD MA, Deputy Administrator

8934 **Jewish Hospital Transplant Center**
200 Abraham Flexner Way
Louisville, KY 40202   502-587-4011
                                  www.jewishhospital.com
An elite group approved to perform five solid organ transplants and has been named a Federally Designated Medicare Heart Lung Kidney Liver and Pancreas Transplant Center.
Robert L Shircliff, President/CEO
Barbara Mackovic, Senior Manager

8935 **National Foundation for Transplants**
5350 Poplar Avenue   901-684-1697
Memphis, TN 38119   800-489-3863
                                  Fax: 901-684-1128
                                  e-mail: info@transplants.org
                                        www.transplants.org
Mission is to reach out to help those who seek a new life through transplantation by providing healthcare and financial support services and patient advocacy for transplant candidates families nationwide.
Jackie D Hancock, President
Connie Gonitzke, Vice President

8936 **National Institute of Allergy and Infectious Diseases (NIAID)**
6610 Rockledge Drive   301-496-2263
Bethesda, MD 20892-6612   Fax: 301-402-0120
                                        www.niaid.nih.gov
Conducts and supports basic and applied research to better understand, treat, and ultimately prevent infectious, immunologic and allergic diseases. Research has led to new therapies, vaccines, di-

agnostic tests, and other technologies that have improved the health of millions of people in the United States and around the world.
Anthony S. Fauci, Director

8937 National Transplant Assistance Fund (NTAF)
150 N. Radnor Chester Rd.   800-642-8399
Radnor, PA 19087   800-642-8399
Fax: 610-353-6106
e-mail: ntaf@transplantfund.org
www.transplantfund.org
Helps to raise funds for transplant and catastrophic injury patients by providing compassionate support education and expertise to them their families and communities.
Lynne Coughl Samson, Executive Director
Fred Kauffman, Managing Director

8938 Organ Procurement and Transplantation Network (OPTN)
700 N 4th Street   804-782-4800
Richmond, VA 23219   888-TXI-NFO1
Fax: 804-782-4994
www.optn.org
A unified transplant network established by the United States Congress under the National Organ Transplant Act (NOTA) of 1984. A unique public-private partnership that links all of the professionals involved in the donation and transplantation system.
Kenneth Andreoni, MD
Carl Berg, Vice President

8939 United Network for Organ Sharing (UNOS)
700 N 4th Street   804-782-4800
Richmond, VA 23219   Fax: 804-782-4817
www.unos.org
Non-profit scientific and educational organization that administers the nation's only Organ Procurement and Transplantation Network (OPTN). Mission is to advance organ availability and transplantation by uniting and supporting our communities.
Walter K Graham, Executive Director
Marcia D Manning, Director of Community Affairs

8940 United Organ Transplant Association (UOTA)
3405 Arlington Avenue
Riverside, CA 92506   e-mail: pres@uota.org
www.uota.org
Non-profit charitable corporation dedicated to providing educational emotional and financial support to pre- and post- transplant patients.
Don Goss, Founder

State Agencies & Associations

Alabama

8941 Alabama Organ Center
500 S 22 Street S   205-731-9200
Birmingham, AL 35233   800-252-3677
Fax: 205-731-9250
e-mail: Rebecca.davis@ccc.uab.edu
alabamaorgancenter.org
A non-profit, independent organ procurement organization (OPO) serving the population of the Southeastern United States.
Devin E Eckhoff, Director
R Alan Hicks MPH CPTC, Associate Director

Arizona

8942 Donor Network of Arizona
201 W Coolidge   602-222-2200
Phoenix, AZ 85013   800-94D-ONOR
Fax: 602-222-2202
e-mail: Contact.Us@dnaz.org
www.dnaz.org
Participates in the equitable distribution of organs, tissues, and corneas for transplant. Also offers donor family support services, community and health care education, and presentations.
Sara Pace Jones, Public Education Contact
Tim Brown, Chief executive officer

Arkansas

8943 Arkansas Regional Organ Recovery Agency
1701 Aldersgate Road   501-907-9150
Little Rock, AR 72205   800-727-6726
Fax: 501-372-6279
e-mail: info@arora.org
www.arora.org
Makes every effort to provide organs and tissues for life-saving and life-enhancing transplantation. Goal will be accomplished through continuous hospital involvement which includes hospital training community involvement andpublic education.
Audrey Brown, Director of Community Education
Boyd Ward, Executive Director

California

8944 California Transplant Donor Network
1000 Broadway   888-570-9400
Oakland, CA 94607   888-570-9400
Fax: 510-444-8501
e-mail: info@ctdn.org
www.ctdn.org
Helps patients in Northern and Central California and Northern Nevada receive organ and tissue transplants. Recovers organs from donors and matches them with the more than 6 000 people who are currently waiting for transplants in this region.
Cynthia Siljestrom, Chief Executive Officer
Sonia Salloum, Community Outreach Coordinator

8945 Golden State Donor Services
1760 Creekside Oaks Drive   916-567-1600
Sacramento, CA 95833   877-401-2546
Fax: 916-567-8300
e-mail: info@gsds.org
www.gsds.org
Support, enhance, and provide for the recovery and allocation of anatomical gifts. Also work to educate the public regarding the critical need for organ and tissue doors.
Katherine Doolittle, Senior Public Education Coordinator
Helen Nelson, Executive Director

8946 LifeSharing Community Organ & Tissue Donation
3465 Camino Del Rio S   619-521-1983
San Diego, CA 92108   Fax: 619-521-2833
e-mail: info@lifesharing.org
www.lifesharing.org
Non-profit unique and creative organ procurement organization that has centers at the University of California at San Diego Medical Center, Green Hospital of Scripps Clinic, Sharp Hospital.
Sharie Shipley, Public Education Contact
Bill Dawson, Chairman of Volunteer Action Committee

8947 One Legacy Transplant Donor Network
221 S Figueroa Street   213-229-5600
Los Angeles, CA 90012   800-786-4077
Fax: 213-229-5601
e-mail: tmone@onelegacy.org
www.onelegacy.org
One Legacy is dedicaated to achieving the donation of life saving and life enhancing organs and tissues for those in need of transplants and to providing a sense of purpose and comfort to those families we serve.
Sandra Walla Blaydow, Human Resources Manager
Thomas Mone, Chief Executive Officer/EVP

Colorado

8948 Donor Alliance
720 S Colorado Boulevard   303-329-4747
Denver, CO 80246   888-868-4747
Fax: 303-321-0366
www.donoralliance.org
In cooperation with others Donor Alliance facilitates the donation and recovery of organs and tissues for people needing transplantation. Donor Alliance is one of 58 not-for-profit organ recovery organizations federally designated by the U.S..
Jennifer Moe, Director of Community Relations/PR
Nancy Williams, Chairman

Connecticut

8949 NorthEast Organ Procurement Organization
80 Seymour Street
860-545-5000
Hartford, CT 06102-5037
Fax: 860-545-5066
www.harthosp.org/NEOPO/index.html
Assures that comprehensive organ and tissue donation services are provided to the community in an efficient and professional manner.
Ginger Van Nostrand, Public Education Contact

Florida

8950 LifeLink of Florida
409 Bayshore Boulevard
813-253-2640
Tampa, FL 33606
800-262-5775
Fax: 813-348-0634
e-mail: info@lifelinkfound.org
www.lifelinkfound.org
Independent, nonprofit community service organization dedicated to the recovery and transplantation of organs and tissues. Operates under the authority of the Social Security Act, and in accordance with the National Organ Transplant Act passed by Congress.
Dennis F Heinrichs, President
Dana L Shires Jr, Chairman of the Board

8951 LifeLink of Southwest Florida
409 Bayshore Boulevard
813-253-2640
Tampa, FL 33906
800-262-5775
Fax: 813-348-0634
e-mail: info@lifelinkfound.org
www.lifelinkfound.org
LifeLink of Southwest Florida and Florida Gulf Coast University joined forces to develop a survey instrument to asss student attitudes and opinions about donation. Worked to conduct and evaluate the impact of the multifaceted education campaign.
Dennis F Heinrichs, President
Dana L Shires Jr, Chairman of the Board

8952 TransLife/Florida Hospital
1560 Orange Avenue
407-644-3770
Winter Park, FL 32789
800-443-6667
Fax: 407-303-2473
www.translife.org
Works closely with hospitals and donor families to coordinate the gift of life in Central Florida. Also a critical link between donors and possible recipients.
Carol Rumsey, Public Education Contact

Georgia

8953 LifeLink of Georgia
2875 Northwoods Parkway
770-225-5465
Norcross, GA 30071
800-544-6667
e-mail: info@lifelinkfound.org
www.lifelinkfound.org/georgia/ga.html
The Foundation attempts to work in a sensitive diligent and compassionate manner with donor families to facilitate the donation of desperately needed organs and tissues for waiting patients.
Dennis F Heinrichs, President
Dana L Shires, Chairman of the Board

Hawaii

8954 Organ Donor Center of Hawaii
1149 Bethel Street
808-599-7630
Honolulu, HI 96813
877-855-0603
Fax: 808-599-7631
e-mail: info@organdonorhawaii.com
www.organdonorhawaii.com
Non-profit organ procurement organization.
Stephen A Kula, Executive Director
Christine L Bogee, Administrative Services Director

Illinois

8955 Regional Organ Bank of Illinois, Inc.
5 Spring Lake Drive
312-431-3600
Chicago, IL 60607
888-307-3668
Fax: 312-803-7643
e-mail: info@robi.org
www.robi.org
ROBI'S mission is to save and enhance the lives of as many people as possible through organ and tissue donation.
Kim McCullough, Public Education Contact

Indiana

8956 Indiana Organ Procurement Organization,
3760 Guion Road
317-685-0389
Indianapolis, IN 46222-1816
888-275-4676
Fax: 317-685-1687
e-mail: info@iopo.org
www.iopo.org
Non-profit organ procurement organization designed to recover and distribute organ and tissues for transplantation.
Sam Davis, Director of Professional Services
Lynn Driver, President and CEO

Iowa

8957 Iowa Donor Network
550 Madison Avenue
319-665-3787
N Liberty, IA 52317
800-831-4131
Fax: 319-665-3788
www.iowadonornetwork.org
Iowa Donor Network is dedicated to serving donow families potentialdonors and candidates doe transplantation through identifying potential donorssupporting and respecting donation decisions and maximizing the recovery of transplantable organs and tissues.
John Watson, Chair
Sara Drobnich, Vice-Chair

Kansas

8958 Midwest Transplant Network & Organ Bank
1900 W 47th Place
913-262-1668
Westwood, KS 66205
Fax: 913-262-5130
e-mail: info@mwob.org
www.mwtn.org
Provides quality transplantation related services that will maximize the availability of organs and tissues to the comunities we serve. Provides procurement services for organ and tissue and laboratory services for HLA.
A. Michael Borkon, MD
Gary Duncan, CEO

Kentucky

8959 Kentucky Organ Donor Affiliates
106 E Broadway
502-581-9511
Louisville, KY 40202
800-525-3456
Fax: 502-589-5157
e-mail: info@kyorgandonor.org
www.kyorgandonor.org
Non-profit organ donor center that retrieves and distributes organs to qualified recipients.

Louisiana

8960 Louisiana Organ Procurement Agency
3545 N. I-10 Service Rd
800-521-4483
Metairie, LA 70002-3626
800-521-GIVE
Fax: 504-837-3587
e-mail: info@lopa.org
www.lopa.org
Non-profit organ procurement organization federally-designated to increase the number of transplantable organs by providing families an opportunity to donate organs and tissues to support these families regardless of their decision.
John Egan, Public Education Contact

Maryland

8961 Transplant Resource Center of Maryland
1730 Twin Springs Road
Baltimore, MD 21227
410-242-7000
800-641-HERO
Fax: 410-242-1871
e-mail: communications@TheLLF.org
www.mdtransplant.org
Provides organ and tissue donation and recovery services hospital donor program development and community education to 42 hospitals and the citizens living in Maryland.
Ann Bromery, Chief Financial Officer
Charles Alexander, President & Chief Executive Officer

Massachusetts

8962 New England Organ Bank Massachusetts
One Gateway Center
Newton, MA 02158
800-446-NEOB
Fax: 617-244-8755
e-mail: info@neob.com
www.neob.org
Independent, not-for-profit agency whose mission is to recover, preserve, and distribute human organs and tissues for transplantation. A federally-designated organ procurement organization for all or part of the six New England states, it serves 177 acute care hospitals and 14 transplant centers.
Sean Fitzpatrick, Public Education Contact

Michigan

8963 Transplantation Society of Michigan
3861 Research Park Drive
Ann Arbor, MI 48108
734-973-1577
800-482-4881
Fax: 734-973-3133
e-mail: info@giftoflifemichigan.org
www.giftoflifemichigan.org
Nonprofit independent corporation certified by Medicare and designated by the Centers for Medicare and Medicaid Services as an organ recovery organization for Michigan.
Tammie Harvermahl, Public Education Contact

Minnesota

8964 LifeSource, Upper Midwest Organ Procurement Organization, Inc.
2550 University Avenue West
St. Paul, MN 55114-1904
651-603-7800
Fax: 651-603-7801
e-mail: info@life-source.org
www.life-source.org
Nonprofit, federally-designated organ procurement organization for the Upper Midwest, managing all organ donation activities in Minnesota.
Jill Halimi, Donor Family Services

Mississippi

8965 Mississippi Organ Recovery
12 River Bend Place
Flowood, MS 39232
601-933-1000
800-690-8878
Fax: 601-933-1006
www.msora.org
Not-for-profit organization coordinates the recovery of human organs for transplantation by working with and providing education to medical professionals donor families and the people of Mississippi.
Kelly Nations, Community Education Coordinator
Kevin Stump, Chief Executive Officer

Missouri

8966 Mid-America Transplant Services
1110 Highlands Plaza Drive E
Saint Louis, MO 63110-3205
314-735-8200
Fax: 314-991-2805
e-mail: info@mts-stl.org
www.mts-stl.org
Community based not-for-profit organ procurement organization dedicated to enhancing the quality of human life. Coordinates the procurement of vital organs tissues and eyes in hospitals throughout its service area.
Diane Brockmeier, COO
Dean F Kappel, President and CEO

Nebraska

8967 Nebraska Organ Retrieval System
8502 W Center Road
Omaha, NE 68124
402-733-1800
877-633-1800
Fax: 402-733-9142
www.NEdonation.org
Responsible for retrieving the proper organs and distrbuting them to the recipients.
Kyle Herber, Executive Director
John Stallabaum, Client Services Manager

Nevada

8968 Nevada Donor Network
2059 E Sahara Avenue
Las Vegas, NV 89104
702-384-7616
Fax: 702-796-4225
e-mail: ksatcher@nvdonor.org
www.nvdonor.org
Improving the quality of human life through the recovery of all available organs and tissues for transplantation education and research while maintaining the dignity of the donors and their families.
Liliana Arredondo, Public Education Coordinator
Ken Richardson, Executive Director

New Jersey

8969 Sharing Network Organ Tissue Donation Services
691 Central Avenue
New Providence, NJ 07974
908-516-5400
800-742-7365
Fax: 908-516-5501
e-mail: tsn@sharenj.org
www.sharenj.org
Federally certified state-approved organ procurement organization responsible for recovering organ and tissue for New Jersey residents currently awaiting transplants.
Vito Pulito, Chair
Bruce I. Goldstein, Vice Chair

New Mexico

8970 New Mexico Donor Services
1609 University Blvd NE
Albuquerque, NM 87102
505-843-7672
877-401-2511
Fax: 505-343-1828
e-mail: info@donatelifenm.org
www.donatelifenm.org
Transplant centers in the service area are: University of New Mexico Hospitals Presbyterian Hospital.
Wayne Dunlap, Interim Executive Director
Maria Sanders, Community Relations

New York

8971 Center for Donation & Transplantation
218 Great Oaks Boulevard
Albany, NY 12203
518-262-5606
800-256-7811
Fax: 518-262-5427
e-mail: dfloeser@cdtny.org
www.cdtny.org
Dedicated to increasing organ and tissue donation by following procurement and equitable distribution of medically suitable organs and tissue for transplantation.
Michael Thiabault, Executive Director
Martin benoit, Director

8972 Finger Lakes Donor Recovery Network
Corporate Woods of Brighton
Rochester, NY 14623
585-272-4930
800-810-5494
Fax: 585-272-4956
e-mail: info@donorrecovery.org
www.donorrecovery.org

Nonprofit organization that covers the Finger Lakes Region Central and Upstate New York for transplant centers.
Diane Ashley, Executive Director
Julius Gene Lattore, Vice Chair

8973 New York Organ Donor Network, Inc
132 West 31st Street   646-291-4444
New York, NY 10001   Fax: 646-291-4600
                                                    www.nyodn.org
The New York Organ Donor Network is dedicated to the recovery of organs and tissues for people in need of life-saving and life-improvving transplants.
Elaine Berg, President/CEO

8974 Upstate New York Transplant Services, Inc.
110 Broadway   716-853-6667
Buffalo, NY 14203   800-227-4771
                                                    Fax: 716-853-6674
                                              e-mail: info@unyts.org
                                                    www.unyts.org
An independent nonprofit organization that encourages and coordinates the donation of human organs and tissue for transplantation.
Richard A Grimm, Chairman
Michael Beecher, Vice Chairman

North Carolina

8975 Life Share of the Carolinas
5000 D Airport Center Parkway   704-512-3303
Charlotte, NC 28208   800-932-4483
                                                    Fax: 704-512-3056
                                      e-mail: lifeshare@carolinas.org
                                              www.lifesharecarolinas.org
Mission is to improve the quality of human life through the provision of organs and tissues for transplantation and to serve our hospitals and their respective communities by rpoviding educational support services which enhance the donation process.
Dan Hayes, Medical Director
David Ugland, Bank Medical Director

Ohio

8976 Life Connection of Ohio
3661 Briarfield Boulevard   419-893-1618
Maumee, OH 43537   800-262-5443
                                                    Fax: 419-893-1827
                                            e-mail: ksteele@lcotro.org
                                            www.lifeconnectionofohio.org
Life Connection of Ohio is committed to serving humanity by ending the wait for organ and tissue transplants in a manner that is beneficial to patients, donor families, health care professionals and the public.
Kara Steele, Director of Community Relations (Toledo)
Cathi Arends, Director of Community Relations (Dayton)

8977 LifeBanc
4775 Richmond Road,   216-752-5433
Cleveland, OH 44128-5343   888-558-LIFE
                                                    Fax: 216-751-4204
                                            e-mail: info@lifebanc.org
                                                    www.lifebanc.org
Non-profit organization that covers all of Northeast Ohio.
Monica Morgan, Public Education Contact

8978 Lifeline of Ohio Organ Procurement Agency, Inc.
770 Kinnear Road   614-291-5667
Columbus, OH 43212   800-525-5667
                                                    Fax: 614-291-0660
                                              www.lifelineofohio.org
Lifeline of Ohio (LOOP) is an independent non-profit organization whose purpose is to promote and coordinate the donation of human organs and tissue dor transplantation.
Roger L Walker, Chairperson
Mark E Brainbridge, Treasurer

8979 Ohio Valley LifeCenter
2925 Vernon Place   513-558-5555
Cincinnati, OH 45219-2430   800-981-5433
                                                    Fax: 513-558-5556
                                          e-mail: info@lifepassiton.org
                                                    www.lifecnt.org
Encourages amd coordinates the donation of human organs and tissues in the Greater Cincinnati area. Provides educational and motivational progams to healthcare professionals regarding their important role in the donation of organs and tissues for transplant.
Mark Sommerville, Public Education Contact
Michael Edwards, Chairman

Oklahoma

8980 Oklahoma Organ Sharing Network
5801 N Broadway
Oklahoma City, OK 73118   888-580-5680
                                                    Fax: 405-840-9748
                                            e-mail: philvs@oosn.org
                                                    www.oosn.org
LifeShare Transplant Donor Services of Oklahoma is committed to providing a better quality of life for those people who require organ or tissue transplantation while respecting and honoring those families who share the gift of life.
Harlan Wright, President

Oregon

8981 Pacific NW Transplant Bank
2611 SW 3rd Avenue   503-494-5560
Portland, OR 97201-4952   800-344-8916
                                                    Fax: 503-494-4725
                                            e-mail: pntb@ohsu.edu
                                                    www.pntb.org
Federally designated nonprofit organ procurement organization serving Oregon southwest Washington and western Idaho.
Mike Seeley, Executive Director
Craig Van De Walker, Director Of Operation

Pennsylvania

8982 Center for Organ Recovery & Education
RIDC Park
Pittsburgh, PA 15238   800-366-6777
                                                    Fax: 412-963-3563
                                            e-mail: hbulvony@core.org
                                                    www.core.org
Continues its efforts to lead the procurement field by becoming a full-service OPO.
Susan A Stuart, President & CEO
Karen Zumba, Executive Adminstratve Director

8983 Gift of Life Donor Program Pennsylvania
401 North 3rd Street   215-557-8090
Philadelphia, PA 19123-3813   888-366-6771
                                                    Fax: 215-963-0587
                                            e-mail: info@donors1.org
                                                    www.donors1.org
Formerly (Delaware Valley Transplant Program) is the region's nonprofit organ and tissue donor program serving eastern half of Pennsylvania, southern New Jersey and the state of Delaware. Also, considered a model program in the United States.
Glen D Moffet, Chair
Gerad J. Fulda, Vice Chair

Tennessee

8984 Mid-South Transplant Foundation, Inc. Tennessee
8001 Centerview Parkway   901-328-4438
Corodova, TN 38018   877-228-LIFE
                                                    Fax: 901-448-8126
                                              www.midsouthtransplant.org
Mission is to provide the option of donation to all families of potential organ donors and to protect their rights and interest throughout the donation process.
Louis G Britt, President
Kenneth D Sellers, Medical Director

8985 Tennessee Donor Services
1600 Hayes Street
Nashville, TN 37203

423-915-0808
888-562-3774
Fax: 901-448-8126
e-mail: info@donatelifetn.org
donatelifetn.org

Mission is to represent the interests of the people of our service area in the formulation of policies procedures and regulations concerning organ donation and transplantation.
Lisa Peoples, Public Education Contact
Jennifer Jenks, Contact

Utah

8986 Intermountain Donor Services
230 S 500 E
Salt Lake City, UT 84102

801-521-1755
800-833-6667
Fax: 801-364-8815
e-mail: debbie@idslife.org
www.idslife.org

Provides high quality organ and tissue procurement services to the medical and public communities. Educating medical professionals and the poublic sector on the benefits of organ and tissue donation.
Alex McDonald, Public Education Director
Tracy C Schmidt, Executive Director

Virginia

8987 LifeNet
1864 Concert Drive
Virginia Beach, VA 23453

75- 46- 476
800-847-7831
Fax: 757-301-6582
e-mail: lifenet@trans.org
www.lifenet.org

An organ procurement agency and the largest full-service tissue bank in the United States providing musculoskeletal and cardiovascular tissues for transplant on a national and international basis.
Becky Lawson, Public Education Contact

8988 Washington Regional Transplant Consortium
7619 Little River Turnpike
Annandale, VA 22003

703-641-0100
866-232-3666
Fax: 703-658-0711
e-mail: contactwrtc@wrtc.org
www.wrtc.org

Recently partnered with fellow Mid-Atlantic Coalition on Donation members and a company called Sports America to sponsor the second annual DeMatha Invitational. WRTC is the official link between organ and tissue donors and the patients who are waiting for transplant.
Sara Idler, Public Education Contact

Washington

8989 LifeCenter Northwest
11245 SE 6th Street
Bellevue, WA 98004

425-201-6563
877-275-5269
Fax: 425-688-7641
e-mail: info@lcnw.org
www.lcnw.org

LifeCenter Northwest Organ Donation Network is a nonprofit organization that facilitates organ donation for a population of over 7.5 million people throughout Washington Montana Alasks and Nothern Idaho. Our mission is to fund education and outreach programs.
Megan Erwin, Vice President Community Relations
Diana Clark, President & CEO

Wisconsin

8990 University of Wisconsin Organ Procurement Organization
University of Wisconsin Hospital and Clinics
600 Highland Ave.
Madison, WI 53972-1735

608-265-0356
Fax: 608-262-9099
e-mail: uwhcopo@uwhealth.org
www.uwhcopo.org

Located within a major academic center and is recognized as one of the most successful organ procurement programs in the nation.
Jill Ellefson, Public Education Contact

8991 Wisonsin Donor Network
638 North 18th Street?
Milwaukee, WI 53233

41- 9-7 61
1 -77 -32 4
Fax: 414-259-8059
e-mail: labinfo@bcw.edu
www.bcw.edu

Recovers organs for transplant as well as provides public and professional education about the tremendous need for organ and tissue donors.
Richard S. Gallaghar, Chairman
Peter D. Zegler, Vice Chair

Foundations

8992 Musculoskeletal Transplant Foundation
125 May Street
Edison, NJ 08837

732-661-0202
800-946-9008
Fax: 732-661-2298
e-mail: information@mtf.org
www.mtf.org

Non-profit service organization dedicated to providing quality tissue through a commitment to excellence in education, research, recovery and care for recipients, donors, and their families.
Bruce W Stroever, President/CEO
Martha Anderson, Executive Vice President

Research Centers

8993 Georgetown University Hospital Transplant Institute
3800 Reservoir Road, NW
Washington, DC 20007

202-444-2000
www.georgetownuniversityhospital.org

Founded to promote health through education, research, and patient care.

Books

8994 History of Organ and Cell Transplantation
Imperial College Press
57 Shelton St., Convent Garden
United Kingdom,

e-mail: edit@icpress.co.uk
www.icpress.co.uk

Covers the areas of modern medical literature.
464 pages Hardcover
ISBN: 1-860942-09-1

8995 Legal and Ethical Aspects of Organ Transplantation
David P T Price, author

Cambridge University Press
40 West 20th Street
New York, NY 10011-4221

212-924-3900
Fax: 212-691-3239
www.cambridge.org/us

A comprehensive analysis of existing laws and policies governing transplantation practices around the world. Examines the meaning of death, cadaver organ procurement policies, use of living donors, trading in human organs, experimental transplant procedures and xenotransplantation.
507 pages Hardcover
ISBN: 0-521651-64-6

8996 Organ Procurement and Transplantation:
Intitute of Medicine, author

National Academies Press
500 Fifth Street NW
Washington, DC 20055

202-334-3313
888-624-8373
Fax: 202-334-2451
www.nap.edu

This book assesses the potential impact of the Final Rule on organ transplantation. Prensents new, original data, and assesses medical

practices, social and economic observations, and other information.
232 pages Hardcover

8997 Organ Transplants from Executed Prisoners:
Louis J Palmer, author

McFarland & Company
960 NC Hwy 88W   336-246-4460
Jefferson, NC 28640   Fax: 336-246-5018
                        e-mail: info@mcfarlandpub.com
                              www.mcfarlandpub.com
A study of the utilitarian creation of death sentence organ removal statutes that would make legal the harvesting of transplantable organs from the cadavers of executed capital murders.
156 pages
ISBN: 0-786406-73-9

8998 Transplantation Ethics
Robert M. Veatch, author

Georgetown University Press
3240 Prospect Street, NW   202-687-5889
Washington, DC 20007   Fax: 202-687-6340
                        e-mail: gupress@georgetown.edu
                              www.press.georgetown.edu
The first complete and systematic account of the ethical and policy controversies surrounding organ transplants.
2000 448 pages Paperback
ISBN: 0-878408-12-2

8999 Twice Dead: Organ Transplants and the Reinvention of Death
Margaret Lock, author

University of California Press
1445 Lower Ferry Road
Ewing, NJ 08618   800-UCB-OOKS
                                 Fax: 800-999-1958
                        www.ucpress.edu/index.html
Raises critically important questions about life and death in the modern world.
429 pages Paperback
ISBN: 0-520228-14-6

9000 US Organ Procurement System: A Prescription for Reform
David L. Kaserman, A.H. Barnett, author

American Enterprise Institute
1150 Seventeenth St, NW   202-862-5800
Washington, DC 20036   Fax: 202-862-7177
                              www.aei.org
Isolates the procurement issue from others to make a compelling and persuasive case for markets in cadaveric organs.
177 pages Paperback
ISBN: 0-844741-71-X

Magazines

9001 Encore: Another Chance for Life
Chronimed Pharmacy
Po Box 59032
Minneapolis, MN 55459-9686   800-888-5753
Published exclusively for transplant patients, their families, and friends, this publication provides a broad look at many issues surrounding transplantation and encourages personal stories and feedback from readers.
Quarterly

9002 Renalife
The American Association of Kidney Patients
100 S. Ashley Drive
Tampa, FL 33260   800-749-2257
                        e-mail: aakpaz@enet.net
Provides articles, news items, and information of interest to kindey patients and their families, individuals, and organizations in the renal health care field.
3 Year

9003 Stadtlanders LifeTIMES
Stadtlanders Pharmacy

600 Penn Center Boulevard
Pittsburgh, PA 15235-5810   800-238-7828
                        www.statlander.com/transplant/#resource
Designed to be an educational, informative and supportive, focusing on a variety of health-care issues of concern to patients (including transplant patients).

Newsletters

9004 Advocate
National Foundation for Transplants
1102 Brookfield Road   901-684-1697
Memphis, TN 38119   800-489-3863
                                 Fax: 901-684-1128
                        e-mail: info@transplants.org
                              www.transplants.org
Judy Strickland, Patient Services Coordinator

9005 Children's Organ Transplant Association (COTA)
2501 COTA Drive   800-366-2682
Bloomington, IN 47403   Fax: 812-336-8885
                        e-mail: cota@cota.org
                              www.cota.org
Provides fundraising assistance to children and young adults needing life-saving transplants and promotes organ, marrow and tissue donation.
Rick Lofgren, President/CEO
Lisa Fulkerson, VP/CFO

9006 New Start News
National Transplant Assistance Fund (NTAF)
3475 West Chester Pike   610-353-9684
Newtown Square, PA 19073   800-642-8399
                                 Fax: 610-353-1616
                        e-mail: ntaf@transplantfund.org
                              www.transplantfund.org
Sidney P. Constien, Editor
Judy Walker, Editor

Web Sites

9007 American Society of Transplantation (AST)
                                 www.a-s-t.org
An organization of transplant professionals dedicated to research, education, advocacy and patient care in transplantation science and medicine.

9008 Association of Organ Procurement Organizations (AOPO)
                                 www.aopo.org
Organization involved in helping people find and obtain the organs they may need for transplantation.

9009 Children's Organ Transplant Association (COTA)
                                 www.cota.org
Not-for-profit national chairty dedicated to helping families and communities raise the necessary funds for transplant expenses.

9010 Donate Life America
                                 www.donatelife.net
A not-for-profit alliance of national organizations and local coalitions across the United States that have joined forces to educate the public about organ, eye and tissue donation, correcting misconceptions about donation and creating a greater willingness to donate.

9011 Georgetown University Hospital Transplant Institute
                                 www.georgetownuniversityhospital.org
Founded to promote health through education, research, and patient care.

9012 Health Resources and Services Administration (HRSA)
                                 www.hrsa.gov
Envisions optimal health for all, supported by a health care system that assures access to comprehensive, culturally competant, quality care. Provides national leadership, program resources and services needed to improve access to culturally competant, quality health care.

9013 Jewish Hospital Transplant Center
                                 www.jewishhospital.com

663

An elite group approved to perform five solid organ transplants and has been named a Federally Designated Medicare Heart, Lung, Kidney, Liver and Pancreas Transplant Center.

9014   MedicineNet

www.medicinenet.com

An online resource for consumers providing easy-to-read, authoritative medical and health information.

9015   National Foundation for Transplants

www.transplants.org

Mission is to reach out to help those who seek a new life through transplantation, by providing healthcare and financial support services and patient advocacy for transplant candidates families nationwide.

9016   National Transplant Assistance Fund (NTAF)

www.transplantfund.org

Helps to raise funds for transplant and catastrophic injury patients by providing compassionate support, education and expertise to them, their families and communities.

9017   Organ Procurement and Transplantation Network (OPTN)

www.optn.org

A unified transplant network established by the United States Congress under the National Organ Transplant Act (NOTA) of 1984. A unique public-prvate partnership that links all of the professionals nvolved in the donation and transplantation system.

9018   Transweb: All About Transplantation and Donation

www.transweb.org

Non-profit educational website serving the world transplant community. Features news and events, real peoples experinces, the top 10 myths about donation, a donation quiz, and a large collection of questions and answers, as well as a reference area with everything from articles to videos.

9019   United Network for Organ Sharing (UNOS)

www.unos.org

Mon-profit, scientific and educational organization that administers the nation's only Organ Procurement and Transplantation Network(OPTN). Mission is to advance organ availability and transplantation by uniting and supporting our communities for the benefit of patients through education, technology and policy development.

9020   United Organ Transplant Association (UOTA)

www.uota.org

Non-profit charitable Corporation dedicated to providing educational, emotional and financial support to pre- and post- transplant patients.

Description

9021 Tuberculosis

Tuberculosis, TB, is an infectious disease caused by mycobacteria. It is spread through the air and normally affects the lungs (pulmonary tuberculosis). Extremely common in the United States early in the twentieth century, tuberculosis declined dramatically after 1950. This trend reversed itself after about 1985, due to immigration, the HIV epidemic, and the development of drug resistance by the germ responsible for the disease.

The usual symptoms of TB infection of the lungs include persistent cough, chest pain and coughing up blood. TB infection can cause weight loss, night sweats and fatigue. Left untreated, TB may spread to the spine, causing bone breakdown with deformity, to the lining of the brain, causing tuberculous meningitis, or, in fact, to any organ of the body (extrapulmonary TB).

People who are otherwise healthy, and who are infected with a strain of mycobacterium that is sensitive to standard drugs, can almost always be cured after 6-9 months of therapy. Persons infected with HIV, because of their lowered resistance to disease, have trouble clearing their TB infection, even if they use effective drugs faithfully. Therefore, they should be treated for one year. Regardless of length of treatment, during this time the germ may become resistant to the drug being used. Therefore treatment includes at least 2 drugs, so that a bacterium that develops resistance to one drug will still be killed by another one. Incomplete or interrupted treatment often leads to drug resistance. Germs that are resistant to multiple drugs may be passed to others, and are now a serious public health menace. Unfortunately, the HIV-infected patient is an ideal breeding ground for drug-resistant TB germs.

Persons with drug-sensitive TB who are otherwise healthy and will cooperate with treatment are generally treated by community physicians. Those with complicated medical status (HIV, drug-resistant organisms) or social difficulties (alcoholism, substance abuse, homelessness) generally require specialized public health clinics that can combine medical expertise with nursing and social outreach support.

Many persons who have been infected by TB keep it successfully contained by their own immune systems. There is some risk of the contained germ, however, even years later, overcoming the body's resistance and causing active disease. The tuberculin skin test (PPD) is used to widely screen certain high-risk populations, particularly those who have been exposed to an infectious individual. Prior, adequately treated infection may be diagnosed by a positive PPD, and is sometimes treated with antibiotics to reduce the risk of future disease.

National Agencies & Associations

9022 American Lung Association
1301 Pennsylvania Avenue NW
Washington, DC 20004
202-785-3355
Fax: 202-452-1805
www.lungusa.org
The mission of the American Lung Association is to prevent lung disease and promote lung health. Founded in 1904 to fight tuberculosis the American Lung Association today fights disease in all its forms, with special emphasis on asthma and tobacco control.
Linn Bilingsly, Director
John F. Emanuel, Secretary

9023 Centers for Disease Control and Prevention National Center for Prevention Services
National Center for Prevention Services
1600 Clifton Road
Atlanta, GA 30333
404-639-8135
800-CDC-INFO
TTY: 888-232-6348
e-mail: cdcinfo@cdc.gov
www.cdc.gov
CDC has been dedicated to protecting health and promoting quality of life through the prevention and control of disease, injury and disability.
Tom Friedan, Director
Ileana Arias, Principle Deputy Director

9024 National Institute of Allergy and Infectious Diseases
6610 Rockledge Drive
Bethesda, MD 20892-6621
301-496-5717
866-284-4107
Fax: 301-402-3573
TTY: 800-877-8339
e-mail: afauci@niaid.nih.gov
www.niaid.nih.gov
Conducts and supports basic and applied research to better understand, treat and ultimately prevent infectious, immunologic and allergic diseases.
Anthony S Fauci MD, Director
H Clifford Lane MD, Acting Deputy Director

9025 New Jersey Medical School: National Tuberculosis Center
225 Warren Street
Newark, NJ 07101-1709
973-972-3270
800-482-3627
Fax: 973-972-3268
www.umdnj.edu/ntbcweb/tbsplash.html
Provides expert medical consultation, trains health care providers and other health related professionals, utilize innovative educational methodologies such as standardized patients, develop linkages with health care delivery systems and collaborate with health care professionals.
Lee B Reichman, Executive Director
Reynard J McDonald, Medical Director

9026 Occupational Safety & Health Administration
200 Constitution Avenue Northwest
Washington, DC 20210
800-321-6742
TTY: 877-889-5627
www.osha.gov
OSHA's mission is to assure the safety and health of America's workers by setting and enforcing standards, providing training, outreach and education, establishing partnerships and encouraging continual improvement in workplace safety and health.
Doug Kalinowski, Director
M. Lucero Oritiz, Chief of Staff

State Agencies & Associations

Alabama

9027 American Lung Association of Alabama
PO Box 3188
Bessemer, AL 35023
205-933-8821
800-LUN-GUSA
Fax: 205-930-1717
e-mail: kperry@alabamalung.org
www.alabamalung.org

Kim Perry, Director of Development

Alaska

9028 American Lung Association of Alaska
500 W International Airport Road   907-276-5864
Anchorage, AK 99518   800-LUN-GUSA
                                         Fax: 907-565-5587
                                  e-mail: mlarson@aklung.org
                                         www.aklung.org

Marge Larson, Director

Arizona

9029 Northern Arizona Branch:Phoenix Area
102 W McDowell Road   602-258-7505
Phoenix, AZ 85003-1299   800-LUN-GUSA
                                         Fax: 602-258-7507
                                  e-mail: infophoenix@lungaz.org
                                         www.lungarizona.org

Nancy Cohrs, Executive Director
Evelyn Frear, Office Manager

9030 Southern Arizona Branch: Tucson Area
2819 E Broadway   520-323-1812
Tuscon, AZ 85716   800-LUN-GUSA
                                         Fax: 520-323-1816
                                  e-mail: infotucson@lungaz.org
                                         www.lungarizona.org

Keith Kaback, Chairman
Heidi Miller, Vice Chairman

Arkansas

9031 American Lung Association of Arkansas
217 W 2nd Street   501-957-0758
Little Rock, AR 72201-1539   Fax: 501-978-5138
                                  e-mail: inquiries@breathehealthy.org
                                         www.lung.org

California

9032 American Lung Association of California
424 Pendleton Way   510-638-LUNG
Oakland, CA 94621-2189   800-LUN-GUSA
                                         Fax: 510-638-8984
                                  e-mail: veronica.cuevas@lung.org
                                         www.lung.org

Linda Hinojosa, Chairman
Laura Keegan Boudreau, Acting CEO

Colorado

9033 American Lung Association of Colorado
5600 Greenwood Plaza Boulevard   303-388-4327
Greenwood Village, CO 80111-2305   800-LUN-GUSA
                                         Fax: 303-377-1102
                                  e-mail: cmichael@lungcolorado.org
                                         www.lung.org

Curt Huber, Executive Director
Connor Michael, Communications Manager

Connecticut

9034 American Lung Association of Connecticut
45 Ash Street   860-289-5401
E Hartford, CT 06108-3272   800-992-2263
                                         Fax: 860-289-5405
                                  e-mail: info@lungne.org
                                         www.lung.org

Margaret LaCroix, Vice President Communications

Delaware

9035 American Lung Association of Delaware
630 Churchmans Rd   302-737-6414
Newark, DE 19806-3280   Fax: 302-737-126
                                  e-mail: llyons@lunginfo.org
                                         www.lung.org

Peter Shanley, Chairman

District of Columbia

9036 American Lung Association of Washington
1301 Pennsylvania Ave NW   202-785-3355
Washington, DC 20004   800-732-9339
                                         Fax: 206-441-3277
                                  e-mail: alaw@alaw.org
                                         www.lung.org

Vivian Echavarria, Chair
Rick Weems, Secretary

9037 American Lung Association of the District of Columbia
1301 Pennsylvania Ave NW   202-785-3355
Washington, DC 20004-2617   Fax: 202-682-5607
                                  e-mail: info@aladc.org
                                         www.lung.org

Jan Morgan, Special Events Director
Phoebe Robinson, Administrative Coordinator

Florida

9038 American Lung Association of Florida
6852 Belfort Oaks Place   904-743-2933
Jacksonville, FL 32216-5216   800-940-2933
                                         Fax: 904-743-2916
                                  e-mail: alaf@lungfla.org
                                         www.lung.org

Michael Diamond, President
Marilin K Glassberg, President-Elect

Georgia

9039 American Lung Association of Georgia
2452 Spring Road   770-434-5864
Smyrna, GA 30080   800-586-4872
                                         Fax: 770-319-0349
                                  e-mail: mail@alaga.org
                                         www.lung.org

Charles J White, Chief Executive Officer
June Deen, VP Public Affairs

Hawaii

9040 American Lung Association of Hawaii
650 Iwilei Road   808-537-5966
Honolulu, HI 96817   Fax: 808-537-5971
                                  e-mail: lung@ala-hawaii.org
                                         www.lung.org

Karen J Lee, President, Executive Director

Illinois

9041 American Lung Association of Illinois-Iowa
55 W Upper Wacker Dr   312-781-1100
Chicago, IL 60601   800-586-4872
                                         Fax: 217-787-5916
                                  e-mail: info@lungil.org
                                         www.lung.org

Harold Wimmer, CEO
Lori Younker, Manager

Indiana

9042 American Lung Association of Indiana: State Office & Support Office
9445 Delegates Row,   317-573-3900
Indianapolis, IN 46240   800-LUN-GUSA
                                         Fax: 317-819-1187
                                  e-mail: info@lungin.org
                                         www.lung.org

Dana Pitts, VP Communications/Marketing

Kansas

9043 **American Lung Association of Kansas**
6701 W 64th Street
Overland Park, KS 66202-2419

913-912-7190
Fax: 866-575-1761
e-mail: menisam@kylung.org
www.lung.org

Judy Keller, Executive Director

Kentucky

9044 **American Lung Association of Kentucky**
4100 Churchman Avenue
Louisville, KY 40209-0067

502-363-2652
800-LUN-GUSA
Fax: 502-363-0222
e-mail: info@kylung.org
www.lung.org

Todd Adams, Development Director
Laura Collins, Executive Assistant

Louisiana

9045 **American Lung Association of Louisiana**
2325 Severn Avenue
Metairie, LA 70001-6918

504-828-5864
800-LUN-GUSA
Fax: 504-828-5867
e-mail: info@louisianalung.org
www.lung.org

Aline Palmisano-Vita, Deputy Executive Director
Thomas P Lotz, Chief Executive Officer

Maine

9046 **American Lung Association of Maine**
122 State Street
Augusta, ME 04330

207-622-6394
800-LUN-GUSA
Fax: 639-426-2919
e-mail: info@lungme.org
www.lung.org

Lee Scott, President of Health Promotion
Edward Miller, Executive Director/SVP

Maryland

9047 **American Lung Association of Maryland**
211 East Lombard St
Baltimore, MD 21202

443-451-4950
Fax: 410-560-0829
e-mail: info@marylandlung.org
www.lung.org

Melina Davis-Martin, President and CEO
Krista Jennings, Chief Operations Officer

Massachusetts

9048 **American Lung Association of Massachusetts**
460 Totten Pond Road
Waltham, MA 02451

781-890-4262
Fax: 781-890-4280
e-mail: info@lungma.org
www.lung.org

Michigan

9049 **American Lung Association of Michigan**
1475 E 12 Mile Road
Madison Heights, MI 48071

248-784-2000
800-543-5864
Fax: 248-784-2008
e-mail: alam@alam.org
www.lung.org

Colette Scholzen, President

Minnesota

9050 **American Lung Association of Minnesota**
490 Concordia Avenue
Saint Paul, MN 55103-2441

651-227-8014
800-LUN-GUSA
Fax: 651-227-5459
e-mail: info@alamn.org
www.lung.org

Bill Westhoff, President

Mississippi

9051 **American Lung Association of Mississippi**
731 Pear Orchard Road
Ridgeland, MS 39158

601-206-5810
800-586-4872
Fax: 601-206-5813
www.lung.org

Greg Wynne, Chairman
Jennifer Cofer, Deputy Executive Director

Missouri

9052 **American Lung Association of Missouri**
1118 Hampton Avenue
Saint Louis, MO 63139

314-645-5505
Fax: 314-645-7128
e-mail: inquiries@breathehealthy.org
www.lung.org

Lori Pickens, Chief Executive Officer
Barry Freedman, VP Community Initiatives

Montana

9053 **American Lung Association of the Northern Rockies: Montana
and Wyoming**
825 Helena Avenue
Helene, MT 59601-3459

406-442-6556
Fax: 406-442-2346
e-mail: ala-nr@ala-nr.org
www.lung.org

Nebraska

9054 **American Lung Association of Nebraska**
8990 W Dodge Rd
Omaha, NE 68114

402-502-4950
Fax: 402-502-3012
e-mail: jegerton@breathehealthy.org
www.lung.org

Nevada

9055 **American Lung Association of Idaho/Nevada**
10615 Double R Boulevard
Reno, NV 89521-7056

775-829-LUNG
800-LUN-GUSA
Fax: 775-829-5850
e-mail: lmartin@lungnevada.org
www.lung.org

Louise Martin, Executive Director
Gwen Bourne, Development Manager - Events

New Hampshire

9056 **American Lung Association of New Hampshire**
1800 Elm St
Manchester, NH 03104

603-369-3977
Fax: 603-369-3978
e-mail: info@nhlung.org
www.lung.org

Jeff Seyler, President & CEO
David Ales, Senior Vice President

New Jersey

9057 **American Lung Association of New Jersey**
1031 Route 22 West
Bridgewater, NJ 08807-3407

908-685-8040
800-LUN-GUSA
Fax: 908-851-2625
e-mail: jgrinwald@lunginfo.org
www.lung.org

John A Rutkowski, President

New Mexico

9058 **New Mexico Branch**
7001 Menaul Boulevard NE
Albuquerque, NM 87110

505-265-0732
800-LUN-GUSA
Fax: 505-260-1739
e-mail: ronh@alanm.org
www.lungusa.org

New York

9059 American Lung Association of Mid New York
155 Washington Avenue   518-465-2013
Albany, NY 12210   Fax: 518-465-2926
e-mail: info@alany.org
www.lung.org

The mission of the American Lung Association and the American Lung Association of New York State is to prevent lung disease and promote lung health. The American Lung Association is the oldest voluntary health organization in the United States.
Deborah Carioto, President
Michael Seilback, Vice President Public Policy

North Carolina

9060 American Lung Association of North Carolina
514 Daniels St.   919-424-6069
Raleigh, NC 27605   800-892-5650
Fax: 919-856-8530
e-mail: lungnc@lungusa.org
www.lung.org

Deborah C. Bryan, President

North Dakota

9061 American Lung Association of North Dakota
212 N 2nd Street   701-223-5613
Bismarck, ND 58502   Fax: 919-856-8530
e-mail: dbryan@lungnc.org
www.lung.org

Deborah C Bryan, VP Advocacy & Donor Value
Mendi Nieters, Regional VP Development

Ohio

9062 American Lung Association of Ohio
1950 Arlingate Lane   614-279-1700
Columbus, OH 43228   800-LUN-GUSA
Fax: 614-279-4940
e-mail: alao@ohiolung.org
www.lung.org

Tracy Ross, President / CEO

Oklahoma

9063 American Lung Association of Oklahoma
1010 E 8th Street   918-747-3441
Tulsa, OK 74120   Fax: 918-747-4629
www.lung.org

Sara Dreiling, Chief Executive Officer
Edward C Rosentel, Chief Financial and Operating Officer

Oregon

9064 American Lung Association of Oregon
7420 SW Bridgeport Road   503-924-4094
Tigard, OR 97224   Fax: 503-924-4120
e-mail: info@lungoregon.org
www.lung.org

Jan Jensen, President
Dana Kaye, Executive Director

Pennsylvania

9065 American Lung Association of Pennsylvania
3001 Old Gettysburg Road   717-541-5864
Camp Hill, PA 17011   800-LUN-GUSA
Fax: 888-415-5757
e-mail: dbrown@lunginfo.org
www.lung.org

South Carolina

9066 American Lung Association of South Carolina
1817 Gadsen Street   803-779-5864
Columbia, SC 29201-2392   800-849-5864
Fax: 803-254-2711
e-mail: alasc@lungsc.org
www.lung.org

South Dakota

9067 American Lung Association of South Dakota
108 E 38th Street   605-336-7222
Sioux Falls, SD 57105   Fax: 803-254-2711
e-mail: shelps@alase.org
www.lung.org

Amanda Strickland, Regional Manager Special Events
Sharon Helps, Regional Manager Programs

Tennessee

9068 American Lung Association of Tennesse
One Vantage Way   615-329-1151
Nashville, TN 37228   800-LUN-GUSA
Fax: 615-329-1723
e-mail: alastaff@alatn.org
www.lung.org

Texas

9069 American Lung Association of Texas
8150 Brookriver Drive   512-467-6753
Dallas, TX 75247-0460   800-252-5864
Fax: 512-467-7621
e-mail: inquiries@breathehealthy.org
www.lung.org

Phillip J Hanson, Senior VP Resource Development
Margaret Crump, Senior VP Community Initiatives

Utah

9070 American Lung Association of Utah
1930 S 1100 E   801-484-4456
Salt Lake City, UT 84106-2317   Fax: 801-484-5461
e-mail: info@utahlung.org
www.lung.org

Vermont

9071 American Lung Association of Vermont
372 Hurricane Lane   802-876-6500
Williston, VT 05495-6196   Fax: 802-876-6505
e-mail: info@vtlung.org
www.lung.org

Erin Hickey, Senior Manager Development
Margaret LaCroix, VP Marketing\Communications

Virginia

9072 American Lung Association of Virginia
9702 Gayton Rd   804-955-4910
Richmond, VA 23238   Fax: 804-267-5634
e-mail: lungva@lungusa.org
www.lung.org

Melina Davis-Martin, President and CEO
Krista Jennings, Chief Operating Officer

West Virginia

9073 American Lung Association of West Virginia
2102 Kanawha Blvd   304-342-6600
East Charleston, WV 25311-3980   Fax: 304-342-6096
e-mail: cfields@lunginfo.org
www.lung.org

Sara Crickenberger, Executive Director

Wisconsin

9074 **American Lung Association of Wisconsin**
13100 W Lisbon Road   262-703-4200
Brookfield, WI 53005-2508   800-586-4872
                                   Fax: 262-781-5180
                                   e-mail: info@lungwi.org
                                   www.lung.org

Susan Gloede Swan, Executive Director
Dona Wininsky, Director of Public Policy

Research Centers

9075 **University of Illinois at Chicago Lions**
2035 W Taylor St   312-355-1715
Chicago, IL 60612   Fax: 312-355-2693
                    www.uic.edu/pharmacy/research/itr
The Institute for Tuberculosis Research is comprised of approximately 30 individuals: biologists chemists pharmacologists and support staff - all working towards a single goal - the discovery of new drugs for tuberculosis.
Scott Franzblau, Director
Lorna Haubrich, ITR General Information

9076 **University of Illinois at Chicago: Institute for Tuberculosis Research**
833 S. Wood Street   312-355-1715
Chicago, IL 60612-7631   Fax: 312-355-2693
                    www.uic.edu/pharmacy/research/itr
Scott Franzblau, Director
Lorna Haubrich, ITR General Information

Support Groups & Hotlines

9077 **National Health Information Center**
PO Box 1133   310-565-4167
Washington, DC 20013   800-336-4797
                                   Fax: 301-984-4256
                                   e-mail: info@nhic.org
                                   www.health.gov/nhic
Offers a nationwide information referral service, produces directories and resource guides.

Pamphlets

9078 **Classification of Tuberculosis and Other Mycobacterial Diseases**
American Lung Association
1740 Broadway   212-315-8700
New York, NY 10019-4315
Chart listing different classes of tuberculosis and other mycobacterial diseases.

9079 **Facts About Tuberculosis**
American Lung Association
1740 Broadway   212-315-8700
New York, NY 10019-4315
Primary public information leaflet on TB as well as on its impact and treatment.
8 pages

9080 **TB Skin Test**
American Lung Association
1740 Broadway   212-315-8700
New York, NY 10019-4315
Primary public information leaflet on the TB skin test.
8 pages

9081 **TB: What You Should Know**
American Lung Association of Connecticut
45 Ash Street   860-289-5401
East Hartford, CT 06108-3294   800-586-4872
                                   Fax: 860-289-5405
                                   www.alact.org
Offers a brief overview of tuberculosis, how transmission is possible, and TB skin testing.
John E Zinn, President/CEO

9082 **This is Mr. TB Germ**
American Lung Association
1740 Broadway   212-315-8700
New York, NY 10019-4315
Lively booklet of drawings and very brief text giving a basic description of TB and its treatments.
20 pages

Web Sites

9083 **American Lung Association**
                                   www.americanlungusa.org
Offers research, medical updates, fund-raising, educational materials and public awareness campaigns relating to lung disease and related disorders.

9084 **Healing Well**
                                   www.healingwell.org
An online health resource guide to medical news, chat, information and articles, newsgroups and message boards, books, disease-related web sites, medical directories, and more for patients, friends, and family coping with disabling diseases, disorders, or chronic illnesses.

9085 **Health Finder**
                                   www.healthfinder.gov
Searchable, carefully developed web site offering information on over 1000 topics. Developed by the US Department of Health and Human Services, the site can be used in both English and Spanish.

9086 **Healthlink USA**
                                   www.healthlinkusa.com
Health information concerning treatment, cures, prevention, diagnosis, risk factors, research, support groups, email lists, personal stories and much more. Updated regularly.

9087 **Helios Health**
                                   www.helioshealth.com
Online resource for your health information. Detailed information about specific health topics, access to expert advice from our Medical Advisory Board, and up-to-date health news.

9088 **MedicineNet**
                                   www.medicinenet.com
An online resource for consumers providing easy-to-read, authoritative medical and health information.

9089 **Medscape**
                                   www.medscape.com
Medscape offers specialists, primary care physicians, and other health professionals the Web's most robust and integrated medical information and educational tools.

9090 **National Institute of Allergy & Inf. Dis.**
                                   www.niaid.nih.gov
NAID is composed of four extramural divisions: the Division of AIDS; the Division of Allergy, Immunology and Transplantation; the Division of Microbology and Infectious Diseases; and the Division of Extramural Activities. In addition, NIAID scientists conduct intramural research in laboratories located in Bethesda, Rockville and Frederick, Maryland, and in Hamilton, Montana.

9091 **WebMD**
                                   www.webmd.com
Information on Tuberculosis, including articles and resources.

Description

9092 **Tuberous Sclerosis**

Tuberous sclerosis is a genetic disorder that causes benign, (non-cancerous) tumors to form in different locations - primarily in the brain, skin, kidneys, heart, lungs and even eyes. The name is derived from tuber-like growths on the brain that become hard. It usually shows itself in infancy or early childhood, and may cause seizures and/or mental retardation. It is inherited through chromosome 9 or 16. Disease severity is highly variable, even within the same family. Those with tuberous sclerosis can have mental retardation as well as seizures.

There are various skin abnormalities that may provide a clue to the diagnosis when an infant or young child exhibits seizures or delayed development. The first is an area of decreased skin pigmentation, called an ash-leaf spot because of its shape. Multiple ash-leaf spots may appear on the trunk and limbs during infancy. At age 3 or 4, tiny red bumps, adenoma sebaceum, resembling acne may appear on the nose and cheeks. Finally, a roughened spot with the consistency of orange peel, shagren patch, may appear over the lower spine.

There is no cure so treatment is based on symptoms and can include anti-epileptic drugs for seizures, removal of skin lesions, treatment of high blood pressure caused by kidney problems, special education and, in some instances, surgery to remove growing tumors.

National Agencies & Associations

9093 **National Tuberous Sclerosis Association**
801 Roeder Road
Sliver Spring, MD 20910

301-562-9890
800-225-6872
Fax: 301-562-9870
e-mail: info@tsalliance.org
www.ntsa.org

A voluntary nonprofit organization that is dedicated to fostering and supporting tuberous sclerosis research; to provide education of the public educators and health care professionals; and to providing support of individuals with tuberous sclerosis.
Kari Luther Carlson, President & Chief Executive Officer
Gail Alexander, Senior Manager of Operations

Support Groups & Hotlines

9094 **National Health Information Center**
PO Box 1133
Washington, DC 20013

310-565-4167
800-336-4797
Fax: 301-984-4256
e-mail: info@nhic.org
www.health.gov/nhic

Offers a nationwide information referral service, produces directories and resource guides.

Books

9095 **Tuberous Sclerosis**
Oxford University Press
2001 Evans Road
Cary, NC 27513

800-451-7556
Fax: 919-677-1303
www.oup-usa.org

A revision offering up-to-date medical information to families, researchers, and professionals on TS.

ISBN: 0-195122-10-0

Newsletters

9096 **NTSA Perspective**
National Tuberous Sclerosis Association
8181 Professional Place
Landover, MD 20785-2226

301-459-9888
800-225-6872
Fax: 301-459-0394
e-mail: ntsa@ntsa.org
www.ntsa.org

Offers the latest research and medical information on tuberous sclerosis to physicians and health care professionals.
Quarterly

Web Sites

9097 **Healing Well**

www.healingwell.com

An online health resource guide to medical news, chat, information and articles, newsgroups and message boards, books, disease-related web sites, medical directories, and more for patients, friends, and family coping with disabling diseases, disorders, or chronic illnesses.

9098 **Health Finder**

www.healthfinder.gov

Searchable, carefully developed web site offering information on over 1000 topics. Developed by the US Department of Health and Human Services, the site can be used in both English and Spanish.

9099 **Healthlink USA**

www.healthlinkusa.com

Health information concerning treatment, cures, prevention, diagnosis, risk factors, research, support groups, email lists, personal stories and much more. Updated regularly.

9100 **Helios Health**

www.helioshealth.com

Online resource for your health information. Detailed information about specific health topics, access to expert advice from our Medical Advisory Board, and up-to-date health news.

9101 **MedicineNet**

www.medicinenet.com

An online resource for consumers providing easy-to-read, authoritative medical and health information.

9102 **Medscape**

www.medscape.com

Medscape offers specialists, primary care physicians, and other health professionals the Web's most robust and integrated medical information and educational tools.

9103 **National Tuberous Sclerosis Association**

www.ntsa.org

NTSA provides information to individuals and families through its family support network, quarterly newsletters, brochures and other printed materials.

9104 **WebMD**

www.webmd.com

Information on Tuberous Sclerosis, including articles and resources.

Description

9105 ## Turner Syndrome

Turner syndrome is a genetic disorder that occurs in 1 in 2,500 to 10,000 live female births. It only affects females because, rather than having two female sex (X) chromosomes, Turner syndrome patients have only one. The disease usually hinders sexual development and produces small stature and varying degrees of mental retardation. There may be associated anomalies such as webbed neck and defects of the heart or aorta, which may occur in up to 25 percent of individuals.

Turner syndrome cannot be cured, but hormonal treatment may give the patient a more normal life. Growth hormone injections can help the patient reach a taller adult height, and estrogen replacement can encourage breast development and other sex characteristics. A few patients will develop menstrual periods spontaneously, and a few have become pregnant; most, however, are infertile. Psychological support for the patient and her family is important.

National Agencies & Associations

9106 **Human Growth Foundation: Turner Syndrome Division**
997 Glen Cove Avenue
Glen Head, NY 11545-1554
800-451-6434
Fax: 516-671-4055
e-mail: hgf1@hgfound.org
www.hgfound.org
A nonprofit, national organization committed to expanding and accelerating research into growth and growth disorders, provides education and support to those affected by growth disorders and their families and fosters the exchange of information.
Pisit PITUKCHEEWANONT,, President
Emily Germain-Lee, Vice President

9107 **MAGIC Foundation for Children's Growth: Turner's Syndrome Division**
6645 W N Avenue
Oak Park, IL 60302-1376
708-383-0808
800-362-4423
Fax: 708-383-0899
e-mail: dianne@magicfoundation.org
www.magicfoundation.org
A national nonprofit organization created to provide support services for the families of children afflicted with a wide variety of chronic and/or critical disorders that affect a child's growth.
Rich Buckley, Chairman
Ken Dickard, Vice Chairman

9108 **Turner's Syndrome Society of Canada**
323 Chapel Street
Ottawa, K1N
613-321-2267
800-465-6744
Fax: 613-321-2268
e-mail: tssincan@web.net
www.turnersyndrome.ca
International society providing support services, educational information and activities to persons with Turner's Syndrome, their families and the professionals who work with them.

9109 **Turner's Syndrome Society of the United States**
11250 W Road
Houston, TX 77065
832-912-6006
800-365-9944
Fax: 832-912-6446
e-mail: tssus@turnersyndrome.org
www.turnersyndrome.org
Through this society members have available a host of informational and support services including consultation services a re-

source center offering access to the most recently published articles on Turner's Syndrome conferences and advocacy.
Cindy Scurlock, Executive Director
Deborah Rios, Member Services Director

State Agencies & Associations

California

9110 **Bay Area Turner Syndrome Society**
Moraga, CA 94556
925-846-0608
e-mail: jenakiko@aol.com
www.turnersyndrome.org

Jennifer Saito, Contact

Colorado

9111 **Turner's Syndrome Society of Rocky Mountain**
Longmount, CO 80501
303-774-0720
e-mail: bpblick@earthlink.net
www.turnersyndrome.org

Brian Blick, President

Florida

9112 **Florida Southwest Turner Syndrome Society**
Orlando, FL 33919
407-859-3131
e-mail: cjubelt@affirmativemanagement.com
www.turnersyndrome.org

Lauren Jubelt, Leader

9113 **Turner's Syndrome Society of South Florida**
5215 N Dixie Highway
Oakland Park, FL 33334
945-815-9100
e-mail: tigger3927@aol.com
www.turnersyndrome.org

Rachel Nowak, Leader

Georgia

9114 **Georgia Atlanta Turner Syndrome Society**
10635 Jones Bridge Road
Alpharetta, GA 30022
770-918-3120
e-mail: jbrownlee@rockdale.org
www.turnersyndrome.org

Judy Brownlee, Contact

Illinois

9115 **Metro Chicago Turner Syndrome Society**
5467 S Ingleside #3E
Chicago, IL 60615
773-667-1364
e-mail: sgfhoff@sbcglobal.net
www.turnersyndrome.org

Susan Hoffman, President

Indiana

9116 **Indiana Chapter Turner Syndrome Society**
2030 S Odell Street
Brownsburg, IN 46112
317-858-9398
e-mail: candjgarland@yahoo.com
www.turnersyndrome.org

Connie Garland, Contact

Iowa

9117 **Turner's Syndrome Society of Iowa**
2615 Meadow Glen Road
Ames, IA 50014-8238
515-292-2757
e-mail: mkepolashek@msn.com
www.turnersyndrome.org

Mary Kay Polashek, Leader

Massachusetts

9118 **Southern New England Turner Syndrome Society**
1034 Maple Street
Mansfield, MA 02048
401-732-2136
e-mail: deb_pomerantz@hotmail.com
www.turnersyndrome.org

Deborah Pomerantz, Leader

Michigan

9119 Michigan Chapter: Southeast
146 Meadow Lane Circle 248-608-6127
Rochester Hills, MI 48307 e-mail: ksemrau@aol.com
www.turnersyndrome.org

Kim Semrau, President

Minnesota

9120 MN Chapter of the Turner Syndrome Society
1531 American Blvd E 952-854-1224
Bloomington, MN 55425 e-mail: jleon101@hotmail.com
www.tssminnesota.org

Julie Leon, Contact

Missouri

9121 Kansas/Missouri- Turner Syndrome Society
Chapter Headquarters
6721 E 127th Street 816-763-9550
Grandview, MO 64030 Fax: 816-763-8884
e-mail: tsskc@hotmail.com
www.tsskc.com

Dennis McKenzie, Co-President
Carolyn McKenzie, Vice-President

9122 Missouri/St. Louis Turner Syndrome Society
8831 Madge 314-963-0565
Brentwood, MO 63144 e-mail: loch5@juno.com
www.turnersyndrome.org

Mary Jo Lochmoeller, Co-President

New Hampshire

9123 Northern New England Turner Society
38 Beaman Street 603-524-6011
Laconia, NH 03246 e-mail: tssnnepa@hotmail.com
www.turnersyndrome.org

Lori Ann Pawlowski, Leader

New Jersey

9124 New Jersey Metroplitan Turner Syndrome Society Association
107 Crabapple Lane 732-217-3021
Franklin Park, NJ 08823 e-mail: tssusnj@turnersyndromenj.com
www.turnersyndrome.org

Laura Fasciano, Contact

New York

9125 Turner Syndrome Support Group of Central New York
476 Ford Hill Road 607-223-4142
Berkshire, NY 13736 e-mail: tlkwwjd@frontiernet.net
www.turnersyndrome.org

Tammy Kozak, President

9126 Turner's Syndrome Society New York - Metro
215 E 95th Street #24M 607-223-4142
New York, NY 10128 e-mail: tlkwwjd@frontiernet.net
www.turnersyndrome.org

Tammy Kozak, Contact

North Carolina

9127 North Carolina Turner Syndrome Society
1223 Pine Springs Drive 828-699-1088
Hendersonville, NC 28739 e-mail: inmydna@charter.net
www.turnersyndrome.org

Cheryl Tuttle, Contact

Ohio

9128 Turner Syndrome Chapter of Ohio
3333 Burnet Avenue ML 5006 513-697-0941
Cincinnati, OH 45229 e-mail: lwestcott@fuse.net
www.turnersyndrome.org

Leslie Westcott, Contact

Oklahoma

9129 Turner Syndrome Chapter of Oklahoma
5904 E Lattimer
Tulsa, OK 74115-6728 918-838-7355
www.turnersyndrome.org

Jean Radtke, Contact

Pennsylvania

9130 Philadelphia Turner Syndrom Society
169 Trappe Lane 215-752-4405
Langhorne, PA 19047 e-mail: wolfepac5@comcast.net
www.turnersyndrome.org

This society covers the 5 surrounding counties of Philadelphia, along with Eastern Pennsylvania, Delaware and Southern New Jersey.

Eileen Wolfe, President

9131 SW Pennsylvania Turner Syndrome Support Gr oup
3110 Westchester 412-767-4321
Pittsburgh, PA 15238 e-mail: fay_larkin@pghcorning.com
www.turnersyndrome.org

Fay Larkin, Contact

Rhode Island

9132 Rhode Island Turner Syndrome Society
24 Turner Street 401-732-2136
Warwick, RI 02886 e-mail: deb_pomerantz@hotmail.com
www.turnersyndrome.org

Debbie Pomerantz, Contact

South Carolina

9133 South Carolina Palmetto Turner Syndrome So ciety
153 Gannet Point Road 843-521-4461
Beaufort, SC 29902 e-mail: auntrobin74@yahoo.com
www.turnersyndrome.org

Robin Butler, Contact

Texas

9134 Turner's Syndrome Society
11250 W Road 832-912-6006
Houston, TX 77065 800-365-9944
Fax: 832-912-6446
e-mail: tssus@turnersyndrome.org
www.turnersyndrome.org

Cindy Scurlock, Executive Director
Deborah Rios, Member Services Director

9135 Turner's Syndrome Society of Texas
11250 W Road 832-912-6006
Houston, TX 77065 800-365-9944
Fax: 832-912-6446
e-mail: tssus@turnersyndrome.org
www.turnersyndrome.org

Cindy Scurlock, Executive Director
Deborah Rios, Member Services Director

Washington

9136 Washington Puget Sound Turner Syndrome Society
12321 22nd Street NE 206-417-6776
Seattle, WA 98125 e-mail: pugetsoundtss@gmail.com
www.turnersyndrome.org

Larin Amos, President

Libraries & Resource Centers

9137 Turner Syndrome Society Resource Center
Turner Syndrome Society of the United States
11250 W Road 832-912-6006
Houston, TX 77065 800-365-9944
Fax: 832-912-6446
e-mail: tssus@turnersyndrome.org
www.turnersyndrome.org

The Turner Syndrome Society of the US creates awareness, promotes research, and provides support for all persons touched by Turner Syndrome.
Cindy Scurlock, Executive Director
Deborah Rios, Member Services Director

Support Groups & Hotlines

9138 National Health Information Center
PO Box 1133   310-565-4167
Washington, DC 20013   800-336-4797
                                                     Fax: 301-984-4256
                                                     e-mail: info@nhic.org
                                                     www.health.gov/nhic
Offers a nationwide information referral service, produces directories and resource guides.

Newsletters

9139 Turner's Syndrome News
Turner's Syndrome Society of the United States
1313 5th Street SE
Minneapolis, MN 55414-4509   800-365-9944
                                                     Fax: 612-379-3619
                                                     www.turner-syndrome-us.org
Includes articles addressing current issues in Turner's Syndrome, updates on national and local activities and letters from girls and women with Turner's syndrome and their families.
Quarterly

Pamphlets

9140 Answers to Some Commonly Asked Questions
Turner's Syndrome Society of the United States
1313 5th Street SE
Minneapolis, MN 55414-4509   800-365-9944
                                                     Fax: 612-379-3619
                                                     www.turner-syndrome-us.org
Offers information on the Society's activities and the role they play in supporting people with Turner's syndrome.

9141 Facing the Challenges of Turner's Syndrome Together
Turner's Syndrome Society of the United States
1313 5th Street SE
Minneapolis, MN 55414-4509   800-365-9944
                                                     Fax: 612-379-3619
                                                     www.turner-syndrome-us.org
A brochure offering information on Turner's syndrome, statistics on how widespread the disease is and the Society's role in conquering this disease and supporting their members.

9142 Facts About Turner's Syndrome
Turner's Syndrome Society of the United States
1313 5th Street SE
Minneapolis, MN 55414-4509   800-365-9944
                                                     Fax: 612-379-3619
                                                     www.turner-syndrome-us.org
Offers statistical and factual information on the disease of Turner's syndrome, causes, symptoms, prevention and treatment.

9143 How to Start a Turner's Syndrome Support Group
Turner's Syndrome Society of the United States
1313 5th Street SE
Minneapolis, MN 55414-4509   800-365-9944
                                                     Fax: 612-379-3619
                                                     www.turner-syndrome-us.org
Offers information to the lay person on how to obtain material from medical professionals, publicity aspects and funding aspects in pertaining to starting a support group.

9144 Turner's Syndrome Society Resource Bibliographies
Turner's Syndrome Society of the United States
1313 5th Street SE
Minneapolis, MN 55414-4509   800-365-9944
                                                     Fax: 612-379-3619
                                                     www.turner-syndrome-us.org

These fact sheets offer information on books, videos and other resources available on Turner's syndrome.

9145 Turner's Syndrome: A Guide for Families
Turner's Syndrome Society of the United States
1313 5th Street SE
Minneapolis, MN 55414-4509   800-365-9944
                                                     Fax: 612-379-3619
                                                     www.turner-syndrome-us.org
Offers information to parents on the causes, symptoms, diagnosis and prognosis of Turner' syndrome, includes resources of where to go for help and support.

9146 Turner's Syndrome: A Personal Perspective
Turner's Syndrome Society of the United States
1313 5th Street SE
Minneapolis, MN 55414-4509   800-365-9944
                                                     Fax: 612-379-3619
                                                     www.turner-syndrome-us.org
A reprint from the Adolescent and Pediatric Gynecology Journal offering a personal account of a woman with Turner's syndrome and her experiences.

9147 Turner's Syndrome: Hows and Whys of the Missing X Chromosome
Human Growth Foundation
977 Glen Cove Avenue   516-671-4041
Glen Head, NY 11545-1554   800-451-6434
                                                     Fax: 516-671-4055
                                                     e-mail: hgf1@hgfound.org
                                                     www.hgfound.org
Provides a brief overview for parents about Turner's Syndrome.
Patricia D Costa, Executive Director

Web Sites

9148 Healing Well
                                                     www.healingwell.com
An online health resource guide to medical news, chat, information and articles, newsgroups and message boards, books, disease-related web sites, medical directories, and more for patients, friends, and family coping with disabling diseases, disorders, or chronic illnesses.

9149 Health Finder
                                                     www.healthfinder.gov
Searchable, carefully developed web site offering information on over 1000 topics. Developed by the US Department of Health and Human Services, the site can be used in both English and Spanish.

9150 Healthlink USA
                                                     www.healthlinkusa.com
Health information concerning treatment, cures, prevention, diagnosis, risk factors, research, support groups, email lists, personal stories and much more. Updated regularly.

9151 Helios Health
                                                     www.helioshealth.com
Online resource for your health information. Detailed information about specific health topics, access to expert advice from our Medical Advisory Board, and up-to-date health news.

9152 Human Growth Foundation
                                                     www.genetic.org
National organization committed to expanding and accelerating research into growth and growth disorders, provides education and support to those affected by growth disorders and their families, and fosters the exchange of information with the medical community.

9153 MAGIC Foundation for Children's Growth: Turner's Syndrome Division
                                                     www.magicfoundation.org
National organization created to provide support services for the families of children afflicted with a wide variety of chronic and/or critical disorders that affect a child's growth.

9154 MedicineNet
                                                     www.medicinenet.com

An online resource for consumers providing easy-to-read, authoritative medical and health information.

9155 Medscape

www.medscape.com

Medscape offers specialists, primary care physicians, and other health professionals the Web's most robust and integrated medical information and educational tools.

9156 Turner's Syndrome Society of the United States

www.turner-syndrome-us.org

Through this society, members have available a host of informational and support services including consultation services, a resource center offering access to the most recently published articles on Turner's syndrome, conferences, advocacy, information and referral services and public relations activities.

9157 WebMD

www.webmd.com

Information on Turner's syndrome, including articles and resources.

Description

9158 # Ulcerative Colitis

Ulcerative colitis is an inflammatory condition of the large bowel, or colon. The cause is unknown, but there is a strong genetic association. First degree relatives have a 3 to 9 percent lifetime risk of the disease, and the illness is much more common in certain racial groups.

Inflammation of the wall of the bowel leads to ulcerations of its surface. Symptoms include weight loss, fatigue, abdominal pain, and diarrhea, which may be bloody. Ulcerative colitis in patients who have a specific antibody in their system (HLA-B27) has a strong association with an arthritis called ankylosing spondylitis. Several kinds of liver and biliary tract disease, inflammation of the eye, and certain characteristic skin rashes may occur.

Treatment depends on the severity of symptoms. Mild cases may respond to simple anti-diarrheal medicines. More severe cases are treated with either rectal or oral forms of 5-ASA, marketed under several trade names. Corticosteroids are sometimes necessary. Disease confined to the rectum can generally be managed with steroid enemas. Extensive disease requires oral steroid medication. Immunosuppressive drugs like azathioprine and 6-mercaptopurine are sometimes given if the disease is resistant to steroids or if steroid side effects are unacceptable. Twenty percent of patients will eventually have their entire colon removed, which cures the disease.

After many years of active ulcerative there is an increased risk of colon cancer. It is usually preceded by warning signs visible on colonoscopy, so physicians generally begin an aggressive surveillance program after 8 to 10 years of disease.

National Agencies & Associations

9159 **American Gastroenterological Association**
4930 Del Ray Avenue   301-654-2055
Bethesda, MD 20814   Fax: 301-654-5920
                            e-mail: member@gastro.org
                                      www.gastro.org
Dedicated to the mission of advancing the science and practice of gastroenterology. As the oldest specialty medical society in the United States the membership includes physicians and scientists who research diagnose and treat disorders.
Anil K. Rustgi, President
Michael H Camillarie, Vice President

9160 **Crohn's & Colitis Foundation of America**
386 Park Avenue S   212-685-3440
New York, NY 10016-8804   800-932-2423
                                    Fax: 212-779-4098
                               e-mail: info@ccfa.org
                                       www.ccfa.org
Supports basic and clinical research into a cure and prevent Crohn's disease and ulcerative colitis; conducts professional and patient education activities; produces public service programs and a wide variety of literature about inflammatory bowel disease.
Maura Breen, Chairperson
Vance Gibbs, General Council

9161 **National Institute of Diabetes and Digestive Disorders**
5 Information Way
31 Center Drive MSC 2560   301-496-3583
Bethesda, MD 20892-3568   800-860-8747
                                    www2.niddk.nih.gov
Offers information and referrals to persons afflicted with ulcerative colitis.
Griffin P. Rodgers, President
Adil Abdalla, Staff

9162 **Reach Out for Youth with Ileitis and Colitis**
84 Northgate Circle   631-293-3102
Melville, NY 11747   e-mail: info@reachourforyouth.org
                               www.reachoutforyouth.org
Provides educational seminars and individual and group support to patients and their families. Fundraising efforts support the Center's programs clinical and laboratory research and purchase of state-of-the-art equipment.
Irwin Maltz, President

9163 **United Ostomy Association**
PO Box 512
Northfield, MN 55057   800-826-0826
                                   Fax: 507-645-5168
                                 e-mail: info@uoaa.org
                                         www.uoa.org
A national network for bowel and urinary diversion support groups in the United States. Its goal is to provide a nonprofit association that will serve to unify and strengthen its member support groups, which are organized for the benefit of people who have, or will have intestinal or urinary diversions and their caregivers.
David Rudzin, President
Susan Burns, Vice Presdient

Support Groups & Hotlines

9164 **National Health Information Center**
PO Box 1133   310-565-4167
Washington, DC 20013   800-336-4797
                                   Fax: 301-984-4256
                                e-mail: info@nhic.org
                                  www.health.gov/nhic
Offers a nationwide information referral service, produces directories and resource guides.

Books

9165 **Alive and Kicking**
Rolf Benirschke Enterprises
PO Box 9922
Rancho Santa Fe, CA 92067-4922   800-571-4770
Football star writes of his struggle with ulcerative colitis.

9166 **Ask Audrey**
7466 Pebble Lane   248-626-6960
West Bloomfield, MI 48322-3521
A compilation of material and the personal story of a medical psychotherapist who has inflammatory bowel disease. Includes practical tips on issues such as handling diarrhea, sexuality, relationships, traveling, coping with hospital stays, ostomies, and TPN.

9167 **IBD Nutrition Book**
John Wiley & Sons
1 Wiley Drive
Somerset, NJ 08873-1222   800-225-5945
Clinical dietitian/nutritionist's overview of the role of diet in IBD, including recipes and meal plans.

9168 **Inflammatory Bowel Disease**
Williams & Wilkins
351 W Camden Street   301-528-4000
Baltimore, MD 21201-7912   800-638-0672
Detailed information on every aspect of IBD. Topics include medical and surgical management, epidemiology, fertility and pregnancy, psychosocial factors, and diagnostic techniques. Written for medical professionals and laypersons who are comfortable with medical terminology.

9169   Treating IBD: A Patient's Guide to the Medical and Surgical Management
Crohn's and Colitis Foundation of America
386 Park Avenue S   212-685-3440
New York, NY 10016-8804   800-932-2423
                                  Fax: 212-779-4098
                              e-mail: info@ccfa.org
                                      www.ccfa.org

Children's Books

9170   You're Bigger Than it
Hotel Dieu Hospital   613-544-3310
Ontario, Canada,
This cartoon book offers a lively, brief introduction to the basics of living with IBD. Contact can be reached at extension 2400.

Magazines

9171   Phoenix Magazine
United Ostomy Association of America
PO Box 512
Northfield, MN 55057   800-826-0826
                                  Fax: 507-645-5168
                              e-mail: info@uoaa.org
                                      www.uoa.org
America's leading ostomy patient magazine providing colostomy, ileostomy, urostomy and continent diversion information, management techniques, new products and much more.
Quarterly
David Rudzin, President

Newsletters

9172   Inner Circle
Reach Out for Youth with Ileitis and Colitis
84 Northgate Circle   631-293-3102
Melville, NY 11747e-mail: reachoutforyouth@reachoutforyouth.org
                              www.reachoutforyouth.org
Newsletter for youth with ileitis and colitis.
Irwin Maltz, President

Pamphlets

9173   Bleeding in the Digestive Tract
Nat'l Digestive Diseases Information Clearinghouse
9000 Rockville Pike   301-496-3583
Bethesda, MD 20892-0001
Informational fact sheet.

9174   Inside Story
Reach Out for Youth with Ileitis and Colitis
84 Northgate Circle   631-293-2102
Melville, NY 11747e-mail: reachoutforyouth@reachoutforyouth.org
                              www.reachoutforyouth.org
Educational brochure for youth with illeitis and colitis.
Irwin Maltz, President

9175   Ulcerative Colitis
National Organization For Rare Disorders
PO Box 8923   203-746-6518
New Fairfield, CT 06812-8923   e-mail: orphan@rarediseases.org
                              www.rarediseases.org
Informational fact sheet.

Web Sites

9176   Crohn's & Colitis Foundation of America
                                      www.ccfa.org
Supports basic and clinical research into a cure and prevent Crohn's disease and ulcerative colitis; conducts professional and patient education activities; produces public service programs and a wide variety of literature about inflammatory bowel disease for patients and their families, professionals and the public; and sponsors chapters nationwide.

9177   Healing Well
                                  www.healingwell.com
An online health resource guide to medical news, chat, information and articles, newsgroups and message boards, books, disease-related web sites, medical directories, and more for patients, friends, and family coping with disabling diseases, disorders, or chronic illnesses.

9178   Health Finder
                                  www.healthfinder.gov
Searchable, carefully developed web site offering information on over 1000 topics. Developed by the US Department of Health and Human Services, the site can be used in both English and Spanish.

9179   Healthlink USA
                                  www.healthlinkusa.com
Health information concerning treatment, cures, prevention, diagnosis, risk factors, research, support groups, email lists, personal stories and much more. Updated regularly.

9180   Helios Health
                                  www.helioshealth.com
Online resource for your health information. Detailed information about specific health topics, access to expert advice from our Medical Advisory Board, and up-to-date health news.

9181   MedicineNet
                                  www.medicinenet.com
An online resource for consumers providing easy-to-read, authoritative medical and health information.

9182   Medscape
                                  www.medscape.com
Medscape offers specialists, primary care physicians, and other health professionals the Web's most robust and integrated medical information and educational tools.

9183   United Ostomy Association
                                      www.uoa.org
A national network for bowel and urinary diversion support groups in the United States. Its goal is to provide a nonprofit association that will serve to unify and strengthen its member support groups, which are organized for the benefit of people who have, or will have intestinal or urinary diversions and their caregivers.

9184   WebMD
                                      www.webmd.com
Information on Ulcerative Colitis, including articles and resources.

Description

9185 ## Visual Impairment

Visual impairment encompasses a wide variety of disorders of the eye. It includes damage to the cornea or retina (macular degeneration or secondary to diabetes), cataracts, glaucoma, muscular imbalance, infections, congenital disorders and those associated with premature birth. Occasionally visual impairment reflects a disease behind the eye, involving some part of the brain that receives and processes images from the eyes.

Visual impairment covers a continuum from decreased visual acuity correctible by refractive means (glasses and contact lenses) to legal blindness, indicating less than 20/200 vision in the better eye, or an extremely limited field of vision. Totally blind represents the complete loss of sight.

Many health problems and eye injuries lead to visual impairment. Half a million Americans are visually impaired, and an additional 50,000 lose their sight each year. Cataracts account for one third of all visual impairments and cause 16 persons to lose their sight every day. Glaucoma causes vision impairment in 2 million persons. One thousand eye injuries resulting in some level of vision impairment occur in the workplace or home each day. Diabetic retinopathy is one of the leading causes of the new cases of blindness. Retinitis pigmentosa, a degeneration of the light-sensing tissue at the back of the eye, also causes vision (especially night vision) deterioration.

Depending on the cause of vision loss, the condition may be fully or partially correctible through surgery or visual aids. Sometimes treatment will not reverse prior losses, but will slow the progression of vision loss. When the visual loss cannot be reversed, a variety of supportive devices and services, improved over the past twenty years, can greatly enhance the person's functional status and quality of life.

Technology has played an increasing role in helping the visually impaired function in their daily lives. Recently, doctors implanted the first artificial retina, and relatively new laser technology allows eye specialists to surgically treat extreme degrees of nearsightedness and astigmatism (blurred vision caused by uneven curvature of the eye).

National Agencies & Associations

9186 **ACB Radio Amateurs**
2200 Wilson Boulevard
Arlington, VA 22201
202-467-5081
800-424-8666
Fax: 703- 46- 508
e-mail: info@acb.org
www.ACB.org
A radio amateur network of blind, visually impaired and sighted members who gather and share common problems and solutions to help members improve radio amateurs in getting started, provides access to educational materials in special media and publishes a newsletter.
Mitch Pomerantz, President
Kim Charlson, First Vice President

9187 **Alliance for Aging Research**
750 17th St.,
Washington, DC 20006
202-293-2856
Fax: 202-785-8574
e-mail: info@agingresearch.org
www.agingresearch.org
Alliance for Aging Research is the nation's leading citizen advocacy organization for improving the health and independence of Americans as they age. It was founded to promote medical and behavioral research into the aging process.
Daniel P Perry, Executive Director
Sarah Rhyne, Executive Coordinator

9188 **American Academy of Ophthalmology**
655 Beach St.
San Francisco, CA 94109-7424
415-561-8500
Fax: 415-561-8533
e-mail: customer_service@aao.org
www.aao.org
Sponsors National Eye Care Project that gives free eye care to the elderly.

9189 **American Association of the Deaf-Blind**
PO Box 2831
Kensington, MD 20891-4500
301-495-4403
Fax: 301-495-4404
TTY: 301-495-4402
e-mail: AADB-Info@aadb.org
www.aadb.org
Promotes better opportunities and services for deaf-blind people. The mission of this organization is to assure that a comprehensive coordinated system of services is accessible to all deaf-blind people, enabling them to achieve their maximum potential.
35-50 pages 600 Members
Jamie McNama Pope, Executive Director
Elizabeth Spiers, Director of Information Services

9190 **American Coucnil of the Blind Impairment**
1155 15th Street NW Suite 1004
Washington, DC 20005
202-467-5081
800-424-8666
Fax: 202-467-5085
e-mail: cindybur@comcast.net
www.acb.org
A network of blind or visually impaired people that offers support and outreach, shares experiences and exchanges information.
Cindy Burgett, President

9191 **American Council of Blind Lions**
148 Vernon Avenue
Louisville, KY 40206
502-897-1472
Fax: 502-721-9929
e-mail: adam148@bellsouth.net
www.acb.org/acbl
The American Council of Blind Lions (ACBL) is a specially chartered Lions club. The goal of this club is to assist other Lions clubs in understanding the issues surrounding people who are blind or visually impaired.
Adam Ruschival, President

9192 **American Council of the Blind**
2200 Wilson Boulevard
Arlington, VA 22201-2706
202-467-5081
800-424-8666
Fax: 703-465-5085
e-mail: info@acb.org
www.acb.org
A national membership organization whose members are visually impaired and fully sighted individuals who are concerned about dignity and well-being of blind people throughout America. Formed in 1961, the Council has become the largest organization of blind individuals.
Mitch Pomerantz, President

9193 **American Foundation for the Blind**
2 Penn Plaza
New York, NY 10121
212-502-7600
800-232-5463
Fax: 888-545-8331
e-mail: afbinfo@afb.net
www.afb.org

AFB is the cause and organization to which Helen Keller dedicated more than 40 years of her life. In addition to being a national information consultative and advocacy resource engaged in a wide variety of initiatives AFB is home to the Helen Keller Arch.
Carl R Augusto, President/CEO
Richard J O'Brien, Chair

9194 American Foundation for the Blind: National Employment Center
2 Penn Plaza   212-502-7600
New York, NY 10121   Fax: 888-545-8331
                                 e-mail: afbinfo@afb.net
                                 www.afb.org
Leads initiatives in the area of employment. Nationally offers consultation, technical assistance and support and undertakes local and national efforts such as training programs and public education in the area of employment. Responds to inquiries from blind and visually impaired people and thier families, service providers and the general public in the region and nationally.
Richard J O'Brien, Chair
John T Bourger, Vice Chair

9195 American Foundation for the Blind: SE National Literacy Center
100 Peachtree Street   404-525-2303
Atlanta, GA 30303   Fax: 646-478-9260
                                 e-mail: literacy@afb.net
                                 www.afb.org
Leads initiatives in the area of literacy. Offers consultation technical assistance and support and undertakes local and national efforts such as training programs and public education in the area of literacy. Offers training and in-service opportunities.

9196 American Optometric Association
243 N Lindbergh Boulevard   314-991-4100
Saint Louis, MO 63141-7881   800-365-2219
                                 Fax: 314-991-4101
                                 e-mail: PHKehoe@aoa.org
                                 www.aoa.org/?
The AOA and affiliates work to provide the public with quality vision and eye care. It sets professional standards helping its members conduct patient care efficiently and effectively. It also lobbies government and other organizations on behalf of the visually impaired population.
Peter H Kehoe, President
Joe E Ellis, Vice President

9197 American Printing House for the Blind
1839 Frankfort Avenue   502-895-2405
Louisville, KY 40206-0085   800-223-1839
                                 Fax: 502-899-2284
                                 e-mail: info@aph.org
                                 www.aph.org
The oldest nonprofit organization of its kind in the US that creates education, workplace and lifestyle products for visually impaired people. This organization promotes the independence of blind persons by providing special media, tools and materials.
Tuck Tinsley III, President
Bob Brasher, Vice President Advisory Services

9198 Assoc. for Education & Rehabilitation of the Blind & Visually Impaired
1703 N Beauregard Street   703-671-4500
Alexandria, VA 22311   877-492-2708
                                 Fax: 703-671-6391
                                 e-mail: lou@aerbvi.org
                                 www.aerbvi.org
The only professional membership organization dedicated to the advancement of education and rehabilitation of blind and visually impaired children and adults.
Lou Tutt, Executive Director
Ginger Croce, Senior Director, Marketing & Office Oper

9199 Associated Services for the Blind
919 Walnut Street   215-627-0600
Philadelphia, PA 19107-5237   Fax: 215-922-0692
                                 e-mail: asbinfo@asb.org
                                 www.asb.org

Limited funding is available to assist aspiring visually impaired users in the purchase of helpful high tech equipment.
Patricia C Johnson, President/CEO
Derby Ewing, Director, Human Services

9200 Association for Macular Diseases
210 E 64th Street   212-605-3719
New York, NY 10065-7480   Fax: 212-605-3795
                                 e-mail: association@retinal-research.org
                                 www.macula.org
A nonprofit corporation to promote education and research in this scarcely-explored field. A nationwide support group for individuals and their families to adjust to the restrictions and changes brought about by macular disease.
Bernard Landou, President
Mary Fern Breheney, Board of Director

9201 Blinded Veterans Association
477 H Street NW   202-371-8880
Washington, DC 20001-2694   800-669-7079
                                 Fax: 202-371-8258
                                 e-mail: bva@bva.org
                                 www.bva.org
The organization seeks and identifies legally blind veterans who need services linking them to appropriate benefits training and opportunities in both the public and the private sectors. It represents blinded veterans before congress.
Paperback
Samuel Huhn, National President
Mark Cornell, National Vice President

9202 Braille Institute of America Library
741 North Vermont Avenue   323-663-1111
Los Angeles, CA 90029-3594   800-272-4553
                                 Fax: 323-663-0867
                                 e-mail: la@brailleinstitute.org
                                 www.brailleinstitute.org
Discs, cassettes, braille, Optacon, home visits, braille writer, reference materials on blindness and other handicaps. Closed-circuit TV, Optacon, braille writer, and large print copier also available. Home visits and cassette books are part of special services offered.
Adama Dyoniziak, Regional Program Director

9203 Canine Companions for Independence
2965 Dutton Ave   707-577-1000
Santa Rosa, CA 95407   800-572-2275
                                 TTY: 707-577-1756
                                 e-mail: info@cci.org
                                 www.cci.org
A non-profit organization that enhances the lives of people with disabilities by providing highly trained assistance dogs and ongoing support to ensure quality partnerships.
Corey Hudson, CEO
Kathy Pierson, Northwest Regional Executive Director

9204 Canine Helpers for the Disabled
5699 Ridge Road   716-433-4035
Lockport, NY 14094   716-433-4035
                                 e-mail: chhdogs@aol.com
                                 www.caninehelpers.org
A non-profit organization devoted to training dogs to assist people with disabilities to lead more independent, secure lives.

9205 Catholic Guild for the Blind Catholic Charities of the Archdiocese of
Catholic Charities of the Archdiocese of New York
65 E. Wacker Place   312-236-8569
Chicago, IL 60601-7463   Fax: 312-236-8128
                                 e-mail: info@guildfortheblind.org
                                 www.second-sense.org
A nonprofit organization under the sponsorship of the Catholic Charities of the Archdiocese of New York. Daily living skills, orientation and mobility training, communication skills and bilingual preparation for high school equivalency diplomas are among things covered.
Kathy Austin, Coordinator of Adult Rehabilitation
Lauri Dishman, Manager of Career Services

9206 Council for Exceptional Children
2900 Crystal Drive 703-620-3660
Arlington, VA 22202 888-232-7733
Fax: 703-264-9494
TTY: 866-915-5000
e-mail: service@cec.sped.org
www.cec.sped.org
Advocates appropriate policies standards and development for individuals with special needs. Provides professional development for special educators.
Stephanie Ineh, Customer Service Manager
Anitra Davis, Senior Customer Services Representative

9207 Council of Citizens with Low Vision International
1155 15th Street NW 714-630-8098
Washington, DC 20005 800-733-2258
e-mail: president@cclvi.org
www.cclvi.org
Affiliated with American Council of the Blind. Promotes the concept that persons with partial sight/low vision are not blind and should have every right to maximize the use of their residual vision.
John Horst, President
Richard Rueda, 1st Vice President

9208 Fidelco Guide Dog Foundation
103 Vision Way 860-243-5200
Bloomfield, CT 06002-0142 Fax: 860-243-7215
e-mail: info@fidelco.org
www.fidelco.org
Fidelco breeds raises trains and places German shepherd guide dogs with men and women who are visually impaired primarily in the Northeast. The pioneer of in-community training in this country the visually impaired individual can remain independent.
Roberta C Kaman, Chairman
George J Salpietro, Executive Director

9209 Fight for Sight
381 Park Avenue S 212-679-6060
New York, NY 10016 Fax: 212-679-4466
e-mail: info@fightforsight.com
www.fightforsight.com
Voluntary health organization that works to conquer defective sight and blindness. Provides grants to accredited medical colleges and institutions to help supply equipment technical assistance and materials for research projects.
Mary Prudden, Executive Director
Kenneth R Barasch MD, President

9210 Foundation Fighting Blindness
7168 Columbia Gateway Drive 410-423-0600
Columbia, MD 21046 800-683-5555
Fax: 410-872-0438
TTY: 410-363-7139
TDD: 800-683-5551
e-mail: info@FightBlindness.org
www.blindness.org
Mission is to drive the research that will provide preventions, treatments, and cures for people affected by retinitis pigmentosa, macular degeneration, Usher syndrome and the entire spectrum of retinal degenerative diseases.
William T Schmidt, CEO

9211 Foundation for Glaucoma Research
251 Post Street 415-986-3162
San Francisco, CA 94108 800-826-6693
Fax: 415-986-3763
e-mail: question@glaucoma.org
www.glaucoma.org
A national organization dedicated to protecting the sight of people with glaucoma through research and education. The Foundation conducts and supports research that contributes to improved patient care and a better understanding of the disease process.
Andrew Jackson, Director of Communications
Thomas M Brunner, President and CEO

9212 Foundation for the Advancement of the Blind
4058 Moore Street 310-301-0344
Los Angeles, CA 90066-5118
Helps blind people attain and retain employment.

9213 Friends-In-Art
4317 Vermont Court 573-445-5564
Columbia, MO 65203 800-424-8666
Fax: 202-467-5085
e-mail: paltschul@centurytel.net
www.friendsinart.com
Aims to enlarge the art experience of blind people encourages blind people to visit museums galleries concerts the theater etc. offers consultation to program planners in establishing accessible art and museum exhibits.
Peter Altschul, President
Gordon Kent, Board Member

9214 Guide Dog Users
4851 N. Cedar Ave.
Fresno, CA 93726-2245 866-799-8436
e-mail: president@gdui.org
www.gdui.org
Promotes the acceptance of blind people and their dogs works for enforcement and expansion of laws admitting guide dogs into public places advocates for quality training and follow-up services.
Laurie Mehta, President
Mary Beth Randall, First Vice President

9215 Guide Dogs for the Blind
PO Box 151200 415-499-4000
San Rafael, CA 94915 800-298-4050
Fax: 415-499-4035
e-mail: information@guidedogs.com
www.guidedogs.com
Offers educational materials, transportation seminars, and newsletters for the blind providing 2 field offices.
Etta Allen, Board Chair
Morgan Watkins, Interim CEO

9216 Helen Keller National Center's National Parent Network
141 Middle Neck Road 516-944-8900
Sands Point, NY 11050-1218 Fax: 516-944-7302
TTY: 516-944-8637
e-mail: hkncinfo@hknc.org
www.hknc.org
Establishes a coalition of state parent organizations to promote the exchange of information among parents of deaf-blind youth. Provides training to parents to develop their legislative advocacy skills, empowers parents and their families to obtain needed services.
Kathy Mezack, Coordinator of Vocational Services

9217 Independent Visually Impaired Enterprises
230 Robinhood Lane
McMurray, PA 15317 e-mail: lengual@concentric.net
www.acb.org
Strives to broaden vocational opportunities in business for the visually impaired. Works to improve rehabilitation facilities for all types of business enterprises and publicizes the capabilities of blind and visually impaired business persons.
Carla Hayes, President

9218 International Agency for the Prevention of Blindness
National Eye Institute
31 Center Drive MSC 2510
Bethesda, MD 20892-3655 301-496-5248
www.nei.nih.gov
Ophthalmic societies and committees for the prevention of blindness whose members include ophthalmologists public health officers nutritionists geneticists and other health workers. Coordinates international research into the causes of impaired vision.
Carl Kupfer, Volunteer
Paul A Sieving, Director

9219 Library Users of America
2200 Wilson Boulevard 202-467-5081
Arlington, VA 22201 800-424-8666
Fax: 703-465-5085
e-mail: info@acb.org
www.acb.org
Provides for chapters in states through the US to encourage the development acquisition and use of technology which enables blind

and visually impaired persons to use printed material independently in library settings and elsewhere.
Barry Levine, President

9220 Lighthouse International Headquarters
111 E 59th Street
New York, NY 10022-1202
212-821-9200
800-821-0500
Fax: 212-821-9707
TTY: 212-821-9713
e-mail: info@lighthouse.org
www.lighthouse.org

A leading resource worldwide on vision impairment and vision rehabilitation. Pioneer in vision rehabilitation services, education, research and advocacy enabling people of all ages who are blind or partially sighted to lead independent and productive lives.
Roger O Goldman, Chairman
Tara A Cortes, President/CEO

9221 Lions World Services for the Blind Lions Clubs International
Lions Clubs International
2811 Fair Park Boulevard
Little Rock, AR 72204
501-664-7100
800-248-0734
Fax: 501-664-2743
e-mail: training@lwsb.org
www.lwsb.org

Lions World Services for the Blind was founded in 1947 to serve people who are blind and visually impaired who needed to learn independent living skills or job training skills that considered the special requirements of their individual visual impairments.
Ramona Sangalli, President and Chief Executive Officer
Larry Morgan, Vice President for Development

9222 Macular Degeneration Foundation
PO Box 515
Northampton, MA 01061-0515
413-268-7660
888-622-8527
e-mail: amdf@macular.org
www.macular.org

The American Macular Degeneration Foundation is committed to the prevention and cure of macular degeneration and offers hope and support to those afflicted and their families.
Chip Goehring, President and Trustee
Mark E Torrey, Vice President and Trustee

9223 National Alliance of Blind Students
2200 Wilson Boulevard
Arlington, VA 22201
202-467-5081
800-424-8666
Fax: 703-465-5085
e-mail: info@acb.org
www.acb.org

Works to facilitate progress toward full accessibility of college programs and facilities provides opportunities for discussion of issues important to students and assists with National Student Seminars.
Rebecca Bridges, President

9224 National Association for Parents of the Visually Impaired
PO Box 317
Watertown, MA 02471-0317
617-972-7441
800-562-6265
Fax: 781-972-7444
e-mail: napvi@perkins.org
www.napvi.org

The only national organization that strives to serve families of children of all ages and ranges with visual loss. It is a community based organization whose members include parents parent organizations agencies and other persons with common objectives.
Susan LaVenture, Executive Director
Doug Halverson, President

9225 National Association for Visually Handicapped
22 West 21st Street
New York, NY 10010
212-889-3141
888-205-5951
Fax: 212-727-2931
e-mail: navh@navh.org
www.navh.org

NAVH ensures that those with limited vision do not lead limited lives. We offer emotional support; training in the use of and access to a wide variety of optical aids and lighting; a large print, nationwide, free-by-mail loan library; large print educational materials;

quarterly newsletter; referrals; self-help groups and educational outreach.
Cesar Gomez, Executive Director

9226 National Association for Visually Hand.
22 W 21st Street
New York, NY 10010
212-889-3141
Fax: 212-727-2931
e-mail: navh@navh.org
www.navh.org

NAVH ensures that those with limited vision do not lead limited lives. We offer emotional support; training in the use of and access to a wide variety of optical aids and lighting and a large print, nationwide, free-by-mail loan library.
Lorraine H Marchi, Founder & CEO
Miriam Rosen, Executive Director

9227 National Association of Blind Educators Sheila Koenig
Sheila Koenig
2200 University Avenue West
St. Paul, MN 55114
651-642-0500
800-652-9000
e-mail: jsanders.nfb@comcast.net
www.nfb.org

Membership organization of blind teachers professors and instructors in all levels of education. Provides support and information regarding professional responsibilities classroom techniques national testing methods and career obstacles.
Judy Sanders, President

9228 National Association of Blind Lawyers Scott LaBarre
Scott LaBarre
1660 S Albion Street
Denver, CO 80222-4046
303-504-5979
Fax: 303-757-3640
e-mail: slabarre@labarrelaw.com
www.nfb.org

Membership organization of blind attorneys law students judges and others in the law field. Provides support and information regarding employment techniques used by the blind, advocacy, laws affecting the blind and current information about the American legal system.
Scott LaBarre, President

9229 National Association of Blind Musicians Linda Mentink
Linda Mentink
6210 Walker Avenue
Lincoln, NE 68507-0952
402-465-5468
e-mail: amy.buresh74@gmail.com
www.nfb.org

Blind persons dedicated to advancing employment and entertainment opportunities in various music fields. Offers support and information regarding copyright publishing promotion and other career details.
Linda Mentik, Chairperson
Amy Buresh, President

9230 National Association of Blind Office Professionals
Lisa Hall
P.O. Box 82055
Columbus, OH 43202-6104
614-935-6965
e-mail: eduffy@pobox.com
www.nfb.org

Membership organization of blind secretaries and transcribers at all levels including medical and paralegal transcription office workers customer-service personnel and many other similar fields. Addresses issues such as technology, accommodation and caregivers.
Lisa Hall, President
Eric Duffy, President

9231 National Association of Blind Students Angela Wolf
Angela Wolf
314 E. Highland Mall Boulevard
Austin, TX 78752-1803
512-323-5444
e-mail: kflores@nfbtx.org
www.nfb.org

For over 30 years this national organization of blind students has provided support information and encouragement to blind college and university students. Leads the way in offering resources in issues such as national testing and accessible textbooks.
Kimberly Flores, President

9232 National Association of Guide Dog Users Priscilla Ferris
Priscilla Ferris

1003 Papaya Drive
Tampa, FL 33619-3714

813-626-2789
800-558-8261
e-mail: president@nagdu.org
www.nagdu.org

Provides information and support for guide dog users and works to secure high standards in guide dog training. Addresses issues of discrimination of guide dog users and offers public education about guide dog use.
Marion Gwizdala, President

9233   National Association to Promote the Use of Braille
Nadine Jacobson
2200 University Avenue West
St. Paul, MN 55114-1819

651-642-0500
800-652-9000
e-mail: nadine.jacobson@visi.com
www.nfb.org

Dedicated to securing improved Braille instruction increasing the number of Braille materials available to the blind and providing information about the importance of Braille in securing independence education and employment for the blind.
Nadine Jacobson, President

9234   National Braille Association
95 Allens Creek Road
Rochester, NY 14618-2513

585-427-8260
Fax: 585-427-0263
e-mail: nbaoffice@nationalbraille.org
www.nationalbraille.org

Provides transcription service for and maintains a depository of braille books.
Diane Spence, President
Jan Carroll, Vice President

9235   National Braille Press
88 Saint Stephen Street
Boston, MA 02115-4302

617-266-6160
888-965-8965
Fax: 617-437-0456
www.nbp.org

The guiding purposes of National Braille Press are to promote the literacy of blind children through braille and to provide access to information that empowers blind people to actively engage in work family and community affairs.
Paul Parravano, Chair
Gayle L Yarnall, Clerk

9236   National Center for Vision and Aging Lighthouse
Lighthouse
111 E 59th Street
New York, NY 10022-1202

212-821-9200
800-829-0500
Fax: 212-821-9707
TTY: 212-821-9713
TDD: 212-821-9713
e-mail: info@lighthouse.org
www.lighthouse.org

The National Center for Vision and Aging provides information on eye conditions and visual impairment of all ages resources education and professionally prepared multimedia and print material for community education lectures.
Roger O Goldman, Chairman
Tara A Cortes, President and Chief Executive Officer

9237   National Center for Vision and Child Development
Lighthouse
111 E 59th Street
New York, NY 10022

212-821-9200
800-829-0500
Fax: 212-821-9707
TTY: 212-821-9713
e-mail: info@lighthouse.org
www.lighthouse.org

Our mission is to overcome vision impairment for people of all ages through worldwide leadership in rehabilitation services education research prevention and advocacy.
Roger O Goldman, Chairman
Tara A Cortes PhD RN, President and Chief Executive Officer

9238   National Diabetes Action Network for the Blind
National Federation of the Blind
1026 East 36th Street
Baltimore, MD 21218-7337

410-645-0632
Fax: 410-685-5653
e-mail: melissa@riccobono.us
www.nfb.org

Leading support and information organization of persons losing vision due to diabetes. Provides personal contact and resource information with other blind diabetics about non-visual techniques of independently managing diabetes and monitoring glucose levels.
Melissa Riccobono, President
Fredric Schroeder, First Vice President

9239   National Eye Institute National Institutes of Health
National Institutes of Health
31 Center Drive MSC 2510
Bethesda, MD 20892-3655

301-496-5248
www.nei.nih.gov

Mission is to discover safe and effective methods to prevent diagnose and treat diseases and disorders of the visual system. In this way the Institute helps to prevent reduce and possibly eliminate blindness and visual impairment.
Paul A Sieving, Director
Carl Kupfer, Volunteer

9240   National Federation of the Blind
1026 East 36th Street
Baltimore, MD 21218

410-645-0632
Fax: 410-685-5653
e-mail: melissa@riccobono.us
www.nfb.org

The largest consumer membership organization for the blind founded in 1940 it has 50 000 members nationwide in 52 affiliates and over 700 local chapters. Provides public education about blindness, support services to the newly blinded and scholarships.
50M Members
Melissa Riccobono, President
Fredric Schroeder, First Vice President

9241   National Federation of the Blind in Computer Science
Curtis Chong
2721 34th Street
Des Moines, IA 50310-4256

515-771-8348
Fax: 515-281-1361
e-mail: michael.NFBI@gmail.com
www.nfb.org

National organization of blind persons knowledgeable in the computer science and technology fields. Works to develop new technologies, to secure access to current technology and to develop new ways of using current or new technologies by the blind.
Curtis Chong, President

9242   National Federation of the Blind: Blind/Deaf Division
Robert Eschbach
9014 East Bellevue Street
Tucson, AZ 85715-5440

520-733-5894
e-mail: krezguy@cox.net
www.nfb.org

Deaf-blind persons working nationally to improve services, training and independence for the deaf-blind. Offers personal contact with other deaf-blind individuals knowledgeable in advocacy, education, employment, technology, discrimination and other issues surrounding deaf-blindness.
Bob Kresmer, President

9243   National Federation of the Blind: Blind Industrial Workers of America
National Federation of the Blind
1026 East 36th Street
Baltimore, MD 21218-4998

410-645-0632
Fax: 410-685-5653
e-mail: melissa@riccobono.us
www.nfb.org

Membership organization of blind persons employed in industrial and manufacturing work or in government job programs for the blind. Dedicated to protecting the rights of blind workers in salary, job stability, advancement and labor issues.
Melissa Riccobono, President

9244   National Federation of the Blind: Human Services Division
Melissa Riccobono
1026 E 36th Street
Baltimore, MD 21218

410-645-0632
e-mail: melissa@riccobono.us
www.nfb.org

Membership organization of blind persons working in counseling personnel psychology social work psychiatry rehabilitation and other social science and human resource fields. Dedicated to im-

681

proving employment opportunities and advancement for blind persons.
Melissa Riccobono, President

9245 National Federation of the Blind: Masonic Square Club
Fred Flowers
1026 East 36th Street   410-645-0632
Baltimore, MD 21218-4766   e-mail: melissa@riccobono.us
                                                    www.nfb.org
Blind individuals committed to sharing of Masonic experiences goals and history.
Melissa Riccobono, President

9246 National Federation of the Blind: Public Employees Division
Ivan Weich
3101 Northeast 87th Avenue   360-576-5965
Vancouver, WA 98662-3009   e-mail: k7uij@panix.com
                                                    www.nfb.org
Organization of blind persons holding local state or federal jobs. Focuses on issues such as changes in governmental hiring and retention practices new job skills needed for the future, government employment downsizing, new electronic means of finding employment and more.
Michael Freeman, President

9247 National Federation of the Blind: Science and Engineering Division
John Miller
3934 Kern Court   925-462-8575
Pleasanton, CA 94588-1920   e-mail: j8miller@soe.ucsd.edu
                                                    www.nfb.org
Blind persons with expertise and experience in fields such as genetics, telecommunications, biology, chemistry, physics and nuclear physics or mechanical electronic and chemical engineering. This is a strong support group to encourage blind persons to excel in science and engineering.
John Miller, President

9248 National Federation of the Blind: Writers Division
Tom Stevens
504 S 57th Street   402-556-3216
Omaha, NE 68106-0809   e-mail: newmanrl@cox.net
                                              www.nfb-writers-division.org
Blind writers in all styles including poetry short story fiction non-fiction magazine writing and theatrical work offer encouragement and support to blind writers and authors. Issues cover various aspects of this business including selling your work.
Robert L Newman, President

9249 National Industries for the Blind
1310 Braddock Place   703-310-0500
Alexandria, VA 22314-1727   Fax: 703-998-8268
                                      e-mail: communications@nib.org
                                                    www.nib.org
A nonprofit organization that represents over 100 associated industries serving people who are blind in thirty-six states. These agencies serve people who are blind or visually impaired and help them to reach their full potential.
Kevin Lynch, President/CEO
Steve Brice, Vice President/CFO

9250 National Library Service for the Blind and Physically Handicapped
Library of Congress
1291 Taylor Street NW   202-707-5100
Washington, DC 20011   888-657-7323
                                              TTY: 202-707-0744
                                              TDD: 202-707-0744
                                              e-mail: nls@loc.gov
                                                    www.loc.gov/nls
Administers a national library service that provides braille and recorded books and magazines on free loan to anyone who cannot read standard print because of visual or physical disabilities who are eligible residents of the United States.
12 pages Quarterly
Frank Kurt Cylke, Director
Michael M Moodie, Research and Development Officer

9251 National Organization of Parents of Blind Children
Barbara Cheadle

1026 East 36th Street   410-645-0632
Baltimore, MD 21218-4998   Fax: 410-685-5653
                                      e-mail: melissa@riccobono.us
                                    www.nfb.org/nfb/Parents_and_Teachers.asp
Support information and advocacy organization of parents of blind or visually impaired children. Addresses issues ranging from help to parents of a newborn blind infant, mobility and Braille instruction, education, social and community participation.
Melissa Riccobono, President

9252 New Eyes for the Needy
549 Milburn Avenue   973-376-4903
Short Hills, NJ 07078   Fax: 973-376-3807
                               e-mail: neweyesfortheneedy@yahoo.com
                                        www.neweyesfortheneedy.org/
Provides new glasses for those with low vision who may not be able to afford them.
Jean Gajano, Executive Director

9253 Prevent Blindess America
211 W Wacker Drive
Chicago, IL 60606-5624   800-331-2020
                                    e-mail: info@preventblindness.org
                                          www.preventblindness.org
Information and referral services provided on specific eye disorders. Publishes literature and supports community screening and testing programs.
Hugh R Parry, President/CEO

9254 Randolph-Sheppard Vendors of America
940 Parc Helene Drive   504-328-6373
Marrero, LA 70072-4104   800-467-5299
                                             Fax: 504-328-6372
                                      e-mail: kim.venable@att.net
                                          www.randolph-sheppard.org
Protects the interests of blind vendors seeks proper implementation of the Randolph-Sheppard Act and encourages facility locations in more visible and profitable areas.
Charles Glaser, President
John Gordon, First Vice President

9255 Recording for the Blind and Dyslexic
20 Roszel Road
Princeton, NJ 08540-6294   866-RFB-D585
                                          www.randolph-sheppard.org
Provides materials for all people who cannot effectively read standard print because of a visual perceptual or other physical disability.

9256 Research to Prevent Blindness
645 Madison Avenue   212-752-4333
New York, NY 10022-1010   800-621-0026
                                             Fax: 212-688-6231
                                      e-mail: inforequest@rpbusa.org
                                                    www.rpbusa.org
National voluntary health foundation supported by foundations corporations and voluntary gifts and bequests from individuals. Established to stimulate basic and applied research into the causes prevention and treatment of blinding eye diseases.
David Weeks, Chairman
Diane S Swift, President

9257 Seeing Eye
PO Box 375   973-539-4425
Morristown, NJ 07963-0375   Fax: 973-539-0922
                                      e-mail: info@seeingeye.org
                                                    www.seeingeye.org
A training school for dogs to guide qualified blind persons.
James A Kutsch, President and Chief Executive Officer

9258 Smith-Kettlewell Eye Research Foundation
2318 Fillmore Street   415-345-2000
San Francisco, CA 94115   Fax: 415-345-8455
                                             TTY: 415-345-2290
                                                    www.ski.org
Dedicated to research on human vision founded to encourage a productive collaboration between the medical clinic and the scientific laboratories.

9259 **Taping for the Blind**
3935 Essex Lane   713-622-2767
Houston, TX 77027-5113   Fax: 713-622-2772
www.tapingfortheblind.org
Records reading material on audiotape copied onto cassettes for use by blind and physically handicapped persons. Promotes increased interest in and use of free audio materials. Books textbooks and technical manuals are recorded and sent to libraries.
Kari Musgrove, Executive Director
Mary Farish Johnston, President

9260 **United States Association for Blind Athletes**
1 Olympic Plaza   719-630-0422
Colorado Springs, CO 80909-3508   Fax: 719-630-0616
e-mail: mlucas@usaba.org
www.usaba.org
Athletic association for blind athletes this association is the national governing body for the United States visually impaired athletes.
Dave Bushland, President
Tracie Foster, Vice President

9261 **Vision World Wide**
5707 Brockton Drive   317-254-1332
Indianapolis, IN 46220-5481   800-431-1739
Fax: 317-251-6588
e-mail: info@visionenhancement.org
www.visionww.org
Believing there is hope when vision fails. It disseminates relevant information on a variety of topics through its information and referral helpline website e-mail announce list and journal Vision Enhancement all designed to encourage and support individuals with vision impairments.
Patricia Price, Editor-In-Chief
William Corbin, Board Chairman

9262 **Washington Ear**
12061 Tech Road   301-681-6636
Silver Spring, MD 20904-2437   Fax: 301-625-1986
e-mail: information@washear.org
www.washear.org
A nonprofit organization providing reading and information services for the blind visually impaired and physically disabled persons who cannot effectively read print see plays watch television programs or view museum exhibits.
Margaret Pfanstiehl, President
George Long, Vice President

9263 **National Federation of the Blind: Blind Merchants Division**
Kevin Worley
1837 S. Nevada Avenue   71- 4-3 23
Colorado Springs, CO 80905-3591   88- 6-1 18
Fax: 303-695-1828
e-mail: kevinworley@blindmerchants.org
www.blindmerchants.org
Membership organization of blind persons employed in either self-employment work or the Randolph-Sheppard vending program. Provides information regarding rehabilitation social security tax and other issues which directly affect blind merchants.
Kevin Worley, President

State Agencies & Associations

Alabama

9264 **Alabama Council of the Blind**
1018 E Street S   256-362-5649
Talladega, AL 35160   e-mail: dart1018@charter.net
www.acbalabama.org
David Trott, President

9265 **National Federation of the Blind: Alabama**
4905 Brooke Court   251-344-7960
Mobile, AL 36618-2708   e-mail: mwkoger21@bellsouth.net
www.nfbofalabama.org
Minnie K Walker, President

Alaska

9266 **National Federation of the Blind: Alaska**
1169 Hess Avenue   907-479-6118
Fairbanks, AK 99709   e-mail: jnhburton@gci.net
www.nfb.org
Jim Burton, President

Arizona

9267 **Arizona Center for the Blind and Visually Impaired**
3100 E Roosevelt Street   602-273-7411
Phoenix, AZ 85008-5036   Fax: 602-273-7410
e-mail: jlamay@acbvi.org
www.acbvi.org
Provides services for individuals to enhance the quality of life of people who are blind or otherwise visually impaired. Services are available to adults who are either legally blind or visually impaired as well as those who have a degenerative eye condition.
Steve Walker, Chair
Stanton Stipes, Vice Chair

9268 **Arizona Industries for the Blind**
515 N 51st Avenue   602-771-9100
Phoenix, AZ 85043   Fax: 602-353-5703
e-mail: LHudspeth@azdes.gov
www.azdes.gov/aib
Arizona Industries for the Blind was established in 1952 to provide employment and training opportunities for Arizonans who are legally blind.
Lorraine Hudspeth, Controller
Letty Cerpa, Senior Accountant

9269 **National Federation of the Blind: Arizona**
9014 E Bellevue Street   520-733-5894
Tucson, AZ 85715-5652   e-mail: krezguy@cox.net
www.nfbarizona.com
Bob Kresmer, President
Vicki Hodges, 1st Vice President

9270 **Region 6 of the National Association for Parents of the Visually Impaired**
Walnut Creek, CA 85282-5724   602-730-8282
e-mail: mebphillips@comcast.net
www.spedex.com/napvi
Susan LaVenture, Executive Director
Julie Urban, President

Arkansas

9271 **Arkansas Lighthouse for the Blind**
6818 Murray Street   510-562-2222
Little Rock, AR 72209-2666   Fax: 501-568-5275
e-mail: bjohnson@arkansaslighthouse.org
www.arkansaslighthouse.org
Pat Smith, President
Jim Shenep, Vice President

9272 **National Federation of the Blind: Arkansas**
2360 Wedington Drive   479-582-0091
Fayetteville, AR 72701-2304   e-mail: tosheeler@cox.net
www.nfb.org
Terry Sheeler, President

California

9273 **Lighthouse for the Blind and Visually Impaired**
Lighthouse Industries
214 Van Ness Avenue   415-431-1481
San Francisco, CA 94102   Fax: 415-863-7568
TTY: 415-431-4572
e-mail: info@lighthouse-sf.org
www.lighthouse-sf.org
The LightHouse promotes the independence, equality and self-reliance of people who are blind or visually impaired through rehabilitation training and relevant services, such as access to employment, education, government, information, recreation and transportation.
Chuck Godwin, Executive Support
Anthony Fletcher, Associate Executive Director and COO

9274 National Federation of the Blind: California
3934 Kern Court
Pleasonton, CA 94588
818-342-6524
877-558-6524
Fax: 818-344-7930
e-mail: nfbcal@sbcglobal.net
http://www.nfbcal.org/

Mary Willows, President
Ever Lee Harriston, Vice President

9275 Northwest Regional Training Center: Canine Companions for Independence
2965 Dutton Avenue
Santa Rosa, CA 95407-0446
707-577-1000
800-572-2275
TTY: 707-577-1756
e-mail: info@cci.org
www.cci.org
Canine Companions for Independence is a non-profit organization that enhances the lives of people with disabilities by providing highly trained assistance dogs and ongoing support to ensure quality partnerships.
Corey Hudson, CEO
Kathy Pierson, Northwest Regional Executive Director

9276 Southwest Regional Training Center: Canine Companions for Independence
124 Rancho del Oro Drive
Oceanside, CA 92057
760-901-4300
800-572-2275
Fax: 760-901-4350
TTY: 760-901-4326
TDD: 760-901-4350
www.cci.org
Canine Companions for Independence is a non-profit organization that enhances the lives of people with disabilities by providing highly trained assistance dogs and ongoing support to ensure quality partnerships.
Linda Valliant, Executive Director
Chuck Contreras, Director of Development

Colorado

9277 National Federation of the Blind: Colorado
2233 W Shepperd Avenue
Littleton, CO 80120
303-778-1130
800-401-4NFB
e-mail: slabarre@labarrelaw.com
www.nfbco.org

Scott LaBarre, President
Kevan Worley, 1st Vice President

Connecticut

9278 National Federation of the Blind: Connecticut
477 Connecticut Boulevard,
East Hartford, CT 06108-3579
860-289-1971
e-mail: aldelucia@nfbct.org
http://www.nfbct.org/

Alfonse DeLucia, President

9279 Prevent Blindness Tri-State
101 Whitney Avenue
New Haven, CT 06510
800-850-2020
e-mail: info@preventblindnesstristate.org
www.preventblindness.org/tristate
Kathryn Garre-Ayars, President & CEO
Maria Giarratana, Grants Manager

Delaware

9280 Delaware Assocation for the Blind Department of Health & Social Services
Department of Health & Social Services
2915 Newport Gap Pike
Wilmington, DE 19801-1526
302-655-2111
888-777-3925
Fax: 302-655-1442
e-mail: contact@dabdel.org
www.dabdel.org

9281 National Federation of the Blind: Delaware
2215 Bradmoor Road
Wilmington, DE 19803-2646
302-652-6761
e-mail: lynne.majewski@gmail.com
www.nfb.org

Lynne Majewski, President

District of Columbia

9282 American Foundation for the Blind: Governmental Relations
1660 L Street, NW
Washington, DC 20036
202-469-6831
Fax: 646-478-9260
e-mail: afbgov@afb.net
www.afb.org
Advocates on behalf of people who are blind or visually impaired before Congress and Executive Branch offices, and participates in advocacy-related coalitions and initiatives nationwide.
Paul W Schroeder, Vice President, Governmental Relations
Barbara Jackson LeMoine, Legislative Assistant

9283 Columbia Lighthouse for the Blind
1825 K Street NW
Washington, DC 20006
301-589-0894
877-324-5252
Fax: 877-595-9228
e-mail: info@clb.org
www.clb.org
Columbia Lighthouse for the blind offers programs and services that enable individuals who are blind or visually impaired to obtain and maintain independence at home, school and in the community.
Anthony Cancelosi, President/CEO

9284 National Federation of the Blind: DC
2354 13th Place, N.E.
Washington, DC 20018-1841   e-mail: callaway.shawn@gmail.com
202-352-1511
www.nfb.org

Shawn M. Callaway, President

Florida

9285 Goodwill Industries-Suncoast
Goodwill Industries-Suncoast
10596 Gandy Boulevard
Saint Petersburg, FL 33702
727-523-1512
888-279-1988
Fax: 727-579-0850
TTY: 727-579-1068
e-mail: gw.marketing@goodwill-suncoast.com
www.goodwill-suncoast.org
A non-profit community based organization whose purpose is to improve the quality of life for people who are disabled, disadvantaged and/or aged. This mission is accomplished through a staff of over 1,200 employees providing independent living skills.
R Lee Waits, President/Chief Executive Officer
Chris Ward, Marketing and Media Relations Manager

9286 National Federation of the Blind: Florida
3708 West Bay to Bay Blvd
Tampa, FL 33629-4266
386-677-6886
888-282-5972
e-mail: president@nfbflorida.org
www.nfbflorida.org

Dan Hicks, President
Gloria Mills Hicks, Treasurer

9287 Southeast Regional Center: Canine Companions for Independence
Anheuser-Busch/SeaWorld Campus
8150 Clarcona Ocoee Road
Orlando, FL 32818-0388
407-522-3300
Fax: 407-522-3347
e-mail: mager@cci.org
www.cci.org
Canine Companions for Independence is a non-profit organization that enhances the lives of people with disabilities by providing highly trained assistance dogs and ongoing support to ensure quality partnerships.
Margaret S Ager, Executive Director
Nancy Baumann, President

9288 Tampa Lighthouse for the Blind
1106 W Platt Street
Tampa, FL 33606-2142
813-251-2407
866-251-2407
Fax: 813-254-4305
e-mail: TLH@tampalighthouse.org
www.tampalighthouse.org
Tampa Lighthouse for the Blind provides comprehensive rehabilitation programs for persons who are blind or visually impaired.
Cliff Olstrom, Executive Director

Georgia

9289 Georgia Industries for the Blind
700 Faceville Highway
Bainbridge, GA 39818-0218   229-248-2666
www.vocrehabga.org
The primary mission of the Georgia Industries for the Blind (GIB) is to provide employment opportunities for people who are visually impaired or blind.

9290 National Federation of the Blind: Georgia
315 Ponce de Leon Avenue   404-371-1000
Decatur, GA 30030   Fax: 404-371-1002
e-mail: gscott@nfbga.org
www.nfb.org

Garrick Scott, President

9291 Southeastern Region: Helen Keller National Center
1003 Virginia Avenue   404-766-9625
Atlanta, GA 30354-1365   Fax: 404-766-3447
TTY: 404-766-2820
e-mail: bc4hknc@aol.com
www.hknc.org

Barbara Chandler, Regional Representative

Hawaii

9292 Division of Vocational Rehabilitation and Services for the Blind
Department of Human Services
601 Kamokila Boulevard   808-692-7715
Kapolei, HI 96707   Fax: 808-692-7727
TTY: 808-692-7715
e-mail: info@hawaiivr.org
www.hawaiivr.org
The American Macular Degeneration Foundation is committed to the prevention and cure of macular degeneration and offers hope and support to those afflicted and their families. The Foundation is a major voice in establishing national research.
Joe Cordova, Administrator

9293 Ho'opono Workshop for the Blind
1901 Bachelor Street   808-586-5286
Honolulu, HI 96817   Fax: 808-586-5288
TTY: 808-586-5269
e-mail: hoopono@hawaiivr.org
www.hawaiivr.org

Dave Eveland, Administrator

9294 National Federation of the Blind: Hawaii
PO Box 4482   808-391-1214
Honolulu, HI 96812   e-mail: nanifife@aol.com
hawaii.nfb.org

Nani Fife, President
Charlene Ota, Vice-President

Idaho

9295 National Federation of the Blind: Idaho
300 Willard Avenue   208-377-9825
Pocatello, ID 83201   Fax: 208-232-5416
e-mail: ElsieLamp@yahoo.com
www.nfbidaho.org

Elsie H Lamp, President

Illinois

9296 Aid to the Aged, Blind or Disabled
Department of Human Services
100 South Grand Avenue, East
Springfield, IL 62762   800-252-8635
TTY: 800-447-6404
www.macular.org/stagency/state_il.html
The American Macular Degeneration Foundation is committed to the prevention and cure of macular degeneration and offers hope and support to those afflicted and their families. The Foundation will be a major voice in establishing the national research agenda for macular degeneration through promoting an alliance among the scientific community, government, and victims of the disease and their families to ensure the prevention and cure of the disease.

9297 Chicago Lighthouse for People Who are Blind and Visually Impaired
1850 W Roosevelt Road   312-666-1331
Chicago, IL 60608-1298   Fax: 312-243-8539
TTY: 312-666-8874
TDD: 312-666-8874
e-mail: helpdesk@chicagolighthouse.org
www.thechicagolighthouse.org
The Chicago Lighthouse is a comprehensive private rehabilitation and educational facility dedicated exclusively to assisting children youth and adults who are blind visually impaired or multi-disabled.
Janet P Szlyk, Executive Director
William L Conaghan, Chairman

9298 Helen Keller National Center Regional Representatives
485 Avenue of the Cities   309-755-0018
E Moline, IL 61244   Fax: 309-755-0025
TTY: 309-755-0018
TDD: 309-755-0021
e-mail: HKNC5LJT@aol.com
www.hknc.org

Laura J Thomas, Regional Representative

9299 National Federation of the Blind: Illinois
6919 W Berwyn Avenue   773-307-6440
Chicago, IL 60656-2040   e-mail: president@nbfofillinois.org
www.nfbofillinois.org

Patti Gregory-Chang, President
Deborah Kent Stein, First Vice-President

Indiana

9300 Bosma Industries for the Blind
8020 Zionsville Road   317-684-0600
Indianapolis, IN 46268-3876   800-362-5463
Fax: 317-684-1946
e-mail: info@bosma.org
www.bosma.org
It is the mission of Bosma Industries for the Blind to enhance opportunities for individuals who are blind or visually impaired to achieve their potential in vocational, economic, social and personal independence.
Lou Moneymaker, CEO
Connie F Campbell, CFO/COO

9301 National Federation of the Blind: Indiana
6010 Winnpeny Lane   317-205-9226
Indianapolis, IN 46220-5253   e-mail: rb15@iquest.net
www.nfb.org

Ron Brown, President

Iowa

9302 National Federation of the Blind: Iowa
2721 34th Street   515-771-8348
Des Moines, IA 50310   e-mail: m.barber@mchsi.com
www.nfb.org

Michael D Barber, President
April Enderton, First Vice-President

Kansas

9303 Kansas Industries for the Blind
425 MacVicar Street   785-296-3211
Topeka, KS 66606   Fax: 785-296-0728

9304 National Federation of the Blind: Kansas
11405 W Grant   913-339-9341
Wichita, KS 67209-3621   e-mail: donnajwood@cox.net
www.nfbks.org

Donna Wood, President
Susan L Stanzel, First Vice President

Kentucky

9305 Kentucky Industries for the Blind
1900 Brownsboro Road   502-893-0211
Louisville, KY 40206-2102   Fax: 502-893-3885

9306 National Federation of the Blind: Kentucky
210 Cambridge Drive
Louisville, KY 40214-2809
502-366-2317
e-mail: cathyj@iglou.com
www.nfbky.org

Cathy Jackson, President
Pamela Roark-Glisson, Vice President

Louisiana

9307 Industries for the Blind and Visually Impaired of Louisiana
PO Box 366
Delhi, LA 71232-0366
318-878-8171

9308 Louisiana Association for the Blind
1750 Claiborne Avenue
Shreveport, LA 71103
318-635-6471
877-913-6471
Fax: 318-635-8902
e-mail: labstore@lablind.com
www.lablind.com

LAB employs people who are blind in manufacturing administrative training and a variety of job positions that match an individual's goals and potential.
Shelly Taylor, President/CEO
Doug Young, Vice President Administration

9309 National Federation of the Blind: Louisana
605 University Boulevard
Ruston, LA 71270-4862
318-251-1511
800-234-4166
e-mail: pallenp@lcb-ruston.com
www.nfbla.org

Pam Allen, President

Maine

9310 Maine Center for the Blind and Visually Impaired
189 Park Avenue
Portland, ME 04102-2909
207-774-6273
Fax: 207-774-0679
e-mail: info@theiris.org
www.theiris.org

Leonard Cole, Chairman
Katherine Ray, Vice Chair

9311 National Federation of the Blind: Maine
33 Morse Avenue
Lewiston, ME 04240-9707
207-212-1455
e-mail: leonproctorjr@yahoo.com
www.nfb.org

Leon Proctor, Jr, President

Maryland

9312 Blind Industries and Services of Maryland
3345 Washington Boulevard
Baltimore, MD 21227
410-737-2600
888-322-4567
Fax: 410-737-2665
www.bism.org

Blind Industries and Services of Maryland provides innovative rehabilitation services training and stable employment opportunities to our state's citizens who are blind or visually impaired.
Don Morris, Chairperson
Walter Brown, Vice-Chairperson

9313 National Federation of the Blind: Maryland
1026 E 36th Street
Baltimore, MD 21218
41- 6-5 06
e-mail: president@nfbmd.org
www.nfbmd.org/

Melissa Riccobono, President
Debbie Brown, First Vice President

Massachusetts

9314 Carroll Center for the Blind
770 Centre Street
Newton, MA 02458-2597
617-969-6200
800-852-3131
Fax: 617-969-6204
TTY: 617-969-6204
e-mail: info@carroll.org
www.carroll.org
Assists blind and visually impaired adults and adolescents to adjust to loss of vision. The goal of this dynamic program is to en-

courage independence, restore self-confidence, prepare for employment and improve the quality of life.
Dina Rosenbaum, Marketing Director

9315 Massachusetts Commission for the Blind
600 Washington St.
Boston, MA 02111-4718
617-748-2000
www.state.ma.us/mcb
Provides services to blind citizens of Massachusetts, enabling them to lead more fulfilling and independent lives. Offers vocational rehabilitation, independent living, social services, home care and respite assistance, radio reading programs and print resources.
Cheryl Standley, Contact
Janet LaBreck, Commissioner

9316 National Federation of the Blind: Massachusetts
140 Wood Street
Somerset, MA 02726-5225
508-679-8543
e-mail: nfbmass@earthlink.net
http://www.nfbmass.org/

Priscilla Ferris, President

9317 New England Region: Helen Keller National Center
152 Lincoln Road
Lincoln, MA 01773
781-259-7100
Fax: 781-259-4014
e-mail: hknc1meb@comcast.net
www.hknc.org

Mary Ellen Barbiasz, Regional Representative
Peg Ouellette, Administrative Assistant

9318 Region 1 of the National Association for Parents of the Visually Impaired
Hudson, MA 06016-9560
860-623-4129
e-mail: sue.rawley@verizon.net
www.spedex.com/napvi

Michigan

9319 Association for the Blind & Visually Impaired
456 Cherry Southeast
Grand Rapids, MI 49503
616-458-1187
800-466-8084
Fax: 616-458-7113
e-mail: abvi@abvimichigan.org
www.abvimichigan.org
To advance the independence of people who are visually impaired and to promote the prevention of blindness.
Richard A Stevens, Executive Director
George Kremer, Director of Rehabilitation Services

9320 Greater Detroit Agency for the Blind and Visually Impaired
16625 Grand River Avenue
Detroit, MI 48227-1419
313-272-3900
Fax: 313-272-6893
e-mail: information@gdabvi.org
www.gdabvi.org
We are a non-profit organization dedicated to preventing blindness reducing the impact of blindness and advocating for those with severe vision loss.
Frederick J Simpson, Chairman
Charles L Cone, Vice Chair

9321 National Federation of the Blind: Michigan
1212 N Foster Avenue
Lansing, MI 48912-3309
517-482-1800
e-mail: f.wurtzel@comcast.net
www.nfbmi.org

Fred Wurtzel, President
Mary Ann Rojek, State Braille Coin Project Coordinator

Minnesota

9322 Duluth Lighthouse for the Blind
4505 W Superior Street
Duluth, MN 55807-2728
218-624-4828
800-422-0833
Fax: 218-624-4479
e-mail: info@lighthousefortheblind-duluth.org
www.lighthousefortheblind-duluth.org
The LightHouse for the blind is a teaching facility providing employment, training and rehab instruction for blind and visually-impaired individuals.
Mary Junnila, Executive Director
Debbie , Book keeper

9323 National Federation of the Blind: Minnesota
100 East 22nd street
Minneapolis, MN 55404-2217 e-mail: joyce.scanlan@earthlink.net
612-872-9363
http://www.nfbmn.org/
Jennifer Dunmann, President

Mississippi

9324 Mississippi Industries for the Blind
2501 N W Street
Jackson, MS 39216-4417
601-984-3200
866-859-4461
Fax: 601-987-3892
e-mail: bcoy@msblind.org
www.msblind.org
The Mississippi Industries for the Blind seeks to provide jobs for the blind and visually-impaired.
Michael Chew, Executive Director
Bob Coy, Sales Manager

9325 National Federation of the Blind: Mississippi
PO Box 1515
Jackson, MS 39215-5431
601-969-3352
e-mail: samgleese@earthlink.net
www.nfbofmississippi.org
rev Sam Gleese, President
Barbara Hadnot, Vice President

Missouri

9326 Alphapointe Association for the Blind
7501 Prospect
Kansas City, MO 64132
816-421-5848
Fax: 816-237-2019
e-mail: sliptak@alphapointe.org.
www.alphapointe.org
The Alphapointe Association for the Blind has a Braille library a Senior Adult Services Program and a dedication to finding employment for the blind and visually-impaired.
Paulette Markel, Chairman
Ken Roberson, Secretary

9327 Kansas City Association for the Blind
1844 Broadway Street
Kansas City, MO 64108-2007
816-333-2173

9328 National Federation of the Blind: Missouri
3910 Tropical Lane
Columbia, MO 65202-6205
573-874-1774
e-mail: info@nfbmo.org
www.nfbmo.org
Gary Wunder, President
Shelia Wright, First Vice President

Montana

9329 National Federation of the Blind: Montana
408 W Sussex Avenue
Missoula, MT 59801
406-546-8546
e-mail: burk.dall@gmail.com
www.mt-blind.org
Daniel Burke, President
Dick Howse, 1st Vice President

Nebraska

9330 National Federation of the Blind: Nebraska
1033 O Street
Lincoln, NE 68508-2468
402-477-7711
866-254-6347
e-mail: amy.buresh@ncbvi.ne.gov
nfbn.inebraska.com
Amy Buresh, President
Jeff Altman, First Vice President

Nevada

9331 National Federation of the Blind: Nevada
1344 N. Jones Boulevard
Las Vegas, NV 89108
702-228-4217
e-mail: realhappygirl1@gmail.com
ww.nfb.org
Terri Rupp, President

9332 Southern Nevada Sightless
1001 N Bruce Street
Las Vegas, NV 89101-1247
702-642-6000
Fax: 702-649-6739
e-mail: info@blindcenter.org
www.blindcenter.org
Neal Marek, Chairman
Veronica Wilson, President/CEO

New Hampshire

9333 National Federation of the Blind: New Hampshire
12 Summer St.
Keene, NH 03431
603-357-4080
e-mail: cemcnabb21@yahoo.com
www.nfbnh.org/
Marie Johnson, President

New Jersey

9334 Bestwork Industries for the Blind
801 E Clements Bridge Road
Runnemede, NJ 08078
856-939-5220
800-370-9560
Fax: 856-939-5022
e-mail: bestwork@bestworkindustries.org
www.bestworkindustries.org
Bestwork Industries for the Blind is dedicated to providing employment opportunities for those with visual impairments.
James Varsaci, Founder

9335 National Federation of the Blind: New Jersey
254 Spruce Street
Bloomfield, NJ 07003
973-743-0075
e-mail: nfbnj@yahoo.com
http://www.nfbnj.org/
Joe Ruffalo, President

New Mexico

9336 National Federation of the Blind: New Mexico
10315 Props dr. NE
Albuquerque, NM 87112
505-268-3895
e-mail: blindart@myfreedombox.com
http://www.nfbnm.org/
Arthur Schreiber, President

9337 New Mexico Industries for the Blind
2200 Yale Boulevard SE
Albuquerque, NM 87106-4212
505-841-8844
888-513-7958
Fax: 505-841-8850
e-mail: Greg.Trapp@state.nm.us
www.state.nm.us/cftb
Greg Trapp, Executive Director
Dallas Allen, Commissioner

9338 State of New Mexico Commission for the Blind
2905 Rodeo Park Drive E
Santa Fe, NM 87505
505-476-4479
888-513-7968
e-mail: Greg.Trapp@state.nm.us
www.state.nm.us/cftb
The mission of the New Mexico Commission for the Blind is to encourage and enable blind citizens to achieve vocational economic and social equality. It provides career preparation and training in the skills of blindness.
Greg Trapp, Executive Director
Arthur A Schreiber, Chairman

New York

9339 Association for the Blind & Visually Impaired of Greater Rochester
422 South Clinton Avenue
Rochester, NY 14620-1198
585-232-1111
www.raen.org
Our mission is to assist people who are blind or visually impaired to achieve their highest level of independence in all aspects of their lives.
A Gidget Hopf, EdD, President/CEO

9340 **Blind Association of Western New York**
1170 Main Street
Buffalo, NY 14209-2331
716-882-1025
e-mail: guildcarebuffalo@jgb.org
www.olmstedcenter.org
Patricia Clabeaux, Chairwomen
Phil Catanese, Vice Chairman

9341 **Blind Work Association**
55 Washington Street
Binghamton, NY 13901-3770
607-724-2428
Fax: 607-771-8045
e-mail: bobh@clarityconnect.com
www.co.tompkins.ny.us

9342 **Central Association for the Blind and Visually Impaired**
507 Kent Street
Utica, NY 13501-2317
315-797-2233
877-719-9996
Fax: 315-797-2244
e-mail: info@cabui.org
www.cabvi.org
Edward P. Welsch, Chairman
James B. Turnbill IV, Vice Chairman

9343 **National Federation of the Blind: New York**
PO Box 205666
Brooklyn, NY 11220-4617
718-567-7821
Fax: 718-765-1843
e-mail: office@nfbny.org
www.nfbny.org
Carl Jacobsen, President
Mindy Jacobson, Vice President

9344 **Northeastern Association of the Blind of Albany**
301 Washington Avenue
Albany, NY 12206-3012
518-463-1211
Fax: 51- 4-3 35
e-mail: info@naba-vision.org
www.naba-vision.org
NABA offers a wide range of services to those with visual impairments from its free vision screening service for children to training and placing legally blind adults in professional employment. Also provides rehabilitation services to seniors with age-related conditions.
Mark J McKarthy, Chair
david P. Quinn, Vice Chairman

9345 **Southern Tier Association for the Visually Impaired**
719 Lake Street
Elmira, NY 14901-2538
607-734-1554
Fax: 607-734-9467
e-mail: info@st-avi.org
www.st-avi.org
Brian Bleiler, President
John Luce, Vice President

North Carolina

9346 **Lions Industries for the Blind**
4126 Berkeley Avenue
Kinston, NC 28504-8321
252-523-1019
Fax: 252-523-7090
e-mail: customerser@lionsindustries.org
www.lionsindustries.com
The Lions Industries for the Blind provides employment opportunities for the blind and visually-impaired.
ray Amette, Executive Director
Marc Camnitz, General Manager

9347 **National Federation of the Blind: North Carolina**
128 Summerlea Drive
Charlotte, NC 28214-1324
704-491-1486
Fax: 704-391-3204
e-mail: tjnc2@carolina.rr.com
http://www.nfbofnc.org/
Gary Ray, President

9348 **Winston-Salem Industries for the Blind**
7730 N Point Drive
Winston-Salem, NC 27106-3310
336-759-0551
800-242-7726
Fax: 336-759-0990
e-mail: info@wsifb.com
www.wsifb.com
The Winston-Salem Industries for the Blind provides employment opportunities for the blind and visually-impaired.
david Byler, Chair
Mike Faircloth, Vice Chairman

North Dakota

9349 **National Federation of the Blind: North Dakota**
301 4th St. East
Williston, ND 58101
701-572-3477
e-mail: diverson@midco.net
www.nfb.org
Duane Iverson, President

Ohio

9350 **Cincinnati Association for the Blind**
2045 Gilbert Avenue
Cincinnati, OH 45202-1490
513-221-8558
888-687-3935
Fax: 513-221-2995
e-mail: info@cincyblind.org
www.cincyblind.org
Persons who are blind visually impaired or print impaired may choose from a wide range of services to help them live more independently. Our services are provided by qualified certified instructors and staff with highly specialized skills.
John Mitchell, Executive Director
Ginny Backschreider, Director of Program services

9351 **Cleveland Sight Center**
1909 E 101st Street
Cleveland, OH 44106-8696
216-791-8118
Fax: 216-791-1101
e-mail: sfriedman@clevelandsightcenter.org
www.clevelandsightcenter.org
Mission is to enable people with vision impairment to reach their full potential and assure that adequate services are available to make a normal life possible.
William L. Spring, Chair
Thomas P. Furnas, Vice Chairman

9352 **Cleveland Skilled Industries**
2239 E 55th Street
Cleveland, OH 44103-4451
216-431-8085
Fax: 216-431-5123

9353 **National Federation of the Blind: Ohio**
P.O. Box 82055,
Columbus, OH 43202-1517
440-775-2216
e-mail: bbpierce@pobox.com
www.nfbohio.org
Duffy Eric, President
Payne Richard, Vice President

Oklahoma

9354 **National Federation of the Blind: Oklahoma**
457 N. Blackwelder Avenue
Edmond, OK 73034
405-600-0695
e-mail: jmassay1@cox.net
www.nfb.org
Jeannie Massay, President

9355 **Oklahoma League for the Blind**
501 N Douglas Avenue
Oklahoma City, OK 73106
405-232-4644
Fax: 405-236-5438
e-mail: swright@newviewoklahoma.org
www.newviewoklahoma.org
The mission of the Oklahoma League for the Blind is to facilitate independence and improve the quality of life for people who are blind or vision impaired by providing employment opportunities and services.
Thomas Larson, Director
Elijha Straw, Business Manager

Oregon

9356 **Blind Enterprises of Oregon**
6540 SE Foster Road
Portland, OR 97206
503-774-6387
Fax: 503-774-0585
e-mail: blindent@aol.com
www.blindenterprises.com
Tami Foss, Executive Director
Bill Smith, Operator

9357   National Federation of the Blind: Oregon
5005 Main Street   541-726-6924
Springfield, OR 97478   800-422-7093
e-mail: admin@mainstreetmontessori.org
www.nfb.org

Carla McQuillan, President

Pennsylvania

9358   Association for the Blind & Visually Impaired of Lehigh County
845 Wyoming Street   610-433-6018
Allentown, PA 18103-2199   Fax: 610-433-4856
e-mail: info@abvi.org
www.abvi.org
The ABVI mission is to strive to be our community's foremost provider and coordinator of preventative, educational, social and rehabilitative programs concerning vision loss. Our goal is to assist each individual and his/her family to achieve their greatest potential.
Kathleen Meckes, Executive Director

9359   Beaver County Association for the Blind
616 Fourth Street   724-843-1111
Beaver Falls, PA 15010   Fax: 724-843-8886
e-mail: bcab@forcomm.net
bcab2.tripoid.com
The Beaver County Association for the Blind conducts educational programs about blindness or vision problems by request and provides opportunities to learn experience share and celebrate in the lives of the blind and visually impaired in Beaver County.
Fay Lentz, Executive Director
Linda Borghi, Controller/Business Manager

9360   Cambria County Association for the Blind and Handicapped
211 Central Avenue   814-536-3531
Johnstown, PA 15902   Fax: 814-539-3270
e-mail: ccabh@ccabh.com
www.ccabh.com
The mission of the Cambria County Association for the Blind and Handicapped is to develop and support an environment for persons with disabilities which promotes vocational and employment training, independence and community involvement through rehabilitative programs.
Richard C Bosserman, President

9361   Chester County Association for the Blind
71 S First Avenue   610-384-2767
Coatesville, PA 19320   Fax: 610-384-8005
e-mail: info@chescoblind.org
www.chescoblind.org

Anita Cavuto, Executive Director
John W Esworthy, President

9362   Delaware County Branch of the Pennsylvania Association for the Blind
100-106 W 15th Street   610-874-1476
Chester, PA 19013   Fax: 610-874-6454
e-mail: delcosce@liberty.org
www.libertynet.org

9363   Greater Wilkes-Barre Association for the Blind
1825 Wyoming Avenue   570-693-3555
Exeter, PA 18643   877-693-3555
Fax: 570-823-4841
e-mail: info@wilkesbarreblind.com
www.wilkesbarreblind.com
Our mission is to address the needs of those with limited vision and we also take an active role in the prevention of blindness.
Ronald V Petrilla, Executive Director
Denise Culver, Office Manager

9364   Indiana County Association for the Blind
31 S 10th Street   724-465-5549
Indiana, PA 15701-2649

9365   Keystone Blind Association
1230 Stambaugh Avenue   724-347-5501
Sharon, PA 16146   800-837-4122
Fax: 724-347-2204
e-mail: kba@keystoneblind.org
www.keystoneblind.org

The Keystone Blind Association is dedicated to maintaining and improving the quality of life for blind and/or visually impaired persons preventing blindness and providing employment opportunities and advocacy for persons who are disabled.
Jonathan G Fister, President/CEO
Perry Templeton, Vice President of Operations

9366   Lancaster County Association for the Blind
244 N Queen Street   717-291-5951
Lancaster, PA 17603-3512   e-mail: info@sfblind.org
www.sfblind.org

Dennis L Steiner, President/CEO
Kay L Macsi, VP Rehabilitation and Education

9367   Montgomery County Association for the Blind
212 N Main Street   215-661-9800
North Wales, PA 19454-3117   Fax: 215-661-9888
e-mail: mcab@mcab.org
www.mcab.org
MCAB's mission is to enhance the quality of life and independence of people coping with blindness and vision impairment through rehabilitation education support and advocacy.
Douglas Yingling, Executive Director
Sharon Zislis, Director of Development

9368   National Federation of the Blind: Pennsylvania
42 South 15th Street   215-988-0888
Philadelphia, PA 19102-2206   Fax: 215-988-0879
e-mail: nfbofpa@att.net
http://www.nfbp.org/

James Antonacci, President

9369   North Central Sight Services
2121 Reach Road   570-323-9401
Williamsport, PA 17701-0292   866-320-2580
Fax: 570-323-8194
e-mail: ncss@ncsight.org
www.ncsight.org
Our agency philosophy focuses on helping people help themselves and emphasizes the abilities and capabilities of the blind and visually impaired people we serve.
Robert B Garrett, President/CEO
Barbara Snauffer, Administrative Assistant

9370   Pittsburgh Vision Services
1800 W Street   412-368-4400
Homestead, PA 15120   800-706-5050
Fax: 412-368-4090
TTY: 412-368-4095
e-mail: info&ref@pghvis.org
www.bvrspittsburgh.org/
Pittsburgh Vision Services is a private non-profit United Way agency whose mission is to reduce the limitations that may result from loss of vision.
Dennis J Farkos, Chairman
louis A Lobes, Vice Chairman

9371   Somerset County Blind Center
748 S Center Avenue   814-445-1310
Somerset, PA 15501   Fax: 814-445-3184
e-mail: rob@somersetblind.org
www.somersetblind.org
The Somerset Blind Center offers a number of services to those who are blind or visually impaired, including work opportunities, eyeglass prescription programs, free vision screenings, and training facilities.
Rob Stemple, Executive Director
Anna Hope, Finance Manager

9372   Tri-County Association for the Blind
1130 S 19th Street   717-238-2531
Harrisburg, PA 17104-2200   Fax: 717-238-0710
e-mail: info@vrocp.org
www.vrocp.org/
The Tri-County Association for the Blind works to improve the quality of life for people who are visually-impaired in the Tri-County region, by helping each person achieve his or her full potential and maximum independence.
Danette Blank, Executive Director
Laurie Thompson, Public Relations/Development Director

9373 **VIABL Services of Northampton County**
845 West Wyoming Street
Allentown, PA 18103
610-433-6018
Fax: 610-866-8730
e-mail: viabl@viablservices.org
www.viablservices.org
Our mission is to promote the social economic and physical self-sufficiency of blind deaf-blind and visually impaired individuals by providing them with the resources and skills needed to live rewarding productive and independent lives.
Jan Leon, Executive Director

9374 **Washington-Greene County Branch for the Pennsylvania Association for Blind**
555 Gettysburg Pike,
Mechanicsberg, PA 17055-3720
71- 7-6 20
Fax: 71- 7-6 20
e-mail: neal.carrigan@pablind.org
www.pablind.org
Neal J Carrigan, President/CEO
Willard D Brown, Vice-President for Finance

9375 **York Industries for the Blind: Division of York County Blind Center**
A Division of York County Blind Center
1380 Spahn Avenue
York, PA 17403-5711
717-848-1690
Fax: 717-845-3889
www.forsight.org
William H Rhinesmith, President

Rhode Island

9376 **IN-SIGHT**
43 Jefferson Boulevard
Warwick, RI 02888
401-941-3322
Fax: 401-941-3356
e-mail: insightri@gmail.com
www.in-sight.org
IN-SIGHT is a private non-profit agency which has been serving the blind and visually impaired since 1925.
Gerard Goulet, President
Eleanor Acton, Director of Communications

9377 **National Federation of the Blind: Rhode Island**
PO Box 14404
East Providence, RI 02914
401-433-2606
Fax: 877-383-3682
e-mail: info@nfbri.org
www.nfbri.org
Richard Gaffney, President

South Carolina

9378 **National Federation of the Blind: South Carolina**
1293 Professional Drive
Myrtle Beach, SC 29577
803-254-3777
e-mail: parnell@sccoast.net
http://www.nfbsc.net/
Parnell Diggs, President

South Dakota

9379 **National Federation of the Blind: South Dakota**
903 Fulton Street
Rapid City, SD 57701
605-791-3939
e-mail: President@nfb-south-dakota.org
www.nfb-south-dakota.org
Kenneth Rollman, President

Tennessee

9380 **Ed Lindsey Industries of the Blind**
4110 Charlotte Avenue
Nashville, TN 37209-3749
615-627-4012
Fax: 615-741-5024
www.elifortheblind.org/
Allen Broughton, Executive Vice President
Patrick Broughton, Administrative Assistant

9381 **National Federation of the Blind: Tennessee**
1226 Goodman Circle West
Memphis, TN 38111-6524
901-452-6596
e-mail: michael.seay@ssa.gov
http://www.nfb-tennessee.org/
Michael Seay, President

Texas

9382 **American Foundation for the Blind**
11030 Ables Lane
Dallas, TX 75229
214-352-7222
Fax: 646-478-9260
e-mail: dallas@afb.net
www.afb.org
Leads initiatives in the areas of aging and education. Nationally offers consultation, technical assistance and support and undertakes local and national efforts such as training programs, public education and coalition building in the areas of aging and elder care.

9383 **American Foundation for the Blind: National Aging Center**
11030 Ables Lane
Dallas, TX 75229
214-352-7222
Fax: 646-478-9260
e-mail: dallas@afb.net
www.afb.org
Leads initiatives in the areas of aging and education. Nationally offers consultaion, technical assistance and support and undertakes local and national efforts such as training programs, public education and coalition building in the areas of aging and education. Responds to inquiries from blind and visually impaired people and their families, service providers and the general public in the region and nationally.

9384 **Dallas Lighthouse for the Blind**
4306 Capitol Avenue
Dallas, TX 75204
214-821-2375
Fax: 214-824-4612
www.dallaslighthouse.org
The Dallas Lighthouse for the Blind provides work opportunities for the blind and visually impaired.
Nancy J Perkins, President/CEO
Gordon Spark, Executive Vice president

9385 **East Texas Lighthouse for the Blind**
500 N Bois D'Arc
Tyler, TX 75702
903-595-3444
888-595-3444
Fax: 903-595-3447
e-mail: customerservice@horizonind.com
www.horizonind.com

9386 **El Paso Lighthouse for the Blind**
200 Washington Street
El Paso, TX 79905
915-532-4495
Fax: 915-532-6338
e-mail: htyler@elp.rr.com
www.lighthouse-elpaso.com
Lighthouse is guided by the unwavering belief that its rehabilitative and employment services can help any person overcome his or her disability and enable them to reach their fullest potential for self-sufficiency and independence.
Harry Tyler, President/CEO
Rusty Hooten, CFO

9387 **Lighthouse for the Blind of Houston**
3602 W Dallas
Houston, TX 77019-0435
713-527-9561
Fax: 713-284-8451
e-mail: houstonlighthouse@houstonlighthouse.org
ww.houstonlighthouse.org
Founded in 1839 the Lighthouse of Houston is a private nonprofit rehabilitation center dedicated to helping blind and visually impaired people live independently.
Gibson M DuTerroil, President

9388 **Lighthouse of the Blind of Fort Worth**
912 W Broadway Street
Fort Worth, TX 76104
817-332-3341
Fax: 817-332-3456
e-mail: plattallen@lighthousefw.org
www.lighthousefw.org
The Lighthouse of the Blind of Fort Worth offers many services including skills assessment orientation and mobilty training assisted employment and senior services.
Dr. Shannon Ship, Chairman
W.B. Zim Zimmerman, Vice Chair

9389 **National Federation of the Blind: Texas**
314 E Highland Mall Boulevard
Austin, TX 78752-3123
512-323-5444
866-636-3289
Fax: 512-420-8160
e-mail: president@nfbtx.org
www.nfb-texas.org
Tommy Craig, President

9390 South Texas Lighthouse for the Blind
PO Box 9697
Corpus Christi, TX 78469
361-883-6553
888-255-8011
Fax: 361-883-1041
e-mail: Regisb@stlb.net
www.stlb.net

Regis Barber, President/CEO
Nicky Ooi, VP/COO

9391 Texas Association of Retinitis Pigmentosa
PO Box 8388
Corpus Christi, TX 78468-8388
361-852-8515
Fax: 361-852-8515
e-mail: tarpmail@homebiz101.com
www.geocities.com/HotSprings/7815
A nonprofit organization based in Texas serving as a national information-sharing center to provide human services to persons with progressive vision loss from retinitis pigmentosa and other retinal degenerative disorders.
Dorothy H Stiefel, Executive Director

9392 Travis Association for the Blind
2307 Business Center Drive
Austin, TX 78764-3297
512-442-2329
Fax: 512-442-5498
e-mail: info@austinlighthouse.org
www.austinlighthouse.org
Travis Association for the Blind (aka Austin Lighthouse) is a service oriented non-profit organization with the mission to assist people who are blind or vision impaired to attain the skills they need to become gainfully employed in the community.
Jerry A Mayfield, Executive Director
Benny Galloway, Chief Financial Officer

9393 West Texas Lighthouse for the Blind
2001 Austin Street
San Angelo, TX 76903-8705
325-653-4231
Fax: 325-657-9367
e-mail: customerservice@lighthousefortheblind.or
www.lighthousefortheblind.org
The West Texas Lighthouse for the Blind is a sheltered facility providing employment for blind and visually impaired individuals.
Steve Cecil, Chairman
Barbara Rogers, Vice Chair

Utah

9394 National Federation of the Blind: Utah
1751 Park St
Salt Lake City, UT 84105-7634
801-631-8108
801-463-6632
Fax: 801-294-6000
e-mail: Baconev@yahoo.com
www.nfbutah.org

Everrete Bacon, President
Cheralyn Bra Creer, First Vice President

9395 Utah Industries for the Blind
PO Box 258
Salt Lake Cty, UT 84110-1258
801-533-9689

Vermont

9396 National Federation of the Blind: Vermont
561 East Hill Rd.
Middlesex, VT 05602
802-272-0087
e-mail: deannaljones@comcast.net
www.nfbvt.org

Franklin Shiner, President

Virginia

9397 National Federation of the Blind: Virginia
3230 Grove Avenue
Richmond, VA 23221
703-319-9226
e-mail: fschroeder@sks.com
www.nfbv.org

Fredric K Schroeder, President
Seville Allen, First Vice President

9398 Virginia Industries for the Blind
1102 Monticello Road
Charlottesville, VA 22902
434-295-5168
Fax: 434-977-0122
e-mail: Robert.Berrang@dbvi.virginia.gov
www.vdbvi.org/vib

Our mission is to be a self-sufficient and self-supporting industry enhance the quality of life for blind and visually impaired individuals through providing gainful employment; and provide opportunities in career development and employment related services.
Robert C Berrang, Deputy Commissioner
Richard C Bohrer, Plant Manager

Washington

9399 Lighthouse for the Blind of Washington
2501 South Plum Street
Seattle, WA 98114
206-322-4200
Fax: 206-329-3397
www.seattlelighthouse.org

Kirk Adams, President
Tami berk, Director

9400 Northwestern Region: Helen Keller National Center
1620 18th Avenue
Seattle, WA 98122-6501
206-324-9120
Fax: 206-324-9159
TTY: 206-324-1133
e-mail: nwhknc@juno.com
www.hknc.org

Dorothy Walt, Regional Representative

9401 Washington State Department of Services for the Blind
402 Legion Way
Olympia, WA 98504-0933
360-725-3830
800-552-7103
Fax: 360-407-0679
e-mail: information@dsb.wa.gov
www.dsb.wa.gov
The Washington State Department of Services for the Blind (DSB) is a state rehabilitation agency that offers assistance to persons who are blind or visually impaired. We also provide various services for employers interested in accomodating or hiring workers with visual impairments.
Bill Palmer, Director

West Virginia

9402 AFB Technology & Employment Center
1000 Fifth Avenue
Huntington, WV 25701
304-523-8651
800-824-2184
Fax: 646-478-9260
e-mail: AFBTECH@afb.net
www.afb.org
AFB Technology runs AFB's CareerConnect and the AFB TECH Product Evaluation Laboratory. Nationally offers consultation, technical assistance and support and undertakes local and national efforts in employment and technology.
Brad Hodges, National Technology Associate

9403 National Federation of the Blind: West Virginia
401 East Olive Street,
Bridgeport, WV 26330
304-622-0626
e-mail: cs.nfbwv@verizon.net
www.nfbwv.org

Charlene Smyth, President

Wisconsin

9404 National Federation of the Blind: Wisconsin
27824 Nuthatch Road
Kendall, WI 54638
608-758-4800
e-mail: johnfritz@centurytel.net
www.nfbwis.org/

John Fritz, President

9405 National Federation of the Blind: Writers
27824 Nuthatch Road
Kendall, WI 54638
608-758-4800
e-mail: johnfritz@centurytel.net
www.nfbwis.org

John Fritz, President

9406 Wiscraft: Wisconsin Enterprises for the Blind
5316 W State Street
Milwaukee, WI 53208-2686
414-778-5800
Fax: 414-778-5805
e-mail: sales@wiscraft.com
www.wiscraft.com
Wiscraft provides long-term supportive employment for people who are blind. It is a manufacturing company that operates as a

non-profit with the clear mission of employing people who are blind by sellng blind-made products and services.
Jim Kerlin, President
Ron Hutchinson, Chair

9407 **National Federation of the Blind: Wyoming**
4808 Ontario Ave. 307-421-8522
Cheyenne, WY 82009-0347 e-mail: kthornbury@bresnan.net
www.nfb.org

Kelly Thornbury, President

Foundations

9408 **Foundation Fighting Blindness**
7168 Columbia Gateway Drive, 410-568-0150
Columbia, MD 21046-2220 800-683-5555
TDD: 800-683-5551
e-mail: info@FightBlindness.org
www.fightblindness.org
For a $25.00 annual membership fee, FFB offers information and referral services for affected individuals and their families as well as for doctors and eye care professionals. The Foundation also provides comprehensive information kits on retinitis pigmentosa, macular degeneration, and usher syndrome. Their newsletter, InFocus, and their e-newsletter, InSight, present articles on coping research updates, and Foundation news. A national conference is usually held every other year.
Gordon Gund, Chairman
Edward H. Gollob, President

9409 **Glaucoma Research Foundation**
251 Post Street 415-986-3162
San Francisco, CA 94108 800-826-6693
Fax: 415-986-3763
e-mail: question@glaucoma.org
www.glaucoma.org
The Glaucoma Research Foundation is a nationa nonprofit dedicated to curing glaucoma. We receive no government funding. Your contribution is tax-deductible as allowed by law.
Thomas M Brunner, President/CEO

Libraries & Resource Centers

9410 **District of Columbia Public Library Librarian for the Deaf Community**
901 G Street North West
Washington, DC 20001 202-727-1111
www.dclibrary.org
Offers reference services through TDD, portable TDD for public use at pay phone, signers for library programs, sign language classes, information about deafness, print and non-print materials for persons who are deaf.
John W Hill, Jr, President
James W Lewis, Vice President

9411 **Alabama Radio Reading Service Network**
WBHM
650 11th Street South 205-934-2606
Birmingham, AL 35233-4530 800-444-9246
Fax: 205-934-5075
e-mail: philip@wbhm.org
www.wbhm.org/ARRS
Services and readings are relayed over the radio to three-quarters of Alabama for the benefit of the visually impaired.
sarah Delia, producer
Will Dahlberg, Manager

9412 **Alabama Regional Library for the Blind and Physically Handicapped**
Alabama Public Library Service

6030 Monticello Drive 334-213-3906
Montgomery, AL 36130-6000 800-392-5671
Fax: 334-213-3993
e-mail: fzaleski@apls.state.al.us
http://statelibrary.alabama.gov
To promote and support equitable access to library and information resources and services to enable all Alabamians to satisfy their educational, working, cultural, and leisure-time interests. These resources and services will be provided through APLS's statewide programs and through direct grants and assistance to libraries and library systems to meet user's needs.
Fara Zaleski, Regional Librarian
Rebecca Mitchell, Director (APLS)

9413 **Houston Love Memorial Library**
212 West Burdeshaw Street 334-793-9767
Dothan, AL 36303 e-mail: bforbus@yahoo.com
www.houstonlovelibrary.org
Offers magnifiers, summer reading programs and more for the blind and physically handicapped. Scanner, software and jaws for windows.
Steve Roy, Chair
Cindy Aman, Board

9414 **Huntsville Subregional Library for the Blind and Physically Handicapped**
P.O. Box 443 256-532-5980
Huntsville, AL 35804 Fax: 256-532-5994
e-mail: bphdept@hpl.lib.al.us
www.hpl.lib.al.us/departments/bph
The Subregional Library for the Blind and Physically Handicapped is located in the Main branch of the Huntsville-Madison County Public Library. It is also part of a Library of Congress administered nationwide network of libraries serving persons who cannot use conventional printed materials.
Joyce Welch, Librarian

9415 **Library and Resource Center for the Blind and Physically Handicapped**
Alabama Institute for Deaf and Blind
205 South Street 256-761-3237
Talladega, AL 35160 800-848-4722
Fax: 256-761-3561
e-mail: lacy.teresa@aidb.state.al.us
http://www.aidb.org
Using federal and state funds, the Resource Center purchases or produces braille textbooks and other necessary materials for students. The Resource Center also loans equipment, like braillewriters, to help students learn alternative methods of communication.
Dr,John Macia, President
Dr. Freida Meichan, Vice President

9416 **Tuscaloosa Subregional Library for the Blind & Physically Handicapped**
1801 Jack Warner Parkway 205-345-5820
Tuscaloosa, AL 35401 Fax: 205-752-8300
e-mail: bjordan@tuscaloosa-library.org
www.tuscaloosa-library.org
Provide talking books to patrons who are unable to use standard print because of a visual or physical limitation. Deliver playback equipment to qualified patrons. Provides reference and referral service to this special population also.
Dr. Horace Allen, Chairman
Dr. Marcia Burke, Vice Chair

9417 **Alaska State Library Talking Book Center**
National Library Services
344 W 3rd Avenue 907-269-6575
Anchorage, AK 99501-2337 800-776-6566
Fax: 907-269-6580
TDD: 907-269-6575
e-mail: tbc@eed.state.ak.us
www.library.state.ak.us
The Alaska State Library Talking Book Center is a cooperative effort between the National Library Service and the Alaska State Li-

brary to provide print handicapped Alaskans with talking book and Braille service.
Bev Griffin, Library Assistant II
Stephanie Schott, Administrative Clerk I

Arizona

9418 Arizona State Braille and Talking Book Library
1030 N 32nd Street
Phoenix, AZ 85008-5108
602-255-5578
800-255-5578
Fax: 602-255-4312
e-mail: btbl@lib.az.us
www.lib.az.us
Closed-circuit TV, summer reading programs, volunteer-produced cassette books, braille writer, films, large-print photocopier and more.
Catherine May, Chair
Ruth Solomon, Vice Chair

9419 Flagstaff City Coconino County Public Library
300 W Aspen Avenue
Flagstaff, AZ 86001-5304
520-779-7670
www.flagstaffpubliclibrary.org
Reference materials on blindness and other handicaps, braille writer, magnifiers and large-print photocopier.

9420 Phoenix Public Library: Special Needs Section
Burton Barr Central Library
1221 North Central Avenue
Phoenix, AZ 85004
602-262-4636
TDD: 602-254-8205
e-mail: specialneeds@phxlib.org
www.phoenixpubliclibrary.org
The Special Needs Center is designed to make the services and resources of the Phoenix Public Library accessible to people with disabilities.
Toni Garvey, City Librarian

Arkansas

9421 Arkansas Regional Library for the Blind and Physically Handicapped
900 W Capitol
Little Rock, AR 72201-1049
501-682-2053
866-660-0885
Fax: 501-682-1529
TDD: 501-682-1002
e-mail: nlsbooks@asl.lib.ar.us
www.asl.lib.ar.us
Public library books in recorded or braille format. Popular fiction and nonfiction books for all ages, books and players are on free loan, sent to patrons by mail and may be returned postage free. Anyone who cannot see well enough to read regular print with glasses on or who has a disability that makes it difficult to hold a book or turn the pages is eligible.
John D Hall, Coordinator

9422 Library for the Blind and Handicapped, Southwest
Columbia County Library
2057 North Jackson St
Magnolia, AR 71754
870-234-0399
866-234-8273
Fax: 870-234-5077
e-mail: lbph@hotmail.com
www.youseemore.com/columbia
The mission of the Columbia County Library is to help the people of our community in their pursuits of information and education , as well as vocational and recreational endeavors, by providing current materials, services, and programs. Our inviting public libraries are the cornerstone of our diverse communities where all people, regardless of age, race, or socio-economic circumstances can experience personal enrichment and literary growth.
Laura Cleaveland, Director
Dana Thornton, Assistant Director

California

9423 Blind Childrens Center
4120 Marathon Street
Los Angeles, CA 90029-3584
323-664-2153
Fax: 323-665-3828
www.blindchildrenscenter.org
The Blind Childrens Center is a family-centered agency which serves children with visual impairments from birth to school-age.

The center-based and home-based programs and services help the children acquire skills and build their independence. The Center utilizes its expertise and experience to serve families and professionals worldwide through support services, education, and research.
Midge Horton, Executive Director
Muriel Scharf, Director Development

9424 Braille Institute Library Services
741 North Vermont Avenue
Los Angeles, CA 90029-3594
323-663-1111
800-808-2555
Fax: 323-662-2440
TDD: 323-660-3880
e-mail: dls@braillelibrary.org
www.braillelibrary.org
The Braille Institute is a non-profit organization whose mission is to eliminate barriers to a fulfilling life caused by blindness and severe sight loss. The Institute provides an environment of hope and encouragement for people who are blind and visually impaired through integrated educational, social and recreational services and programs.
Henry C. Chang, Librarian

9425 California State Library Braille and Talking Book Library
National Library Service
PO Box 942837
Sacramento, CA 94237-0001
916-654-0640
800-952-5666
Fax: 916-654-1119
e-mail: btbl@library.ca.gov
www.library.ca.gov
Library services in braille and recorded formats. Free to residents of Northern California who are unable to read ordinary print on hold a printed book.
Michael Marlin, Manager
Mary Jane Kayes, Outreach Coordinator

9426 Fresno County Public Library: Talking Book Library for the Blind
2420 Mariposa Street
Fresno, CA 93721-3640
559-488-3217
800-742-1011
Fax: 559-488-1971
TDD: 559-488-1642
e-mail: wendy.eisenberg@fresnolibrary.org
www.fresnolibrary.org/tblb
We provide books and magazines on cassette tape and in Braille to people of all ages who are blind, visually impaired, or have physical disabilities preventing the reading of standard print.
Karen Bosch Cobb, County Librarian
Wendy Eisenberg, Librarian

9427 San Francisco Public Library for the Blind and Print Disabled
100 Larkin Street
San Francisco, CA 94102-4733
415-557-4253
TTY: 415-557-4433
e-mail: citylibrarian@sfpl.org
www.sfpl.lib.ca.us
Foreign-language books on cassette, children's books on cassettes and more.
Luis Herrera, City Librarian
Marcia Schneider, Chief, Communications/Adult Services

9428 San Jose State University Library
1 Washington Square
San Jose, CA 95192-0001
408-924-1000
www.library.sjsu.edu
Information on physical disabilities, accessibility and learning disabilities.

Colorado

9429 Boulder Public Library
1001 Arapahoe Avenue
Boulder, CO 80302-1326
303-441-3100
Fax: 303-442-1808
e-mail: ask@boulder.lib.co.us
www.boulder.lib.co.us
Offers braille books, cassettes, talking books, large print photocopier, large print books and more for the visually impaired.
Tony Tallent, Library & Arts Director

9430 Colorado Talking Book Library
201 East Colfax Ave.   303-727-9277
Denver, CO 80203-8101   800-685-2136
Fax: 303-727-9281
e-mail: ctbl.info@cde.state.co.us
www.cde.state.co.us
Take advantage of the services offered by the Colorado Talking Book Library (CTBL). CTBL provides postage-free recorded, braille, and large print library materials to eligible residents in Colorado.
Debbi MacLeod, Director

Connecticut

9431 Connecticut State Library for the Blind and Physically Handicapped
198 W Street   860-721-2020
Rocky Hill, CT 06067-3554   800-842-4516
Fax: 860-721-2056
e-mail: lbph@cslib.org
www.cslib.org/lbph.htm
Free audio cassettes and braille books and magazines along with reference materials on blindness and other handicaps. Necessary playback equipment for eligible residents of Connecticut.
Carol Taylor, Director

Delaware

9432 Delaware Division of Libraries: Library for the Blind and Physically Handicapped
43 South DuPont Highway   302-739-4748
Dover, DE 19901   800-282-8676
Fax: 302-739-6787
TDD: 302-739-4847
e-mail: john.phillos@state.de.us
www.state.lib.de.us
Since 1971, the Delaware Library for the Blind and Physically Handicapped has provided books in Braille and audio books on record and cassette for the blind and physically handicapped residents of Delaware.
John Phillos, Librarian

District of Columbia

9433 Council of Families with Visual Impairment
American Council of the Blind
1155 15th Street NW   202-467-5081
Washington, DC 20005   800-424-8666
Fax: 202-467-5085
e-mail: info@acb.org
www.acb.org
Members are sighted parents of blind or visually impaired children. Offers a forum for support and outreach, sharing of experiences in parent-child relationships, and educational and cultural information about child development. Monitors developments in technical and legislative arenas.
Melanie Brunson, Executive Director

9434 DC Public Library Adaptive Services Division
901 G Street NW, Room 215   202-727-2142
Washington, DC 20001   Fax: 202-727-1129
TTY: 202-727-2255
TDD: 202-727-1129
e-mail: lbph.dcpl@dc.gov
www.dclibrary.org
The DC Public Library has a special Adaptive Technology Program to help older adults, the deaf, and those with visual and physical disabilities use library materials and resources.
Venetia V. Demson, Librarian

9435 National Library Service for the Blind and Physically Handicapped
1291 Taylor Street,   202- 70- 510
Washington, DC 20011   Fax: 202-707-0712
TDD: 202-707-0744
e-mail: raj@loc.gov
www.loc.gov/nls
The NLS, Library of Congress, administers the free programs that loans recorded and braille books and magazines, music scores in

braille and large print, and specially designed playback equipment to residents of the United States who are unable to read or use standard print materials due to visual or physical impairment.
Yealuri Rathan Raj, Librarian

Florida

9436 Brevard County Libraries: Talking Books Library
2725 Judge Fran Jamieson Way   32- 6-3 20
Viera, FL 32940-7781   Fax: 32- 9-2 63
e-mail: dmartin@brev.org
www.brev.org
The Talking Books/Homebound Services has many devices and special materials to assist blind, physically handicapped and/or homebound citizens to access library services.
Debra A. Martin, Librarian

9437 Broward County Talking Book Library
100 S Andrews Avenue   954-357-7555
Fort Lauderdale, FL 33301-1830   Fax: 954-577-20
e-mail: talkingbooks@browardlibrary.org
www.broward.org/library/talkingbooks
Reference materials on blindness and other handicaps, closed-circuit TV, Talking Book cassettes, print/Braille and descriptive videos.
William Forbes, Librarian

9438 Florida Bureau of Braille and Talking Book Library Services
421 Platt Street   386-239-6000
Daytona Beach, FL 32114-2803   800-226-6075
Fax: 386-239-6069
e-mail: mike.gunde@dbs.fldoe.org
dbs.myflorida.com/library/index.php
The Florida Bureau of Braille and Talking Book Library Services provides information and reading materials needed by Florida residents who are unable to use standard print as the result of visual, physical, or reading disabilities.
Michael Gunde, Librarian

9439 Hillsborough County Talking Book Library
Jan Kaminis Platt Regional Library
900 N ashley drive   813-273-3652
Tampa, FL 33602-1214   TTY: 813-273-3610
TDD: 813-273-3610
e-mail: talkingbooks@hillsboroughounty.org
www.hcplc.org
This free program provides recorded and braille books and magazines to people who are blind, visually impaired or physically handicapped.
Ann Palmer, Librarian
Ann Palmer, Librarian

9440 Jacksonville Public Library
303 North Laura Street
Jacksonville, FL 32202
904-630-2665
http://jpl.coj.net
Discs, cassettes, reference materials on blindness and other handicaps and children's books on cassettes.
Dr Brenda Simmons Hutchins, Chairperson
Erin Skinner, Vice Chair

9441 Lee County Talking Books Library
13240 North Cleveland Avenue, #5-6   239-995-2665
North Ft. Myers, FL 33903-4855   800-854-8195
Fax: 239-995-1681
TDD: 2399952665
e-mail: talkingbooks@leegov.com
www.lee-county.com/library
Talking Books are books and magazines that are recorded for people who need to hear their reading. The books are played on special players provided free by the National Library Service for the Blind and Physically Handicapped.
Sheldon Kaye, Librarian

9442 Miami Dade Talking Book Library
Miami Dade Public Library System

101 W flagler street
Miami, FL 33130

305- 37- 266
800-451-9544
Fax: 305-757-8401
TDD: 305-474-7258
e-mail: talkingbooks@mdpls.org
www.mdpls.org

The Talking Books Library loans books and magazines on cassette tapes or in Braille FREE by mail to persons who have difficulty seeing or using standard small print.
Raymond Santiago, Director
Barbara Moyer, Librarian

9443 Orange County Library System: Orlando Public Library
101 E Central Boulevard
Orlando, FL 32801-2462

407-835-7323
Fax: 407-425-6779
www.ocls.info

The library's collection consists of a wide variety of print materials, including fiction, nonfiction, world languages, genealogy, and special materials that comprise the Florida and Disney collections. The library also has audiovisual materials and electronic resources to meet customer needs.
Mary Anne Hodel, Library Director/CEO

9444 Palm Beach County Library Annex: Talking Books
Mil-Lake Plaza
3650 Summit Blvd.
West Palm Beach,, FL 33406

561-233-2600
888-780-5151
Fax: 561-233-2627
e-mail: talkingbooks@pbclibrary.org
www.pbclibrary.org

The Talking Books Library is a special service of the Palm Beach County Library and a part of the Library of Congress National Library Service for the Blind and Physically Handicapped.
Pat Mistretta, Librarian

9445 Pinellas Talking Book Library for the Blind and Physically Handicapped
1330 Cleveland Street
Clearwater, FL 33755-5103

727-441-9958
86- 6-9 95
Fax: 727-441-9068
TDD: 727-441-3168
www.pplc.us/tbl/

The Pinellas Talking Book Library's mission is to encourage and support reading by providing free library services to Pinellas County residents for whom conventional print is a barrier. The Pinellas Talking Book Library is part of a nationwide network of cooperating libraries serving people who have difficulty using or reading regular print.
Marilyn Stevenson, Access Services Librarian

9446 Sub Regional Talking Book Library
1755 Edgewood Avenue West
Jacksonville, FL 32208-7206

904-765-5588
Fax: 904-768-7822
TDD: 904-768-7822
e-mail: jerryco@j.net

Susan V Arthur, Librarian
Laurie Baumgardner, Librarian

9447 West Florida Public Library: Talking Book Library
239 North Spring Street
Pensacola, FL 32502-4822

850-436-5060
Fax: 850-436-5039
e-mail: talkingbooks@ci.pensacola.fl.us
www.cityofpensacola.com/library

As a subregional Talking Book Library, the Pensacola Public Library offers free service by mail to blind and physically handicapped adults and children who have difficulty reading ordinary print or holding or turning the pages of a book.
Rodney L Kendig, Chairman
Dr. Rebecca Temple, Vice Chairman

Georgia

9448 Albany Library for the Blind and Physically Handicapped
Dougherty County Public Library
1180 Washington Avenue
Macon, GA 31201

478-744-0840
800-805-7613
Fax: 478-744-0840
e-mail: lbph@docolib.org
www.docolib.org/libblind.html

The Library for the Blind and Physically Handicapped provides resources to individuals who are blind, visually impaired, physically handicapped or learning disabled in a thirteen-county area.
Kathryn Sinquefield, Librarian

9449 Atlanta Metro Subregional Library
1800 Century Place
Atlanta, GA 30345

404-235-7200
800-248-6701
Fax: 404-756-4618
e-mail: glass@georgialibraries.org
www.georgialibraries.org/public.glass

Through Georgia's Regional Library for the Blind and Physically Handicapped and cooperating local libraries, Georgians have access to a free national library program that offers books and magazines on cassette tape and in Braille.
Linda B Stetson, Director

9450 Augusta Regional Library Talking Book Center
425 James Brown Boulevard
Augusta, GA 30901

706-821-2625
Fax: 706-724-5403
e-mail: talkbook@ecgrl.org
www.ecgrl.public.lib.ga.ua/lbph.htm

Through the Georgia Library for Accessible Services, Georgians have access to a free national library program that offers books and magazines on cassette tape and in Braille.
Gary Swint, Librarian

9451 Bainbridge Subregional Library for the Blind and Physically Handicapped
Southwest Georgia Regional Library
301 South Monroe Street
Bainbridge, GA 39819-4029

229-248-2680
800-795-2680
Fax: 229-248-2670
TDD: 229-248-2665
e-mail: lbph@swgrl.org
www.swgrl.org

The library houses a large collection of recorded materials as well as reference materials.
Susan S. Whittle, Director

9452 Columbus Library for Accessible Services (CLASS)
The Columbus Public Library
3000 Macon Road
Columbus, GA 31906-2201

706-243-2686
800-652-0782
Fax: 706-243-2710
e-mail: sbarnes@cvrls.net
www.thecolumbuslibrary.org

CLASS serves as one of the Georgia subregional distribution centers for books and magazines on audiocassettes published by the National Library Service for the Blind and Physically Handicapped.
Suzanne Barnes, Librarian

9453 Georgia Library for Accessible Services (GLASS)
1800 Century Place
Atlanta, GA 30345-3803

404-235-7200
800-248-6701
Fax: 404-756-4618
e-mail: glass@georgialibraries.org
www.georgialibraries.org

Georgians have access to a free national library program that offers books and magazines on cassette tape and in Braille. These materials are provided by the Library of Congress, National Library Service for the Blind & Physically Handicapped (NLS),), to eligible persons with a visual or physical disability. All reading material and playback equipment is sent to borrowers and returned by postage-free mail.
Linda B Stetson, Director

9454 Hall County Library System: East Hall Branch and Special Needs Library
2434 Old Cornelia Highway
Gainesville, GA 30507

770-532-3311
Fax: 770-531-2502
TDD: 770-531-2530
e-mail: kevans@hallcountylibrary.org
www.hallcountylibrary.org/ehmap.htm

The East Hall Branch and Special Needs Library goal is to provide excellent service to those with disabilities including the blind, handicapped, mobility impaired and deaf.
Kathy Evans, Branch Manager

9455 Middle Georgia Subregional Library for the Blind and Physically Handicapped
Washington Memorial Library
1180 Washington Avenue 478-744-0877
Macon, GA 31201-1790 800-805-7613
Fax: 478-744-0840
e-mail: mgrltbc2@bibblib.org
www.co.bibb.ga.us/library/TBC.htm
Books, magazines, newspapers, radio programs and various publications are available. Assistive technology equipment is also available at the library.
Thomas Jones, Director
Karen Monroe, Finance Officer

9456 Oconee Regional Library for the Blind and Physically Handicapped
801 Bellevue Avenue 478-275-5382
Dublin, GA 31040 800-453-5541
Fax: 478-275-3821
e-mail: wdaniel@ocrl.org
www.laurens.public.lib.ga.us
Through the Georgia Library for Accessible Services and cooperating local libraries, Georgians have access to a free national library program which offers braille and recorded materials.
Wanda Daniel, Librarian

9457 Rome Subregional Library for People with Disabilities
205 Riverside Parkway NE 706-236-4618
Rome, GA 30161-2911 888-263-0769
Fax: 706-236-4631
TDD: 706-236-4618
e-mail: dhickman@rome-lpd.org
www.rome-lpd.org
Provides free library service to the disabled in eleven counties of Northwest Georgia.
Delana Hickman, Coordinator

9458 Special Needs Library of Northeast Georgia
Athens-Clarke County Regional Library
2025 Baxter Street 706-613-3655
Athens, GA 30606-6331 800-531-2063
Fax: 706-613-3660
TDD: 706-613-3655
e-mail: specialneedslibrary@athenslibrary.org
www.clarke.public.lib.ga.us/specneeds
The Special Needs Library of Northeast Georgia provides free library services for patrons with visual, physical, and reading disabilities.
Claudia L. Markov, Librarian

9459 Subregional Library for the Blind and Physically Handicapped
Live Oak Public Libraries, Thunderbolt Branch
2002 Bull Street 912-652-3600
Savannah, GA 31401 800-342-4455
Fax: 912-354-5534
e-mail: stokesl@liveoakpl.org
www.liveoakpl.org
Library for the blind and physically handicapped.
LaTrelle Mobley, Manager

9460 Three Rivers Regional Library
Brunswick-Glynn County Regional Library
208 Gloucester Street 912-267-1212
Brunswick, GA 31520-5324 866-833-2878
Fax: 912-267-9597
e-mail: bransom@trrl.org
www.threerriverslibraries.org
The Talking Book Center serves 12 counties with over 1200 patrons. The center provides talking books which are recorded at a slower speed which requires the use of a special player.
Betty D. Ransom, Librarian

9461 Valdosta Talking Book Library
South Georgia Regional Library
300 Woodrow Wilson Drive 229-333-0086
Valdosta, GA 31602-2592 800-246-6515
Fax: 229-333-7669
e-mail: djernigan@sgrl.org
www.sgrl.org

The Talking Book Center is available to blind persons with visual difficulty or physical handicaps which prevent them from using printed material.
Diane Jernigan, Librarian

9462 Hawaii State Library for the Blind and Physically Handicapped
402 Kapahulu Avenue 808-733-8444
Honolulu, HI 96815 800-559-4096
Fax: 808-733-8449
TDD: 808-733-8444
e-mail: olbcirc@librarieshawaii.org
www.librarieshawaii.org
The Library for the Blind and Physically Handicapped serves as the regional library and machine lending agency for the blind and physically disabled throughout the state and the outlying Pacific Islands in cooperation with the Library of Congress and the National Library Service for the Blind and Physically Handicapped.
Fusako Miyashiro, Librarian

9463 Idaho Commission for Libraries Talking Book Service
325 West State Street 208-334-2150
Boise, ID 83702-6072 800-458-3271
Fax: 208-334-4016
TDD: 800-377-1363
e-mail: talkingbooks@libraries.idaho.gov
http://libraries.idaho.gov/tbs
The Idaho Talking Book Service provides books and magazines in cassette format for individuals who are unable to read standard print.
Sue Walker, Librarian

9464 Catholic Guild for the Blind
65 E. Wacker Place 312-236-8569
Chicago, IL 60601 Fax: 312-236-8128
e-mail: info@guildfortheblind.org
www.second-sense.org
The Guild's adult rehabilitation services include a program geared towards seniors experiencing new vision loss called New Visions. This program promotes independence within the home and community by providing participants with the information, techniques, and tools they need to successfully adjust to their new lives with impaired sight. Two workshop series are available to beginners or to those ready for more advanced topics.
David J Tabak, Executive Director
Polly Abbott, Manager Adult Rehabilitation Services

9465 Illinois State Library Talking Book and Braille Service
401 East Washington 217-782-9435
Springfield, IL 62701-1207 800-665-5576
Fax: 217-558-4723
TDD: 888-261-7863
The Illinois State Library Talking Book and Braille Service plays a supporting rols for the Illinois Network of Libraries Serving the Blind and Physically Handicapped.

9466 Mid-Illinois Talking Book Center
125 Tower Drive 217-224-6619
Burr Ridge, IL 60527 800-426-0709
Fax: 217-224-9818
e-mail: info@illinoistalkingbooks.org
www.illinoistalkingbooks.org
We provide free library service for anyone unable to read regular print because of low vision, blindness, or a physical disability. We provide recorded and Braille books and popular magazines. There are over 60,000 titles available including popular fiction and non-fiction, bestsellers, classics, history, biographies, children's books and more.
Karen Bershe, Director
Valerie Brandon, PR/Outreach Coordinator

9467 Shawnee Library System: Southern Illinois Talking Book Center
607 South Greenbriar Road
Carterville, IL 62918
618-985-8375
800-445-2665
Fax: 618-985-4211
TDD: 618-985-8375
e-mail: imsastaff@imsa.lib.il.us
www.imsa.lib.il.us/

The Talking Book Program is a free library service for anyone who has difficulty reading print or holding books and turning pages due to any visual or physical limitation or medically diagnosed reading disability. Participants are loaned cassette players along with unabridged books and magazines on tape and in Braille.
Diana Brawley Sussman, Director/Librarian

9468 Skokie Accessible Library Services
Skokie Public Library
5215 Oakton Street
Skokie, IL 60077-3634
847-673-7774
Fax: 847-673-7797
e-mail: anthe@skokie.library.info
www.skokie.lib.il.us

Library services for people with disabilities, including electronic aids, materials in special formats, programs and special services, and access to the North Suburban Library System.
Carolyn A Anthony, Director

9469 Voices of Vision Talking Book Center
125 Tower Drive
Burr Ridge, IL 60527
630-208-0398
800-426-0709
Fax: 630-208-0399
e-mail: info@illinoistalkingbooks.org
www.illinoistalkingbooks.org.

Voices of Vision is part of a statewide and national network of libraries which provide the talking book and braille service. We provide free library service to persons unable to read or use conventional print material due to a visual or physical disability. There is no cost to eligible readers.
Karen Odean, Director

Indiana

9470 Bartholomew County Public Library
National Library Services
536 Fifth Street
Columbus, IN 47201
812-379-1255
800-685-0524
Fax: 812-791-75
e-mail: talkingbooks@barth.lib.in.us
www.barth.lib.in.us

Talking Books for the Blind and Physically Handicapped is a free library service for visually or physically challenged persons of all ages. Anyone who is unable to use regular printed materials as the result of a temporary or permanent visual or physical limitation is eligible.
Sharon Thompson, Librarian

9471 Evansville-Vanderburgh County Public Library
200 SE Martin Luther King Jr Blvd
Evansville, IN 47713
812-428-8200
Fax: 812-428-8397
www.evpl.org

The Evansville-Vanderburgh County Public Library, an essential provider of shared information and a core community service, promotes reading, lifelong learning, and economic vitality through its resources, services and programs to the residents of Vanderburgh County.
Mike Russ, President
Brenda Schiedler, Vice President

9472 Indiana Talking Book & Braille Library
315 West Ohio Street
Indianapolis, IN 46202
317-232-3697
800-622-4970
e-mail: lbph@statelib.lib.in.us
www.in.gov/library/tbbl.htm

The TBBL provides large print books, braille books, and books on tape to Indiana residents who are unable to read regular print.
Roberta L Brooker, Interim Director

9473 Lake County Public Library
1919 W 81st Street
Merrillville, IN 46410
219-769-3541
Fax: 219-769-0690
www.lcplin.org/

Talking books provides cassette books, descriptive videos, magazines and large print books to people who are blind and physically handicapped. Materials are sent through the mail and the service is free to those who qualify.
Renee Lewis, Director

Iowa

9474 Iowa Department for the Blind
524 Fourth Street
Des Moines, IA 50309-2364
515-281-1333
800-362-2587
Fax: 515-281-1263
TTY: 515-281-1355
e-mail: information@blind.state.ia.us
www.blind.state.ia.us/?

Our program offers the specialized, integrated services that blind and severely visually impaired Iowans need to live independently and work competitively.
Allen Harris, Director

Kansas

9475 CKLS Headquarters
1409 Williams Street
Great Bend, KS 67530-4090
620-792-4865
800-362-2642
Fax: 620-793-7270
e-mail: jswan@ckls.org
www.ckls.org

Offers direct services to rural residents and those who need special services because of disability.
Chris Rippel, Department Head Continuing Education
Kathy Rippel, Department Head

9476 Manhattan Subregional Library of the Kansas Talking Books Service
629 Poyntz Avenue
Manhattan, KS 66502-6006
785-776-4741
800-432-2796
Fax: 785-776-1545
e-mail: annp@manhattan.lib.ks.us
www.manhattan.lib.ks.us

Books and magazines in braille and recorded format and playback equipment are provided to any Kansas citizen residing in the twelve county area of the North Central Kansas Libraries System who is unable to use standard print as a result of temporary or permanent visual or physical impairments.
Ann Pearce, Department Manager
Wandean Rivers, Assistive Technology Center Instructor

9477 Northwest Kansas Library System
Northwest Kansas Library System
2 Washington Square
Norton, KS 67654
785-877-5148
800-432-2858
Fax: 785-877-5697
www.nwkls.mykansaslibrary.org/

The Kansas Library Network for the Blind and Physically Handicapped, in cooperation with the Library of Congress, National Library Service for the Blind and Physically Handicapped, provides library services and materials to Kansans unable to use conventional print.
Leslie Bell, Director
Clarice Howard, BPH Librarian

9478 South Central Kansas Library System
321A North Main Street
South Hutchinson, KS 67505
620-663-3211
800-234-0529
Fax: 313-663-9797
e-mail: phawkins@sckls.info
www.sckls.info/

Summer reading programs, braille writer, magnifiers, closed-circuit TV, large-print photocopier, cassette books and magazines, children's books on cassette, home visits and other reference materials on blindness and other handicaps.
Paul Hawkins, Director
Tram Nguyen, Technology Services Coordinator

9479 Talking Books Service
Topeka and Shawnee County Public Library

1515 SW 10th Avenue

Topeka, KS 66604-1304

785-580-4530
800-432-2925
Fax: 785-580-4530
e-mail: tbooks@tscpl.lib.ks.us
www.tscpl.org/services/talkingbooks

Summer reading programs, braille writer, magnifiers, closed-circuit TV, large-print photocopier, cassette books and magazines, children's books on cassette, home visits and other reference materials on blindness and other handicaps.

Suzanne Bundy, Librarian

9480 Wichita Public Library

223 S Main

Wichita, KS 67202

316-261-8500
Fax: 316-262-4540
TDD: 316-262-3972
e-mail: admin@wichita.lib.ks.us
www.wichita.lib.ks.us

Talking books provides cassette books, descriptive videos, magazines adn large print books to people who are blind and physically handicapped. Materials are sent through the mail and the service is free to those who qualify.

Brad Reha, Talking Books Manager

Kentucky

9481 Kentucky Talking Book Library

PO Box 537

Frankfort, KY 40602-0537

502-564-8300
800-372-2968
Fax: 502-564-5773
e-mail: katherine.kimball@ky.gov
www.kdla.ky.gov

Our mission is to provide library service to individuals who have a visual or physical disability that prevents them from using standard print materials. We send books on tape and Braille books through the mail at no cost to our patrons.

Katherine K. Adelberg, E-Rate Coordinator,Field Services
Jackie Arnold, Local Records Regional Administrator

9482 Louisville Talking Book Library for the Blind and Physically Handicapped

301 York Street

Louisville, KY 40203-2205

502-574-1611
www.lfpl.org/tbl

The Louisville Talking Book Library offers recorded books and other materials to eligible visually and physically handicapped Jefferson County, KY residents. All recorded books & equipment may be sent to borrowers and returned by postage-free mail.

Linda Atzinger, Supervisor Accessibility Services

9483 Northern Kentucky Talking Book Library

502 Scott Boulevard

Covington, KY 41011

859-962-4095
866-491-7610
Fax: 859-962-4096
www.kenton.lib.ky.us

Our library provides books and magazines on specially recorded cassettes for people who are visually impaired and/or physically handicapped and live in Boone, Campbell, Carroll, Gallatin, Grant, Kenton, Owen and Pendleton counties.

Dave Schroeder, Director

Louisiana

9484 State Library of Louisiana

701 N 4th Street

Baton Rouge, LA 70802

225-342-4913
Fax: 225-219-4804
e-mail: admin@state.lib.la.us
www.state.lib.la.us

Talking books provides cassette books, descriptive videos, magazines and large print books to people who are blind and physically handicapped. Materials are sent through the mail and the service is free to those who qualify.

Maine

9485 Bangor Public Library

145 Harlow Street

Bangor, ME 04401-4900

207-947-8336
Fax: 207-945-6694
e-mail: bplill@bpl.lib.me.us
www.bpl.lib.me.us

Summer reading programs, braille writer, magnifiers, closed-circuit TV, large-print photocopier, cassette books and magazines, children's books on cassette, home visits and other reference materials on blindness and other handicaps.

Barbara McDade, Director

9486 Cary Library

107 Main Street

Houlton, ME 04730-2196

207-532-1302
Fax: 207-532-4350
www.cary.lib.me.us

Summer reading programs, braille writer, magnifiers, closed-circuit TV, large-print photocopier, cassette books and magazines, children's books on cassette, home visits and other reference materials on blindness and other handicaps.

Linda Faucher, Librarian

9487 Lewiston Public Library

200 Lisbon Street

Lewiston, ME 04240-7203

207-513-3004
Fax: 207-784-3011
TTY: 207-784-3123
e-mail: lplweb@lplonline.org
www.lplonline.org

Summer reading programs, braille writer, magnifiers, closed-circuit TV, large-print photocopier, cassette books and magazines, children's books on cassette, home visits and other reference materials on blindness and other handicaps.

Rick Speer, Director
Jake Paris, Adult Services Librarian

9488 Maine State Library

64 State House Station

Augusta, ME 04333-0064

207-287-5650
800-452-8793
Fax: 207-287-5624
www.state.me.us/msl

Large Print Books is a service through Outreach Services for residents of Maine who are certified as visually impaired and public libraries who serve the visually impaired.

Chris Boynton, Outreach/Special Services Coordinator
Alan Fecteau, Media Coordinator

9489 Portland Public Library

5 Monument Square

Portland, ME 04101-4072

207-871-1700
Fax: 207-871-1715
e-mail: reference@portland.lib.me.us
www.portlandlibrary.com

Portland Public Library's Outreach Services brings library resources to those who are unable to visit the library in person. For people living in nursing homes or assisted living facilities, or for those confined to home due to illness or disability, the library will deliver print and audio books right to your doorstep.

Stephen J Podgajny, Director

9490 Waterville Public Library

73 Elm Street

Waterville, ME 04901-6027

207-872-5433
Fax: 207-873-4779
www.watervillelibrary.org

Summer reading programs, braille writer, magnifiers, closed-circuit TV, large-print photocopier, cassette books and magazines, children's books on cassette, home visits and other reference materials on blindness and other handicaps.

Sarah Sugden, Director

Maryland

9491 American Action Fund for Blind Children and Adults

1800 Johnson Street, Suite 100

Baltimore, MD 21230

410-659-9315
e-mail: actionfund@actionfund.org
www.actionfund.org

Our mission is to assist blind persons in securing reading matter, to educate the public about blindness, to give aid to the deaf-blind, to provide specialized aids and appliances to the blind, to give consultation to governmental and private agencies serving the blind, to offer assistance to older blind persons, to offer services to blind children and their parents, and to do any other lawful thing which it can to improve the quality of life for blind persons.

Barbara Loos, President
Ramona Walhof, First Vice President

9492 Disability Resource Center of Montgomery County Public Libraries
Rockville Library
21 Maryland Avenue   240-777-0311
Rockville, MD 20850   TTY: 240-773-3556
e-mail: county.council@montgomerycountymd.gov
www.montgomerycountymd.gov
The Disability Resource Center (DRC) is the focal point within the Montgomery County Public Libraries (MCPL) for library and literacy services to people with disabilities, their families, caretakers and professionals.
Kay Bowman, Agency Manager

9493 International Braille and Technology Center for the Blind
National Federation of the Blind
1026 East 36th Street   410-645-0632
Baltimore, MD 21218-4998   Fax: 410-685-5653
e-mail: melissa@riccobono.us
www.nfb.org
A comprehensive and complete evaluation and demonstration center for assistive technology used by the blind worldwide. Includes all Braille, synthetic speech, print-to-speech scanning, internet and portable devices and programs. Available for tours by appointment to blind persons, employers, technology manufacturers, teachers, parents and those working in the assistive technology field.
Melissa Riccobono, President

9494 Maryland State Library for the Blind and Physically Handicapped
415 Park Avenue   410-230-2424
Baltimore, MD 21201   800-964-9209
Fax: 410-333-2095
TTY: 800-934-2541
www.lbph.lib.md/us
The basic mission of the Maryland State Library for the Blind and Physically Handicapped is to provide comprehensive library services to the eligible blind and physically handicapped residents of the State of Maryland.
Jill Lewis, Director

9495 Prince George's County Memorial Library: Talking Book Center
6532 Adelphi Road   301-699-3500
Hyattsville, MD 20782-2098   TTY: 301-808-2061
e-mail: kathleen.teaze@pgcmls.info
www.prge.lib.md.us
Talking books provides cassette books, descriptive videos, magazines and large print books to people who are blind and physically handicapped. Materials are sent through the mail and the services are free to those who qualify.
Kathleen Teaze, Director

Massachusetts

9496 Caption Center
125 Western Avenue   617-492-9225
Allston, MA 02134-1008   Fax: 617-562-0590
Provides closed captioning for videos, including training, safety, instructional and educational films. Maintains a consumer information service for overcoming communications barriers in the workplace.
Lori Kay, Co-Director
Tom Apone, Co-Director

9497 Laboure College Library
2120 Dorchester Avenue   617-296-8300
Boston, MA 02124-5617   e-mail: library@laboure.edu
www.laboure.edu
Offers information on physical disabilities, independent living, peer counseling and advocacy.
Maryann O'Toole, Director

9498 Perkins Braille and Talking Book Library
175 N Beacon Street   617-924-3434
Watertown, MA 02472-2751   800-852-3133
Fax: 617-972-7315
TTY: 617-972-7690
e-mail: Info@Perkins.org
www.perkins.org

The Perkins Braille & Talking Book Library, funded in part by the Massachusetts Board of Library Commissioners, provides free services to Massachusetts residents of any age who are unable to read traditional print materials due to a visual or physical disability.
Kim Charlson, Director

9499 Talking Book Library at Worcester Public Library
3 Salem Square   508-799-1655
Worcester, MA 1608-2074   800-762-0085
Fax: 508-799-1676
e-mail: talkbook@cwmars.org/talkingbook
www.cwmars.org/talkingbook
Adapted computers, braille embosser, magnifiers, closed circuit TV, large print books, cassette books and magazines, children's books on cassette, reference materials on blindness and other disabilities. Summer reading programs.
James L Izatt, Librarian

Michigan

9500 Detroit Subregional Library for the Blind and Physically Handicapped
Detroit Public Library
3666 Grand River Avenue   313-833-5494
Detroit, MI 48208   Fax: 313-325-97
TDD: 313-833-5492
e-mail: dmiddle@detroitpubliclibrary.org
www.detroit.lib.mi.us
Talking books along with talking book machines are available to eligible residents who live in a 14 ZIP code area of Detroit and Highland Park. Loans of the books and machines are made to individuals and to institutions such as schools, nursing homes and senior residences. Over 45,000 books are available. Magazines available in recorded format include Ebony, Good Housekeeping, and Sports Illustrated.
Dori V. Middleton, LBPH Specialist

9501 Grand Traverse Area Library for the Blind and Physically Handicapped
322 6th Street   616-935-6520
Traverse City, MI 49684-2414   Fax: 616-922-0904
TDD: 616-922-0901

Evelyn Welty

9502 Kent County Library for the Blind
775 Ball Avenue NE   616-336-3250
Grand Rapids, MI 49503-1397   Fax: 616-336-3256
e-mail: kdlem@lakeland.lib.mi.us
Summer reading programs, braille writer, magnifiers, closed-circuit TV, large-print photocopier, cassette books and magazines, children's books on cassette, home visits and other reference materials on blindness and other handicaps.
Claudya Muller, Librarian

9503 Library of Michigan Service for the Blind
PO Box 30007   517-373-5614
Lansing, MI 48909-7507   Fax: 517-735-65
e-mail: sbph@michigan.gov
www.michigan.gov/sbth
Braille writer, magnifiers, closed circuit TV, large print photocopier, cassette books and magazines, children's books on cassette, reference materials on blindness and other handicaps. Books on cassette and braille books and cassette players will be loaned and sent through the mail at no charge. For blind and those physically unable to read standard print or turn the pages.
Susan Thinault, Manager

9504 Macomb Library for the Blind and Physically Handicapped
35891 South Gratiot   586-226-5072
Clinton Township, MI 48035-1132   Fax: 810-286-0634
TDD: 8102869940
e-mail: macbld@libcoop.net
www.cmpl.org/MLBPH/?
Summer reading programs, braille writer, closed-circuit TV, cassette books and magazines, children's books on cassette, reference materials on blindness and other handicaps.
Beverlee Babcock, Librarian

9505 Midwestern Michigan Library Cooperative
G4195 West Pasadena Avenue
Flint, MI 48504
810-732-1120
Fax: 810-321-15
www.mideasteRN.lib.mi.us
Roger Mendell, Director

9506 Muskegon County Library for the Blind
635 Ottawa Street
Muskegon, MI 49442-1016
616-724-6248
Fax: 616-724-6675
TDD: 616-722-4103
Summer reading programs, braille typewriter, magnifiers, closed-circuit TV, large-print photocopier, cassette books and magazines, children's books on cassette, home visits and other reference materials on blindness and other handicaps, The Reading Edge, Perkins Brailler and large print books.
Linda Clapp, Librarian

9507 Northland Library Cooperative
220 W. Clinton St.
Charlevoix, MI 49720-2892
231-855-2206
Fax: 517-354-3939
e-mail: webmaster@nlc.lib.mi.us
www.nlc.lib.mi.us/
Summer reading programs, braille writer, magnifiers, closed-circuit TV, large-print photocopier, cassette books and magazines, children's books on cassette, home visits and other reference materials on blindness and other handicaps.
Catherine Glomski, Librarian

9508 Oakland County Library for the Visually and Physically Impaired
1200 N Telegraph Road
Pontiac, MI 48341-1032
248-858-5050
800-774-4542
Fax: 248-858-9313
e-mail: lVPi@co.oakland..mi.us
www.co.oakland.mi.us/lVPi
Free cassette book service to eligible visually or physically impaired Oakland County residents; demonstrations, CCTV and hand held magnifiers and a large print collection.
David Conklin, Head Librarian

9509 St. Clark County Library for the Blind and Physically Handicapped
210 McMorran Boulevard
Port Huron, MI 48060-4014
810-982-3600
800-272-8570
Fax: 810-987-7327
e-mail: lbph@sccl.lib.mi.us
www.sccl.lib.mi.us/LBPH.aspx
Offers library services to the blind and visually impaired.
Jackie Skinner, Librarian

9510 Upper Peninsula Library for the Blind and Physically Handicapped
1615 Presque Isle Avenue
Marquette, MI 49855-2811
906-228-7697
Fax: 906-285-27
e-mail: uproc.lib.mi.us
www.michigan.gov/sbth
Summer reading programs, braille writer, magnifiers, closed-circuit TV, large-print photocopier, cassette books and magazines, children's books on cassette, home visits and other reference materials on blindness and other handicaps.
Susan Thinault, Manager

9511 Washtenaw County Library for the Blind and Physically Disabled
PO Box 8645
Ann Arbor, MI 48107-8645
734-971-6059
Fax: 734-971-3892
e-mail: lbpd@co.washtennaw.mi.us
comnet.org/cgi-bin/helpnet/viewitem?290+
Book lovers club.adaptive technology,cassette equipment, cassette books and magazines, described videos, low vision aids reference and referral services.
Margaret Wolfe, Cordinator

9512 Wayne County Regional Library for the Blind and Physically Handicapped
41365 Vincenti Court
Novi, MI 48375-5310
248-536-3100
888-968-2737
Fax: 248-536-3098
TDD: 313-326-3008
e-mail: werlbph@tln.lib.mi.us
www.tln.lib.mi.us
Summer reading programs, braille writer, magnifiers, closed-circuit TV, large-print photocopier, cassette books and magazines, children's books on cassette, home visits and other reference materials on blindness and other handicaps.
Pat Klemans, Librarian

Minnesota

9513 Duluth Public Library
City of Duluth Department
520 W Superior Street
Duluth, MN 55802-1578
218-730-4200
Fax: 218-233-15
e-mail: webmail@duluthmn.gov
www.duluth.lib.mn.us
Adapted access to Apple computer, adapted toys and adapted library equipment.
Randall Deth Kelly, Director

9514 Minnesota Library for the Blind
1500 Highway 36 West
Roseville, MN 55113
507-333-4828
800-722-0550
Fax: 507-333-4832
e-mail: mn.lbph@state.mn.us
www.education.state.mn.us
Summer reading programs, braille writer, magnifiers, closed-circuit TV, large-print photocopier, cassette books and magazines, children's books on cassette, home visits and other reference materials on blindness and other handicaps.
Catherine Durivage, Director

Mississippi

9515 Christian Resource for People Who Are Blind
Care Ministries Inc
PO Box 1830
Starkville, MS 39760-1830
662-323-4999
800-366-2232
e-mail: careministries@bellsouth.net
www.careministries.org
Offers braille and large print books and cassettes for the visually impaired.
B J LeJeune, Director

9516 Mississippi Library Commission
3881 Eastwood Drive
Jackson, MS 39211-7328
601-432-4486
800-647-7542
Fax: 601-961-4113
TDD: 601-354-6411
e-mail: mslib@mic.lib.ms.us
www.mlc.lib.ms.us
Summer reading programs, braille writer, magnifiers, closed-circuit TV, large-print photocopier, cassette books and magazines, children's books on cassette, home visits and other reference materials on blindness and other handicaps.
Larry Mc Millan, Director

Missouri

9517 Adriene Resource Center for Blind Children
Assembly of God Center for Blind
1445 Boonville Avenue
Springfield, MO 65802
417-862-2781
Fax: 417-625-20
e-mail: info@ag.org
www.blind.ag.org
Offers braille and cassette lending library, braille and cassette Sunday school materials for all ages, braille and cassette periodicals and resource assistance, and resources for blind children and children of blind parents.
Paul Weingariner, Director
Caryl Weingariner, Co-Director

9518 Assemblies of God National Center for the Blind
1445 Boonville Avenue 417-831-1964
Springfield, MO 65802 Fax: 417-627-66
e-mail: blind@ag.org
Offers braille and cassette lending library, braille and cassette Sunday school materials for all ages, braille and cassette periodicals and resource assistance, and resources for blind children and children of blind parents.
Paul Weingariner, Director

9519 Church of the Nazarene
Nazarene Publishing House
PO Box 419527 816-931-1900
Kansas City, MO 64141-6527 800-877-0700
e-mail: NPH@direct.nph.com
www.nph.com
Offers braille and large print books. Also offers a lending library and cassettes for the blind.

9520 Lutheran Library for the Blind
Lutheran Church - Missouri Synod
1333 S Kirkwood Road 314-965-9000
Saint Louis, MO 63122-7295 800-248-1930
Fax: 314-996-1016
e-mail: infocenter@lems.org
www.lcms.org
Offers braille and large print books and cassettes for the blind and visually impaired.

9521 Whitney Library for the Blind: Assemblies of God
1445 N Boonville Avenue 417-862-2781
Springfield, MO 65802-1894 800-641-4310
Fax: 417-862-5881
www.gospelpublishing.com
Offers braille and cassette lending library, braille and cassette Sunday school materials for all ages, braille and cassette periodicals and resource assistance.
Paul Weingariner, Librarian

9522 Wolfner Memorial Library for the Blind
PO Box 387 573-751-8720
Jefferson City, MO 65102-387 800-392-2614
Fax: 573-526-2985
TDD: 800-347-1379
e-mail: wolfner@sos.mo.gov
www.sos.mo.gov/wolfner
Summer reading programs, braille writer, closed circuit TV, large print photocopier, cassette books and magazines, children's books on cassette, home visits and other reference materials on blindness and other handicaps.
Richard J Smith, Director Wolfner Library
Debbie Musselman, Administrative Program Coordinator

Montana

9523 Montana State Library
1515 E 6th Avenue 406-444-3009
Helena, MT 59620-1800 Fax: 406-444-0266
home.montanastatelibrary.org/?
Summer reading programs, braille writer, magnifiers, closed-circuit TV, large-print photocopier, cassette books and magazines, children's books on cassette, home visits and other reference materials on blindness and other handicaps.
Darlene Staffeldt, Director

Nebraska

9524 Nebraska Library Commission Talking Book and Braille Services
1200 N Street, Suite 120 402-471-4038
Lincoln, NE 68508-2023 800-742-7691
e-mail: nlc.talkingbook@nebraska.gov
www.nlc.nebraska.gov/tbbs
Free loan of books and magazines on flash cartridge, cassette, and in Braille, including children's materials, along with specially designed playback equipment. Summer reading program for children and young adults, Braille embossing, closed circuit TV, large-print copier. Reference materials on blindness and other disabilities.
David Oertli, Director
Kay Goehring, Reader Services Coordinator

9525 North Platte Public Library
120 W 4th Street 308-535-8036
North Platte, NE 69101-3901 Fax: 308-535-8296
e-mail: library@ci.north-platte.ne.us
www.ci.north-platte.ne.us/library
Summer reading programs, braille writer, magnifiers, closed-circuit TV, large-print photocopier, cassette books and magazines, children's books on cassette, home visits and other reference materials on blindness and other handicaps.
Cecelia Lawrence, Library Director

Nevada

9526 Las Vegas Clark County Library District
7060 W. Windmill Lane
Las Vegas, NV 89113-5256 702-734-7323
www.lvccld.org
Summer reading programs, braille writer, magnifiers, closed circuit TV, large-print photocopier, cassette books and magazines, children's books on cassette, home visits and other reference materials on blindness and other handicaps.
Daniel Walters, Executive Directors

9527 Nevada State Library and Archives
100 North Stewart Street 775-684-3360
Carson City, NV 89701-4285 800-922-2880
Fax: 775-684-3330
TDD: 775-687-8338
e-mail: nslref@clan.lib.nv.us
www.nsla.nevadaculture.org
Summer reading programs, braille writer, magnifiers, closed-circuit TV, large-print photocopier, cassette books and magazines, children's books on cassette, home visits and other reference materials on blindness and other handicaps.
Kevin E Putnam, Librarian

New Hampshire

9528 New Hampshire State Library
117 Pleasant Street 603-271-3429
Concord, NH 03301-3852 Fax: 603-271-8370
e-mail: talking@lilac.nhsh.lib.nh.us
www.nh.us
Summer reading programs, braille writer, magnifiers, closed-circuit TV, large-print photocopier, cassette books and magazines, children's books on cassette, home visits and other reference materials on blindness and other handicaps.
Eileen Keim, Librarian

9529 Voices for the Blind
PO Box 781 603-332-9355
Barrington, NH 3825
Tape library and depository for people with visual and learning disabilities. Recording services available by request.
Connie Hindman, Director

New Jersey

9530 New Jersey Library for the Blind and Handicapped
2300 Stuyvesant Avenue 609-530-4000
Trenton, NJ 08618-3226 800-792-8322
Fax: 609-530-6384
TDD: 877-882-5593
e-mail: nglbh@njstatelib.org
www2.njstatelib.org/lbh/index.htm
Summer reading programs, large print, cassette, braille books and magazines, children's books on cassette and brailles and other reference materials on blindness and other handicaps.
Deborah Toomey, Director

New Mexico

9531 New Mexico State Library for the Blind and Physically Handicapped
National Library Services

1209 Camino Carlos Rey
Santa Fe, NM 87507

505-476-9770
800-456-5515
Fax: 505-476-9776
e-mail: lbph@state.nm.us
www.nmstatelibrary.org/lbph?

Summer reading programs, braille writer, magnifiers, closed-circuit TV, large-print photocopier, cassette books and magazines, children's books on cassette, home visits and other reference materials on blindness and other handicaps.
John Mugford, Library Manager

New York

9532 Choice Magazine Listening
85 Channel Drive
Port Washington, NY 11050-2216

516-883-8280
888-724-6423
Fax: 516-944-6849
e-mail: choicemag@aol.com
www.choicemagazinelistening.org

A free recorded spoken word magazine anthology for anyone college level and older unable to read large print because of visual or physical handicaps. Produced on special speed cassette format, playable on free library of congress player.
Sondra Mochson, Editor

9533 JGB Cassette Library International
Jewish Guild for the Blind
15 W 65th Street
New York, NY 10023-6601

212-769-6331
Fax: 212-769-6266
e-mail: bemass@aol.com

Summer reading programs, braille writer, magnifiers, closed-circuit TV, large-print photocopier, cassette books and magazines, children's books on cassette, home visits and other reference materials on blindness and other handicaps.
Bruce Massis

9534 Nassau Library System
900 Jerusalem Avenue
Uniondale, NY 11553-3039

516-292-8920
Fax: 516-481-4777
e-mail: nls@lilrc.org
www.nassaulibrary.org/?

Summer reading programs, braille writer, magnifiers, closed-circuit TV, large-print photocopier, cassette books and magazines, children's books on cassette, home visits and other reference materials on blindness and other handicaps.
Dorothy Pruyear, Librarian

9535 New York State Talking Book & Braille Library, New York State Library, DOE
Empire State Plaza, CEC
Albany, NY 12230-0001

518-474-5935
800-342-3688
Fax: 518-486-2142
e-mail: tbbl@mail.nysed.gov
www.nysl.nysed.gov/tbbl/

Books on audio cassette, cassette players, braille books, summer reading programs, braille writer, magnifiers, closed-circuit TV, large-print photocopier, cassette books and magazines, children's books on cassette, reference materials on blindness and other disabilities. Library is part of the National Service Network serving those with print disabilities. Available: audio and braille books sent post-free by mail, euipment loans, services to schools and institutions. Serves 55 New York counties.
Sharon B. Phillips, Program Director

9536 Suffolk Cooperative Library System
627 N Sunrise Service Road
Bellport, NY 11713-9000

631-286-1600
Fax: 631-286-1647
gateway.suffolklibrarysystem.org

Talking books services.
Julie Klauber, Adjunct Professor

9537 Xavier Society for the Blind
154 E 23rd Street
New York, NY 10010-4501

212-473-7800
800-637-9193
Fax: 212-473-7801
e-mail: info@xaviersocietyfortheblind.org
www.XavierSocietyfortheBlind.org

Provides spiritual and inspirational reading material to visually impaired persons in suitable format: Braille, large print and cassette, throughout the USA and Canada. Services provided by way of regular periodicals which are non-returnable, and through our lending library where books are returned. All services are provided free of charge, and interested persons can write or phone.
Fr. John R. Sheehan, SJ, Chairman
Margie Montenegro, Client Services Representative

North Carolina

9538 North Carolina Library for the Blind
1841 Capital Boulevard
Raleigh, NC 27635

919-733-4376
888-388-2460
Fax: 919-733-6910
TDD: 919-733-1462
e-mail: nclbph@ncdcr.gov
statelibrary.ncdcr.gov/lbph

A general interest library offering books and magazines at no cost in large print, in braille on audio cassette for anyone who cannot use regular print in North Carolina due to physical or visual disability. Summer reading programs, braille writer, magnifiers, closed circuit TV, large print photocopier, cassette books and magazines, children's books on cassette, digital, cartridges and large print and other reference materials.
Carl Keehn, Director

North Dakota

9539 North Dakota State Library Services for the Disabled
North Dakota State Library
604 E Boulevard Avenue
Bismarck, ND 58505-800

701-328-4622
800-843-9948
Fax: 701-328-2040
TDD: 800-892-8622
e-mail: statelib@nd.gov
www.library.nd.gov

Stella Cone, Regional Librarian

9540 Services for the Visually Impaired
8720 Georgia Avenue
Silver, MD 20910

301-589-0894
Fax: 301-589-7281
www.servicesvi.org

Eligible readers of North Dakota receive library service from the regional library in Pierre, South Dakota.
Betty Bender

Ohio

9541 Case Western Reserve University
10900 Euclid Avenue
Cleveland, OH 44117-2620

216-368-2000
www.cwru.edu

Research in electrical stimulation and rehabilitation technology.
Barbara R. Snyder, President
W. A. Bud Baeslack III, Executive Vice President

9542 Ohio Regional Library for the Blind and Physically Handicapped
800 Vine Street
Cincinnati, OH 45202

513-369-6999
800-528-0335
Fax: 513-369-3111
TDD: 513-369-6072
www.cincinatilibrary.org/main/lb.asp

Summer reading programs, braille writer, magnifiers, closed-circuit TV, large-print photocopier, cassette books and magazines, children's books on cassette, home visits and other reference materials on blindness and other handicaps.
Donna Foust, Librarian

9543 State Library of Ohio Talking Book Program
274 E First Avenue
Columbus, OH 43201-3673

614-644-6895
800-686-1531
Fax: 614-995-2186
winslo.state.oh.us/services

A machine-lending agency for the visually impaired.
Roger Verney, Head Supervisor

Oklahoma

9544 Oklahoma Library for the Blind and Physically Handicapped
300 NE 18th Street
Oklahoma City, OK 73105-3212

405-521-3514
Fax: 405-214-82
www.state.ok.us/~library

Summer reading programs, braille writer, magnifiers, closed-circuit TV, large-print photocopier, cassette books and magazines, children's books on cassette, home visits and other reference materials on blindness and other handicaps.
Geraldine Adams, Director

9545 Tulsa City: County Library System
400 Civic Center 918-596-7977
Tulsa, OK 74103-3830 Fax: 918-596-7990
www.tulsalibrary.org
Summer reading programs, braille writer, magnifiers, closed-circuit TV, large-print photocopier, cassette books and magazines, children's books on cassette, home visits and other reference materials on blindness and other handicaps.
Ellen Ontko, Librarian

Oregon

9546 Oregon State Library
250 Winter Street NE 503-378-4243
Salem, OR 97301-3950 800-452-0292
Fax: 503-588-7119
TDD: 503-378-4276
www.oregon.gov/osl
Summer reading programs, braille writer, magnifiers, closed-circuit TV, large-print photocopier, cassette books and magazines, children's books on cassette, home visits and other reference materials on blindness and other handicaps.
Jim Scheppke, Head Librarian

Pennsylvania

9547 Carnegie Library of Pittsburgh
4724 Baum Boulevard 412-687-2440
Pittsburgh, PA 15213-1321 800-242-0586
Fax: 412-687-2442
e-mail: lbph@carneigelibrary.org
www.clpgh.org/clp/LBPH
Provides on loan recorded books and magazines, large print books, and described videos to Western Pennsylvannia residents unable to use standard printed materials due to visual, physical, or physically-based reading disabilities. Also loans special cassette and disc machines; does not loan equipment to play described videos. Information about disabilities and related agencies is also available.
Sue Murdock, Director
Kathleen Kappel, Assistant Director

9548 Free Library of Philadelphia
919 Walnut Street 215-925-3213
Philadelphia, PA 19107-5237 Fax: 215-928-0856
e-mail: flpblind@library.phila.gov
Summer reading programs, braille writer, magnifiers, closed-circuit TV, large-print photocopier, cassette books and magazines, children's books on cassette, home visits and other reference materials on blindness and other handicaps.
Vickie Lange Collins, Librarian

Rhode Island

9549 Rhode Island Department of State Library for the Blind and Physically Handicapped
1 Capitol Hl 401-277-2726
Providence, RI 02908-5803 Fax: 401-277-4195
e-mail: richard@dsl.rhilinet.gov
Offers information and services for the visually impaired including reference materials, braille printers, braille writers, large-print books and more.
Richard Ledue, Librarian

South Carolina

9550 South Carolina State Library
PO Box 11469 803-734-8666
Columbia, SC 29202-0821 Fax: 803-734-8676
TDD: 803-734-7298
e-mail: guynell@leo.scsl.state.sc.us
www.state.sc.us/scsl

Summer reading programs, braille writer, magnifiers, closed-circuit TV, large-print photocopier, cassette books and magazines, children's books on cassette, home visits and other reference materials on blindness and other handicaps.
Guynell Williams, Librarian

South Dakota

9551 South Dakota State Library
800 Governors Drive 605-773-3131
Pierre, SD 57501-2235 Fax: 605-734-50
TDD: 605-773-4950
e-mail: daRN@stlib.state.sd.us
www.sdstatelibrary.com
Summer reading programs, braille writer, magnifiers, closed-circuit TV, large-print photocopier, cassette books and magazines, children's books on cassette, home visits and other reference materials on blindness and other handicaps.
Daniel Boyd, Librarian

Tennessee

9552 LRC for Students with Disabilities
MSU Library Reference Department
Memphis State University 901-678-2208
Memphis, TN 38152-0001 800-669-2267
Fax: 901-678-3070
www.memphis.edu
Information on physical disabilities, blindness and visual impairments.
Ross Johnson, Reference Librarian

9553 Tennessee Library for the Blind and Physically Handicapped
National Library Services
403 7th Avenue N 615-741-3915
Nashville, TN 37243-1409 800-342-3308
Fax: 615-532-8856
e-mail: tlbph@mail.state.tn/sos/statelib/LBPH/
www.state.tn.us
Offers free public library services to those unable to hold, read, or turn the pages of books and magazines due to physical or visual impairment. Collections include books and magazines in large print, braille and audio format. Players loaned for the audio books and magazines. All items are delivered and returned via the US Postal Service free matter mailing.
Ruth Hemphill, Director
Janie Murphee, Assistant Director

Texas

9554 Houston Public Library Access Center
500 McKinney Street 832-393-1313
Houston, TX 77002-2534 Fax: 832-931-83
e-mail: website@hpl.lib.tx.us
www.houstonlibrary.org
Offers Kurzweil Reading Machine 400, closed-circuit TV, braille writer, reference materials on visual impairments and other handicaps.
Heidi Miller, Supervisor

9555 Texas State Library
1201 Brazos Street 512-463-5460
Austin, TX 78711-2927 800-252-9605
Fax: 512-936-0685
TDD: 512-463-5449
e-mail: dale.propp@tsl.state.tx.us
www.tsl.state.tx.us
Summer reading programs, braille writer, magnifiers, closed-circuit TV, large-print photocopier, cassette books and magazines, children's books on cassette, home visits and other reference materials on blindness and other handicaps.
Dale Propp, Librarian

9556 Texas State Library: Talking Book Program
1201 Brazos Street 512-463-5460
Austin, TX 78711-2927 800-252-9605
Fax: 512-936-0685
e-mail: tbp.services@tsl.state.tx.us
www.tsl.state.tx.us

Part of the free National Library Services. Provides equipment and books in alternate formats to qualified individuals who cannot read standard print. Certified applications required. Disabilities and information referral services available.
Ava Smith, Librarian
Dina Abramson, Disabilities/Information Referral

Utah

9557 Utah State Library Division
Program for the Blind and Disabled
250 North 1950 West, Suite A
Salt Lake City, UT 84116-7901

801-715-6789
800-662-5540
Fax: 801-715-6767
TDD: 801-715-6721
e-mail: blind@utah.gov
http://blindlibrary.utah.gov

Library providing services to individuals with visual impairments who cannot read standard print.
Bessie Y. Oakes, Director

Vermont

9558 Vermont Department of Libraries Special Services Unit
109 State Street
montpelier, VT 05609

80- 8-8 32
800-479-1711
Fax: 802-828-2199
e-mail: ssu@mail.dol.state.vt.us
dol.state.vt.us

Summer reading programs, braille writer, magnifiers, closed-circuit TV, large-print photocopier, cassette books and magazines, children's books on cassette, home visits and other reference materials on blindness and other handicaps.
Theresa Faust, Librarian

Virginia

9559 Arlington County Department of Libraries
1015 N Quincy Street
Arlington, VA 22201-4603

703-228-5959
Fax: 703-358-5962
TDD: 703-358-6320
www.library.arlingtonva.us/

Summer reading programs, braille writer, magnifiers, closed-circuit TV, large-print photocopier, cassette books and magazines, children's books on cassette, home visits and other reference materials on blindness and other handicaps.
Roxanne Barnes, Librarian

9560 Central Rappahannock Regional Library
1201 Caroline Street
Fredericksburg, VA 22401-3701

540-372-1144
Fax: 540-373-9411
TDD: 540-371-9165
e-mail: nschiff@hq.crrl.org

Offers reference materials on blindness and other disabilities.
Nancy Schiff, Librarian

9561 Division for the Visually Handicapped
2900 Crystal Drive
Arlington, VA 22202

703-620-3660
888-232-7733
Fax: 703-264-9494
TTY: 866-915-5000
e-mail: service@cec.sped.org
www.cec.sped.org

Members are teachers, college faculty members, administrators, supervisors and others concerned with the education and welfare of visually handicapped and blind children and youth. This is a division of the Council For Exceptional Children.
Stephanie Ineh, Customer Service Manager
Anitra Davis, Senior Customer Services Representative

9562 Fairfax County Public Library
12000 Government Center Parkway
Fairfax, VA 22035-0012

703-660-6943
Fax: 703-765-5893
TDD: 703-660-8524
e-mail: sjapikse@leo.vsla.edu
www.co.fairfax.va.us.

Summer reading programs, braille writer, magnifiers, closed-circuit TV, large-print photocopier, cassette books and magazines, children's books on cassette, home visits and other reference materials on blindness and other handicaps.
Jeanette Studley, Librarian

9563 Hampton Subregional Library for the Blind
4207 Victoria Blvd.
Hampton, VA 23669-4243

75- 7-7 11
Fax: 75- 7-7 11
www.hamptonpubliclibrary.org

Summer reading programs, braille writer, magnifiers, closed-circuit TV, large-print photocopier, cassette books and magazines, children's books on cassette, home visits and other reference materials on blindness and other handicaps.
Douglas Perry, Director

9564 Newport News Public Library System
110 Main Street
Newport News, VA 23601-4105

757-591-4858
Fax: 757-591-7425
e-mail: shalswin@leo.vsla.edu
www.newport-news.va.us

Summer reading programs, braille writer, magnifiers, closed-circuit TV, large-print photocopier, cassette books and magazines, children's books on cassette, home visits and other reference materials on blindness and other handicaps.
Sue Balswin, Librarian

9565 Roanoke City Public Library System
2607 Salem Tpke NW
Roanoke, VA 24017-5333

540-853-2648
Fax: 540-853-1030

Summer reading programs, braille writer, magnifiers, closed-circuit TV, large-print photocopier, cassette books and magazines, children's books on cassette, home visits and other reference materials on blindness and other handicaps.
Rebecca Cooper, Librarian

9566 Staunton Public Library: Talking Book Center
1291 Taylor Street,
Washington, DC 20011-3229

20- 7-7 51
20- 7-7 07
Fax: 540-332-3906
e-mail: talkingbook@ci.staunton.via.us
www.loc.gov/nls

Sub-regional library for those who are unable to use standard print materials due to visual, physical, or reading disability.
Oakley Pearson, Librarian

9567 University Library Services
Virginia Commonwealth University
901 Park Avenue
Richmond, VA 23284-2033

804-828-1105
Fax: 804-828-0150
www.ucu.edu

Library services for the visually disabled.
Sally Jacobs, Reference Librarian

9568 Virginia Beach Public Library
936 Independence Boulevard
Virginia Beach, VA 23455-6006

757-460-7518
Fax: 757-460-6741
e-mail: vb311@vbgov.com
vbgov.com/libraries

Summer reading programs, braille writer, magnifiers, closed-circuit TV, large-print photocopier, cassette books and magazines, children's books on cassette, home visits and other reference materials on blindness and other handicaps.
Susan Head, Librarian

Washington

9569 Washington Talking Book & Braille Library
2021 9th Avenue
Seattle, WA 98121

206-615-0400
Fax: 206-615-0437
TTY: 206-615-0418
e-mail: wtbbl@spl.lib.wa.us
www.wtbbl.org

Summer reading programs, braille writer, magnifiers, closed-circuit TV, large-print photocopier, cassette books and magazines, children's books on cassette, home visits and other reference materials on blindness and other handicaps.
Danielle Miller, Director

9570 Cabell County Public Library
455 9th Street   304-528-5700
Huntington, WV 25701-1417   Fax: 304-285-5701
                                   e-mail: tbooks@cabell.libwv.us
                                             www.cabell.lib.wv.us
Summer reading programs, braille writer, magnifiers, Arkenstone
reader/scanner, cassette books and magazines, children's books on
cassette, home visits and other reference materials on blindness
and other handicaps.
Judy K Ruke, Director
Angela Strait, Assistant Director

9571 Kanawha County Public Library
1900 Kanawha Boulevard E   304-558-2041
Charleston, WV 25305-2609   800-642-9021
                                     Fax: 304-558-2044
                                       kanawha.lib.wv.us
Summer reading programs, braille writer, magnifiers, closed-circuit TV, large-print photocopier, cassette books and magazines,
children's books on cassette, home visits and other reference materials on blindness and other handicaps.
Francis Fesenmainer, Librarian

**9572 Ohio County Public Library Services for the Blind and Physically
Handicapped**
52 16th Street   304-232-0244
Wheeling, WV 26003-3671   Fax: 304-232-6848
                             e-mail: llnicholson@hotmail.com
Lori Nicholson, Subregional Librarian BIPH

9573 Parkersburg and Wood County Public Library
3100 Emerson Avenue   304-420-4587
Parkersburg, WV 26104-2414   800-642-8674
                                       Fax: 304-420-4589
                               e-mail: raitzb@hp9k.park.lib.wv.us
                                           parkersburg.lib.wv.us
Services for the bind and physically handicapped.
Michael Hickman

9574 West Virginia Library Commission
1900 Kanawha Boulevard E   304-558-2041
Charleston, WV 25305-0009   800-642-9021
                                     Fax: 304-558-2044
                             e-mail: web_one@wvlc.lib.wv.us
                                     librarycommission.lib.wv.us
Summer reading programs, braille writer, magnifiers, closed-circuit TV, large-print photocopier, cassette books and magazines,
children's books on cassette, home visits and other reference materials on blindness and other handicaps.
Francis Fesenmainer, Librarian

9575 West Virginia School for the Blind
301 E Main Street   304-822-4800
Romney, WV 26757-1828   Fax: 304-822-3377
                             e-mail: cjohn@access.mountain.net
Summer reading programs, braille writer, magnifiers, closed-circuit TV, large-print photocopier, cassette books and magazines,
children's books on cassette, home visits and other reference materials on blindness and other handicaps.
Cynthia Johnson, Librarian

9576 Brown County Library
P.O box 23600   920-448-4035
Green Bay, WI 54305-5194   Fax: 920-448-4036
                                          www.co.brown.wi.us
Summer reading programs, braille writer, magnifiers, closed-cir-
cuit TV, large-print photocopier, cassette books and magazines,
children's books on cassette, home visits and other reference mate-
rials on blindness and other handicaps.
Moyninhan Jr Patrick, Chair
Lund Thomas, Vice Chair

9577 Wisconsin Regional Library for the Blind Talking Book Program
813 W Wells Street   414-286-3045
Milwaukee, WI 53233-1436   800-242-8822
                                        Fax: 414-286-3102
                                        TDD: 414-286-3548
                                     e-mail: mvalne@mpl.org
                                     www.regionallibrary.wi.gov
Circulates recorded materials, playback equipment and braille ma-
terials to print-handicapped Wisconsin residents.
Marsha Valance, Regional Librarian

9578 Wyoming Services for the Visually Disabled
State Department of Education
2300 Capitol Avenue Hathaway Buildi   307-777-7690
Cheyenne, WY 82002-50   Fax: 307-776-34
                                              www.k12.wy.us
Eligible readers of Wyoming receive library service from the re-
gional library in Salt Lake City, Utah.
Duane Edmonds, Chairman
Ruby Calvert, Vice Chairman

Research Centers

9579 Baylor College of Medicine: Cullen Eye Institute
6565 Fannin   713-798-6100
Houston, TX 77030-2703   800-229-5676
                                        Fax: 713-798-4231
                                     e-mail: ant@bcm.edu
                                          www.bcm.edu/eye
Research activities focus on restoring vision and preventing blind-
ness through a better understanding of the disease.
Dan B Jones, Professor and Chair
Milton Boniuk, Professor

9580 BermanGund Laboratory for the Study of Retinal Degenerations
Massachusetts Eye & Eye Infirmary
243 Charles Street   617-573-3600
Boston, MA 02114-3002   Fax: 617-733-44
                             e-mail: directors@meei.harvard.edu
                     www.masseyeandear.org/research/ophthalmo
The Berman-Gund Laboratory for the Study of Retinal Degenera-
tions of Harvard Medical School continues multidisciplined re-
search on retinitis pigmentosa, Usher syndrome, macular
degeneration, and other related degenerative diseases of the retina.
Eliot L. Berson, M.D.,, Director
Eric A. Pierce, M.D., Ph.D.,, Associate Director

9581 Braille Institute Desert Center
70-251 Ramon Rd   760-321-1111
Rancho Mirage, CA 92270-5203   800-212-4533
                                        Fax: 760-321-9715
                               e-mail: dc@brailleinstitute.org
                                       www.brailleinstitute.org
Dedicated to providing blind and visually impaired men women
and children with the training programs and services they need to
enjoy productive lives. Services offered include child development youth programs library services and adult education.
Leslie E Stocker Jr, President
Sally H Jameson, VP of Programs and Services

9582 Braille Institute Orange County Center
527 N Dale Avenue   714-821-5000
Anaheim, CA 92801-4899   Fax: 714-527-7621
                               e-mail: oc@brailleinstitute.org
                                       www.brailleinstitute.org
Offers services publications information and programs to blind
and visually impaired persons.
Sheila F Daily, Orange County Regional Director
Gene Mathiowetz, Assistant Regional Director

**9583 Braille Institute Santa Barbara Center Braille Institute of Los
Angeles**
Braille Institute of Los Angeles

2031 De La Vina Street 805-682-6222
Santa Barbara, CA 93105-3895 800-272-4553
Fax: 805-687-6141
e-mail: sb@brailleinstitute.org
www.brailleinstitute.org
Offers classes type library services and information for persons
with visual impairments.
Angela Nowlin, Assistant Regional Director
Michael Lazarovits, Santa Barbara Regional Director

9584 Braille Institute Sight Center
741 N Vermont Avenue 323-663-1112
Los Angeles, CA 90029 800-272-4553
Fax: 323-663-0867
e-mail: la@brailleinstitute.org
www.brailleinstitute.org/los_angeles
Offers help programs services and information to the blind and vi-
sually impaired children and adults.
Dr Henry C Chang, Director of Library Services
Anita Wright, Los Angeles Regional Program Director

9585 Braille Institute Youth Center
741 N Vermont Avenue 323-663-1112
Los Angeles, CA 90029-1381 800-272-4553
Fax: 323-663-0867
e-mail: la@brailleinstitute.org
www.brailleinstitute.org/los_angeles
Offers various youth programs and services for the blind and visu-
ally impaired youngster.
Leslie E Stocker Jr, President
Sally H Jameson, Vice President of Programs and Services

9586 Braille Textbook Assignment Service National Braille Association
National Braille Association
95 Allens Creek Road 585-427-8260
Rochester, NY 14618-2537 Fax: 585-427-0263
e-mail: nbaoffice@nationalbraille.org
www.nationalbraille.org
National Braille Association, founded in 1945, is a non-profit organization dedicated to providing continuing education to those
who prepare braille, and to providing braille materials to persons
who are visually impaired.
Jan Carroll, President
David W Shaffer, Executive Director

9587 Carroll Center for the Blind
770 Centre Street 617-969-6200
Newton, MA 02458-2597 800-852-3131
Fax: 617-969-6204
TTY: 617-969-6204
e-mail: info@carroll.org
www.carroll.org
The Carroll Center serves the needs of blind and visually-impaired
persons by providing rehabilitation, skills training, and educational opportunities to achieve independence, self-sufficiency,
and self-fulfillment and by educating the public regarding the potential of persons who are blind and visually-impaired.
Joseph Abely, President
Brian Charlson, Director of Computer Training Services

9588 Clearinghouse for Specialized Media and Translation
California Department of Education/CSMT
1430 N Street 916-445-5103
Sacramento, CA 95814 Fax: 916-323-9732
e-mail: csmt@cde.ca.gov
www.cde.ca.gov/re/pn/sm
Assists schools and students in the identification and acquisition
of textbooks reference books and study materials in aural media,
braille, large print, and electronic media access technology.
Tom Torlakson, State Superintendent of Public Instructi
Jonn Paris-Salb, Administrator

9589 Clovernook Center for the Blind and Visually Impaired
7000 Hamilton Avenue 513-522-3860
Cincinnati, OH 45231-5240 888-234-7156
Fax: 513-728-3946
www.clovernook.org
Innovative programs including community living support and a
youth initiative with a focus on developing the skills people with
visual impairments need to become independent in the community.

An array of employment services help individuals maximize their
earning potential and job satisfaction, both on site in our manufacturing center and in the local job market.
Robin L Usalis, President/CEO
Jacqueline L Conner, VP of Multi-State Center East

9590 Dean A McGee Eye Institute
608 Stanton L Young Boulevard 405-271-6060
Oklahoma City, OK 73104-5065 800-787-9012
Fax: 405-271-4442
www.dmei.org
The Dean McGee Eye Institute is the first center in Oklahoma to offer a new treatment for dry eyes that can last up to a year and frees
patients from time-consuming warm compresses and lubricating
eye drops. The LipiFlow Thermal Pulsation System combines pre-
cisely administered heat and pressure to open and clear clogged oil
glands in the eyelids, allowing lubricating oils to flow naturally
again.
Edward L. Gaylord, Professor and Chair
Gregory L. Skuta, MD, President

9591 Emory University: Laboratory for Ophthalmic Research
1365B Clifton Road, N.E.
Atlanta, GA 30322-1013 404-778-2020
www.eyecenter.emory.edu
Various studies into the aspects of blindness.
Timothy W. Olsen, MD, Chair/Director
Joy H. Bell, Director of Public Relations

9592 Florida Ophthalmic Institute
7106 NW 11th Pl 352-331-2020
Gainesville, FL 32605-3157 Fax: 352-331-2019
e-mail: afn22025@gmail.com
www.sites.google.com/site/flophthalmicin
Nonprofit organization that understands and treats ocular diseases
including glaucoma.
Norman S Levy MD, Director
Trudy K. Ramjattan, MD, Surgeon

9593 Glaucoma Laser Trabeculoplasty Study Sinai Hospital of Detroit
Sinai Hospital of Detroit
6767 W Outer Drive 313-966-3256
Detroit, MI 48235-2899 Fax: 313-966-4296
Examines the effectiveness and safety of the treatments of glau-
coma.
Hugh Beckman, Chairman

9594 Glaucoma Research Foundation
251 Post Street 415-986-3162
San Francisco, CA 94108 800-826-6693
Fax: 415-986-3763
e-mail: question@glaucoma.org
www.glaucoma.org
Our mission is to prevent vision loss from glaucoma by investing in
innovative research, education, and support with the ultimate goal
of finding a cure.
Thomas M Brunner, Chief Executive Officer/President
Nancy Graydon, Executive Director of Development

9595 Harvard University Howe Laboratory of Ophthalmology
Massachusetts Eye & Ear Infirmary
243 Charles Street
Boston, MA 02114-3002 617-523-7900
www.masseyeandear.org
Established in 1926, the Howe Laboratory is comprised of investigators working on both basic research, focused on retinal development, structure and function in various organisms, and
translational research, focused on developing treatments for glaucoma and conditions affecting the cornea.
Dr. Mack Cheney, Director
Wendy Williams, Associate Director

9596 Helen Keller International
352 Park Avenue S 212-532-0544
New York, NY 10010 877-535-5374
Fax: 212-532-6014
e-mail: info@hki.org
www.hki.org

Nonprofit organization for the blind.
Kathy Spahn, President/CEO
Shawn K Baker, VP/Regional Director-Africa

9597   Helen Keller National Center for Deaf/Blind Youths and Adults
141 Middle Neck Road   516-944-8900
Sands Point, NY 11050-1299   Fax: 516-944-7302
                                        TTY: 516-944-8637
                                e-mail: hkncinfo@hknc.org
                                        www.hknc.org
We enable all those who are deaf-blind to live and work in the community of their choice. We provide comprehensive vocational rehabilitation training at our headquarters in NY and assistance with job and residential placements when training is completed.
Joseph McNulty, Executive Director

9598   Institute for Visual Sciences
1 E 71st Street   212-305-2919
New York, NY 10021-4102
Ophthalmology with emphasis on the development of care for the eye.
Melissa Mount, Executive Director

9599   Institute of Ophthalmology and Visual Scie nce New Jersey Medical School
New Jersey Medical School
PO Box 1709   973-972-2036
Newark, NJ 07101-2425   Fax: 973-723-94
                                e-mail: churchbf@umdnj.edu
                                        www.njms.rutgers.edu
The Institute comprises ophthalmic surgeons, researchers, ophthalmic surgeons-in-training, administrators, and ancillary staff (such as ophthalmic technicians). We are dedicated to providing outstanding compassionate patient care, teaching current and future providers of eye care, and developing cures for blindness. This site provides comprehensive information on our faculty members, eye-care professionals, patient-care services, research, residency training programs, and continuing education cu
Marco A Zarbin, MD, PhD, FACS, Chair
Robert D. Fechtner, Professor

9600   Jerusalem Center for Multi-Handicapped Blind Children
350 7th Avenue   212-279-4070
New York, NY 10001-7903   Fax: 212-279-4043
                                e-mail: info@keren-or.org
                                        keren-or.org
Maintains the Keren-Or Center for the Multiply Handicapped Blind Child in Jerusalem for rehabilitation and training. Funds acquired through contributions bequests and legacies.
Madelyn Cohen, Executive Director
Tamara Silberberg, Director Keren-Or Center

9601   Johns Hopkins University: Dana Center for Preventive Ophthalmology
Wilmer Ophthalmology Institute
600 N Wolfe Street
Baltimore, MD 21287-0001   410-955-2777
                        www.hopkinsmedicine.org/wilmer/danacente
Research at the Dana Center focuses on national and international public health prevention of blinding eye disease.
Harry A Quigley, Director

9602   New Beginnings: The Blind Children's Center
4120 Marathon Street   213-664-2153
Los Angeles, CA 90029-3505   800-222-3566
The purpose of the Center is to turn initial fears into hope. Helps children and their families become independent by creating a climate of safety and trust. Children learn to develop self confidence and to master a wide range of skills. Services include an infant stimulation program, educational preschool, interdisciplinary assessment services, family services, correspondence program, toll free national hotline and a publication and research service.

9603   New Beginnings: The Blind Children's Cente
4120 Marathon Street   323-664-2153
Los Angeles, CA 90029   800-222-3566
                                        Fax: 323-665-3828
                                www.blindchildrenscenter.org
The purpose of the Center is to turn initial fears into hope. Helps children and their families become independent by creating a cli-

mate of safety and trust. Children learn to develop self confidence and to master a wide range of skills. Services include an infant stimulation program educational preschool interdisciplinary assessment services family services correspondence program toll free national hotline and a publication and research service.

9604   Oregon Health Sciences University: Elk's Children's Eye Clinic
Casey Eye Institute
3375 SW Terwilliger Boulevard   503-494-3000
Portland, OR 97239-4197   Fax: 503-494-5347
                                        www.ohsucasey.com
Our mission at the Casey Eye Institute is to provide excellent eye care in a quality cost-effective environment that combines education research clinical leadership and service to the community.
Earl Palmer, Director

9605   Reader-Transcriber Registry National Braille Association
National Braille Association
3 Townline Circle   716-427-8260
Rochester, NY 14623-2537
Certified braillists fill requests for college textbooks and other technical works through this service of the National Braille Association.

9606   Smith-Kettlewell Eye Research Institute
2318 Fillmore Street   415-345-2000
San Francisco, CA 94115-1821   Fax: 415-345-8455
                                        www.ski.org

Dedicated to research on human vision. The Institute was founded to encourage a productive collaboration between the medical clinic and scientific laboratory. Research is conducted with clinical studies which relate directly to the diagnosis and treatment of eye diseases the development of devices and vocational programs to aid the partially sighted and basic research to understand how the eye and brain work for both the clinical and rehabilitation programs.
Arthur Jampolsky, Executive Director
Ruth S Poole, COO

9607   University of Illinois Eye and Ear Infirma ry
1855 W Taylor Street   312-996-6591
Chicago, IL 60612-7242   Fax: 312-996-7770
                                e-mail: eyeweb@uic.edu
                                        www.uic.edu/com/eye
Offers help support information and research for persons with vision problems including Retinitis Pigmentosa.
Dr. Rohit Verma, Department Chair
Elmer Tu, Director of Cornea Service

9608   University of Illinois at Chicago Lions of Illinois Eye Research Institute
UIC Eye Center
1905 W Taylor Street   312-996-1466
Chicago, IL 60612-7245   Fax: 312-355-4248
                                www.uic.edu/com/eye/Lions
Visual impairments and blindness research including glaucoma studies.
Janet Szlyk, President
Julie Daraska, Secretary

9609   University of Miami: Bascom Palmer Eye Institute
Department of Ophthalmalogy
900 NW 17th Street   305-326-6000
Miami, FL 33136-1015   800-329-7000
                                        Fax: 305-326-6306
                        www.bpei.med.miami.edu/site/default.asp
Clinical and basic research into blindness and visual impairments.
John G Clarkson, Dean Emeritus

9610   Visually Impaired Center
1422 W Court Street   810-767-4014
Flint, MI 48503   Fax: 810-767-0020
                                e-mail: info@vicflint.org
                                        www.vicflint.org
A private non-profit agency which offers special programs and some very practical help to people who are blind or partially sighted. Offers rehabilitation low vision aids orientation and mobility vocational training reading and information recreation counseling services volunteer services and community awareness.
Fharon Reigle, Director

9611 Warren Grant Magnuson Clinical Center National Institute of Health
National Institute of Health
9000 Rockville Pike   301-496-4000
Bethesda, MD 20892   800-411-1222
                                  Fax: 301-480-9793
                                  TTY: 866-411-1010
                           e-mail: prpl@mail.cc.nih.gov
                                       www.cc.nih.gov

Established in 1953 as the research hospital of the National Institutes of Health. Designed so that patient care facilities are close to research laboratories so new findings of basic and clinical scientists can be quickly applied to the treatment of patients. Upon referral by physicians patients are admitted to NIH clinical studies.
John I Gallin, Director
David Henderson, Deputy Director for Clinical Care

9612 Yale University: Vision Research Center
330 Cedar Street   203-785-5687
New Haven, CT 06510-3218   800-395-7949
                                  Fax: 203-785-7401
                           e-mail: sarah.gelo@yale.edu
                               visionresearch.med.yale.edu

Vision including studies on growth and development.
Bruce Shields, Chair
Sarah Gelo, Administrator

Kansas

9613 Kansas Services for the Blind and Visually Impaired
Social Rehabilitation Services
915 SW Harrison   785-368-7471
Topeka, KS 66612-2445   800-547-5789
                                  Fax: 785-368-7467
                                  TTY: 785-368-7478
                             e-mail: rehab@srs.ks.gov
                       www.srskansas.org/rehab/text/SBVI.htm

Instructional employment oriented services for blind adults.
Laura Howard, Deputy Secretary and Chief Financial Off
Theresa Addington, Accounting and Administrative Operations

Support Groups & Hotlines

9614 1-800-BRAILLE
Braille Institute
741 N Vermont Avenue   323-663-1111
Los Angeles, CA 90029-3594   800-272-4553
                                  Fax: 323-663-0867
                          e-mail: la@brailleinstitute.org
                                www.brailleinstitute.org

A toll free information and referral service where callers can obtain information about community programs and referrals to organizations serving the blind in their local areas.
Lester M. Straussman, Director
James B. Boyle, Boardmember

9615 AFB Toll-Free Hotline
American Foundation for the Blind
2 Penn Plaza   212-502-7600
New York, NY 10121-2018   800-232-5463
                                  Fax: 888-545-8331
                              e-mail: afbinfo@afb.net
                                       www.afb.org

Supplies information on visual impairment and blindness, answers queries regarding AFB services, products, publications, technology, the Careers and Technology Information Bank (a national data bank) and much more.
Carl R. Augusto, President & CEO
Rick Bozeman, CFO

9616 American Foundation for the Blind Information Center
11 Penn Plaza   212-502-7600
New York, NY 10001   800-232-5463
                                  Fax: 212-502-7777
                              e-mail: afbinfo@afb.net
                                       www.afb.org

Nationally recognized information clearinghouse on blindness and visual impairment. Serves people who are blind or visually impaired, professionals in the field of blindness and visual impairment — including the staff at AFB, business and government organizations and the general public. Provides a toll-free information line available 24 hours a day, online information and referral services, professional library and archival services.

9617 Aurora of Central New York
518 James Street   315-422-7263
Syracuse, NY 13203   Fax: 315-422-4792
                                  TTY: 315-422-9746
                                  TDD: 315-422-9746
                       e-mail: auroracny@auroraofcny.org
                                   www.auroraofcny.org/

Professional counseling services to assist individuals and their families deal with the trauma of hearing or vision loss.
Earleen Foulk, President Board of Directors
Debra Chaiken, Executive Director

9618 Carroll Center for the Blind
770 Centre Street   617-969-6200
Newton, MA 2458-2597   800-852-3131
                                  Fax: 617-969-6204
                                       www.carroll.org

We have developed many methods for people with low vision to learn the skills to be independent in their homes, in class settings, and in their work places. Our services for the blind include vision rehabilitation services, vocational and transition programs, assistive technology training, educational support and recreation opportunities for individuals who are visually impaired of all ages
Dina Rosenbaum, VP Marketing

9619 Department of Ophthalmology Information Line
Illinois Eye & Ear Infirmary
1855 W Taylor Street m/c 648   312-996-6500
Chicago, IL 60612-7242   Fax: 312-996-7770
                              e-mail: eyeweb@uic.edu
                                   www.uic.edu/com/eye/

Offers eye clinic and physician referrals to persons suffering from vision disorders as well as offers emergency information.
Dimitri Azar, Director

9620 Job Opportunities for the Blind
National Federation of the Blind
200 E Wells St   410-659-9314
Baltimore, MD 21230-4998   Fax: 410-685-5653
                                  e-mail: nfb@nfb.org
                                       www.nfb.org

A specialized service that provides free support, resources and information to blind persons seeking employment and to employers interested in hiring the blind. A partnership program with the US Department of Labor, this is the most successful program of it's kind in helping blind persons find competitive work.
Anthony Cobb, Dircetor

9621 National Association for Parents of the Visually Impaired
Watertown, MA 2471   617-972-7441
                                       800-562-6265
                                  Fax: 617-972-7444
                          e-mail: napvi@perkins.org
                                       www.napvi.org

Susan Laventure, Executive Director

9622 National Center for Sight
National Society to Prevent Blindness
211 Wacker Drive   312-363-6001
Chicago, IL 60606   800-331-2020
                                  Fax: 312-363-6052

A toll-free line offering information on a broad range of vision, eye health and safety topics including sports eye safety, lazy eye, diabetic retinopathy, glaucoma, cataracts, children's eye disorders, and more.

9623 National Eye Health Education Program
1855 W Taylor Street   312-996-6590
Chicago, IL 60612-7242   800-786-3937
                                  Fax: 312-996-9967
                                       www.uic.edu

Offers information and support for persons with vision disorders, including Retinitis Pigmentosa.
Mary Go, Supervisor

9624 National Health Information Center
PO Box 1133
Washington, DC 20013
310-565-4167
800-336-4797
Fax: 301-984-4256
e-mail: info@nhic.org
www.health.gov/nhic
Offers a nationwide information referral service, produces directories and resource guides.

9625 National Service Dog Center
Delta society
875 124th Avenue, NE
Bellevue, WA 98005
425-679-550
Fax: 425-679-5539
e-mail: info@petpartners.org
www.petpartners.org
Pet Partners is the leader in demonstrating and promoting positive human-animal interaction to improve the physical, emotional and psychological lives of those we serve.
Brenda Bax, Chair
Mary Craig, Vice Chair/Treasurer

9626 PXE International
4301 Connecticut Avenue NW
Washington, DC 20008-2369
202-362-9599
Fax: 202-966-8553
e-mail: info@pxe.org
www.pxe.org
Initiates, funds and conducts research; provides support for individuals and families affected by pseudoxanthoma elasticum; and provides resrouces for healthcare professionals.
Sharon Terry, CEO
Terry Dermaid, Executive Director

9627 Recorded Periodicals
Associated Services for the Blind
919 Walnut Street
Philadelphia, PA 19107-5237
215-627-0600
Fax: 215-922-0692
e-mail: asbinfo@asb.org
www.asb.org
A subscription service of Associated Services for the Blind, these periodicals provide 21 magazines through this subscription service. A magazine list can be sent, in both large print and on audio cassette.
Richard Forsythe, Director
David Goldfield, Computer Instructor

9628 Recording for the Blind Helpline
20 Roszel Road
Princeton, NJ 08540-6294
609-750-1830
800-221-4792
e-mail: PrincetonStudio@LearningAlly.org
www.learningally.org
An organization dedicated to helping people with print disabilities.
Andrew Friedman, President & CEO
Jim Halliday, Executive VP

9629 Vision Use in Employment
Carroll Center for the Blind
770 Centre Street
Newton, MA 02458-2597
617-969-6200
800-852-3131
Fax: 617-969-6204
www.carroll.org
We have developed many methods for people with low vision to learn the skills to be independent in their homes, in class settings, and in their work places. Our services for the blind include vision rehabilitation services, vocational and transition programs, assistive technology training, educational support and recreation opportunities for individuals who are visually impaired of all ages
Joseph Abely, President
Diana Rosenbaum, Director of Marketing

9630 Washington Connection
American Council of the Blind
1155 15th Street NW
Washington, DC 20005-2706
202-467-5081
800-424-8666
Fax: 202-467-5085
e-mail: info@acb.org
www.acb.org

Coverage of issues affecting blind people via legislative information, participates in law-making, legislative training seminars and networking of support resources across the US.
Melanie Brunson, Executive Director

Books

9631 AFB Directory of Services for Blind/Vis. Impaired Persons in the US & Canada
AFB Press: American Foundation for the Blind
11 Penn Plaza
New York, NY 10001
212-502-7600
800-232-3044
Fax: 212-502-7774
e-mail: afbdirectory@afb.net
www.afb.org/store
Provides the most comprehensive collection of information available on services for blind and visually impaired individuals. Over 800 pages of revised and updated information on more than 1,500 agencies and 45 new indexes. Includes complete descriptions of services offered by organizations and web sites and e-mail addresses. Available online on a subscription basis.

9632 APH Catalog of Accessible Books for People Who are Visually Impaired
American Printing House for the Blind
1839 Frankfort Avenue
Louisville, KY 40206-3148
502-895-2405
800-223-1839
Fax: 502-895-1509
e-mail: info@aph.org
Offers thousands of selections and publishers of large type and braille books for persons with visual impairments.

9633 Access to Mass Transit for Blind & Visually Impaired Travelers
AFB Press: American Foundation for the Blind
11 Penn Plaza
New York, NY 10001
212-502-7600
800-232-3044
Fax: 212-502-7774
www.afb.org/store
Addresses several travel issues vital to the independence of blind and visually impaired persons from serveral perspectives — those of the blind and visually impaired persons who use mass transit, orientation and mobility instructors and transportation professionals. Focusing on national and international issues, this information filled manual covers approaches to making mass transit available in several cities in the US and Canada, the United Kingdom and Japan.
192 pages Paperback
ISBN: 0-891281-66-5

9634 An Orientation and Mobility Primer for Families and Young Children
American Foundation for the Blind
11 Penn Plaza
New York, NY 10001-2018
212-502-7600
800-232-5463
Fax: 212-502-7777
Practical information for helping a child learn about his or her environment right from the start. Covers sensory training, concept development and orientation skills.
48 pages Papberback
ISBN: 0-891281-57-6

9635 Art Beyond Sight: Resource Guide to Art, Creativity and Visual Impairment
AFB Press: American Foundation for the Blind
11 Penn Plaza
New York, NY 10001
212-502-7600
800-232-3044
Fax: 212-502-7774
www.afb.org/store
AFB and Art Education for the Blind have joined together to co-publish this one-of-a-kind resource that provides vital information on all aspects of exploring art and creativity by people who are blind or visually impaired. Includes a section of reproducible pages for classroom or workshop activities.
504 pages Paperback
ISBN: 0-891288-50-3

9636 Art and Science of Teaching Orientation to the Visually Impaired
AFB Press: American Foundation for the Blind

11 Penn Plaza
New York, NY 10001
212-502-7600
800-232-3044
Fax: 212-502-7774
www.afb.org/store

Updated and comprehensive description of the techniques of teaching orientation and mobility, presented along with strategies for sensitive and effective teaching. Such factors as individual needs, environmental features and ethical issues are discussed in this important text.

200 pages Paperback
ISBN: 0-891282-59-9

9637   Beginning with Braille: Balanced Approach to Literacy
AFB Press: American Foundation for the Blind
11 Penn Plaza
New York, NY 10001
212-502-7600
800-232-3044
Fax: 212-502-7774
www.afb.org/store

Exciting resource from a skilled practitioner, this book provides a wealth of effective activitoes for promoting literacy at the early stages of braille instruction. The text includes creative and practical strategies for designing and delivering quality braille instruction and offers teacher-friendly suggestions for many areas, such as reading aloud to young children, selecting and making early tactile books and teaching tactile and hand movement skills. Tips on lessons and worksheets.

ISBN: 0-891283-23-4

9638   Behavioral Vision Approaches for Persons with Physical Disabilities
William V. Padula, author
Optometric Extension Program Foundation
1921 E. Carnegie Ave., Suite 3-L
Santa Ana, CA 92705-5510
949-250-8070
Fax: 949-250-8175
e-mail: smc.oep@worldnet.att.net
www.oepf.org

A discussion of the behavioral vision/neuro-motor approach to providing directions for prescriptive and therapeutic services for the visually handicapped child or adult.

197 pages
ISBN: 0-943599-04-0
Beverly Roberts, President
Gregory Kitchener, O.D., Vice President

9639   Blindness and Early Childhood Development
AFB Press: American Foundation for the Blind
11 Penn Plaza
New York, NY 10001
212-502-7600
800-232-3044
Fax: 212-502-7774
www.afb.org/store

Reviews knowledge of motor and locomotor development, language and cognitive processes and social, emotional and personality development. It is a classic resource for teachers and those who work with children who are blind or visually impaired.

384 pages Paperback
ISBN: 0-891281-23-1

9640   Braille Book Bank: Music Catalog
National Braille Association
95 Allens Creek Road, 1-202
Rochester, NY 14618
585-427-8260
Fax: 585-427-0263
e-mail: NBAOffice@nationalbraille.org
www.nationalbraille.org

Offers hundreds of musical titles in print form, braille and on cassette.

62 pages

9641   Building Blocks: Foundations for Learning for Young Blind & Vis. Impaired Children
AFB Press: American Foundation for the Blind
11 Penn Plaza
New York, NY 10001
212-502-7600
800-232-3044
Fax: 212-502-7774
www.afb.org/store

Available in English and Spanish, this work presents the essential components of a successful early intervention program, including collaboration with family members, positive relationships between parents and professionals, public education, and attention to

important programming components such as space exploration, braille readiness, orientation and mobility, play, cooking and music. VHS video also available.

149 pages Paperback
ISBN: 0-891281-87-8

9642   Burns Braille Transcription Dictionary
AFB Press: American Foundation for the Blind
11 Penn Plaza
New York, NY 10001
212-502-7600
800-232-3044
Fax: 212-502-7774
www.afb.org/store

A handy, portable guide that is a quick reference for anyone who needs to check print-to-braille and braille-to-print meanings and symbols. This easy-to-use listing provides readers with the essential alphabet, contractions, punctuation and signs and symbols for braille, as well as brief descriptions of rules for thier use. Organized into four clear sections aimed at providing information at a glance, this valuable tool is an ideal reference for teachers, rehabilitation professionals and others.

96 pages Paperback
ISBN: 0-891292-32-7

9643   Business Owners Who Are Blind or Visually Impaired
AFB Press: American Foundation for the Blind
11 Penn Plaza
New York, NY 10001
212-502-7600
800-232-3044
Fax: 212-502-7774
www.afb.org/store

Demonstrates the wide range of careers and talents that can be pursued by persons with visual impairments. Each profile features a successful individual who has acomplised his or her dream of business ownership and who shares important insights. Available in paperback, audio cassette or ASCII disk.

148 pages
ISBN: 0-891283-24-2

9644   Career Perspectives: Interviews with Blind & Visually Impaired Professionals
AFB Press: American Foundation for the Blind
11 Penn Plaza
New York, NY 10001
212-502-7600
800-232-3044
Fax: 212-502-7774
www.afb.org/store

Profiles of 20 successful archivers who describe in their own words what it takes to pursue and attain professional success in a sighted world. From all around the country and representing a wide range of professions, including law, science, journalism, management and medicine, the blind and visually impaired individuals featured serve as role models for others who wnat to follow career paths.

96 pages Paperback
ISBN: 0-891281-70-3

9645   Childhood Glaucoma: A Reference Guide for Families
NAPVI
PO Box 317
Watertown, MA 02471-0317
617-972-7441
800-562-6265
Fax: 617-972-7444
e-mail: napvi@perkins.org
www.napvi.org

Susan LaVenture, Executive Director

9646   Communication Skills for Visually Impaired
Charles C Thomas Publisher
2600 S 1st Street
Springfield, IL 62704-4730
217-789-8980
Fax: 217-789-9130
e-mail: books@ccthomas.com
www.ccthomas.com

322 pages
ISBN: 0-398066-92-2

9647   Concept Development for Visually Impaired Children: Resource Guide
AFB Press: American Foundation for the Blind
11 Penn Plaza
New York, NY 10001
212-502-7600
800-232-3044
Fax: 212-502-7774
www.afb.org/store

710

Program for integrating such concepts as body imagery, gross motor movement, posture and tactile discrimination into the curriculum from kindergarten on.
80 pages Paperback
ISBN: 0-891280-18-9

9648 **Coping with Vision Loss**
Bill Chapman, EdD, author
Hunter House Publishing
PO Box 2914   510-865-5282
Alameda, CA 94501   800-266-5592
                                                   Fax: 510-865-4295
                                    e-mail: ordering@hunterhouse.com
                                                   www.hunterhouse.com
Maximizing what you can see and do. The Author explains the five leading causes of vision loss, and how to use new skills and vision aids.
2001 304 pages Paperback
Cristina Sverdrup, Customer Service Manager

9649 **Development of Social Skills by Blind and Visually Impaired Students**
AFB Press: American Foundation for the Blind
11 Penn Plaza   212-502-7600
New York, NY 10001   800-532-3044
                                                   Fax: 212-502-7774
                                                   www.afb.org/store
Examination of the social interactions of children with visual impairments, theory and research are combined to explore how these children can be helped to succeed socially. Innovative practical strategies are provided for educators, researchers and families on how to assist children in the development of social skills. Qualitative ethnographic approaches demonstrate how classroom teachers can work effectively with individual children and present valuable insights about children's interactions.
232 pages Paperback
ISBN: 0-891282-17-3

9650 **Early Focus: Working with Young Children Who Are Blind or Visually Impaired**
AFB Press: American Foundation for the Blind
11 Penn Plaza   212-502-7600
New York, NY 10001   Fax: 212-502-7777
                                                   www.afb.org/store
Early intervention has increasingly been recognized as critical in the development and growth of children with visual impairments and other disabilities. Federal regulations have mandated early indentifacation and assesment, underscoring its importance for children's well being. This revised and updated edition of Early Focus provides the important information you need to know including serving culturally diverse families with children who have multiple disabilities and practical tips.
376 pages Paperback
ISBN: 0-891282-15-7

9651 **Encyclopedia of Blindness and Vision Impairment**
Facts on File
11 Penn Plaza   212-967-8800
New York, NY 10001   800-322-8755
                                                   Fax: 800-678-3633
Designed to provide both laymen and professionals with concise, practical information on the second most common disability in the US.
340 pages Hardcover

9652 **Equals in Partnership: Basic Rights for Families of Children with Blindness**
NAPVI
PO Box 317   617-972-7441
Watertown, MA 02471-0317   800-562-6265
                                                   Fax: 617-972-7444
                                       e-mail: napvi@perkins.org
                                                   www.napvi.org

Susan LaVenture, Executive Director

9653 **Essential Elements in Early Intervention: Visual Impairment & Multiple Disability**
AFB Press: American Foundation for the Blind

11 Penn Plaza   212-502-7600
New York, NY 10001   800-232-3044
                                                   Fax: 212-502-7774
                                                   www.afb.org/store
Latest comprehensive resource from an outstanding early childhood specialist, this guide provides a range of information on effective early intervention with young children who are visually impaired and have other disabilities.
503 pages Paperback
ISBN: 0-891283-05-6

9654 **Eye and Your Vision**
Dr Lorrain H Marchi, author
National Association for Visually Handicapped
22 W 21st Street   212-889-3141
New York, NY 10010-6904   Fax: 212-727-2931
                                                   e-mail: navh@navh.org
                                                   www.navh.org
A large booklet offering information, with illustrations, on the eye. Includes information on protection of eyesight, how the eye works and vision disorders.
19 pages $5.00 n/members
Lorraine Marchi LHD, Founder/CEO
Cesar Gomez, Executive Director

9655 **First Steps**
Blind Children's Center
4120 Marathon Street   213-664-2153
Los Angeles, CA 90029-3584   Fax: 213-665-3828
                                                   e-mail: info@blindcntr.org
                                                   www.blindcntr.org
A handbook for teaching young children who are visually impaired. Designed to assist students, professionals and parents working with children who are visually impaired.
203 pages

9656 **Foundations of Education**
AFB Press: American Foundation for the Blind
11 Penn Plaza   212-502-7600
New York, NY 10001   800-232-3044
                                                   Fax: 212-502-7774
                                                   www.afb.org/store
Complete revision of landmark text. Comprehensive compilation of state-of-the-art information is the essential resource on educating visually impaired students, the essential theory forming the knowledge base, and methodology of teaching visually impaired students in all areas.
2000
ISBN: 0-891283-49-8

9657 **Foundations of Orientation and Mobility**
AFB Press: American Foundation for the Blind
11 Penn Plaza   212-502-7600
New York, NY 10001   800-232-3044
                                                   Fax: 212-502-7774
                                                   www.afb.org
Updated and revised, this new edition of the field's founding classics includes current research fom a variety of disiplines, an international perspective, and expanded contents on low vision, aging, multiple disabilities, accessibility, program design and adaptive technology from more than 30 eminent subject experts. Divided into four main sections, the book explores every of Orientation and Mobility learning and instruction.
800 pages Hardcover
ISBN: 0-891289-46-1

9658 **Foundations of Rehabilitation Counseling with Persons Who Are Blind/Visually Imp.**
AFB Press: American Foundation for the Blind
11 Penn Plaza   212-502-7600
New York, NY 10001   800-232-3044
                                                   Fax: 212-502-7774
                                                   www.afb.org/store
Rehabilitation professionals have long recognized that the needs of people who are blind or visually impaired are unique and require a special knowledge and expertise for the provision and coordination of effective rehabilitation services. Contributions to this text from more than 25 experts provide essential information on subjects as functional, medical, vocational and phychological assess-

ments, demographic and cultural issues, pacement and employment issues, and the rehabilitation team.
464 pages Hardcover
ISBN: 0-891289-45-3

9659 Get a Wiggle On
American Alliance For Health, Phys. Ed. & Dance
1900 Association Drive   703-476-3400
Reston, VA 20191-1598   800-213-7193
www.aahperd.org/
Gives teachers and parents practical suggestions for helping blind and visually impaired infants grow and learn like other children.
80 pages
ISBN: 0-883140-77-2

9660 Guide to Independence for the Visually Impaired and Their Families
Demos Medical Publishing
386 Park Avenue S   212-683-0072
New York, NY 10016-8804   800-532-8663
Fax: 212-683-0118
e-mail: orderdept@demopub.com
www.demosmedpub.com
This first comprehensive, hands-on book for the newly visually impaired and their families presents detailed instructions to deal with emotional reactions and fioght depression; contact organizations and get information; obtain federal and other types of financial aid; use the other senses more effectively; adapt their homes and do household chores; handle paperwork and become socially active.
248 pages Paperback
ISBN: 0-939957-61-2
Dr. Diana M Schneider, President

9661 Guidelines and Games for Teaching Efficient Braille Reading
AFB Press: American Foundation for the Blind
11 Penn Plaza   212-502-7600
New York, NY 10001   800-232-3044
Fax: 212-502-7774
www.afb.org/store
Based on research in the areas of rapid reading and precision teaching, these effective guidelines and games represent a unique adaptation of a general reading program to the needs of braille readers.
116 pages Paperback
ISBN: 0-891281-05-3

9662 Hammond Large Type World Atlas
American Map-Langensceidt Publishing Group
15 Tyger River Drive   864-486-0214
Duncan, SC 29334   800-432-6277
Fax: 888-773-7979
www.hammondmap.com
100 maps.

ISBN: 0-816159-11-4

9663 Handbook for Itinerant and Resource Teachers of Blind Students
National Federation of the Blind
1800 Johnson Street   410-659-9314
Baltimore, MD 21230-4998   Fax: 410-685-5653
e-mail: subscribe@diabetes.nfb.org
www.nfb.org
The Handbook provides help to teachers, school administrators or other school personnel that have experience with blind or visually impaired students. The Handbook devotes 45 pages to Braille and how to teach Braille for parents and teachers; other chapters iclude law, physical education, fitting in socially, testing and evaluation, home economics, daily living skills and more.
533 pages Softcover
Eileen Ley, Director of Publishing
Elizabeth Lunt, Editor

9664 Health Care Professionals Who are Blind or Visually Impaired
AFB Press: American Foundation for the Blind
11 Penn Plaza   212-502-7600
New York, NY 10001   800-232-3044
Fax: 212-502-7774
www.afb.org/store
Exciting career possibilities for people who are visually impaired as well as those who are sighted. Inspirational profiles of 15

sucessful role models. Written in an accesible, easy-to-read style, this book documents the stories and stategies of professionals ranging from a forensic psychiatrist to a radiology dark room technician. Information on technology and tactics that are used to perform demanding jobs are also included. Available in paperback, audio casette, or ASCII disk.
2001 166 pages
ISBN: 0-891283-88-9

9665 I Keep Five Pairs of Glasses in a Flower Pot
Henrietta Levner, author
National Association for Visually Handicapped
22 W 21st Street   212-889-3141
New York, NY 10010-6904   Fax: 212-727-2931
e-mail: navh@navh.org
www.navh.org
A short story, printed in 18 point type, is the saga of one womans struggle with low vision.
Lorraine Marchi LHD, Founder/CEO
Cesar Gomez, Executive Director

9666 If Blindness Comes
National Federation of the Blind
1800 Johnson Street   410-659-9314
Baltimore, MD 21230-4998   Fax: 410-685-5653
e-mail: subscribe@diabetes.nfb.org
www.nfb.org
An introduction to issues relating to vision loss and provides a positive, supportive philosophy about blindness. It is a general information book which includes answers to many common questions about blindness, information about services and programs for the blind and resource listings.
Eileen Ley, Director of Publishing
Elizabeth Lunt, Editor

9667 Independence Without Sight or Sound: Suggestions for Practitioners
AFB Press: American Foundation for the Blind
11 Penn Plaza   212-502-7600
New York, NY 10001   800-232-3044
Fax: 212-502-7774
www.afb.org/store
Written in a personal and informal style, this practical guidebook covers the essential aspects of communicating and working with deaf-blind persons. Full of valuable information on subjects such as how to talk with deaf-blind people, adapt orientation and mobility techniques for deaf-blind travelers, and interact with deaf-blind individuals socially, this useful manual also contains a substantial resource section detailing sources of information and adapted equipment. Also available in braille.
193 pages Paperback
ISBN: 0-891282-46-7

9668 Jewish Heritage for the Blind
1655 E 24th Street   718-338-4999
Brooklyn, NY 11229-2401   800-995-1888
Offers large print traditional prayer books for the High Holy days, festivals, fast days and daily rituals for those finding it difficult or impossible to read small print.

9669 Kernel Book Series
National Federation of the Blind
1800 Johnson Street   410-659-9314
Baltimore, MD 21230-4998   Fax: 410-685-5653
e-mail: subscribe@diabetes.nfb.org
www.nfb.org
A series of books written by the blind themselves. Each book is a collection of articles and stories about the real life experiences of blind persons. These books help educate the blind and the sighted alike about a positive philosophy regarding blindness.
Eileen Ley, Director of Publishing
Elizabeth Lunt, Editor

9670 King James Bible: Large Print
Science Products
PO Box 888
Southeastern, PA 19399-0888   800-888-7400
24 point type easily seen with 20/200 acuity. Makes bible reading for children easier too.

9671 Knotholes are for Seeing: Therapy Through Poetry, Prose & Other Writings
Business of Living Publications
PO Box 8388   512-852-8515
Corpus Christi, TX 78468-8388

ISBN: 1-879518-08-2

9672 Large Print American Heritage Dictionary
Houghton Mifflin Harcourt
222 Berkeley Street   617-351-5000
Boston, MA 02116   800-888-7400
                               www.hmco.com
More than 35,000 easy to read entries for those who prefer large type.

ISBN: 0-395929-32-6

9673 Legislative Handbook for Parents
NAPVI
PO Box 317   617-972-7441
Watertown, MA 02471-0317   800-562-6265
                               Fax: 617-972-7444
                    e-mail: napvi@perkins.org
                               www.spedex.com
Written by parents for parents in dealing with legislative processes that ultimately affect their children's lives.
Susan LaVenture, Executive Director

9674 Library Resources for the Blind and Physically Handicapped
National Library Service for the Blind
1291 Taylor Street NW   202-707-5100
Washington, DC 20542-0002   Fax: 202-707-0712
                               www.loc.gov/nls

9675 Low Vision: Reflections of the Past, Issues for the Future
AFB Press: American Foundation for the Blind
11 Penn Plaza   212-502-7600
New York, NY 10001   800-232-3044
                               Fax: 212-502-7774
                               www.afb.org/store
Research report based on a multiphase survey of professionals. Identifies important trends that will shape the field of low vision services into the next century. Designed for administrators, policy planners and university instructors, as well as for direct service providers, Low Vision includes overview papers by six eminent leaders in the low vision field.
181 pages Paperback
ISBN: 0-891282-18-1

9676 Madness of Usher's: Coping with Vision & Hearing Loss
Richard A. Lewis, Dorothy H. Stiefel, author
Business of Living Publications
PO Box 8388   512-852-8515
Corpus Christi, TX 78468-8388
Paperback
ISBN: 1-879518-06-6
Dorothy H Stiefel, Author

9677 Mainstreaming & the American Dream: Soc. Logical Perspectives on Parental Coping
AFB Press: American Foundation for the Blind
11 Penn Plaza   212-502-7600
New York, NY 10001   800-232-3044
                               Fax: 212-502-7774
                               www.afb.org/store
Based on in-depth interviews with parents and professionals, this research monograph presents a sociological framework for looking at the needs and aspirations of parents of blind and visually impaired children.
256 pages Paperback
ISBN: 0-891281-91-6

9678 Mainstreaming the Visually Impaired Child
NAPVI
PO Box 317   617-972-7441
Watertown, MA 02471-0317   800-562-6265
                               Fax: 617-972-7444
                    e-mail: napvi@perkins.org
                               www.napvi.org

A unique, informative guide for teachers and educational professionals that work with the visually impaired.
Susan LaVenture, Executive Director

9679 Making Life More Livable: Adaptations for Living at Home After Vision Loss
AFB Press: American Foundation of the Blind
11 Penn Plaza   212-502-7600
New York, NY 10001   800-232-3044
                               Fax: 212-502-7774
                               www.afb.org/store
Essential guide for adults experiencing vision loss and an invaluable resource for their family and friends. Full of practical tips and illustrated by numerous photographs, this easy-to-use resource shows how people who are visually impaired can continue living independent, productive lives at home on their own. Useful general guidelines and room-by-room specifics provide simple and effective solutions for making homes accessible and everyday activities doable for visually impaired individuals.
132 pages Cassette avail.
ISBN: 0-891281-15-0

9680 Occupational Therapy Practice Guidelines for Adults with Low Vision
American Occupational Therapy Association
4720 Montgomery Lane   301-652-2682
Bethesda, MD 20824-1220   Fax: 301-652-7711
                               TDD: 800-377-8555
                               www.aota.org

25 pages
ISBN: 1-569001-50-2

9681 Perkins Activity and Resource Guide: A Handbook for Teachers
Perkins School for the Blind Publications
175 N Beacon Street   617-924-3434
Watertown, MA 02472-2790   Fax: 917-926-2027
This is a comprehensive, two volume guide with over 1,000 pages of activities, resources and instructional strategies for teachers and parents of students with visual and multiple disabilities.

9682 Preschool Learning Activities for the Visually Impaired Child
NAPVI
PO Box 317   617-972-7441
Watertown, MA 02471-0317   800-562-6265
                               Fax: 617-972-7444
                    e-mail: napvi@perkins.org
                               www.napvi.org
This guide for parents offers games and activities to keep visually impaired children active during the preschool years.
Susan LaVenture, Executive Director

9683 Prescriptions for Independence: Working with Older People Who Are Visually Imp.
AFB Press: American Foundation for the Blind
11 Penn Plaza   212-502-7600
New York, NY 10001   800-232-3044
                               Fax: 212-502-7774
                               www.afb.org/store
Easy-to-read manual on how older persons with visual impairments can pursue their interests and activities in community residences, senior centers, long-term care facilities and other community settings. Topics covered include signs of vision loss, recreation, personal care, orientation and mobility and modifications in the environment.
87 pages Paperback
ISBN: 0-891282-44-0

9684 Providing Services for People with Vision Loss: Multidisciplinary Perspective
Resources For Rehabilitation
22 Bonad Road   781-368-9094
Winchester, MA 01890   Fax: 781-368-9096
                    e-mail: info@rfr.org
                               www.rfr.org
A collection of articles by ophthalmologists and rehabilitation professionals, including chapters on operating a low vision service, starting self-help programs, mental health services, aids and techniques that help people with vision loss.
136 pages
ISBN: 0-929718-02-X

9685 Psychoeducational Assessment of Visually Impaired Students
Pro-Ed, Inc.
8700 Shoal Creek Boulevard   512-451-3246
Austin, TX 78757-6897   800-897-3202
Fax: 800-397-7633
e-mail: info@proedinc.com
www.proedinc.com
Professional reference book that addresses the problems specific to assessment of visually impaired children. Of particular value to the practitioner are the extensive reviews of available tests, including ways to adapt those not designed for use with the visually handicapped.
140 pages Paperback
Lindy Jordaan, Marketing Coordinator

9686 Resources Family Centered Intervention for Infants, Toddlers & Preschoolers
Hope
1856 N 1200 E   435-245-2888
North Logan, UT 84341   Fax: 435-245-2888
Describes children with vision impairment in terms of characteristics, needs, and parent concerns.
Hardcover

9687 Show Me How: Manual for Parents Preschool Visually Impaired & Blind Children
AFB Press: American Foundation for the Blind
11 Penn Plaza   212-502-7600
New York, NY 10001   800-232-3044
Fax: 212-502-7774
www.afb.org/store
Practical guide for parents, teachers and others who help preschool children attain age-related goals. Includes activities for growing and learning, building self-concept, moving around, playing, perfecting daily living skills and developing sensory awareness. It also covers such issues as observing safety precautions, choosing appropriate toys and facilitating relationships with playmates.
56 pages Paperback
ISBN: 0-891281-13-4

9688 Starting Points
Blind Children's Center
4120 Marathon Street   213-664-2153
Los Angeles, CA 90029-3584   Fax: 213-665-3828
Basic information for the clasroom teacher of 3 to 8 year olds whose multiple disabilities include visual impairment.
160 pages

9689 Tactile Graphics
AFB Press: American Foundation for the Blind
11 Penn Plaza   212-502-7600
New York, NY 10001   800-232-3044
Fax: 212-502-7774
www.afb.org/store
Easy-to-read encyclopedia handbook on translating visual information into a three-dimensional form that the blind and visually impaired persons can understand. This heavily illustrated guide covers theory, techniques, materials and step-by-step instructions for educators, rehabilitators, graphic artists, museum and busines personnel, employers and anyone involved in producing tactile material for visually impaired persons.
544 pages Paperback
ISBN: 0-891281-94-0

9690 Teachers Who Are Blind or Visually Impaired
AFB Press: American Foundation for the Blind
11 Penn Plaza   212-502-7600
New York, NY 10001   800-232-3044
Fax: 212-502-7774
www.afb.org/store
First volume in the Jobs That Matter series, this book profiles 18 visually impaired individuals who have successfully fulfilled their dreams of becoming teachers. These engaging individuals demonstrate how visually impaired teachers can be effective in their jobs and achieve classroom sucess and satisfaction. Available in paperback, audio cassette or braille.
1998 176 pages
ISBN: 0-891283-06-4

9691 Textbook Catalog
National Braille Association
95 Allens Creek Road 1-202   585-427-8260
Rochester, NY 14618   Fax: 585-427-0263
www.nationalbraille.org
Lists hundreds of scholarly, college and professional textbooks offered in large print, braille or on cassette for visually impaired readers.
80 pages

9692 To Love This Life: Quotations by Helen Keller
AFB Press: American Foundation for the Blind
11 Penn Plaza   212-502-7600
New York, NY 10001   800-232-3044
Fax: 212-502-7774
www.afb.org/store
Beautiful and moving souvenir of one of the world's most admired women. This memorable collection of quotations from Helen Keller brings words of wisdom, courage and inspiration from a remarkable individual who above all wanted to make a difference in the lives of her fellow men and women. The thought captured here — many from unpublished letters and speeches — offer profound statements on the meaning of being human and on life in all its complexity. Available in hardcover and audio cassette.
2000 118 pages
ISBN: 0-891283-47-1

9693 Unseen Minority: Social History of Blindness in the US
Frances A. Koestler, author
David McKay Company/AFB Press, Distributor
11 Penn Plaza   412-741-1398
New York, NY 10001   800-232-3044
Fax: 412-741-0609
e-mail: afborder@abdintl.com
www.afb.org
Lively narrative, peppered with anecdotes, recounts how the blind overcame discrimination to gain full participation in the social, educational, economic and legislative spheres. Here are the gripping stories: Why it took a century for braille to become a universal medium in English, how america's first school for the blind began with a chance encounter on a Boston street, and how the talking book came into existence.
573 pages Hardcover
ISBN: 0-679505-39-3

9694 Vision and Aging: Crossroads for Service Delivery
AFB Press: American Foundation for the Blind
11 Penn Plaza   212-502-7600
New York, NY 10001   800-232-3044
Fax: 212-502-7774
www.afb.org/store
This overview of the service delivery systems in the aging and blindness fields covers the essential issues concerning vision loss among older persons in this country, the growth of visual impairment among the increasing number of elderly people in the US, and the policy and service questions that will demand national attention throughout this and the coming decades.
392 pages Paperback
ISBN: 0-891282-16-5

9695 Visual Aids and Informational Material
National Association for Visually Handicapped
22 W 21st Street   212-889-3141
New York, NY 10010-6904   Fax: 212-727-2931
e-mail: navh@navh.org
www.navh.org
A large reference guide offering a list of visual aids and resources for persons with visual impairments.
65 pages
Lorraine Marchi LHD, Founder/CEO
Cesar Gomez, Executive Director

9696 Visual Handicaps and Learning
Pro-Ed, Inc.
8700 Shoal Creek Boulevard   512-451-3246
Austin, TX 78757-6897   800-897-3202
Fax: 800-397-7633
e-mail: info@proedinc.com
www.proedinc.com

This text covers a range of topics associated with visual impairment, from past practices to up-to-date research, and from legal responsibilities to personal beliefs, without losing sight of the individual child.

180 pages
ISBN: 0-890795-15-0
Lindy Jordaan, Marketing Coordinator

9697   Visual Impairment: An Overview
AFB Press: American Foundation for the Blind
11 Penn Plaza   212-502-7600
New York, NY 10001   800-232-3044
                                       Fax: 212-502-7774
                                         www.afb.org/store

Down-to-earth look at the common forms of vision loss and their impact on the individual. Explains the different aspects of visual impairment, describes adaptive techniques and devices and provides information on available resources and services in a conscise and easy-to-understand manner for professionals and visually impaired people and their families.

56 pages Paperback
ISBN: 0-891281-74-6

9698   Walking Alone and Marching Together
Floyd Matson, author

National Federation of the Blind
1800 Johnson Street   410-659-9314
Baltimore, MD 21230-4998   Fax: 410-685-5653
                       e-mail: subscribe@diabetes.nfb.org
                                              www.nfb.org

The history of the organized blind movement, this book spans more than 50 years of civil rights, social issues, attitudes and experiences of the blind. Published in 1990, it has been read by thousands of blind and sighted persons and is used in colleges, libraries and programs across the country as an important tool in understanding blindness and it's impact on both personal lives and the society at large.

1100 pages
Eileen Ley, Director of Publishing
Elizabeth Lunt, Editor

9699   Webster Large Print Dictionary
Random House
1745 Broadway, 15-3   212-782-9000
New York, NY 10019   800-888-7400
                                        www.randomhouse.com

Ten point type, more than 60,000 word entries and illustrations.

880 pages
ISBN: 0-375722-32-7

9700   What Museum Guides Need to Know: Access for Blind & Visually Impaired Visitors
AFB Press: American Foundation for the Blind
11 Penn Plaza   212-502-7600
New York, NY 10001   800-232-3044
                                       Fax: 212-502-7774
                                         www.afb.org/store

Provides practical, easy-to-use guidelines on how to greet and help blind and visually impaired museum goers. With numerous photographs taken at the High School Museum of Art and the Atlanta Historical Society, this handbook also covers aesthetics and visual impairment, legal requirements for accessibility, resources, a training outline for museum requirements for accessibility, a bibliography on art and museum access for blind and visually impaired persons, and guidelines for preparing media.

64 pages Paperback
ISBN: 0-891281-58-4

Children's Books

9701   Belonging
Dial Books
375 Hudson Street
New York, NY 10014-3658   212-366-2000
                                        www.penguingroup.com

Meg attended special schools for the blind until she was ready for high school. She decided that she wanted to go to a regular high school. She and her mother practiced her walks to school and stud-ied the layout of the building prior to school starting, but Meg was unprepared for the trip when there were 1,500 students. She adjusted quickly to the crowds and the pace of the new school.

200 pages Hardcover
ISBN: 0-803705-30-1

9702   Beside Me
Leader Dogs For The Blind
1039 S. Rochester Road   248-651-9011
Rochester Hills, MI 48307   888-777-5332
                                       Fax: 248-651-5812
                                       TTY: 248-651-3713
                          e-mail: leaderdog@leaderdog.org
                                          www.leaderdog.org

Marion became blind as an adult. She was totally dependent on her parents to move around and go places she wanted to be. Marion decided to go to the leader-dog program and learn to use a leader dog. Particularly she wanted the independence she would need to go to college. Marion enrolled at the Leader-Dog-For-The-Blind Program in Rochester, Michigan. After weeks of training she was given a German Shepherd named Heidi. Marion and Heidi trained together until they were a team and ready.

Films

9703   Guide Dog Goes to School
William Morrow and Company
105 Madison Avenue   212-889-3050
New York, NY 10016-7418   800-843-9389
                          william-morrow-co.1.searchbook.net

Cinderena is a golden retriever. As a puppy Cindy is outgoing and not afraid of things in her environment. This disposition is ideal for a guide dog to the blind, and Cindy is selected to be in a program for guide dogs. Follow Cindy as we focus on the guide dog training.

51 pages Hardcover
ISBN: 0-688068-44-8

9704   How Do You Kiss a Blind Girl?
Charles C Thomas Publisher
2600 S First Street   217-789-8980
Springfield, IL 62704-4730   Fax: 217-789-9130
                             e-mail: books@ccthomas.com
                                          www.ccthomas.com

Focuses, in a humorous way, on the attitudes toward persons with visual impairments.

126 pages
ISBN: 0-398052-62-X

9705   Living with Blindness
Franklin Watts Grolier
90 Old Sherman Tpke   203-797-3500
Danbury, CT 06816-0001   800-621-1115
                                       Fax: 203-797-3197
                                            www.grolier.com

Shows how persons with visual impairments and blindness can overcome their disability and lead productive lives.

32 pages Grades 5-7
ISBN: 0-531108-43-0

9706   Man Who Sang in the Dark
Eth Clifford, author

Houghton, Mifflin & Company
1 Beacon Street   617-725-5000
Boston, MA 02108-3107

The story of a girl and a man who is blind and how they both come to an understanding about certain prejudices.

Grades 3-5

9707   Out of the Corner of My Eye
American Foundation for the Blind
15 W 16th Street   212-502-7600
New York, NY 10011-6301   Fax: 212-502-7777

A personal account of students' vision loss and subsequent adjustment that is full of practical advice and cheerful encouragement, told by an 87 year old retired college teacher who has maintained her independence and zest for life.

ISBN: 0-891281-93-2

9708   She'll Never Walk Alone
Leader Dog For The Blind

1964 Park Street
306-565-8211
Regina, SK, S4P 3G4,
Leader dogs for the blind require many weeks of training before
they are ready to work with the blind individual. Two courses, basic and advanced, are provided for each dog.
Films

Magazines

9709 Access World: Technology and People with Visual Impairments
AFB Press: American Foundation for the Blind
11 Penn Plaza
212-502-7600
New York, NY 10001
800-232-3044
Fax: 212-502-7774
e-mail: afbdirectory@afb.net
www.afb.org/store
Comprehensive and reader friendly online magazine covering every aspect of assistive technology and visual impairment.
Bimonthly

9710 Blind Educator
National Federation of the Blind
1800 Johnson Street
410-659-9314
Baltimore, MD 21230-4998
Fax: 410-685-5653
e-mail: subscribe@diabetes.nfb.org
www.nfb.org
The articles in this newsletter are written by people who are blind.
Blind people can teach. In fact, this newsletter captures a glimpse
of the range of subjects and grade levels in which blind people are
engaged.
Eileen Ley, Director of Publishing
Elizabeth Lunt, Editor

9711 Braille Forum
Penny Reeder, author

American Council of the Blind
1155 15th Street NW
202-467-5081
Washington, DC 20005-2706
800-424-8666
Fax: 202-467-5085
e-mail: info@acb.org
www.acb.org
Offered in large print, braille, half speed cassette, via email and on
the website.
32 pages 10x/year
Sharon Lovering, Editor

9712 Braille Monitor
National Federation of the Blind
1800 Johnson Street
410-659-9314
Baltimore, MD 21230-4998
Fax: 410-685-5653
e-mail: subscribe@diabetes.nfb.org
www.nfb.org
The leading publication in the blindness field, with a circulation of
30,000, this publication addresses issues of concern to the blind
and the philosophy and activities of the National Federation of the
Blind.
100 pages Monthly
Eileen Leyrce, Director of Publishing
Elizabeth Lunt, Editor

9713 Dialogue Magazine
Blindskills
PO Box 5181
503-581-4224
Salem, OR 97304-0181
800-860-4224
Fax: 503-518-0178
e-mail: blindsci@teleport.com
www.teleport.com
Publishes quarterly magazine in braille, large-type, cassette and
disk of news items, fiction and articles of special interest.
Quarterly

9714 Future Reflections
Barbara Cheadler, author

National Federation of the Blind
1800 Johnson Street
410-659-9314
Baltimore, MD 21230-4998
Fax: 410-685-5653
e-mail: subscribe@diabetes.nfb.org
www.nfb.org

National magazine written specifically for parents and educators
of blind children. Each issue addresses various topics important to
blind children, their families and to school personnel.
Quarterly
Eileen Ley, Director of Publishing
Elizabeth Lunt, Editor

9715 Illinois Braille Messenger
Illinois Council of the Blind
PO Box 1336
217-523-4967
Springfield, IL 62705-1336
888-698-1862
Fax: 217-523-4302
e-mail: icb@fgi.net

Quarterly
Laura Booker, Editor

9716 Journal of Vision Rehabilitation
Media Productions & Marketing
2440 O Street
402-474-2676
Lincoln, NE 68510-1125
Multidisciplinary journal containing articles and papers dealing
with low vision, its evaluation, instrumentation and rehabilitation.

9717 Journal of Visual Impairment & Blindness
AFB Press: American Foundation for the Blind
11 Penn Plaza
212-502-7600
New York, NY 10001
800-232-3044
Fax: 212-502-7774
www.afb.org/store

Peer-reviewed journal reporting on the cutting-edge research, innovative practice and news on all aspects of visual impairment.
Available online, on cassette and ASCII disk.
10 Issues

9718 Recorded Periodicals
Associated Services for the Blind
919 Walnut Street
215-627-0600
Philadelphia, PA 19107-5237
Fax: 215-922-0692
e-mail: asbinfo@asb.org
www.asb.org

A subscription service of Associated Services for the Blind, this
service provides 26 recorded magazines for blind and visually impaired individuals.
Audio Cassette
Patricia C Johnson, President/CEO

9719 Review
AER
206 N Washington Street
703-823-9690
Alexandria, VA 22314-2528
Fax: 703-823-9695
The Association's practice-oriented journal.

9720 Tactic
Clovernook Ctr. for the Blind & Visually Impaired
7000 Hamilton Avenue
513-522-3860
Cincinnati, OH 45231-5240
888-224-7156
Fax: 513-728-3946
www.clovernook.org

Quarterly
Jeffrey D Brasie, President

9721 Vision Enhancement Journal
Vision World Wide
5707 Brockton Drive
317-254-1332
Indianapolis, IN 46220-5481
800-733-2258
Fax: 317-251-6588
e-mail: info@visionww.org
www.visionww.org

Leading International publication providing information and resources for people with vision loss. Journal is available in large
print, audio cassette and computer disk.
68-78 pages Quarterly
Patricia Price, President/Managing Editor

9722 Vision World Wide
5707 Brockton Drive
Indianapolis, IN 46220-5481
317-254-1332
800-733-2258
Fax: 317-251-6588
e-mail: info@visionww.org
www.visionww.org

Believing there is hope when vision fails. It disseminates relevant information on a variety of topics through its information and referral helpline, website, e-mail announce list and journal Vision Enhancement, all designed to encourage and support individuals with vision loss, family memebers, professionals who serve them. Aims to enhance everyday living so as to maintain an independent lifestyle. It also serves as a consumer protection against misrepresentation and fraud.
72-78 pages Quarterly
Patricia Price, President/Managing Editor

9723 Voice of the Diabetic
National Federation of the Blind
1800 Johnson Street
Baltimore, MD 21230-4998
410-659-9314
Fax: 410-685-5653
e-mail: subscribe@diabetes.nfb.org
www.nfb.org

The leading publication in the diabetes field. Each issue addresses the problems and concerns of diabetes, with a special emphasis for those who have lost vision due to diabetes. Available in print and on cassette.
30 pages Quarterly
Eileen Ley, Director of Publishing
Elizabeth Lunt, Editor

Newsletters

9724 ACB Reports
American Council of the Blind
1155 15th Street NW
Washington, DC 20005-2706
202-467-5081
800-424-8666
Fax: 202-467-5085
e-mail: info@acb.org
www.acb.org

Radio news feature program for radio information services.
Monthly
Melanie Brunson, Executive Director

9725 AER Report
AER
4600 Duke Street
Alexandria, VA 22304
703-823-9690
877-492-2708
Fax: 703-823-9695
www.aerbvi.org

Contains organizational news, conference dates and information concerning services to visually impaired people.
28 pages BiMonthly
Jackie Fairbarns, Assistant Director

9726 AFB News
American Foundation for the Blind
11 Penn Plaza
New York, NY 10001-2018
212-502-7600
800-232-5463
Fax: 212-502-7777

National newsletter for general readership about blindness and visual impairments featuring people, programs, services and activities.
12 pages Quarterly

9727 Aging and Vision News
National Center for Vision and Aging
800 2nd Avenue
New York, NY 10017
212-808-0077
800-334-5497
3x Year

9728 Awareness
NAPVI
PO Box 317
Watertown, MA 02471-0317
617-972-7441
800-562-6265
Fax: 617-972-7444
e-mail: napvi@perkins.org
www.napvi.org

Newsletter offering regional news, sports and activities, conferences, camps, legislative updates, book reviews, audio reviews, professional question and answer column and more for the visually impaired and their families.
Quarterly
Susan LaVenture, Executive Director

9729 Braille Book Review
National Library Service for the Blind
1291 Taylor Street NW
Washington, DC 20542-0002
202-707-5100
Fax: 202-707-0712
www.loc.gov/nls

New braille books and product news.
BiMonthly

9730 Bulletin
National Association for Visually Handicapped
22 W 21st Street
New York, NY 10010-6904
212-889-3141
Fax: 212-727-2931
e-mail: navh@navh.org
www.navh.org

Annual report offering information on association activities and events, conferences, vision aids and resources for the visually impaired.
Lorraine Marchi LHD, Founder/CEO
Cesar Gomez, Executive Director

9731 DVH Quarterly
University of Arkansas At Little Rock
2801 S University Avenue
Little Rock, AR 72204-1000
501-296-1815
Fax: 501-663-3536

Offers information on upcoming events, conferences and workshops on and for visual disabilities. Book reviews, information on the newest resources and technology, educational programs, want ads and more.
Quarterly
Bob Brasher, Editor

9732 Eye Research News
645 Madison Avenue
New York, NY 10022-1010
212-752-4333
800-621-0026
Fax: 212-688-6231
e-mail: inforequest@rpbusa.org
www.rpbusa.org

Newsletter on the latest development in eye research
Annual
David Weeks, Chairman
Diane S Swift, President

9733 Focus
Visually Impaired Center
1422 West Court Street
Flint, MI 48503
810-767-4014
Fax: 810-767-0020
e-mail: info@vicflint.org
www.vicflint.org

Newsletter offering information for the visually impaired person in the forms of legislative and law updates, ADA information, support groups, hotlines, and articles on the newest technology in the field.
Quarterly
Laurie MacArthur, Executive Director

9734 Gleams Newsletter
Glaucoma Research Foundation
251 Post Street
San Francisco, CA 94108
415-986-3162
800-826-6693
Fax: 415-986-3763
e-mail: question@glaucoma.org
www.glaucoma.org

It includes information about glaucoma, new treatments, updates on research findings, and more.
3x/year
Thomas M Brunner, President/CEO
Andrew Jackson, Director Communications

9735 Guide Dog Foundation for the Blind Newsletter
371 E Jericho Turnpike
Smithtown, NY 11787-2976
631-265-2121
800-548-4337
Fax: 631-361-5192
e-mail: info@guidedog.org
www.guidedog.org

This organization relies on voluntary public contributions to provide persons with blindness the gift of second sight through the eyes of a guide dog. This nonprofit organization furnishes guide dogs, free of charge, to qualified people who seek independence, mobility and companionship.
Wells B Jones CAE CFRE, CEO
Michelle Lavitt, Marketing Manager

9736 Guide Dog News
Guide Dogs for the Blind
PO Box 151200
San Rafael, CA 94915
415-499-4000
800-298-4050
Fax: 415-499-4035
e-mail: information@guidedogs.com
www.guidedogs.com

About graduates, volunteers and donors of Guide Dogs for the Blind.
Quarterly
Etta Allen, Board Chair
Morgan Watkins, Interim CEO

9737 Guideway
Guide Dog Foundation for the Blind
371 E Jericho Turnpike
Smithtown, NY 11787-2976
631-265-2121
800-548-4337
Fax: 631-361-5192
e-mail: info@guidedog.org
www.guidedog.org

Offers updates and information on the foundation's activities and guide dog programs. In print form but is also available on cassette.
6 pages Monthly
Wells B Jones CAE CFRE, CEO
Michelle Lavitt, Marketing Manager

9738 Hearsay
Radio Information Service
600 Forbes Avenue
Pittsburgh, PA 15282
412-488-3944
Fax: 412-488-3953
e-mail: info@readingservice.org
www.readingservice.org

Newsletter for persons interested in radio reading services.
Quarterly

9739 Hub
SPOKES Unlimited
415 Main Street
Klamath Falls, OR 97601
541-883-7547
Fax: 541-885-2469
www.spokesunlimited.org

Newsletter on rehabilitation, peer counseling, blindness, visual impairments, information and referral.
Meg Graf, Resource Librarian

9740 InSight
Foundation Fighting Blindness
11435 Cronhill Drive
Owings Mill, MD 21117-2220
410-568-0150
800-683-5555
Fax: 410-363-2393
TDD: 410-363-7139
e-mail: info@fightblindness.org
www.fightblindness.org

The Foundation Fighting Blindness newsletter, delivered to members monthly. The major emphasis is to report on research and science news, and FDA approved clinical trials around retinal degenerative diseases.
20 pages 3 per year
William T. Schmidt, CEO

9741 Lion
Lions Clubs International
300 W 22nd Street
Oak Brook, IL 60523-8815
312-571-5466

Publication for the blind.

9742 Listen Up
Recording for the Blind & Dyslexic (RFB&D)
20 Roszel Road
Princeton, NJ 08540-6294
609-452-0606
800-221-4792
Fax: 609-987-8116
e-mail: custserv@rfbd.org
www.rfbd.org

RFB&D's bi-monthly newsletter for members.

9743 Long Cane News
American Foundation for the Blind
15 W 16th Street
New York, NY 10011-6301
212-502-7600
800-232-5463
Fax: 212-502-7777

Semiannual

9744 Musical Mainstream
National Library Service for the Blind
1291 Taylor Street NW
Washington, DC 20542-0002
202-707-5100
Fax: 202-707-0712

Articles selected from print music magazines.
Quarterly

9745 NAVH UPDATE
National Association for Visually Handicapped
22 W 21st Street
New York, NY 10010-6904
212-889-3141
Fax: 212-727-2931
e-mail: navh@navh.org
www.navh.org

This newsletter offers vision news, medical updates, assistive device information, resources and more for the visually impaired.
4 pages Quarterly
Lorraine Marchi LHD, Founder/CEO
Cesar Gomez, Executive Director

9746 NLS News
National Library Service for the Blind
1291 Taylor Street NW
Washington, DC 20542-0002
202-707-5100
Fax: 202-707-0712

Newsletter on current program developments.
Quarterly

9747 NLS Update
National Library Service for the Blind
1291 Taylor Street NW
Washington, DC 20542-0002
202-707-5100
Fax: 202-707-0712

Newsletter on the services volunteer activities.
Quarterly

9748 NOAH News
National Organization for Albinism
PO Box 959
E. Hampsted, NH 03826-0959
603-887-2310
800-473-2310
Fax: 603-887-2310
www.albinism.org

BiAnnually

9749 Newsline for the Blind
National Federation of the Blind
1800 Johnson Street
Baltimore, MD 21230-4998
410-659-9314
Fax: 410-685-5653
e-mail: subscribe@diabetes.nfb.org
www.nfb.org

Nation's only digital talking newspaper service for the blind. Allows the blind to read the full text of leading national and local newspapers by using a touch-tone telephone. Service is free of charge and available 24 hours a day, 7 days per week.
Eileen Ley, Director of Publishing
Elizabeth Lunt, Editor

9750 Open Windows
Sunday School Board of the Southern Baptists
127 9th Avenue N
Nashville, TN 37234-0001
800-458-2772

Guide for personal devotions on audio cassette tape, using Bible references, devotional readings, and prayer calendar of popular Open Windows devotional guide for visually handicapped adults.
Quarterly

9751 Personal Reader Update
Personal Reader Department
9 Centennial Drive   978-977-2000
Peabody, MA 01960-7906   800-343-0311
                                     Fax: 978-977-2437
Offers information on new services, assistive devices and technology for the blind.

9752 Prevent Blindness America News
Prevent Blindness America
211 West Wacker Drive, Suite 1700   847-843-2020
Chicago, IL 60606   800-331-2020
                                     www.preventblindness.org
Offers information and articles on eye safety, programs, and services of the Society.
Quarterly

9753 RP Messenger
Texas Association of Retinitis Pigmentosa
PO Box 8388   361-852-8515
Corpus Christi, TX 78468-8388   Fax: 361-852-8515
A bi-annual newsletter offering information on Retinitis Pigmentosa.
BiAnnual

9754 Raised Dot Computing Newsletter
Raised Dot Computing
211 S Paterson Street   608-257-9595
Madison, WI 53703-3789
Discusses braille computer techniques and devices for blind persons.

9755 SCENE
Braille Institute
741 N Vermont Avenue   213-663-1111
Los Angeles, CA 90029-3594   800-272-4553
                                     www.brailleinstitute.org
Offers information on the organization, question and answer column, articles on the newest technology and more for visually impaired persons.
Paul J Porelli, Managing Editor

9756 Smith-Kettlewell Technical File
Smith-Kettlewell Eye Research Foundation
2232 Webster Street   415-561-1619
San Francisco, CA 94115-1821   Fax: 415-561-1610
Quarterly

9757 Student Advocate
National Alliance of Blind Students
1155 15th Street NW, Suite 1004   202-467-5081
Washington, DC 20005   800-424-8666
                            e-mail: president@acbstudents.org
                                     www.acbstudents.org
A communication forum covering issues of concern to postsecondary students who are blind.

Cammie Vloedman, President
Olivia Norman, First Vice President

9758 Talking Book Topics
National Library Services For The Blind
1291 Taylor Street NW   202-707-5100
Washington, DC 20542-0002   Fax: 202-707-0712
Offers hundreds of listings of books, fiction and nonfiction, for adults and children on cassette. Also offers listings on foreign language books on cassette, talking magazines and reviews.
Bimonthly

9759 Tarheel Talk
North Carolina Library for the Blind

1841 Capital Boulevard   919-733-4376
Raleigh, NC 27635   888-388-2460
                                     Fax: 919-733-6910
                                     TDD: 919-733-1462
                                e-mail: nclbph@ncdcr.gov
                                  statelibrary.ncdcr.gov/lbph
Quarterly
Carl Keehn, Director

9760 The Macula Foundation Manhattan Eye, Ear & Throat Hospital
American Macular Degeneration Foundation
8th Floor 210 East 64th St.   212-605-3777
New York, NY 10021-0515   Fax: 212-605-3795
                        e-mail: foundation@retinal-research.org
                                  www.macular.org/spotlite.html
Newsletter of the American Macular Degeneration Foundation, a nationwide support group for individuals and their families to adjust to the restrictions and changes brought about by macular disease.
Quarterly
Nikolai Stevenson, President
Walter Ross, VP

9761 The Pioneer Projects and Programs Periodic al
TelecomPioneers
930 15th St. 12th Floor
Denver, CO 80202   303-571-1200
                                  www.pioneersvolunteer.org
Monthly

9762 Viva Vital News
5016 Silk Oak Drive   941-371-2153
Sarasota, FL 34232-5410
Membership service organization offering information for veterans and is an affiliate of the American Council of the Blind.

9763 Voice of Vision
GW Micro
310 Racquet Drive   219-483-3625
Fort Wayne, IN 46825-4229   Fax: 219-489-2608
                            e-mail: webmaster@gwmicro.com
                                     www.gwmicro.com
Offers product reviews, product announcements, tips for making systems or applications more accessible, or explanations of concepts of interest to any computer user or would-be computer user. This association newsletter is available in braille, in large print, on audio cassette and on 3.5 or 5.25 IBM format diskette.
Quarterly

9764 What's Line
Alabama Regional Library for the Blind
6030 Monticello Drive   334-213-3906
Montgomery, AL 36130-6000   800-392-5671
                                     Fax: 334-213-3993
                            e-mail: fzaleski@apls.state.al.us
                                  http://statelibrary.alabama.gov
Informational 4 page newsletter in large print. Also available in braille and e-text formats.
4 pages Quarterly
Fara Zaleski, Division
Rebecca Mitchell, Director

Pamphlets

9765 About Children's Vision: Guide for Parents
National Association for Visually Handicapped
22 W 21st Street   212-889-3141
New York, NY 10010-6904   Fax: 212-727-2931
                                  e-mail: navh@navh.org
                                     www.navh.org
Offers a better understanding of the normal and possible abnormal development of a childs eyesight.
Lorraine Marchi LHD, Founder/CEO
Cesar Gomez, Executive Director

9766 Age Related Macular Degeneration
National Association for Visually Handicapped

22 W 21st Street
New York, NY 10010-6904

212-889-3141
Fax: 212-727-2931
e-mail: navh@navh.org
www.navh.org

Describes various conditions which affect the macular area and how to best maximize the use of residual peripheral vision.
Lorraine Marchi LHD, Founder/CEO
Cesar Gomez, Executive Director

9767   Are You Looking for a Few Good Workers?
AFB Press: American Foundation for the Blind
11 Penn Plaza
New York, NY 10001

212-502-7600
800-232-3044
Fax: 212-502-7774
www.afb.org/store

Helpful pamphlet explores both the importance and the advantage of hiring workers who are blind or visually impaired. Designed for human resource and other professionals responsible for hiring, it answers critical questions about hiring blind or visually impaired applicants. This enlightening guide to employment practices relating to these individuals offers insights on interviewing, job performance, tax incentives for businesses, insurance issues and more.
7 pages Pack of 20
ISBN: 0-891283-60-9

9768   BVA Bulletin
Blinded Veterans Association
477 H Street NW
Washington, DC 20001-2694

202-371-8880
800-669-7079
Fax: 202-371-8258
e-mail: bva@bva.org
www.bva.org

The Bulletin informs blinded veterans, their families, and those of the general public with an interest in BVA issues, about the organization. The publication includes current information relating to technology for the blind, legislation affecting blinded veterans, and news about the people who have overcome the challenges of blindness and are doing amazing work in their lives.
32 pages Quarterly
Thomas Miller, Executive Director
Stuart Nelson, Coordinator Public Relations

9769   Books are Fun for Everyone
National Library Service for the Blind
1291 Taylor Street NW
Washington, DC 20542

202-707-5100
Fax: 202-707-0712

9770   Braille Alphabet and Numbers
AFB Press: American Foundation for the Blind
11 Penn Plaza
New York, NY 10001

212-502-7600
800-232-3044
Fax: 212-502-7774
www.afb.org/store

Embossed with the braille alphabet and numbers, this 9 x 4 inch display card includes an explanation of braille and a short history of its development.
Pack of 25
ISBN: 0-891281-98-3

9771   Braille Literacy: Blind Persons, Families, Prof. & Producers of Braille
AFB Press: American Foundation for the Blind
11 Penn Plaza
New York, NY 10001

212-502-7600
800-232-3044
Fax: 212-502-7774
www.afb.org/store

Vigorous defece of the use of braille and an explanation of the importance of positive attitudes toward it that states: Braille is an assertion of equality between blind and sighted persons with respect to written communication. For everyone who uses or teaches braille and is interested in its future.
12 pages Pack of 25
ISBN: 0-891289-28-3

9772   Braille: An Extraordinary Volunteer Opportunity
National Library Service for the Blind
1291 Taylor Street NW
Washington, DC 20542-0002

202-707-5100
Fax: 202-707-0712

9773   Cataracts
National Eye Institute, Information Office

31 Center Drive MSC 2510
Bethesda, MD 20892-2510

301-496-5248
e-mail: 2020@nei.nih.gov
www.nei.nih.gov

Provides information about this common condition and its treatment.

9774   Classification of Impaired Vision
National Association for Visually Handicapped
22 W 21st Street
New York, NY 10010-6904

212-889-3141
Fax: 212-727-2931
e-mail: navh@navh.org
www.navh.org

Describes various degrees of impaired vision.
Lorraine Marchi LHD, Founder/CEO
Cesar Gomez, Executive Director

9775   Communicating with People Who Have Trouble Hearing & Seeing: A Primer
National Association for Visually Handicapped
22 W 21st Street
New York, NY 10010-6904

212-889-3141
Fax: 212-727-2931
e-mail: navh@navh.org
www.navh.org

Line drawings that depict problems for those with both deficiencies.
Lorraine Marchi LHD, Founder/CEO
Cesar Gomez, Executive Director

9776   Dancing Cheek to Cheek
Blind Children's Center
4120 Marathon Street
Los Angeles, CA 90029-3584

213-664-2153
Fax: 213-665-3828

Discusses beginning social, play and language interactions.
33 pages

9777   Diabetes, Vision Impairment and Blindness
AFB Press: American Foundation for the Blind
11 Penn Plaza
New York, NY 10001

212-502-7600
800-232-3044
Fax: 212-502-7777
www.afb.org/store

Presentation of how chronic diabetes affects vision and how diabetes can be managed at home by blind and visually impaired individuals.
32 pages
ISBN: 0-891289-02-0

9778   Diabetic Retinopathy
National Association for Visually Handicapped
22 W 21st Street
New York, NY 10010-6904

212-889-3141
Fax: 212-727-2931
e-mail: navh@navh.org
www.navh.org

Describes types of this disease and methods of treatment.
Lorraine Marchi LHD, Founder/CEO
Cesar Gomez, Executive Director

9779   Directory of Radio Reading Services
Radio Information Service
600 Forbes Avenue
Pittsburgh, PA 15282

412-488-3944
Fax: 412-488-3953
e-mail: info@readingservice.org
www.readingservice.org

Annually

9780   Don't Lose Sight of Age-Related Macular Degeneration
National Eye Institute, Information Office
31 Center Drive MSC 2510
Bethesda, MD 20892-2510

301-496-5248
e-mail: 2020@nei.nih.gov
www.nei.nih.gov

9781   Don't Lose Sight of Cataracts
National Eye Institute, Information Office
31 Center Drive MSC 2510
Bethesda, MD 20892-2510

301-496-5248
e-mail: 2020@nei.nih.gov
www.nei.nih.gov

9782   Don't Lose Sight of Glaucoma
National Eye Institute, Information Office

31 Center Drive MSC 2510   301-496-5248
Bethesda, MD 20892-2510   e-mail: 2020@nei.nih.gov
www.nei.nih.gov

9783   **Eye-Q Test**
National Association for Visually Handicapped
22 W 21st Street   212-889-3141
New York, NY 10010-6904   Fax: 212-727-2931
e-mail: navh@navh.org
www.navh.org
Five questions and answers to assist in knowing more about vision.
Lorraine Marchi LHD, Founder/CEO
Cesar Gomez, Executive Director

9784   **Facts: Books for Blind and Physically Handicapped Individuals**
National Library Service for the Blind
1291 Taylor Street NW   202-707-5100
Washington, DC 20542-0002   Fax: 202-707-0712
www.loc.gov
Annual

9785   **Facts: Music for Blind and Physically Handicapped Individuals**
National Library Service for the Blind
1291 Taylor Street NW   202-707-5100
Washington, DC 20542-0002   Fax: 202-707-0712
www.loc.gov
Annual

9786   **Facts: Playback Machines and Accessories Provided on Free Loan**
National Library Service for the Blind
1291 Taylor Street NW   202-707-5100
Washington, DC 20542-0002   Fax: 202-707-0712
www.loc.gov

9787   **Facts: Sources for Purchase of Cassette & Disc Players From NLS**
National Library Service for the Blind
1291 Taylor Street NW   202-707-5100
Washington, DC 20542-0002   Fax: 202-707-0712
www.lov.gov

9788   **Family Guide to Vision Care**
American Optometric Association
243 N Lindbergh Boulevard   314-991-4100
Saint Louis, MO 63141-7881   Fax: 314-991-4101
www.aoanet.org
Offers information on the early developmental years of your vision, finding a family optometrist and how to take care of your eyesight through the learning years, the working years and the mature years.

9789   **Family Guide: Growth & Development of the Partially Seeing Child**
National Association for Visually Handicapped
22 W 21st Street   212-889-3141
New York, NY 10010-6904   Fax: 212-727-2931
e-mail: navh@navh.org
www.navh.org
Offers information for parents and guidelines in raising a partially seeing child.
Lorraine Marchi LHD, Founder/CEO
Cesar Gomez, Executive Director

9790   **General Facts and Figures on Blindness**
National Society to Prevent Blindness
500 Remington Road
Schaumburg, IL 60173-5624   800-331-2020

9791   **General Interest Catalog**
National Braille Association
3 Townline Circle   716-427-8260
Rochester, NY 14623-2537
Lists hundreds of titles of fiction and non-fiction books offered in large print, braille or on cassette to visually impaired readers.
19 pages

9792   **Glaucoma**
Foundation For Glaucoma Research
490 Post Street   415-986-3162
San Francisco, CA 94102-1409

Offers information on what glaucoma is, the causes, treatments, types of glaucoma, eye exams and prevention.

9793   **Glaucoma: Sneak Thief of Sight**
National Association for Visually Handicapped
22 W 21st Street   212-889-3141
New York, NY 10010-6904   Fax: 212-727-2931
e-mail: navh@navh.org
www.navh.org
A pamphlet describing the disease, treatment and medications.
Lorraine Marchi LHD, Founder/CEO
Cesar Gomez, Executive Director

9794   **Guide Dog Foundation Flyer**
Guide Dog Foundation for the Blind
371 E Jericho Turnpike   631-265-2121
Smithtown, NY 11787-2976   800-548-4337
Fax: 631-361-5192
e-mail: info@guidedog.org
www.guidedog.org
Offers information on the programs and services provided by the foundation.
Wells B Jones CAE CFRE, CEO
Michelle Lavitt, Marketing Manager

9795   **Guidelines for Comprehensive Low Vision Care**
National Association for Visually Handicapped
22 W 21st Street   212-889-3141
New York, NY 10010-6904   Fax: 212-727-2931
e-mail: navh@navh.org
www.navh.org
A description of the proper method to conduct a low vision evaluation.
Lorraine Marchi LHD, Founder/CEO
Cesar Gomez, Executive Director

9796   **Guidelines for Helping Deaf/Blind Persons**
Helen Keller National Center for Deaf/Blind
111 Middle Neck Road   516-944-8900
Sands Point, NY 11050-1299   Fax: 516-944-7302
TTY: 516-944-8637
e-mail: hkncinfo@rcn.com
www.hknc.org
Pamphlet offering information on how persons should interact with deaf/blind individuals. Includes drawings of the one hand manual alphabet.
Joseph McNulty, Executive Director

9797   **Heart to Heart**
Blind Children's Center
4120 Marathon Street   213-664-2153
Los Angeles, CA 90029-3584   Fax: 213-665-3828
Parents of blind and partially sighted children talk about their feelings.
12 pages

9798   **Heartbreak of Being a Little Bit Blind**
National Association for Visually Handicapped
22 W 21st Street   212-889-3141
New York, NY 10010-6904   Fax: 212-727-2931
e-mail: nvah@navh.org
www.navh.org
Summary of what it means to have impaired vision with illustrations. Free for members.
Lorraine Marchi LHD, Founder/CEO
Cesar Gomez, Executive Director

9799   **Helen Keller**
AFB Press: American Foundation for the Blind
11 Penn Plaza   212-502-7600
New York, NY 10001   800-232-3044
Fax: 212-502-7774
www.afb.org/store
Brief biography that focuses on the major events of Helen Keller's life, from her birth in Tuscumbia, Alabama on June 27, 1880 to her death in Connecticut on June 1, 1968.
6 pages Pack of 25
ISBN: 0-891282-03-3

9800   **How Does a Blind Person Get Around?**
AFB Press: American Foundation for the Blind

11 Penn Plaza   212-502-7600
New York, NY 10001   800-232-3044
     Fax: 212-502-7774
     www.afb.org/store
Offers information on daily living as a blind person.

9801 How to Develop a Self-Help Group for Elders Losing Eyesight
National Association for Visually Handicapped
22 W 21st Street   212-889-3141
New York, NY 10010-6904   Fax: 212-727-2931
     e-mail: navh@navh.org
     www.navh.org
The pioneer for development of self-help groups, using the NAVH model, this publication is designed to help start and facilitate self-help groups.
Lorraine Marchi LHD, Founder/CEO
Cesar Gomez, Executive Director

9802 How to Use Your Low Vision Glasses
National Association for Visually Handicapped
22 W 21st Street   212-889-3141
New York, NY 10010-6904   Fax: 212-727-2931
     e-mail: navh@navh.org
     www.navh.org
A line drawing showing the correct way to benefit from low vision glasses.
Lorraine Marchi LHD, Founder/CEO
Cesar Gomez, Executive Director

9803 Information on Glaucoma
Foundation for Glaucoma Research
490 Post Street   415-986-3162
San Francisco, CA 94102-1409

9804 Information on Macular Degeneration
American Council of the Blind
1155 15th Street NW   202-467-5081
Washington, DC 20005-2706   800-424-8666
     Fax: 202-467-5085
     e-mail: info@acb.org
     www.acb.org
Melanie Brunson, Executive Director

9805 It's All Right to Be Angry
National Association for Visually Handicapped
22 W 21st Street   212-889-3141
New York, NY 10010-6904   Fax: 212-727-2931
     e-mail: navh@navh.org
     www.navh.org
A helpful pamphlet describing reactions to learning to live with vision impairment.
Lorraine Marchi LHD, Founder/CEO
Cesar Gomez, Executive Director

9806 Large Print Loan Library Catalog
National Association for Visually Handicapped
22 W 21st Street   212-889-3141
New York, NY 10010-6904   Fax: 212-727-2931
     e-mail: navh@navh.org
     www.navh.org
Listing of over 9,000 commercially published and NAVH large print books available through NAVH on a loan basis. Includes a limited selection of titles available for purchase.
Lorraine Marchi LHD, Founder/CEO
Cesar Gomez, Executive Director

9807 Learning to Play
Blind Children's Center
4120 Marathon Street   213-664-2153
Los Angeles, CA 90029-3584   Fax: 213-665-3828
Discusses how to present play activities to the visually impaired preschool child.
12 pages

9808 Let's Eat
Blind Children's Center
4120 Marathon Street   213-664-2153
Los Angeles, CA 90029-3584   Fax: 213-665-3828
Teaches competent feeding skills to children with visual impairments.
28 pages

9809 Low Vision Questions and Answers
AFB Press: American Foundation for the Blind
11 Penn Plaza   212-502-7600
New York, NY 10001   800-232-3044
     Fax: 212-502-7774
     www.afb.org/store
What does low vision mean? What do low vision services cost? What diseases cause low vision? Answers to these and other questions are presented in a straightforward yet comprehensive format. Photographs show how objects appear to people with low vision, what low vision devices look like, and how they are used.
21 pages Pack of 25
ISBN: 0-891281-96-7

9810 Magnifier
Macular Degeneration Foundation
PO Box 9752   408-260-1335
San Jose, CA 95157-0752   888-633-3937
     www.eyesight.org
Large-font publication.

9811 Magnifier Highlights
Independent Living Aids
200 Robbins Lane
Jericho, NY 11753-2341   800-537-2118
     Fax: 516-752-3135
     e-mail: indlivaids@aol.com
     www.independentliving.com
Full line of magnifiers, ranging from high-powered vision aids to instruments and accessories
Marvin Sandler, President

9812 Move with Me
Blind Children's Center
4120 Marathon Street   213-664-2153
Los Angeles, CA 90029-3584   Fax: 213-665-3828
A parent's guide to movement development for visually impaired babies.
12 pages

9813 Music Is for Everyone
National Library Service for the Blind
1291 Taylor Street NW   202-707-5100
Washington, DC 20542-0002   Fax: 202-707-0712

9814 Parenting Preschoolers: Raising Young Blind & Visually Impaired Child
AFB Press: American Foundation for the Blind
11 Penn Plaza   212-502-7600
New York, NY 10001   800-232-3044
     Fax: 212-502-7774
     www.afb.org/store
Why is my baby so quiet? Why does my child seem slower than other children? What will happen when my child goes to school? This primer provides practical answers to the questions most freqently asked by parents and gives advice on what to expect, how to adapt to the child's situation and needs, and what to look for in early education programs.
28 pages Pack of 25
ISBN: 0-891289-98-4

9815 Patient's Guide to Visual Aids and Illumination
National Association for Visually Handicapped
22 W 21st Street   212-889-3141
New York, NY 10010-6904   Fax: 212-727-2931
     e-mail: navh@navh.org
     www.navh.org
A reference booklet offering information on aids for the visually impaired.
Lorraine Marchi LHD, Founder/CEO
Cesar Gomez, Executive Director

9816 Puppy Walker Brochure
Guide Dog Foundation for the Blind
371 E Jericho Turnpike   631-265-2121
Smithtown, NY 11787-2976   800-548-4337
     Fax: 631-361-5192
     e-mail: info@guidedog.org
     www.guidedog.org

Offers information on being a volunteer puppy walker family.
Wells B Jones CAE CFRE, CEO
Michelle Lavitt, Marketing Manager

9817   Reaching, Crawling, Walking-Let's Get Moving
Blind Children's Center
4120 Marathon Street   213-664-2153
Los Angeles, CA 90029-3584   Fax: 213-665-3828
Orientation and mobility for visually impaired preschool children.
24 pages

9818   Reading is for Everyone
National Library Service for the Blind
1291 Taylor Street NW   202-707-5100
Washington, DC 20542-0002   Fax: 202-707-0712

9819   Reading with Low Vision
National Library Service for the Blind
1291 Taylor Street NW   202-707-5100
Washington, DC 20542-0002   Fax: 202-707-0712

9820   Reference and Information Services from NLS
National Library Service for the Blind
1291 Taylor Street NW   202-707-5100
Washington, DC 20542-0002   Fax: 202-707-0712

9821   Resource List for Persons with Low Vision
American Council of the Blind
1155 15th Street NW   202-467-5081
Washington, DC 20005-2706   800-424-8666
                                                    Fax: 202-467-5085
                                                 e-mail: info@acb.org
                                                       www.acb.org

Melanie Brunson, Executive Director

9822   Seeing Eye to Eye: An Administrator's Guide
AFB Press: American Foundation for the Blind
11 Penn Plaza   212-502-7600
New York, NY 10001   800-232-3044
                                                    Fax: 212-502-7774
                                                    www.afb.org/store
Visual impairment often has a profound impact on a child's ability
to learn language and basic communication concepts. This
easy-to-read booklet explains the student's needs and the practical
services essential for helping them become literate and successful.
An ideal tool for administrators and educators, it includes clear explanations of common terminology, the impact of visual impairment on learning, specialized services for visually impaired
students, and in-service training for teachers.
72 pages Pack of 10
ISBN: 0-891283-59-5

9823   Selecting a Program
Blind Children's Center
4120 Marathon Street   213-664-2153
Los Angeles, CA 90029-3584   Fax: 213-665-3828
A guide for parents of infants and preschoolers with visual impairments.
28 pages

9824   Standing on My Own Two Feet
Blind Children's Center
4120 Marathon Street   213-664-2153
Los Angeles, CA 90029-3584   Fax: 213-665-3828
A step-by-step guide to designing and constructing simple, individually tailored adaptive mobility devices for preschool-age children who are visually impaired.
36 pages

9825   Talk to Me
Blind Children's Center
4120 Marathon Street   213-664-2153
Los Angeles, CA 90029-3584   Fax: 213-665-3828
A language guide for parents of deaf children.
11 pages

9826   Talk to Me II
Blind Children's Center
4120 Marathon Street   213-664-2153
Los Angeles, CA 90029-3584   Fax: 213-665-3828

A sequel to Talk To Me, available in English and Spanish.
15 pages

9827   Talking Books for Senior Adults
National Library Service for the Blind
1291 Taylor Street NW   202-707-5100
Washington, DC 20542-0002   Fax: 202-707-0712

9828   Touch the Baby: Blind & Visually Impaired Children as Patients
American Foundation for the Blind
11 Penn Plaza   212-502-7600
New York, NY 10001-2018   800-232-3044
                                                    Fax: 212-502-7774
                                                    www.afb.org/store
How-to manual for health care professionals working in hospitals,
clinics and doctors' offices that teaches the special communication
and touch-related techniques needed to prevent blind and visually
impaired patients from withdrawing from healthcare staff and the
outside world. includes how to talk to infants and how to signal to
children that a procedure may cause discomfort.
13 pages Pack of 25
ISBN: 0-891281-97-5

9829   Volunteer at Your Braille and Talking Book Library
National Library Service for the Blind
1291 Taylor Street NW   202-707-5100
Washington, DC 20542-0002   Fax: 202-707-0712
Brochure

9830   What Do You Do When You See a Blind Person — and What Don't You Do?
AFB Press: American Foundation for the Blind
11 Penn Plaza   212-502-7600
New York, NY 10001   800-232-3044
                                                    Fax: 212-502-7774
                                                    www.afb.org/store
Examples of real-life situations that teach sighted persons how to
interact effectively with blind persons. Topics covered include
how to help someone across the street, how not to distract a guide
dog and how to take leave of a blind person.
8 pages Pack of 25
ISBN: 0-891281-95-9

9831   Wings for the Future
American Printing House for the Blind
1839 Frankfort Avenue   502-895-2405
Louisville, KY 40206-3148   800-223-1839
                                                    Fax: 502-895-1509
                                                 e-mail: info@ahp.org
This booklet offers an introduction to the American Printing
House For The Blind's programs, services, tools, aids and more.
13 pages

9832   Without Sight and Sound
Helen Keller National Center for Deaf/Blind
111 Middle Neck Road   516-944-8900
Sands Point, NY 11050-1299   Fax: 516-944-7302
                                                    TTY: 516-944-8637
                                              e-mail: hkncinfo@rcn.com
                                                       www.hknc.org
Pamphlet offering facts, causes, types and descriptions of
deaf/blindness.
Joseph McNulty, Executive Director

9833   You Seem Like a Regular Kid to Me
AFB Press: American Foundation for the Blind
11 Penn Plaza   212-502-7600
New York, NY 10001   800-232-3044
                                                    Fax: 212-502-7774
                                                    www.afb.org/store
An interview with Jane, a blind child, allows other children to understand what it's like to be blind. Jane explains how she gets
around, takes care of herself, does her school work, spends her leisure time and even pays for things when she can't see money. Photographs show Jane engaged in various activities.
16 pages Pack of 25
ISBN: 0-891289-21-6

Audio & Video

9834 Adult Bible Study
Sunday School Board of the Southern Baptists
127 9th Avenue N
Nashville, TN 37234-0001   800-458-2772
Unabridged Sunday School lessons recorded on audio cassette as printed in Adult Bible Study.
Quarterly

9835 Aging and Vision: Declarations of Independence
AFB Press: American Foundation for the Blind
11 Penn Plaza   212-502-7600
New York, NY 10001   800-232-3044
                                     Fax: 212-502-7774
                                       www.afb.org/store
Very personal look at five older people who have successfully coped with visual impairment and continue to lead active, satisfying lives. Their stories are not only inspirational, they also provide paractical, down-to-earth suggestions for adapting to vision loss later in life.
18 Minutes VHS
ISBN: 0-891282-20-3

9836 Bible Alliance
PO Box 621   941-748-3031
Bradenton, FL 34206-0621   e-mail: aurora@auroraministries.org
                                     www.careministries.org
Offers the Christian bible on cassettes in over 52 languages for those finding it impossible to read small print.

9837 Blindness: A Family Matter
AFB Press: American Foundation for the Blind
11 Penn Plaza   212-502-7600
New York, NY 10001   800-232-3044
                                     Fax: 212-502-7774
                                       www.afb.org/store
Frank exploration of the effects of an individual's visual impairment on other members of the family and how family members can play a positive role in the rehabltation process. Features three families whose success stories provide advice and encouragement, as well as interviews with newly blinded adults currently involved in a rehabilitation program. Also available in PAL.
23 Minutes VHS
ISBN: 0-891282-22-X

9838 Braille Documents
Metrolina Sight Services
704 Louise Avenue   704-372-3870
Charlotte, NC 28204-2128   e-mail: braille@charlotte.infi.net
                                       www.careministries.org
This production shop creates Braille and large-print documents.

9839 Brief Encounters of the Right Kind: How to Make Your Point in 10 Minutes or Less
AFB Press: American Foundation for the Blind
11 Penn Plaza   212-502-7600
New York, NY 10001   800-232-3044
                                     Fax: 212-502-7774
                                       www.afb.org/store
Humorous and instructional tour through the do's and don'ts of lobbying at the local, state and national levels. Three seasoned lobbyists discuss how professionals, families, consumers and volunteer advocates can use their expert knowledge to influence public policy. A Toolkit for Advocates, the accompanying manual, complements the video by providing a summary of the legislative process and key points on how to meet successfully with legislators.
VHS & PAL
ISBN: 0-891282-83-1

9840 Destination Unlimited
Leader Dog For The Blind
1964 Park Street   306-565-8211
Regina, SK, S4P 3G4,
This is a documentary about Leader-Dog-For-The-Blind Program. The needs of various people and how their dog fulfills their needs are shown. In addition, the overall leader-dog program is reviewed. This training program would be of interest to many teenagers.
Films

9841 Employed Ability: Blind Persons on the Job
AFB Press: American Foundation for the Blind
11 Penn Plaza   212-502-7600
New York, NY 10001   800-232-3044
                                     Fax: 212-502-7774
                                       www.afb.org/store
Blind and visually impaired people from a wide variety of occupations talk about career opportunities and their experiences in the workplace. Employers and coworkers are also interviewed and speak openly about supervising and working alongside visually impaired employees.
14 Minutes VHS
ISBN: 0-891282-24-6

9842 Focused On: Importance and Need for Skills
AFB Press: American Foundation for the Blind
11 Penn Plaza   212-502-7600
New York, NY 10001   800-232-3044
                                     Fax: 212-502-7774
                                       www.afb.org/store
Provides an overview of the importance of social competence and details the course of social skills development in children in general and in children who are blind or visually impaired in particular. This study guide examines both the development of social skills in general and how this process applies to children who are blind or who have visual impairments.
VHS & PAL
ISBN: 0-891283-25-0

9843 Hand in Hand: It Can Be Done
AFB Press: American Foundation for the Blind
11 Penn Plaza   212-502-7600
New York, NY 10001   800-232-3044
                                     Fax: 212-502-7774
                                       www.afb.org/store
One hour introduction to working effectively with individuals who are deaf-blind. Designed as both an overview and a reinforcer of the self-study text, this video can be used as a whole or in sections for parents and regular educators, as well as in the community. Includes a discussion guide. Available in audioscribed or open captioned VHS and PAL.

ISBN: 0-891283-25-0

9844 Heart to Heart
Blind Children's Center
4120 Marathon Street   213-664-2153
Los Angeles, CA 90029-3584   Fax: 213-665-3828
Parents of blind and partially sighted children talk about their feelings.
Videotape

9845 Helen Keller in Her Story
AFB Press: American Foundation for the Blind
11 Penn Plaza   212-502-7600
New York, NY 10001   800-232-3044
                                     Fax: 212-502-7774
                                       www.afb.org/store
Patty Duke, who portrayed the young Helen Keller on stage and on screen in The Miracle Worker, introduces this Oscar-winning documentary about the extraordinary lives of Ms. Keller, her teacher Anne Sullivan Macy and her friend and companion Polly Thompson. Includes vintage still photographs as well as early movie footage and newsreel footage.
VHS & PAL
ISBN: 0-891282-25-4

9846 Let's Eat
Blind Children's Center
4120 Marathon Street   213-664-2153
Los Angeles, CA 90029-3584   Fax: 213-665-3828
Teaches competent feeding skills to children with visual impairments.
Videotape

9847 Making the Most of Early Communication: Strategies for Supporting Communication
AFB Press: American Foundation for the Blind

11 Penn Plaza
New York, NY 10001

212-502-7600
800-232-3044
Fax: 212-502-7774
www.afb.org/store

Demonstrates selected interventions to assist infants and toddlers with multiple disabilities, including vision and hearing loss, in developing early communication and other skills. Emphasizing the critical importance of early intervention, this video is designed to help service providers and families create effective communication straegies that encourage cognitive development and funtional abilities in young children with multiple disabilities and those who are deaf-blind. 37 minutes.
VHS & PAL
ISBN: 0-891282-96-3

9848   New What Do You Do When You See a Blind Person?
AFB Press: American Foundation for the Blind
11 Penn Plaza
New York, NY 10001

212-502-7600
800-232-3044
Fax: 212-502-7774
www.afb.org/store

Engaging remake of the 1971 classic brings a fresh perspective on how to interact comfortably with someone who is visually impaired. The entertaining experiences of Mark Johnson, a computer programmer who is blind, and Dave Simon, a computer salesman who is not, show the simple ways to provide assistance, if it is needed, to someone who is blind or visually impaired. 16 minutes.
VHS & PAL
ISBN: 0-891283-13-7

9849   Oh, I See
AFB Press: American Foundation for the Blind
11 Penn Plaza
New York, NY 10001

212-502-7600
800-232-3044
Fax: 212-502-7774
www.afb.org/store

Lively and entertaining video provides practical suggestions on helping students who are blind and visually impaired adapt to the mainstream classroom. The modifacations shown can easily be used by teachers, students, or anyone working with blind and visually impaired students. Seven minutes.
VHS & PAL
ISBN: 0-891282-52-1

9850   Out of Left Field
AFB Press: American Foundation for the Blind
11 Penn Plaza
New York, NY 10001

212-502-7600
800-232-3044
Fax: 212-502-7774
www.afb.org/store

Illustrates how youngsters who are blind or visually impaired are integrated with their sighted peers in a variety of recreational and athletic activites. 17 minutes.
VHS & PAL
ISBN: 0-891282-28-9

9851   Profiles in Aging and Vision
AFB Press: American Foundation for the Blind
11 Penn Plaza
New York, NY 10001

212-502-7600
800-232-3044
Fax: 212-502-7774
www.afb.org/store

Can be used on its own or in conjunction with the text, this is an informative overview of the common eye conditions that affect older people, with a detailed description of the vision-related services that help older people who are visually impaired continue to lead independent lives. Experienced professionals provide valuable information on crucial issues, and older visually impaired persons offering their own revealing perspectives. 33 minutes.
VHS
ISBN: 0-891289-48-8

9852   Reaching Out: A Creative Access Guide for Designing Exhibits & Cultural Programs
AFB Press: American Foundation for the Blind
11 Penn Plaza
New York, NY 10001

212-502-7600
800-232-3044
Fax: 212-502-7774
www.afb.org/store

Video and accompanying manual are a creative package for making information on cultural programs and facilities accessable to people who are blind or visually impaired. Created especially for libraries, museums, historical societies, outdoor cultural facilities, corporations and everyone whose mission involves providing information to the community, this video offers practical design and program solutions. 22 minutes.
VHS & PAL
ISBN: 0-891289-49-6

9853   Seven Minute Lesson
AFB Press: American Foundation for the Blind
11 Penn Plaza
New York, NY 10001

212-502-7600
800-232-3044
Fax: 212-502-7774
www.afb.org/store

Introduction to the basic techniques used when acting as a sighted guide for a person who is blind or visually impaired.
VHS & PAL
ISBN: 0-891282-29-7

9854   Solutions for Everyday Living for Older People with Visual Impairments
AFB Press: American Foundation for the Blind
11 Penn Plaza
New York, NY 10001

212-502-7600
800-232-3044
Fax: 212-502-7774
www.afb.org/store

Presents a positive and helpful view of how older people who have lost some or all of their vision can continue to lead satisfying lives within supportive environments. This engaing video shows how staff members in continuing care communities and other living settings for older people can help residents function as independently as possible. Different types of vision loss are explained, and simple solutions are offered for carrying out everyday activities. 34 minutes.
VHS & PAL
ISBN: 0-891288-52-X

9855   Strategies for Community Access: Braille & Raised Large Print Facility Signs
AFB Press: American Foundation for the Blind
11 Penn Plaza
New York, NY 10001

212-502-7600
800-232-3044
Fax: 212-502-7774
www.afb.org/store

Brief and effective advocacy tool that can be used to educate architects, planners, facility managers, sign makers and consumers about the value of accessible signs. Topics covered include ADA requirements for accessible signs, samples of signs designed to be compatible with an organization's interior design, demonstrations of how blind and print signs are a cost-effective way to provide access. Reproducible fact sheets on ADA signage guidelines are enclosed. Seven minutes.
VHS & PAL
ISBN: 0-891282-56-4

9856   Understanding Braille Literacy
AFB Press: American Foundation for the Blind
11 Penn Plaza
New York, NY 10001

212-502-7600
800-232-3044
Fax: 212-502-7774
www.afb.org/store

Motovational and intructional video covers all aspects of a successful braille education program. Teachers and students demonstate how braille is learned and used from preschool through high school and describes how braille skills contribute to literacy, independence, mastry of academic skills and successful education experiences in the regular classroom. Parents, classroom teachers and school administrators also speak out about the importance of braille. 25 minutes.
VHS & PAL
ISBN: 0-891282-61-0

9857   We Can Do it Together: Mobility for Students with Multiple Disabilities
AFB Press: American Foundation for the Blind

11 Penn Plaza | 212-502-7600
New York, NY 10001 | 800-232-3044
| Fax: 212-502-7774
| www.afb.org/store

Illustrates a transdisiplinary team approach to teaching orientation and mobility to students with severe visual and multiple impairments, covering both adapted communication systems that are used to teach mobility skills and basic indoor mobility in the school. For mobility instructors, administrators, teachers of visually impaired and severely disabled students, occupational, physical and speech therapists and parents. Discussion guide included, 13 minutes.

VHS & PAL
ISBN: 0-891282-13-0

9858 What Can Baby See? Vision Tests & Intervention Strategies for Infants

AFB Press: American Foundation for the Blind
11 Penn Plaza | 212-502-7600
New York, NY 10001 | 800-232-3044
| Fax: 212-502-7774
| www.afb.org/store

Presents common vision tests and methods of gathering information that can be used with infants and very young children to help indentify visual impairments that require early intervention services. Effective ways of working with families and early intervention strategies for encouraging infants with multiple disabilities to use their vision in functional ways are demonstrated to help families and service providers contribute to children's growth and development.

VHS & PAL
ISBN: 0-891282-99-8

Web Sites

9859 ACB Government Employees

www.acb.org

Concerns of the organization include recruitment, placement and advancement of blind and visually impaired employees.

9860 ACB Radio Amateurs

www.acb.org

A radio amateur network of blind, visually impaired and sighted members who gather and share common problems and solutions to help members improve radio amateurs in getting started, provides access to educational materials in special media and publishes a directory for the visually impaired.

9861 ACB Social Service Providers

www.acb.org

Information on blind and visually impaired social workers, social service professionals, students pursuing careers in social work, and other interested persons.

9862 American Blind Lawyers Association

www.acb.org

Information on law school admission tests and bar exams, private sector and government employment relations and specialized work techniques for the blind and visually impaired.

9863 American Council of Blind Lions

www.acb.org

Information concerning Club activities in the field of work for the blind and encourages blind people to join Lions Clubs and other civic activities.

9864 American Council of the Blind

www.acb.org

Information for the visually impaired and fully sighted individuals who are concerned about the dignity and well-being of blind people throughout America.

9865 American Foundation for the Blind

www.afb.org

Our web site unique in that it combines state-of-the-art features, an attractive visual environment and an accessible design for people with all types of disabilities. Features include a searchable database of vision services nationwide, community message boards and the largest collection of Helen Keller memorbilia on the web. It

meets the stringent AAA guidelines of the Web Accessibility Initiative of the World Wide Web Consortium, established to help organizations build accessible websites.

9866 American Printing House for the Blind

www.aph.org

This organization promotes the independence of blind persons by providing special media, tools and materials needed for education and life.

9867 Blinded Veterans Association

www.bva.org

Offers two main service programs without cost to blinded veterans. Field service program provides counseling to veterans and families, and information on benefits and rehabilitation.

9868 Braille Revival League

www.acb.org

Information for people to read and write in braille, advocates for mandatory braille instruction in educational facilities for the blind, strives to make available a supply of braille materials from libraries and printing houses and more.

9869 Council of Families with Visual Impairment

www.acb.org

Offers support and outreach, shares experiences in parent/child relationships, exchanges educational, cultural and medical information about child development and more.

9870 Fidelco Guide Dog Foundation

www.fidelco.org

Fidelco breeds, raises, trains, and places German shepherd guide dogs with men and women who are visually impaired, primarily in the Northeast.

9871 Friends-In-Art

www.acb.org

Offers consultation to program planners in establishing accessible art and museum exhibits and presents Performing Arts Showcases.

9872 Guide Dog Foundation for the Blind

www.guidedog.org

Furnishes guide dogs, free of charge, to qualified people who seek independence, mobility and companionship.

9873 Guide Dog Users

www.acb.org

Promotes the acceptance of blind people and their dogs, works for enforcement and expansion of laws admitting guide dogs into public places, advocates for quality training and follow-up services.

9874 Healing Well

www.healingwell.com

An online health resource guide to medical news, chat, information and articles, newsgroups and message boards, books, disease-related web sites, medical directories, and more for patients, friends, and family coping with disabling diseases, disorders, or chronic illnesses.

9875 Health Finder

www.healthfinder.gov

Searchable, carefully developed web site offering information on over 1000 topics. Developed by the US Department of Health and Human Services, the site can be used in both English and Spanish.

9876 Healthlink USA

www.healthlinkusa.com

Health information concerning treatment, cures, prevention, diagnosis, risk factors, research, support groups, email lists, personal stories and much more. Updated regularly.

9877 Helios Health

www.helioshealth.com

Online resource for your health information. Detailed information about specific health topics, access to expert advice from our Medical Advisory Board, and up-to-date health news.

9878 Independent Visually Impaired Enterprises

www.acb.org

Information on rehabilitation facilities for all types of business enterprises and publicizes the capabilities of blind and visually impaired business persons.

9879 **Library Users of America**

www.acb.org

Provides for chapters in states through the US to encourage the development, acquisition and use of technology which enables blind and visually impaired persons to use printed material independently in library settings and elsewhere.

9880 **Lighthouse International**

www.lighthouse .org

Offers information about vision impairment and vision rehabilitation, and provides referrals to services and support groups nationwide.

9881 **MedicineNet**

www.medicinenet.com

An online resource for consumers providing easy-to-read, authoritative medical and health information.

9882 **Medscape**

www.medscape.com

Medscape offers specialists, primary care physicians, and other health professionals the Web's most robust and integrated medical information and educational tools.

9883 **National Alliance of Blind Students**

www.acb.org

Works to facilitate progress toward full accessibility of college programs and facilities, provides opportunities for discussion of issues important to students and assists with National Student Seminars.

9884 **National Association for Visually Hand.**

www.navh.org

NAVH ensures that those with limited vision do not lead limited lives. We offer emotional support; training in the use of and access to a wide variety of optical aids and lighting; a large print, nationwide, free-by-mail loan library; large print educational materials; quarterly newsletter; referrals; self-help groups and educational outreach.

9885 **National Association of Blind Educators**

www.nfb.org

Provides support and information regarding professional responsibilities, classroom techniques, national testing methods and career obstacles. Publishes The Blind Educator, national magazine specifically for blind educators.

9886 **National Association of Blind Lawyers**

www.nfb.org

Provides support and information regarding employment, techniques used by the blind, advocacy, laws affecting the blind, current information about the American Bar Association and other issues for blind lawyers.

9887 **National Association of Blind Secretaries and Transcribers**

www.nfb.org

Addresses issues such as technology, accomodation, career planning and job training.

9888 **National Association of Blind Students**

www.nfb.org

Provides support, information and encouragement to blind college and university students.

9889 **National Association of Blind Teachers**

www.acb.org

Works to advance the teaching profession for blind and visually impaired people, protects the interest of teachers, presents discussions and solutions for special problems encountered by blind teachers and publishes a directory of blind teachers in the US.

9890 **National Association of Guide Dog Users**

www.nfb.org

Provides information and support for guide dog users and works to secure high standards in guide dog training. Addresses issues of discrimination of guide dog users and offers public education about guide dog use.

9891 **National Association to Promote the Use of Braille**

www.nfb.org

Provides information about the importance of Braille in securing independence, education and employment for the blind.

9892 **National Braille Association**

www.nationalbraille.org/

Provides transciption service for, and maintains a depository of, braille books.

9893 **National Federation of the Blind: Blind/Deaf Division**

www.nfb.org

Offers personal contact with other deaf-blind individuals knowledgeable in advocacy, education, employment, technology, discrimination and other issues surrounding deaf-blindness.

9894 **National Federation of the Blind**

www.nfb.org

Provides public education about blindness, support services to the newly blinded, scholarships, publications about blindness, adaptive equipment for the blind, advocacy services, Newsline for the Blind, assistive technology information and Job Opportunities for the Blind.

9895 **National Federation of the Blind in Computer Science**

www.nfb.org

New technologies, to secure access to current technology and to develop new ways of using current or new technologies by the blind.

9896 **National Federation of the Blind: Blind Merchants Division**

www.nfb.org

Provides information regarding rehabilitation, social security, tax and other issues which directly affect blind merchants. Serves as advocacy and support group.

9897 **National Federation of the Blind: Human Services Division**

www.nfb.org

Organization of blind persons working in counseling, personnel, psychology, social work, psychiatry, rehabilitation and other social science and human resource fields. Provides resources regarding blindness-related techniques and methods used in these fields.

9898 **National Federation of the Blind: Masonic Square Club**

www.nfb.org

Blind individuals committed to sharing of Masonic experiences, goals and history.

9899 **National Federation of the Blind: Music Division**

www.nfb.org

Offers support and information regarding copyright, publishing, promotion and other career details.

9900 **National Federation of the Blind: Public Employees Division**

www.nfb.org

Focuses on issues such as changes in governmental hiring and retention practices, new job skills needed for the future, government employment downsizing, new electronic means of finding public sector jobs, self-advocacy and career planning strategies.

9901 **National Federation of the Blind: Science and Engineering Division**

www.nfb.org

This is a strong support group to encourage blind persons in pursuit of these careers, many of which have been considered not possible for the blind in the past.

9902 **National Federation of the Blind: Writers Division**

www.nfb.org

Covers various aspects of this business, including selling your work, publishing, technology, motivation and discovering writing and publishing resources.

9903 **National Library Service for the Blind**

www.loc.gov/nls

Administers a national library service that provides braille and recorded books and magazines on free loan to anyone who cannot read standard print because of visual or physical disabilities who are eligible residents of the United States or American citizens living abroad.

9904 **National Organization of Parents of Blind Children**

www.nfb.org

Addresses issues ranging from help to parents of a newborn blind infant, mobility and Braille instruction, education, social and community participation, development of self-confidence and other vital factors involved in the growth of a blind child.

9905 National Organization of the Senior Blind

www.nfb.org

Provides support and information to other blind seniors. Issues include concerns such as remaining active in community and social life, maintaining private homes or living in retirement communities or nursing homes, learning the techniques used by the blind, independently caring for oneself and maintaining a positive approach to vision loss.

9906 Randolph-Sheppard Vendors of America

www.acb.org

Protects the interests of blind vendors, seeks proper implementation of the Randolph-Sheppard Act and encourages facility locations in more visible and profitable areas.

9907 Vision World Wide

www.visionww.org

Aims is to enhance everyday living so as to maintain an independent lifestyle. It also serves as a consumer protection against misrepresentation and fraud.

9908 Visually Impaired Data Processors International

www.acb.org

Provides for the exchange of work technique ideas and works with agencies to increase the availability of braille and recorded materials.

9909 Visually Impaired Piano Tuners International

www.acb.org

Works to preserve, advance and enrich the skilled professional piano tuning for competent, well-trained blind and visually impaired persons.

9910 Visually Impaired Veterans of America

www.acb.org

Promotes the rights of visually impaired veterans to receive all benefits, encourages research and development of new products for blind people.

9911 WebMD

www.webmd.com

Information on Blindness and Visual Impairments, including articles and resources.

Description

9912 **War Syndromes**

War syndromes have plagued soldiers for centuries. Though symptoms may vary, soldiers may become affected by various postulated physiological diseases as well as psychological illnesses. Agent Orange and the Gulf War Syndrome are two of the conditions still prevalent today.

Agent Orange is the common name for a mix of chemicals developed by the military. It was first used during the Vietnam War to destroy vegetation that concealed the enemy. During the war, soldiers were exposed heavily to this chemical; years later, many of them contracted a variety of conditions. There has been an intense controversy about whether Agent Orange caused these conditions, with medical scientists, patients, politicians and advocacy groups all involved.

Among the conditions sometimes attributed to Agent Orange exposure are a variety of cancers, an acne-like skin condition called chloracne, neurological diseases, repeated infections, sterility, and birth defects in the children of exposed persons.

To further understand this condition, the Department of Veterans Affairs has been established a registry of Vietnam veterans concerned that they may have been exposed to Agent Orange. Veterans who suspect their symptoms are related to this exposure can contact the Department's Medical Administrative Services to request the Agent Orange Registry Examination, a complete health evaluation. The Department offers service-connected compensation for those veterans who develop a condition believed to be related to exposure to Agent Orange.

Gulf War Syndrome, GWS, or Persian Gulf War Syndrome is a constellation of illnesses experienced by 5,000 to 80,000 US veterans after returning from the Persian Gulf Wars in the 1990's and 2000's. Symptoms are predominately neurologic and consist of impaired cognition, with problems of attention, memory, reasoning, insomnia, depression and headaches. Complaints of muscle and joint pain, gastrointestinal difficulties, vertigo and weakness are also common. As veterans resumed family life, various birth defects were added to the list. The cause of GWS is unknown.

A 1997 study funded by the Centers for Disease Control shows that Gulf War personnel are more likely than others to report depression, syptoms similar to post-traumatic stress disorder, chronic fatigue, cognitive difficulties, bronchitis, asthma, fibromyalgia, alcohol abuse, anxiety and sexual dysfunction.

Many causes of GWS have been suggested, but none have been definitely identified or eliminated. These include: effects of chemical and/or biological weapons; exposure to pesticides; smoke from oil well fires; air-borne contamination from munitions plants destroyed in Iraq, exposure to depleted uranium used as a material in some US munitions and exposure to volatile solvents used in the normal course of equipment maintenance. None of these exposures have been convincingly linked to a cause of the illness.

Given the range of reported GWS effects, treatment is highly individualized and symptomatic. A number of specialized support groups and websites have been established by members of the Persian Gulf War Community.

National Agencies & Associations

9913 **Advocacy for the Gulf War Children**
1692 6th Road   308-795-2319
St Libory, NE 68872
Gives listings of names and addresses of families with children with gulf war syndrome.

9914 **Agent Orange Registry Department of Veterans Affairs**
Department of Veterans Affairs
810 Vermont Avenue NW   202-233-4000
Washington, DC 20420   800-827-1000
                                   www.va.gov
Offers a computerized index of examinations of Vietnam veterans who were worried that they may have been exposed to chemical herbicides which might be causing a variety of ill effects. Services available to any veteran, male or female, who had active military service.

9915 **Centers for Disease Control**
1600 Clifton Road   404-639-3311
Atlanta, GA 30333   800-232-4636
                              Fax: 404-639-3435
                              TTY: 888-232-6348
                        e-mail: cdcinfo@cdc.gov
                                   www.cdc.gov
Offers reprints from the CDC Health Status of Vietnam veterans and the Journal of the American Medical Association. Also offers reports from the Centers for Disease Control Vietnam Experience Study, which was a multidimensional assessment of the health of Vietnam War veterans.
William H Gimson, Chief Operating Officer
John Tibbs, Director

9916 **National Veterans Services Fund**
209 West Ave   203-656-0003
Darien, CT 06820-0465   800-521-0198
                              Fax: 203-656-1957
                        e-mail: philvet@NVSF.org
                                   www.nvsf.org
Supports and informs those who were exposed to the defoliant Agent Orange or dioxin while serving the US in the conflict in Vietnam. The organization has developed a detailed exposure survey form to collect information on exposed veterans.
Phil Kraft, President/Treasurer
Cathie Green Stansell, Vice President

9917 **VA Data Processing Center**
1615 E Woodward Street   512-389-5380
Austin, TX 78772-0001
Helps veterans register after receiving the Agent Orange examination.

State Agencies & Associations

Alabama

9918 **Gulf War Veterans of Alabama**
2344 Glendale Avenue   205-265-7723
Montgomery, AL 36107   e-mail: 76163 1323@compuserve.com
Don Reeves
Shannon Reeves

9919 Veterans Administration Medical Center: Alabama
3701 Loop Road E   205-554-2000
Tuscaloosa, AL 35404   888-269-3045
                                               Fax: 205-554-2034
                                               www.tuscaloosa.va.gov
The Tuscaloosa VA Medical Center (TVAMC) is located in West
Alabama, where the facility is situated on a beautiful campus of
125 acres with 25 major buildings. TVAMC provides primary care,
long-term health care and mental health care services to eligible
Veterans in the VA Southeast Network (Veterans Integrated Ser-
vice Network [VISN 7]. The Tuscaloosa VA Medical Center pro-
vides access to secondary and tertiary care services.
Maria R. Andrews, MS, FACHE, Director
Paula Stokes, CTRS, CPM, M.Ed,, Associate Director

9920 Veterans Association Medical Center
700 S 19th Street   205-933-8101
Birmingham, AL 35233   866-487-4243
                                               Fax: 205-933-4484
                                               www.birmingham.va.gov
The Birmingham VA Medical Center is a 313-bed acute tertiary
care facility located in the historic Southside district of the city.
The facility provides acute tertiary medical and surgical care to
veterans of Alabama and surrounding states. We provide health
care services to eligible veterans in the VA Southeast Network Veterans Integrated Service Network
Thomas Smith, FACHE, Director
Phyllis Smith, MBA, FACHE, Associate Director

Alaska

9921 Alaska Gulf War Syndrome Referral Coordinator
23740 Sunny Glen Drive   907-696-8688
Eagle River, AK 99577   Fax: 907-696-8688
                                               e-mail: mcclure@alaska.net

Larry McClure

9922 Alaska VA Healthcare System
Outpatient Clinic
1201 North Muldoon Road   907-257-4700
Anchorage, AK 99504   888-353-7574
                                               Fax: 907-257-6774
                                               www.alaska.va.gov
The Alaska VA Healthcare System (AVAHS) offers primary, spe-
cialty, and mental health outpatient care. Services are provided
through a Joint Venture with the United States Air Force on nearby
Elmendorf Air Force Base, as well as through purchased care ar-
rangements with the community hospitals. The facility also features a comprehensive Homeless Veteran Service, consisting of a
Domiciliary Residential Rehabilitation Program, Veterans Industries, Compensated Work Therapy Transitional Residence Pr
Susan M. Yeager, Director
Greg Puckett, Associate Director

Arizona

9923 Phoenix VA Healthcare System
Carl T. Hayden VA Medical Center
650 E Indian School Road   602-277-5551
Phoenix, AZ 85012   800-554-7174
                                               www.phoenix.va.gov
The Phoenix VA Health Care System proudly serves Veterans in
central Arizona at its main medical center and outpatient VA
Health Care Clinics.
Sharon Helman, Director
Lance E Robinson, MS, FACHE,, Associate Director

**9924 Veterans Adm. Medical Center: Tucson Southern Arizona VA
Health Care System**
Southern Arizona VA Health Care System
3601 S 6th Avenue   520-792-1450
Tucson, AZ 85723   800-470-8262
                                               Fax: 520-629-1818
                                               www.tucson.va.gov
The VA Medical Center located at Tucson Arizona is the "Flagship" for the Southern Arizona VA Health Care System
(SAVAHCS), which serves over 170,000 veterans located in eight
counties in Southern Arizona and one county in Western New Mexico. This 285-bed hospital provides training, primary care and
sub-specialty health care in numerous medical areas for eligible

Veterans.SAVAHCS has specialized and numerous unique treat-
ment programs to better serve its patients such as: The South
Western Blin
Jonathan Gardner, Director
Jennifer S Gutowski, MHA, FACHE, Associate Director

Arkansas

**9925 Central Arkansas Veterans Healthcare Syste Eugene J. Towbin
Healthcare Center**
Eugene J. Towbin Healthcare Center
2200 Fort Roots Drive
North Little Rock, AR 72114-1706   501-257-1000
                                   www.va.gov/directory/guide/facility.asp?
The Central Arkansas Veterans Healthcare System (CAVHS), a
flagship Department of Veterans Affairs (VA) healthcare provider,
is one of the largest and busiest VA medical centers in the country.
Its two hospitals, located in Little Rock and North Little Rock, an-
chor a broad spectrum of inpatient and outpatient healthcare services, ranging from disease prevention through primary care, to
complex surgical procedures, to extended rehabilitative care. This
System serves as a teaching facility for mor

9926 Gulf War Veterans of Arkansas
11127 Eglia Valley Drive   501-225-9347
Little Rock, AR 72212
Lydia Pace

9927 Veterans Adm. Medical Center: Fayetville
2300 Ramsey Street   910-488-2120
Fayetteville, AR 28301   800-771-6106
                                               www.fayettevillenc.va.gov
The Fayetteville Veterans Affairs Medical Center (VAMC) is a
general medicine, surgery and mental health facility. The
Fayetteville VAMC is a Complexity Level 2 Medical Center and is
authorized 58 general medical, surgical, and mental health beds. It
also maintains a 69-bed long-term care unit. The medical center
serves Veterans in 19 counties in southeastern North Carolina and
two counties in northeastern South Carolina.
Elizabeth Goolsby, Director
James Galkowski, PA-C, FACHE, Associate Director

California

9928 California Association of Persian Gulf Veterans
Santa Cruz, CA 95063   408-476-6684
                                               Fax: 415-227-0848
                                               e-mail: CAGulfVets@aol.com

Erika Lundholm

9929 Northern California Association of Persian Gulf Veterans
9141 East Stockton Boulevard   916-684-1693
Elk Grove, CA 95624   Fax: 916-684-1693
                                               e-mail: NCAPGV@aol.com

Debbie Judd

9930 Sacramento Veterans Center
1111 Howe Avenue   916-566-7430
Sacramento, CA 95825   877-927-8387
                                               Fax: 916-566-7433
                                   www.va.gov/directory/guide/facility.asp?
Michael Miracle, Team Leader
Edna Gabaldon, Counselor

9931 San Francisco VA Medical Center
4150 Clement Street   415-221-4810
San Francisco, CA 94121   877-487-2838
                                               Fax: 415-750-2185
                                               www.sanfrancisco.va.gov
SFVAMC has several National Centers of Excellence in the areas
of Epilepsy Treatment; Cardiac Surgery; Post Traumatic Stress
Disorder; HIV; and Renal Dialysis. It has many other nationally
recognized programs including: the Parkinson's Disease Re-
search, Education, and Clinical Center; the Hepatitis C Research
and Education Center; the Mental Illness Research & Education
Clinical Center; and the Western Pacemaker and AICD
Surveillance Program.
C. Diana . Nicoll, M.D., Ph.D., M.P, Acting Medical Center Director
Karen A rnold, MA, RD, Acting Associate Director

9932 Sepulveda Ambulatory Care Center
16111 Plummer Street   818-891-7711
North Hills, CA 91343   800-516-4567
                                   Fax: 818-895-9559
                                www.losangeles.va.gov
The VA Greater Los Angeles Healthcare System is the largest, most complex healthcare system within the Department of Veterans Affairs. It is one component of the VA Desert Pacific Healthcare Network (VISN22) offering services to veterans residing in Southern California and Southern Nevada.
Donna M. Beiter, RN, MSN, Director
Christopher Sandles, Assistant Director

9933 VA Northern California Health Care System
10535 Hospital Way   916-843-7000
Mather, CA 95655   800-382-8387
                                   Fax: 916-843-9001
                         e-mail: Robin.Jackson2@va.gov
                             www.northerncalifornia.va.gov
David G. Mastalski, Interim Director
Donna Iatarola, RN, MSN, Associate Director, Patient Care Service

9934 Veterans Adm. Medical Center: Livermore
4951 Arroyo Road   925-373-4700
Livermore, CA 94550   800-455-0057
                                   Fax: 925-449-6522
                                 www2.va.gov/directory
The VA Palo Alto Health Care System (VAPAHCS) consists of three inpatient facilities located at Palo Alto, Menlo Park, and Livermore. VAPAHCS is a teaching hospital, providing a full range of patient care services with state-of-the-art technology as well as education and research. Comprehensive health care is provided in areas of medicine, surgery, psychiatry, rehabilitation, neurology, oncology, dentistry, geriatrics, and extended care.
Elizabeth Joyce Freeman, FACHE, Director
Gloria Martinez, RN, MS, Associate Director for Patient Care & Nu

9935 Veterans Administration Medical Center: Fresno
2615 E. Clinton Avenue   559-228-6933
Fresno, CA 93703   888-826-2838
                                   Fax: 559-487-5399
                                     www.fresno.va.gov
VACCHCS consists of 1 inpatient facility located in Fresno (Fresno Medical Center), plus 3 outpatient clinics in Merced, Oakhurst and Tulare. We are expanding to better serve Veterans in Central California! VACCHCS mission is to honor America's Veterans by providing exceptional health care that improves their health and well-being. VACCHCS is a teaching hospital, providing a full range of services, with state-of-the-art technology as well as education and researc
Joanne Krumberger RN, FACHE, Director
Susan Shyshka FACHE, Associate Director

9936 Veterans Affairs Medical Center: Loma Linda
11201 Benton Street   909-825-7084
Loma Linda, CA 92357   800-741-8387
                                   Fax: 909-422-3106
                                   www.lomalinda.va.gov
Since 1977, VA Loma Linda Healthcare System has been improving the health of the men and women who have so proudly served our nation. We consider it our privilege to serve your health care needs in any way we can. Services are available to more than 67,000 Veterans living in a 2-county area of San Bernardino and Riverside.
Barbara Fallen, RD, MPA, FACHE, Director
Prachi V. Asher, FACHE, Assistant Director

9937 West Los Angeles Medical Center
11301 Willshire Boulevard   310-478-3711
Los Angeles, CA 90073   Fax: 310-268-3494
                                www.losangeles.va.gov
The VA Greater Los Angeles Healthcare System is the largest, most complex healthcare system within the Department of Veterans Affairs. It is one component of the VA Desert Pacific Healthcare Network (VISN22) offering services to veterans residing in Southern California and Southern Nevada.
Donna M. Beiter, RN, MSN, Director
Christopher Sandles, Assistant Director

Colorado

9938 Veterans Adm. Medical Center: Grand Junction
2121 N Avenue   970-242-0731
Grand Junction, CO 81501   866-206-6415
                                   Fax: 970-244-1303
                                www.grandjunction.va.gov
The Grand Junction VA Medical Center (VAMC) serves 37,000 veterans residing on the Western Slope. The VAMC consists of one facility located in the city of Grand Junction; a Community Based Outpatient Clinic (CBOC) in Montrose, serving the southwestern Colorado counties; and a telehealth outreach clinic in Craig, serving northwestern Colorado and southwestern Wyoming. The VAMC operates 53 beds comprised of 23 acute care and 30 Transitional Care Unit beds. The VAMC provides primary and secondary c
Patricia A. Hitt, MS, Acting Director Grand Junction VA Medica
Randal France, M.D, Chief Psychiatry Service/ Int. Chf. of S

Connecticut

9939 Gulf War Veterans of Connecticut: New England Chapter
8 Frances Lane   860-623-1456
Windsor Locks, CT 6096   Fax: 860-292-1849
                          e-mail: DIANEDULKA@aol.com
Diane Dulka

Delaware

9940 Veterans Adm. Medical Center: Wilmington VA Medical Center
Wilmington VA Medical Center
1601 Kirkwood Highway   302-994-2511
Wilmington, DE 19805   Fax: 302-633-5591
                                   www.va.gov/directory
The Wilmington VA Medical Center is a member of the Veterans Integrated Service Network 4 which includes 9 other facilities in Philadelphia, Coatesville, Lebanon, Wilkes-Barre, Altoona, Butler, Clarksburg, Erie, and Pittsburgh. The hospital has an approved authorized/operating bed capacity of 60. Also included within the hospital is a 60-bed Community Living Center for extended care. Both are accredited by the Joint Commission on Accreditation of Healthcare Organizations.

District of Columbia

9941 Disabled American Veterans National Service Headquarters
807 Maine Avenue SW   202-554-3501
Washington, DC 20024   Fax: 202-554-3581
                                        www.dav.org
Serves America's disabled veterans and their families. Direct services include legislative advocacy professional counseling about compensation pension educational and job training programs and VA health care. Also offers assistance in applying for those programs.
Arthur H Wilson, National Adjutant
David G Gorman, Executive Director

9942 US Veteran's Administration
810 Vermont Avenue NW   202-273-5400
Washington, DC 20420   Fax: 202-273-4877
                                 www2.va.gov/directory
Provides a wide range of services for those who have been in the military and their dependents as well as offering information on driver assessment and education programs.
Louise R Van Diepen MS CGP, Chief of Staff
Patricia Van MHA BS, Assistant Deputy Policy/Planning

9943 Veterans Adm. Medical Center: Washington
50 Irving Street NW   202-745-8000
Washington, DC 20422   877-328-2621
                                   Fax: 202-754-8530
                                www.washingtondc.va.gov
The Washington DC VA Medical Center's employees and volunteers take great pride in serving Veterans of the national capital area. Capitol Excellence is our number one priority. From the Executive Office to the mailroom, from the canteen to the warehouse, whether offering you medical services, prosthetic devices, or a warm meal, every staff member and volunteer here is charged with

the responsibility of providing an environment of respect, courtesy and concern.
Brian A. Hawkins, MHA, Medical Center Director
Bryan C. Matthews, MBA, Associate Medical Center Director

Florida

9944 Desert Storm Justice Foundation: Florida
10 Marlow Road   813-635-3261
Frostproof, FL 33843-9321   Fax: 813-635-3261
e-mail: BillCarpenter@cjewel.com
William Carpenter

9945 Desert Storm Veterans of Florida
Titusville, FL 32782   407-269-3453
e-mail: GulfVet@Metrolink.net
Kevin Knight

9946 Veterans Adm. Medical Center: Bay Pines
10000 Bay Pines Boulevard   727-398-6661
Bay Pines, FL 33744   888-820-0230
Fax: 727-398-9442
www.baypines.va.gov
Since 1933, Bay Pines VA Healthcare System has been improving the health of the men and women who have so proudly served our nation. We consider it our privilege to serve your health care needs in any way we can. Our services are available to Veterans living in a ten county catchment area in west central Florida.
Suzanne M. Klinker, Medical Center Director
Kristine Brown, MPH, Associate Director

9947 Veterans Adm. Medical Center: Gainesville
1601 SW Archer Road   352-376-1611
Gainesville, FL 32608-1197   800-324-8387
Fax: 352-374-6113
www.northflorida.va.gov
In addition to our medical centers in Gainesville and Lake City, we offer services in three satellite outpatient clinics and several community-based outpatient clinics across North Florida and South Georgia.Patient-centered integrated health care organization for veterans providing excellent health care, research, and education; an organization where people choose to work; an active community partner; and a back-up for National emergencies..
Thomas Wisnieski, MPA, FACHE, Director
Nicklous J Ross, Associate Director

9948 Veterans Adm. Medical Center: Lake City
Lake City Veterans Administration Medical Center
619 S Marion Avenue   386-755-3016
Lake City, FL 32025-5808   800-308-8387
Fax: 386-758-3209
www.northflorida.va.gov
In addition to our medical centers in Gainesville and Lake City, we offer services in three satellite outpatient clinics and several community-based outpatient clinics across North Florida and South Georgia.Patient-centered integrated health care organization for veterans providing excellent health care, research, and education; an organization where people choose to work; an active community partner; and a back-up for National emergencies..
Thomas Wisnieski, MPA, FACHE, Director
Nicklous J Ross, Associate Director

9949 Veterans Adm. Medical Center: Miami
1201 NW 16th Street   305-575-7000
Miami, FL 33125   888-276-1785
Fax: 305-575-3232
www.miami.va.gov
The Miami VA is an accredited comprehensive medical provider, providing general medical, surgical, inpatient and outpatient mental health services, the Miami VA Healthcare System includes an AIDS/HIV center, a prosthetic treatment center, spinal cord injury rehabilitative center, and Geriatric Research, Education, and Clinical Center (GRECC). The Miami VA Healthcare System is recognized as a Center of Excellence in Spinal Cord Injury Research, Substance Abuse Treatment and is a recognized Chest
Paul M. Russo, Director
Mark E. Morgan, Associate Director

9950 Veterans Adm. Medical Center: St. Petersburg
Bay Pines VA Medical Center
10000 Bay Pines Boulevard   727-398-6661
Bay Pines, FL 33744   888-820-0230
Fax: 727-398-9442
www.baypines.va.gov
Since 1933, Bay Pines VA Healthcare System has been improving the health of the men and women who have so proudly served our nation. We consider it our privilege to serve your health care needs in any way we can. Our services are available to Veterans living in a ten county catchment area in west central Florida.
Suzanne M. Klinker, Medical Center Director
Kristine Brown, MPH, Associate Director

9951 Veterans Adm. Medical Center: Tampa
Tampa Veterans Administration Medical Center
13000 Bruce B Downs Boulevard   813-972-2000
Tampa, FL 33612   Fax: 813-972-7673
www.va.gov/visn8/tampa
Richard A Silver, Medical Center Director
Thomas E Bowen, Chief of Staff

9952 Vietnam Veterans of Brevard The Vietnam And All Veterans Of Brevard
The Vietnam And All Veterans Of Brevard
1125 W King Street   321-690-0805
Cocoa, FL 32922-0929   Fax: 321-690-0106
e-mail: BVagianos@cfl.rr.com
www.vietnamandallveteransofbrevard.com
Bill Vagianos, President
Don Wassmer, Vice President

9953 West Palm Beach VA Medical Center
7305 N Military Trail   561-422-8262
West Palm Beach, FL 33410-6400   800-972-8262
Fax: 561-422-8613
www.westpalmbeach.va.gov
The West Palm Beach VA Medical Center consists of one VHA facility located at 7305 N. Military Trail, West Palm Beach, Florida. The medical center is a general medical, psychiatric and surgical facility. It is a teaching hospital, providing a full range of patient care services, with state-of-the-art technology as well as education and limited research. Comprehensive healthcare is provided through primary care and long-term care in the areas of dentistry, extended care, medicine, neurology, onco
Charleen R. Szabo, FACHE, Medical Center Director
Cristy McKillop, FACHE, MHA, Medical Center Associate Director

Georgia

9954 Charlie Norwood VA Medical Center
950 15th Street Downtown   706-733-0188
Augusta, GA 30904   800-836-5561
Fax: 706-823-3934
www.augusta.va.gov
The Charlie Norwood VA Medical Center is a two-division Medical Center that provides tertiary care inmedicine, surgery, neurology, psychiatry, rehabilitation medicine, and spinal cord injury. The Downtown Division is authorized 155 beds (58 medicine, 37 surgery, and 60 spinal cord injury). The Uptown Division, located approximately three miles away, is authorized 315 beds (68 psychiatry, 15 blind rehabilitation and 40 medical rehabilitation. In addition, a 132-bed Restorative/Nursing Home C
Robert U. Hamilton, MHA, FACHE, Medical Center Director
Richard Toby Rose, Associate Director

9955 Gulf War Veterans of Georgia
307 Adair Street   404-373-3741
Decatur, GA 30030   Fax: 404-377-3741
e-mail: 70711 3174@compuserve.com
Paul Sullivan

9956 VA Southeast Network: Georgia
3700 Crestwood Parkway NW   678-924-5700
Duluth, GA 30096-5585   Fax: 678-924-5757
www.southeast.va.gov
The VA Southeast Network proudly serves veterans in the tri-state area which includes Alabama, Georgia, and South Carolina. Treating veterans and providing excellent health care at medical centers and community-based outpatient clinics is our focus.

9957 Veterans Adm. Medical Center: Decatur Atlanta VA Medical Center

Atlanta VA Medical Center
1670 Clairmont Road   404-321-6111
Decatur, GA 30033   Fax: 404-728-7733
www.atlanta.va.gov
The Atlanta VA Medical Center (VAMC), located on 26 acres in Decatur, is one of eight medical centers in the VA Southeast Network. It is a teaching hospital, providing a full range of patient care services complete with state-of-the-art technology, education, and research.
Leslie B. Wiggins, Medical Center Director
Thomas Grace, Associate Medical Center Director

9958 Veterans Adm. Medical Center: Dublin Carl Vinson VA Medical Center

Carl Vinson VA Medical Center
1826 Veterans Boulevard   912-272-1210
Dublin, GA 31021   800-595-5229
Fax: 912-277-2717
e-mail: Frank.Jordan@va.gov
www.dublin.va.gov
Since 1948, Carl Vinson VA Medical Center has been improving the health of the men and women who have so proudly served our nation. We consider it our privilege to serve your health care needs in any way we can. Services are available to veterans living in the Middle Georgia area.
John S. Goldman, Director
Gerald M. DeWorth, Associate Director

Hawaii

9959 Veterans Adm. Medical Centery: Honolulu VA Pacific Islands Health Care System

VA Pacific Islands Health Care System
459 Patterson Road   808-433-0600
Honolulu, HI 96819-1522   800-214-1306
Fax: 808-433-0390
www.hawaii.va.gov
The VA Pacific Islands Health Care System (VAPIHCS) Honolulu provides a broad range of medical care services, serving an estimated 127,600 veterans throughout Hawaii and the Pacific Islands. The VAPIHCS provides outpatient medical and mental health care through a main Ambulatory Care Clinic on Oahu (Honolulu) and through five Community Based Outpatient Clinics (CBOCs) on the neighboring islands including: Hawaii (Hilo and Kona), Maui, Kauai, and Guam. Traveling clinicians also provide episodi
William F. Dubbs, M.D., Acting Director
Brandon K. Yamamoto, Acting Associate Director

Idaho

9960 Idaho Persian Gulf Veterans

2055 Sotuh Colorado Street   208-344-3028
Boise, ID 83706
Vaughn Kidwell

9961 Veterans Adm. Medical Center: Boise Boise VA Medical Center

Boise VA Medical Center
500 W Fort Street   208-422-1000
Boise, ID 83702   866-437-5093
Fax: 208-422-1326
www.boise.va.gov
Boise VAMC's Primary Service Area has a radius of approximately 160 miles with an estimated veteran population of 94,000. The Boise VAMC, within VISN 20, provides highly sophisticated primary and secondary care with some tertiary services. The Boise VA Medical Center also operates a Community Based Outpatient Clinic (CBOC) in Twin Falls, Idaho and Caldwell, Idaho and an Extension Clinic in Burns, Oregon. A behavioral Health Clinic is located in Salmon, Idaho. A Vet Center and Veterans Benefits
Wayne Tippets, Director

Illinois

9962 Captain James A. Lovell Federal Health Car e Center

North Chicago VA Medical Center

3001 Green Bay Road   847-688-1900
North Chicago, IL 60064   800-393-0865
Fax: 847-578-3806
www.lovell.fhcc.va.gov
The Captain James A. Lovell Federal Health Care Center (FHCC) is a first-of-its-kind partnership between the U. S. Department of Veterans Affairs and the Department of Defense (DoD), integrating all medical care into a fully-integrated federal health care facility with a single combined VA and Navy mission.
Patrick L. Sullivan, Director
Captain Jos Acosta, MC, USN, Director/Commanding Officer

9963 Desert Storm Justice Foundation: Illinois

Rural Route 4   618-457-2621
Carbondale, IL 62901
Shan Now

9964 Edward J Hines Jr VA Hospital

5000 South 5th Avenue   708-202-8387
Hines, IL 60141   Fax: 708-202-7998
e-mail: hineswebmaster@va.gov
www.hines.va.gov
Edward Hines, Jr. VA Hospital, located 12 miles west of downtown Chicago on a 147-acre campus, offers primary, extended and specialty care and serves as a tertiary care referral center for VISN 12. Specialized clinical programs include Blind Rehabilitation, Spinal Cord Injury, Neurosurgery, Radiation Therapy and Cardiovascular Surgery. The hospital also serves as the VISN 12 southern tier hub for pathology, radiology, radiation therapy, human resource management and fiscal services.
Joan Ricard, Director
Carol A. Gouty, M.S.N.,PhD, Associate Director for Patient Care Serv

9965 Jesse Brown VA Medical Center

820 S Damen Avenue   312-569-8387
Chicago, IL 60612   888-569-5282
www.chicago.va.gov
The Jesse Brown VA Medical Center consists of a 200-bed acute care facility and four community based outpatient clinics (CBOCs). Jesse Brown VAMC provides care to approximately 58,000 enrolled veterans who reside in the City of Chicago and Cook County, Illinois, and in four counties in northwestern Indiana. In FY10, the medical center had over 8100 inpatient admissions and 560,000 outpatient visits. A budget of over $355 million supports approximately 2,000 full-time equivalent staff, including
Michelle Y. Blakely, FACHE, Associate Director for Operations
Ronald J. Fought, RN, Associate Director for Patient Care

9966 VA Great Lakes Health Care System

11301 W. Cermak Road   708-492-3900
Hines, IL 60154-5000   Fax: 708-492-3948
www.visn12.va.gov
The VA Great Lakes Health Care System, a group of seven VA medical centers and over thirty VA clinics, is dedicated to providing a comprehensive health care package to America's veterans. VA Great Lakes serves veterans who reside in northwestern Indiana, northern Illinois, Wisconsin and the Upper Peninsula of Michigan. Our Mission is to serve the health care needs of America's veterans.

9967 VA Illinois Health Care System

1900 E Main Street   217-554-3000
Danville, IL 61832-5198   800-320-8387
Fax: 217-554-4552
www.danville.va.gov
Since 1898, our buildings, facilities, patients, and missions have changed, but remaining constant is VA Illiana Health Care System's endeavor in improving the health of the men and women who have so proudly served our nation. Being the 8th oldest VA facility, we consider it our privilege to serve your health care needs in any way we can. Services are available to more than 150,000 veterans living in the surrounding 34-county areas of Illinois and Indiana.
Emma Metcalf, MSN, RN, Director
Diana Carranza, Associate Director

9968 Veterans Adm. Medical Center: Marion Marion VA Medical Center

Marion VA Medical Center

2401 W Main Street
Marion, IL 62959
618-997-5311
www.marion.va.gov

The VA Medical Center in Marion, Illinois, is a general medical and surgical facility that operates 55 acute care beds and a 60 bed Community Living Center. Ten Outpatient Clinics that provide primary care and behavioral medicine services are located in Harrisburg; Carbondale; Effingham; and Mt. Vernon, IL; Paducah; Hanson; Owensboro; and Mayfield, Kentucky; Vincennes and Evansville, IN.
Frank Kehus, Associate Director
Rose Burke, Acting Associate Director, Patient Care/

9969 Veterans Adm. Medical Center: Northport North Chicago VA Medical Center
3001 Green Bay Road
847-688-1900
North Chicago, IL 60064
Fax: 847-578-3806
www.northchicago.va.gov

Indiana

9970 VA Northern Indiana Health Care System Marion Campus
1700 E 38th Street
765-674-3321
Marion, IN 46953-4589
800-360-8387
Fax: 765-677-3124
www.northernindiana.va.gov

Originally constructed as the Marion branch of the National Home for Disabled Volunteer Soldiers, VANIHCS Marion Campus has been improving the health of the men and woman who have so proudly served our nation since 1889. The Marion Campus has 75 acute psychiatry beds and a 150 bed nursing home care unit, as well as primary care, medical and surgical specialty care and mental health clinics. The Marion Campus also offers programs for Mental Health Intensive Case Management, Post-Traumatic Stress
Denise M. Deitzen, Medical Center Director
Helen Rhodes MPA, RN, Associate Director for Operations

9971 Veterans Adm. Medical Center: Fort Wayne
2121 Lake Avenue
260-426-5431
Fort Wayne, IN 46805
800-360-8387
Fax: 260-460-1336
www.northernindiana.va.gov

Since 1950 VANIHCS Fort Wayne Campus has been improving the health of the men and woman who have so proudly served our nation. The Fort Wayne campus has a 26 bed medical center providing acute medical and surgical services, as well as primary care, medical and surgical specialty care and mental health clinics. Fort Wayne Campus also offers programs for the treatment of disorders such as Post-Traumatic Stress Disorder (PTSD) and Substance Abuse Treatment Program (SATP).
Denise M. Deitzen, Medical Center Director
Ajay Dhawan MD FACHE, Chief of Staff

Iowa

9972 Cedar Rapids Persian Gulf Veterans, Spouses and Children
909-28th Street Southeast 1
319-366-0756
Cedar Rapids, IA 52403
Mary Shears

9973 Des Moines Division: VA Central Iowa Health Care System
3600 30th Street
515-699-5999
Des Moines, IA 50310-5774
800-294-8387
Fax: 515-699-5862
www.centraliowa.va.gov

The VA Central Iowa Health Care System (VACIHCS) operates a Veterans Health Administration (VHA) medical facility in Des Moines, with Community Based Outpatient Clinics (CBOCs) in Mason City, Fort Dodge, Knoxville, Marshalltown and Carroll. The medical center provides acute and specialized medical and surgical services, residential outpatient treatment programs in substance abuse and post-traumatic stress and a full range of mental health and long-term care services, as well as sub-acute and r
Donald Cooper, Director
Susan Martin, Associate Director for Resources and Ope

9974 Knoxville Division: VA Central Iowa Health Care System
1515 W Pleasant Street
641-842-3101
Knoxville, IA 50138
800-816-8878
Fax: 515-699-5862
www.centraliowa.va.gov/visitors/Knoxvill

Features: Primary Ambulatory Care, Mental Health, Prescriptions: Routine prescriptions processed through the mail or My HealtheVet
Donald Cooper, Director
Susan Martin, Associate Director for Resources and Ope

9975 Veterans Adm. Medical Center: Iowa City
601 Highway 6 W
319-338-0581
Iowa City, IA 52246-2208
800-637-0128
Fax: 319-339-7171
www.iowacity.va.gov

Since 1952, the Iowa City VA Health Care System has been improving the health of the men and women who have so proudly served our nation. We consider it our privelege to serve your health care needs in any way we can. Services are available to more than 184,000 veterans living in 50 counties in Eastern Iowa, Western Illinois and Northern Missouri.
Barry Sharp, Medical Center Director
Timothy McMurry, Associate Director for Operations

Kansas

9976 Veterans Adm. Medical Center: Leavenwoth Dwight D. Eisenhower VA Medical Center
Dwight D. Eisenhower VA Medical Center
4101 4th Street Trafficway
913-682-2000
Leavenworth, KS 66048-5055
800-952-8387
Fax: 913-758-4149
www.leavenworth.va.gov

Since 1886, the staff of the Dwight D. Eisenhower VA Medical Center has been serving veterans. Today, we proudly serve our nation's veterans with excellent health care as part of the VA Eastern Kansas Health Care System (VAEKHCS). We consider it our privilege to serve your health care needs in any way we can.
A. Rudy Klopfer, Director
John M Moon, Associate Director

9977 Veterans Adm. Medical Center: Topeka Colmery O'Neil VA Medical Center
Colmery O'Neil VA Medical Center
2200 SW Gage Boulevard
785-350-3111
Topeka, KS 66622
800-574-8387
Fax: 785-350-4336
www.leavenworth.va.gov

VA Eastern Kansas Health Care System's primary service area consists of 39 counties in Kansas and Missouri. Veteran population in these counties totals over 104,000. VAEKHCS provides care to approximately 36,000 veterans.
A. Rudy Klopfer, Director
John M Moon, Associate Director

9978 Veterans Adm. Medical Center: Wichita Robert J. Dole Department Of VA Medical
Robert J. Dole Department Of VA Medical Center
5500 East Kellogg Ave
316-685-2221
Wichita, KS 67218
888-878-6881
Fax: 316-651-3666
www.wichita.va.gov

For 75 years, the Dole VA Medical and Regional Office Center has been honored to serve Kansas area veterans. The Center provides a full range of primary and specialty acute and extended care services to 30,000 veterans in 59 counties of Kansas.
Kevin Inkley, MA, Interim Medical Center Director
Vicki Bondie, MBA, Associate Director

Kentucky

9979 Carol and Dr. James W Stutts
108 Whispering Hills Drive
606-986-3267
Berea, KY 40403
e-mail: cstutts@kih.net

9980 National Association of State Directors of Veterans Affairs
Kentucky Department of Veteran Affairs

107 S. West Street
Alexandria, VA 22314

334-242-5075
Fax: 334-353-5072
e-mail: les.beavers@ky.gov
www.nasdva.net

The National Association of State Directors of Veterans Affairs (NASDVA) is an organization with a history dating back to 1946. In the aftermath of World War II many veterans earned State and Federal benefits which required coordinated efforts to assure that veterans received these entitlements. Thus, states developed a Department or Agency specifically to manage veterans' affairs and carry out the responsibility for veteran services and program.

W. Clyde Marsh, President
Terry Schow, Senior Vice President

9981 Veterans Adm. Medical Center: Lexington Lexington VA Medical Center
Lexington VA Medical Center
1101 Veterans Drive
Lexington, KY 40502

859-281-4900
859-233-4511
www.lexington.va.gov

The Lexington Veterans Affairs Medical Center is a fully accredited, two-division, tertiary care medical center with an operating bed complement of 199 hospital beds. Acute medical, neurological, surgical and psychiatric inpatient services are provided at the Cooper Division, located adjacent to the University of Kentucky Medical Center. Other available services include: emergency care, medical-surgical units, acute psychiatry, ICU, progressive care unit, (includes Cardiac Cath Lab) ambulatory s

Pamala Thompson, RN, MSA, MSN,, Interim Medical Center Director
Michael M Young, Acting Associate Director

9982 Veterans Adm. Medical Center: Louisville Louisville VA Medical Center
Louisville VA Medical Center
800 Zorn Avenue
Louisville, KY 40206

502-287-4000
800-376-8387
Fax: 502-287-6225
www.louisville.va.gov

Robley Rex Veterans Affairs Medical Center improves the health of our veterans and other eligible patients by providing a continuum of care through an integrated health care delivery system.

Wayne L. Pfeffer, MHSA, FACHE, Medical Center Director
Douglas V Paxton, Sr, Associate Director / Operations

Louisiana

9983 Alexandria VA Healthcare System
Alexandria VA Medical Center
2495 Shreveport Highway
Pineville, LA 71360

318-466-4000
800-375-8387
Fax: 318-483-5029
www.alexandria.va.gov

Service Recovery is used at our facility to improve customer service and is a critical process in organizations that excel in service to their customers. It identifies a service failure, effectively resolves a service problem, classifies its root cause(s), and yields data that can be integrated with other sources of performance measurement to assess and improve the service system. It entails making a person feel whole by staff demonstrating politeness, concern and candor.

Martin J. Traxler, Medical Center Director
Yolanda Sanders-Jackson, Associate Director

9984 Southeast Louisiana Veterans Health Care S ystem
New Orleans VA Medical Center
1601 Perdido Street
New Orleans, LA 70112

504-568-0811
800-935-8387
Fax: 504-589-5210
www.neworleans.va.gov

Southeast Louisiana Veterans Health Care System (SLVHCS) provides quality, compassionate, safe health care to Veteran patients throughout 23 parishes in southeast Louisiana. In the aftermath of Hurricane Katrina, the New Orleans VAMC was devastated. SLVHCS reorganized to meet the needs of Veterans and now consists of eight community-based clinics located in New Orleans, Slidell, Hammond, St. John Parish, Houma, Franklin, Bogalusa

and Baton Rouge. Ninety percent of patients live within 30 minutes
Julie A. Catellier, Director
Jimmy Murphy, Associate Director

9985 Veterans Adm. Medical Center: Shreveport Overton Brooks VA Medical Center
Overton Brooks VA Medical Center
510 E Stoner Avenue
Shreveport, LA 71101

318-221-8411
800-863-7441
Fax: 318-424-6156
www.shreveport.va.gov

The Overton Brooks VAMC and our associated CBOC's (Community Based Outpatient Clinics) are part of the South Central Health Care Network, VISN 16. VISN stands for Veterans Integrated Service Network, and is one of 22 VISN's in the U.S. Department of Veterans Affairs. VISN 16 provides comprehensive inpatient and outpatient health care, and limited nursing home and domiciliary care, to eligible veterans of the U.S. Armed Services. health care services are provided through a network of medical cent

Shirley M. Bealer, Medical Center Director
Erik J. Glover, Associate Medical Center Director

Maine

9986 Veterans Adm. Medical Center: Augusta Togus VA Medical Center
Togus VA Medical Center
1 VA Center
Augusta, ME 4330

207-623-8411
866-590-2976
Fax: 207-623-5792
TTY: 800-829-4833
TDD: 800-829-4833
e-mail: togus.query@vba.va.gov
www.benefits.va.gov/togus

Dale Denners, Regional Office Director

Maryland

9987 Fort Howard VA Outpatient Clinic
9600 N Point Road
Fort Howard, MD 21052

410-477-1800
800-351-8387
Fax: 410-477-7177
www.maryland.va.gov/facilities/Fort_Howa

Health Care Services: Anticoagulation AC,Arthritis,Dermatology,Medication Management, Mental Health, Nutrition, Podiatry, Post Traumatic Stress, Primary Care, Pulmonary, Social Work, Telemental Health, Women's Health
Dennis H Smith, Director

9988 Loch Raven VA Community Living & Rehabilit ation Center
3900 Loch Raven Boulevard
Baltimore, MD 21218

410-605-7000
Fax: 410-605-7900
www.maryland.va.gov/facilities/LochRaven

The Loch Raven VA Community Living & Rehabilitation Center specializes in providing rehabilitation and post-acute care for patients in the VA Maryland Health Care System. The center coordinates the delivery of rehabilitation services, including physical therapy, occupational therapy, kinesiotherapy and recreation therapy, to achieve the highest level of recovery and independence for Maryland's Veterans.

9989 Maryland Group
8725 Fairhaven Place
Jessup, MD 20794
Nancy Kaplan

301-725-4269

9990 VA Capitol Health Care Network
849 International Drive
Linthicum, MD 21090

410-691-1131
Fax: 410-684-3189
www.va.gov/visn5

The VA Capitol Health Care Network (VISN 5) was established in October 1995, and serves Veterans from economically and demographically diverse areas within Maryland, the District of Columbia, and portions of Virginia, West Virginia, and Pennsylvania.

Fernando O. Rivera, MBA, FACHE, Network Director
Guy B. Richardson, MHSA, FACHE, Deputy Network Director

9991 VA Maryland Health Care System Perry Point VA Medical Center
Perry Point VA Medical Center
Perry Point, MD 21902
410-642-2411
800-949-1003
Fax: 410-642-1161
www.maryland.va.gov

The Perry Point VA Medical Center provides a broad range of inpatient, outpatient and primary care services. As the largest inpatient facility in the VA Maryland Health Care System, the medical center provides inpatient medical, intermediate and long-term care programs, including nursing home care, rehabilitation services, geriatric evaluation and management, respite care, chronic ventilator care and hospice care.
Dennis H Smith, Director
Dorothy M Snow, Chief of Staff

9992 Veterans Adm. Medical Center: Baltimore
10 N Greene Street
Baltimore, MD 21201
410-605-7000
800-463-6295
Fax: 410-605-7901
www.maryland.va.gov/facilities/Baltimore

As a modern health care facility, the Baltimore VA Medical Center offers Veterans state-of-the-art technology and clinical services. The medical center is home to the world's first filmless radiology department, which allows health care providers to have nearly instant access to patient radiology images.

Carol Nizzardini, Chief Nurse Executive
Dennis H Smith, Director

Massachusetts

9993 Persian Gulf Era Veterans
24 Beacon Street
Boston, MA 02133
617-329-8149
e-mail: jagmedic@pgev.org
www.pgev.org

The general consensus is that VA is planning to use the materials generated from the pending IOM report on Chronic Multisymptom Illness Volume 9 to create a ICD code for sick Gulf War vets. Its uncertain if this is broad sweeping or badly managed science to produce a faulty definition based on psychiatry.
VenusVal Hammack, Executive Director

9994 VA Boston Healthcare System: Jamaica Plain Jamaica Plain Campus
Jamaica Plain Campus
150 S Huntington Avenue
Jamiaca Plain, MA 02130
617-232-9500
800-865-3384
Fax: 617-278-4508
www.boston.va.gov

VA Boston Healthcare System's consolidated facility consists of the Jamaica Plain campus, located in the heart of Boston's Longwood Medical Community; the West Roxbury campus, located on the Dedham line; and the Brockton campus, located 20 miles south of Boston in the City of Brockton.
Vincent Ng, Acting Director
Michael E Charness, Chief of Staff

9995 VA Boston Healthcare System: West Roxbury West Roxbury Campus
West Roxbury Campus
1400 VFW Parkway
W Roxbury, MA 02132
617-323-7700
800-865-3384
www.boston.va.gov

VA Boston Healthcare System's consolidated facility consists of the Jamaica Plain campus, located in the heart of Boston's Longwood Medical Community; the West Roxbury campus, located on the Dedham line; and the Brockton campus, located 20 miles south of Boston in the City of Brockton.
Vincent Ng, Acting Director
Susan MacKenzie, Associate Director

9996 VA New England Health Care System
200 Springs Road
Bedford, MA 01730
781-687-2000
800-838-6331
Fax: 781-687-3470
www.newengland.va.gov

Bedford VA is a long-term care facility specializing in geriatric and psychiatric care. Comprehensive health services include mental health, medicine, psychiatry, physical medicine, dentistry, geriatrics and ambulatory care.
Christine Croteau, Acting Hospital Director
Bob Colpitts, Acting Associate Director

9997 Veterans Adm. Medical Center: Brockton Brockton Campus
Brockton Campus
940 Belmont Street
Brockton, MA 02301
508-583-4500
800-865-3384
Fax: 700-885-1000
www.boston.va.gov

VA Boston Healthcare System's consolidated facility consists of the Jamaica Plain campus, located in the heart of Boston's Longwood Medical Community; the West Roxbury campus, located on the Dedham line; and the Brockton campus, located 20 miles south of Boston in the City of Brockton.
Vincent Ng, Acting Director
Michael E Charness, Chief of Staff

Michigan

9998 Detroit VA Medical Center John D. Dingell VA Medical Center
John D. Dingell VA Medical Center
4646 John R Street
Detroit, MI 48201
313-576-1000
800-511-8056
Fax: 313-576-1025
www.detroit.va.gov

Since 1939, this VA facility has been improving the health of the men and women who have so proudly served our nation. In 1996, the medical center moved from its original location in Allen Park, Michigan to the current location in Detroit. The John D. Dingell VAMC is one of the newest VA facilities in the country. It's our privilege to serve your health care needs in any way we can. Services are available to more than 330,000 Veterans living in Wayne, Oakland, Macomb, and St. Clair counties.
Pamela J Reeves, Director
Basim Dubaybo, Chief of Staff

9999 International Advocacy for Gulf War Syndrome
2297 Westfield Drive
Niles, MI 49102
616-684-5903
e-mail: DSVETERAN1@juno.com
Brian Martin

10000 Oscar G. Johnson VA Medical Center
Iron Mountain VA Medical Center
325 E H Street
Iron Mountain, MI 49801
906-774-3300
800-215-8262
Fax: 906-779-3188
www.ironmountain.va.gov

OGJVAMC is a primary and secondary level care facility with 17 acute care beds, 13 in the medical/surgical ward and 4 in the intensive care unit (ICU). The main facility provides limited emergency and acute inpatient care, and collaborates with larger VA Medical Centers in Milwaukee and Madison, WI, to provide higher-level emergency and specialty care services. OGJVAMC also provides rehabilitation and extended care, including palliative and hospice care, in its 40-bed Community Living Center.
James W. Rice, Medical Center Director
William J. Caron, PT, MHA, FACHE, Associate Director

10001 Veterans Adm. Medical Center: Ann Arbor Ann Arbor Healthcare System
Ann Arbor Healthcare System
2215 Fuller Road
Ann Arbor, MI 48105
734-769-7100
800-361-8387
Fax: 734-845-3245
www.annarbor.va.gov

The main hospital campus located in Ann Arbor serves as a referral center for specialty care and operates 105 acute care beds and 40 Community Living Center (extended care) beds. More than 500,000 outpatient visits were made at our facilities in fiscal year

2012; there were nearly 6,000 inpatient episodes of care provided in the hospital and extended care center.
Robert P. McDivitt, FACHE, Director
Randall E. Ritter, Associate Director

10002 Veterans Adm. Medical Center: Battle Creek
Battle Creek VA Medical Center
5500 Armstrong Road   269-966-5600
Battle Creek, MI 49037   888-214-1247
                                  Fax: 269-966-5483
                                  www.battlecreek.va.gov
The medical center offers a wide variety of health care services, which includes both inpatient and outpatient care. Once eligibility has been determined, each patient enrolling for care is assigned to a primary care provider and team, who provides continuous and coordinated care.
Mary Beth Skupien, Director
Edward Dornoff, Associate Director

10003 Veterans Adm. Medical Center: Saginaw Aleda E. Lutz VA Medical Center
Aleda E. Lutz VA Medical Center
1500 Wiess Street   989-497-2500
Saginaw, MI 48602   800-406-5143
                                  Fax: 989-321-4903
                                  www.saginaw.va.gov
Since 1950, the Aleda E. Lutz VA Medical Center has been improving the health of the men and women who have so proudly served our nation. We consider it our privilege to serve your health care needs in any way we can. Services are available to more than 31,000 veterans living in the Central and Northern 35 counties of Michigan's Lower Peninsula.
Peggy Kearns, Medical Center Director
Stephanie Young, Associate Director

Minnesota

10004 Desert Storm Justice Foundation: Minnesota
Buhl, MN 55713   218-258-3685
Jeff Zakula

10005 Veterans Adm. Medical Center: Minneapolis Minneapolis VA Medical Center
Minneapolis VA Medical Center
1 Veterans Drive   612-725-2000
Minneapolis, MN 55417   866-414-5058
                                  Fax: 612-725-2049
                                  www.minneapolis.va.gov
Minneapolis VA Health Care System (VAHCS) is a teaching hospital providing a full range of patient care services with state-of-the-art technology, as well as education and research. Comprehensive health care is provided through primary care, tertiary care and long-term care in areas of medicine, surgery, psychiatry, physical medicine and rehabilitation, neurology, oncology, dentistry, geriatrics and extended care.
Patrick J. Kelly, Director
Erik J. Stalhandske, Associate Director

10006 Veterans Adm. Regional Office: St. Paul
1 Federal Drive Fort Snelling   612-970-5415
Saint Paul, MN 55111   800-827-1000
                                  Fax: 612-970-5415
                                  e-mail: VBCINQ@VBA.VA.GOV
                                  www.va.gov/directory/guide/facility.asp?
St. Paul VA Regional Office will be accessible and responsive as we provide timely, accurate, and cost-effective service to veterans and their families. We will earn the respect and trust of veteran and their families by exceeding expectations and achieving excellence in the delivery of benefits and services. May we always keep our country's promise.

Mississippi

10007 G.V Montgomery VA Medical Center
1500 E Woodrow Wilson Drive   601-362-4471
Jackson, MS 39216   800-949-1009
                                  Fax: 601-364-1359
                                  www.jackson.va.gov
This medical center provides primary, second and tertiary medical, neurological and mental health inpatient care. Services include

hemodialysis, sleep studies, substance abuse treatment, post traumatic stress disorder (PTSD), hematology/oncology, and rehabilitation programs. Both primary and specialized outpatient services are available, including such specialized programs as: ambulatory surgery, spinal cord injury, neurology, infectious disease, substance abuse, PTSD, readjustment counseling,
Joe D. Battle, Medical Center Director
Bryan C. Matthews, Acting Associate Director

10008 South Central VA Health Care Network
715 S. Pear Orchard Road,   601-206-6900
Ridgeland, MS 39216   800-639-5137
                                  Fax: 601-206-7018
                                  www.visn16.va.gov
This medical center provides primary, second and tertiary medical, neurological and mental health inpatient care. Services include hemodialysis, sleep studies, substance abuse treatment, post traumatic stress disorder (PTSD), hematology/oncology, and rehabilitation programs. Both primary and specialized outpatient services are available, including such specialized programs as: ambulatory surgery, spinal cord injury, neurology, infectious disease, substance abuse, PTSD, readjustment counseling,
Joe D. Battle, Medical Center Director
Bryan C. Matthews, Acting Associate Director

10009 VA Gulf Coast Veterans Health Care System
400 Veterans Avenue   228-523-5000
Biloxi, MS 39531   800-296-8872
                                  Fax: 228-523-5719
                                  www.biloxi.va.gov
Since 1932, VA Gulf Coast Veterans Health Care System has been improving the health of the men and women who have so proudly served our nation. The VA Gulf Coast Veterans HCS is privileged to serve over 50,000 veterans. Additionally, it provides support to readjustment counseling centers and VA National Cemeteries along the Gulf Coast. The Health Care System is a part of VISN 16, South Central VA Health Care Network.
Anthony L. Dawson, MHA, FACHE, Director
Nancy Weaver, MBA, VHA-CM, Associate Director

10010 Veterans Adm. Regional Office: Jackson
1600 E Woodrow Wilson Avenue   601-364-7000
Jackson, MS 32916   800-827-1000
                                  Fax: 601-364-7007
                                  www.benefits.va.gov/jackson
The Department of Veterans Affairs provides a variety of services and benefits to honorably discharged veterans of the U.S. Military and their dependents. The purpose of this Web page is to assist Mississippi veterans, their dependents and survivors, in contacting the nearest VA facility to inquire about their veterans benefits or health care services.

Missouri

10011 John J. Pershing VA Medical Center
John J. Pershing VA Medical Center
1500 N Westwood Boulevard   573-686-4151
Poplar Bluff, MO 63901   888-557-8262
                                  Fax: 573-778-4559
                                  www.poplarbluff.va.gov
The John J. Pershing VA Medical Center, located in Poplar Bluff, Missouri, provides primary care to veterans throughout 29 counties of Southeast Missouri and Northeast Arkansas. Approximately 50,000 veterans live in our service area and about 40 percent of them receive care at our Medical Center annually. Our facility is comprised of 18 general medicine beds and 40 extended care beds. Tertiary care support is provided by VA Medical Centers in St. Louis and Columbia, Missouri; Memphis, Tennessee;
Marj Hedstrom, Medical Center Director
Vijayachandr Nair, MD, Chief of Staff

10012 VA Heartland Network
1201 Walnut Street   816-701-3000
Kansas City, MO 64106   Fax: 816-221-0930
                                  www.visn15.va.gov
The VA Heartland Network is one of twenty-two Veterans Integrated Service Networks (VISN) located throughout the United States. The VA Heartland Network also known as VISN 15, provides health care services to veterans in Kansas and Missouri, as well as parts of Illinois, Indiana, Kentucky and Arkansas.

10013 Veterans Adm. Medical Center: Columbia Harry S. Truman Memorial
Harry S. Truman Memorial
800 Hospital Drive   573-814-6000
Columbia, MO 65201-5297   800-349-8262
                                   Fax: 573-814-6600
                                        www.columbiamo.va.gov
Truman VA in Columbia, Missouri, serves 44 counties in Missouri as well as Pike County, Illinois, and is one of seven medical center facilities in the VA Heartland Network, a Veterans Integrated Service Network (VISN).
Sallie Houser-Hanfelder, FACHE, Director
Robert Ritter, FACHE, Associate Director

10014 Veterans Adm. Medical Center: Kansas City Kansas City VA Medical Center
Kansas City VA Medical Center
4801 Linwood Boulevard   816-861-4700
Kansas City, MO 64128   800-525-1483
                                   Fax: 816-922-3303
                                        www.kansascity.va.gov
Opening in 1952, the Kansas City VA Medical Center has a rich legacy of providing quality care to the men and women who have proudly served our nation — America's heroes. We consider it an honor and privilege to serve the health care needs of our Veterans.
Kent D. Hill, Medical Center Director
Kevin Inkley, Associate Director

10015 Veterans Adm. Regional Office: St. Louis John Cochran Division
John Cochran Division
915 N Grand Boulevard   314-652-4100
Saint Louis, MO 63106   800-228-5459
                                   Fax: 314-289-6557
                                        www.stlouis.va.gov
The VA St. Louis Health Care System provides inpatient and ambulatory care in medicine, surgery, psychiatry, neurology, and rehabilitation, and many other subspecialty areas. It is a two-division facility that serves veterans and their families in east central Missouri and southwestern Illinois. The John Cochran Division, named after the late Missouri congressman, is located in midtown St. Louis and has all of the medical center's operative surgical capabilities, the ambulatory care unit, intensi
Rimaann O. Nelson, RN,, Medical Center Director
Marc A. Magill, Deputy Medical Center Director

Montana

10016 Veterans Adm. Medical Center: Fort Harrison
VA Montana Health Care System
3687 Veterans Drive   406-442-6410
Fort Harrison, MT 59636   877-468-8387
                                   Fax: 406-477-7916
                                        www.montana.va.gov
Fort Harrison (Helena) is a 48-bed acute care, medical-surgical facility that offers a broad range of acute, chronic, and specialized inpatient and outpatient services for both male and female veterans. Specialty care includes internal medicine, gerontology, neurology, dermatology, cardiology, palliative care, pain management, medical oncology, surgery (general, vascular, laparoscopic, endoscopic), urology, orthopedics, plastic, ophthalmology, ENT, podiatry, gynecology, chiropractic care, psych
Christine Gregory, Director
Vicki Thennis, Interim Associate Director

10017 Veterans Adm. Medical Center: Miles City
210 S Winchester   406-874-5600
Miles City, MT 59301   877-468-8387
                                   Fax: 406-874-5696
                                        www.va.gov/directory/guide/facility.asp?
The Miles City Division of the VA Montana Healthcare System is located in southeastern Montana in Miles City. Headquarters for the VA Montana Healthcare System is located at the Ft. Harrison facility in Helena. Services at Miles City include a community based outpatient clinic and a 30 bed Nursing Home Care Unit. Some specialty clinics are also available. The VA Montana Healthcare System provides care to over 19,000 veterans annually.

Nevada

10018 Veterans Adm. Medical Center: Las Vegas VA Southern Nevada Healthcare System
VA Southern Nevada Healthcare System (VASNHS)
6900 North Pecos Road   702-791-9000
North Las Vegas, NV 89086   877-252-4866
                                   Fax: 702-636-3027
                                        www.lasvegas.va.gov
Since 1972, VA Southern Nevada Healthcare System has been improving the health of the men and women who have so proudly served our nation. We consider it our privilege to serve your health care needs in any way we can. Services are available to more than 240,000 Veterans living in our catchment area.
Isabel M Duff, Acting Director
Ramu Komanduri, M.D., Chief of Staff

10019 Veterans Adm. Medical Center: Reno VA Sierra Nevada Health Care System
VA Sierra Nevada Health Care System
975 Kirman Avenue   775-786-7200
Reno, NV 89502   888-838-6256
                                   Fax: 775-328-1464
                                        www.reno.va.gov
The VA Sierra Nevada Health Care System (VASNHCS), Reno, Nev., provides primary and secondary care to a large geographical area that includes 20 counties in northern Nevada and northeastern California.
Kurt W Schlegelmilch, M.D., FAC, Director
Steven E Brilliant, M.D., FACP, Chief of Staff

New Hampshire

10020 Veterans Adm. Medical Center: Manchester Manchester VA Medical Center
Manchester VA Medical Center
718 Smyth Road   603-624-4366
Manchester, NH 03104   800-892-8384
                                   Fax: 603-626-6579
                                        www.manchester.va.gov
Mission: Honor America's Veterans by providing exceptional health care that improves their health and well-being.
Tammy A. Krueger, BS, Acting Medical Center Director
Andrew J. Breuder, MD, MPH, FACPM, Chief of Staff

New Jersey

10021 Veterans Adm. Medical Center: East Orange East Orange Campus
East Orange Campus
385 Tremont Avenue   973-676-1000
E Orange, NJ 07018   Fax: 973-395-7062
                                        www.newjersey.va.gov
The Department of Veterans Affairs New Jersey Health Care System (VANJHCS) is a consolidated facility comprised of two main campuses, one in East Orange, the corporate office located in Northeastern New Jersey within the greater New York metropolitan area, and one in Lyons, 22 miles to the west of the East Orange Campus. The System's Diabetes Education, Pulmonary Rehabilitation, Prosthetics, Homeless Outreach Programs, and others have been recognized for outstanding achievement both within the D
Kenneth H Mizrach, Director
Steven L Lieberman, Chief of Staff

10022 Veterans Adm. Medical Center: Lyons Lyons Campus
Lyons Campus
151 Knollcroft Road   908-647-0180
Lyons, NJ 07939   Fax: 908-647-3452
                                        www.newjersey.va.gov
Primary care is emphasized at the VANJHCS. Veterans are assigned their own health care providers whom they see on a regular basis. Access to a wide variety of specialists is available through the primary providers. In addition to general medical, psychiatry, and long-term care, a full range of medical and surgical subspecialty care is provided to veterans of the VANJHCS in a variety of special programs as listed below. Because the VANJHCS is dedicated to developing programs that meet all veteran
Kenneth H Mizrach, Director
Steven L Lieberman, Chief of Staff

New Mexico

10023 Veterans Adm. Medical Center: Albuquerque New Mexico VA Health Care System
New Mexico VA Health Care System
1501 San Pedro Drive SE   505-265-1711
Albuquerque, NM 87108-5153   800-465-8262
                                 Fax: 505-256-2855
                                 www.albuquerque.va.gov
The NMVAHCS is a leader in the provision of rural health care, opening its first VA-staffed community based outpatient clinic (CBOC) in Farmington, New Mexico, followed by clinics in Artesia, Gallup, Raton, Silver City, Rio Rancho and Santa Fe. In recent years, the NMVAHCS has contracted with Health Net Federal Services and Ben Archer Health Center to provide Veterans access to clinics throughout New Mexico and southwest Colorado.
George Marnell, Director
Pamela Crowell, Associate Director

New York

10024 Brooklyn Campus of the VA NY Harbor Health care System
Brooklyn Campus
800 Poly Place   718-836-6600
Brooklyn, NY 11209   Fax: 718-567-4082
                                 www.nyharbor.va.gov
The NY Harbor Healthcare System is always improving the health of the men and women who have so proudly served our nation. We consider it our privilege to serve your health care needs in any way we can. Services are available to veterans living in the 5 boroughs of New York City.
Martina A. Parauda, Director
Veronica J. Foy, Associate Director, Facilities & Human R

10025 Gulf War Veterans of Long Island, NY
100 Robinson   516-289-1580
E Patchogue, NY 11772   Fax: 516-447-5871
                                 e-mail: DStormMom@aol.com
Jackie Olsen

10026 Persian Gulf Veterans
212 Garfield Avenue   716-385-4097
E Rochester, NY 14445-1314   Fax: 716-924-2161
Beverly Place

10027 VA Helathcare Network: Upstate New York
113 Holland Avenue   518-626-7327
Albany, NY 12208-8980   Fax: 518-626-7333
                                 www.visn2.va.gov
VA Health Care Upstate New York (VISN 2) is composed of five VA medical centers and 29 community based outpatient clinics. We provide comprehensive inpatient and outpatient health care to eligible Veterans.
David J. West, MSHA, FACHE, Network Director
Lawrence H Flesh, M.D., Chief Medical Officer

10028 VA NY/NJ Veterans Healthcare Network
130 W Kingsbridge Road   718-741-4110
Bronx, NY 10468   Fax: 718-741-4141
                                 www2.va.gov/directory/guide/facility.asp
Veterans Integrated Service Network 3 serves the wide diversity of needs for the greater New York and New Jersey veteran population. The Network provides care in some of the most urban settings in the nation as well as in sprawling suburban and rural areas. A full range of services is provided with each medical center emphasizing primary care complimented by specialized care. Additional services are provided in 30 community based outpatient clinics. VA's network of facilities includes; VA Medica
Michael A Sabo, Network Director

10029 Veterans Adm. Medical Center: Albany Samuel S. Stratton: VA Medical Center
Samuel S. Stratton: VA Medical Center
113 Holland Avenue   518-626-5000
Albany, NY 12208   800-223-4810
                                 Fax: 518-626-5500
                                 www.albany.va.gov

The Stratton VA Medical Center opened in 1951 and serves Veterans in 22 counties of upstate New York, western Massachusetts and Vermont.
Linda W. Weiss MS, FACHE, Director
Donald W Stuart, Associate Dirctor Albany VA Medical Cent

10030 Veterans Adm. Medical Center: Batavia VA Western New York Healthcare System
VA Western New York Healthcare System at Batavia
222 Richmond Avenue   585-297-1053
Batavia, NY 14020   888-823-9656
                                 Fax: 716-344-3305
                                 www.buffalo.va.gov/batavia.asp
The Batavia facility opened its doors in 1933. It provides geriatric and rehabilitation services, separate residential post traumatic stress disorder units for men and women, and outpatient services. In 1995, a New York State Veterans Home was built on the Batavia grounds making additional extended care available.
Brian G. Stiller, Director
Jason C. Petti, Associate Medical Center Director

10031 Veterans Adm. Medical Center: Bath Bath VA Medical Center
Bath VA Medical Center
76 Veterans Avenue   607-664-4000
Bath, NY 14810   877-845-3247
                                 Fax: 607-664-4511
                                 www.bath.va.gov
The Medical Center, founded in 1878 as a Grand Army of the Republic Soldiers and Sailors Home has proudly served Veterans for more than 130 years. The facility provides a full range of patient care services. We also provide primary and mental health care through clinics in Coudersport, Elmira, Mansfield and Wellsville.

Michael J. Swartz, Medical Center Director
Kenneth P. Piazza, Associate Director

10032 Veterans Adm. Medical Center: Buffalo
3495 Bailey Avenue   716-834-9200
Buffalo, NY 14215   800-532-8387
                                 Fax: 716-862-8759
                                 www.buffalo.va.gov
The Buffalo VA Medical Center opened in 1950 and provides medical, surgical, mental health and long term care services through a range of inpatient and outpatient programs. It is the main referral center for cardiac surgery, cardiology and comprehensive cancer care for central and western New York and northern Pennsylvania.
Brian G. Stiller, Director
Jason C. Petti, Associate Medical Center Director

10033 Veterans Adm. Medical Center: Montrose Franklin Delano Roosevelt Campus
Franklin Delano Roosevelt Campus
2094 Albany Post Road   914-737-4400
Montrose, NY 10548   800-269-8749
                                 Fax: 914-788-4244
                                 e-mail: complaint@jointcommission.org
                                 www.hudsonvalley.va.gov
Our vision is to be a patient-centered, integrated health care organization for Veterans providing excellent health care, research, and education; an organization where people choose to work; an active community partner; and a back up for national emergencies.
Gerald F Culliton, Director
Joanne J. Malina, M.D., Chief of Staff

10034 Veterans Adm. Medical Center: New York New York Campus
New York Campus
423 E 23rd Street   212-686-7500
New York, NY 10010   Fax: 718-567-4082
                                 www.nyharbor.va.gov
The NY Harbor Healthcare System is always improving the health of the men and women who have so proudly served our nation. We consider it our privilege to serve your health care needs in any way we can. Services are available to veterans living in the 5 boroughs of New York City.
Martina A. Parauda, Director
Veronica J. Foy, Associate Director, Facilities & Human R

10035 Veterans Adm. Medical Center: Northport Northport VA Medical Center
Northport VA Medical Center
79 Middleville Road   516-261-4400
Northport, NY 11768   800-551-3996
                                    Fax: 631-754-7933
                                    www.northport.va.gov
The Northport Veterans Affairs Medical Center is always improving the health of the men and women who have proudly served our nation. We consider it our privilege to serve your health care needs in any way we can. Services are available to veterans living in the Long Island area of New York.
Philip C Moschitta, Director
Edward J. Mack, MD, Chief of Staff

10036 Veterans Adm. Medical Center: Syracuse Syracuse VA Medical Center
Syracuse VA Medical Center
800 Irving Avenue   315-425-4400
Syracuse, NY 13210   800-792-4334
                                    Fax: 315-425-4375
                                    www.syracuse.va.gov
The Syracuse VA Medical Center, part of VA Health Care Upstate New York opened its doors on June 14, 1953. The Medical Center utilizes state-of-the-art technology to provide a full range of patient care services, education and research.
Judy Hayman, Ph.D., Acting Medical Center Director
William H Marx, DO, FACS, Chief of Staff

10037 Veterans Affairs Medical Center Canandaigua
Canandaigua VA Medical Center
400 Fort Hill Avenue   716-394-2000
Canandaigua, NY 14424   800-204-9917
                                    Fax: 716-393-8328
                                    e-mail: Laurie.Guererri@va.gov
                                    www.canandaigua.va.gov
The Canandaigua VA Medical Center, part of VA Health Care Upstate New York is located in the heart of the Finger Lakes region, 30 miles southeast of Rochester in Canandaigua, New York. Providing inpatient and outpatient care to veterans living in upstate New York since 1933, the Medical Center provides numerous health care programs and services.
Craig S. Howard, Director
Margaret Owens, Associate Director

North Carolina

10038 Charles George Veterans Affairs Medical Center
1100 Tunnel Road   828-298-7911
Asheville, NC 28805   800-932-6408
                                    Fax: 828-299-2563
                                    www.asheville.va.gov
The Extended Care and Rehabilitation Program at VAMC Asheville is composed of the following areas:Physical Medicine and Rehabilitation, Extended Care Center, Home and Community Care, Hospice and Palliative Care
Cynthia Breyfogle FACHE, Medical Center Director
David A Pattillo MHA FACHE, Associate Medical Center Director

10039 Desert Storm Veterans of North Carolina
739 E Haggard Avenue   910-584-5038
Ellon College, NC 27224
Kevin Treiber

10040 Veterans Adm. Medical Center: Durham Durham VA Medical Center
Durham VA Medical Center
508 Fulton Street   919-286-0411
Durham, NC 27705   888-878-6890
                                    Fax: 919-286-6825
                                    www.durham.va.gov
Since 1953, Durham Veterans Affairs Medical Cetner has been improving the health of the men and women who have so proudly served our nation. We consider it our privilege to serve your health care needs in any way we can. Services are available to more than 200,000 veterans living in a 26-county area of central and eastern North Carolina.
DeAnne M Seekins, Director
John D Shelburne, M.D. Ph.D, Chief of Staff

10041 Veterans Adm. Medical Center: Fayetville Fayettville VA Medical Center
Fayettville VA Medical Center
2300 Ramsey Street   910-488-2120
Fayetteville, NC 28301   800-771-6106
                                    Fax: 910-822-7093
                                    e-mail: james.neal@va.gov
                                    www.fayettevillenc.va.gov
Since 1940, the Fayetteville VA Medical Center (VAMC) has improved the health of the men and women who have so proudly served our nation. We consider it our privilege to serve your health care needs in any way we can. Medical, mental health, women's health care and specialty services are available to more than 157,000 veterans living in a 21-county area of North Carolina and South Carolina.
Elizabeth Goolsby, Director
James James Galkowski, PA-C, F, Associate Director

10042 Veterans Adm. Medical Center: Salisbury W.G. Hefner VA Medical Center
W.G. Hefner VA Medical Center
1601 Brenner Avenue   704-683-9000
Salisbury, NC 28144   800-469-8262
                                    Fax: 704-638-3395
                                    www.salisbury.va.gov
Inpatient services include acute medicine, cardiology, surgery, psychiatry and physical medicine and rehabilitation, as well as sub-acute and extended care. Primary and specialized outpatient services are provided at the medical center complex and the community based outpatient clinics. Services are also provided at the Veterans Outreach Centers Centers in Greensboro and Charlotte. Contractual extended care is provided through an extensive residential care treatment program and a community nursi
Kaye Green, FACHE, Director
Linette Baker, MPA, Associate Director

North Dakota

10043 Fargo VA Healthcare System
Fargo VA Medical.Regional Office Center
2101 N Elm Street   701-232-3241
Fargo, ND 58102   800-410-9723
                                    Fax: 701-239-3705
                                    e-mail: margaret.wheelden@va.gov
                                    www.fargo.va.gov
Since 1929, VAMC Fargo has been improving the health of the men and women who have so proudly served our nation. We consider it our privilege to serve your health care needs in any way we can. Services are available to more than 89,000 veterans living in North Dakota, Minnesota, and South Dakota.
Michael J. Murphy, FACHE, Center Director
Dale DeKrey, Associate Director for Operations and Re

Ohio

10044 Chalmers P. Wylie VA Ambulatory Care Cente r
Chalmers P. Wylie Outpatient Clinic
420 N James Road   614-257-5200
Columbus, OH 43219-1278   888-615-9448
                                    Fax: 614-257-5460
                                    e-mail: vhacoswebteam@va.gov
                                    www.columbus.va.gov
The Chalmers P. Wylie VA Ambulatory Care Center (VA ACC) has been improving the health of the men and women who have so proudly served our nation. We consider it our privilege to serve your health care needs in any way we can. From surgery to diagnostics, fitness to rehabilitation, depend on us for care.
Darwin Goodspeed, Director
Laura E Ruzick, FACHE, Associate Director

10045 Persian Gulf War Veterans of Western Pennsylvania, W Virginia and NE Ohio
600 North Market Street   216-426-3203
East Palestine, OH 44413   Fax: 216-426-3309
Barry M Walker

10046 VA Healthcare System Of Ohio
11500 Northlake Drive
Cincinnati, OH 45249

513-247-4621
Fax: 513-247-4620
e-mail: visn10webmaster@med.va.gov
www.visn10.va.gov

Each VISN 10 medical facility respects the patient's right to make decisions about his or her care, treatment and services, and to involve the patient's family in care, services, and treatment decisions to the extent permitted by the patient or surrogate decision-maker.

10047 Veterans Adm. Medical Center: Chillicothe Chillicothe VA Medical Center
Chillicothe VA Medical Center
17273 State Route 104
Chillicothe, OH 45601

740-773-1141
800-358-8262
Fax: 740-773-1141
e-mail: vhacllwebmaster@va.gov
www.chillicothe.va.gov

The Chillicothe VA Medical Center provides acute and chronic mental health services, primary and secondary medical services, a wide range of nursing home care services, specialty medical services as well as specialized women Veterans health clinics. The facility is an active ambulatory care setting and serves as a chronic mental health referral center for VA Medical Centers in southern Ohio and parts of West Virginia and Kentucky.
Wendy Hepker, Medical Center Director
Keith Sullivan, FACHE, Associate Medical Center Director

10048 Veterans Adm. Medical Center: Cincinnati Cincinnati VA Medical Center
Cincinnati VA Medical Center
3200 Vine Street
Cincinnati, OH 45220

513-861-3100
888-267-7873
Fax: 513-475-6500
e-mail: vhacinwebmasters@va.gov
www.cincinnati.va.gov

Cincinnati VAMC consists of 2 divisions located in Cincinnati, Ohio and Fort Thomas, Kentucky. Provides services to 17 counties in Ohio, Kentucky, and Indiana. Cincinnati VAMC has an active affiliation with the University of Cincinnati College of Medicine. Referral site for neurosurgery. PTSD Residential Programs for Men & Women. PTSD/Traumatic Brain Injury Residential Program. Iraq/Afghanistan Clinic Veterans Mobile Health Unit
Linda D Smith, Director
David E. Ninneman, RA, Associate Director

10049 Veterans Adm. Medical Center: Cleveland Louis Stokes VA Medical Center
Louis Stokes VA Medical Center
10701 E Boulevard
Cleveland, OH 44106

216-791-3800
877-838-8262
Fax: 216-421-3217
e-mail: cleveland.webmaster@va.gov
www.cleveland.va.gov

The Louis Stokes Cleveland VA Medical Center is one of five facilities constituting the VA Healthcare System of Ohio. A full range of primary, secondary and tertiary care services are offered at the Cleveland VA Medical Center to an eligible Veteran population covering 24 counties in Northeast Ohio. Care is provided to more than 105,000 Veterans each year through an inpatient tertiary care facility (Wade Park), 13 Multi-Specialty Clinics, Vet Centers, and numerous community-based contract nursin
Susan Fuehrer, Director
Darwin Goodspeed, Associate Director

10050 Veterans Adm. Medical Center: Dayton Dayton VA Medical Center
Dayton VA Medical Center
4100 W 3rd Street
Dayton, OH 45428

937-268-6511
800-368-8262
Fax: 937-262-2179
TTY: 800-829-4833
e-mail: 552webmaster@va.gov
www.dayton.va.gov

The Dayton VAMC is a state of the art teaching facility that has been serving Veterans for 146 years, having accepted its first patient in 1867. The Dayton VA Medical Center provides a full range of health care through medical, surgical, mental health (inpatient and outpatient), home and community health programs, geriatric

(nursing home), physical medicine and therapy services, neurology, oncology, dentistry, and hospice.
Glenn Costie, Medical Center Director
Mark Murdock, Associate Director

10051 Veterans and Families Support Network Ohio
5488 State Route 7
New Waterford, OH 44445

216-457-0641
Fax: 216-457-1923
e-mail: VFSN@delphi.com

Gina Brown

Oklahoma

10052 American Veterans Justice Foundation
3908 NW Santa Fe
Lawton, OK 73505

405-355-3811
e-mail: dwolf@sirinet.net

Dannie Wolf

10053 Jack C. Montgomery VA Medical Center
Dayton VA Medical Center
1011 Honor Heights Drive
Muskogee, OK 74401

918-577-3000
888-397-8387
Fax: 918-680-3648
www.muskogee.va.gov

Our Community-Based Outpatient Clinic in Tulsa is also named after a Native American. On May 27, 2008, the Tulsa Clinic was re-dedicated as the Ernest Childers VA Outpatient Clinic after Ernest Childers, a WWII Veteran and Medal of Honor recipient.
James R. Floyd, FACHE, Director
Inez Reitz, Acting Associate Medical Center Director

10054 Veterans Adm. Medical Center: Oklahoma City
Oklahoma City VA Medical Center
921 NE 13th Street
Oklahoma City, OK 73104

405-456-1000
866-835-5273
Fax: 405-270-1560
www.oklahoma.va.gov

The Oklahoma City VAMC is a tertiary care facility, classified as a Clinical Referral Level III facility (VA complexity level rating of 1b). The Oklahoma City VAMC is a teaching hospital, providing a full range of patient care services, with state-of-the-art technology as well as education and research. Comprehensive health care is provided through primary care, tertiary care, and long-term care in areas of medicine, surgery, psychiatry, physical medicine and rehabilitation, neurology, oncology
Daniel L. Marsh, Director
Debra Colombe, Acting Associate Medical Center Director

Oregon

10055 Northwest Network
3710 SW U.S. Veterans Hospital Rd.
Portland, OR 97239

503-220-8262
800-949-1004
Fax: 360-737-1405
e-mail: Daniel.Herrigstad@va.gov
www.visn20.med.va.gov

The Portland VA Medical Center (PVAMC) is a 303-bed consolidated facility with two main divisions. The medical center serves as the quaternary referral center for Oregon, Southern Washington, and parts of Idaho for the U.S. Department of Veterans Affairs. The Portland VAMC is located atop Marquam Hill on 28.5 acres overlooking the city of Portland. In addition to comprehensive medical and mental health services, the Portland VAMC supports ongoing research and medical education, including nati
John E. Patrick, MBA, Director
David Stockwell, MHA, Deputy Director of Administration and Fi

10056 Northwest Vets for Peace
811 E Burnside Street
Portland, OR 97214

503-656-9785
e-mail: NWVP@teleport.com

Marvin Simmons

10057 Veterans Adm. Medical Center: Roseburg VA Roseburg Healthcare System
VA Roseburg Healthcare System
913 NW Garden Valley Boulevard
Roseburg, OR 97471

541-440-1000
800-549-8387
Fax: 541-440-1225
e-mail: visn20webmaster@va.gov
www.roseburg.va.gov

The VA Roseburg Healthcare System (VARHS) consists of one Veterans Health Administration (VHA) facility located in Roseburg, OR, and four Community Based Outpatient Clinics (CBOC). The Roseburg campus consists of 200 acres and 32 buildings. VARHS offers primary care and hospital services in medicine, surgery and mental health for the 62,000 veterans who reside in Central and Southern Oregon and Northern California.
Carol Bogedain, Director
Steven J Broskey, Associate Director

10058 Veterans Adm. Medical Center: White City VA S Oregon Rehabilitation Center
VA Southern Oregonrehabilitation Center & Clinics
8495 Crater Lake Highway   541-826-2111
White City, OR 97503   800-809-8725
                                   Fax: 541-830-3500
          www.va.gov/directory/guide/facility.asp?
The SORCC provides a residential program with a two-fold mission of providing bio-psychosocial rehabilitation and long-term health maintenance. The SORCC offers an appropriate level of care for Veterans who do not require acute hospitalization or nursing home care but who cannot adequately provide for themselves in the community, and therefore need residential support. The SORCC adheres to Patient Centered Care Methodologies and Philosophy and provides safety, shelter, and food in a therapeutic,
Pam Harris, Human Resources Assistant

10059 Veterans Adm. Regional Office: Portland Portland VA Medical Center
Portland VA Medical Center
3710 SW US Veterans Hospital Road 503-220-8262
Portland, OR 97239   800-949-1004
                                   Fax: 503-273-5319
          e-mail: Daniel.Herrigstad@va.gov
                  www.portland.va.gov
The Portland VA Medical Center (PVAMC) is a 303-bed consolidated facility with two main divisions. The medical center serves as the quaternary referral center for Oregon, Southern Washington, and parts of Idaho for the U.S. Department of Veterans Affairs. The Portland VAMC is located atop Marquam Hill on 28.5 acres overlooking the city of Portland. In addition to comprehensive medical and mental health services, the Portland VAMC supports ongoing research and medical education, including nati
John E. Patrick, MBA, Director
Tom Anderson, MD, Chief of Staff

10060 Veterans Administration Domicillary
8495 Crater Lake Highway   541-826-2111
White City, OR 97503   Fax: 541-830-3519
          e-mail: David.Schwing@med.va.gov
                  www1.va.gov/domiciliary

Pennsylvania

10061 Erie VA Medical Center
135 E 38th Street Blvd.   814-868-8661
Erie, PA 16504   800-274-8387
                                   Fax: 814-860-2120
          e-mail: vhaeriweb@va.gov
                  www.erie.va.gov
Today, Erie VAMC is recognized as one of the top-performing medical centers in the delivery of high-quality health care. My goal is to assist in accelerating the improvements in service provided by our facility to the veterans we serve. These improvements are tracked in three important areas: the satisfaction veterans experience, the quality of the service we provide, and the efficiency with which we provide care and services to you. I am committed to making sure you have access to these service
Michael D Adelman MD, Director
Melissa Sundin, Associate Director

10062 Pennsylvania Gulf War Veterans
RR 3   814-226-4084
Clarion, PA 16214   e-mail: kjsmith@penn.com
Kenneth J Smith, President
Daniel J Meck, VP

10063 VA Pittsburgh Healthcare System: University Drive Division
University Drive   412-822-3578
Pittsburgh, PA 15240   866-482-7488
                                   Fax: 412-688-6121
          e-mail: vhapthwebmanager@va.gov
                  www.va.gov/pittsburgh
Terry Gerigk Wolf, Director
Rajiv Jain MD, Chief of Staff

10064 VA Stars & Stripes Healthcare Network
1010 Delafield Road   412-688-6000
Pittsburgh, PA 15240   866-482-7488
                                   Fax: 412-784-3724
          e-mail: vhapthwebmanager@va.gov
                  www.visn4.va.gov
VA Pittsburgh Healthcare System (VAPHS) is a two-campus, integrated healthcare system that proudly serves the Veteran population throughout the tri-state area of Pennsylvania, Ohio and West Virginia. VAPHS consists of two clinical care facilities in Pittsburgh as well as five community based outpatient clinics.
Michael E Moreland FACHE, Network Director
Carla Acre Sivek, MSW, Deputy Network Director

10065 Veterans Adm. Medical Center: Philadelphia
Philadelphia VA Medical Center
University & Woodland Avenues   215-823-5800
Philadelphia, PA 19104   877-626-2500
                                   Fax: 215-823-6007
                                   www.va.gov

10066 Veterans Adm. Medical Center: Coatesville
Coatesville VA Medical Center
1400 Black Horse Hill Road   610-384-7711
Coatesville, PA 19320   800-290-6172
          e-mail: VHACOAWebOperations@va.gov
                  www.coatesville.va.gov
Coatesville VA Medical Center is an integrated health care system dedicated to providing the best in care and services to our nation's Veterans. The hospital offers health care that is continuously improving, patient-centered, data-driven and team-based and includes mental health care, primary care, geriatrics and extended care, specialty and women's health care, and pharmacy and social work services, and more for both inpatients and outpatients. Additionally, the medical center operates communi
Gary W. Devansky, MHA, Director
Jonathan Eckman, P.E, Associate Director

10067 Veterans Adm. Medical Center: Lebanon Lebanon VA Medical Center
Lebanon VA Medical Center
1700 S Lincoln Avenue   717-272-6621
Lebanon, PA 17042   800-409-8771
                                   Fax: 717-228-5907
          e-mail: douglas.etter@va.gov
                  www.lebanon.va.gov
VAMC MISSION AND VISION: Honor America's Veterans by providing exceptional health care that improves their health and well-being. To be a patient-centered integrated health care organization for Veterans providing excellent health care, research, and education; an organization where people choose to work; an active community partner; and a back-up for national emergencies.
Robert W Callahan Jr, Director
Robin C. Aube-Warren, Associate Director

10068 Veterans Adm. Medical Center: Pittsburg VA Pittsburgh Healthcare System
VA Pittsburgh Healthcare System
University Drive   412-822-3578
Pittsburgh, PA 15240   866-482-7488
                                   Fax: 412-365-4213
          e-mail: vhapthwebmanager@va.gov
                  www.pittsburgh.va.gov
VA Pittsburgh Healthcare System (VAPHS) is a two-campus, integrated healthcare system that proudly serves the Veteran population throughout the tri-state area of Pennsylvania, Ohio and West Virginia. VAPHS consists of two clinical care facilities in Pittsburgh as well as five community based outpatient clinics.
Terry Gerigk Wolf, Director
Ali Sonel, MD, Chief of Staff

10069 Wilkes-Barre VA Medical Center
1111 E End Boulevard
Wilkes-Barre, PA 18711
570-824-3521
877-928-2621
Fax: 570-821-7278
www.wilkes-barre.va.gov
For over 50 years, VAMC Wilkes-Barre has been improving the health of the men and women who have so proudly served our nation. We consider it our privilege to serve your health care needs in any way we can. Services are available but not limited to veterans living in 18 counties in Pennsylvania and one county in New York.
Margaret B. Caplan, Director
Joseph F. Sharon, Interim Associate Director

Rhode Island

10070 Veterans Adm. Medical Center: Providence Providence VA Medical Center
Providence VA Medical Center
830 Chalkstone Avenue
Providence, RI 02908-4799
401-273-7100
866-363-4486
Fax: 401-457-3370
www.providence.va.gov
The Providence VA Medical Center is dedicated to providing high quality comprehensive outpatient and inpatient health care to Veterans residing in Rhode Island and southeastern Massachusetts. Each veteran who comes to the Medical Center for care is assured personalized care by a team of health care providers. A Primary Care Provider coordinates each patient's medical care, patient education needs and referrals to any of the medical centers 32 subspecialty clinics. The Medical Center's Ambulatory
Vincent Ng, Director
Erin Clare Sears, Associate Director

South Carolina

10071 Ralph H. Johnson VA Medical Center
109 Bee Street
Charleston, SC 29401-5799
843-577-5011
888-878-6884
Fax: 843-937-6100
e-mail: kevin.abel@va.gov
www.charleston.va.gov
The Ralph H. Johnson VA Medical Center serves more than 53,000 Veterans in 22 counties along the South Carolina and Georgia coastline in our main medical center or one of six community-based outpatient clinics.
Carolyn L. Adams, Director
Mr. Scott R Isaacks, MBA, FAAMA, Associate Director

10072 William Jennings Bryan Dorn VA Medical Center
6439 Garners Ferry Road
Columbia, SC 29209
803-776-4000
800-293-8262
Fax: 803-695-6739
www.columbiasc.va.gov
The William Jennings Bryan Dorn VA Medical Center (VAMC) opened in 1932 at its current location. Dorn VAMC is a 216 authorized bed facility (204 operating as of November 2012), which includes acute medical, surgical, psychiatric, and long-term care. The hospital provides primary, secondary, and some tertiary care. In 2012, the medical center served over 73,690 uniques Veterans during FY 2012. There were 906,858 (not unique) outpatient visits and a total of 4,821 inpatient treated.
Carolyn L. Adams, MS, Interim Medical Center Director
David L. Omura, DPT, MHA, MS, Associate Director

South Dakota

10073 Sioux Falls VA Healthcare System
2501 W 22nd Street
Sioux Falls, SD 57105-5046
605-336-3230
800-316-8387
Fax: 605-333-6878
e-mail: daniel.deblock@va.gov
www.siouxfalls.va.gov
Healthcare for eligible veterans.The Sioux Falls VA Health Care System includes a 98-bed medical center and five Community Based Outpatient Clinics. It provides inpatient and outpatient care for Veterans in eastern South Dakota, southwestern Minnesota, and northwestern Iowa. Services include primary and specialty medical care, mental health services, and rehabilitation. Affiliated

with The Sanford School of Medicine of the University of South Dakota, it supports residency programs in internal me
Sandra L. Horsman, Acting Director
Sara Ackert, MS, Associate Director

10074 VA Black Hills Health Care System- Fort Meade Campus
113 Comanche Road
Fort Meade, SD 57741
605-347-2511
800-743-1070
Fax: 605-347-7171
e-mail: BlackHillsVAFOIA.gov@va.gov
www.blackhills.va.gov
VA Black Hills Health Care System provides primary and secondary medical and surgical care, along with residential rehabilitation treatment program (RRTP) services, extended nursing home care and tertiary psychiatric inpatient services for Veterans residing in South Dakota, portions of Nebraska, North Dakota, Wyoming and Montana. Care is delivered through the Fort Meade and Hot Springs VA Medical Centers, as well as through a number of community based outpatient and rural outreach clinics.
Stephen R. DiStasio, FACHE, Director
C.B. Alexander, FACHE, Associate Director

10075 VA Black Hills Health Care System- Hot Springs Campus
500 N 5th Street
Hot Springs, SD 57747
605-745-2000
800-764-5370
Fax: 605-745-2091
e-mail: BlackHillsVAFOIA.gov@va.gov
www.blackhills.va.gov
VA Black Hills Health Care System provides primary and secondary medical and surgical care, along with residential rehabilitation treatment program (RRTP) services, extended nursing home care and tertiary psychiatric inpatient services for Veterans residing in South Dakota, portions of Nebraska, North Dakota, Wyoming and Montana. Care is delivered through the Fort Meade and Hot Springs VA Medical Centers, as well as through a number of community based outpatient and rural outreach clinics.
Stephen R. DiStasio, FACHE, Director
C.B. Alexander, FACHE, Associate Director

Tennessee

10076 Mountain Home VA Medical Center
Corner of Lamont & Veterans Way
Mountain Home, TN 37684
423-926-1171
877-573-3529
Fax: 423-979-3519
e-mail: mouwebmaster@va.gov
www.mountainhome.va.gov
Since 1903, James H. Quillen VA Medical Center has been improving the health of the men and women who have so proudly served our nation. We consider it our privilege to serve your health care needs in any way we can. Services are available to more than 170,000 veterans living in a 41-county area of Tennessee, Virginia, Kentucky, and North Carolina.
Charlene S. Ehret, FACHE, Director
Daniel B. Snyder III, P.E., MBA, Associate Director

10077 Persian Gulf Information Network
PO Box 10160
Clarksville, TN 37042
931-674-1518
Fax: 615-431-5222
e-mail: pgin@knightwave.com
www.home.att.net/~vetcenter/vetgrps.htm
Paul Lyons

10078 Tennessee Valley Healthcare System- Nashville Campus
1310 24th Avenue, South
Nashville, TN 37212-2637
615-327-4751
800-228-4973
Fax: 615-321-6350
www.tennesseevalley.va.gov
TVHS provides ambulatory care, primary care, and secondary care in acute medicine and surgery, specialized tertiary care, transplant services, spinal cord injury, outpatient care, and a full range of extended care and mental health services. The Nashville Campus is the only VA facility that supports all solid organ transplant programs, including total in-house kidney and bone marrow transplants. The Alvin C. York Campus is a network referral center for mental health services, geriatrics, and ext
Juan A. Morales, RN, MSN, Health System Director
Gary Trende, Chief Operating Officer, Nashville Camp

10079 Tennessee Valley Healthcare System- Alvin C. York (Murfreesboro) Campus
3400 Lebanon Pike
Murfreesboro, TN 37129

615-867-6000
800-876-7093
Fax: 615-225-4901
e-mail: TVHWebmaster@va.gov
www.tennesseevalley.va.gov

TVHS has active affiliations with two local institutions. The Alvin C. York Campus is primarily affiliated with Meharry Medical College, with active residency programs in oral surgery, psychiatry, general internal medicine, occupational medicine, preventive medicine, geriatric medicine, and family practice. The Nashville Campus is primarily affiliated with the Vanderbilt University School of Medicine with active residency programs in all major medical and surgical specialties and sub-specialties
Juan A. Morales, RN, MSN, Health System Director
Suzanne Jen, Chief Operating Officer, Murfreesboro

10080 VISN 9: VA Mid South Healthcare Network
1801 W End Avenue
Nashville, TN 37203

615-695-2200
Fax: 615-321-2721
e-mail: VISN9FOIA@va.gov
www.visn9.va.gov

VA MidSouth Healthcare Network (VISN 9) is committed to providing high quality, innovative, comprehensive, and compassionate care. VISN 9's goal is to ensure access for all enrolled veterans to the right care, at the right time, and at the right place to better serve Veterans in Huntington, West Virginia, Tennessee, Kentucky, and surrounding areas.

10081 Veterans Adm. Medical Center: Murfreesboro
3400 Lebanon Road
Murfreesboro, TN 37130

615-893-1360
Fax: 615-898-4872

10082 Veterans Adm. Medical Center: Memphis
1030 Jefferson Avenue
Memphis, TN 38104

901-523-8990
800-636-8262
www.memphis.va.gov

Since 1922, VAMC Memphis has been improving the health of the men and women who have so proudly served our nation. We consider it our privilege to serve your health care needs in any way we can. Services are available to more than 196,000 veterans living in a 53-county area of western Tennessee, northern Mississippi, and northwest Arkansas.
Jimmy H. McGlawn, MPH, Interim Medical Center Director/CEO
Douglas D. Southall, FACHE, Assistant Medical Center Director

10083 Veterans Adm. Medical Center: Muskogee
3400 Lebanon Pike
Murfreesboro, TN 37129

615-867-6000
Fax: 615-225-4901
www.tennesseevalley.va.gov

10084 Veterans Adm. Medical Center: Nashville
1310 24th Avenue S
Nashville, TN 37212

615-327-4751
800-228-4973
Fax: 901-577-7306
www.tennesseevalley.va.gov

TVHS has active affiliations with two local institutions. The Alvin C. York Campus is primarily affiliated with Meharry Medical College, with active residency programs in oral surgery, psychiatry, general internal medicine, occupational medicine, preventive medicine, geriatric medicine, and family practice. The Nashville Campus is primarily affiliated with the Vanderbilt University School of Medicine with active residency programs in all major medical and surgical specialties and sub-specialties
Juan A. Morales, RN, MSN, Health System Director
Gary Trende, Chief Operating Officer, Nashville Camp

10085 Veterans Affairs Medical Center
1030 Jefferson Avenue
Memphis, TN 38104

901-523-8990
800-636-8262
Fax: 901-577-7251
www.memphis.va.gov

Since 1922, VAMC Memphis has been improving the health of the men and women who have so proudly served our nation. We consider it our privilege to serve your health care needs in any way we can. Services are available to more than 196,000 veterans living in

a 53-county area of western Tennessee, northern Mississippi, and northwest Arkansas.
Jimmy H. McGlawn, MPH, Interim Medical Center Director/CEO
Douglas D. Southall, FACHE, Assistant Medical Center Director

10086 Veterans Affairs Medical Center, Memphis, Tennessee
1030 Jefferson Avenue
Memphis, TN 38104

901-523-8990
Fax: 901-577-7251
www.memphis.va.gov

Since 1922, VAMC Memphis has been improving the health of the men and women who have so proudly served our nation. We consider it our privilege to serve your health care needs in any way we can. Services are available to more than 196,000 veterans living in a 53-county area of western Tennessee, northern Mississippi, and northwest Arkansas.
Jimmy H. McGlawn, MPH, Interim Medical Center Director/CEO
Douglas D. Southall, FACHE, Assistant Medical Center Director

Texas

10087 Amarillo VA Health Care System
6010 Amarillo Boulevard W
Amarillo, TX 79106

806-355-9703
800-687-8262
Fax: 806-354-7860
e-mail: AMARILLOFOIA@VA.GOV
www.amarillo.va.gov

The Amarillo VA Health Care System, a division of the Southwest VA Health Care Network (VISN 18), provides primary specialty, and extended care of the highest quality to veterans throughout the Texas and Oklahoma panhandles, eastern New Mexico, and southern Kansas. Approximately 25,000 patients are treated annually. The health care system maintains 55 acute care inpatient beds for general medical, surgical, and intensive care. Geriatric and extended care is provided in the 120-bed skilled nursin
Andrew M. Welch, MHA, FACHE, Director
Gerald Darnell, Pys.D., Associate Director

10088 Austin Outpatient Clinic
7901 Metropolis Drive
Austin, TX 78744

512-823-4000
Fax: 512-389-6545
www.centraltexas.va.gov/locations/Austin

The clinic is 184,000 square feet - the largest, free-standing VA outpatient clinic in the nation. The clinic will offer expanded services for oncology; chemotherapy; ear, nose and throat; orthopedic services; minor surgeries; urology; gastroenterology; an endoscopy suite, and additional space for the Women's Clinic and all current services.
Russell E Lloyd, Associate Director of Resources
William F Harper, MD, FACP, Chief of Staff

10089 Central Texas Veterans Health Care System
1901 Veterans Memorial Drive
Temple, TX 76504

254-778-4811
800-423-2111
e-mail: Deborah.Meyer@va.gov
www.centraltexas.va.gov

The Central Texas Veterans Health Care System (CTVHCS), accredited by the Joint Commission, is comprised of two large Department of Veterans Affairs (VA) medical centers located in Temple and Waco, one stand-alone outpatient clinic in Austin, four community based outpatient clinics located in Brownwood, Bryan/College Station, Cedar Park, and Palestine plus a rural outreach clinic in La Grange. The system is one of the largest integrated health care systems in the United States and provides a ful
Russell E Lloyd, Associate Director of Resources
William F Harper, MD, FACP, Chief of Staff

10090 El Paso VA Health Care Center
5001 N Piedras
El Paso, TX 79930-4211

915-564-6100
800-672-3782
Fax: 915-564-7920
www.elpaso.va.gov

The El Paso VA Health Care System serves Veterans in far Southwest Texas and Doa Ana County, New Mexico. The El Paso VA Health Care System (VAHCS) includes the main health care facility located adjacent to William Beaumont Army Medical Center (WBAMC) on Ft. Bliss, Texas, and two VA-staffed Community Based Outpatient Clinics (CBOC) - one in Las Cruces, New Mexico, the second in east El Paso. The VAHCS provides primary and specialized ambulatory care services at its main campus with consultants

John A. Mendoza, Director
Elizabeth Lowery, Associate Director

10091 Michael E. DeBakey VA Medical Center
2002 Holcombe Boulevard 713-791-1414
Houston, TX 77030-4298 800-553-2278
Fax: 713-794-7218
e-mail: vhahoupublicaffairs@va.gov
www.houston.va.gov
Awarded re-designation for Magnet Recognition for Excellence in Nursing Services in 2008, the Michael E. DeBakey VA Medical Center serves as the primary health care provider for almost 130,000 veterans in southeast Texas. Veterans from around the country are referred to the MEDVAMC for specialized diagnostic care, radiation therapy, surgery, and medical treatment including cardiovascular surgery, gastrointestinal endoscopy, nuclear medicine, ophthalmology, and treatment of spinal cord injury and

Adam C. Walmus, M.H.A., F.A.C.H, Medical Center Director
Bryan T. Bayley, M.H.A., F.A.C.H, Deputy Medical Center Director

10092 Operation Desert Shield/Desert Storm
Odessa, TX 79760 915-368-4667
Fax: 915-580-7451

Vic Sylvester

10093 Persian Gulf Veterans of America
San Antonio, TX 78280 210-666-4409
e-mail: KathyPGVA@aol.com

Kathy Hughes

10094 South Texas Veterans Health Care System
7400 Merton Minter 210-617-5300
San Antonio, TX 78229 877-469-5300
www.southtexas.va.gov
South Texas Veterans Health Care System (STVHCS) is comprised of two inpatient campuses: the Audie L. Murphy Memorial VA Hospital in San Antonio and the Kerrville VA Hospital in Kerrville, Texas. STVHCS serves one of the largest primary service areas in the nation and is part of the VA Heart of Texas Veterans Integrated Service Network (VISN 17), with offices located in Arlington, Texas. With an FY12 budget for STVHCS of $605 million and more than 3,400 employees, South Texas provides health ca

Marie L. Weldon, Director
Wade Vlosich, Associate Director

10095 VA Heart of Texas Health Care Network Dallas VA Medical Center
Dallas VA Medical Center
4500 S Lancaster Road 214-742-8387
Dallas, TX 75216 800-849-3597
Fax: 214-857-1171
www.northtexas.va.gov
VANTHCS provides comprehensive health services through primary, tertiary and long-term care in many areas like medicine, surgery, mental health and rehabilitation. The 853-bed system has a Spinal Cord Injury Center, Domiciliary Care Program and Community Living Center with a dedicated hospice unit. In 2009, a Fisher House was established on the Dallas campus to provide no-cost temporary lodging in a home-like setting for families of Veterans or active duty military personnel undergoing treatment

Jeffery L. Milligan, Director
Peter Dancy, Associate Director

10096 Veterans Adm. Medical Center: Big Spring
300 Veterans Boulevard 432-263-7361
Big Spring, TX 79720-5500 800-472-1365
Fax: 432-264-4834
www.bigspring.va.gov
The West Texas VA Health Care System (WTVAHCS) proudly serves Veterans in 33 counties across 53,000 square miles of rural geography in West Texas and Eastern New Mexico. The George H. O'Brien, Jr. VA Medical Center is located in Big Spring, Texas and the six Community Based Outpatient Clinics (CBOC's) that comprise the remainder of the health care system are located in Abilene, TX, Stamford, TX, San Angelo, TX, Odessa, TX, Fort

Stockton, TX, and Hobbs, NM. Two Vet Centers also provide services a

Andrew M. Welch, Interim Director
Kenneth Allensworth, Associate Director

10097 Veterans Adm. Medical Center: Dallas
4500 S Lancaster Road 214-742-8387
Dallas, TX 75216 800-849-3597
Fax: 214-857-1171
www.northtexas.va.gov
VA North Texas Health Care System (VANTHCS) is a progressive health care provider in the heart of Texas. Poised as VA's second largest health care system, we serve over 113,000 Veterans and deliver 1.4 million outpatient episodes of care each year to Veterans in 38 Texas counties and two counties in southern Oklahoma. We have 4,700 employees and 1,700 community volunteers who are driven by the passion to serve at Dallas VA Medical Center, Sam Rayburn Memorial Veterans Center, Fort Worth Outpatie

Jeffery L. Milligan, Director
Peter Dancy, Associate Director

10098 Veterans Adm. Medical Center: Kerrville
3600 Memorial Boulevard 830-896-2020
Kerrville, TX 78028 866-487-7653
www.southtexas.va.gov

The Kerrville VA Hospital (KVAH), located 65 miles northwest of San Antonio, provides primary care, some specialty care, geriatric evaluation and management, palliative care, and long-term care services with a Community Living Center. The Satellite Clinic Division (SCD) offer primary care and some specialty care while sharing resources with each other and their respective communities. When required, Veterans are referred to ALMMVAH or KVAH for specialty care including medicine, surgery, neurop

Marie L. Weldon, Director
Joe A. Perez, Assistant Director

10099 Veterans Adm. Medical Center: Marlin
1016 Ward Street 254-883-3511
Marlin, TX 76661 Fax: 254-883-9240
www.southtexas.va.gov

10100 Veterans Adm. Medical Center: San Antonio
7400 Merton Minter Boulevard 210-617-5300
San Antonio, TX 78229 877-469-5300
www.southtexas.va.gov
South Texas Veterans Health Care System (STVHCS) is comprised of two inpatient campuses: the Audie L. Murphy Memorial VA Hospital in San Antonio and the Kerrville VA Hospital in Kerrville, Texas. STVHCS serves one of the largest primary service areas in the nation and is part of the VA Heart of Texas Veterans Integrated Service Network (VISN 17), with offices located in Arlington, Texas. With an FY12 budget for STVHCS of $605 million and more than 3,400 employees, South Texas provides health ca

Marie L. Weldon, Director
Wade Vlosich, Associate Director

10101 Veterans Adm. Medical Center: Temple
1901 Veterans Memorial Drive 254-778-4811
Temple, TX 76504 800-423-2111
Fax: 254-771-4588
e-mail: Deborah.Meyer@va.gov
www.centraltexas.va.gov

The Central Texas Veterans Health Care System (CTVHCS), accredited by the Joint Commission, is comprised of two large Department of Veterans Affairs (VA) medical centers located in Temple and Waco, one stand-alone outpatient clinic in Austin, four community based outpatient clinics located in Brownwood, Bryan/College Station, Cedar Park, and Palestine plus a rural outreach clinic in La Grange. The system is one of the largest integrated health care systems in the United States and provides a ful

Russell E Lloyd, Associate Director of Resources
William F Harper, MD, FACP, Chief of Staff

10102 Waco VA Medical Center
4800 Memorial Drive 254-752-6581
Waco, TX 76711 800-423-2111
e-mail: Deborah.Meyer@va.gov
www.centraltexas.va.gov

745

The Central Texas Veterans Health Care System (CTVHCS), accredited by the Joint Commission, is comprised of two large Department of Veterans Affairs (VA) medical centers located in Temple and Waco, one stand-alone outpatient clinic in Austin, four community based outpatient clinics located in Brownwood, Bryan/College Station, Cedar Park, and Palestine plus a rural outreach clinic in La Grange. The system is one of the largest integrated health care systems in the United States and provides a ful
Russell E Lloyd, Associate Director of Resources
William F Harper, MD, FACP, Chief of Staff

10103 West Texas VA Health Care System
300 Veterans Boulevard — 432-263-7361
Big Spring, TX 79720 — 800-472-1365
Fax: 432-264-4834
www.bigspring.va.gov
The West Texas VA Health Care System (WTVAHCS) proudly serves Veterans in 33 counties across 53,000 square miles of rural geography in West Texas and Eastern New Mexico. The George H. O'Brien, Jr. VA Medical Center is located in Big Spring, Texas and the six Community Based Outpatient Clinics (CBOC's) that comprise the remainder of the health care system are located in Abilene, TX, Stamford, TX, San Angelo, TX, Odessa, TX, Fort Stockton, TX, and Hobbs, NM. Two Vet Centers also provide services a
Andrew M. Welch, Interim Director
Kenneth Allensworth, Associate Director

Utah

10104 VA Salt Lake City Health Care System
500 Foothill Drive — 801-582-1565
Salt Lake City, UT 84148 — 800-613-4012
Fax: 801-584-1289
www.saltlakecity.va.gov
The George E. Wahlen Department of Veterans Affairs Medical Center is a mid-sized affiliated tertiary care facility with 121 authorized active beds. It is a teaching facility, providing a full range of patient care services, with state-of-the-art technology as well as education and research. Comprehensive health care is provided through primary care, tertiary care, and long-term care in areas of medicine, surgery, psychiatry, physical medicine and rehabilitation, neurology, oncology, dentistry,
Steven W. Young, FACHE, Director
Warren E. Hill, Associate Director

Vermont

10105 White River Junction VA Medical Center
215 N Main Street — 802-295-9363
White River Junction, VT 05009 — 866-687-8387
Fax: 802-296-6354
www.whiteriver.va.gov
The White River Junction VA Medical Center (WRJ VAMC) is responsible for the delivery of health care services to eligible Veterans in Vermont and the 4 contiguous counties of New Hampshire. These services are delivered at the Medical Center's main campus located in White River Junction, Vermont, and at its seven Outpatient Clinics (Bennington, Brattleboro, Colchester, Newport, and Rutland, Vermont; Keene and Littleton, New Hampshire). The White River Junction VA is closely affiliated with the Ge
Deborah Amdur, Director
Danielle S Ocker, RN, BSN, Associate Director

Virginia

10106 Desert Storm Justice Foundation: Virginia
Alexandria, VA 22309 — 703-550-1346
Fax: 703-550-1346

10107 Gulf War Veterans of Virginia
Chesapeake, VA 23320 — 757-988-3PGW
Ted Myers, President

10108 Veterans Adm. Medical Center: Hampton Hampton VA Medical Center
Hampton VA Medical Center

100 Emancipation Drive — 757-722-9961
Hampton, VA 23667 — 888-869-6060
Fax: 757-723-6620
www.hampton.va.gov
The Hampton VAMC is a tertiary care, Complexity Level 2 hospital. Hampton VAMC provides comprehensive primary and specialty care in medicine, surgery, and psychiatry. The Medical Center is geographically positioned among one of the largest DoD active duty and military retiree populations in the United States. As a result, the Medical Center has seen a 7% increase among Veterans seeking VA care. The Hampton VAMC recently opened a state-of-the-art Women's Clinic designed to provide gender speci
Michael H. Dunfee, MHA, Medical Center Director
Benita K. Miller, MHA, FACHE, Associate for Operations Director

10109 Veterans Adm. Medical Center: Richmond Hunter Holmes McGuire VA Medical Center
Hunter Holmes McGuire VA Medical Center
1201 Broad Rock Boulevard — 804-675-5000
Richmond, VA 23249 — 800-784-8381
Fax: 804-675-5581
www.richmond.va.gov
Since 1946, the Richmond VAMC has been improving the health of the men and women who have so proudly served our nation. We consider it our privilege to serve your health care needs in any way we can. Services are available to more than 200,000 veterans coming from 52 cities and counties covering 22,515 miles of central and southern Virginia and parts of northern North Carolina.
John A. Brandecker, Director
David P. Budinger, FACHE, Associate Director for Operations

10110 Veterans Adm. Medical Center: Roanoke Roanoke Vet Center
Roanoke Vet Center
350 Albemarle Avenue SW — 540-342-9726
Roanoke, VA 24016 — 877-927-8387
Fax: 540-857-2405
www.va.gov

Lynn McGhee, Team Leader
John Whitlock, Counselor

10111 Veterans Adm. Medical Center: Salem Salem VA Medical Center
Salem VA Medical Center
1970 Roanoke Boulevard — 540-982-2463
Salem, VA 24153 — 888-982-2463
Fax: 540-983-1096
www.salem.va.gov
Since 1934, Salem VAMC has been improving the health of the men and women who have so proudly served our Nation. We consider it our privilege to serve your health care needs in any way we can. Services are available to more than 112,500 Veterans living in a 26-county area of southwestern Virginia.
Miguel H LaPuz, MD, MBA, Director, SAMVAMC
Rebecca J. Stackhouse, FACHE, VHA-, Associate Director

Washington

10112 Persian Gulf Veterans of Washington
13523 202nd Street E — 360-893-2480
Graham, WA 98338 — Fax: 360-893-3998
e-mail: amehl@ix.netcom.com

10113 VA Puget Sound Health Care Network
1660 S Columbian Way — 206-762-1010
Seattle, WA 98108 — 800-329-8387
Fax: 206-764-2224
www.pugetsound.va.gov
With a reputation for excellence, innovation and extraordinary care of our Nation's heroes, VA Puget Sound strives to lead the nation in terms of quality, efficiency and public service through its proven record of innovation and extraordinary care of Veterans. As the primary referral site for VA's northwest region, VA Puget Sound provides care for Veteran populations encompassing Alaska, Montana, Idaho and Oregon.
Michael J. Murphy, FACHE, Director
Michael Tadych, Deputy Director

10114 Veterans Adm. Medical Center: Spokane Spokane VA Medical Center
Spokane VA Medical Center

4815 N Assembly Street
Spokane, WA 99205-6197

509-434-7000
800-325-7940
Fax: 509-434-7119
www.spokane.va.gov

The Spokane VA Medical Center is dedicated to providing quality health care services to veterans. In carrying out this mission, the VAMC focuses on providing primary and secondary care, with emphasis on preventive health and chronic disease management.

10115 Veterans Adm. Medical Center: Tacoma Tacoma Vet Center
Tacoma Vet Center
4916 Center Street
Tacoma, WA 98409

253-565-7038
877-927-8387
Fax: 253-565-4981
www.va.gov

Robert Ramsey, Team Leader
George Rippon, Counselor

10116 Veterans Adm. Medical Center: Walla Walla Johnathan M. Wainwright Memorial VA MC
Johnathan M. Wainwright Memorial VA Medical Center
77 Wainwright Drive
Walla Walla, WA 99362

509-525-5200
888-687-8863
Fax: 509-527-3452
www.wallawalla.va.gov

Since 1921, the Jonathan M. Wainwright Memorial VA Medical Center (Walla Walla VAMC) has been improving the health of the men and women who have so proudly served our nation. We consider it our privilege to serve your health care needs in any way we can. Services are available to Veterans living in eastern Washington and Oregon and western Idaho. We pride ourselves in giving the best care - anywhere!

West Virginia

10117 Veterans Adm. Medical Center: Beckley
Beckley VA Medical Center
200 Veterans Avenue
Beckley, WV 25801

304-255-2121
877-902-5142
Fax: 304-255-2431
www.beckley.va.gov

Beckley VAMC is a 40-bed general medical and surgical care facility with a 50-bed community living center. The medical center is a Joint Commission accredited, rural access facility. The community living center offers skilled nursing care, post-acute rehabilitation and restorative care, palliative care, and respite care for eligible Veterans. The medical center also operates a home based primary care program.
Karin L McGraw, Director
J. Brian Nimmo, Associate Director

10118 Veterans Adm. Medical Center: Clarksburg Louis A. Johnson VA Medical Center
Louis A. Johnson VA Medical Center
One Medical Center Drive
Clarksburg, WV 26301

304-623-3461
800-733-0512
Fax: 304-626-7026
www.clarksburg.va.gov

The Louis A. Johnson VA Medical Center exists to serve the veteran through the delivery of timely quality care by staff who demonstrate outstanding customer service, the advancement of health care through research, and the education of tomorrow's health care providers.
Beth M. Brown, MS, FACHE, VHA-C, Medical Center Director
Judy T. Finley, MBA, Associate Director

10119 Veterans Adm. Medical Center: Huntington
1540 Spring Valley Drive
Huntington, WV 25704

304-429-6741
800-827-8244
Fax: 304-429-6713
www.huntington.va.gov

Since 1932, VAMC Huntington has been improving the health of the men and women who have so proudly served our nation. We consider it our privilege to serve your health care needs in any way we can. Services are available to veterans living in southwestern West Virginia, southern Ohio, and eastern Kentucky.
Edward H Seiler, Medical Center Director
Pamela G Smith, Associate Medical Center Director

10120 Veterans Affairs Medical Center: Martinsburg
510 Butler Avenue
Martinsburg, WV 25405

304-263-0811
800-817-3807
Fax: 304-262-7448
www.martinsburg.va.gov

Since 1944, the Martinsburg VA Medical Center has been improving the health of the men and women who have so proudly served our nation. We consider it our privilege to serve your health care needs in any way we can. Services are available to more than 126,000 veterans living in 22 counties in Western Maryland, West Virginia, South Central Pennsylvania, and Northwest Virginia.
Ann R. Brown, FACHE, Medical Center Director
Timothy J. Cooke, Associate Medical Center Director

Wisconsin

10121 Clement J. Zablocki Veterans Affairs Medical Center
5000 W National Avenue
Milwaukee, WI 53295-1000

414-384-2000
Fax: 414-382-5321
e-mail: vhamiwwebmaster@va.gov
www.milwaukee.va.gov

The Clement J. Zablocki VA Medical Center is located on 125 acres on the western edge of Milwaukee and part of VA Integrated Services Network 12 (VISN 12), which includes facilities in Iron Mountain, MI; Tomah and Madison, WI, and North Chicago, Hines, and Chicago. The Medical Center delivers primary, secondary, and tertiary medical care in 168 care acute operating beds and provides over 500,000 visits annually through an extensive outpatient program. The nursing home care unit of 113 beds offer
Robert H. Beller, FACHE, Medical Center Director
James McLain, Deputy Medical Center Director

10122 Gulf War Veterans of Wisconsin
33 University Square
Madison, WI 53715

608-250-9645
e-mail: gulfwarwisc@geocities.com
Anthony Hardie

10123 MidWest Gulf War Veterans Association
Pewaukee, WI 53072

414-695-8694
Fax: 414-695-8694
e-mail: mrlbrty@execpc.com

Robert Schramm

10124 Veterans Adm. Medical Center: Tomah
500 E Veterans Street
Tomah, WI 54660

608-372-3971
800-872-8662
www.tomah.va.gov

VAMC Tomah has been improving the health of the men and women who have so proudly served our nation. We consider it our privilege to serve your health care needs in any way we can. Services are available to veterans living in a Western/Central area of Wisconsin.
Mario V. DeSanctis, FACHE, Medical Center Director
David Huffman, M.S., Associate Director

10125 William S. Middleton Memorial Veterans Hospital
2500 Overlook Terrace
Madison, WI 53705-2286

608-256-1901
888-478-8321
Fax: 608-280-7096
www.madison.va.gov

The Madison VA Hospital is one of seven facilities that comprise Veterans Integrated Services Network 12 which is administratively headquartered at Hines, IL, and includes facilities in Illinois, Wisconsin, and Michigan.
Judy K. McKee, FACHE, Director
John Rohrer, Associate Director

Wyoming

10126 Veterans Adm. Medical Center: Cheyenne
2360 E Pershing Boulevard
Cheyenne, WY 82001

307-778-7550
888-483-9127
Fax: 307-778-7336
www.cheyenne.va.gov

Cheyenne VAMC Police Service is responsible for providing a safe and secure environment for all patients, staff, and visitors to the property. The Police Service is on-duty and available for the facility/Staff 24/7/365 with professionally trained and conscientious officers.

Cynthia McCormack, RN, PhD, Medical Center Director
Paul L Roberts, Medical Center Associate Director

10127 Veterans Adm. Medical Center: Sheridan
1898 Fort Road   307-672-3473
Sheridan, WY 82801   866-822-6714
                                                                   Fax: 307-672-1900
                                    e-mail: sheridanwebmaster@va.gov
                                                            www.sheridan.va.gov
Since April 1922, the Sheridan VAMC has been a mental health care and primary care facility for men and women who have served their country. In 1898 the grounds that are now the Sheridan VAMC were set aside by President William McKinley to be a military fort. The fort was named after Brigadier General Ranald Slidell Mackenzie. The first troops to the fort in 1901 were Buffalo Soldiers who used the fort for rest and retraining. By World War I, the fort was closed and ready for demolition. Ho

Debra L. Hirschman, Director
Michele Beach, Associate Director/Chief Business Offic

Libraries & Resource Centers

10128 American GI Forum NVOP
611 N. Flores   210-212-4088
San Antonio, TX 78205   Fax: 210-223-4970
                                           e-mail: nvopweb@agif-nvop.org
                                                             www.agif-nvop.org
Our Mision is to establish and maintain a comprehensive community service agency with a diversified funding source that will serve the needs of veterans, their families, and other needy individuals of the community.

10129 COPIN Foundation
2644 North Avenue   716-283-5622
Niagara Falls, NY 14305   Fax: 716-283-5721

10130 Kennedy-Krieger Institute
707 N Broadway   443-923-9200
Baltimore, MD 21205   800-873-3377
                                                                   Fax: 443-923-9405
                                                            www.kennedykrieger.org
Kennedy Krieger Institute is an internationally recognized institution dedicated to improving the lives of individuals with disorders of the brain, spinal cord, and musculoskeletal system through Patient Care, Research and Professional Training, Special Education and Community. We at the Kennedy Krieger Institute dedicate ourselves to helping children and adolescents with disorders of the brain, spinal cord and musculoskeletal system achieve their potential and participate as fully as possible i

Jennifer Accardo, M.D., Neurologist
Adrianna Amari, Ph.D., Training and research coordinator

10131 Shriver Center University Affiliated Program
Eunice Kennedy Shriver Center
200 Trapelo Road   781-642-0001
Waltham, MA 02452-6319   e-mail: shriver.center@umassmed.edu
                                                            www.umassmed.edu/shriver
The Eunice Kennedy Shriver Center has a four-decade history of pioneering research, education, and service for people with intellectual and developmental disabilities (IDD) and their families. Founded in 1970, the Center was one of twelve original Intellectual and Developmental Disabilities Research Centers (IDDRCs) established by US Congress at that time and also one of the earliest-established University Centers of Excellence in Developmental Disabilities (UCEDD). The Center was named after Mr

William McIlvane, Director
Charles Hamad, Associate Director

10132 Veterans Benefits Clearinghouse
38 Dudley Street   617-541-8846
Roxbury, MA 02119-1707

Support Groups & Hotlines

10133 National Health Information Center
Washington, DC 20013   310-565-4167
                                                                    800-336-4797
                                                            Fax: 301-984-4256
                                                      e-mail: info@nhic.org
                                                            www.health.gov/nhic
The National Health Information Center (NHIC) is a health information referral service sponsored by the Office of Disease Prevention and Health Promotion. NHIC puts health professionals and consumers who have health questions in touch with those organizations that are best able to provide answers. Using a database that contains descriptions of health-related organizations, NHIC staff refer people to the most appropriate resource. Spanish language information specialists are available.

DeSanctis, FACHE

10134 National Veterans Services Fund
Darien, CT 06820-0465   203-656-0003
                                                                    800-521-0198
                                                            Fax: 203-656-1957
                                                  e-mail: NatVetSvc@aol.com
                                                                    www.nvsf.org
NVSF, Inc. provides an integrated program of services managed by veterans that include the following: a national hotline for veterans and their families that responds to hundreds of inquiries each month from throughout the country; an extensive repository of free information on topics ranging from the history of the Agent Orange lawsuit to the most recent Gulf War legislation; a special fund that offers limited emergency economic assistance and relief for families in crisis; business partnership

Phil Kraft, President

Books

10135 An Assessment of Technical Issues Raised in RW Haley's Critique of Health Studies
Gus Haggstrom, author
Rand Corporation
1776 Main Street   310-393-0411
Santa Monica, CA 90407-2138   Fax: 310-393-4818

ISBN: 0-833027-52-2

10136 Gulf War and Health
National Academy Press
500 5th Street NW   202-334-3313
Washington, DC 20055   888-624-8373
                                                                   Fax: 202-334-2793
                                                       e-mail: zjones@nas.edu

Lyla M Hernandez, Editor
Merwyn R Greenlick, Editor

10137 Natural Attenuation for Groundwater Remediation
National Academy Press
500 5th Street NW   202-334-3313
Washington, DC 20055   888-624-8373
                                                                   Fax: 202-334-2793
                                                       e-mail: zjones@nas.edu

10138 Yes, You Can
Demos Medical Publishing
386 Park Avenue S   212-683-0072
New York, NY 10016   Fax: 212-683-0118
                                             e-mail: orderdept@demospub.com
                                                            www.demosmedpub.com

112 pages
ISBN: 1-888799-48-x
Dr. Diana M Schneider

Newsletters

10139 Agent Orange Briefs
Department of Veterans Affairs
810 Vermont Avenue NW
Washington, DC 20420-0002   202-233-4000

Designed to answer questions regarding Agent Orange and related matters. This fact sheet series is prepared and updated annually.
Monthly

10140 Agent Orange Review
Department of Veterans Affairs
810 Vermont Avenue NW   202-233-4000
Washington, DC 20420-0002
Published periodically to provide information on Agent Orange to concerned veterans and their families. The most recent issues include updated information about Federal government studies and activities related to Agent Orange and the Vietnam experience.

Pamphlets

10141 Agent Orange Anxiety: The Human Response to Possable Oncogenicity and Mutagencity
National Veterans Services Fund
PO Box 2465   203-656-0003
Darien, CT 06820-0465   800-521-0198
Fax: 203-656-1957
e-mail: NatVetSvc@optonline.net
www.angelfire.com/ct2/natvetsvc

10142 Agent Orange Fact Sheet: A Historical Perspective
Veterans Of The Vietnam War
805 South Township Boulevard   570-603-9740
Pittston, PA 18640-3327   Fax: 570-603-9741
www.vvnw.org
Fact sheet designed to bring an awareness of Agent Orange and related herbicides to the American public, includes a bibliography for the professional.
10 pages

10143 Agent Orange and Birth Defects
Veterans Health Adminstration
810 Vermont Avenue Northwest   202-273-8580
Washington, DC 20420-3517   Fax: 202-273-9080
www.tpromo2.com/usvi/index2.htm
Letters to the editor, New England Journal of Medicine articles.

10144 Agent Orange and Chloracme
National Veterans Services Fund
PO Box 2465   203-656-0003
Darien, CT 06820-0465   800-521-0198
Fax: 203-656-1957
e-mail: NatVetSvc@optonline.net
www.angelfire.com/ct2/natvetsvc

10145 Agent Orange and Hodgkin's Disease
Veterans Health Administration
810 Vermont Avenue Northwest   203-273-8580
Washington, DC 20420-3517   Fax: 203-273-9080
www.tpromo2.com/usvi/index2.htm

10146 Agent Orange and Mutiple Myeloma
National Veterans Services Fund
PO Box 2465   203-656-0003
Darien, CT 06820-0465   800-521-0198
Fax: 203-656-1957
e-mail: NatVetSvc@optonline.net
www.angelfire.com/ct2/natvetsvc

10147 Agent Orange and Non-Hodgkin's Lymphoma
Veterans Health Administration
810 Vermont Avenue   203-273-8580
Washington, DC 20420-3517   Fax: 203-273-9080
www.tpromo2.com/usvi/index2.htm

10148 Agent Orange and Peripheral Neuropathy
Veterans Health Administration
810 Vermont Avenue   203-273-8580
Washington, DC 20420-3517   Fax: 203-273-9080
www.tpromo2.com/usvi/index2.htm

10149 Agent Orange and Porphyria Cutanea Tarda
National Veterans Services Fund

PO Box 2465   203-656-0003
Darien, CT 06820-0465   800-521-0198
Fax: 203-656-1957
e-mail: NatVetSvc@optonline.net
www.angelfire.com/ct2/natvetsvc

10150 Agent Orange and Prostate Cancer
National Veterans Services Fund
PO Box 2465   203-656-0003
Darien, CT 06820-0465   800-521-0198
Fax: 203-656-1957
e-mail: NatVetSvc@optonline.net
www.angelfire.com/ct2/natvetsvc

10151 Agent Orange and Respiratory Cancers
National Veterans Services Fund
PO Box 2465   203-656-0003
Darien, CT 06820-0465   800-521-0198
Fax: 203-656-1957
e-mail: NatVetSvc@optonline.net
www.angelfire.com/ct2/natvetsvc

10152 Agent Orange and Soft Tissue Sarcomas
National Veterans Services Fund
PO Box 2465   203-656-0003
Darien, CT 06820-0465   800-521-0198
Fax: 203-656-1957
e-mail: NatVetSvc@optonline.net
www.angelfire.com/ct2/natvetsvc

10153 Agent Orange and Spina Bifida
National Veterans Services Fund
PO Box 2465   203-656-0003
Darien, CT 06820-0465   800-521-0198
Fax: 203-656-1957
e-mail: NatVetSvc@optonline.net
www.angelfire.com/ct2/natvetsvc

10154 Agent Orange: It is Part of Your Life
National Veterans Services Fund
PO Box 2465   203-656-0003
Darien, CT 06820-0465   800-521-0198
Fax: 203-656-1957
e-mail: NatVetSvc@optonline.net
www.angelfire.com/ct2/natvetsvc

10155 Brief History of the Agent Orange Lawsuit
National Veterans Services Fund
PO Box 2465   203-656-0003
Darien, CT 06820-0465   800-521-0198
Fax: 203-656-1957
e-mail: NatVetSvc@optonline.net
www.angelfire.com/ct2/natvetsvc

10156 Case Control Study: Soft-Tissue Sarcomas and Exposure to Phenoxyacetic Acids
National Veterans Services Fund
PO Box 2465   203-656-0003
Darien, CT 06820-0465   800-521-0198
Fax: 203-656-1957
e-mail: NatVetSvc@optonline.net
www.angelfire.com/ct2/natvetsvc

Case control study: soft-tissue sarcoma and exposure to phenoxyacetic acids or chlorophenols.

10157 Children of Vietnam Veterans: Complex Concerns and Innovative Solutions
National Veterans Services Fund
PO Box 2465   203-656-0003
Darien, CT 06820-0465   800-521-0198
Fax: 203-656-1957
e-mail: NatVetSvc@optonline.net
www.angelfire.com/ct2/natvetsvc

7 pages

10158 Dioxin, A Case in Point
National Veterans Services Fund
PO Box 2465   203-656-0003
Darien, CT 06820-0465   800-521-0198
Fax: 203-656-1957
e-mail: NatVetSvc@optonline.net
www.angelfire.com/ct2/natvetsvc

10159 Enviromental Chloracne
National Veterans Services Fund
PO Box 2465   203-656-0003
Darien, CT 06820-0465   800-521-0198
                                       Fax: 203-656-1957
                        e-mail: NatVetSvc@optonline.net
                           www.angelfire.com/ct2/natvetsvc

10160 History of the Agent Orange Litigation
National Veterans Services Fund
PO Box 2465   203-656-0003
Darien, CT 06820-0465   800-521-0198
                                       Fax: 203-656-1957
                        e-mail: NatVetSvc@optonline.net
                           www.angelfire.com/ct2/natvetsvc

10161 List of Agent Orange-Related Illnesses Recognized By the VA
National Veterans Services Fund
PO Box 2465   203-656-0003
Darien, CT 06820-0465   800-521-0198
                                       Fax: 203-656-1957
                        e-mail: NatVetSvc@optonline.net
                           www.angelfire.com/ct2/natvetsvc

10162 List of Diseases Accepted by the VA for Presumptive Service-Connection
National Veterans Services Fund
PO Box 2465   203-656-0003
Darien, CT 06820-0465   800-521-0198
                                       Fax: 203-656-1957
                        e-mail: NatVetSvc@optonline.net
                           www.angelfire.com/ct2/natvetsvc
List of diseases accepted by the VA for presumptive service-connection that are associated with exposure to certain herbicide agents including Agent Orange.

10163 Relation of Soft-Tissue Sarcome, Malignant Lymphoma & Colon Cancer
National Veterans Services Fund
PO Box 2465   203-656-0003
Darien, CT 06820-0465   800-521-0198
                                       Fax: 203-656-1957
                        e-mail: NatVetSvc@optonline.net
                           www.angelfire.com/ct2/natvetsvc
Relation to soft-tissue sarcomas, malignant lymphoma and colon cancer to phenoxy acids, chlorphenois and other agents.

10164 Spina Bifida Benefits Guide
National Veterans Services Fund
PO Box 2465   203-656-0003
Darien, CT 06820-0465   800-521-0198
                                       Fax: 203-656-1957
                        e-mail: NatVetSvc@optonline.net
                           www.angelfire.com/ct2/natvetsvc
4 pages

Audio & Video

10165 Agent Orange Videotapes
Regional Learning Resources Service
915 N. Grand Boulevard   314-652-4100
St. Louis, MO 63106
Produces several Agent Orange videotape programs that explain what Agent Orange is, where, when and how it was used, why persons are concerned about exposure to it and what VA and other departments and agencies are doing in response to these concerns. These videotapes are maintained at all VA medical centers across the country.

Web Sites

10166 Gulf War Syndrome Database
                          www.louisville.edu/library/ekstrom
This is a substantial database of relevant documents and studies kept by University of Louisville, Ekstrom Library.

10167 Gulf War Veteran Resource Pages
                                       www.gulfweb.org

This page is administered by Gulf War veterans and provides a great range of information on a variety of Gulf War-related items, including GWS. The site includes many links to other groups interested in GWS and to GWS studies.

10168 Healing Well
                                       www.healingwell.com
An online health resource guide to medical news, chat, information and articles, newsgroups and message boards, books, disease-related web sites, medical directories, and more for patients, friends, and family coping with disabling diseases, disorders, or chronic illnesses.

10169 Health Finder
                                       www.healthfinder.gov
Searchable, carefully developed web site offering information on over 1000 topics. Developed by the US Department of Health and Human Services, the site can be used in both English and Spanish.

10170 Healthlink USA
                                       www.healthlinkusa.com
Health information concerning treatment, cures, prevention, diagnosis, risk factors, research, support groups, email lists, personal stories and much more. Updated regularly.

10171 Heatlhcentral.com
                                       www.healthcentral.com
The HealthCentral Network has a collection of owned and operated web sites and multimedia affiliate properties providing timely, in-depth, trusted medical information, personalized tools and resources for people seeking to manage and improve their health.

10172 Helios Health
                                       www.helioshealth.com
Online resource for your health information. Detailed information about specific health topics, access to expert advice from our Medical Advisory Board, and up-to-date health news.

10173 InteliHealth
                                       www.intelihealth.com
InteliHealth's mission is to empower people with treusted solutions for healthier lives. They accomplish this by providing credible information fromt he most trusted sources.
Brian Berkenstock, Writer/Editor

10174 MedicineNet
                                       www.medicinenet.com
Medicine Net is an online healthcare media publishing company. It provides easy-to-read, in-depth, authoritative medical information for consumers via its robust, user-friendly, interactive web site.

10175 Medscape
                                       www.medscape.com
Medscape offers specialists, primary care physicians, and other health professionals the Web's most robust and integrated medical information and educational tools.

10176 National Veterans Services Fund
                                       www.nvsf.org
Supports and informs those who were exposed to the defoliant Agent Orange, or dioxin, while serving the US in the conflict in Vietnam.

10177 Office of the Special Assistant for Gulf War Illnesses
                                       www.gulflink.osd.mil
This is a page sponsored by the Defense Department's Special Assistant for Gulf War Illnesses. It provides information on and linkes to Federal and State-funded studies of Gulf War Illnesses.

10178 WebMD
                                       www.webmd.com
Information on Agent Orange related injuries, including articles and resources.

Description

10179 Wilson's Disease

Wilson's disease is a rare genetic disorder that results from an inability to adequately excrete copper. In the United States, approximately one person in 40,000 has this condition. The resulting accumulation of copper in the body's tissues and organs leads to disease of the brain and liver, and to a lesser extent, the kidney and red blood cells. The disease is genetic; if two carriers have children, the disease would have a 1 in 4 chance of being passed on.

Build-up of copper in the liver causes a hepatitis-like illness with loss of appetite, low grade fever, abdominal discomfort and jaundice. If not detected and treated, this process can lead to cirrhosis and fatal liver failure. In 40 to 50 percent of patients, the illness affects the brain and can include unsteadiness, tremors, slurred speech and intellectual deterioration. Copper rings may appear in the eye in up to 10 percent of patients. Although they do not cause any symptoms, their appearance may help establish the diagnosis.

In untreated Wilson's, the disease is fatal, generally before the age of 30. Continual, lifelong treatment is mandatory for any patient with confirmed Wilson's disease, whether symptomatic or not. The critical therapy is to administer a drug that helps the body release its copper stores. D-penicillamine is the most common such drug. Some patients have required liver transplantation.

National Agencies & Associations

10180 American Liver Foundation
39 Broadway
New York, NY 10006

212-668-1000
212-483-8179
Fax: 212-483-8179
e-mail: info@liverfoundation.org
www.liverfoundation.org

Our mission is to facilitate, advocate and promote education, support and research for the prevention, treatment and cure of liver disease.
Rick Smith, President/CEO
Newton Guerin, COO

10181 United Liver Foundation
11646 W Pico Boulevard
Los Angeles, CA 90064

213-445-4204

Foundation offering information public awareness materials support and medical research for persons suffering from liver diseases.

10182 Wilson's Disease Association
5572 North Diversey Blvd
Milwaukee, WI 53217

414-961-0533
866-961-0533
Fax: 330-264-0974
e-mail: info@wilsonsdisease.org
www.wilsonsdisease.org

Serves as a communications support network for individuals affected by Wilson's disease; distributes information to professionals and the public; makes referrals; and holds meetings.
8 pages
Mary L. Graper, President
Stefanie F. Kaplan, Vice President

Foundations

10183 Hepatitis B Foundation
3805 Old Easton Road
Doylestown, PA 18902

215-489-4900
Fax: 215-489-4313
e-mail: info@hepb.org
www.hepb.org

We are dedicated to finding a cure and improving the quality of life for those affected by hepatitis B worldwide. Our commitment includes funding focused research, promoting disease awareness, supporting immunization and treatment initiatives, and serving as the primary source of information for patients and their families, the medical and scientific community, and the general public.

Joel Rosen, Chair
Timothy Block, PhD, Founder/President

Support Groups & Hotlines

10184 National Health Information Center
PO Box 1133
Washington, DC 20013

240-453-8280
800-336-4797
Fax: 240-453-8282
e-mail: info@nhic.org
www.health.gov/nhic

Offers a nationwide information referral service, produces directories and resource guides.

Pamphlets

10185 Wilson's Disease
American Liver Foundation
1425 Pompton Avenue
Cedar Grove, NJ 07009

800-465-4837
Fax: 973-256-3214
e-mail: info@liverfoundation.org
www.liverfoundation.org

A brochure offering information on the causes, symptoms and treatments of Wilson's Disease.
Rick Smith, President & CEO

Web Sites

10186 Healing Well

e-mail: webmaster@healingwell.com
www.healingwell.com

An online health resource guide to medical news, chat, information and articles, newsgroups and message boards, books, disease-related web sites, medical directories, and more for patients, friends, and family coping with disabling diseases, disorders, or chronic illnesses.
Peter Waite, MS, MA, Founder/Editor

10187 Health Finder
PO Box 1133
Washington, DC 20013-1133

e-mail: healthfinder@nhic.org
www.healthfinder.gov

Searchable, carefully developed web site offering information on over 1000 topics. Developed by the US Department of Health and Human Services, the site can be used in both English and Spanish.

10188 Healthlink USA

www.healthlinkusa.com

Health information concerning treatment, cures, prevention, diagnosis, risk factors, research, support groups, email lists, personal stories and much more. Updated regularly.

10189 Helios Health

www.helioshealth.com

Online resource for your health information. Detailed information about specific health topics, access to expert advice from our Medical Advisory Board, and up-to-date health news.

10190 MedicineNet

www.medicinenet.com

751

An online resource for consumers providing easy-to-read, authoritative medical and health information.

10191 Medscape
Corporate Headquarters
111 8th Avenue
New York, NY 10011   212-624-3700
                                      www.medscape.com
Medscape offers specialists, primary care physicians, and other health professionals the Web's most robust and integrated medical information and educational tools.
Kate Hahn, Media Relations
Tony G Holcombe, President

10192 WebMD
                                      www.webmd.com
Information on Wilson's disease, including articles and resources.

National Agencies & Associations

10193 ABLEDATA
8630 Fenton Street   301-608-8998
Silver Spring, MD 20910   800-227-0216
Fax: 301-608-8958
TTY: 301-608-8912
e-mail: abledata@macrointernational.com
www.abledata.com
Provides objective information on assistive technology and rehabilitation equipment available from domestic and international
sources to consumers, organizations, professionals, and caregivers within the United States.
Katherine Belknap, Project Director
Steve Lowe, Assistant Project Manager

**10194 ABLEDATA-REHAB DATA Alliance for Technology Access
(ATA)**
8630 Fenton Street   301-608-8998
Silver Spring, MD 20910   800-227-0216
Fax: 301-608-8958
TTY: 301-608-8912
e-mail: abledata@macrointernational.com
www.abledata.com
National organization dedicated to providing access to technology
for people with disabilities through its coalition of 45 commu-
nity-based resource centers in 34 states and the Virgin Islands.
Each center provides information, awareness and training.
Katherine Belknap, Project Director
Juanita Hardy, Information Specialist

10195 Access Unlimited
570 Hance Road
Binghamton, NY 13903   800-849-2143
Fax: 607-669-4595
e-mail: tom@accessunlimited.com
www.accessunlimited.com
We celebrate the rich diversity of our customers' needs by creating
products that allow easy access to any vehicle, from cars and vans
to trucks and SUVs. We believe that adaptive equipment should be
unobtrusive and should meet the needs of its user with a minimum
of modification to vehicle or lifestyle. We believe every person
should be able to choose the vehicle they like best, regardless of
their disability. Access Unlimited products empower people with
disabilities to regain control of thei
Tom Cole, Owner

10196 American Academy of Pediatrics
141 NW Point Boulevard   847-434-4000
Elk Grove Village, IL 60007-1098   800-433-9016
Fax: 847-434-8000
www.aap.org
To attain optimal physical, mental, and social health and well-be-
ing for all infants, children, adolescents, and young adults.
Thomas K. McInerny, President
Errol T Alden MD FAAP, Executive Director

10197 American Association for the Advancement of Science
1200 New York Avenue NW   202-326-6400
Washington, DC 20005   Fax: 202-371-9526
e-mail: webmaster@aaas.org
www.aaas.org
The non-profit AAAS is open to all and fulfills its mission to advance science and serve society through initiatives that include
science policy, international programs, science education, and
public understanding of science.
William Press, Chair
Phillip A. Sharp, President

10198 American Association of People with Disabilities
2013 H Street, NW   202-457-0046
Washington, DC 20006   800-840-8844
Fax: 866-536-4461
TTY: 202-457-0046
www.aapd.com
The American Association of People with Disabilities is the nation's largest disability rights organization. We promote equal opportunity, economic power, independent living, and political
participation for people with disabilities. Our members, including

people with disabilities and our family, friends, and supporters,
represent a powerful force for change.
Mark Perriello, President/CEO
Henry Claypool, Executive VP

10199 American Autoimmune Related Diseases Association
22100 Gratiot Avenue   586-776-3900
East Detroit, MI 48021   Fax: 586-776-3903
e-mail: aarda@aarda.org
www.aarda.org
Dedicated to the eradication of autoimmune diseases and the alleviation of suffering and the socioeconomic impact of
autoimmunity through fostering and facilitating collaboration in
the areas of education, public awareness, research, and patient services in an effective, ethical and efficient manner.
Stanley M Finger PhD, Chairman
Virginia T Ladd, President/Executive Director

**10200 American Bar Association Commission on Mental and Physical
Disability Law**
1050 Connecticut Ave. N.W.   202-662-1000
Washington, DC 20036   800-285-2221
Fax: 202-442-3439
e-mail: campdl@americanbar.org
www.americanbar.org
The Commission's mission is to promote the ABA's commitment to
justice and the rule of law for persons with mental, physical, and
sensory disabilities and to promote their full and equal participation in the legal profession.
John W Parry, Director
Laurel G. Bellows, President

10201 American Camp Association
5000 State Road 67 N   765-342-8456
Martinsville, IN 46151-7902   800-428-2267
Fax: 765-342-2065
www.acacamps.org
Formerly the American Camping Association, a community of
camp professionals who have joined together to share the knowl-
edge and experience and to ensure the quality of camp programs.
Tisha Bolger, President
Melanie Lock Herman, Treasurer

10202 American Counseling Association
5999 Stevenson Avenue
Alexandria, VA 22304   800-347-6647
Fax: 703-823-0252
e-mail: ryep@counseling.org
www.counseling.org
A not-for-profit, professional and educational organization that is
dedicated to the growth and enhancement of the counseling profession. Represents professional counselors in various practice
settings.
Marcheta Evans, President
Richard Yep, Executive Director

10203 American Foundation for The Blind
2 Penn Plaza   212-502-7600
New York, NY 10121   800-232-5463
Fax: 888-545-8331
e-mail: afbinfo@afb.net
www.afb.org
AFB's priorities include broadening access to technology; elevating the quality of information and tools for the professionals who
serve people with vision loss by providing them and their families
with relevant and timely resources.
Carl R Augusto, President/CEO
Rick Bozeman, Chief Financial Officer

10204 American Institute for Preventive Medicine
30445 NW Highway   248-539-1800
Farmington Hills, MI 48334   800-345-2476
Fax: 248-539-1808
e-mail: aipm@healthylife.com
www.healthylife.com
An award winning, internationally recognized authority on th development and implementation of health promotion, wellness,

medical self-care, and disease management programs and publications.
Larry Chapman, President
Dee Edington, Director

10205 American Institute for Preventive Medicine
30445 NW Highway   248-539-1800
Farmington Hills, MI 48334   800-345-2476
                                               Fax: 248-539-1808
                                    e-mail: aipm@healthylife.com
                                              www.healthylife.com
The institute provides health promotion programs disease management guides and self-care publications to hospitals HMOs corporations and government agencies. Programs are designed to lower health care costs, decrease absenteeism and improve productivity.
Larry Chapman, President
Dee Edington, Director

10206 American Organ Transplant Association
PO Box 418   713-344-2402
Stilwell, KS 66085   Fax: 281-617-4274
                                    e-mail: aotaonline@gmail.com
                                                www.aotaonline.org
Helps patients with free transportation to and from their transplant center, many times hundreds of miles away. Also provides transplant patients and their loved ones with resources regarding transplantation.
Pamela H Terry, Board President
Kenneth Klingensmith, Immediate Past Board President

10207 American Red Cross National Headquarters
2025 E Street NW   202-303-5000
Washington, DC 20006   800-733-2767
                                                    www.redcross.org
The nation's premier emergency response organization that aids victims of devastating natural disasters; community services that help the needy; support and comfort for military members and their families; the collection, processing and distribution of lifesaving blood and blood products; educational programs that promote health and safety; and international relief and development programs.
Gail J McGovern, President/CEO
Bonnie McElveen-Hunt, Chairman

10208 American Rehabilitation Counseling Association
5999 Stevenson Avenue
Alexandria, VA 22304-3300   800-347-6647
                                               Fax: 800-473-2329
                                               TTY: 703-823-6862
                                               TDD: 7038236862
                                 e-mail: webmaster@counseling.org
                                                 www.counseling.org
Mission of ARCA is to enhance the development of persons with disabilities throughout their life span and to promote excellence in the rehabilitation counseling professional.
Colleen Logan, President
Richard Yep, Executive Office

10209 American Society of Dermatology
Port St Lucie, FL 34984   561-873-8335
                                               Fax: 561-344-8388
                                                      www.asd.org
The mission of this organization is to facilitate optimal dermatologic care being available to all citizens of this country by preserving, promoting and enhancing the private practice of dermatology. It shall represent its members in those scientific, educational, socioeconomic and legislative areas that affect the practice of dermatology and shall endeavor to cooperate with other organizations of similar purpose.
W Gerald Klinger MD, President
Don Printz, MD, Secretary

10210 Americas Association for the Care of Children
Boulder, CO 80306-2154
                                                     303-527-2742
                                                www.aaccchildren.net
Americas Association for the Care of the Children (AACC) is the brain child of Deborah Young together with 2 friends that have been in the child care field for over 30 years. AACC is a non-profit, 501(c)3 and the umbrella organization for Programma Integral

Educando con Amor y Tenura (PIEAT). PIEAT is located in Nicaragua. In the United States AACC partners with Companeras, in Nepal with Hands in Nepal, in Kenya with Mama Beth's orphanage, feeding center and school, and in Bhutan with the Royal
Judi Jackson, President
Doreen Trees, Vice President

10211 Asbestos Information Association/North America
1745 Jefferson Davis Highway   703-412-1150
Arlington, VA 22202   Fax: 703-412-1586
                                       e-mail: aiabjpigg@aol.com
Founded to represent the interests of the asbestos industry and to collect and disseminate information about asbestos and asbestos products with emphasis on safety health and environmental issues.

10212 Beach Center on Disability
University of Kansas
1200 Sunnyside Avenue   785-864-7600
Lawrence, KS 66045   Fax: 786-864-7605
                                    e-mail: beachcenter@ku.edu
                                                www.beachcenter.org
The Beach Center on Disability is a multi-disciplinary research and training center committed to making a significant and sustainable positive difference in the quality of life of individuals and families affected by disability and the professionals who support them. Its staff of approximately 40 professors, researchers, educators, doctoral students, and support personnel carry out research, technical assistance, and undergraduate, masters, and doctoral training. Its staff focuses on families, f
Ann Turnbull, Co-Founder, Co-Director, Distinguished P
Rud Turnbull, Co-Founder, Co-Director, Distinguished P

10213 Breaking New Ground Resource Center
2255 S University Street   765-494-5088
W Lafayette, IN 47907   800-825-4264
                                               Fax: 765-496-1356
                                    e-mail: bng@enc.purdue.edu
                            www.ninds.nih.gov/find_people/voluntary_
Has become internationally recoginzed as the primary source for information and resources on rehabilitation technology for persons working in agriculture.
Prof William Field, Project Leader

10214 Center for Children with Chronic Illness and Disability
University of Minnesota School of Public Health
2525 Chicago Avenue   612-813-6000
Minneapolis, MN 55404   e-mail: Get.Well@childrensmn.org
                                                www.childrensmn.org
Serving as Minnesota's children's hospitalSM since 1924, we provide 347 staffed beds at our two hospital campuses in St. Paul and Minneapolis. An independent, not-for-profit health care system, Children's provides care through more than 12,000 inpatient visits and more than 200,000 emergency room and other outpatient visits each year.
Alan L. Goldbloom, MD, Chief Executive Officer
David A. Brumbaugh, SPHR, Vice President Human Resources

10215 Center for Chronic Disease Prevention and Centers for Disease Control
1600 Clifton Road   404-639-3311
Atlanta, GA 30333   800-232-4636
                                               TTY: 888-232-6348
                                        e-mail: cdcinfo@cdc.gov
                                                       www.cdc.gov
Chronic diseases such as heart disease cancer and diabetes are the leading causes of death and disability in the United States. These diseases account for 7 of every 10 deaths and affect the quality of life of 90 million Americans.
Richard E Besser, Director

10216 Center for Developmental Disabilities University of South Carolina
8301 Farrow Road   803-935-5231
Columbia, SC 29208   Fax: 803-935-5059
                                e-mail: steve.wilson@uscmed.sc.edu
                                            www.uscm.med.sc.edu/cdrhome
The vision of The Center for Developmental Disabilities is to work as a team to create a quality environment in which the following

values are embraced: Everyone is treated with dignity and respect. Individual strengths and abilities are recognized.

10217 Center for Disability Resources
University of South Carolina
8301 Farrow Road 803-935-5231
Columbia, SC 29208 Fax: 803-935-5059
e-mail: steve.wilson@uscmed.sc.edu
www.uscm.med.sc.edu/cdrhome
To enhance the well-being and quality of life of persons with disabilities and their families. Collaborates with persons with disabilities and their families to develop new knowledge and best practices, train leaders, and effect systems change.

10218 Center for Disease Control and Prevention
1600 Clifton Rd
Atlanta, GA 30333 800-232-4636
TTY: 888-232-6348
e-mail: cdcinfo@cdc.gov
www.cdc.gov
To collaborate to create the expertise, information, and tools that people and communities need to protect their health - through health promotion, prevention of disease, injury and disability, and preparedness for new health threats.
Thomas R Frieden MD MPH, Director

10219 Center for Health Research
Kaiser Permanente Northwest
3800 N Interstate Avenue
Portland, OR 97227-1098 503-335-2400
e-mail: information@kpchr.org
www.kpchr.org
Conducts professionally independent, public domain research and idsseminates its findings in the scholarly literature and scientific community.
Mary L Durham PhD, Director
Donald R Freel, Executive Director COO

10220 Center for Medical Consumers
239 Thompson Street 212-674-7105
New York, NY 10012 e-mail: centerformedicalconsumers@gmail.com
www.medicalconsumers.org
A non-profit advocacy organization that was founded with the philosophy: Whenever long-term drug therapy, elective surgery, or any other major treatment is prescribed, the question of whether the treatment has been proven safe and effective should come up.
Arthur Aaron Levin MPH, Director
Maryann Napoli, Associate Director

10221 Center for Universal Design North Carolina State University
North Carolina State University
Campus Box 7701 919-515-8302
Raleigh, NC 27695-8613 800-647-6777
Fax: 919-515-8951
e-mail: nilda_cosco@ncsu.edu
www.design.ncsu.edu
National research information and technical assistance center that evaluates develops and promotes accessible and universal design in housing buildings outdoor and urban environments and related products.
Nilda Cosco PhD, Education Specialist
Leslie Young, Director of Design

10222 Child Center
3995 Marcola Road 541-726-1465
Springfield, OR 97477 Fax: 541-726-5085
e-mail: info@thechildcenter.org
www.thechildcenter.org
To provide individualized, diagnostic, therapeutic and educational services for the emotional and behavioral problems children exhibit in the home, school and community; provide integreated community based psychiatric and support services that are child centered, family driven and culturally competent
Jeffrey Miller, President
Chris Dunnington, Vice President

10223 Children's Hospice International
1101 King Street 703-684-0330
Alexandria, VA 22314 800-242-4453
Fax: 703-684-0226
e-mail: info@chionline.org
www.chionline.org

To ensure medical, psychological, social and spiritual support to all children with life-threatening conditions and their families by providing a network of resources and care.
Ann Armstrong-Dailey, Founding Director/CEO
Richard Larkin, Secretary/Treasurer

10224 Children's National Medical Center
111 Michigan Avenue NW 202-476-5000
Washington, DC 20010 888-884-2327
TTY: 800-855-1155
e-mail: tbear@childrensnational.org
www.childrensnational.org
The only exclusive provider of pediatric care in the metropolitan Washington area and is the only freestanding children's hospital between Philadelphia, Pittsburgh, Norfolk, and Atlanta; the leader in the development and application of innovative new treatments for childhood illness and injury.
Kurt Newman MD, President/CEO
Roberta Alessi, Senior VP

10225 Christian Horizons
25 Sportsworld Crossing Road 519-650-0966
Kitchener, ON N2P 0 866-362-6810
Fax: 519-650-8984
e-mail: info@christian-horizons.org
www.christian-horizons.org
Empowers individuals with exceptional needs, enabling them to embrace their God-given potential and enjoy hope and opportunity in everyday living.
Nigel Wilford, Chair
Greg Wilson, Secretary

10226 Clearinghouse on Disability Information Office of Special Education & Rehab Svcs
US Department of Education
550 12th Street SW 202-245-7307
Washington, DC 20202-2550 Fax: 202-245-7636
TTY: 202-205-5637
TDD: 2022055637
e-mail: customerservice@inet.ed.gov
www.health.gov/nhic/NHICScripts/Entry.cf
Provides information to people with disabilities or anyone requesting information by doing research and providing documents in response to inquiries. Information provided includes areas of federal funding for disability-related programs.
Carolyn Corlett, Contact

10227 Council for Learning Disabilities (CLD)
11184 Antioch Road 913-491-1011
Overland Park, KS 66210 Fax: 913-491-1012
e-mail: CLDInfo@cldinternational.org
www.cldinternational.org
The Council for Learning Disabilities (CLD) is an international organization that promotes evidence-based teaching, collaboration, research, leadership, and advocacy. CLD is comprised of professionals who represent diverse disciplines and are committed to enhancing the education and quality of life for individuals with learning disabilities and others who experience challenges in learning.
Slivana Watson, President
Steve Chamberlain, President Elect

10228 Disabled & Alone: Life Services for the Handicapped
1440 Broadway 212-532-6740
New York, NY 10018 800-995-0066
Fax: 212-532-3588
e-mail: info@disabledandalone.org
www.disabledandalone.org
A non-profit organization established to help families provide a secure future for their loved ones with a disability. Also believes that no person should have to live his life in loneliness and isolation because of a disability.
Leslie D Park, Chairman
Lee Alan Ackerman, Executive Director

10229 Distance Education and Training Council
1601 18th Street NW 202-234-5100
Washington, DC 20009 Fax: 202-332-1386
e-mail: brianna@detc.org
www.detc.org

A voluntary, non-governmental, educational organization that operates a nationally recognized accrediting association, the DETC Accrediting Commission.
Michael P Lambert, Executive Director
Patrice Wall, General Information

10230 Educational Equity Center at The Academy for Educational Development
71 Fifth Avenue   212-243-1110
New York, NY 10003   Fax: 212-627-0407
e-mail: lcolon@aed.org
www.edequity.org
A national non-profit organization promoting educational excellence for children.
Merle Froschl, Co-Director
Barbara Sprung, Co-Director

10231 Equal Opportunity Employment Commission
131 M Street NE   202-663-4900
Washington, DC 20507   TTY: 202-663-4494
e-mail: info@eeoc.gov
www.eeoc.org
The U.S. Equal Employment Opportunity Commission (EEOC) is responsible for enforcing federal laws that make it illegal to discriminate against a job applicant or an employee because of the person's race, color, religion, sex (including pregnancy), national origin, age (40 or older), disability or genetic information. It is also illegal to discriminate against a person because the person complained about discrimination, filed a charge of discrimination, or participated in an employment discrimina
Jacqueline A Berrien, Chair
Constance S. Barker, Commissioner

10232 Estate Planning for the Disabled
2232 W Avenue 133   510-352-4127
San Leandro, CA 94577-1050   Fax: 510-352-4127
e-mail: EFM@EFMOODY.com
www.efmoody.com
Counsels and assists parents of children with special needs to develop viable estate plans, letters of intent, wills and special needs trusts. EPD will work with the appropriate professionals and agencies to help put together an effective comprehensive plan.

10233 Extensions for Independence
555 Saturn Boulevard   619-618-2154
San Diego, CA 92154   866-632-7149
Fax: 866-632-7149
e-mail: info@mouthstick.net
www.mouthstick.net
Designer and manufacturer of home and office related equipment for the functional independence of the most physically challenged.
Arthur Heyer, President

10234 Favarh
225 Commerce Drive   860-693-6662
Canton, CT 06019-1099   Fax: 860-693-8662
www.favarh.org
Provides a variety of programs and services to adults with developmental, physical or mental disabilities and their families, throughout the Farmington Valley communities of Avon, Burlington and more.
Stephen Morr MPA, Executive Director

10235 Federation for Children with Special Needs
529 Main Street   617-236-7210
Boston, MA 02129   800-331-0688
Fax: 617-241-0330
e-mail: fcsninfo@fcsn.org
www.fcsn.org
Provides information, support, and assistance to parents of children with disabilities, their professional partners and their communities. Committed to listening to and learning from families, and encouraging full participation in community life by all people, especially those with disabilities.
Rich Robison, Executive Director
Sara Miranda, Associate Executive Director

10236 Florida Disabled Outdoor Association
2475 Apalachee Parkway   850-201-2944
Tallahassee, FL 32301   Fax: 850-201-2945
www.fdoa.org
Enriches lives through accessible inclusive recreation and active leisure for all.
David Jones, Director
Laurie LoRe-Gussak, Execcutive Director

10237 Goodwill Industries International
15810 Indianola Drive   301-530-6500
Rockville, MD 20855   800-741-0186
Fax: 301-530-1516
TTY: 301-530-9759
e-mail: contactus@goodwill.org
www.goodwill.org
Enhances the dignity and quality of life of individuals, families and communities by eliminating barriers to opportunity and helping people in need reach their fullest potential through the power of work.
Jim Gibbons, President/CEO
Bill J Kacal, Chair

10238 HEATH Resource Center
George Washington University
2134 G Street NW   202-939-9329
Washington, DC 20052-0001   800-544-3284
Fax: 202-994-3365
e-mail: AskHEATH@gwu.edu
www.heath.gwu.edu
Serves as a national clearinghouse on postsecondary education for individuals with disabilities.
Dr Lynda West, Principal Investigator
Dr Joel Gomez, Co-Principal Investigator

10239 Health Care For All
30 Winter Street   617-350-7279
Boston, MA 02108   Fax: 617-451-5838
TTY: 617-350-0974
e-mail: aslemmer@hcfama.org
www.hcfama.org
HCFA seeks to create a consumer-centered health care system that provides comprehensive, affordable, accessible, culturally competent, high quality care and consumer education for everyone, especially the most vulnerable.
Amy Whitcomb Slemmer, Executive Director

10240 International Association for the Study of Pain
1510 H Street NW   202-524-5300
Washington, DC 20005-4955   Fax: 202-524-5301
e-mail: iaspdesk@iasp-pain.org
www.iasp-pain.org
Brings together scientists, clinicians, health care providers, and policy makers to stimulate and support the study of pain and to translate that knowledge into improved pain relief worldwide.
Kathy Kreiter, Executive Director
Janet Brangman, Executive Assistant

10241 International Council on Disability
1012 14th Street NW   202-347-0102
Washington, DC 20005   Fax: 202-347-0315
e-mail: info@usicd.org
www.usicd.org
To promote the rights and full participation of persons with disabilities through global engagement and United States foreign affairs.
Marca Bristo, President
Barbara LeRoy, Secretary

10242 LAUNCH Department of Special Education
Department of Special Education
Commerce, TX 75428   903-886-5932
Provides resources for learning disabled individuals coordinates efforts of other local state and national LD organizations acts as a communication channel for people with learning disabilities through a monthly newsletter and provides programs.

10243 Learning Disabilities Association of America
4156 Library Road
Pittsburgh, PA 15234-1349
412-341-1515
888-300-6710
Fax: 412-344-0224
e-mail: info@ldaamerica.org
www.ldaamerica.org
To create opportunities for success for all individuals affected by learning disabilities and to reduce the incidence of learning disabilities in future generations.
Patricia Lillie, President
Andrea Turkheimer, Director Resource/Referral/Education

10244 Learning How
1583 Sulphur Spring Road
Baltimore, MD 21227
410-242-7100
Fax: 410-242-5246
e-mail: info@learninghow.com
www.learninghow.com
To provide educational materials for parents, teachers, and daycare providers that will encourage the learning process and help children reach their fullest potential.

10245 Life Development Institute
18001 N 79th Avenue
Glendale, AZ 85308
623-773-2774
866-736-7811
Fax: 623-773-2788
e-mail: info@life-development-inst.org
www.lifedevelopmentinstitute.org
LDI's mission to inspire individuals to experience success while optimizing their potential for an enhanced quality of life in a challenging and supportive learning environment. LDI is a nonprofit private organization based in Glendale Arizona.
Rob Crawford, CEO
Veronica Crawford, Vice President

10246 Lions Quest
300 W 22nd Street
Oak Brook, IL 60523-8842
630-571-5466
Fax: 630-571-5735
e-mail: matthew.kiefer@lionsclub.org
www.lions-quest.org
To empower and support adults throughout the world to nuture caring and responsibility in young people.
Matthew Kiefer, Manager
Michael Di Maria, Educational Program Specialist

10247 Lymphatic Research Foundation
40 Garvies Point Road
Glen Cove, NY 11542
516-625-9675
Fax: 516-625-9410
e-mail: lrf@lymphaticresearch.org
www.lymphaticresearch.org
A not-for-profit organization whose mission is to advance research of the lymphatic system and to find the cause of and cure for lymphatic diseases, lymphedema, and related disorders.
Roy E. Reichbach, Executive Director
Phillip Braginsky, Chair

10248 MedEscort International ABE International Airport
ABE International Airport
PO Box 8766
Allentown, PA 18105-8766
610-792-3111
800-255-7182
Fax: 610-791-9189
e-mail: service@medescort.com
www.medescort.com
Offers specially trained escorts for individuals who cannot travel alone due to age or disability.
David M Stein DO, Medical Director
Sherry L Sefcik RN/BSN, Senior Flight Nurse

10249 MedicAlert Foundation International
2323 Colorado Avenue
Turlock, CA 95382-2018
888-633-4298
Fax: 800-863-3429
e-mail: customer_service@medicalert.org
www.medicalert.org
We protect the health and well-being of more than 4 million members worldwide through our trusted emergency support network. We educate emergency responders and medical personnel - our partners in everyday emergency situations. And we communicate your health information, your wishes, and your directives to ensure you receive the best care possible
Andrew B Wigglesworth, President/CEO
Karen M. Lamoree, COO

10250 Mental Health Services Training Center
University of Maryland
3700 Koppers Street
Baltimore, MD 21227
410-646-7758
Fax: 410-646-7849
e-mail: wbaysmor@psych.umaryland.edu
www.trainingcenter.umaryland.edu
Formerly the Mental Health Services Training Collaborative, assists Mental Hygiene Administration in planning, organizing and implementing conference and training activities to support the continued growth and development of the public mental health system.
Eileen Hansen MSSW, Director
Wendy Baysmore MSHSA, Assistant Director

10251 National Association of Councils on Developmental Disabilities
1825 K Street NW
Washington, DC 20006
202-506-5813
Fax: 202-506-5846
e-mail: info@nacdd.org
www.nacdd.org
Serves as the national voice of State and Territorial Councils on Dvelopment Disabilities. Supports Councils in implementing the Developmental Disabilities Assistance and Bill of Rights Act and promoting the interests and rights of people with developmental disabilities and their familes.
Claire Mantonya, President
Brett Cunnigham, VP

10252 National Center for Family-Centered Care
695 Park Avenue
New York, NY 10021
212-772-4000
Fax: 212-452-7475
e-mail: gmallon@hunter.cuny.edu
www.hunter.cuny.edu/socwork/nrcfcpp//tra
Goals are to promote implementation of a family-centered care approach for children with special health care needs.
Karen Lawrence

10253 National Chronic Pain Outreach Association
Millboro, VA 24460
540-862-9437
Fax: 540-862-9485
e-mail: ncpoa@cfw.com
www.chronicpain.org
Purpose is to lessen the suffering of people with chronic pain by educating pain sufferers, health care professionals, and the public about chronic pain and its management.

10254 National Clearinghouse of Rehabilitation Training Materials
Utah State University
6524 Old Main Hill
Logan, UT 84322-6524
866-821-5355
Fax: 435-797-7537
e-mail: ncrtm@usu.edu
www.ncrtm.org
Offers reference materials on rehabilitation for professionals and the disabled.
Jared Schultz, Principal Investigator
Joshua Southwick, Interim Director

10255 National Council on Disability
1331 F Street NW
Washington, DC 20004
202-272-2004
Fax: 202-272-2022
TTY: 202-272-2074
e-mail: ncd@ncd.gov
www.ncd.gov
The National Council on Disability is an independent federal agency that works with the President and Congress to increase the inclusion independence and empowerment of Americans with disabilities. They are involved in policy making issues.
Jonathan Young, Ph.D., Chairman
Aaron Bishop, Executive Director

10256 National Council on Independent Living
1710 Rhode Island Avenue NW   202-207-0334
Washington, DC 20036   877-525-3400
                                Fax: 202-207-0341
                                TTY: 202-207-0340
                                e-mail: ncil@ncil.org
                                www.ncil.org
A membership organization that advanced independent living and the rights of people with disabilities through consumer-driven advocacy.
Kelly Buckland, Executive Director
Dan Kessler, President

10257 National Digestive Diseases Information Clearinghouse
2 Information Way
Bethesda, MD 20892-3570   800-891-5389
                                Fax: 703-738-4929
                                TTY: 866-569-1162
                                e-mail: nddic@info.niddk.nih.gov
                                www.digestive.niddk.nih.gov
An information dissemination service of the National Institute of Diabetes and Digestive and Kidney Diseases that was established to increase knowledge and understanding about digestive diseases among people with these conditions and their families, health care professionals, and the general public.
Griffin P Rodgers MD MACP, Director

10258 National Dissemination Center for Children
1825 Connecticut Ave NW   202-884-8200
Washington, DC 20009   800-695-0285
                                Fax: 202-884-8441
                                TTY: 202-884-8200
                                e-mail: nichcy@aed.org
                                www.nichcy.org
Provides information to the nation on: disabilities in children and youth; programs and services for infants, children, and youth with disabilities; IDEA, the nation's special education law; No Child Left Behind, the nation's general education law; and research-based information on effective practices for children with disabilities.

10259 National Endowment for the Arts: Office for Accessability
1100 Pennsylvania Avenue NW   202-682-5400
Washington, DC 20506   TTY: 202-682-5496
                                e-mail: webmgr@arts.endow.gov
                                www.nea.gov
Since 1957, the YAI Network has been providing hope and opportunity to people of all ages with developmental disabilities and their families. Our organization includes more than 450 programs and serves more than 20,000 people every day.
Stephen E. Freeman, CEO
Thomas A. Dern, COO

10260 National Institute for People with Disabilities
460 W 34th Street
New York, NY 10001-2382   212-273-6100
                                www.yai.org
To create hope and opportunity for people with developmental and learning disabilities and their families.
Philip H Levy PhD, President/CEO

10261 National Institute of Child Health and Human Development
31 Center Drive   301-496-5133
Bethesda, MD 20892   800-370-2943
                                Fax: 866-760-5947
                                TTY: 888-320-6942
                                e-mail: NICHDInformationResourceCenter@mail.nih.
                                www.nichd.nih.gov
The NICHD was initially founded to realize a vision: to support the world's best minds in investigating human development throughout the entire life process, focusing on understanding developmental disabilities, including intellectual and developmental disabilities (IDDs), and illuminating important events that occur during pregnancy.
Alan E Guttmacher, Director

10262 National Institute of Disability and Rehabilitation Research
US Department of Education

400 Maryland Avenue SW   202-245-7640
Washington, DC 20202   Fax: 202-245-7323
                                TTY: 202-245-7316
                                www.ninds.nih.gov/find_people/government
provides leadership and support for a comprehensive program and research related to the rehabilitation of individuals with disabilities. All of the programmatic efforts are aimed at improving the lives of individuals with disabilities from birth through adulthood.

10263 National Job Accommodation Network
Morgantown, WV 26506-6080   304-293-7186
                                800-526-7234
                                Fax: 304-293-5407
                                TTY: 877-781-9403
                                e-mail: jan@askjan.org
                                www.askjan.org
The JAN is an international information service for people with disabilities and their employers. They have information about implementation of workplace accommodations as well as resources to promote an awareness of functional limitations.
Anne Hirsh, Co-Director
Louis Orslene, Co-Director

10264 National Legal Center for the Medically Dependent & Disabled
50 S Meridian Street   317-632-6245
Indianapolis, IN 46204-3537
Committed to defending the rights of vulnerable persons threatened by infanticide, euthanasia, assisted suicide, non-voluntary withdrawal/withholding of essential medical treatment and care and discrimination in health care financing.
Marilyn Bove, President

10265 National Network of Learning Disabled Adults
808 N 82nd Street   602-941-5112
Scottsdale, AZ 85257
Provides information and referral for LD adults involved with or in search of support groups and networking opportunities.

10266 National Organization for Rare Disorders
55 Kenosia Avenue   203-744-0100
Danbury, CT 06810-1968   800-999-6673
                                Fax: 203-798-2291
                                TDD: 203-797-9590
                                e-mail: orphan@rarediseases.org
                                www.rarediseases.org
The National Organization for Rare Disorders(NORD) a 501(c)3 organization is a unique federation of voluntary health organizations dedicated to helping people with rare orphan diseases and assisting the organizations that serve them.
Peter L. Saltonstall, President & CEO
Russell Teagarden, Senior Vice President of Medical and Sci

10267 National Organization on Disability
77 Water Street   646-505-1191
New York, NY 10005   Fax: 646-505-1184
                                e-mail: info@nod.org
                                www.nod.org
The National Organization on Disability (NOD) is a private, non-profit organization that promotes the full participation of America's 56 million people with disabilities in all aspects of life.
Carol Glazer, President
Aleysha Anderson, Administrative Assistant

10268 National Parent Network on Disabilities
1130 17th Street NW   202-434-8686
Washington, DC 20036   Fax: 202-638-7299
                                www.npnd.org
To provide a presence and national voice for all families of children, youth and adults with disabilities.
Linda Shepard, Executive Director
Jill Foss, Office Manager

10269 National Rehabilitation Information Center
8400 Corporate Drive   301-459-5900
Landover, MD 20785   800-346-2742
                                Fax: 301-459-4263
                                TTY: 301-459-5984
                                e-mail: naricinfo@heitechservices.com
                                www.naric.com

One of the three components of the office of Special Education and Rehabilitative Services. Mission is to generate, disseminate and promote new knowledge to improve the options available to disabled persons. The ultimate goal is to allow these individuals to perform their regular activities in the community and to bolster society's ability to provide full opportunities and appropriate supports for its disabled citizens.
Mark Odum, Director

10270 North American Society for Pediatric Gastroenterology, Hepatology & Nutrition
Flourtown, PA 19031   215-233-0808
                                      Fax: 215-233-3918
                      e-mail: naspghan@naspghan.org
                                      www.naspghan.org
To advance understanding of normal development, physiology and pathophysiology of diseases of the gastrointestinal tract and liver in children, improve quality of care by fostering the dissemination of this knowledge through scientific meetings, professional and public education, and policy development, and serve as an effective voice for members and the profession.
Margaret K Stallings, Executive Director
Kim Rose, Director of Membership

10271 Office of Civil Rights
US Department of Education
S/OCR, Room 7428   202-647-9295
Washington, DC 20520-1100   800-421-3481
                                      Fax: 202-647-4969
                                      TTY: 877-521-2172
                        e-mail: socr_direct@state.gov
                                  www.state.gov/s/ocr/
To ensure equal access to education and to promote educational excellence throughout the nation through vigorous enforcement of civil rights.
Russlynn Ali, Assistant Secretary

10272 Office of Policy Planning and Legislation
200 Independence Avenue SW   202-619-0257
Washington, DC 20201-0004   877-696-6775
                        www.hhs.gov/about/referlst.html
Administers grants to the states for social services under Title XX of the Social Security Act to welfare recipients and others likely to become welfare recipients.
G Barry Nielsen, Director

10273 Office of Special Education Programs
Department of Education
400 Maryland Avenue SW
Washington, DC 20202   202-245-7459
                      www2.ed.gov/about/offices/list/osers
Dedicated to improving results for infants, toddlers, children and youth with disabilities ages birth through 21 by providing leadership and financial support to assist states and local districts.
Melody Musgrove, Director
Bill Wolf, Acting Deputy Director

10274 Office on Smoking and Health
Centers for Disease Control and Prevention
4770 Buford Highway   404-639-3311
Atlanta, GA 30341-3717   800-232-4636
                                      TTY: 888-232-6348
                          e-mail: tobaccoinfo@cdc.gov
                            www.cdc.gov/tobacco/osh/index.htm
The leading federal agency for comprehensive tobacco prevention and control, the Office develops, conducts, and supports strategic efforts to protect the public's health from the harmful effects of tobacco use.
Tim McAfee MD MPH, Director

10275 Option Institute International Learning & Training Center
2080 S Undermountain Road   413-229-2100
Sheffield, MA 01257   800-714-2779
                                      Fax: 413-229-8931
                  e-mail: participantsupport@option.org
                                      www.option.org
Offers self improvement and personal growth workshops and seminars that provide practical tools and strategies to help people worldwide to live happier, more confident, more empowered and

more fulfilling lives, and enjoy gratifying relationships and careers.
Barry Neil Kaufman, Co-Founder/Co-Director
Samahria Kaufman, Co-Founder/Co-Director

10276 Pediatric Neurology Georgetown University Hospital
Georgetown University Hospital
3800 Reservoir Road NW
Washington, DC 20007   202-444-2000
                          www.georgetownuniversityhospital.org
provides a wide range of consultative services, neurodiagnostic studies and therapies for children with neurodevelopmental disorders.
Cesar Santos MD, Chief

10277 People-to-People Committee for the Handicapped
Washington, DC 20036-8131   301-774-7446
Individuals concerned about the circumstances of handicapped people throughout the world. Disseminates information acts as a consultant in promoting exchange activities coordinates special assistance projects in developing countries and more.
David Brigham, Chairman

10278 President's Committee on the Employment of People with Disabilities
200 Constitution Avenue NW   202-693-6000
Washington, DC 20210   866-633-7365
                                      Fax: 202-693-7888
                                      TTY: 877-889-5627
                          e-mail: webmaster@dol.gov
                                      www.dol.gov
Independent federal agency to facilitate the communication coordination and promotion of public and private efforts to empower Americans with disabilities through employment.
Seth D. Harris, Secretary of Labour
Ana M. Ma, Chief of Staff

10279 Rehabilitation International
25 E 21st Street   212-420-1500
New York, NY 10010   Fax: 212-505-0871
                                      e-mail: ri@riglobal.org
                                      www.riglobal.org
RI and its members work to protect the rights of people with disabilities, including ensuring access to and the improvement of crucial services for persons with disabilities and their families
Jan A. Monsbakken, President
Megan Brinster, Development/Program Officer

10280 Rehabilitation Services Administration
US Department of Education
1125 15th Street, NW   202-730-1843
Washington, DC 20005-2800   Fax: 202-730-1843
                                      TTY: 202-730-1516
                                      e-mail: dds@dc.gov
                      www.dc.gov/DC/DDS/Rehabilitation+Service
Oversees grant programs that help individuals with physical or mental disabilities to obtain employment and live more independently through the provision of such supports as counseling, medical and psychological services, job training and other individualized services.
Lynnae M Ruttledge, Commissioner

10281 Social Security Administration Office of Public Inquiries
Office of Public Inquiries
Windsor Park Building
Baltimore, MD 21235   800-772-1213
                                      TTY: 800-325-0778
                                      www.ssa.gov
Administers old age survivors and disability insurance programs under Title II of the Social Security Act. Also administers the federal income maintenance program under Title XVI of the Social Security Act. Maintains networks of local/regional offices.
Michael J Astrue, Commissioner
James A Winn, Chief of Staff

10282 US Department of Justice
950 Pennsylvania Avenue NW   202-514-2000
Washington, DC 20530-0001   e-mail: askdoj@usdoj.gov
                                      www.usdoj.gov

759

To enforce the law and defend the interests of the United States according to the law; to ensure public safety against threats foreign and domestic; to provide federal leadership in preventing and controlling crime; to seek just punishment for those guilty of unlawful behavior; and to ensure fair and impartial administration of justice for all Americans.
Eric Holder, Attorney General
James Cole, Deputy Attorney General

10283 US Department of Transportation
1200 New Jersey Avenue SE
Washington, DC 20590
202-366-4000
866-377-8642
TTY: 800-877-8339
e-mail: dot.comments@dot.gov
www.dot.gov
Serves the United States by ensuring a fast, safe, efficient, accessible and convenient transportation system that meets the vital national interests and enhances the quality of life of the American people, today and into the future.
Anthony Foxx, Secretary of Transportation
John D. Porcari, Deputy Secretary of Transport

10284 US Office of Personnel Management
1900 E Street NW
Washington, DC 20415
202-606-1800
TTY: 202-606-2532
e-mail: General@opm.gov
www.opm.gov
Recruiting, retaining and honoring a world-class workforce to serve the American people.
Elaine Kaplan, Acting Director

10285 World Institute on Disability
3075 Adeline Street
Berkeley, CA 94703-1520
510-225-6400
Fax: 510-225-0477
TTY: 510-225-0478
e-mail: wid@wid.org
www.wid.org
WID's mission in communities and nations worldwide is to eliminate barriers to full social integration and increase employment, economic security, and health care for persons with disabilities
Anita Shafer Aaron, Executive Director
Rebecca Palmer, Executive Assistant

State Agencies & Associations

Alabama

10286 Division of Rehabilitation: Montgomery
Montgomery, AL 36111-0586
334-281-8780
Marilyn Bove, President

Alaska

10287 Client Assistance Program: Anchorage
3330 Arctic Boulevard
Anchorage, AK 99503
907-333-2211
800-478-1234
Fax: 907-565-1000
e-mail: akpa@dlcak.org
www.home.gci.net/~alaskacap
James Shine, President
Julie Renwick, Vice President

Arizona

10288 HPV Support Groups: Arizona
7331 E Osborn Drive
Scottsdale, AZ 85251-6422
602-994-8330
800-223-2159
e-mail: sthf@home.com

Arkansas

10289 Disability Rights Center of Arkansas
1100 N University
Little Rock, AR 72207
501-296-1775
800-482-1174
Fax: 501-296-1779
e-mail: panda@advocacyservices.org
www.arkdisabilityrights.org

Protection and advocacy system for people with disabilities in Arkansas.
Traci Perrin, President

California

10290 Disability Rights California
1831 K Street
Sacramento, CA 95811
916-504-5800
800-776-5746
Fax: 916-504-5801
TTY: 800-719-5798
e-mail: services@disabilityrightsca.org
www.disabilityrightsca.org
Mission is to advance the rights of Californians with disabilities.
Catherine Blakemore, Executive Director
Andrew Murdryk, Deputy Director

Colorado

10291 Disability Careers
5760 E Evans Avenue
Denver, CO 80222-5305
303-757-3070
Fax: 303-757-3392
This is a non profit corporation that provides employee and employer services. Founder and Executive Director Ted Pavakis is a former commercial real estate broker with multiple sclerosis.

10292 Legal Center for People with Disabilities and Older People
455 Sherman Street
Denver, CO 80203
303-722-0300
800-288-1376
Fax: 303-722-0720
TTY: 303-722-3619
e-mail: tlcmail@thelegalcenter.org
www.thelegalcenter.org
An independent public interest non-profit specializing in civil rights and discrimination issues. We protect the human, civil and legal rights of people with mental and physical disabilities, people with HIV, and older people throughout Colorado.
Mary Anne Harvey, Executive Director
Peter Lindquist, President

Connecticut

10293 Office of Protection and Advocacy for Persons with Disabilities
60B Weston Street
Hartford, CT 06120-1551
860-297-4300
800-842-7303
TTY: 860-297-4380
www.ct.gov
To advance the cause of equal rights for persons with disabilities and their families by: increasing the ability of individuals, groups and systems to safeguard rights; exposing instances and patterns of discrimination and abuse; seeking individual and systemic remediation when rights are violated; increasing public awareness of unjust situations and of means to address them; and empowering people with disabilities and their families to advocate effectively.

Delaware

10294 Client Assistance Program: Delaware
13 SW Front Street
Milford, DE 19963-1900
302-422-6744
Marilyn Bove, President

District of Columbia

10295 Client Assistance Program: District of Columbia
Rehabilitation Services Administration
605 G Street NW
Washington, DC 20001-3705
202-727-0977
Jim Tolbert, Director

10296 Information Protection & Advocacy Center for Handicapped Individuals
Center for Handicapped Individuals
4455 Connecticut Avenue NW
Washington, DC 20008-2328
202-966-8081
Marilyn Bove, President

Florida

10297 Disability Rights: Florida
2728 Centerview Drive
Tallahassee, FL 32301

850-488-9071
800-342-0823
Fax: 850-488-8640
TDD: 800-346-4127
e-mail: info@advocacycenter.org
www.disabilityrightsflorida.org

To advance the quality of life, dignity, equality, self-determination, and freedom of choice of persons with disabilities through collaboration, education, advocacy, as well, as legal and legislative issues.
Catherine Piecora, Chair
Minerva Bailey, Vice-Chair

10298 North Florida: HPV Support Group
126 Salem Court
Tallahassee, FL 32301-2810

850-877-3183

Georgia

10299 Division of Rehabilitation Service
148 Andrew Young Int'l Blvd NE
Atlanta, GA 30303-1751

404-232-3910
TTY: 404-232-3911
e-mail: rehab@dol.state.ga.us
www.vocrehabga.org

Operates five integrated and interdependent programs that share a primary goal — to help people with disabilities to become fully productive members of society by achieving independence and meaningful employment.

Hawaii

10300 Protection & Advocacy Agency
1132 Bishop Street
Honolulu, HI 96813-9607

808-949-2922
800-882-1057
Fax: 808-949-2928
TTY: 808-949-2922
e-mail: info@hawaiidisabilityrights.org
www.hawaiidisabilityrights.org

Hawaii Disability Rights Center is the State of Hawaii's designated client assistance program and designated protection and advocacy system for people with disabilities.
Gary L Smith, Executive Director

Idaho

10301 Co-Ad
4477 Emerald St
Boise, ID 83706-2017

208-336-5353
800-632-5125
Fax: 208-336-5396
TTY: 208-336-5353
e-mail: coadinc@cableone.net
www.users.moscow.com

Marilyn Bove, President

Illinois

10302 Illinois Client Assistance Program
Illinois Department of Human Services
100 N 1st Street
Springfield, IL 62702

800-641-3929
TTY: 800-447-6404
e-mail: dhs.cap@illinois.gov
www.dhs.state.il.us

Helps people with disabilities receive quality services by advocating for their interests and helping them identify resources, understand procedures, resolve problems, and protect their rights in the rehabilitation process, employment and home services.

Indiana

10303 Indiana Protection and Advocacy Services
4701 N Keystone Avenue
Indianapolis, IN 46205

800-622-4845
TTY: 800-838-1131
e-mail: kpedevilla@ipas.in.gov
www.in.gov/ipas

To protect and promote the rights of individuals with disabilities, through empowerment and advocacy.
Karen Pedevilla, Education/Training Director

Iowa

10304 Client Assistance Program: Iowa Division o n Persons with Disabilities
Division on Persons with Disabilities
Lucas State Office Building
Des Moines, IA 50310

515-281-3656
800-652-4298
Fax: 515-242-6119
TTY: 800-652-4298
e-mail: dhr.disabilities@iowa.gov
www.humanrights.iowa.gov/pd/text_version

The Division of Persons with Disabilities exists to promote the employment of Iowans with disabilities and reduce barriers to employment by providing information, referral, assessment and guidance, training, and negotiation services to employers and citizens with disabilities.
Marilyn Bove, President

Kansas

10305 Disability Rights Center of Kansas
635 SW Harrison
Topeka, KS 66603-3726

785-273-9661
877-776-1541
Fax: 785-273-9414
TTY: 877-335-3725
e-mail: rocky@drckansas.org
www.icdri.org

A public interest legal advocacy agency empowered by federal law to advocate for the civil and legal rights of Kansans with disabilities.
Rocky Nichols MPA, Executive Director
Debbie White, Deputy Director

Kentucky

10306 Client Assistance Program: Kentucky
275 E Main Street
Frankfort, KY 40621

502-564-4440
800-633-6283
e-mail: vanessa.denham@ky.gov
www.ovr.ky.gov

David Beach, Executive Director
Jane Smith, Director of Program Services

Louisiana

10307 Advocacy Center
8325 Oak Street
New Orleans, LA 70118

504-522-2337
800-960-7705
Fax: 504-522-5507
TTY: 855-861-3577
e-mail: advocacycenter@advocacyla.org
www.advocacyla.org

Serves people with disabilities and senior citizens.
Lois Simpson, Executive Director

Maine

10308 Disability Rights Center: Maine
24 Stone St
Augusta, ME 04330-2007

207-626-2774
800-452-1948
Fax: 207-621-1419
e-mail: advocate@drcme.org
www.drcme.org

To enhance and promote the equality, self-determination, independence, productivity, integration, and inclusion of people with disabilities through education, strategic advocacy and legal intervention.
Kim Moody, Executive Director
Kristin Aiello, Managing Attourney

Maryland

10309 Client Assistance Program: Maryland
Maryland State Department of Education

2301 Argonne Drive
Baltimore, MD 21218

410-554-9442
888-554-0334
Fax: 410-554-9362
TTY: 410-554-9360
e-mail: cap@dors.state.md.us
www.dors.state.md.us

Helps individuals who have concerns or difficulties when applying for or receiving rehabilitation services funded under the Rehabilitation Act.
Beth Lash, Director

Massachusetts

10310 Client Assistance Program: Massachusetts
250 Washington Street
Boston, MA 02108-1518

617-727-7440
800-322-2020
e-mail: james.aprea@state.ma.us
www.mass.gov

If you have a disability and want to work but are having trouble getting vocational rehabilitation services, or want a lifestyle which is more self-reliant but are having trouble getting independent living services, contact the Client Assistance Program (CAP).
Barbara E Lybarger Esq, Director

10311 Merrimack Valley HPV Support Group Holy Family Hospital
Holy Family Hospital
70 E Street
Methuen, MA 01844-4597

978-687-0156

10312 Neurosurgical Service
Massachusetts General Hospital
55 Fruit Street
Boston, MA 02114

617-726-2937
e-mail: Referral@Neurosurgery.MassGeneral.org
neurosurgery.mgh.harvard.edu

Uses a multidisciplinary approach to provide a complete range of services for the diagnosis, treatment and rehabilitation of patients with neurological disorders.

Michigan

10313 Client Assistance Program: Michigan
Michigan Protection and Advocacy Service
4095 Legacy Parkway
Lansing, MI 48911-7508

517-487-1755
800-292-5896
Fax: 517-487-0827
e-mail: molson@mpas.org
www.mpas.org

Assists people who are seeking or receiving services from Michigan Rehabilitation Services, Consumer Choice Programs, Michigan Commission for the Blind, Centers for Independent Living, and Supported Employment and Transition Programs.
Mark R Lezotte, President

10314 Commission for the Blind
201 N Washington 2nd Floor
Lansing, MI 48909

517-373-2062
800-292-4200
Fax: 517-335-5140
TDD: 517-373-4025
e-mail: heibeckc@michigan.gov
www.michigan.gov/mcb

To provide opportunity to individuals who are blind or visually impaired to achieve employability and/or function independently in society.
Patrick Cannon, Director

Minnesota

10315 Minnesota Disability Law Center
430 1st Avenue N
Minneapolis, MN 55401-1780

612-334-5970
Fax: 612-334-5755
TTY: 612-332-4668
www.mndlc.org

Addresses the unique legal needs of Minnesotans with disabilities. Provides free civil legal assistance to individuals with disabilities statewide on legal issues related to their disabilities.
Cathy Madouken, Executive Director
Lisa Cohen, Deputy Director of Operations

Mississippi

10316 Mississippi Client Assistance Program
Mississippi Society for Disabilities
Jackson, MS 39296

601-362-2585
800-962-2400
Fax: 601-982-1951
www.icdri.org

A federal grant to the State of Mississippi to provide advocacy services for clients and client applicants of the Office of Vocational Rehabilitation, Vocational Rehabilitation for the Blind, and the Independent Living programs.
Johnny McGinn, Director

Missouri

10317 Missouri Protection and Advocacy Services
925 S Country Club Drive
Jefferson City, MO 65109

573-893-3333
866-777-7199
Fax: 573-893-4231
TDD: 800-735-2966
e-mail: mopasjc@embarqmail.com
www.moadvocacy.org

To protect the rights of individuals with disabilities by providing advocacy and legal services.
Joe Wrinkle, Chair
Lawrence O. Daniels, Vice-Chair

Montana

10318 Disability Rights Montana
1022 Chestnut Street
Helena, MT 59601

406-449-2344
800-245-4743
Fax: 406-449-2418
TDD: 406-449-2344
e-mail: advocate@disabilityrightsmt.org
www.disabilityrightsmt.org

Protects and advocates for the human, legal, and civil rights of Montanans with disabilities while advancing dignity, equality, and self-determination.
Bernadette Franks-Ongoy, Executive Director
Alexandra Volkerts, Staff Attourney

Nebraska

10319 Client Assistance Program: Nebraska Division of Rehabilitative Services
Division of Rehabilitative Services
301 Centennial Mall S
Lincoln, NE 68509

402-471-3656
800-742-7594
e-mail: victoria.rasmussen@cap.ne.gov
www.cap.state.ne.us

The Nebraska Client Assistance Program is a free service to help you find solutions if you are having problems with any of the following programs: Vocational Rehabilitation, Nebraska Commission for the Blind and Visually Impaired or Centers for Independent Living.

10320 Omaha HPV Support Group: PP of Omaha
Planned Parenhood
4610 Dodge Street
Omaha, NE 68132-3234

402-397-2739
www.aad.org

Nevada

10321 Client Assistance Program: Nevada
2800 E Saint Louis Avenue
Las Vegas, NV 89104

775-684-3849
800-633-9879
Fax: 775-684-3850
TTY: 800-326-6868
e-mail: InternetHelp@nvdetr.org
www.detr.state.nv.us

Designed to assist individuals with disabilities resolve problems they may experience with any of Nevada's rehabilitation programs.
Maureen Cole, Rehabilitation Administrator

New Hampshire

10322 Client Assistance Program: New Hampshire
Governor's Commission for the Handicapped
57 Regional Drive 603-271-2773
Concord, NH 03301-8518 800-852-3405
Fax: 603-271-2837
e-mail: disability@nh.gov
www.nh.gov/disability/about/cap.htm

CAP provides information about vocational rehabilitation services; advises you of your rights and responsibilities; investigate your complaint; helps resolve problems with your vocational plan; and represents you at administratove reviews and fair hearings.
John Richards, Executive Director

New Jersey

10323 Disability Rights New Jersey
210 S Broad Street 609-292-9742
Trenton, NJ 08608 800-922-7233
Fax: 609-777-0187
TTY: 609-633-7106
e-mail: adocate@drnj.org
www.drnj.org

To protect, advocate for and advance the rights of persons with disabilities in pursuit of a society in hich persons with disabilities exercise self-determination and choice, and are treated with dignity.
Walter A. Woodberry, Chair
Kathleen F. Wood, Vice Chair

New Mexico

10324 Protection and Advocacy System of Alburque rque
1720 Louisiana Boulevard NE 505-256-3100
Albuquerque, NM 87110-7070 800-432-4682
Fax: 505-256-3184
e-mail: info@drnm.org
www.drnm.org

Disability Rights New Mexico - DRNM - is a private, non-profit organization whose mission is to protect, promote and expand the rights of persons with disabilities.
Marilyn Bove, President

New York

10325 Client Assistance Program: NY State Commission of Quality of Care
Advocacy Bureau
One Commerce Plaza
Albany, NY 12234-2810 518-459-6422
800-222-5627
Fax: 518-473-6296
e-mail: accesadm@mail.nysed.gov
www.acces.nysed.gov/vr/do/cap.htm

The Client Assistance Program (CAP) is a statewide network of skilled advocates that assist New Yorkers with disabilities in getting the training, equipment and services needed for employment.

Marilyn Bove, President

10326 March of Dimes Foundation
1275 Mamaroneck Avenue
White Plains, NY 10605 914-997-4488
www.marchofdimes.com

We help moms have full-term pregnancies and research the problems that threaten the health of babies
Jennifer L Howse, President/CEO

North Carolina

10327 North Carolina Client Assistance Program
805 Ruggles Drive 919-855-3600
Raleigh, NC 27603-2806 800-215-7227
Fax: 919-715-2456
e-mail: nccap@dhhs.nc.gov
www.cap.state.nc.us

Helping people understand and access rehabilitation services.
John Marens, Director
Sharon Wisner, Client Advocate

North Dakota

10328 Client Assistance Program: North Dakota
400 East Broadway 701-328-2950
Bismarck, ND 58501-1208 800-472-2670
Fax: 701-328-3934
TDD: 707-328-8968
e-mail: panda@nd.gov
www.ndpanda.org/cap

Assists clients and client applicants of North Dakota Vocational Rehabilitation services, Tribal Vocational Rehabilitation, or Independent Living services.

Ohio

10329 Cincinnati HPV Support Group: PP of Cincin nati
Planned Parenthood
PO Box 12407
Cincinnati, OH 45212-0407 513-357-7300
www.dermconsultants.com

10330 Disability Rights Center at Ohio Legal Rights Service
50 W Broad Street 614-466-7264
Columbus, OH 43215-5923 800-282-9181
TTY: 614-728-2553
www.disabilityrightsohio.org

To protect and advocate, in partnership with people with disabilities, for their human, civil and legal rights.
Kalpana Yalamanchili, Chair

10331 Richland County HPV Support Group
Mansfield, OH 44907-3881
419-525-3075
www.skinpatient.com

10332 Technology Resource Center
2140 Arbor Boulevard 937-294-8086
Dayton, OH 45439

Oklahoma

10333 Client Assistance Program: Oklahoma Office of Handicapped Concerns
Oklahoma Ofice of Handicapped Concerns
2401 NW 23rd 405-521-3756
Oklahoma City, OK 73107-5106 Fax: 405-522-6695
e-mail: Marilyn.Burr@ohc.state.ok.us
www.icdri.org

Marilyn Bove, President

10334 Oklahoma City HPV Support Group: PP of Cen tral Oklahoma
Planned Parenthood of Central Oklahoma
Oklahoma City, OK 73103-1415
405-528-0221
www.aad.org

Oregon

10335 Resources for Seniors and People with Disabilities
Department of Human Services
500 Summer Street NE 503-947-5811
Salem, OR 97301-1097 800-282-8096
Fax: 503-378-2897
TTY: 800-282-8096
e-mail: spd.web@state.or.us
www.oregon.gov

To secure economic, social, legal and political justice for individuals with disabilities through systems change
Dr Bruce Goldberg, Director
Margaret Carter, Deputy Director Human Services Program

Pennsylvania

10336 Client Assistance Program: Philadelphia
1515 Market Street
Philadelphia, PA 19102
215-557-7112
888-745-2357
Fax: 215-557-7602
TDD: 215-557-7112
e-mail: info@equalemployment.org
www.equalemployment.org
Ensuring that vocation rehabilitation is open and responsive to your needs. Provides information and advice about rehabilitation programs; to advise you of your legal rights and responsibilities; to help resolve probelms that may arise while you are seeking services from rehabilitation programs; to help you pursue administrative and legal remedies to protect your rights.
Stephen S Pennington, Executive Director
Jamie C Ray- Leonetti, Assistant Director

Rhode Island

10337 Rhode Island Disability Law Center
275 Westminster Street
Providence, RI 02903-3434
401-831-3150
800-733-5332
Fax: 401-274-5568
TTY: 401-831-5335
e-mail: info@ridlc.org
www.ridlc.org
Provides free legal assistance to persons with disabilities. Services include individual representation to protect rights or to secure benefits and services; self-help information; educational programs; and administrative and legislative advocacy.

South Carolina

10338 South Carolina Protection & Advocacy System for the Handicapped
3710 Landmark Drive
Columbia, SC 29204-4034
803-782-0639
866-275-7273
TTY: 866-232-4525
e-mail: info@pandasc.org
www.pandasc.org

Marilyn Bove, President

10339 Tri County HPV Support Group
Mt Pleasant, SC 29465-1997
843-884-7333
www.aad.org

South Dakota

10340 South Dakota Advocacy Services
221 S Central Avenue
Pierre, SD 57501
605-224-8294
800-658-4782
Fax: 605-224-5125
TTY: 800-658-4782
e-mail: sdas@sdadvocacy.com
www.sdadvocacy.com
To protect and advocate the rights of South Dakotans with disabilities through legal, administrative, and other remedies.

Tennessee

10341 Disability Law & Advocacy Center of Tennessee
2416 21st Avenue S
Nashville, TN 37212
615-298-1080
800-342-1660
Fax: 615-298-2046
e-mail: gethelp@dlactn.org
www.dlactn.org
Advocates for the rights of Tennesseans with disabilities to ensure they have an equal opportunity to be productive and respected members of the society.
Jerry Gonzalez, Chair
Shalani Rose, Vice Chair

Texas

10342 Dallas/Ft.Worth Metroplex HPV Support Group
8215 Westchester Drive
Dallas, TX 75225-6116
214-363-6733

10343 Disability Rights Texas
Advocacy Inc
2222 W Braker Lane
Austin, TX 78758-1024
512-454-4816
866-362-2851
Fax: 512-323-0902
www.advocacyinc.org
Protecting and advocating the rights of Texans with disabilities - because all people have dignity and worth.
Mary Faithfull, Executive Director

Utah

10344 Legal Center for People with Disabilities
205 North 400 West
Salt Lake City, UT 84103-3076
801-363-1347
800-662-9080
Fax: 801-363-1437
www.disabilitylawcenter.org
We enforce and strengthen laws that protect the opportunities, choices and legal rights of people with disabilities in Utah.
Kevin Murphy, President
Barbara M. Campbell, Senior VP

Vermont

10345 Citizen Advocacy of Burlington
Chase Mill 1 Mill Street
Burlington, VT 05401
802-655-0329
Marilyn Bove, President

10346 Client Assistance Program: Vermont Ladd Hall
Ladd Hall
57 N Main Street
Rutland, VT 05701-8409
802-775-0021
800-769-7459
Fax: 802-775-0022
e-mail: nbreiden@vtlegalaid.org
www.icdri.org

Marilyn Bove, President

Virginia

10347 Richmond HPV Support Group: Fan Free Clini c
Fan Free Clinic
PO Box 5669
Richmond, VA 23220-0669
804-358-6343
www.ashastd.org

10348 Virginia Office for Protection and Advocacy
1910 Byrd Avenue
Richmond, VA 23230
804-225-2042
800-552-3962
Fax: 804-662-7057
e-mail: general.vopa@vopa.virginia.gov
www.vopa.state.va.us
Helps with disability-related problems like abuse, neglect, and discrimination. Also help people with disabilities obtain services and treatment.
Coleen Miller, Executive Director
Eric Berthiaume, Administrator

Washington

10349 Seattle HPV Support Group
Seattle, WA 98103-1171
425-619-7190
www.aad.org

10350 Washington State Client Assistance Program
2531 Rainer Avenue S
Seattle, WA 98144-9510
206-721-5999
800-544-2121
Fax: 206-721-5980
TTY: 888-721-6072
e-mail: info@washingtoncap.org
www.washingtoncap.org
Jerry Johnson, Director
Bob Huven, Rehabilitation Coordinator

West Virginia

10351 Northcentral West Virginia HPV Support Group
Monongalia County Health Department

453 Van Voorhis Road
Morgantown, WV 26505-3408

304-598-5100

10352 West Virginia Advocates
1207 Quarrier Street
Charleston, WV 25301

304-346-0847
800-950-5250
Fax: 304-346-0867
e-mail: contact@wvadvocates.org
www.wvadvocates.org

Protects and advocates for the human and legal rights of persons with disabilities.
Clarice Hausch, Executive Director
Barbara Criner, Administrative Director

Wisconsin

10353 Governor's Committee for People with Disabilities
Wisconsin Department of Health Services
1 W Wilson Street
Madison, WI 53703

608-261-7816
Fax: 608-266-3386
TTY: 888-701-1251
e-mail: sarah.lincoln@wisconsin.gov
www.dhs.wisconsin.gov/Disabilities/Physi

In 1948, a Governor's Committee was established with one goal: to improve employment opportunities for people with disabilities.
Sarah Lincoln, Director

Wyoming

10354 Wyoming Protection & Advocacy System
7344 Stockman Street
Cheyenne, WY 82009

307-632-3496
Fax: 307-638-0815
e-mail: wypanda@wypanda.com
www.wypanda.com

To establish, expand, protect and enforce the human and civil rights of persons with disabilities through administrative, legal, and other appropriate remedies.
Mary Carson Barks, President
Jeanne A Thobro, CEO

Libraries & Resource Centers

Alabama

10355 Horizons Schools
2018 15th Avenue South
Birmingham, AL 35205

205-322-6606
800-822-6242
Fax: 205-322-6605
www.horizonsschool.org

The Horizons School offers a non-degree postsecondary program specifically designed to facilitate personal, social and career independence for students with mild learning disabilities and other mild handicapping conditions.
Don Lutomski, President
Bayard Tynes, Treasurer

Arizona

10356 Life Development Institute
18001 N 79th Avenue
Glendale, AZ 85308

623-773-2774
866-736-7811
Fax: 623-773-2788
e-mail: info@life-development-inst.org
www.lifedevelopmentinstitute.org

Make the special wishes of children with life-threatening or terminal illnesses come true.
Rob Crawford, CEO
Veronica Crawford, Vice President

California

10357 Center for Adaptive Learning
3227 Clayton Road
Concord, CA 94519

925-827-3863
Fax: 925-827-4080
e-mail: info@c4al.org
www.centerforadaptivelearning.org

Committed to creating and maintaining a living and working environment for neurologically impaired individuals, which will promote dignity and support a sense of community. The CAL program provides each participant with an individual program for growth. CAL is committed to maintaining the highest quality of living possible, which will allow each client to develop a sense of pride, to augment self-esteem and to foster a sense of self-worth.
Robert L. Edwards, President
Barry Chinn, VP

10358 Independence Center
3640 S Sepulveda Boulevard
Los Angeles, CA 90034

310-202-7102
Fax: 310-202-7180
e-mail: judym@independencecenter.com
www.independencecenter.com

A mainstreamed transitional residential program for young adults (18-30) with learning disabilities. Program highlights include training in independent living, social and vocational skills, counseling and more.
Judith Maizlish, Executive Director
Gloria Ogletree, Administrative Director

Connecticut

10359 Chapel Haven
1040 Whalley Avenue
New Haven, CT 06515

203-397-1714
Fax: 203-937-2466
e-mail: admissions@chapelhaven.org
www.chapelhaven.org

Providing an array of lifelong individualized support services for adults (18+) on the autism spectrum and those with developmental and social disabilities, enabling them to lead independent and productive lives.
Betsey Parlato, CEO/Executive Director

District of Columbia

10360 ERIC Clearinghouse on Disabilities and Gifted Education
ERIC Project
C/O Computer Sciences Corporation
Washington, DC 20008

800-538-3742
Fax: 703-620-4334
TTY: 703-264-9449
www.eric.ed.gov

The ERIC mission is to provide a comprehensive, easy-to-use, searchable, Internet-based bibliographic and full-text database of education research and information. The simple version of that is that it provides an enormous amount of print materials online, for easy access to important research and journal materials.
Cheryl Racey, Director

Georgia

10361 Creative Community Services (CCS)
4487 Park Drive
Norcross, GA 30093

770-469-6226
866-618-2823
Fax: 770-469-6210
e-mail: info@ccsgeorgia.org
www.ccsgeorgia.org

Provides therapeutic foster care services for children and home-based support for adults with developmental disabilities. CCS improves the quality of life for children, adults and families through its community-based support and services. CCS gives both kids and adults hope by encouraging independent living resulting in involved, engaged citizens and community members.
Nicolette Lee, President
Henri Munyengano, Secretary

Massachusetts

10362 Berkshire Center
18 Park Street
Lee, MA 01238

413-243-2576
Fax: 413-243-3351
www.berkshirecenter.org

The College Internship Program at the Berkshire Center provides individualized, post-secondary academic, internship and independent living experiences for young adults with Asperger's Syndrome and other Learning Differences.
Lucy Gosselin MSBM, Program Director

Minnesota

10363 National Resource Library on Youth with Disabilities
University of Minnesota
Minneapolis, MN 55455
612-626-3087
800-276-8642
Fax: 612-626-2134
TTY: 612-624-3939
e-mail: kdwb-var@umn.edu
www.peds.umn.edu

Offers comprehensive sources of information related to adolescents, disability and transition. The database contains bibliographic, programs, training/education and technical assistance files for the medical community, families, parents and children with chronic illnesses.
Peggy Mann Reinhart, Director
Elizabeth Latts, Resource Coordinator

New Hampshire

10364 Camp Allen
56 Camp Road
Bedford, NH 03110-6606
603-622-8471
Fax: 603-626-4295
e-mail: mary@campallennh.orgg
www.campallennh.org

Camp Allen welcomes about 600 campers each summer. They are persons of all ages with special needs and extraordinary challenges, including cerebral palsy, autism, muscular dystrophy, Down syndrome, and other developmental disabilities.
Sebastian Grasso, President & CEO
Thomas Aites, Treasurer

New Jersey

10365 HealthyWomen
157 Broad Street
Red Bank, NJ 07701
877-986-9472
Fax: 732-530-3347
e-mail: info@healthywomen.org
www.healthywomen.org

Independent health information source for women whose mission is to educate, inform and empower women to make smart health choices for themselves and their families.
Elizabeth Battaglino Cahill, RN, Executive Director
Erin Graves, Director of Marketing & Communications

New York

10366 Center for Medical Consumers
239 Thompson Street
New York, NY 10012
212-674-7105
Fax: 212-674-7100
e-mail: centersformedicalconsumers@gmail.com
www.medicalconsumers.org

A non-profit advocacy organization that was founded with the philosophy of: Whenever long-term drug therapy, elective surgery, or any other major treatment is prescribed, the question of whether the treatment has been proven safe and effective should come up. And the prescribing physician should be expected to cite the relevant studies.
Arthur Aaron Levin MPH, Director
Maryann Napoli, Associate Director

Support Groups & Hotlines

10367 Behavioral Pediatrics Program
KDWP Variety Family Center
200 Oak Street SE
Minneapolis, MN 55455-2002
612-626-4260
800-276-8642
Fax: 612-624-0997
TTY: 612-624-3939
www.peds.umn.edu/pedsadol

Behavioral Pediatrics Staff help children, teen and their families with a wide variety of behavioral concerns including adjustment to coping with chronic illness. Treatments vary depending on the age, developmental state and needs of each child and family. Often, children are taught to self-regulate their behavior.
Daniel Kohen MD, Director

10368 Childrens Hospice International
1101 King Street
Alexandria, VA 22314
703-684-0330
800-242-4453
Fax: 703-684-0226
e-mail: info@chionline.org
www.chionline.org

To ensure medical, psychological, social and spiritual support to all children with like-threatening conditions and their families by providing a network of resources and care.
Ann Armstrong Dailey, Founding Director/CEO
Richard Larkin, Secretary/Treasurer

10369 Fetal Alcohol Network
KDWP Variety Family Center
200 Oak Street SE
Minneapolis, MN 55455-2002
612-626-4260
800-276-8642
Fax: 612-624-0997
TTY: 612-624-3939
e-mail: kdwb-var@umn.edu
www.peds.umn.edu/peds-adol

Staff provide assessment, intervention and consultation regarding the physical, developmental learning, behavioral and emotional well-being of children and individuals affected by prenatal exposure to alcohol and drugs.
Daniel Kohen MD, Director

10370 Foundation for Hospice and Homecare
3801 Vanesta Drive
Manhattan, KS 66503
785-537-0688
800-748-7474
Fax: 785-537-1309
e-mail: cnolte@hcandh.org
www.homecareandhospice.org

We aim to be the premier non-profit Homecare & Hospice provider of compassionate, quality affordable health, wellness and support services. To be committed to preserving hope, dignity and independence in the sheltering embrace of a home environment.
Lowell Kohlmeier, Chair
Judine Mecseri, Director of Program Operations

10371 Friends Health Connection
New Brunswick, NJ 08903
732-418-1811
800-483-7436
Fax: 732-249-9897
e-mail: info@friendshealthconnection.org
www.friendshealthconnection.org

Enhances mind, body and soul through our personalized support network and dynamic educational and motivational programs. Works with hospitals and other nonprofit organizations to complement their program offerings and connect people with resources and support that can enrich their lives.

10372 Genetic Alliance
4301 Connecticut Avenue NW
Washington, DC 20008
202-966-5557
Fax: 202-966-8553
e-mail: info@geneticalliance.org
www.geneticalliance.org

Improves health through the authentic engagement of communities and individuals. The goal is to build capacity within the genetics community. Transform health through genetics and promote an environment of openness centered on the health of individuals, families, and communities.
Sharon F Terry, President/CEO
Greg Biggers, Entrepeneur-in-residence

10373 KDWB Family Resource Center
200 Oak Street SE
Minneapolis, MN 55455-2002
612-626-3087
800-276-8642
Fax: 612-624-0997
TTY: 612-624-3939
e-mail: kdwb-var@umn.edu
www.peds.umn.edu/peds-adol

A place families can visit to learn about their child's chronic illness or disability, identify psychological and developmental issues, and link-up with program and community resources. Information will be available by telephone and via the web site.
Elizabeth Latts, Resource Coordinator

10374 KDWB Variety Family Canter
200 Oak Street SE
Minneapolis, MN 55455-2002

612-626-3087
800-276-8642
Fax: 612-624-0997
TTY: 612-624-3939
e-mail: kdwbvar@umn.edu
www.peds.umn.edu/pedsadol/

University-Community pertnership that provides family-centered services that promote physical, emotional, psychological and social health and well being for children and youth at risk, including children and youth with disabilities. The Center is dedicated to teaching, research, outreach, and community services.
Peggy Mann Reinhart, Director
Elizabeth Latts, Resource Coordinator

10375 National Association for Home Care
228 Seventh Street SE
Washington, DC 20003

202-547-7424
Fax: 202-547-3540
e-mail: exec@nahc.org
www.nahc.org

Promotes the concepts of hospice, a philosophy of health care which is expressed through the provision of a variety of medical and nonmedical services to terminally ill patients and their families.
Val J. Halamandaris, President
Andrea Devoti, Chair

10376 National Family Caregivers Association
10400 Connecticut Avenue
Kensington, MD 20895-3944

301-942-6430
800-896-3650
Fax: 301-942-2302
e-mail: info@thefamilycaregiver.org
www.thefamilycaregiver.org

Educates, supports, empowers and speaks up for the more than 65 million Americans who care for loved ones with a chronic illness or disability or the frailties of old age. Reaches across the boundaries of diagnosis, relationships and life stages to help transform family caregivers' lives by removing barriers to health and well being
Suzanne Mintz, President/CEO

10377 National Health Information Center
Washington, DC 20013

310-565-4167
800-336-4797
Fax: 301-984-4256
e-mail: info@nhic.org
www.health.gov/nhic

Offers a nationwide information referral service, produces directories and resource guides.

10378 National Parent to Parent Support and Information System
3805 Presidential Parkway
Atlanta, GA 30340

770-451-5484
Fax: 770-458-4091
e-mail: info@p2pga.org
www.p2pusa.org

NPPSIS is a nonprofit organization established to support, strengthen, and empower families through one-on-one parent contacts. They link families nationally whose children have special health care needs and rare disorders. They provide parents with heath care information, resources and referrals to allow them to identify appropriate services.
Dana Yarbrough, President
Debra S. Tucker, Executive Director

10379 Okizu Foundation Camps
16 Digital Drive
Novato, CA 94949-6115

415-382-9083
Fax: 415-382-8384
e-mail: info@okizu.org
www.okizu.org

This foundation runs family camp programs for children who have cancer and their families, and for children who have or had a parent with cancer.
Suzie Randall, Executive Director
Heather Ferrier, Asst. Executive Director

10380 Parent to Parent of New York State
500 Balltown Road
Schenectady, NY 12304-2247

518-381-4350
800-305-8817
Fax: 518-393-9607
e-mail: staciap2p@verizon.net
www.parenttoparentnys.org

Parent to Parent programs provide informational and emotional support to parents who have a child, adolescent or adult family member with special needs. Offers an important connection for a parent who is seeking support for special disability issues, by matching him or her with a trained veteran parent who has already been there. Because the two parents share so many common concerns and interests, the support given and received is often uniquely meaningful. Also helps families locate information
Jenni Austen, Regional Coordinator
Holly Bartczak, Coordinator

10381 Pediatric Psychology
KDWP Variety Family Center
200 Oak Street SE
Minneapolis, MN 55455-2002

612-626-4260
800-276-8642
Fax: 612-624-0997
TTY: 612-624-3939
e-mail: kdwbvar@umn.edu
www.peds.umn.edu/pedsadol

Staff provide assessment, intervention and consultation regarding the physical, developmental, learning, behavioral and emotional well-being of children and individuals affected by prenatal exposure to alcohol and drugs.
Daniel Kohen MD, Director

10382 STAR Center for Family Health
KDWB University Pediatrics Family Center
200 Oak St, SE,
Minneapolis, MN 55455-2002

612-626-4260
Fax: 612-624-0997
TTY: 6126243939
e-mail: kdwb-var@umn.edu
www.peds.umn.edu/peds-adol/

Helps children, youth and families develop new and enhanced ways of coping with stress, learn strategies for adjusting to living with a chronic illness, and discover new ways of finding health, balance and well-being.
Lavon Anderson, M.A., Administrator
Linda Boche, Executive Secretary to Division Director

10383 U Special Kids
KDWB Variety Family Center
200 Oak Street SE
Minneapolis, MN 55455-2002

612-626-3081
800-276-8642
Fax: 612-624-0997
TTY: 6126243939
e-mail: uspclkid@umn.edu
www.peds.umn.edu/peds-adol/

A program that provides care coordinators for children with complex medical conditions. A team of health care providers advocates for children and their families within the health care system.
Anne Kelly MD, Director

10384 Visiting Nurse Association of America
601 Thirteenth St NW
Washington, DC 20005

202-384-1420
888-866-8773
Fax: 202-384-1444
e-mail: webadmin@vnaa.org
www.vnaa.org

The VNAA will support, promote and advance nonprofit providers of home and community-based healthcare, hospice and health promotion services to ensure quality care for their communities.
Mary B. DeVeau, Chair
Ellen Rothberg, Vice Chair

10385 Well Spouse Association
63 W Main Street
Freehold, NJ 07728

800-838-0879
e-mail: support@wellspouse.org
www.wellspouse.org

This association is a nonprofit national self-help organization serving the well spouse of the chronically ill. Members help each other develop coping and survival skills through local support

groups (including bereavement), letter and telephone networks, and personal outreach and a quarterly newsletter.
Lawrence Bocchiere, President
Gerald Bishop, Board Chair

Books

10386 A History of Childhood and Disability
Philip Safford and Elizabeth Safford, author

Teachers College Press
1234 Amsterdam Avenue 212-678-3929
New York, NY 10027 Fax: 212-678-4149
e-mail: tcpress@tc.columbia.edu
www.teacherscollegepress.com
This book presents an interdisciplinary perspective on children considered exceptional and how services have evolved in reponse to their diverse neeeds.
1996 352 pages
ISBN: 0-807734-85-3

10387 Art of Getting Well
David Spero, RN, author

Hunter House Publishing
1515 1/2 Park Street 510-865-5282
Alameda, CA 94501 800-266-5592
Fax: 510-865-4295
e-mail: ordering@hunterhouse.com
www.hunterhouse.com
A five step plan for maximazing health when you have a chronic illness.
224 pages Paperback

10388 Assisstive Technology for Young Children: A Guide to Family-Centered Services
Sharon Lesar Judge and Howard P Parette, author

Brookline Books
PO Box 1209 617-734-6772
Brookline, MA 02445 800-666-2665
Fax: 617-734-3952
www.brooklinebooks.com
Explores the wide range of considerations involved in evaluating children's needs, selecting and prescribing devices, and training children, families, and teachers to use the technology.
1998 Softcover
ISBN: 1-571290-51-6

10389 Awaking to Disability
Volcano Press
PO Box 270 209-296-3445
Volcano, CA 95689-0270 800-879-9636
Fax: 209-296-4995
e-mail: sales@volcanopress.com
www.volcanopress.com
From the disability activist whose columns have been avidly followed by readers of the Albuquerque Journal and Miami Herald comes this revealing compedium of her thoughts. It offers a perspective for parents of children with disabilites, or for newly disabled people.
1997 288 pages
ISBN: 1-884244-14-9

10390 Blood Pressure Book: How to Get it Down & Keep it Down
Bull Publishing
PO Box 1377 303-545-6350
Boulder, CO 80306 800-676-2855
Fax: 303-545-6354
www.bullpub.com
Provides basic information on the causes and treatment of high blood pressure includes check up charts and illustrations that will help readers find out where they stand and lead them to practical advice tailored to their own needs.
1996
ISBN: 0-923521-97-6

10391 Building Partnerships in Hospital Care
Bull Publishing

PO Box 1377
Boulder, CO 80306 800-676-2855
Fax: 303-545-6354
www.bullpub.com
Aims to desensetize patients and families to their fears of illness, hospital machinery and authority figures at the same time resensitize institution weary professionals to the feelings, instincts and emotions that brought them into the field in the first place.
304 pages
ISBN: 0-923521-07-0

10392 Child of Mine: Feeding with Love and Good Sense
Bull Publishing
PO Box 1377
Boulder, CO 80306 800-676-2855
www.bullpub.com
Parents need to learn how to provide a nutritionally wholesome diet, but they also need to know how to feed in a way that nurtures a child's senses of autonomy and trust in themselves and their bodies.
470 pages
ISBN: 0-923521-51-8

10393 Childhood Emergencies: What to Do A Quick Refrence Guide
Bull Publishing
PO Box 1377
Boulder, CO 80306 800-676-2855
www.bullpub.com
Handy book contains clear and quick referance for most common injuries including cuts and wounds, broken bones, abdominal pain, burns, toothaches, convulsion, eye and ear injuries, abrasions, bites insect and animal, bleeding, choking, seizures, freezing and frostbite, CPR, etc.
44 pages
ISBN: 0-923521-62-3

10394 Chiropractor's Self-Help Back and Body Book
Samuel Homola, DC, author

Hunter House Publishers
1515 1/2 Park Street 510-865-5282
Alameda, CA 94501 800-266-5592
e-mail: ordering@hunterhouse.com
www.hunterhouse.com
How to relieve common aches and pains at home and on the job.
2002 320 pages Paperback
ISBN: 0-897933-76-6

10395 Choose the Right Long Term Care
NOLO
950 Parker Street
Berkeley, CA 94710-2524 800-728-3555
Fax: 800-645-0895
e-mail: cs@nolo.com
www.nolo.com
You can use this book to figure out how to choose a nursing home, or find a viable alternative. Covers how to get the most out of Medicare and other benefit programs.
336 pages
ISBN: 0-873375-15-7
Ralph Warner, Executive Chairman & Co-Founder
Bob Dubow, CEO

10396 Chronic Physical Illness
S. Newman, E. Steed, K. Mulligan, author

McGraw-Hill Companies
Returns Department
Dubuque, IA 52002 877-833-5524
Fax: 609-308-4484
e-mail: pbg.ecommerce_custserv@mcgraw-hill.com
www.mcgraw-hill.com
Provides an overview of self-management in chronic physical illness, theoretical and conceptual background, and examines issues related to the delivery of self-management. Discussion of a range of chronic conditions including: asthma, coronary artery disease, heart failure, COPD, hypertension, diabetes and rheumatoid ar-

thritis. Authored by a number of leading international experts in the diseases they discuss. Hardcover also available for $136.95.
2008 240 pages
ISBN: 0-335217-86-9

10397 Directory of Health Grants
Research Grant Guides
PO Box 1214 561-795-6129
Loxahatchee, FL 33470-1214 Fax: 561-795-7794
1000 foundation profiles.
Second edition
ISBN: 0-945078-19-6

10398 Directory of Social Service Grants
Research Grant Guides
PO Box 1214 561-795-6129
Loxahatchee, FL 33470-1214 Fax: 561-795-7794
1100 foundation profiles.
Second edition
ISBN: 0-945078-18-8

10399 Disabled Woman's Guide to Pregnancy and Birth
Judith Rogers OTR, author
Demos Medical Publishing
11 W 42nd Street 212-683-0072
New York, NY 10036 800-532-8663
Fax: 212-683-0118
e-mail: info@demosmedpub.com
www.demosmedpub.com
Based on the experiences of ninety women with disabilities who chose to have children. Contains in-depth interviews with women with 22 different types of disabilities and with a total of 143 pregnancies.
528 pages
ISBN: 1-932603-08-8
Dr. Diana M Schneider, President

10400 Family Interventions Throughout Chronic Illness and Disability
Springer Publishing Company
536 Broadway 212-431-4370
New York, NY 10012-3955 Fax: 212-941-7842
e-mail: marketing@springerpub.com
www.springerpub.com
This book provides usable methods for professionals to help families deal with the reality of chronic illness of disability of a family member. Included at the end of each section are study questions and suggested activities for those working with the disabled, as well as for students.
336 pages Hardcover
ISBN: 0-826155-80-1
Annette Imperati, Marketing Director

10401 Get Fit While You Sit: Easy Workouts From Your Chair
Charlene Torkelson, author
Hunter House Publishing
1515 1/2 Park Street
Alameda, CA 94501 510-865-5282
800-266-5592
e-mail: ordering@hunterhouse.com
www.hunterhouse.com
A total body workout that can be done right from your chair, anywhere. Perfect for office workers, travelers, and those with age-related movement limitations or special conditions.
Paperback
ISBN: 0-897932-53-0

10402 Good Bones: Complete Guide to Building and Maintaining the Healthiest Bones
Barbara Luke, author
Bull Publishing
PO Box 1377
Boulder, CO 80306 800-676-2855
Fax: 303-545-6354
www.bullpub.com
Examines 17 major risks in bone health with women. Author offers nutrional advice and preventative nutritional advice and

prevenative measures in this comprehensive and scientifically sound guide for woman of all ages.
192 pages
ISBN: 0-923521-44-5

10403 Grants for Organizations Serving People with Disabilities
Research Grant Guides
PO Box 1214
Loxahatchee, FL 33470-1214 Fax: 561-795-7794
800 foundation profiles, including funding for all types of nonprofits. Also two key articles on winning grant strategies.
Tenth edition
ISBN: 0-945078-17-X

10404 Habits Not Diets: Secret to Lifetime Weight Control
James M Ferguson MD, Cassandra Ferguson, author
Bull Publishing
PO Box 1377 303-545-6350
Boulder, CO 80306 800-676-2855
Fax: 303-545-6354
www.bullpub.com
This sensible approach puts the emphasis on how to eat rather than what. Uses the cognitive aspects of weight management including thinking skills, stress management and problem solving to help analyze individual eating habits , break undesirable patterns and establish new ones.
352 pages
ISBN: 0-923521-70-7

10405 Health
Sage Publications
2455 Teller Road 805-499-9774
Thousand Oaks, CA 91320 800-818-7243
Fax: 805-499-0871
e-mail: journals@sagepub.com
www.sagepublications.com
A interdisciplinary and international journal committed to the social and cultural study of health, illness and medicine with a particular focus on the changing place of health matters in modern society and in public onsciousness.
Quarterly

10406 I Can't Chew Cookbook
J Randy Wilson, author
Hunter House Publishing
1515 1/2 Park Street 510-865-5282
Alameda, CA 94501 800-266-5592
Fax: 510-865-4295
e-mail: ordering@hunterhouse.com
www.hunterhouse.com
Delicious soft-diet recipes for people with chewing, swallowing and dry-mouth disorders.
224 pages Paperback
ISBN: 0-897934-00-8

10407 Informed Woman's Guide to Breast Health
Kerry McGinn RN, author
Bull Publishing
PO Box 1377 303-545-6350
Boulder, CO 80306 800-676-2855
Fax: 303-545-6354
www.bullpub.com
Covers all elements of self-examination, mammography, medical exams and tests; includes new information about the genes BRCA 1 and BRCA 2, possible early predictors of cancer

ISBN: 0-923521-61-5

10408 Insider's Guide to HMOs
Penguin Putnam
PO Box 999
Bergenfield, NJ 07621-0903 800-526-0275
Fax: 800-227-9604

ISBN: 0-452276-91-8

10409 Journel to Pain Relief
Phyllis Berger, author
Hunter House Publishing
PO Box 2194
Alameda, CA 94501   510-865-5282
                                     800-266-5592
                                     Fax: 510-865-4295
                e-mail: ordering@hunterhouse.com
                              www.hunterhouse.com
Hands-on guide to breakthroughs in pain treatment.
2007 288 pages Paperback
Cristina Sverdrup, Customer Service Manager

10410 Joy of Laziness
Peter Axt, PhD, Michaela Axt-Gardermann, author
Hunter House Publishing
1515 1/2 Park Street
Alameda, CA 94501   510-865-5282
                                     800-266-5592
                                     Fax: 510-865-4295
                e-mail: ordering@hunterhouse.com
                              www.hunterhouse.com
Explains that every human being has a limited amount of energy at
his or her disposal.
160 pages Paperback
ISBN: 0-897934-01-5
Cristina Sverdrup, Customer Service Manager

10411 Just Like Everyone Else
World Institute on Disability
510 16th Street, Suite 100
Oakland, CA 94612-1520   510-763-4100
                                     Fax: 510-763-4109
                                     TTY: 510-208-9493
                                     e-mail: wid@wid.org
                                     www.wid.org
Provides perspective, inspiration and information about the Inde-
pendent Living Movement and the Americans with Disabilities
Act.
16 pages
Kathy Martinez, Executive Director

10412 Laurel's Kitchen Caring: Recipes for Everyday Home Caregiving
Ten Speed Press
PO Box 7123
Berkeley, CA 94707-0123   510-559-1600
                                     800-841-2665
                                     Fax: 510-524-4588
                      e-mail: order@tenspeed.com
                              www.tenspeed.com
A cookbook tailored to the nutritional needs of recovering patients
as well as morale booster, caregiving primer, and resource book.
1997 158 pages
ISBN: 0-898159-51-2

10413 Living a Healthy Life with Chronic Conditions
Kate Lorig, Halsted Holman, David Sobel, author
Bull Publishing
PO Box 1377
Boulder, CO 80306   303-545-6350
                                     800-676-2855
                                     Fax: 303-545-6354
                                     www.bullpub.com
Full of tips, suggestions, and strategies to deal with chronic illness
and common symptoms, such as fatigue, pain, shortness of breath,
disability, and depression. Encourages readers to develop individual approaches to setting goals, making decisions, and finding resources and support so they are able to do the things they want, and
need, to accomplish.
292 pages
ISBN: 1-933503-01-1

10414 Maximize Your Body Potential
Joyce D Nash PhD, author
Bull Publishing
PO Box 1377
Boulder, CO 80306   303-545-6350
                                     800-676-2855
                                     Fax: 303-545-6354
                                     www.bullpub.com

Using selftests, checklists, and fill-in forms, shows readers how to
make a committment, how to set realistic goals, and how to design
an individualized exercise and eating program.
640 pages
ISBN: 0-923521-71-4

10415 Menopause Without Medicine
Linda Ojeda, author
Hunter House Publishing
1515 1/2 Park Street
Alameda, CA 94501   510-865-5282
                                     800-266-5592
                                     Fax: 510-865-4295
                e-mail: ordering@hunterhouse.com
                              www.hunterhouse.com
Provides complete information on the symptoms of menopause -
hot flashes, sexual changes, deperssion and osteoporosis - and how
to alleviate them.
400 pages Paperback
ISBN: 0-897934-05-3

**10416 Nolo's Guide to Soc. Security Disability: Getting and Keeping
Your Benefits**
David Morton MD, author
NOLO
950 Parker Street
Berkeley, CA 94710-2524   800-728-3555
                                     Fax: 800-645-0895
                                     e-mail: cs@nolo.com
                                     www.nolo.com
The essential book for anyone dealing with a long-term or permanent disability. Written both for first-time applicants and existing
recipients of Social Security disability, this guide demystifies the
program and tells you everything you need to know about qualify-
ing and applying for benefits, maintaining your benefits, and
appealing the denial of a claim.
512 pages
ISBN: 1-413311-04-4

**10417 Ostomy Book: Living Comfortably with Colostomies, Ileostomies
and Urostomies**
Barbara Dorr Mullen, Kerry Anne McGinn, author
Bull Publishing
PO Box 1377
Boulder, CO 80306   303-545-6350
                                     800-676-2855
                                     Fax: 303-545-6354
                                     www.bullpub.com
For people who have a colostomy, ileostomy or urinary diversion
(utostomy), either permanent or temporary, as well as for family,
friends and health professionals.

ISBN: 0-933503-13-4

**10418 Psychological Management of Chronic Pain: A Treatment
Manual**
Springer Publishing Company
536 Broadway   212-431-4370
New York, NY 10012-3955   Fax: 212-941-7842
This volume provides the clinician with a practical guide to help
clients manage and alleviate problems associated with chronic
pain and places an emphasis on the cognitive components of treatment. The manual illustrates a time-limited, thera-
pist-guide/self-management program.
1996 80 pages Softcover
ISBN: 0-826161-12-X

10419 Self Help: Your Strategy for Living with COPD
Bull Publishing
PO Box 1377
Boulder, CO 80306   800-676-2855
                                     Fax: 303-545-6354
                                     www.bullpub.com
Contains vital information for patients suffering from asthma, em-
physema, or chronic bronchitis. Colorful charts, graphs and illus-
trations highlight major concepts and help make the booklet user
friendly.
1997 32 pages
ISBN: 0-923521-40-2

10420 ShapeWalking

Marilyn Bach, PhD, Lorie Schleck, author

Hunter House Publishing
1515 1/2 Park Street
Alameda, CA 94501
510-865-5282
800-266-5592
Fax: 510-865-4295
e-mail: ordering@hunterhouse.com
www.hunterhouse.com

An easy low cost total fitness program that is suited for exercisers of all levels.
144 pages Paperback
ISBN: 0-897933-73-5

10421 Social Security, Medicare and Government Pensions

Dorothy Matthews Berman, author

NOLO
950 Parker Street
Berkeley, CA 94710-2524
800-728-3555
Fax: 800-645-0895
e-mail: cs@nolo.com
www.nolo.com

Gets you the most out of your retirement benefits
496 pages
ISBN: 1-413310-97-9

10422 Strength Training for Seniors

Michael Fekete, CSCS; ACE, author

Hunter House Publishing
PO Box 2194
Alameda, CA 94501
510-865-5282
800-266-5592
Fax: 510-865-4295
e-mail: ordering@hunterhouse.com
www.hunterhouse.com

How to rewind your biological clock. Reduce a person's biological age by 10-20 years.
2006 160 pages Paperback
Cristina Sverdrup, Customer Service Manager

10423 Succeeding Against the Odds: Strategies and Insights from the Learning Disabled

Jeremy P Tarcher
5858 Wilshire Boulevard
Los Angeles, CA 90036-4521
213-935-9980

Filled with information on adults with learning disabilities, including the hidden handicaps, the definition of learning disabilities, and characteristics of individuals with learning disabilities. The book also looks at the responsibility of preparing for adulthood, and includes information for parents and teachers.
Lex Frieden, Program Director

10424 Taking Care of Caregivers

D Jeanne Roberts MA, author

Bull Publishing
PO Box 1377
Boulder, CO 80306
303-545-6350
800-676-2855
Fax: 303-545-6354
www.bullpub.com

Covers the needs of caregivers; their feelings; stress management techniques; communication; grief; sharing and support

ISBN: 0-923521-09-7

10425 Tax Options and Strategies for People with Disabilities

Demos Vermande
386 Park Avenue S
New York, NY 10016-8804
212-683-0072
800-532-8663
Fax: 212-683-0118
e-mail: info@demospub.com

1996 288 pages
ISBN: 0-939957-85-

10426 Teens Face to Face with Chronic Illness

Asthma and Allergy Foundation of America
1233 20th Street NW
Washington, DC 20036-2330
202-466-7643
800-727-8462
Fax: 202-466-8940
www.aafa.org

Young people easily relate to this book, which uses anecdotes from teens dealing with chronic illness. Teens address issues such as peer pressure and feeling different.
129 pages Paperback

10427 The Personal Care Attendant Guide: The Art of Finding, Keeping, or Being One

Katie Rodriguez Banister, author

Program Development Associates
5620 Business Avenue
Cicero, NY 13039-9576
315-452-0643
800-543-2119
Fax: 315-452-0710
e-mail: info@disabilitytraining.com
www.disabilitytraining.com/pcgb.html

To live independently, many people with chronic illness and/or disabilitiy hire a personal attendant to assist with day-to-day tasks. Finding a qualified caregiver can be challenging, but not impossible. The Guide teaches readers how to find a competent caregiver, and gives prospective attendants vital information and real-life examples to help them succeed. Includes easy-to-use forms and worksheets to make the search easy and organized, anecdotes, and resources.
2007 160 pages

10428 Time for Healing: Relaxation for Mind and Body

Bull Publishing
PO Box 1377
Boulder, CO 80306
800-676-2855
Fax: 303-545-6354
www.bullpub.com

Helps and guides listeners release tension and acheive deep muscular relaxation, heightened self-awareness and total relaxation.

10429 Understanding Addiction

Elizabeth Connell Henderson MD, author

University Press of Mississippi
3825 Ridgewood Road
Jackson, MS 39211
601-432-6205
800-737-7788
www.upress.state.ms.us

A concise overview of this complex affliction for all those affected by addiction — addicts, family members, and even employers
224 pages Paperback
ISBN: 1-578062-40-9

10430 Understanding Anemia

Ed Uthman, MD, author

University Press of Mississippi
3825 Ridgewood Road
Jackson, MS 39211
601-432-6205
www.upress.state.ms.us

Gently builds upon elementary knowledge of biology to provide the general reader with a fairly sophisticated understanding of the various causes of anemia, of the methods used to make diagnoses, and of the principles of treatment.
160 pages Paperback
ISBN: 1-578060-39-9

10431 Understanding Child Sexual Abuse

Edward L Rowan, MD, author

University Press of Mississippi
3825 Ridgewood Road
Jackson, MS 39211
601-432-6205
Fax: 601-432-6217
www.upress.state.ms.us

For those looking to comrephend and to prevent child sexual abuse, a succinct guidebook of advice and resources.
96 pages Paperback
ISBN: 1-578068-07-X

10432 Understanding Cosmetic Laser Surgery

Robert Langdon, MD, author

University Press of Mississippi
3825 Ridgewood Road
Jackson, MS 39211
601-432-6205
Fax: 601-432-6217
www.upress.state.ms.us

A description of the processes and procedures available in cosmetic laser surgery.
112 pages
ISBN: 1-578065-87-9

10433 Understanding Dental Health

Francis G Serio, DMD; MS, author

University Press of Mississippi
3825 Ridgewood Road   601-432-6205
Jackson, MS 39211   Fax: 601-432-6217
                                   www.upress.state.ms.us
A user-friendly manual on the basics of dental health.
128 pages Paperback
ISBN: 1-578060-10-9

10434 Understanding Dietary Supplements

Jenna Hollenstein, author

University Press of Mississippi
3825 Ridgewood Road   601-432-6205
Jackson, MS 39211   Fax: 601-432-6217
                                   www.upress.state.ms.us
A handy guide to the evaluation and use of vitamins, minerals,
herbs, botanicals, and more.
96 pages Paperback
ISBN: 1-578069-81-5

10435 Understanding Stuttering

Nathan Lavid, MD, author

University Press of Mississippi
3825 Ridgewood Road   601-432-6205
Jackson, MS 39211   Fax: 601-432-6217
                                   www.upress.state.ms.us
Insight into an ailment that impairs more than sixty million in the
world population.
112 pages Paperback
ISBN: 1-578065-73-9

10436 Understanding Your Learning Disability

Cheri Warner, author

Ohio State University at Newark
1179 University Drive
Newark, OH 43055   740-366-3321
                                   newark.osu.edu
Provides tips for students based on the author's experience as a
Learning Disability Specialist. Offers definitions, characteristics,
and suggestions related to reading, math, note taking, test taking,
social interactions, and organizational strategies.

10437 Writing from Within

Bernard Selling, author

Hunter House Publishers
1515 1/2 Park Street   510-865-5282
Alameda, CA 94501   800-266-5592
                                   Fax: 510-865-4295
                         e-mail: ordering@hunterhouse.com
                                   www.hunterhouse.com
A guide to creativity and life story writing
320 pages Paperback
ISBN: 0-897932-17-2

10438 Yes, You Can!: Go Beyond Physical Adversity and Live Life to Its Fullest

Janis Dietz PhD, author

Demos Medical Publishing
11 W 42nd Street   212-683-0072
New York, NY 10036   800-532-8663
                         e-mail: info@demosmedpub.com
                                   www.demosmedpub.com
Based on the premise that life should be lived to the fullest extent
possible, disability or no disability.
102 pages Paperback
ISBN: 1-888799-48-x

Children's Books

10439 Are You Tired Again?...I Understand: An Activities Workbook for Children

Marilyn W Deutsch PhD, author

Western Psychological Services

12031 Wilshire Boulevard   310-478-2061
Los Angeles, CA 90025-1251   800-648-8857
                                   Fax: 310-478-7838
                         e-mail: customerservice@wpspublish.com
                                   www.wpspublish.com
This reassuring activity and coloring book is for children with a
chronically ill parent—children who often feel guilty, neglected,
lonely, helpless, and afraid. It gives these youngsters the tools they
need to work through their feelings, while gently explaining why
Mom isn't getting better, why she's always tired, and how the family can still enjoy life and function as a family. It can be used with
individuals or with support groups.

10440 In the Hospital

Peter Alsop, Bill Harley, author

Compassion Books
7036 State Highway 80 S   828-675-5909
Burnsville, NC 28714-7569   800-970-4220
                                   Fax: 828-675-9687
                         e-mail: heal2grow@aol.com
                                   www.compassionbooks.com
Wonderful songs and entertaining stories dealing with being sick,
being different, being scared and finding strength and hope.
Audiotape/Book
Bruce Greene, Director

10441 Zink the Zebra

Gareth Stevens, Inc
330 West Olive Street   414-332-3520
Milwaukee, WI 53212-3952   800-542-2595
                                   Fax: 414-336-0156
                         e-mail: info@gspub.com
                                   www.garethstevens.com
Zink is a zebra with spots instead of stripes. Here is an inspiring
and touching tale about being different in ways that don't matter
and shouldn't get in the way when it comes to making friends and
enjoying companionship and respect. Written by 11-year-old
Kelly Weil in the last year of a battle she bravely fought, but ultimately lost, against cancer.
1997
ISBN: 0-836816-26-9

Magazines

10442 Advance: for Directors in Rehabilitation

Merion Publications
2900 Horizon Drive   215-265-7812
King of Prussia, PA 19406-2651   800-355-5627
                         rehabilitation-director.advanceweb.com
An informational magazine designed to provide a balance of mate-
rial concerning all aspects of a rehabilitation manager's job.
Scott Huelskamp, Editor
Johnathan Bassett, Senior Associate Editor

10443 Closing the Gap

526 Main Street   507-248-3294
Henderson, MN 56044   Fax: 507-248-3810
                         e-mail: info@closingthegap.com
                                   www.closingthegap.com
Strives to provide parents and educators alike, the information and
training necessary to locate, compare, and implement assistive
technology.
BiMonthly
Budd Hagen, Co-Founder
Connie Kneip, VP/General Manager

10444 Exceptional Parent Magazine

209 Harvard Street   617-730-5800
Brookline, MA 02446-5005   800-852-2884
                                   Fax: 617-730-8742

Lex Frieden, Program Director

Newsletters

10445 Asbestos Watch

PO Box 1483   301-243-5864
Baltimore, MD 21203-1483   Fax: 301-243-5234

A national nonprofit organization dedicated to the education of the public to the hazards of asbestos exposure. The association developed programs of public education and consults with victims of asbestos exposure, school boards, building owners, government agencies, and others interested in identifying asbestos hazards and developing control programs.
Annual

10446 Chronic Pain Letter
Dolak
Old Chelsea Station   718-797-0015
New York, NY 10011
Brings current information on the management of chronic pain to the sufferer and the health professional.

Dorothy Fabian, Circulation Manager

10447 Health Facts
Center for Medical Consumers
237 Thompson Street   212-674-7105
New York, NY 10012-1017   Fax: 212-674-7100
                                                 www.medicalconsumers.org
Analyses of topics such as cancer, nutrition, depression, exercise, prescription drugs and nonmedical therapies.
6 pages Monthly

10448 In Confidence
American Health Information Management Association
233 N Michigan Avenue, 21st Floor   312-233-1100
Chicago, IL 60601   800-621-6828
                                                 Fax: 312-233-1090
                                                 e-mail: info@ahima.org
                                                 www.ahima.org
Provides medical, legal and other professionals with a forum to exchange ideas and share knowledge about the confidentiality of health information and people's rights to privacy.
12 pages BiMonthly
Linda Kloss, Chief Executive Officer
Becky Perry, Executive Vice President & CFO

10449 Johns Hopkins Health Insider
Intelihealth
960C Harvest Drive
Blue Bell, PA 19422
                                                 800-988-1127
                                                 Fax: 800-676-3299
                                                 e-mail: service@jhinsider.com
                                                 www.jhinsider.com
Expert advice and information from America's leading health institution. The most authoritative, cutting-edge health information available today, straight from the leading specialists and experts.
David B Hellmann MD, Associate Editor
Linda A Lewandowski PhD, RN, Associate Editor

10450 Learning Disability Quarterly
Council for Learning Disabilities
11184 Antioch Road   913-491-1011
Overland Park, KS 66210   Fax: 913-491-1012
                                                 e-mail: CLDInfo@ie-events.com
                                                 www.cldinternational.org

Caroline Dunn, President
Monica Lambert, President Elect

10451 Lifelines
Disabled & Alone/Life Services for the Handicapped
61 Broadway   212-532-6740
New York, NY 10006   800-995-0066
                                                 Fax: 212-532-3588
                                                 e-mail: info@disabledandalone.org
                                                 www.disabledandalone.org

8 pages Quarterly
Leslie D Park, Chairman
Lee Alan Ackerman BA, Executive Director

10452 Lymphatic Research Matters
Lymphatic Research Foundation
40 Garvies Point Road   516-625-9675
Glen Cove, NY 11542   Fax: 516-625-9410
                                                 e-mail: lrf@lymphaticresearch.org
                                                 www.lymphaticresearch.org

Reporting information about LRF activities and current research. The newsletters are sent to registrants in our data base: patients, their families, the scientific community and health care providers.
Bi-Annual
Jacqueline Reinhard, Executive Director
Wendy Chaite, Esq., Founder

10453 Mainstay
Well Spouse Association
63 W Main Street   732-577-8899
Freehold, NJ 7728   800-838-0879
                                                 Fax: 732-577-8644
                                                 e-mail: info@wellspouse.org
                                                 www.wellspouse.org
The Well Spouse Association quarterly newsletter featuring articles written by WSA members.

10454 NHF Head Lines
National Headache Foundation
820 N Orleans   312-274-2650
Chicago, IL 60610   888-643-5552
                                                 Fax: 312-640-9049
                                                 e-mail: info@headaches.org
                                                 www.headaches.org
Up-to-date information on the latest developments in headache treatment; breaking news about newly-approved drugs; reviews of topical books; reader's mail feature, where the nation's leading medical experts answer questions about headaches; and a list of support group meetings where you can learn how to make a positive change in your life.
Bimonthly
Robert R Dalton, Executive Director

10455 National Networker
National Network of Learning Disabled Adults
808 N 82nd Street   602-941-5112
Scottsdale, AZ 85257-3850
For adults with learning disabilities.
Quarterly
Lex Frieden, Program Director

10456 Orphan Disease Update
National Organization for Rare Disorders
PO Box 8923   203-746-6518
New Fairfield, CT 06812-8923   800-999-6673
                                                 Fax: 203-756-6481
                                                 e-mail: orphan@rarediseases.org
                                                 www.rarediseases.org
Information about rare disorders for families with similar disorders.

10457 VSA Arts
JFK Center for the Performing Arts
1300 Connecticut Avenue NW   202-628-2600
Washington, DC 20036-1715   800-933-8721
                                                 Fax: 202-737-0725
                                                 TDD: 202-737-0645
                                                 e-mail: info@vsarts.org
                                                 www.vsarts.org
VSA arts is an international, nonprofit organization dedicated to promoting artistic excellence and providing educational opportunities through the arts for children and adults with disabilities. The Creative Spirit is a quarterly newsletter that features VSA arts special events throughout the world, interviews with artistd and articles relating to disability and the arts.
8 pages
D Dixon, CEO
S Datton-Kumins, Writer/Research Coordinator

10458 Wheel Life News
University of Virginia, Rehab Engineering Centers
3363 University Station   804-924-0311
Charlottesville, VA 22903
Features tie downs and other adaptive technology for persons with disabilities.

10459 Worklife: A Publication of Employment and People with Disabilities
Office of Disability Employment Policy

200 Constitution Avenue NW
Washington, DC 20210

202-693-7880
Fax: 202-693-7888
TDD: 202-376-6205

Quarterly

Pamphlets

10460 Campus Opportunities for Students with Learning Differences
Judith & Stephen Crooker, author

Octameron Associates
PO Box 2748
Alexandria, VA 22301

703-836-5480
Fax: 703-836-5650
e-mail: octameron@aol.com
www.octameron.com

Tells learning disabled students what questions to ask when selecting a school, how to prepare for the more rigorous academic schedule and when to get special assistance.
36 pages
ISBN: 1-575090-52-x

10461 Issues in Independent Living
Independent Living Research Utilization
2323 S Shepherd Drive
Houston, TX 77019-7024

713-520-0232
Fax: 713-520-5785

This booklet is a report of the National Study Group on the Implications of Health Care Reform for Americans with Disabilities and Chronic Health Conditions.
30 pages
Lex Frieden, Program Director

10462 OSERS News in Print: Office of Special Education & Rehabilitative Services
US Department of Education
400 Maryland Avenue SW
Washington, DC 20202-0001

202-205-8241
800-872-5327
www.ed.gov

Provides information, research, and resources in the area of special learning needs.
Quarterly
Lex Frieden, Program Director

Audio & Video

10463 Assisting Parents Through the Mourning Process
Hope
55 E 100 N
Logan, UT 84321-4648

435-752-9533
Fax: 435-752-9533

Describes the mourning process experienced by some parents of children with disabilities and ways in which the professional can help them through the process.
20 minutes

10464 No Fears, No Tears
Leora Kuttner, PhD, author

Fanlight Productions
4196 Washington Street
Boston, MA 02131-1731

617-469-4999
800-937-4113
Fax: 617-469-3379
e-mail: fanlight@fanlight.com
www.fanlight.com

Dr. Leora Kuttner explores the effects of childrens pain management.
1985 28 Minutes

10465 No Fears, No Tears: 13 Years Later
Leora Kuttner, PhD, author

Fanlight Productions
4196 Washington Street
Boston, MA 02131-1731

617-469-4999
800-937-4113
Fax: 617-469-3379
e-mail: fanlight@fanlight.com
www.fanlight.com

Dr. Leora Kutner explores the effects of childrens pain management therapies 13 years after their use.
1998 47 Minutes
ISBN: 1-572952-77-6

Web Sites

10466 Access Unlimited

www.accessunlimited.com

Assists educators, health care providers and parents in discovering how personal computers help children and adults with disabilities compensate for some of the barriers imposed by their conditions.

10467 American Academy of Pediatrics

www.aap.org

Committed to the attainment of optimal physical, mental and social health and well-being for all infants, children, adolescents and yound adults.

10468 American Association for the Advancement of Science

www.aaas.org

An international non-profit organization dedicated to advancing science around the world by serving as an educators, leader, spokesperson and professional association.

10469 American Bar Association Commission

www.abanet.org/disability

10470 American Camp Association

www.acacamps.org

Enriching the lives of children, youth and adults through the camp experience.

10471 American Counseling Association

www.counseling.org

Dedicated to the growth and development of the counseling profession and those who are served.

10472 American Institute for Preventive Medicine

www.healthylife.com

An award winning, internationally recognized authority on the development and implementation of health promotion, wellness, medical self-care and disease management programs and publications.

10473 American Organ Transplant Association

www.aotaonline.org

To help transplant patients lead happy, productinve lives by helping them obtain and sustain transplantation.

10474 American Red Cross

www.redcross.org

In addition to domestic disaster relief, the American Red Cross offers compassionate services in five other areas: community services that help the needy; support and comfort for military members and their families; the collection, processing and distribution of lifesaving blood and blood products; educational programs that promote health and safety; and international relief and development programs.

10475 American Self-Help Group Clearinghouse

www.selfhelpgroups.org

A keyword-searchable database of over 1,100 national, international, model and online self-help support groups for addictions, bereavement, health, mental health, disabilities, abuse, parenting, caregiver concerns and many other stressful life situations.

10476 American Society of Dermatology

www.asd.org

A non-partisan professional association of dermatologists across the country whose mission is to facilitate optimal dermatologic care being available to all citizens of this country by preserving, promoting and enhancing the private practice of dermatology.

10477 Americas Association for the Care of the Children

www.aaccchildren.net

To promote support for those who are involved in early childhood care and education through educational programs and projects, including among other things, citizen exchange programs, global communication networks, and resource assistance to participating communities.

10478 Beach Center on Families and Disability

www.beachcenter.org

Makes a significant and sustainable difference in the quality of life of families and individuals affected by disability and of those who are closely involved with them.

10479 Center for Chronic Disease Prevention and Health Promotion

www.cdc.gov/nccdphp

The forefront of the nation's efforts to prevent and control chronic diseases. Leads efforts that promote health and well-being through prevention and control of chronic diseases.

10480 Center for Developmental Disabilities

www.centerfor.com

Committed to its mission of helping children and adults with differing abilities achieve their dreams by overcoming barriers to living, working, learning and enjoying recreational opportunities in the community of their choice.

10481 ChiroWeb.com

www.chiroweb.com

Chiropractic news source for chiropractors, students, patients and health care professionals. Over 7,000 articles are available.

10482 Commission on Accreditation of Rehabilitation Services

www.carf.org

An independent, nonprofit accreditor of health and human services that promotes the quality, value and optimal outcomes of services through a consultative accreditation process that centers on enhancing the lives of the persons served.

10483 Disabled & Alone/Life Services for the Handicapped

www.disabledandalone.org

A non-profit organization established to help families provide a secure future for their loved ones with a disability. Believes that no person should have to live his life in loneliness and isolation because of a disability.

10484 Discovery Health

www.health.discovery.com

A large website covering various health topics; such as male and female health, senior health, children's health, mental health, alternative medicine, nutrition, fitness, and more.

10485 Educational Equity Center at AED

www.edequity.org

EEC at AED is an outgrowth of Educational Equity Concepts, a national not-for-profit organization with a 22-year history of promoting educational excellence for all children.

10486 Federation for Children with Special Needs

www.fcsn.org

Provides information, support, and assistance to parents with children with disabilities, their professional partners, and their communities.

10487 Healing Well

www.healingwell.com

A social network and support community for patients, caregivers, and families coping with the daily struggles of diseases, disorders and chronic illness.

10488 Health Care For All

www.hcfa.org

HCFA seeks to create a consumer-centered health care system that provides comprehensive, affordable, accessible, culturally competent, high quality care and consumer education for everyone, especially the most vulnerable.

10489 Health Finder

www.healthfinder.gov

A government website that contains information and tools to help you and those you care about stay healthy.

10490 Health on the Net Foundation

www.hon.ch

Promotes and guides the deployment of useful and reliable online health information, and its appropriate and efficient use.

10491 Healthcentral.com

www.healthcentral.com

Empower millions of people to improve and take control of their health and well-being.

10492 Healthlink USA

www.healthlinkusa.com

Discussion forum for treatments, symptoms and causes of 700 health conditions, diseases and topics.

10493 Helios Health

www.helioshealth.com

Online resource for your health information. Detailed information about specific health topics, access to expert advice from our Medical Advisory Board, and up-to-date health news.

10494 Life Development Institute

www.lifedevelopmentinst.org

Serving men and women between the ages of 18-30 who have Asperger's Syndrome, ADHD, learning disabilities, anxiety, depression and other disorders

10495 MedicineNet

www.medicinenet.com

An online resource for consumers providing easy-to-read, authoritative medical and health information.

10496 Medscape

www.medscape.com

Medscape offers specialists, primary care physicians, and other health professionals the Web's most robust and integrated medical information and educational tools.

10497 Medtronic

www.medtronic.com

Medtronic is changing the face of chronic disease. By working closely with physicians around the world, they create therapies to help patients do things they never thought were possible.

10498 National Clearinghouse of Rehabilitation Training Materials

www.ncrtm.org

The mission of the NCRTM is to advocate for the advancement of best practice in rehabilitation counseling through the development, collection, dissemination, and utilization of professional knowledge, information and skill.

10499 National Council on Disability

www.ncd.gov

The National Council on Disability is an independent federal agency that works with the President and Congress to increase the inclusion, independence and empowerment of Americans with disabilities.

10500 National Organization for Rare Disorders (NORD)

www.rarediseases.org

Serves as a clearinghouse for information about rare disorders and brings together families with similar disorders for mutual support; fosters communication among rare disease voluntary agencies, Government agencies, industry, scientific researchers, academic institutions, and concerned individuals; and encourages and promotes research and education on rare disorders and orphan drugs.

10501 Office of Special Education and Rehabilitative Services

www2.ed.gov/osers

The Office of Special Education and Rehabilitative Servics (OSERS) is committed to improving the results and outcomes for people with disabilities of all ages.

10502 WebMD

www.webmd.com

General information, including articles.

10503 World Institute on Disability

www.wid.org

A public policy center that is run by persons with disabilities. Conducts research, public education, and advocacy campaigns.

National Agencies & Associations

10504 A Kid Again
777-G Dearborn Park Lane
Columbus, OH 43085

614-797-9500
800-543-9735
Fax: 614-797-9600
e-mail: customerservice@akidagain.org
www.akidagain.org

Enriches the lives of children with life threatening illnesses and their families by providing year round fun-filled group activities and destination events by fostering joy, laughter, normalcy and supportive networking opportunities. Includes regional chapters.
Jeffrey Damron, CFRE, CEO
Kathy Derr, Director of Programs and Volunteers

10505 A Wish with Wings, Inc.
3817 Alamo Ave
Fort Worth, TX 76107

817-469-9474
Fax: 817-275-6005
e-mail: wish@awishwithwings.org
www.awishwithwings.org

Grants the wishes of Texas children with life-threatening diseases.
Pat Skaggs, Founder
Judy Youngs, Executive Director

10506 BASE Camp Children's Cancer Foundation
140 N Orlando Avenue
Winter Park, FL 32789-3679

407-673-5060
Fax: 407-673-5095
e-mail: email@basecamp.org
www.basecamp.org

Supports children and their families who are facing the challenge of living with cancer or other life-threatening hematological illnesses. Offers year round programs, monthly overnight camps, support groups, and weekly events.
Terri Jones, President/Founder
Cindy Whitaker, Parent & Program Coordinator

10507 Believe In Tomorrow Children's Foundation
6601 Frederick Road
Baltimore, MD 21228

410-744-1984
800-933-5470
Fax: 410-744-1984
e-mail: info@believeintomorrow.org
www.believeintomorrow.org

Formerly Grant-A-Wish Foundation, this Foundation provides exceptional hospital and retreat housing services to critically ill children and their families. The Foundation also believes that keeping families together during a child's medical crisis, and that the gentle caring environment is crucial.
Brian R Morrison, Founder
Richard E McCready, Chairman

10508 Camp Good Days
1332 Pittsford-Mendon Road
Mendon, NY 14506

585-624-5555
800-785-2135
Fax: 585-624-5799
www.campgooddays.org

A non-profit organization that provides a camping experience and more for children and adults facing the toughest challenges of life. Accepts the wishes of terminal ill children through age eighteen.
Gary Mervis, Founder/Chairman
Wendy Bleier-Mervis, Executive Director

10509 Children's Wish Foundation International
8615 Roswell Road
Atlanta, GA 30350-7526

770-393-9474
800-323-9474
Fax: 770-393-0683
e-mail: arthurs@childrenswish.org
www.childrenswish.org

Committed to bringing joy and happiness to seriously ill children throughout the world and this dedication has created special experiences for children around the globe. Our commitment is also developing hospital enrichment programs.
Linda Dozoretz, Executive Director
Jacque Niles, Director of Program Services

10510 Cure Our Children Foundation
711 S Carson Street
Carson City, NV 89701

310-355-6046
Fax: 310-454-9592
e-mail: barry@cureourchildren.org
www.cureourchildren.org

Support medical approaches to treatment of Ewings Sarcoma. Alternate and complimentary treatment information is provided only for use in conjunction with traditional approaches.
Barry Sugarman, President

10511 Dream Come True
Lehigh Valley, PA 18002

610-865-3475
Fax: 610-865-4710
e-mail: RVasko@aol.com
www.dreamcometrue.org

Seeks to fulfill the dreams of children ages 4 - 17 who are seriously, chronically and terminally ill and whom live in the Lehigh Valley area. Includes regional offices.
Rayann Vasko, Director
Jeane Hockenbury, President

10512 Dream Factory, Inc.
National Headquarters
120 W Broadway
Louisville, KY 40202

502-561-3001
800-456-7556
Fax: 502-561-3004
e-mail: dfinfo@dreamfactoryinc.org
www.dreamfactoryinc.org

Grants wishes to children and young adults ages 3 - 18 with a critical or chronic illness.
Janice Harris, President
Mark Whitworth, Vice President

10513 Dream Foundation
1528 Chapala Street
Santa Barbara, CA 93101

805-564-2131
Fax: 805-564-7002
www.dreamfoundation.org

Enhances the quality of life for individuals and families battling terminal illnesses ages 18 and over.
Thomas Rollerson, Founder/President
Carol Brown, Chief Operating Officer

10514 Fairygodmother Foundation
550 W Webster Avenue
Chicago, IL 60614

773-388-1160
Fax: 773-883-3656
e-mail: info@fairygodmother.org
www.fairygodmother.org

Our wish granting program brings joy to the lives of adults (18 and older) and loved ones in their time of greatest need by turning dreams into reality. In the process of fulfilling wishes, we create an opportunity for peace, closure and a sense of belonging.
Lena Clement, Program Director

10515 Friends of Karen
118 Titicus Road
North Salem, NY 10560

914-277-4547
e-mail: info@friendsofkaren.org
www.friendsofkaren.org

Provides financial, emotional and advocacy support to children with life-threatening illnesses and their families.
Judith Factor, Executive Director
Nancy Mariano, Regional Director

10516 Give Kids the World Village
210 S Bass Road
Kissimmee, FL 34746

407-396-1114
800-995-KIDS
Fax: 407-396-1207
e-mail: dream@gktw.org
www.gktw.org

A 70-acre non-profit resort in Central Florida that creates magical memories for children with life-threatening illnesses and their families. GKTW provides accommodations at its whimsical resort, donated attractions, tickets, meals and more for a week-long stay.
Pamela Landwirth, President
Tabrei Scott, VP

10517 High Hopes Foundation of New Hampshire, Inc.
301 Daniel Webster Highway
Merrimack, NH 03054

603-429-1010
800-639-6804
Fax: 603-429-0037
e-mail: info@highhopesnh.net
highhopesfoundation.org

Grants wishes for severely and chronically ill children and young adults ages 3-18 who live in New Hampshire.
Jacque Yinger, Founder
Rachel Camer McMeen, Director

10518 Hopes & Dreams Foundation, Inc.
517 Cedarbrook Road   215-264-2859
Southampton, PA 18966 e-mail: info@hopesanddreamsfoundation.org
www.hopesanddreamsfoundation.org
For children and young adults with disabilities such as down syndrome and other specific challenges. Helps to promote education and community involvement through social activities.
Vick Franklin, President

10519 Kidd's Kids
220 E Las Colinas Boulevard   972-432-8595
Irving, TX 75039   866-541-5437
Fax: 214-853-5212
e-mail: derrick@kiddlive.com
www.kiddskids.com
Founded by nationally syndicated morning show personality Kidd Kraddick. Provides chronically ill and/or physically challenged children between the ages of 5 to 12 with an unforgettable adventure.
Toby Wilson, President
Dr. Kevin Wylie, Vice President

10520 Kids Incorporated
9300 Old Keene Mill Road   703-455-5437
Burke, VA 22015-4277   Fax: 703-440-9208
www.jcambellinc.com
Grants wishes to gravely ill children 16 years and younger. Children older than 16 are sometimes eligible depending on child's situation and the availability of resources.
John Campbell, President

10521 Kids Wish Network
4060 Louis Avenue   727-937-3600
Holiday, FL 34691   888-918-9004
Fax: 727-937-3688
e-mail: info@kidswishnetwork.org
www.kidswishnetwork.org
A nationally recognized charitable organization dedicated to infusing hope creating happy memories and improving the quality of life for children. The Network also fulfills the wishes of children ages 3 to 18 with life threatening medical conditions.
Karen Pelle, President
Andy Gottlieb, Treasurer

10522 Magic Moments
2112 11th Ave S   205-638-9372
Birmingham, AL 35205   Fax: 205-939-6717
e-mail: info@magicmoments.org
www.magicmoments.org
Grants wishes to children 4 to 19 living or being treated in Alabama who have chronic life-threatening diseases or who have severe trauma (burn, spinal cord or head trauma).
Joyce T. Spielberger, Executive Director
Susan J. Driggers, Director of Development

10523 Make-A-Wish Foundation of America
4742 N. 24th Street   602-279-9474
Phoenix, AZ 85016-4862   800-722-9474
Fax: 602-279-0855
e-mail: mawfa@wish.org
www.wish.org
A national organization that grants wishes for children with terminally or life threatening diseases and who are 18 years of age or younger. Includes regional chapters.
David Williams, President/CEO

10524 Marty Lyons Foundation, Inc.
326 W 48th Street   212-977-9474
New York, NY 10036   Fax: 212-977-1752
e-mail: mac@martylyonsfoundation.org
www.martylyonsfoundation.org
A national organization that grants wishes of children between the ages of three and seventeen who have life-threatening diseases or terminal illnesses. Those interested can submit applications for their wish fulfillment.
Marty Lyons, Chairman
Richard A. Miller, President

10525 New Hope for Kids Wish Program
205 E. SR 436   407-331-3059
Fern Park, FL 32730   Fax: 407-331-3063
e-mail: information@newhopeforkids.org
www.newhopeforkids.org
Grants wishes to children ages 3-18 who have been diagnosed with a life-threatening illness.
Dave Joswick, Executive Director
Dana Duffie, Office Manager

10526 Rainbow Connection
621 W University   248-601-9474
Rochester, MI 48307   877-649-4743
Fax: 248-601-0086
e-mail: info@rainbowconnection.org
www.rainbowwishconnection.org
Make the special wishes of children with life-threatening or terminal illnesses come true.
L. Brooks Patterson, Founder
Mary Grace McCarter, Executive Director

10527 Special Wish Foundation
1250 Memory Lane   614-258-3186
Columbus, OH 43209   800-486-9474
Fax: 614-258-3518
e-mail: info@spwish.org
www.spwish.org
A Special Wish Foundation Inc. is a non-profit charitable organization dedicated to granting the wishes of children under the age of 21 who have been diagnosed with a life-threatening disorder.
Laura Marchetta, Contact/Chicago Chapter
Patti Piening, Contact/Cincinnati

10528 Starlight Foundation
2049 Century Park E   310-479-1212
Los Angeles, CA 90067-1035   800-274-7827
e-mail: info@starlight.org
www.starlight.org
A non-profit organization dedicated to brightening the lives of seriously ill children and their families.
Jacqueline Hart-Ibrahim, CEO
Dvorah Waldman, VP Global Brand & Alliances

10529 Sunshine Foundation National Headquarters
1041 Mill Creek Drive   215-396-4770
Feasterville, PA 19053   Fax: 215-396-4774
e-mail: philly@sunshinefoundation.org
www.sunshinefoundation.org
Answers the dreams of seriously ill physically challenged and abused children aged three to eighteen whose families cannot fulfill their requests due to financial strain that the child's illness may cause.
Kate Sample, President
Pamela Vasserman, Director of Development

10530 Vision Foundation
8901 Strafford Circle   865-357-4603
Knoxville, TN 37923-1567   Fax: 865-690-9322
e-mail: gordon@visionfoundation.net
www.visionfoundation.net
Offers counseling support groups seminars and transportation for the blind providing 600 members.
Gordon Adams, Executive Director/President
Hank Brink, Vice President

10531 Wish Upon A Star
Visalia, CA 93278   559-733-7753
800-821-6805
Fax: 559-733-0962
e-mail: info@wishuponastar.org
www.wishuponastar.org
A non-profit law enforcement effort designed to grant the wishes of children afflicted with high-risk and life threatening illnesses.
Wally Nelson, President
Carmen Perez, Executive Director

10532 Wishing Star Foundation
139 S Sherman
Spokane, WA 99202
509-744-3411
Fax: 509-744-3414
e-mail: paulan@wishingstar.org
www.wishingstar.org

Grants wishes to children with life threatening illnesses. Ages 3-21 in Eastern Washington and all of Idaho.
Paula Nordgaarden, M.Ed. MSW, Executive Director
Sarah Carpenter, Program Director

10533 Wishing Well Foundation USA, Inc.
3000 W Esplanade Avenue
Metairie, LA 70002
504-841-0001
888-663-9474
e-mail: wellfoundation@bellsouth.net
www.wishingwellusa.org/home0.aspx

To bring joy to children with life threatening illnesses by providing them with their fondest wish in life.
Elwin Lebeau, President

Foundations

10534 Angelwish, Inc.
Rutherford, NJ 07070
201-672-0722
Fax: 201-672-0733
e-mail: info@angelwish.org
www.angelwish.org

Provides the public with an easy way to grant wishes to the millions of children that are living with HIV/AIDS around the world. Infected or affected by the disease, their opportunities for a normal childhood are virtually impossible. By harnessing the power of the Internet, Angelwish helps donors add a ray of hope to their lives.
Shimmy Mehta, Founder/CEO
Tom Fuller, Director

10535 Chef David's Kids
1100 E Oakland Park Boulevard
Fort Lauderdale, FL 33334
954-594-1024
e-mail: chefdavidmitchell@gmail.com
www.chefdavidskids.com

Helps children afflicted with any form of terminal illness such as cancer, leukemia, and pediatric HIV. Also helps neglected and abused children.
Chef David Mitchell, Founder/Director of Operations
Laurie Amber, National Hospital Events Director

10536 Children's Wish Foundation of Canada
1101 Kingston Rd
Pickering, ON L1V 1-7J7
905-427-5353
800-267-9474
Fax: 905-427-0536
e-mail: on@childrenswish.ca
www.childrenswish.ca

Works with the community to provide children living with high risk life threatening illnesses the opportunity to realize their most heartfelt wish.
Chris Kotsopoulos, Director
Jeannette Wakelin, Chair

10537 Dreams Come True
6803 Southpoint Parkway
Jacksonville, FL 32216
904-296-3030
Fax: 904-296-4244
www.dreamscometrue.org

Grants the dreams of children with life-threatening illnesses.
Jeffrey Conn, President
Eddie Allen, Managing Director

10538 Dreams for Seniors Charity Inc
512 Court Street
Pekin, IL 61554
309-353-7300
Fax: 309-353-7311
e-mail: info@dreamsforseniorscharity.org
www.dreamsforseniorscharity.org

Dreams for Seniors Charity (Dreams for Seniors) is a 501(c)(3) non-profit organization focused on celebrating seniors, granting their wishes and making dreams come true.
Debbie Davison, President/Founder

10539 Jason's Dreams for Kids Foundation, Inc.
20 Monmouth Street
Red Bank, NJ 07701
732-758-0060
Fax: 732-758-0070
e-mail: jasonsdreams@comcast.net
www.jasonsdreamsforkids.com

Devoted to granting wishes to children diagnosed with life-threatening illnesses. Holds a variety of fundraising events to meet the cost of fulfilling these childrens' wishes.

10540 Little Star Foundation
256 Rancho Milagro Way
Hesperus, CO 81326
800-543-6565
e-mail: info@littlestar.org
www.littlestar.org

Provides lifetime opportunities for children with cancer to enhance the quality of their lives.
Andrea Jaeger, Co-Founder & President

10541 Starlight Children's Foundation
2049 Century Park E
Los Angeles, CA 90067
310-479-1212
e-mail: info@starlight.org
www.starlight.org

Helps seriously ill children and their families cope with their pain, fear and isolation through entertainment, education and family activities.
Jacqueline Hart-Ibrahim, CEO
Dvorah Waldman, VP Global Brand & Alliances

10542 Sunshine Dreams for Kids
300 Wellington St
London, Ontario, N6B 2-5A9
519-642-0990
800-461-7935
Fax: 519-642-1201
e-mail: info@sunshine.ca
www.sunshine.ca

Grants dreams to children who are between the ages of 3 and 19 who are challenged by severe physical disabilities or life threatening illnesses.
Patrick DeMeester, MBA, President
Adam Jean, Treasurer

10543 United Special Sportsman Alliance
7864 Shotwell Lane
Pittsville, WI 54466
715-884-2256
800-518-8019
Fax: 715-884-7388
www.childswish.com

A dream wish granting charity that specializes in sending critically ill and disabled youth on the outdoor adventure of their dreams.
Brigid O'Donoghue, CEO/Founder
Ron Johnson, President

National Agencies & Associations

10544 Children's Hospice International
1101 King Street   703-684-0330
Alexandria, VA 22314   800-24C-HILD
e-mail: info@chionline.org
www.chionline.org
This organization was founded to provide a network of support and care for children with life threatening conditions and their families. The hospice is a team effort which provides medical, psychological, social and spiritual expertise in the US and abroad.
Ann Armstrong-Dailey, Founding Director/CEO
Rebecca Brant, Director

10545 Childrens Hospice International
1101 King Street   703-684-0330
Alexandria, VA 22314   800-242-4453
Fax: 703-684-0226
e-mail: info@chionline.org
www.chionline.org
To ensure medical, psychological, social and spiritual support to all children with like-threatening conditions and their families by providing a network of resources and care.
Ann Armstrong Dailey, Founding Director/CEO
Richard Larkin, Secretary/Treasurer

10546 Compassionate Friends
900 Jorie Blvd   630-990-0010
Oak Brook, IL 60523-3696   877-969-0010
Fax: 630-990-0246
e-mail: nationaloffice@compassionatefriends.org
www.compassionatefriends.org
A national organization that gives support to people who have experienced the death of a child. Offers monthly support meetings to get through the difficult times and learn how to cope.
Patricia Loder, Executive Director
Terry Novy, Chapter Services Coordinator

10547 HOSPICELINK Hospice Education Institute
Hospice Education Institute
3 Unity Square   207-255-8800
Machiasport, ME 04655-0098   800-331-1620
Fax: 207-255-8008
e-mail: info@hospiceworld.org
www.hospiceworld.org
Provides educational and informational services to health professionals and the public on subjects such as hospice care, death and dying and bereavement counseling.

10548 Helping Other Parents in Normal Grief
Underwood Memorial Hospital
509 N Broad Street
Woodbury, NJ 08096   856-845-0100
www.umhospital.org
Offers support to newly bereaved parents through trained parents who have suffered a similar loss and resolved their grief.
Eileen K. Cardile, RN, MS, CNA, President/CEO
John Graham, FACHE, Executive Vice President/COO

10549 National Association for Home Care and Hospice
228 7th Street SE   202-547-7424
Washington, DC 20003-4306   Fax: 202-547-3540
e-mail: hospice@nahc.org
www.nahc.org
Promotes the concepts of hospice, a philosophy of health care which is expressed through the provision of a variety of medical and nonmedical services to terminally ill patients and their families.
Val J. Halamandaris, President
Andrea Devoti, Chair

10550 National Hospice & Palliative Care Organization
1731 King Street   703-837-1500
Alexandria, VA 22314   800-646-6460
Fax: 703-837-1233
e-mail: nhpco_info@nhpco.org
www.nhpco.org
The nation's only advocate for terminally ill patients and their families. Founded in 1978, the NHPCO is the only organization devoted to hospice in the United States. Support is included from state hospice organizations, patients, families, communities, provider program members and professional/volunteer members. Represents hospice care interests to Congress, regulatory agencies, courts, voluntary organizations and the public.
J. Donald Schumacher, PsyD, President/CEO
Galen Miller, PhD, Executive Vice President

10551 National Hospice & Palliative Care Organiz ation
1731 King Street   703-837-1500
Alexandria, VA 22314   800-646-6460
Fax: 703-837-1233
e-mail: nhpco_info@nhpco.org
www.nhpco.org
The nation's only advocate for terminally ill patients and their families. Founded in 1978, the NHPCO is the only organization devoted to hospice in the United States. Support is included from state hospice organizations, patients, families and communities.
J. Donald Schumacher, President/CEO
Galen Miller, Executive Vice President

10552 National Institute for Jewish Hospice
732 University Street   516-791-9888
North Woodmere, NY 11581   800-446-4448
Fax: 516-791-6999
e-mail: mlamm@nijh.org
www.nijh.org
Serves as a resource center that seeks to help terminal patients and their families deal with their grief by providing information on traditional Jewish views on death, dying and managing the loss of a loved one.
Shirley Lamm, Executive Director
Maurice Lamm, Founder/President

10553 Share Pregnancy and Infant Loss Support, Inc.
The National Share Office
402 Jackson Street   636-947-6164
St. Charles, MO 63301   800-821-6819
Fax: 636-947-7486
e-mail: info@nationalshare.org
www.nationalshare.org
Serving those whose lives have been touched by the tragic death of a baby through pregnancy loss, stillbirth or the first few months of life.
Cathie Lammert, Executive Director
Rose Carlson, Program Director

10554 Wrap Myself in a Rainbow Compassion Books
Compassion Books
7036 State Highway 80 S   828-675-5909
Burnsville, NC 28714-7569   800-970-4220
Fax: 828-675-9687
e-mail: bruce@compassionbooks.com
www.compassionbooks.com
This is a collection of poignant songs and sensitive guided images that validates and transforms loss with hope. Side I is guided meditation Side II delivers powerful performances of Over The Rainbow, Rainbow Connection and Bring Rainbows to Children.
Audio Cassette
Bruce Greene, Director
Karen Walker, Staff

Support Groups & Hotlines

10555 Bereavement Group for Children
Corstone Center
250 Camino Alto   415-338-6161
Mill Valley, CA 94941-2535   Fax: 415-338-6165
e-mail: info@corstone.org
www.corstone.org
The CorStone Center for Personal Resilience (CPR) develops and implements resilience-based interventions and research initiatives to improve the health, education, and self-sufficiency of marginalized adults and youth around the world.
Steve Leventhal, Executive Director
Brenda Rivas-Camarena, Program Coordinator

10556 Grief & Loss Support Group
First Love Outreach Ministries

Milwaukee, WI 53206

414-263-1323
Fax: 414-263-1148
e-mail: zelodius@aol.com
www.firstlovelifecoaching.com

Pr Zelodius Morton, CEO

10557 National Hospice Helpline
1731 King Street
Alexandria, VA 22314

703-837-1500
800-646-6460
Fax: 703-837-1233
e-mail: nhpco_info@nhpco.org
www.nhpco.org

Offers more information on hospice in general and offers referrals to a hospice program in your area.
J. Donald Schumacher, President & CEO
Galen Miller, Executive VP

10558 Rainbows for All God's Children
1360 Hamilton Parkway
Itasca, IL 60143

847-952-1770
800-266-3206
Fax: 847-952-1774
e-mail: info@rainbows.org
www.rainbows.org

A support program for children who have suffered a significant loss in their lives due to death, divorce or any other painful transition.
Bob Thomas, Executive Director
Laurie Olbrisch, Executive VP

Books

10559 A Good Death: Conversations with East Londoners
Lesley Cullen and Michael Young, author

Routledge
270 Madison Avenue
New York, NY 10016

212-216-7800
800-634-7064
Fax: 212-563-2269
e-mail: orders@taylorandfrancis.com
www.routledge.com

Based on a survey in East London and provides a wide range of fascinating and helpful insights into all aspects of experiencing death and surviving grief. The voices in the book are those of people who have managed to cope despite being under the shadow of impending death. Their experience could be a comfort to anybody in a similar situation. A Good Death is intended for people who are dying, and for student doctors, nurses, and social workers.
272 pages
ISBN: 0-415137-97-3

10560 Anatomy of Bereavement
Beverly Raphael, author

Rowman & Littlefield Publishers, Inc.
15200 NBN Way
Blue Ridge Summit, PA 17214

717-794-3800
800-462-6420
Fax: 717-794-3803
e-mail: orders@rowman.com
customercare@rowman.com

In this comprehensive book, Dr. Raphael describes all the stages of mourning and healing.
454 pages Softcover
ISBN: 1-568212-70-4

10561 Bereaved Children: A Support Guide for for Parents And Professionals
Earl A. Grollman, author

Beacon Press
25 Beacon Street
Boston, MA 02108-2824

617-742-2110
Fax: 617-723-3097
www.beacon.org

Comprehensive guide that helps children and teens cope with the loss of a loved one.
256 pages
ISBN: 0-807023-07-5

10562 Bereaved Parent
Harriet Sarnoff Schiff, author

Penguin USA

375 Hudson Street
New York, NY 10014

212-366-2372
800-847-5515
Fax: 212-366-2933
e-mail: insidesales@us.penguingroup.com
www.penguingroup.com

Supportive advice for bereaved parents and professionals who work with them.
146 pages
ISBN: 0-140050-43-4

10563 Concerning Death: A Practical Guide for the Living
Earl A. Grollman, author

Beacon Press
25 Beacon Street
Boston, MA 02108-2824

617-742-2110
Fax: 617-723-3097
www.beacon.org

A guide for people to learn how to cope with death and dying, and the many decisions involved in the process.
265 pages
ISBN: 0-807027-65-0

10564 Conversations At Midnight
William Morrow & Company/Order Department
39 Plymouth Street
Fairfield, NJ 07004-1633

973-227-7200
800-821-1513

Herbert Kramer is dying of cancer. For him, as for everyone someday, death is now an unavoidable companion. This book tells how Herb learns to acknowledge this presence and come to terms with human mortality. This book is a powerful way to look at death and to deal with losing a loved one.
256 pages Hardcover
ISBN: 0-688120-84-9

10565 Death and the Quest for Meaning
Stephen Strack & Herman Feifel, author

Rowman & Littlefield Publishers, Inc.
4501 Forbes Blvd., Suite 200
Lanham, MD 20706

800-462-6420
www.rowmanlittlefield.com

This work covers all aspects of the study of death and dying and the care of the bereaved.
Hardcover
ISBN: 0-765700-14-x

10566 Death: The Final Stage of Growth
Elisabeth Kubler-Ross, author

Simon & Schuster
1230 Avenue of the Americas
New York, NY 10020

212-698-7000
www.simonandschuster.com

This books shows readers how to come to terms with death as a part of human development, and how death can provide us with a key meaning of human existence.
208 pages

10567 Difference in the Family
Penguin Putnam
PO Box 999
Bergenfield, NJ 07621-0903

201-387-0600
800-526-0275
Fax: 800-227-9604

A frank chronicle of the grief, rage and guilt everyone in a family suffers after a death, and the adjustments each make to cope.
Helen Featherstone, Editor

10568 Dying and Disabled Children
Haworth Press
10 Alice Street
Binghamton, NY 13904-1580

607-722-5857
800-429-6784
Fax: 607-722-0012
www.haworthpress.com

In this sensitive and compassionate look at terminally ill and disabled children, professionals from the medical community examine the stresses faced by their parents and siblings. They address crucial element of communication in dealing with a child's serious illness. Ethical decision making, learning to recognize the child's suffering, and talking to children about death are honestly and clearly discussed.
153 pages Hardcover
ISBN: 0-866567-59-0

10569 For Those Who Live: Helping Children Cope with Death of a Brother or Sister
Centering Corporation
7230 Maple Street
Omaha, NE 68134
402-553-1200
866-218-0101
Fax: 402-553-0507
e-mail: danni@centeringcorp.com
www.centering.org
Deals with the grieving family as a whole and offers references for further help.
122 pages
Kathy LaTour, Editor

10570 Grief, Dying and Death: Clinical Intervention for Caregivers
Research Press
2612 N Mattis Avenue
Champaign, IL 61822-1053
217-352-3273
800-519-2707
Fax: 217-352-1221
e-mail: rp@researchpress.com
www.researchpress.com
In this comprehensive manual, the author provides both the theoretical background and the practical treatment interventions necessary for working with those who are bereaved or dying. Important topics such as anticipatory grief, postdeath mourning and the stress of grief are described in detail. Grief reactions, both normal and abnormal, as well as their causes are analyzed. Special attention is given to grief caused by death of a child or spouse, death by suicide, and children's grief.
488 pages Softcover
ISBN: 0-878222-32-4

10571 Helper's Journey
Dr. Dale G. Larson, author
Research Press
Dept. 11W
Champaign, IL 61826
217-352-3273
800-519-2707
Fax: 217-352-1221
e-mail: orders@researchpress.com
www.researchpress.com
This groundbreaking work, written for both professional and volunteer caregivers, provides exercises, activities and specific strategies for more successful caregiving, increased personal growth and effective stress management. In this thoughtfully written book, Dr. Larson explores the theory and practice of helping. He includes numerous case examples and verbatim disclosures of fellow caregivers that powerfully convey the joys and sorrows of the helpers journey.
292 pages Softcover
ISBN: 0-878223-44-4

10572 On Death & Dying
Dr. Elizabeth Kubler-Ross, author
MacMillan Publishing Company
175 Fifth Avenue
New York, NY 10010
646-307-5151
e-mail: customerservice@mpsvirginia.com
www.macmillan.com
Offers a new perspective on the terminally ill by refocusing on the patient as a human being and teacher, in hopes of learning from him or her about the final stages of life.
277 pages Paperback

10573 On Death and Dying
MacMillan Publishing Company
175 Fifth Avenue
New York, NY 10010
646-307-5151
A wonderful book offering information on how to deal and cope with death and dying.
Paperback

10574 Recovery from Bereavement
Rowman & Littlefield Publishers, Inc.
4501 Forbes Blvd.
Lanham, MD 20706
717-794-3800
800-462-6420
Fax: 717-794-3803
e-mail: orders@rowman.com
www.rowmanlittlefield.com

Outstanding authorities on loss and bereavement discuss the factors that play a role in successful recovery.
344 pages Softcover
ISBN: 1-568213-61-1

10575 Talking About Death - A Dialog Between Parent and Child
Earl A. Grollman, author
Beacon Press
25 Beacon Street
Boston, MA 02108-2824
617-742-2110
Fax: 617-723-3097
e-mail: bp_information@beacon.org
www.beacon.org
A compassionate guide for children and adults. Also includes listings of resources and organizations.
128 pages

10576 Treatment of Complicated Mourning
Dr. Therese A. Rando, author
Research Press
Dept. 11W
Champaign, IL 61826
217-352-3273
800-519-2707
Fax: 217-352-1221
e-mail: orders@researchpress.com
www.researchpress.com
This is the first book to focus specifically on complicated mourning, often referred to as pathological, unresolved, or abnormal grief. It provides caregivers with practical therapeutic strategies with and specific interventions that are necessary when traditional grief counseling is insufficient. The author provides critically important information on the prediction, identification, assessment, classification and treatment of complicated mourning.
768 pages Hardcover
ISBN: 0-878223-29-0

10577 What Helped Me When My Loved One Died
Beacon Press
25 Beacon Street
Boston, MA 02108-2824
617-742-2110
Fax: 617-723-3097
www.beacon.org

Children's Books

10578 Aarvy Aardvark Finds Hope
Donna O'Toole, author
Centering Corporation
7230 Maple Street
Omaha, NE 68134
402-553-1200
866-218-0101
www.centering.org
A best selling, illustrated, read-aloud story of the pain and sadness of loss and the hope of grief recovery.
80 pages Paperback
Janet Sieff, Executive Director

10579 Badger's Parting Gifts
Susan Varley, author
Compassion Books, Inc.
7036 State Highway 80 South
Burnsville, NC 28714-7569
828-675-5909
800-970-4220
Fax: 828-675-9687
e-mail: orders@compassionbooks.com
www.compassionbooks.com
A story of the death of old Badger. As the animals talk about Badger they remember the gift of skills and kindnesses he taught them.
23 pages Paperback
Bruce Greene, Director

10580 Compassion Books, Inc.
7036 State Highway 80 South
Burnsville, NC 28714-7569
828-675-5909
800-970-4220
Fax: 828-675-9687
e-mail: orders@compassionbooks.com
www.compassionbooks.com
Hand picked resources to help people through loss, grief and changes of all kinds. Carry over 400 books and videos on death and

dying, bereavement and change, comfort and healing, hope and much more.
Bruce Greene, VP

10581 Fire in My Heart: Ice in My Veins

Enid Samuel Traisman, author

Compassion Books, Inc.
7036 State Highway 80 South   828-675-5909
Burnsville, NC 28714-7569   800-970-4220
    Fax: 828-675-9687
e-mail: orders@compassionbooks.com
www.compassionbooks.com
A fill in scrapbook/journal to help teenagers experiencing a loss express feelings, sort out their thoughts and gather memories.
70 pages Paperback
Bruce Greene, Director

10582 Gentle Willow: A Story for Children About Dying

Joyce C. Mills, PhD, author

Magination Press (American Psychological Assoc.)
750 First Street NE   202-336-5500
Washington, DC 20002-4242   800-374-2721
    TDD: 202-336-6123
e-mail: order@apa.org
www.apa.org
This book is written for children who may not survive their own illness or for children who know them. This tender and touching tale helps address feelings of disbelief, anger, and sadness, along with love and compassion.
2003 32 pages Hardcover
ISBN: 1-591470-71-7
Melba Vasquez, PhD, President

10583 Great Change
Compassion Books, Inc.
7036 State Highway 80 S   828-675-5909
Burnsville, NC 28714-7569   800-970-4220
    Fax: 828-675-9687
e-mail: orders@compassionbooks.com
www.compassionbooks.com
In this deeply moving Native American story, grandmother uses nature to explain death, the great change, to a grieving granddaughter.
32 pages Hardcover
Bruce Greene, Director

10584 Let's Talk About When A Parent Dies
Rosen Publishing Group's PowerKids Press
29 E 21st Street   212-777-3017
New York, NY 10010   800-237-9932
    Fax: 888-436-4643
e-mail: customerservice@rosenpub.com
www.rosenpublishing.com
This book guides children through the grieving process in a language they can understand. Recommended for grades K-4.

ISBN: 0-823923-09-6
Elizabeth Weitzman, Author

10585 Nana Upstairs and Nana Downstairs
Compassion Books
7036 State Highway 80 S   828-675-5909
Burnsville, NC 28714-7569   800-970-4220
    Fax: 828-675-9687
e-mail: heal2grow@aol.com
www.compassionbooks.com
This charming picture book recognizes that even after a family member dies the love connections continue in heart and home.
32 pages Paperback
Bruce Greene, Director

Magazines

10586 Compassion Books Catalog
Compassion Books

7036 State Highway 80 South   828-675-5909
Burnsville, NC 28714-7569   800-970-4220
    Fax: 828-675-9687
e-mail: orders@compassionbooks.com
www.compassionbooks.com
More than 400 books and videos to help with serious illness, death and dying, and losses of all kinds.
32 pages
Bruce Greene, VP

Pamphlets

10587 Approaching Grief

Richard Deitrick/Ann Armstrong Dailey, author

Children's Hospice International
1101 King Street   703-684-0330
Alexandria, VA 22314   800-242-4453
    e-mail: info@chionline.org
www.chionline.org
Delves into the different stages of grief, guilt, depression, fear and anger. Also tells how children approach grief and ways in which to help your children get past the sorrow.
Ann Armstrong-Dailey, Founding Director/CEO
Rebecca Brant, Director

10588 Pregnancy After a Loss
Abbott Northwestern Hospital Parent Education
800 E 28th Street-Chicago Avenue   612-863-4000
Minneapolis, MN 55407
This booklet is written by a group of parents that have experienced a pregnancy after a loss, sensitively written with suggestions for coping with the fears and anxieties of the new pregnancy.

10589 Pregnancy Heartbreak: Unfulfilled Promises
Abbott Northwestern Hospital Parent Education
800 E 28th Street-Chicago Avenue   612-863-4000
Minneapolis, MN 55407
This handbook is written for parents who had to face the reality of the diagnosis and birth of a baby with life-threatening conditions.

Audio & Video

10590 Encounters with Grief
Fanlight Productions
C/O Icarus Films   718-488-8642
Brooklyn, NY 11201   800-876-1710
    Fax: 718-488-8642
e-mail: info@fanlight.com
www.fanlight.com
A mother who lost her teenage son, a woman widowed in her sixties and a man whose wife died at fifty-two discuss the emotional upheaval that followed and their moving perspectives on the process of recovery.
1992 13 Minutes
ISBN: 1-572950-91-9

10591 Grave Words: Tools for Discussing End of Life Choices

Maren Monson, MD, author

Fanlight Productions
C/O Icarus Films   718-488-8900
Brooklyn, NY 11201   800-876-1710
    Fax: 718-488-8642
e-mail: info@fanlight.com
www.fanlight.com
Blends humor, music and insightful interviews to confront the issues that arise in discussions between physicians and healthcare providers and patients about end-of-life care decisions.
1996 25 Minutes
ISBN: 1-572952-24-5

10592 Pitch of Grief

Eric Strange, author

Fanlight Productions

C/O Icarus Films
Brooklyn, NY 11201

718-488-8900
Fax: 718-488-8642
e-mail: info@fanlight.com
www.fanlight.com

Explores the process of grieving through interviews with four bereaved men and women, and is helpful to not only the grieving person, but for others within the family who have faced the loss of a loved one.
1985 28 Minutes
ISBN: 1-572950-18-8

10593 There Was a Child
Fred Simon, author

Fanlight Productions
C/O Icarus Film
Brooklyn, NY 11201

718-488-8642
800-876-1710
Fax: 718-488-8642
e-mail: orders@fanlight.com
www.fanlight.com

Demonstrates the impact that losing a pregnancy, or the birth of a stillborn child, has had on three mothers and a father. Validates the emotions of parents who feel alone with their loss, while helping health care workers and families to give appropriate, meaningful support.
1991 32 Minutes
ISBN: 1-572950-48-X

10594 We Will Remember
Compassion Books, Inc.
7036 State Highway 80 South
Burnsville, NC 28714-7569

828-675-5909
800-970-4220
Fax: 828-675-9687
e-mail: orders@compassionbooks.com
www.compassionbooks.com

A video meditation that uses the beauty of natural photography, soothing music and gentle words to give permission and encouragement in using the memories of the past for healing in the present.
11 minutes
Bruce Greene, Director

10595 When the Bough Breaks
Fanlight Productions
4196 Washington Street
Boston, MA 02131-1731

617-469-4999
800-937-4113
Fax: 617-469-3379
e-mail: fanlight@fanlight.com
www.fanlight.com

Based on the real story of a patient who experienced a stillbirth, these ten vignettes dramatically recreate her interactions with health care providers during the final weeks of pregnancy. Study guide included.
1992 71 Minutes
ISBN: 1-572951-08-7

Web Sites

10596 Compassionate Friends

www.compassionatefriends.org
Gives support to people who have experienced the death of a child.

10597 Hospice Association of America

www.nahc.org
Promotes the concepts of hospice, a philosophy of health care which is expressed through the provision of a variety of medical and nonmedical services to terminally ill patients and their families.

10598 National Hospice & Palliative Care Organization

www.nhpco.org
The nation's only advocate for terminally ill patients and their families. Founded in 1978, the NHPCO is the only organization devoted to hospice in the United States. Support is included from state hospice organizations, patients, families, communities, provider program members and professional/volunteer members. Represents hospice care interests to Congress, regulatory agencies, courts, voluntary organizations and the public.

10599 Share Pregnancy and Infant Loss Support, Inc.

www.nationalshare.org
Offers studies, information, statistics, help and support to parents who have suffered the loss of a child.

B

D

E

H

J

K

Kansas City Support Group: National Ataxia Foundation, 1439

Kansas Department of Health & Environment Bureau of Family Health, 8620

Kansas Department of Health & Environment Epidemiology & Disease Prevention: HIV, 264

Kansas Industries for the Blind, 9303

Kansas Services for the Blind and Visually Impaired, 9613

Kansas State University: Terry C Johnson Center for Basic Cancer Research, 2208

Kansas University Medical Center: Cystic Fibrosis Center, 3003

Kansas/Missouri- Turner Syndrome Society, 9121

Kathy's Hats: A Story of Hope, 2361

Keep Quit, 8203

Keep it Simple, 8204

Keeping the Balance, 5753

Kellogg Cancer Care Center Evanston Hospital, 2199

Kemo Shark, 2362

Kendall Demonstration Elementary School Curriculum Guides, 4391

Kennedy Krieger Institute, 3465

Kennedy Krieger Institute - Down Syndrome, 3475

Kennedy-Krieger Institute, 10130

Kent County Health Department, 8634

Kent County Library for the Blind, 9502

Kent Waldrep National Paralysis Foundation Main Office, 7817

Kentucky Alliance for the Mentally Ill, 5949

Kentucky Association of the Deaf, 4207

Kentucky Cancer Program, 2210

Kentucky Chapter of the Myasthenia Gravis Foundation of America, 6579

Kentucky Hemophilia Foundation, 4839

Kentucky IMPACT, 6047

Kentucky Industries for the Blind, 9305

Kentucky Organ Donor Affiliates, 8959

Kentucky Talking Book Library, 9481

Kentucky University: Cystic Fibrosis Center, 3005

Keon Paschal Perry Sickle Cell Anemia Disease Awareness, 7469

Kernel Book Series, 9669

Ketogenic Diet: A Treatment for Epilepsy, 7352

Kettering-Scott Magnetic Resonance Laboratory, 8090

Key Elements of Dementia Care, 903

Keys for Networking: Kansas FFCMH, 5946

Keys to Parenting the Child with Autism, 1647

Keystone Blind Association, 9365

Kid, 5579

A Kid Again, 10504

Kid's 1st Cookbook: Delicious-Nutritious Treats to Make Yourself, 2363

Kid's Corner, 3388

Kid-Friendly Parenting with Deaf and Hard of Hearing Children, 4392

Kidd's Kids, 10519

Kidneeds, 5546

Kidney & Urology Foundation of America, 5504

Kidney Association of South Florida, 5473

Kidney Beginnings: A Patient's Guide to Li ving with Reduced Kidney Function, 5549

Kidney Cooking, 5550

Kidney Disease Institute, 5536

Kidney Disease: A Guide for Patients and Their Families, 5580

The Kidney Foundation of Canada, 5067

Kidney Transplant: A New Lease on Life, 5581

Kidneys for Kids, 5582

Kids Incorporated, 10520

Kids Wish Network, 10521

Kids and Alcohol: Get High on Life, 8321

Kids and Drugs: A Handbook for Parents & Professionals, 8453

Kids on the Block Arthritis Programs, 1144

Kids with Heart National Association for Children's Heart Disorders, 2839

Kidscope, 2063

Kindey Beginnings: The Magazine, 5557

King County Crisis Clinic, 384

King James Bible: Large Print, 9670

King Midas, 4668

King Midas Videotape, 4669

King Midas With Selected Sentences in ASL, 4523

Kiss the Candy Days Good-bye, 3373

Kits for Adults with Epilepsy, 7372

Knollwoodpark Hospital Sleep Disorders Cen, 7624

Knollwoodpark Hospital Sleep Disorders Center, 7623

Knotholes are for Seeing: Therapy Through Poetry, Prose & Other Writings, 9671

Know Your Brain, 4105

Knoxville Division: VA Central Iowa Health Care System, 9974

Kosair Childrens Cystic Fibrosis Center, 3006

Krannert Institute of Cardiology, 4746

Kuakini Parkinson Disease (PD) Information & Referral, 6901

L

LAC/USC Imaging Science Center, 3889

LAUNCH Department of Special Education, 10242

LD Alert Card, 8816

LD Awareness Packet, 8817

LD Child and the ADHD Child, 1511

LD: Diagnosis & Treatment, 8824

LD: Facts for Kids, 8825

LIAFLine Newsletter, 928

LINK, 1049

LINK Directory Information, 5097

LODAT: Brain Tumor Support Group, 1930

LRC for Students with Disabilities, 9552

LaRabida Children's Hospital: Developmental Disabilities & Delays, 3466

Label Reading and Shopping, 3408

Laboratory of Dermatology Research Memorial Sloane-Kettering Cancer Center, 7516

Laboure College Library, 9497

Lake County Public Library, 9473

Lancaster County Association for the Blind, 9366

Landon Center on Aging University of Kansas Medical Center, 81

Langley Porter Psychiatric Institute University of California, 6019

Language, Speech and Hearing Services in the Schools, 4571

Laparoscopy and Hysteroscopy, 5409

Laradon Services for Children and Adults w ith Developmental Disabilities, 6037

Large Print American Heritage Dictionary, 9672

Large Print Loan Library Catalog, 9806

Las Vegas Clark County Library District, 9526

Last in Line, 6097

Late Onset Community Newsletter, 8751

Late Onset Tay-Sachs Disease Medical Bibliography, 8743

Late Onset Tay-Sachs Fact Sheet, 8753

Late Stage Care, 941

Late-Deafened Adults: A Selected Annotated Bibliography, 4627

Latex Allergy, 1355

Laugh at Your Muscles, 3744

Laurel's Kitchen Caring: Recipes for Everyday Home Caregiving, 10412

Lawyers Concerned for Lawyers, 7992, 8567

Lead Line, 8346

Leaders Link, 1325

Leading Age, 24

Leading National Publications of and for Deaf People, 4628

Leading Self-Help Groups: Report on Workshop for Leaders of Groups, 2430

Learning Among Children with Spina Bifida, 7790

Learning Disabilities Association of America, 1495, 10243

Learning Disabilities and the Person with Spina Bifida, 7773

Learning Disabilities in Children with Hydrocephalus, 5098

Learning Disability Quarterly, 10450

Learning How, 10244

Learning Problems & the Child with TS, 8880

Learning to Communicate: The First Three Years Videotape, 4670

Learning to Fall: the Blessings of an Imperfect Life, 1044

Learning to Hear Again, 4393

Learning to Live Drug Free: A Curriculum Model for Prevention, 8205

Learning to Live Well with Diabetes, 3339

Learning to Live with Neuromuscular Desease: A Message to Parents, 6549

Learning to Play, 9807

Learning to See: American Sign Language as a Second Language, 4394

Learning to Sign in my Neighborhood, 4524

Learning to be Independent and Responsible, 1681

Least Restrictive Environment: The Paradox of Inclusion, 4395

Lee County Talking Books Library, 9441

Lee the Rabbit with Epilepsy, 7359

Legal Center for People with Disabilities, 10344

Legal Center for People with Disabilities and Older People, 10292

Legal Plans, 942

Legal Rights for the Deaf and Hard of Hearing, 4396

Legal Rights of Hearing-Impaired People, 4397

Legal and Ethical Aspects of Organ Transplantation, 8995

Legal and Financial Issues for Families, 4106

Legislative Handbook for Parents, 9673

Lehigh Valley Chapter of the American Association of Kidney Patients, 5515

Lehigh Valley Sickle Cell Support Group, 7470

Les Turner Amyotrophic Lateral Sclerosis Foundation, 1038

Les Turner Research Laboratory Northwestern University Medical School, 1026

Lessons in Laughter: The Autobiography of a Deaf Actor, 4398

Let Community Employment Be the Goal for Individuals with Autism, 1648

Let Me Hear Your Voice A Family's Triumph Over Autism, 1649

Let's Be Friends, 4671

Let's Breathe Sarcoidosis Support Group, 7086

Let's Eat, 9808, 9846

Let's Learn About Deafness, 4399

Let's Solve the Smokeword Puzzle, 8454

Let's Talk, 8455

Let's Talk About Alcohol Abuse, 8206

Let's Talk About Depression, 6222

Let's Talk About Drug Abuse, 8322

Let's Talk About Having Asthma, 1313

Let's Talk About Having Lyme Disease, 8807

Let's Talk About When A Parent Dies, 10584

Let's Talk About When Someone You Love Has Alzheimer's Disease, 917

Let's Talk Facts About Childhood Disorders, 6151

Lethal Secrets: The Psychology of Donor Insemination, 5343

Letter to a Friend Whose Child is Newly Diagnosed with Cancer, 2431

Letter to a Woman Alcoholic, 8456

Letting Go of the Need to Control, 8457

Leukemia & Lymphoma Society Chapter: New York City, 2111

Leukemia & Lymphoma Society: Orange, Riverside, And San Bernadino Counties, 2037

Leukemia & Lymphoma Society: Suncoast Chapter, 2057

Leukemia & Lymphoma Society: Tennessee Chapter, 2143

Leukemia & Lymphoma Society: Westchester/ Hudson Valley Chapter, 2112

Leukemia Research Foundation, 2200

Leukemia and Lymophoma Society: National Capital Area Chapter, 2152

Leukemia and Lymphoma Society, 1999, 2495

Leukemia and Lymphoma Society Chapter: New York City, 2113

Leukemia and Lymphoma Society: Southern Florida Chapter, 2058

Leukemia and Lymphoma Society: Alabama Chapter, 2017

Leukemia and Lymphoma Society: Central Florida Chapter, 2059

Leukemia and Lymphoma Society: Central New York Chapter, 2114

Leukemia and Lymphoma Society: Central Ohio Chapter, 2123

M

O

S

X

Y

Z

Navajo Nation Office of Special Education & Rehabilitation Services (OSERS), 6036

Neurofibromatosis Association of Arizona, 6643

New Mexico Chapter of the Myasthenia Gravis Foundation of America, 6589

Northern Arizona Branch:Phoenix Area, 9029

Office of Chronic Disease Prevention and Nutrition Services, 6707

Office of Womens And Childrens Health: Alabama Department of Health, 8590

Phoenix Area Support Group: National Ataxi a Foundation, 1416

Phoenix Public Library: Special Needs Section, 9420

Phoenix VA Healthcare System, 9923

Prader-Willi Syndrome Arizona Association, 7014

Prader-Willi Syndrome Arizona Association: Phoenix Area, 7013

RESOLVE of Valley of the Sun, 5257

Ruth E Golding Clinical Pharmacokinetics Laboratory, 8104

Scleroderma Foundation: Arizona Chapter, 7175

Southern Arizona Brain Tumor Support Group, 1807

Southern Arizona Branch: Tucson Area, 9030

Southwest Association for Education in Biomedical Research, 2169

Spina Bifida Association of Arizona, 7720

St. Joseph's Hemophilia Center, 4919

Teratology OTIS, 1734

Tucson Interfaith HIV/AIDS Network (TIHAN), 241

Tucson Support Group: National Ataxia Foundation, 1417

United Cerebral Palsy of Central Arizona, 2575

United Cerebral Palsy of Southern Arizona, 2576

University of Arizona Cancer Center, 2170

Veterans Adm. Medical Center: Tucson Southern Arizona VA Health Care System, 9924

Arkansas

AARP Arkansas State Office: Little Rock, 31

Alzheimer's Arkansas Programs and Services, 660

Alzheimer's Association: Western Arkansas Chapter, 661

American Cancer Society: Arkansas, 2022

American Diabetes Association: Arkansas, 3112

American Lung Association of Arkansas, 5682

American Lung Association of Arkansas, 9031

Arkansas Association of the Deaf, 4201

Arkansas Chapter of the Myasthenia Gravis Foundation of America, 6570

Arkansas Cystic Fibrosis Center Arkansas Children's Hospital, 2977

Arkansas Department of Health AIDS Prevention Program, 242

Arkansas Department of Health: SIDS Information & Counseling Program, 8591

Arkansas FFCMH Jane Burgan, 5918

Arkansas Lighthouse for the Blind, 9271

Arkansas Regional Library for the Blind and Physically Handicapped, 9421

Arkansas Regional Organ Recovery Agency, 8943

Arthritis Foundation: Arkansas Chapter, 1082

Brain Injury Association of Arkansas, 3947

Brain Injury Association of Arkansas Helpl ine, 4010

Central Arkansas Veterans Healthcare Syste Eugene J. Towbin Healthcare Center, 9925

Disability Rights Center of Arkansas, 10289

Gulf War Veterans of Arkansas, 9926

Health Resource, 2023

Hemophilia Foundation of Arkansas, 4827

John L McClellan Memorial Veterans' Hospital Research Office, 4745

Juvenile Diabetes Research Foundation: Northwest Arkansas Branch, 3113

Library for the Blind and Handicapped, Southwest, 9422

Lions World Services for the Blind Lions Clubs International, 9221

Lupus Foundation of America: Arkansas Chapter, 5775

NAMI Arkansas, 5919

NNFF Arkansas Affilaite, 6644

National Federation of the Blind: Arkansas, 9272

National Kidney Foundation of Arkansas, 5459

National Multiple Sclerosis Society: Arkansas Chapter, 6340

Office of Alcohol and Drug Abuse Prevention, 8019

Prader-Willi Arkansas Association Prader-Willi Syndrome Association, 7015

RESOLVE Affiliate of Northwest Arkansas, 5258

Research and Training Center for Persons Who are Deaf or Hard of Hearing, 4245

United Cerebral Palsy of Central Arkansas, 2577

Veterans Adm. Medical Center: Fayetville, 9927

California

1-800-BRAILLE, 9614

AARP California State Office: Pasadena, 32

AARP California State Office: Sacramento, 33

AEGIS AIDS Education Global Information System, 371

AIDS Clinical Trials Unit CARES Clinic, 308

AIDS.ORG, 178

ALS Association Free Standing Support Groups, 1035

ALS Association: Bay Area Chapter, 982

ALS Association: Greater Los Angeles Chapter, 983

ALS Association: Greater Sacramento Chapter, 984

ALS Association: Greater San Diego CIO, 985

ALS Center at UCSF, 1022

ASTHMA Hotline, 593

Adopt-A-Special-Kid America, 5250

Adult Research Opportunities, 309

Advocates 4 Health: Tick-borne Disease Self-Help Group, 8796

Aids, Medicine and Miracles, 243

Alcohol Drug Treatment Referral, 8119

Alcohol Research Group Public Health Institute, 8077

Alta Bates Summit Medical Center, 6012

Alzheimer's Association San Diego/Imperial Chapter, 662

Alzheimer's Association: California Central Chapter: Ventura County Office, 663

Alzheimer's Association: Greater North Valley Chapter, 665

Alzheimer's Association: Greater Sacramento, 664

Alzheimer's Association: Los Angeles Chapter, 666

Alzheimer's Association: Monterey County Chapter, 667

Alzheimer's Association: North Bay Chapter, 668

Alzheimer's Association: Orange County Chapter, 669

Alzheimer's Association: Riverside/San Bernardino Counties Chapter, 670

Alzheimer's Association: San Francisco Bay Area Chapter, 671

Alzheimer's Association: Santa Barbara Central Coast Chapter, 672

Alzheimer's Association: Santa Cruz County Chapter, 673

Alzheimer's Disease Center: University of California, Davis, 846

American Academy of Ophthalmology, 9188

American Association of Gynecologic Laproscopists, 3654

American Cancer Society Santa Clara County / Silicon Valley / Central Coast Region, 2024

American Cancer Society: Central Los Angeles, 2025

American Cancer Society: East Bay/Metro Region, 2026

American Cancer Society: Fresno/Madera Counties, 2027

American Cancer Society: Inland Empire, 2028

American Cancer Society: Orange County, 2029

American Cancer Society: Sacramento County, 2030

American Cancer Society: San Diego County, 2031

American Cancer Society: San Francisco County, 2032

American Cancer Society: San Jose Prostate Cancer Support Group, 2286

American Cancer Society: Santa Maria Valley, 2033

American Cancer Society: Sonoma County, 2034

American Chronic Pain Association, 2506

American Chronic Pain Association, 2802

American Diabetes Association: California, 3114

American Liver Foundation Greater Los Angeles Chapter, 5607

American Liver Foundation Northern CA Chapter, 5608

American Liver Foundation San Diego Chapte r, 5609

American Lung Association of California, 5683

American Lung Association of California, 9032

Amyotrophic Lateral Sclerosis Toll Free Hotline, 1037

Arthritis Foundation: Northern California Chapter, 1083

Arthritis Foundation: San Diego Area Chapter, 1084

Arthritis Foundation: Southern California Chapter, 1085

Asian & Pacific Islander Wellness Center Community HIV/AIDS Services, 187

Asian and Pacific Island Wellness Center, 188

Association for the Cure of Cancer of the Prostate, 1985

Asthma and Allergy Foundation of America: Southern California Chapter, 570

Asthma and Allergy Foundation of America: Southern California Chapter, 1267

Autism Research Institute, 1552

Autism Society of California, 1562

Bay Area LE Foundation, 5776

Bay Area Turner Syndrome Society, 9110

Bees-Stealy Research Foundation, 4726

Bereavement Group for Children, 1808

Bereavement Group for Children, 10555

Blind Childrens Center, 9423

Braille Institute Desert Center, 9581

Braille Institute Library Services, 9424

Braille Institute Orange County Center, 9582

Braille Institute Santa Barbara Center Braille Institute of Los Angeles, 9583

Braille Institute Sight Center, 9584

Braille Institute Youth Center, 9585

Braille Institute of America Library, 9202

Brain Injury Association of California Hel pline, 4011

Brain Tumor Society, 1809

Brain Tumor Support Group: Duarte, 1810

Brain Tumor Support Group: Fresno, 1811

Brain Tumor Support Group: Fullerton, 1812

Brain Tumor Support Group: Newport Beach, 1813

Brain Tumor Support Group: Orange, 1814

Brain Tumor Support Group: Redding, 1815

Brain Tumor Support Group: Sacramento, 1816

Brain Tumor Support Group: San Diego, 1817

Brain Tumor Support Group: San Francisco, 1818

Brain Tumor Support Group: Santa Barbara, 1819

Brain Tumor Support Group: Stanford, 1820

Brain Tumor Support Group: Westlake Village, 1821

Brain Tumor/Pituitary Patient Support Group, 1822

Breast Cancer Action, 1987

Burnham Institute Cancer Center The Burnham Institute for Medical Resear, 2171

CCFA California: Greater Los Angeles Chapter, 2893

California Ambassador: National Ataxia Foundation, 1418

California Association of Persian Gulf Veterans, 9928

California Collaborative Treatment Group CCTG Data Center, 244

California Department of Health Services Office of Aids, 245

California Institute for Medical Research, 6893

California Lyme Disease Association, 8793

California SIDS Program, 8592

California State Library Braille and Talking Book Library, 9425

California Teratogen Information Service UC San Diego School of Medicine Dept of, 1728

California Transplant Donor Network, 8944

California Women's Commission on Alcohol and Drug Dependencies, 8020

Cancer Control Society and Cancer Book House, 2035

Cancer Federation, 2162

Cancer Prevention Institute of California, 2172

Cancer Support Community, 2290

Cancervive, 2291

Canine Companions for Independence, 9203

Celiac Disease Foundation, 2531

Center for AIDS Prevention Studies AIDS Research Institute University of C, 310

Center for Adaptive Learning, 10357

Center for Cancer Survival, 2292

Center for Interdisciplinary Research in Immunology and Diseases at UCLA, 311

Centers for AIDS Research: North-Central California, 312

Centers for AIDS Research: USCD Center for AIDS Research, 313

Centers for AIDS Research: University of California, Los Angeles, 314

Central California Chapter National Multiple Sclerosis Society, 6341

Central California Chapter of the National Hemophilia Foundation, 4828

Children Affected by AIDS Foundation, 195

Children Living with Illness, 1823

Children of Deaf Adults, 4269

Children's Gaucher Research Fund, 3887

Children's Hospital of Los Angeles, 2978

Children's Hospital of Orange County, 2975

Children's Liver Association for Support S ervices, 5630

Childrens Hospital at Oakland, 2979

City of Hope Comprehensive Cancer Research Center, 2173

City of Hope National Medical Center Beckman Research Institute, 2036

City of Hope National Medical Center Drug Discover/AIDS Group, 315

Clearinghouse for Specialized Media and Translation, 9588

Coalition for Pulmonary Fibrosis, 5672

Cocaine Anonymous: World Service Office, 7985

Collaborative Medicine Center, 2293

Commonwealth Cancer Help Program, 2294

Comprehensive Gaucher Treatment Center at Tower Hermatology Oncology, 3888

Continuum, 199

Cooley's Anemia Foundation (CAF): California, 2848

Cystic Fibrosis Center: Cedars-Sinai Medical Center, 2980

Cystic Fibrosis Center: University of California at San Francisco, 2981

Cystic Fibrosis Research, 2982

Department of Alcohol and Drug Programs, 8021

Departments of Neurology & Neurosurgery: University of California, San Francisco, 7920

Diabetes Control Program, 3258

Diabetes Society, 3297

Diabetes Society of Santa Clara Valley, 3115

Disability Rights California, 10290

Down Syndrome Association of Los Angeles, 3435

Dream Foundation, 10513

Drug Abuse Resistance Education of America, 7986

Dwarf Athletic Association of America, 3905

Eczema Association for Science and Education, 566

Eczema Association for Science and Education, 7509

Enzymology Research Laboratory Dept. of Veterans Affairs Medical Center, 5732

Epilepsy Foundation of Northern California, 7314

Ernest Gallo Clinic and Research Center, 8083

Estate Planning for the Disabled, 10232

Extensions for Independence, 10233

Families Anonymous, 7988

Family Caregiver Alliance/National Center on Caregiving, 3941

Foundation for Glaucoma Research, 9211

Foundation for the Advancement of the Blind, 9212

Fresno County Public Library: Talking Book Library for the Blind, 9426

Friday Night Live, 8122

General Clinical Research Center: University of California at LA, 4739

Geraldine Brush Cancer Research Institute California Pacific Medical Center, 2174

Glaucoma Research Foundation, 9409

Glaucoma Research Foundation, 9594

Glendale Adventist Medical Center Brain Tumor Support Group, 1824

Golden State Donor Services, 8945

Guide Dog Users, 9214

Guide Dogs for the Blind, 9215

HIV/Hepatitis C in Prison (HIP) Committee, 205

HIV/Hepatitis C in Prison (HIP) Committee, 5002

Harbor-South Bay Orange County Chapter of the American Assoc. of Kidney Patients, 5460

Heads Up!, 1825

Hear Center, 4236

Hearing Education and Awareness for Rocker s, 4177

Heart Research Foundation of Sacramento, 4743

Heart Touch™ Project, 208

Hemophilia Association of San Diego County, 4829

Hemophilia Center of the Huntington Hospital, 4896

Hemophilia Foundation of Northern California, 4830

Hemophilia Foundation of Southern California, 4831

House Ear Institute, 4180

Ida and Joseph Friend Cancer Resource Center, 2175

Independence Center, 10358

International Association of Cancer Victors and Friends, 2302

International Association of Laryngectomees, 1998

International Skeletal Dysplasia Registry Medical Genetics Institute, 3914

International Spinal Cord Regeneration Center, 7816

Jane & Terry Semel Institute for Neuroscie nce & Human Behavior, 6018

Jodi House, 4012

John Douglas French Alzheimer's Foundation, 650

John Tracy Clinic, 4183

John Tracy Clinic on Deafness, 4273

Jonsson Comprehensive Cancer Center University of California At Los Angeles, 2176

Juvenile Diabetes Research Foundation: Bakersfield Chapter, 3116

Juvenile Diabetes Research Foundation: Inl and Empire Chapter, 3117

Juvenile Diabetes Research Foundation: Los Angeles Chapter, 3118

Juvenile Diabetes Research Foundation: Nor thern California Inland Chapter, 3119

Juvenile Diabetes Research Foundation: Ora nge County Chapter, 3120

Juvenile Diabetes Research Foundation: San Diego Chapter, 3121

Juvenile Scleroderma Network, 7203

Kaiser Foundation Research Institute, 316

LAC/USC Imaging Science Center, 3889

Langley Porter Psychiatric Institute University of California, 6019

Leukemia & Lymphoma Society: Orange, Riverside, And San Bernadino Counties, 2037

Leukemia and Lymphoma Society: Greater Los Angeles Chapter, 2040

Leukemia and Lymphoma Society: Greater Sacramento Area Chapter, 2039

Leukemia and Lymphoma Society: Northern California Chapter, 2041

Leukemia and Lymphoma Society: Orange, Riverside, And San Bernadino Counties, 2042

Leukemia and Lymphoma Society: San Diego/Hawaii Chapter, 2038

Leukemia and Lymphoma Society: Tri-County Chapter, 2043

LifeSharing Community Organ & Tissue Donation, 8946

Lighthouse for the Blind and Visually Impaired, 9273

Little People of America, 3907

Loma Linda University Sleep Disorders Clinic, 7625

Los Angeles Alliance Against Parkinson's Disease, 6859

Los Angeles Chapter of the American Association of Kidney Patients, 5461

Los Angeles County Department of Health Services, 246

Los Angeles Orthopaedic Hospital, 4899

Los Angeles Support Group: National Ataxia Foundation, 1419

Lupus Foundation of America: California Chapter, 5777

Marijuana Anonymous: World Services, 7993

Marin Institute, 8091

MedicAlert Foundation International, 10249

Memorial Miller Children's Hospital Cystic Fibrosis Center, 2983

NAMI California, 5920

Narcotics Anonymous World Service Office, 7995

National Association to Advance Fat Acceptance, 6698

National Brain Tumor Foundation, 1794

National Brain Tumor Society, 1795

National Federation of the Blind: California, 9274

National Federation of the Blind: Science and Engineering Division, 9247

National Fibromyalgia Association, 3722

National Health Federation, 2044

National Hepatitis C Coalition, 5006

National Hydrocephalus Foundation, 5064

National Kidney Foundation of Northern California, 5462

National Kidney Foundation of Southern California, 5463

National Multiple Sclerosis Society Channel Islands Chapter, 6343

National Multiple Sclerosis Society: Silicon Valley Chapter, 6344

National Multiple Sclerosis Society: Southern California Chapter, 6342

National Parkinson Foundation: California Office, 6860

National Parkinson Foundation: Orange County Chapter, 6861

National Sarcoidosis Family Aid and Research Foundation, 7081

National Spinal Cord Injury Association: Los Angeles Chapter, 7826

National Spinal Cord Injury Association: San Diego County Chapter, 7825

Neuro-Oncology Information and Support Group, 1826

Neurofibromatosis Support Network, 6673

Neuroscience Institute Brain Tumor Hotline, 1827

Neurosciences Institute of the Neurosciences Research Program, 863

New Beginnings: The Blind Children's Cente, 9603

New Beginnings: The Blind Children's Center, 9602

Northern California Association of Persian Gulf Veterans, 9929

Northern California Chapter National Multiple Sclerosis Society, 6345

Northern California Support Group: National Ataxia Foundation, 1420

Northstate Parkinson's Chapter, 6862

Northwest Regional Training Center: Canine Companions for Independence, 9275

Okizu Foundation Camps, 10379

One Legacy Transplant Donor Network, 8947

Orange County Chapter National Multiple Sclerosis Society, 6346

Orange County Chapter of the ALS Association, 986

Orange County Support Group: National Ataxia Foundation, 1421

Osteoporosis Center Memorial Hospital/Advanced Medical Diagn, 6795

Parents Helping Parents A Family Resource Center, 8696

Parkinson Association of the Sacramento Valley, 6863

Parkinson Network of Mount Diablo, 6864

Parkinson's Disease Association of San Die go (PDASD), 6897

Parkinson's Institute, 6856

Parkinson's Resource Organization, 6892

Patient Services, 1828

Pediatric AIDS Foundation, 227

Pediatric Cancer Research Laboratory Children's Hospital of Orange County, 2177

Peninsula Support & Education Group for Parents of Children with Brain Tumors, 1829

Prader-Willi California Foundation, 7016

Preventive Medicine Research Institute, 4752

Project Inform, 229

Project Inform Hotline, 387

RESOLVE of Greater Los Angeles, 5259

RESOLVE of Greater San Diego, 5260

RESOLVE of Northern California, 5261

RRTC on Aging with a Disability Los Amigos Research and Education Instit, 7846

Rebecca and John Moores UCSD Cancer Center, 2178

Redding Chapter of the American Association of Kidney Patients, 5464

Region 6 of the National Association for Parents of the Visually Impaired, 9270

Regional Cancer Foundation, 2045

Research Institute of Palo Alto Medical Foundation, 585

Brain Injury Association of Colorado, 3948
Brain Injury Association of Colorado Helpline, 4013
Brain Tumor Resource and Vital Encouragement, 1836
CCFA Rocky Mountain Chapter, 2894
CO Center for AIDS Research: University Colorado Health Sciences Center/CFAR, 249
Centers for AIDS Research: University of Colorado Health Sciences Center, 324
Colorado Brain Tumor Support Group, 1837
Colorado Cancer Research Program, 2186
Colorado Chapter National Hemophilila Foun dation, 4832
Colorado Chapter of the American Association of Kidney Patients, 5466
Colorado FFCMH, 5922
Colorado Parkinson Foundation, 6865
Colorado SIDS Program, 8595
Colorado Talking Book Library, 9430
Colordao Department of Health and Environment, 8596
Denver Childrens Hospital, 2985
Denver Support Group: National Ataxia Foundation, 1423
Disability Careers, 10291
Donor Alliance, 8948
FFCMH: Denver/Aurora Chapter, 5923
International Hearing Dog, 4181
Jimmie Heuga Center, 6425
Juvenile Diabetes Research Foundation: Colorado Springs Chapter, 3123
Juvenile Diabetes Research Foundation: Roc ky Mountain Chapter, 3124
Laradon Services for Children and Adults w ith Developmental Disabilities, 6037
Legal Center for People with Disabilities and Older People, 10292
Little Star Foundation, 10540
Lung Facts, 5737
Lupus Foundation of Colorado, 5778
Mile High Down Syndrome Association, 3436
Mountain-Plains AIDS Education and Training Center (MPAETC), 250
Myasthenia Gravis Association of Colorado, 6606
NNFF Colorado Chapter, 6645
National Alliance for the Mentally Ill of Colorado, 5924
National Association of Blind Lawyers Scott LaBarre, 9228
National Federation of the Blind: Blind Merchants Division, 9263
National Federation of the Blind: Colorado, 9277
National Jewish Center for Immunology, 5733
National Jewish Center for Immunology and Respiratory Medicine, 584
National Jewish Division of Immunology, 1283
National Jewish Medical and Research Center, 5673
National Kidney Foundation of Colorado, Idaho, Montana, and Wyoming, 5481
National Kidney Foundation of Colorado/Idaho/Montana/Wyoming, 5497
National Kidney Foundation of Colorado/Idaho/Montana/Wyoming, 5535
National Kidney Foundation of Colorado: Idaho, Montana, and Wyoming, 5467
National MS Society: Colorado Chapter, 6348
National Native American AIDS Prevention Center, 221
National Stroke Association, 5121
National Stroke Association, 7914
Neurofibromatosis Foundation: Colorado, 6672
No. Colorado FFCMH, 5925
Prader-Willi Colorado Association, 7017
RESOLVE of Colorado, 5262
Rocky Mountain CFIDS/FMS Association, 3731
Scleroderma Foundation: Colorado Chapter, 7179
Spina Bifida Association of Colorado, 7722
Turner's Syndrome Society of Rocky Mountain, 9111
United Cerebral Palsy of Colorado, 2591
United States Association for Blind Athletes, 9260
University of Colorado Cancer Center, 2187
University of Colorado: General Clinical Research Center, Pediatric, 3281
Veterans Adm. Medical Center: Grand Junction, 9938

Western Slope Chapter of the American Association of Kidney Patients, 5468

Connecticut

Alzheimer's Association: Connecticut Chapter, 677
Alzheimer's Association: South Central Connecticut Chapter, 678
American Cancer Society: Connecticut, 2048
American Diabetes Association: Connecticut, 3125
American Epilepsy Society, 7310
American Liver Foundation: Connecticut Chapter, 5611
American Lung Association of Connecticut, 5685
American Lung Association of Connecticut, 9034
American Lyme Disease Foundation, 8797
Arthritis Foundation: Southern New England Chapter, 1087
Arthritis Foundation: Southern New England Chapter, 1118
Autism Society of Connecticut, 1564
Brain Injury Association of Connecticut, 3949
Brain Injury Association of Connecticut Helpline, 4014
CCFA Central Connecticut Chapter, 2895
CCFA Northern Connecticut Affiliate Chapter, 2896
Chapel Haven, 10359
Connecticut Alcohol and Drug Abuse Commission, 8023
Connecticut Brain Tumor Support Group, 1838
Connecticut Chapter of the ALS Association, 988
Connecticut Chapter of the Myasthenia Gravis Foundation of America, 6571
Connecticut Department of Health Services AIDS Programs, 251
Connecticut Down Syndrome Congress, 3437
Connecticut Pregnancy Exposure Information Service, 1742
Connecticut SIDS Alliance, 8597
Connecticut State Library for the Blind and Physically Handicapped, 9431
Cornelia de Lange Syndrome Foundation, 1720
Exceptional Cancer Patients/ECaP, 2296
Families United For CMH, Inc., 5926
Favarh, 10234
Fidelco Guide Dog Foundation, 9208
Gulf War Veterans of Connecticut: New England Chapter, 9939
International Lawyers in Alcoholics Anonymous, 8124
Juvenile Diabetes Research Foundation: Fai rfield County Chapter, 3127
Juvenile Diabetes Research Foundation: Greater New Haven Chapter, 3126
Juvenile Diabetes Research Foundation: Nor th Central CT and Western MA, 3128
Leukemia and Lymphoma Society: Connecticut Chapter, 2049
Leukemia and Lymphoma Society: Fairfield County Chapter, 2050
Lupus Foundation of America: Connecticut Chapter, 5779
Lupus Network, 5771
Lyme Disease Foundation, 8792
Motor Neuron Disease Clinic University of Connecticut Health Center, 1028
NNFF Connecticut Chapter, 6646
National Alliance for the Mentally Ill of Connecticut, 5927
National Federation of the Blind: Connecticut, 9278
National Kidney Foundation of Connecticut, 5469
National MS Society: Greater Connecticut Chapter, 6349
National Organization for Rare Disorders, 8735
National Organization for Rare Disorders, 10266
National Organization for Rare Disorders (NORD), 3698
National Organization for Rare Disorders (NORD), 3886
National Organization for Rare Disorders (NORD), 8582
National Spinal Cord Injury Association: Connecticut Chapter, 7827
National Veterans Services Fund, 9916

National Veterans Services Fund, 10134
NorthEast Organ Procurement Organization, 8949
Northwestern Connecticut AIDS Project, 252
Office of Protection and Advocacy for Persons with Disabilities, 10293
Prader-Willi Connecticut Association, 7018
Prevent Blindness Tri-State, 9279
RESOLVE of Fairfield County, 5263
RESOLVE of Greater Hartford, 5264
Raynaud's Foundation, 7071
Reflex Sympathetic Dystrophy Syndrome Association (RSDSA), 2806
Renfrew Center of Connecticut, 3562
SIDS Program: Connecticut Department of Health, 8598
Spina Bifida Association of Connecticut, 7723
Sudden Infant Death Syndrome (SIDS) Network, 8585
Terri Gotthelf Lupus Research Institute, 5847
Tourette Syndrome Clinic Yale Child Study Center, 8848
United Cerebral Palsy of Eastern Connecticut, 2592
United Cerebral Palsy of Greater Hartford, 2593
United Cerebral Palsy of Southern Connecticut, 2594
University of Connecticut Health Center, 2986
University of Connecticut Osteoporosis Center, 6797
Yale University Comprehensive Cancer Center, 2188
Yale University Cystic Fibrosis Research Center, 2987
Yale University: Behavioral Medicine Clinic, 6192
Yale University: Ribicoff Research Facilities/CT Mental Health Center, 6193
Yale University: Vision Research Center, 9612

Delaware

Alliance for the Mentally Ill in Delaware (AMID), 5928
Alzheimer's Association: Delaware Chapter, 679
American Cancer Society: Delaware, 2051
American Diabetes Association: Delaware, 3129
American Lung Association of Delaware, 5686
American Lung Association of Delaware, 9035
Autism Society of Delaware, 1565
Brain Injury Association of Delaware, 3950
Brain Injury Association of Delaware Helpl ine, 4015
Client Assistance Program: Delaware, 10294
Delaware Assocation for the Blind Department of Health & Social Services, 9280
Delaware Department of Health and Social Services, 253
Delaware Division of Alcoholism, Drug Abuse and Mental Health, 8024
Delaware Division of Libraries: Library for the Blind and Physically Handicapped, 9432
Delaware FFMCH, 5929
Juvenile Diabetes Research Foundation: Del aware, 3130
Leukemia and Lymphoma Society: Delaware Chapter, 2052
Lupus Foundation of America: Delaware Chapter, 5780
Mental Health Association of Delaware, 5930
National Federation of the Blind: Delaware, 9281
National MS Society: Delaware Chapter, 6350
Pediatric Brain Tumor Support Group, 1839
Prader-Willi Delaware Association, 7019
SIDS Information & Counseling: Division of Public Health, 8599
Sarcoidosis Support Group Delaware, 7095
Spina Bifida Association of Delaware, 7724
United Cerebral Palsy of Delaware, 2595
Veterans Adm. Medical Center: Wilmington VA Medical Center, 9940

District of Columbia

AAA Foundation for Traffic Safety, 7971
AIDS United, 177
ALS Association National Office, 980
ARC The ARC of the United States, 3427
Agent Orange Registry Department of Veterans Affairs, 9914

Washington DC Metropolitan Area Support Group, 1841

Whitman Walker Clinic AIDS/Medical Services Programs, 326

Florida

AARP Florida State Office: St. Petersburg, 35

ALS Association: Florida Chapter, 990

ALS Association: Florida Chapter East Coast Regional Office, 991

Alcohol and Drug Abuse Program Department Of Children And Families, 8026

Alzheimer's Association: Broward County Chapter, 681

Alzheimer's Association: East Central Florida Chapter, 682

Alzheimer's Association: Florida Gulf Coast Chapter, 683

Alzheimer's Association: Greater Miami Chapter, 684

Alzheimer's Association: Greater Orlando Area Chapter, 685

Alzheimer's Association: Greater Palm Beach Area Chapter, 686

Alzheimer's Association: Northeast Florida, 687

Alzheimer's Association: Northern Central Florida Chapter, 688

Alzheimer's Association: Northwest Florida Chapter, 689

Alzheimer's Association: Southwest Florida Chapter, 690

Alzheimer's Association: Tampa Bay Chapter, 691

Alzheimer's Association: Volusia/Flagler Branch, 692

Alzheimer's Association: West Central Florida Chapter, 693

Alzheimer/Parkinson Association of Indian River County, 6866

American Association of Kidney Patients, 5452

American Association of Kidney Patients, 5472

American Cancer Society: Florida, 2056

American Diabetes Association: Northeast F lorida/Southeast Georgia, 3133

American Diabetes Association: Seattle, 3134

American Diabetes Association: South Coast Regional/Central Florida, 3135

American Hemochromatosis Society, 3781

American Liver Foundation Gulf Coast Chapter, 5612

American Lung Association of Florida, 5688

American Lung Association of Florida, 9038

American Society of Dermatology, 10209

Angels in the Sun Brain Tumor Support Group, 1842

Arthritis Foundation: Florida Chapter, Gulf Coast Branch, 1089

Association of Birth Defect Children Birth Defect Research for Children, 563

Association of Birth Defect Children Birth Defect Research for Children, 1262

Asthma and Allergy Foundation of America: Florida Chapter, 571

Autism Society of Greater Orlando, 1567

BASE Camp Children's Cancer Foundation, 10506

Birth Defect Research for Children, 1717

Brain Injury Association of Florida, 3951

Brain Injury Association of Florida, 4016

Brain Tumor Support Group, 1843

Brave Kids, 3890

Brevard County Libraries: Talking Books Library, 9436

Broward County Talking Book Library, 9437

CCFA Florida Chapter, 2897

Central Florida Chapter, 6352

Chef David's Kids, 10535

Children's Medical Services Program: Florida SIDS Program, 8606

Choices for Work Program Goodwill Industries-Suncoast, 3952

Coconut Creek Eating Disorders Support Group, 3582

Comprehensive Pediatric Hemophilia Center University of South Florida, 4882

Cystic Fibrosis Center: All Children's Hospital, 2989

Department of Epidemiology and Health Policy Research: University of Florida, 327

Desert Storm Justice Foundation: Florida, 9944

Desert Storm Veterans of Florida, 9945

Disability Rights: Florida, 10297

Dreams Come True, 10537

East Central Florida Chapter of the Myasthenia Gravis Foundation of America, 6574

Endometriosis Association, 3656

Endometriosis Reseach Center and Women's Hospital, 3665

Epilepsy Association of Big Bend, 7315

Epilepsy Foundation of South Florida, 7316

Epilepsy Services Foundation, 7317

Epilepsy Services of North Central Florida, 7318

Epilepsy Services of Northeast Florida, 7319

Epilepsy Services of Southwest Florida, 7320

Florida Alliance for the Mentally Ill, 5933

Florida Ambassador: National Ataxia Foundation, 1424

Florida Association of the Deaf, 4203

Florida Brain Tumor Association, 1844

Florida Brain Tumor Support Group, 1845

Florida Brain Tumor Support Group: Deerfield Beach, 1846

Florida Bureau of Braille and Talking Book Library Services, 9438

Florida Department of Health, 8607

Florida Department of Health Bureau of HIV/AIDS, 255

Florida Disabled Outdoor Association, 10236

Florida FFCMH: Tampa Chapter, 5934

Florida Gulf Coast Chapter National Multiple Sclerosis Society, 6353

Florida Heart Research Institute, 4736

Florida Hemophilia Association, 4833

Florida Institute for Family Involvement (FIFI), 6038

Florida Ophthalmic Institute, 9592

Florida SIDS Alliance, 8608

Florida Southwest Turner Syndrome Society, 9112

Gilda's Club: South Florida, 2300

Give Kids the World Village, 10516

Gold Coast Down Syndrome Organization, 3438

Goodwill Industries-Suncoast, 36

Goodwill Industries-Suncoast, 3439

Goodwill Industries-Suncoast, 5689

Goodwill Industries-Suncoast, 6354

Goodwill Industries-Suncoast, 6867

Goodwill Industries-Suncoast, 7828

Goodwill Industries-Suncoast, 9285

Greater Daytona Area Parkinson Support Group, 6898

HEALTHSOUTH Rehabilitation Hospital of Tal lahassee, 7848

Hillsborough County Talking Book Library, 9439

Hollywood Area Brain Tumor Support Group, 1847

International Society of Dermatology, 7510

Iron Overload Diseases Association, 3793

Jacksonville Public Library, 9440

Juvenile Diabetes Research Foundation: Cen tral Florida Chapter, 3136

Juvenile Diabetes Research Foundation: Flo rida Sun Coast Chapter, 3137

Juvenile Diabetes Research Foundation: Gre ater Palm Beach County Chapter, 3138

Juvenile Diabetes Research Foundation: Nor th Florida Chapter, 3139

Juvenile Diabetes Research Foundation: Sou th Florida Chapter, 3140

Juvenile Diabetes Research Foundation: Tam pa Bay Chapter, 3141

Kidney Association of South Florida, 5473

Kids Wish Network, 10521

Lee County Talking Books Library, 9441

Leukemia & Lymphoma Society: Suncoast Chapter, 2057

Leukemia and Lymphoma Society: Southern Florida Chapter, 2058

Leukemia and Lymphoma Society: Central Florida Chapter, 2059

Leukemia and Lymphoma Society: Northern Florida Chapter, 2060

Leukemia and Lymphoma Society: Palm Beach Area Chapter, 2061

LifeLink of Florida, 8950

LifeLink of Southwest Florida, 8951

Lupus Foundation of America: Northeast Florida Chapter, 5781

Lupus Foundation of America: Northwest Florida Chapter, 5782

Lupus Foundation of America: Southeast Florida Chapter, 5783

Lupus Foundation of America: Suncoast Chapter, 5784

Lupus Foundation of America: Tampa Area Chapter, 5785

Lupus Foundation of Florida, 5786

MSWorld, 6429

Manattee County Office Epilepsy Services of Southwest Florida, 7321

Metabolic Research Institute, 3278

Miami Childrens Hospital Division of Pulmonology, 2990

Miami Comprehensive Hemophilia Center Jackson Medical Towers, 4903

Miami Dade Talking Book Library, 9442

Miami Project to Cure Paralysis, 7844

Mount Sinai Medical Center, 4749

Multiple Sclerosis Foundation, 6333

NNFF Florida Chapter, 6647

National Association of Guide Dog Users Priscilla Ferris, 9232

National Federation of the Blind: Florida, 9286

National Kidney Foundation of Florida, 5474

National Multiple Sclerosis Society: North Florida Chapter, 6355

National Parkinson Foundation, 6853

National Parkinson Foundation Hotline, 6899

National Spinal Cord Injury Support Goups, 7851

National Spinal Cord Injury Support Groups, 7854

Nemours Childrens Clinic, 2991

New Hope for Kids Wish Program, 10525

North Florida: HPV Support Group, 10298

Northwest Florida Support Group: National Ataxia Foundation, 1425

Orange County Library System: Orlando Public Library, 9443

Palm Beach County Library Annex: Talking Books, 9444

Parent Education Network (PEN) Project Health, 6039

Parkinson Association of Greater Daytona Beach, 6868

Parkinson Association of Southwest Florida, 6869

Pembroke Pines Parkinson Support Group, 6900

Pensacola Brain Injury TBI/ABI Support Group, 3953

Pinellas Talking Book Library for the Blind and Physically Handicapped, 9445

Positive Voices, 256

Prader-Willi Florida Assocation, 7020

Prader-Willi Syndrome Association (USA), 7012

PraderWilli Syndrome Association, 7048

RESOLVE Affiliate of Central Florida, 5266

RESOLVE of North Florida, 5267

RESOLVE of South Florida, 5268

Rambaugh-Goodwin Institute for Cancer Research, 2192

Renfrew Center of Miami, 3563

Renfrew Center of South Florida, 3564

Sarasota Area Brain Tumor Support Group, 1848

Scleroderma Foundation: Southeast Florida Chapter, 7181

Scoliosis Association, 7246

South Florida Chapter National Multiple Sclerosis Society, 6356

South Florida Chapter of the American Association of Kidney Patients, 5475

South Florida Gold Coast Chapter of the Myasthenia Gravis Foundation of America, 6575

South Palm Beach County Chapter of NFP, 6870

Southeast Parkinson Disease Association, 6871

Southeast Regional Center: Canine Companions for Independence, 9287

Spina Bifida Association of Florida Space Coast, 7725

Spina Bifida Association of Jacksonville, 7726

Spina Bifida Association of Tampa, 7727

Sub Regional Talking Book Library, 9446

Sunshine Chapter of the American Association of Kidney Patients, 5476

TPN: The Perspective Network, 3944

Tallahassee Memorial Diabetes Center, 3265

Georgia

Hawaii

Alcohol and Drug Abuse Division Department of Health, 8028
Alzheimer's Association: Honolulu Chapter, 701
Alzheimer's Association: West Hawaii Chapter, 702
American Cancer Society: Hawaii, 2065
American Diabetes Association: Hawaii, 3145
American Lung Association of Hawaii, 5691
American Lung Association of Hawaii, 9040
Autism Society of Hawaii, 1569
Brain Injury Association of Hawaii, 3954
Brain Injury Association of Hawaii, 4017
Division of Vocational Rehabilitation and Services for the Blind, 9292
Hawaii Department of Health: Communicable Disease Division, 258
Hawaii Department of Health: Family Health Division, 8612
Hawaii Down Syndrome Congress, 3441
Hawaii Families As Allies (HFAA), 6041
Hawaii Lupus Foundation, 5789
Hawaii Parkinson Association Gwendolyn A Montibon President, 6873
Hawaii State Library for the Blind and Physically Handicapped, 9462
Hemophilia Foundation of Hawaii Kapiolani Medical Center, 4835
Ho'opono Workshop for the Blind, 9293
Juvenile Diabetes Research Foundation: Haw aii Chapter, 3146
Kuakini Parkinson Disease (PD) Information & Referral, 6901
NAMI: The Local Affiliate of the National Alliance for the Mentally Ill, 5936
National Federation of the Blind: Hawaii, 9294
National Kidney Foundation of Hawaii, 5480
National MS Society: Hawaii Chapter, 6358
Organ Donor Center of Hawaii, 8954
Pacific Health Research Institute, 2196
Prader-Willi Hawaii Association, 7022
Protection & Advocacy Agency, 10300
RESOLVE of Hawaii, 5270
United Cerebral Palsy of Hawaii, 2609
University of Hawaii: Cancer Research Center, 2197
Veterans Adm. Medical Centery: Honolulu VA Pacific Islands Health Care System, 9959

Idaho

AARP Idaho State Office: Meridian, 39
Alzheimer's Association: Greater Idaho Chapter, 703
Alzheimer's Association: Northern Idaho Chapter, 704
American Cancer Society: Idaho, 2066
American Lung Association of Idaho, 5692
Autism Society of Treasure Valley, 1570
Brain Injury Association of Idaho, 3955
Co-Ad, 10301
Department of Health and Welfare Department Of Health And Welfare, 8029
FFCMH: Idaho Chapter, 5937
Hemophilia Foundation of Idaho, 4836
Idaho Alliance for the Mentally Ill, 5938
Idaho Commission for Libraries Talking Book Service, 9463
Idaho Department of Health and Welfare, 8613
Idaho Department of Health and Welfare The STD/AIDS Program, 259
Idaho Persian Gulf Veterans, 9960
NNFF Idaho Chapter, 6649
National Federation of the Blind: Idaho, 9295
National MS Society: Idaho Division, 6359
Prader-Willi Idaho Association, 7023
United Cerebral Palsy of Idaho, 2610
Veterans Adm. Medical Center: Boise Boise VA Medical Center, 9961

Illinois

AARP Illinois State Office: Chicago, 40
AIDS Legal Council of Chicago, 260
ARRISE, 1551
Academy for Eating Disorders, 3545
Academy for Eating Disorders, 3575

Adult Down Syndrome Center of Lutheran General Hospital, 3452
Aid to the Aged, Blind or Disabled, 9296
Alzheimer's Association: Central Illinois Chapter, 705
Alzheimer's Association: East Central Illinois Chapter, 706
Alzheimer's Association: Four Rivers Chapter, 707
Alzheimer's Association: Greater Illinois Chapter, 708
Alzheimer's Association: Greater Illinois Chapter: Carbondale Office, 709
Alzheimer's Association: Land of Lincoln Chapter, 710
Alzheimer's Disease and Related Disorders Association, 647
American Academy of Dermatology, 7503
American Academy of Orthopaedic Surgeons, 2505
American Academy of Orthopaedic Surgeons, 7243
American Academy of Pediatrics, 10196
American Academy of Sleep Medicine, 2718
American Association of Diabetes Educators, 3097
American Board of Dermatology American Society for Dermatologic Surger, 7504
American Brain Tumor Association, 1792
American Brain Tumor Association, 3937
American Brain Tumor Association Patient Line, 4018
American Cancer Society: Illinois, 2067
American College of Allergy, Asthma & Immunology, 561
American Dental Association Department of Library Services, 7978
American Dermatological Association University of Iowa Hospital and Clinics, 7505
American Diabetes Association: Greater Ill inois, 3147
American Diabetes Association: Northern Il linois, 3148
American Dietetic Association, 562
American Dietetic Association, 3546
American Dietetic Association, 3779
American Hearing Research Foundation, 4156
American Homes for the Aging: Midwest Regional Office, 711
American Liver Foundation Illinois Chapter, 5613
American Lung Association Help Line, 5736
American Lung Association of Illinois, 5693
American Lung Association of Illinois-Iowa, 9041
American Pain Society, 2803
American Society for Dermatologic Surgery, 7506
American Society for Gastrointestinal Endoscopy, 3785
American Society for Surgery of the Hand, 2507
American Society of Colon and Rectal Surgeons, 1982
American Society of Plastic and Reconstructive Surgeons, 7507
Arthritis Foundation: Greater Chicago Chapter, 1091
Arthritis Foundation: Greater Illinois Chapter, 1092
Arthritis Foundation: Northwestern Ohio Chapter, 1113
Association of Halfway House Alcoholism Programs of North America, 7980
Association of Late-Deafened Adults, 4160
Association of Professional Sleep Societies, 7609
Autism Society of Illinois, 1571
Baxter Hyland Division, 4821
Benjamin B Greenfield National Alzheimer's Center, 648
Better Existence with HIV, 189
Brain Injury Association of Illinois, 3956
Brain Injury Association of Illinois Helpline, 4019
Brain Research Foundation, 1801
Brain Tumor Support Group, 1854
CANDU Parent Group, 6042
CCFA Illinois: Carol Fisher Chapter, 2899
Cancer and Leukemia Group B, 2198
Captain James A. Lovell Federal Health Car e Center, 9962
Catholic Guild for the Blind, 9464
Catholic Guild for the Blind Catholic Charities of the Archdiocese of, 9205
Center for Digestive Disorders: Central, 3788

Center for Narcolepsy Research at the University of Illinois at Chicago, 7617
Central Brain Tumor Registry of the US, 1803
Chicago Area Support Group: National Ataxia Foundation, 1428
Chicago Department of Health, 261
Chicago Lighthouse for People Who are Blind and Visually Impaired, 9297
Chicago Metro Support Group: National Ataxia Foundation, 1429
Chicagoland Chapter of the American Association of Kidney Patients, 5482
Citizens Alliance for VD Awareness, 7410
Clinical Research Center Northwestern Center for Clinical Researc, 335
Cognitive Neurology and Alzheimer's Disease Center, 851
Comer Children's Hospital at the Universit, 2995
Comer Children's Hospital at the University of Chicago, 2994
Compassionate Friends, 8580
Compassionate Friends, 10546
Cooley's Anemia Foundation (CAF): Illinois Oakbrook Towers, 2849
Cystic Fibrosis Center: Childrens Memorial Hospital, 2996
Cystic Fibrosis Center: Park Ridge Lutheran General Children's Hospital, 2997
David T Siegel Institute for Communicative Disorders, 4233
Department of Alcoholism and Substance Abuse, 8030
Department of Ophthalmology Information Line, 9619
Depression and Bipolar Support Alliance, 6194
Dermatology Foundation, 2160
Dermatology Foundation, 7508
Desert Storm Justice Foundation: Illinois, 9963
Division on Endocrinology Northwestern University Feinberg School, 3271
Dreams for Seniors Charity Inc, 10538
Easter Seals, 1721
Easter Seals, 2563
Easter Seals, 7715
Edward J Hines Jr VA Hospital, 9964
Fairygodmother Foundation, 10514
Gastro-Intestinal Research Foundation, 3802
Gastrointestinal Research Foundation, 3806
Hands Organization: Advocacy Network for the Deaf and Hearing Impaired, 4175
Helen Keller National Center Regional Representatives, 9298
Hemophilia Foundation of Illinois, 4837
Ileitis and Colitis Educational Foundation, 2884
Illinois Alliance for the Mentally Ill, 5939
Illinois Association of the Deaf, 4205
Illinois Church Action on Alcohol Problems, 8031
Illinois Client Assistance Program, 10302
Illinois Department of Public Health: Division of Infectious Diseases, 262
Illinois Federation of Families, 5940
Illinois Midwest Neurofibromatosis, 6650
Illinois Spina Bifida Association, 7729
Illinois State Library Talking Book and Braille Service, 9465
Illinois Teratogen Information Service (IT IS), 1743
International Association for Chronic Fatigue, 2719
International Association of Eating Disorders Professionals, 3554
International Pelvic Pain Society Women's Medical Plaza, 2805
International Pelvic Pain Society Women's Medical Plaza, 3659
Jesse Brown VA Medical Center, 9965
Juvenile Diabetes Research Foundation: Gre ater Chicago Chapter, 3149
KALEIDOSCOPE, 6043
Kellogg Cancer Care Center Evanston Hospital, 2199
LaRabida Children's Hospital: Developmental Disabilities & Delays, 3466
Les Turner Amyotrophic Lateral Sclerosis Foundation, 1038
Les Turner Research Laboratory Northwestern University Medical School, 1026
Let's Breathe Sarcoidosis Support Group, 7086

Indiana

Vision World Wide, 9261

Iowa

AARP Iowa State Office: Des Moines, 42
Alzheimer's Association: Big Sioux Chapter, 714
Alzheimer's Association: East Central Iowa Chapter, 715
Alzheimer's Association: Greater Iowa Chapter, 716
Alzheimer's Association: Heart of Iowa Chapter, 717
American Cancer Society: Iowa, 2071
American Diabetes Association: Cedar Rapid s District, 3154
American Lung Association of Iowa, 5695
Arthritis Foundation: Iowa Chapter, 1094
Autism Society of Iowa, 1573
Blank Childrens Hospital Pediatric Pulmonology Clinic, 3001
Brain Injury Alliance of Iowa Helpline, 4021
Brain Injury Association of Iowa, 3958
CCFA Iowa Chapter, 2901
Cedar Rapids Persian Gulf Veterans, Spouses and Children, 9972
Center for Disabilities and Development, 3455
Client Assistance Program: Iowa Division o n Persons with Disabilities, 10304
Department of Public Health: Division of Substance Abuse and Health, 8034
Des Moines Division: VA Central Iowa Health Care System, 9973
FFCMH: Iowa Chapter, 5944
Gilda's Club: Quad Cities, 2299
Great Plains Regional Hemophilia Center University of Iowa Hospitals, 4886
Greater Iowa Chapter Alzheimer's Association Quadcity Office, 718
Iowa Brain Tumor Support Group, 1858
Iowa Chapter of the Association of Kidney Patients, 5485
Iowa Department for the Blind, 9474
Iowa Donor Network, 8957
Iowa Federaion of Families for Children's Mental Health (FFCMH), 6046
Iowa Oncology Research Association, 2206
Iowa SIDS Alliance, 8618
Iowa SIDS Program Iowa Department of Public Health, 8619
Juvenile Diabetes Research Foundation: Eas tern Iowa Chapter, 3155
Juvenile Diabetes Research Foundation: Gre ater Iowa Chapter, 3156
Kidneeds, 5546
Knoxville Division: VA Central Iowa Health Care System, 9974
Lupus Foundation of America: Iowa Chapter, 5794
NAMI Iowa: National Alliance on Mental Illness, 5945
NNFF Iowa Chapter, 6657
National Center for Voice and Speech: Univ ersity of Iowa, 4187
National Federation of the Blind in Computer Science, 9241
National Federation of the Blind: Iowa, 9302
National MS Society: Iowa Chapter, 6362
Neurological Center of Iowa, 1859
Orthopaedic Biomechanics Laboratory Shriners Hospital for Crippled Children, 2688
Pediatric Allergy & Pulmonary Division University of Iowa Healthcare, 3002
People Against Cancer, 2072
Prader-Willi Iowa Association, 7026
Quad Cities Brain Tumor Support Group, 1860
RESOLVE Affiliate of Iowa, 5273
Spina Bifida Association of Iowa, 7731
Turner's Syndrome Society of Iowa, 9117
University of Iowa Birth Defects and Genetic Disorders Unit, 1737
University of Iowa College of Medicine, 7924
University of Iowa Mental Health Clinical Research Center, 6252
University of Iowa Teratogen Information Service, 1755
University of Iowa: Diabetes Research Center, 3282

University of Iowa: Holden Comprehensive Cancer Center, 2207
University of Iowa: Iowa Cardiovascular Center, 4762
Veterans Adm. Medical Center: Iowa City, 9975

Kansas

AARP Kansas State Office: Topeka, 43
ALS Association: Keith Worthington Chapter, 995
ALS Association: Keith Worthington Chapter Central/Western Kansas Branch, 996
Alcohol and Drug Abuse Services, 8035
Alzheimer's Association: Heart of America Chapter, 719
Alzheimer's Association: Sunflower Chapter, 720
American Academy of Environmental Medicine, 560
American Cancer Society: Kansas City, 2073
American Diabetes Association: Kansas, 3157
American Lung Association of Kansas, 5696
American Lung Association of Kansas, 9043
American Lung Association of Missouri, 5705
American Organ Transplant Association, 10206
American Stroke Foundation, 7916
Arthritis Foundation: Kansas Chapter, 1095
Arthritis Foundation: Western Missouri, Greater Kansas City, 1103
Association for Neuro-Metabolic Disorders, 3694
Autism Society of Kansas Autism Society of America, 1574
Beach Center on Disability, 10212
Brain Injury Association of Kansas and Greater Kansas City, 3959
Brain Injury Association of Kansas and Greater Kansas City Helpline, 4022
CKLS Headquarters, 9475
Council for Learning Disabilities (CLD), 10227
Disability Rights Center of Kansas, 10305
Foundation for Hospice and Homecare, 10370
Gray Matters Support: Kansas City, 1861
Headstrong Brain Tumor Support Group, 1862
Kansas Association of the Deaf, 4206
Kansas Department of Health & Environment Bureau of Family Health, 8620
Kansas Department of Health & Environment Epidemiology & Disease Prevention: HIV, 264
Kansas Industries for the Blind, 9303
Kansas Services for the Blind and Visually Impaired, 9613
Kansas State University: Terry C Johnson Center for Basic Cancer Research, 2208
Kansas University Medical Center: Cystic Fibrosis Center, 3003
Keys for Networking: Kansas FFCMH, 5946
Landon Center on Aging University of Kansas Medical Center, 81
Leukemia and Lymphoma Society: Mid-America Chapter, 2074
Leukemia and Lymphona Society: Kansas Chapter, 2075
Lupus Foundation of America: Heartland Chapter, 5795
Manhattan Subregional Library of the Kansas Talking Books Service, 9476
Midwest Transplant Network & Organ Bank, 8958
NAMI Kansas: Kansas' Voice on Mental Illness, 5947
National Federation of the Blind: Kansas, 9304
National Kidney Foundation of Kansas and Western Missouri, 5486
National MS Society: Mid-America Chapter, 6363
National MS Society: South Central & West Kansas Division, 6364
Neurofibromatosis Kansas and Central Plains, 6659
Northeast Kansas Parkinson Association, 6874
Northwest Kansas Library System, 9477
Parkinson Association of Greater Kansas City, 6875
Region VII Office Program: Consultants for Maternal and Child Health, 8641
SIDS Network of Kansas, 8621
South Central Kansas Library System, 9478
St. Joseph Medical Center Cystic Fibrosis Care and Teaching Center, 3004
Talking Books Service, 9479
United Cerebral Palsy of Kansas, 2622

University of Kansas Allergy and Immunology Clinic, 589
University of Kansas Cray Diabetes Center, 3283
University of Kansas Kidney and Urology Research Center, 5541
Veterans Adm. Medical Center: Leavenwoth Dwight D. Eisenhower VA Medical Center, 9976
Veterans Adm. Medical Center: Topeka Colmery O'Neil VA Medical Center, 9977
Veterans Adm. Medical Center: Wichita Robert J. Dole Department Of VA Medical, 9978
Wichita Medical Research & Education Foundation, 1740
Wichita Public Library, 9480

Kentucky

AARP Kentucky State Office: Louisville, 44
ALS Association: Kentucky CIO, 997
Academy of Doctors of Audiology, 4150
Alzheimer's Association: Lexington/ Bluegrass Chapter, 721
Alzheimer's Association: Louisville Chapter, 722
Alzheimer's Disease Center Kentucky University, 841
American Cancer Society: Kentucky, 2076
American Council of Blind Lions, 9191
American Diabetes Association: Kentucky, 3158
American Lung Association of Kentucky, 5697
American Lung Association of Kentucky, 9044
American Printing House for the Blind, 9197
Arthritis Foundation: Kentucky Chapter, 1096
Autism Chapter of Bluegrass Chapter, 1575
Autism Society of Western Kentucky, 1576
Brain Injury Alliance of Kentucky, 4023
Brain Injury Association of Kentucky, 3960
Carol and Dr. James W Stutts, 9979
Client Assistance Program: Kentucky, 10306
Department of Public Health: Adult and Child Health Division, 8622
Diabetes Exercise and Sports Association, 3099
Division of Substance Abuse: Department of Mental Health, 8036
Dream Factory, Inc., 10512
Henry Vogt Cancer Research Institute James Graham Brown Cancer Center, 2209
Jewish Hospital Transplant Center, 8934
Juvenile Diabetes Research Foundation: Kentuckiana Chapter, 3159
KY Partnership For Families and Children, 5948
Kentucky Alliance for the Mentally Ill, 5949
Kentucky Association of the Deaf, 4207
Kentucky Cancer Program, 2210
Kentucky Chapter of the Myasthenia Gravis Foundation of America, 6579
Kentucky Hemophilia Foundation, 4839
Kentucky IMPACT, 6047
Kentucky Industries for the Blind, 9305
Kentucky Organ Donor Affiliates, 8959
Kentucky Talking Book Library, 9481
Kentucky University: Cystic Fibrosis Center, 3005
Kosair Childrens Cystic Fibrosis Center, 3006
Leukemia and Lymphoma Society: Kentucky Chapter, 2077
Louisville Talking Book Library for the Blind and Physically Handicapped, 9482
Lovelace Respiratory Research Institute, 5538
Meningioma/Benign Brain Tumor Support Group, 1863
National Anxiety Foundation, 6185
National Federation of the Blind: Kentucky, 9306
National Kidney Foundation of Kentucky, 5487
National MS Society: Kentucky Chapter, 6365
National Spinal Cord Injury Association: Derby City Area Chapter, 7832
Northern Kentucky Talking Book Library, 9483
Parents Resource Institute for Drug Education, 8075
Prader-Willi Kentucky Association, 7027
RESOLVE of Kentucky, 5274
SIDS Network of Kentucky, 8623
Spina Bifida Association of Kentucky, 7732
USA Deaf Sports Federation, 4198
University of Kentucky: Children Cancer Study Group, 2211

Frederick Cancer Research Center, 2215
Friends Medical Science Research Center, 8085
Friends of Libraries for Deaf Action USA, 4223
Genetic and Rare Diseases Information Center, 3695
Goodwill Industries International, 10237
Health Resources and Services Administration (HRSA), 8933
Hearing Loss Association of America, 4178
Hemophilia Foundation of Maryland, 4841
Hepatitis Foundation International, 5003
Hydrocephalus Association, 5069
Hydrocephalus Association Hydrocephalus Association, 5062
Immune Deficiency Foundation, 209
Immune Deficiency Foundation, 568
Impotents Anonymous, 5179
Indian Health Service, 7991
Institute of Psychiatry and Human Behavior: University of Maryland, 6017
International Agency for the Prevention of Blindness, 9218
International Braille and Technology Center for the Blind, 9493
Job Opportunities for the Blind, 9620
Johns Hopkins Brain Tumor Education Group, 1870
Johns Hopkins University: Asthma and Allergy Center, 1282
Johns Hopkins University: Behavioral Pharmacology Research Unit, 8089
Johns Hopkins University: Center for Communication Programs, 338
Johns Hopkins University: Dana Center for Preventive Ophthalmology, 9601
Johns Hopkins University: Scleroderma Center, 7207
Johns Hopkins University: Sleep Disorders Francis Scott Key Medical Center, 7622
Johns Hopkins University: Sydney Kimmel Comprehensive Cancer Center, 2216
Joslin Center at University of Maryland Medicine, 3261
Juvenile Diabetes Research Foundation: Mar yland Chapter, 3167
Kennedy Krieger Institute, 3465
Kennedy Krieger Institute - Down Syndrome, 3475
Kennedy-Krieger Institute, 10130
Learning How, 10244
Leukemia and Lymphoma Society: Maryland Chapter, 2081
Little People's Research Fund (LPRF), 3908
Loch Raven VA Community Living & Rehabilit ation Center, 9988
MD/DC/Delaware Chapter of Myasthenia Gravis Foundation of America, 6572
MD/DC/Delaware Chapter of Myasthenia Gravis Foundation of America, 6573
MD/DC/Delaware Chapter of Myasthenia Gravis Foundation of America, 6580
Maryland Group, 9989
Maryland National Spinal Cord Injury Association Support Group Network, 7849
Maryland Psychiatric Research Center, 6248
Maryland SIDS Information & Counseling Program, 8630
Maryland State Alcohol and Drug Abuse Administration, 8039
Maryland State Library for the Blind and Physically Handicapped, 9494
Mental Health America, 6183
Mental Health Services Training Center, 10250
Mt. Washington Pediatric Clinic, 3469
NIH Clinical Center, 6023
NIH Osteoporosis and Related Bone Diseases - National Resource Center, 6762
NIH Osteoporosis and Related Bone Diseases - National Resource Center, 6765
NIH Osteoporosis and Related Bone Diseases - National Resource Center, 6793
NIH/National Institute of Neurological Disorders and Stroke, 7611
National Advisory Allergic and Infectious Disease Council, 1265
National Alliance for the Mentally Ill: Maryland, 5953
National Arthritis and Musculoskeletal & Skin Diseases Information Clearinghouse, 1078

National Arthritis and Musculoskeletal & Skin Diseases Information Clearinghous, 7511
National Association for Children of Alcoholics, 7996
National Association of the Deaf, 4185
National Cancer Institute, 2002
National Center for the Prevention of SIDS, 8694
National Clearinghouse for Alcohol and Drug Information, 8000
National Clearinghouse for Alcohol and Drug Information, 8074
National Coalition for Cancer Survivorship, 2004
National Diabetes Action Network for the Blind, 3102
National Diabetes Action Network for the Blind, 9238
National Diabetes Information Clearinghous e, 3263
National Diabetes Information Clearinghous e, 5453
National Digestive Diseases Information Clearinghouse, 2929
National Digestive Diseases Information Clearinghouse, 3794
National Digestive Diseases Information Clearinghouse, 10257
National Eye Institute National Institutes of Health, 9239
National Family Caregivers Association, 10376
National Federation of Families for Children's Mental Health, 1500
National Federation of the Blind, 9240
National Federation of the Blind: Blind Industrial Workers of America, 9243
National Federation of the Blind: Human Services Division, 9244
National Federation of the Blind: Maryland, 9313
National Federation of the Blind: Masonic Square Club, 9245
National Foundation for Cancer Research, 2005
National Foundation for Cancer Research Hotline, 2306
National Foundation for Cancer Research National Foundation for Cancer Research, 2217
National Heart, Lung & Blood Institute, 5119
National Heart, Lung & Blood Institute, 7911
National Heart, Lung and Blood Institute, 4722
National Institute of Allergy and Infectious Diseases, 569
National Institute of Allergy and Infectious Diseases, 2721
National Institute of Allergy and Infectious Diseases, 7412
National Institute of Allergy and Infectious Diseases, 9024
National Institute of Allergy and Infectious Diseases (NIAID), 8936
National Institute of Arthritis & Musculoskeletal Skin Diseases, 2512
National Institute of Arthritis and Musculoskeletal and Skin Disease (NIAMS), 1079
National Institute of Arthritis and Musculoskeletal and Skin Disease (NIAMS), 2509
National Institute of Arthritis and Musculoskeletal and Skin Disease (NIAMS), 7512
National Institute of Child Health and Human Development, 3476
National Institute of Child Health and Human Development, 3909
National Institute of Child Health and Human Development, 6763
National Institute of Child Health and Human Development, 7011
National Institute of Child Health and Human Development, 8733
National Institute of Child Health and Human Development, 10261
National Institute of Diabetes & Digestive & Kidney Diseases, 4
National Institute of Diabetes & Digestive & Kidney Diseases, 5454
National Institute of Diabetes and Digestive Disorders, 9161
National Institute of Diabetes, Digestive & Kidney Diseases, 2886
National Institute of Diabetes, Digestive & Kidney Diseases, 3103

National Institute of Mental Health, 5905
National Institute of Neurological Disorders and Stroke, 1558
National Institute of Neurological Disorders and Stroke, 1796
National Institute of Neurological Disorders and Stroke, 6334
National Institute of Neurological Disorders and Stroke, 6852
National Institute of Neurological Disorders and Stroke, 7313
National Institute of Neurological Disorders and Stroke, 7912
National Institute of Neurological Disorders and Stroke, 8734
National Institute of Neurological Disorders and Stroke, 8845
National Institute of Neurological Disorders and Stroke (NINDS), 3697
National Institute of Neurological Disorde rs and Stroke, 7913
National Institute on Aging Information Center, 2007
National Institute on Deafness and other Communication Disorders, 4191
National Kidney Foundation of Maryland, 5491
National Kidney and Urologic Diseases Information Clearinghouse, 2008
National Kidney and Urologic Diseases Information Clearinghouse, 5174
National Library of Medicine, 303
National MS Society: Maryland Chapter Hunt Valley Business Center, 6368
National Organization of Parents of Blind Children, 9251
National Prevention Information Network CDC NPIN, 222
National Prevention Resource Center CSAP Division of Communications Programs, 8094
National Rehabilitation Information Center, 2565
National Rehabilitation Information Center, 10269
National Spinal Cord Injury Association: Metropolitan Washington Chapter, 7818
National Tuberous Sclerosis Association, 9093
National Volunteer Training Center for Sub CSAP Division of Communications Programs, 8097
National Volunteer Training Center for Substance Abuse Prevention, 8096
Neurofibromatosis, 6671
Neurofibromatosis: Mid-Atlantic, 6661
New York Obesity/Nutrition Research Center, 6704
Office of Applied Studies Substance Abuse & Mental Health Services, 8005
Office of Substance Abuse Prevention, 8006
Office of Women's Services Substance Abuse & Mental Health Services, 8007
Osteogenesis Imperfecta Foundation, 6764
Osteogenesis Imperfecta Foundation, 6769
PDQ, 2309
Parents Supporting Parents of MD, 5954
Parents of Children with Down Syndrome, 3480
Parkinson Support Groups of America, 6903
Pediatric Adolescent Gastroesophageal Reflux Association, 3796
Pediatric/Adolescent Gastroesophageal Reflux Association, 3588
Prince George's County Memorial Library: Talking Book Center, 9495
Pulmonary Hypertension Association, 4723
Pulmonary Hypertension Association, 4782
Pulmonary Hypertension Association, 5122
Pulmonary Hypertension Association, 5676
RADAR Network National Clearinghouse for Alcohol & Dru, 8099
SIDS Information and Referral Hotline, 8697
Schizophrenia Research Branch: Division of Clinical and Treatment Research, 6250
Services for the Visually Impaired, 9540
Sickle Cell Disease Association of America, 7450
Sjogren's Syndrome Foundation, 7486
Social Security Administration Office of Public Inquiries, 10281
Spina Bifida Association of Maryland, 7734
Spina Bifida Association of the Eastern Shore, 7735
St. Joseph's Medical Center, 3565

Substance Abuse and Mental Health Services Administration, 8014

Sudden Infant Death Syndrome Alliance, 8586

Sudden Infant Death Syndrome Institute of the University of Maryland, 8692

Telecommunications for the Deaf, 4196

Transplant Resource Center of Maryland, 8961

United Cerebral Palsy of Central Maryland, 2626

United Cerebral Palsy of Prince Georges & Montgomery Counties, 2627

United Cerebral Palsy of Southern Maryland, 2628

University of Maryland Center for Research, Grants & Contracts, 339

University of Maryland Center for Studies Family Studies Depatrment, 340

University of Maryland Center for Studies of Cerebrovascular Disease & Stroke, 7925

University of Maryland: Department of Pediatrics, 3472

University of Maryland: Medical Biotechnology Center, 341

Urban Cardiology Research Center, 4774

Urology Care Foundation, 5211

VA Capitol Health Care Network, 9990

VA Maryland Health Care System Perry Point VA Medical Center, 9991

Veterans Adm. Medical Center: Baltimore, 9992

Warren Grant Magnuson Clinical Center, 592

Warren Grant Magnuson Clinical Center, 1142

Warren Grant Magnuson Clinical Center, 2218

Warren Grant Magnuson Clinical Center, 3294

Warren Grant Magnuson Clinical Center, 4775

Warren Grant Magnuson Clinical Center, 5544

Warren Grant Magnuson Clinical Center, 5735

Warren Grant Magnuson Clinical Center National Institute of Health, 9611

Washington DC Metropolitan Area Brain Tumor Support Group, 1871

Washington Ear, 9262

Weight-Control Information Network National Institutes of Health, 3561

Weight-control Information Network, 6701

White Lung Association, 5678

Workplace Program CSAP Division of Communication Programs, 8015

Massachusetts

AARP Massachusetts State Office: Boston, 47

AIDS Support Group of Cape Cod, 374

ALS Association: Massachusetts Chapter, Wakefield Office, 998

Affiliated Children's Arthritis Centers of New England, 1127

Alzheimer's Association: Massachusetts Chapter, 731

Alzheimer's Association: Western Regional Office: Massachusetts Chapter, 732

Alzheimer's Disease Center: Boston University, 844

American Cancer Society: Boston, 2082

American Cancer Society: Central New England Region-Weston MA, 2083

American Diabetes Association: Boston, 3168

American Lung Association of Massachusetts, 5701

American Lung Association of Massachusetts, 9048

American Society of Adults with Pseudo-Obstruction, 3787

Arthritis Foundation: Massachusetts Chapter, 1098

Association of Gastrointestinal Motility D isorders, 3581

Asthma and Allergy Foundation of America: New England Chapter, 573

Asthma and Allergy Foundation of America: New England Chapter, 1269

Attention Deficit Information Network, 1499

Autism Society of Massachusetts, 1580

Autism Treatment Center of America, 1555

Autism Treatment Center of America: Son-Rise Program, 1556

Baystate Medical Center Wesson Memorial Unit, 3013

Berkshire Center, 10362

BermanGund Laboratory for the Study of Retinal Degenerations, 9580

Boston Hemophilia Center Fegan 5 Children's Hospital, 4876

Boston Sickle Cell Center Boston Medical Center, 7456

Boston University Arthritis Center, 1129

Boston University Cancer Research Center, 2219

Boston University Center for Human Genetics, 1727

Boston University Laboratory of Neuropsychology, 8078

Boston University Medical Campus General Clinical Research Center, 1130

Boston University University Medical Center, 7204

Boston University, Whitaker Cardiovascular Institute, 4728

Brain Injury Association of Massachusetts, 3963

Brain Injury Association of Massachusetts Helpline, 4026

Brain Tissue Resource Center McLean Hospital, 1802

Brain Tumor Patient and Caregiver Support Group, 1872

Brain Tumor Society, 1793

Brain Tumor Support Group: Lahey, 1873

Brain Tumor Support Group: Worcester, 1874

Brigham and Women's Hospital: Center for Neurologic Diseases, 6423

Brigham and Women's Hospital: Rheumatology Immunology, and Allergy Division, 1278

Brigham and Women's Orthopedica and Arthritis Center, 1131

CAPP National Parent Resource Center, 1718

CCFA New England Chapter: Massachusetts, 2905

California Center for Population Research, 5307

Cape Cod Chapter National Parkinson Foundation, 6877

Caption Center, 9496

Carroll Center for the Blind, 9314

Carroll Center for the Blind, 9587

Carroll Center for the Blind, 9618

Center for AIDS Research: Harvard Medical School, Division of AIDS, 342

Center for Blood Research Harvard Medical School/CBR, 343

Centers for AIDS Research: University of Massachusetts Medical School, 344

Childrens Hospital Immunology Division Children's Hospital, 1279

Childrens Hospital Medical Center Cystic Fibrosis Center, 3014

Client Assistance Program: Massachusetts, 10310

Cooley's Anemia Foundation (CAF): Massachusetts Chapter, 2851

Cystic Fibrosis Worldwide, 2973

Cystic Firbrosis Center: Tufts New England Medical Center, 3015

Dana Farber Cancer Institute National Drug Discovery Group for AIDS Treatment, 345

Dana-Farber Institute: Department of Biostatistics and Computational Biology, 2220

David H. Koch Institute for Integrative Ca ncer Research, 2221

Developmental Medicine Center (DMC), 3460

Developmental Medicine Center Children's Hospital Boston, 346

Division of Substance Abuse, 8040

Eaton-Peabody Laboratory of Auditory Physiology, 4234

Facioscapulohumeral Muscular Dystrophy Soc iety (FSH Society), 6515

Federation for Children with Special Needs, 1722

Federation for Children with Special Needs, 10235

Fertility and Women's Health Care Center, 5309

Framingham Heart Study, 4737

General Clinical Research Center at Beth Israel Hospital, 4738

Harris Center for Education and Advocacy in Eating Disorders, 3578

Harvard Clinical Nutrition Research Center, 6702

Harvard Cocaine Recovery Project, 8087

Harvard Throndike Laboratory Harvard Medical Center, 4741

Harvard University Howe Laboratory of Ophthalmology, 9595

Health Care For All, 10239

Hydrocephalus Foundation, 5063

Joslin Diabetes Center, 3277

Juvenile Diabetes Research Foundation: New England/Bay State Chapter, 3169

Laboure College Library, 9497

Lupus Foundation of America: Massachusetts Chapter, 5800

Macular Degeneration Foundation, 9222

Mass./New Hampshire Chapter of the Myasthenia Gravis Foundation of America, 6581

Mass./New Hampshire Chapter of the Myasthenia Gravis Foundation of America, 6587

Massachusetts Alliance for the Mentally Ill, 5955

Massachusetts Alzheimers Disease Research Center, 859

Massachusetts Chapter of the MG Foundation, 6582

Massachusetts Commission for the Blind, 9315

Massachusetts Department of Health HIV/AIDS Bureau, 267

Massachusetts Down Syndrome Congress, 3443

Massachusetts Eating Disorder Association, 3566

Massachusetts General Departments of Neurology and Neurosurgery, 7922

Massachusetts General Hospital, 3016

Massachusetts General Hospital: Harvard Cutaneous Biology Research Center, 7517

Massachusetts State Association of the Deaf, 4209

Massachusetts Sudden Infant Death Syndrome Boston City Hospital, 8690

Merrimack Valley HPV Support Group Holy Family Hospital, 10311

Myasthenia Gravis: Massachusetts Chapter, 6583

National Association for Parents of the Visually Impaired, 9224

National Association for Parents of the Visually Impaired, 9621

National Braille Press, 9235

National CFIDS Foundation, 2723

National Eating Disorders Screening Program, 3559

National Federation of the Blind: Massachusetts, 9316

National Kidney Foundation of MA/RI/NH/VT, 5492

National Kidney Foundation of MA/RI/NH/VT, 5499

National Kidney Foundation of MA/RI/NH/VT, 5518

National Kidney Foundation of MA/RI/NH/VT, 5532

National MS Society: Central New England Chapter, 6378

National MS Society: Massachusetts Chapter, 6369

National Parkinson Foundation:Cape Cod Chapter, 6878

National Scoliosis Foundation, 7245

National Spinal Cord Injury Association, 7834

National Spinal Cord Injury Association: Greater Boston Chapter, 7835

National Tay-Sachs and Allied Disease Association, 3699

National Tay-Sachs and Allied Diseases Association (NTSAD), 8736

National Tay-Sachs and Allied Diseases Association (NTSAD), 8737

National TaySachs & Allied Diseases, 8740

Neurofibromatosis: New England, 6662

Neurological Support Group of St. Luke's Hospital, 1875

Neurosurgical Service, 10312

New England AIDS Education & Training Center (NEHEC), 268

New England AIDS Education and Training Center, 224

New England Area Support Group: National Ataxia Foundation, 1434

New England Hemophilia Association, 4842

New England Medical Center: ALS Laboratory, 1031

New England Organ Bank Massachusetts, 8962

New England Region: Helen Keller National Center, 9317

New England Regional Genetics Group, 1733

Northeast Parkinson's and Caregivers, 6879

Option Institute, 2722

Option Institute, 3726

Option Institute, 6188

Option Institute International Learning & Training Center, 10275

Option Istitute Learning and Training Center, 5908

PALS Support Groups, 1749

Parent Education/Support Group, 1876

Parent Professional Advocacy League, 1726

Parent Professional Advocacy League, 6048
Pediatric Crohn's and Colitis Association, 2887
Pediatric Pulmonary Unit Massachusetts General Hospital, 8691
Perkins Braille and Talking Book Library, 9498
Persian Gulf Era Veterans, 9993
Prader-Willi New England Association, 7028
RESOLVE of the Bay State, 5276
Region 1 of the National Association for Parents of the Visually Impaired, 9318
Region I Office Program: Consultants for Maternal and Child Health, 8631
Rhode Island Hemophilia Foundation, 4861
SIDS Support Group, 8698
Safe Homes, 8012
Scleroderma Foundation, 7173
Scleroderma Foundation: New England Chapter, 7184
Scleroderma Foundation: New England Chapter, 7185
Scleroderma Foundation: New England Chapter, 7190
Scleroderma Foundation: New England Chapter, 7196
Scleroderma Foundation: New England Chapter, 7200
Scleroderma Support Groups, 7221
Screening For Mental Health, 6189
Shriver Center University Affiliated Program, 10131
Sleep Disorders Unit Beth Israel Deaconess Medical Center, 7656
Sleep Research Foundation, 7660
Society for Surgery of the Alimentary Tract, 3797
Southern New England Turner Syndrome Society, 9118
Spina Bifida Association of Massachusetts, 7736
Students Against Destructive Decisions, 8013
Talking Book Library at Worcester Public Library, 9499
Traditional Tibetan Healing, 6432
Tufts Medical Center, 4924
United Cerebral Palsy of Berkshire County, 2629
United Cerebral Palsy of MetroBoston, 2630
United Scleroderma Foundation, 7072
University of Massachusetts Memorial Medical Center, 3017
University of Massachusetts: Diabetes and Endocrinology Research Center, 3284
VA Boston Healthcare System: Jamaica Plain Jamaica Plain Campus, 9994
VA Boston Healthcare System: West Roxbury West Roxbury Campus, 9995
VA New England Health Care System, 9996
VALT Support Group (Vital Active Life After Trauma), 4027
Veterans Adm. Medical Center: Brockton Brockton Campus, 9997
Veterans Benefits Clearinghouse, 10132
Vision Use in Employment, 9629

Michigan

AARP Michigan State Office: Lansing, 48
ALS Association: Michigan Chapter, 999
ALS Association: West Michigan Chapter, 1000
Alzheimer's Association: East Central Michigan Chapter, 733
Alzheimer's Association: Greater Michigan Chapter, 734
Alzheimer's Association: Greater Michigan Chapter: Upper Peninsula Region, 735
Alzheimer's Association: Michigan Great Lakes Chapter: West Shore Region, 736
Alzheimer's Association: Mid-Michigan Chapter, 737
Alzheimer's Association: Northeast Michigan Chapter, 738
Alzheimer's Association: Northwest Michigan Chapter, 739
American Autoimmune Related Diseases Association, 183
American Autoimmune Related Diseases Association, 4777
American Autoimmune Related Diseases Association, 10199
American Diabetes Association: Michigan, 3170
American Institute for Preventive Medicine, 10204
American Institute for Preventive Medicine, 10205
American Liver Foundation Michigan Chapter, 5615
American Lung Association of Michigan, 5702

American Lung Association of Michigan, 9049
American Motility Society, 3782
Apnea Identification Program Children's Ho spital of Michigan, 8632
Arthritis Foundation: Michigan Chapter Chapter and Metro Detroit, 1099
Association for Children's Mental Health, 5956
Association for the Blind & Visually Impaired, 9319
Asthma and Allergy Foundation of America: Michigan Chapter, 574
Asthma and Allergy Foundation of America: Michigan Chapter, 1270
Autism Society of Michigan, 1581
Autoimmune Diseases Association, 5769
Brain Injury Association of Michigan, 3964
Brain Injury Association of Michigan Helpline, 4028
Brain Tumor Networking Club, 1877
Brain Tumor Support Group for Patients & Families, 1878
Brain Tumor Support Group: Ann Arbor, 1879
Brain Tumor Support Group: West Bloomfield, 1880
CCFA Michigan Chapter: Farmington Hills, 2906
Client Assistance Program: Michigan, 10313
Commission for the Blind, 10314
Council on Education of the Deaf College of Education, 4168
Detroit Subregional Library for the Blind and Physically Handicapped, 9500
Detroit Support Group: National Ataxia Foundation, 1435
Detroit VA Medical Center John D. Dingell VA Medical Center, 9998
Dynamic Rehab, 3939
East Lansing Cystic Fibrosis Center Michigan State University, 3018
Eastern Michigan Hemophilia Center St. Joseph Hospital, 4883
Genesee County Health Department, 8633
Gershenson Radiation Oncology Center Barbara Ann Karmanos Cancer Institute, 2222
Gilda's Club: Grand Rapids, 2297
Glaucoma Laser Trabeculoplasty Study Sinai Hospital of Detroit, 9593
Grand Traverse Area Library for the Blind and Physically Handicapped, 9501
Great Lakes Chapter of the Myasthenia Gravis Foundation of America, 6584
Greater Detroit Agency for the Blind and Visually Impaired, 9320
Greater Grand Rapids Pediatric Hemophilia Program, 4887
Hemophilia Foundation of Michigan, 4843
Henry Ford Hospital: Hypertension and Vascular Research Division, 5126
Hydrocephalus Support Group of Michigan Children's Hospital of Michigan, 5070
International Advocacy for Gulf War Syndrome, 9999
International Hearing Society, 4182
International Hearing Society, 4272
JIMHO Affiliated Centers (Justice in Mental Health Organization), 5957
Juvenile Diabetes Research Foundation: Metropolitan Detroit/SE Michigan, 3171
Juvenile Diabetes Research Foundation: Wes t Michigan Chapter, 3172
Kalamazoo Center for Medical Studies Michigan State University, 3019
Kent County Health Department, 8634
Kent County Library for the Blind, 9502
Leukemia and Lymphoma Society: Michigan Chapter, 2084
Library of Michigan Service for the Blind, 9503
Lupus Foundation of America: Michigan Lupus Foundation, 5801
Lyme Alliance, 8798
Macomb Library for the Blind and Physically Handicapped, 9504
Meyer L Prentis Comprehensive Cancer Cente Barbara Ann Karmanos Cancer Institute, 2224
Meyer L Prentis Comprehensive Cancer Center of Metropolitan Detroit, 2223
Michigan Alliance for the Mentally Ill, 5958
Michigan Alzheimer's Disease Research Center, 861
Michigan Chapter: Southeast, 9119
Michigan Deaf Association, 4210

Michigan Department of Community Health, 8635
Michigan Department of Community Health HIV/AIDS Prevention & Intervention Secti, 269
Michigan Hand Center, 2511
Michigan Kidney Foundation, 5493
Michigan State University Hemophilia Comprehensive Care Clinic, 4904
Midwestern Michigan Library Cooperative, 9505
Motor Neuron Disease Program University of Michigan Health System, 1029
Muskegon County Library for the Blind, 9506
Myasthenia Gravis Association, 6585
NF Support Group of West Michigan, 6669
National Federation of the Blind: Michigan, 9321
National MS Society: Michigan Chapter, 6370
Northland Library Cooperative, 9507
Oakland County Health Division: SIDS Project, 8636
Oakland County Library for the Visually and Physically Impaired, 9508
Office of Substance Abuse Services Department of Public Health, 8041
Oscar G. Johnson VA Medical Center, 10000
PRIDE Youth Programs, 8009
Patient Advocates for Advanced Cancer Treatments (PAACT), 2164
Prader-Willi Michigan Association, 7029
RESOLVE of Michigan, 5277
Rainbow Connection, 10526
Regional Hemophilia Treatment Center Children's Hospital of Michigan, 4914
Rehabilitation Institute of Michigan, 3998
SIDS LEAD: Children's Special Health Care Services, 8637
Scleroderma Foundation: Michigan Chapter, 7186
Spina Bifida Association of Grand Rapids, 7737
Spina Bifida Association of Upper Peninsula Michigan, 7738
Spina Bifida and Hydrocephalus Association of Southwestern Michigan, 7739
St. Clark County Library for the Blind and Physically Handicapped, 9509
Transplantation Society of Michigan, 8963
United Cerebral Palsy of Metropolitan Detroit, 2631
United Cerebral Palsy of Michigan, 2632
University of Michigan Communicative Disorders Clinic, 4259
University of Michigan Hemophilia Center, 4930
University of Michigan Michigan Gastrointestinal Peptide Research Ctr., 3809
University of Michigan Montgomery: John M. Sheldon Allergy Society, 590
University of Michigan Nephrology Division, 5542
University of Michigan Pulmonary and Critical Care Division, 4763
University of Michigan Reproductive Sciences Program, 5312
University of Michigan: Alcohol Research Center, 8109
University of Michigan: Cancer Center Cancer Research Committee, 2225
University of Michigan: Cardiovascular Med icine, 4764
University of Michigan: Cystic Fibrosis Center, 3020
University of Michigan: Division of Hypertension, 5129
University of Michigan: Kresge Hearing Research Institute, 4260
University of Michigan: Mental Health Research Institute, 6026
University of Michigan: National Cooperative Drug/AIDS Group, 347
University of Michigan: Orthopaedic Research Laboratories, 1141
University of Michigan: Psychiatric Center, 8110
Upper Peninsula Library for the Blind and Physically Handicapped, 9510
Veterans Adm. Medical Center: Ann Arbor Ann Arbor Healthcare System, 10001
Veterans Adm. Medical Center: Battle Creek, 10002
Veterans Adm. Medical Center: Saginaw Aleda E. Lutz VA Medical Center, 10003
Visually Impaired Center, 9610
Washtenaw County Library for the Blind and Physically Disabled, 9511

Wayne County Regional Library for the Blind and Physically Handicapped, 9512
Wayne State University Center for Health Research, 348
Wayne State University Center for Molecular Medicine and Genetics, 2226
Wayne State University: CS Mott Center for Human Growth and Development, 1739
Wayne State University: Comprehensive Sickle Cell Center, 7468
Wayne State University: Gurdjian-Lissner Biomechanics Laboratory, 3992
Wayne State University: University Women's Care, 5314
William T Gossett Parkinson's Disease Center, 6896

Minnesota

AARP Minnesota State Office: Saint Paul, 49
ALS Association: Minnesota Chapter, 1001
African American Family Services, 7972
Alzheimer's Association: Minnesota/Dakotas, 740
Alzheimer's Disease Center Mayo Clinic Mayo Medical School, 842
American Academy of Neurology, 6276
American Academy of Neurology: Tourette Syndrome, 8844
American Cancer Society: Duluth, 2085
American Cancer Society: Mendota Heights Mendota Heights, 2086
American Cancer Society: Rochester, 2087
American Cancer Society: Saint Cloud, 2088
American Diabetes Association: Minnesota, 3173
American Liver Foundation Minnesota Chapte r, 5616
American Lung Association of Minnesota, 5703
American Lung Association of Minnesota, 9050
American Pancreatic Association, 3783
Anna Westin Foundation, 3547
Arthritis Foundation: North Central Chapter, 1100
Autism Society of Minnesota, 1582
Behavioral Pediatrics Program, 10367
Brain Injury Alliance of Minnesota, 4029
Brain Injury Association of Minnesota, 3965
CCFA Minnesota Chapter, 2907
Center for Children with Chronic Illness and Disability, 10214
Chemical Dependency Program Division Department of Human Services, 8042
Dads and Daughters, 3549
Dentists Concerned for Dentists, 8043
Desert Storm Justice Foundation: Minnesota, 10004
Down Syndrome Association of Minnesota, 3444
Duluth Lighthouse for the Blind, 9322
Duluth Public Library, 9513
Emotional Health Anonymous, 6049
Fairview-University Hemophilia & Thrombosis Center, 4885
Fetal Alcohol Network, 10369
Hazelden, 7990
Hear Now: Starkey Hearin Foundation, 4176
Hemophilia Foundation of Minnesota and the Dakotas, 4844
Immunization Action Coalition, 5004
Impotence Information Center, 5178
International Diabetes Center at Nicollet, 3276
Juvenile Diabetes Research Foundation: Min nesota Chapter, 3174
KDWB Family Resource Center, 10373
KDWB Variety Family Canter, 10374
Lawyers Concerned for Lawyers, 7992
Leukemia and Lymphoma Society: Minnesota Chapter, 2089
LifeSource, Upper Midwest Organ Procurement Organization, Inc., 8964
Lupus Foundation of America: Minnesota Chapter, 5802
MN Chapter of the Turner Syndrome Society, 9120
Mayo Clinic and Foundation Mayo Foundation, 6512
Mayo Clinic and Foundation: Division of Allergic Diseases, 583
Mayo Clinic: Department of Neurology, 1027
Mayo Comprehensive Cancer Center, 2227
Mayo Comprehensive Hemophilia Center Mayo Clinic, 4902

Melpomene Institute for Women's Health Research, 5310
Minnesota AIDS Project AIDSLine, 385
Minnesota Alliance for the Mentally Ill, 5959
Minnesota Ambassador: National Ataxia Foundation, 1436
Minnesota Association for Children's Mental Health, 5960
Minnesota Department of Health: AIDS/STD Prevention Service, 270
Minnesota Disability Law Center, 10315
Minnesota Library for the Blind, 9514
Minnesota Obesity Center, 6703
Minnesota State Chapter of the Myasthenia Gravis Foundation of America, 6586
Minnesota Sudden Infant Death Center Minneapolis Children's Medical Center, 8638
Myasthenia Gravis Foundation, 6567
National Association of Blind Educators Sheila Koenig, 9227
National Association of Epilepsy Centers, 7312
National Association to Promote the Use of Braille, 9233
National Ataxia Foundation, 1412
National Federation of the Blind: Minnesota, 9323
National Kidney Foundation Serving Minneso ta, Dakotas & Iowa Division Office, 5520
National Kidney Foundation of Minnesota, 5494
National MS Society: Minnesota Chapter, 6371
National Marrow Donor Program, 2009
National Resource Library on Youth with Disabilities, 10363
Neurofibromatosis, 6639
Neurofibromatosis: Minnesota, 6663
PACER Center, 6050
Parkinson Association of Minnesota, 6880
Pediatric Psychology, 10381
Prader-Willi Minnesota Association, 7030
RESOLVE of Minnesota, 5278
STAR Center for Family Health, 10382
Schulze Diabetes Institute, 3264
Scleroderma Foundation: Minnesota Chapter, 7187
Spina Bifida Association of Minnesota, 7740
Spinal Cord Society, 7823
Twin Cities Area Support Group: National Ataxia Foundation, 1437
U Special Kids, 10383
United Cerebral Palsy of Central Minnesota, 2633
United Cerebral Palsy of Minnesota, 2634
United Ostomy Association, 2889
United Ostomy Association, 3800
United Ostomy Association, 9163
United Ostomy Associations of America Advocacy Hotline, 2311
University of Minnesota Department of Psychiatry, 6027
University of Minnesota Masonic Cancer Center, 2228
University of Minnesota: Cystic Fibrosis Center, 3021
University of Minnesota: Hypertensive Research Group, 5130
University of Minnesota: Program on Alcohol/Drug Control, 8111
Veterans Adm. Medical Center: Minneapolis Minneapolis VA Medical Center, 10005
Veterans Adm. Regional Office: St. Paul, 10006

Mississippi

Alzheimer's Association: Mississippi Chapter, 741
Alzheimer's Foundation of the South: Mississippi Division, 742
American Cancer Society: Jackson, 2090
American Diabetes Association: Mississippi, 3175
American Lung Association of Mississippi, 5704
American Lung Association of Mississippi, 9051
Arthritis Foundation: Mississippi Chapter, 1101
Brain Injury Association of Mississippi, 3966
Brain Injury Association of Mississippi Helpline, 4030
Christian Resource for People Who Are Blind, 9515
Division of Alcohol & Drug Abuse: Mississippi, 8044

Division of Alcohol & Drug Abuse: South Department of Mental Health, 8045
G.V Montgomery VA Medical Center, 10007
Leukemia and Lymphoma Society: Mississippi Chapter, 2091
Lupus Foundation of America: Mississippi Chapter, 5803
Mississippi Alliance for the Mentally Ill, 5961
Mississippi Area Support Group: National Ataxia Foundation, 1438
Mississippi Client Assistance Program, 10316
Mississippi Department of Public Health: STD/HIV Prevention Program, 271
Mississippi Families as Allies, 5962
Mississippi Hemophilia Foundation, 4845
Mississippi Industries for the Blind, 9324
Mississippi Library Commission, 9516
Mississippi Organ Recovery, 8965
Mississippi SIDS Alliance, 8639
Mississippi State Department of Health and Child Health Services, 8640
National Federation of the Blind: Mississippi, 9325
National Kidney Foundation of Mississippi, 5495
National Multiple Sclerosis Society: Alaba ma-Mississippi Chapter, 6372
South Central VA Health Care Network, 10008
University of Mississippi Medical Center, 3022
VA Gulf Coast Veterans Health Care System, 10009
Veterans Adm. Regional Office: Jackson, 10010

Missouri

AARP Missouri State Office: Kansas City, 50
ALS Association: Keith Worthington Chapter Central Missouri Branch Office, 1002
ALS Association: St. Louis Regional Chapter, 1003
APDA Center for Advanced Parkinson Disease Research, 6904
Adriene Resource Center for Blind Children, 9517
Alphapointe Association for the Blind, 9326
Alzheimer's Association: Mid-Missouri Chapter, 743
Alzheimer's Association: Northwest Missouri-Chapter, 744
Alzheimer's Association: Southwest Missouri Chapter, 745
Alzheimer's Association: St. Louis Chapter, 746
Alzheimer's Disease Research Center Washington University School of Medicine, 849
American Cancer Society: Saint Louis, 2092
American Diabetes Association: Missouri, 3176
American Liver Foundation Greater Kansas City Chapter, 5617
American Lung Association of Eastern Missouri, 5706
American Lung Association of Missouri, 9052
American Lung Association: Kansas City Office, 5707
American Optometric Association, 9196
Arthritis Foundation: Eastern Missouri Chapter, 1102
Assemblies of God National Center for the Blind, 9518
Asthma and Allergy Foundation of America: Greater Kansas City Chapter, 1271
Asthma and Allergy Foundation of America: St. Louis Chapter, 575
Asthma and Allergy Foundation of America: St. Louis Chapter, 1272
Autism Society of Gateway Chapter, 1583
Brain Cancer Support Group, 1881
Brain Injury Association of Missouri, 3967
Brain Injury Association of Missouri Helpline, 4031
Brain Tumor Support Group: Kansas City, 1882
Brain Tumor Support and Networking Group, 1883
CCFA Mid-America Chapter: Kansas, 2902
CCFA Mid-America Chapter: Missouri, 2908
Cancer Research Center, 2229
Canine Assistance for the Disabled CADI, 4164
Central Institute for the Deaf, 4229
Central Missouri Regional Arthritis Center Stephen's College Campus, 1132
Children's Mercy Hospital Children's Mercy Hospitals & Clinics, 3023
Church of the Nazarene, 9519
Fabry Support & Information Group, 3702

Montana

Nebraska

Nevada

New Hampshire

American Diabetes Association: New Hampshire, 3185

American Lung Association of New Hampshire, 5711

American Lung Association of New Hampshire, 9056

Arthritis Foundation: Northern New England Chapter, 1122

Autism Society of New Hampshire, 1586

Brain Injury Association of New Hampshire, 3969

Brain Injury Association of New Hampshire, 4033

Brain Injury/Brain Tumor Support Group, 1885

Camp Allen, 10364

Client Assistance Program: New Hampshire, 10322

Dartmouth Medical School: Microbiology Department, 3663

Dartmouth-Hitchcock Medical Center - Genetics and Development, 3458

Granite State FFCMH, 5970

High Hopes Foundation of New Hampshire, Inc., 10517

Juvenile Diabetes Research Foundation: New England/New Hampshire Chapter, 3186

National Alliance for the Mentally Ill: New Hampshire, 5971

National Alliance for the Mentally Ill: New Hampshire, 6054

National Federation of the Blind: New Hampshire, 9333

New Hampshire Cancer Pain Initiative, 2098

New Hampshire Chapter NSCIA, 7836

New Hampshire Cystic Fibrosis Care Teaching and Research Center, 3028

New Hampshire Department of Health and Human Services, 276

New Hampshire Lupus Foundation, 5809

New Hampshire SIDS Program, 8648

New Hampshire State Library, 9528

Norris Cotton Cancer Center Dartmouth-Hitchcock Medical Center, 2232

Northern New England Turner Society, 9123

Office of Alcohol and Drug Abuse Prevention, 8050

RESOLVE of New Hampshire, 5281

Sleep Disorders Center Dartmouth Hitchcock Medical Center, 7637

Sleep/Wake Disorders Center: Hampstead Hospital, 7665

Veterans Adm. Medical Center: Manchester Manchester VA Medical Center, 10020

Voices for the Blind, 9529

New Jersey

AARP New Jersey State Office: Princeton, 55

Alcohol Disease Foundation, 8076

All Access Mental Health, 5972

Alzheimer's Association: Greater New Jersey Chapter, 754

Alzheimer's Association: South Jersey Chapter, 755

American Anorexia Bulimia Association: New Jersey Chapter, 3567

American Auditory Society, 4155

American Cancer Society: New Jersey, 2099

American Council for Headache Education, 6277

American Diabetes Association: New Jersey, 3187

American Headache Society, 6278

American Lung Association of New Jersey, 5712

American Lung Association of New Jersey, 9057

American Society of Transplantation (AST), 8929

Angelwish, Inc., 10534

Arthritis Foundation: New Jersey Chapter, 1105

Asthma and Allergy Foundation of America: Southeast Pennsylvania Chapter, 1273

Asthma and Allergy Foundation of America: Southern Pennsylvania Chapter, 577

Autism Society of Southwest New Jersey, 1587

Bestwork Industries for the Blind, 9334

Brain Injury Alliance of New Jersey, 4034

Brain Injury Association of New Jersey, 3970

Brain Tumor Support Group: New Jersey, 1886

Brain Tumor Support Group: Toms River, 1887

CCFA New Jersey Chapter, 2909

CanHelp, 2100

Central New Jersey Brain Tumor Support Group, 1888

Christ Hospital Hepatitis C Support Group, 5009

Christopher & Dana Reeve Foundation Paralysis Resource Center, 7812

Community Mental Health Foundation, 5973

Congenital Heart Information Network, 2838

Cooley's Anemia Foundation (CAF): New Jersey Chapter, 2852

Department of Health, 8051

Disability Rights New Jersey, 10323

Division of Narcotic and Drug Abuse Control, 8052

Eating Disorders Association of New Jersey, 3584

Epilepsy Foundation of New Jersey, 7322

Friends Health Connection, 10371

Garden State Chapter of the Myasthenia Gravis Foundation of America, 6588

Garrett Mountain Chapter of the American Association of Kidney Patients, 5500

Greater New York Pull-Thru Network, 5212

HealthyWomen, 10365

Helping Other Parents in Normal Grief, 10548

Huxley Insititute-American Schizophrenic Association, 6247

Hydrocephalus Parents Support Group, 5075

Institute of Ophthalmology and Visual Scie nce New Jersey Medical School, 9599

Jason's Dreams for Kids Foundation, Inc., 10539

Juvenile Diabetes Research Foundation: Cen tral Jersey Chapter, 3189

Juvenile Diabetes Research Foundation: Mid -Jersey Chapter, 3190

Juvenile Diabetes Research Foundation: Roc kland County/Northern New Jersey, 3191

Juvenile Diabetes Research Foundation: South Jersey Chapter, 3188

Leukemia and Lymphoma Society: Northern New Jersey Chapter, 2101

Leukemia and Lymphoma Society: Southern New Jersey Chapter, 2102

Lupus Foundation of America: New Jersey Chapter, 5810

Lupus Foundation of America: South Jersey Chapter, 5811

Lyme Disease Network, 8799

Lyme Disease Network of New Jersey, 8801

Meadowlands Chapter of the American Association of Kidney Patients, 5501

Monmouth Medical Center: Cystic Fibrosis & Monmouth Medical Center, 3030

Monmouth Medical Center: Cystic Fibrosis & Pediatric Pulmonary Center, 3029

Multiple Sclerosis Association of America, 6332

Musculoskeletal Transplant Foundation, 8992

Nadeene Brunini Comprehensive Hemophilia Care Center, 4907

National Federation of the Blind: New Jersey, 9335

National MS Society: Greater North Jersey Chapter, 6379

National MS Society: Mid-Jersey Chapter, 6380

National Sarcoidosis Resource Center, 7082

National Women's Health Resource Center, 5306

National Women's Health Resource Center, 8770

National Womens Health Resource Center, 3662

Neuromuscular and ALS Center The Clinical Academic Building, 1030

New Eyes for the Needy, 9252

New Jersey Alliance for the Mentally Ill, 5974

New Jersey Department of Health: Child Health Program, 8649

New Jersey Department of Health: Division of AIDS Prevention & Control, 277

New Jersey Institute of Technology Center for Biomedical Engineering, 3915

New Jersey Library for the Blind and Handicapped, 9530

New Jersey Medical School, 3031

New Jersey Medical School: National Tuberculosis Center, 9025

New Jersey Metroplitan Turner Syndrome Society Association, 9124

New Jersey Parkinson's Disease Information Center, 6906

New Jersey Pregnancy Risk Information Service, 1748

New Jersey SIDS Alliance, 8650

New Jersey Woman AIDS Network, 278

Northern New Jersey Chapter of the American Association of Kidney Patients, 5502

Parent Project: Muscular Dystrophy, 6506

Parkinson Alliance, 6881

Prader-Willi New Jersey Association, 7033

RESOLVE of New Jersey, 5282

Recording for the Blind Helpline, 9628

Recording for the Blind and Dyslexic, 9255

Renfrew Center of Northern New Jersey, 3568

Rutgers University Center of Alcohol Studies, 8102

Rutgers University: Controlled Drug- Delivery Research Center, 8103

SIDS Center of New Jersey, 8651

Sarcoidosis Support Group: New Jersey, 7096

Seeing Eye, 9257

Sharing Network Organ Tissue Donation Services, 8969

Sleep Disorders Center: Newark Beth Israel Medical Center, 7651

Spina Bifida Association of the Tri-State Region, 7743

United Cerebral Palsy of Hudson County, 2640

United Cerebral Palsy of Morris-Somerset, 2641

United Cerebral Palsy of New Jersey, 2642

Veterans Adm. Medical Center: East Orange East Orange Campus, 10021

Veterans Adm. Medical Center: Lyons Lyons Campus, 10022

Well Spouse Association, 10385

Women's AIDS Network Women and Children's Service Program, 236

World Ostomy and Continence Nurses Society, 2890

New Mexico

AARP New Mexico State Office: Sante Fe, 56

ALS Association: New Mexico CIO, 1006

Alzheimer's Association: New Mexico Chapter, 756

American Cancer Society: New Mexico, 2103

American Diabetes Association: New Mexico, 3192

American Lung Association of New Mexico, 5713

Autism Society of New Mexico, 1588

Brain Injury Alliance of New Mexico, 4035

Brain Injury Association of New Mexico, 3971

Hemophilia Foundation of New Mexico, 4849

Juvenile Diabetes Research Foundation: Albuquerque, 3193

Leukemia and Lymphoma Society: Mountain States Chapter, 2104

Lovelace Medical Foundation, 5537

Lupus Foundation of America: New Mexico Chapter, 5812

National Federation of the Blind: New Mexico, 9336

National Kidney Foundation of New Mexico, 5503

National MS Society: Rio Grande Division, 6381

Navaho Nation K'E Project Children and Families Advocacy Corp, 5975

Navajo Nation K'E Project: Shiprock Children & Families Advocacy Corp, 5976

Navajo Nation Office Special Education & R ehabilitation Services, 6055

New Mexico Alliance for the Mentally Ill, 5977

New Mexico Branch, 9058

New Mexico Donor Services, 8970

New Mexico Health Department: Public Health Division, 279

New Mexico Industries for the Blind, 9337

New Mexico SIDS Information and Counseling Program, 8652

New Mexico State Library for the Blind and Physically Handicapped, 9531

Overeaters Anonymous World Service Office, 6699

People Living Through Cancer Support Groups, 1889

Protection and Advocacy System of Alburque rque, 10324

RESOLVE of New Mexico, 5283

Spina Bifida Association of New Mexico, 7744

State of New Mexico Commission for the Blind, 9338

Substance Abuse Bureau, 8053

Ted R Montoya Hemophilia Program University of New Mexico, 4920

University of New Mexico General Clinical Research Center, 3286

North Carolina

Sickle Cell Anemia Foundation, 7448
Spina Bifida Association of North Carolina, 7748
Triangle Area Sarcoidosis Support Group, 7098
UNC Cystic Fibrosis Center Department of
    Pediatrics, 3039
University of North Carolina Sarcoidosis Support
    Group, 7100
University of North Carolina UNC Lineberger
    Comprehensive Cancer Center, 2251
University of North Carolina at Chapel Hill Division
    of Speech & Hearing, 4262
Veterans Adm. Medical Center: Durham Durham VA
    Medical Center, 10040
Veterans Adm. Medical Center: Fayettville Fayettville
    VA Medical Center, 10041
Veterans Adm. Medical Center: Salisbury W.G.
    Hefner VA Medical Center, 10042
Wake Forest University: Arteriosclerosis Research
    Center, 5133
Wake Forest University: Cerebrovascular Research
    Center, 7927
Western Michigan University School of Medi cine,
    3040
Winston-Salem Industries for the Blind, 9348
Wrap Myself in a Rainbow Compassion Books,
    10554

North Dakota

AARP North Dakota State Office: Bismarck, 60
Alzheimer's Association: Fargo/Moorhead Regional
    Center, 770
American Cancer Society: North Dakota, 2121
American Diabetes Association: Nashville, 3207
American Diabetes Association: North Dakota, 3208
American Lung Association of North Dakota, 5716
American Lung Association of North Dakota, 9061
Autism Society of North Dakota, 1591
Brain Injury Association of North Dakota, 4040
Client Assistance Program: North Dakota, 10328
Division of Alcoholism & Drug Abuse: Department
    of Human Services, 8056
Fargo VA Healthcare System, 10043
Healthy Weight Network, 3553
MeritCare Children's Hospital Down Syndrome
    Outpatient Service, 3468
ND FFCMH Region II, 6058
ND Region V FFCMH Chapter-Federation of Fa
    milies for Children's Mental Health, 6059
ND Region VII FFCMH-Federation of Families for
    Children's Mental Health, 6060
National Federation of the Blind: North Dakota, 9349
National MS Society: Dakota Chapter, 6392
North Dakota Alliance for the Mentally Ill, 5982
North Dakota Association of the Deaf, 4213
North Dakota Comprehensive Hemophilia Center,
    4908
North Dakota FFCMH, 5983
North Dakota Hemostasis and Thrombosis Treatment
    Center, 4909
North Dakota SIDS Alliance, 8659
North Dakota SIDS Management Program, 8660
North Dakota State Library Services for the Disabled,
    9539
Prader-Willi North Dakota Association, 7036
St. Alexius Medical Heart and Lung Clinic, 3041

Ohio

1st Capital FFCMH, 5984
A Kid Again, 10504
AARP Ohio State Office: Columbus, 61
ALS Association: Northeast Ohio Chapter, 1009
ALS Association: Western Ohio Chapter, 1010
Alzheimer's Association: Canton Chapter, 771
Alzheimer's Association: Central Ohio Chapter, 772
Alzheimer's Association: Clark/Champaign, Miami
    Valley Chapter, 773
Alzheimer's Association: Cleveland Area Chapter,
    774
Alzheimer's Association: Greater Cincinnati Chapter,
    775

Alzheimer's Association: Greater East Ohio Chapter:
    Greater Youngstown Office, 776
Alzheimer's Association: Miami Valley Chapter, 777
Alzheimer's Association: Northwest Ohio Chapter,
    778
Alzheimer's Association: West Central Ohio Chapter,
    779
American Cancer Society: Ohio, 2122
American Diabetes Association: Ohio, 3209
American Lung Association of Ohio, 5717
American Lung Association of Ohio, 9062
American Sickle Cell Anemia, 7446
Arthritis Foundation: Central Ohio Chapter, 1111
Arthritis Foundation: Northeastern Ohio Chapter,
    1112
Arthritis Foundation: Ohio River Valley Chapter,
    1114
Arthritis Foundation; Great Lakes Region,
    Northeastern Ohio, 1115
Autism Society of Greater Cincinnati, 1592
Autism Society of Ohio Tri-County Chapter, 1593
Blick Clinic for Developmental Disabilities, 3454
Brain Injury Association of Ohio, 3975
Brain Injury Association of Ohio, 4041
Brain Tumor Support Group: Cincinnati, 1898
Bureau on Alcohol Abuse and Recovery Ohio
    Department of Health, 8057
Bureau on Drug Abuse: Ohio Department of Health,
    8058
CCFA Central Ohio Chapter, 2917
CCFA Northeast Ohio Chapter, 2918
CCFA Southwest Ohio Chapter, 2919
Case Western Reserve University, 9541
Case Western Reserve University: Bolton Brush
    Growth Study Center, 3913
Case Western Reserve University: Center on Aging
    and Health, 77
Case Western Reserve University: Cystic Fibrosis
    Center, 3042
Case Western Reserve University: Ireland Cancer
    Center, 2252
Center for ALS and Related Diorders The Cleveland
    Clinic DepartmentOf Neurol, 1025
Center for Research in Sleep Disorders Affiliated
    with Mercy Hospital, 7618
Center for Sleep & Wake Disorders: Miami Valley
    Hospital, 7619
Centers for AIDS Research: Case Western University,
    360
Central Ohio Chapter of the National Hemophilia
    Foundation, 4853
Central Ohio Support Group: National Ataxia
    Foundation, 1444
Chalmers P. Wylie VA Ambulatory Care Cente r,
    10044
Child & Adolescent Behavioral Health, 6061
Children's Hospital Hemophilia Treatment Center,
    4878
Children's Hospital Research Foundation, 2253
Cincinnati Association for the Blind, 9350
Cincinnati HPV Support Group: PP of Cincin nati,
    10329
Cleveland Clinic Lerner Research Institute, 4731
Cleveland Hearing and Speech Center, 4232
Cleveland Sight Center, 9351
Cleveland Skilled Industries, 9352
Clinical Research Center: Pediatrics Children's
    Hospital Research Foundation, 5625
Clovernook Center for the Blind and Visually
    Impaired, 9589
Columbus Center of the National Multiple Sclerosis
    Society, 6393
Columbus Children's Hospital: Cystic Fibrosis
    Center, 3043
Columbus Children's Research Institute, 580
Comprehensive Sickle Cell Center Children's
    Hospital Research Foundation, 7458
Congenital Heart Disease Anomalies Support,
    Education & Resources CHASER, 4733
Disability Rights Center at Ohio Legal Rights
    Service, 10330
District Board of Health: Mahoning County, 8661
Division Of Developmental and Behavioral
    Pediatrics, 1730

Down Syndrome Association of Greater Cinci nnati,
    3446
Down Syndrome Association of Greater Cinci nnati,
    3477
FES Information Center WO Walker Industrial
    Rehabilitation Cent, 7814
First Ohio Chapter: FFCMH, 6062
JamesCare For Life Support Groups & Services, 2303
Jane and Richard Thomas Center for Down
    Syndrome, 3464
Juvenile Diabetes Research Foundation/JDRF, 3210
Juvenile Diabetes Research Foundation: Akr
    on/Canton Chapter, 3212
Juvenile Diabetes Research Foundation: Gre ater
    Cincinnati Chapter, 3213
Juvenile Diabetes Research Foundation: Mid-Ohio
    Chapter, 3211
Juvenile Diabetes Research Foundation: Tol
    edo/Northwest Ohio Chapter, 3214
Kettering-Scott Magnetic Resonance Laboratory,
    8090
Leukemia and Lymphoma Society: Central Ohio
    Chapter, 2123
Leukemia and Lymphoma Society: Northern Ohio
    Chapter, 2124
Leukemia and Lymphoma Society: Southern Ohio
    Chapter, 2125
Lewis H Walker MD: Cystic Fibrosis Center, 3044
Life Connection of Ohio, 8976
LifeBanc, 8977
Lifeline of Ohio Organ Procurement Agency, Inc.,
    8978
Lupus Foundation of America: Greater Ohio Chapter,
    5823
Mahoning-Shenango Chapter of the Myasthenia
    Gravis Foundation of America, 6594
Medical College of Toledo: Cancer Research
    Division, 2254
Miami Valley Ohio Chapter of the American
    Association of Kidney Patients, 5511
Mitral Valve Prolapse Program of Cincinnati Support
    Group, 4779
National Association of Blind Office Professionals,
    9230
National Federation of the Blind: Ohio, 9353
National Kidney Foundation of Ohio, 5512
National MS Soceity: Western Ohio Chapter The
    Woolpert Building, 6394
National MS Society: Northeast Ohio Chapter, 6396
National MS Society: Northwest Ohio Chapter, 6397
National MS Society: Southwestern Ohio/Northern
    Kentucky, 6395
National Reye's Syndrome Foundation, 5633
North East Ohio Support Group National Ataxia
    Foundation, 1445
Northern Ohio Chapter of the National Hemophilia
    Foundation, 4854
Northwest Ohio Hemophilia Association, 4855
Northwest Ohio Hemophilia Treatment Center, 4911
Northwest Ohio Sleep Disorders Center Toledo
    Hospital, 7628
Ohio Alliance for the Mentally Ill, 5985
Ohio Ambassador: National Ataxia Foundation, 1446
Ohio Chapter of the Myasthenia Gravis Foundation of
    America, 6595
Ohio Department of Health, 8662
Ohio Department of Health: Division of Preventive
    Medicine, 282
Ohio Regional Library for the Blind and Physically
    Handicapped, 9542
Ohio Sleep Medicine Institute, 7629
Ohio State University Clinical Pharmacology
    Division, 8098
Ohio State University Comprehensive Cancer Center,
    2255
Ohio State University General Clinical Research
    Center, 2256
Ohio State University Laboratory of Psychobiology,
    3997
Ohio State University Neuroscience Program, 864
Ohio State University Otological Research
    Laboratories, 4240
Ohio University Therapy Associates: Hearing, Speech
    and Language Clinic, 4241
Ohio Valley LifeCenter, 8979

Pediatric Pulmonary Center The Children's Medical Center of Dayton, 3045
Persian Gulf War Veterans of Western Pennsylvania, W Virginia and NE Ohio, 10045
Prader-Willi Ohio Association, 7037
RESOLVE of Ohio, 5288
Rainbow Alliance of the Deaf, 4193
Richland County HPV Support Group, 10331
SIDS Network of Ohio, 8663
Scleroderma Foundation: Ohio Chapter, 7193
Sleep Disorders Center Bethesda Oak Hospital, 7635
Sleep Disorders Center Ohio State University Medical Center, 7639
Sleep Disorders Center: Cleveland Clinic Foundation, 7645
Sleep Disorders Center: Kettering Medical Center, 7649
Sleep Disorders Center: St. Vincent Medical Center, 7653
Southwest Ohio Brain Tumor Support Group, 1899
Southwestern Ohio Chapter of the National Hemophilia Foundation, 4856
Special Wish Foundation, 10527
Spina Bifida Association of Canton, 7749
Spina Bifida Association of Central Ohio, 7750
Spina Bifida Association of Cincinnati, 7751
Spina Bifida Association of Greater Dayton, 7752
Spina Bifida Association of Northwest Ohio, 7753
State Library of Ohio Talking Book Program, 9543
Support Group for Parents of Children with Brain Tumors, 1900
Technology Resource Center, 10332
The Cancer Prevention Institute, 2257
Turner Syndrome Chapter of Ohio, 9128
United Cerebral Palsy of Central Ohio, 2658
United Cerebral Palsy of Cincinnati, 2659
United Cerebral Palsy of Greater Cleveland, 2660
United Cerebral Palsy of Greater Dane, 2661
University Alzheimer Center UHC: Case Western Reserve University, 869
University Treatment Center of University Hospitals of Cleveland, 4928
University of Cincinnati Adult Hemophilia Treatment Program, 4929
University of Cincinnati College of Medicine Division of Pediatrics, 3046
University of Cincinnati Department of Pathology & Laboratory Medicine, 4761
VA Healthcare System Of Ohio, 10046
Veterans Adm. Medical Center: Chillicothe Chillicothe VA Medical Center, 10047
Veterans Adm. Medical Center: Cincinnati Cincinnati VA Medical Center, 10048
Veterans Adm. Medical Center: Cleveland Louis Stokes VA Medical Center, 10049
Veterans Adm. Medical Center: Dayton Dayton VA Medical Center, 10050
Veterans and Families Support Network Ohio, 10051
West Central Ohio Hemophilia Center Childens Medical Center, 4932
World Hypertension League, 5068

Oklahoma

AARP Oklahoma State Office: Edmond, 62
Alzheimer's Association: Oklahoma Chapter, 780
American Association of Kidney Patients: Tulsa Chapter, 5513
American Cancer Society: Oklahoma, 2126
American Diabetes Association: Oklahoma, 3215
American Lung Association of Oklahoma, 5718
American Lung Association of Oklahoma, 9063
American Veterans Justice Foundation, 10052
Arthritis Foundation: Oklahoma Chapter, 1116
Autism Society of Central Oklahoma, 1594
Brain Injury Association of Oklahoma, 3976
Brain Injury Association of Oklahoma Helpl ine, 4042
CCFA Oklahoma Chapter, 2920
Client Assistance Program: Oklahoma Office of Handicapped Concerns, 10333
Dean A McGee Eye Institute, 9590
Jack C. Montgomery VA Medical Center, 10053

Juvenile Diabetes Research Foundation: Cen tral Oklahoma Chapter, 3216
Juvenile Diabetes Research Foundation: Tul sa Green County Chapter, 3217
Leukemia and Lymphoma Society: Oklahoma Chapter, 2127
Myasthenia Gravis Support Group, 6607
Natalie Warren Bryant Cancer Center St. Francis Hospital, 2258
National Federation of the Blind: Oklahoma, 9354
National Kidney Foundation of Oklahoma, 5514
National MS Society: Oklahoma Chapter, 6398
Neuroscience Institute at Mercy Hospital, 6674
Oklahoma Alliance for the Mentally Ill, 5986
Oklahoma Ambassador: National Ataxia Foundation, 1447
Oklahoma Association of the Deaf, 4214
Oklahoma Chapter of the Myasthenia Gravis Foundation of America, 6596
Oklahoma Chapter of the National Hemophilia Foundation, 4857
Oklahoma City HPV Support Group: PP of Cen tral Oklahoma, 10334
Oklahoma Comprehensive Hemophilia Diagnostic Treatment Center, 4912
Oklahoma Department of Health: AIDS Division, 283
Oklahoma Department of Mental Health and Substance Abuse Services, 8059
Oklahoma League for the Blind, 9355
Oklahoma Library for the Blind and Physically Handicapped, 9544
Oklahoma Lupus Association, 5824
Oklahoma Medical Research Foundation, 1138
Oklahoma Medical Research Foundation Immunobiolgy & Cancer Research, 2259
Oklahoma Medical Research Foundation: Cardiovascular Research Program, 4750
Oklahoma Organ Sharing Network, 8980
Oklahoma State Department of Health: Maternal and Child Health Services, 8664
Parkinson Foundation of the Heartland Oklahoma Branch, 6884
Prader-Willi Oklahoma Association, 7038
RESOLVE of Oklahoma, 5289
Samuel Roberts Noble Foundation Biomedical Division, 2260
Tulsa City: County Library System, 9545
Tulsa Unified FFCMH, 5987
Turner Syndrome Chapter of Oklahoma, 9129
United Cerebral Palsy of Oklahoma, 2662
University of California Northern Comprehensive Sickle Cell Center, 7465
University of Oklahoma: Cystic Fibrosis Center, 3047
University of Oklahoma: Health Sciences Ce nter, 4263
Veterans Adm. Medical Center: Oklahoma City, 10054

Oregon

AARP Oregon State Office: Clackamas, 63
ALS Association: Oregon & SW Washington CIO, 1011
ALS Association: Oregon & SW Washington CIO, 1020
Aging and Alzheimer's Disease Center Oregon Health Sciences University, 839
Alzheimer's Association: Cascade/Coast Chapter, 782
Alzheimer's Association: Columbia-Willamet Chapter, 781
Alzheimer's Association: Mary's Peak Chapter, 783
Alzheimer's Association: Mid-Willamette Chapter, 784
American Cancer Society: Oregon, 2128
American Diabetes Association: Oregon, 3218
American Lung Association of Oregon, 5719
American Lung Association of Oregon, 9064
American Tinnitus Association, 4159
Asthma and Allergy Foundation of America: Oregon Chapter, 576
Asthma and Allergy Foundation of America: Oregon Chapter, 1274
Autism Society of Oregon, 1595
Blind Enterprises of Oregon, 9356

Brain Injury Alliance of Oregon, 4043
Brain Injury Association of Oregon, 3977
Brain Tumor Education & Support Group, 1901
Cascade AIDS Project Hotline, 379
Center for Health Research, 10219
Central Oregon Brain Tumor Support Group, 1902
Child Center, 10222
Comprehensive Stroke Center of Oregon University of Oregon Health Sciences Cen, 7919
Dogs for the Deaf, 4173
Fanconi Anemia Research Foundation, 2847
Hemophilia Foundation of Oregon, 4858
Juvenile Diabetes Research Foundation: Ore gon/SW Washington Chapter, 3219
Leukemia and Lymphoma Society: Oregon Chapter, 2129
NAMI-Oregon, 5988
NNFF Oregon Affiliate Kaiser Permanente Northwest, 6665
National Consortium on Deaf-Blindness, 4188
National Federation of the Blind: Oregon, 9357
National MS Society: Oregon Chapter, 6399
National Psoriasis Foundation, 7513
Northwest Network, 10055
Northwest Vets for Peace, 10056
Office of Alcohol and Drug Abuse Programs, 8060
Oregon Association of the Deaf, 4215
Oregon Department of Human Resources Health Division HIV Program, 284
Oregon Department of Human Services, 8665
Oregon Family Support Network, 5989
Oregon Health & Science University, 3048
Oregon Health Sciences University, 6912
Oregon Health Sciences University Oregon Hearing Research Center Tinnitus Clinic, 4242
Oregon Health Sciences University: Elk's Children's Eye Clinic, 9604
Oregon State Library, 9546
Pacific NW Transplant Bank, 8981
Parkinsons Resources of Oregon, 6885
Prader-Willi Oregon Association, 7039
Psoriasis Research Institute, 7519
RESOLVE of Oregon, 5290
Regional Resource Center on Deafness Western Oregon State College, 4243
Resources for Seniors and People with Disabilities, 10335
Scleroderma Foundation: Oregon Chapter, 7194
United Cerebral Palsy of Oregon & SW Washington, 2663
Veterans Adm. Medical Center: Roseburg VA Roseburg Healthcare System, 10057
Veterans Adm. Medical Center: White City VA S Oregon Rehabilitation Center, 10058
Veterans Adm. Regional Office: Portland Portland VA Medical Center, 10059
Veterans Administration Domicillary, 10060
Willamette Valley Support Group: National Ataxia Foundation, 1448

Pennsylvania

AARP Pennsylvania State Office: Harrisburg, 64
AIDS Library of Philadelphia, 302
ALS Association: Greater Philadelphia Chapter, 1012
ALS Association: Western Pennsylvania Chapter, 1013
ALS Clinic at Penn Neurological Institute ALS Association Greater Philadelphia Cha, 1023
Abramson Cancer Center of the University of Pennsylvania, 2261
Adult Congenital Heart Association, 2837
Albert Einstein Medical Center Hemophilia Program, 4874
Allegheny Singer Research Institute West Penn Allegheny Health System, 2262
Alzheimer's Association: Delaware Valley Chapter, 785
Alzheimer's Association: Greater Mid-Ohio, 787
Alzheimer's Association: Greater Pennsylvania Chapter: SW Regional Office, 786
Alzheimer's Association: Laurel Mountains Chapter, 788

Alzheimer's Association: Northeast Pennsylvania Chapter, 789

Alzheimer's Association: Northwest Pennsylvania Chapter, 790

Alzheimer's Association: South Central Pennsylvania Chapter, 791

Alzheimer's Disease Center Pennsylvania University School of Medicine, 843

American Anorexia Bulimia Association of Philadelphia, 3571

American Cancer Society: Harrisburg Capital Area Unit, 2130

American Cancer Society: Philadelphia, 2131

American Cancer Society: Pittsburgh, 2132

American Diabetes Association: Pennsylvania, 3220

American Diabetes Association: Western Pennsylvania, 3221

American Liver Foundation Delaware Valley Chapter, 5620

American Liver Foundation Western Pennsylvania, 5621

American Lung Association of Pennsylvania, 9065

American Respiratory Alliance of Western Pennsylvania, 5720

Arthritis Foundation: Central Pennsylvania Chapter, 1117

Associated Services for the Blind, 9199

Association for the Blind & Visually Impaired of Lehigh County, 9358

Association of Hydrocephalus Education Advocacy & Discussion (AHEAD), 5060

Autism Society of Greater Harrisburg, 1596

Beaver County Association for the Blind, 9359

Bockus Research Institute Graduate Hospital, 4727

Brain Injury Association of Pennsylvania, 3978

Brain Tumor Community Group, 1903

Brain Tumor Support Group: Johnstown, 1904

Brain Tumor Support Group: Philadelphia, 1905

Brain Tumor Support Group: Pittsburgh, 1906

Breathe Pennsylvania, 5721

Burger King Cancer Caring Center, 1989

CCFA Philadelphia/Delaware Valley Chapter, 2921

CCFA Western Pennsylvania/West Virginia Chapter, 2922

Cambria County Association for the Blind and Handicapped, 9360

Carnegie Library of Pittsburgh, 9547

Center for Organ Recovery & Education, 8982

Centers for AIDS Research: University of Pennsylvania, 361

Chemical People Project Public Television Outreach Alliance, 7984

Chester County Association for the Blind, 9361

Children of Aging Parents, 86

Children's Hospital of Philadelphia, 3456

Childrens Hospital of Philadelphia Hemophilia Program, 4879

Client Assistance Program: Philadelphia, 10336

Cystic Fibrosis Center: Polyclinic Medical Center, 3049

Delaware County Branch of the Pennsylvania Association for the Blind, 9362

Delaware Valley Chapter of the National Hemophilia Foundation, 4859

Delware Valley Brain Tumor Support Group at Jefferson, 1907

Department of Reproductive Genetics: Magee Women's Hospital, 1729

Diabetes Education and Research Center The Franklin House, 3269

Dial-a-Hearing Screening Test, 4271

Down Syndrome Center of Western Pennsylvania, 3461

Dr. Gertrude A Barber National Institute, 3463

Dream Come True, 10511

Drug and Alcohol Programs Department Of Health, 8061

Eastern Cooperative Oncology Group, 2263

Epilepsy Foundation of Western Pennsylvania, 7324

Erie VA Medical Center, 10061

Foundation for Children with AIDS, 203

Foundation for Dignity, 1997

Fox Chase Cancer Center, 2264

Free Library of Philadelphia, 9548

Geisinger Wyoming Valley Medical Center: Sleep Disorders Center, 7621

Gift of Life Donor Program Pennsylvania, 8983

Greater Wilkes-Barre Association for the Blind, 9363

Hahnemann University Hospital, Orthopedic Wellness Center, 1134

Hahnemann University Laboratory of Human Pharmacology, 8086

Hahnemann University Likoff Cardiovascular Institute, 4740

Hahnemann University Lupus Study Center Hahnemann University Medical Center, 5846

Hahnemann University, Krancer Center for Inflammatory Bowel Disease Research, 2930

Hahnemann University: Division of Surgical Research, 5125

Hemophilia Center of Central Pennsylvania Penn State Milton S Hershey Medical Cent, 4892

Hepatitis B Foundation, 5007

Hepatitis B Foundation, 10183

Hopes & Dreams Foundation, Inc., 10518

Hospital of the University of Pennsylvania, 7921

Hospital of the University of Pennsylvania University of Pennsylvania, 6511

Hydrocephalus Association of Philadelphia, 5071

Hysterectomy Educational Resources & Services (HERS) Foundation, 3658

Hysterectomy Educational Resources & Services (HERS) Foundation, 5253

Independent Visually Impaired Enterprises, 9217

Indiana County Association for the Blind, 9364

Intestinal Disease Foundation, 5207

Juvenile Diabetes Research Foundation: Ber ks County Chapter, 3223

Juvenile Diabetes Research Foundation: Central Pennsylvania Chapter, 3222

Juvenile Diabetes Research Foundation: Nor thwestern Pennsylvania Chapter, 3224

Juvenile Diabetes Research Foundation: Phi ladelphia Chapter, 3225

Juvenile Diabetes Research Foundation: Wes tern Pennsylvania, 3226

Keystone Blind Association, 9365

Lancaster County Association for the Blind, 9366

Learning Disabilities Association of America, 1495

Learning Disabilities Association of America, 10243

Lehigh Valley Chapter of the American Association of Kidney Patients, 5515

Lehigh Valley Sickle Cell Support Group, 7470

Leukemia and Lymphoma Society: Central Pennsylvania Chapter, 2133

Leukemia and Lymphoma Society: Eastern Pennsylvania Chapter, 2134

Leukemia and Lymphoma Society: Western Pennsylvania/West Virginia Chapter, 2135

Lupus Foundation of America: Central Pennsylvania Chapter, 5825

Lupus Foundation of America: Northeast Pennsylvania Chapter, 5826

Lupus Foundation of America: Northwestern Pennsylvania Chapter, 5827

Lupus Foundation of America: Western Pennsylvania Chapter, 5828

Lupus Foundation of Philadelphia, 5829

Lysosomal Disease Center at the University of Pittsburgh, 3700

MedEscort International ABE International Airport, 10248

Medical College of Pennsylvania Center for the Mature Woman, 6794

Medical College of Pennsylvania: Eastern Psychiatric Institute, 6020

Montgomery County Association for the Blind, 9367

Myasthenia Gravis Association of Western Pennsylvania, 6597

National Federation of the Blind: Pennsylvania, 9368

National Kidney Foundation of Delaware Valley, 5516

National Kidney Foundation of Western Pennsylvania, 5517

National MS Society: Central Pennsylvania Chapter, 6400

National MS Society: Greater Delaware Valley Chapter, 6401

National Mental Health Consumer's Self-Help Clearinghouse, 6014

National Mental Health Consumers' Self- Help Clearinghouse, 6015

National Organization for Hearing Research, 4192

National Tay-Sachs Association: Delaware Valley (NTSAD-DV), 8739

National Transplant Assistance Fund (NTAF), 8937

North American Society for Pediatric Gastroenterology and Nutrition, 3795

North American Society for Pediatric Gastroenterology, Hepatology & Nutrition, 10270

North Central Sight Services, 9369

Parents Involved Network, 5990

Parkinson Chapter of Greater Pittsburgh, 6886

Parkinson Council, 6887

Pediatric Cancer Foundation of the Lehigh Valley, 1908

Pediatric Pulmonary and Cystic Fibrosis Center, 3050

Penn Center for Sleep Disorders: Hospital of the University of Pennsylvania, 7630

Pennsylvania Alliance for the Mentally Ill, 5991

Pennsylvania Chapter of the Myasthenia Gravis Foundation of America, 6598

Pennsylvania Department of Health Bureau of Family Health, 8666

Pennsylvania Department of Health: Bureau of HIV/AIDS, 285

Pennsylvania Educational Network for Eating Disorders, 3572

Pennsylvania Gulf War Veterans, 10062

Pennsylvania State University Artificial Heart Research Project, 4751

Philadelphia Biomedical Research Institute, 7461

Philadelphia Department of Public Health: AIDS Program, 286

Philadelphia Turner Syndrom Society, 9130

Pittsburgh Vision Services, 9370

Prader-Willi Pennsylvania Association, 7040

Pregnancy Healthline: Pennsylvania Hospital, 1750

Pregnancy Safety Hotline, 1752

Presbyterian-University Hospital: Pulmonary Sleep Evaluation Center, 7631

RESOLVE of Philadelphia, 5291

RESOLVE of Pittsburgh, 5292

RESOLVE of Southcentral Pennsylvania, 5293

Recorded Periodicals, 9627

Renfrew Center of Bryn Mawr, 3573

Renfrew Center of Philadelphia, 3574

SIDS of Pennsylvania, 8667

SW Pennsylvania Turner Syndrome Support Gr oup, 9131

Sarcoidosis Treatment and Research Center Thomas Jefferson University Hospital, 7084

Scleroderma Foundation: Western Pennsylvania Chapter, 7195

Shriners Hospital for Children, 7839

Sickle Cell Disease Association of America Philadelphia/Delaware Valley Chapter, 7473

Sleep Disorders Center Lankenau Hospital, 7638

Sleep Disorders Center: Community Medical Center, 7646

Sleep Disorders Center: Crozer-Chester Medical Center, 7647

Sleep Disorders Center: Good Samaritan Medical Center, 7648

Sleep Disorders Center: Medical College of Pennsylvania, 7650

Sleep and Chronobiology Center: Western Psychiatric Institute and Clinic, 7662

Somerset County Blind Center, 9371

Spina Bifida Association of Central Pennsylvania, 7754

Spina Bifida Association of Delaware Valley, 7755

Spina Bifida Association of Greater Pennsylvania, 7756

Spinal Cord Injury Program at Harmarville Rehabilitation Center, 7840

Sunshine Foundation National Headquarters, 10529

Temple University Clinical Research Center Office of Clinical Research, 362

Temple University FELS Institute for Cancer Research, 2265

Temple University Speech and Hearing Science Laboratories, 4252

Temple University: Section of Auditory Research, 4253

Thomas Jefferson University Hospital, 7212

Thomas Jefferson University Ischemia-Shock, 4000

Thomas Jefferson University Ischemia-Shock Research Center, 3999

Thomas Jefferson University: Sleep Disorders Center, 7667

Thomas Jefferson University: Cardenza Foundation for Hematologic Research, 4923

Thomas Jefferson University: Center for Research in Medical Education, 363

Thomas Jefferson University: Daniel Baugh Institute, 1735

ToughLove International, 8126

Tri-County Association for the Blind, 9372

Understanding Sarcoidosis Self-Help Group, 7099

United Cerebral Palsy Central PA, 2664

United Cerebral Palsy of Beaver, Butler & Lawrence Counties, 2665

United Cerebral Palsy of Northwestern Pennsylvania, 2666

United Cerebral Palsy of Pennsylvania, 2667

United Cerebral Palsy of Philadelphia Vicinity, 2668

United Cerebral Palsy of Pittsburgh, 2669

United Cerebral Palsy of South Central Pennsylvania, 2670

United Cerebral Palsy of Southern Alleghenies Region, 2671

United Cerebral Palsy of Southwestern Pennsylvania, 2672

United Cerebral Palsy of Western Pennsylvania, 2673

University of Pennsylvania Diabetes and Endocrinology Research Center, 3287

University of Pennsylvania Institute on Aging, 84

University of Pennsylvania Muscle Institut e, 4766

University of Pennsylvania: Depression Research Unit, 6190

University of Pennsylvania: Harrison Department of Surgical Research, 3810

University of Pennsylvania: Penn Lung Center, 3051

University of Pittsburgh, 6913

University of Pittsburgh, 7216

University of Pittsburgh Cancer Institute, 2266

University of Pittsburgh Cystic Fibrosis Center: Children's Hospital, 3052

University of Pittsburgh: Department of Molecular Genetics and Biochemistry, 3288

University of Pittsburgh: Human Energy Research Laboratory, 4767

University of Pittsburgh: Western Psychiatric Institute & Clinic, 6029

VA Pittsburgh Healthcare System: University Drive Division, 10063

VA Stars & Stripes Healthcare Network, 10064

VIABL Services of Northampton County, 9373

Veterans Adm. Medical Center: Philadelphia, 10065

Veterans Adm. Medical Center: Coatesville, 10066

Veterans Adm. Medical Center: Lebanon Lebanon VA Medical Center, 10067

Veterans Adm. Medical Center: Pittsburg VA Pittsburgh Healthcare System, 10068

WFS' New Life Program, 8127

WM Krogman Center for Research in Child Growth and Development, 3916

Washington-Greene County Branch for the Pennsylvania Association for Blind, 9374

Western Pennsylvania Chapter of the National Hemophilia Foundation, 4860

Wilkes-Barre VA Medical Center, 10069

York Industries for the Blind: Division of York County Blind Center, 9375

Rhode Island

Alzheimer's Association: Rhode Island Chapter, 792

American Cancer Society: Rhode Island, 2136

American Diabetes Association: Rhode Island, 3227

American Lung Association of Rhode Island, 5722

American Narcolepsy Association, 7607

Autism Society of Rhode Island, 1597

Brain Injury Association of Rhode Island, 3979

Brain Injury Association of Rhode Island H elpline, 4044

Brain Tumor Support Group: Providence, 1909

Brown University Division of Biology and Medicine, 2267

Center for Alcohol & Addiction Studies Brown University, 8079

Centers for AIDS Research: Brown University, 364

Children's Neurodevelopment Center, 3457

Division of Substance Abuse: Department of Mental Health and Hospitals, 8062

Hemophilia Center of Rhode Island Rhode Island Hospital, 4893

Hydrocephalus Association of Rhode Island, 5072

IN-SIGHT, 9376

Leukemia and Lymphoma Society: Rhode Island Chapter, 2137

Lupus Foundation of America: Rhode Island Chapter, 5830

Narcolepsy Network, 7670

National Alliance for the Mentally Ill of Rhode Island (NAMI), 5992

National Federation of the Blind: Rhode Island, 9377

National MS Society: Rhode Island Chapter, 6402

Parent Support Network of Rhode Island, 6063

RESOLVE of the Ocean State, 5294

Rhode Island Association of the Deaf, 4216

Rhode Island Brain & Spine Tumor Foundation, 1910

Rhode Island Department of Health, 8668

Rhode Island Department of Health: Division of Disease Prevention & Control, 287

Rhode Island Department of State Library for the Blind and Physically Handicapped, 9549

Rhode Island Disability Law Center, 10337

Rhode Island Hospital: Cystic Fibrosis Center, 3053

Rhode Island Scleroderma Support Group, 7220

Rhode Island Turner Syndrome Society, 9132

Roger Williams Clinical Cancer Research Center, 2268

Sleep Disorders Center: Rhode Island Hospital, 7652

Spina Bifida Association of Rhode Island, 7757

United Cerebral Palsy of Rhode Island, 2674

Veterans Adm. Medical Center: Providence Providence VA Medical Center, 10070

South Carolina

AARP South Carolina Office: Columbia, 65

Agromedicine Program Medical University of South Carolina, 7514

Alzheimer's Association: Low Country Chapter, 793

Alzheimer's Association: Mid-State South Carolina Chapter, 794

Alzheimer's Association: Upstate South Carolina Chapter, 795

American Cancer Society: South Carolina, 2138

American Diabetes Association: South Carolina, 3228

American Lung Association of South Carolina, 5723

American Lung Association of South Carolina, 9066

Autism Society of South Carolina, 1598

Brain Injury Association of South Carolina, 3980

Brain Tumor Support Group: Charleston, 1911

Brain Tumor Support Group: Florence, 1912

Carolinas Support Group: National Ataxia National Ataxia Foundation, 1449

Center for Developmental Disabilities University of South Carolina, 10216

Center for Disability Resources, 10217

Children's Center for Cancer and Blood Disorders, 2269

Division of Perinatal Systems Mills Jarret Complex, 8669

Federation of Families of South Carolina, 6064

Hemophilia Association of South Carolina, 4862

Interdisciplinary Program in Cell and Molecular Pharmacology, 8088

James R Clark Memorial Sickle Cell Foundation, 7452

Juvenile Diabetes Research Foundation: Low Country Chapter, 3230

Juvenile Diabetes Research Foundation: Palmetto Chapter, 3229

Leukemia and Lymphoma Society: South Carolina Chapter, 2139

Leukemia and Lymphoma Society: South/West, 2140

Lupus Foundation of America: South Carolina Chapter, 5831

Lyme Disease Network of South Carolina, 8802

Medical University of South Carolina, 1135

Medical University of South Carolina Health Services Administration, 365

Medical University of South Carolina Medical University of South Carolina, 7209

Medical University of South Carolina: Cystic Fibrosis Center, 3054

Medical University of South Carolina: Division of Rheumatology & Immunology, 1136

NAMI-SC: National Alliance on Mental Illness: South Carolina, 5993

NNFF South Carolina Chapter, 6666

National Association for Continence, 5208

National Federation of the Blind: South Carolina, 9378

National Kidney Foundation of South Carolina, 5519

National MS Society: South Carolina Branch, 6403

Prader-Willi South Carolina Association, 7041

RESOLVE of South Carolina, 5295

Ralph H. Johnson VA Medical Center, 10071

Richland Memorial Comprehensive Pediatric Hemophilia Center, 4915

Scleroderma Foundation: South Carolina Chapter, 7197

South Carolina Commission on Alcohol and Drug Abuse, 8063

South Carolina Department of Health & Environmental Control, 288

South Carolina Palmetto Turner Syndrome So ciety, 9133

South Carolina Protection & Advocacy System for the Handicapped, 10338

South Carolina State Library, 9550

Tri County HPV Support Group, 10339

William Jennings Bryan Dorn VA Medical Center, 10072

South Dakota

American Cancer Society: South Dakota, 2141

American Lung Association of South Dakota, 5724

American Lung Association of South Dakota, 9067

Autism Society of Black Hills, 1599

Cancer Support Group, 1913

Division of Alcohol & Drug Abuse: South Dakota, 8064

Juvenile Diabetes Research Foundation: Sio ux Falls Chapter, 3231

NAMI South Dakota, 5994

National Federation of the Blind: South Dakota, 9379

Parkinson Association of South Dakota, 6888

Sioux Falls VA Healthcare System, 10073

South Dakota Advocacy Services, 10340

South Dakota Department of Health, 8670

South Dakota State Library, 9551

Teratogen and Birth Defects Information Project, 1754

VA Black Hills Health Care System- Fort Meade Campus, 10074

VA Black Hills Health Care System- Hot Springs Campus, 10075

Tennessee

AARP Tennessee State Office: Nashville, 66

ALS Association: Middle Tennessee Chapter, 1015

Alzheimer's Association: Eastern Tennessee Chapter, 796

Alzheimer's Association: Highland Rim Chapter, 797

Alzheimer's Association: Memphis Area Office, 798

Alzheimer's Association: Middle Tennessee Chapter, 799

Alzheimer's Association: Northeast Tennessee Chapter, 800

Alzheimer's Association: Southeast Tennessee Chapter, 801

American Cancer Society: Tennessee, 2142

American Diabetes Association: Nashville, 3232

American Diabetes Association: Tennessee, 3233

American Liver Foundation Midsouth Chapter, 5622

Texas

Kent Waldrep National Paralysis Foundation Main Office, 7817
Kidd's Kids, 10519
LAUNCH Department of Special Education, 10242
Leukemia and Lymphoma Society: North Texas Chapter, 2145
Leukemia and Lymphoma Society: South/West Texas Chapter, 2146
Leukemia and Lymphoma Society: Texas Gulf Coast Chapter, 2147
Lighthouse for the Blind of Houston, 9387
Lighthouse of the Blind of Fort Worth, 9388
Lone Star Chapter of the American Association of Kidney Patients, 5526
Lone Star Chapter of the National Hemophilia Foundation, 4864
Lupus Foundation of America: North Texas Chapter, 5835
Lupus Foundation of America: South Central Texas Chapter, 5836
Lupus Foundation of America: Texas Gulf Coast Chapter, 5837
Lupus Foundation of America: West Texas Chapter, 5838
Mended Hearts, 4778
Menninger Clinic: Department of Research, 6021
Methodist Hospital Sleep Center Winona Memorial Hospital, 7626
Michael E. DeBakey VA Medical Center, 10091
Mothers Against Drunk Driving (MADD), 7994
National Association of Blind Students Angela Wolf, 9231
National Federation of the Blind: Texas, 9389
National Kidney Foundation of North Texas, 5527
National Kidney Foundation of Southeast Texas, 5528
National Kidney Foundation of Texas, 5529
National Kidney Foundation of West Texas, 5523
National Kidney Foundation of the Texas Coastal Bend, 5530
National MS Society: North Central Texas Chapter, 6407
National MS Society: Panhandle Chapter, 6408
National MS Society: Southern Texas, 6409
National MS Society: West Texas Division, 6410
National MS Socisty: Southeast Texas Chapter, 6411
National Ovarian Cancer Coalition, 2010
Neuromuscular Treatment Center: Univ. of Texas Southwestern Medical Center, 6426
North Texas Comprehensive Pediatric Hemophilia Center, 4910
North Texas FFCMH, 5997
North Texas Support Group: National Ataxia Foundation, 1451
Northwest Texas Chapter of the Myasthenia Gravis Foundation of America, 6601
Operation Desert Shield/Desert Storm, 10092
Persian Gulf Veterans of America, 10093
Prader-Willi Texas Association, 7043
Presbyterian Hospital of Dallas, 6914
RESOLVE of Central Texas, 5297
RESOLVE of Dallas/Fort Worth, 5298
RESOLVE of Houston, 5299
RESOLVE of South Texas, 5300
RRTC on Community Integration of Persons with TBI, 3973
Region VI Office Program Consultants for Maternal and Child Health, 8676
Rio Grande Chapter: NSCIA Rio Vista Rehabilitation Hospital, 7841
Roy M and Phyllis Gough Huffington Center on Aging, 83
San Antonio Bexar County FFCMH, 5998
San Antonio Cancer Institute, 2274
Santa Rosa Medical Center, 3470
Scleroderma Foundation: Bluebonnet Chapter, 7199
Sickle Cell Anemia Association of Austin: Marc Thomas Chapter, 7472
Sickle Cell Association of the Texas Gulf Coast, 7464
Sleep Medicine Associates of Texas, 7659
South Texas Brain Tumor Foundation Support Group, 1920
South Texas Lighthouse for the Blind, 9390
South Texas Veterans Health Care System, 10094
SouthWestern Medical Center, 4917
Southwest Foundation for Biomedical Research, 2275

Southwest SIDS Research Institute, 8677
Spina Bifida Association of Austin, 7759
Spina Bifida Association of Dallas, 7760
Spina Bifida Association of Texas, Gulf Coast, 7761
Stroke Clubs International, 7930
Taping for the Blind, 9259
Texas Alliance for the Mentally Ill, 5999
Texas Ambassador: National Ataxia Foundation, 1452
Texas Association of Retinitis Pigmentosa, 9391
Texas Association of the Deaf, 4217
Texas Association on Mental Retardation, 3449
Texas Central Chapter of the National Hemophilia Foundation, 4865
Texas Children's Allergy and Immunology Clinic, 587
Texas Childrens Cystic Fibrosis Care Center, 3060
Texas Commission on Alcohol and Drug Abuse Department Of State Health, 8066
Texas Department of Health: Bureau of HIV and STD Prevention, 292
Texas FFCMH, 6000
Texas Heart Institute St Lukes Episcopal Hospital, 4757
Texas Mining and Reclamation Association, 5909
Texas Neurofibromatosis Foundation, 6675
Texas State Library, 9555
Texas State Library: Talking Book Program, 9556
Texas Tech University Tarbox Parkinson's Disease Institute, 6894
The Alzheimer's Disease & Memory Disorders Center, 866
Travis Association for the Blind, 9392
Tri-Services Military Cystic Fibrosis Center, 3061
Turner Syndrome Society Resource Center, 9137
Turner's Syndrome Society, 9134
Turner's Syndrome Society of Texas, 9135
Turner's Syndrome Society of the United States, 9109
United Cerebral Palsy of Greater Houston, 2677
United Cerebral Palsy of Metropolitan Dallas, 2678
United Cerebral Palsy of Tarrant County, 2679
United Cerebral Palsy of Texas, 2680
University of Texas General Clinical Research Center, 3290
University of Texas HSC at San Antonio, 6915
University of Texas Health Science Center, 7218
University of Texas Health Science Center Neurophysiology Research Center, 8114
University of Texas Mental Health Clinical Research Center, 6191
University of Texas Sleep/Wake Disorders Center, 7668
University of Texas Southwestern Medical, 5628
University of Texas Southwestern Medical Center, 5627
University of Texas Southwestern Medical Center at Dallas, 591
University of Texas Southwestern Medical Center at Dallas, 4771
University of Texas Southwestern Medical Center/Sickle Cell Management, 7467
University of Texas at Austin: Drug Synamics Institute, 8115
University of Texas at Dallas Callier Center for Communication Disorders, 4264
University of Texas: MD Anderson Cancer Center, 2276
University of Texas: Medical Branch at Galveston Cancer Center, 2277
University of Texas: Southwestern Medical Center at Dallas, Immunodermatology, 7526
VA Data Processing Center, 9917
VA Heart of Texas Health Care Network Dallas VA Medical Center, 10095
VIVA!, 7852
Veterans Adm. Medical Center: Big Spring, 10096
Veterans Adm. Medical Center: Dallas, 10097
Veterans Adm. Medical Center: Kerrville, 10098
Veterans Adm. Medical Center: Marlin, 10099
Veterans Adm. Medical Center: San Antonio, 10100
Veterans Adm. Medical Center: Temple, 10101
Waco VA Medical Center, 10102
West Texas Lighthouse for the Blind, 9393
West Texas VA Health Care System, 10103

Utah

AARP Utah State Office: Midvale, 68
Allies with Families, 6067
Alzheimer's Association: Utah Chapter, 815
American Cancer Society: Utah, 2148
American Diabetes Association: Utah, 3242
American Lung Association of Utah, 5727
American Lung Association of Utah, 9070
Arthritis Foundation: Utah/Idaho Chapter, 1121
Brain Injury Alliance of Utah, 4046
Brain Injury Association of Utah, 3983
Brigham Young University Cancer Research Center, 2278
Cancer Wellness House, 1921
Department of Social Services: Division of Substance Abuse, 8067
Huntsman Cancer Institute University of Utah School of Medicine, 2279
Intermountain Donor Services, 8986
Legal Center for People with Disabilities, 10344
Lupus Foundation of America Utah Chapter, 5839
National Clearinghouse of Rehabilitation Training Materials, 10254
National Federation of the Blind: Utah, 9394
National Kidney Foundation of Utah, 5531
National MS Society: Utah State Chapter, 6412
Prader-Willi Utah Association, 7044
Pregnancy Risk Line, 1751
RESOLVE of Utah, 5301
United Cerebral Palsy of Utah, 2681
University of Utah Intermountain Cystic Fibrosis Center, 3062
University of Utah Rocky Mountain Center for Occupational & Environmental Health, 5734
University of Utah Utah Genome Depot University of Utah, 6514
University of Utah: Artificial Heart Research Laboratory, 4772
University of Utah: Cardiovascular Genetic Research Clinic, 4773
University of Utah: Center for Human Toxicology, 8116
Utah Alliance for the Mentally Ill, 6001
Utah Chapter of the National Hemophilia Foundation, 4866
Utah Department of Health, 8678
Utah Department of Health: Bureau of Communicable Disease Control, 293
Utah Industries for the Blind, 9395
Utah SIDS Alliance, 8679
Utah State Intermountain Chapter of the Myasthenia Gravis Foundation of America, 6602
Utah State Library Division, 9557
Utah Support Group: National Ataxia Foundation, 1453
VA Salt Lake City Health Care System, 10104
Veterans Affairs Medical Center: Research Service, 3293

Vermont

AARP Vermont State Office: Montpelier, 69
ALS Clinical Department of Neurology, 1024
Alcohol and Drug Abuse Programs of Vermont Department Of Health, 8068
Alzheimer's Association: Vermont Chapter, 816
American Cancer Society: Vermont, 2149
American Diabetes Association: Vermont, 3243
American Lung Association of Vermont, 9071
Autism Society of Vermont Autism Society of America, 1602
Brain Injury Association of Vermont, 3984
Brain Injury Association of Vermont Helpli ne, 4047
Citizen Advocacy of Burlington, 10345
Client Assistance Program: Vermont Ladd Hall, 10346
Lupus Foundation of America: Vermont Chapter, 5840
Medical Center Hospital of Vermont Cystic Fibrosis Center, 3063
National Federation of the Blind: Vermont, 9396
National MS Society: Vermont Division, 6413

RESOLVE of Vermont, 5302
University of Vermont Cancer Center University of Vermont, 2280
University of Vermont: Office of Health Promotion Research, 368
Vermont Alliance for the Mentally Ill, 6002
Vermont Department of Health: Health Surveillance HIV/AIDS/STD/TB Program, 294
Vermont Department of Health: SIDS Information and Counseling Program, 8680
Vermont Department of Libraries Special Services Unit, 9558
Vermont FFCMH, 6003
Vermont FFCMH, 6068
Vermont Pregnancy Risk Information Service, 1757
Vermont Regional Hemophilia Center, 4931
White River Junction VA Medical Center, 10105

Virginia

AABA Support Group, 3579
AARP Virginia State Office: Richmond, 70
ACB Radio Amateurs, 9186
Al-Anon Alateen Family Group Hotline, 8118
Al-Anon Family Group Headquarters, 7973
Alateen Al-Anon Family Group Headquarters, 7974
Allergy & Asthma Network Mothers of Asthmatics, 557
Allergy & Asthma Network Mothers of Asthmatics, 1259
Allergy & Asthma Networks Hotline, 1287
Alzheimer's Association: Central Virginia Chapter, 817
Alzheimer's Association: Greater Richmond Chapter, 818
Alzheimer's Association: National Capital Area Chapter, 819
Alzheimer's Association: Piedmont-Valley Area Chapter, 820
Alzheimer's Association: Roanoke Salem Chapter, 821
Alzheimer's Association: Southeastern Virginia Chapter, 822
Alzheimer's Association: Southside Virginia Chapter, 823
American Academy of Audiology, 4152
American Academy of Otolaryngology: Head, 4153
American Association for the Study of Liver Diseases, 5604
American Cancer Society: Virginia, 2150
American Council of the Blind, 9192
American Counseling Association, 6179
American Counseling Association, 10202
American Diabetes Association, 3098
American Diabetes Association National Center, 3296
American Diabetes Association: Richmond, 3244
American Diabetes Association: Virginia, 3245
American Lung Association of Virginia, 5728
American Lung Association of Virginia, 9072
American Psychiatric Association, 5890
American Psychiatric Association, 6180
American Rehabilitation Counseling Association, 10208
American Thyroid Association, 8769
Arlin J Brown Information Center, 2151
Arlington County Department of Libraries, 9559
Arthritis Foundation: Virginia Chapter, 1123
Asbestos Information Association/North America, 10211
Assoc. for Education & Rehabilitation of the Blind & Visually Impaired, 9198
Association of Organ Procurement Organizations (AOPO), 8930
Auditory-Verbal International, 4161
Autism Society of Northern Virginia, 1603
Brain Injury Association, 3938
Brain Injury Association of America's National Family Helpline, 3985
Brain Injury Association of Virginia, 3986
Brain Injury Association of Virginia Helpline, 4048
Brain Tumor Support Group: Richmond, 1922
CAPCOM, 4163
CCFA Greater Washington DC/Virginia Chapter, 2926

Cancer Research Foundation of America, 2281
Central Rappahannock Regional Library, 9560
Cerebral Palsy of Virginia, 2682
Children's Hospice International, 10223
Children's Hospice International, 10544
Childrens Hospice International, 10368
Childrens Hospice International, 10545
Council for Exceptional Children, 1493
Council for Exceptional Children, 9206
Desert Storm Justice Foundation: Virginia, 10106
Division for the Visually Handicapped, 9561
Donate Life America, 8932
Down Syndrome Association of Hampton Roads, 3450
Eastern Virginia Medical School Children's Hospital of The King's Daught, 3064
Fairfax County Public Library, 9562
Food Allergy and Anaphylaxis Network, 567
Gulf War Veterans of Virginia, 10107
Hampton Subregional Library for the Blind, 9563
Hemophilia Association of the Capital Area, 4867
International Brain Injury Association, 3942
International Council on Infertility Information Dissemination, 5254
International Society for the Study of Dissociation, 6244
Juvenile Diabetes Research Foundation: Gre ater Blue Ridge Chapter, 3246
Keon Paschal Perry Sickle Cell Anemia Disease Awareness, 7469
Kids Incorporated, 10520
Leukemia and Lymphoma Society: National Capital Area Chapter, 2152
Library Users of America, 9219
LifeNet, 8987
Lupus Foundation of America: Eastern Virginia Chapter, 5841
Mental Health America, 5898
Mental Health America Resource Center, 5899
Migraine Awareness Group: A National Understanding for Migraineurs, 6281
Myasthenia Gravis Support Group: Virginia/ West Virginia, 6610
Myositis Association, 1077
National Alliance On Mental Illness, 6184
National Alliance for the Mentally Ill, 5901
National Alliance for the Mentally Ill, 6246
National Alliance of Blind Students, 9223
National Association of Alcoholism and Drug Abuse Counselors, 7998
National Association of State Directors of Veterans Affairs, 9980
National Association of State Mental Health Program Directors, 5902
National Captioning Institute, 4186
National Chronic Pain Outreach Association, 10253
National Crime Prevention Council, 8002
National Federation of the Blind: Virginia, 9397
National Fibromyalgia Partnership (NFP), 3723
National Hospice & Palliative Care Organiz ation, 10551
National Hospice & Palliative Care Organization, 10550
National Hospice & Palliative Care Organization (NHPCO), 219
National Hospice & Palliative Care Organization (NHPCO), 2006
National Hospice Helpline, 2308
National Hospice Helpline, 10557
National Industries for the Blind, 9249
National Kidney Foundation of Virginia, 5533
National MS Society: Blue Ridge Chapter, 6414
National MS Society: Central Virginia Chapter, 6415
National MS Society: Hampton Roads Chapter, 6416
National Mental Health Association, 6186
National Mental Health Information Center, 6187
National Women's Health Information Center, 3560
Newport News Public Library System, 9564
Old Dominion Area Chapter: NSCIA, 7842
Organ Procurement and Transplantation Network (OPTN), 8938
PACCT, 6069
PACCT of Roanoke Valley, 6070
Parkinson Foundation of the National Capitol Area, 6889

RESOLVE Helpline, 3668
RESOLVE of Alabama, 5256
RESOLVE of the Washington Metro Area, 5265
RESOLVE: The National Infertility Association, 5255
Registry of Interpreters for the Deaf, 4194
Richmond HPV Support Group: Fan Free Clini c, 10347
Richmond Support Group, 3589
Roanoke City Public Library System, 9565
SIDS Mid-Atlantic, 8681
Sarcoidosis Self-Help Group: Virginia, 7094
Scleroderma Foundation: Greater Washington DC Chapter, 7180
Scleroderma Foundation: Greater Washington DC Chapter, 7201
Sickle Cell Anemia Research Foundation, 7463
Speech Simulation Research Foundation, 4248
Substance Abuse Services Office of Virginia, 8069
United Network for Organ Sharing (UNOS), 8939
United Virginia Chapter of the National Hemophilia Foundation, 4868
University Library Services, 9567
University of Virginia School of Medicine Cystic Fibrosis Center, 3065
University of Virginia: General Clinical Research Center, 1285
University of Virginia: Hypertension and Atherosclerosis Unit, 5132
Valley Brain Tumor Support Group, 1923
Veterans Adm. Medical Center: Hampton Hampton VA Medical Center, 10108
Veterans Adm. Medical Center: Richmond Hunter Holmes McGuire VA Medical Center, 10109
Veterans Adm. Medical Center: Roanoke Roanoke Vet Center, 10110
Veterans Adm. Medical Center: Salem Salem VA Medical Center, 10111
Virginia Alliance for the Mentally Ill, 6004
Virginia Association of the Deaf, 4218
Virginia Beach Public Library, 9568
Virginia Chapter of the Myasthenia Gravis Foundation of America, 6603
Virginia Commonwealth University: Massey Cancer Center, 2282
Virginia Commonwealth University: Rehab Research and Training Center, 4006
Virginia Department of Health: Division of HIV, STD, and Pharmacy Services, 295
Virginia Industries for the Blind, 9398
Virginia Office for Protection and Advocacy, 10348
Virginia SIDS Alliance, 8682
Virginia SIDS Program: Virginia Department of Health, 8683
Washington Regional Transplant Consortium, 8988
World Federation for Mental Health, 5911

Washington

AARP Washington State Office: Seattle, 71
ALS Association: Evergreen Chapter, 1019
Alzheimer's Association Autopsy Assistance Network, 875
Alzheimer's Association: Inland Northwest Chapter, 824
Alzheimer's Association: Western & Central Washington Chapter, 825
Alzheimer's Disease Center: Washington University, 848
American Cancer Society: Washington, 2153
American Diabetes Association: Seattle, 3247
American Diabetes Association: Washington, 3248
American Liver Foundation Pacific Northwest Chapter, 5623
American Lung Association of Washington, 5729
Arthritis Foundation: Washington/Alaska Chapter, 1124
Asthma and Allergy Foundation of America: Washington State Chapter, 579
Autism Society of Washington, 1604
BABES Network-YWCA, 377
Benaroya Research Institute Virginia Mason Medical Center, 3268
Bleeding Disorder Foundation of Washington, 4869
Brain Cancer Support Group: Port Orchard, 1924

Brain Cancer Support Group: Seattle, 1925
Brain Injury Association of Washington, 3987
Brain Injury Association of Washington Hel pline, 4049
Brain Injury Resource Center, 4050
CCFA Washington State Chapter, 2927
Cancer Information Service, 2289
Centers for AIDS Research: University of Washington, Harborview Medical Center, 369
Children's Hydrocephalus Support Group, 5074
Common Voice for Pierce County Parents, 6071
Dunshee House, 380
Epilepsy Foundation of North West Washington, 7325
Fred Hutchinson Cancer Research Center, 2283
Gluten Intolerance Group: GIG, 2529
HIV Prevention Trials Unit University of Washington/Seattle HPTU Si, 370
Health Information Network, 206
Health Information Network for Women and AIDS, 207
Hepatitis Education Project, 5008
Hepatitis Education Project, 5010
Hope Heart Institute, 4744
Inland Empire Bleeding Disorders, 4870
International Association for the Study of Pain, 2804
Juvenile Diabetes Research Foundation: Sea ttle Chapter, 3250
Juvenile Diabetes Research Foundation: Seattle Guild, 3249
Juvenile Diabetes Research Foundation: Spo kane County Area Chapter, 3251
King County Crisis Clinic, 384
LifeCenter Northwest, 8989
Lighthouse for the Blind of Washington, 9399
Lupus Foundation of America: Pacific Northwest Chapter, 5842
Mental Illness Research and Education Institute, 6022
Multifaith Works, 214
NAMI Washington (National Alliance for the Mentally Ill of Washington), 6005
National Association for Native American Children of Alcoholics, 7997
National Eating Disorders Association, 3558
National Federation of the Blind: Public Employees Division, 9246
National MS Society: Greater Washington Chapter, 6417
National MS Society: Inland Northwest Chapter, 6418
National Service Dog Center, 9625
Northwest AIDS Education and Training Center (AETC), 296
Northwestern Region: Helen Keller National Center, 9400
Pacific NW Support Group, 7090
Pacific Northwest Chapter of the Myasthenia Gravis Foundation of America, 6604
Persian Gulf Veterans of Washington, 10112
Prader-Willi Washington Association, 7045
Puget Sound Blood Center, 4913
Region X Office Program Consultants for Maternal and Child Health, 8684
SIDS Foundation of Washington, 8685
SIDS Northwest Regional Center, 8686
Scleroderma Foundation: Evergreen Chapter, 7202
Seattle HPV Support Group, 10349
Seattle Support Group: National Ataxia Foundation, 1454
Solomon Park Research Institute, 1032
Spina Bifida Association of Washington State, 7762
United Cerebral Palsy of Pierce County, 2683
University of Washington, 6916
University of Washington Department of Speech & Hearing Sciences, 4265
University of Washington Diabetes: Endocrinology Research Center, 3291
University of Washington: Cystic Fibrosis Center, 3066
University of Washington: Experimental Education Unit, 3473
VA Puget Sound Health Care Network, 10113
Veterans Adm. Medical Center: Spokane Spokane VA Medical Center, 10114
Veterans Adm. Medical Center: Tacoma Tacoma Vet Center, 10115

Veterans Adm. Medical Center: Walla Walla Johnathan M. Wainwright Memorial VA MC, 10116
Virginia Mason Brain Tumor Support Group, 1926
Virginia Mason Medical Center Neuroscience Institute, 1034
Washington Ambassador National Ataxia Foundation, 1455
Washington Department of Health: Division of HIV/AIDS Prevention Services, 297
Washington Department of Social and Health Services, Alcohol and Drug Prog., 8070
Washington FFCMH, 6006
Washington Leukemia and Lymphoma Society: Alaska Chapter, 2154
Washington Puget Sound Turner Syndrome Society, 9136
Washington State Client Assistance Program, 10350
Washington State Department of Services for the Blind, 9401
Washington Talking Book & Braille Library, 9569
Wenatchee Valley Brain Tumor Support Group, 1927
Wishing Star Foundation, 10532

West Virginia

AARP West Virginia Office: Charleston, 72
AFB Technology & Employment Center, 9402
Alzheimer's Association: Greater Mid-Ohio Valley Chapter, 826
Alzheimer's Association: N Central West Virginia Chapter, 827
Alzheimer's Association: South West Virginia Chapter, 828
American Cancer Society: West Virginia, 2155
American Diabetes Association: West Virginia, 3252
American Lung Association of West Virginia, 5730
American Lung Association of West Virginia, 9073
Autism Services Center, 1553
Autism Services Center, 1607
Autism Socity of West Virginia, 1605
Brain Injury Association of West Virginia, 3988
Brain Injury Association of West Virginia Helpline, 4051
Brain Tumor Support Group: Southern West Virginia, 1928
Cabell County Public Library, 9570
Health Science Library, 3260
Hemophilia Association of the Huntington Area, 4891
Hemophilia Center of West Virginia University Health Sciences Center, 4894
Juvenile Diabetes Research Foundation: Hun tington Chapter, 3253
Kanawha County Public Library, 9571
Mountain State/Parents/Children/ Adolescents Network, 6007
NAMI West Virginia, 6008
National Association of Therapeutic Wilderness Camps, 5903
National Autism Hotline Autism Services Center, 1619
National Federation of the Blind: West Virginia, 9403
National Job Accommodation Network, 10263
Northcentral West Virginia HPV Support Group, 10351
Office of Maternal, Child & Family Health, 8687
Ohio County Public Library Services for the Blind and Physically Handicapped, 9572
Parkersburg and Wood County Public Library, 9573
The West Virginia Autism Training Center Marshall University, 1616
Veterans Adm. Medical Center: Beckley, 10117
Veterans Adm. Medical Center: Clarksburg Louis A. Johnson VA Medical Center, 10118
Veterans Adm. Medical Center: Huntington, 10119
Veterans Affairs Medical Center: Martinsburg, 10120
West Virginia Advocates, 10352
West Virginia Department of Health & Human Resources, 298
West Virginia Division of Alcohol & Drug Abuse, 8071
West Virginia Library Commission, 9574
West Virginia School for the Blind, 9575
West Virginia University Cystic Fibrosis Center, 3067

West Virginia University: Mary Babb Randolph Cancer Center, 2284

Wisconsin

AARP Wisconsin State Office: Madison, 73
AIDS Network, 171
ALS Association: Southeast Wisconsin Chapter, 1021
About Kids GI Disorders, 3580
Alzheimer's Association: Greater Wisconsin Chapter, 829
Alzheimer's Association: Indianhead Chapter, 830
Alzheimer's Association: Lake Superior Chapter, 831
Alzheimer's Association: Midstate Wisconsin Chapter, 832
Alzheimer's Association: North Central Wisconsin Chapter, 833
Alzheimer's Association: Northeast Wisconsin Chapter, 834
Alzheimer's Association: South Central Wisconsin Chapter, 835
Alzheimer's Association: Southeast Wisconsin Chapter, 836
American Academy for Cerebral Palsy and Developmental Medicine, 2561
American Academy of Allergy, Asthma & Immunology, 559
American Academy of Allergy, Asthma & Immunology, 1260
American Association of Children's Residential Centers, 5888
American Cancer Society: Wisconsin, 2156
American Diabetes Association: Wisconsin, 3254
American Liver Foundation Wisconsin Chapter, 5624
American Lung Association of Wisconsin, 5731
American Lung Association of Wisconsin, 9074
Anxiety Disorders Center University of Wisconsin, 6016
Arthritis Foundation: Wisconsin Chapter Foundation, 1125
Autism Society of Wisconsin, 1606
Brain Injury Alliance of Wisconsin, 4052
Brain Injury Association of Wisconsin, 3989
Brain Tumor Support Group: John Sierzant Lutheran Hospital, Gunderson Clinic, 1929
Brown County Library, 9576
CCFA Wisconsin Chapter, 2928
Children's Brittle Bone Foundation, 6767
Clement J. Zablocki Veterans Affairs Medical Center, 10121
Cyclic Vomiting Syndrome Association, 3789
Down Syndrome Association of Wisconsin, 3451
Eau Claire Hemophilia Center, 4884
Endometriosis Association International, 3657
FASST, Friends & Survivors Standing Together, 3940
Governor's Committee for People with Disabilities, 10353
Great Lakes Hemophilia Foundation, 4871
Grief & Loss Support Group, 10556
Gulf War Veterans of Wisconsin, 10122
Gundersen Clinic Comprehensive Hemophilia Treatment Center, 4889
Hematology Treatment Center of the Great Lakes Hemophilia Foundation, 4890
Infant Death Center of Wisconsin, 8688
International Foundation for Functional Gastrointestinal Disorders (IFFGD), 2885
International Foundation for Functional Gastrointestinal Disorders, 3792
International Foundation for Functional Gastrointestinal Disorders (IFFGD), 5206
Juvenile Diabetes Research Foundation: Gre ater Madison Chapter, 3256
Juvenile Diabetes Research Foundation: Nor theast Wisconsin Chapter, 3257
Juvenile Diabetes Research Foundation: Southeastern Chapter, 3255
Kids with Heart National Association for Children's Heart Disorders, 2839
LODAT: Brain Tumor Support Group, 1930
Leukemia and Lymphoma Society: Wisconsin Chapter, 2157
Lupus Foundation of America: Wisconsin Chapter, 5843

Wyoming

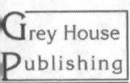

2013 Title List

Visit **www.greyhouse.com** for Product Information, Table of Contents and Sample Pages

General Reference

America's College Museums
American Environmental Leaders: From Colonial Times to the Present
An African Biographical Dictionary
An Encyclopedia of Human Rights in the United States
Constitutional Amendments
Encyclopedia of African-American Writing
Encyclopedia of the Continental Congress
Encyclopedia of Gun Control & Gun Rights
Encyclopedia of Invasions & Conquests
Encyclopedia of Prisoners of War & Internment
Encyclopedia of Religion & Law in America
Encyclopedia of Rural America
Encyclopedia of the United States Cabinet, 1789-2010
Encyclopedia of War Journalism
Encyclopedia of Warrior Peoples & Fighting Groups
From Suffrage to the Senate: America's Political Women
Nations of the World
Political Corruption in America
Speakers of the House of Representatives, 1789-2009
The Environmental Debate: A Documentary History
The Evolution Wars: A Guide to the Debates
The Religious Right: A Reference Handbook
The Value of a Dollar: 1860-2009
The Value of a Dollar: Colonial Era
This is Who We Were: A Companion to the 1940 Census
This is Who We Were: The 1910s
This is Who We Were: The 1950s
US Land & Natural Resource Policy
Weather America
Working Americans 1770-1869 Vol. IX: Revol. War to the Civil War
Working Americans 1880-1999 Vol. I: The Working Class
Working Americans 1880-1999 Vol. II: The Middle Class
Working Americans 1880-1999 Vol. III: The Upper Class
Working Americans 1880-1999 Vol. IV: Their Children
Working Americans 1880-2003 Vol. V: At War
Working Americans 1880-2005 Vol. VI: Women at Work
Working Americans 1880-2006 Vol. VII: Social Movements
Working Americans 1880-2007 Vol. VIII: Immigrants
Working Americans 1880-2009 Vol. X: Sports & Recreation
Working Americans 1880-2010 Vol. XI: Inventors & Entrepreneurs
Working Americans 1880-2011 Vol. XII: Our History through Music
Working Americans 1880-2012 Vol. XIII: Education & Educators
World Cultural Leaders of the 20th & 21st Centuries

Business Information

Complete Television, Radio & Cable Industry Directory
Directory of Business Information Resources
Directory of Mail Order Catalogs
Directory of Venture Capital & Private Equity Firms
Environmental Resource Handbook
Food & Beverage Market Place
Grey House Homeland Security Directory
Grey House Performing Arts Directory
Hudson's Washington News Media Contacts Directory
New York State Directory
Sports Market Place Directory
The Rauch Guides – Industry Market Research Reports
Sweets Directory by McGraw Hill Construction

Health Information

Comparative Guide to American Hospitals
Complete Directory for Pediatric Disorders
Complete Directory for People with Chronic Illness
Complete Directory for People with Disabilities
Complete Mental Health Directory

Diabetes in America: A Geographic & Demographic Analysis
Directory of Health Care Group Purchasing Organizations
Directory of Hospital Personnel
HMO/PPO Directory
Medical Device Register
Obesity in America: A Geographic & Demographic Analysis
Older Americans Information Directory
Pharmaceutical Industry Directory

Statistics & Demographics

America's Top-Rated Cities
America's Top-Rated Small Towns & Cities
America's Top-Rated Smaller Cities
American Tally
Ancestry & Ethnicity in America
Comparative Guide to American Hospitals
Comparative Guide to American Suburbs
Profiles of America
Profiles of... Series – State Handbooks
The Hispanic Databook

Education Information

Charter School Movement
Comparative Guide to American Elementary & Secondary Schools
Complete Learning Disabilities Directory
Educators Resource Directory
Special Education

Financial Ratings Series

TheStreet.com Ratings Guide to Bond & Money Market Mutual Funds
TheStreet.com Ratings Guide to Common Stocks
TheStreet.com Ratings Guide to Exchange-Traded Funds
TheStreet.com Ratings Guide to Stock Mutual Funds
TheStreet.com Ratings Ultimate Guided Tour of Stock Investing
Weiss Ratings Consumer Box Set
Weiss Ratings Guide to Banks & Thrifts
Weiss Ratings Guide to Credit Unions
Weiss Ratings Guide to Health Insurers
Weiss Ratings Guide to Life & Annuity Insurers
Weiss Ratings Guide to Property & Casualty Insurers

Bowker's Books In Print® Titles

Books In Print®
Books In Print® Supplement
American Book Publishing Record® Annual
American Book Publishing Record® Monthly
Books Out Loud™
Bowker's Complete Video Directory™
Children's Books In Print®
Complete Directory of Large Print Books & Serials™
El-Hi Textbooks & Serials In Print®
Forthcoming Books®
Law Books & Serials In Print™
Medical & Health Care Books In Print™
Publishers, Distributors & Wholesalers of the US™
Subject Guide to Books In Print®
Subject Guide to Children's Books In Print®

Canadian General Reference

Associations Canada
Canadian Almanac & Directory
Canadian Environmental Resource Guide
Canadian Parliamentary Guide
Financial Services Canada
Governments Canada
Libraries Canada
The History of Canada

Grey House Publishing
4919 Route 22, PO Box 56, Amenia NY 12501-0056 | (800) 562-2139 | www.greyhouse.com | books@greyhouse.com